TEXTBOOK OF Medicine

Dr. P. D. Howdle
Dept. of Medicine
St. James's Hospital
Leeds LS9 7TF
U.K.

TEXTBOOK OF Medicine

Edited by

R. L. Souhami MD FRCP

Kathleen Ferrier Professor of Clinical Oncology;
Consultant Physician, University College and Middlesex
School of Medicine, London, UK

J. Moxham MD FRCP

Consultant Physician, King's College Hospital;
Senior Lecturer, King's College School of Medicine
and Dentistry; Honorary Senior Lecturer, National Heart
and Lung Institute, London, UK

Churchill Livingstone
EDINBURGH LONDON MELBOURNE AND
NEW YORK 1990

CHURCHILL LIVINGSTONE
Medical Division of Longman Group UK Limited

Distributed in the United States of America by
Churchill Livingstone Inc., 1560 Broadway, New York,
N.Y. 10036, and by associated companies, branches
and representatives throughout the world.

First published 1990

ISBN 0-443-03434-6

Artwork drawn by Chapman Bounford and Associates, London

British Library Cataloguing in Publication Data
Textbook of medicine.
 1. Medicine
 I. Souhami, Robert L. (Robert Leon) II. Moxham, J.
 610

Library of Congress Cataloging in Publication Data
Textbook of medicine / edited by R. L. Souhmai, J. Moxham.
     p. cm.
  1. Internal medicine. I. Souhami, Robert L. II. Moxham, J.
(John)
  [DNLM: 1. Disease. 2. Medicine. WB 100 T3535]
 RC46.T353 1990
 616—dc20

Printed in Great Britain by
Butler & Tanner Ltd, Frome and London

Preface

This new textbook is intended to provide a comprehensive account of clinical medicine incorporating the language and ideas of modern medical science. The rate of growth in the understanding of mechanisms of disease is greater than at any previous period and there has been a corresponding change in the content and form of the pre-clinical teaching of medical science. Many students now undertake basic science degree courses before starting their clinical training. We believe that the new understanding of cellular and physiological processes illuminates medical practice and makes it more exciting and less arbitrary.

The main emphasis of the textbook is clinical, giving a full description of the presentation, investigation and treatment of disease. We have attempted to interpret these clinical aspects by reference to the underlying mechanisms whenever possible. The text is primarily intended for undergraduate students of medicine, but we hope and anticipate that it will be of value to postgraduates and health care professionals in many fields.

As our understanding of disease has advanced in the industrialised world, so doctors are now faced with the illnesses of an ageing population. These may not be cured but can be alleviated or, sometimes, prevented. We have included sections on epidemiology and on the particular problems of disease in the elderly. Worldwide, infection continues to pose a formidable challenge and air travel means that doctors all over the world must have a working knowledge of the common tropical diseases. The comprehensive chapter 'Infectious, tropical and parasitic diseases' is designed for doctors in training and practising in this country and overseas. The chapter on nutrition deals with the problems of the elderly and the poor in the indus-trialised world as well as malnutrition in economically depressed countries. Other general chapters cover genetics, principles of cancer treatment and immunology, all of which are of relevance to every aspect of medical practice. Drugs are the mainstay of medical treatment and for this reason we have included chapters on the principles of drug use as well as the management of drug overdose and addiction.

The range and depth of specialist medical knowledge required for a book of this type has led us to select our authors from medical schools throughout the United Kingdom. They have been chosen because of their acknowledged reputation both in scientific and clinical medicine. In addition to writing their own chapters, our authors have contributed by scrutinising those sections of other chapters which concern their area of expertise. In this way we have tried to achieve a consistency of approach. The difficulty we faced was how to incorporate so much information into a manageable text. We believe that much can be achieved by simple and effective illustration. This textbook contains numerous diagrams, graphs and charts of a style and content which are intended to capture the reader's interest and imagination.

Undergraduates will find all they need in this book. It is not, however, a syllabus – it contains more knowledge than is required for the final examinations in the UK. All of us who have contributed to the text would be pleased to receive suggestions which will help the book change and develop in future editions.

London
1990

RLS
JM

Acknowledgements

The enormous task of producing this book has been immeasurably lightened by the help we have had from the team at Churchill Livingstone to whom we express our gratitude for their enthusiasm and dedication.

In Gillian Thornton we found someone who could not only read the writing of all the contributors, but who was unerringly accurate in preparing the innumerable drafts of word processor text. Trevor Bounford and his team, Chapman Bounford and Associates developed the diagrams, often from primitive sketches, and coped cheerfully with many subsequent alterations. They all have our warmest thanks.

Together with the individual contributors, we wish to thank the following for their assistance with individual chapters; Dr Christopher Bass (Chapter 11); Dr Michèle Clement (Chapter 26); Dr Timothy Dornan (Chapter 18); Dr Jeremy Gibb (Chapter 23); Dr Clive Handler (Chapter 13); Dr David Isenberg (Chapter 24); and Dr Michael McDowell (Chapter 1).

London
1990

RLS
JM

Contributors

David C Anderson MD FRCP FRCPE MRCPath
Professor of Endocrinology, University of Manchester; Honorary Consultant Physician, Hope Hospital, Salford, Manchester, UK

Eric R Beck BSc FRCP
Consultant Physician in General Medicine and Gastroenterology, Whittington Hospital; Honorary Senior Clinical Lecturer in Medicine, University College and Middlesex School of Medicine, London, UK

John F Costello MD FRCP
Consultant Physician, King's College Hospital; Director, Department of Thoracic Medicine, King's College School of Medicine and Dentistry, London, UK

John Cunningham DM FRCP
Consultant Nephrologist and Honorary Senior Lecturer, The London Hospital and Medical College, London, UK

Adrian L W F Eddleston DM FRCP
Professor of Liver Immunology and Vice Dean, Faculty of Medicine; Consultant Physician, King's College School of Medicine and Dentistry, London, UK

Edwin A M Gale MA FRCP
Senior Lecturer in Medicine, Department of Diabetes and Metabolism, St Bartholomew's Hospital, London, UK

John Goldstone FFARCS
Research Fellow and Registrar, Department of Thoracic Medicine, King's College School of Medicine and Dentistry, London, UK

Brian Hazleman MA FRCP
Consultant Rheumatologist and Director, Rheumatology Research Unit, Addenbrooke's Hospital; Honorary Consultant, Strangeways Research Laboratories; Associate Lecturer, Department of Medicine, University of Cambridge; Fellow, Corpus Christi College, Cambridge, UK

Jeremy Holmes MA MRCP FRCPsych
Consultant Psychiatrist/Psychotherapist, North Devon District Hospital, Barnstaple, North Devon, UK

Cameron T C Kennedy FRCP
Consultant Dermatologist and Clinical Teacher, Bristol Royal Infirmary, Bristol Children's Hospital and Southmead Hospital, Bristol, UK

David C Linch FRCP
Professor of Clinical Haematology, University College and Middlesex School of Medicine, London, UK

Richard G Long MD FRCP
Consultant Physician and Gastroenterologist, City Hospital; Clinical Teacher, University of Nottingham, Nottingham, UK

Thomas J McManus MRCOG
Consultant in Genitourinary Medicine, King's College School of Medicine and Dentistry, London, UK

John P Monson MD FRCP
Senior Lecturer in Metabolism and Endocrinology, London Hospital and Medical College; Honorary Consultant Physician, London Hospital, London, UK

John Moxham MD FRCP
Consultant Physician, King's College Hospital; Senior Lecturer, King's College School of Medicine and Dentistry; Honorary Senior Lecturer, National Heart and Lung Institute, London, UK

Peter W Overstall FRCP
Consultant in Geriatric Medicine, General Hospital, Hereford, UK

John H L Playfair DSc PhD
Professor of Immunology, University College and Middlesex School of Medicine, London, UK

Alan Richens MSc PhD FRCP
Professor of Pharmacology and Therapeutics, University of Wales College of Medicine, Cardiff, UK

Phillip A Routledge MD FRCP
Reader in Clinical Pharmacology, University of Wales College of Medicine; Honorary Consultant Physician, South Glamorgan Health Authority; Director, Welsh National Poisons Unit and Consultant Toxicologist, Welsh Office, Cardiff, UK

John W Scadding MD FRCP
Consultant Neurologist, The National Hospital for
Nervous Diseases; Senior Lecturer, Institute of
Neurology, Queen Square, London, UK

Thomas Sherwood MA FRCP FRCR
Professor of Radiology, University of Cambridge,
Cambridge, UK

Robert L Souhami MD FRCP
Kathleen Ferrier Professor of Clinical Oncology;
Consultant Physician, University College and Middlesex
School of Medicine, London, UK

Andrew Tomkins FRCP
Senior Lecturer in Clinical Nutrition, London School of
Hygiene and Tropical Medicine; Honorary Consultant
Physician, Hospital for Tropical Diseases and University
College Hospital, London, UK

Dan Tunstall Pedoe FRCP DPhil
Senior Lecturer and Consultant Cardiologist, St
Bartholomew's and Homerton Hospitals, London, UK

Nicholas J Wald DSc FFCM FRCP
Professor and Director, Department of Environmental
and Preventive Medicine, Medical College, St
Bartholomew's Hospital, London, UK

J Malcolm Walker MD MRCP
Consultant Cardiologist, University College and
Middlesex Hospital, London, UK

Mark H Wansbrough-Jones FRCP
Consultant Physician and Senior Lecturer in
Communicable Diseases, St George's Hospital and
Medical School, London, UK

Robin M Winter BSc MRCP
Consultant Clinical Geneticist, Kennedy Galton Centre,
Northwick Park Hospital, Middlesex, UK

Stephen G Wright MRCP
Senior Lecturer, Department of Clinical Sciences,
London School of Hygiene and Tropical Medicine;
Honorary Consultant Physician, Hospital for Tropical
Diseases, London, UK

Contents

The Epidemiological Approach

INTRODUCTION

Epidemiology is the study of the incidence, distribution and determinants of diseases in human populations with a view to identifying their causes and effecting their prevention.

Epidemiology and clinical medicine are linked, but there is an important distinction between the two. Clinical medicine is concerned with people who already have a disease; it seeks to understand how the disease progresses, what its effects are and how it can be treated. Epidemiology seeks to understand the antecedents of a disease and identify its causes, so making possible its prevention. As such, epidemiology is concerned with populations, which necessarily include not only individuals who have the disease in question but also those who do not, thereby permitting the calculation of the *rate* of occurrence of the disease and hence the study of factors that influence that rate. Clues to what those factors are may be obtained by seeing:

1. whether the disease is more common in one place than in another
2. whether its frequency has changed over time or
3. whether this differs in people with and without certain characteristics.

Epidemiology has also extended its field of interest directly into areas relevant to clinical medicine, such as clinical trials and the quantitative interpretation of diagnostic or screening tests (p. 9).

Like a detective, the epidemiologist must usually deduce the factors responsible for causing a disease from naturally occurring circumstances over which he has no control. He asks, for example, 'Why is coronary heart disease so much more common in the United States than it is in Japan?

Does the risk change when Japanese people migrate to the US? Is cholesterol (the principal substance in the atheromatous lesions in the coronary arteries) present in different concentrations in the blood of the Japanese and Americans? And, within each country, is there an association between serum cholesterol concentration and the risk of coronary heart disease? Is there any evidence that serum cholesterol is not associated with the risk of heart disease?' The work of the epidemiologist thus mostly involves observation and interpretation. Only insofar as he conducts clinical or prophylactic trials is the epidemiologist an experimental scientist.

Epidemiology relies on pathology and clinical medicine to define and understand disease patterns, and on statistics to quantify the frequency of disease and the size of the associations with possible aetiological factors.

CAUSE OF A DISEASE

A cause of a disease is a factor that is *associated* with the disease, such that if the intensity or frequency of the factor in a population is changed, the frequency of the disease also changes.

It is important to note that not all associations are causal. For example, alcohol consumption is associated with lung cancer because cigarette smokers tend to drink more alcohol than non-smokers and smoking is itself associated with lung cancer. The alcohol–lung cancer association is said to be an indirect one whereas the smoking–lung cancer association is direct and causal. This is supported by noting that the risk of lung cancer varies according to cigarette consumption in persons with a similar alcohol intake but does *not* vary according to alcohol intake in persons with a similar cigarette consumption.

There can be more than one cause of a disease so that, for example, exposure to arsenic, asbestos or nickel can each independently cause lung cancer.

Not everyone exposed to a specific cause of a disease will automatically develop that disease. For example, not everyone exposed to the tubercle bacillus will develop pulmonary tuberculosis (it is not a *sufficient* cause) and non-smokers can also develop lung cancer (smoking is not a *necessary* cause). Whether a particular individual develops a disease after such exposures will depend on the interplay of several factors, including, for example, exposure to other agents, the influence of factors as yet unidentified, constitutional differences and also the play of chance.

Establishing causality

The most direct way to determine causality is by experiment – adding or withholding the factor and observing whether the frequency of the disease changes. However, such an experiment often cannot be done in humans when investigating a toxic substance; removal of the factor may not be possible, the necessary scale of intervention may be too large or the duration of observation too long, or this too may be considered unethical. In such circumstances, causality needs to be inferred from observational studies. This can be done in two stages:

1. determine that an association between an exposure and a disease is a real one, i.e. unlikely to have arisen by chance
2. assess whether the association is one of cause and effect.

A *real association* is most likely to be detected if:

1. the magnitude of the association is large
2. the study includes a large number of subjects
3. variations in other factors affecting the rate of the disease (which introduce extraneous variability or 'noise' into the system) can be minimised.

A real association between a factor and a disease must either be causal or due to bias. Bias can arise in two ways:

1. *Observer bias.* An apparent association between a disease and a study factor may be due to systematic measurement error so that, for example, subjects with the disease are recorded as having more, or less, of the study factor than unaffected subjects even when no such difference exists. This may occur, for example, because an observer who believes that the factor does cause the disease is more likely to diagnose the disease in an individual he knows to have been exposed to the factor. Such observer bias can be avoided by ensuring that the observer who diagnoses the disease is *blind* as to the presence or absence of the factor.
2. *Presence of a confounding factor,* i.e. a factor that is associated with both the disease and the study factor. Thus, in the above example involving lung cancer and alcohol consumption, the confounding factor was cigarette smoking.

The magnitude of an association provides an indication of whether the association is causal; big differences are less likely to have been produced by bias than small differences. Establishing causality is facilitated by knowledge of the sequence of events involved; it is always a *necessary* condition of a causal association for the causal factor to precede

---

Summary 1 Criteria and evidence for inferring causality between exposure to a factor and a disease.

Essential criteria

- A real association between the factor and the disease, that is, an association that is unlikely to be due to chance.
- Exposure to the factor precedes the occurrence of the disease.
- The association cannot be reasonably explained by bias, either through systematic measurement error or through the effect of one or more confounding factors.
- The causal explanation is biologically plausible.

Additional evidence

- Demonstration of a dose-response relationship between the factor and the disease in studies of individuals.
- The demonstration of reversibility; elimination or reduction in the intensity of exposure to the factor is associated with a reduction in the risk of disease.
- The distribution and frequency of the disease in different places and in different groups and over time follows the distribution and intensity of exposure to the factor.
- Support from animal or *in vitro* laboratory experimental evidence.

---

the effect. This is often clear (e.g. with the association between smoking and lung cancer) but, at other times, it is uncertain. Thus, for example, two equally plausible explanations could apply to the association found between low serum retinol and cancer: either the low serum retinol precedes the cancer and therefore may cause it, or the presence of cancer exerts metabolic effects that lower serum retinol. Only appropriate epidemiological enquiry (a prospective study, p. 5) can determine which explanation is correct. Once the sequence of events is known, it is usually possible to conclude that an association is causal if bias can be excluded, provided the causal explanation is biologically plausible and there is no seriously conflicting evidence.

A causal explanation for an association is supported by the following:

1. a dose–response relationship between exposure and the disease
2. demonstrating that reduction in exposure produces a reduction in the incidence of the disease
3. observing that the variation in the distribution of disease in different places, at different times and in different groups of people, is related to corresponding variations in the distribution of the causal factor.

The above definition of the cause of a disease stresses the central importance of *why* disease occurs rather than how it progresses after it has occurred. In epidemiology, the notion of cause is thus concerned with origins of disease rather than mechanisms. The clinician might regard the cause of diabetes as being a relative lack of insulin; the epidemiologist would wish to know what factors influenced this lack. Both views are correct; to treat diabetes it need only be regarded as a lack of insulin, but to prevent it, it is necessary to understand the factors which led to this lack.

EPIDEMIOLOGICAL ENQUIRY

Epidemiological enquiry initially involves finding clues that will help identify the causes of disease. Such clues can arise from many sources, for example from clinical observation, from inferences drawn from knowledge of the biology involved, or from a more formal description of the epidemiology of the disease concerned. From such observations and inferences, a hypothesis may emerge that a particular disease is caused by a particular exposure. Following such *descriptive* epidemiological studies, two types of investigation can be undertaken – *analytical* epidemiological studies and, in special circumstances, *intervention* (or experimental) studies.

DESCRIPTIVE STUDIES

Descriptive studies involve answering three questions.

1. How does the risk of developing a disease vary over *time*?
2. How does it vary from *place to place*?
3. How does it vary with respect to certain characteristics of the *individuals*, such as age, sex or occupational group?

Incidence and prevalence

Answering these questions requires quantitative measures of the risk of developing a disease. This is done by estimating the incidence or prevalence of the disease in question, both of which involve counting the number of individuals in a defined population with that disease (the numerator) and dividing by the total population (the denominator) so that disease rates can be determined.

The *incidence* of a disease is the number of new cases occurring in a specified period of time and in a defined population. The *prevalence* of a disease is the number of cases of a disorder present at a given point in time in a defined population.

The prevalence of a disease changes according to the product of its incidence and duration. The duration of a disease will be shortened if it either kills the patient or remits completely. Thus, a condition with a high incidence and low prevalence could be either a common disease which has a high fatality rate (e.g. lung cancer) or a common disease with a high remission rate (e.g. measles). A disease with a low incidence and a high prevalence will be a chronic disease with a low fatality rate and a low remission rate (e.g. rheumatoid arthritis).

Age standardisation

The prevalence and incidence of a disease are usually strongly dependent on age; e.g. the incidences of lung cancer and coronary heart disease are relatively high in the elderly and low in the young. When comparing incidence or prevalence across different communities, it can therefore be misleading to compare the overall rates directly, since one population may have a larger number of elderly people. One approach to this problem is to compare rates in specific age groups, although such a comparison across a whole range of specific age groups is usually unwieldy since it does not yield a single summary figure. However, such a summary figure can be obtained by *age standardisation*, in which the age-specific rates of the study population are applied to a standard population (direct standardisation). Alternatively, the age-specific rates for a standard population can be applied to the numbers of individuals in the study population in each age group to derive an *expected* number of deaths for the study population that is compared with the *observed* number (indirect standardisation). This ratio multiplied by 100 is known as the *standardised mortality ratio*, and it provides a single and widely used index that enables one to compare disease or mortality rates in different populations. In expectation, the two methods should yield the same result. In practice, however, this is not always the case; in smaller studies, indirect standardisation is usually the preferred method.

Life expectancy

Another important summary measure for comparing death rates within and between countries over time is *life expectancy*. It is calculated by considering a hypothetical group of, say, 1000 individuals at a given age and applying to the group the age-specific death rates of the population for each year of age until the whole group are estimated to have died. Expectation of life is calculated as the total number of person-years of life lived by the group divided by the number in the group, i.e. the average number of years an individual is expected to live. The calculation assumes that the current death rates will remain unchanged for the lifetime of the group (which, of course, they will not), but expectation of life is a useful single index of *current* death rates.

Use of descriptive studies

Descriptive epidemiological studies are useful not only because they sometimes suggest clues as to the causes of disease, but also because they enable assessment of the burden (in both economic and health terms) of different diseases in different communities. The study of immigrants is especially helpful. For example, the Japanese have a high incidence of stomach cancer but this declines substantially in Japanese migrants moving to the US, the incidence rates approximating to those of the indigenous Americans. The age-specific incidence rates of colon cancer among the Japanese immigrants increase towards those experienced by native Americans. There is evidently an important cause of stomach cancer in Japan that is relatively absent in the US. Similarly, an important cause of colon cancer appears to be present in the US but relatively absent in Japan.

The Epidemiological Approach

Once a hypothesis has been produced that a particular disease is caused by a particular exposure, the epidemiology of the exposure can be described in much the same way as the epidemiology of the disease to see whether the two are correlated with respect to time and place, and whether they tend to occur together in certain groups of people within the same community. Descriptive studies can thus serve as tests of a hypothesis as well as a means of generating aetiological clues.

ANALYTICAL STUDIES

Once descriptive epidemiological studies have pointed to a possible association between an exposure and a disease, the hypothesis can be explored further through analytical studies specially designed to investigate directly the risk of a disease in relation to a given exposure. It is simplest to consider first the measures of risk used and then the usual study designs employed.

Measures of risk used in analytical studies

Incidence rates (or mortality rates) in two groups of people, say, among smokers and non-smokers, can be compared in two ways.

1. The *relative risk* of a disease in relation to a particular exposure is the incidence of a disease among exposed persons divided by the incidence among unexposed persons.
2. The *absolute excess risk* of a disease in relation to a particular exposure is the incidence of the disease among exposed persons minus the incidence among non-exposed persons.

The relative risk is useful in judging the strength of an association between exposure and disease, and hence whether the association might be causal. If it is causal, the absolute excess risk is a direct measure of how much disease the exposure causes in a particular population. It thus estimates the preventive effect of removing the exposure from the population and is therefore of public health importance. The absolute excess risk depends on the underlying risk of the disease concerned in the unexposed members of a particular population and cannot automatically be generalised to other populations.

Table 1.1 shows the relative and absolute excess risks of mortality from lung cancer, other cancers, chronic bronchitis and cardiovascular disease in heavy cigarette smokers and non-smokers. Smoking is strongly associated with lung cancer and chronic bronchitis, as evidenced by their high relative risks (25.1 and 38.0 respectively) but it is much less strongly associated with ischaemic heart disease (relative risk 1.9). However, because lung cancer and chronic bronchitis are rare in non-smokers, while ischaemic heart disease is common, smoking causes fewer excess deaths from chronic bronchitis and lung cancer (241 and 111 deaths per 100 000 per year respectively) than from ischaemic heart disease (379 deaths per 100 000 per year). If the incidence of a common disease is increased only two

Summary 2   Types of epidemiological enquiry

Descriptive studies
Studies of the variation in the incidence of a disease according to time, place and person.

Analytical studies
Studies specially designed to investigate directly the risk of disease in relation to a given exposure.

Intervention studies
Experiments on humans designed to test the efficacy and safety of medical procedures or medications.

or three times the final number of deaths can be greater than if a rare disease is increased by as much as, say, 30 times. Another, related measure of risk is the *attributable proportion*. This is the proportion of cases of a disease that can be attributed to an exposure.

A simple hypothetical (but realistic) example illustrates each measure of risk. In a population of 100 000 men aged 45–54 years, 30% (30 000) are smokers; and the risk of dying from coronary heart disease (CHD) is 3 per 1000 per year among smokers and 1 per 1000 per year among non-smokers. The number of deaths from CHD per year is thus 90 ($3/1000 \times 30\,000$) among smokers; and 70 ($1/1000 \times 70\,000$) among non-smokers, giving a total of 160 CHD deaths overall.

The relative risk of death from CHD in smokers compared to non-smokers is 3/1000 divided by $1/1000 = 3$.

The absolute excess risk in smokers is 3/1000 minus $1/1000 = 2/1000$, i.e. smoking causes 2 deaths from CHD per 1000 people each year.

If no-one smoked, there would be 100 deaths (100 000 $\times$ 1/1000) each year instead of 160, so that 60 out of the 160 observed deaths are attributable to smoking. The proportion of deaths attributable to smoking in this population is therefore 60/160 or 38%. To estimate the attributable proportion one need not know the absolute death rates in

Table 1.1   Relative and absolute excess risks of deaths from selected causes associated with heavy cigarette smoking (25 or more cigarettes per day) by British male physicians.*

Cause of death	Annual death rate per 100 000		Relative risk	Absolute excess risk death rate (per 100 000 per year)
	Non-smokers	Heavy cigarette smokers		
Lung cancer	10	251	25.1	241
Chronic bronchitis and emphysema	3	114	38.0	111
Ischaemic heart disease	413	792	1.9	379
All causes	1317	2843	2.16	1526

*From Doll R and Peto R, 1976 Mortality in relation to smoking: 20 years' observations on male British doctors. Brit. med J 1976; ii: 1525–36.

Summary 3   Quantitative measures of risk

- *Incidence* The number of new cases of a disorder occurring in a defined population in a specified period of time (e.g. 5/1000 persons/year).
- *Prevalence* The number of cases of a disorder present in a defined population at a given time (e.g. 5/1000 persons).
- *Relative risk* The incidence among exposed individuals divided by the incidence among unexposed individuals.
- *Absolute excess risk* The incidence among exposed individuals minus the incidence among unexposed individuals.
- *Attributable proportion* The proportion of cases of a disease that can be attributed to a given exposure.

Table 1.2   Simple 2×2 table used in epidemiological studies to show the exposed and unexposed individuals who do and do not develop disease

	Disease	No disease	
Exposed	a	b	a + b
Not exposed	c	d	c + d
	a + c	b + d	

smokers and non-smokers, simply the relative risk, r, and the prevalence of the exposure, p, so that:

$$\text{Attributable proportion} = \frac{p(r-1)}{p(r-1)+1}$$

which, in our example $= \dfrac{0.3\,(3-1)}{0.3\,(3-1)+1} = \dfrac{0.6}{1.6} = 38\%$

Clearly, the attributable proportion will vary from one population to another depending on the prevalence and extent of exposure.

Study designs used in analytical studies

Analytical epidemiological studies are either prospective or retrospective.

Prospective studies

In a *prospective study* (also called a longitudinal or cohort study) we take a group of individuals and categorise them according to whether or not they are, or have been, exposed to a certain factor. We then follow the groups for a period of time, often many years, and record the number who do and do not develop the disease of interest.

A simple 2×2 table of the number of individuals involved can be constructed to show the exposed and unexposed individuals who do and do not develop disease (Table 1.2).

The rates of disease in exposed subjects $(a/a+b)$ and in unexposed subjects $(c/c+d)$ are then determined. The first divided by the second is the *relative risk* (r). Thus,

$$r = \frac{\dfrac{a}{a+b}}{\dfrac{c}{c+d}}$$

Exposed individuals are then r times more likely than unexposed individuals to develop disease. A value of r that is statistically significantly greater than, or less than, 1 is evidence of an association.

The second rate subtracted from the first is the *absolute excess risk* (e per 100). Thus,

$$e = \frac{a}{a+b} - \frac{c}{c+d}$$

Exposed individuals then have a risk of e per 1000 in excess of that experienced by unexposed individuals.

The figures in the hypothetical (but realistic) study of smoking and lung cancer discussed on page 4 may be used to illustrate the design of a prospective study.

Both the 30 000 smokers and 70 000 non-smokers in the initial population of 100 000 are followed up for, say, 10 years. During this time, there are 42 new cases of lung cancer among the smokers. The rate of disease in exposed subjects is thus

$$\frac{42}{30\,000} = \frac{14}{10\,000}$$

There are 7 new cases among the non-smokers. The rate of disease in non-exposed subjects is thus

$$\frac{7}{70\,000} = \frac{1}{10\,000}$$

$$\text{Relative risk (r)} = \frac{\dfrac{14}{10\,000}}{\dfrac{1}{10\,000}} = 14$$

$$\text{Absolute excess risk} =$$

$$\frac{14}{10\,000} - \frac{1}{10\,000} = \frac{13}{10\,000} \text{ per ten years}$$

$$= 1.3/10\,000 \text{ per year}$$

The main advantages of prospective (or longitudinal) studies are: the knowledge that the exposure preceded the occurrence of the disease; the ability to obtain a direct estimate of the incidence of the disease in the exposed and the unexposed groups (allowing both the relative risk and absolute excess risk to be estimated directly); and the ability to detect unsuspected associations.

The main disadvantages of longitudinal studies when studying chronic disorders such as cardiovascular disease and cancer are: their long duration (many years); their large

The Epidemiological Approach

> **Summary 4   Study designs: prospective (cohort) studies**
>
> A group of individuals who are categorised according to whether they have or have not been exposed to a certain factor are followed up over a period of time and the incidence of the disease or diseases of interest recorded according to the assigned exposure.
>
> *Advantages*
> - Exposure known to precede development of the disease.
> - Direct estimate of incidence, in both exposed and non-exposed groups.
> - Permits the study of many diseases so that unsuspected associations can be identified.
>
> *Disadvantages*
> - Long duration (decades).
> - Large size (thousands of individuals).
> - High financial cost.

size (thousands of individuals); and therefore their financial cost. For a rare disease, few cases may develop even in a large study of this type.

Retrospective studies

In a *retrospective study* (also called a case-control study) we take a sample of individuals who have the disease (cases) and another sample who do not (controls). The prevalence of exposure in those with the disease and in those without it is determined retrospectively, usually by the administration of a questionnaire.

In a retrospective study, we cannot estimate the relative risk directly because the proportions of diseased and non-diseased subjects sampled from the population are different and unknown. However, if the disease being studied is rare, a simple approximation solves the problem. Referring to the 2×2 table on page 5, for a prospective study,

$$\text{the relative risk (r)} = \frac{\dfrac{a}{a+b}}{\dfrac{c}{c+d}}$$

Now, since the disease is rare, a and c are much smaller than b and d, so that:

$$a+b \simeq b, \text{ and } \quad \frac{a}{a+b} \simeq \frac{a}{b}$$

$$c+d \simeq d, \text{ and } \quad \frac{c}{c+d} \simeq \frac{c}{d}$$

Therefore,

$$\text{the relative risk (r)} \simeq \frac{\dfrac{a}{b}}{\dfrac{c}{d}} = \frac{ad}{bc}$$

For a retrospective study, let s_1 and s_2 be the fraction of the individuals with and without the disease sampled from the underlying population to yield, respectively, the number of cases and controls in the study. Then:

$$\text{relative risk (r)} = \frac{\dfrac{as_1}{bs_2}}{\dfrac{cs_1}{ds_1}} = \frac{as_1}{bs_2} \times \frac{ds_2}{cs_1} = \frac{ad}{bc}$$

i.e. the cross products of the 2×2 table. The unknown sampling fractions s_1 and s_2 conveniently cancel out. An example is shown in Table 1.3.

The main advantages of retrospective studies are that they are: quick; require relatively small numbers; and are hence reasonably economical. They are sometimes the only feasible way to conduct an analytical epidemiological study of a rare disease.

Their main disadvantages are: the difficulty, in certain studies, of determining whether the exposure preceded the inception of the disease; and avoiding bias. For example, sick people may be more likely to recall a past exposure than healthy controls.

Table 1.3   Example of a retrospective study: lung cancer and cigarette smoking.*

Smoking habits	Cases (lung cancer)	Controls (no lung cancer)	
Cigarette smokers	647	622	1269
Non-smokers	2	27	29
Total	649	649	1298

$$\text{Relative risk (r)} = \frac{647 \times 27}{622 \times 2} = 14.0$$

*From Doll R, Hill A B, 1952 The study of the aetiology of carcinoma of the lung. Brit Med J 1952; ii: 1271–86.

> **Summary 5   Study designs: retrospective (case/control) studies**
>
> A sample of individuals who already have the disease of interest (cases) and a sample of similar individuals who do not have the disease (controls) are compared to see if their exposure to the factor under study is or has been different.
>
> *Advantages*
> - Quick.
> - Relatively small numbers are adequate.
> - Economical.
>
> *Disadvantages*
> - Sometimes there is uncertainty as to whether the exposure preceded the inception of the disease.
> - It can sometimes be more difficult to avoid bias than with prospective studies.

INTERVENTION STUDIES

Methodological issues

Intervention studies resemble prospective studies in that subjects are followed up to determine their outcome. They differ in that some action or intervention is performed rather than only observing what takes place naturally. Intervention studies are experiments on humans in which something is done to an experimental group and the observed outcome compared with a control group which is not subjected to the intervention. If a difference in outcome between the two groups is demonstrated that is considered unlikely to be due to bias and unlikely to have arisen by chance, cause and effect can be inferred.

In general, three types of control groups can be used:

1. *Historical controls*: patients with the same disorder seen in the past before the use of the new intervention
2. *Geographical controls*: patients with the same disorder seen at another hospital or clinic where the new intervention is not provided
3. *Randomised controls*: concurrent patients chosen at random to be controls while other patients from the same population are chosen at random to receive the new intervention. It is the allocation to receive or not receive the new intervention, say a new treatment, that is conducted at random, not the group of patients for the study. The latter are, rather, often a special subset, e.g. those with a particular complication, those in a particular age group, or those thought likely to comply with the treatment.

Historical and geographical controls

The use of historical and geographical controls is usually unsatisfactory because like is probably not being compared with like. The introduction of a new type of treatment may itself alter the selection of patients referred for the treatment. For example, patients with early disease may start coming from other centres to receive the new treatment. Past patients may have been referred to hospitals at a different stage of the disease and this alone will influence their survival or remission rate. They are also likely to have received different treatments apart from the new one under study and this would have influenced their outcomes. Similar biases affect the use of geographical controls.

Randomised controls

In randomised studies, on the other hand, allocation to treatment is decided at random, and so the study and control groups will, on average, be alike. Randomisation, thus removes *allocation bias*. *Observer bias* (where the assessment of response to treatment is influenced by knowledge of treatment group) can be avoided by a single (or observer) blind design. Bias due to patients knowing that they are in a particular treatment (because of the psychological or *placebo* effect or because it would influence habits

> **Summary 6   Study designs: intervention studies**
>
> A substance is administered to, or a procedure conducted on, an experimental group and the observed outcome compared to a control group that is not subjected to the intervention.
>
> Three types of control groups can be employed:
>
> *Historical controls* – affected patients seen before the new intervention.
>
> *Geographical controls* – affected patients seen at another unit which does not have the new intervention.
>
> *Randomised controls* – intervention is randomly assigned to concurrent patients in the same population.
>
> *Advantages of a randomised trial*
> - Avoids selection bias that may arise through patients with a better (or worse) prognosis being allocated the new intervention.
> - Any subject or observer bias can be removed by making the trial double-blind.

that may themselves affect prognosis) can be avoided by a double blind design in which neither observers nor patients know the treatment allocation. Provided sufficient numbers of patients are entered into the trial to avoid chance differences between the treatment and control groups, any observed differences must be due to the new treatment.

To avoid bias some researchers match treated and untreated patients retrospectively on factors known to influence prognosis, rather than allocate patients on a random basis. This is usually inadequate, however, because it can only allow for factors that are known to be related to prognosis. In practice, there are important selective factors relating to both being offered and complying with treatment, and to prognosis, which are usually not known. Matching cannot overcome this problem (one cannot match for unknown factors) but randomisation can.

The statistical analysis of randomised trials should be done by comparing outcome in all the subjects originally allocated to each of the treatment groups, including non-compliers (referred to as an *intention-to-treat* analysis), rather than by comparing outcome only in patients from each group who actually completed treatment (*treatment received* analysis). It is only with the intention-to-treat analysis that bias can be avoided. Bias could easily be introduced by an actual treatment analysis, e.g. because the more symptomatic patients with a poorer prognosis may be less likely to adhere to the one treatment than the other, particularly if it has side-effects that exacerbate the symptoms from the disease itself, such as nausea. Poor compliance on an intention-to-treat analysis will obviously reduce the ability of the trial to detect a treatment effect if one does exist (as the trial will have little statistical power and may yield inconclusive results), but it will not be biased as may be the case with the treatment received analysis.

Ethical issues

Observational studies represent one of the most innocent forms of medical investigation. In observational studies in which data are obtained from existing medical records, the only ethical issue of concern is maintaining the confidentiality of the records. If the data are obtained by interviewing subjects, the questions asked and the manner of working should be designed in such a way as to avoid causing anxiety.

In an intervention study, however, there is the further ethical concern that patients must not be harmed, either by adverse effects of a new treatment or by withholding a treatment which might have been of benefit. Investigators are naturally enthusiastic about the possible benefits of a new 'treatment' with which they have been associated and are often understandably unwilling to carry out a controlled experiment to test its effects. However, it is important to be objective, since many supposedly beneficial treatments have been introduced, which have been found subsequently to be of little or no value and sometimes even to be harmful; it is always possible that the initial impression of benefit may be due to bias or chance. Assessing the level of certainty over the benefits and risks of a new intervention thus requires dispassionate judgement. This is not always easy, as may be seen in the varying practice of clinicians, some of whom avoid a new treatment through scepticism of its value or possibly even fear of its risks, while others offer it because of their conviction that it is effective. In such circumstances, a formal clinical trial is both a practical and an ethical way of organising the diversity in clinical practice so that the uncertainty can be resolved. New medical procedures are best evaluated early, before they become universally and uncritically accepted.

PREVENTION

Epidemiology, with its emphasis on identifying the antecedents of disease, offers the opportunity for disease prevention. Different preventive measures can be applied at different stages in the natural history of the disease.

Primary prevention

Primary prevention is the prevention of the future occurrence of a disorder in unaffected individuals by removing a cause, e.g. preventing lung cancer by avoiding smoking or preventing an infectious disease by increasing host resistance, either by general measures (e.g. nutrition) or by specific measures (e.g. immunisation).

Secondary prevention

Secondary prevention is the prevention of overt (clinical) cases of a disorder through screening and early detection followed by appropriate intervention, e.g. breast cancer screening by mammography.

The treatment of clinical disease, while not normally regarded as prevention, is sometimes referred to as *tertiary prevention*, as effective treatment of overt disease can often prevent disability and pain resulting from the disease.

PRIMARY PREVENTION

General measures

The prevention of disease through general social and economic changes that improve nutrition, increase living standards, lead to smaller families and reduce overcrowding, is extremely important, even if the precise social and economic factors causally involved are difficult to identify. The expectation of life in most countries tends to be positively associated with economic performance as judged, for example, by the gross national product (GNP) per person (Fig. 1.1) although above a certain GNP (about $5000 per person in 1983) the relationship is weak and other factors must operate. Past improvements in life expectancy in developed countries have been largely accomplished by general measures such as those that led to the primary prevention of common infectious diseases; mortality from infectious diseases had thus greatly decreased before the availability of specific methods of prevention or treatment such as vaccination or antibiotics. Some infectious diseases, however, have increased in recent years, particularly venereal diseases such as non-gonococcal urethritis and recently the acquired immune deficiency syndrome (AIDS).

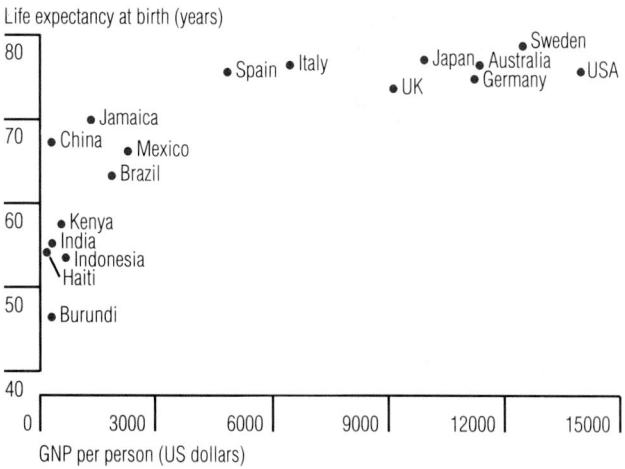

Fig. 1.1 Expectation of life versus gross national product (1983). (Source: World Bank.)

Specific measures

With the notable exception of AIDS, the major challenge today in the industrialised countries of the world is the prevention of illness due to non-infectious diseases by modification of *specific* cultural and personal patterns of behaviour such as the change in specific dietary components (e.g. lower fat intake), increases in the level of physical activity, reduction in the use of alcohol and the avoidance of tobacco. It has been estimated that the adoption throughout western countries of a diet reducing serum cholesterol levels by 10% would reduce coronary heart disease (CHD) mortality by at least 20%. Since CHD is the leading cause of death in such countries, this would result in a considerable reduction in mortality, approximately equivalent in numbers to the complete eradication of all cases of lung cancer in men and of breast cancer in women. Also important, particularly among young adults, is the problem of death and injury from accidents, especially road accidents.

In general, society can exert an influence on health in various ways, for example by legislation on driving and alcohol consumption, and on the prevention of pollution of air, soil and water; by encouraging the alteration of the composition and quality of the food we eat; by influencing choice through financial incentives (increasing the tax on cigarettes); and by applying engineering principles to build safety into the design of motor vehicles, equipment, buildings and highways.

SECONDARY PREVENTION

Secondary prevention is achieved through screening. *Screening* is the identification, among apparently healthy individuals, of those who are sufficiently at risk from a specific disorder to justify a subsequent diagnostic test or procedure or, in certain circumstances, direct preventive action.

Screening represents a radical departure from traditional medicine in that it is usually concerned with the detection of disorders at an asymptomatic stage before an individual is prompted to seek medical attention. Indeed, it involves seeking out asymptomatic individuals among people who are not receiving any type of medical attention. The early detection of disease is only worthwhile for disorders which lend themselves to effective intervention and hence prevention. The identification of either trivial or untreatable conditions may cause anxiety with no useful result, and would therefore not be suitable diseases for screening.

Screening may take the form of a simple inquiry, such as determining whether a pregnant woman has an affected close male relative, when offering antenatal screening for a sex-linked recessive disorder such as Duchenne muscular dystrophy; or, it may take the form of a special test such as maternal serum alpha-fetoprotein estimation when screening for neural tube defects.

Parameters of a screening test

The performance of screening tests as well as diagnostic tests is characterised by three measures which should be known before the test is used in practice:

1. The *detection rate* (or *sensitivity*) of a test is the proportion of affected individuals with positive test results (Table 1.4).
2. The *false-positive rate* of a test is the proportion of unaffected individuals with positive test results. This is sometimes given as the *specificity* which is the false-positive rate expressed as a percentage subtracted from

100; so that, for example, a false-positive rate of 3% is the same as a specificity of 97%.
3. The *odds of being affected given a positive result* is the ratio of the number of affected to unaffected individuals among those with positive test results.

The odds of being affected given a positive result depend on the prevalence of the disorder, as well as on the detection rate and the false positive rate. Figure 1.2 shows a hypothetical flow diagram used to estimate the consequences of two screening tests offered in sequence followed by a diagnostic test. In each case, the detection rate and false-positive rate of each test is applied to the number of affected and unaffected subjects (considered separately) to yield the number of true positives and false positives at each stage of the screening and diagnostic process. The ratio of one to the other gives the odds of being affected given a positive result; in our example, this is 169:11 (about 15 to 1) after the diagnostic test. (This ratio is also known as the *predictive value positive* when expressed as a proportion, i.e. 15/16 or 94%.)

The prevalence of the disorder being screened for has an important influence on the results of screening. The more common the disorder, the more likely it is that a positive test result will be associated with that disorder (the higher the odds of being affected given a positive result). Thus, with a common disorder, a screening test with a relatively poor detection rate and false positive rate might be acceptable, but the same test might be unacceptable where the disorder is rarer. The detection rate and false-positive rate characterise the ability of an investigation to identify or exclude a particular disorder. They are not affected by the prevalence of the disorder. The probability that a positive test result will be associated with the disorder in question is dependent on the prevalence of the disorder in the setting in which screening is carried out, i.e. the odds of being affected given a positive result is a function of the prevalence of the condition as well as the detection rate and false-positive rate.

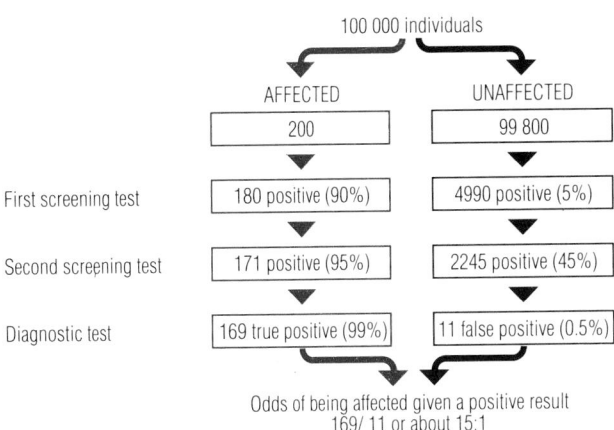

Fig. 1.2 Hypothetical flow-diagram used to estimate the consequences of a screening programme. (From: Cuckle and Wald in Wald N J (ed) 1984 Antenatal and neonatal screening. Oxford University Press, Oxford.)

1

Table 1.4 Definition of detection rate and false-positive rate of a qualitative test

Test result	Affected	Unaffected	Total
Positive	a	b	a + b
Negative	c	d	c + d
Total	a + c	b + d	

$$\text{Detection rate (sensitivity)} = \frac{a}{a+c}$$

$$\text{False-positive rate (1 - specificity)} = \frac{b}{b+d}$$

Table 1.4 provides a complete description of the detection and false-positive rates for a test which yields *qualitative* (or categorical) results such as cervical smear examinations when screening for cancer of the cervix, or karyotype determinations when making a diagnosis of a chromosome abnormality. It does not provide a complete description for quantitative tests or enquiries that yield results as a continuous variable, such as the measurement of blood pressure when screening for stroke or serum alpha-fetoprotein measurement when screening for spina bifida. In such cases, the detection rate and false positive rate vary according to the cut-off level chosen. These rates can be determined by reference to frequency distributions of the test variable for affected and unaffected subjects. For example, the use of, say, cut-off level A in Figure 1.3 will have a detection rate given by the area under the curve for affected subjects above cut-off level A; the false-positive rate is given by the area under the curve for unaffected subjects above the same cut-off level. In this example the higher the cut-off level (say, B or C) the lower the detection rate and the lower the false-positive rate.

Requirements for a worthwhile screening programme

Before screening can provide an effective means of disease prevention certain criteria need to be fulfilled. A knowledge of the disorder being screened for, including its prevalence and natural history, is needed to ensure that the disease is sufficiently common and serious to represent an important medical problem. An effective remedy must be available. The performance of the screening test should be known in terms of its detection rate for the disorder concerned and in terms of its false-positive rate. The screening test must be simple, cheap, acceptable and safe, and facilities must be available or could be made available to provide the screening service and the consequent remedy. The whole process from initial screening to application of the remedy must be ethical and regarded as desirable and offering value for money. Table 1.5 provides a summary of the

Table 1.5 Requirements for a worthwhile screening programme*

Factor	Requirement
Disorder	Well defined
Prevalence	Known
Natural history	Medically important disorder for which there is an effective remedy available
Financial	Cost effective
Facilities	Available or easily installed
Ethical	Procedures following a positive result are generally agreed and acceptable both to the screening authorities and to the patients
Test	Simple and safe
Test performance	Detection rate and false-positive rates known, i.e. distributions of test values in affected and unaffected individuals known, extent of overlap sufficiently small and a suitable cut-off level defined

* Modified from: Cuckle and Wald in Wald N J (ed) 1984 Antenatal and neonatal screening. Oxford University Press, Oxford.

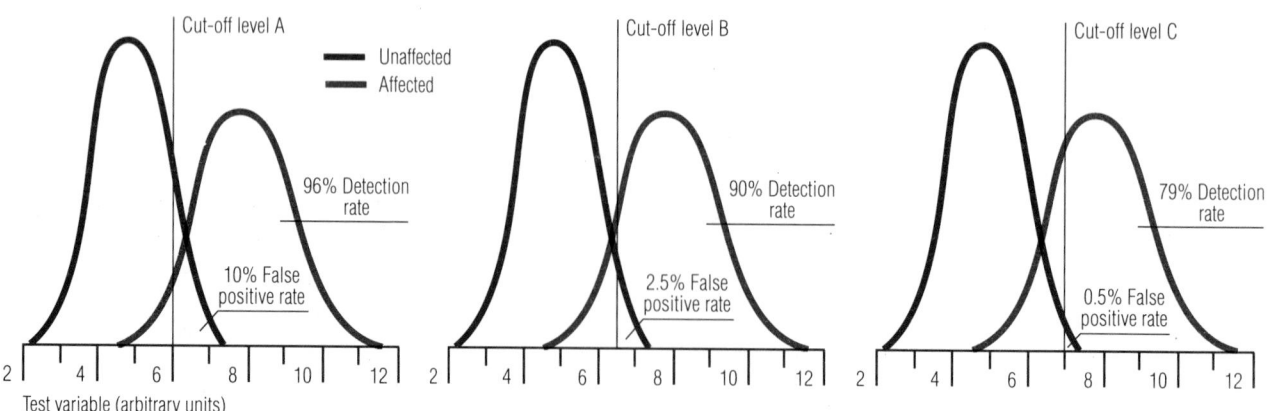

Fig. 1.3 Hypothetical example of the detection rate and false-positive rate of a screening test at three different cut-off levels. (Modified from: Cuckle and Wald in Wald NJ (ed) 1984 Antenatal and neonatal screening, Oxford University Press, Oxford.)

Table 1.6 Examples of worthwhile screening procedures

Disorder	Initial screening test or enquiry	Subsequent test	Approximate proportion of disease preventable
Antenatal screening			
Down's syndrome	Maternal age and maternal serum alpha-fetoprotein, unconjugated oestriol and human chorionic gonadotrophin	Amniocentesis and fetal karyotype	60%
Open neural tube defects	Maternal serum alpha-fetoprotein	Amniotic fluid alpha-fetoprotein and acetylcholinesterase, and ultrasound	90%
β-thalassaemia	Red cell mean corpuscular volume	Haemoglobin electrophoresis, DNA analysis	95%
Screening in infancy			
Congenital hypothyroidism (cretinism)	Neonatal serum thyroid stimulating hormone and/or thyroxine	Repeat screening tests	95%
Phenylketonuria	Neonatal serum phenylalanine	Repeat screening test and serum tyrosene	95%
Adult screening			
Mortality from cancer of the cervix	Age (over 25 years)	Cervical smear	80%
Mortality from cancer of the breast	Age (over 40–50 years)	Mammogram	40%
Mortality from cerebrovascular disease	Age (over 40–50 years)	Diastolic blood pressure above 100 mmHg	50%

requirements of a worthwhile screening programme and Table 1.6 lists screening programmes that, in general, meet these requirements. Potentially worthwhile screening programmes can fail through being badly implemented; cervical cytology, for example, is often carried out widely in younger women but infrequently in older women who are at higher risk.

Summary 7   Secondary prevention of disease: screening

Secondary prevention is prevention through screening and early detection and/or early intervention.

Screening is the identification, among apparently healthy individuals, of those who are sufficiently at risk from a specific disorder to justify a subsequent diagnostic test or procedure, or in certain circumstances, direct intervention.

Terms used in screening:
- *Detection rate* (*sensitivity*) is the proportion of affected individuals with a positive result.
- *False-positive rate* is the proportion of unaffected individuals with a positive result.
  (False-positive rate is 100 minus specificity expressed as a percentage, e.g. a false-positive rate of 3% is the same as a *specificity* of 97%.)
- *Odds of being affected given a positive result* is the ratio of affected to unaffected individuals among those with a positive result.
  (Expressed as a proportion, this is also called the *predictive value positive*, e.g. a 4:1 odds is the same as a predictive value of 4/5 or 80%.)

PATTERNS OF MORTALITY AND MORBIDITY

A useful description of the pattern of mortality and morbidity in a country can often be obtained by national organisations concerned with the collection of vital statistics. The Office of Population Censuses and Surveys (OPCS) in the UK and similar offices in other countries play a crucial role in providing the intelligence needed for effective public health and the appropriate allocation of resources for medical care.

Obtaining reliable information on the extent of disease in the low income countries referred to loosely as 'the developing world' is difficult. The data used below has been drawn from publications from the World Bank and from the 'The Health of Nations' published by the Open University in the UK.

ENGLAND AND WALES

The pattern of mortality and morbidity in England and Wales is fairly typical of that of an economically rich western nation.

Mortality

The introduction of death registration was a landmark in the development of epidemiology. It permitted the quantitative assessment of the frequency of fatal disease, both over time and between different geographical regions. The UK was one of the first countries to collect mortality

11

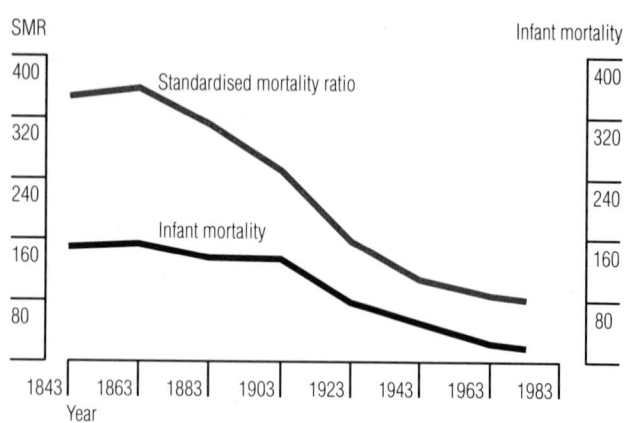

Fig. 1.4   Standardised mortality ratios (SMR) and infant mortality in England and Wales, 1843–1973. Standardised mortality ratios are for all causes, 1950–52 = 100. Infant mortality = deaths under one year of age per 1000 live births. (Source: OPCS.)

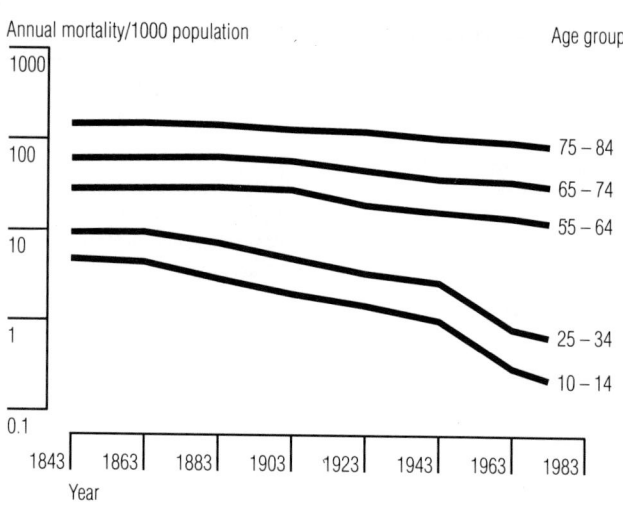

Fig. 1.5   Age specific mortality in England and Wales, 1843–1973. (Source: OPCS.)

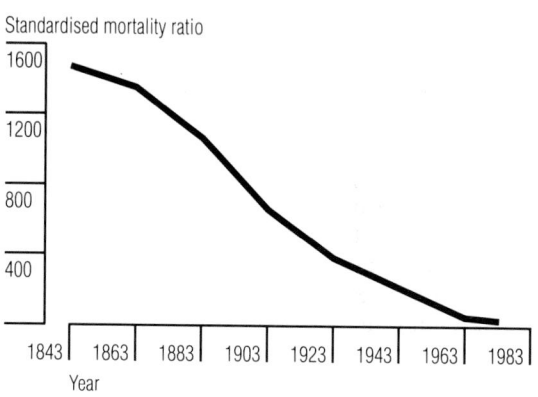

Fig. 1.6   Mortality from tuberculosis in England and Wales, 1850–1980. (1950–52 = 100. Source: OPCS.)

Fig. 1.7   Expectation of life from birth in England and Wales, 1840–1980. (Source: OPCS.)

statistics routinely, and annual figures have been produced since 1838. Figure 1.4 shows that the standardised mortality ratio (SMR) fell steeply from the middle of the 19th century and that infant mortality has declined rapidly from the beginning of the current century. Figure 1.5 shows the reduction in selected age-specific death rates from 1843 to 1973. There has been a decline in all age groups with the greatest percentage reductions in the relatively young. For example, there has been a 90% reduction in mortality in persons aged 25–34, compared to a reduction of 38% in those aged 75–84 years. The most important reason for the decline in mortality in the young is the decline in mortality from infectious diseases. Figure 1.6 shows the decline in the standardised mortality ratio for tuberculosis from about 1500 in the mid-1850s to 60 in recent years. Most of this reduction occurred well before the introduction of specific medical interventions such as the use of antibiotics, immunisation or the use of special investigative techniques such as X-ray. It has, instead, been largely due to the improvement in living standards, particularly in housing conditions and nutrition.

With the reduction in age-specific death rates, the expectation of life has increased. From birth, it is now about 78 years in women and 72 in men, compared to 42 and 40 years respectively in the middle of the 19th century (Fig. 1.7).

The major causes of death vary considerably according to age. In the first four weeks of life the main causes are those associated with prematurity, congenital malformations and complications of birth. The main causes of death during the remaining part of the first year of life are infectious diseases, congenital malformations, sudden infant death syndrome and accidents. Table 1.7 shows the age-specific death rates in 1984 in England and Wales for selected causes of death.

Accidents are the major cause of death in both children (1–14 years) and young adults (15–34 years), with road traffic accidents accounting for about half of these. In adults aged 35–54 (both sexes combined), ischaemic heart

Table 1.7 Death rates per million population from selected causes by age and sex in England and Wales, 1984

Cause	Sex	under 1 year	1–4	5–14	15–24	25–34	35–44	45–54	55–64	65–74	75–84	85 and over
All causes	M	10 800	474	256	776	878	1 662	5 493	17 177	44 362	99 740	211 306
	F	8 539	371	179	301	494	1 116	3 406	9 484	23 899	61 741	168 987
Lung cancer	M	–	–	–	0	8	72	499	2 288	5 309	7 837	7 163
	F	–	–	–	1	4	36	213	842	1 424	1 517	1 207
Breast cancer	F	–	–	–	2	42	216	649	1 028	1 336	1 795	3 183
Colorectal cancer	M	–	–	–	1	7	48	196	612	1 453	2 780	4 442
	F	–	–	–	1	6	35	148	433	973	1 899	3 590
All other cancers	M	47	71	46	79	132	290	938	2 814	6 696	12 944	19 861
	F	56	49	42	49	130	299	842	2 051	3 829	6 431	9 485
Ischaemic heart disease	M	–	–	–	5	52	402	2 176	6 777	15 557	29 358	49 278
	F	–	–	–	2	11	61	417	2 025	6 760	16 960	36 762
Cerebrovascular disease	M	13	2	1	9	26	81	276	1 051	4 138	12 379	29 212
	F	16	2	3	8	27	70	228	751	3 076	11 436	32 300
Other circulatory diseases	M	75	7	7	21	34	71	259	910	2 954	8 494	24 317
	F	66	12	5	13	19	47	156	542	1 792	6 429	26 440
Accidents, injury, violence etc.	M	232	136	122	520	452	430	463	474	629	1 332	3 158
	F	168	83	59	129	124	162	229	283	459	1 103	3 159
Chronic obstructive lung disease	M	36	5	8	14	12	24	123	797	3 102	8 502	15 945
	F	20	8	3	9	9	15	87	408	928	1 678	3 348

Source: OPCS

disease is the major cause of death, followed by cancer and cerebrovascular disease. The death rate in men has levelled since about 1920, but that in women has continued to decline. Both ischaemic heart disease and lung cancer have increased rapidly during this century; both are more common in men than in women. Mortality from these two diseases is the main reason for the fact that, among the 55–74 year old age group, the death rate from all causes in men is about twice that in women (see Table 1.7). The rise in lung cancer mortality during this century (see Ch. 9, Fig. 9.6) is particularly striking, not only on account of its magnitude but also because it is almost all caused by smoking. Although some of the increase must be due to improvements in diagnosis, the differences in lung cancer mortality between the sexes indicate that this alone could not explain the rise.

Taking men and women of all ages together, about a quarter of deaths are caused by ischaemic heart disease, a quarter by cancer, an eighth by strokes, and a further eighth by obstructive lung disease and pneumonia, leaving three-eighths attributable to other causes (Fig. 1.8). The distribution of cancer deaths according to the organ affected is shown in Chapter 9, Figure 9.5.

About half of all deaths are sudden and unexpected; about one-fifth are prolonged.

In all societies, there are inequalities in health. Figure 1.9 shows the death rates in England and Wales in 1971, classified according to social class. This system of categorising the population according to occupation was devised by the Registrar General in 1875, and has been continued

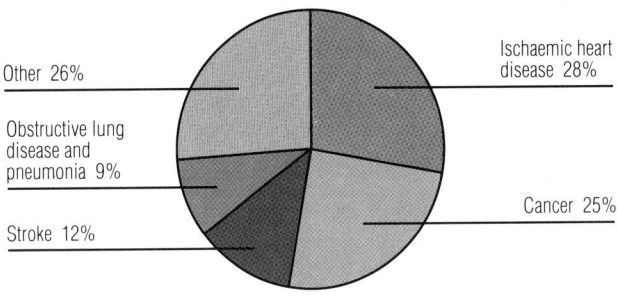

Fig. 1.8 Causes of death in England and Wales, 1984. (Source: OPCS.)

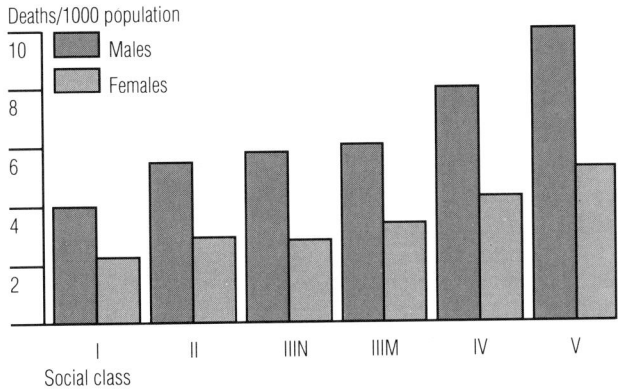

Fig. 1.9 Death rates by social class in England and Wales, 1971. (Source: OPCS.)

ever since. According to this system, there are five social classes, with class three divided into two sub-classes. These are:

I. professional
II. semi-professional
III. skilled – subdivided into non-manual (IIIN) and manual (IIIM)
IV. semi-skilled
V. unskilled.

The proportions of the population of each of the six categories in 1971 were 5%, 18%, 12%, 38%, 18% and 9% respectively. The differences in mortality among social classes illustrates the extent to which mortality in Western countries is due to differences in life style and environmental factors. As Figure 1.9 shows, the mortality of social class V in 1971 was about two and a half times greater than that in social class I. For accidents in children under 14 years of age, the difference was over eightfold. Nearly all diseases are more common in social classes IV and V than in I and II, e.g. there are large differences in mortality from ischaemic heart disease and lung cancer, reflecting differences in smoking habit and diet detween the social classes. Some diseases, however, are more common in social classes I and II, e.g. breast cancer, multiple sclerosis, malignant melanoma and Hodgkin's disease. This observation suggests some interesting aetiological hypotheses – such as the possible link between melanoma and sudden episodes of sunbathing among fair-skinned persons able to afford holidays in the sun.

Morbidity

There are four main sources of information on the extent of illness in the population:

1. hospital statistics on the number of episodes of hospital illness and bed occupancy rates (counted as discharges from hospital and deaths in hospital)
2. registration of all newly diagnosed cases of cancer
3. general practitioner consultation rates
4. self-reported illness in population surveys.

Figure 1.10 shows bed occupancy rates according to disease. Mental disorders account for nearly half of inpatient hospital days mainly because these admissions tend to be long-term. Figure 1.11 shows the general practitioner consultation rates according to major disease groups. Consultation rates are, for nearly all conditions, higher for women than for men.

THE DEVELOPING WORLD

The pattern of disease in the developing world is quite different from that of the economically rich western nations. Apart from malaria and certain disorders specific to particular regions, it is similar to that found in the UK in the early part of the 19th century. Infectious disease accounts for the major burden of mortality in developing countries; infant mortality rates are some ten times greater

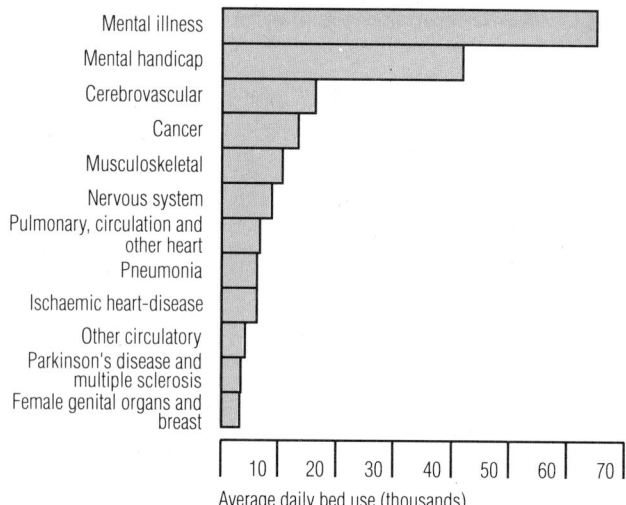

Fig. 1.10   Average daily hospital bed use according to disease in England, 1983. (Source: DHSS/OPCS.)

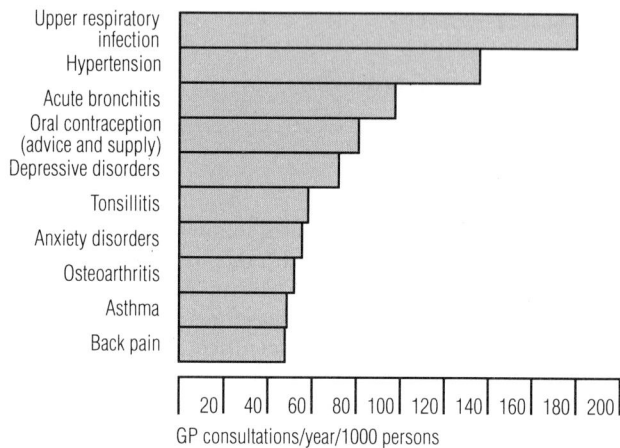

Fig. 1.11   General practitioner consultation rates in England and Wales, 1981–2. (Source: OPCS.)

than those now seen in rich countries (Fig. 1.12); and the expectation of life in developing countries is nearly half that seen today in industrialised countries (Fig. 1.1).

The main cause of disease in the economically poor countries of the world – home to three-quarters of the world's four and a half billion inhabitants – is poverty and, unfortunately, most of the poor countries in the world are remaining poor. In addition, some diseases typical of industrial societies are being exported to the poorer countries. A prime example is lung cancer through the introduction of cigarette smoking, so that this formerly relatively rare cancer is now the commonest cancer in the world.

A useful way to compare the relative importance of different diseases in different countries is to calculate, for each disease, the years of life lost due to deaths from that particular disease. A disease that kills a person at age 60 results in that person losing fewer years of life than a person

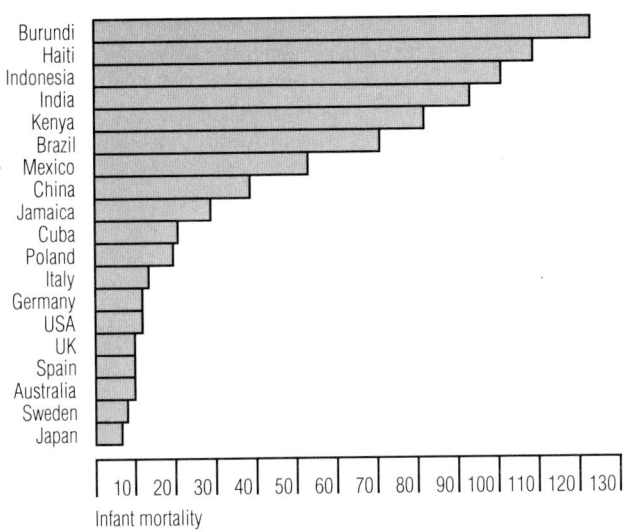

Infant mortality

Fig. 1.12   Infant mortality (deaths under one year of age per 1000 live births) for selected countries, 1983. (Source: World Bank.)

Table 1.8   Years of life lost by men between ages of 1 and 70 due to accident, circulatory diseases and cancer in Ghana and Canada in 1967

| | Years of life lost (% total) | |
Cause of death	Ghana	Canada
Accidents	3	39
Circulatory diseases	4	24
Cancer	1	16
Total	8	79

(Adapted from Table 3.1 in The Health of Nations, 1985, Open University Press.)

Table 1.9   Major causes of years of life lost in Ghana

Disease	Years of life lost (% total)
● Perinatal disorders	24
Pregnancy complications	(1.6)
Congenital malformations	(1.9)
Prematurity	(9.1)
Birth injury	(6.0)
Neonatal tetanus	(3.7)
Neonatal respiratory disorders	(1.6)
● Malaria	15
● Malnutrition and gastroenteritis	10
● Sickle-cell disease	6
● Measles	6
● Pneumonia	6
Total	67

(Adapted from Table 3.2 in The Health of Nations, 1985, Open University Press.)

who dies at, say, 20. Table 1.8 compares the years of life lost from three diseases (accidents, circulatory disease and cancer) which are important causes of mortality in the industrialised world, with the years of life lost through these diseases in the developing world. Two representative countries, namely Ghana and Canada, have been used for comparison. It may be seen that, while these three diseases account for only 8% of years of life lost in Ghana, they account for 79% in Canada.

In Ghana, the major causes of years of life lost are quite different (Table 1.9). Six groups of diseases account for two-thirds of life lost, namely perinatal disorders, malaria, malnutrition and gastroenteritis, sickle cell disease, measles and pneumonia. Malaria is judged to be among the most serious health problems in many parts of tropical Africa and has been estimated to cause over one million deaths a year. Sickle cell disease affects about 1 in 400 Africans and about 1 in 10 people of African descent carry the gene. Measles, while not a typical tropical disease, is an important cause of mortality in the developing world; the reason for the high case fatality from this disease in these countries is not understood. It may be due to the reduced host defences in children suffering from malnutrition and other infections, or it may be due to the fact that measles in the developing world occurs at a young age when the susceptibility to the disease may be greater.

Diarrhoeal disease is another important cause of morbidity and mortality in the developing world. In 1975, an estimated 500 million episodes of diarrhoea in children in Asia, Africa and Latin America caused 5–18 million deaths. The problem is largely due to the vicious cycle arising from contaminated water and food and malnutrition. Poorly nourished children are more liable to get diarrhoea, contaminate the water supplies and thereby infect others. In the developing world, it is from this vicious cycle that the greatest disease burden arises, rather than from diseases more generally regarded as 'tropical' such as schistosomiasis, leishmaniasis, leprosy and onchocerciasis.

About a billion people in the developing world are infested by worms. Surveys in Sri Lanka, Bangladesh and Venezuela indicate that over 90% of 6-year-old children are affected. The commonest worm infestations are hookworm and roundworm (ascariasis).

The burden of disease from respiratory illness is largely due to the same infections that arise (or arose before satisfactory control measures were introduced) in industrial countries – mainly pneumonia, whooping cough, influenza, measles, TB and diphtheria. Overall, the important difference between the developing world and the industrialised countries lies not so much in the types of diseases that occur as in the frequency and impact that they have.

Within developing countries, there are important geographical differences in the distribution of disease. These tend to reflect the local ecological conditions. For example, malaria is transmitted by certain kinds of mosquito; and transmission of schistosomiasis (bilharzia) depends on passage of the parasite from urine or faeces through certain kinds of water snail, in which the parasites develop and then emerge in a form than can reinfect people. The prevalence of these two parasitic diseases therefore depends upon a combination of circumstances favourable to the existence of the mosquito and water snail respectively. Many parasitic diseases are restricted to certain locations, e.g. Chagas' disease is confined to South America and sleeping sickness, transmitted by the tsetse fly, is restricted to Africa.

Disease problems in the Third World cannot be solved by building hospitals with their costly infrastructure of staff and equipment. The greatest need is for simple measures, such as ensuring the supply and quality of food, the provision of clean water, effective sewerage systems and the control of fertility. The World Bank has estimated that the cost of providing clean water to all those in need would be about $260 billion which, although a vast sum, is only about one half of one year's global expenditure on military arms.

The importance of education in improving the health of the world cannot be overestimated. Much of the difficulty in the introduction of measures designed to improve health is due to cultural or religious obstacles which may take the form of traditional practices that are deeply ingrained. In a poor country, people obtain long-term security in large families so that birth control, while of benefit to the community, may not be of help to the individual. Social and cultural changes must progress together with economic development in a way that is sensitive and responsive to all the relevant issues. Few would doubt that the rich industrialised countries of the world have an obligation to provide a lead but, to be effective, they will need to recognise the cultural and political obstacles to the prevention of disease as well as the economic ones.

FURTHER READING

Ahlbom A, Norell S 1984 Introduction to modern epidemiology. Epidemiology Resources Ltd, Chestnut Hill, Maine. *A short, handy textbook*

Doll R, Peto R 1984 The causes of cancer. Oxford University Press, Oxford. *A good example of how epidemiology can identify causes of diseases*

MacMahon B, Pugh T F 1970 Epidemiology: principles and methods. Little, Brown and Company, Boston. *A good basic textbook of epidemiology*

Mausner J S, Bahn A K 1974 Epidemiology: an introductory text. W B Saunders, Philadelphia. *A monograph presenting the concepts of modern epidemiology in a quantitative manner.*

McKeown T 1984 The role of medicine. Blackwell, Oxford. *A short book dealing with concepts of health and disease, and the role of medicine in influencing our health.*

The U205 Course Team 1985 The health of nations. The Open University Press, Milton Keynes. *OUP coursebook examining contemporary and historical patterns of health and disease in the UK and the rest of the world.*

ACKNOWLEDGEMENT

The author is grateful to Kiran Nanchahal for her help in computer programming in connection with the preparation of the data and figures in this chapter; and to Michael McDowall for providing the OPCS data.

The Clinical Approach to Diagnosis and Investigation

INTRODUCTION

The theme of this chapter is the doctor-patient consultation and relationship. This relationship has always been regarded as the cornerstone of medical practice and is the basis of the concept of clinical freedom, by which is meant the freedom of the doctor to act independently in the best interests of the patient. If it is to be acceptable and effective, such freedom demands responsibility – awareness of the effects of clinical actions on other patients and colleagues and on the utilisation of finite resources. The most apolitical doctor cannot ignore the political aspects of his work. He must be aware, for example, that, as a hospital specialist, he will lead a multidisciplinary team with a considerable annual expenditure. Doctors must therefore try to make the best use of advances in high technology medicine and involve themselves in decisions about allocation of resources in collaboration with other members of the health care team.

Although the relationship between a doctor and patient is essentially private, the increasing complexity of medical practice sometimes means that decisions about clinical management are best made jointly with other specialties. Wards and clinics are shared by gastroenterologists and gastrointestinal surgeons, rheumatologists and orthopaedic surgeons, endocrinologists and gynaecologists. For many years, the contribution of the nursing and paramedical staff was taken for granted, often with little direct formal contact with clinicians. It is now clear, however, that the best care is given if doctor, nurse, physiotherapist, occupational therapist and social worker meet regularly to discuss their patients' problems. Colleagues in investigative departments, such as radiology and pathology, and those involved in therapeutic measures, such as the microbiologist advising on antibiotic choices and policies, the pharmacist, clinical pharmacologist or dietician, are some of those regularly involved in making clinical decisions.

The presenting complaint

The most common way a patient presents to a doctor is with symptoms. His usual motive and expectation is the relief of that symptom, a wish for an explanation for it, and reassurance to allay the anxiety it may be creating.

An asymptomatic patient may also seek medical advice for secondary prevention of disease. He may have participated in a screening programme, for example at school or at work, and been found to be at risk. Increasing awareness of the importance of early presymptomatic diagnosis – e.g. because of the improved prognosis if illness (such as cancer or hypertension) is detected early in its development – and of the increasing availability of effective and relatively trouble-free treatment, is changing the pattern of patients' approach to their doctors. Occasionally, the patient may present with a seemingly trivial symptom as an excuse for a 'check-up', perhaps as a result of recent illness in another family member or friend.

Whatever the reason for the consultation, doctors also have a responsibility for the primary prevention of illness and to give advice on general health measures such as diet, smoking, alcohol, drugs, occupational hazards, physical fitness and contraception.

THE PROCESS OF DIAGNOSIS

The traditional sequence of the consultation is as follows:

1. Establish a data base, by history-taking and physical examination.
2. Synthesis, or interpretation, of the data base into either a *problem list* or *differential diagnosis*.
3. Investigations, which will add to the data base, may then be undertaken to confirm or refute a diagnosis, or to document the effects of a known disease. Since investigation may often be invasive, uncomfortable for

2

the patient and expensive, it is always essential to consider how the outcome of an investigation will influence or alter the *management* of a patient. The term management thus embraces both investigation and treatment of the patient.

History-taking

Many sequences of questioning and listening are advocated in history-taking. The hardest skill to acquire is the ability to reconcile the often haphazard and rambling fashion in which a patient gives the history (which may contain valuable information) with the need to fit the history into a pattern. Both practice and skill are required to elicit a history within a reasonable time and without asking too many leading questions (in which case the patient's answers may reflect his wish to please the doctor rather than the true situation). For the same reason, attempts to substitute questionnaires or interactive computer interviewing programmes have had only a limited success. Their value has mainly been in healthy population screening, such as pre-employment examinations, or where there are barriers of language or culture, as with certain immigrant groups.

The history will usually be recorded under the following headings:

1. *Presenting complaints and duration.* These should be documented in detail.
2. *Past history.* The past history is usually chronologically recorded and should try to differentiate *inactive problems*, which are unlikely to be of immediate relevance to the present problem (e.g. tonsillectomy in childhood), and *active problems*, which continue, or are likely to recur intermittently (e.g. hypertension, diabetes, asthma or duodenal ulcer).
3. *Personal history* (or system review) inquires into body functions and habits, such as weight, appetite, bowel habit, micturition, menstruation and sleep. A more or less detailed dietary history may be required, together with a record of smoking and alcohol consumption. Sexual practices should also be discussed in view of the increasing importance of sexually transmitted diseases, and methods of contraception recorded.
4. *Drug history* merits particular enquiry. It is often incomplete, partly because of use of self-prescribed over-the-counter remedies being overlooked or unrecorded.
5. *Family history* is important (and can be succinctly recorded by a genetic tree). The health or illnesses of the genetically unrelated spouse or partner are also relevant because of both disease transmission and the effect it may have on the relationship.
6. *Travel, pets and animals, recreations and occupation history.* These are all self-explanatory parts of the medical history. The patient's occupation may not only reveal contact with known and potential industrial hazards but also forms an important part of the social history.
7. *Social history.* Employment and unemployment influ-

ence a patient's income and may frustrate ambitions, leading to physical symptoms of stress. Poor living conditions are well recognised determinants of disease prevalence and often play a part in individual illnesses.

Population projections indicate that, by the year 2000, half the population of the UK will be beyond retirement age. The problems of retirement, and the increasing disabilities of old age, will thus make enormous demands on family, community and commercial resources (Ch.10). The elderly patient may be reluctant to seek help and it is therefore important to inquire whether they make use of services such as home helps, meals-on-wheels, dining clubs, geriatric visitors and day centres, and voluntary agencies.

A useful open-ended question to ask is, 'What do you think is wrong with you?'. It can be very difficult to anticipate the fears patients may have about their symptoms and the illnesses they think they may signify. For example, a healthy young woman in her twenties, who presents with occasional constipation, may be afraid that she has cancer of the bowel. It may not occur to the doctor to reassure her that this is not the case, as the diagnosis would hardly enter his mind. However, her unspoken fear might undo the benefit derived from an otherwise sympathetic approach and sensible advice. Open-ended questions may also create an opportunity to find out how much the patient wants to know about his illness, or whether he wishes others to be informed.

In addition to avoiding or minimising direct or leading questions, it is essential to be careful with the use of medical terminology when taking a history. Several studies have demonstrated the misconceptions and confusions that can arise from the patient's (improper) use of seemingly common terms like dizzy, giddy, palpitations, angina, indigestion and dyspepsia. The doctor, in using these terms to record the patient's symptom, will be making an interpretation which may not only be erroneous but may also preclude further inquiry. If the patient uses these words, it is essential to obtain more detail and to ask the patient to describe the symptom clearly. Another potential error is for the doctor to make an instant translation of the patient's symptoms when recording them. For example, if the patient complains of chest pain but the doctor records it as angina, further questions tend to pursue only this possibility. This may have important consequences, as the interpretation of the symptoms will, to some extent, influence the clinical examination to follow. The doctor should be open to further interpretation at all stages of investigation and management until a diagnosis is made.

Other difficulties in history taking arise from more general communication problems. The intelligence of the patient, his age, socio-economic group, regional or ethnic origin may all create barriers to understanding.

Physical examination

There is no one 'correct' order in which physical examination should be carried out. A topographical ('head-to-

toe'), or system-by-system approach is equally valid, and most doctors construct their own system which tends to be a compromise between the two. Examination is rarely undertaken without using clues from the history as a guide, even in the comatose or confused patient. As in history-taking, examination of the affected system must be accompanied by a comprehensive examination of the rest of the patient. The recording of base-line observations (which may initially be normal) is crucial in most medical emergencies where management is guided by changes in these. For example, changes in pulse and blood pressure are an important determinant in treating gastrointestinal haemorrhage, changes in jugular venous pressure in monitoring diuretic or intravenous therapy, and level of consciousness and other neurological signs in the management of stroke or subarachnoid haemorrhage.

Physical examination is not a ritual; the tendency to find only what you are seeking must be avoided. The more curiosity with which the doctor carries out the examination the more rewarding it will be. With practice and experience, the time spent will shorten, thereby allowing a more detailed examination of certain systems where appropriate. The physical examination of particular systems is discussed in the relevant chapters.

Differential diagnosis

After the history-taking and physical examination have been carried out, the patient's problems are reformulated as a *differential diagnosis*, i.e. a statement of the possible causes of the complaint. To this may be added a *problem list*. Construction of a problem list and a differential diagnosis should not be regarded as alternatives but, rather, as complementary.

Differential diagnosis is a problem-solving activity dependent on past experience and knowledge. Common conditions can be diagnosed with confidence unless their presentation is highly atypical. The clinician's experience of less common, or specialised, conditions may be limited and possibly misleading if his experience is based on unusual or atypical cases.

Problem list

A problem list is of particular help to the medical student who has not yet acquired detailed medical knowledge and therefore has difficulty in suggesting a list of diagnoses which may explain the clinical features. A problem list is much less restrictive than a differential diagnosis, since it leaves the next stage of diagnosis open. It also leads to the patient being considered as a whole person and not just a collection of diseases (Table 2.1). Social problems, which may be the main cause of admission of an elderly patient or a barrier to his discharge, are documented. The patient's (or his family's) emotional responses to illness (especially if chronic) may need to be identified to enable subsequent successful management; a problem list will draw attention to this.

Table 2.1   The use of a problem list.

A woman of 78 is admitted with a haematemesis. The following active and inactive problems are identified:

Problems

Active	Inactive
Acute blood loss	Cholecystectomy
Hypotension	Appendicectomy
Aspirin ingestion	
Osteoarthritis of knees	
Social isolation	
Chronic asthma	

Differential diagnosis

Acute gastric erosion
Peptic ulceration
Other causes of upper gastrointestinal bleeding

The differential diagnosis leads to appropriate investigations (e.g. endoscopy) but the problem list also identifies wider issues in management.

The problem list records both *active* problems and past or *inactive* problems. The list will draw attention to the potential hazards of treatment of an active problem; for example, treatment with corticosteroids in a patient who also has the inactive problem of healed peptic ulcer may convert it to an active problem. Alternatively, the patient presenting with the active problem of abdominal pain and vomiting may have the inactive problem of past appendicectomy. Recognition of this not only excludes appendicitis as a cause of the pain, but also introduces the possibility of intestinal obstruction due to adhesions.

A problem list enables a flexible approach, such that several problems may combine into a single problem or diagnosis as a result of further information. For example, the initial problems of nausea and upper abdominal pain will reveal themselves as aspects of the single problem of cholestasis following the appearance of pruritus and jaundice. Abdominal ultrasound scanning may then show dilated intrahepatic bile ducts and a stone in the common bile duct. The active problem is thus extrahepatic cholestasis due to obstructing gallstones. Successful surgery will mean that the problem becomes inactive but it is recorded, nonetheless, during any subsequent illness. The problem could of course become active again as a result of stricture formation in the common bile duct or retained gallstones in the biliary tree.

Diagnostic aids

Apart from discussion and reference to books, other aids to rapid and accurate diagnosis have been developed. Several studies of computer aided diagnosis have been undertaken. The frequency of specific symptoms and signs in a disease are recorded, and the probabilities of the different possible diagnoses can be given. With a little more mathematical sophistication, numerical weighting can be applied to the individual symptoms or signs. For example, in a model based on the diagnosis of peptic ulcer, a correct diagnosis

The Clinical Approach to Diagnosis and Investigation

of ulcer could be made with over 90% confidence if the patient answered four key questions affirmatively. The computer can also indicate further discriminating questions to be asked, or physical signs to be elicited. The model can be extended to include the results of investigations and then to indicate which further investigations will be of value in discriminating between diagnoses.

An alternative approach has been to devise algorithms, or branching diagnostic trees, based on a pathophysiological understanding of the presenting symptoms or signs (Fig. 2.1). Such systems can be used as a guide for inexperienced doctors or paramedical workers in poor countries enabling them to achieve rapid diagnoses, often inexpensively, by indicating the few investigations of relevance.

Fig. 2.1 Diagnostic algorithm for dysphagia. Pharyngeal causes are shown above and oesophageal causes below. (From Beck E, Francis J, Souhami R L 1982 Tutorials in differential diagnosis, 2nd edn. Churchill Livingstone, Edinburgh)

A study in East Africa has shown that paramedicals, using such a system, could diagnose common, locally prevalent, conditions such as tuberculosis more accurately and rapidly than trained doctors.

Similarly, statistical techniques based on probabilities using data from large numbers of patients can be used to devise a prognostic index. This is particularly useful in diseases which have varied manifestations and prognoses, and where the effects of treatment are difficult to evaluate. Examples are the staging systems used in cancer, which clearly define patients with a good or bad prognosis. The management of non-malignant conditions of uncertain prognosis, e.g. acute pancreatitis and Crohn's disease, has also been improved by such prognostic indices. As with diagnosis, algorithms can be used to formulate a uniform management policy for specific clinical situations, and adjusted to local needs and resources.

Investigation

Investigations are undertaken to help make decisions about diagnosis or treatment. Clinical medicine has been greatly enhanced by advances in the technology of diagnostic specialities, but one must not lose sight of the fact that these techniques represent means rather than ends. The clinician must be aware of both their scope and their limitations. In making judicious use of what is available, he must collaborate closely with specialist colleagues in medicine, pathology and imaging. The revolution in diagnostic imaging in recent years has had a major impact on the practice of medicine and is discussed in a separate section of this chapter (p. 23).

Investigations may also be required to establish the extent or severity of a disease, to detect its complications, to assess the likelihood of remission or relapse, or to give prognostic information. A doctor is sometimes concerned that he might be considered negligent if he has not requested a particular test, even if it would not have influenced his clinical action. Nevertheless, the clinical usefulness of the test should always be the basis for investigation, not medico-legal considerations. An economic argument for comprehensive investigation is sometimes made in wealthy countries, the aim being speed in diagnosis and the shortest possible stay in an expensive hospital bed. Many unnecessary tests may be done and normal results obtained, with a sprinkling of unexpected abnormalities. The problem is that these abnormalities may then generate further, frequently unrewarding, investigations. Thus, such an approach to investigation is not necessarily economical and may result in poor clinical decisions. Some investigations are, however, carried out as routine because laboratory equipment is automated and, in requesting a single common biochemical or haematological test, many others are automatically performed.

It is important when selecting appropriate investigations to be able to judge both their sensitivity and their specificity. These two attributes may be in conflict but, as long as one understands this, one or other type of test may be selected for a particular purpose, or both used in com-plementary fashion. In the diagnosis of giant cell (temporal) arteritis, for example, the ESR is nearly always raised, making this a very sensitive test for the diagnosis. However, the ESR is also raised in many other inflammatory or neoplastic disorders which might enter the differential diagnosis, giving the test poor specificity. In contrast, the histological appearances seen with temporal artery biopsy are highly specific and are not seen in any other unrelated condition. Biopsy may, however, give a false negative result and has the disadvantage of being invasive and relatively expensive. In everyday practice, a typical history and physical findings associated with an ESR greater than 100 mm/hour would therefore be accepted as diagnostic, and biopsy restricted to cases where there was diagnostic difficulty.

THE AIMS OF TREATMENT

Prevention and cure

Ideally, prevention is the best form of cure. Preventative medicine in the general population, despite its earlier success in combatting infectious diseases by improved living conditions and immunisation, has not yet made great inroads into the degenerative and malignant diseases that have replaced them as the major causes of morbidity, at least in the developed world. Individual prevention may be relevant in the relatives of index patients with inherited disorders, such as colonic carcinoma and familial polyposis, or coronary artery disease in the hyperlipidaemias. In many patients, the expectation of permanent cure can be high, e.g. in the antibiotic treatment of a pneumococcal pneumonia, or replacement therapy in hypothyroidism. The aims in treating an individual patient thus depend on the nature of the disease and the stage it has reached. This must be explained to the patient and an attempt made to reconcile the proposed approach with his expectations. While one must not remove hope, it is both unkind and counterproductive to make unreasonable claims for the treatment proposed.

Palliation

The aim of treatment may be only palliative if the patient has disseminated cancer, advanced multiple sclerosis or crippling rheumatoid arthritis. Nevertheless, the skilful anticipation and alleviation of the patient's symptoms is rewarding to both the patient and the clinical team. The practices initiated by the hospice movement in terminal care and pain relief (Ch. 9) have now been introduced in the hospital and domiciliary setting, often under the supervision of a hospice-trained nurse. The patient deteriorating from an incurable condition must be given as much attention as someone with an acute and curable illness. Medical staff may find difficulty in talking to such patients and discussing their fears and expectations. Furthermore, while they understandably get satisfaction from seeing a patient's disease go into remission – be it severe asthma, left ventricular failure, or fulminating ulcerative colitis – this should be tempered by the knowledge that, though healing has been achieved, relapse or recurrence is probable.

The diseases prevalent in advanced industrialised nations, where the proportion of middle-aged and elderly in the population is increasing, tend not to be curable. It is true that cure can now be achieved in some diseases which in the past were lethal. This is particularly true of infections such as meningococcal meningitis, pneumococcal pneumonia and tuberculosis, and surgery can now cure some patients of cancer, and of structural abnormalities such as hernias or congenital heart lesions. However, in the ageing population, cures are rare, and the main objective of treatment (both medical and surgical) tends to be the relief of symptoms rather than removal of the underlying disease. Insulin for the control of diabetes mellitus, total hip replacement for arthritis, H_2-receptor blockers for peptic ulcer, and medical and surgical treatment for angina pectoris, are all examples of excellent long-term treatments. In the elderly, 'treatment' may also consist of the use of social services to allow patients to return to an independent existence.

'Complementary' medicine

Some patients become dissatisfied with conventional medicine, especially when there is an over-readiness to prescribe on the part of the doctor, and a lack of time to listen and talk. Patients also expect to be relieved of symptoms, and reassurance that there is nothing seriously wrong may not be enough. For both these and other reasons, such as when a patient has a serious disease for which there is no cure, the patient may seek alternative opinions, not necessarily within conventional medicine. He may turn instead to 'alternative' or 'complementary' medicine. The lack of validation and the extravagant claims made by the exponents of alternative medicine have led to deep scepticism from within the medical profession. Few of these forms of treatment have been submitted to the rigours of a controlled trial; and when such a study was done comparing homeopathic and conventional treatment in patients with rheumatoid arthritis, the latter was shown to be more effective. The techniques of acupuncture and osteopathy have attracted medical interest in recent years, but their role in treatment remains ill-defined. Some of these approaches to treatment are dangerous both in themselves (e.g. the use of laetrile for cancer) and because they delay diagnosis. Often what helps the patient is the interest and attention he receives and which he may feel is lacking from conventional doctors.

Constraints on treatment

A treatment decision requires an appraisal of the quality, as well as the prolongation, of life that treatment may achieve. This is shown by the difference in approach to an advanced lymphoma in a 35-year-old compared to a 75-year-old patient. Intensive chemotherapy for the younger patient has the aim of cure and justifies the toxicity. In the older patient, cure is less likely and intensive treatment therefore less appropriate. Therapeutic decisions of this kind are often made in conjunction with other members of the clinical team, the patient and the family.

Financial constraints may limit resources for expensive treatment. This is shown by the unsatisfied demand for dialysis and transplantation for the treatment of chronic renal failure. Other, less dramatic, deficiencies exist in the areas of mental and physical handicap and psychogeriatrics.

THE DOCTOR-PATIENT RELATIONSHIP

For a patient to have confidence in his doctor, he must feel that confidentiality will apply in all their dealings. In recent years, the question of who should have access to medical records has become an important area for debate in the growing public awareness of, and involvement in, medical ethics. For practical purposes, the principle of confidentiality has not as yet been eroded although vigilance is required, especially with the use of computerised record systems.

With complex and technical problems, the patient cannot be involved as an entirely equal partner in making decisions. Some patients in fact seem pleased to relinquish responsibility for their treatment, while others say that they would like to know everything. Knowing how much to tell patients, and when, is a skill acquired slowly and with practice. This is particularly true when breaking bad news, such as a diagnosis of cancer. It is valuable to keep a record of such conversations in the case notes, so that those talking to the patient at a later date can see what has already been said. It should be remembered that the patient may not have as clear a memory of what was said as the doctor or his notes indicate. This may be because of genuine difficulty in comprehending what was said, but may also be due to an inability to come to terms with it. Such 'denial' may be of the whole or only part of the conversation. Further quiet discussion is therefore always necessary. It is sometimes helpful if another member of the team is present on the first occasion, so that the patient has someone readily available to talk to at a later date.

Conflicts of interest

Situations can arise where the patient's interests conflict with those of others. An example is the right of parents to know when a daughter, who is still a minor, seeks contraceptive advice from her GP, even if the girl requests that they are not informed. Similarly, a doctor employed in an occupational health capacity by organisations or companies may face a conflict between the interests of an employee, whom he sees as a patient and who expects the usual confidentiality between patient and doctor to prevail, and his employers, who may expect the doctor's loyalty to be towards them. Employees should be aware, or made aware, that the doctor-patient relationship is somewhat different in these situations. Similarly, prisoners only have access to medical care through the prison doctor, who is employed by the Home Office and thus, again, has potentially divided loyalties.

Conflict between the patient's interests and those of his family may arise in attempting to return a severely disabled patient to his home. The patient's dearest wish may be to be at home, but the effects on family life may be disastrous.

A particular and unavoidable ethical problem arises in the doctor-patient relationship when a patient (or, in the case of organ donation for transplantation, a relative) is asked to participate in an action of no direct benefit to himself. For example, the patient may be asked to help in bedside teaching, or to have a clinical photograph or video recording made of his condition. More difficult issues arise in relation to participation in research. Trials of a new therapy, where the patient is randomly allocated to a treatment, require full explanation to be given and informed consent obtained. The manner in which consent is obtained, both in such trials and in everyday practice, has been the subject of considerable discussion. Should one, for example, indicate every conceivable mishap which might occur as a result of treatment? Such a policy might add considerably to the anxieties of patients. In the United Kingdom, practical ethical issues, especially those involving research, are now regularly discussed and resolved by hospital based ethics committees which have lay representation. Helpful guidelines on many such problems have been prepared for such local and national committees by the Royal College of Physicians, the Medical Research Council and various associations representing workers in the field of transplantation, cancer research and other areas of specialist practice.

DIAGNOSTIC IMAGING

The last 20 years have seen major advances in our ability to demonstrate disease processes by imaging methods. Doctors have a particular responsibility to understand the power and the limitations of the new techniques involved, and should always remember that investigation is an adjunct to diagnosis and does not replace careful clinical assessment. This section outlines the uses and limitations of some of the most important imaging techniques.

Wilhelm Röntgen's brilliant chance discovery of X-rays, in 1895, opened up an entirely new method of looking at the living human organism. Within months X-ray pictures were being taken in many European centres. Methods have been refined since then, so that exposures now take not minutes but milliseconds; foggy pictures have been replaced by sharp images; and temperamental apparatus has given way to today's sophisticated engineering. Röntgen would still, however, recognise the essentials of his technique in the standard X-ray rooms, but might have difficulty elsewhere in a present-day radiology department,

with the radically new ways of making images of the human body which have arisen in the second half of the 20th century – radionuclides in the 1950s, ultrasound in the 1960s, computed tomography in the 1970s, and magnetic resonance in the 1980s.

X-ray pictures

X-ray pictures or radiographs are *tissue absorption maps* – two-dimensional representations of what happens when an X-ray beam passes through a three-dimensional part and irradiates a photographic film behind it. The film is developed and usually viewed directly as a negative. Thus, on a chest X-ray, the ribs are white (dense or opaque) because X-rays are absorbed by high atomic number elements such as calcium; the lungs are almost black (radiolucent) since air is a poor absorber, and everything else is grey (water-dense). Muscle, blood, urine and collagen, for example, are all water-dense to X-rays and cannot be distinguished by their absorption characteristics on a film. The lungs thus show some grey structures within them such as blood vessels which are water-dense. X-ray maps are best regarded as *interface maps* – their landscapes can only be made out where different absorbers are up against one another. Thus, the kidneys (water-dense) can often be seen on an abdominal radiograph because fat (composed of low atomic number elements, and hence radiolucent) acts as a perinephric marker. Similarly, a hiatus hernia (water-dense to air interface) is easily seen on a chest X-ray (Fig. 2.2).

Radiographs are at the cheap end of an expensive market; in the UK, for example, a chest X-ray costs £10. With complex radiographic examinations, however, the cost may rise steeply; an inpatient arteriogram will amount to several hundred pounds (Table 2.2).

Fig. 2.2 There is a large mass behind the heart on this film (overpenetrated on purpose): a hiatus hernia (large arrows). Note also the normal junction line where the two lungs almost meet anteriorly (small arrows).

2

Computed tomography

Computed tomography (CT) is a further development of standard X-ray techniques. In the latter, the photographic film placed behind a patient for obtaining a standard radiograph is a fairly poor sensor of photons. It also means that a complex three-dimensional structure is imaged 'flat', i.e. compressed by superimposition into a two-dimensional summation picture. For this reason, most X-ray examinations involve two separate views taken at right angles, to help reconstruct the part in three dimensions. In CT examinations, however, a fan beam of X-rays is made to

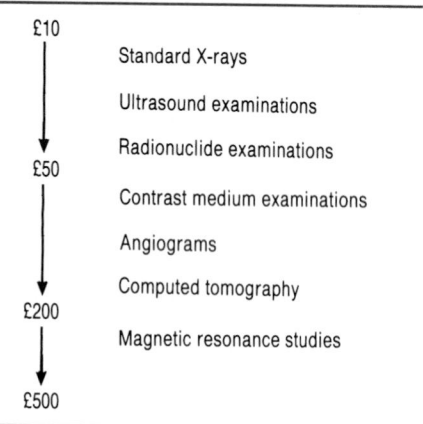

Table 2.2 Order of costs for imaging tests in the United Kingdom.

£10
↓
£50
↓
£200
↓
£500

Standard X-rays

Ultrasound examinations

Radionuclide examinations

Contrast medium examinations

Angiograms

Computed tomography

Magnetic resonance studies

traverse just one section of the body, so that a slice is obtained. An array of scintillation counters (a better sensor than photographic film) is used to record the radiation emerging. A computer then reconstructs a detailed cross-sectional view from the multiple recordings (Fig. 2.3). However, the essential characteristic of CT pictures is still, as with radiographs, that of a tissue absorption map.

Radiographs vs. CT sections

A standard X-ray of, say, the abdomen is a single summation picture. Abnormal calcareous lesions (e.g. renal stones) can be seen, and abnormal radiolucent features (e.g. gaseous distension of bowel loops) made out. If a mass is present, for example, in the retroperitoneum, it may displace normal landmarks of fat and so become visible. An anterior, intraperitoneal mass is much less likely to be detected on X-ray examination. An abdominal radiograph is readily obtainable and comparatively cheap in developed countries.

A CT examination is much less straightforward. It requires 10–20 sections to cover the abdomen, rising to 20–30 if the pelvis is to be included. Each single CT slice contains much more data than can be compressed on the grey scale of a photograph and so a television monitor is necessary to extract the wealth of structural information. The detailed picture of *in vivo* cross-sectional anatomy

Fig. 2.3 A computed tomograph (CT) scan of abnormal kidneys after intravenous contrast medium has been given. There is patchy renal atrophy: note how close some calyces (arrowed bottom right) are to the renal surface. This is the picture of renal papillary necrosis following chronic analgesic abuse. The centre arrow indicates the left renal vein curving over the aorta to reach the inferior vena cava (normal anatomy).

thus obtained is at present unrivalled; abnormal masses, for example, are readily seen, wherever they are. However, access to CT, even in developed countries, is limited, and a CT examination costs £100–200, compared with £10–20 for an abdominal radiograph.

Such simple comparisons do not tell the complete story, however. A CT examination can be used as the single outpatient test to refute or confirm a suspected abdominal mass. A series of other, less certain, investigations may require days in hospital, add to the patient's discomfort and also be more expensive. Even a simple test, if it has an equivocal result that leads on to other investigations, is not cheap.

Contrast media

Standard radiographs can reveal much more if the organ in question is first opacified, e.g. the stomach with a barium meal. Two main classes of contrast media are used.

Enteral contrast media

Barium sulphate is harmless if swallowed, as the insoluble suspension passes through the gut unabsorbed. Present-day barium meals and barium enemas make much use of so-called *double contrast techniques* where the wall of the bowel is coated with a thin layer of barium and the gut lumen distended with gas. Defects in the wall can then be easily seen (Ch. 16).

Parenteral contrast media

Benzoic acid derivatives incorporating three iodine atoms (for radio-opacity) are the standard agents for urography and angiography (Fig. 2.4). Minor variations in chemical make-up can adapt these derivatives for other uses, e.g. for opacifying the biliary tree.

Considerable amounts of the standard urographic/angiographic compounds can be injected safely, but hazards do exist. Reactions to contrast media are ill understood and potentially life-threatening events, occurring without warning in otherwise fit patients. No contrast medium examination should therefore be requested without good clinical reason.

Contrast is cleared by the kidneys. Patients in renal failure, and also infants, cannot therefore readily cope with a large contrast medium load, and such examinations should only be used with great caution in these individuals. The clinician should discuss the investigation with the radiologist if there is doubt over indications and risks in particular patients.

Fig. 2.4 Leg venogram showing clot in many veins. Contrast medium injected from the foot courses along the periphery of veins, outlining the clot in the centre (arrow). Arteriographic and venographic techniques generally use multiple views in sequence.

Ultrasound

Ultrasound pictures are two-dimensional sections as in CT, but depend on quite different tissue properties, viz. reflection of high-frequency sound waves. For practical purposes, these pictures may be regarded as *collagen maps*. As in all sectional techniques, great care is needed to build up a correct three-dimensional notion of the organ under examination by means of multiple contiguous slices. The interpretation of ultrasound maps is often more difficult

than that of CT pictures, as they appear less immediately life-like, and are also more dependent on the individual operator.

A two-plane ultrasound picture can gain an important additional dimension (time) by recording signals continuously on a television monitor. The movement of the fetus *in utero*, of the heart valves, or of the leaves of the diaphragm can be studied in this way, thus providing an insight into functional events. The few still images returned to the clinician as the end result of an ultrasound examination are second best to seeing the image in real time.

At the frequencies and intensities used in diagnostic work, ultrasound appears to be harmless. Medical ultrasound was pioneered in the field of obstetrics, and monitoring the progress of pregnancy remains one of its most frequent uses. Fluid-solid interfaces (in the sense of reflective surfaces) are shown clearly: gallstones (Fig. 2.5) and heart valves as well as the fetus in its liquor are thus all good ultrasound candidates. When an abdominal swelling is discovered, ultrasound can determine whether or not this is a fluid mass, e.g. an abscess or a cyst.

The Doppler principle can be made use of for flow studies, generally over vessels which are placed superficially.

The cost of an ultrasound examination varies from £20 to £50, depending on the range and complexity of the clinical questions posed. It is thus more expensive than plain X-rays but cheaper than CT.

Fig. 2.5 Ultrasound scan of gallbladder containing three small gallstones (arrow). The black lines running down from them through the tissues behind the gallbladder are 'acoustic corridors', where the stones have prevented sound transmission.

Radionuclides

Radionuclides are natural tools of very diverse diagnostic capability. When used in scanning (a better term is *scintigraphy*) they can provide *tissue emission maps*, the usual purpose of which is to give a picture of the function of an organ or system. These functional events can also be used to answer topographical questions. In skeletal scintigraphy, for example, a chemical in the metabolic turnover of bone (e.g. diphosphonate) is labelled with the radionuclide technetium, injected intravenously, and the bone scintigram recorded on a gamma camera some hours later. Areas of increased bone turnover, as in metastases or fractures, will appear as areas of increased activity (Fig. 2.6).

The method is capable of much functional and technical sophistication. In suspected pulmonary emboli, for example, perfusion and ventilation of the lungs can be studied simultaneously by following both small labelled particles (injected intravenously) into the pulmonary arterial bed, and a labelled gas (inhaled) into the acini (Ch. 14, p. 504). Similarly, uptake of an isotopic tracer by the kidney will give a functional, quantitative map of the organ (Ch. 21, p. 797). The transport of the same or another agent down the ureters can then be monitored to determine if the kidney is obstructed. Isotopes can also be used to label cells and study their distribution. For example, the patient's red cells can be labelled, reinjected and followed in order to locate an internal bleeding point. White blood cells may also be labelled and reinjected, to localise an inflammatory lesion (Ch. 12, Fig. 12.2). Tomographic techniques, following injection of isotopically-labelled material, can be used to obtain high resolution images. This is termed *emission tomography*.

Radiation hazards of scintigraphy are generally slight, certainly much less than those of X-ray techniques. Many different radionuclide methods are available, with varying costs. In general, standard scintigrams are in a middle range of cost, i.e. more expensive than plain radiographs but cheaper than angiograms or CT. In the UK, the cost of a bone scintigram is about £30, comparable to that of an ultrasound examination.

Magnetic resonance

The technique of magnetic resonance, currently undergoing rapid development, attempts to produce images based on tissue biochemistry, using whole body cross-sectional slice techniques familiar from CT (Fig. 2.7). The patient is placed in a strong magnetic field and subjected to radiofrequency pulses. The manner in which the magnetic axes of protons align and realign themselves under these influences is then studied and translated into tissue maps. The method appears to be harmless, and promises much; but it is very expensive, even more so than CT at present (Table 2.2).

Hazards in radiology

Contrast medium reactions and indiscriminate overuse of diagnostic investigations are two important dangers in radiology. Radiation risks make up a third hazard of obvious concern, because each time a patient is exposed to X-rays there is a possibility of harm.

At the low exposures to ionising radiation involved in diagnostic radiology, the possibility of a harmful outcome is a chance event, dependent on whether or not the ionising radiation hits a specific sensitive target in a dividing cell. The hazard of inducing a carcinoma from a diagnostic X-ray examination is approximately 1 in 10 000 from an absorbed dose of 0.01 Gy (10 mGy).

The gonads are often used as examples of radiosensitive tissues. The great majority of radiation received by them derives from natural sources, amounting to about 1 mGy per year on average. Diagnostic X-rays add about 0.2 mGy to this gonad dose per year to a person in the United Kingdom. This represents a comparatively low diagnostic

Fig. 2.6 Bone scan. A. Normal bone scan. Note symmetrical uptake.
B. Multiple metastases. Multiple 'hot spots' can be seen in skull, shoulder girdle, ribs and pelvis.

Fig. 2.7 Magnetic resonance image of brain. This is a T1 weighted sagittal view of a normal brain, taken through the midline at 1.5 tesla.

X-ray burden among Western countries, deriving from a rate of about 400 X-ray examinations per 1000 people per year. The risks in question are therefore small but must, nevertheless, be taken into account by a doctor requesting an X-ray examination, and weighed against the benefit to be expected from the investigation.

FURTHER READING

British Medical Journal Editorial 1989. Central nervous system clinical algorithms. Endocrine system clinical algorithms. British Medical Journal reprints. *Problem-solving and management algorithms, each accompanied by an essay.*

Evans K T, Gravelle I H, Roberts G M, Hayward C 1987 Clinical radiology for medical students, 2nd edn. Butterworths, London. *Everything and more that the student needs in radiology.*

Knill-Jones R P 1987. Diagnostic systems as an aid to clinical decision making. British Medical Journal 295: 1392–1396.

Macartney E J 1987 Diagnostic logic. British Medical Journal 295: 1325–1331.

    The above two articles from a series of eight, the volume entitled 'Logic in medicine'. The first includes a discussion of the weighting of symptoms in relation to their discriminating value.

McCarthy M 1982. Epidemiology and policies for health planning. King Edward's Hospital Fund for London. *A well-illustrated monograph, containing a broad range of health statistics. Each chapter briefly describes needs, followed by evidence for the effectiveness of prevention and treatment.*

Royal College of Physicians 1989. Guidelines on the practice of ethics committees in medical research involving human subjects, 2nd edn. Royal College of Physicians, London. *A brief, well-written guide used as a model by most ethics committees.*

Clinical Pharmacology

3

DRUG REGULATION AND DEVELOPMENT

The importance of drug regulation has grown with the rapid increase in the number of therapeutic agents developed over the last 50 years. Increased efficacy of new compounds is often associated with a risk of serious adverse effects.

The United Kingdom Medicines Act (1968)

In the late 1950's, thalidomide was introduced as a new hypnotic drug and was widely used in Europe in all types of patient, including pregnant women. In 1961 an epidemic of appalling proportions occurred in which hundreds of the babies were born with limb abnormalities (phocomelia). The connection with thalidomide administration was soon realised and the drug was hastily withdrawn. The nature of this adverse reaction and the public pressure which it provoked resulted in the formation, in the United Kingdom, of the Committee on Safety of Drugs (the Dunlop Committee) in 1965, and the consequent development of strict legislation concerning all aspects of drug manufacture, testing and selling. This legislation is contained in the United Kingdom Medicines Act (1968). Most countries have comparable systems of vetting and approval.

Licensing authority

The United Kingdom Medicines Act is administered by the Medicines Central Agency. Together with the Health Ministers, the Medicines Division acts as the *Licensing Authority*. If a pharmaceutical company wishes to market a new product, it requires a *Product Licence*, and this is given only if the Licensing Authority is satisfied of its safety, quality and efficacy. It is illegal for a medicinal product to be sold without a product licence.

A number of advisory committees exist to ensure the Licensing Authority performs its duties properly. The Medicines Commission, established immediately the Medicines Act came into force, was charged by Section 4 of the Act to set up five committees, usually referred to as *Section 4 Committees*. The Committee on Safety of Medicines (CSM), which replaced the Dunlop Committee, is now the best known of these. It reviews all applications for Clinical Trials Certificates (p. 30) and Product Licences for new products (i.e. a new drug or new formulation). Its most publicised activity, however, is in reviewing adverse drug reactions, and it has in recent years often been criticised over decisions to withdraw the Product Licence of a number of drugs.

When the Medicines Act was introduced, a *Product Licence of Right* was given to every product already on the market, as it would have been impossible to review all 36 000 of them simultaneously. The Committee on Review of Medicines (CRM) has the less than exciting task of reviewing all these products, a task to be completed by 1990. As a result of its activities, many products have been taken off the market, while those which remain have been given a full Product Licence.

The main task of the British Pharmacopoeia Commission is to maintain the *British Pharmacopoeia*, or list of approved drugs. Only drugs listed here can be sold as generic products and have the abbreviation *BP* in parentheses after their name.

Four sub-committees have also been established to provide expert advice to the Section 4 Committees. One of these, the Safety, Efficacy and Adverse Reactions Sub-committee (SEAR) is concerned with the collection and evaluation of information on adverse reactions through the Yellow Card system (p. 39).

Developing new drugs

Virtually all new drugs are developed within the pharmaceutical industry because of the enormous financial

---

Summary 1　Drug development

Synthesis/isolation of new substance

Animal studies
　Pharmacological/toxicological studies

Clinical trials
　Phase 1　Pharmacological tests in healthy volunteers (20–50)
　Phase 2　Tested in patients (50–300). Collection of data on efficacy and safety
　Phase 3　Formal, larger-scale trials (250–1000 or more). Efficacy, safety and comparison with other drugs in same therapeutic class
　Phase 4　Post-marketing studies on a much larger population of patients (2000–10 000 or more)

investment (about £50 million for a new product in 1985), and considerable amount of work involved. Because a patent taken out on a new compound lasts for only 17 years, the 10–12 years (or longer) required for most drugs to reach the stage of a Product Licence erodes the patent life alarmingly. The industry therefore has to look very carefully at the likely returns on its investment over the short period that it alone can market the drug under patent. Developing drugs for less common diseases becomes unattractive under these circumstances.

Apart from the basic chemistry and pharmacology required to develop a new drug, a large amount of toxicological data from animal testing is also required from the pharmaceutical company to satisfy the CSM that the drug is unlikely to cause serious adverse reactions in man. If it is so satisfied, the Committee will grant a Clinical Trials Exemption (CTX) or Clinical Trials Certificate (CTC), both of which allow the drug to be tested in patients. In the UK, a CTX or CTC is not required for studies in healthy volunteers, however, and thus it is normal for initial tolerance and pharmacokinetic data to be available before an application is made to the CSM.

Clinical trials are usually divided into four phases. In phase 1, healthy volunteer studies are performed. If the results are satisfactory, a small number of patients are given the drug to discover whether the pharmacological effect shown in animals also occurs in man (phase 2). In the third phase, formal and larger-scale clinical trials are performed, in order to confirm the drug's therapeutic benefit, evaluate its adverse effects and compare it with existing drugs in the same therapeutic class. At this point, assuming that the results are satisfactory, an application will be made for a Product Licence so that marketing and promotion of the drug can begin. Post-marketing studies (phase 4) examine its effect on a much larger population of patients.

Monitoring adverse reactions

Following the thalidomide tragedy, the Government set up a voluntary system for reporting suspected adverse reactions (better called *adverse events*, as a cause-effect relationship has yet to be established at this stage). This is known as the Yellow Card system (because of the colour

of the cards used for the reports). Initially, the system was monitored by the Dunlop Committee, but is now the responsibility of the CSM and SEAR sub-committee. If a doctor or dentist sees an unusual or serious reaction to an old drug, or any suspected reaction to a new one (new drugs are marked with an inverted triangle in the British National Formulary (BNF)), he or she is encouraged to fill in a card and send it to the Medicines Division or one of the Regional Monitoring Centres to be assessed by medical assessors. A substantial data bank is thereby accumulated and analysed monthly for associations between adverse events and individual drugs, e.g. venous thrombosis and the contraceptive pill. The main shortcomings of the Yellow Card system are that less than a quarter of registered doctors and dentists use it (the 15 000 reports received in 1985 represent only a small proportion of adverse events occurring); and the lack of case control. The system has therefore seldom identified a new association, but has nevertheless been invaluable in confirming a suspected reaction.

Several other systems of monitoring have been suggested or are under trial and pharmaceutical companies are, in addition, being encouraged (and may in the future be required), to set up a system of post-marketing surveillance. These systems monitor every patient receiving the new drug together with a matched control, and therefore have a much greater power to detect a novel adverse reaction. Nevertheless, large numbers of patients will need to be given a drug before rare adverse reactions (e.g. those occurring only once in 10 000 patients), can be detected by any system.

Controlling prescribing

While free enterprise leads to a dynamic and healthy pharmaceutical industry, it also leads to the promotion of excessive numbers of similar drugs, as one company vies with another for its share of the lucrative markets. Cephalosporin antibiotics, benzodiazepines and β-adrenoceptor blocking drugs are three such examples. In order to rationalise prescribing, most hospitals and many general practitioners have compiled their own restricted lists. In 1985, however, the Government decided that this voluntary limitation was not happening fast enough and, in order to curb escalating drug costs, introduced the NHS Limited List. At present, this covers mild to moderate pain-killers, indigestion remedies, laxatives, cough and cold remedies, vitamins, tonics and benzodiazepine drugs. An Advisory Committee keeps the list under review and may recommend its extension to other therapeutic classes.

PHARMACODYNAMICS AND PHARMACOKINETICS

Pharmacodynamics is the study of the action of drugs on the body, while *pharmacokinetics* describes the action of the body on the drug (i.e. the process by which it absorbs, distributes and eliminates the drug).

Pharmacokinetics has benefitted from advances in chemistry which allow the accurate and sensitive determination of even tiny quantities of drugs in biological fluids. Pharmacodynamics, on the other hand, is still in its infancy, as it has proved difficult to measure accurately the effects of drugs on the body. However, because drugs are prescribed not for their pharmacokinetic behaviour but for their pharmacodynamic activity, much effort is now being directed towards improving measurement of drug action.

PHARMACODYNAMICS

There are three major ways by which a drug can produce pharmacological effects:

1. by combination with specific receptors
2. by alteration of physiological enzyme processes
3. by direct physical or chemical action.

Interaction with specific receptors

An increasing number of drugs are being discovered to act through receptors on the cell surface or within the cell. When this combination of a drug with a receptor provokes a biological response, the drug is known as an *agonist*. According to the receptor occupancy theory, the intensity of the pharmacological effect (E) is directly proportional to the number of receptors combined with the drug molecule; thus, the relation between intensity of effect and drug concentration (D) is given by a rearrangement of the law of mass action.

$$E = \frac{E_{max} \cdot D}{K_D + D} \qquad \textbf{3.1}$$

where E_{max} is the maximum response and K_D is the dissociation constant of the reaction between drug and receptor site. When the intensity of pharmacological action is plotted as a proportion of maximum response against drug concentration, the relationship in Equation 3.1 results in a rectangular hyperbolar (Fig. 3.1A). Logarithmic transformation of drug concentration results in a sigmoid shape to the curve, with a log-linear relationship in its central portion (Fig. 3.1B). Most drugs exert their action on the log-linear portion of their dose response curve; maximum drug effect is rarely advisable because of the risk of other adverse effects of the drug. The dissociation constant, K_D,

is a measure of the reversibility of the drug-receptor interaction and is low when the interaction is slowly reversible. It is also the concentration at which half the maximum response of the agonist is seen and is thus a measure of drug 'potency'. The E_{max}, on the other hand, is a measure of drug 'efficacy'. The lower the K_D the greater the potency. It is thus possible to have a drug which is more potent than another but less efficacious. Thiazide diuretics, for example, are more potent than frusemide since they usually produce their effects at lower molar drug concentrations; but they are less efficacious since their maximum diuretic effect is lower.

Antagonists are drugs which will combine with the receptor site to prevent another agent from producing its maximal effect. If the antagonist produces some activity, it is termed a partial agonist. If it has no efficacy of its own, but merely prevents the activity of an agonist at the receptor site, it is termed a full antagonist. When this antagonism is competitive, the dose response relationship of the agonist is shifted to the right in a parallel fashion. Non-competitive antagonists reduce the number of receptors available for binding of agonists by irreversibly binding to receptors. Maximum efficacy is therefore reduced and the dose response relationship, although shifted to the right, is shifted in a non-parallel fashion. Some examples of receptors, their agonists and antagonists are shown in Table 3.1.

Alteration of physiological enzyme processes

The vast majority of drugs acting in this way inhibit (rather than stimulate) enzyme processes either competitively or non-competitively. Thus, neostigmine competitively inhibits the enzyme cholinesterase, which allows the buildup of concentrations of acetylcholine which, in turn, enhances neuromuscular transmission in myasthenia gravis. The dose response relationship of such drugs often resembles those of drugs acting at receptor sites.

Most monoamine oxidase inhibitors (e.g. phenelzine) inhibit this enzyme irreversibly and only when new enzyme has been synthesised does the effect of these drugs wear off. Similarly, it is probable that the action of some cytotoxic agents is due to intermediate products to which they are metabolised, and which inhibit enzymes responsible for synthesis of DNA and RNA.

Figure 3.1 Relationship between drug effect and drug concentration A on linear scale and **B** on logarithmic scale.

Clinical Pharmacology

Table 3.1   Receptor types and their agonists and antagonists

Receptor type	Natural agonist	Some effects of agonist	Other agonists	Antagonists
Adrenergic				
α_1	Noradrenaline	Contraction of vascular smooth muscle	Phenylephrine	Prazosin
α_2	Noradrenaline	Inhibition of noradrenaline release at presynaptic receptors in CNS	Clonidine	Yohimbine
β_1	Adrenaline	Increased cardiac inotropism and chronotropism	Dobutamine	Atenolol
β_2	Adrenaline	Relaxation of bronchial, vascular and uterine smooth muscle	Salbutamol	Propranolol (also β_1)
Cholinergic				
Muscarinic	Acetylcholine	Decreased heart rate	Carbachol	Atropine
Nicotinic	Acetylcholine	Neuromuscular transmission	Nicotine	Tubocurarine
Dopaminergic	Dopamine	Renal vasodilatation	Bromocriptine	Metoclopramide
Histaminergic				
H_1	Histamine	Contraction of bronchial smooth muscle	–	Chlorpheniramine
H_2	Histamine	Stimulation of gastric acid secretion	–	Cimetidine Ranitidine
Serotonergic	5-hydroxytryptamine	Contraction of vascular smooth muscle	–	Ketanserin
Opioid	β-endorphins, enkephalins	Modulation of pain perception	Morphine	Naloxone

Direct physical or chemical actions

Bulk purgatives and osmotic diuretics are examples of this mechanism of action. Chelating agents combine chemically with heavy metals to produce less active chelates which are eventually excreted. Local and general anaesthetics, which are highly lipid soluble, appear to change the properties of neuronal membranes and discourage depolarisation by a physical action.

PHARMACOKINETICS

Before a drug can exert a biological effect, it must be absorbed or directly introduced into the body; distribute through body tissues to its site of action; and, finally,

be eliminated from the body either by metabolism and subsequent excretion of the metabolites, or by direct excretion of unchanged drug. These biological processes are often termed *drug disposition*, and *pharmacokinetics* is the mathematical description of these biological events.

When a drug is introduced directly into the circulation (i.e. by intravenous administration), its concentration in plasma declines in an exponential fashion as shown in Figure 3.2. This process is known as *first order elimination*. A fixed proportion of the drug present in the plasma is eliminated per unit time, but the total amount of drug removed per unit time falls. The time necessary for the drug concentration to fall to half of its original value is constant and is known as the half-life of elimination of the drug. Transformation of drug concentration to its natural

Figure 3.2   Time course of decline of plasma drug concentrations A on a linear and **B** on a logarithmic scale after intravenous injection of 1 g of drug (V_d =10 l, K =0.347–1 h, $t_{1/2}$ elim =2 h, plasma clearance =3.47 l/h).

logarithm results in a linear decline with time, and the slope of the line is the elimination rate constant (K). This is related to the half-life ($t_{1/2}$) of the drug in the following fashion:

$$K = \frac{0.693}{t_{1/2}} \qquad \textbf{3.2}$$

where 0.693 is the natural logarithm of 2. When common logarithms ($\log_{10}$) are used (Fig. 3.2), the slope of the line is

$$-\frac{K}{2.303}.$$

Apparent volume of distribution

The apparent volume of distribution (V_d) is a measure of the proportion of drug present in the plasma relative to the rest of the body at any particular time. It is calculated by dividing the dose of the drug administered intravenously, by the concentration at zero time (C_0) (Fig. 3.2). Although this measure has no direct anatomical significance, it does reflect tissue uptake of the drug. Thus, tricyclic antidepressants, which are avidly taken up by tissues, have a very high apparent distribution volume (over 1000 litres in a normal adult); while drugs which remain principally in the intravascular space, such as heparin, have a distribution volume of around 7 litres in the normal adult.

Drug clearance

Clearance (Cl) is the best measure of the efficiency of elimination of a drug. It is defined as the volume of plasma cleared of the drug per unit time, and can be calculated from the equation:

$$Cl = V_d . K \qquad \textbf{3.3}$$

or from the equation:

$$Cl = \frac{D}{AUC} \qquad \textbf{3.4}$$

where ÁUC is the area under the plasma concentration curve from time O to infinity. Equations 3.3 and 3.4 show that, unlike the elimination rate constant K (and thus also the half-life of elimination), clearance is not dependent on the volume of distribution of the drug. The total plasma clearance of drug is the sum of the clearances by· metab-

olism and excretion. Some drugs (e.g. phenytoin, ethanol and salicylate) undergo concentration-dependent metabolism sometimes known as capacity-limited or *saturation kinetics*. For these drugs, clearance falls with rising drug concentration. The fall in drug concentration is not log-linear with time, and a true half-life of elimination cannot be calculated.

Absorption and bioavailability

When drugs are given by the oral route they are often absorbed in a first order fashion, so that the plasma concentration rises exponentially to a peak when absorption rate equals distribution or elimination rate and then declines (Fig. 3.3). However, it must be remembered that at the time of peak concentration, absorption is still not complete and continues for some time after this. *Bioavailability* is defined as the proportion of the drug reaching the systemic circulation when administered by any route other than the intravenous route. (By the intravenous route, bioavailability is of course 100%.) The bioavailability of a drug can be calculated by dividing the area under the plasma concentration curve produced after administration by a given route, by the area under the curve produced using the intravenous route. Bioavailability after oral administration may be less than 100% either because the drug is not completely absorbed from the gastrointestinal tract, or because it is metabolised in the gut (e.g. isoprenaline), the liver (e.g. propranolol) or the lung (e.g. noradrenaline) before it can reach the systemic circulation. The reduced bioavailability in these situations is due to presystemic (or *first-pass*) elimination and such drugs are termed high clearance compounds.

Steady state pharmacokinetics

Most drugs are not given as a single dose but are administered on a regular basis. This may result in accumulation of drug depending on the frequency of administration and the half-life of the compound. Eventually, a *steady state* situation will be achieved when the rate of drug administration is equal to the rate of drug elimination. Fifty percent of the steady state concentration will be achieved in one half-life, 75% in two half-lives and so on, so that it takes approximately five half-lives to reach steady state

Figure 3.3 Time course of plasma drug concentrations after repeated oral administration of the same oral dose at 12 hourly intervals. The drug has a $t_{1/2}$ elim of 12 hours and is described by a two-compartment open model.

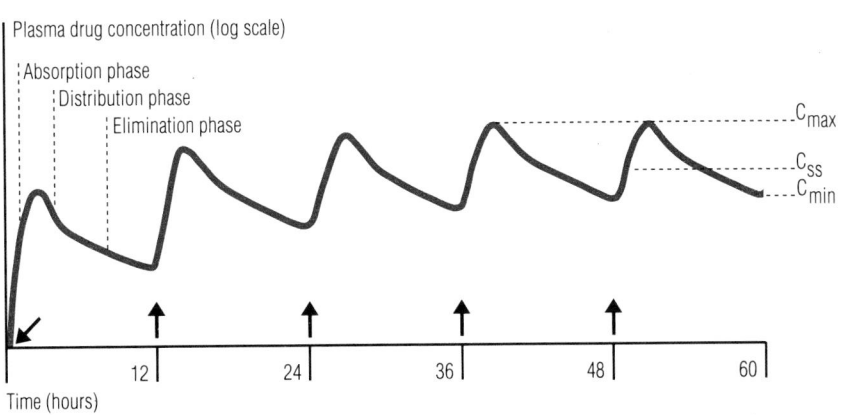

Clinical Pharmacology

3

(Fig. 3.3). Thus, for warfarin ($t_{1/2} = 36$ hours), steady state will take over a week to achieve; and a similar period will be required for the plasma concentration to decline to undetectable levels after the drug has been discontinued. The steady state concentration (C_{ss}) is defined as the average plasma concentration of drug during the dosage interval; and is calculated using the equation:

$$C_{ss} = \frac{D.F}{Cl. Tau} \qquad 3.5$$

where D is the dosage, Cl the clearance (l/min), Tau is the time interval between doses and F the bioavailability of the drug after the particular route of administration. It is evident from this equation that, if the total dose of drug given per day remains the same, C_{ss} will remain constant, although if larger doses are given at less frequent intervals, the difference between C_{max} and C_{min} (the peak and trough plasma concentrations) will increase. These fluctuations may be important if the adverse effects of the drug are related to peak concentrations, or if there is a threshold concentration below which drug effect is not obtained. For this reason, heparin (which has a short half-life and whose concentration would therefore fluctuate markedly after intermittent intravenous administration), is normally given by continuous intravenous infusion. The longer the half-life of the drug, the longer the interval that can elapse between doses for any given difference between peak and trough concentrations. It is also clear from Equation 3.5 that this steady state concentration (C_{ss}) will be directly proportional to the dose administered under first order conditions. For drugs with saturation kinetics (e.g. phenytoin), where the clearance falls with increasing dosage, the relationship between steady state concentration and dose will be curvilinear, so that increases in dose will produce disproportionate increases in circulating drug concentrations and a risk of toxicity.

Multicompartment models

When the natural logarithm ($\log_e$) of drug concentrations is measured against time, a relationship with two or more linear portions may be obtained. The simplest example is the two-compartment open model shown in Figure 3.3. Each portion has its own rate constant with the early com-

ponent normally due to distribution of the drug throughout the tissues. This means firstly, that the circulating plasma concentration may fall rapidly after administration of a drug so that a loading dose may be necessary to achieve and maintain an effective circulating drug concentration. Secondly, blood samples taken during the distribution phase will tend to overestimate the steady state concentration of drug. Thirdly, estimates of clearance made using data which do not contain sufficient sampling points soon after drug administration may underestimate the area under the curve (AUC) by missing the distribution phase, and therefore tend to overestimate drug clearance.

Absorption

Drugs are usually given by the alimentary route, and must therefore pass through the bowel wall in order to enter the bloodstream. This occurs by four different mechanisms:

1. *Passive diffusion*, which involves diffusion down a concentration gradient from the gut into the bloodstream. For this to occur, the drug must dissolve in the gastrointestinal fluids, traverse the cell membrane and enter the bloodstream. The rate at which it does so depends on both the concentration gradient and the lipid solubility of the drug. This is the most important mechanism of absorption for most drugs.
2. *Active transport*, a less important mechanism by which some drugs, because of their resemblance to naturally occurring substances, utilise existing transport systems. Thus, alpha methyl dopa and levodopa are absorbed by the active process responsible for absorption of the amino acid tyrosine.
3. *Filtration through pores*, a route generally limited to molecules of molecular weight less than 100 (e.g. urea), as most drugs are too large to traverse the pores between cells.
4. *Endocytosis*, by which drugs or particles are engulfed by cells in the bowel wall. This is of relatively little importance to drug absorption.

Factors affecting absorption

Absorption is affected by the chemical nature and formulation of the drug, as well as the physiological characteristics of the absorption site. Thus, some drugs cannot be administered orally because they are broken down by gastrointestinal enzymes (e.g. the polypeptide, insulin) or because they are unstable at extremes of pH (e.g. benzyl penicillin at gastric pH). Most drugs are either weak acids or weak bases and thus exist in two forms in solution – as ions or as undissociated molecules. The equilibrium between these forms is determined by the pK of the drug (the pH at which 50% of the drug is ionised) and the pH of the medium in which the drug is dissolved. At the low pH encountered in the stomach, a weakly acidic drug exists mainly in its undissociated form, and is thus more lipid soluble, and will tend to be more easily absorbed. Basic drugs, on the other hand, are largely ionised at low pH and exist predominantly in the undissociated form only in the

---

Summary 2 Clinical pharmacokinetics

- A drug, once introduced into the body, takes five half-lives to reach steady state concentration.

- For drugs undergoing first-order elimination, the concentration at steady state is directly proportional to the dose and inversely proportional to the clearance.

- For drugs with saturation kinetics, increased doses cause reduced clearance and therefore disproportionate increases in steady-state drug concentration.

- Clearance is independent of the volume of distribution, whereas the $t_{1/2}$ elimination is not.

34

alkaline media of the small bowel. Despite these considerations, however, both acidic and basic drugs tend to be absorbed predominantly in the small intestine, because they are there for longer and because the inner surface of the intestine provides a much greater absorptive area than does the stomach. A few basic drugs have a pK much greater than the highest pH reached in the intestine, and therefore remain ionised throughout the gastrointestinal tract and are poorly absorbed.

Formulation factors are important in determining the rate and extent of drug absorption. Most drugs consist not only of an active agent but also of diluents, granulating and binding agents, lubricants and disintegrating agents, any of which may have a marked effect on absorption. Particle size of the active constituent may also be important, and sustained or delayed release preparations will also delay absorption rate.

Gastrointestinal motility affects the rate of absorption. Delays in gastric emptying rate will generally result in delayed rate of drug absorption although the extent of absorption is normally unchanged. *Food* has a variable effect. Some drugs (e.g. propranolol) have greater bioavailability in the presence of food because of reduced pre-systemic elimination, whereas others (e.g. rifampicin) are more poorly absorbed. Such factors may be important in determining the times of administration of drugs.

The *route of administration* is also important. A number of alternatives to the oral route exist. Drugs may be given by:

1. *Intramuscular injection*, either to speed the onset of effects or to enhance bioavailability when the oral route is suboptimal. Use of the intramuscular route can, however, cause local pain and some drugs (such as phenytoin and diazepam) are poorly and variably absorbed when administered in this way, because of poor solubility at tissue pH. Absorption rate varies with the muscle group used (it is usually faster from the deltoid than from the vastus or gluteus muscles) and may be slow in situations of poor tissue perfusion (e.g. shock).

2. *Rectal administration* can sometimes be used but, because the haemorrhoidal veins drain partly into the portal tract, presystemic elimination is not completely avoided. The suppository may also be variably retained or have poor and erratic absorption.

3. *Buccal administration* can completely avoid pre-systemic elimination and is used for drugs (e.g. glyceryl trinitrate) which are rapidly metabolised after the oral route. Unfortunately, not all such drugs can rapidly penetrate the buccal mucosa and enter the systemic circulation.

4. *Transdermal administration* is an alternative to the buccal route for drugs such as glyceral trinitrate or the antihistamine, hyoscine. The latter is used for motion sickness but, when given by the oral route, may be ineffective due to delayed gastric emptying associated with nausea. The rate of absorption varies with the site of skin used and the extent of absorption is limited, so that only very potent drugs (effective dose < 10 mg)

can be usefully administered by this route. Absorption is normally rapid but membranes are being developed to control the rate.

5. *Intrapulmonary route* Some drugs, and all anaesthetic gases, are administered by the intrapulmonary route. Non-gaseous compounds are difficult to introduce into the lungs. Only 10% of a drug administered by press-urised aerosol (or up to 15% if administered by nebu-liser) actually enters the lungs; the remainder is deposited in the buccal cavity and subsequently swallowed.

Distribution

If drug distribution did not occur, only those drugs with an action within the vascular compartment would provoke biological effects. Like absorption, distribution is dependent on the physicochemical characteristics of the drug as well as upon biological factors.

The major physicochemical properties determining drug distribution are lipid solubility and (if the drug is a weak electrolyte) the degree of dissociation (ionisation) in tissues. Highly lipid soluble drugs are generally distributed throughout all fluid compartments and, because they can cross lipid membranes readily, can reach most organs including the brain. Poorly lipid soluble drugs are normally able to enter the interstitial fluid but, if they are weak electrolytes, only the undissociated form can penetrate the cells and then only to a limited extent, depending on the lipid-water partition coefficient.

Biological factors determining the distribution of drugs in the body include the degree of both plasma protein binding and of uptake by tissue, either by binding or by active transport mechanisms. The blood contains approximately 180 g of protein, half of which is albumin. Albumin is thus the most abundant single protein in the plasma and, because of its structure, is able to reversibly bind many drugs by Van der Waals forces, hydrogen bonds or hydrophobic bonds. However, its binding capacity is relatively limited and it has been estimated that only 200 mg of drug of average molecular weight (300) would be bound to albumin in plasma if there were only one binding site available on each albumin molecule. For some drugs, there may be more than one binding site and the binding capacity will be relatively greater. Major sites of binding are the so-called site one (warfarin site), which also binds the endogenous compound bilirubin; and site two (diazepam site) – the site at which the endogenous amino acid tryptophan also binds. Drugs may bind to either or both of these sites and can competitively displace each other.

The relationship between the serum albumin concentration and the proportion of two drugs in the free (unbound) form is shown in Figure 3.4. It can be seen that the differences in protein binding are likely to be relatively small over the range of serum albumin concentrations seen in health. In situations of hypoalbuminaemia, however, even small further decreases in serum albumin concentration may cause marked increases in the proportion of drug free in the plasma.

3

It has recently become apparent that another plasma protein, α_1-acid glycoprotein (orosomucoid) also binds drugs, particularly those of a basic nature. Although its plasma concentration is much lower than (c. 2%) that of albumin, its affinity for drugs is high and some drugs (e.g. lignocaine, erythromycin and disopyramide) may bind appreciably more to this protein than to albumin. Because of its low concentration, however, its binding capacity is relatively limited and, for several drugs, protein binding falls with increasing drug concentration.

The tissues also contain proteins which combine with drugs (60% of the total exchangeable body albumin is outside the vascular compartment); while body fat can serve as an important reservoir for lipid soluble agents such as thiopentone. Finally, active transport mechanisms – such as the uptake of adrenergic neurone blocking drugs by the adrenergic neurone – may also contribute to high tissue concentrations of a drug. Extensive tissue binding tends to result in the drug having a large apparent volume of distribution (V_d), since the majority of the drug is outside the intravascular space.

Metabolism

The liver is the main organ of metabolism of drugs although some may also occur in the gastrointestinal tract, lung, blood or kidney. Metabolism is particularly of lipid soluble drugs which can more readily enter cells in order to be metabolised and are also prevented by their lipid solubility from being excreted unchanged by the kidney. The routes of metabolism are relatively non-specific and are shared by a variety of drugs. In most instances, more water-soluble metabolites (which are more easily excreted by the kidney) are produced. It has been suggested that, without metabolism, a lipid soluble drug would have a half-life of around 30 days and, if it were also reversibly bound to tissues, its half-life might be as great as 100 years!

There are two groups of metabolic reactions: phase 1 and phase 2 reactions:

1. *Phase 1 reactions* involve the enzyme mono-oxygenase situated in the smooth endoplasmic reticulum of cells with metabolic function, especially the liver. These are called cytochrome P_{450} enzymes and are responsible for oxidation, reduction, hydrolysis and dealkylation of drugs with the relevant molecular structure. A given drug may be metabolised by one or more of these routes to produce generally more water soluble (and thus biologically active) metabolites.

2. *Phase 2 reactions* are conjugation reactions of more water soluble molecules to the drug or metabolite. Conjugation with glucuronide (glucuronidation) is the commonest pathway, but conjugation can also occur with sulphate, amino acids such as glutathione, or acetylcoA (acetylation). Most of these conjugated metabolites (except for some acetylated compounds) are biologically inactive. Although most metabolic processes are controlled by environmental factors, acetylation is under genetic control – 45% of the United Kingdom population are slow acetylators and the remainder either intermediate or fast acetylators. Approximately 10% of the British population have a reduced ability to hydroxylate several drugs (e.g. debrisoquine, nortriptyline and phenformin) and this may lead to an increased risk of adverse reactions to drugs metabolised by this route.

Excretion

The vast majority of drugs must first be metabolised to more water soluble compounds before they can be excreted in the urine. Those drugs (e.g. cimetidine, digoxin, aminoglycosides, lithium, cephalosporins, penicillins, atenolol and chlorpropamide) which are largely excreted unchanged, tend to be relatively water soluble drugs which are not appreciably bound to plasma proteins and can therefore enter the glomerular filtrate. Lipid soluble drugs may also enter the glomerular filtrate, provided they are not extensively plasma protein bound, but they then readily pass back through the proximal tubular cells into the bloodstream by passive diffusion down a concentration gradient. Only when they have been metabolised to more water soluble compounds will they have difficulty in passing back through the renal tubular cells and therefore be excreted in the urine. Weak electrolytes can also be actively secreted in the proximal renal tubules – weak bases sharing one mechanism and weak acids another. And there is some evidence for an active transport system promoting the excretion of digoxin in the distal renal tubule.

Drugs may also be excreted in the bile, normally as conjugates and particularly if they have a high molecular weight. The drug may, however, be reabsorbed from the intestine, either directly or after deconjugation by intestinal microflora, to create an enterohepatic cycle. This may reduce the clearance of the drug and thus prolong its effect.

CAUSES OF PHARMACODYNAMIC VARIABILITY

Altered sensitivity to a particular drug concentration at its effector site (pharmacodynamic variability) may occur in several situations, but the effects of disease and other

---

Summary 3 Drug disposition

Absorption Most drugs are administered by the alimentary route. Absorption from the gut occurs via passive diffusion (main mechanism), active transport, filtration through pores, or endocytosis.

Distribution Depends on the drug's ability to penetrate cells and bind to plasma proteins and on tissue uptake (cell protein binding or active transport). In the plasma, acidic drugs bind to albumin. Basic drugs may also bind to α_1-acid glycoprotein.

Metabolism The liver is the main site of the metabolism of drugs. Phase I metabolic reactions involve oxidation, reduction, hydrolysis and dealkylation of the drug. Phase II reactions involve conjugation reactions (e.g. with glucuronic acid) to form generally more water soluble compounds.

Excretion Almost all drugs must be metabolised to more water soluble compounds before excretion in the urine.

---

factors on pharmacodynamics are difficult to predict. The very young and elderly appear to have an increased sensitivity to several drugs, particularly those affecting the central nervous system. An increased sensitivity to drugs acting on the central nervous system is also seen in patients with chronic renal and liver disease. The elderly appear also to have less adaptable homeostatic mechanisms and are therefore more prone to drug induced postural hypotension or hypothermia. Hyperthyroid patients are more sensitive to the effects of digoxin and oral anticoagulants.

Information in this field is limited because of difficulties in accurately measuring drug effects, but great care should be exercised in prescription of drugs to the very young, the very old, and patients with chronic renal or liver disease.

CAUSES OF PHARMACOKINETIC VARIABILITY

Absorption

Drug absorption is normally such an efficient process, that it is rare to see differences in the extent of absorption of most modern formulations of drugs, even in the presence of extensive bowel resection. Reduction in absorption may, however, occur in severe malabsorption syndromes or in severe diarrhoea and differences in bowel motility may affect the rate (although not the extent) of absorption. Gastric emptying is slow and erratic in the very young and in adults who are shocked or in pain. In such circumstances (e.g. in myocardial infarction), threshold concentrations for drug effect may not be achieved rapidly, or at all, and the drug may have to be given by an alternative, non-alimentary route.

Distribution

Drug distribution may be altered by changes in regional blood flow in disease: the volume of distribution of lignocaine, for example, appears to be lower in patients with cardiac failure. Protein binding also determines drug distribution. Albumin concentrations are low in the neonate, begin to decline over the age of 40, and are reduced during pregnancy. Severe hypoalbuminaemia also occurs in neph-

rotic syndrome (Fig. 3.4) and chronic liver disease. In patients with chronic renal failure, the proportion of drug in the free form is greater than would be expected from the reduction in serum albumin alone, indicating either structural changes in albumin or the presence of endogenous inhibitors of binding.

Alpha$_1$-acid glycoprotein (AAG) is reduced in neonates and in pregnancy, but tends to be normal in healthy elderly individuals. It is markedly increased in patients with rheumatoid arthritis and other inflammatory diseases, including chronic renal disease, after myocardial infarction, and in cancer. As with albumin, it may be reduced in patients with nephrotic syndrome or chronic liver disease. Concomitant changes in plasma protein binding also occur – the effects depending on the relative strength of binding of the drug to these proteins and on the disease state in question (Fig. 3.5) – which may alter the amount bound to free drug. Thus, the total plasma concentration of drug (free + bound), which is generally used as an index of drug concentration, may not always reflect the free (presumably active) concentration. Therapeutic ranges for total drug may therefore need to be altered in diseases where plasma protein binding is affected.

Metabolism

Drug metabolism may be diminished at the extremes of age. Neonates have a reduced capacity for phase 1 and most phase 2 reactions: impaired glucuronidation of chloramphenicol, for example, may lead to grey baby syndrome in the neonate. In the elderly, impairment of drug metabolism is only slight and tends to be overshadowed by changes in pharmacodynamic response. Dietary and environmental factors, such as smoking, may affect the rate of drug metabolism; and chronic liver disease may be associated with an impairment of metabolism, particularly of phase 1 pathways. In liver disease, the serum albumin concentration correlates roughly with the degree of impairment of drug metabolism (i.e. the lower the albumin the more severe the impairment). The effect of impairment of metabolism in liver disease will be greater for those drugs with extensive presystemic metabolism. The bioavailability of propranolol is much greater in patients with chronic liver disease not because of better absorption

Figure 3.4 Relationship between the percentage of diazepam and theophylline free in plasma and plasma albumin concentration in different disorders. See text for details.

Figure 3.5 Relationship between the percentage of lignocaine free in plasma and plasma AAG concentration in several disease states and in neonates.

Clinical Pharmacology

> **Summary 4   Causes of pharmacokinetic variability**
>
> *Absorption*
>   Extent of absorption rarely affected
>   Bowel motility may affect rate
>
> *Distribution*
>   Alteration of regional blood flow in disease
>   Altered protein binding e.g. hypoalbuminaemia in nephrotic
>   syndrome
>
> *Metabolism*
>   Diminished in neonates and the elderly
>   Dietary and environmental factors e.g. smoking
>   Liver disease
>
> *Excretion*
>   Immature renal function in neonates
>   Impaired in renal disease

(absorption is virtually complete in health) but because it cannot be efficiently metabolised on its first passage through the liver.

The metabolism of high clearance drugs given intravenously is dependent upon the delivery of the drug to the liver. Thus, because liver blood flow falls in heart failure and shock, the clearance of lignocaine, propranolol and several other high clearance drugs is impaired. Hepatic cirrhosis has a similar effect, due in part to a reduction in the liver's intrinsic metabolic capacity, but also because of intra- and extra-hepatic shunting of blood past the liver cells and a consequent reduction in effective liver blood flow.

Excretion

Neonates have a reduced glomerular filtration rate relative to their body surface area, and their active tubular secretory mechanisms are also not fully developed. These processes mature relatively rapidly and are fully functional after 6–12 months, but glomerular filtration rate begins to fall again over the age of 40 (the renal tubular secretory mechanisms appear to be less affected by age). Thus, the dose of digoxin or gentamicin (drugs excreted predominantly by glomerular filtration) may need to be reduced in the elderly or very young. Renal disease is associated predominantly with a fall in glomerular filtration rate, with active renal tubular secretion mechanisms less markedly affected. Measurement of serum creatinine or creatinine clearance is therefore useful in calculating the optimum dose of drugs excreted predominantly by glomerular filtration (e.g. the aminoglycoside antibiotics); but it is of less value in the case of drugs such as penicillins, which are actively secreted at the proximal renal tubule.

ADVERSE REACTIONS

It has been estimated that approximately 5% of all hospital admissions are due to adverse reactions to a drug; one in ten of patients admitted for other reasons will develop an adverse reaction to a drug while in hospital; and perhaps 1 in 1000 deaths in hospital are due to an adverse reaction to a drug. Adverse reactions are equally common in general practice. The drug groups most commonly associated with adverse reactions are antihypertensive drugs, anticoagulants, antirheumatic drugs (particularly the non-steroidal anti-inflammatory drugs), cytotoxic drugs, corticosteroids and digoxin.

Although adverse reactions can affect all systems of the body, they are most often described in the skin and central nervous system (where detection tends to be easier). The very young (i.e. under one year of age) and the elderly are particularly at risk; and women appear to be at greater risk than men, although the reason for this is unknown. Patients with a history of allergy, or who have had a drug reaction in the past, are more likely to develop further reactions even to a drug in some other therapeutic group. The presence of disease, particularly heart failure, or liver or renal disease predisposes to a risk of adverse reactions, as may genetic factors, such as enzyme deficiencies.

Types of adverse drug reaction

Adverse reactions have been classified into two major types:

Type A

The most common type is the *dose-dependent adverse reaction (type A)* which is an 'augmentation' or 'accentuation' of a known pharmacological effect of the drug – not necessarily always the wanted effect. Thus, beta sympathomimetic agents can cause increased tremor – a recognised pharmacological effect of the drug, but one which may limit its use in bronchodilator therapy. Type A reactions account for about 75% of all adverse reactions and, because they are often insidious in onset, may go unrecognised for some time. They may thus produce considerable morbidity but the mortality from type A reactions is generally low. They may occur because of altered pharmacokinetic or pharmacodynamic factors and are therefore commonest in those diseases (e.g. renal and liver disease) where these are affected.

Type B

Type B reactions are not dependent on the dose given, but are unpredictable or 'bizarre' reactions to a drug, which may be present only in tiny concentrations. Because of their lack of predictability and their often acute onset, they have a higher mortality than type A reactions; but the morbidity is relatively low if the patient survives the initial event. Like type A reactions, type B reactions can be related to pharmacokinetic or pharmacodynamic factors. There are many ingredients in medications other than the active compound and reactions may occur to the preservative, filler, dye, binder or solubilising agent in the tablet or injection. Type B reactions may occur because individual subjects metabolise the drug through a novel pathway

Summary 5   Types of adverse reaction

Type A: Dose-dependent. Account for 75% of all adverse reactions. Cause considerable morbidity but mortality is low. Can sometimes be treated by dose reduction rather than cessation of treatment.

Type B: Non-dose-dependent, unpredictable. Higher mortality, but lower morbidity if patient survives. Type B reactions may be related to, e.g. hereditary enzyme deficiencies or allergic mechanisms. Usually treated by discontinuing treatment immediately.

which produces a toxic metabolite. In other cases, the presence of hereditary enzyme deficiencies may predispose the patient to the toxic effects of drugs or their metabolites. Thus, haemolysis caused by dapsone and other oxidising agents is commoner in patients with glucose-6-phosphate dehydrogenase (G6PD) deficiency. Similarly, many agents can precipitate an attack of acute intermittent porphyria (p. 781) in those carrying a gene for this disorder.

Type B reactions are also often related to allergic mechanisms, and may involve any or all of the forms of antibody mediated or cell mediated tissue damage. Thus, anaphylaxis may occur due to immediate (Type I) hypersensitivity associated with cell bound IgE, after administration of drugs such as penicillin. Cell surface (Type II hypersensitivity) damage may occur as a result of the combination of methyldopa with red cell membranes and subsequent haemolysis. Toxic immune complexes may be formed in patients receiving gold or penicillamine, with subsequent renal or skin toxicity by a Type III hypersensitivity mechanism. Cell mediated (Type IV) tissue damage is thought to be the mechanism of the relatively common (but usually mild) rash associated with ampicillin therapy, or the more serious erythoderma sometimes associated with drugs such as gold.

Diagnosis and management of adverse reactions

Diagnosis

It is rarely possible to make a diagnosis of drug induced adverse reaction with complete certainty. Erythema multiforme, for example, may be caused either by an infective agent or by the antibiotic with which the patient was being treated. It is therefore necessary to weigh up all pieces of circumstantial evidence carefully before making the diagnosis. This includes taking a *full drug history* (which is helpful in many cases), remembering that patients may not consider over-the-counter remedies, or even the oral contraceptive pill, as medicines or drugs. The brand names of the agents may also be important, since different pharmaceutical formulations may contain different dyes, binders, fillers, preservatives or lubricants, and reactions may therefore occur after only some formulations of a particular drug.

Physical examination provides only limited information. Some physical signs may be directly attributable to drug therapy, for example blue discolouration of the skin associated with amiodarone therapy is rarely caused by disease. Similarly, an eruption occurring at a fixed site on the skin may suggest a drug-induced fixed drug eruption. But in most cases, the organs affected have a limited number of responses to noxious stimuli. *Biochemical tests* are also of limited value, but measurement of plasma drug concentration may help to confirm the suspicion of a dose dependent (type A) adverse reaction. In some cases, measurement of metabolic phenotype may also be of help. It is extremely rare, for example, for patients who are fast acetylators to develop drug induced lupus erythematosus after hydralazine therapy.

Probably the most helpful indication of the drug responsible for the adverse reaction is the *time course* relative to drug treatment, particularly the rate of resolution of symptoms on stopping a specific drug. Subsequent re-exposure associated with a recurrence of the symptoms or signs gives the strongest evidence of causation; but it is rarely ethically justifiable to rechallenge the patient, unless his need for the drug outweighs the potential risk of the adverse reaction.

Management

The treatment of adverse reactions will depend on the type and severity of the reaction in question and the availability of alternative agents. The only choice with most type B reactions is to stop the suspected drug completely. With type A reactions, it is sometimes possible to reduce the dose to prevent the unwanted effects whilst still obtaining therapeutic benefit. If an adverse reaction does occur, the patient's medical notes and prescription chart should be clearly marked with an eye-catching label to indicate the nature and date of the reaction. Failure to do so may result in a patient being re-exposed to a drug to which he has previously had severe reactions. Any serious adverse reaction should also be reported to the Committee on Safety of Medicines using a 'yellow card' (p. 29). In addition, even minor adverse reactions to drugs which have been recently introduced (marked with an inverted black triangle in the British National Formulary) should be reported.

Prevention of adverse reactions

It must be remembered that although drugs provide enormous benefit to patients, all are potentially toxic and should be used selectively, particularly in those patients at greatest risk of adverse reactions, i.e. the very young, very old and those with severe disease. The risk of developing an adverse reaction appears to increase disproportionately with increasing number of drugs prescribed concomitantly. Prescriptions should therefore be reviewed and drug therapy rationalized at frequent intervals. When a drug is prescribed, the prescription should be written legibly, in block letters, and preferably using the approved name. Failure to do so may lead to errors in prescribing. In some cases, the risk of adverse reactions to certain drugs is such that they should be avoided if at all possible. There are

Table 3.2 Drugs to avoid during pregnancy or breast-feeding

	Pregnancy	Breast-feeding
Antibiotics	Tetracyclines Sulphonamides Aminoglycosides Trimethoprim Rifampicin	Tetracyclines Sulphonamides Isoniazid Chloramphenicol
Antithyroids	All, including radioiodine	All, including radioiodine
Analgesics	Opiates NSAIDs	Opiates
Anticoagulants	Warfarin	Phenindione
Antineoplastics	Most	Most
Antidiabetics	Hypoglycaemics	Use with caution
Androgens	All, also oestrogens and high dose progestogens	All, also high dose oestrogens and progestogens
Miscellaneous	Vitamin D and its analogues Live vaccines	Lithium Anthraquinone laxatives and phenolphthalein

particular dangers during pregnancy or breast-feeding, when certain drugs may cause an adverse reaction in the foetus or breast-fed child (Table 3.2).

DRUG INTERACTIONS

Drug interactions have been recognised for over 100 years and are described under the classical headings of antagonism, synergism or potentiation. Many of these interactions are beneficial and have been used to therapeutic advantage; but unwanted or adverse interactions also account for 10–20% of all adverse reactions to drugs. Those of clinical importance (the actual number of interactions may be much larger than this) usually occur in drugs with a relatively low margin between safety and toxicity (i.e. a narrow 'therapeutic ratio'). Thus, they are most often described with oral anticoagulants, anticonvulsants, antidepressants or antihypertensive drugs (Table 3.3). As with adverse reactions in general, the risk of developing an adverse interaction increases disproportionately with the number of drugs prescribed concomitantly; and the mechanisms of interaction are also similar, in that both pharmacodynamic and pharmacokinetic interactions may occur. Interactions may also take place, however, before the drugs even enter the body, and these have been termed 'pharmaceutical' interactions.

Pharmaceutical interactions

Interactions may occur prior to the drug entering the body when drugs are mixed together for infusion, or when a

Table 3.3 Drug interactions of clinical importance

Drug (A)	May interact with (B)	Effect of interaction	Mechanism
Warfarin	Cholestyramine	Reduced anticoagulant effect of A	Impaired absorption and increased elimination of A NB long term R may cause impaired vit K absorption and enhance anticoagulant effect
	Barbiturates Carbamazepine Rifampicin	Reduced anticoagulant effect of A	Induction of metabolism of A
	Cimetidine Sulphonamides Erythromycin Metronidazole Mefenamic acid Azapropazone Phenylbutazone Amiodarone Ketoconazole Sulphinpyrazone Chloramphenicol	Increased anticoagulant effect of A	Inhibition of metabolism of A
	Salicylates Clofibrate Bezafibrate D Thyroxine L Thyroxine Stanozolol Danazol	Increased anticoagulant effect of A	Pharmacodynamic potentiation of anticoagulant effect
	Oral contraceptives Vitamin K	Reduced anticoagulant effect of A	Pharmacodynamic antagonism of anticoagulant effect

drug interacts with the infusion material itself. Guides to intravenous mixture are available, and should be consulted before compounds are given by intravenous infusion or mixed together. In general terms, it is advisable to avoid adding drugs to infusion fluids unless absolutely necessary and certainly to avoid adding more than one drug if at all possible. Infusion fluids particularly likely to be associated with pharmaceutical incompatibilities include blood and blood products, amino acid and lipid solutions, mannitol and sodium bicarbonate.

Pharmacodynamic interactions

Pharmacodynamic interaction occurs where one drug alters the response to another by interacting either at the receptor site or at a different site to enhance or diminish the primary drug effect.

Some of the important receptors, their function and the drugs which interact with them are shown in Table 3.1. As described earlier, agonists provoke a response whereas antagonists compete with agonists to prevent the response

Table 3.3 Drug interactions of clinical importance (cont.)

Drug (A)	May interact with (B)	Effect of interaction	Mechanism
Phenytoin	Isoniazid Cimetidine Chloramphenicol Sulphonamides	Increased effect or toxicity of A	Inhibition of metabolism of A
	Carbamazepine	Reduced effect of A	Induction of metabolism of A
Carbamazepine	Isoniazid Verapamil Erythromycin	Increased effect or toxicity of A	Inhibition of metabolism of A
Oral contraceptives	Barbiturates Phenytoin Carbamazepine Primidone Rifampicin	Reduced effect of A	Induction of metabolism of A
	Antibiotics		? Interruption of enterohepatic recycling of A
Theophylline	Cimetidine Erythromycin	Increased effect of A	Inhibition of metabolism of A
Digoxin	Quinidine Verapamil	Increased effect of A	? Reduced renal excretion
	Potassium-losing diuretics	Increased effect of A	Pharmacodynamic potentiation by hypokalaemia induced by B
Beta-blockers	Cimetidine	Increased effect of A	Inhibition of metabolism of A
	Verapamil	Increased effect of A	Pharmacodynamic potentiation
	NSAIDs	Reduced hypotensive effect of A	Unclear, ? sodium retention
Angiotensin converting enzyme (ACE) inhibitors	NSAIDs	Reduced hypotensive effect of A	Unclear, ? sodium retention
Diuretics	NSAIDs	Reduced diuretic effect of A	Unclear
Lithium carbonate	Thiazide diuretics	Increased effect of A	Increased renal tubular absorption
Azathioprine Mercaptopurine	Allopurinol	Increased effect of A	Inhibition of metabolism of A
Methotrexate	Aspirin NSAIDs	Increased effect of A	Inhibition of renal tubular secretion of A
Cyclosporin	Erythromycin	Increased effect of A	? Inhibition of metabolism of A
	Phenytoin	Reduced effect of A	? Reduced absorption of A
Zidovudine (AZT)	Paracetamol	Increased toxicity of A	Unknown

Clinical Pharmacology

3

occurring. Partial agonists initiate a minor response but, by occupying a significant fraction of the receptors, they antagonise the action of more potent agonists. Nalorphine, for example, is a partial antagonist but may add to the respiratory depression produced by opiates; whereas naloxone, while having no efficacy itself, antagonises the pharmacological effects of most opiates. Many pharmacodynamic interactions occur when the physician forgets that a drug known to be acting at one receptor may also act at another. Thus, antihistamines, phenothiazines and tricyclic antidepressants may have muscarinic anticholinergic activity in addition to their desired pharmacological effects; and administration of two or more of these agents – particularly in the elderly – may lead to pronounced anticholinergic symptoms and signs.

Pharmacodynamic interaction may also occur when two drugs act at different sites, e.g. the interaction of digoxin and diuretics. Here, hypokalaemia induced by diuretics leads to a reduction of potassium reabsorption in the kidney, which may potentiate the effects of digoxin on the heart.

Pharmacokinetic interactions

Absorption

Drugs may interact with each other to prevent either the rate or the extent of absorption of another compound. Drugs which increase gastric emptying (e.g. metoclopramide) will increase the rate of absorption of many drugs, so that the peak concentration of that drug will tend to be higher. The opposite effect is achieved by agents, such as the anticholinergic compound propantheline, which diminish gastric emptying. These changes are likely to be more important after single dose administration in a situation where threshold concentration for drug effect exists, e.g. for analgesics. Under these circumstances (particularly if the rate of elimination of the drug is high), a delay in absorption may result in an inability to reach therapeutic drug concentrations.

The extent of absorption of a drug may be impaired by the presence of another through the formation of chelates, ion pairs or complexes. Ion exchange resins such as cholestyramine and colestipol combine with warfarin, thyroxine and digitalis glycosides to impair absorption. Similarly, the calcium, magnesium or aluminium ions in antacids or milk may interact with tetracycline. In most cases, these interactions can be prevented by ensuring a time interval of at least two hours between administration of the two compounds. In the case of warfarin and digitoxin, however, cholestyramine or colestipol may also affect enterohepatic recirculation and reduce concentrations of these drugs, even if they are administered after absorption has been completed.

Distribution

Drugs may compete for both plasma protein binding sites, and for active transport processes in the body. The importance of plasma protein binding displacement interactions has been much exaggerated. For most drugs, only the drug free in plasma is available for metabolism. Thus, an increase in the percentage of free drug will result in a concomitant increase in total clearance and the rapid return of the free (biologically active) drug concentration to its original value. (The net result is a lower total drug concentration, but a larger percentage of this is in the free form.) The temporary increase in free drug concentration is only likely to be important if the drug is normally highly protein bound (e.g. greater than 90%) and has a low apparent volume of distribution. If the displacing agent is given by a rapid intravenous injection, the increase in free drug concentration of the displaced agent may also be important, but clinically significant examples of this interaction are difficult to find. For those few drugs which are relatively efficiently cleared by the liver, drug displacement interactions could (in theory) result in permanent increases in the free drug concentration, since metabolism is not limited to free drug but also extends to bound drug, which is effectively stripped from its plasma binding sites and metabolised. However, no clinically important examples of such an interaction have yet been described. At present, whenever significant clinical interactions have been shown to be associated with protein binding displacement, other mechanisms – such as competition for metabolism – have been shown to be the major causes of the interaction. It is therefore possible that plasma protein binding displacement merely reflects the physicochemical similarities of the two compounds which leads to their competing for transport or metabolic processes.

Inhibition of active transport of one drug by another can result in significant interactions. The adrenergic neurone blocking drugs guanethidine, bethanidine and debrisoquine are all substrates for the amine pump, which normally takes up noradrenaline into the adrenergic nerve endings. Drugs which inhibit this process (e.g. tricyclic antidepressants and chlorpromazine) may antagonise the antihypertensive effect of these drugs. Blocking of the amine pump may also potentiate the pressor effect of directly acting sympathomimetics such as noradrenaline or phenylephrine.

Metabolism

Metabolism of drugs by the hepatic mono-oxygenase system can be stimulated by compounds in cigarette smoke and a variety of other drugs (Table 3.4). Enzyme induction

Table 3.4 Some drugs causing induction of drug metabolism

- Barbiturates and primidone
- Carbamazepine
- Cigarette smoking
- Dichloralphenazone
- Phenytoin
- Rifampicin

42

is related to an increase in the amount of cytochromes present, and may therefore take 7–14 days to develop fully, and a similar lag period to wear off after the inducing agent is discontinued. This time lag tends to disguise any causal relationship between the drug interaction and administration of the inducing agent. Furthermore, if the dose of the active drug has been increased to maintain adequate effects, marked increases in drug concentration and toxic effects may be seen when induction wears off.

Other agents can impair the metabolism of concomitantly administered drugs, either by competing for metabolism or in a non-competitive manner (Table 3.5). Cimetidine is an interesting example in that although not itself metabolised (it is largely excreted unchanged in the urine), it inhibits the metabolism of drugs by the liver. Since the effect of enzyme inhibitors is generally direct, the lag time for this effect to occur is shorter than with enzyme inducers, and the effects disappear more quickly after discontinuation. Allopurinol has little effect on drugs metabolised by the mono-oxygenase pathway but, by inhibiting xanthine oxidase, can impair the metabolism of azathioprine and 6-mercaptopurine and potentiate their toxicity.

Table 3.5 Some drugs causing inhibition of drug metabolism

- Allopurinol
- Amiodarone
- Cimetidine
- Erythromycin
- Isoniazid
- Ketoconazole
- Metronidazole
- Monoamine oxidase inhibitors
- Sulphonamides

Excretion

It is unlikely that drug-induced changes in glomerular filtration rate will markedly alter the excretion of other drugs by the kidney. However, drugs which alter urinary pH may have a marked effect on the renal clearance of weak bases or acids, because of the effects on passive reabsorption in the proximal tubule. The administration of bicarbonate, for example, may enhance the removal of weak acids (such as phenobarbitone and aspirin) by

increasing the proportion of drug in the ionised form in the urine, thus preventing passive reabsorption. Similarly, acidification of the urine (using ammonium chloride) reduces tubular reabsorption of weak bases such as amphetamine – an effect which has been used in overdose to enhance renal excretion.

Acidic drugs may compete with each other for the active renal tubular secretory pathway – salicylates and thiazides may potentiate the toxicity of methotrexate in this way. No clinically important interactions involving basic drugs at this site have been reported. Quinidine and verapamil may compete with digoxin for an active tubular secretory mechanism in the distal convoluted tubule. This may result in digoxin toxicity, although quinidine also displaces digoxin from binding sites in tissues and this could also contribute to the interaction.

THERAPEUTIC DRUG MONITORING

Therapeutic drug monitoring refers to the measurement of drug concentrations in plasma to aid in optimising drug efficacy and reducing the risk of toxicity.

The ideal way to monitor drug therapy is, of course, to measure wanted and unwanted effects directly; and where good measures of these exist (e.g. in anticoagulant therapy) measurement of plasma drug concentrations has a very limited role. There are, however, situations in which drug efficacy or toxicity are more difficult to measure, and both here, and where the drug is being given prophylactically to prevent serious events (e.g. antiepileptic and anti-arrhythmic drugs) therapeutic drug monitoring may have a role to play (Table 3.6). Measurement of plasma (or urine) drug concentration is also of value in detecting overdose (either deliberate or accidental) and in monitoring compliance with therapy in patients who may not be responding normally to the drug.

For therapeutic drug monitoring to be of value in optimising therapeutic benefit, the drug should work by a reversible mechanism without development of tolerance to the therapeutic effect. The possibility of accumulation of active metabolites which are not detected by the drug assay must also be considered. Procainamide, for example, is

Table 3.6 Drug concentrations associated with optimal efficacy in most patients

	Usual half-life (h)	Usual therapeutic plasma concentrations	Toxic concentration	Principal route of elimination
Digoxin	30–40	1.3–2.6 nmol/l	>2.6 nmol/l	Renal excretion
Gentamicin	2	Trough <2 mg/l Peak 4–8 mg/l	Trough >2 mg/l Peak >12 mg/l	Renal excretion
Lithium	7–20	0.6–1.4 mmol/l	>1.5 nmol/l	Renal excretion
Phenytoin	20–60	Plasma 40–80 μmol/l Saliva 4–8 μmol/l	>80 μmol/l >8 μmol/l	Hepatic metabolism
Theophylline	4–16	Plasma 55–110 μmol/l Saliva 35–70 μmol/l	>110 μmol/l >70 μmol/l	Hepatic metabolism

metabolised to N-acetylprocainamide which also has anti-arrhythmic activity, and should also therefore be measured.

Sample collection

Unlike many endogenous compounds, such as creatinine, which are produced at a continuous rate, drugs are normally administered at fixed intervals and the plasma concentration will therefore vary markedly with time after administration. Early after administration, the plasma concentration may be affected by the rate of gastric emptying. While if there is extensive distribution of the drug, early samples may be higher than the average, or steady state, drug concentration during the dosage interval, and may not accurately reflect the concentration at the site of action of the drug. It is therefore preferable to wait at least eight hours after administration of an oral dose of digoxin, or twelve hours after lithium, before sampling. If peak levels are important, samples should be taken two to three hours after a conventional tablet or later if a sustained-release formulation has been administered; or a half to one hour after intramuscular injection. In most cases, however, a trough concentration taken just before the next dose will correlate most closely with the steady state drug concentration.

Since it takes approximately five half-lives before steady state is achieved, sampling before this time will tend to underestimate the subsequent steady state concentration and is only indicated if toxicity due to accumulation of the drug is possible. Details of sampling time, change in dose, and last administration of the dose, should always be given on the assay request form to enable the plasma concentration to be interpreted correctly.

Total drug concentrations are normally measured and these generally mirror the free plasma concentration. This may not be true in diseases where changes in plasma protein binding of drugs are likely, such as hepatic and renal disease. For some drugs (e.g. phenytoin and theophylline), the saliva drug concentration may be a closer reflection of the free plasma drug concentration; and in young children, saliva collection (stimulated by a drop of citric acid solution on the tongue) may avoid venepuncture.

SPECIFIC DRUGS

Anticonvulsants

Phenytoin metabolism shows saturation rather than first order kinetics, so that clearance falls with increasing dose and the risk of toxicity increases. Half-life also increases with increasing dose and so it will take longer for steady state to be achieved. Most patients tend to be given too small a dose of phenytoin, but therapeutic drug monitoring has reduced the tendency to prescribe a second anti-epileptic drug in many patients who initially received sub-therapeutic doses. Therapeutic monitoring of other anticonvulsants is of limited value except in the identification of poor compliance.

Antiarrhythmics

Because of their serious toxicity and the narrow margin between therapeutic and toxic doses, monitoring of several antiarrhythmic drugs may help to reduce adverse effects and improve response. The half-life of most anti-arrhythmics is short but that of amiodarone is around 30–45 days. A loading dose is therefore necessary to achieve early therapeutic concentrations of this drug, and prolonged monitoring will help to detect accumulation of amiodarone and its major (and possibly toxic) metabolite, desethylamiodarone.

Digoxin

The plasma digoxin concentration is one of the determinants of toxicity of the drug, particularly the non-cardiovascular toxicity, causing lassitude, depression and anorexia. Monitoring is particularly important in patients with reduced renal function (e.g. in the elderly) and will also help to identify poor compliance.

Theophylline

Patients vary greatly in metabolic clearance of this potentially toxic bronchodilator, and adjustment of dose is facilitated by measurement of plasma theophylline concentrations.

Antibiotics

The aminoglycosides are the most frequently monitored antibiotics. The risk of ototoxicity can be reduced by preventing excessive plasma drug concentrations, but the nephrotoxic effects of the drug are less closely related to the plasma concentration, so that renal function must also be carefully monitored during therapy.

Lithium

Lithium is used in the treatment of hypomania and, because toxicity may occur insidiously (p. 54), therapeutic monitoring is essential.

FURTHER READING

Davies D M (ed) 1985 Textbook of adverse drug reactions, 3rd edn. Oxford University Press, Oxford. *Reference source for adverse reactions*

Gibaldi M 1984 Biopharmaceutics and clinical pharmacokinetics, 3rd edn. Lea and Febiger, Philadelphia. *A clear, relatively non-mathematical introduction to pharmacokinetics*

Hansten P D 1989 Drug interactions, 6th edn. Lea and Febiger, Philadelphia. *A comprehensive reference source for drug interactions*

Speight T M (ed) 1987 Avery's drug treatment, 3rd edn. Churchill Livingstone, Edinburgh. *A large text covering most aspects of clinical pharmacology and drug treatment*

Turner P, Richens A, Routledge P A 1986 Clinical pharmacology, 5th edn. Churchill Livingstone, Edinburgh. *A concise introductory guide to clinical pharmacology*

Drug Overdose, Poisoning and Drug Addiction

4

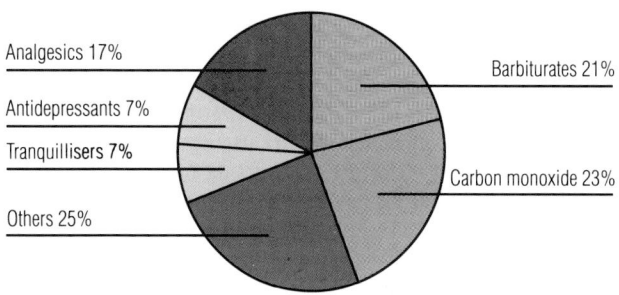

Fig. 4.1 **Drugs involved in fatal poisoning episodes.**

DRUG OVERDOSE

Modern society is so dependent upon chemicals that it is not surprising that many people are exposed to these agents, either deliberately or accidentally. Approximately 4000 people die each year of poisoning in England and Wales, a quarter of them of carbon monoxide poisoning. Approximately two-thirds of the remaining deaths occur outside hospital, so that hospital mortality due to poisoning is relatively low. Nevertheless, more than 100 000 patients are admitted to hospital in England and Wales each year due to poisoning, so that patients with accidental poisoning or drug overdose account for 10% of all acute admissions. Toxic compounds may be ingested or inhaled either accidentally or deliberately by the individual or may be administered accidentally or deliberately by another individual. This forms the basis for a classification of poisoning incidents separating them into broad epidemiological categories. The major causes of deaths from poisoning are shown in Figure 4.1.

Accidental poisoning

Although accidental poisoning can occur at any age, it is much more likely to occur in children under five years of age (Fig. 4.2). Peak incidence is around two years, when children have just become independently mobile. Boys, perhaps because they are more adventurous, appear to be more at risk. This contrasts with other categories of poisoning in which women seem to be involved more often than men. Fortunately, the mortality from accidental poisoning is relatively small, although all such deaths are particularly tragic. While death from carbon monoxide poisoning predominates, there are approximately 20 acci-

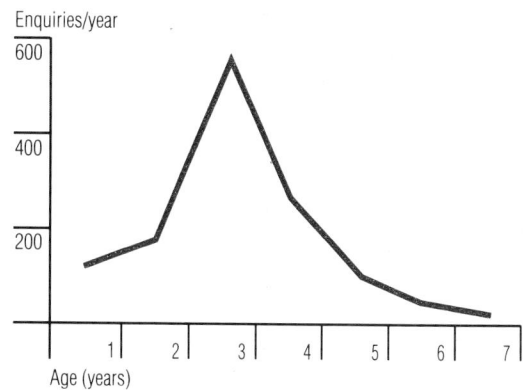

Fig. 4.2 **The relationship between age and the incidence of accidental poisoning in children.** Figures are based on enquiries concerning accidental poisoning made to the Welsh National Poisons Unit in 1984.

45

4

dental deaths per year from other agents, particularly tricyclic antidepressants, aspirin and barbiturates. The incidence of accidental poisoning in childhood is partly determined by availability. Poisoning by cough and cold remedies is commoner in the winter and spring, by herbicides and pesticides in the summer months, and by berries and seeds in the autumn. Another factor may be the degree of supervision of the child since incidents appear to occur more often at times of family crisis, when supervision is likely to be less strict.

Deliberate self-poisoning

Deliberate self-poisoning is commoner in adults who, unlike children, ingest medicinal agents more readily than they do household chemicals and other non-medicinal compounds. Women are more often involved than men in deliberate self-poisoning, and the vast majority of instances are not intended to be ultimately fatal, although some, unfortunately, are. Generally they represent a response to an apparently insoluble personal predicament (Ch. 11). Some have definite suicidal intent, attempt to conceal their overdose and may therefore die outside hospital. Patients who successfully commit suicide tend to be older and may have been recently divorced or bereaved, may be living alone, suffering from a physical illness, unemployed or abusers of alcohol.

Non-accidental poisoning

Non-accidental poisoning generally involves children and is a form of child abuse. The parents of such children may have suffered child abuse or deprivation themselves, and often have marital or financial problems or difficulties in managing the child at the time of the non-accidental poisoning episode. A thorough history and examination of the child may sometimes help to identify this form of poisoning.

Homicidal poisoning

Although often featured in novels and plays, homicidal poisoning is very uncommon. When it does happen, it is often caused by a close relative or friend and generally involves the use of poisons producing chronic, rather than acute, symptoms. Such a situation may lead to difficulty in diagnosis.

DIAGNOSIS OF POISONING

It is impossible to identify by laboratory tests every agent to which an individual might be exposed. A full history and clinical examination is therefore as much an integral part of the diagnosis as it is in other causes of disease. Since the subject may be unwilling or unable to give a history on presentation, it is important to talk to relatives or friends of the individual, to the general practitioner, or to the ambulancemen who brought him into hospital. Particular difficulties are encountered with the patient who is found alone and unconscious and in which poisoning is just one of the differential diagnoses.

The first priority in the unconscious patient is maintenance of vital functions – the airway, ventilation and cardiovascular function. When this has been ensured, the question arises as to whether the patient is poisoned. Other causes of unconsciousness are discussed in Chapter 23. In deep coma due to drug overdose, the pupillary reflexes are often preserved, whilst the oculovestibular responses (e.g. 'doll's eye response') are absent. Focal neurological signs are rare in overdose and, unless they can be accounted for by previous pathology, these should alert the clinician to the possibility of another cause, particularly if preceded by a history of trauma, headache, nausea and vomiting or recent personality change. Papilloedema due to drug overdose is rare, unless the overdose has been associated with cerebral hypoxia and oedema.

It is rare for poisoned patients to show no improvement in consciousness level by 12 hours after admission. In those who do not do so, some other pathology should be suspected.

Clinical examination

It is sometimes possible to identify the poison by the clinical signs on examination, although it may be more difficult if the patient has taken several agents. In the unconscious subject, it may be more useful to use the 'head to toe' scheme of examination, which is used in the assessment of the patient who is unconscious from other causes. The most helpful clinical signs which implicate particular toxins are shown in Tables 4.1A and B.

Eyes

Pupillary dilatation occurs in poisoning with anticholinergic drugs such as the tricyclic antidepressants, anti-Parkinsonian agents, antihistamines and phenothiazines. Pupillary dilatation is also seen with agents which stimulate the sympathetic nervous system such as amphetamines, LSD and theophyllines. Unequal pupils are occasionally seen in poisoning and are not necessarily related to previous eye disease or focal neurological causes. Strabismus is not uncommon in poisoned patients, particularly in carbamazepine poisoning. Papilloedema however is rare, except as a result of methanol, carbon monoxide or glutethimide poisoning. Nystagmus may be caused by agents affecting the central nervous system, and particularly by phenytoin.

Mouth

Acneiform lesions around the buccal cavity may suggest solvent abuse, and the characteristic odour of solvent or alcohol may be present on the breath. Examination of the oral cavity may reveal ulceration due to corrosion by acids or alkalis. The mouth may be abnormally dry because of anticholinergic compounds, and increased salivation may

Table 4.1A Physical signs suggestive of overdose or poisoning: head and neck

Sign	Possible cause
Dilated pupils	Tricyclic antidepressants Anticholinergics Sympathomimetics
Strabismus	Carbamazepine
Nystagmus	Phenytoin Carbamazepine
Papilloedema	Methanol Carbon monoxide Glutethimide
Perforated nasal septum	Cocaine abuse
Acneiform rash	Solvent abuse
Erythema/burns	Corrosives
Mouth dryness	Anticholinergics
Hypersalivation	Parasympathomimetics

Table 4.1B Physical signs suggestive of overdose or poisoning: trunk and limbs

Sign	Possible cause
Bronchospasm	Irritant gases NSAIDs
Pulmonary oedema	Irritant gases Opiates Aspirin
Tachycardia	Anticholinergics Sympathomimetics
Bradycardia	Beta-blockers Verapamil Digoxin
Hypotension	Many agents
Hypertension	Clonidine MAOIs
Needle tracks	Drugs of addiction
Absent bowel sounds	Anticholinergics
Bladder distension	Anticholinergics
Hypothermia	Phenothiazines
Hyperthermia	Salicylates Anticholinergics Sympathomimetics MAOIs
Hyperreflexia	Anticholinergics Sympathomimetics Opiates
Blisters	Barbiturates Carbon monoxide Occasionally other hypnotics
Extensor plantar response	Anticholinergics

be seen in subjects who have taken agents which stimulate the parasympathetic nervous system, e.g. carbamate insecticides and anticholinesterases.

Chest

Chest wheeze may be caused by inhalation of irritant compounds; pulmonary oedema can also be caused by these agents or by ingestion of some drugs such as opiates or aspirin. Auscultation of the heart may reveal a tachycardia in association with poisoning due to anticholinergic compounds, salicylates or drugs stimulating the sympathetic nervous system. Bradycardia, on the other hand, may be caused by verapamil, beta-blockers or drugs stimulating the parasympathetic nervous system. Cardiac arrhythmias may be associated with hypoxia, but are particularly troublesome in patients who have taken tricyclic antidepressants, drugs stimulating the sympathetic nervous system, phenothiazines or quinine. Hypotension can be caused by many agents, but hypertension is rarer and generally associated with poisoning by monoamine oxidase inhibitors or clonidine which, in overdose, may act like alpha-adrenoreceptor agonists.

Abdomen

Examination of the abdomen may reveal absent bowel sounds or bladder enlargement, suggesting the possibility of anticholinergic poisoning. Rectal examination should be performed and may reveal melaena due to poisoning by iron, non-steroidal anti-inflammatory agents or other agents which cause damage to the gut mucosa. The rectal temperature should be recorded at the same time, using a low reading thermometer. This may reveal hypothermia (e.g. with phenothiazine poisoning) or hyperthermia (in poisoning by salicylates, anticholinergic compounds or drugs stimulating the sympathetic nervous system).

Skin

The hands and arms should be examined for needle tracks which may indicate drug abuse; such lesions may also be present on the lower limbs. Blisters over the bony prominences may be seen on the upper limbs, but are commoner on the lower limbs. Although they are most often seen in patients who have taken barbiturate overdose, they are by no means diagnostic, even of a drug-induced coma; they may, for example, occur after hypoxia.

Neuromuscular

Examination of the upper (as well as lower) limbs normally reveals hypotonia and hyporeflexia in poisoning, but anticholinergic drugs, some opiates and drugs stimulating the sympathetic nervous system may cause hypertonia, hyperreflexia and, occasionally, myoclonus. Anticholinergic compounds may also produce an extensor plantar response which is usually bilateral.

Convulsions may be caused directly by a variety of compounds including the anticholinergic agents and drugs stimulating the sympathetic nervous system, opiates, mefenamic acid and isoniazid, or may be secondary to hypoxia or hypoglycaemia associated with overdose. Dystonic reactions are much less commonly seen, and are generally related to poisoning with drugs with anti-dopaminergic activity such as metoclopromide, the phenothiazines and butyrophenones.

Laboratory investigations

Routine laboratory investigations are sometimes helpful in identification of the drug ingested.

Urine

The urine should be examined both macroscopically and microscopically, and by ward urinalysis. A specimen should also be stored for possible future analysis even if this is not indicated initially. Red discolouration of the urine may be caused by rifampicin or phenindione, and haematuria by drugs affecting haemostasis or clotting, or by drugs causing haemolysis, such as chlorates. Drugs which contain methylene blue (e.g. some commercial analgesics) may colour the urine blue or, more commonly, green; a greyish discolouration of the urine may indicate poisoning due to phenols or cresols. Microscopic haematuria or albuminuria may be the first sign of renal damage; crystalluria can occur with primidone and some of the sulphonamides.

Blood

A brown discolouration of venous blood may indicate methaemoglobinaemia, which can be caused by oxidising agents such as dapsone. Pink discolouration of the plasma indicates haemolysis which, if not due to poor venepuncture technique, may be related to drug induced haemolysis.

The urea and electrolytes are only rarely of diagnostic value. Hypokalaemia can be caused by theophylline and drugs stimulating the sympathetic nervous system, or may indicate potassium loss due to diuretic or purgative overdose. Hyperkalaemia is sometimes seen in digoxin overdose, the degree of hyperkalaemia often reflecting the severity of the overdose. Reduction in the serum bicarbonate may indicate metabolic acidosis and should be followed by arterial blood gas analysis. The alcohols and glycols, as well as aspirin, may cause metabolic acidosis. Finally, profound hypoglycaemia may indicate overdose with oral hypoglycaemic agents, or be secondary to overdose with alcohols, salicylates or paracetamol. Not all of these investigations are indicated in every case of poisoning and clinical judgement must be used in deciding which will give useful diagnostic or prognostic information. As with urine, it may be useful to take blood and store it for possible future reference.

Specific tests

An increasing number of compounds can now be detected specifically in either urine (which tends to be more useful since it concentrates the drug or its metabolites) or in blood. The availability of such tests does not, however, automatically justify their use. Toxicological analyses should not be used as a substitute for sound clinical judgement and, before a test is ordered, the physician should ask himself whether the result will alter his management of a particular case.

PRINCIPLES OF MANAGEMENT OF POISONING

The most important aspect of managing poisoned patients is general supportive measures to prevent complications rather than specific therapy to treat the particular poison, since the latter are not always available.

Supportive management

Maintenance of respiratory function

Maintenance of an adequate airway and respiration is the first priority in an unconscious patient, since many early deaths due to poisoning are due to airway obstruction. Dentures should be removed, the tongue pulled forward and the mouth and pharynx cleared of saliva and vomitus. If the patient has no cough reflex, a cuffed endotracheal tube is necessary to protect the lungs; in other cases, a short oropharyngeal tube should be inserted. The patient is then moved into a semi-prone position and, if there is any suspicion of inadequate ventilation, oxygen should be administered; assisted ventilation may be necessary.

In less urgent circumstances, arterial blood gas analysis is the best guide to assessing adequacy of ventilation. Drugs which stimulate respiration (e.g. doxapram) should be used cautiously in poisoned patients, since they may provoke convulsions or cardiac arrhythmias. The 'shock lung syndrome' (adult respiratory distress syndrome, ARDS; see p. 518) may appear at about 24 hours. The patient begins to hyperventilate but remains hypoxic, and develops a respiratory and metabolic acidosis. A chest X-ray may show changes similar to pulmonary oedema and, in severe cases, the lung fields may be completely obscured. The aetiology is unknown, but assisted ventilation using positive end expiratory pressure (PEEP) may help to support the patient through this severe complication. The treatment of aspiration pneumonia is discussed on p. 475.

Maintenance of circulatory function

Maintenance of circulatory function is the next priority. Hypotension and reduced peripheral perfusion may be caused by several mechanisms including:

1. depression of the vasomotor centre
2. a direct cardio-depressant action
3. increased venous capacitance, leading to reduced venous return to the heart and a consequent fall in cardiac output

4. increased capillary permeability resulting in a reduced circulating blood volume.

If the hypotension does not respond to elevation of the foot of the bed, a central venous pressure line should be inserted. If the venous pressure is low, the blood volume should be increased using a plasma expander, such as haemacell. If the hypotension does not respond to the correction of hypovolaemia, dopamine or dobutamine by intravenous infusion may restore the blood pressure; low dose dopamine may prevent subsequent acute renal failure.

Consideration should then be given to any possible specific means (e.g. charcoal haemoperfusion) to remove the poison; this may restore the blood pressure to normal. Cardiac arrhythmias, which may be a direct effect of the drug or a result of hypoxia and acidosis, may also contribute to hypotension by reducing cardiac output. It is important to correct the predisposing causes before considering specific anti-arrhythmic therapy, since many of these agents may further reduce the cardiac output. The choice of an anti-arrhythmic agent is generally based upon the arrhythmia rather than the specific toxin.

Prevention of complications

Good nursing care of the unconscious patient will help to prevent further complications. A particular problem is skin and muscle compression injuries. The bladder can sometimes be emptied by firm suprapubic pressure but, if it is markedly distended, catheterisation may be necessary, particularly when measurement of urine production is required. The level of consciousness should be monitored (a convenient classification is shown in Table 4.2). If the level of consciousness fails to improve after 12 hours, a search should be made for neurological complications of the overdose or an alternative diagnosis of the coma. Cerebral oedema is the most life-threatening complication of overdose, and may be caused by hypoxia, hypoglycaemia, hypercapnia or hypotension. It is particularly likely to occur after cardio-respiratory arrest and may respond to the use of dexamethasone or mannitol. Convulsions may also be secondary to hypoxia or cerebral oedema, but otherwise are generally shortlived and do not always require specific therapy. If necessary, intravenous diazepam may be used, but if the patient is vomiting, temporary intu-

bation and mechanical ventilation may be necessary to prevent aspiration pneumonia.

Gastrointestinal bleeding or paralytic ileus may be seen in patients with drug overdose. Insertion of a nasogastric tube and regular emptying of the stomach help to reveal bleeding early and also to prevent the aspiration pneumonia or acute gastric dilatation sometimes seen with paralytic ileus.

Measures to prevent further drug absorption

Gastric emptying

It is occasionally possible to reduce further absorption of the drug from the gut by emptying the stomach, either by inducing emesis or by gastric lavage. These procedures are only indicated if the amount of poison taken is likely to cause serious symptoms, and are of little value if the material ingested has already left the stomach. They should thus only be attempted when less than four hours has elapsed since ingestion of the toxin, although they may still be worthwhile if the time of ingestion is unknown or if the overdose itself is associated with delayed gastric emptying (e.g. with salicylates, mefenamic acid, opiates and drugs with anticholinergic activity, such as tricyclic anti-depressants).

Emesis and lavage are contraindicated in patients who have taken corrosive agents, unless the danger of systemic toxicity associated with a corrosive agent is greater than the risk of local damage. Lavage and emesis are also usually contraindicated after oral ingestion of petroleum distillates, because of the risk of aspiration pneumonia; and emesis is unlikely to be effective after treatment with drugs with antiemetic properties (e.g. metoclopramide). It should not be performed in patients whose consciousness is impaired, because of the delay in action of ipecacuanha and the risk of aspiration pneumonia in a subsequently unconscious individual.

Gastric lavage

Gastric lavage is the preferred method of emptying of the stomach in adults. In the unconscious patient, a cuffed endotracheal tube must always be inserted first. Lavage should be done in the left lateral position in a bed or trolley which has been raised at the foot. A large-bore Jaques

---

Table 4.2 Assessment of level of consciousness (Edinburgh Method)

Grade	Degree of consciousness
Grade 0	Fully conscious
Grade 1	Drowsy but able to obey commands
Grade 2	Responds only to pain
Grade 3	Responds only to maximal painful stimuli
Grade 4	Completely unresponsive to any stimuli

Summary 1 Prevention of further drug absorption

- Gastric lavage may prevent further absorption of drug, if performed sufficiently early
- Emesis induced by syrup of ipecacuanha is the preferred method of emptying the stomach in conscious children
- Emptying the stomach by either lavage or emesis should not be performed if the airway cannot be protected
- Activated charcoal prevents further absorption of many drugs, if administered sufficiently early

Drug Overdose, Poisoning and Drug Addiction

4

stomach tube (external diameter c. 14 mm) is introduced into the stomach and the gastric contents removed. Aliquots of water warmed to body temperature are then introduced and removed until the returned fluid is clear of particles.

Emesis

Emesis is generally the preferred method in children provided there are not contraindications, with syrup of ipecacuanha the most reliable agent. This will produce vomiting in 70% of individuals within 20 minutes. A repeated dose after this time will be effective in most of those patients who did not vomit initially. Salt and water should not be used to produce emesis, since death may occur from hypernatraemia. This is particularly likely in small children.

Oral adsorbents

Activated charcoal is being used increasingly in the treatment of poisoning as it may reduce the absorption of many drugs (Table 4.3). It is most effective with agents with high toxicity at low dose, since ten times as much charcoal as drug is required to provide adequate adsorption onto the charcoal; the charcoal must be given early after the overdose to achieve maximum efficacy. It is of little value in adsorbing organic solvents, lithium, cyanide, corrosive agents and iron. A dose of 50–100 g can be administered either orally or, in an adult, by nasogastric tube. Oral adsorbents such as activated charcoal are of particular value in accidental poisoning in children, since these cases normally present early enough for the adsorbent to be effective.

In iron poisoning, desferrioxamine is the preferred method to prevent further absorption of iron present in the stomach.

Table 4.3 Drugs for which charcoal may prevent absorption

Hypnotics and tranquillisers	Cardiovascular drugs
Phenobarbitone	Digoxin
	Disopyramide
Antidepressants	Mexiletene
Amitriptyline	Pindolol
	Quinidine
Analgesics	Sotalol
Aspirin	
Dextropropoxyphene	**Respiratory drugs**
Indomethacin	Aminophylline
Mefenamic acid	
Paracetamol	**Antidiabetic drugs**
Phenylbutazone	Chlorpropamide
	Tolbutamide
Anticonvulsants	
Carbamazepine	**Diuretics**
Phenytoin	Frusemide
Valproate	
	Others
Antibiotics	Cimetidine
Tetracycline	Paraquat
Trimethoprim	Thallium

Antidotes

The Ancient Persians believed that a stone found in the stomach of ruminants, when ground and added to their drink, would act as an antidote to all poisons. This was known as the 'Bezoar stone' and was probably as ineffective as the 'universal antidote' (two parts activated charcoal, one part tannic acid, and one part magnesium oxide) still listed in pharmacopoeias today. In fact, there are only direct antidotes to about 5% of poisons, so that supportive therapy remains the mainstay of treatment for the vast majority of patients, including those where an antidote exists.

Antidotes work in several different ways:

1. They may speed the metabolism of a toxin. For example, thiosulphate speeds the metabolism of cyanide by providing sulphur to combine with cyanide and form non-toxic thiocyanate which is then excreted in the urine.
2. If a compound is only toxic once it has been metabolised, antidotes may be used to reduce the rate at which the metabolite is produced. Thus, ethanol is used in poisoning by methanol and ethylene glycol to reduce the rate of production of toxic aldehydes and acids from the latter compounds.
3. For those toxins in which the toxicity is receptor mediated, an antagonist which competes for a receptor occupation may be useful, e.g. the use of beta-agonists in the treatment of beta-adrenoceptor blocking drug overdose.
4. If the toxin is competing with a natural substrate, a compound which allows the natural substrate's concentration to increase so that it can competitively displace the poison from the receptor site is also useful. This is the method by which inhibitors of acetyl cholinesterase reverse some of the features of anticholinergic poisoning.
5. Antidotes may combine with the poison to form an inactive compound. Thus, specific anti-digoxin antibody (Fab) fragments combine with digoxin to produce an inert complex which can be excreted more rapidly via the kidney.

The availability of a specific antidote does not necessarily justify its routine use. Many are toxic in their own right and should only be used if the severity of the poisoning merits their administration. In general they are most useful early on in the course of poisoning.

Enhancement of drug elimination

Methods to enhance drug elimination are of limited value in the treatment of overdose. All the methods listed below are generally only effective when the volume of distribution of the drug is relatively small. This is because drug removal can only occur from the 'central' (intravascular) compartment, which must therefore contain a reasonable proportion of the total body burden of the compound. Each method has its particular advantages and disadvantages but most are used on only a small proportion of the total number of patients admitted with poisoning (Table 4.4).

Forced diuresis

Forced diuresis can be used to enhance the elimination of those drugs excreted predominantly in an unchanged form by the kidney. It acts in part by increasing the glomerular filtration rate but also, more importantly, by reducing the tubular reabsorption of unchanged drug. This is dependent partly on renal tubular flow, but also on the degree of ionisation of the drug in the tubular fluid. For weak acids, alkalinisation of the tubular fluid by administration of bicarbonate will result in a greater proportion of the drug existing in the ionised, poorly lipid soluble, form. It is thus unable to diffuse back across the lipid membrane of the tubular cell and be reabsorbed. Conversely, acidification of the urine by administration of ammonium chloride, arginine or lysine hydrochloride will increase the ionisation of some basic drugs, thereby reducing reabsorption from the tubular fluid back into the systemic circulation. Renal excretion of these compounds is therefore enhanced.

Alkaline diuresis has been used in the treatment of pheno-barbitone, barbitone and salicylate poisoning since all are weak acids with a relatively low volume of distribution and are substantially excreted unchanged in the urine, at least in overdose. Digoxin, although also excreted unchanged in the urine, is not effectively removed by forced diuresis, partly because it is not a weak acid or base, and partly because its volume of distribution in the body is so large. *Forced acid diuresis* has been used to enhance removal of phencyclidine (the active ingredient of 'angel dust'), amphetamine and the closely related appetite suppressant fenfluramine.

Forced diuresis should only be used in patients with good cardiac and renal function since fluid overload can lead to water intoxication, pulmonary oedema or severe electrolyte and acid-base disturbances. A careful assessment of fluid status is therefore necessary, and unconscious patients will require catheterisation. Intravenous frusemide is used to maintain the fluid output around 500 ml per hour. In forced alkaline diuresis, sufficient sodium bicarbonate (1.2% solution) is given to maintain the urine pH between 7.0 and 8.0; in forced acid diuresis, the pH is maintained between 5 and 6.5 with oral ammonium chloride. Urine pH should be monitored at least half-hourly and electrolytes every 2–4 hours.

Dialysis

Dialysis (peritoneal or haemodialysis) is useful in removing drugs which have low plasma protein binding, poor lipid solubility and relatively low volume of distribution. It is generally reserved for those cases where other methods of removal are contraindicated. Salicylates, phenobarbitone and barbitone, methanol, isopropanol, ethylene glycol and lithium are effectively removed by this process. Haemodialysis is normally the most effective of the two approaches.

Table 4.4 Techniques used to enhance drug elimination

Forced diuresis	Haemoperfusion
Alkaline	Barbiturates
Barbitone	Carbamazepine
Phenobarbitone	Chloroquine
Phenoxyacetate herbicides	Glutethimide
Salicylates	Meprobamate
	Methaqualone
Acid	Phenytoin
Amphetamine	Salicylates
Fenfluramine	Theophylline
Phencyclidine	
	Enteral adsorbants
Dialysis	Charcoal
Barbitone	Amitriptyline
Ethanol	Carbamazepine
Ethylene glycol	Dapsone
Isopropanol	Dextropropoxyphene
Lithium	Digitoxin
Methanol	Nadolol
Phenobarbitone	Nortriptyline
Salicylates	Phenobarbitone
	Quinine
	Sotalol
	Theophylline
	Cholestyramine
	Digitoxin
	Phenprocoumon
	Warfarin

Haemoperfusion

Haemoperfusion involves the passage of arterial blood through an extracorporeal column of activated charcoal or ion-exchange resin. This method effectively removes a number of drugs where the lipid solubility or plasma protein binding reduces the efficacy of removal by dialysis techniques, but a low volume of distribution is still required. Haemoperfusion is therefore useful in severe poisoning with barbiturates, including the short-acting barbiturates which are not removed effectively by haemodialysis, and with the non-barbiturate hypnotics such as glutethimide, ethchlorvynol, meprobamate, methaqualone and chloral derivatives (e.g. chloral hydrate). Fortunately, all these agents are used less frequently as hypnotics in medical practice than they once were. Haemoperfusion using resin columns is particularly effective in removing theophylline and, to a lesser extent, salicylates. Complications of the procedure include thrombocytopenia, bleeding and possible infection, so haemoperfusion should only be used in patients with severe poisoning who fail to improve despite supportive management and who have developed, or are at high risk of developing, complications of the overdose.

Enteral removal

Enteral removal of drugs is the most recent approach to the enhancement of the elimination of poisons. It relies upon the ability of some non-absorbed agents either to remove drugs which have been excreted in the bile but would have been reabsorbed in the gut, or to directly remove drugs from the splanchnic circulation. Charcoal is the most widely used enteral adsorbent, and markedly enhances the rate of removal of phenobarbitone, digitoxin, theophylline and dapsone. It is given as an initial loading dose of 50 g followed by repeated doses of 20–60 g every 4–12 hours, together with a laxative to prevent constipation. Oral cholestyramine (an anion-binding resin) increases the rate of removal of digitoxin, warfarin and some other coumarin anticoagulants. This procedure, being non-invasive, is normally free from major adverse effects.

Support services

The number of toxins is so great that it is impossible for a clinician to be familiar with all the details of management of each one. In the United Kingdom and Eire, Poisons Information Services have therefore been established in several major cities. Details of the facilities provided by these and other centres which provide information services in poisoning are shown in the appendix to this chapter.

When the patient has recovered from the overdose, he should undergo thorough psychiatric and, if necessary, social assessment (Ch. 11, p. 211). There appears to be a poor correlation between the medical severity of the overdose and the severity of any underlying psychiatric illness. Opinions differ as to whether psychiatric assessment need always be performed by a trained psychiatrist but, if there is any doubt about the patient's state of mind, specialist psychiatric assessment is essential. The general practitioner also plays an important role in supporting the patient once he has left hospital, and a telephone call to the family doctor on discharge of the patient will often prevent future difficulties. Finally, voluntary services often provide useful emotional and practical support to the patient at risk, and details of these local organisations should be made available.

MANAGEMENT OF SPECIFIC DRUG OVERDOSE

The drugs most commonly involved in acute poisoning are hypnotics and tranquillisers, antidepressants and analgesics.

Hypnotics and tranquillisers

Barbiturates

The incidence of barbiturate poisoning has declined markedly over the past ten years. However, this group of compounds is associated with high mortality and still accounts for the largest number of deaths of any drug group.

Diagnosis

In overdose, the barbiturates produce an impaired level of consciousness and, in severe cases, hypotension and respiratory depression. Approximately 5% of patients have bullous lesions on the extremities, particularly over the extensor surfaces, but these are not specific to barbiturate overdose and can also occur (although less frequently) with other drugs.

Barbiturates can be detected in the urine. Although their plasma concentrations can also be measured, these tend to correlate poorly with the severity of the overdose, partly because of other confounding drugs such as alcohol, and partly because of tolerance, particularly in those taking the drug chronically. Plasma concentrations are therefore of limited value in the management of a particular case, although very high concentrations in the presence of grade 4 coma and other complications of overdose may indicate the need to enhance the removal of the drug.

Management

Gastric lavage should be performed if tablets have been taken less than four hours previously, or if the time of ingestion in an unconscious patient is unknown. General supportive management is all that is required in most cases, with particular attention to respiration and cardiovascular function. However, even with these measures, the mortality in grade 4 coma is about 5% and procedures to enhance drug elimination and reduce the duration of coma may be considered in such subjects, particularly if complications of overdose are already present. Forced alkaline diuresis has been used to enhance the removal of phenobarbitone and barbitone because these drugs are mainly excreted unchanged in the urine. This procedure is relatively inefficient, however, and has been largely replaced by the use of charcoal haemoperfusion which effectively removes most barbiturates, even those (e.g. many of the short and intermediate acting compounds) that are relatively highly protein bound and eliminated by hepatic metabolism. Repeated doses of activated charcoal given by mouth through a nasogastric tube can reduce the half-life of phenobarbitone from over 100 hours to less than 20 hours. Since this procedure is relatively non-invasive, it may replace the use of haemoperfusion for phenobarbitone poisoning, particularly in centres where the latter facility is not available. Activated charcoal has not yet been shown to enhance the elimination of any of the other barbiturates.

Summary 2   Management of barbiturate poisoning

- Barbiturate poisoning is now relatively rare but has a significant mortality

- Gastric lavage should be performed if within four hours of ingestion

- Supportive care is the most important aspect of treatment

- Charcoal haemoperfusion is effective in enhancing elimination of phenobarbitone, barbitone and other barbiturates and should be considered in severe poisoning

- Activated charcoal may prevent absorption of phenobarbitone and repeated doses may enhance elimination of drug already absorbed

Benzodiazepines

It is fortunate that benzodiazepines are relatively safe in overdose, since they are involved in almost half of the drug overdoses in the United Kingdom. There are a small number of fatal cases each year in which a benzodiazepine is the only drug identified, but they also potentiate the effects of other CNS-depressant drugs and can thus contribute to fatal outcome.

Diagnosis

The major effects in overdose are on the central nervous system and include drowsiness, ataxia, dysarthria and nystagmus. Coma then supervenes, although it is rarely greater than grade 2 unless other agents have been ingested. Recovery is normally within 24 hours, although flurazepam and flunitrazepam may cause deeper and more prolonged coma, and clonazepam has been associated with cyclical coma. Lorazepam causes only modest central nervous system depression but can be associated with restlessness and hallucinations, particularly in children. Respiratory depression occurs rarely in benzodiazepine overdose, although it may occur in patients with pre-existing respiratory disease, particularly with flunitrazepam. Cardiovascular effects are also generally mild although slight hypotension may occur. Flunitrazepam may cause more profound hypotension and a sinus bradycardia. Bullous skin lesions have been reported, but are much rarer than after barbiturate overdose. The short-acting agent triazolam has recently been associated with several deaths after overdose.

Management

The management of benzodiazepine overdose is supportive. Methods to enhance the elimination of the parent compound or its active metabolites do not have a place in the management of overdose, and the vast majority of patients will recover with no permanent sequelae. Antagonists of benzodiazepines (e.g. flumazenil) may be helpful in the diagnosis of mixed overdose, or in avoiding the need for ventilatory support in severe poisoning. They should be used with caution, however, since they may precipitate benzodiazepine withdrawal in dependent individuals.

Summary 3   Management of benzodiazepine poisoning

- Benzodiazepine poisoning is common but death is rare, unless other potentiating agents (e.g. alcohol) have also been taken
- Flurazepam, flunitrazepam and triazolam may cause deeper coma than the other agents
- Management is generally supportive
- Flumazenil, a specific benzodiazepine antagonist may help in the diagnosis of mixed overdose

---

Non-barbiturate, non-benzodiazepine hypnotics

Non-barbiturate, non-benzodiazepine hypnotics were once widely used but have now been largely replaced by benzodiazepines. Isolated overdoses of these agents still occur however. A number of more specific effects may be seen in addition to the central nervous depression common to all of these agents.

Methaqualone can cause hypertonia, myoclonus, hyperflexia, extensor plantar responses and occasionally papilloedema. Pulmonary oedema, coma and convulsions have also been reported. Supportive measures are normally sufficient, but charcoal haemoperfusion is indicated in severely poisoned patients.

Glutethimide may cause fluctuating coma, convulsions and acute respiratory failure. Pulmonary oedema and cerebral oedema may also occur and papilloedema may be a sign of severe overdose. Charcoal haemoperfusion is indicated in severe overdose, together with management of specific complications.

Chloral hydrate and its relatives (e.g. dichloralphenazone) may cause gastrointestinal irritation, haematemesis and subsequent oesophageal stricture. Cardiac arrhythmias are a particular problem with this group of agents but generally respond well to beta-blockers. Haemodialysis may remove the active metabolite, trichlorethanol, but charcoal haemoperfusion is probably more effective and may be helpful in very seriously poisoned patients.

Chlormethiazole is often used in alcoholic patients, although its value is not proven and it may be dangerous when taken in overdose together with alcohol. Increased salivation is a particular problem which may increase the risk of aspiration pneumonia, and regular oropharyngeal aspiration may be necessary.

Meprobamate is still used in the treatment of anxiety, and particularly with muscle spasm. Signs of overdose are muscular incoordination and weakness and central nervous system depression. In severe cases, pulmonary oedema may be seen. Haemodialysis may be useful in severe overdose, but haemoperfusion appears to be more effective.

Antidepressants

Antidepressants, particularly those in the tricyclic group, are commonly taken in overdose and are particularly dangerous. They are the commonest cause of death in children aged under ten years and, in contrast to the situation with barbiturates, adult mortality is also rising.

Tricyclic antidepressants

The tricyclic antidepressants act by blocking the uptake of noradrenaline by neurones both peripherally and in the central nervous system. They also have an anticholinergic effect and, in overdose, may have direct actions on the heart.

Diagnosis

The first signs of tricyclic antidepressant poisoning are usually the anticholinergic effects. These include dryness of the mouth and initial stimulation of the central nervous

4

system followed by depressant effects. In severe overdose, muscle hypertonia, hyperreflexia and extensor plantar responses are followed by hypotonia and hyporeflexia; convulsions may also occur. Other anticholinergic features are warm dry skin, pupillary dilatation, urinary retention and, in severe cases, paralytic ileus. Depression of respiration may be associated with hypoxia and respiratory and metabolic acidosis. Hypothermia may also occur, and respiratory complications such as aspiration and ARDS (p. 518) can further compromise tissue perfusion.

The most life-threatening complication of tricyclic antidepressant poisoning is cardiotoxicity. Tricyclic antidepressants resemble quinidine in their action on the heart, producing a decrease in myocardial contractility, prolongation of the PR interval and widening of the QRS complex. In severe cases, the T wave may disappear and the ECG may resemble ventricular tachycardia. Severe ventricular arrhythmias occur in a small proportion of patients, particularly in the early stages, and the ECG should therefore be monitored preferably even before emptying the stomach.

Management

The stomach should be emptied if more than 250 mg of drug has been taken by an adult, and correspondingly less in a child. This may be of value for up to 12 hours in overdose, because of delayed gastric emptying induced by the anticholinergic effects of the drug. After emptying the stomach, activated charcoal should be given to prevent further absorption of drug in the gastrointestinal tract. Repeated administration of charcoal may have only a modest effect on the half-life of amitriptyline, but be slightly more effective in removing its active metabolite, nortriptyline. Other methods of removal are unlikely to be of value in the treatment of overdose with tricyclic antidepressants, since these agents have such a large volume of distribution that only a small proportion of the drug is present in the blood.

Convulsions associated with tricyclic antidepressant poisoning may be related to anoxia and will sometimes respond to adequate oxygenation, although they may require treatment with anticonvulsants such as diazepam. Physostigmine has been used to reverse the central nervous effects, but its effect is short-lived and may precipitate convulsions, ventricular tachyarrhythmias and increased

salivary and bronchial secretions. It is therefore rarely used.

Arrhythmias and hypotension may respond to correction of acidosis, hypoxia, hypothermia and hypovolaemia. Antiarrhythmic agents should be used cautiously since they may further worsen already impaired myocardial contractility, but positive inotropes (e.g. dobutamine) may be necessary to correct the hypotension.

Monoamine oxidase inhibitors

The monoamine oxidase inhibitors (MAOIs) are much less frequently taken in overdose than tricyclic antidepressants. They produce features of increased sympathetic activity, with hyperexcitability and hyperreflexia followed by coma and convulsions. A sinus tachycardia is often present, but the patient may be either hypertensive or hypotensive. Hyperthermia, or more rarely hypothermia, has been reported. The agitation may require treatment with a sedative agent such as diazepam, while hypotension may respond to replacement of the circulating blood volume. Sympathomimetic agents (e.g. dopamine and dobutamine) should be avoided if possible, since they may lead to a severe hypertensive crisis. Severe hypertension should be treated with an alpha-blocker such as phentolamine.

Lithium carbonate

Lithium carbonate is widely used in the prophylaxis of manic-depressive psychosis. It has a low therapeutic ratio, and signs of toxicity are most often due to excessive therapeutic doses.

Diagnosis

Nausea, vomiting and diarrhoea are often the first signs of overdose, followed by dysarthria, ataxia, drowsiness, confusion, coma and convulsions. Renal impairment and nephrogenic diabetes insipidus may occur, and liver damage has also been reported. Cardiotoxicity may be first indicated by ECG findings of non-specific ST segment depression, T wave inversion, atrioventricular block, and prolongation of the QRS and QT intervals.

Management

Rehydration is important, but hypernatraemia (which may indicate nephrogenic diabetes insipidus) may require that dextrose solutions be given until the serum sodium and osmolality become normal. Hypokalaemia should also be treated. Toxicity correlates relatively well with the plasma lithium level. Concentrations greater than 5 mmol/l may indicate the need for active elimination of the lithium. Forced diuresis is of little value in this condition, and carries the risk of fluid overload, particularly if renal failure occurs. Peritoneal dialysis is more effective, but haemodialysis is better still in removing lithium. Because of the relatively large volume of distribution of the drug, plasma lithium concentrations may increase by up to two-fold

---

> **Summary 4   Overdose of tricyclic antidepressants**
>
> - Tricyclic antidepressant poisoning is common and life-threatening.
>
> - Anticholinergic signs predominate in the early stages but coma may supervene
>
> - Direct cardiotoxicity may result in ventricular tachycardia or ventricular fibrillation. The ECG should be monitored until recovery
>
> - Gastric lavage may be effective up to 12 hours after overdose and activated charcoal may prevent further drug absorption

shortly after the end of the dialysis. Repeated dialyses may therefore be necessary to maintain the serum lithium level below 1.5 mmol/l. Levels above this may be associated with toxicity.

Other antidepressants

Mianserin is a tetracyclic compound with only weak peripheral anticholinergic activity. It appears to be less likely to cause cardiotoxicity, convulsions or respiratory depression than the tricyclic compounds. Maprotiline is similar to mianserin in its effects, but is more toxic in overdose. In both cases, treatment is supportive.

Analgesics

The dangers of analgesics are not widely appreciated. After the hypnotic agents, analgesics are the second commonest group of drugs involved in overdosage in adults and, in children, salicylates are the second commonest cause of drug-related death.

Salicylates

Salicylate overdose is responsible for approximately 200 deaths each year in the United Kingdom. Toxicity is related to marked acid-base and electrolyte disturbance. In addition to being acids themselves, salicylates also increase circulating lactic and pyruvic acid concentrations by interfering with normal carbohydrate metabolism. Stimulation of fat metabolism causes increased production of β-hydroxybutyric and acetoacetic acids, and increased protein metabolism results in increased circulating amino acids. Impairment of reabsorption of these amino acids, by competition with the salicylate for active tubular reabsorption, produces amino-aciduria and increased fluid loss due to the effect of this solute load. Fluid loss is worsened by the vomiting associated with salicylate overdose, and by the uncoupling of oxidative phosphorylation which causes hyperpyrexia and increased sweating. Stimulation of the respiratory centre by salicylates causes a respiratory alkalosis which partly offsets the metabolic acidosis but causes further bicarbonate depletion, electrolyte loss and dehydration.

Diagnosis

The clinical features of salicylate overdose are agitation, tinnitus and deafness, increased sweating and hyperventilation; nausea and vomiting and epigastric pain may also be present. Respiratory alkalosis may occur initially but is quickly followed, particularly in children, by a metabolic acidosis associated with increased production of lactate, pyruvate and ketones. There may be hypokalaemia and hypo- or, more rarely, hyperglycaemia. Impaired clotting factor and platelet function are sometimes seen, but bleeding is rare. Pulmonary oedema can also occur even in the presence of hypovolaemia and is usually caused by increased pulmonary capillary permeability.

Summary 5 Salicylate poisoning

- Salicylate poisoning is serious because of the derangement of acid-base and electrolyte balance (metabolic acidosis, respiratory alkalosis and dehydration)
- Coma is rare except as a terminal event, and agitation and restlessness, tinnitus, deafness and hyperventilation are characteristic
- Emptying the stomach is indicated up to 24 hours after overdose in adults, and activated charcoal may prevent further absorption
- Correction of acid-base abnormalities and dehydration is usually sufficient in mild to moderate poisoning; forced alkaline diuresis, haemoperfusion or haemodialysis may be necessary in severe poisoning

---

Management

Treatment of salicylate overdose involves emptying of the stomach, either by gastric aspiration in the adult or induction of emesis in a child. Activated charcoal can be administered after emptying the stomach but may have limited value, partly because an optimum ratio of charcoal to the mass of drug ingested cannot be attained, and partly because the tablets may form a large mass in the stomach which is difficult to remove or adsorb. Emesis or gastric lavage may be of value up to 12 and possibly up to 24 hours after ingestion, because salicylates may cause pylorospasm and delayed gastric emptying.

Correction of any acid-base abnormalities and rehydration should be sufficient to prevent problems in mild or moderate cases of salicylate poisoning. Patients whose blood salicylate level is greater than 700 mg/l should be considered for forced alkaline diuresis. Potassium supplements may be necessary to achieve adequate urinary alkalinisation but, if this cannot be attained without increasing the blood pH to greater than 7.5, haemodialysis or haemoperfusion may prove necessary. The latter procedures are generally the treatment of choice for severely poisoned patients or in those in whom forced alkaline diuresis is contraindicated. Pulmonary oedema may occur due to fluid overload or as a direct consequence of the drug. In the former, the pulmonary artery pressure will be raised but this will be normal in the latter and ventilation with positive end expiratory pressure may be helpful in such patients.

Other non-steroidal anti-inflammatory drugs

Salicylates form one group of non-steroidal anti-inflammatory drugs (NSAIDs) but there are five other groups which can be classified according to chemical structure. These are:

1. *The arylalkanoic acids*, which include phenyl propionic acid derivatives like ibuprofen, the naphthyl propionic acid derivatives such as naproxen, and the phenyl acetic acid derivatives such as fenclofenac
2. *The anthranilic acids*, which include the fenamates (mefenamic acid and flufenamic acid)

55

4

3. *The pyrazalone group of compounds*, e.g. azapropazone and phenylbutazone
4. *The cyclic acetic acids*, which include indomethacin, sulindac and tolmetin
5. *The oxicams*, at present represented by piroxicam.

Diagnosis

The arylalkanoic acids, like all NSAIDs, cause headache, nausea and epigastric discomfort, but coma is rare with these agents. Gastrointestinal bleeding has been reported and bronchospasm is a rare complication of overdose. Poisoning with anthranilic acids (e.g. mefenamic acid) is more serious and, in addition to the gastrointestinal features associated with arylalkanoic acid overdose, severe haemorrhagic enterocolitis may occur. Central nervous system effects are also commoner and may include convulsions. Overdose with pyrazolones can produce gastrointestinal and central nervous system toxicity and hepatic and renal damage have also been seen. In addition to the above, the cyclic acetic acids also produce coma, while piroxicam has been associated with coma and convulsions.

Management

The stomach should be emptied if appropriate. Early administration of charcoal will reduce the absorption of some of the anthranilic and cyclic acetic acids, and may also be of benefit in poisoning with other groups of NSAIDs. Although there is no definite evidence that histamine-2-receptor antagonists (e.g. ranitidine) protect against gastrointestinal haemorrhage, they are often administered prophylactically. Convulsions occurring with overdose are generally short-lived but can be treated with diazepam if necessary. The blood pressure should also be measured regularly and hypotension corrected to prevent subsequent acute renal failure.

Paracetamol

Paracetamol is a remarkably safe drug in therapeutic doses but in overdose may cause fatal hepatic necrosis and is responsible for approximately 200 deaths per year. Toxicity of paracetamol in overdose is related to the metabolism of the drug. In therapeutic doses, approximately 90% of the drug is conjugated with glucuronide or sulphate, with only 10% oxidised by the mixed function oxidase system. The latter pathway produces a highly reactive intermediate compound which is normally conjugated with glutathione and subsequently excreted. In overdose, however, the glucuronidation and sulphation pathways cannot metabolise such a high proportion of the drug so that more is oxidised. The availability of glutathione is not sufficient to detoxify all the intermediate product produced which instead binds to macromolecules in the liver cell, causing necrosis.

Diagnosis

The clinical features of paracetamol overdose are initially mild and consist of nausea, vomiting and epigastric pain.

Liver damage normally shows itself clinically around three days, although the one-stage prothrombin time (INR) is often prolonged in such patients as early as 24 hours after the overdose, even before the liver enzymes have started to rise. Liver damage may occur with as little as 15 g of paracetamol and, although individuals vary in their sensitivity to the drug, those with liver disease or on enzyme-inducing drugs may be more susceptible. In severe overdose, metabolic acidosis, hypoglycaemia, hypotension and cardiac arrhythmias have been described. Acute renal failure has also been reported which, although generally associated with severe liver damage, has also been seen in the absence of severe liver toxicity. Renal function and electrolytes should therefore be measured daily. Finally, there have been very rare reports of pancreatitis associated with severe paracetamol poisoning. Patients may have a raised serum amylase concentration, but this may be related to inability to clear amylase because of liver damage and does not necessarily indicate pancreatic damage.

Management

Initial treatment is the induction of emesis or gastric lavage within six hours of tablet ingestion. Plasma paracetamol concentration should also be checked and, if it is greater than a given concentration (shown in Fig. 4.3) an antidote should be administered. Antidotal therapy should also be used without waiting for the plasma paracetamol concentration if the overdose has been taken at least eight hours previously, since the efficacy of the antidotes declines markedly with time.

Acetylcysteine is a glutathione precursor which can be given orally, but is generally given intravenously because it causes severe vomiting after the oral route. Acetylcysteine appears to have some efficacy up to 16 hours after overdose, and even up to 24 hours after a large overdose. Oral methionine is also recommended, but is probably ineffective 12 hours or more after an overdose; since patients may be vomiting as a result of the paracetamol ingestion, it may also be difficult to retain in the stomach. Anaphylactoid reactions have been reported after the use of acetylcysteine, in which case the infusion may have to be discontinued

Fig. 4.3 Plasma paracetamol concentrations above which antidotal treatment for poisoning is required.

and methionine used instead. The anaphylactoid reaction (urticaria and bronchospasm) has been more serious in patients who have been inadvertently given an overdose of acetylcysteine, so that the dose of this antidote should be checked carefully.

Blood sugar should be measured and any abnormality treated. The one-stage prothrombin time (INR) should be measured daily. An INR of three or more at 48 hours indicates the likelihood of liver failure in which case the patient should be commenced on a low protein diet and oral lactulose to help to remove nitrogenous compounds from the gut. Vitamin K may reduce the INR but this is often ineffective and fresh frozen plasma may be necessary to prevent haemorrhagic complications. Even if severe liver damage does occur, the mortality is still only around 5% with good supportive management (p. 637).

Opiates

Opiates are used not only as narcotic analgesics but also as constituents of some cough suppressants, antidiarrhoeal products (e.g. diphenoxylate) and veterinary tranquillisers. The opiate most often involved in poisoning is dextropopoxyphene. Opiates are being increasingly misused in society for their effects on mood, administered intravenously as well as orally.

Diagnosis

Respiratory depression is the commonest cause of death in opiate overdose. The pupils are often pin-point. Depression of the central nervous system eventually leads to coma and convulsions. The muscles may be hypotonic, but muscular twitching and hyperreflexia have been described. Hypotension is common and hypertension has been described after pentazocine overdose. Finally, non-cardiogenic pulmonary oedema may occur, particularly in methadone overdose.

Management

If the opiate has been taken orally, gastric emptying may be of value for up to 12 hours because of opiate-induced delay in gastric emptying. Naloxone is effective in reversing the symptoms of opiate overdose with all compounds except buprenorphine, which is a partial agonist and not completely antagonised. Repeated doses may be necessary because of the short half-life of naloxone, and, in severe overdose with long-acting agents, such as dihydrocodeine and methadone, naloxone by continuous infusion may be required. In buprenorphine poisoning, naloxone may have only limited benefit and, if doxapram fails to stimulate respiration sufficiently, assisted ventilation may be necessary. Naloxone may precipitate acute opiate withdrawal, with abdominal pain, diarrhoea and pilo-erection. However, the dangers of opiate overdose are such that the doctor should not be deterred from using adequate doses of naloxone in poisoned patients.

Anticonvulsants

The incidence of psychiatric abnormalities is higher in epileptics than in the non-epileptic population. The availability of anticonvulsants to some epileptic patients results in their being taken relatively frequently in overdose. Barbiturates and primidone (which is converted into phenobarbitone and phenylethylmalonamide) are the most toxic anticonvulsants (p. 52).

Phenytoin

In the United Kingdom, phenytoin is the most widely prescribed anticonvulsant. Acute overdosage leads to ataxia, dysarthria, horizontal nystagmus, drowsiness and, in severe cases, coma. Respiratory depression is a rare but potentially serious complication, which is generally only seen after massive overdose. The stomach should be emptied within four hours of ingestion and the use of activated charcoal will help to prevent the absorption of any phenytoin still left in the gastrointestinal tract. Because phenytoin is highly protein bound, only charcoal haemoperfusion will effectively remove the drug from the circulation. This should, however, be reserved for patients with severe overdose. Rarely, cases of permanent cerebellar damage with persistent ataxia after phenytoin overdose have been described.

Carbamazepine

Carbamazepine is widely used for the treatment of generalised and partial seizures. The drug is structurally similar to tricyclic antidepressants, and overdose can be associated with anticholinergic effects including dry mouth, hyperreflexia and generalised convulsions. Nystagmus, diplopia, ataxia, hypotension and respiratory depression have been noted, and cardiac conduction disturbances may also occur. The stomach should be emptied if appropriate, and activated charcoal administered to prevent further absorption of drug. Repeated doses of charcoal have been shown to speed the elimination of drug in normal volunteers and may be effective in severe overdose. Effective removal of drug by haemoperfusion has also been reported.

Summary 6 Management of opiate poisoning

- Opiate poisoning is a common, serious medical emergency
- Naloxone reverses the effects of all opiates (except buprenorphine) if given in sufficient dose, since it is a competitive antagonist
- The short half-life of naloxone necessitates repeated doses or even constant infusion in treatment of opiates with long half-lives of elimination (e.g. dihydrocodeine and methadone)
- The association between intravenous opiate abuse and infection (hepatitis B and HIV) should be recognised, and appropriate safe-guards taken

---

4

Sodium valproate

Sodium valproate poisoning is associated with coma and respiratory depression. The drug is rapidly absorbed, and supportive measures form the mainstay of treatment.

Cardiovascular drugs

Overdose with cardiovascular drugs is relatively rare, which is fortunate because of their toxic effects, particularly on cardiac contractility.

Antihypertensives

Not surprisingly, the major toxic adverse effect of antihypertensive drugs in overdose is hypotension. With clonidine, hypotension is often associated with bradycardia but in occasional patients, severe hypertension caused by the drug's partial alpha-agonist activity is a major problem. Bradycardia often responds to atropine, and alpha-adrenergic blocking drugs have been used to treat the hypertension. Beta-receptor blocking agents also cause bradycardia and hypotension and, like clonidine, can cause drowsiness, coma and convulsions in overdose. In severe hypotension, glucagon increases cardiac output by a mechanism separate from beta-receptor stimulation. Beta-agonists, such as isoprenaline or prenalterol, are also effective, although large amounts may have to be given by intravenous infusion to competitively antagonise the beta-blockade. Beta-2 agonists (e.g. salbutamol) may be necessary if bronchospasm is present, and the blood sugar should be monitored to detect and treat hypoglycaemia.

Calcium antagonists, such as verapamil, may also cause severe hypotension and bradycardia and, in the case of verapamil, conduction abnormalities may also be seen. If atropine is ineffective in treating the bradycardia, calcium gluconate (10–20 ml of a 10% solution) may be required.

Digitalis glycosides

Poisoning with the digitalis glycosides is a rare, but potentially very serious, problem. Nausea, vomiting and diarrhoea are early features, but the major life-threatening complications are hypotension and cardiac conduction disturbances with brady- and tachyarrhythmias. Hyperkalaemia is often present and mirrors roughly the severity of the overdose. This should be treated with glucose and insulin, or a sodium resonium ion exchange resin, or by haemodialysis if necessary. Digoxin is predominantly excreted by the renal route, and a good urine output should be maintained. Digitoxin is excreted by metabolism with marked enterohepatic recirculation of the drug. Repeated doses of activated charcoal or cholestyramine will speed up elimination of the drug. Continuous monitoring of cardiac rhythm is essential; bradyarrhythmias may require temporary cardiac pacing. Ventricular tachyarrhythmias often respond to lignocaine, but phenytoin has been used in resistant cases. Digoxin-specific fab antibody fragments have recently been used with success in the treatment of digoxin poisoning. In the UK, the National Poisons

Information Service can be consulted for information on their availability and applicability to specific cases (see Appendix).

Respiratory drugs

Theophylline

Theophylline is the respiratory drug most often taken in overdose; it causes central nervous system stimulation, hallucinations and convulsions. A sinus tachycardia may be followed by supraventricular and ventricular arrhythmias with hypokalaemia (often profound), metabolic acidosis and pancreatitis.

The stomach should be emptied to prevent further absorption, and charcoal left in the stomach. The metabolic abnormalities should be treated appropriately, while convulsions may respond to diazepam administered intravenously. Supraventricular and ventricular arrhythmias may respond to the use of beta-1 adrenergic blockers (e.g. metoprolol), but the metabolic abnormalities may only respond to agents which also possess beta-2 agonist activity (e.g. propranolol). Beta-blockers should be used extremely cautiously in asthmatic patients, because of the risk of precipitating bronchospasm. In such patients, verapamil has been used successfully to treat arrhythmias. Haemoperfusion is one of the most efficient ways of enhancing the removal of theophylline from the circulation. It should be considered in severely poisoned patients, particularly those with major arrhythmias, hypotension or convulsions. Repeated enteral administration of charcoal has recently been shown to markedly reduce the half-life of elimination of theophylline and should be considered if haemoperfusion facilities are not readily available.

Ephedrine, salbutamol and terbutaline

Ephedrine, salbutamol and terbutaline are generally safer than theophylline in overdose, but can cause all the same features in severe cases. Treatment is broadly similar to that of theophylline overdose; again, beta-blockers must only be used with extreme care in asthmatic subjects.

Drugs with anticholinergic activity

In addition to tricyclic antidepressants, many drugs have anticholinergic activity, including some used to suppress gastrointestinal motility (e.g. propantheline), some antiparkinsonian drugs (e.g. amantidine and orphenadrine) and some antihistamines (eg chlorpheniramine and promethazine). The effects of these drugs are similar to those caused by overdosage with tricyclic antidepressants, but they are less likely to cause arrhythmias.

Physostigmine may antagonise the central effects for a short period but may itself produce convulsions and hypersalivation; although physostigmine has been used to treat ventricular arrhythmias, it may also itself induce ventricular tachycardia. Treatment of overdose is otherwise supportive.

Antidiabetic drugs

Poisoning with antidiabetic drugs and insulin produce all the features of hypoglycaemia (Ch. 20, p. 774). If the patient is uncooperative, intramuscular glucagon may be used temporarily to treat the hypoglycaemia, until it is possible to infuse intravenous dextrose; but glucagon is ineffective once glycogen stores are exhausted. Prolonged glucose administration may be necessary after overdose of oral hypoglycaemic agents. Severe hypoglycaemia has been treated with diazoxide which inhibits insulin release and raises circulating plasma catecholamines. At the dose used (1.25 mg/kg over one hour every six hours), it rarely produces hypotension. Once hypoglycaemia has been corrected, the stomach should be emptied if appropriate; activated charcoal will help to prevent further absorption of chlorpropamide and tolbutamide.

Metabolic acidosis may occur after sulphonylurea poisoning, but is more common after poisoning with metformin. Oral antidiabetic drugs may also cause haematemesis and melaena, so patients should be examined carefully for signs of gastrointestinal bleeding. Pulmonary oedema has also been recorded. None of the methods to enhance drug elimination has yet been shown to be effective in treatment of oral antidiabetic drug poisoning.

Antibiotics

The penicillins and cephalosporins are generally safe in overdose.

Sulphonamides may cause bone marrow depression and renal damage (and haemolysis in glucose-6-phosphate dehydrogenase deficient patients). Maintenance of a high urine output and alkalinisation of the urine may prevent sulphonamide-induced renal damage, by preventing crystallisation of the drug in the renal tubule. Calcium folinate may help to reverse bone marrow depression induced by sulphonamide or trimethoprim.

Isoniazid is used in the treatment of tuberculosis and can, in overdose, cause central nervous symptoms with coma and convulsions. Pyridoxine can be used to treat or prevent both convulsions and the metabolic abnormalities; it should be given in a dose of 1 g for every gram of isoniazid ingested.

Rifampicin is routinely used for the treatment of tuberculosis. Overdose may be associated with the so-called 'red man syndrome' in which the skin is discoloured orange (although this colour can be removed by washing). Treatment is usually supportive. Although most patients recover completely, occasional deaths have been reported, presumably from cardiac arrhythmias.

Antimalarials

Quinine

Although rarely used for malaria prophylaxis, quinine is the antimalarial agent most often taken in overdose and also the one most likely to cause serious toxicity. In the United Kingdom, it has been most often prescribed for 'night cramps'. Many incidents of poisoning occur in children who ingest tablets belonging to another member of the family. Early symptoms of overdose are similar to those of aspirin, with nausea, vomiting, bowel disturbances, tinnitus and deafness. Initial respiratory stimulation may be followed by respiratory depression and respiratory arrest. Like its close relative quinidine, quinine can cause brady- and tachyarrhythmias, with death from ventricular fibrillation. Its effect on vision is dramatic. Visual acuity is initially impaired, and this may progress to constriction of visual fields or even complete blindness. Retinal examination reveals retinal oedema, optic atrophy and constricted retinal arteries. Most patients recover vision, although some are left with permanent visual field defects.

The management of quinine poisoning is supportive. Stellate ganglion block has been used to treat the visual impairment but, since quinine toxicity is likely to be direct on the retina, it is not surprising that this procedure (which carries its own complications) appears to be of limited efficacy. As quinine has a large volume of distribution and is predominantly metabolised by the liver, methods to enhance elimination are of limited value, but repeated oral charcoal may be beneficial.

Chloroquine

Chloroquine is widely used as prophylaxis against malaria and can be purchased without prescription. Its toxicity is similar to that of quinine and management of overdose is therefore similar. Chloroquine is also predominantly metabolised by the liver and has a high volume of distribution; thus, none of the techniques for enhancing removal appear to be effective..

Anticoagulants

The major risk of oral anticoagulant poisoning is haemorrhage; this occurs several days after the overdose because of the delayed effect of these agents. Vitamin K should be administered intravenously and may be necessary for up to a week. Repeated administration of cholestyramine will enhance the removal of warfarin and phenprocoumon and also reduce the length of time for which Vitamin K is required.

POISONING WITH GASES AND VOLATILE LIQUIDS

Carbon monoxide

Carbon monoxide is still the most common cause of fatal poisoning in the United Kingdom, despite the substitution of natural gas for coal gas in general use. Deaths occur either accidentally (often by inhalation of fumes during fires), or deliberately, from inhalation of car exhaust fumes in a confined space. Methylene chloride, which is widely used in paint removers, is metabolised by the body to

4

carbon monoxide and causes symptoms identical to those of direct carbon monoxide exposure.

Diagnosis

The early symptoms of chronic or acute exposure are headache, mental agitation, nausea and vomiting. The characteristic cherry-pink colour of the skin is rarely present during life, but the patient is not cyanosed, despite considerable hypoxia because of the production of carboxyhaemoglobin. Cerebral oedema and myocardial ischaemia or infarction may also occur.

Management

Oxygen should be given in as high a concentration as possible. Hyperbaric oxygen is even more effective in severe cases, but is not always immediately available, and transfer to this facility should not interrupt the treatment of severely poisoned patients. Oxygen should be administered until the carboxyhaemoglobin concentration in blood falls below 15%; this may take up to two days.

Most patients who die of carbon monoxide poisoning do so before they reach hospital; those who do arrive in hospital usually survive. Unfortunately, permanent neuropsychiatric sequelae may be seen, including intellectual and personality deterioration, Parkinsonism and, in rare cases, akinetic mutism. These severely affected patients often show areas of low density in the area of the globus pallidus when computerised tomography of the brain is performed.

Irritant vapours and gases

Carbon disulphide, hydrogen sulphide, sulphur dioxide, hydrochloric acid and ammonia are all highly irritant to the eyes and respiratory tract. Cough and chest pain may be followed by dyspnoea, bronchospasm, haemoptysis and pulmonary oedema.

Management

Treatment is supportive, with bronchodilators for bronchospasm, oxygen for hypoxia and, in severe cases, assisted ventilation (with PEEP if pulmonary oedema is present). Steroids, diuretics and antibiotics have been used but, since the complications are direct effects of the gas, they are unlikely to be of benefit. The metabolic acidosis may improve with adequate oxygenation but if this fails, sodium bicarbonate may have to be administered. The eyes should be carefully examined with fluorescein, and ophthalmological advice should be sought if corneal abrasions are present.

Cyanide

Cyanide may be inhaled in the form of hydrogen cyanide. Symptoms appear within a few minutes, firstly with headache, agitation, confusion leading to coma, cardiovascular

collapse and respiratory arrest. Cyanide may also be taken orally in which case symptoms may occur much later, particularly if food in the stomach delays gastric emptying.

Management

Oxygen in high concentrations should be administered and assisted ventilation performed if necessary. Dicobalt edetate is the treatment of choice, but this may cause hypotension and chest pain on intravenous administration, and should therefore only be used if the diagnosis is certain. It acts by forming inert complexes with cyanide, thus preventing the cyanide-induced inhibition of cellular oxidising enzymes. Thiosulphate acts as a sulphur donor to allow conversion of cyanide to thiocyanate via the enzyme rhodanase. Amyl- and sodium nitrites convert haemoglobin to methaemoglobin, which chelates the cyanide ion. Amyl nitrite can be given by inhalation, but it is much less effective than sodium nitrite by intravenous injection. The latter is often given with intravenous sodium thiosulphate as together they have synergistic action in the treatment of poisoning by cyanide. They are generally used if there is no response to dicobalt edetate, or if the latter is not immediately available.

Hydrocarbons

Poisoning with hydrocarbons is nearly always accidental, generally from industrial or domestic exposure, but also increasingly from solvent abuse.

Aliphatic hydrocarbons

In general, the aliphatic hydrocarbons appear to be less toxic than the aromatic group. The shorter chain aliphatic hydrocarbons are volatile so that poisoning is generally from inhalation. High concentrations of the gas may cause asphyxia and the butane in lighter fluid has been used to produce euphoria by solvent abusers. Coma may occur, with death from respiratory depression or ventricular fibrillation. Renal and liver damage may occur if the patient survives, and pulmonary and cerebral oedema have also been reported. Inhaled hydrocarbons may also produce myopathies, neuropathies, and permanent neuropsychiatric damage, although some of these effects may be related to additives to the hydrocarbon. Ingestion of liquid aliphatic hydrocarbons can produce effects similar to the above, either due to a systemic effect or, more likely, to aspiration of the low surface tension solvents. Pyrexia, cough and hyperpnoea may be followed by basal crackles in the chest, consolidation and collapse involving predominantly the middle and lower zones of the lung.

Treatment of solvent inhalation or ingestion is generally supportive. Gastric lavage or emesis should not be performed after ingestion because of the risk of chemical pneumonitis. There is no evidence that steroids and antibiotics are effective in the pulmonary complications but, in severe cases, ventilatory support may enable the patient to recover.

Chlorinated aliphatic hydrocarbons

Chlorinated aliphatic hydrocarbons are widely used as solvents in industry. In addition to the effects described with other hydrocarbons, the chlorinated aliphatics are also more likely to produce hepatic and renal damage (particularly carbon tetrachloride and chloroform), and blood dyscrasias, including haemolytic anaemia and aplastic anaemia. Methylene chloride is metabolised by the body to carbon monoxide and its systemic toxicity is that of this metabolite, although it is itself locally corrosive. It has been suggested that acetylcysteine may inhibit the metabolism of chlorinated hydrocarbons to reactive intermediate metabolites and thereby reduce hepatotoxicity if given early.

Aromatic hydrocarbons

Aromatic hydrocarbons are less often involved in poisoning. Benzene is the most toxic of these agents and, in acute overdose, produces effects similar to those of the aliphatic hydrocarbons. Chronic exposure, however, may lead to blood dyscrasias and lymphomas, and leukaemias have also been described. Toluene and xylene are similar in structure and effects to, but less toxic than, benzene. Any marrow toxicity described with these substances is probably related to benzene contamination. Benzene contamination is probably also responsible for the haematological problems sometimes seen with chronic petrol inhalation.

OVERDOSE WITH ALCOHOLS

Ethanol (ethyl alcohol)

Ethanol is the alcohol most often taken in overdose. It is found as a solvent in some cosmetic and antiseptic preparations, as well as being a constituent of alcoholic drinks. Beers contain 3–6%, table wines 10–12% and spirits 40–50% alcohol by volume. Its major toxicity is related to its central nervous depressant effects; the loss of the gag reflex may result in aspiration of stomach contents. Alcohols inhibit gluconeogenesis and may cause profound hypoglycaemia, particularly in children. Blood ethanol concentrations give a rough guide to the severity of overdose, but may be misleading because of tolerance in chronic alcohol users. Severe intoxication with stupor and marked incoordination is generally associated with blood concentrations above 3000 mg/l, but the author has had a lucid conversation with an outpatient whose blood concentration was 4200 mg/l.

Management

The stomach should be emptied if large quantities have been taken within four hours of presentation, but the airway must be protected. Alcohol metabolism shows Michaelis-Menten kinetics, and metabolism is saturated and zero-order even at low doses. Although haemodialysis will remove alcohol efficiently, it is only indicated in severe and complicated cases of poisoning. Fructose accelerates the metabolism of alcohol, but it can potentiate the metabolic acidosis already caused by the alcohol and may therefore be dangerous in overdose. Intravenous dextrose may be necessary to treat hypoglycaemia. The problems of alcoholism are discussed on page 73.

Methanol

Methanol is much more toxic than ethanol and is used widely both as a solvent and to denature alcohol (methylated spirits is 5% methyl alcohol and 95% ethanol). The mode of toxicity is not clear, but accumulation of formaldehyde and formic acid is partly responsible. As little as 10 ml of methanol may cause serious symptoms. The initial features are only those of mild inebriation, but eight or more hours later the patient may develop abdominal pain and vomiting, dilated and unreactive pupils, a metabolic acidosis and, sometimes, signs of cerebral oedema. The optic disc is at first hyperaemic and then becomes oedematous; vision is progressively lost.

Management

The stomach should be emptied within four hours of methanol ingestion, and intravenous sodium bicarbonate used to correct any metabolic acidosis. Diazepam is indicated if convulsions are a problem. Ethanol competitively inhibits the metabolism of methanol to formaldehyde and formic acid, and is used in less serious poisoning. Haemodialysis may be necessary if the blood methanol concentration exceeds 500 mg/l or if clinical deterioration is occurring despite the other measures used. Haemodialysis also removes ethanol, so that ethanol administration during this procedure has to be increased. Visual impairment often remains permanent, although prompt treatment reduces the severity of this problem.

Isopropanol (isopropyl alcohol)

Isopropanol is found in rubbing agents, sterilising fluids and disinfectants, window cleaning fluids and some aftershave lotions. Features of poisoning resemble those of ethyl alcohol poisoning but, because some of it is metabolised to acetone, ketonuria and a characteristic smell of acetone on the breath may be observed.

Management

The stomach should be emptied within four hours of ingestion, but treatment is otherwise symptomatic. Haemodialysis will remove isopropyl alcohol but is normally only indicated in severe poisoning.

Ethylene glycol

Antifreeze solutions contain ethylene glycol, a solvent which is sweet-tasting and therefore not unpleasant to

4

drink. Death may occur after ingesting as little as 100 ml of ethylene glycol which, like alcohols, is metabolised by alcohol dehydrogenase. Central nervous system toxicity is similar to alcohol overdose, but ophthalmoplegias, papilloedema and subsequent optic atrophy may also occur and the patient may become comatose and develop convulsions. Around 12 hours after the overdose, respiratory and cardiovascular complications are seen, together with a metabolic acidosis, hypocalcaemia and hyperkalaemia. If the patient survives this phase, he may develop acute renal failure after approximately 24 hours.

Ethylene glycol is not itself toxic but is metabolised by alcohol dehydrogenase to aldehydes, glycolates, oxalates and lactate which are responsible for the toxic features.

Management

The stomach should be emptied within four hours of ingestion, and arterial blood gases and serum calcium measured. The metabolic acidosis may respond to intravenous bicarbonate, and calcium gluconate may be necessary to treat any hypocalcaemia. Like methanol, ethylene glycol metabolism can be inhibited by administration of alcohol in doses sufficient to attain blood ethanol concentrations between 1000 and 2000 mg/l. In severe cases (normally those in whom ethylene glycol concentrations are greater than 500 mg/l and whose clinical condition is deteriorating despite other measures), haemodialysis is necessary to remove ethylene glycol metabolites. Ethanol administration may also be necessary for up to four days after the overdose to reduce its production. Dialysis may be required for treatment of renal failure.

POISONING WITH CORROSIVE AGENTS

Fortunately, poisoning with corrosive agents is rare, and most incidents are accidental rather than deliberate. The majority of agents produce local tissue damage by protein denaturation, but some (e.g. paraquat) also have serious systemic toxicity. The patterns of damage with acids and alkalis are different and are therefore discussed separately.

Acids

Acids produce severe pain on ingestion. They may cause asphyxia from epiglottal oedema and, although oesophageal damage has been described, they are more likely to cause gastric perforation, particularly in the region of the antrum. Late stricture formation is also a possibility.

Lavage or emesis should not be performed unless the agents also have serious systemic toxicity. Any metabolic acidosis should be treated with intravenous bicarbonate, but weak alkalis should not be given by mouth. Endoscopy is of limited value in the acute phase, and may cause perforation; in later stages, however, it may be helpful in identifying stricture formation. Corticosteroids have been

---

> **Summary 7 Acid poisoning**
>
> - Acid ingestion may cause local corrosion, asphyxia due to oedema of the glottis and perforation of the stomach (less commonly the oesophagus)
> - Metabolic acidosis and renal failure may also occur
> - Lavage should not be performed unless the agent has severe systemic toxicity
> - Late stricture formation may occur but the value of corticosteroids in preventing this complication is not proven

used to prevent stricture formation, but their value is unclear.

Phenol (carbolic acid) can cause systemic toxicity as well as local corrosion. Haemolysis, renal failure, coma and convulsions, myocardial damage and metabolic acidosis may occur, and early gastric lavage is indicated, provided the airway can be protected. Cresols (methylphenols) have similar effects and treatment is therefore as for phenol poisoning.

Formic acid is used in kettle de-scalers and de-staining solutions. It too can produce a metabolic acidosis, intravascular haemolysis and renal failure, as well as local corrosion; gastric lavage is therefore indicated early after ingestion. As with phenols, aspiration into the lung may cause haemorrhagic tracheobronchitis and the airway must therefore be protected during lavage.

Alkalis

Corrosion by alkalis (e.g. drain and oven cleaners) is generally more severe than by acids and is more likely to cause serious oesophageal, as well as gastric, damage. Treatment is identical to acid ingestion; lavage should not be performed. The risks of perforation should always be considered if endoscopy is performed but it may be useful in identifying alkalis in tablet form which may adhere to the oesophagus (e.g. Clinitest tablets and some denture cleaners).

Bleaches

Most bleaches contain sodium hypochlorite (up to 10%) which may produce corrosion in large or concentrated doses, and laryngeal oedema due to chlorine liberation. The stomach should be emptied and sodium thiosulphate solution (2%) left to prevent further chlorine liberation. The sodium load resulting from ingestion of large amounts of bleach can cause hypernatraemia and hyperchloraemic acidosis.

Disinfectants

Although phenols and cresols have been largely replaced by dichlorometaxylenol in disinfectants, corrosive effects may occur after large or concentrated doses. Metabolic acidosis, coma, myocardial and renal damage and laryngeal oedema may also occur after severe overdose, and the stomach should therefore be emptied and the metabolic abnormalities corrected. Some disinfectants also contain isopropanol (discussed on p. 61).

POISONING WITH INSECTICIDES, HERBICIDES, FUNGICIDES AND RODENTICIDES

Insecticides

The organochlorine group of insecticides (e.g. DDT) have now largely been replaced by safer compounds because of the persistence of the former in the environment. The safer compounds now in use include the organophosphorus and carbamate insecticides.

Organophosphates

The organophosphates act as inhibitors of cholinesterase in man, causing symptoms of excessive cholinergic activity with vomiting, abdominal pain, sweating and hypersalivation. These are followed by muscle fasciculation, diarrhoea, convulsions and coma. Plasma cholinesterase activity, measured in several centres throughout the UK, is useful in the diagnosis of both organophosphate and carbamate insecticide poisoning. Severe toxicity is associated with a reduction in plasma cholinesterase activity to around 10% of normal. Treatment consists of atropine to antagonise the cholinergic (muscarinic) effects. Large doses (up to 30 mg in 24 hours) may be necessary until there are signs of atropinisation (dry skin, tachycardia, dilated pupils and dry mouth). Within the first 24 hours, use of an oxime (e.g. pralidoxime) will help to reactivate cholinesterase. A clear airway must be maintained and assisted ventilation may be necessary.

Carbamate insecticides

Carbamate insecticides produce identical symptoms and atropine is again the treatment of choice. However, because these compounds have a reversible effect on cholinesterase, their duration of action is much shorter and pralidoxime is contraindicated in poisoning with these agents.

Herbicides

The five major groups of herbicides are: chlorates, triazines, bipyridilium herbicides, dinitro compounds and phenoxyacetic acids.

Chlorates

The chlorates are powerful oxidising agents which can produce haemolysis, methaemoglobinaemia, haemorrhagic gastroenteritis and, in severe cases, renal failure. Treatment consists of emptying the stomach (if appropriate) and methylene blue to reverse methaemoglobinaemia.

Triazines

Triazine herbicides (e.g. simazine) appear to be relatively non-toxic and serious human poisoning has not been reported.

Bipyridilium herbicides (paraquat)

The bipyridilium herbicides, particularly paraquat, are extremely toxic. Not only can they cause local corrosion, but systemic absorption leads to renal and liver damage and later progressive pulmonary fibrosis. Diquat causes similar toxicity although pulmonary fibrosis seems to be slightly less likely to occur. Treatment consists of gastric lavage with care because of the corrosive effects of the toxin. Fuller's earth or bentonite is left in the stomach as an adsorbent for paraquat and magnesium sulphate or mannitol is used to purge the gut and remove any remaining material. Finally, haemodialysis and haemoperfusion have been tried in an attempt to remove the body burden of drug, but there is no evidence that either has any effect on the mortality, particularly when the more concentrated solutions (e.g. Gramoxone) are ingested.

Dinitro compounds

Dinitro compounds (e.g. dinitroorthocresol) are generally used in the form of washes for fruit trees. They cause yellow staining of the skin but can be absorbed subcutaneously and produce toxicity by uncoupling oxidative phosphorylation. This results in pyrexia, hyperpnoea and tachycardia with subsequent sweating, thirst, dehydration and collapse. Treatment consists of preventing severe pyrexia and replacement of electrolytes and fluid. Pentachlorophenol acts similarly to the dinitro compounds, but does not produce yellow discolouration of the skin.

Phenoxyacetic acids

The phenoxyacetic herbicides are probably the most widely used herbicides. They are relatively non-toxic unless large doses have been ingested; signs of cholinergic hyperactivity are then evident resulting in coma and occasionally ventricular arrhythmias. The stomach should be emptied if appropriate, contaminated clothing should be removed and the skin washed with soap and water. With 2-4-D and mecoprop, forced alkaline diuresis may enhance their rate of removal and should be considered in severely poisoned patients.

Fungicides

Organic and inorganic mercurials, organotin derivatives and dithiocarbamates are all used as fungicides in industry and horticultural practice. Organotin compounds are poorly absorbed from the gastrointestinal tract and therefore have low toxicity and dithiocarbamates are also relatively non-toxic.

4

Organic mercurials

Inhalation or ingestion of organic compounds can produce severe corrosion and irritation of the respiratory tract. The central nervous system toxicity of these compounds consists of tremor, and memory and psychiatric disturbances together with visual impairment leading, in some cases, to blindness. The chelating agent, dimercaprol, may reduce the systemic toxicity.

Inorganic mercurials

Inorganic mercurial fungicides (e.g. mercuric chloride) are also predominantly corrosive. Inorganic mercury salts are sometimes present in disc batteries, and severe local corrosion or systemic mercury toxicity can occur. Treatment of inorganic mercurial toxicity includes gastric lavage, adequate analgesia and treatment of any complications. Mercurous chloride and mercuric oxide (the most commonly used agents) are poorly absorbed and, although corrosive, systemic toxicity is unlikely. If albuminuria occurs, however, significant absorption may have taken place and plasma mercury concentration should be measured. Treatment is as for organic mercurials.

Metallic mercury

Ingestion of metallic mercury is of no major consequence, and if related to a broken thermometer, the greatest danger is from any broken glass which may have been swallowed. However, intramuscular injection of metallic mercury may cause systemic toxicity, and intravenous injection has resulted in pulmonary embolus.

Rodenticides

Many rodenticides contain warfarin or related coumarin anticoagulants and, unless taken in huge amounts, generally cause few symptoms. If the INR does rise, vitamin K should be administered as for warfarin overdose. Alphachloralose is a hypnotic agent related to the chloral hypnotics and can cause drowsiness and coma if taken in large amounts by children. Treatment is as for chloral hydrate overdose. Chloroacetic acid derivatives are only used as rodenticides for commercial purposes but are highly toxic. They can be absorbed subcutaneously and orally and produce muscle twitching, tremor, cardiac arrhythmias, convulsions and coma. Cyanides are sometimes used as rabbit killers.

Arsenic is sometimes used as a rodenticide and also as a timber treatment. Symptoms of overdose are similar to those of tetanus. Sensory stimuli should be minimised by nursing in a darkened room; convulsions should be treated with diazepam. In severe cases, neuromuscular blockers may be needed to paralyse the patient while ventilation is supported mechanically.

POISONOUS PLANTS AND FUNGI

Although the number of plants that have been suggested to be poisonous is extremely high, many of these contain only small amounts of toxins and generally do not cause severe poisoning. They can be classified into those:

1. producing cholinergic (nicotinic) stimulation
2. producing cholinergic (muscarinic) stimulation
3. with anticholinergic activity
4. with gastrointestinal activity
5. with effects on the heart
6. with convulsant activity
7. with hallucinogenic effects
8. with dermatological effects
9. with toxicity on other organs.

Plants with cholinergic (nicotinic) activity

Alkaloids similar to nicotine are found in the hemlock (coniine) and laburnum (cytisine). Nausea and vomiting may be followed in severe poisoning by confusion, hallucinations, convulsions and finally coma and respiratory arrest. Treatment for severe poisoning is as for nicotine. The stomach should be emptied and activated charcoal administered. Monitoring of fluid and electrolytes and adequate replacement therapy, together with measures to assist the respiration and cardiovascular functions are generally only necessary in severe poisoning (rarely caused by laburnum).

Plants with cholinergic (muscarinic) activity

Plants with cholinergic activity include the clitocybe and inocybe fungi. Ingestion produces increased perspiration, abdominal pain and visual disturbances. Treatment is with atropine.

Plants with anticholinergic activity

Plants with anticholinergic activity include the deadly nightshade (*Atropa belladonna*), the thorn apple and henbane. In addition to atropine these plants may contain hyoscine and hyoscyamine. The symptoms are similar to those caused by drugs with anticholinergic activity (e.g. tricyclic antidepressants). Neostigmine is sometimes used to counteract the peripheral anticholinergic effects, but treatment with physostigmine is rarely necessary or indicated.

Plants with gastrointestinal toxicity

Oxalates present in some plants can cause local gastrointestinal irritation and painful ulceration of the mouth if chewed by children. These include the household plants, dumbcane (dieffenbachia) and some of the monstera and philodendron species. Other plants contain irritant resins and saponins (e.g. arum, taxus, bryonia, and daphne mezereum), which can cause severe vomiting and diarrhoea. Delayed gastrointestinal symptoms can be caused by the beans of the Abrus species (e.g. Ricinus and Robinia) as these contain compounds which can impair RNA synthesis. Solanum species also produce delayed gastrointestinal symptoms; these include potatoes which have been allowed to sprout, and woody and black nightshades. Treatment is supportive, with replacement of fluids and electrolyte loss.

Plants causing cardiovascular disturbances

Digitalis glycosides are found not only in the foxglove but also in lily of the valley (Convallaria). Treatment is as for digitalis poisoning. The aconitine present in the monksfoot and delphinium may cause bradycardias and muscular weakness.

Plants with convulsant activity

Cicuta virosa (cowbane) and *Oenanthe crocata* (hemlock water dropwort) contain potent alcohols with effects similar to picrotoxin in antagonising the central nervous inhibitory effects of γ-amino butyric acid. In severe cases, nausea, vomiting and hypersalivation are followed by convulsions and respiratory failure. *Oenanthe crocata* is sometimes eaten in the United Kingdom because its roots are mistakenly felt to be edible; nine deaths have occurred in this century. Convulsions can be controlled with either short-acting barbiturates or diazepam; respiration may require support until the effects of the toxin wear off.

Strychnine is an alkaloid present in the seeds of the tree *Strychnos nux-vomica*, native to India. It is used predominantly as a rodenticide and produces severe muscular spasms which may respond to short-acting barbiturates or to diazepam. Sensory stimulation should be minimised, since it may provoke convulsions; assisted ventilation may also be necessary. Once convulsions have been controlled, the stomach should be emptied and charcoal left inside. Acute renal failure and hepatic necrosis may occur after strychnine poisoning.

Plants with hallucinogenic effects

In addition to those anticholinergic agents with hallucinogenic effects, there are several other hallucinogens in plants and fungi. These include the psilocin and psilocybin in psilocybes (magic) mushrooms, the tetrahydrocannabinols in cannabis, and the ibotinic acid and muscimol found in *Amanita muscaria*. Tranquillisers may be necessary if the patient is a risk to himself or to others, and adequate supervision must be given until the hallucinations subside.

Plants which cause dermatological toxicity

Plants contain substances which can either cause direct chemical irritation (e.g. histamine and oxalic acid) or delayed hypersensitivity reactions (e.g. *Primula obconica*, the hogweeds, which can produce photoallergic dermatitis, and several other species). Treatment is symptomatic.

Plants with toxicity on other organs

The lectins present in the seeds of *Ricinus communis* not only cause delayed gastrointestinal tract symptoms but may also lead to liver and lung damage. Ricin is the most potent toxin known to man and was probably the toxin used in the assassination of a Bulgarian diplomat in London several years ago. At autopsy, a small metallic sphere just 1.25 mm in diameter was found in the calf of the victim; at most it could have contained about 250 micrograms of ricin. Management is purely supportive.

Severe liver damage can also be caused by the phallotoxins and amatoxins found in *Amanita phalloides* and some of the other Amanita species. Vomiting, abdominal pain and diarrhoea often occur 6–12 hours after ingestion, while albuminuria, haematuria, renal failure and liver failure may occur around 2–3 days later. Treatment consists of emptying the stomach and replacement of any fluid loss caused by the diarrhoea and vomiting. Specific antidotes are of unproven value, but thioctic acid and high doses of penicillin may be of value in preventing the liver and renal damage.

POISONOUS ANIMALS

Adder evenomation

The adder, *Vipera berus*, is the only indigenous poisonous snake in Western Europe. Only 50% of those bitten develop signs of evenomation which may occur either immediately, with shock, vomiting and explosive diarrhoea, or several hours later. The initial collapse may be due to activation of the kinin system; the later shock is more often due to hypovolaemia, caused by increased capillary permeability and fluid loss into the swollen limb, and direct cardiotoxicity of the venom.

Management

Treatment includes reassurance since shock may be exacerbated by the fear of impending toxicity. The limb should be kept still, but a ligature should not be used unless there is likely to be a delay of more than half-an-hour between the patient having been bitten and transfer to hospital. If a ligature is used, it should only be tight enough to prevent venous return but not to obstruct arterial inflow. The patient should be admitted and observed for at least a day after the bite. Pulse and blood pressure should be recorded, together with urinary output and fluid losses from diarrhoea and vomiting. Local swelling should also be noted and the white cell count, urea and electrolytes should be measured each day.

The use of Zagreb antivenom should be considered if

65

4

hypotension persists, ECG signs occur, the white count rises markedly to above 20 000/mm³ or, in an adult, severe swelling has extended up the limb within two hours after the bite. Anaphylactic reactions to the antivenom occur in 1% of patients and so antivenom should only be used when the indications described above are present. A history of asthma or allergy is a relative contraindication to its use. Antivenom is given by slow intravenous infusion and is stopped at the first signs of allergic reaction. Adrenaline solution must be drawn up prior to administration of the antivenom and given intramuscularly if a reaction occurs, (intravenously in the case of a severe reaction).

Deaths from adder bite are extremely rare, but local tissue necrosis may be severe, particularly in adults.

Fish evenomation

In the United Kingdom, the only venomous fish regularly found are the Weever fish (*Trachinus vipera*) which is found around the coast in the summer months, and the Lion fish (an aquarium species). Both contain heat labile venom in their spiny dorsal fins, which causes severe local pain. Some individuals develop hypotension, and myocardial and respiratory depression.

Management

Treatment of Weever fish sting is to remove any barbs and clean the wound, immersing the limb in water as hot as can be tolerated without discomfort to destroy the toxin. The wound should be examined at a later stage for signs of secondary infection.

Treatment for Lion fish sting is similar although the symptoms are usually less severe.

Venomous invertebrates

The Portuguese man of war (Physalia) is the only poisonous jellyfish found around the coasts of the United Kingdom. Its sting contains substances capable of releasing histamine and other kinins. Local pain is common, but more serious symptoms include abdominal pain, dyspnoea, hypotension, muscular paralysis and convulsions.

Management

The wound should be bathed in vinegar solution (4–6% acetic acid), and any tentacles still adherent to the wound removed with adhesive tape.

Arthropod evenomation

Wasp and bee stings contain amines, kinins, peptides and enzymes which cause local pain, erythema and swelling. Systemic effects are rare, unless the stings are extremely numerous or the subject is hypersensitive, in which case even a single sting may kill. Initial symptoms are generalised urticaria, flushing, dizziness, bronchospasm, col-

lapse and coma. Serum sickness may occur a week or more after the initial sting.

Management

The sting should be removed, taking care not to squeeze it and inject more venom. Severe pain may respond to local anaesthetic or aspirin. Anaphylaxis should be treated immediately with adrenaline (0.5–1 ml of a 0.1% solution). Severe respiratory tract obstruction may be caused by stings in the mouth, even in those patients who are not hypersensitive. In allergic individuals, specific venoms have been used in increasing doses to produce desensitisation.

Poisonous seafoods

Seafood may contain bacteria (e.g. vibrio, salmonella) or viruses (e.g. hepatitis A); toxicity may also occur as a result of contamination by dinoflagellates or decomposition by bacteria.

Antemortem infestation by dinoflagellates of certain subtropical fish (such as groupers and snappers) may occur but, in the UK, contamination most commonly involves shellfish, such as mussels, oysters, scallops and clams. The dinoflagellates contain neurotoxins (e.g. saxitoxin) which can cause nausea, vomiting and diarrhoea, followed by circumoral paraesthesiae, ataxia, muscular weakness and, in severe cases, respiratory paralysis.

Treatment is symptomatic, with respiratory and cardiovascular support.

Postmortem contamination of some oily fish such as mackerel, skipjack and tuna, sardines and pilchards by Proteus bacteria may result in production of histamine and other unidentified toxins which produce urticaria, flushing, abdominal pain, nausea, vomiting and diarrhoea and, in some cases, bronchospasm. The effects occur around four hours after ingestion, last only a few hours and are seldom very severe.

Treatment is symptomatic. Prevention involves keeping the raw fish frozen or on ice to prevent decomposition by bacteria.

POISONING BY METALS

Iron

Although mortality from iron poisoning has fallen in recent years, it remains one of the most dangerous metals in overdose. Children are particularly sensitive to its effects and develop toxicity at lower serum iron concentrations. Abdominal pain, nausea and vomiting are often followed by gastrointestinal bleeding, encephalopathy, metabolic acidosis, pulmonary oedema, acute renal failure and liver failure. A serum iron level greater than 5 mg/l (90 μmol/l) in a child, or greater than 8 mg/l (145 μmol/l) in an adult, within four hours of the overdose, is associated with an increased likelihood of severe poisoning.

> **Summary 8   Iron poisoning**
>
> ● Children are particularly sensitive to the toxicity of iron
>
> ● Abdominal pain, nausea and vomiting may be followed by gastrointestinal haemorrhage, encephalopathy and renal and hepatic failure
>
> ● Severe poisoning is normally associated with plasma concentrations (4 hours after ingestion) greater than 5 mg/l in children and 8 mg/l in adults
>
> ● Gastric lavage with desferrioxamine and intramuscular and intravenous desferrioxamine should be given in severe iron poisoning

Management

The stomach should be emptied if more than 15 tablets have been ingested within the previous four hours. Desferrioxamine (2 g/l of warm water) should be used as lavage fluid, and a further 5 g per 50 ml water left in the stomach after lavage. X-ray of the abdomen will reveal whether or not the tablets have been removed. If the patient has clinical evidence of severe iron poisoning, desferrioxamine should also be administered both intramuscularly (2 g per 10 ml water) and by slow intravenous infusion (15 mg/kg per hour to a maximum of 80 mg/kg in 24 hours, to prevent hypotension induced by the desferrioxamine). With prompt treatment, the mortality should be less than 5% in severe cases.

Heavy metal poisoning

Heavy metals can cause acute or chronic symptoms, depending upon the dose and duration of exposure. Acute ingestion of most heavy metals will cause gastroenteritis. Generalised convulsions may also be seen, particularly with lead poisoning, and renal failure and cardiac arrhythmias have also been recorded. Inhalation of heavy metal fumes may cause chemical pneumonitis and, in severe cases, pulmonary oedema and a syndrome known as 'Metal Fume Fever' may occur several hours after the inhalation of some metallic oxides.

Chronic effects of heavy metal exposure are similar but milder. Chronic gastrointestinal symptoms have been recorded together with central nervous system effects, particularly after exposure to lead, manganese and mercury. Lead, thallium, bismuth and arsenic can also produce peripheral neuropathy and renal damage may be caused by gold, lead, cadmium and mercury. Inhalation of heavy metal fumes can cause pulmonary fibrosis, particularly with beryllium, cadmium, tungsten, titanium and cobalt. An emphysematous picture has been seen with cadmium, and an asthma-like syndrome may occur as a result of sensitivity to chromium, vanadium and platinum. Nickel, chromium, cobalt, platinum and beryllium may also cause skin sensitisation and subsequent dermatitis.

Diagnosis of heavy metal poisoning is helped by taking a full occupational history. Clinical examination may reveal specific signs of poisoning, such as the blue line on the gums in chronic mercury poisoning or the raindrop pigmentation of the skin in arsenic poisoning. Toxicological examination of the urine, blood, or hair and nail clippings may help in diagnosis, although this often has to be performed in specialised centres.

Management

Treatment consists of preventing further exposure to the heavy metal, treatment of the complications of poisoning, and chelation therapy to enhance the elimination of the metal already absorbed. It must be remembered, however, that most chelating agents have their own toxicity and should only be used when their benefits are likely to outweigh the risks of their use. Sodium calcium edetate is the treatment of choice for lead poisoning. It must be given by slow intravenous infusion. Dimercaprol is effective in severe mercury, as well as arsenic, poisoning. Penicillamine is the treatment of choice for copper poisoning and has the advantage that it may be given by mouth. Finally, Prussian Blue has been used successfully in the treatment of thallium poisoning.

DRUG DEPENDENCE (GENERAL)

Addiction to illicit drugs, especially opiates, is a source of widespread medical and social concern. There are three main reasons for this. Firstly, there has been an epidemic increase in opiate abuse over the past fifty years. In 1936, there were about 500 known addicts in the United Kingdom (of whom one-quarter were doctors); by the mid-1970s this figure had risen to 6000; and in 1983, following the introduction to the UK of cheap heroin, the number of known addicts was estimated to be at least 50 000 (Fig. 4.4). Secondly, the impact of opiate addiction has profound

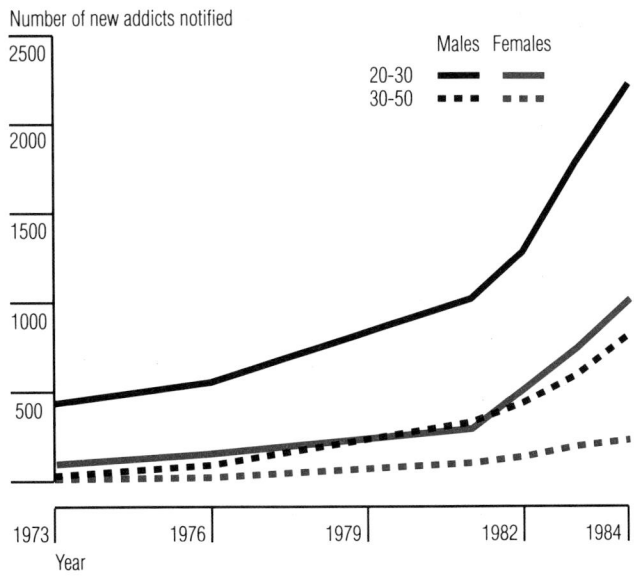

Fig. 4.4   **The number of new opiate addicts registered in England and Wales, 1973–1984.**

4

medical and social consequences. Within five years, ten per cent of addicts will have died from drug-related causes. Thirdly, 'drug addiction' is a microcosm of a much wider problem.

Addiction in its widest sense is an integral feature of society: the medical consequences of addiction to alcohol, tranquillising drugs and tobacco are, numerically, far more serious than those caused by opiates. Drug addicts and 'drug pushers' can be seen as the 'folk devils' of such a society. Caricatured as wicked parasites living in amoral squalor, they illustrate the process of projection at a social level, in which a negative aspect of society (in this case, endemic addiction) is split off and attributed to an alien group.

Nature and causes of drug dependence

In the past, definitions of drug abuse have concentrated on a contrast between the harmful and the beneficial effects of drugs, thus dividing drugs into 'good' drugs (prescribed by doctors) and 'bad' ones (self-administered by addicts). This distinction does not take account of the fact that almost all drugs, even when medically prescribed, have harmful effects and can be misused; analgesics and tranquillisers are the best examples of this. Conversely, opiates can be of great benefit in the treatment of severe pain. Another outmoded distinction is that made between psychological and physiological addiction. There is a continuum between mild psychological need and overwhelming physiological compulsion; any firm separation of the two is inevitably artificial. Current definitions of drug dependence are based on the interaction between the individual and the drug leading to a compulsion to take it:

1. in order to experience its psychic effects and/or
2. to avoid the unpleasant effects of its withdrawal (abstinence syndrome).

There is no single cause of drug addiction. The prevalence of addiction is determined by:

1. the *availability* of the drug. The greater the availability, the greater prevalence of addiction. In Hong Kong, where heroin is widely available, 8–10 per cent of the adult male population is addicted
2. the *accessibility* of the drug. This explains the relative commonness of drug addiction among doctors and nurses, and in inner-city and coastal areas
3. the *susceptibility* of individuals to addiction or misuse.

Treatment for drug addiction is equally multifaceted and involves a combination of physical, psychological and social rehabilitation.

OPIATE ADDICTION

Causes

The most important cause of opiate addiction is its availability. Susceptible individuals expose themselves to the drug, either because they inhabit a subculture in which drug taking is prevalent, or because they are psychologically vulnerable due to family difficulties, depression or boredom. The pharmacological features of opiates – tolerance and withdrawal syndrome – ensure the establishment of a habit, and social, as well as physiological factors, then maintain the addiction and make rehabilitation difficult.

Biochemical factors

The discovery in 1977 of the encephalin neurotransmitters was a major advance in the understanding of opiate addiction. Endorphins are naturally occurring, opiate-like substances which mediate pain and other sensations in the mid-brain. It is possible that individuals susceptible to addiction may be deficient in endorphins. Both opiates and endorphins reduce the amount and effects of other cerebral neurotransmitters such as acetylcholine. This has led to the 'supersensitivity' theory of withdrawal syndrome, which postulates that addicted individuals have reduced amounts of transmitter reaching post-synaptic receptors. Stopping the drug then results in a sudden increase in transmitter and stimulation of the already supersensitive receptor.

Psychological factors

Drugs can be administered ('dropped') by injection ('fixing') either sub-cutaneously ('skin-pop') or intravenously ('mainline'); or by smoking ('chasing the dragon'). All these methods are powerful reinforcers in the Pavlovian sense:

1. *primary* reinforcement from both the pleasure ('buzz') and removal of withdrawal symptoms.
2. *secondary* reinforcement from the associated rituals of administration, e.g. filling the needle.
3. *social* reinforcement from fellow-addicts.

Psychiatric factors

Opiate addiction is more likely to be a cause than a consequence of psychiatric illness. 'Loners' may well be suffering from anxiety and depressive symptoms which they are trying vainly to treat with opiate drugs. Hospitalised addicts (as opposed to the generality of addicts) tend to be suffering from personality disorder and to have difficulty in forming close relationships. Addicts are caught in a vicious circle in which their primary relationship comes to be with the drug, which is felt to be more accessible, reliable and instantly gratifying than a person. There is some evidence that family discord and alcoholism is commoner in the childhood histories of addicts than in controls. The anxiety associated with the early stages of opiate withdrawal may mirror early childhood experiences of separation from desired, but inaccessible, parents.

Social factors

There is no particular social class preponderance for opiate addiction.

Presentation

Addiction to opium and its derivatives, morphine and heroin (diacetyl morphine), can be considered as a model of drug addiction in general. The physical signs which should arouse suspicion of opiate abuse are listed in Table 4.5. Addicts present to doctors in one of four ways:

1. With infective complications of self-administered injections, e.g. septic abscess at injection site or septicaemia, infectious hepatitis or manifestations of HIV.
2. With confusion or unconsciousness due to overdose of the drug, deliberate or accidental.
3. Wanting, or apparently wanting, help with their habit.
4. With a withdrawal syndrome. This consists of a craving for the drug together with physiological features which include rhinorrhoea, lacrimation, yawning, perspiration, irritability, gooseflesh, nausea, diarrhoea, cramps, muscle pains, tachycardia, flushing and involuntary movements. It is not life-threatening and the symptoms begin to recede at about 72 hours after last taking the drug.

Opiate users are heterogeneous; only a minority correspond to the social stereotype of the addict. Lifestyles can be divided into four types:

'*Stables*'. Addicts in whom the habit exists with a fairly conventional life, e.g. regular employment, family and marriage.

'*Junkies*'. Here, the addict inhabits a drug subculture in which all activities – social, financial, sexual – are subsidiary to the need to obtain drugs.

'*Loners*'. The addict is socially isolated and inhabits a solitary world of addiction.

'*Two-worlders*'. These contain elements of stables and junkies, often leading a 'normal' life at work but returning to a 'junkie' world when not working.

Management

Legal requirements

In the UK, any doctor attending a patient who is known, or suspected, to be addicted to opiates is required to inform the Home Office Drug Branch. The controlled drugs morphine and diamorphine (heroin) may be prescribed by any doctor for the treatment of terminal illness; only specially licensed doctors are permitted to prescribe them for the maintenance of addiction. Other opiates, such as methadone, may be prescribed by any doctor for the management of withdrawal syndrome, but this should be done only with great constraint and in an emergency. The entire prescription must be in the doctor's own handwriting, and amounts must be written in both words and figures.

General management

Drug abusers may not be open about their habit, which should be suspected in unexplained cases of psychosis, sepsis, serum hepatitis or HIV infection. Scapegoating should be avoided, and drug users should be treated with the same concern and courtesy as any other patient. At the same time, caution should be exercised: addicts may take prescription pads and syringes, and exaggerate their drug needs in order to obtain drugs which are then sold. In an initial interview, the patient should have a urine screen to confirm that he is a user, and blood should also be tested for hepatitis B and HIV (the latter normally with the patient's consent). Whenever possible, he should then be referred for specialist help. Occasionally, withdrawal symptoms have to be treated and a dose of methadone given equivalent to the average daily intake which the doctor calculates is being used. The usual dose is between 20 and 70 mg of methadone. Typical detoxification schedules are given in Table 4.6. Where heroin intake is low, diphenoxylate and chlormethiazole can be used. Prescriptions should be on a daily basis for not more than two days. A clear management policy should be instituted and explained to the patient.

Table 4.5 History and examination of suspected opiate abuser

History
Previous contact with a prescribing doctor or clinic
History of recent use (doses, frequency, legal, illegal)
Assessment of demands or requests
Assessment of withdrawal symptoms
Current legal problems

Examination
Injection sites: needle marks, tracks, bruises, thrombosed veins, abscesses, skin ulcers
Arterial spasm or gangrene (caused by, e.g. dipipanone, cyclizine)
Jaundice from hepatitis A or B
Emaciation

Investigation
Urine for drug assays
Liver function tests
Hepatitis A and B serology
HIV test (with consent)

Table 4.6 A typical detoxification schedule for opiate addiction

10 day detoxification (volume kept at 25 ml)
Methadone 25 mg/day – 2 days
             15 mg/day – 2 days
             8 mg/day – 2 days
             4 mg/day – 2 days
             2 mg/day – 2 days

28 day detoxification (volume kept at 25 ml)
Methadone 30 mg/day – 4 days
             25 mg/day – 3 days
             20 mg/day – 4 days
             13 mg/day – 3 days
             10 mg/day – 4 days
             6 mg/day – 3 days
             3 mg/day – 7 days

4

Treatment of medical complications of addiction

The main medical complications of addiction are septicaemia (p. 229), hepatitis (p. 648), endocarditis (p. 420) and HIV infection (p. 250).

Rehabilitation

In the UK, all regions have drug clinics to which the addict should be referred. Here, he may be offered an oral methadone maintenance programme in the hope, not always realised, of reducing use of illicit drugs. An attempt is made to form a rapport with the user. After establishing a baseline habit, the addict is gradually withdrawn from the drug over a 10 week period either as an outpatient or, more rapidly, as an inpatient. Withdrawal is an essential, but by no means sufficient, aspect of treatment. Addicts exposed to enforced abstinence, e.g. in prison, almost always relapse when released. Psychotherapeutic and social help are also needed if the addict is to remain drug-free. Group methods are particularly important and perhaps the most effective form of treatment is the residential self-help approach, in which ex-addicts help those desiring withdrawal. In the UK, the organisations known as Synanon and Phoenix House are examples of this method. Not all addicts can tolerate their stringent approach and firm setting of limits, but such is the physiological power of heroin that an equally strong psychological force is needed to overcome it.

ADDICTION TO NON-OPIATES

Dependence on non-opiate drugs has become a major health problem in recent years. The changing pattern of dependence is shown in Figure 4.5.

Barbiturates

In the 1960's, the prescription of barbiturates as hypnotics and tranquillisers created about 100 000 barbiturate addicts. Subsequent voluntary restrictions on prescribing mean that, as a group, barbiturate addicts now comprise a small number of older patients (mostly women) who are relics of the barbiturate era, and a number of young multiple drug users for whom barbiturates are one of a number of drugs in their repertoire.

The effects of barbiturates are similar to those of alcohol, viz. intoxication, ataxia and depression of consciousness. Respiratory depression due to overdose is a frequent cause of death. A *withdrawal syndrome* occurs in which convulsions are common. This should be controlled by pentobarbitone (short-acting) 4–6 hourly. Withdrawal should be carried out slowly over several weeks.

Benzodiazepines

Benzodiazepines have now replaced barbiturates both in popularity and as a cause for widespread addiction.

A

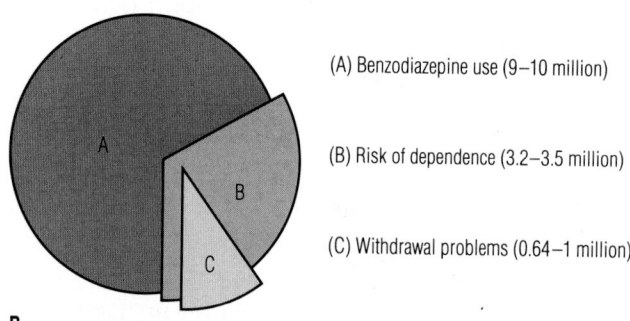

(A) Benzodiazepine use (9–10 million)

(B) Risk of dependence (3.2–3.5 million)

(C) Withdrawal problems (0.64–1 million)

B

Fig. 4.5 **Changing patterns of consumption of non-opiate drugs in the United Kingdom. A.** Prescriptions for sedatives/tranquillisers and hypnotics, 1974–1985. **B.** Current benzodiazepine use and dependence in the UK. In one year, (A) 9–10 million people use benzodiazepines. (B) Of these, 3.2–3.5 million use them for more than four months and are at risk of dependence. (C) Of these, 0.64–1 million are likely to suffer withdrawal problems.

Although the three million annual prescriptions cause less mortality than barbiturates (as they do not produce respiratory depression), they are undoubtedly an important source of morbidity. The ill-effects of benzodiazepines include lethargy, irritability, reduced sexual drive, and feelings of depersonalisation. There is an increased incidence of road traffic accidents in benzodiazepine-takers. A withdrawal syndrome occurs in patients who have taken more than 20 mg daily over six weeks; the symptoms

---

Summary 9   Symptoms of benzodiazepine withdrawal

- Insomnia
- Anxiety
- Depression
- Outbursts of anger
- Muscular pains
- Tremor
- Headache
- Nausea, weight loss, anorexia

- Sweating
- Tiredness
- Perceptual abnormalities
  Visual disturbance
  Depersonalisation
  Vertigo
- Fits
- Psychosis

include painful sensations in the limbs, anxiety, insomnia, depression and convulsions. The symptoms of minor affective disorder (often self-limited), for which benzodiazepines are initially prescribed, may also then become part of a withdrawal syndrome which can be mistaken for the original illness and lead to further prescriptions. Like barbiturates, benzodiazepines are best withdrawn in a slowly reducing dosage over several weeks. Rapid withdrawal may need to be carried out in hospital.

Stimulants

Amphetamines and cocaine do not appear to cause physiological dependence, but produce a psychosis which is clinically very similar to paranoid schizophrenia. Tactile hallucinations in particular are a feature of cocaine intoxication. Withdrawal from amphetamines often leads to a severe state of depression.

Hallucinogens

The effects of hallucinogenic drugs like LSD (lysergic acid diethylamide) and 'magic mushrooms' were popularised by the writer Aldous Huxley and enjoyed a brief vogue in the treatment of schizophrenia in the 1960s. They produce a toxic psychosis characterised by vivid hallucinations and delusions. Prolonged psychosis may be precipitated by taking LSD in susceptible individuals. 'Flash-backs' may occur for several months after an LSD 'trip'. There is *in vitro* (but not *in vivo*) evidence that LSD produces chromosomal abnormalities.

Cannabis

Cannabis, like alcohol, appears to have few harmful effects if taken in moderation. Ten per cent of all young people have tried cannabis at some time, and 25% of students use it at least once a week. In some cultures and subcultures (e.g. Rastafarians), regular cannabis use, especially among males, is the rule. The active principle is THC (tetrahydrocannabinol) which is sometimes used as an antiemetic in terminal care. As with LSD, excessive use (or occasional use in susceptible subjects) produces a psychosis, and a withdrawal syndrome may occur. It has been suggested that regular use of cannabis may produce a state of apathy or *amotivational syndrome*.

Solvent abuse

Inhalation of solvents such as toluene and acetone (used as vehicles for glue and other agents) produces a temporary state of euphoria. Glue-sniffing is common in certain youth subcultures. It is dangerous: an appreciable mortality has been recorded from direct cerebral damage as well as asphyxia due to the use of polythene bags to concentrate the vapour. Morbidity includes hepatitis, renal damage, cardiac arrhythmias, polyneuropathy and aplastic anaemia.

ALCOHOLISM

Alcohol is a major cause of medical and psychiatric morbidity worldwide (Table 4.7). In the UK, a 200% increase in alcohol consumption since 1950 (Fig. 4.6) has been accompanied by a 25-fold increase in admissions for alcoholism to psychiatric hospitals between 1960 and 1980. About 20% of admissions to medical wards are due to alcohol or alcohol-related diseases. Forty per cent of male attenders at hospital casualty departments have drink-related problems (p. 644).

Table 4.7 Alcohol consumption and alcoholism in the United Kingdom (population 55 million)

Alcohol consumption	Estimated numbers
Regular drinkers	36 M
Heavy drinkers	2 M
Problem drinkers	700 000
Addicted drinkers	200 000

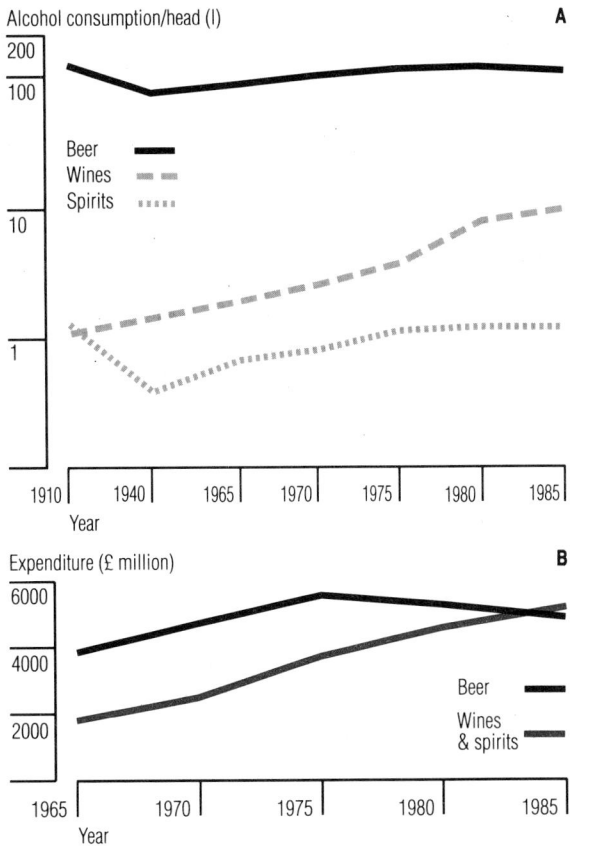

Fig. 4.6 Trends in alcohol consumption and expenditure in the United Kingdom. **A.** Alcohol consumption, 1916–1986. **B.** Consumer expenditure on alcohol, 1950–1985.

Drug Overdose, Poisoning and Drug Addiction

Definitions

There are two main problems about definitions of alcoholism, one practical, the other conceptual. Firstly, 90% of the adult population drink alcohol and it is difficult to make definite distinctions between 'normal' heavy drinking, problem drinking and alcoholism. Secondly, the very attempt to define alcoholism assumes the existence of a disease called 'alcoholism', and this medical model of a personal and social problem may be used by individuals and societies to absolve themselves of responsibility. Some criteria for alcohol dependence are given in Table 4.8. Two important levels of alcoholism require definition, problem drinking and alcohol dependence.

Table 4.8 Criteria of alcohol dependence

- More than 80 g of alcohol consumed daily
- Tolerance: blood alcohol levels greater than 150 mg/100 ml
- Withdrawal symptoms
- Continued drinking in spite of psychological, social, and physical problems
- Abnormal blood tests

Problem drinking

The WHO defines alcoholism as drinking that causes emotional, social or physical damage to the individual. Problem drinkers may suffer from all three, for example: anxiety or depression related to alcohol; divorce, unemployment or financial difficulties; and gastritis or physical trauma associated with drinking.

Alcohol dependence

The essential feature of alcohol dependence is the development of a *withdrawal syndrome* when the drug is removed. The dependent alcoholic will drink, usually early in the day, in order to stave off withdrawal symptoms such as nausea, tremor, sweating or agitation. Other features of alcohol dependence include:

1. *Narrowing of the drinking repertoire.* The ordinary drinker's consumption varies from day to day. The dependent alcoholic has a daily drinking routine which must be followed.
2. *Predominance of drinking over other activities.* For the alcoholic, drink, even if it is clearly damaging his life, comes first.
3. *Tolerance.* The capacity of the dependent individual to drink large quantities of alcohol is an expression of physiological tolerance.

Presentation: the hidden alcoholic

Alcoholics have to be very ill or very brave to complain of their condition directly. Only about 10% of alcoholics in the community are in contact with psychiatric services,

---

Summary 10 Some presentations of undeclared alcohol abuse (should raise 'index of suspicion')

Psychological	Physical
Memory lapses	Gastrointestinal symptoms
Depression	Dyspepsia
Anxiety	Pain
Outbursts of unprovoked anger	Nausea
Suicide attempts	Haematemesis
Morbid jealousy	Neurological symptoms
Paranoia	Tremor
Acute confusional state (DTs)	Paraesthesia
Unpredictability	Muscular weakness
	Unexplained fits

Social
Marital difficulties
Problems at work
Accidents at home or on the roads
Delinquency, crime
Violence

---

while about half are known to other agencies such as general practitioners, social services or parish priests. The remainder are unknown and untreated. Doctors need a high 'index of suspicion' if they are to diagnose these hidden alcoholics correctly. The following factors should alert the examining doctor:

1. unexplained gastrointestinal complaints, recurrent gastritis
2. complaints of anxiety and depression or panic attacks without obvious external precipitants
3. social difficulties, e.g. marital disruption, absenteeism from work, minor crime
4. unexplained accidents, e.g. recurrent head injuries
5. smelling of alcohol at unexpected times, e.g. in morning surgery
6. single males over 40, socially isolated females
7. certain occupations, e.g. publicans, journalists, doctors
8. unexplained macrocytosis on a full blood count, or elevated liver enzyme values on liver function tests.

Where alcoholism is suspected, a detailed alcohol history should be taken. Vague questions, such as 'How much do you drink?', are unlikely to be informative, while positive answers to two or more of the CAGE questions (Table 4.9) suggest a drinking problem. A detailed account of a typical 'drinking day' is required. Alcohol intake is measured in units. One unit equals half-a-pint of beer, quarter-of-a-

Table 4.9 The CAGE questions*

- Have you ever felt you ought to cut down on your drinking?
- Have people annoyed you by criticising your drinking?
- Have you ever felt bad or guilty about your drinking?
- Have you ever had a drink first thing in the morning to steady your nerves or get rid of a hangover (eye-opener)?

* Positive answers to two or more of these suggests a drinking problem.

pint of strong lager, one 'short' or one glass of wine. Regular intake of six units or more per day puts men at risk of alcohol dependence. Women need half as much (i.e. three units per day) for half as long (e.g. as little as two years) for dependency to occur. The patient should be asked when he last had a day without a drink; about the longest period without a drink in the preceding five years; about withdrawal symptoms ('Do you ever feel shaky or nauseated in the mornings?'); about blackouts ('Do you ever forget what happened to you while drinking?'). A 'drink diary' in which the patient records his drinking behaviour for a week can be a useful aid to history-taking. Raised serum γ-glutamyl transpeptidase (γ-GT) and increased mean corpuscular volume (MCV) are useful supportive evidence of abnormal drinking and are also helpful in monitoring progress. A blood alcohol concentration may confirm suspicions of recent excessive intake.

Aetiology

Mutually interacting genetic, psychological and cultural factors underlie alcoholism. Adoption studies show that adopted children of alcoholics are four times as likely to develop alcoholism as adopted children of non-alcoholics. The biochemical mediator of an inherited tendency to alcoholism is unknown: however, active alcohol dehydrogenase leading to higher (and unpleasant) acetaldehyde levels has been postulated as protective against alcoholism.

Psychological factors (Table 4.10) operate in two ways in alcoholism.

1. *Imitation learning*. An individual's tendency to drink follows that of his subculture, parents and peer group. This explains, for example, the high levels of alcoholism among the Irish and Scots, as compared with Jews. Occupational factors associated with an increased risk of alcoholism are listed in Table 4.10.
2. *Alleviation of unpleasant feelings*. Alcohol reduces unpleasant feelings such as social anxiety and guilt.

Each time an individual drinks he reinforces his experience of reduction of unpleasant mood ('drowning your sorrows'). Family disruption is a common experience in the history of alcoholics. Where attachment figures are unreliable, the alcoholic will cling (however self-destructively) to 'the bottle' for security in preference to people.

The true aetiology should be distinguished from the reasons for drinking offered by the patient, as the alcoholic's explanation of why he drinks is often a rationalisation. The alcohol addict drinks because of his physiological state of addiction.

Physical complications

The physical complications of alcoholism are shown in Table 4.11. They include liver disease, neurological syndromes (including peripheral neuropathy, cerebellar degeneration, myopathy and convulsions), cardio-

Table 4.10 Occupational factors associated with risk of alcoholism

Factor	Examples of occupations affected
Availability of alcohol	Workers in the drink trade, caterers, business executives
Social pressure to drink	Coal miners, seamen, medical students, journalists
Freedom from supervision	Company directors, lawyers, GPs
Separation from normal social or sexual relationships	Commercial travellers, seamen, oil-rig workers, service personnel
Strains, stresses, and hazards	Coal miners, doctors, military personnel, actors, saxophonists
Very high or low income	Doctors, the unemployed
Collusion by colleagues	Doctors, workers in the drink trade

Table 4.11 Physical complications of alcoholism

Symptom	Differential diagnosis
Neuropsychiatric	
Trembling	Anxiety state
Sweating	Epilepsy
Insomnia	
Headaches	
Blackouts	
Inability to concentrate	
Confusion	
Fits	
Burning legs	
Gastrointestinal	
Indigestion	Peptic ulcer
Vomiting	Gall-stones
Heartburn	Viral hepatitis
Diarrhoea	
Jaundice	
Bleeding	
Cardiorespiratory	
Palpitations	Ischaemic heart disease
Chest pain	
Pneumonia	
Musculoskeletal	
Repeated injuries	Accidents
Gout	
Backache	
Hormonal and metabolic	
Reduced libido	Cushing's syndrome
Breast swelling (males)	Breast tumour
Obesity	Diabetes mellitus
Infertility	
Polyuria and polydipsia	
Pregnancy	
Repeated stillbirths	
Congenital lesions	

4

myopathy, pulmonary tuberculosis, anaemia, hypo-glycaemia and pancreatitis. Children of alcoholic mothers may be born with a syndrome of low birth-weight and developmental retardation known as the *fetal alcohol syndrome*.

Psychiatric complications

There are three levels of severity at which psychiatric complications of alcoholism occur. In the initial stages, the patient may present with minor psychiatric symptoms of panic attacks, anxiety, depressions or sexual difficulties. The alcoholic addict will develop delirium tremens and sometimes alcoholic hallucinosis. Prolonged and severe alcohol addiction leads to alcohol-related dementia including Korsakoff psychosis. For a detailed discussion of the neurological complications of alcoholism, see Chapter 23.

Delirium tremens (DTs). This is a late and potentially fatal manifestation of the alcohol withdrawal syndrome. It usually starts at night, 48 hours after alcohol intake has stopped, and the patient experiences fear, restlessness and tactile or visual hallucinations. Paranoid delusions are common. He is disorientated in time and place, tremulous and may develop a fever, tachycardia and hypertension. It is common in general hospital wards either because the patient has been admitted in a state of unexplained confusion, or because admission for some other reason (e.g. a surgical condition) produces the withdrawal from alcohol that initiates the DTs.

The management of DTs includes: sedation with chlor-diazepoxide, chlormethiazole or chlorpromazine; parenteral vitamin B administration; and correction of electrolyte imbalance.

Alcoholic hallucinosis. Alcoholics may experience auditory hallucinations, usually derogatory or persecutory, in the presence of clear consciousness (consciousness is always clouded in DTs). These usually stop when drinking ceases but occasionally persist, suggesting coexisting schizophrenia and alcoholism.

Morbid jealousy. Alcohol is a frequent cause of a syndrome of morbid jealousy, in which an individual (usually male) becomes convinced that his spouse is unfaithful.

Wernicke-Korsakoff syndrome. Wernicke's encephalopathy is characterised by an acute onset of nystagmus, ocular palsy and ataxia, usually accompanied by confusion and apathy. The underlying pathology is multiple haemmorhages around the ventricles (particularly the third and fourth) due to thiamine deficiency, of which alcoholism is the commonest cause. It may be followed by a chronic syndrome of dementia known as Korsakoff psychosis, characterised by impairment of short-term memory, a variable degree of global intellectual deficit, and the covering up of memory impairment by plausible conversation known as *confabulation*.

Alcoholic brain damage. Generalised intellectual impairment, associated with demonstrable abnormalities on CAT scanning (e.g. flattening of sulci, widening of ventricles) is a long-term consequence of prolonged alcohol addiction.

Treatment

The outcome of treatment for alcoholism (Table 4.12) depends less on the nature of the treatment than on the social situation and personality of the patient. Addicts with stable family and employment and a good personality do best. The impulsive or psychopathic drinker lacking home, family or job has a very poor prognosis for sobriety.

The aim of treatment should almost always be abstinence. Any doctor who attempts to help alcoholics must be prepared for disappointment as relapses ('slips') are common. A combination of limit-setting and acceptance is needed in all of the following treatment approaches.

Table 4.12 Outcome of treatment for alcoholism

Outcome	1 year (%)	2 year (%)
Improved	25	35
Still drinking	53	43
Dead	1	3
Lost to follow-up	21	19

Psychotherapy

A supportive relationship, either with a spouse, peer (e.g. through Alcoholics Anonymous), or a professional helper is probably essential. Formal psychotherapy or social help should be conditional on sobriety, on the principle that whatever an alcoholic's problems (and they will be many) drink makes them worse. Wherever possible, the spouse and family should be included in any psychotherapy programme.

Inpatient treatment

Brief admission for 'drying-out', or longer admission to a therapeutic community with group therapy can help maintenance of sobriety. Patients who need admission are by definition more disturbed, and the long-term prognosis is therefore often poor.

Drug treatment

Drug treatment for withdrawal syndrome is discussed above. In addition, disulfiram (Antabuse) reacts with alcohol to produce acetaldehyde, producing unpleasant feelings of flushing and nausea. Some patients find it helpful to have this internal 'chemical fence' to discourage drinking.

Alcoholics Anonymous

Alcoholics Anonymous (AA) is a worldwide self-help organisation for alcoholics run by ex-alcoholics. It offers a structured personal and group psychotherapy programme aimed at sobriety. An important feature of AA is that it provides a social life that is not based on pubs or drinking.

Not all alcoholics can accept its quasi-religious ideology, but those that do benefit greatly. A parallel organisation, Al-Anon, offers support to the families of alcoholics.

'Shop-front'/'dry house' programmes

The 'skid-row' alcoholic has usually lost everything – job, home, family, possessions, friends – through drinking, and special facilities are needed for this group of patients (about 10% of alcoholics). These include non-threatening 'drop-in' day centres, after-care hostels, and long-term medical and social support.

Prevention

The above treatments reach only a proportion of alcoholics. There is a direct relationship between per capita consumption and the price and availability of alcohol. As the real cost of alcohol has fallen steadily in the UK over the past decade, so per capita alcohol consumption and hence alcoholism rates have risen accordingly (Fig. 4.6). Governments, through pricing policies and licensing laws, can have a direct effect on alcoholism rates. Well-funded education programmes are also needed to alert the public to the dangers of alcohol. In the UK, organisations such as 'Drinkwatch' aim to promote sensible drinking patterns (e.g. 'halves' rather than pints; alternating soft and alcoholic drinks) among potential alcoholics.

FURTHER READING

Dreisbach R H 1983 Handbook of poisoning: prevention, diagnosis and treatment. Lange, Los Altos, California. *A small, but relatively comprehensive handbook on poisoning.*

Edwards G 1987 Treatment of drinking problems: a guide for the helping professions. Blackwell, Oxford. *A helpful, common-sense approach.*

Edwards G 1987 Drug scenes. Royal College of Psychiatrists, London. *A good guide to the problems and management of opiate addiction.*

Proudfoot A T 1982 Diagnosis and management of acute poisoning. Blackwell, Oxford. *An excellent textbook of the clinical aspects of acute poisoning.*

Vale J A, Meredith T J (eds) 1981 Poisoning diagnosis and treatment. Update Books, London. *A well-illustrated overview of clinical toxicology.*

Vale J A, Meredith T J 1985 A concise guide to the management of poisoning. Churchill Livingstone, Edinburgh. *A handy reference source for the management of poisoning.*

APPENDIX

Information, analytical and clinical services in the United Kingdom and Eire.

National Poisons Information Service		*Other Centres*	
Belfast	(0232) 240503	Birmingham ★⁺	(021) 554 3801
Cardiff ★⁺	(0222) 709901	Leeds	(0532) 430715
Dublin ⁺	(0001) 745588	Newcastle ★	(0632) 325131
Edinburgh	(031) 229 2477		
	(031) 228 2441		
	(SPIB Viewdata)		
London ⁺	(01) 635 9191	★ Poisons Treatment Unit	
	(01) 407 7600	⁺ 24 hour Toxicological Analysis	

Physical and Environmental Causes of Disease

5

DISORDERS DUE TO HEAT AND COLD

Heat produced by metabolism is lost mainly through the skin and, to a lesser extent, through the gut, urine and breath. Inadequate heat loss leads to sweating and vasodilatation. Cold produces cutaneous vasoconstriction and shivering which results in increased muscle metabolism. In moving from a cold to a hot climate, acclimatisation occurs over a period of 1–2 weeks; this process is not well understood. There is increased sweating and the salt content of sweat diminishes. Aldosterone secretion increases, at least at first, causing a low urinary sodium with loss of potassium.

HEAT EXCESS

Three syndromes due to excess heat occur: heat cramps, heat exhaustion and heatstroke.

Heat cramps

Spasms of painful muscular contraction may occur with sudden rises in temperature during strenuous activities such as long-distance running, or during work in very hot environments (mines, boiler rooms or direct sunlight). Muscles of the legs and arms are usually affected, typically after the exertion or heavy work is over. There is usually hyponatraemia, and severe cramps may be accompanied by a rise in creatine phosphokinase and evidence of rhabdomyolysis. Part of the pathogenesis appears to be due to replacement of fluid and salt loss by water with too low a salt content; the condition is preventable by drinking fluids containing 0.25% saline.

Heat exhaustion

Heat exhaustion or heat collapse is the commonest syndrome and is especially likely to occur in individuals exposed to a hot environment for a few days, before they are acclimatised. The very young and the elderly (especially those on diuretics) are particularly likely to be affected. The syndrome is due in part to salt and water loss, and in part to a failure of circulatory adaptation to heat.

When water loss predominates, there is intense thirst and weakness, fatigue, agitation and confusion. Haemoconcentration occurs with a rise in haematocrit and blood urea. With salt depletion, there are muscle cramps, headaches, vomiting and myalgia. Usually, salt and water depletion occur together, and the patient has a normal temperature, and appears pale and clammy.

The disorder is treated by rest and oral fluids containing salt; it is seldom necessary to administer intravenous fluids.

Heatstroke

Heatstroke is a serious and sudden disease which may be fatal unless treated urgently. It is due to a failure of thermoregulation, resulting in a rapid rise in body temperature. The patient is usually elderly, often with underlying disease such as cardiac failure, diabetes, obesity or alcoholism. Atropine-like drugs, beta-blockers, phenothiazines and diuretics predispose to the syndrome. Heatstroke can also occur in fit men working in hot environments, and there are some clinical differences in these cases.

Typically the patient develops headache, dizziness and faintness, and abdominal pain and delirium may occur. Sweating stops and the body temperature rises rapidly (and may reach 43°C). Hypotension, renal failure and rhabdomyolysis may occur; the latter is especially common in heatstroke following severe exertion. Sweating may continue in this form of heatstroke.

On examination, the skin is hot and usually dry, and the patient exhibits tachypnoea and flaccidity. Coma and shock are grave signs. The blood shows leucocytosis and respiratory alkalosis (but may be acidotic in the exertional

77

5

form), the urea is raised and hypokalaemia and hyperphosphataemia occur. Myocardial necrosis may give ST changes and even an infarction pattern on the ECG. Liver function tests are abnormal, and acute renal failure may occur. Disseminated intravascular coagulation is present in mild degree in the elderly, but may be severe in exertional heatstroke.

Management

Treatment is of the utmost urgency. The patient must be cooled as quickly as possible. The most effective way is immersion in very cold water, the skin being rubbed to increase the efficiency of cooling. An alternative is to blow cold air over dampened skin. Core temperature must be monitored using a rectal thermometer. Hypotension can be treated with small quantities of saline, with care to avoid circulatory overload. Hypoglycaemia, if present, can be treated with glucose, and severe acidosis by sodium bicarbonate.

More serious complications, such as acute renal failure and disseminated intravascular coagulation, are treated in the usual way (Chapters 21 and 25).

HYPOTHERMIA

Hypothermia is a common problem mainly affecting the elderly population, in whom the response to cold may be defective (p. 166). Hypothermia contributes to the excess mortality of the elderly during winter months. It occurs when the deep body temperature falls below 35°C. As the mouth temperature may fluctuate depending upon the ambient air temperature, it is best to use a rectal thermometer when monitoring hypothermia patients. Because the ordinary clinical thermometer does not read below 35°C, a low-reading thermometer is also necessary.

Aetiology

Hypothermia may be due simply to an age-related impaired thermoregulatory response to a cold environment (Ch. 10, p. 166). In the majority of patients, however, there is an associated underlying pathological cause, including any cause of autonomic dysfunction (p. 167). Hypothyroidism and hypopituitarism are both associated with hypothermia, and the risk is also higher in immobile or demented patients, or in the presence of an acute illness such as bronchopneumonia. There is a clear association between phenothiazines and impairment of temperature regulation, and hypothermia may also be precipitated by sedative drugs, such as hypnotics and alcohol.

Prevalence

Accurate figures for the prevalence of hypothermia are hard to obtain. In the UK, death certificates mentioning hypothermia as a main or contributory cause of death amount to about 300 per year, but this is likely to be an underestimate. Doctors are sometimes reluctant to enter hypothermia on a death certificate since this will automatically involve the coroner in the case. A survey carried out in London between January and April, 1975, found that of patients over the age of 65 admitted to hospital through the Accident and Emergency Department, 3.6% were hypothermic – a much higher incidence than previously suspected.

Clinical features

Hypothermic patients typically live alone in poor housing with impaired mobility. A typical case would be that of an old person who gets out of bed in the middle of the night to go to the lavatory, falls, and then lies all night on the cold floor in thin night-clothes until discovered the next morning by a neighbour.

The skin has a greyish look due to a combination of vasoconstriction and cyanosis; the face may appear puffy, resembling myxoedema. The diagnosis is often first suspected during examination, when it is found that the patient's skin feels cold in normally warm areas, such as the axilla or the abdomen. The patient is often confused, since drowsiness and loss of consciousness occur when the temperature falls below 32°C. Shivering is absent below this temperature; instead, there is increased skeletal muscle tone with neck stiffness and abdominal rigidity. The heart rate is slowed and the ECG may show a prolonged PR interval and J waves (Fig. 5.1). Respirations are slow and shallow, and there may be hypoxia and hypercapnia. Acute pancreatitis is often found at necropsy, but this is only rarely diagnosed in life.

Impaired renal and respiratory function may lead to a raised blood urea or bicarbonate. Blood sugar levels may be raised, but do not indicate diabetes mellitus, and will fall as the temperature returns to normal. Serum aspartate aminotransferase and creatinine kinase may be raised due to muscle damage.

Figure 5.1 Electrocardiogram showing J wave (arrowed) in a hypothermic patient.

Management

The lower the deep body temperature, the higher the mortality; this is about 50% overall. The high mortality is because many hypothermic patients have a serious underlying illness. Patients with mild hypothermia (core temperature 32–35°C) should be wrapped in a space blanket and nursed in a side ward where the ambient temperature is 25–30°C. The patient's temperature should be allowed to rise *gradually*, at a rate of about 0.5°C per hour, as fast surface rewarming carries the risk of hypotension. For this reason, the patient's pulse and blood pressure must be monitored. If the blood pressure drops, the space blanket should be removed or the room temperature lowered so that the patient is temporarily cooled. A broad-spectrum antibiotic is usually given parenterally because broncho-pneumonia is nearly always present, even if not clinically apparent. Oxygen is not usually necessary unless there are signs of hypoxaemia, and intravenous fluids are not normally needed (except possibly for underlying illness). The ECG should be monitored, since both brady-arrhythmias and ventricular fibrillation may occur. The patient is at serious risk of developing a pressure sore and must be nursed on a suitable mattress (such as the Nuclearform) and turned regularly.

When the deep body temperature is below 32°C, a more aggressive approach to resuscitation is sometimes advocated – although there is little evidence that this reduces mortality. These measures include positive pressure ventilation to correct hypoxia, measurement of central venous pressure, and active rewarming using a radiant heat cradle over the torso or warmed intravenous fluids.

Thyroid hormones should not normally be given to hypothermic patients. If there is very good clinical or laboratory evidence of the presence of hypothyroidism, then tri-iodothyronine (5 μg) may be given by slow intravenous injection every 12 hours.

RADIATION SICKNESS

Ionising irradiation is of two broad types: photons (gamma and X-rays) and particulate (alpha and beta particles). Radiation dose is defined in a variety of ways. The energy deposited *in a tissue* is measured in Gray (Gy; 1 Gy = 1 J/kg). Since different types of radiation have different tissue effects, a unit called the Sievert (SV) is sometimes used to weight the radiation dose. Particulate radiations are absorbed according to their mass and energy, but do not penetrate deeply into tissues (see also Chapter 9, p. 150).

Exposure

Exposure to ionising irradiation comes about in three ways:

1. *Background irradiation.* We are exposed to approximately 2–3 mSV per year from solar and geological irradiation in the form of photons. Of this, 80% is in the form of radon.
2. *Medical exposure.* The therapeutic uses of ionising irradiation are described in Chapter 9. Accidental exposure of patients or staff has been rare since the advent of stringent precautions following the radiation-induced damage to skin and eyes in the early days of therapeutic and diagnostic radiation.

3. *Military and industrial irradiation.* The atomic bombs dropped on Hiroshima and Nagasaki later led to numerous cases of acute leukaemia and other cancers. Fallout from nuclear tests has increased annual background radiation by 1%. Industrial accidents also occur, the most dramatic example of which has been the ingestion of radium by radium dial painters from 1920–1926, resulting in a great increase in risk of bone sarcoma and cancer of the air sinuses of the skull. The recent accident in the nuclear power station at Chernobyl in the USSR resulted in many deaths due to acute radiation exposure, and an increase in background radiation over a wide geographical area.

Tissue damage

The tissue-damaging effect of ionising irradiation is probably related mainly to damage to DNA, leading to strand breakage and impaired reproductive integrity of the cell. Following whole-body exposure, there are certain tissues which are damaged acutely by relatively low doses:

1. *Bone marrow.* This can regenerate after exposure to 10 Gy, but above this dose permanent aplasia may occur. The white count and platelet count begin to fall within 10 days of exposure.
2. *Intestine.* Doses of 10 Gy or over cause severe loss of crypt cells leading to loss of villi and extensive ulceration.
3. *Skin.* Erythema occurs at doses below 10 Gy. At 20 Gy, the skin starts to desquamate and ulcerate.
4. *Lung.* Above 10 Gy in a single fraction, pneumonitis occurs and is increasingly severe with increase in dose.

Long-term changes include glomerular loss and interstitial nephritis, infertility, pulmonary fibrosis, neuronal loss and gliosis, intestinal stricture and hepatic fibrosis. The development of cancers occurs after a latent interval of several years.

Clinical features

After acute whole-body exposure, the clinical features depend on the received dose. The syndromes mentioned below represent the components due to each tissue. Clearly, in many cases, the full clinical picture will be due to a mixture of damage to several organs.

Following an initial period of nausea and vomiting (sometimes with parotid swelling), the patient may be relatively well for 7-10 days and then develop a *syndrome of haematological failure*. There is depression of the white count and platelets, with infection, bruising and bleeding. At the same time, *skin reactions* occur with desquamation, alopecia and ulceration. If the dose is above 15 Gy, the *gastrointestinal syndrome* may predominate and be the first sign of toxicity. In a patient with severe leucopenia, severe diarrhoea and fluid loss is followed by septicaemia from gut bacteria. This is almost always fatal. Higher doses of radiation (25–60 Gy) cause cardiovascular collapse and shock.

Management

Management is supportive. Anti-emetics are given in the acute phase, and fluid losses from diarrhoea are replaced. Blood platelets and antibiotics are used during the phase of myelosuppression and infection. Allogeneic bone-marrow transplantation may help the minority of patients for whom there is a donor, and in whom the haematological toxicity is the major life-threatening complication.

Accidental exposure to radionuclides is treated according to the isotope. Potassium iodide is given for ^{131}I ingestion, and soluble phosphate for ^{32}P overdose. Overdose with bone-localising isotopes (caesium, radium, strontium) is treated with EDTA and large doses of oral calcium.

Prognosis

With adequate treatment, most patients will survive with exposures up to 10 Gy. Above this dose, bone-marrow failure and the intestinal syndrome are usually fatal.

DISORDERS DUE TO EXTREMES OF BAROMETRIC PRESSURE

ALTITUDE SICKNESS

The effects of reduced barometric pressure result from the low partial pressure of oxygen and reduced oxygen-carrying capacity of the blood. Figure 5.2 shows this relationship. Because of the sigmoid shape of the oxygen-

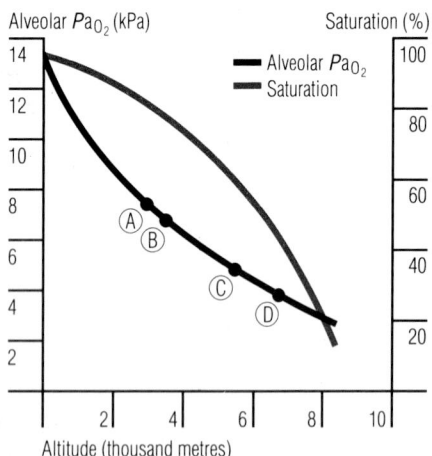

Figure 5.2 Effect of altitude on alveolar Pa_{O_2} and oxygen saturation. Because of the steep slope of the oxygen dissociation curve, increasing altitude above 5000 metres causes a precipitous fall in saturation. In an unacclimatised person, acute changes occur at: (A) 3000 metres (10 000 feet) – slightly impaired memory and judgement, increased heart rate, abdominal cramps, nausea and diarrhoea; (B) 3500 metres (12 000 feet) – headache, nausea, diminished visual acuity, and possible pulmonary oedema; (C) 5500 metres (18 000 feet) – impaired consciousness after several hours in many people; and (D) 6750 metres (22 000 feet) – loss of consciousness.

dissociation curve, oxygen saturation is reasonably well maintained until an altitude of 5000 metres. A precipitous fall in saturation then occurs with increasing height. Commercial aircraft are maintained at a pressure equivalent to 2500 metres, so that no additional oxygen is needed unless a patient has severe cardiac or respiratory disease. If there is a loss of pressurisation (to pressure levels below that obtained at 5000 metres), extra oxygen is made available through masks.

There are three recognised syndromes of altitude sickness: acute altitude sickness, acute pulmonary oedema and chronic altitude sickness.

Acute altitude (mountain) sickness

The syndrome of acute altitude sickness occurs in unacclimatised individuals who ascend rapidly to heights in excess of 2500 metres. People who are unfit or elderly and patients with respiratory and cardiac disease are especially prone.

The symptoms are headache, dyspnoea, malaise, nausea, vomiting, abdominal pain and diarrhoea. The symptoms slowly subside over a week if not relieved by oxygen or by descent. Respiratory alkalosis is present, and acetozolamide can alleviate some of the symptoms by causing renal bicarbonate excretion and partially reversing the alkalosis.

Acute pulmonary oedema

Rapid ascent to heights greater than 3000 metres may provoke the sudden onset of acute pulmonary oedema. Hypoxia is the cause, but the pathogenesis is unclear. The symptoms usually begin 5–36 hours after ascent; acute dyspnoea, haemoptysis and widespread crackles in the lungs occur. Pathologically, there is acute oedema and a 'hyaline' membrane in bronchioles of unknown cause. Treatment is with oxygen and diuretics.

Chronic altitude (mountain) sickness

Individuals who have lived for many years at altitudes above 4000 metres may develop polycythaemia, with very high values of haemoglobin (in excess of 20 g/dl) and a chronic insensitivity of the respiratory centre to hypoxia. Such individuals hypoventilate and develop a raised P_{CO_2}. There is central cyanosis, with cough, headache and giddiness. These symptoms are similar to those found in polycythaemia rubra vera and are due to the decreased cerebral blood flow (a consequence of the raised haematocrit) and to the hypoxia. Not all people living at high altitude develop this syndrome which appears in part to be an excess response to decreased inspired P_{O_2}. The syndrome can only be treated by descent to a lower altitude.

INCREASE IN BAROMETRIC PRESSURE

An increase in barometric pressure is encountered in diving or in mining.

Breathhold diving

During a breathhold dive the body directly encounters the increased pressure (one atmosphere for every 33 feet descent). The breathhold causes a rise in $P\text{CO}_2$ and a falling $P\text{O}_2$. The main respiratory stimulus is the raised $P\text{CO}_2$, so that hyperventilation *before* diving leads to a serious lack of stimulus to breathe (due to CO_2 depletion). This may cause fatal loss of consciousness from hypoxia (which does not cause an irresistible urge to breathe and thus terminate the dive). As the diver surfaces, decompression lowers $P\text{O}_2$ and again may cause loss of consciousness.

Decompression sickness

Deep diving and tunnel (caisson) work places a diver under an increased barometric pressure. If this is air, the nitrogen dissolved in blood ($P\text{N}_2$) increases and, on rapid decompression, forms bubbles which come out of solution in small blood vessels. Ischaemia results, causing pain in joints, spinal cord injury, chest pain, cyanosis, confusion, visual defects, paralysis and fits. Minor confusion occurs with lesser degrees of decompression injury.

Treatment is by recompression followed by very gradual decompression over days.

Air embolism

Occasionally, a scuba diver breathing air may hold his breath while ascending rapidly, without breathing out. The gas expands in the lung and may rupture it, causing air embolism with cerebral vascular occlusion leading to paralysis, fits and visual disturbance. Rapid recompression is necessary. Air embolism is a common cause of death in these divers.

DROWNING AND NEAR-DROWNING

There are considerable differences in the osmotic pressure of salt water (5% NaCl), fresh water (0% NaCl) and plasma (0.9% NaCl). It has been suggested that, when large amounts of salt water are aspirated into the lung, water may be sucked into the alveoli from pulmonary capillary plasma, causing death from pulmonary oedema. When fresh water is aspirated, however, large volumes may pass into the pulmonary circulation causing haemolysis and consequent potassium release, which may lead to cardiac arrest. In fact, in all cases, death usually results from acute reflex laryngospasm, causing asphyxia, most of the water entering the lungs only during the last few moments of life.

Resuscitation from near-drowning

A patient who is nearly drowned needs urgent resuscitation. The basic techniques are the same as for any 'sudden death', but the physiology of drowning raises special issues.

In both fresh- and sea-water drowning, abdominal aspiration must be performed once a cuffed endotracheal tube is in place. Large volumes of water tend to be swallowed during drowning. Similarly, ventilation with positive end expiratory pressure is required, once in hospital, to attempt to reinflate atelectatic and waterlogged lungs.

Sea-water drowning is often associated with cardiac arrest produced by the rapid absorption of Ca^{2+} and Mg^+ into the blood. Treatment by basic life support is frequently effective in sea-water drowning, if begun within five minutes. Fresh-water drowning may produce massive intravascular haemolysis. It is associated with ventricular fibrillation and hyperkalaemia, which can be difficult to treat. Survival after fresh-water drowning during warm weather is unusual, but survival (with normal cerebral function) has been recorded in children, even after 30 minutes immersion, particularly in low-temperature water. Apart from the usual life-support measures, exchange transfusion and repeated DC defibrillation may be required, with cardiopulmonary resuscitation maintained for hours if necessary.

Sudden death due to a combination of vagal slowing of the heart and intense peripheral vasoconstriction may occur in previously fit individuals who dive into cold water.

ELECTRIC SHOCK

Injury following electric shock depends on the voltage and current. Sudden death is less likely below 1000 volts. Alternating current appears to be much more dangerous than direct, since it produces muscle spasm and is more likely to stop the heart. The direction of flow is also important, as flow from hand to hand or hand to foot traverses the heart. At high voltage, the body heats up as the current flows. This heating is much more severe in a small cross-sectional area (fingers) than in a large one (trunk), and burns and charring are thus mostly found in the hands. Burns occur at the skin, and arcing of the current may ignite clothing, causing further burns.

Clinical features

With high voltage, cardiac arrest occurs. Cardiac resuscitation is essential, as is a careful assessment for burns which may manifest themselves later. Arrhythmias may recur for up to two days after resuscitation.

Intestinal perforation, and liver and gall bladder injury may occur. There may be cerebral and spinal cord damage, and peripheral nerves may be permanently damaged. Spinal cord injury may have a delayed onset, with paraplegia or a tabes-dorsalis-like syndrome. Acute muscle necrosis may result in renal failure.

Treatment

After resuscitation, the cardiac rhythm must be monitored for two days after the last rhythm disturbance. Renal failure

5

due to rhabdomyolysis must be treated. A surgical assessment must be made of burns and charring, and peripheral circulation. Debridement, fasciotomy and even amputation may be necessary.

An extreme example of high-voltage injury is a lightning strike. Cardio-pulmonary resuscitation is essential as described above. Rhabdomyolysis and burns are treated in the same way as in other electric-shock injury. With effective resuscitation, over half the victims will survive.

FURTHER READING

Howard J, Tyrer F H 1987 Textbook of occupational medicine. Churchill Livingstone, Edinburgh. *A comprehensive and very readable textbook describing environmental and work hazards.*

Raffle P A B, Lee W R, McCallum R I, Murray R 1987 Hunter's diseases of occupations. Hodder and Stoughton, London. *A traditional and comprehensive text covering the entire field of occupational medicine.*

The Genetic Basis of Disease

6

In the Western World, chronic diseases with a substantial genetic component occur in 5–10% of the adult population. Furthermore, more than one in 50 babies have a recognisable congenital anomaly at birth, many of which will have a genetic cause. Genetic disorders and malformations account for around 30% of paediatric hospital admissions and up to 50% of deaths under the age of 15 years. The relative frequency of the different types of genetic disorders in the United Kingdom is shown in Figure 6.1.

In certain populations, specific genetic disorders are of such high incidence as to represent significant public health problems. Examples are the thalassaemias in Mediterranean and Oriental populations, and sickle cell anaemia and other haemoglobinopathies in Afro-Caribbean populations. The incidence of affected homozygotes with these disorders can be as high as one in 50 births in some areas. Worldwide, over 200 000 individuals homozygous for a serious haemoglobinopathy are born each year.

DNA, GENES AND CHROMOSOMES

The basic unit of inheritance is the *gene*. A gene is a length of *deoxyribonucleic acid* (DNA) which codes for a specific protein.

The DNA molecule is a double helix, i.e. it is formed from two interwoven strands. Each strand consists of a chain of nucleotides, and each nucleotide is made up of a deoxyribose sugar and a nitrogenous base. There are four possible nitrogenous bases: adenine (A), thymine (T), guanine (G) and cytosine (C). The deoxyribose sugars link to form the backbone of each strand, and the bases on each strand face each other and pair by hydrogen bonding. The base pairing is specific: adenine always pairs with thymine and guanine with cytosine. The specific base pairing allows DNA molecules to be copied precisely when cells divide.

A sequence of bases coding for a gene is sometimes divided into coding regions (exons) and non-coding regions (introns). DNA is *transcribed* by synthesising a single strand *ribonucleic acid* (RNA) molecule, using one of the DNA strands as a template. The resultant *messenger* RNA (m-RNA) molecule is processed, to splice out the non-coding regions, and to modify each end, and then migrates into the cytoplasm where it directs the synthesis of a specific protein by a process known as *translation*. This process involves the interaction of the m-RNA with both *ribosomes* in the cytoplasm and a series of molecules known as *transfer* RNA (t-RNA) (Fig. 6.2). t-RNA is a specialised molecule, to which can be attached a specific amino acid. Each t-RNA carries a three-base coding region, which pairs specifically with a corresponding sequence of three bases on the m-RNA. The sequence of three bases is known as a *codon* and is specific for each amino acid. The sequence of codons makes up the *genetic code*. There are also three codons which determine the end of a protein; these are known as *stop codons*.

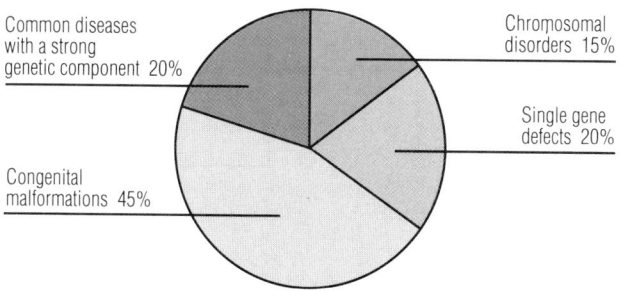

Fig. 6.1 The relative frequencies of different types of genetic disorder in the United Kingdom.

Common diseases with a strong genetic component 20%

Congenital malformations 45%

Chromosomal disorders 15%

Single gene defects 20%

The Genetic Basis of Disease

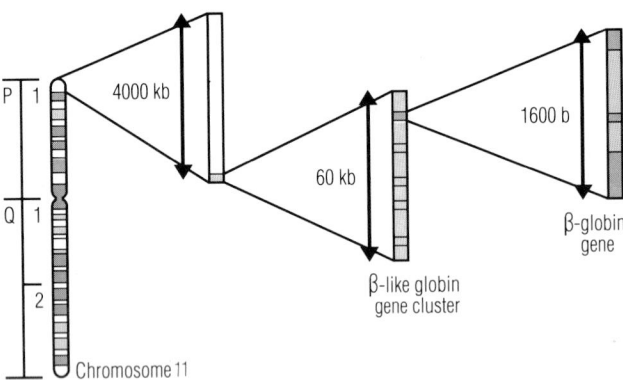

Fig. 6.2 DNA transcription and translation (after Emery 1984). See text for details.

A gene may occupy a sequence of one to tens of kilobases (one kilobase = 1000 base pairs), depending on the length of the resultant protein and the number of introns in the gene. A *chromosome* consists of a continuous molecule of DNA coding for many thousands of genes. In a chromosome, DNA is intricately coiled and combined with proteins, including *histones*, which results in a compact structure that can be seen with a light microscope. Often, special stains are used, which create a pattern of light and dark bands. These band patterns are specific for each chromosome, and reflect their macrostructure. Figure 6.3 demonstrates the relative size of a gene, in relation to a chromosome band and the chromosome itself.

Fig. 6.3 The size of a gene relative to a chromosome and chromosome band, illustrated by the β-globin gene. This is situated on chromosome 11 in band 11p15.5, which may contain around 4000 kb. The gene itself is around 1600 base pairs long and is part of a cluster of similar genes, the β-like globin gene cluster.

WAYS OF LOOKING AT GENES

There are three basic steps in the analysis of the sequences of DNA that make up genes (Fig. 6.4):

1. *Use of restriction enzymes.* Restriction enzymes, which originate from bacteria, cut double stranded DNA at specific base sequences. The distance between such restriction enzyme recognition sites may range from one to tens of kilobases, so that the genome is cut into fragments of differing sizes.

2. *Electrophoresis and Southern blotting.* Fragments generated using restriction enzymes can be separated by electrophoresis on an agarose gel. The fragments are then denatured (i.e. the double stranded DNA separates into single stranded molecules) and a mirror image of the pattern of fragments is made onto nitrocellulose paper by a process known as Southern blotting.

3. *Use of DNA probes.* At this stage, single stranded fragments of DNA have been separated according to size, and fixed onto the nitrocellulose filter paper. A gene probe must now be used to identify the sequences of individual genes present in specific bands. A gene probe is a radioactively labelled single stranded length of DNA whose sequence is specific for a particular gene, or length of chromosome. It is sometimes made using m-RNA coding for a specific protein, by a process known as reverse transcription. The single

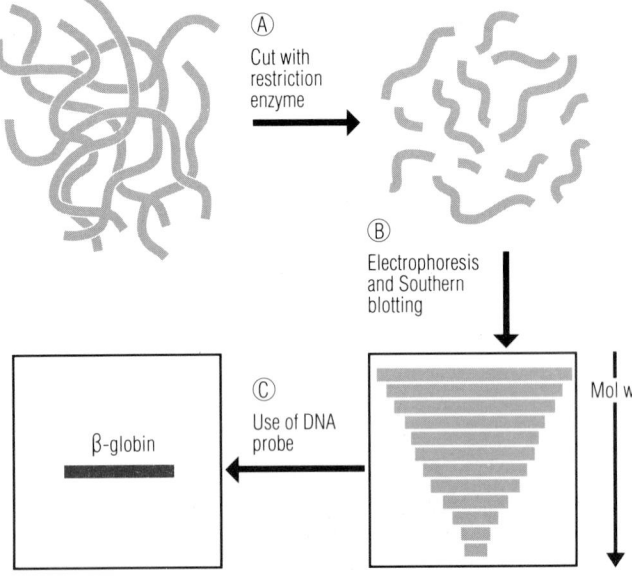

Fig. 6.4 DNA analysis. (A) DNA is cut at specific points by restriction enzymes into different sized fragments. (B) these fragments are separated by electrophoresis on an agarose gel and blotted onto nitrocellulose paper (Southern blotting). Specific genes cannot be visualised at this stage. (C) a radioactive DNA probe is used to locate a specific gene. The position of the gene on the gel depends on the size of the DNA fragment in which it is contained.

stranded probe recognises complementary sequences of DNA on the Southern blot, and anneals to them. Autoradiography can be used to locate the position of the gene probe, which will mark the position of all similar sequences on the Southern blot. If a gene-specific probe has been used, only a few bands will be seen on the autoradiograph, according to how many restriction enzyme recognition sites there are within the gene itself. Different restriction enzymes will generate different patterns, using the same probe. The position of the various restriction enzyme cutting sites within the gene can be inferred, and a *restriction map* produced.

Restriction fragment length polymorphism

The restriction enzyme cutting sites in and around genes are variable, as a common, harmless base change may create or destroy a cutting site. Thus, in some individuals, different patterns may be seen on Southern blotting using the same restriction enzyme and the same gene probe. This is because the gene in question will be contained in

Fig. 6.5 Restriction fragment length polymorphism. (1) shows the two alleles (A and B) of a gene at a specific locus. The alleles are represented by the coloured blocks on each of the two chromosomes. The arrows indicate restriction enzyme recognition sites. In allele A, there is an extra site in the middle of the gene so that, when a DNA sample from this individual is cut with the restriction enzyme and a Southern blot made, three bands will be seen (2). The largest band represents allele B and the two smaller bands allele A. (3) shows a pedigree where alleles A and B are being passed from generation to generation. Allele B causes an autosomal dominant disorder (e.g. Huntington's chorea) in this family so that the restriction fragment length polymorphism can be used to track the abnormal gene.

fragments of different lengths according to the presence or absence of specific cutting sites. Such *restriction fragment length polymorphisms* (RFLPs) are extremely important because they act as genetic markers, allowing abnormal genes to be tracked through families (Fig. 6.5).

TYPES OF SINGLE GENE MUTATION

At the molecular level, there are many mechanisms that can give rise to a malfunctioning gene (Table 6.1). The haemoglobinopathies best illustrate the full range of molecular defects which can occur.

Table 6.1 Molecular mechanisms of single gene mutation, illustrated by the haemoglobinopathies

Abnormality of DNA	Effect	Example
Deletion of gene	Diminished or absent protein, depending on the number of genes involved	Most forms of α-thalassaemia
Point mutation (i.e. single base change)	Substitution of a single amino acid in the protein	Sickle cell anaemia, Hb E, C and many other examples
	Creation of a stop codon leading to a short protein chain	Hb McKees Rocks, some forms of β-thalassaemia
	Removal of a stop codon, leading to an elongated protein chain	Hb Constant Spring (α-chain).
	Alteration of splicing signal	Some forms of α- and β-thalassaemia
Insertion or deletion of a number of nucleotides that are not a multiple of three	Frame-shift mutation	Hb Cranston, Tak and Wayne Some forms of β-thalassaemia
Fusion of genes	Absence of normal product and presence of a new protein resulting from the fused genes	Lepore haemoglobins involving β- and δ-globin chains (β-thalassaemias)

CHROMOSOME STUDIES

Chromosomes are usually visualised during mitosis, at metaphase (p. 87). At this stage, they consist of two identical *chromatids*, joined together at the *centromere*. The position of the centromere is specific for each chromosome. In some chromosomes (1–3) the centromere is close to the centre of the chromosome (metacentric); in others (13–15, 21–22) it is near one end (acrocentric); while in the remaining chromosomes, the centromere is somewhere in between these two extremes (sub-metacentric). By convention, all chromosomes are divided by the centromere into a short arm (p) and a long arm (q).

Chromosome banding

Like other cell structures, chromosomes must be stained in order to visualise them with the light microscope. Using various methods, a pattern of bands can be produced, which is specific for each chromosome. A number of staining techniques are commonly used:

1. G (*Giemsa*) *banding* is the most widely used technique. Light and dark bands are produced.
2. Q (*quinacrine*) *banding* requires a fluorescent microscope. The band patterns are similar to G-banding. Certain chromosome structures, e.g. the long arm of the Y, are particularly well stained.
3. R (*reverse*) *banding* produces a negative image of G-banding.
4. T (*telomere*) *banding* preferentially stains the telomeres (ends of the chromosomes).
5. C (*centromere*) *banding* stains centromeric regions.

Band nomenclature

The banding pattern is specific for each chromosome, and a convention exists for labelling each band. The long and short arms are divided into regions by particularly prominent bands (landmark bands) (Fig. 6.6). Within each region, individual bands are numbered from the centromere distally and landmark bands are included in the distal region they demarcate. Thus, in Figure 6.6, band 1q32 means band 2 in region 3 of the long arm (q) of chromosome 1.

Types of chromosome abnormality

Chromosome abnormalities can be divided into those involving the number of chromosomes, and those involving breakage or rearrangement.

Abnormalities in chromosome number

The normal diploid number of chromosomes in humans is 46. Individuals with chromosome counts that are not multiples of the normal haploid number (23) are said to be aneuploid. A fetus can receive higher multiples of the haploid number of chromosomes to give 69 ($\times$ 3) or 92 ($\times$ 4) chromosomes. Such triploid or tetraploid fetuses usually miscarry early.

If individuals carry one extra chromosome, they are said to be trisomic for the chromosome concerned. Very occasionally, an individual can have two extra chromosomes (double trisomy). Monosomy describes the situation where one chromosome is missing. In liveborn children, it is virtually only seen for the sex chromosomes, giving monosomy X (Turner's syndrome, p. 90).

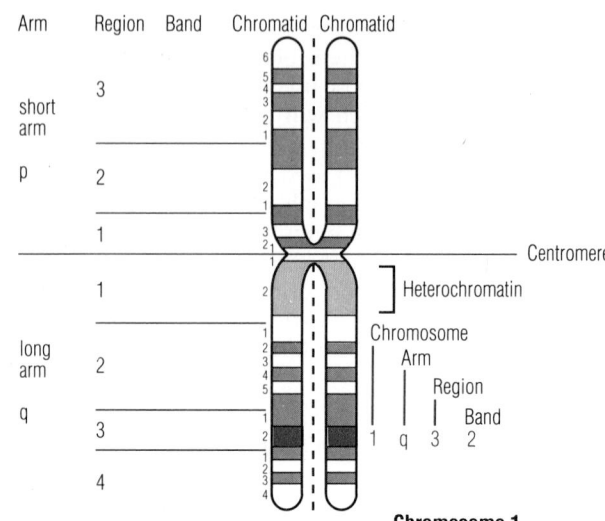

Fig. 6.6 Chromosome nomenclature, using chromosome 1 as an example.

Translocation, deletion and insertion

Breakage of chromosomes can result in loss of material (*deletion*), exchange of material between two non-identical chromosomes (*reciprocal translocation*), inversion of a segment of chromosome (*pericentric inversions* involve the centromere, *paracentric inversions* do not), and joining of the two ends of the same chromosome (to give a *ring chromosome*). Horizontal splitting of the centromere can result in a chromosome with identical long and short arms, an *isochromosome*. A translocation between the long arms of two acrocentric chromosomes, joined at the centromere, is known as a *Robertsonian translocation*. These possibilities are illustrated in Figure 6.7.

Fig. 6.7 Types of chromosome aberration. (A) Two normal non-homologous chromosomes. (B) A reciprocal translocation between the two chromosomes. Note that material has been exchanged between the short arms. (C) A pericentric inversion of the large chromosome. Breaks have occurred in the long and short arms and the middle segment of the chromosome has become inverted. (D) A deletion. The top part of the large chromosome has been lost. (E) An isochromosome. The small chromosome consists of two identical short arms due to mis-division after replication. (F) A ring chromosome. Both ends of the small chromosome have joined to form a ring.

Karyotype nomenclature

The convention in karyotype nomenclature is to give the number of chromosomes first, followed by the types of sex chromosomes, followed by the types of any additional, missing or abnormal chromosomes. Thus, for example:

1. 46,XX – normal female
2. 45,X – Turner's syndrome
3. 47,XY + 21 – male with trisomy 21
4. 69,XXY – triploidy, XXY sex chromosome complement
5. 45,X/46,XX – mosaic Turner's syndrome

For inversions or translocations, the numbers of the chromosomes involved are given in brackets (with the chromosome with the lowest number first). This is followed by the bands or regions involved in further brackets. Symbols are used to indicate the type of re-arrangement involved. Thus, 46,XX,t(9:21)(q11:p11) karyotype means that chromosome 9 has broken at band q11 and chromosome 21 has broken at band p11. The small letter, t (for translocation), indicates that material has been exchanged between the two chromosomes.

CELL DIVISION

Mitosis

Division of somatic cells is known as *mitosis*. This is divided into four stages (Fig. 6.8). Between cell divisions, in *interphase*, the chromosomes are extremely elongated and cannot be seen with the light microscope.

1. *Prophase.* As a preparation for cell division, the chromosomes replicate, to give the classical structure with two chromatids, and they begin to condense.
2. *Metaphase.* The chromosomes line up at the centre of the cell.

3. *Anaphase.* Each chromosome separates longitudinally at the centromere, and the two chromatids pass to opposite poles of the cell.
4. *Telophase.* Two new daughter cells are created by the formation of a nuclear envelope around each new set of chromosomes.

Meiosis

During the production of gametes, the normal diploid complement of 46 chromosomes must be reduced to the haploid number of 23 in the gametes by the process known as *meiosis*. During meiosis, there is the independent assortment of maternally and paternally derived genes in the different gametes of an individual. This is brought about by two separate means:

1. Different gametes receive different combinations of maternally and paternally derived chromosomes.
2. There is an exchange of genetic material between the two members of an homologous pair of chromosomes, known as *crossing over*. This process results in the creation of a chromosome containing part of the maternal and part of the paternal member of an homologous pair, known as a *recombinant* chromosome. Without crossing over, alleles on the same chromosome would always be inherited en bloc.

Crossing over takes place during the first step of meiosis (meiosis I) which is divided into prophase, metaphase, anaphase and telophase, as in mitosis. However, meiosis I differs in that homologous members of a pair of chromosomes line up and exchange genetic material during prophase, while at anaphase, each member chromosome passes to an opposite pole without division at the centromere. Meiosis I is known as *reduction division*, because it results in the formation of two daughter cells containing 23 chromosomes, each of which has two chromatids that may not be identical because of crossing over.

The second step, meiosis II, is similar to mitosis except that each 'parent' cell now has only 23 chromosomes (each with two chromatids), and each 'daughter' cell contains 23 chromatids at telophase. Fusion of parental gametes at fertilisation restores the diploid number of chromosomes.

| Prophase | Metaphase | Anaphase | Telophase |

Mitosis

Meiosis I

Meiosis II

Fig. 6.8   Mitosis and meiosis: see text for details.

LOCI, ALLELES AND SEGREGATION

The genes determining a particular trait are situated at identical points or *loci* on each member of a homologous pair of chromosomes. The two genes on each chromosome at a particular locus may not be identical, and are known as *alleles*. If two alleles at a locus are identical, the individual is said to be *homozygous* at that locus; if the alleles are not identical, the individual is said to be *heterozygous*. The chance of a child inheriting one particular allele from a heterozygous parent is 1 in 2 (50%). For autosomal loci, if both parents are heterozygous, the chance of a child being

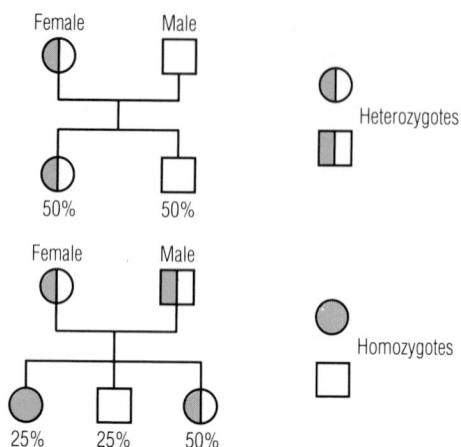

Fig. 6.9A   Inheritance of alleles at autosomal loci.

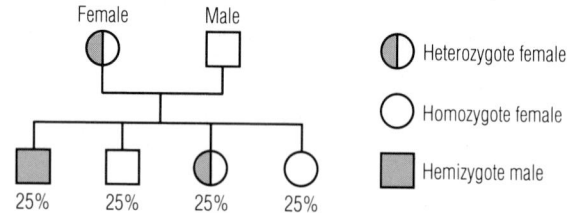

Fig. 6.9B   Inheritance of alleles at X-linked loci.

Fig. 6.10A   Autosomal recessive inheritance with first cousin parents. The boy at the bottom of the pedigree is homozygous for an abnormal gene inherited from the great-grandmother through both parents. The double line indicates consanguinous marriage.

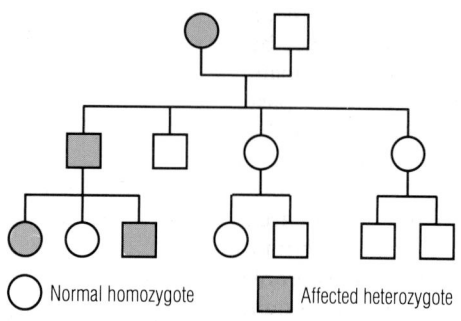

Fig. 6.10B   Autosomal dominant inheritance. Note that the disease is passed on from parent to child and that both males and females are affected. There is also transmission of the disease from father to son.

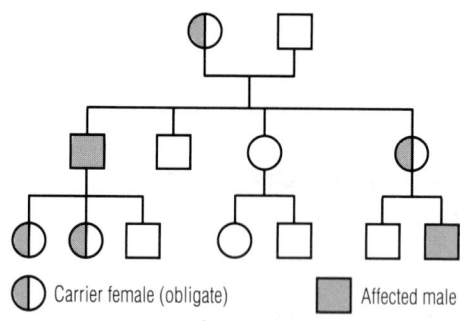

Fig. 6.11   X-linked recessive inheritance. Note that half of the sons of a carrier female are affected and half of the daughters are carriers. All the daughters of an affected male are carriers and all the sons are normal, because a male passes on his one X chromosome to his daughters and his Y chromosome to his sons.

homozygous for one particular allele is 1 in 4 (25%) (Fig. 6.9A).

If a locus is on the X chromosomes, males can only carry one allele (because they only have one X chromosome). They are said to be *hemizygous* for a particular allele. All daughters of a male hemizygous for an abnormal gene will receive that gene; on the other hand, none of the sons will receive the abnormal gene (because a male must pass on a Y chromosome to his sons, and not an X). Each time a heterozygous female has a child, there is a 50% chance it will be a boy, and if it is a boy, a 50% chance that he will be affected. Likewise there is a 50% chance of a girl and a 50% chance she will be heterozygous (Fig. 6.9B).

Dominant and recessive inheritance

Disorders where it is only necessary to carry one abnormal allele in order for an individual to be affected are said to be dominant. In autosomal dominant disorders, the abnormal gene is carried on a non-sex chromosome; in X-linked disorders, the gene is carried on the X chromosome.

In recessive inheritance, an individual is only affected if he does not carry a normal allele at all. For autosomal recessive inheritance, affected individuals will be homozygous for the abnormal allele and both of the parents will be heterozygote carriers. In X-linked recessive disorders, males hemizygous for the abnormal allele will be affected, whereas heterozygous females will be unaffected.

Typical pedigree patterns are shown in Figures 6.10 and 6.11.

New mutation, penetrance and gene expression

Abnormal alleles have to arise somewhere in a pedigree by the process of *new mutation*. Sometimes this can be inferred in a case where an affected individual for an autosomal dominant disorder has normal parents. However, many autosomal dominant disorders also display *incomplete penetrance* or *reduced expression*. This means the gene carriers sometimes show no signs, or only a few minor signs, of the condition. The two phenomena are therefore important in the context of genetic counselling.

If a person has an autosomal dominant disorder, but there is no family history, both parents must be examined very carefully in order to determine whether either of them carries the abnormal gene. If they do not carry the gene, the chance of them having a further affected child will be very small (as this would require two, unconnected, new mutations). On the other hand, if one parent shows very minor signs of the condition, recurrence risk would be 50% for a further affected child.

Gene maps and linkage

The presence of loci close to one another on chromosomes leads to the phenomenon of linkage. The closer together loci are on a chromosome, the lower the probability that a crossover will take place between them during meiosis I, and the higher the probability that two alleles inherited from the parent will be passed on *together* to an offspring. Linkage between loci can be studied in suitable families by looking at the joint inheritance of specific traits, and an estimate can be made of the distance separating the loci.

These family studies are informative for linkage but do not give information about the chromosomes on which the loci are situated. This problem is known as *gene assignment* and can be tackled by a number of different methods such as somatic cell hybrids. Using these methods, a human gene map is being constructed giving information about the assignment of various loci and their distance from other loci on the same chromosome.

CHROMOSOME DISORDERS

Frequency of chromosomal disorders

About 7 per 1000 babies are born with detectable chromosomal anomalies. Of these, 3 per 1000 will have sex chromosome anomalies, 1.5 per 1000 autosomal trisomies (mainly Down's syndrome) and the remaining 2.5 per 1000 will have chromosomal rearrangements. Most of the latter are balanced, i.e. no genetic material is lost.

Of the autosomal trisomies, only trisomy 21 (Down's syndrome) cases are likely to survive into adulthood. The sex chromosome anomalies will frequently present with infertility or amenorrhoea. Unbalanced chromosomal rearrangements usually cause severe physical and mental handicap. However, balanced rearrangements have no effect on the carrier, although they predispose to recurrent miscarriage and children with unbalanced chromosome complements. An unbalanced karyotype means that there is duplication or deletion of some genetic material.

Down's syndrome

Between 1 in 700–1000 live births have Down's syndrome. The characteristic physical features are well described in paediatric texts and are present at birth, allowing immediate clinical diagnosis in most cases (Fig. 6.12). The head is foreshortened (brachycephaly) and there are usually three fontanelles. The eyes have an upward slant and crescents of skin are present covering the inner canthi (epicanthic folds). Brushfield spots are commonly seen on the iris. These are small white spots, situated around the outer third of the iris. The nasal bridge is flat and the tongue protruberant and deeply furrowed. A single transverse palmar crease is present on the hand, together with a short, incurved fifth finger (clinodactyly). A wide gap is present between the first and second toes, often with a longitudinal palmar crease. Hypotonia and delayed development are universal. Congenital heart defects (particularly A-V canal defects) and duodenal atresia can occur. It is essential that the chromosomal type of a Down's syndrome child is obtained. There are three possibilities (Table 6.2):

1. In about 95% of cases, there is an extra, free-lying chromosome 21. This form of Down's syndrome is associated with increased maternal age. The risk at a maternal age of 37 years is one in 250, at 40 years one in 100, and at 45 years one in 40.
2. In 2–3% of Down's syndrome cases, there is a chromosome translocation, usually involving Robertsonian translocation. The parents of such individuals must be checked to see whether they carry a balanced translocation.
3. The remaining Down's cases are mosaic. In these

Fig. 6.12 Down's syndrome.

cases, the degree of mental retardation can vary according to the proportion of abnormal cells.

The recurrence risks for Down's syndrome are set out in Table 6.3.

Table 6.2 Chromosomal types of Down's syndrome

Types of Down's syndrome	Chromosome complement	Comment
Standard trisomy 21	47,XX, +21 or 47,XY, +21	Approximately 95% of Down's syndrome children
Translocation Down's syndrome	e.g. 46,XY, −14, +t(14:21) 46,XX, −21, +t(21q:21q)	In about 2–3% of cases, an extra chromosome 21 is attached to another chromosome. It is essential to examine the chromosomes of the parents, as one may carry a balanced translocation
Mosaic Down's syndrome	e.g. 46,XX/47,XX, +21	Can be demonstrated in about 2–3% of cases

Table 6.3 Recurrence risks for Down's syndrome

Type of Down's syndrome	Risk to sibs of affected patient	Risk to other relatives (excluding offspring of an affected patient)
Standard trisomy 21		
Mother <40 years old	1%	Probably similar to
Mother >40 years old	Population risk	population risk
Translocation Down's (Parents have normal chromosomes)	Population risk	Population risk
Translocation Down's (One parent carries the translocated chromosome)		
Mother carries 14:21 translocation	10%	Depends on chromosomes of relative
Father carries 14:21 translocation	2%	Depends on chromosomes of relative
Either parent carries 21:21 translocation	100%	Depends on chromosomes of relative
Mosaic Down's	Population risk	Population risk

Sex chromosome abnormalities

Klinefelter's syndrome

Klinefelter's syndrome (47,XXY) occurs in about one in 1000 males. Adult individuals tend to have eunuchoid proportions with female fat distribution and gynaecomastia. The testes are small. Pituitary gonadotrophins are raised

and androgen production is low. Affected individuals are sterile, as they produce no sperm. Androgen therapy may help to improve libido and encourage the development of male secondary sexual characteristics. Intelligence is usually normal, although mild to moderate retardation may be seen.

XYY males

About one in 1500 males are XYY, i.e. they have an extra Y chromosome. Such individuals are physically normal although they tend to be tall. Although an increased tendency to psychopathic behaviour has been reported, prospective studies have shown that the majority of affected individuals lead normal lives.

Turner's syndrome

The incidence of Turner's syndrome (45,X) is one in 5000 births. Affected individuals are short, tend to have a web of skin on the lateral borders of the neck (Fig. 6.13), and may have other physical abnormalities such as a broad chest with wide-spread nipples and an increased carrying angle at the elbows. Coarctation of the aorta can occur. The vagina and internal genitalia are normally formed, but the ovaries consist of simple streaks of fibrous tissue without ovarian follicles, so that primary amenorrhoea is

Fig. 6.13 Turner's syndrome, 45,XO, showing characteristic facies, webbing of the neck, absent breast development and widely spaced nipples.

the rule. Treatment consists of oestrogen replacement around puberty to promote the development of secondary sexual characteristics.

47,XXX females

Females with a chromosome constitution 47,XXX have no physical abnormalities. However, primary and secondary amenorrhoea may occur, and IQ is 20–30 points below average, so that mental retardation is more common than in the general population. Nevertheless, the majority of affected females (about 70–80%) have normal intelligence.

Chromosome aberrations and cancer

Cytogenetic analysis of any malignant cell will frequently reveal a non-specific chromosome abnormality. However, there are certain malignancies where a characteristic abnormality is found; in others, the development of a specific

Table 6.4 Chromosome aberrations in different types of malignancies

Chromosome aberration present in tumour cells only	Malignancy	Comment
t(9:22)	Chronic myeloid leukaemia	These are characteristic changes. c-myc and c-abl oncogenes are on chromosomes 8 and 9. Immunoglobulin genes are on chromosomes 2, 14 and 22.
t(8:2)	Burkitt's lymphoma	
t(8:14)	Burkitt's lymphoma	
t(8:22)	Burkitt's lymphoma	
t(8:21)	Acute myeloblastic leukaemia	Loci involved uncertain
Trisomy 12	Chronic lymphocytic leukaemia	Good prognosis
inv (16)	Acute non-lymphocytic leukaemia	Good prognosis
Complex rearrangements	Acute non-lymphocytic leukaemia	Poor prognosis
Constitutional chromosome abnormality predisposing to specific cancers		
del(13q)	Retinoblastoma	Deletion may be submicroscopic and only revealed by DNA studies.
del(11p)	Wilms' tumour	Deletion may be submicroscopic and only revealed by DNA studies.
Trisomy 21 (Down's syndrome)	Acute lymphocytic anaemia	

chromosome change can be of prognostic significance (Table 6.4). In the case of Burkitt's lymphoma and chronic myeloid leukaemia, the chromosome translocations are known to bring together the loci for immunoglobulin genes and specific oncogenes (see p. 142). In other cases, the precise nature of the genetic change is not known. Occasionally, an individual with a specific chromosome abnormality will be predisposed to develop particular types of cancer (Table 6.4).

Genetic disorders predisposing to chromosome breakage

A group of single gene disorders exists, which result in an increased tendency to chromosome breakage, due to abnormalities of DNA repair after damage by agents such as ultraviolet light and radiation. These disorders, most of which are autosomal recessive, also predispose to malignancies (Table 6.5).

Table 6.5 Genetic disorders predisposing to chromosome breakage

Disorder	Clinical features
Fanconi's anaemia	Short stature, radial defects, patches of skin hyperpigmentation, pancytopenia, malignancies
Ataxia telangiectasia	Telangiectasia of conjunctiva, face and ears, ataxia, malignancies
Bloom syndrome	Short stature, facial telangiectasia, immunodeficiency, leukaemia
Xeroderma pigmentosum	Skin freckles and carcinomata, sensitivity to uv light, sometimes mental retardation

SINGLE GENE DISORDERS

Sir Archibald Garrod first put forward the concept of an 'inborn error of metabolism' in 1908 after studying alkaptonuria, a familial disorder in which patients excrete large amounts of homogentisic acid. This led to the concept that an enzyme controlling a metabolic step can be missing or reduced, leading to failure of production of essential metabolites further down the metabolic chain (e.g. in albinism) or accumulation of toxic substrates of the enzyme (e.g. in alkaptonuria and phenylketonuria) (Fig. 6.14).

Today, McKusick's catalogue of genetic disorders lists over 2000 defects involving every organ system. Only a few important groups of disorders are described here.

Aminoacidopathies

Defects in the metabolism of amino acids include a form of congenital hypothyroidism, albinism, disorders of the urea cycle and organic acid metabolism, as well as the disorders described below.

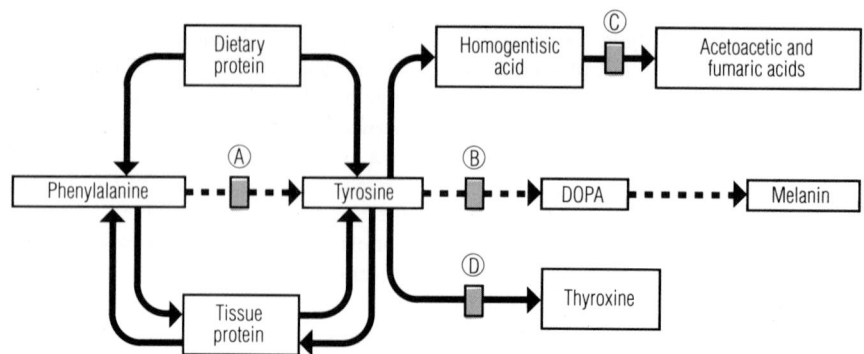

Fig. 6.14   Partial metabolic pathway of phenylalanine, tyrosine and related compounds showing position of 'metabolic blocks' caused by enzyme deficiencies. (A) Deficiency of phenylalanine hydroxylase results in an inability to metabolise phenylalanine, leading to phenylketonuria. Dietary tyrosine prevents albinism and hypothyroidism. (B) Tyrosinase deficiency leads to an inability to produce melanin, thus causing albinism. (C) Deficiency of homogentisic acid oxidase leads to the accumulation of homogentisic acid, and hence to alkaptonuria. (D) Deficiency of any one of several enzymes at this point means that thyroxine cannot be synthesised. The result is familial hypothyroidism.

Phenylketonuria

Phenylketonuria is an autosomal recessive disorder affecting about one in 10 000 infants at birth. It is usually caused by a defect of the enzyme phenylalanine hydroxylase, which converts phenylalanine to tyrosine. The most common clinical presentation, now rarely seen, is vomiting in early infancy, with eczema, depigmentation of skin and hair, hypertonia, seizures, and mental retardation developing during the first years of life. Fortunately, screening at birth is now widely available. This involves placing a drop of blood, obtained within the first few days of life, onto a filter paper and using a bacterial inhibition assay to measure phenylalanine levels in the so-called *Guthrie test*. Affected infants can be treated by giving an artificial diet low in phenylalanine until at least eight years of age. If dietary control is strict, prognosis for mental development is good.

Females with phenylketonuria run a very high risk of having abnormal children, unless a strict diet is reintroduced throughout pregnancy. Their children do not have phenylketonuria themselves, but the abnormal metabolites cross the placenta during pregnancy and affect the developing fetus. Microcephaly, cardiac defects and mental retardation are common.

Phenylketonuria is a heterogenous disorder; the most common form results from a mutation at the phenylalanine hydroxylase locus itself. However, a rarer form due to a defect in dihydropteridine reductase has been described. This enzyme is essential for the recycling of the cofactor, tetrahydrobiopterine.

Homocystinuria

Homocystinuria is an autosomal recessive disorder and affects one in 200 000 infants. It is due to a defect of cystathionine β-synthase and leads to the accumulation of homocysteine, methionine and other metabolites. Clinical manifestations include lens dislocation, mental retardation, osteoporosis and thrombosis of arteries and veins. Affected individuals tend to be long and thin, making Marfan's syndrome part of the differential diagnosis. Treatment involves a low methionine diet, and pyridoxine treatment in that proportion of patients who are vitamin B_6 responsive.

Cystinosis

Cystinosis should be distinguished from cystinuria (Table 6.6). The precise biochemical abnormality is not known, but there are abnormally high intracellular levels of free cystine, which lead to crystal deposition in the kidneys, conjunctiva, bones and leucocytes. Presentation is in childhood with photophobia and crystalline deposits in the conjunctiva, and the effects of renal tubular malabsorption (Fanconi's syndrome). Renal failure can occur before the age of ten years. Inheritance of cystinosis is autosomal recessive.

Alkaptonuria

Alkaptonuria is a rare autosomal recessive disorder due to a defect in the enzyme homogentisic acid oxidase (Fig. 6.14). Homogentisic acid, a byproduct of the metabolism of tyrosine and phenylalanine, cannot be metabolised, and so accumulates in the body tissues and is excreted in increased quantities in the urine. Classically, the urine turns dark on standing, and the sweat may be black, but these findings are not invariable. The homogentisic acid and resultant polymers also stain cartilage and other connective tissue; ochronosis is the name given to the generalised blue/grey pigmentation that results and is best seen in the cartilage of the ear and the sclerae. It can also be seen in the tendons of the hands, through the overlying skin, in older patients.

The main clinical problem in alkaptonuria is arthritis, which affects the hips, knees, shoulders and spine. Onset is unusual before middle age. Radiological changes include narrowing and calcification of the intervertebral discs, together with some fusion of the vertebral bodies. Rarer complications include an increased incidence of ischaemic heart disease, calcification of the cardiac valves, and

Table 6.6 Transport disorders

Disorder	Site	Metabolites affected	Clinical features	Inheritance
Intestinal disaccharidase deficiency	Small intestine	Maltose, sucrose, lactose	Abdominal pain and distension, diarrhoea	Autosomal recessive
Hypophosphataemic rickets	Renal tubules	Phosphates	Rickets (vitamin D-resistant)	X-linked dominant
Hartnup disease	Renal tubules	Amino acids (mono-amino-monocarboxylic group)	Red, scaly facial rash, ataxia	Autosomal recessive
Cystinuria	Renal tubules, small intestine	Cystine, ornithine, arginine, lysine	Renal stones	Autosomal recessive
Nephrogenic diabetes insipidus	Renal tubules	Insensitivity to ADH	Polyuria, polydipsia	X-linked dominant

occasionally arterial aneurysms. Treatment is symptomatic.

Transport disorders

The transport of metabolites across cell membranes often involves specific binding sites and transport proteins. Mutations can disrupt these mechanisms and result in a group of disorders characterised by the failure of essential metabolites to enter the appropriate body compartments. Some important disorders are outlined in Table 6.6.

Storage disorders

Macromolecules in the body are often in a perpetual state of accumulation and breakdown. Thus, if an enzyme

Table 6.7 Storage disorders

Type	Example	Symptoms
Glycogen storage disorders	8 types including: Von Gierke's disease (glucose-6-phosphate deficiency) Pompe's disease (acid maltase deficiency)	Hepatomegaly, hypoglycaemia, muscle weakness, cardiac failure. (Symptoms vary according to type).
Sphingolipidoses	Niemann-Pick disease Gaucher's disease Krabbe's disease Metachromatic leukodystrophy	Hepatosplenomegaly (in some), progressive neurological deterioration
Gangliosidoses	Tay-Sachs disease	Progressive blindness and neurological deterioration
Mucopolysaccharidoses	At least 8 types including: Hurler's syndrome Hunter's syndrome Maroteaux-Lamy syndrome Morquio syndrome	Hepatosplenomegaly, abnormal bones (dysostosis multiplex), corneal clouding, mental deterioration

needed to break down a macromolecule is deficient, increased accumulation occurs, leading to a variety of symptoms according to the type of molecule and the site involved. Storage material usually accumulates in the lysosomes. Several examples are given in Table 6.7.

Connective tissue disorders

The main protein of connective tissue is collagen. There are at least four different types of collagen, each with its own functions (Table 6.8). Defects of collagen synthesis can cause a wide variety of disorders (Table 6.9). Some of these have been characterised at the molecular level, and

Table 6.8 Types of collagen and their functions

Type	Function
I	Major collagen in skin, tendon, bones, heart valves and scar tissue
II	Major collagen in cartilage
III	Found mainly in blood vessels and intestine; also in skin
IV	Found mainly in basement membranes

Table 6.9 Connective tissue disorders

Disorder	Clinical features
Ehlers-Danlos syndrome (At least 8 distinct forms)	Hyperextensible skin, loose joints, 'cigarette paper' scars, easy bruising, rupture of blood vessels, internal viscera etc.
Osteogenesis imperfecta (At least 4 distinct forms)	Multiple fractures of bones, blue sclerae, hyperextensible skin, easy bruising
Cutis laxa (Several different forms)	Loose skin, premature aged appearance, hernias, diverticulae and emphysema
Marfan's syndrome	Tall stature, span greater than height, loose joints, dislocated lens of eyes, aortic and mitral incompetence, dissection and aneurysms of the aorta

6

various collagen probes are available for precise diagnosis. The specific collagen chain abnormality can sometimes be deduced from the clinical features (Table 6.9). Thus, some forms of osteogenesis imperfecta are caused by abnormalities of type I collagen; while type III collagen deficiency can result in a form of Ehlers-Danlos syndrome, with thin, atrophic skin and a tendency to spontaneous rupture of blood vessels and other internal organs. Defects of the connective tissue protein elastin are thought to cause the different forms of cutis laxa. Both collagen and elastin are abnormal in pseudoxanthoma elasticum (Ch. 13, Table 13.27).

MULTIFACTORIAL DISORDERS

Many common malformations, some diseases, and many normal traits are said to have a *multifactorial* origin.

This means that both genetic and environmental factors contribute to their aetiology. Furthermore, the genetic component is thought to be due to several genes acting together, so-called *polygenic* inheritance. The inheritance of height is a good example of a trait determined by multifactorial inheritance. The genetic component is determined by several genes, and final height correlates between parents and children. Nevertheless, environmental factors (such as nutrition) can play an important role. The contribution of the many factors involved results in a Gaussian (normal) distribution of height in the general population.

Common malformations

There are many clues which suggest that a common malformation has a multifactorial origin:

1. After one affected family member, the risk to other first degree relatives is usually in the range 1–5%, depending on the condition.
2. The presence of additional affected family members increases the risk to subsequent offspring.
3. Where a condition can have varying degrees of severity (for example cleft lip, with or without cleft palate), risks are higher for relatives of an individual with a more severe malformation.
4. If there is a sex difference in incidence, risks are greater for relatives of an affected individual of the least commonly affected sex.
5. The risk declines rapidly as one passes from first to second degree relatives.

It is thought that everyone inherits a *liability* to a particular malformation. The degree of liability can vary in different individuals and families, according to the number of adverse genes and environmental factors present. If the liability exceeds a given threshold, the malformation is manifested. Individuals from families where there is more than one affected member will, on average, have a higher liability, as will relatives of more severely affected individuals. Similarly, where a condition is less common in a

Table 6.10 Recurrence risk (%) in some common multifactorial malformations

Condition	Normal parent		Affected parent
	Risk of second affected child	Risk of third affected child	Risk of affected child
Cleft palate alone	2	8	7
Cleft lip ± cleft palate	4	10	4
Neural tube defect	4	10	4
Club foot	3	10	3
Dislocation of hip	6	10	12
Congenital heart disease (varies with type)	1–4	5–10	1–10
Hirschsprung's disease (long segment):			
Male index case	8	–	–
Female index case	14	–	–
Pyloric stenosis:			
Male index case	3	–	4
Female index case	7	–	13

particular sex, affected persons of that sex must carry a greater liability, as will their relatives.

Some common multifactorial malformations with their recurrence risks are given in Table 6.10.

Common diseases, genetic markers and disease association

Many common diseases, e.g. the common allergies, and some forms of epilepsy, have been proposed as candidates for multifactorial inheritance. As more research is carried out into these conditions, heterogeneity is recognised and subtypes are defined. Subdivision is aided by the identification of genetic markers, which may indicate that a major contribution to the disorder is being made by a gene on a specific chromosome. These genetic markers are particular blood groups, tissue types or restriction fragment length polymorphisms at specific gene loci which are found to occur more commonly in individuals with the disorder (Table 6.11).

A good example of the complex interaction between environmental factors and genetic loci is provided by the various possible causes of atheroma. A proportion of patients with early onset atherosclerosis show abnormalities of lipoproteins or lipoprotein receptors which are determined by various gene loci. In some patients, a single gene defect (e.g. of the cell membrane low-density lipoprotein receptors) can strongly predispose to atheroma. In the majority of cases, however, factors such as diet, smoking and high blood pressure may play the pre-

Table 6.11 Some common disorders of multifactorial origin, with possible genetic markers

Disorder	Marker	Status of marker studies
Insulin dependent diabetes mellitus	HLA haplotypes e.g. B8, B15, DW3, DW4	Established
Coeliac disease	HLA-A1-B8-DW3	Established
Ankylosing spondylitis Reiter's disease Anterior uveitis	HLA-B27	Established
Non-insulin dependent diabetes	Polymorphism around insulin gene	Probable
Peptic ulceration	Blood group O	Established
Atherosclerosis	Apolipoprotein A-1	Established
	Polymorphism around insulin gene	Probable
	Low density lipoprotein receptors	Established

dominant role, with minor abnormalities of the lipoproteins merely providing an extra predisposition.

Linkage disequilibrium and pleiotropy

There are two possible explanations for the association of a genetic marker and a specific disease; linkage disequilibrium and pleiotropy.

Linkage disequilibrium. If a genetic marker (e.g. a restriction fragment length polymorphism) is extremely closely linked to a disease locus, specific marker alleles may not be separated from the disease allele by recombination over the generations and an *association* will be observed in random individuals. This is known as linkage disequilibrium. It should be noted that linkage disequilibrium is a special case, observed only with very close linkage. In most cases of linkage, recombination over many generations will mean that a particular marker allele will not necessarily be associ-

ated with the disease in individuals picked at random.

Pleiotropy. The allele at the marker locus itself may predispose an individual to develop the disease, due to some function of the gene. Some of the disorders associated with specific HLA types may be examples of a pleiotropic effect. For example, a specific HLA type may predispose to infection with specific viruses, leading to some forms of insulin dependent diabetes mellitus.

MANAGEMENT OF GENETIC DISORDERS

Screening

The treatment of many genetic disorders is often most successful if the disorder is diagnosed in an early, presymptomatic stage. In addition, the prevention of genetic disease by genetic counselling and prenatal diagnosis requires the identification of asymptomatic gene carriers. For these reasons, genetic screening programmes have been developed. Depending on the nature and frequency of the condition, screening can involve the entire population, subgroups of the population (for example, particular ethnic groups), or specific families in which a genetic disorder is known to be segregating (Table 6.12).

Treatment of genetic disorders

It is not yet possible to replace missing or defective genes; although it may be possible to isolate and replicate a gene in the laboratory, it is much more difficult to ensure that a replacement gene reaches the correct tissue, and is properly regulated.

There are, however, a number of treatment strategies for genetic disorders which aim to ameliorate the phenotypic effects. Many common malformations of multifactorial or chromosomal origin can be corrected surgically; while a variety of treatments have been devised for single gene disorders (Table 6.13).

Table 6.12 Screening for genetic disorders

Disease	Group screened	Method	Purpose
Phenylketonuria	Total population of neonates	Guthrie test	Early dietary treatment of affected homozygotes
Hypothyroidism	Total population of neonates	TSH levels from dried blood spot	Early thyroxine therapy
Sickle cell anaemia and other haemoglobinopathies	Offspring of heterozygote mothers (total population of neonates in some regions)	Haemoglobin electrophoresis	Prophylaxis and early treatment of complications. Prevention by counselling and prenatal diagnosis.
Tay-Sachs disease	Individuals of Ashkenazi Jewish extraction	Carrier detection by serum enzyme analysis	Prenatal diagnosis where both parents are heterozygous
Adult-onset polycystic renal disease	Relatives of affected individuals	Renal ultrasound, blood pressure, gene tracking in families using DNA probes	Early treatment of hypertension and renal failure
Multiple endocrine adenomatosis	Relatives of affected individuals	Calcitonin, urinary VMA, gene tracking in families using DNA probes	Early treatment of endocrine tumours

The Genetic Basis of Disease

Table 6.13 Therapy for single gene disorders*

Treatment	Disorder
Replacement therapy	
Replacement of deficient protein	Haemophilias
	Diabetes
Replacement of deficient vitamin or co-enzyme:	
Vitamin B$_{12}$	Methylmalonicacidaemia (some types)
Vitamin D	Vitamin D-resistant rickets
Biotin	Biotinidase deficiency
Replacement of deficient metabolite:	
Cortisone	Adrenogenital syndrome
Thyroxine	Congenital hypothyroidism
Organ or cell replacement:	
Kidney	Polycystic renal disease
Bone marrow	Immunodeficiencies
	Osteoporosis
Blood transfusion	Thalassaemias
Amelioration therapy	
Restriction of substrates in diet:	
Phenylalanine	Phenylketonuria
Methionine	Homocystinuria
Galactose	Galactosaemia
Drug therapy to remove harmful metabolites:	
Penicillamine	Wilson's disease
Cholestyramine	Hypercholesterolaemia
Iron chelating agents	Thalassaemias
Avoidance of harmful drugs or dietary factors	G6PD deficiency
	Porphyria
Preventive therapy	
Removal of potentially malignant tissues	Polyposis coli
Removal of site of destruction of diseased cells (e.g. spleen)	Spherocytosis

*After Emery 1984

Genetic counselling

Most doctors will be faced at some stage with questions about the risk of a genetic disorder in patients or their families. Straightforward situations, such as Down's syndrome or neural tube defect, can be dealt with by the non-specialist; but complex problems, involving the diagnosis of rare disorders or the use of carrier detection tests and linkage studies, require a specialist opinion.

Whatever the problem, there are a number of essential steps in genetic counselling:

1. *Detailed family history.* At least a three generation pedigree should be taken and details of racial background and consanguinity (i.e. whether parents have common ancestors) obtained.

2. *Accurate diagnosis in affected family members.* An accurate diagnosis in affected family members must be made. This should include both a pathological diagnosis (established where possible from original notes and investigations) and an assessment of any genetic subgroup of the disorder.

3. *Ancillary tests.* Chromosome analysis, DNA marker studies or other carrier detection tests may need to be carried out, according to the nature of the problem.

4. *Risk assessment.* For single gene disorders, risk assessment is sometimes straightforward, providing a correct diagnosis is available. For example, the recurrence of risk for a couple who have had one child with phenylketonuria is one in four, because phenylketonuria is autosomal recessive. However, difficulties arise where a disorder has different inheritance types (e.g. retinitis pigmentosa) and with X-linked disorders, where carrier detection tests may need to be applied, new mutations have to be considered and risks must be modified to allow for normal sons in the pedigree. In addition, disorders with a late age of onset (such as Huntington's chorea) or of variable expression (such as tuberose sclerosis) can present problems that may require a specialist opinion. Where linked DNA probes are used, risk assessment can become complex. If a condition is caused by a chromosomal abnormality or is multifactorial, empirical risks derived from follow-up studies must be used.

5. *Prenatal diagnosis.* The availability of prenatal diagnostic tests (Table 6.14) has to be assessed and any possible risks to the mother or fetus weighed against the risk of fetal abnormality.

6. *Communicating risks.* Having marshalled all the facts, sufficient time must be set aside to discuss the risks in detail with the patient. A non-directive approach should be taken, whereby objective risks are given and discussed in detail, in the light of the severity of the condition, and the availability and reliability of prenatal diagnosis. These factors may be crucial in the final decision of the parents.

It is best to give the risks as a proportion (i.e. one in two; one in 100 etc.) and to emphasise that a one in 20 risk of a child being affected means that 19 times out of 20 the child will not be affected. In order to put the risks into perspective, it is also worth pointing out that over one in 50 children are born with significant abnormalities at birth. In comparison to these background risks, a genetic risk of one in 20 is generally regarded as low, and those of greater than one in 10 as relatively high. However, the perception of an 'unacceptable' risk will depend on a large number of factors. The severity of the condition and the availability of treatment will obviously affect the willingness of a couple to have further children. For example, a one in 20 risk of a child with isolated cleft lip and palate will often be seen as acceptable, whereas the same risk for a child with severe, untreatable mental retardation may seem too high.

7. *Sympathy and understanding.* If a couple have given birth to an abnormal child, the genetic counselling clinic is often the place where considerable feelings of guilt are expressed. Alternatively, there may be an understandable tendency to blame poor medical care or environmental factors for the abnormalities. Time should be set aside to discuss all these feelings in a sympathetic and under-

Table 6.14 Techniques of prenatal diagnosis

Procedure	Timing	Types of disorder detected
Villus biopsy	Transcervical 9–11 weeks Transabdominal 12–16 weeks	Cytogenetic abnormalities Enzyme defects Single gene defects (DNA probes)

Maternal α-fetoprotein	16–19 weeks	α-fetoprotein
		  Raised: neural tube defects
		  Lowered: Down's syndrome
		           Edwards' syndrome
		(N.B. These are screening tests; diagnosis must be confirmed by further investigation)

Amniocentesis	16–20 weeks	Cytogenetic abnormalities Enzyme defects Neural tube defects Single gene defects (DNA probes)

Ultrasound	From 16 weeks	Anatomical defects
		  Neural tube/hydrocephalus
		  Body wall defects
		  Limb reduction defects
		  Hydrops
		  Major urinary anomaly
		  Bone dysplasias
		  Cardiac defects
		  Craniofacial anomalies

Fetoscopy/ cordocentesis	16–20 weeks	Fetal blood sample
		  Clotting disorders
		  Haemoglobinopathies
		  Cytogenetic abnormalities
		Fetal skin biopsy
		  Epidermolysis bullosa
		  Ichthyosis
		  Albinism
		Fetal liver biopsy
		  Urea cycle enzyme defects
		Fetal visualisation
		  Craniofacial defects
		  Digital defects
		  Genital defects

standing manner, as they are part of the normal reaction to the birth of an abnormal child. Guilt and blame are usually the result of lack of information. Once a couple have been fully informed of the nature and causes of a child's problems, they can be helped to accept the fact that many genetic abnormalities are unavoidable.

Successful genetic counselling requires a combination of communication skills, detailed genetic knowledge, and a sound clinical background in both adult and paediatric medicine, if couples are to be helped to make the most appropriate decisions about childbearing. It is this combination that makes the practice of clinical genetics so rewarding.

FURTHER READING

Emery A E H 1984 An introduction to recombinant DNA. John Wiley, London. *An excellent review of the impact of DNA techniques on all branches of medicine*

Harper P S 1988 Practical genetic counselling, 3rd edn. John Wright & Sons, Bristol. *A comprehensive introduction to the problems of clinical genetics*

McKusick V A 1988 Mendelian inheritance in man, 8th edn. The Johns Hopkins Press, London. *A catalogue of all known single gene disorders in man*

The Immunological Basis of Disease

The immune system exists in order to recognise and eliminate infectious micro-organisms. Its normal working is unobtrusive and can be detected only by cellular or serological changes. However, there are five circumstances in which it comes to the attention of the doctor:

1. *Inadequate immunity.* Immunity may be inadequate either because a particular micro-organism is difficult or impossible to eliminate, which leads to persistent infection, or because, in a particular patient, some part of the immune system is deficient, either intrinsically or as a result of medical treatment. In this case, normally mild infections may become severe or fatal, and normally non-pathogenic organisms may cause unusual symptoms (opportunistic infection). Improved immune function may be brought about by vaccination, by immunostimulants, or by replacement therapy, depending on the circumstances.
2. *Hypersensitivity.* In the process of responding to a foreign organism, immune mechanisms may produce side-effects which damage normal host tissue. Reactions of this type are collectively known as hypersensitivity and can affect virtually any organ, the skin, joints and kidneys being especially vulnerable.
3. *Autoimmunity.* The normal ability of the immune system to discriminate foreign or 'non-self' material from 'self' may break down, leading to autoimmunity. Again, almost any organ can be affected, but autoimmunity is particularly common within the endocrine system.
4. *Immunosuppression.* It is sometimes desirable for foreign material *not* to be eliminated, e.g. in a blood transfusion or a kidney graft. Immunology therefore has an important contribution to make to the practice of transplantation, in minimising and/or *suppressing* the rejection response. Immunosuppression may also

be required for severe autoimmunity or hypersensitivity.
5. *Immunological techniques.* Finally, it should be mentioned that the extremely sensitive and precise discriminatory power of antibodies to recognise molecules of all kinds is made use of in the measurement of hormone levels etc by *immunoassay*, and in blood and tissue *typing*. Another special use of antibodies may be in the targeting of drugs etc on particular cells.

THE IMMUNE SYSTEM

The identification and management of the conditions mentioned above would be very hazardous without some understanding of the underlying mechanisms. This section summarises the essential information, but it must be remembered that research into immunology proceeds at an ever-increasing rate and many aspects are still controversial.

It is useful to distinguish between natural and adaptive immune mechanisms.

Natural immunity is based on ever-present and relatively unchanging elements such as *phagocytic cells*, together with *complement* and other tissue and serum factors.

Adaptive immunity is based on the special properties of *lymphocytes*, which include a high degree of specificity of individual cells for individual foreign molecules or *antigens*, rapid proliferation to expand a small specific population and the retention of specific *memory*. The term *immune response* is used to describe the events of adaptive immunity.

Another convenient distinction is between *cellular* and *humoral* immunity. The principal units of function in the immune system are a variety of cells and the molecules they secrete into the blood or extracellular fluids. The principal units of recognition are *receptors* carried by these cells; some of these recognise foreign material, and thus represent the actual interface between *self* and *non-self*, while some recognise other cells and allow them to *interact*.

The Immunological Basis of Disease

Fig.7.1 **Natural and adaptive immunity: The principal cells and molecules of the immune system and their interactions.** PMN = polymorphonuclear leucocyte, M = mast cell, Mac = macrophage, APC = antigen presenting cell, NK = natural killer cell. T cells: T^H = helper, T^C = cytotoxic, T^S = suppressor. IFN-γ = gamma interferon, IL-1 = interleukin 1, IL-2 = interleukin 2, HF = helper factor(s), SF = suppressor factor(s). Cells and molecules with high antigen specificity are printed in red. Red arrows indicate secretion of molecules.

Most cell-cell interactions are ultimately carried out by soluble factors called *cytokines*, usually acting only at close range.

The principal components of the natural and adaptive immune systems are shown in Figure 7.1, which also emphasises the number of important interactions between the two.

NATURAL IMMUNITY

Natural immune mechanisms are responsible for a great deal of resistance to infection, and deficiencies in them can be extremely serious.

Skin

The intact skin and mucous membranes constitute a barrier to the entry of many micro-organisms, which have to rely on injuries, insect bites etc in order to gain access to the body. However, some micro-organisms can penetrate these barriers by means of specific attachment and penetration mechanisms.

Antimicrobial secretions

Numerous anti-microbial substances (e.g. unsaturated fatty acids) are secreted onto the skin or into other secretions (e.g. lysozyme). Of particular importance in viral infections are the *interferons*, a family of molecules made by a variety of cells, which lead to the blocking of viral replication.

Phagocytosis

Once in the tissues, many micro-organisms are rapidly *phagocytosed* by polymorphonuclear leucocytes (PMN) or macrophages. Some bacteria (e.g. pneumococci) can resist phagocytosis by virtue of their capsules, while others (e.g. staphylococci) release toxins that destroy the phagocytes. Certain bacteria, fungi and protozoa can survive within phagocytic cells, to give rise to chronic infection and, often, chronic inflammation, but the majority of organisms are killed by a combination of acid pH, oxygen metabolites (e.g. hydrogen peroxide) and various cytotoxic proteins. Although it is over a century since the discovery of phagocytosis, the exact nature of the recognition between the phagocyte and its prey is still not properly understood.

Complement system

A second line of defence is the *complement* system (Fig. 7.2). This is a series of 20 serum proteins activated in succession to give three important effects:

1. the release of small peptides that stimulate inflammation and attract phagocytes
2. the deposition of a component (C3b) on microbial membranes which promotes their phagocytosis by virtue of attachment sites for C3b on phagocytic cells
3. the activation of lytic components which puncture cell membranes.

This activation 'cascade' can be triggered by numerous microbial surfaces, notably by the endotoxins of Gram-negative bacteria and, together with phagocytic cells, constitutes a rapid, integrated defence system against many bacteria, viruses, fungi etc. However, as will be seen (p. 106), both phagocytosis and other complement functions can be greatly enhanced by the presence of *antibody*. Also, many of the inflammatory effects of complement operate via *mast cells* which, scattered throughout the tissues, respond rapidly to injury to all kinds. Here, again, antibody can augment mast cell activation, sometimes to dangerous levels, as in allergies (p. 110).

Macrophage and PMN secretions

Not all killing is intracellular. With large targets, e.g. worms, and perhaps also with tumour cells, the secretion of toxic molecules by macrophages or PMN may contribute to killing. Macrophages are particularly active in this respect, and more than 80 secreted products have been

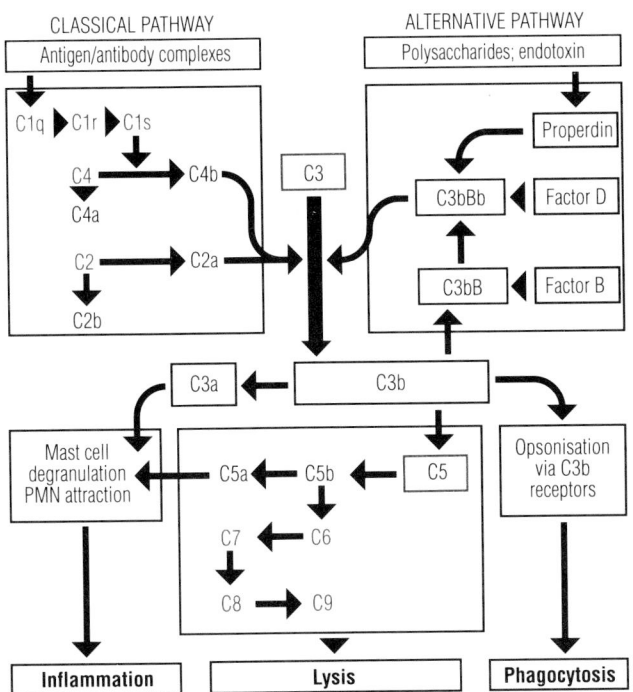

CLASSICAL PATHWAY
Antigen/antibody complexes

ALTERNATIVE PATHWAY
Polysaccharides; endotoxin

Fig. 7.2 Complement activation pathways. Components normally present in serum are shown outlined in red. Note the central role of C3→C3b conversion in both classical and alternative pathways.

identified, of which the most important are lysozyme, some complement components, oxygen metabolites, interferon, and a variety of cytotoxic proteins. In the case of tumours, *natural killer (NK) cells* are also thought to play a part, though exactly what lineage (macrophage or lymphocyte) these cells belong to, and how they function, has not yet been worked out.

ADAPTIVE IMMUNITY

The adaptive immune system represents a great advance over natural immune mechanisms in terms of both precision and flexibility. It is based on the *lymphocyte*, a type of cell found essentially only in vertebrates (whereas natural immunity is also found in invertebrates and, indeed, in the earliest life forms); by virtue of its *specificity* for individual chemical shapes or antigens and its extensive proliferative capacity, this cell confers on the animal the property of *memory* of particular infections. This, in turn, forms the basis for the frequently observed immunity to reinfection and the efficacy of vaccines. In both cases, a small *primary response* is followed, on subsequent contact with the same micro-organisms, by a greatly augmented, and biologically more effective, *secondary response*.

Lymphocytes are of two main kinds and give rise to two corresponding types of immune response:

1. B (bone-marrow derived) lymphocytes give rise to the *antibody-mediated (B)* immune response.

2. T (thymus-derived) lymphocytes give rise to the cell-mediated (T) immune response.

However, some T lymphocytes are also involved in antibody formation and in the complex regulation of all immune mechanisms, including many 'natural' ones. The T lymphocyte can thus be regarded as the central cell of the whole adaptive system.

THE GENETIC AND MOLECULAR BASIS OF ADAPTIVE IMMUNITY

The specificity of lymphocytes for individual antigens is mediated by specific surface *receptors*, which are complementary to and 'recognise' small portions of the antigenic molecule. B cells use, as their receptors, antibody molecules essentially identical to those they secrete when stimulated. T cell receptors are smaller, but more complex, since they recognise not only portions of antigen but also normal molecules found on the surface of cells with which they interact. These molecules, known as *class I* and *class II major histocompatibility antigens*, are of great importance in normal immune responses and also, unfortunately, in transplant rejection.

Three sets of highly polymorphic genes code for these recognition molecules (Fig. 7.3). They are spread over several chromosomes, but the amino acid sequences of the proteins they code for show a degree of homology that suggests they have all evolved from a single precursor gene. These proteins are:

1. the antibody, or immunoglobulin (Ig) molecule
2. the T cell receptor
3. the major histocompatibility antigens (HLA in man).

Antibody genes

The antibody genes are found on three separate chromosomes; two code for light (L) chains (kappa and lambda type) and one for heavy (H) chains. Each gene consists of four main regions:

1. V (variable)
2. D (diversity)
3. J (joining)
4. C (constant)

separated by untranslated introns. The V region contains several hundred copies, each slightly different, of a gene coding for the variable region of the antibody molecule; parts of the latter (the 'hypervariable regions') are responsible for antigen recognition, and thus specificity. The C region is much larger for heavy chains than for light chains because it includes, in tandem, the genes for all the immunoglobulin classes and subclasses (IgM, IgG etc; see p. 102).

In B lymphocytes, but not in other cells, rearrangement of DNA occurs so that particular V and D genes are brought next to a particular J gene. The RNA transcribed from this is further spliced, so that the VDJ and one of the C regions are brought together to code for a complete

101

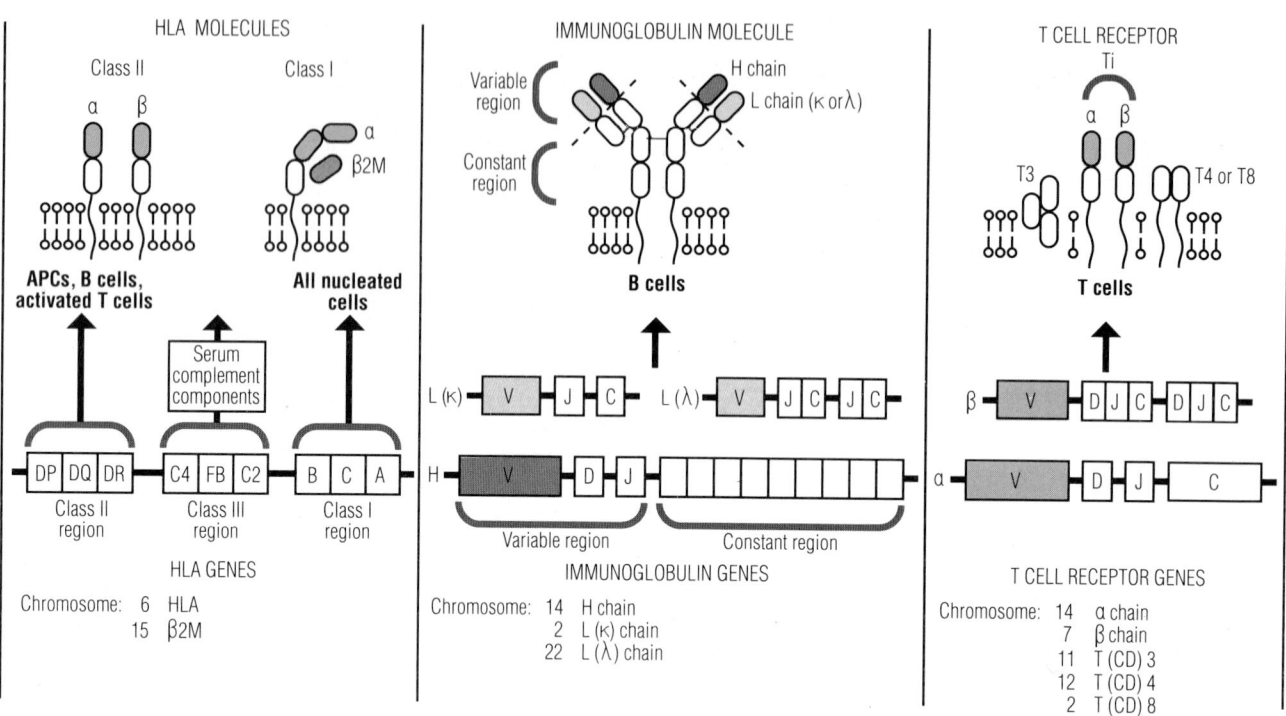

Fig. 7.3. Genes and molecules involved in immune recognition. The genes are shown in the centre, the molecules they code for at the top, inserted in the plasma membrane of the respective cells. Domains showing high variability and involved in antigen recognition are shown in red. Note that T and CD are alternative nomenclatures for T cell surface molecules, but the CD terminology also applies to molecules on other types of cell. APC = antigen-presenting cell; H = heavy; L = light.

polypeptide chain. Finally, two identical H chains and two identical L chains (either both kappa or both lambda) are disulphide-bonded and glycosylated, to form the antibody molecule, which is now ready either for secretion into the blood, or insertion into the B lymphocyte membrane as a specific receptor.

Individual B lymphocytes and their progeny retain transcription of the same V gene, but can switch from one C gene to another, usually in the direction IgM→IgG. The enormous diversity of V genes ensures that an antibody molecule can be produced to fit virtually any shape of antigenic determinant. How this diversity is generated has been the subject of heated controversy, but it is now agreed that the combinatorial possibilities of one heavy and two kinds of light chain plus, within each chain, a number of different V, D, and J genes, to which is added the occasional mutation, are sufficient to code for about 10^8 different antibody specificities.

Genetic differences between antibody molecules are known as *isotypic* if they reside in the constant region (the various classes and subclasses are thus isotypes), and as *idiotypic* if they reside in the hypervariable regions; the idiotype of an antibody is the portion which is unique to that variable region, and may include either the antigen combining site itself or the adjacent regions. There are also allelic differences known as *allotypes*, which enable the antibody molecules of one individual to be distinguished from those of another, just as with blood groups on the red cells.

The antibody molecule

The antibody or *immunoglobulin* (Ig) molecule is ideally suited to its function of promoting the removal of foreign antigens. Its basic structure is seen in antibodies of the IgG class (Fig.7.4).

The N-terminal half is composed of H and L chains and is responsible for binding to antigen (Fab portions); the C-terminal half (Fc portion), which consists of heavy chains alone, determines the *class* of antibody and is responsible for the biological functions of the molecule.

1. *IgG.* In the case of IgG, these functions include activation of complement, attachment to phagocytic cells, passage into the tissues, and transport across the placenta. The four IgG subclasses vary somewhat in these functions, while the other classes of Ig show more substantial differences.
2. *IgM* is a large molecule confined to the bloodstream, but very efficient at activating complement and agglutinating foreign material by virtue of its 10 combining sites.
3. *IgA* is secreted into, and can survive, in such locations as the eyes, nose, gut, and urine.
4. *IgE* attaches to mast cells and causes them to release the contents of their granules, which lead to increases in local vascular permeability and the changes of acute inflammation.
5. *IgD* is found mainly on B lymphocyte membranes, where it may have a role in triggering their responses.

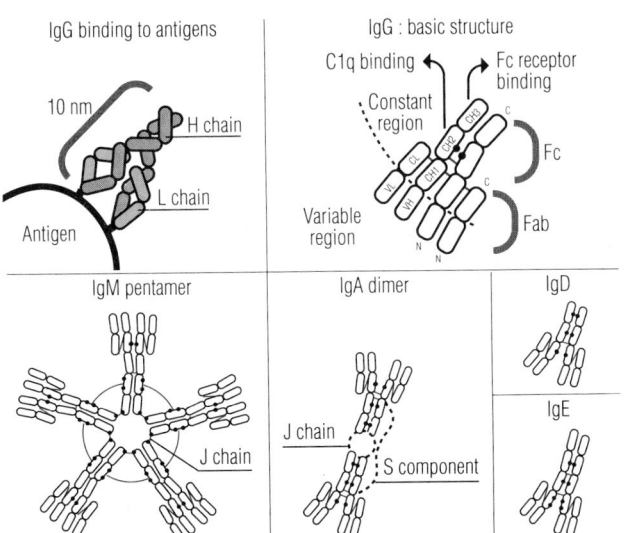

Fig. 7.4 Antibody structure and function: the five classes of immunoglobulins showing their main structural and functional differences. The basic domains of about 110 amino acids are shown as ellipsoids. Except in the top left figure, interchain disulphide bonds are in red (intrachain disulphide bonds are not shown). J chain = joining chain, which stabilises the pentameric and dimeric structure of IgM and IgA respectively; S component = secretory component, which allows IgA to be secreted and to avoid digestion by proteolytic enzymes. L chains are shown in red, and H chains in grey. Solid black circles represent carbohydrate side-chains. C1q = the first component of complement.

The properties of the various Ig classes and subclasses are summarised in Table 7.1.

The T cell receptor

The T cell receptor is a two-chain (alpha and beta) molecule, rather like a shortened immunoglobulin. In this case, DNA rearrangement occurs only in T lymphocytes. However, the T cell receptor has a more complicated combining site than antibody, and recognises combinations of small foreign peptides and molecules of the major histocompatibility complex (MHC; see below and Fig.7.5).

Associated with the T cell receptor are smaller molecules, named T3, T4, and T8 after the monoclonal antibodies which were first used to identify them, and these also play a part in cell-cell interaction. Their main practical value is that the corresponding monoclonal antibodies can be used to identify different kinds of T lymphocytes (p. 105).

The major histocompatibility complex

The important set of genes comprising the major histocompatibility complex (MHC) is so named because, in all higher animals, it dominates transplant rejection responses (p. 114). However, its normal function is to control cell-cell interactions in adaptive immunity (see below). The human MHC is known as HLA and its genes lie on the short arm of chromosome 6. They are grouped in two sets, referred to as class I and class II, each set containing three genetic loci, each of which has a large number of alleles coding for HLA antigens (Fig.7.3). The genes for certain complement components also lie within the MHC, but their products are quite unrelated to class I and class II molecules.

Class II HLA molecules are two-chain (alpha and beta) structures somewhat resembling the T cell receptor. Class I molecules consist of a larger alpha chain and a small beta chain known as beta-2-microglobulin whose gene lies on a different chromosome and shows no variability. In order for a T lymphocyte to respond to a foreign antigen, its receptor must interact with both the antigen and an HLA molecule.

Class I antigens (i.e. alleles at the A, B and C loci) are expressed on all nucleated cells (two from each locus on diploid cells), and are mainly concerned with the recognition of viral antigens by cytotoxic T cells (p. 107). Class II antigens (alleles at the DP, DQ, and DR loci) are expressed on a more limited range of cells, namely those with which T lymphocytes are required to interact – principally antigen-presenting cells, B lymphocytes, and certain other T lymphocytes – and are concerned with the initiation and control of the immune response (p. 106).

Quite apart from their importance in matching transplants, certain HLA antigens are associated with particular

Table 7.1 Classes and subclasses of immunoglobulin and their major features

Class	Subclass	Mol wt (sedimentation coefficient)	Normal serum level (g/l)	Functions Complement	Opsonisation
IgM		900 000 (19S)	0.5–2	+	
IgG	G1	150 000 (7S)	9	+	+
	G2	150 000 (7S)	3	+	
	G3	170 000 (7S)	1 } 7–19	+	+
	G4	150 000 (7S)	0.5		+
IgA	A1	160 000 (7S) or a dimer of	3	Protects mucous surfaces	
	A2	320 000 (11S)	0.5 } 0.8–5		
IgE		190 000 (7S)	50 ng/l	Mast cell activation	
IgD		180 000 (7S)	30 mg/l	B cell surface receptor	

Table 7.2 Major HLA-associated diseases

Disease type	Disease	Associated HLA antigen			
		DR	B	C	A
Joints	Ankylosing spondylitis		27(87)		
	Reiter's		27(37)		
	Juvenile RA		27		
	Rheumatoid arthritis	4(6)			
Skin	Psoriasis			W6(13)	1
	Alopecia		12		
	Behçet's		5		
Gut	Ulcerative colitis		5		
	Atrophic gastritis		7		
	Haemochromatosis		14		
	Coeliac disease	3(11)	8		
	Chronic active hepatitis	3(14)	8		
Endocrine and autoimmune	Addison's	3(6)	8*		
	IDDM	3(5) 4(7)	8(10)		
	Sjögren's	3(10)	8		
	Graves'	3(4)	8		
	Hashimoto's	5(3.2)			
	Myaesthenia gravis		8(4)		
Cancer	Thyroid	3(3), 1(6)			
CNS	Multiple sclerosis	2(5)	7		
	Narcolepsy	2			
Other	Allergies				23

The boxes denote the major HLA-associated diseases associated with particular alleles. The numbers refer to alleles at the various loci (B27, DR3, B8 etc.), and the numbers in brackets indicate the risk of developing the disease (if known) relative to the rest of the population.
*210H-ase gene linked to HLA-B

diseases (Table 7.2). Sometimes, as with antigen B27 and ankylosing spondylitis, this association is so strong as to be of value in diagnosis; more often, however, it is only relative. The combination of B8 and DR3 is associated with a variety of autoimmune diseases, and possible reasons for this are discussed on page 113. Figure 7.5 illustrates the probable interactions involved.

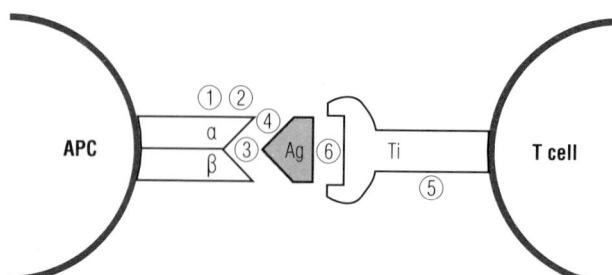

Fig.7.5 HLA and disease: a simplified scheme to show the probable interactions between antigen, HLA molecules and the T cell receptor. The numbers indicate points at which abnormalities may lead to unduly high or low responses to a foreign antigen, and so predispose to disease. (1) General high or low responsiveness associated with particular HLA combinations. (2) Linkage disequilibrium between HLA and other disease-associated genes. (3) Failure of an antigen to associate with a particular HLA molecule. (4) Suppressor-inducing epitopes on an antigen. (5) Lack of a specific T cell receptor for an antigen. (6) Resemblance between an antigen and particular HLA molecule.

LYMPHOCYTES

Like all other haemopoietic cells, lymphocytes originate from stem cells in the bone marrow; unlike other cells, however, they have the ability to leave and re-enter the circulation repeatedly. This facilitates the contact between a foreign antigen and the tiny minority of lymphocytes specific for it, which would otherwise be a very rare event. Differentiation and maturation of lymphocytes, and most of their functions, are carried out in specialised *lymphoid organs*.

Lymphoid organs

Primary

The B lymphocytes complete their maturation in the *bone marrow*, but T lymphocytes require passage through the *thymus* where, under the influence of peptide hormones probably secreted by epithelial cells, they acquire full immunocompetence. At the same time, they appear to 'learn' to recognise the individual's own HLA specificities and to avoid self-reactivity.

Secondary

The secondary lymphoid organs contain mature lymphocytes and are strategically placed where foreign antigens are likely to be encountered: *lymph nodes* for antigens in the tissues, the *spleen* for those in the blood, *Peyer's patches* for the small intestine, *tonsils* and *adenoids* for the nose, mouth and pharynx. The structure of secondary lymphoid tissue is best seen in the lymph node, where the cortex contains mainly B lymphocytes, and the paracortex T lymphocytes, while antibody-secreting plasma cells are found in the medulla. Other lymphoid organs show a similar demarcation, which is also seen in the aggregates of lymphocytes that can develop wherever there is a focus of infection. The lymphoid tissues of the gut and lungs behave, to a certain extent, autonomously, in that particular B cells (largely IgA-secreting) and T cells recirculate selectively through them. They are sometimes referred to as the *mucosal immune system* (Fig.7.6).

Lymphocyte subpopulations and markers

B lymphocytes are identified by the possession of surface Ig, usually detected by immunofluorescent staining with anti-Ig sera. T lymphocytes lack surface Ig, but conveniently form 'rosettes' when centrifuged lightly with sheep red blood cells. However, using these two techniques, about 10% of blood lymphocytes still cannot be classified; these are referred to as *null*.

Among T lymphocytes, the use of monoclonal antibodies against the T3, T4, and T8 molecules (p. 106), combined with immunofluorescence, makes it possible to identify subpopulations with important functional differences. In general, T4 is found on *helper* T lymphocytes, T8 on *cytotoxic* and *suppressor* lymphocytes, and T3 on all types (Fig.7.7). Further subdivision can be made using other antibodies (Table 7.3).

Fig. 7.6 Lymphocyte recirculation. In this stylised diagram, blood vessels (arterial side only shown) are in red, lymphatics in black. LN = Lymph node; MLN = mesenteric lymph node; PP = Peyer's patch; IEL = Intra-epithelial lymphocytes; LP = Lamina propria.

Fig. 7.7   T and B lymphocyte differentiation markers. Diagram shows the principal stages in the T and B cell lineages, with some of the surface and cytoplasmic molecules that help to differentiate them. Tdt = terminal deoxynucleotidyl transferase (possibly involved in receptor gene rearrangement); E = receptor for sheep erythrocytes (= CD2); Ti = T cell receptor for antigen; T^H = T helper cell; T^C, T^S = cytotoxic or suppressor T cell; T^M, B^M = T or B memory cell; IL-2R = receptor for interleukin 2 (= CD25); TFR = transferrin receptor; M = cytoplasmic IgM heavy chain; CR2 = complement receptor (= CD21); CD20 = a useful B cell marker, possibly involved in triggering. Note: CD3, CD4, CD6, and CD8 are also known as T3, T4, T6, and T8. Antigen-specific receptor molecules are shown in red.

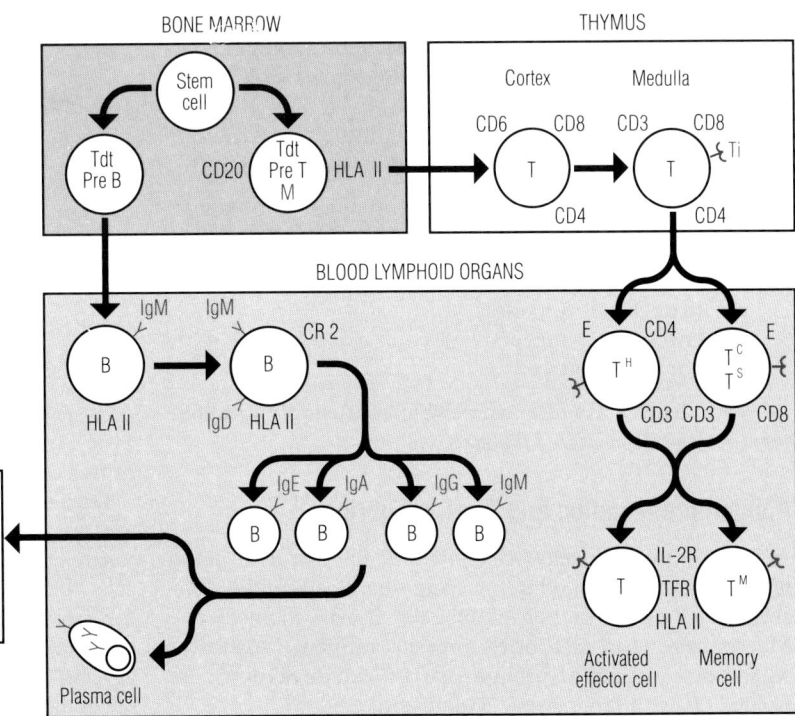

Table 7.3 Some useful lymphocyte markers and their functional significance*

Cell type	Standard name*	Other names	Distribution and functional significance
T lymphocyte	Ti		Receptor for antigens
	CD3	T3	All T cells
	CD2	T11	Receptor for sheep rbc
	CD4	T4	Helper cells, HIV receptor
	CD8	T8	Cytotoxic/suppressor cells
	CD5	T1	Thymocytes
	CD25	Tac	Receptor for IL-2 (activated cells)
B lymphocyte	Ig		Receptor for antigens
	CD25	Tac	Receptor for IL-2
		IL4 receptor	
		IL5 receptor	Involved in 'help'
		IL6 receptor	
	CD21	C3d receptor	Receptor for C3 and EB virus
	CD5	T1	? Autoimmune B cells

*CD numbers refer to 'clusters of differentiation', a nomenclature which has now become standard.

THE IMMUNE RESPONSE

The term 'immune response' covers all responses of lymphocytes to antigen, whether involving T or B cells or both. All immune responses have certain features in common.

1. *Presentation*, i.e. the requirement for antigens to be *presented* by specialised cells.
2. *Selection* of lymphocytes whose receptors are specific for determinants on the antigen.
3. *Clone formation*: proliferation of these lymphocytes to form a *clone* of cells with identical specificity. This process was predicted by Burnet in his clonal selection theory of 1959, but received full confirmation only recently, with the development of methods of growing clones of T and B cells in culture.
4. *Differentiation*. Interactions between lymphocytes leading to their differentiation into effector cells.
5. The generation of *memory*.
6. *Regulation*, i.e. control of the magnitude and duration of the response by various regulatory mechanisms.

On the basis of the type of effector cell generated, immune responses can be classified into three types:

1. antibody responses
2. cytotoxic T cell responses
3. responses involving activation of macrophages and other non-specific cells.

Types 2 and 3 are often somewhat confusingly lumped together as *cell-mediated immunity*.

Antigen presentation and T cell triggering

Antigen presenting cells (APC) include the dendritic cells of spleen and lymph nodes, the Langerhans cells of the skin and related cells in other organs, and B cells themselves. Macrophages can also often present antigen, especially when some degree of preliminary antigen breakdown is needed, as with large or particulate antigens.

When APC make contact with specific lymphocytes, they secrete a protein known as interleukin-1 (IL-1) and perhaps other factors, which cause lymphocytes to proliferate. In the case of T4 (helper) cells, recognition of class II MHC molecules, as well as antigen, is required, so that only cells expressing these can act as APC. In the case of cytotoxic (T8) cells (p. 107), antigen is recognised in association with class I MHC molecules. In both cases, other soluble mediators are required for proliferation and expansion of the specific clone of T cells, notably interleukin 2 (IL-2), which is made by T helper cells and for which activated T cells of all types express surface receptors. The half-life of IL-2 is very short (due in part to serum inhibitors), so that its action is highly localised and predominantly restricted to antigen-specific cells.

The antibody response

Both B and T cells are required for the antibody response. The exceptions are some large polymeric antigens (e.g. bacterial capsular polysaccharides), which stimulate B cells directly and are known as *T-independent*. With all other antigens, B cells are triggered to proliferate by interaction between their surface Ig and the antigen, plus factors secreted by the APC; however, they require additional signals from T helper cells in order to differentiate into plasma cells and secrete antibody. These signals consist of non-antigen-specific cytokines, principally the *interleukins* 1–6. The T helper cells also need antigen to be presented, in this case in association with MHC class II molecules.

During T-dependent responses, some B lymphocytes are retained in *germinal centres* instead of differentiating 'terminally' into plasma cells; these are called *memory B cells*. These, together with memory T cells, form the basis for the vigorous *secondary response* that follows subsequent exposures to the same antigen. Typical features of secondary, as compared to primary, responses are: more rapid onset, higher level of antibody, higher average affinity, and relatively more IgG.

Antibody is predominantly effective against micro-organisms free in the blood or tissue spaces; in practice, this means viruses in their extracellular stage and many bacteria. Pneumococcal pneumonia is a good example of a disease in which a rapid antibody response can make the difference between life and death. The predominant role of antibody, in such cases, is to improve phagocytosis by virtue of the attachment of the Fab portion to the microbe and the Fc portion to Fc receptors on phagocytic cells; this process is known as *opsonisation*.

The cytotoxic T cell response

The cytotoxic T cell response is mainly useful against viruses in their intracellular stage, though it unfortunately also contributes to transplant rejection. The final effector cell is a T cell, usually of T8 phenotype, which recognises viral antigens on the surface of infected cells in association with class I MHC molecules. Rather like a B cell, it usually requires help from T helper cells for clonal proliferation, in this case mainly in the form of IL-2. The mechanism by which cytotoxic T cells act is not exactly known, but it involves contact with the virus-infected cell which is subsequently destroyed by lysis.

T cell–macrophage interactions

The third group of responses is somewhat more het-erogeneous and includes all those in which a specifically activated T cell modifies the function of another, non-specific, cell via the secretion of soluble molecules collectively known as *cytokines*. Table 7.4 shows the best-known of these. Many of the cytokines act on macrophages, to improve their ability to terminate, or at least control, infection by intracellular bacteria such as mycobacteria, and several important fungi and protozoa. However, there are also lymphokines that affect eosinophils, NK cells, other lymphocytes (e.g. IL-2), haemopoietic precursors in the bone marrow, osteoclasts, and even mucus secretion. In all these types of response, memory resides entirely in the specific T cells.

Regulation of immune responses

Both T and B cells require specific antigens for triggering, so that *elimination of antigen* constitutes the most effective way of terminating a response. However, there are other ways in which a prolonged response can be damped down, presumably as an attempt to limit hypersensitivity and autoimmunity (pp. 110–114). These include the stimulation of suppressor T cells and the production of anti-idiotypic antibodies. Suppressor T cells resemble cytotoxic T cells in their usual phenotype (T8), and appear to use similar receptors, but their triggering requirements are not clear. They may be antigen-specific, idiotype-specific, or non-specific, and they act by inhibiting, and possibly sometimes killing, specific T or B cells. Antibody itself can also regulate antibody production, and this too may be idiotype-

Table 7.4 The major cytokines and their functions

Cytokine*	Other names	Principal cellular source	Principal effects
IL-1	LAF	APC	T cell proliferation; fever etc. (as TNF)
IL-2	TCGF	T	T, B proliferation
IL-3	Multi-CSF	T	T, B, mast cell growth
IL-4	BCGF 1	T	T, B proliferation
IL-5	BCGF 2	T	Eosinophil growth; B differentiation
IL-6	BSF2	T	B differentiation; acute-phase proteins
IFN-α	Type I	Mac	Anti-viral
IFN-β		Fibroblast	Anti-viral
IFN-γ	Type II	T	Anti-viral; MHC; activates macrophages
GCSF			Granulocyte growth and maturation
MCSF			Monocyte growth and maturation
GMCSF			As GCSF and MCSF
TNF (TNF-α)	Cachectin	Mac	{ Anti-tumour; vascular damage;
LT (TNF-β)		T	anti-viral; PMN activation; bone absorption; etc.

IL = interleukin; IFN = interferon; TNF = tumour necrosis factor; LT = lymphotoxin; CSF = colony-stimulating factor; APC = antigen presenting cell;
Mac = macrophage; MHC = major histocompatibility complex

7

specific or antigen-specific. In general, IgG antibodies are more inhibitory than IgM.

TOLERANCE

Immune responses are not normally triggered by the body's own antigens; this is known as *self-tolerance* and is thought to be due to a combination of several mechanisms including:

1. the elimination of self-reactive lymphocytes in the primary lymphoid organs (thymus and bone marrow)
2. suppressor T cells, specific for self-antigens
3. antigen-receptor interactions that lead to unresponsiveness instead of responsiveness.

None of these mechanisms is fully understood, and they clearly are not foolproof because *auto-antibodies* (antibodies against self) are quite often found (pp. 112–114).

The same mechanisms are apparently also responsible for the unresponsiveness to foreign antigens found in special circumstances and also known as *tolerance*. This can occur with:

1. very *large* amounts of antigen
2. an *immature* or compromised immune system
3. antigens that for any reason are not properly *presented*
4. antigens absorbed through the *gut* (of particular interest in relation to food allergies).

The induction of tolerance against foreign MHC antigens is one of the aims of research into transplant rejection (pp. 114–115).

IMMUNODEFICIENCY

Like any other intricate mechanism, the immune system can be defective in a number of ways. Deficiencies of immunity can be classified as *primary* (i.e. cause unknown) or *secondary* to some known cause such as infection, cancer, malnutrition, drugs or X-radiation. Alternatively, they can be described in terms of the component which is faulty, the most important being defects of phagocytic cells, of complement, of B cells and antibody, and of T cells, or combinations of these (Table 7.5).

Phagocytic cell deficiencies

Polymorphonuclear leucocytes (PMN) are especially prone to genetic deficiencies usually involving particular enzymes; examples are *chronic granulomatous disease* (CGD) in which the generation of oxygen metabolites does not occur, and deficiencies of myeloperoxidase, G6PD, pyruvate kinase and other enzymes. There is also a defect of phagosome-lysosome fusion known as Chediak-Higashi syndrome. In general, PMN defects are associated with recurrent bacterial (especially staphylococcal), and fungal infections.

Complement deficiencies

Almost any of the complement components may be absent or reduced, the most serious (but extremely rare), being C3 and the commonest, C2. Defects of the (lytic) components of C5–8 are associated mainly with Neisserial (meningococcal and gonococcal) infection, suggesting that lysis is not a major killing mechanism for most other organisms, and that phagocytosis is more important overall. Deficiencies of the 'classical' components (C1, C2 or C4) are associated with an increased risk of immune complex disease, because this pathway plays a role in reducing the size of complexes. An interesting defect is that of a C1 inhibitor associated with hereditary angioneurotic oedema. There is also a poorly characterised deficiency of a serum opsonising activity apparently distinct from complement.

Antibody deficiencies

The newborn baby relies on IgG transferred across the placenta, and is protected from common infections for about six months. Any delay thereafter in endogenous Ig synthesis may lead to recurrent pyogenic infection. Occasionally, the synthesis of IgA is selectively reduced or absent, often in association with allergies or autoimmune disease. Sometimes, all Ig classes are affected (*common variable immunodeficiency*). More rarely, B lymphocytes are absent altogether, leading to agammaglobulinaemia. When inherited on the X chromosome, this is known as Bruton's disease. Pneumonia is the commonest presenting condition, but repeated infections can occur almost anywhere. Treatment is by immunoglobulin replacement and, where appropriate, antibiotics.

T cell deficiencies

AIDS, in which the virus infects T helper cells using the T4 molecule as receptor, represents the extreme end of the spectrum of T cell deficiency. However, a mild lowering of T cell is probably quite common, particularly during other virus infections, such as measles. Very rarely, absence of the thymus leads to a total lack of T cells; if associated with absence of the parathyroids, this is known as the Di George syndrome. Severe T cell deficiency leads to fatal infections with micro-organisms of all kinds, including normally nonpathogenic *opportunists*, such as cytomegalovirus, pseudomonas, pneumocystis and candida, and also, in some cases, to the development of tumours. Treatment is unsatisfactory, but bone marrow and/or thymus grafting have had some success.

Combined deficiencies

In *severe combined immunodeficiency* syndromes (SCID) both antibody and T cells are affected in various proportions. Sometimes, the defect appears to be in an enzyme of the purine salvage pathway, such as adenosine deaminase (ADA) or purine nucleoside phosphorylase (PNP), and, in these cases, replacement of the missing

Table 7.5. Some immunodeficiency syndromes

System affected	Syndrome	Clinical effects
Primary		
Antibody	Hypogammaglobulinaemia	Bacterial infections
	Transient (neonatal)	Bacterial infections
	Congenital X-linked (Bruton's disease)	Bacterial infections
	Selective IgA	Gut infection; allergies
	Selective IgM	Septicaema
T cells	Thymic aplasia (Di George)	Viral infections
	PNP deficiency	Viral infections
	Ataxia telangiectasia	Viral infections
	Wiskott-Aldrich syndrome	Viral infections
T and B cells	Common variable	Childhood infection
	Severe combined	Childhood infection
	ADA deficiency	
Myeloid cells	Chronic granulomatous disease	Abscesses; granulomas
	Chediak-Higashi syndrome	Pneumonia
	MPO, G6PD, deficiency*	Pneumonia
Complement	C1,2,4 deficiency	Immune complex disease
	C3 deficiency	Infection
	C5,6,7,8,9 deficiency	Neisserial infection
Other	Opsonisation defect	Infection
Secondary		
Antibody	Splenectomy	Pyogenic infections
	Myeloma, CLL*	
	Cyclophosphamide	
	Malnutrition	
	Nephrotic syndrome	
T cells	AIDS	Pneumocystis; TB; Kaposi's sarcoma
	Hodgkin's disease	Fungal infections; TB
	Azathioprine (Imuran)	CMV
	Cyclosporin A	Infections rare
	Measles, CMV, IM*	
	Malnutrition: zinc	
Myeloid cells	Steroids	
	Gentamycin	
	Malnutrition: iron, zinc	

MPO = myeloperoxidase; G6PD = glucose 6 phosphate dehydrogenase; CLL = chronic lymphatic leukaemia; CMV = cytomegalovirus; IM = infectious mononucleosis.

enzyme is a practical possibility. There are a number of very rare syndromes in which immunodeficiency is found alongside abnormalities of the CNS (e.g. ataxia telangiectasia), of platelets (Wiskott-Aldrich syndrome) or of the entire haemopoietic system (reticular dysgenesis).

IMMUNOPATHOLOGY

It is disturbing to realise that a number of unpleasant, dangerous, and even fatal conditions can be due to the activity of the immune system, whose function is normally to protect life and health. In evolutionary terms, however, these conditions are evidently less of a threat to survival than is infectious disease; in other words, immunopathology is the price paid for the possession of a vigorous immune system.

Immunopathological reactions are usually classified in terms of the *mechanism* responsible for the damage. This is the basis of the Gell and Coombs classification shown in Table 7.6 and used throughout this book. An alternative approach would be a classification based on the *antigen* concerned. This has the virtue of clearly distinguishing responses to foreign antigens from those to self antigens, the former being essentially 'normal' responses that have got out of hand, the latter being inherently abnormal. Responses to foreign antigens are loosely referred to as *hypersensitivity*, and to self antigens as *autoimmunity*; however, as will be seen, there is a substantial overlap.

The Immunological Basis of Disease

Table 7.6   Immunopathological mechanisms (the Gell & Coombs classification)

Type	Mediators	Result	Examples
Hypersensitivity			
I	IgE, mast cells	Allergy Anaphylaxis	Hay fever Bee sting
II	Ig bound to cell-surface antigens	Phagocytosis Cytotoxicity Lysis	Transfusion Rh disease Autoimmune diseases
III	Ag-ab complexes, PMN, complement	Vascular damage	SLE Post-streptococcal glomerulonephritis
IV	T cells, macrophages	Granuloma Oedema	TB Contact sensitivity
Other mechanisms (Designated IIa or V)	Ig bound to hormone receptors	Stimulation Blocking	Graves' disease Myxoedema
	Cytokines	Vascular damage	Gram-negative shock

HYPERSENSITIVITY

The word hypersensitivity was coined over 100 years ago, to describe differences in immune status detectable by skin testing. A patient immune to (that is, recovered from) a disease, who is subsequently injected intradermally with an appropriate antigen, might show an *immediate* reaction (a wheal and flare within minutes), a slower *acute* reaction (swelling and redness within hours), or a *delayed* reaction (swelling and redness two days or more after the injection). Later work established that the immediate and acute reactions were a sign that the patient possessed antibody to the antigen in question, while the delayed reaction indicated the presence of specific memory T cells. Skin testing is still widely used in diagnosis, but, confusingly, a positive result may be either good or bad for the patient depending on circumstances; a knowledge of the underlying mechanism is thus essential.

Anaphylaxis and allergy

The commonest forms of hypersensitivity are hay fever and other allergies, up to 15% of the population being affected to some degree. The crucial steps in the allergic response are:

1. the formation of *IgE antibody* specific to the inducing antigen or 'allergen'
2. binding of this antibody to *mast cells* and basophils
3. attachment of further molecules of the allergen to the cell-bound IgE
4. degranulation of the mast cells and release of a number of *mediators* with a variety of inflammatory effects.

The symptoms of allergy depend partly on the type of mediators released, but mainly on the site at which it occurs.

The serum IgE level, which normally constitutes only a few millionths of total Ig, is regulated partly by T cells and also by genetic factors, including HLA. The level is usually raised in allergic subjects, but why individual patients often make high levels of IgE to only a single allergen is not clear.

Mast cells are found in most organs and there is a special subpopulation in the mucosa of the gut and the lung. Together with basophils, these cells have very high affinity receptors for the Fc region of IgE. If two molecules of IgE bound to a mast cell or basophil are cross-linked by a molecule of antigen, membrane changes occur, leading to Ca^{2+} influx, a fall in intracellular cAMP, and release of mediators. The same result can also be produced by stimulation of adrenergic receptors by noradrenalin or cholinergic receptors by acetylcholine; β receptor stimulation has the opposite effect.

The main effect of the released mediators is to increase vascular permeability and to cause bronchial constriction. *Histamine* has both of these effects, while the *leukotrines* and *prostaglandins* tend to bring about one or other of them. There are also some important chemotactic molecules which attract other cells, such as PMN, eosinophils and platelets, to the site of inflammation. Eosinophils may play a regulatory role in allergic reactions, by releasing molecules that counteract many of the mast cell products. Allergic responses may be localised to the site of entry of the allergen, e.g. the nose and eyes in hay fever, the bronchi in asthma, and the skin in eczema. When allergens enter the circulation, as with insect venoms or injected drugs, the reaction may be widespread and lead to vascular collapse, vomiting and even death; this is known as *systemic anaphylaxis* and calls for immediate treatment with adrenalin. For localised allergies, treatment consists of removing the cause if possible, or the use of drugs that inhibit mast cell degranulation in one way or another. Numerous desensitisation regimes are in use and these undoubtedly work sometimes; however, why this is so has not been definitely shown.

It is worth noting that, while asthma is frequently allergic, there are numerous other contributory factors. In addition, some chemicals, e.g. anaesthetics, can cause mast cells to degranulate in the absence of IgE antibodies; the resulting reactions are called *anaphylactoid*, the key difference being that, unlike true anaphylactic reactions, they can occur without previous exposure to the inciting agent.

One may well wonder why such unpleasant and alarming reactions should have evolved at all and, indeed, whether the IgE class of antibody has any useful function. However if we accept that acute inflammation is valuable in increasing the local availability of blood components such as antibody, complement and PMN, it is not surprising that an antibody has evolved which enhances and accelerates this in an antigen-specific fashion. A particularly important case may be intestinal worm infections, where contact between potentially cytotoxic cells and their target would normally be extremely limited.

Antibody-mediated cytotoxic hypersensitivity

Antibody-mediated cytotoxic hypersensitivity refers to reactions in which antibody attached to a cell surface leads to damage by complement and/or by PMN or other Fc-receptor-bearing cytotoxic cells. This is of course one of the predominant mechanisms by which antibody destroys infectious micro-organisms and, in the majority of cases, is purely beneficial. Because of the specificity of antibody, the damage is normally focussed on the foreign organism, but ill-effects to the host can result in two particular situations:

1. when the foreign cell is one whose destruction is not desirable, such as a blood transfusion or an organ graft
2. when the antibody is directed not against foreign but against *self*-antigens. It follows that most type II 'hypersensitivity' reactions are, in fact, aspects of either transplant rejection (p. 114) or autoimmunity (p. 112). They are dealt with more fully in these sections.

Immune complexes and disease

Damage to tissues or blood vessels by the deposition of antigen-antibody complexes is a very important cause of disease but, as with the type II reactions noted above, there is nothing inherently abnormal in the formation of such complexes; indeed, without them, antibody would be useless. Millions of antigen-antibody complexes are removed from the blood and tissues every day in normal health, chiefly by phagocytic cells, but partly also by the solubilising effect of complement. It is only when such clearance is inadequate that complexes become deposited elsewhere and cause disease.

Pathogenesis

The commonest reasons for inadequate clearance and thus deposition of complexes are *persistent* antibody responses, for example chronic infections, inhalation of antigens in special occupations, or (in the days before antibiotics), passive immunotherapy with foreign serum. A special case is when the antibody is directed against *self*-antigens, which obviously can never be totally eliminated. Such auto-immune reactions are considered on pages 112–114.

The mechanism of damage is essentially the same for all immune complex-mediated diseases. The activation of complement releases the inflammatory peptides, C3a and C5a, generating local vascular permeability, the attraction of platelets, basophils and PMN, microthrombus formation and PMN degranulation; it is the lysosomal enzymes released by the PMN that do most of the damage. Complexes tend to deposit in sites of turbulent blood flow or of filtration, such as the renal glomerulus, but it is probable that the nature of the antigen is also important; thus, anti-DNA complexes (for example in systemic lupus erythematosus), are especially prone to deposit in the glomerulus, and anti-Ig complexes (for example in rheumatoid arthritis) in the joints. However, very widespread complex deposition, as used to be seen in *serum sickness*, can affect both sites.

Investigation

A variety of techniques are available for detecting immune complexes; most laboratories use a combination of tests that depend on the size of the complex (such as precipitation with polyethylene glycol), and on the ability of the antibody in the complex to bind complement (CIq binding assays). However, except in bacterial endocarditis, the level of complexes in the serum *per se* is not usually of much diagnostic value. On the other hand, when tissue biopsies are available, the demonstration of Ig and/or complement in a particular site can be most informative; a striking example of this is the difference between the linear deposition of anti-glomerular basement membrane complexes of Goodpasture's syndrome (an autoimmune disease), and the more granular appearance of immune-complex glomerulonephritis, which may be due to a variety of infections, such as hepatitis B virus, streptococci, and malaria, to drugs or to an auto-antigen such as DNA.

Delayed-type and cell-mediated hypersensitivity

Delayed-type hypersensitivity

As already mentioned, a delayed-type hypersensitivity (DTH) skin test indicates the presence of T cell-mediated immunity to the antigen in question, the best known example being the Mantoux (tuberculin) test for previous exposure to tuberculosis. The changes in the skin include: contact between the antigen and circulating specific T lymphocytes of helper type; release of cytokines by the latter; and the consequent accumulation and activation of non-specific cells, particularly monocytes, in the vicinity. Most of these steps can also be reproduced in tissue culture, and it is assumed that they represent the 'cell-mediated' changes that would take place at the site of the actual re-infection, e.g. in the lung for tuberculosis. DTH tests are useful for diagnosis of a number of infections, particularly those involving chronic intracellular organisms. They can also be of prognostic value, e.g. in leprosy, where strong DTH correlates with effective immunity to the bacterium, but also with tissue damaging and truly immuno-pathological reactions.

Other forms of delayed reaction

The relationship between cell-mediated immunity, DTH, and resistance to infection is, however, more complicated than this. In the first place, very similar changes can be found in *contact sensitivity*, an eczematous skin reaction to, e.g. dyes, metals and plants, which has no beneficial value. In addition, there are other forms of delayed reaction where the cellular changes are somewhat different. These range from the slightly earlier (24-hour) Jones-Mote response, in which vascular changes and basophil accumulation are more prominent, to the much slower-developing granulomatous and necrotic lesions originally noted by Koch. It is assumed that different T cells and cytokines are responsible for these different patterns of response, about which there is still much to be learned.

Granuloma formation

In terms of immunopathology, *granuloma* formation is the most serious manifestation of cell-mediated hypersensitivity. A granuloma is a solid mass of macrophages, some of which may fuse to form *giant cells*, while others become specialised for protein synthesis (the *epithelioid cells*). Eosinophils are often prominent, as are lymphocytes. The latter include the T cells, whose lymphokines initiate and maintain the lesion, though there is evidence that T cells can also suppress granuloma formation.

The clash of interests faced by the cell-mediated immune system is illustrated by the deposition of eggs in the liver during the worm disease schistosomiasis. In the absence of a cellular reaction (e.g. in T cell-deficient mice) enzymes secreted by the eggs (in a vain attempt to escape into the intestine) lead to damage and destruction of liver tissue. A granulomatous reaction around each egg, with ultimate fibrosis and calcification, protects liver function but can result in cirrhosis with portal hypertension, oesophageal varices and fatal haematemesis. It is evident that protective cell-mediated immunity and type IV hypersensitivity are two sides of the same coin.

Anti-receptor antibodies

Although not part of Gell and Coombs' original classification, antibodies against cell-surface receptors for hormones can cause important pathological effects in one of two ways:

1. by blocking the binding of the natural hormone and thus preventing cell stimulation
2. by actually mimicking the action of the hormone and leading to over-stimulation of the cell.

Such antibodies are of course auto-antibodies, and both types are found in thyroid disease (p. 692).

Lymphocytes themselves can also be inhibited or stimulated in a similar way by antibodies against their own surface receptors. An example would be the ability of anti-idiotype antibodies to trigger a B lymphocyte, by combining with its antigen-binding site in the same manner as antigen. Such idiotype-anti-idiotype interactions form the basis for artificial manipulations of the immune response with exciting prospects for the future.

AUTOIMMUNITY

Perhaps even more alarming than hypersensitivity is the idea that the immune system should actually react against the host's own antigens. In fact, given the range and genetic complexity of the various receptors involved and the underlying similarity between the proteins, carbohydrates etc. of which the cell membranes of mammals and micro-organisms are composed, it is amazing that autoimmunity is avoided so successfully in most people. Details of particular autoimmune diseases will be found in the relevant chapters, this section being concerned with the general principles underlying self-tolerance and its breakdown in autoimmunity.

Self-tolerance

It is clearly impossible to prevent the *genes* for a self-antigen and an antibody which recognises it occurring in the same individual; one has only to consider the blood group AB child of an A father and B mother, who will inherit the genes for both anti-B and anti-A but must not make either of these antibodies. The mechanisms preventing this appear to be a combination of clonal elimination of lymphocytes, suppressor T cells, receptor-blocking, and anti-idiotypic interactions (p. 108). Which of these mechanisms is most effective depends partly on the antigen in question. Thus, for example, antigens present in high concentrations, such as the blood groups or serum albumin, may lead to clonal elimination; whereas, in normal individuals, B lymphocytes are demonstrably present against thyroglobulin, of which there are only trace amounts in the serum. With T lymphocytes, the situation is more complicated, since part of their normal triggering involves recognition of self MHC molecules (p. 106). However, recent work with cultured monoclonal T cells suggests that fully self-reactive T cells also exist in normal individuals. This implies an important role for *regulatory* mechanisms in maintaining self-tolerance, and suggests that, when autoimmunity does develop, it is these that may have failed. However, with a few exceptions, our present understanding of the aetiology of human autoimmune diseases consists largely of tantalising glimpses.

Experimental autoimmunity

Much has been learned of the aetiology of autoimmunity from animal models. There is a strong genetic element in susceptibility to many autoimmune diseases; this involves several different genetic loci, one of which is usually the MHC. Autoimmunity can often be induced in normal animals by the injection of *cross-reacting antigens*, which carry both foreign and self determinants (as do some micro-organisms), and also by the injection of molecules that *polyclonally activate* lymphocytes, such as bacterial endotoxins. There is frequently an increased tendency to auto-immunity in older animals and in females, suggesting a role for endocrine factors. Most importantly, it has been shown that the production of *auto-antibodies* and the induction of organ damage with loss of function (autoimmune *disease*) by no means always go together.

Classification of autoimmune diseases

The traditional classification of human autoimmune diseases is based on the site affected, ranging from highly localised damage to single organs, frequently endocrine glands (*organ-specific*), to multi-site disease with lesions disseminated throughout the blood vessels, kidney, skin and joints (*non-organ-specific*). Generally speaking, the pathological mechanisms in organ-specific disease are of the cytotoxic or anti-receptor type, while non-organ-specific disease is due to immune complex deposition (p. 111). Table 7.7 lists some common autoimmune diseases in these two categories. Interestingly, the organ-specific as well as the non-organ-specific diseases tend to be grouped in individuals or families; an example of the latter is the association of anti-DNA and anti-Ig (rheumatoid factor) antibodies in connective tissue diseases, such as rheumatoid arthritis, SLE and Sjögren's syndrome, and of the former, the association of antibodies to stomach, thyroid, and other endocrine organs.

It must be emphasised that the finding of an auto-antibody in a patient does not mean that it is the cause of the presenting disease; it may be purely secondary, such as the anti-cardiolipin (Wasserman) antibodies in syphilis. Nor does the absence of detectable auto-antibodies rule out an autoimmune cause; it may be a purely T cell-mediated disease. The strongest evidence for a direct link between auto-antibodies and disease comes when the symptoms can be transferred by antibody, as can occur in the newborn babies of mothers with thyrotoxicosis or myaesthenia gravis.

The influence of HLA

Autoimmune diseases make up the largest group of conditions associated with particular HLA phenotypes (p. 103 and Table 7.2). The B8-DR3 combination is particularly interesting, in view of the range of quite different organ-specific diseases to which it is linked; it has been suggested that people with this combination are immu-

Table 7.7 Major autoimmune diseases

Category	Area affected	Disease	Auto-antibodies found
Organ-specific	Thyroid	Hashimoto's Graves'	Thyroglobulin TSH receptor
	Stomach	Atrophic gastritis Pernicious anaemia	Parietal cells Intrinsic factor
	Adrenal	Addison's	Adrenal cell
	Pancreas	Juvenile diabetes	Islet cells
	Liver	Chronic active hepatitis	Smooth muscle; LSP
	Gut	Ulcerative colitis	Colon antigen (?)
	Skin	Pemphigus	Desmosomes
	Blood	AIHA ITP	Red cells Platelets
	Nerve-muscle	Myasthenia gravis	Acetylcholine receptor
	Salivary gland, eye, joints	Sjögren's syndrome	Salivary cells and ducts
	Kidney, lung	Goodpasture's syndrome	Basement membrane
	Liver, salivary gland	Primary biliary cirrhosis	Mitochondrial
Non-organ-specific	Joints Lung Blood Skin Kidney	Rheumatoid arthritis Polymyositis Scleroderma SLE	IgG (→Immune complexes) DNA (→Immune complexes) Red cells, platelets

LSP = liver-specific protein; AIHA = autoimmune haemolytic anaemia; ITP = idiopathic thrombocytopenic purpura; SLE = systemic lupus erythematosus.

The Immunological Basis of Disease

nologically 'high responders' to a variety of antigens. In the case of ankylosing spondylitis, actual cross-reaction between the B27 molecule and an antigen on certain enterobacteria, such as *Klebsiella* and *Yersinia*, may be an element in the disease.

A second aspect of HLA is the finding of class II molecules on the cells of affected organs where they are not normally expressed, the most striking example being the thyroid in Graves' and Hashimoto's disease. It remains to be established whether this anomalous expression is a primary phenomenon leading to presentation of self-antigens to T cells, or whether it is secondary to T cell infiltration and release of mediators such as interferon.

TRANSPLANTATION

The understanding of transplant rejection began in 1900, when Landsteiner discovered the ABO blood groups and put blood transfusion on a rational footing. Donor and patient had to be matched so that no antigens were present in the donor that were absent in the recipient: apparent exceptions turned out to be due to other 'minor' antigenic systems. However, almost 50 years passed before it was realised that tissue transplants obeyed similar rules, with the MHC playing the dominant role, and a still unknown number of minor histocompatibility antigens making their contribution to rejection.

Here, however, the parallel with blood transfusion ends because:

1. a blood transfusion is rejected purely by *antibody*, while, with most organ and tissue grafts, *cell-mediated* immunity also plays a crucial part
2. the degree of complexity and polymorphism at the MHC are such that matching of donor and recipient are seldom perfect; thus, the resulting rejection response usually has to be suppressed by drugs or other means.

HLA typing and matching

Class I antigens (A,B and C) are typed using monospecific antisera and complement in a micro-cytotoxic assay. Of the class II antigens, those at the DQ and DR locus can be typed in the same way, but DP antigens seem to be recognised only by T lymphocytes and are typed by *mixed lymphocyte reactions* (MLR). For convenience, B lymphocytes from a blood sample are normally used, since those cells carry all the class I and class II antigens of the individual. All MHC alleles are expressed *co-dominantly*, so that it should be possible to detect two antigens at each locus, unless the patient happens to be homozygous for one of them. Because of the large number of alleles at each locus, the number of possible permutations is enormous (at least 10^{13}), but some alleles are very rare so that, in practice, the chance of a perfect match between unrelated people is around 1 in 10^5. This chance is higher in relatives, rising to 1 in 4 in siblings and, of course, 1 in 1 in identical twins. Retrospective studies on large groups of kidney-grafted patients suggest that class II matching is the most important.

Two questions of very great interest arise in connection with the MHC: why is the MHC so polymorphic, and why do individuals react so strongly to foreign MHC antigens? Current thinking relates this to the need to maintain self-recognition in a world where parasitic micro-organisms can change their antigens rapidly in an attempt to mimic the antigens of their host; much, however, remains to be understood.

Mechanisms of rejection

The mechanisms of transplant rejection (Fig.7.8) depend to some extent on the tissue concerned. Transplants introduced via the circulation, such as blood and bone marrow, are highly vulnerable to the lytic and phagocytic actions of antibody. Skin grafts are destroyed by purely cell-mediated reactions, probably a combination of cytotoxic T cells and activated macrophages. Well-vascularised organs, such as the kidney and heart, are susceptible to damage by both mechanisms: antibody against MHC class I or ABO blood group antigens on the vascular endothelium leads to platelet and PMN accumulation and vascular obstruction; while T cells infiltrate and damage the organ much as they

Fig. 7.8 Transplant rejection and immunosuppression. Donor cells and molecules are shown in red. On the right are the principal mechanisms by which the recipient recognises and responds to donor antigens. APC = antigen-presenting cell; Endo = vascular endothelium; Mac = macrophage; T^H and T^C = helper and cytotoxic T cells; IL-2 = interleukin 2; HF = helper factors; IFN-γ = gamma interferon. Immunosuppression: (1) Removal of HLA class II bearing cells (organ culture; anti-HLA class II antibodies). (2) Blocking of recognition (anti-HLA class II antibodies). (3) Elimination of specific lymphocytes (antigen suicide; anti-idiotype antibodies). In addition to these specific mechanisms, there are also non-specific means of suppressing rejection: irradiation; anti-lymphocyte antibodies; cytotoxic drugs, e.g. azathioprine; anti-T cell agents, such as cyclosporin A; and anti-inflammatory drugs, e.g. steroids.

do a skin graft. Liver grafts are unusual, in that HLA matching seems to make no difference.

Bone marrow transplants pose an additional problem because they contain competent T lymphocytes which can react against the HLA antigens of the recipient – the *graft versus host* (GVH) reaction. GVH disease is frequently fatal, but progress has been made in developing methods for removing T cells from the transplanted marrow, e.g. using monoclonal anti-T cell antibodies.

Prevention of rejection

Apart from HLA matching, the mainstay of management of transplant patients is immunosuppression. Many drugs can suppress one or other aspect of the immune response; indeed, screening for immunosuppression is an important part of the testing of new drugs, and it was in this way that the dramatic effects of *cyclosporin A* (CSA) were discovered. Cyclosporin A is rapidly becoming the drug of choice for transplantation, and perhaps also for severe autoimmune diseases; it acts by selectively suppressing activated T lymphocytes, mainly by blocking cytokine production. Other drugs, still widely used, are antiproliferative agents such as *azathioprine* (Imuran) which kill dividing cells, including lymphocytes, and corticosteroids, such as *prednisone*, which act mainly by depressing macrophage function. All these drugs have the unwelcome side-effect of rendering the patient susceptible to infection. In addition, the antiproliferative drugs can cause agranulocytosis and thrombocytopaenia (by inhibiting cell division in the bone marrow), unless carefully monitored.

There is currently considerable research into methods of inducing antigen-specific immunosuppression, i.e. *tolerance*. The rather unexpected beneficial effect of pre-operative blood transfusion on kidney graft survival may be an example of tolerance, perhaps due to the induction of antibodies that block T cell-HLA recognition. Another approach is to use anti-idiotype antibodies (p. 102 and p. 107). With some tissues, it may be possible to remove all class II MHC antigen-bearing cells from the graft before transplantation, so that the host T cells are not triggered. This has produced promising results with endocrine grafts, for example of the parathyroid and pancreas.

IMMUNOLOGICAL TECHNIQUES

Antibodies are highly discriminatory and highly sensitive in their reactions with antigens. This makes them valuable reagents for typing cells or micro-organisms, and for detecting very small amounts of materials such as hormones. Antigen-antibody interactions can be visualised by the use of a fluorescent dye, a radioisotope or a specific enzyme attached to the antigen or the antibody. In the case of tissue sections, *immunofluorescence* is commonly used to identify the sites to which a particular antiserum binds, e.g. in autoimmune diseases. For hormone estimation, *radioimmunoassay* can be used. Here, the unknown sample is allowed to compete with the binding of a standard antibody/labelled antigen mixture. Enzyme-linked (ELISA) assays, in which an enzyme (such as peroxidase) which induces a colour change in its substrate is used in place of the radioisotope, are increasingly popular because of their cheapness and safety.

At present, considerable hopes are attached to the use of monoclonal antibodies as reagents for 'finding' particular antigens *in vivo* and directing other compounds to the site. Examples would be the localisation of tumours by isotope-labelled antibody, or the anti-tumour effect of antibodies coupled to cytotoxic drugs, such as ricin molecules. The same idea can be applied in reverse, by using a toxic preparation of antigen to seek out and destroy lymphocytes whose receptors recognise the antigen.

FURTHER READING

Bibel D J 1988 Milestones in immunology. Springer-Verlag. *A fascinating history of immunology since the first vaccine (1798) with excerpts from classic papers.*

Chapel H, Heaney M 1989 Essentials of clinical immunology, 2nd edn. Blackwell Scientific Publications, Oxford. *The best short textbook of clinical immunology, predominantly systems-based.*

Fudenburg H H, Stites D P, Caldwell J L, Wells J V 1984 Basic and clinical immunology, 5th edn. Lange Medical Publications, Los Altos. *An excellent multi-author volume, one of the few to combine basic and clinical aspects.*

Lachman P J, Peters D K, Rosen F S, Walport M J, 1990 Clinical aspects of immunology, 5th edn. Blackwell Scientific Publications, Oxford. *The bible of British clinical immunology, now with an Anglo-American editorial panel. A massive and authoritative reference book.*

Playfair J H L 1987 Immunology at a glance, 4th ed, Blackwell Scientific Publications, Oxford. *A simple illustrated introduction to the subject.*

Roitt I M 1988 Essential immunology, 6th edn. Blackwell Scientific Publications, Oxford. *An up-to-date and stimulating textbook, including many experimental details.*

Nutrition in Clinical Medicine

FOOD AND ITS USE

Nutrition is the process by which food is eaten and utilised by the body. It is a dynamic process, crucial to the maintenance of normal function of tissues and organs as well as enabling activity and growth. This chapter is concerned with the ways in which nutrient supplies – especially energy – are utilised, and how dietary factors and deficiencies may produce specific clinical syndromes or contribute to the development of disease.

Energy

Without energy, maintenance of metabolic processes, physical activity and growth could not occur. The majority of dietary energy is needed for pumping ions across cell membranes, e.g. in red blood cells, cardiac muscle or intestinal epithelium. Classically, energy expenditure is measured as the basal metabolic rate (BMR) first thing in the morning in a resting subject in a relaxed frame of mind having last eaten the previous evening. More recent methods measure energy expenditure in free-living adults using stable isotopes.

The energy requirement of an individual subject depends primarily on body size and composition; but age, physical activity, environmental temperature and physiological state (whether pregnant, lactating or suffering from systemic infection) are also important. Energy expenditure may be considerably increased in situations of metabolic stress such as pyrexia and burns. Energy is expressed as kilocalories (kcal) or kilojoules (kJ); (one kcal = 4.18 kJ). Energy requirements are highest – on a body weight basis or by comparison with 'lean body mass' – in infants and young children. Energy expenditure starts to drop in the twenties and declines steadily thereafter into old age. Because the factors affecting energy requirement vary considerably between individuals, it is impossible to give an exact ideal nutrient intake; but there are clearly differences in daily energy expenditure between adults with different lifestyles (Table 8.1). Table 8.2 shows how this expenditure is partitioned between different activities; and Table 8.3 the energy required for various physical activities. As the total time in each 24 hours spent in such activities is often rather short, significant increases in energy expen-

Table 8.1 Average daily energy expenditure in various lifestyles

Occupation (age in years)	Expenditure in kcal (MJ)	
	Men	Women
Retired elderly (65 +)	2300 (9.5)	1900 (7.8)
Housewife (25–45)	–	2200 (9.0)
Office worker (20–50)	2500 (10.4)	2100 (8.6)
Laboratory technician (20–50)	2800 (11.7)	2200 (9.0)
Factory worker (20–45) (Heavy industry)	3200 (13.2)	2400 (9.9)
Labourer (20–45) (Heavy physical work)	3600 (14.8)	–

Table 8.2 Breakdown of average daily energy expenditure in clerks and miners

	Clerks		Miners	
	kcal	MJ	kcal	MJ
Sleep	500	2	500	2
Work	900	4	1750	7
Non-work activity	1400	6	1400	6
Total	2800	12	3650	15

117

8

Table 8.3 Average energy expenditure in various degrees of physical activity

Degree of activity	Expenditure (kcal/min)
Minimal (e.g. sitting, slow walking)	1
Moderate (e.g. walking, gardening)	5
Intermediate (e.g. swimming, brisk walking)	7
Heavy (e.g. digging, squash, running)	10

diture are hard to sustain. This is particularly frustrating for people who work intensively at weight reduction by increasing their physical activity. However, there are indications that energy expenditure remains elevated for 12–24 hours after vigorous exercise, and even resting energy expenditure may be increased by fitness.

Energy is required for growth, and measurements of weight gain or height gain are useful indicators of dietary insufficiency. During the first few weeks of catch-up growth from severe protein-energy malnutrition (PEM), the energy cost of weight gain is about 5 kcal/g. Thereafter, it becomes more energy expensive to lay down tissue, as fat rather than protein is stored.

Almost all components of the diet – fat, carbohydrate, protein and alcohol – provide energy. In the UK, fat and carbohydrate each provide between 40% and 50% of dietary energy whereas, in developing countries, the proportion from fat may be less than 15% and from carbohydrates more than 75%. The proportion of energy from protein is around 10% in an average UK diet. If protein is given without sufficient energy – for example in parenteral feeding regimes using amino acid solutions alone, or in athletes in training on very high protein diets – a large proportion is used up in oxidation. This also occurs in certain synthetic micro-diets providing 400 kcal/day or less, where protein is supplied in otherwise adequate quantities, but without adequate calories. At least some of the resulting weight loss is due to loss of body protein as it is oxidised.

Protein

Nearly all body tissues exist in a dynamic state of synthesis and breakdown, allowing growth, repair and atrophy to occur. The basic component of the tissues in this process is protein. There has in the past been considerable debate about the relative efficiency of proteins from different sources in promoting tissue growth – with vegetable protein often rated lower than that from animal products. The important factor is the presence or otherwise in the protein of the nine essential amino acids (those which cannot be synthesised by the body and must therefore be provided in the diet). If one or more are in low concentration then the food is less efficient at building protein (i.e. more has to be eaten). Dietary proteins are usually scored for their efficiency in comparison with whole egg or milk protein. However, it is important to remember that foodstuffs with a low score such as maize (which scores 47% because of low levels of tryptophan) or beans (which score 47% because of low levels of sulphur-containing amino acids) may complement each other in terms of amino acid level. A maize/beans mix – which is eaten by millions of people all over the world – has a score of 57%, i.e. this diet is not really 'protein limiting' provided there is enough of it.

Adequate protein intake can be achieved either by eating more of the cereals or by increasing the intake of foods with a higher protein score. The protein content of some common foods is shown in Table 8.4. Most of the world's population (i.e. those in developing countries) practises the cereals strategy. Their diet is, of necessity, very bulky because of the high viscosity and low energy density of most cereal porridges (Fig. 8.1). Nutritionists have, in the past, tended to overemphasise the need for increased high protein foodstuffs. It is true that there are some cereals, such as cassava, with very low protein content, but most populations take a mixed vegetarian diet well balanced with respect to protein and energy. The major problem is that millions of people do not get enough of it.

There is considerable debate as to how much protein we require; but a useful strategy in all nutritional states is to consider the nitrogen balance – the difference between the dietary intake and obligatory losses of nitrogen (e.g. in the urine, faeces, sweat and sputum). Positive balance is achieved when intake exceeds losses, such as occurs in normal infant and child growth or during recovery from malnutrition in adulthood. Negative balance occurs when losses exceed intake, as in systemic infection or diarrhoea,

Table 8.4 The protein content of some common foods

Protein source	Proportion of energy from protein (%)
Poor	
Cassava	3.3
Cooked bananas (plantains)	4.0
Sweet potatoes (*Ipomoea batatas*)	4.4
Taros	6.8
Adequate	
Irish potatoes	7.6
Rice (home-pounded)	8.0
Maize (wholemeal)	10.4
Millet (*Setaria italica*)	11.6
Sorghum (*Sorghum vulgare*)	11.6
Wheat flour (medium extraction)	13.2
Millet (*Pennisetum glaucum*)	13.6
Good	
Groundnuts (peanuts)	18.8
Cows' milk (3.5% fat)	21.6
Beans and peas	25.6
Beef (lean)	38.4
Cows' milk (skimmed)	40.0
Soya bean	45.2
Fish, fatty	45.6
Fish, dried	61.6

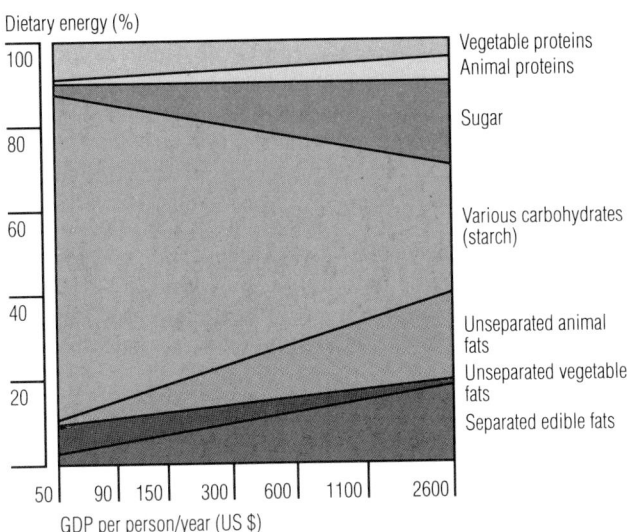

Dietary energy (%)

GDP per person/year (US $)

Fig. 8.1 Breakdown of total dietary energy related to income (GDP of countries).

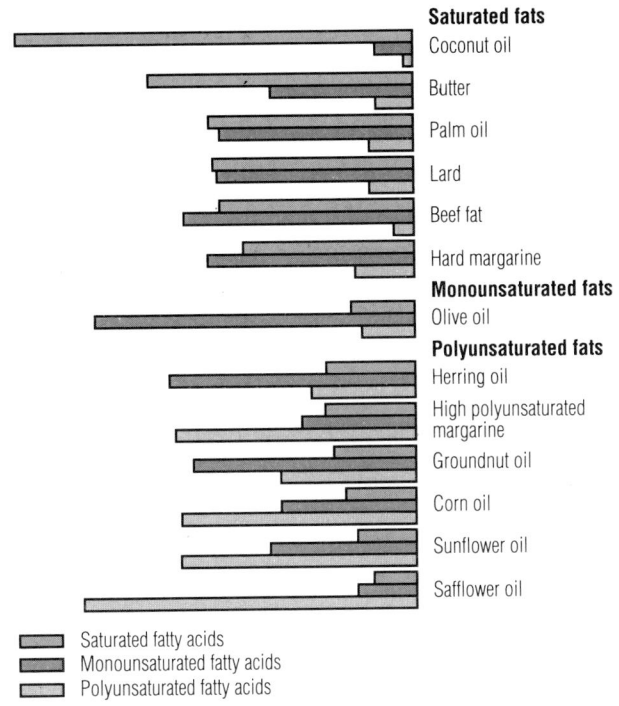

Fig. 8.2 Fatty acid composition of some common fats and oils.

or when dietary intake is reduced. The greatest requirements for protein (relative to body weight) occur among young infants. Those less than three months of age require about 2.5 g protein/kg body weight/day, and the older infant (9–12 months age) requires 1.5 g protein/kg body weight/day. Children need less than infants but more than adults. Rates of protein synthesis vary with age, being highest in the newborn and declining with time (Table 8.5).

Fat

The term 'fat' covers a range of chemicals. Fats provide the chief store of energy in the subcutaneous tissue, are important in the development of all cell membranes and some tissues, and are essential components of some hormones. The most common storage fats are the *triglycerides*. These are esters of glycerol and three fatty acids, which exist in a variety of forms according to the length of the carbon chain and the degree of saturation. This affects their solubility in water (shorter chain triglycerides are more soluble), fluidity and melting point. Vegetable oils have a greater proportion of polyunsaturated fats and are more fluid than the more saturated fats from animal sources, which are often hard (Fig. 8.2). *Phospholipids* – esters of glycerol with two fatty acids – are important for stability of cell membranes and deficiency may therefore affect satisfactory psychomotor development. *Cholesterol* is the most important sterol. It is the precursor of the bile acids (which are essential for mixed micelle formation in the intestinal absorption of fat) as well as of adrenal and sex hormones and vitamin D. Cholesterol is also linked to the development of atheroma.

Lipoproteins are the chemical complexes, formed by the triglycerides, phospholipids and cholesterol with proteins, that circulate in the blood. These lipoproteins can be sep-

arated by electrophoresis or according to density on ultra-centrifugation (p. 777).

The body is remarkably efficient at synthesising triglycerides, sterols, and phospholipids. Many populations whose diet provides only 15% of total energy as fat, yet are able to lay down good stores of subcutaneous fat. Requirements for essential fatty acids are rather low and deficiency is therefore uncommon. However, low fat diets are often less palatable which sometimes limits dietary intake and may lead to malnutrition. Low fat diets may also limit the absorption of carotene (the precursor of vitamin A found in green leafy vegetables). Fats provide twice as much energy per unit weight as protein or carbohydrate, and are thus useful sources of energy in diets designed to increase the rate of weight gain, e.g. in malnourished children. Conversely, a reduction in the fat content of the diet is a relatively efficient way to lose weight. The potential of a combination of reducing total dietary fat and increasing the ratio of polyunsaturated to saturated fats in the prevention of coronary heart disease is currently being investigated.

Micronutrients

Deficiencies of individual vitamins result in specific biochemical and clinical responses, but vitamins are also involved in metabolism in more general ways. Folate, for example, is necessary for cell division and the transfer of methyl groups in protein synthesis; thus, a deficiency may impair tissue repair or growth, even if dietary energy and protein are adequate. Thiamine is important in carbo-

8

hydrate metabolism, and lactic acidosis may occur in deficiency states. A number of trace elements, such as zinc, are important in protein metabolism; deficiency of zinc is associated with an increased energy requirement for deposition of lean tissue. Children receiving nutrient supplements for protein-energy malnutrition grow more slowly relative to the number of calories given, if they are not also supplemented with zinc. Severe individual micronutrient deficiencies may have recognizable clinical features, but even marginal deficiencies may affect metabolism of protein and energy.

Eating enough

Any set of standards for child growth – made up from subjects living in a clean environment with an abundance of food, such as the National Child Health Statistics (NCHS) Standards from North American children – show a considerable range in rates of gain in weight and stature. There are also considerable differences in dietary intake among such children; and this is also true among healthy adults who are not excessively over- or underweight. Furthermore, an individual in his thirties who continues eating the same amount of food that he ate in his late teens is likely to become overweight. In each case, the difference in nutritional status is the result of a balance between energy intake and energy expenditure. There are several physiological and pathological states which affect this.

Early infancy

In the young infant, nutritional requirements for protein are particularly high in relation to body weight (Table 8.5). Breast milk certainly provides enough protein for at least the first four months, and also has immunological advantages over cows' milk. Cows' milk formulae, while nutritionally adequate, are frequently dangerous when prepared under unhygienic conditions, as in many poor families in developing countries.

Table 8.5 Variation in rate of protein synthesis with age

Age group	Body weight (kg)	Total body protein synthesis (g/kg body weight/day)
Newborn (premature)	2.0	15.0
Infant	9.0	7.0
Young adult	70.0	3.0
Elderly	55.0	2.0

Later infancy and early childhood

Nutritional requirements are also high in infants over four months of age, when children often begin to receive solid foods in addition to breast milk. In developing countries, the growth rate frequently falters at this stage – either because the energy given is not enough (the energy density

of weaning foods in traditional societies is often low); or because there is so much gut infection (there is abundant evidence that mucosal damage is severe in this age group) that the food is not so well absorbed. Specific nutrient deficiencies (e.g. zinc, protein, folate) may also play a role.

Later childhood and adolescence

Nutritional requirements for protein and energy are usually met in older children, but there tend to be micronutrient deficiencies (e.g. of iron, folate and zinc), which may lead to anaemia, impaired intellectual performance and short stature.

Pregnancy

The nutritional stress of pregnancy is created by the need to produce both an infant and a placenta, plus some maternal fat stores. The generally accepted idea of a 9–12 kg weight gain during pregnancy requires (on the assumption of 5 kcal/g weight gain) an increased dietary intake of 150 kcal/day during the first trimester, and about 300 kcal/day thereafter, including extra protein (Table 8.6). Several studies show that the baby is rather small at birth if this is not achieved. Among women in the UK, there is evidence of decreased birth weight in those with low energy and protein intakes, a situation found especially among Asian immigrants. There are also increased demands on maternal stores, especially of iron, zinc and folate. However, despite such considerable increases in requirement, there are populations of women in developing countries with rather poor diets and very unfavourable lifestyles who yet produce babies of reasonable weight. Similarly, there are many women in the UK who date their obesity from their pregnancy. The reason for these findings is the markedly increased efficiency of metabolism during pregnancy so that dietary energy is stored more easily.

Table 8.6 Average weight gain during pregnancy

| | Increase in weight (g) | | | |
	Up to 10 weeks	20 weeks	30 weeks	40 weeks
Fetus, placenta and liquor	55	720	2530	4750
Uterus and breasts	170	765	1170	1300
Blood	100	600	1300	1250
Fat	325	1915	3500	4000
Total gain	650	4000	8500	12 000

Lactation

The need to produce breast milk (up to 800 kcal/day) for many months has obvious nutritional implications. Some of this can be provided from maternal stores laid down in pregnancy, but an additional 500 kcal intake and extra protein is often recommended. Again, many women are able to produce adequate volumes of breast milk despite poor dietary intakes. However, when maternal nutritional status is severely decreased, there is a corresponding decrease in the volume and nutritional content of the milk. It is thus essential to improve the diet and lifestyle of women in developing countries if breast-feeding is to be promoted. A high proportion of women in the UK on the other hand eat more than they need during lactation and pregnancy.

Recommended daily allowances

In view of the considerable variation in nutrient metabolism between both population groups and individuals, accurate nutritional recommendations are difficult to make. The *recommended daily allowance* (RDA) is the level of intake of nutrient at which nobody would be deficient; (there are various tables available). The RDA is thus set to prevent undernutrition but may, if adhered to slavishly, contribute to overnutrition. The term *safe level* is also sometimes used – usually for nutrients where accurate measurements of requirements have not been performed.

Food patterns in the UK

There is currently an increased awareness of the importance of diet in the prevention of coronary thrombosis, hypertension and colon cancer. The National Advisory

Committee on Nutrition Education (NACNE) proposed that a healthy diet should contain no more than 35% of energy from fat, that dietary fibre should increase to 25 g daily, that salt intake should be reduced by about 30% and that total energy intake should maintain body weight within normal levels (Fig. 8.3). Various District Health Authorities in the UK have sought to implement policies such as these within hospitals, although these have not always been successful due to the conservatism of caterers and the apathy of medical staff. The Coronary Prevention Group seeks to publicise the NACNE recommendations which are summarised in Table 8.7.

Table 8.7 Summary of proposals for dietary change to lower disease prevalence*

Nutrient	Current intake	Proposals
Energy	Increasing prevalence of obesity in UK indicates excessive intake.	Energy intake such as to keep body weight within healthy limits (BMI 20–26).
Fat	Above 40% of energy taken in the form of fat.	Reduce, such that intake is <35% of energy intake.
Saturated fats	About 18% of energy taken in form of saturated fat.	Reduce such that <15% of energy intake comes from saturated fats.
Polyunsaturated fats	About 4% of energy taken in form of polyunsaturates.	Increase to >5% of energy from polyunsaturates.
Fibre	About 15 g daily	Increase to above 25 g
Sugar	Very variable	Reduce by 10%
Salt	Very variable	Reduce by 10%
Alcohol	Very variable	Not more than 4 alcohol units per day

*National Advisory Committee on Nutrition Education, 1983; DHSS Diet and Cardiovascular Disease, 1984. BMI =Body Mass Index =weight/height².

ASSESSMENT OF NUTRITIONAL STATUS

The body is made up of lean body mass (the bony framework, muscle and dense connective tissue), adipose tissue and water. In weight terms, the composition of the constituents is 16% protein, 10–25% fat in men (15–30% in women), 5% minerals, 1% carbohydrate and the rest water (about 60%). This total body water is either in the cells (intracellular water, 35%) or in the vascular system and tissues (extracellular water, 25%). Measurement of nutritional status seeks to determine how these body compartments compare with one another and whether nutrient deficiencies or excesses are affecting the function of tissues.

Anthropometry

Measurements of weight in childhood can be compared with the weight of a child of the same age in tables of reference standards (thus, for example, a child's weight for

A Today's average UK diet

B The 'new' diet

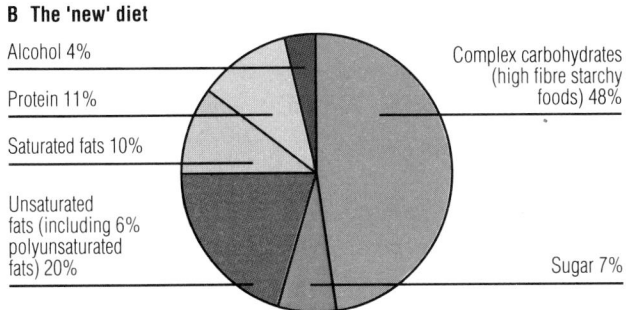

Fig. 8.3 Composition of an average UK diet, compared with that recommended by NACNE.

8

its age may be 70% of the standard. See Table 8.8). The standards recommended by the World Health Organisation are those of the National Centre for Health Statistics (NCHS) which are based on the measurements of a large number of North American children. There are obvious objections to their use in that populations throughout the world are often lighter. However, genetic factors seem relatively unimportant in causing these population differences, since children from well-off parents (who tend to be fed well and have any illnesses treated rapidly and effectively), are generally indistinguishable from the NCHS standards, regardless of their ethnic group. Similar NCHS standards exist for height, and an index of thinness can be expressed by calculating a child's weight as a proportion of that expected for a child of that height.

Among adults the range of body proportion is considerable. This can be expressed in a number of ways:

1. As a weight as a percentage of ideal body weight from tables constructed from life assurance tables, or
2. As the body mass index (BMI = weight/height^2).
3. The mid-arm circumference (MAC) relates closely to weight/height measurements though the sensitivity and specificity of this method for screening for thinness varies according to whether there has been very recent weight loss (presumably mainly loss of fat) or whether the loss has been over a longer period (presumably loss of fat and skeletal muscle). Nevertheless, plastic strips to measure MAC using coloured bands have been used with great success in screening for children with severe PEM in developing countries (Table 8.9).
4. A reasonable measurement of body fat can be made from measurement of skin fold thickness using Harpenden calipers, which apply a constant spring loaded pressure to the fold. Skin folds may be measured at biceps, triceps, subscapular and supra-iliac; but the first and last of these sites give greater variability. Despite the apparent simplicity of this measurement there is considerable variation both between observers and within the same observer, so that skin fold thickness may be best kept as a research tool rather than a routine clinical method.
5. Functional tests of muscle, such as dynamometry and measurement of the response to electrical stimulation, are said to measure muscle mass; but results are only abnormal when the level of nutrition is very poor.
6. Urinary creatinine, on the other hand, is a very reliable index of muscle mass and is a useful marker for completeness of 24 hour urine collections.

Table 8.8 Assessment of nutritional status: body size, protein and fat

Method	Comments
Body size	
Weight and height	
Weight as % of standard weight/age in children	A child who is chronically underweight (compared to international standards) may still achieve good rates of weight gain.
Weight as % ideal body weight in adults	Weight varies by 0.5–1.0 kg/day in healthy adult subjects.
Weight/height^2 (BMI) in teenagers and adults	BMI is difficult to interpret in the elderly – use length of humerus as index of height
Degree and rate of weight loss	More than 10% loss usually indicates PEM
Protein	
Mid-arm circumference (MAC) Use the absolute value in children age 1–5 years because there is little change with age In adults there is considerable variation but <22 cm usually indicates loss of muscle mass	Use the % of standard MAC for age in children
Urinary creatinine/height Use 24 hour urine collection which indicates how much muscle mass is present	Creatinine excretion is affected by pyrexia. Incomplete 24 hour collections invalidate the method.
Plasma concentrations of hepatic export proteins (e.g. albumin, pre-albumin, retinol binding globulin, thyroid binding globulin, transferrin)	All are affected by dietary intake in 2 weeks prior to test. 'Leak' of proteins (e.g. albumin in intestinal disease) may occur. Acute and chronic infections may decrease synthesis of the export proteins. Plasma albumin of <35 g/l or plasma transferrin of <1.5 g/l usually indicates PEM
Tests of cellular immunity In vitro lymphocyte studies or skin tests	Considerable amount of laboratory work. No more sensitive than anthropometry.
Fat	
Skin fold thickness Measured at mid-triceps, subscapular and supra-iliac sites and expressed as absolute values or percentage of standard	Considerable sources of error in repeat measurements by different observers. Triceps skin fold thickness is the least variable.

Table 8.9 Mid-arm circumference (MAC) in children aged 12–60 months

MAC (cm)	Level of nutrition
More than 14	Normal
12.5–14	Mild/moderate protein-energy malnutrition
Less than 12.5	Severe protein-energy malnutrition

Biochemical

A series of proteins produced by the liver may be used in the assessment of protein status, namely albumin, pre-albumin, transferrin, retinol binding globulin and thyroid binding globulin. These indicators are of limited value on their own because they are affected by short term energy intake as well as by protein stores. However, low levels (of albumin in particular) suggest decreased synthesis due to poor dietary intake, increased metabolism as in systemic infection, or a leak of protein as occurs, for example, in intestinal disease. Table 8.8 shows the tests available to assess individual nutrients.

Cellular immunity is depressed in severe protein-energy malnutrition (PEM), and selective T cell function tests can thus be used to monitor nutritional status; although this is rather laborious. A total lymphocyte count of $<2.0 \times 10^6/1$ is suggestive of impaired function.

PRIMARY NUTRITIONAL DISORDERS

PROTEIN-ENERGY MALNUTRITION

The term *protein-energy malnutrition* (PEM) is used to describe a variety of clinical syndromes which result from a diet inadequate with respect to both energy and protein. It is often accompanied by micronutrient deficiencies, electrolyte imbalance and metabolic disorders. When it occurs in the UK, it is usually precipitated by a severe illness (e.g. gastro-intestinal disease, or surgery); in developing countries, it is the result of a poor diet due to social and economic deprivation, often exacerbated by the added stress of infection (especially diarrhoea and measles). Indeed, the presence of infection is so common in children with PEM that the term *malnutrition/infection syndrome* is often used to describe the condition. Classification of the severe clinical syndromes of PEM (Table 8.10) depends on the child's weight calculated as a percentage of the median international standard for a child of the same age. Milder grades of PEM also exist according to weight/age. Undernourished children may be further classified according to whether, or to what degree, they are short for their age (*stunting*); alternatively they may be underweight and thin, i.e. a low weight/height (*wasting*, see Table 8.11 and Fig. 8.4). The inference is that children who are stunted are likely to have been deprived of an adequate diet for

Table 8.10 Classification of severe protein-energy malnutrition

Weight for age*	With oedema	Without oedema
60–80%	Kwashiorkor	Undernutrition
Less than 60%	Marasmic kwashiorkor	Marasmus

* Weight as % of standard (NCHS) weight of child of that age

Table 8.11 Classification of stunting and wasting

Degree	Stunting (height/age)	Wasting (weight/height)
Normal	Over 95	Over 90
Mild	87.5–95	80–90
Moderate	80–87.5	70–80
Severe	Less than 80	Less than 70

* Weight (or height) as percentage of standard (NCHS) weight of child of that age

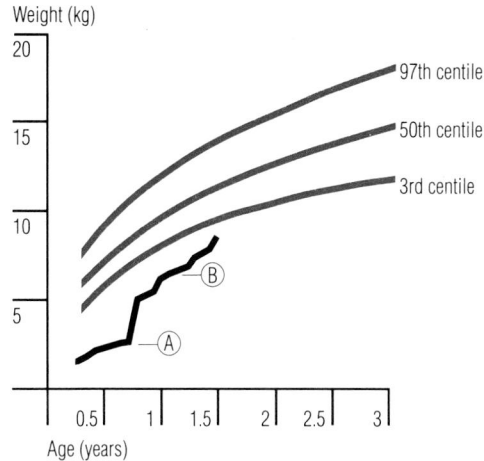

Fig. 8.4 Growth chart of a severely malnourished child. A. Start of nutrition rehabilitation. **B.** After discharge from nutrition rehabilitation centre.

many months (sufficient to cause linear growth retardation). The child who is wasted has lost body tissues, often, though not always, because of a recent infection or poor diet, for example due to harvest failure.

PEM in children

PEM is the end result of several processes. Thus, a child may become marasmic because of total lack of food in a famine, or because he has severe giardiasis, intestinal parasites or tuberculosis. A child may develop kwashiorkor at the time he is weaned off the breast and has to rely instead on rather inadequate quantities of solid food. It was this aspect of the history that first stimulated the suggestion that kwashiorkor was due to lack of dietary protein. However, there is only limited evidence that dietary differences explain why some children develop kwashiorkor and others become marasmic; kwashiorkor is often precipitated by measles and intestinal infection.

Marasmus

In marasmus, there is loss of both lean tissue and subcutaneous fat with characteristic wrinkling of the skin. This is sometimes difficult to differentiate from dehydration. The child is usually very cachectic, and has long eyelashes and lanugo hair on the forearms despite loss of hair on the head. However, the child is generally alert. The plasma albumin is usually maintained but plasma sodium and potassium levels are low.

Kwashiorkor

The main feature of kwashiorkor is oedema which conceals the loss of lean tissue. The oedema usually starts in the legs but may extend to the trunk and head. There is often an associated scaly cracking of the skin and some children have discoloured or orange hair. The liver is sometimes enlarged, as it becomes infiltrated with fat which cannot be removed because of inadequate production of lipoproteins (see Ch. 20, p. 778). Plasma albumin is low, as are plasma sodium and potassium. The low plasma potassium indicates a reduction in total body potassium, due to the loss of muscle mass. The low plasma sodium, however, is misleading, as it is due to an excess of body water. The total body sodium is in fact elevated.

Several factors contribute to the development of oedema. A decrease in plasma albumin decreases colloid osmotic pressure; while an increase in the generation of free radicals by infection (from systemic or intestinal pathogens, or toxins such as aflatoxin) can damage the capillaries sufficiently to cause them to leak fluid into the tissues. The deleterious effects are greatest in children with impaired scavenging mechanisms for free radicals, due to a deficiency of zinc, copper and vitamin A.

Associated deficiencies

Zinc deficiency is common in severe PEM, and may account for the skin lesions and impaired cellular immunity. Vitamin A deficiency is frequently precipitated by PEM, probably because of lack of synthesis of retinol binding globulin by the liver; and anaemia often occurs as a consequence of folate and/or iron deficiency and systemic infection (especially malaria). Cellular immunity is frequently depressed, thus permitting infections such as tuberculosis to become rampant. Antibody production is also impaired, but to a lesser extent, so that even severely malnourished children generally produce satisfactory levels of antibodies following immunisation. However, the general reduction in immunity is a key factor in the development of bacterial overgrowth syndromes in the intestine, pneumonia and septicaemia. The decreased heat production in PEM is often severe enough to cause hypothermia and prevents a pyrexial response to infection.

Specific organ changes

There is atrophy of the lining of the alimentary tract causing hypochlorhydria and flattening of intestinal villi. Nearly all children are heavily colonised by intestinal parasites and bacteria. Renal function is often impaired, leading to difficulties in excreting sodium and water. Experimental studies show marked affects of PEM on brain size and psychomotor development; but longitudinal studies of severely malnourished children show that the social environment is more important than nutrient deficiency in determining subsequent intellectual achievement.

Management

Several principles should be followed:

1. Resuscitation for dehydration (in most cases using oral rehydration therapy).
2. Antibiotics (such as procaine penicillin or chloramphenicol) should be given for systemic infections, together with treatment for malaria.

3. Nutritional therapy depends on the introduction of special feeds providing maintenance requirements (100 kcal/kg body weight and 3 g protein/kg body weight). This should be accompanied by mineral mixes (especially potassium and zinc). In children with kwashiorkor, maintenance requirements are given until the oedema is cleared, then energy intakes are increased. In marasmic children, the intake can be increased earlier, until – ideally – about 200 kcal/kg body weight/day are given (Table 8.12). Table 8.13 shows some mixes which can be given during different stages of nutritional rehabilitation.

Table 8.12 Predicted rate of weight gain* in malnourished child weighing 7 kg

Total intake (kcal/day)	Excess (kcal/day)	Weight gain (g/day)	Days to gain 3000 g
700	0	0	–
760	60	10	300
820	120	20	150
940	240	40	75
1180	480	80	38
1660	960	160	19

* Assuming maintenance requirements of 100 kcal/kg/body weight/day

Table 8.13 Suitable high energy/protein mixes for children with severe protein-energy malnutrition

Type of milk (g)	Sugar (g)	Oil (g)	Water (ml)
Dried skimmed milk 86	67	86	811
Evaporated milk 443	67	52	488
Lactogen 183	14	43	813
Complan 100	67	71	812
Cows' milk 885	67	56	42

PEM in adults

PEM in adults is surprisingly common in medical and surgical practice. Inadequate intake is the most important factor, whether due to psychological factors (such as anorexia nervosa), pain (oral or intestinal cancer), nausea/vomiting (liver metastases, chemotherapy, gastrointestinal disease) or fever (which often causes anorexia). Nutrient intakes are often reduced drastically among those who can only take fluids. Nutrient requirements may be considerably increased by sepsis. Energy expenditure increases by at least 10% for every 1°C rise in body temperature, and muscle protein is mobilised to provide amino acid precursors for the inflammatory response. Infection also increases the production of acute phase proteins such as C-reactive protein; but levels of plasma albumin may decrease, due to decreased synthesis by the liver and

Table 8.14 Assessment of causes of protein-energy malnutrition in adults

Food intake	Energy and protein intakes can be assessed by dietitian using memory recall or direct weighing. Reasons for decrease can be assessed by clinical history.
Nutrient requirements	Assessment of inflammatory response by measurement of body temperature and C-reactive protein.
Malabsorption	Use degree of steatorrhoea to assess energy losses approximately if unable to measure faecal energy losses directly.
Nutrient losses	Estimates of faecal protein losses can be made approximately from measurement of stool blood/mucus losses.

increased catabolism of the circulatory albumin. Any cause of malabsorption may cause a serious decrease in absorption of protein and energy. Disease of the lower small intestine and colon may cause serious leakage of endogenous protein and protein loss in blood. A checklist for nutritional assessment is given in Table 8.14. An approximate nitrogen balance can be obtained by measurement of urinary urea (the form in which 80% of urinary nitrogen is excreted).

VITAMIN DEFICIENCIES

A checklist for the methods of assessment of vitamin deficiencies is given in Table 8.15. The important food sources of the various vitamins are shown in Table 8.16, and their roles in the body in Table 8.17.

Vitamin A deficiency

Vitamin A deficiency leads to night blindness and xerophthalmia (damage to the conjunctiva): it also affects the immune system – increasing the prevalence of respiratory infections and diarrhoea – and the formation of epithelium in the sweat glands, lung and gut. It may also contribute to the high rates of child mortality in certain populations, particularly among poor communities where dietary intakes of carotene (the dietary precursor of vitamin A) are low, and where the availability of the nutrient may be further reduced by intestinal parasites and diarrhoea. Vitamin A deficiency sometimes complicates inflammatory bowel disease, coeliac disease and cirrhosis. Measles is an important precipitatory factor because of its effect (a) directly on the conjunctiva, where it increases the local requirement for vitamin A needed to repair the damaged conjunctiva; and (b) indirectly, by its effect on synthesis of retinol binding protein which carries vitamin A from the liver stores to the eye.

Night blindness alone is easily reversible, but xerosis (the dry appearance of the conjunctiva) and Bitot's spots (heaped up desquamated cells causing flecks on the conjunctiva) are signs that, unless treatment is started soon, the lesion may progress to irreversible corneal ulceration.

Table 8.15 Assessment of nutritional status: vitamins*

Vitamin	Method	Comment
A	Clinical	Night-blindness is a good indicator. Corneal lesions are very late stage findings.
	Plasma carotene	Marked increase after dietary intake.
	Plasma retinol	Sensitive indicator of liver stores.
Thiamine	Clinical	Neuropathy and optic atrophy are late stage findings.
	Erythrocyte transketolase	Sensitive but rapidly altered by amount of dietary thiamine.
Riboflavin	Clinical	Mouth lesions are nonspecific.
	Erythrocyte glutathione reductase	Difficult to know physiological significance of low enzyme levels.
Niacin	Clinical	Glossitis, stomatitis, dermatitis.
	Urinary n-methyl-nicotinamide/creatine excretion	Sensitive. Difficult assay.
Folate	Serum folate	Marked changes after dietary intake.
	Erythrocyte folate	Sensitive assay of body stores.
B$_{12}$	Plasma vitamin level	Sensitive assay of body stores
C	Clinical	Specific but occur at late stage only.
	Plasma or leucocyte ascorbate	Sensitive. Rapid response to diet.
D	Clinical Plasma alkaline phosphatase	Rickets, osteomalacia. Nonspecific. Sensitivity may be improved by isoenzyme analysis.
	Plasma 25-hydroxycholecalciferol	Very specific.
	Bone marrow histology	Specific.
E	Plasma or erythrocyte tocopherol	Sensitive and specific.
K	Prothrombin time	Nonspecific, as it is influenced by hepatocellular dysfunction

*Pyridoxine is omitted as this is not a routine assay.

In those areas where dietary vitamin A intake cannot be increased by horticulture and nutrition education programmes, the administration of vitamin A capsules

(100 000 IU every six months) will largely prevent xerophthalmia. Vitamin A capsules should not, however, be given to pregnant women because of their teratogenic effect. Breastfeeding tends to prevent vitamin A deficiency. In established xerophthalmia, retinol palmitate (100 000 IU) is given intramuscularly.

Thiamine deficiency

Thiamine is an essential factor in many glycolytic pathways and is especially important for proper function of the peripheral nervous system and the heart. Deficiency can cause a peripheral neuropathy, especially in the legs, with ataxia and optic atrophy. Although this syndrome was described classically among prisoners on an inadequate, predominantly polished rice diet, most cases in the UK occur in malnourished alcoholics. Such patients may develop two additional syndromes. In *Wernicke's encephalopathy* nuclear or supranuclear ophthalmoplegia occurs with nystagmus, pupillary abnormalities, aphasia and mental confusion. In *Korsakoff's psychosis* a confused state characterised by memory loss and confabulation develops. Cardiac beri-beri (a high-output cardiac failure) sometimes occurs, particularly in populations who change to eating rice which is highly milled as this process removes the thiamine.

Diagnosis is usually made on clinical history and examination, but elevated levels of erythrocyte transketolase activity and blood pyruvate occur. Thiamine (100 mg) may be given intravenously or orally, followed by repeated doses of 20 mg three times daily. Cardiac beri-beri improves rapidly, but nutritional neuropathies tend to recover only partially, especially if present for a long time.

Niacin (nicotinic acid and nicotinamide) deficiency

Nicotinic acid occurs in many plant and animal foods and can also be synthesised from tryptophan. Nicotinic acid deficiency tends to occur in those who eat a monotonous maize diet (which is low in tryptophan), such as occurred in a considerable proportion of the poor whites of the southern states of the USA earlier this century. The resulting deficiency syndrome, *pellagra*, was initially thought to be infectious.

Pellagra often starts with any one of a sore mouth, mild diarrhoea or confusion. (Before 1960, up to 10% of acute psychiatric admissions in Southern India were attributable to confusion due to pellagra.) The full clinical syndrome of 'dermatitis, diarrhoea and dementia' is not striking, except in well-established cases. The skin lesions are initially erythematous, but dry, cracked appearances then occur, especially in areas exposed to the sun, producing 'Casal's necklace' around the neck. There may be villus atrophy in the small intestine and malabsorption. If untreated, later stage deficiency may cause severe encephalopathy and spasticity. Pellagra is rare in the UK, but may occur in malabsorption syndromes such as coeliac disease, in patients treated with isoniazid, in Hartnup disease, in the carcinoid syndrome, in patients with very low protein

diets, or in conditions giving rise to considerable loss of protein such as the nephrotic syndrome. Deficiency responds rapidly to daily doses of nicotinic acid (500 mg).

Riboflavin deficiency

Riboflavin deficiency occurs whenever a diet is continually deficient in legumes, pulses and animal products. It may thus accompany PEM or alcoholism and is especially liable to occur during pregnancy. The main lesions are mucosal dryness and cracking around the mouth, ears and eyelids, with the genital region also affected. Red blood cells are affected, causing a normochromic anaemia.

Diagnosis is usually on clinical grounds but can be confirmed by reduced glutathione reductase activity in red blood cells. Lesions respond fairly quickly to riboflavin (6 mg daily).

Pyridoxine deficiency

Pyridoxine deficiency occurs in malabsorption syndromes, alcoholism and secondary to drug toxicity (especially isoniazid), but rarely as a primary deficiency disorder. Clin-

Table 8.16 Vitamins and their important food sources.

Vitamin	Food sources
A	Carotenoids (esp. β-carotene), in carrots, dark green leafy vegetables, pumpkin, mango. Preformed vitamin A, in fish oils, liver, eggs, margarine.
Thiamine (B$_1$)	Fortified wheat flour (much of the thiamine in flour is removed by milling, but is then replaced in most flours), fortified breakfast cereals, milk, eggs, yeast extract, fruit.
Riboflavin (B$_2$)	Milk, cheese, eggs, fortified breakfast cereals, liver, kidney, whole grain cereals.
Nicotinic acid	Liver, kidney, milk, cheese, eggs, beef, chicken, pork, yeast extract, instant coffee, peas, beans.
Pyridoxine (B$_6$)	Liver, meat, fish, whole grain cereals, milk, peanuts
Folate	Liver, kidney, green leafy vegetables, peas, beans, oranges, bananas.
Cobalamine (B$_{12}$)	Liver, kidney, fish, beef, pork, lamb, eggs, cheese.
Ascorbic acid (C)	Oranges, lemons, potatoes, green vegetables, fortified fruit drinks.
D	Fortified milk (e.g. evaporated), fatty fish, fortified margarine, eggs, liver.
E	Vegetable oils, wholegrain cereals, eggs, margarine.
K	Vegetables, peas, beans, liver.

ically, there is mental confusion, glossitis, dry skin lesions and peripheral neuropathy. There are also a number of rare metabolic disorders in which pyridoxine deficiency is associated with infantile convulsions and sideroblastic anaemia. Pyridoxine deficiency is popularly believed to be a cause of pre-menstrual syndrome but there is no scientific evidence of this.

Treatment of deficiency in adults is by 5–20 mg doses daily. Excess leads to neurotoxicity.

Folate deficiency

Folate deficiency occurs in those whose diet lacks fresh vegetables or meat, or in which the vitamin is destroyed by overcooking. It may also occur secondary to upper small bowel malabsorption; in situations of increased requirements (i.e. pregnancy or any haemolytic condition); or in patients taking anti-folate drugs (e.g. methotrexate, trimethoprim). The main effect is to slow the rate of DNA synthesis, thus limiting the regeneration of new cells. Megaloblastic anaemia, buccal lesions, villus atrophy and impaired fetal development also occur.

Diagnosis is suggested by red cell macrocytosis and the presence of megaloblastic erythropoiesis; while red blood cell folate levels distinguish it from vitamin B_{12} deficiency. Folic acid 5 mg daily rapidly improves the clinical features.

Vitamin B_{12} deficiency

Vitamin B_{12} deficiency (see also Ch. 25, p. 1046) occurs in those who lack intrinsic factor as a result of: autoimmune gastric atrophy or gastric resection, malabsorption due to ileal disease, bacterial overgrowth syndromes, or (rarely) infection with *Diphyllobothrium latum*. It sometimes also occurs in vegans. The resulting impaired DNA synthesis particularly affects the bone marrow, so that the main effect of vitamin B_{12} deficiency is a megaloblastic anaemia. It also causes optic atrophy and subacute combined degeneration of the cord. Neurological signs may occur without haematological effects. Hyperpigmentation of the palms is described in coloured skins.

The serum vitamin B_{12} is the only reliable indicator of deficiency. Vitamin B_{12} should be given as 1000 mg intramuscularly, monthly for the first six months. Thereafter, four times per year is usually enough.

Vitamin C deficiency

Scurvy was well-known among those on long distance sea voyages for centuries, until the cause became known. In the eighteenth century, Lind carried out a controlled trial treating scurvy with citrus fruits and using mouthwashes of dilute vinegar or sea water as a control. Complete recovery occurred in the treated group but none in the controls and oranges and lemons were distributed among the British Royal Navy in 1747.

Today, deficiencies occur among the elderly – especially those on a 'tea and toast' diet – and among food faddists. It may also occur in young children during the first years of life when requirements are high. The clinical features of tiredness, hyperkeratosis of the hair follicles, petechial haemorrhages and bleeding gums are only present in severe deficiency: bleeding gums in malnourished children are more usually due to poor oral hygiene than to vitamin deficiency. The classical features of infantile scurvy – irritability, pain on moving the legs, and tenderness and enlargement of costochondral epiphyses together with megaloblastic anaemia – are now rarely seen.

Diagnosis is by measurement of leucocyte ascorbate content, but as leucocytes are rapidly renewed, normal levels are usually acquired within a few days of eating a hospital diet. Ascorbic acid 100 mg three times per day is rapidly effective in clinical deficiency. There is no consistent scientific evidence that large doses of vitamin C are effective in the prevention or treatment of the common cold.

Vitamin D deficiency

Vitamin D deficiency occurs among those who fail to produce enough in their skin (from the precursor 7-dehydrocholesterol in response to uv light), or who have inad-

Table 8.17 Role of vitamins in the body

Vitamin	Function
A	Maintenance of mucosal surfaces; production of mucus; immune system and retinal function
Thiamine (B_1)	Metabolism of carbohydrate to provide energy; maintenance of cardiac muscle and peripheral nerves.
Riboflavin (B_2)	Control of intracellular oxidation; maintenance of skin, especially around the mouth.
Nicotinic acid	Utilisation of energy from food; maintenance of skin, especially in light-exposed areas.
Pyridoxine (B_6)	Metabolism of amino acids, especially tryptophan to nictonic acid.
Folate	Cell multiplication, in the blood and mucosa.
Cobalamine (B_{12})	Cell multiplication, esp. blood cells; control of fatty acid synthesis in myelin sheaths of nerves.
Ascorbic acid (C)	Maintenance of connective tissue; stimulates iron absorption
D	Maintenance of calcium and phosphate levels in the blood; control of absorption of dietary calcium and movement of calcium between blood and bone.
E	Contributes to anti-oxidant capacity of body; important in maintenance of erythrocyte membranes in neonates.
K	Control of blood clotting.

equate dietary intake. In the UK, the high risk group are immigrant Asians who tend not to expose themselves to the limited sunlight available. Although they do eat fatty fish (a good source of vitamin D), their consumption of vitamin D fortified foods, e.g. margarine, is low, and the high phytate content (in chapatti flour) of the diet further decreases its bioavailability. The result of vitamin D deficiency is rickets (in children) or osteomalacia (in adults), both of which produce bony deformities (beading of the costochondral junctions – the 'rickety rosary') and bowing of the legs (Ch. 19, p. 735). In adults, there may be radiological lesions, such as stress fracture lines in the pelvis, femurs and scapulae.

Diagnosis is by estimation of 25-hydroxycholecalciferol (25-OH-D3) levels in plasma. The main management is through prevention, especially in ante-natal and child welfare clinics with a high proportion of immigrant Asians. Vitamin drops should be prescribed prophylactically for high risk groups. Vitamin D deficiency secondary to disease is discussed with its management in Chapter 19.

Vitamin E deficiency

Vitamin E deficiency occurs in low birth weight infants, malabsorption syndromes (especially cystic fibrosis) and abetalipoproteinaemia. Deficiency permits free radical damage to a number of membranes such as red blood cells (causing haemolytic anaemia) and nerve cells (causing ataxia and peripheral neuropathy). These conditions are exacerbated if extra nutrients, such as linoleic acid and iron, are given without vitamin E. There is no consistent scientific evidence of any effect of vitamin E on athletic success, sexual potency or atheroma. The only indication for therapy is if the level of plasma tocopherol is shown to be low in an appropriate clinical setting. Deficiency can be treated by 200 mg daily doses in adults.

Vitamin K deficiency

This may occur in neonates because placental transfer is limited and breast milk is often deficient: it also occurs in obstructive jaundice and certain malabsorption syndromes (see pp. 640 and 583). The result is hypothrombinaemia and bleeding, which is rapidly reversed by injections of vitamin K (phytomenadione).

Trace elements

The precise role of trace elements in health is uncertain but zinc deficiency appears important. Zinc, and probably also copper, are important in protecting cell membranes against free radical damage. Deficiency is seen most clearly in the congenital disorder *acrodermatitis enteropathica*, which is characterised in children by a scaly skin rash, secondary bacterial and fungal infection, diarrhoea and severe growth faltering. All are rapidly reversed by zinc therapy. Deficiencies are also seen in children with severe PEM and were formerly seen in patients receiving parenteral nutrition without sufficient trace element mixes.

Summary 1	Vitamin deficiency syndromes
Vitamin	*Deficiency syndrome*
A	Night blindness; xerophthalmia
Thiamine	Wernicke's encephalopathy; Korsakoff's psychosis
Niacin	Pellagra
Riboflavin	Mucosal lesions
Pyridoxine	Glossitis; neuropathy
Folate	Megaloblastosis; villus atrophy
B_{12}	Megaloblastosis; neuropathy
C	Scurvy
D	Rickets; osteomalacia
K	Hypoprothrombinaemia

Iodine deficiency

Most iodine deficiency is due to low levels in the soil and water. There are many regions in the world e.g. Nepal, Peru and Bangladesh where iodine intakes are so low ($<50–75$ mg/day) that thyroid function is impaired. There is a high prevalence of cretinism in neonates in these regions, which may present as deaf mutism, mental retardation and ataxia with the characteristic morphological features of thickened facial appearance, stunted stature and enlarged tongue. The brain damage is irreversible if not treated early. It is now also realised that the poor intellectual performance and deafness (without any unusual morphological features) found in many children in iodine deficient areas is due to marginal iodine deficiency. This may be partially reversible. In some areas, an already limited iodine availability is made worse by the consumption of goitrogens, e.g. certain brassicas, cassava or soya beans. The extent of the problem can be assessed by measuring the prevalence of goitre (enlargement of the thyroid gland) which is particularly common among adolescents and pregnant women. Measurements of urinary iodide and iodine/thiocyanate levels can determine if the problem is primary dietary iodine deficiency (low iodine) or a result of a dietary goitrogen (high thiocyanate).

Richer people in goitrous areas generally obtain enough iodine by eating food (e.g. fish) brought in from other areas; but the main strategy is to iodise salt. Where this is impractical, injections of iodised oil (lipiodol) may be given, especially to women of childbearing age. A single dose (5 ml) will usually last for up to five years. Oral doses (400 mg) of iodine preparations may provide enough to last for two years.

VITAMIN EXCESS

In addition to the variety of illnesses now attributed to vitamin deficiency, there are also several toxicological syndromes associated with vitamin excess (Table 8.18).

Vitamin A

Toxicity occasionally occurs acutely in children given large doses (e.g. 200 000 IU) of vitamin A intramuscularly. It takes the form of irritability, and even convulsions, as a result of increased intracranial pressure. Recovery occurs within a few days. It is extremely rare if the vitamin is given orally, but chronic headache accompanied by bone marrow depression and hepatosplenomegaly has been described in children given excessive oral doses. Vitamin A toxicity should be distinguished from hypercarotenaemia which may follow consumption of excessive quantities of mangos or carrots. In the latter condition, the sclera become yellow and the skin hyperpigmented, but it is not usually associated with any dysfunction.

Pyridoxine

Pyridoxine toxicity has been occurring more frequently in recent years due to its use – successful or otherwise – in the alleviation of severe premenstrual syndromes (depression and fluid retention). A peripheral neuropathy is likely if the daily dose exceeds 500 mg. Some cases have neurological abnormalities e.g. peripheral neuropathy, which persist even after stopping the drug.

Vitamin C

Toxicity occurs among those who take large doses of vitamin C in the unfounded belief that it will prevent the common cold or cancer. Doses above 2 g/day may cause abdominal discomfort and osmotic diarrhoea. There is increased urinary oxalate excretion – which may predispose to oxalate stones – and some evidence of damage to the intestinal epithelium.

Vitamin D

Vitamin D toxicity occurred in the UK after World War II in some children given too much fortified milk. (The quantities added are now more strictly controlled). Mild forms of vitamin D toxicity are characterised by weakness, weight loss and growth failure. Severe forms cause nephrocalcinosis, radiological changes in the epiphyses and mental retardation.

OBESITY

Everybody who is obese must necessarily be eating more than he or she needs; but it is not clear in every case why this is so.

Causes

There are obvious causes of obesity such as a history of compulsive eating between meals and during the night. Many people eat excessively in response to stress or lack of satisfaction in their lives. A sympathetic request for a two-week diary of everything the patient eats may be very revealing; but most obese people underestimate their intake and so a brief history in the outpatient clinic will usually fail to give an accurate assessment. A careful history taken by a dietitian is often invaluable.

Obesity may be the result of an obvious decrease in energy expenditure due to a change in lifestyle (e.g. to a more sedentary job) or an injury or arthritis which limits mobility. However, in the majority of obese individuals it seems that intake and expenditure problems occur together.

The metabolism of food energy has been studied in detail over the last 20 years, and the evidence to date would suggest that some individuals are more prone to weight gain than others with a similar energy intake.

1. Certain thin people eat more than fat people.
2. When volunteers are given extra calories some put on weight faster than others.
3. Prolonged, severe dieting may lead to an adaptive decrease in energy expenditure.
4. Obese people appear to have a decreased thermogenic response to stimulation by norepinephrine; this persists even when they have lost weight.
5. Studies with certain genetic strains of experimental animals provide strong evidence for a metabolic basis for obesity (attributed to differences in brown fat content). However, a number of studies, including whole body calorimetry, have not produced convincing evidence for a metabolic basis for obesity in man. There are occasional obese subjects with hypothyroidism or hypothalamic lesions, but these are rare. Nevertheless, the improved energy efficiency during pregnancy and lactation, and the weight gain that some experience while on the contraceptive pill, do point to some form of hormonal control of energy metabolism.

Whatever the nature of the metabolic processes which cause obesity, there is little doubt that a variety of metabolic

Table 8.18 Main consequences of vitamin toxicity

Vitamin	Symptoms of toxicity
A	Headache, convulsions, muscular stiffness, hepatomegaly, teratogenic effects.
Thiamine (B₁)	Not described.
Riboflavin (B₂)	Not described.
Nicotinic acid	Vasodilatation.
Pyridoxine (B₆)	Peripheral neuropathy
Folate	Not described.
Cobalamine (B₁₂)	Not described.
Ascorbic acid (C)	Increased urinary oxalate
D	Hypercalcaemia, renal failure
E	Nausea
K	Hyperbilirubinaemia

8

Table 8.19 Metabolic changes in obesity

Glucose tolerance	Decreased
Plasma insulin	Increased
Sensitivity to insulin	Decreased
Response to starvation:	
production of ketone bodies	Decreased
plasma free fatty acids	Increased
Plasma triglycerides	Increased
Plasma cholesterol	Increased
Plasma uric acid	Increased
Sensitivity to growth hormone	Decreased
Urinary 17-hydroxycorticoids	Increased

consequences occur, including an increased risk of diabetes mellitus and atheroma (Table 8.19).

Assessment

Before any advice is given it is important to assess how fat the patient is. The body mass index (BMI = weight/height^2) is an objective index of size by which the level of risk of morbidity and mortality can be estimated from graphs derived from insurance company data (Table 8.20 and Fig. 8.5). 'Acceptable weights' are in the range BMI 20–25; obesity is anything above BMI 30. This index may

Table 8.20 Classification of Body Mass Index (Quetelet Index)

Grade	W/H^2	Description
0	19–25	Normal range of weight
I	26–29	Overweight
II	30–39	Obesity
III	40 or more	Severe or morbid obesity

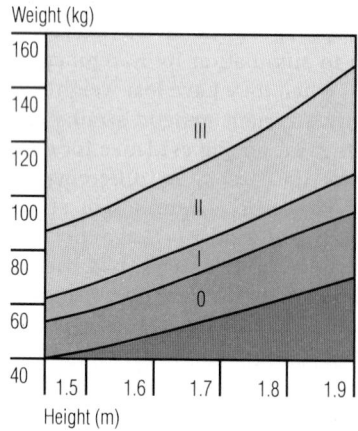

Fig. 8.5 Grades of obesity as measured using the body mass index (BMI = weight/height^2). Grade 0 is the desirable range, and grade III morbid obesity.

also be used in children and adolescents but, as there are some age effects, it is best to compare their measurements with the National Centre for Health Statistics (NCHS) data.

Why diet?

There are many thousands of people in the UK who seem to themselves and/or to other people to be excessively fat. A number of studies – among school-children, army recruits or housewives – show that, as a nation, we are indeed much heavier than in previous decades. At the same time, a considerable proportion of the population is on diets of various types – many of them low calorie 'crash' diets. Before the doctor recommends or condemns such approaches to weight reduction, it is important to consider the social and medical implications of obesity (Table 8.21).

There are three main reasons why people wish to lose weight:

1. Self-esteem. Mass media images of 'thin is beautiful' foster the idea held by many that they would be more attractive if they were thinner.
2. A concern that life should be lived to the full, unaffected by the diseases associated with obesity, such as coronary thrombosis, arthritis and gallstones.
3. A crisis response to a medical condition which requires weight reduction for its improvement (e.g. an operation which has been postponed until weight is lost).

Most people succeed at weight reduction without help from others. Many are helped by a variety of group approaches. The failures consult dietitians and/or doctors.

Table 8.21 Advantages of weight reduction

- Reduction in blood pressure
- Lowered risk of coronary thrombosis
- Improved pulmonary function
- Reduction in pain from osteoarthritis and lower back pain
- Decrease in venous thrombosis
- Less risk of gallstones and gout
- Reduction in fatigue/increase in energy
- Increased self-esteem, increased social gregariousness, better 'body image'
- Improved sexual relationships

How to reduce weight

1. Of the three factors – food intake, metabolism and exercise – affecting weight gain or loss, *food intake* is quantitatively the most important. Food energy intake needs to be reduced by about 500 kcal/day for recognisable weight loss (i.e. more than 0.5 kg per week) to occur. Most people – patients and doctors included – want rapid results, and more severe dietary restriction,

e.g. an intake of less than 600 kcal/day may be used. This undoubtedly leads to weight loss, but a high proportion of the initial loss is water. In addition, there is likely to be loss of body nitrogen from breakdown of skeletal muscle. There has been a vogue in recent years for 'nitrogen sparing modified fasts' in which high protein/low calorie formula feeds are given. These may help the patient to remain in positive nitrogen balance, and are a successful means of weight reduction in the short term; but the long-term benefit is very uncertain, partly because of an adaptive decrease in energy expenditure. There are many people in their forties who are still struggling to control their body weight on a relatively low energy intake having attempted many very low calorie diets in their twenties and thirties. The current vogue for such diets (300 kcal/day) may well die out as more and more people find that they regain weight rapidly once they return to their customary diet. Undoubtedly the best approach to weight loss is to reduce customary intake by 500–1000 kcal/day and to set realistic long-term goals. Advice from a dietitian is frequently useful in setting diets and identifying previously unrecognised sources of high energy foods, especially fats and alcohol.

2. *Exercise* should be encouraged, primarily to increase energy expenditure, but also because it increases fitness and well-being, and may of itself be a useful diversion from thinking about the unpleasantness of dieting. It is also possible that the thermogenic effect of a meal is increased after exercise. People taking regular exercise generally have less illness and longer lives.

3. Many obese people have emotional problems, but formal psychiatric treatment is not particularly effective in most cases. *A positive, caring and supportive approach* by the dietitian or doctor is often invaluable in assisting the obese patient regain his confidence – a key factor in success. Continuity of visits and regular supervision is essential in achieving this. It is striking how many patients' emotional crises seem to lessen as they lose weight.

4. *Appetite suppressants* are of very limited value. Fenfluramine and diethylpropion have been tried, but individual responses vary greatly and, as they are drugs to which it is possible to become habituated, they should not be prescribed.

5. *Thyroxine* is initially effective, but the rate of weight loss always slows as endogenous thyroid hormone ceases to be produced and thyroxine should not, therefore, be prescribed.

6. *Jaw-wiring* – when liquids only are taken – has been used by some with success; but many find that the weight lost is rapidly regained once the wires are removed, and damage to teeth and gums is common.

7. Some particularly unfortunate individuals have severe obesity (BMI >40). Such patients have usually tried – and failed – every diet possible, usually because they cannot sustain the effort. In the past, a jejunoileal bypass operation was often performed, but this has now been abandoned because of severe side effects (diarrhoea, liver disease, arthritis and osteomalacia). The main *surgical approach* is now the vertical banded gastroplasty, in which the stomach is stapled to reduce its size, thus inducing satiety at an early stage of the meal. This appears to be both effective and relatively safe; however, it does not cure hunger completely and selection of patients for this procedure requires very careful consideration.

FOOD SENSITIVITY

The clinical importance of food allergy is difficult to assess as little is known of the scientific basis for hypersensitivity to food, there have been few controlled clinical trials of exclusion diets, and the mechanisms by which they work are not understood. A variety of foods have been implicated in food intolerance (Table 8.22).

Table 8.22 Foods associated with food intolerance*

Food	% of cases
Milk	25
Egg	22
Nuts/peanuts	12
Fish/shellfish	12
Wheat/flour	6
Chocolate	5
Artificial colours	3
Pork/bacon	3
Chicken	3
Tomato	3
Soft fruit	3
Cheese (but not milk)	3

*From: Truswell AS 1986 ABC of nutrition.

A number of food allergies are associated with immunological reactions – usually an IgE response. A radio allergosorbent test (RAST) may detect antibodies in plasma against a specific food protein, but there is little correlation between the clinical features and the results of a variety of RAST tests. Skin tests of purified antigens may detect an urticarial response within a few minutes of intradermal inoculation, but positive skin tests do not correlate well with sensitivity reactions in other organs, such as lungs and the gastrointestinal tract. In short, there is as yet no defined mechanism in most cases of food sensitivity and very few laboratory tests are of any use. Management therefore depends on careful history taking and a critical approach to elimination diets.

Clinical symptoms

The major clinical symptoms associated with food sensitivity are shown in Table 8.23.

8

Table 8.23 Symptoms in 100 patients with food intolerance*

Symptom	Number of patients affected
Asthma	58
Gastrointestinal	41
Eczema	37
Urticaria	35
Rhinorrhoea	31
Angio-oedema	8

*From: Truswell AS 1986 ABC of nutrition.

Eczema

Exacerbations of eczema are frequently associated with reactions against eggs and milk. Infantile eczema is sometimes improved by withdrawing eggs and cows' milk products; and families with a strong history of eczema are advised to breast-feed as long as possible, and delay the introduction of eggs and cows' milk. Dietary manipulation in older children and adults is also worth trying but is often disappointing, and must be supervised.

Gastrointestinal symptoms

The classical and best defined gastrointestinal hypersensitivity syndrome is coeliac disease (p. 584). The onset of this condition is sometimes precipitated by a gut infection (especially in children). Transient gluten intolerance following mucosal damage from giardiasis or rotavirus infections may sometimes occur.

A more frequent problem is cows' milk protein intolerance. Here, mucosal damage permits access to mucosal lymphocytes which become sensitised to the dietary protein. Subsequent exposure then produces a severe response in which lymphokines are released, damaging enterocytes. Villus atrophy occurs and malabsorption develops. There is also some evidence of exacerbation of symptoms of ulcerative colitis by cows' milk; and it is sometimes suggested – though reliable evidence is lacking – that infantile colic is caused by dietary factors transmitted across breast milk or contained in cows' milk.

Many patients with severe intestinal infections complain of a relapse of diarrhoea in the convalescent period after eating certain foods (e.g. chocolate, alcohol, coffee, certain fruits). Their symptoms differ from irritable bowel syndrome (IBS) in which abdominal pain dominates. There are no specific patterns of food intolerance in IBS.

Migraine

Migraines sometimes appear to be precipitated by foods such as chocolate, cheese, red wine, nitrates, cows' milk and wheat. Some of these contain amines or stimulate histamine release which may produce an effect on cranial arteries.

Respiratory tract responses

Respiratory tract responses – including excessive production of tears, nasal secretions, sneezing and asthma – may all be related to environmental factors, e.g. chemical sprays, cosmetics and food or plant pollens; but eggs, cows' milk and chocolate may also precipitate symptoms. Recent studies suggest that a variety of food preservatives, including tartrazine and sulphur dioxide, may also be responsible.

Urticaria

Acute or chronic urticaria may occur in response to eggs, fish (particularly shellfish) and cows' milk, as well as certain fruit, wine and cheese.

Management of food sensitivity

If the patient suffers a reaction each time exposure to the allergen occurs, the latter should be easily identifiable. However, in the case of the general system symptoms described above, identification of the allergen is more difficult. There are two approaches:

1. exclude a suspected allergen for at least four weeks and then re-introduce it (this is mostly satisfactory where the condition is mild); or
2. work out an elimination diet (one based on lamb, rice and pears is sometimes effective) as advised by a dietitian. Then re-introduce a potential allergen every two weeks and observe the response.

MALNUTRITION IN DISEASE STATES

Weight loss and deficiency of individual nutrients are common in a variety of illnesses and frequently occur after major surgery (Table 8.24). There are a multiplicity of factors leading to nutritional deficiency in disease.

Dietary intake

Decreased appetite is the commonest cause of weight loss. In patients who have lost weight it is often helpful to ask a dietitian to take a careful history of the recent food intake. Modern microcomputer software programmes can process data on energy, protein, fat, fibre, iron intake, etc. very quickly, and certain patterns may emerge. For example, patients with malabsorption often avoid fat; adolescents with early forms of anorexia nervosa may become very fussy over food; and painful abdominal conditions (e.g. pancreatitis) may cause the patient to avoid solid foods altogether. In addition to identifying the specific food items avoided, the strictness with which a patient keeps to a diet should also be assessed. In all cases, patients' relatives should be interviewed to corroborate the dietary history. Dietary diaries kept by patients, relatives or nursing staff can be very valuable.

Table 8.24 Factors causing weight loss in surgical patients

Reduced appetite
Anxiety, pain
Infection and sepsis
Drugs e.g. anaesthetics, chemotherapy
Radiotherapy, metabolic disturbances

Reduced intake of nutrients
Difficulty in feeding
Inability to sit up or use arms
Damage to CNS and impaired consciousness
Damage to upper alimentary tract
Inadequate provision by medical/nursing staff

Increased need for nutrients
Raised energy expenditure
Metabolic response to injury
Increased protein synthesis

Replacement for extraneous losses
Haemorrhage
Serous exudates, especially after burns
Fistulae and sinuses

Maldigestion

Following partial gastrectomy, food may not be completely digested in the small bowel. Short-term maldigestion may complicate intestinal infection (such as with rotavirus or giardiasis) as a result of impaired hydrolysis of lactose due to temporary lactase deficiency. The presence of undigested lactose in the intestinal lumen causes severe osmotic diarrhoea, and a consequent loss of some nutrients.

Malabsorption

This term is often used to describe steatorrhoea (excessive fat in the faeces), but carbohydrate and vitamin malabsorption are also important. The mechanisms of malabsorption are described in Chapter 16. With some nutrients, such as iron, folate and vitamin B_{12}, malabsorption may present as a clinical deficiency syndrome with excessive losses of dietary protein and energy in the faeces. However, metabolic balance studies show that weight loss in some malabsorption patients is due more to a decrease in dietary intake, than to malabsorbed nutrients.

Increased nutrient requirements

Energy requirements are often increased in pyrexial conditions – usually about 10% increase for every 1°C in body temperature. The rate of protein synthesis (e.g. of acute phase reactant proteins or antibodies) is also increased in systemic infections. As nutrient intakes are often decreased rather than increased during infection, these processes lead to energy deficiency. There may be mobilisation of muscle protein for oxidation as a fuel and thus increased urinary losses of nitrogen. At the present time, various chemical messengers – such as interleukins and prostaglandins – are thought to control all of these processes; but it has not yet proved possible to reverse them successfully by pharmacological means.

Losses of endogenous nutrient

Losses of albumin, electrolytes and blood may occur in intestinal diseases, particularly those such as Crohn's disease or ulcerative colitis where the mucosa is 'leaky'. Systemic infection may also lead to loss of zinc and other minerals in the urine.

NUTRITION SUPPORT

Many patients leave hospital weighing considerably less than when they came in. This can be regarded as a form of PEM, if the body weight is less than 80% of the ideal weight for a person of that height or the BMI is less than 20. The majority of cases of PEM are the result of poor appetite due to illness and the experience that eating tends to make the pain and diarrhoea worse. The reasons for PEM should always be investigated.

Severe degrees of PEM delay wound healing and recovery of muscle tone after an operation, and may increase susceptibility to infection. Adults with a BMI below 16 have three times the postoperative mortality of better nourished patients. The striking changes in body composition from partial starvation in illness are shown in Figure 8.6. It is better to avoid PEM than treat it and it is essential to make a nutritional assessment of every patient. If any of the criteria for PEM are present, some form of nutrition support, such as dietetic supplements, enteral feeding or parenteral feeding can be used to prevent further deterioration (Table 8.25). In deciding which technique of nutrition support to use, it is often advisable to use a nutrition team – comprising a physician or surgeon with special experience in clinical nutrition, a nutrition nurse/technician and a dietitian, together with strong support from the pharmacy – as a focal point for discussion.

Fig. 8.6 Body composition of a man in health and after partial starvation.

8

Illness associated with nausea and abdominal pain	Intestinal disease
Gastrointestinal disease	Malabsorption
Malignancy	Inflammatory bowel disease
Chemotherapy	Fistulae
Inability to eat	**Increased requirements**
Coma	Burns
Weakness	Sepsis
	Trauma

Enteral feeding

Many patients find hospital food unappetising even when they feel relatively well. In such cases, it may be possible to increase energy and protein intake by snacks provided by the diet kitchen between main meals; and food and drink may be fortified by a range of supplements available from the dietician (Table 8.26). A 24 hour calorie count performed by the dietitian is a good way of monitoring intake. If solid food is not well accepted, it is often possible to give liquid feeds for sipping. A considerable range of commercially prepared feeds are available, presented as 200 ml cartons (Table 8.27). These should be served chilled and their volumes recorded accurately.

If the intake is still not satisfactory, a fine-bore silastic tube may be passed per-nasally. Enteral feeding solutions are passed down the tube at controlled rates from a reservoir situated above the patient's head. Small battery operated pumps can control the exact flow rate but they

Table 8.26 Examples of commercially available nutritional supplements

Commercial name	Nutrient source	Nutrient content
Maxipro	Whey protein	Protein 88 g/100g Energy 390 kcal/100 g
Maxijul/Caloreen	Maltodextrin powder	Carbohydrate 96 g/100 g Energy 375 kcal/100 g
Prosparol	Peanut oil	Energy 450 kcal/100 g

Table 8.27 Examples of commercially available enteral feeds

Name	Osmolality (mosmol/kg)	Non-protein energy/nitrogen (kcal/gN)
Ensure	380	149
Ensure Plus	460	140
Clinifeed	255	142
Special feeds		
Osmolite	Lactose and gluten free	
Enrich	Lactose and gluten free plus fibre	

are not essential. The commercially available enteral feeds are made up from a variety of protein sources including casein, soya and mixtures of amino acids, with glucose polymers and triglycerides added to increase the energy content. Most feeds provide about 1 kcal/ml and have an osmolality of 280–420 mosmol/kg. Low lactose and cows' milk-free feeds are available. Flavour and consistency vary considerably and a tasting session is generally advisable before prescribing large quantities. The feeds should be started in small volumes, and no more than 1000 ml given in the first 24 hours – otherwise diarrhoea may develop. The volume is then increased to the desired amount (probably a maximum of 2500 ml/day). The feed should be stopped for one hour before meals and continued throughout the night.

Enteral feeding can be performed at home: the reservoir bottles and lines should be changed every 24 hours to avoid the risk of contamination of feeds but the silastic tubes can remain in situ for several weeks. Even so, complications of enteral feeding occasionally occur and should be anticipated. Oesophagitis caused by the tubes is rare with modern silastic tubing, but the tube may be misplaced and an X-ray should be performed before feeding is commenced. A few patients suffer abdominal distension and pain, and the volume infused should then be decreased. Diarrhoea is best controlled by codeine phosphate (30–60 mg tds) or imodium (2–4 mg tds).

Parenteral feeding

If enteral feeds cannot be given (e.g. due to severe ileus) then parenteral feeding is an option, but the dangers of infection and metabolic problems with this method are considerable. There are various commercial preparations; these should be mixed in a three litre bag system in sterile laminar airflow conditions in the pharmacy.

The regime used varies with the patient's clinical condition (Table 8.28). In general, regimes 1–4 are administered through a central venous catheter. Where central venous access is impossible, regime 5 may be used, administered through a butterfly needle on the back of the hand or forearm. The site of this needle should be changed every 24–48 hours to avoid thrombophlebitis.

A number of metabolic complications may occur in patients receiving parenteral nutrition (Table 8.29).

1. Hyperglycaemia is common in patients with severe surgical stress (e.g. burns and trauma) and sepsis, but it is usually possible to control the plasma glucose levels with carefully monitored insulin. Rebound hypoglycaemia may occur if intravenous feeding is abruptly halted.
2. Metabolic acidosis is rare if fructose and excessive quantities of amino acids are avoided.
3. Parenteral feeding, especially with lipid solutions, has been blamed for hepatic abnormalities. However, most patients receiving parenteral feeding have many other potential causes for hepatic damage and there is rarely

Table 8.28 Standard parenteral nutrition regimes*

Composition	Regimen 1 (central line)	Regimen 2 (central line)	Regimen 3 (central line)	Regimen 4 (central line)	Regimen 5 (peripheral)
Nitrogen (g)	9.4	9.4	13.5	14.1	9.4
Carbohydrate (g)	200	200	250	350	240
Fat (g)	50	100	100	100	100
Non-protein energy (kcal)	1350	1800	2000	2400	1900
Sodium (mmol)	80	80	122.5	122.5	80
Potassium (mmol)	60	60	80	80	60
Calcium (mmol)	5	5	5	5	5
Magnesium (mmol)	5	7	8	8	7
Zinc (μmol)	100	100	100	100	100
Phosphate (mmol)	27.5	27.5	37.5	37.5	35
Chloride (mmol)	85	85	107.5	107.5	108
Trace elements (Additrace) (ml)	10	10	10	10	10
Vitilipid N Adult (ml)	10	10	10	10	10
Solivito N (vial)	1	1	1	1	1
Volume of feed (ml)	2560	2560	2540	2540	3050

*Regimen 1 is indicated for a patient of weight 35–54 kg; regimen 2, 46–59 kg; and regimens 3–5, 60–75 kg.

any indication for parenteral nutrition to be stopped on account of mild biochemical changes.

4. Fat is metabolised more favourably than glucose by septic patients.
5. Patients with respiratory failure should not receive large glucose loads because of their impaired ability to excrete the extra CO_2 produced.
6. Mineral and electrolyte abnormalities occur variously according to the underlying diverse processes. Fortunately, deficiencies can be made up relatively easily during preparation of the three litre bag which contains the feeding solutions.

Table 8.29 Metabolic complications in patients receiving parenteral nutrition

- Hyperglycaemia
- Rebound hypoglycaemia
- Electrolyte and mineral imbalance
- Metabolic acidosis
- Disturbed liver function
- Raised plasma CO_2

Monitoring nutrition support

The measurements available for monitoring nutrition support are shown in Table 8.30.

Regular measurements of weight are necessary but are difficult to perform in the very sick without special bed balances. Changes in body weight may indicate alterations in fluid balance rather than an increase in lean body mass.

Plasma proteins are useful indicators of progress in nutrition support, but are subject to considerable change by underlying disease processes. *Glucose* should be measured regularly.

Plasma phosphate levels may decrease rapidly and even precipitate cardiac arrhythmia if nutrition support is given rapidly in large quantities to a severely malnourished subject who has previously received very little dietary intake. Most modern amino acid solutions, however, have sufficient phosphate to avoid this.

A low plasma *sodium* is often present in severely malnourished subjects. Total body sodium, however, is often high and extra sodium should only be given with great caution.

An approximate assessment of urinary *nitrogen* loss can be obtained by measurement of the 24 hour urinary urea excretion, corrected according to the formula

$$\text{Nitrogen (g/24 h)} = \text{urinary urea (mmol/l)} \times \text{urine volume (l)} \times 0.028 \times 6/5.$$

This formula allows for the conversion of mmol of urea to grams of nitrogen and corrects for the fact that urea accounts for approximately five-sixths of total urinary nitrogen loss.

The previously high prevalence of infection has been reduced by the three litre bag system, but high standards of nursing and medical care of the lines are essential if sepsis is to be prevented. Different types of intravenous catheters are available – the best are those tunnelled subcutaneously (e.g. Hickman). Blood samples should never be taken from this line as the clot at the tip is a major

Table 8.30 Measurements for monitoring nutrition support

- Anthropometric: weight, mid-arm muscle circumference (MAC)
- Plasma proteins: albumin, transferrin, retinol binding globulin
- Minerals and electrolytes: uric acid, phosphate, sodium, potassium, zinc
- Nitrogen balance: corrected 24 hour urinary urea excretion
- Glucose

source of infection. Specialist texts should be referred to before any central venous feeding is attempted, to reduce the complications of catheter insertion, which include pneumothorax, central vein thrombosis, nerve injury, haematoma and arrhythmias. Similarly, only staff trained in the care of central venous feeding lines should be allowed to touch them; and aseptic changing of sets and meticulous care of the catheter entry site should be emphasised. Efforts to reduce infection rates are particularly important among immunocompromised patients.

Parenteral feeds are made up from mixtures of L-form amino acids to which glucose (20%) or lipid emulsions (10% or 20%) are added as energy sources. An ideal calorie to nitrogen ratio is around 150:1. Electrolytes, minerals and vitamins are then added to this basic solution. If large quantities of glucose are given, the patient may become hyperglycaemic; this is best managed by subcutaneous insulin administered by a pump. Considering the relative costs, risks and nutritional benefit from total parenteral nutrition (TPN) it seems best to confine its use to those who need it for at least two weeks; anything less is not really justified.

NUTRITION AS A COFACTOR IN DISEASE

There are several diseases in which dietary factors are implicated. In many cases, this has been demonstrated in experimental studies in animals, or limited intensive biochemical studies of dietary manipulation in human volunteers. Dietary fat in coronary heart disease and dietary salt in hypertension are two good examples. However, the importance of such single factors in human disease is not clear-cut, because most studies have not allowed for the degree of variance in other cofactors (e.g. cigarette smoking in coronary heart disease and genetic factors in hypertension).

Hypertension

International comparisons show a direct relationship between sodium intake and blood pressure. There is a threshold effect of additional salt in volunteers, with those on very high doses showing an increased blood pressure. However, there are also important cofactors including family history, stress, obesity and potassium intake which may obscure the relationship in an individual. In the UK, the average daily intake in adults is 150 mmol of sodium (equivalent to about 20 g NaCl). This is more than twice the amount associated with lower rates of hypertension experimentally.

Atheroma

International comparisons of mortality rates from coronary heart disease (CHD) show that rates are highest in populations with the highest fat intakes. This is true even when

the effects of obesity, hypertension, cigarette smoking, diabetes, stress and family history are allowed for. The major risk factors for the development of atheroma are high levels of plasma cholesterol and low density lipoproteins (VLDL). Consumption of fat in the saturated form is particularly likely to increase both VLDL and cholesterol. Diets in which fats are consumed mainly in the unsaturated form lead to lowering of these levels. In practice, saturated fats are present in butter, lard, sausages, meat pies, pastries and chocolates; while unsaturated fats predominate in margarines prepared from maize, sunflower or soya. Not all margarines are unsaturated – those which contain coconut oil (used in many hospital canteens in the UK), for example, are highly saturated. It should be remembered that plasma cholesterol indicates the production of cholesterol by the liver; cholesterol-containing foods (such as eggs) do not necessarily increase the synthesis of cholesterol in the liver.

In the UK, only a relatively minor proportion of the population have a high plasma cholesterol and VLDL; why only some people respond to a high fat diet in this way is unknown.

Two main dietary strategies have been proposed to reduce CHD mortality in the UK.

1. Encourage everybody to eat less fat. This is the approach recommended by the National Advisory Committee for Nutrition Education (NACNE). At the present time, the population eats over 45% of its daily energy in the form of fat; they should be encouraged to eat less fat (say 35% of energy) and eat more starch and carbohydrates.
2. Screen high risk groups (e.g. men between 35 and 55 years of age) for plasma cholesterol and VLDL, and select out those with high levels for individual dietary counselling. The second approach is perhaps the more logical, but has not been widely adopted because of administrative and financial constraints.

The best advice is to eat fat in as unsaturated form as possible. Certain polyunsaturated fats – such as eicosapentaenoic acid present in cod-liver oil, mackerel and pilchards – tend to inhibit thrombosis and should be particularly encouraged. Increasing dietary fibre intake may also reduce plasma cholesterol. Obesity is often associated with high levels of plasma cholesterol and triglycerides; and successful weight reduction by moderately or severely obese subjects is followed by a decreased risk of mortality from CHD.

Diabetes

Non-insulin dependent diabetes (Type II) is closely linked with diet, although there are some populations (e.g. the Pima Indians of N. America) in which the disease is so common that genetic factors are presumably involved. In nearly every society, those who are overweight and whose diet is high in fat and low in dietary fibre have a significantly increased risk of diabetes. The current epidemics in middle income countries, as they eat more polished rice and white

Summary 2	Nutrition as a cofactor in disease
Disease	*Associated dietary factors*
Hypertension	High sodium intake
Atheroma	High consumption of saturated fats; obesity; insufficient fibre (all lead to high cholesterol and VLDL)
Diabetes (Type II)	High fat, low fibre
Oesophageal cancer	Preservatives e.g. nitrosamines; dietary deficiencies e.g. zinc, carotenoids, retinol. Also alcohol, mycotoxins
Stomach cancer	Nitrosamines (derived from nitrates in diet); fat
Cancer of large intestine	High protein and fat; low fibre
Gallstones	High cholesterol due to obesity, high sugar, low fibre
Cirrhosis	Alcohol
Liver cancer	Aflatoxins (in badly stored cereals)
Pancreatitis	PEM
Dental caries	Sugar in prolonged contact with teeth
Urinary calculi (oxalate)	High phosphate

bread, are striking. The benefits conferred by dietary fibre are probably due to its effects on gastric emptying and the rate of carbohydrate hydrolysis.

Gastrointestinal disease

There are striking differences in the prevalence of cancer of the oesophagus, stomach and large intestine between populations on different diets. A variety of carcinogens such as nitrosamines (which are widely available in preserved food such as pickled foods, continental sausage and certain types of fish), together with dietary deficiencies (e.g. of zinc, carotenoids and retinol) appear to be associated with cancer of the oesophagus. Other toxins include alcohol (especially from spirits), silica derived from grinding cereals (as in parts of China) and mycotoxins (e.g. in Transkei, South Africa).

Cancer of the stomach may also be associated with high levels of dietary nitrosamines. There is evidence that high levels of dietary nitrates (both in food and in water) may be converted into nitrites by the gastric microflora. The nitrites then react with amino acids to form nitrosamines which are carcinogenic in experimental studies. When gastric acidity is low – as in the elderly and those with pernicious anaemia – there is greater opportunity for bacterial metabolism of nitrates to nitrites and this may account for the higher incidence of gastric cancer in these subjects. Other dietary factors, such as fat, have been implicated in explaining the changes in stomach cancer rates observed among Japanese migrating to the USA.

High rates of cancer of the large intestine have been associated with diets high in fat and protein and low in dietary fibre. A series of carcinogens are produced as a result of bacterial metabolism of endogenous bile salts and dietary fat; and it may be that the prolonged contact between carcinogen and mucosa in subjects with a low fibre diet accounts for the high rate of large bowel cancer in some communities.

Gallstones

The deposition of cholesterol to form gallstones depends on the relative concentrations of total bile salts, lecithin and cholesterol. The fine balance between these is affected by obesity, high dietary sugar intake and low dietary fibre intake but the precise mechanisms of the imbalance or of the formation of gallstones are not clear.

Liver disease

The most important association between dietary factors and liver disease is that between alcohol and cirrhosis. However, mycotoxins may also affect the liver: aflatoxins – which are widely prevalent in cereals kept under poor storage conditions – may be a factor in causing primary liver cell cancer and may also contribute to the development of the fatty liver in kwashiorkor. Temporary PEM in children does not account for the high prevalence of cirrhosis in developing countries; hepatitis B infection seems to be the major cause.

Pancreatic disease

Chronic pancreatitis is found frequently among populations where PEM is rife. Periods of undernutrition may cause stasis of exocrine juices within the pancreas, leading to acinar cell destruction and loss of digestive function. Pancreatic calcification often follows.

Dental caries

There has been a marked decrease in dental caries among children in certain social groups in the UK over the last twenty years. This has been associated with: an increase in the use of fluoride (in toothpaste, in drinking water or as tablets); reduced consumption of sticky sweets; and possibly also an increased prevalence of cleaning the teeth. Dental caries occur when *Streptococcus viridans* adheres to the tooth and metabolises sugar into lactic acid. All sugars can act as substrate; thus 'natural' sugars, such as fructose, are just as cariogenic as sucrose. The most important factor is the length of time that sugar-containing foods remain in contact with the tooth; adhesive foods are thus particularly damaging.

Urinary calculi

Calcium or oxalate stones are sometimes precipitated in the urinary tract as a result of increased dietary intake. Oxalate stones are those most frequently associated with

8

dietary factors, occurring most commonly in populations with high phosphate intakes. In Thailand, for example, oxalate calculi occur most commonly in the rural populations, where the high phosphate intakes associated with a predominantly vegetarian diet contrast with the lower phosphate intakes of the better off, urban families. Oxalate stones may also be precipitated by dehydration in extremely hot climates.

NUTRITIONAL FACTORS IN HEALTH PROMOTION

There is increasing public awareness of the importance of attention to lifestyle in avoiding the development of disease. In the UK, many of the diseases – coronary artery disease, hypertension, lung cancer, cancer of the large intestine, gallstones, diabetes, irritable colon syndrome and varicose veins – that now cause premature death or years of discomfort were far less prevalent a hundred or so years ago, and are rare today in developing countries. The reasons for the differences in disease patterns between communities are complex but some factors, such as cigarette smoking, obesity and lack of exercise, are clearly implicated. This should be emphasised by both GPs and community health programmes in routine medical examinations and screening of high risk groups.

There is now a reasonable consensus that the risk of developing certain diseases is reduced if the diet contains:

1. sufficiently few calories to avoid obesity (BMI > 30)
2. less than 35% of energy in the form of fat
3. more than 25 g of fibre daily
4. about 30% less salt than in the average UK diet
5. 50% less sugar than in the average UK diet
6. daily alcohol consumption less than four units of alcohol for men and three for women.

To achieve this overall change in diet it is necessary to increase the consumption of wholegrain cereals, pasta and vegetables such as potatoes. The introduction of numerous diet and health magazines over the last ten years means that appropriate menus and dietary information are readily available. Some of this information is conflicting and many community dietitians produce booklets designed to clarify the situation.

In recent years, there have been many claims of an association between many commercial food additives and cancer, food allergy, skin conditions and behaviour disorders. These include preservatives (such as nitrates, chromates, sulphur dioxide), emulsifiers (such as lecithin), antioxidants, colourants (such as tartrazine) and flavourings (Table 8.31). While the quantitative degree to which any of these contributes to disease in man is unknown, it is probably minimal compared with the risks associated with current dietary levels of fat, fibre, salt and sugar.

Table 8.31 Food additives in the UK diet

Type of additive	Example
Colourants	Synthetic e.g. tartrazine, amaranth Naturally occurring e.g. β-carotene, beetroot red, chlorophyll
Flavourings	Monosodium glutamate
Thickening agents	Pectin, guar gum, carboxymethyl-cellulose
Emulsifiers	Lecithin
Preservatives	Nitrates, sulphur dioxide, propionate
Antioxidants	Tocopherols
Sweeteners	Sorbitol, inositol

There are, in addition, specific disorders associated with nutrient deficiencies. Thus, neural tube defects are associated with folate deficiency; coronary heart disease is associated with dietary selenium deficiency in some communities; and iron deficiency is associated with poor intellectual performance at school. Unfortunately, it is difficult to obtain rigorous proof for some of these associations and even more difficult to evaluate critically the value of dietary additions. This leaves much scope for those favouring approaches such as micronutrient therapy in micro doses, megadoses of vitamins etc. The proliferation of 'health consultants' and 'nutrition counsellors' in the UK and elsewhere reflects public anxieties about food and health fuelled by intensive information in the media. The wise clinician will respect this anxiety, ensure that he or she is as well informed as possible on new developments and – at all times – maintain the same critical approach to the claims of the health stores as to the claims made for new pharmaceuticals.

FURTHER READING

Dickerson J W T, Lee H A 1986 Nutrition in the clinical management of disease, 2nd edn. Edward Arnold, London. *A comprehensive textbook of a range of disease states in which nutrition is involved.*

Eastwood M A, Passmore R 1986 Human nutrition and dietetics, 8th edn. Churchill Livingstone, Edinburgh. *Still the classic textbook of human nutrition.*

Garrow J S 1988 Obesity and related disorders. Churchill Livingstone, Edinburgh. *A personal account of in-depth studies of obese subjects by a single author. Stimulating and instructive.*

Manuel P D, Tomkins A M, Walker-Smith J A 1986 Infections of the gastrointestinal tract. Churchill Livingstone, Edinburgh. *An account of the interaction of gut immunology, infection and malnutrition.*

Silk D B A 1983 Nutritional support in hospital practice. Blackwell Scientific Publications, Oxford. *A scientific review of the principles of nutrition support, with a strong emphasis on practical management.*

Truswell A S 1986 ABC of nutrition. British Medical Association, London. *A well-illustrated series of articles first published as weekly reviews in the British Medical Journal.*

Cancer Medicine

Each year in the United Kingdom there are approximately 220 000 new cases of cancer. Almost one-third of the population will develop cancer during their lifetime and 70% of these will die of the disease – 150 000 deaths a year. As a cause of mortality, cancer is second only to cardiovascular disease. It is most common in the elderly: the age-specific incidence rates for men and women are shown in Figure 9.1. The frequency of cancer and the increasing complexity of management mean that every clinician must have a firm grasp of the principles of diagnosis, investigation and treatment. In recent years, the approach has been changing rapidly as a consequence of fundamental advances in cancer biology, increasing accu-

racy in diagnosis and staging, and major developments in the use of radiotherapy and chemotherapy. At the same time, clinicians have developed a better awareness of the problems faced by patients who are incurable, and professional attitudes have changed in the direction of more open discussion with patients. Cancer medicine therefore demands a combination of a high degree of technical competence and a sympathetic insight into the feelings of the patients; it is this double challenge which makes it a most rewarding part of medical practice.

INCIDENCE AND EPIDEMIOLOGY

Incidence means the proportion of a defined population developing a disease in a stated period of time; *prevalence* is the proportion which has the condition at a single point in time. *Crude* incidence or prevalence rates refer to a whole population and *specific* rates to selected groups, for example those defined by age or sex.

The age-specific incidence rates of some cancers are shown in Figures 9.2 to 9.4. It can be seen that adeno-carcinomas in women have quite different age-specific incidence rates. Cancer of the breast increases rapidly in incidence before the menopause, and at a slightly slower rate thereafter (Fig. 9.2). Uterine and ovarian cancer also show an increasing incidence premenopausally but the rate does not rise in later life. Gut cancers (Fig. 9.3), on the other hand, show no relation to the menopause but rise rapidly in incidence in old age in both sexes. The biphasic age-specific incidence of Hodgkin's disease (Fig. 9.4) contrasts markedly with the findings in adeno-carcinoma. Lung cancer is at present more common in men. Cancer is the second main cause of death in childhood, with acute lymphoblastic leukaemia accounting for nearly half the deaths.

The commonest sites of cancer in the West are lung, skin, large bowel, prostate, stomach and rectum in men; and breast, large bowel, skin and lung in women. The mortality rates are, however, different from incidence rates (Fig. 9.5), with skin cancer having a low mortality rate and

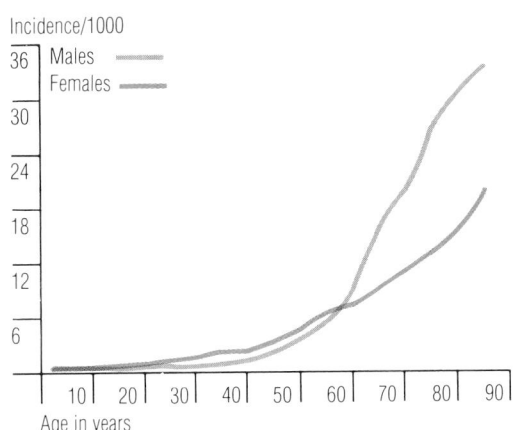

Fig. 9.1 Age-specific incidence of cancer (England 1984).

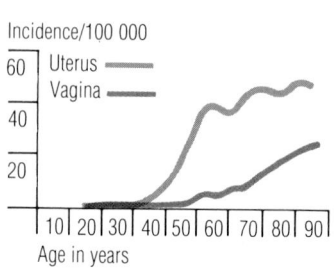

Fig. 9.2 Age-specific incidence of carcinomas of the breast, ovary, uterus and vagina (England 1984). Note change in rate of increase in adenocarcinoma of the breast, ovary and uterus at the time of the menopause.

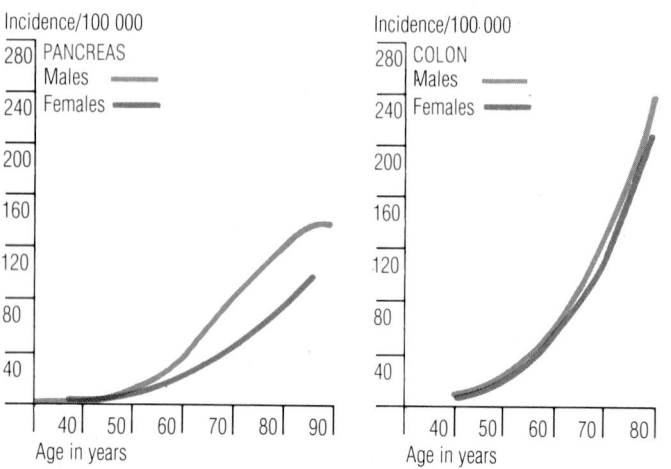

Fig. 9.3 Age-specific incidence of adenocarcinoma of the pancreas and colon (England 1984).

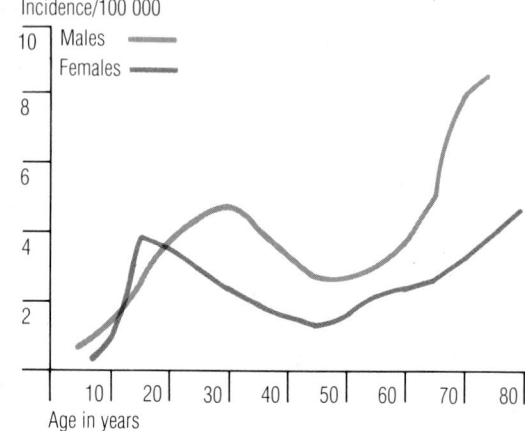

Fig. 9.4 Age-specific incidence of Hodgkin's disease (England 1984).

lung cancer a very bad prognosis. However, the relative incidence of cancers is changing with time. For example, the incidence of lung cancer has been rising rapidly since the mid–1960s, especially in women; while that of stomach cancer has been falling for both men and women (Fig. 9.6). The rise in incidence of lung cancer is undoubtedly due to smoking, but the reason for the decline in stomach cancer is not clear.

Cancer incidence varies in different countries (Table 9.1) and this variation may provide insights into aetiology. Carcinoma of the oesophagus has a high incidence in an area extending from the Caspian Sea to Central Asia and the Far East; it is also more common in the Transkei. In these areas, it has an incidence 200 times that found in the UK. In Japan, gastric carcinoma is 30 times more common than it is in the UK, but pancreatic cancer is much rarer. The reasons for these variations are as yet unknown, but dietary

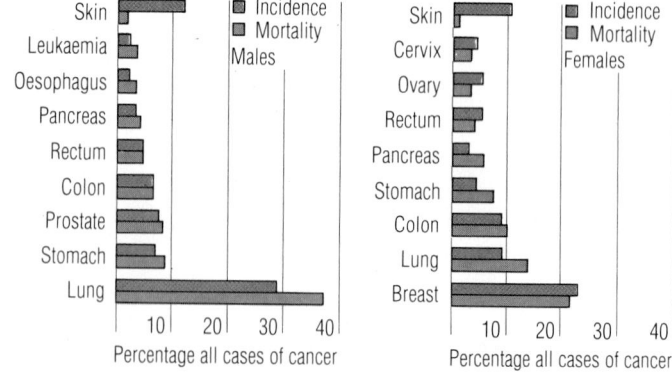

Fig. 9.5 Incidence and mortality of common cancers in men and women in England and Wales. Note that while skin cancer is common, its mortality is low. Cancer of the lung is common and accounts for a large number of total cancer deaths.

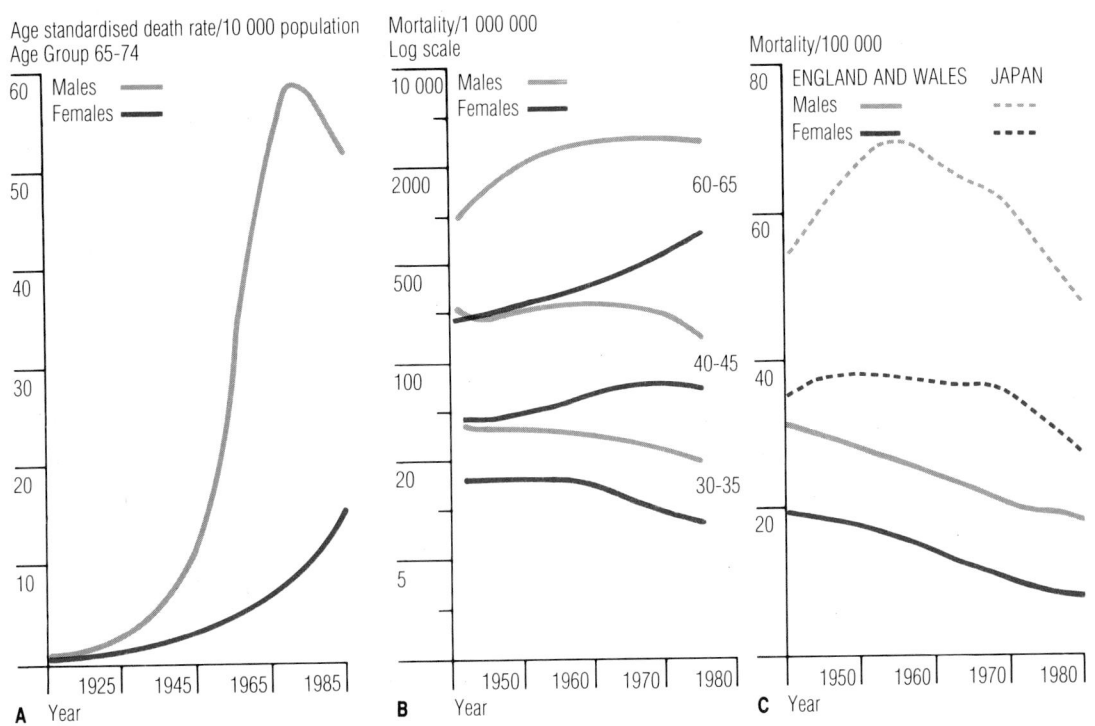

Fig. 9.6 Cancer of the lung and stomach. A. Cancer of the lung – age-standardised death rate/10 000 in age group 65–74, 1905–85 in the UK. **B.** Cancer of the lung – mortality 1940–80 for different age groups. **C.** Cancer of the stomach – change in mortality in England and Wales and in Japan, 1940–1980.

Table 9.1 Geographical incidence of cancer

Cancer	High incidence	Low incidence	Ratio (high:low)
Oesophagus	Transkei, Kazakhstan	Holland	200:1
Liver	Mozambique	UK	100:1
Nasopharynx	Far East (China)	Europe	100:1
Stomach	Japan	UK	3:1

and nutritional factors are suspected to play a part. The migration of populations has helped to determine how much of the geographical variation is genetic and how much is environmental. When Japanese people settle in the USA, the incidence of cancers in their offspring resembles that of the adopted country – the high incidence of gastric cancer falls, and the lower incidence of cancers of the breast, colon, ovary, and prostate rises. These findings suggest that environmental, rather than genetic, causes account for most of the observed differences between countries.

AETIOLOGY

Evidence suggesting aetiological factors in cancer has come from epidemiological and laboratory investigation. It is probable that, for many types of neoplasm, an interaction of genetic and environmental factors is responsible for the development of a cancer.

Chemical carcinogens

The frequency of scrotal carcinoma in chimney sweeps was noted by Sir Percivall Pott in 1775, and the high incidence of bladder cancer in dye workers in 1895. The mechanisms of action of chemical carcinogens have been intensively studied. There are several classes of experimental carcinogens which are possible causes in humans:

1. *Polycyclic hydrocarbons* are formed from combustion of organic compounds. They are present in cigarette smoke, soot, car exhaust fumes and some foods. Dibenzanthracene was one of the first to be shown to be carcinogenic. Others are listed in Table 9.2. The carcinogenic effect is thought to result from a reaction with bases in cellular DNA.
2. *Aromatic amines and azo dyes*, such as beta naphthylamine and benzidine, are metabolised to an active form. In the case of beta naphthylamine, this is then glucuronated in the liver and excreted in the urine where glucuronidases liberate the carcinogen in the bladder.
3. *Nitrosamines* are formed when nitrites in food are converted to nitrates which react with amines in food. The substances can cause stomach cancer experimentally.

Cancer Medicine

4. *Alkylating agents*, such as those used in cancer treatment, bind to DNA. Use of these drugs in cancer has been associated with the development of secondary malignancies.

5. *Organic toxins* include the best studied example aflatoxin, produced by the mould *Aspergillus flavus* growing on grain. This substance has been suggested as an aetiological agent in liver cancer in Africa, but the hepatitis B virus is perhaps a more important agent.

When carcinogens act on a cell, they may cause a permanent change which predisposes to cancer – a process known as *initiation*. Other agents can then produce transient changes which lead, with continued exposure, to cancer; this is known as *tumour promotion*. This two-stage process has been shown in some experimental cancers, where mutagens act as initiators and hormones or dietary constituents act as promoters.

Table 9.2 Chemical carcinogens

Class	Example	Source
Polycyclic hydrocarbons	Dibenzanthracene	Smoke, cigarettes
Aromatic amines	Beta naphthylamine	Aniline dyes
Azo dyes	Dimethylamino-benzene	Butter yellow
Nitrosamines	Dimethylnitrosamine	? Food
Toxins	Aflatoxin	*Aspergillus flavus*
Alkylating agents	Melphalan	Drug treatment of cancer
Chromates		Industrial exposure
Asbestos		Insulation and heating installations

Irradiation

The carcinogenic effect of ionising irradiation was indicated by the skin cancers that developed on the hands of early radiologists, and by the increased frequency of acute and chronic leukaemia, breast and thyroid cancer in Hiroshima during the 30 years after the atom bomb was dropped. The mechanism of carcinogenesis is probably related to the chromosomal damage caused by X-rays. It seems likely that 'background' ionising irradiation does not contribute greatly to common cancers in humans.

Ultraviolet light probably plays a role in the development of skin cancers. This is seen most clearly in the autosomal recessive disorder, xeroderma pigmentosum, where a defective DNA repair mechanism is associated with the early development of skin cancers on skin exposed to sunlight. Malignant melanoma and other skin cancers are uncommon in black people but are particularly frequent in fair-skinned Celts. In Australia, skin cancers are common among the non-indigenous population and increase in incidence in the north nearer the Equator.

Viruses

Ribonucleic acid (RNA) viruses can cause a variety of cancers in animals. These viruses contain a gene which codes for the enzyme reverse transcriptase, which is produced in the infected cell and results in the cellular synthesis of DNA complementary to the viral RNA and thus to the production of more viruses. For this reason they are called *retroviruses*. Tumours caused by these viruses include avian erythroblastosis, rat sarcoma, feline leukaemia and murine leukaemia. The insertion of the viral genome into DNA leads to malignant transformation, but the steps involved are not yet clear. A growth-factor receptor is encoded by the erythroblastosis-B virus (v-erb B): a phosphokinase by Rous sarcoma virus (sis). The relationship between these gene products and cancer remains to be elucidated and promises to be one of the most fruitful areas of cancer research. Until recently, RNA viruses had not been shown to cause cancer in humans. There is now strong evidence that an RNA virus is involved in the development of some forms of T cell leukaemia and lymphoma (human T cell leukaemia virus, HTLV types 1 and 2). Another virus, the human immunodeficiency virus (HIV), is the cause of the Acquired Immune Deficiency Syndrome (AIDS) in which there is a greatly increased frequency of skin sarcoma and B cell lymphoma. These tumours are probably not caused by the virus but are, rather, a consequence of oncogenesis in patients with greatly reduced immunity.

Research into RNA viruses led to the discovery that the viral oncogenes had homologues in normal cellular DNA. These cellular *proto-oncogenes* appear to code for products very similar to those produced by the equivalent virus. Indeed, it is probable that the viral oncogene sequence was originally acquired during evolution from cellular DNA. These findings have led to the search for increased expression of cellular oncogenes in human cancers, for the gene products, and for the link between carcinogenesis and oncogene activation.

There is strong circumstantial evidence implicating DNA viruses in the pathogenesis of some malignant neoplasms. For example, Epstein-Barr virus (EBV) was first isolated from cells from a case of Burkitt's lymphoma. The virus causes proliferation of normal human B lymphocytes; EBV-coded proteins are found in Burkitt's lymphoma cell lines; and African children with the lymphoma have high titres of antibody to viral antigens. Despite this evidence, however, it is not clear if the virus is a cause of the lymphoma or whether other oncogenic stimuli produce the cancer in infected cells. Infection with two other DNA viruses has been linked to cancer: Herpes simplex II (HSV II) with cervical carcinoma and cytomegalovirus (CMV) with Kaposi's sarcoma. In both these cases the evidence is inconclusive.

Although uncommon in the West, hepatoma is a common cancer in Africa. Infection with hepatitis B virus

(HBV) is associated with its development both in Africa and in Europe. Hepatoma is particularly likely to occur in chronic active hepatitis associated with HBV, and in alcoholic cirrhosis where there is evidence of previous HBV infection. Cancer of the uterine cervix is increasing in frequency in young women. Recent evidence suggests that human papilloma virus may be associated with this disease, possibly as a sexually transmitted infection.

Genetic factors

Numerous *inherited*, rare, genetic abnormalities predispose to the development of malignancy (Table 9.3). These syndromes include examples of autosomal dominant and recessive inheritance, and X-linked disorders. The relationship between the genetic abnormality and carcinogenesis is unclear. Inherited chromosomal abnormalities may also predispose to cancer (Table 9.3). The most common is Down's syndrome (trisomy-21), where there is an increased incidence of acute leukaemia. Apart from these disorders (where there is an identifiable syndrome and inheritance) there is a less well-defined tendency for cancers to affect some families more frequently than they would by chance. These cancers are common cancers of adults but occur at an early age. In these families more than 25% of siblings are affected and one person may develop more than one tumour.

Acquired genetic abnormalities are frequently found in cancer cells with transposition and deletion of genetic material. These abnormalities are sometimes consistent, such as the translocation from chromosome 22 in chronic granulocytic leukaemia, and the reciprocal translocation involving chromosome 8 in Burkitt's lymphoma. Cells from acute leukaemia and solid tumours frequently show translocations and deletions of chromosomes of a less consistent pattern, but the relationship of these abnormalities to the development of cancer is not understood.

TUMOUR GROWTH AND DEVELOPMENT

Some tumours exhibit properties which imply that they have arisen as a result of clonal expansion caused by an oncogenic event in a single cell. Lymphomas, for example, usually show restriction to one type of surface immunoglobulin light chain; and studies in individuals who are heterozygotes for the enzyme glucose-6-phosphate dehydrogenase have shown that tumours contain only one form of the enzyme. Whether all cancers are monoclonal in origin is not known, and development of some carcinomas in a polyclonal field of premalignant change remains a possibility. Even if many tumours are monoclonal, heterogeneity of structure and function arises during the course of tumour growth. Cells from a tumour are diverse with respect to resistance to damage by irradiation or cytotoxic drugs, surface antigen expression, growth rate, and expression of biochemical markers such as embryonic proteins or peptide hormones. The mech-

Table 9.3 Inherited genetic abnormalities and malignancy

Inherited disorder	Cancer
Skin disorders	
Neurofibromatosis (AD)	Sarcoma Phaeochromocytoma Medullary carcinoma of thyroid
Tylosis palmaris (AD) (keratosis of palms and soles)	Oesophageal cancer
Peutz-Jehger's syndrome (AD)	Intestinal and ovarian cancer
Immune deficiency	
X-linked agammaglobulinaemia (XLR)	Lymphoma
Wiscott-Aldrich syndrome (XLR)	Lymphoma
Ataxia telangiectasia (AR)	Lymphoma and stomach cancer
X-linked lymphoproliferative syndrome (XLR)	Lymphoma
Gut disorders	
Polyposis coli (AD)	Colonic carcinoma
Gardner's syndrome (AD)	Colonic carcinoma Duodenal carcinoma Many other tumours
Neurological disorders	
Tuberose sclerosis (AD)	Glioma
Retinal/cerebellar angiomatosis (von Hippel-Lindau syndrome) (AD)	Hypernephroma Phaeochromocytoma Ependymoma
Other syndromes	
Bloom's syndrome (AR) (short stature, telangiectasia)	Leukaemia Many other cancers
Hemihypertrophy	Wilm's tumour Hepatoblastoma
Fanconi's anaemia (AR) (skeletal abnormality, patchy pigmentation, mental retardation)	Acute leukaemia
Multiple enchondromata (S) (Ollier's syndrome)	Chondrosarcoma
Chromosomal abnormalities	
Down's syndrome (trisomy 21)	Acute leukaemia
Klinefelter's syndrome (47, XXY)	Breast cancer
Aniridia-Wilm's syndrome (11p⁻)	Wilm's tumour
Mosaicism (45XO/46XY)	Gonadoblastoma
13q⁻ (multiple malformations)	Retinoblastoma

AD	Autosomal dominant	XLR	X-linked recessive
AR	Autosomal recessive	S	Sporadic

9

anism of acquisition of this diversity is ill understood, but heterogeneity within tumours presents a formidable problem for treatment.

In normal tissues, self-renewing stem cells replenish a proliferating population of cells which follow a pathway of differentiation resulting in a mature tissue (Fig. 9.7). Cell death is balanced by formation of precursors, and the tissue is static in size or else grows and diminishes in response to such external controls as hormonal environment. This model of tissue growth can be applied to tumours but it is not certain whether, in cancer, renewal comes from a small stem-cell population. In cancers, the restraint on growth is disrupted so that sustained expansion of the tumour occurs.

For clinically detectable cancers, the kinetics of growth appear to be exponential and the rate of tumour doubling varies widely. In Burkitt's lymphoma, the doubling time of visible tumour may be as short as one to two days, in contrast to 100–400 days for some squamous carcinomas and adenocarcinomas. It seems unlikely that growth is exponential from the beginning of the cancer, since this would imply very long subclinical growth periods for some tumours (Fig. 9.8). Cancers are clinically apparent after about 32 doublings, and lethal after 36–38. It is possible that tumours grow more rapidly when they are very small and slow progressively as they enlarge (Gompertzian growth). If true, this may have implications for therapy, since the more rapidly dividing small tumour might be more susceptible to chemotherapy.

During growth, the tumour becomes vascularised and lymphatic drainage is established. Cells more than 150 μm from a capillary are relatively hypoxic, and such cells are resistant to radiotherapy. They are also exposed to a lower concentration of cytotoxic agents. The vascularisation may be insufficient to sustain viability and areas of necrosis and haemorrhage are frequently found in large cancers. The process of vascularisation allows tumour cells to penetrate blood and lymphatic channels, and thence to metastasise to regional lymph nodes and distant sites.

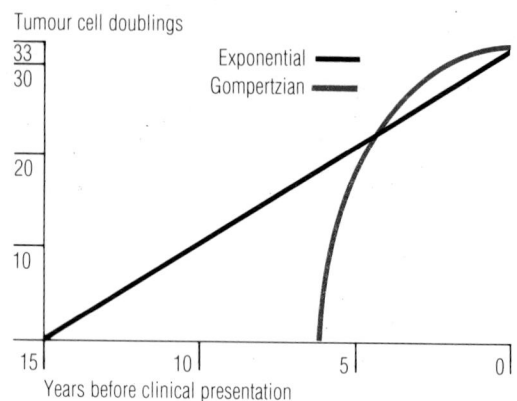

Fig. 9.8 Diagrammatic representation of exponential and Gompertzian growth.

Metastasis

Metastasis is a remarkable process and one which is still very poorly understood. The risk of metastases increases as tumours become larger. The metastatic cells have to survive the processes of circulation, passage across the capillary wall, and establishment in tissues. Only a few cells are likely to survive and the precise location of a metastasis is probably due in part to chance. Nevertheless, clinical patterns of blood-borne metastasis are apparent: gut cancers spread through the portal venous system to the liver; ovarian cancers seed into the peritoneal space; breast cancer has a predilection for bones of the axial skeleton; sarcomas characteristically spread to the lungs.

PATHOLOGY

The major categories of malignant tumours are:

1. *carcinomas* which arise from ectoderm or endodermal cells;
2. *sarcomas* which arise from mesodermal cells making up bone and connective tissue;
3. *leukaemias and lymphomas* which arise in cells of the bone marrow and immune system.

The distinction between benign and malignant neoplasms is based histologically on the cellular pleomorphism, frequent mitoses and tissue invasion which are characteristic of malignancy. The clinical manifestations of malignancy are tissue infiltration and lymphatic and blood-borne metastasis.

The degree of differentiation of a tumour is often an important guide to prognosis and therefore to therapy. Poorly differentiated carcinomas, for example of the breast and ovary, have a worse prognosis than well-differentiated tumours. This is due in part to an association with a more rapid growth rate and more early and widespread metastases. About 5% of cancers present as metastases where the primary site of the tumour is unknown. The histology

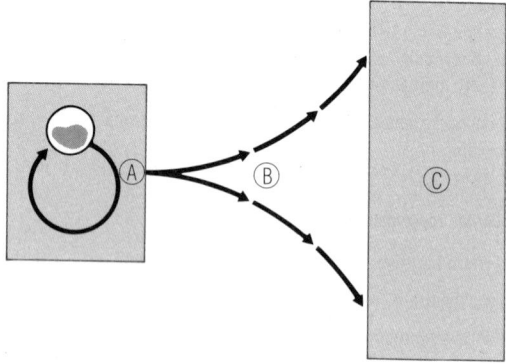

Fig. 9.7 Diagrammatic representation of cellular proliferation in a tumour. A. Pluripotent self-renewing stem cell. **B.** Proliferative compartment in which cell number increases but gradually loses reproductive potential. **C.** Mature tissue.

is usually a poorly differentiated carcinoma often with features suggestive of adenocarcinoma, but the pathologist may find the tumour difficult to classify.

In recent years, there have been major developments in histological diagnosis and classification of malignancy. The development of monoclonal antibodies has led to a greater precision in diagnosis by using immunocytochemical methods. Many anaplastic tumours can now be diagnosed as epithelial tumours, melanomas or lymphomas by using antibodies against epithelial antigens, and antigens associated with melanoma, leucocytes or T and B lymphocytes. The correct identification of lymphoma will lead to important changes in management of a patient (Fig. 9.9). Many antibodies will not bind to antigens on formalin-fixed and paraffin-embedded sections, and require fresh tissue. Other specialised investigations can be carried out on fresh tumour tissue – measurement of hormone receptor content (e.g. oestrogen and progesterone receptors) for example, which may be of importance in prognosis and in deciding treatment. Using immunocytochemical techniques, the

presence of such substances as alphafetoprotein can be detected in the tumour. In germ cell tumours, when preoperative measurement of tumour markers has not been made, this may be helpful in indicating that a relapse is likely to be associated with the appearance of this marker in the blood (Fig. 9.12). The increasing complexity and versatility of histopathological diagnosis means that it is now essential for there to be close collaboration between clinician and pathologist before specimens are obtained.

Ultrasound and computerised tomography (CT) scanning now allow accurate needle biopsy and aspiration cytology of hitherto inaccessible intra-abdominal and intrathoracic tumours. Cytological diagnosis does have some limitations; in the diagnosis of lymphoma, for example, it may be difficult to distinguish tumour cells from normal reactive lymphocytes. For this reason, histological diagnosis is preferred, especially in situations in which there is clinical doubt about the diagnosis.

CLINICAL FEATURES

Cancers cause symptoms due to the local spread of the primary tumour, and as a result of metastasis and of metabolic and remote effects of the malignancy.

Symptoms due to local disease

The primary tumour is clinically silent either until it becomes a visible painless lump which the patient notices (this is a common presentation of breast cancer and Hodgkin's disease and other lymphomas) or until it impinges on surrounding tissues. Thus, carcinoma of the lung will cause increasing bronchial narrowing, with breathlessness, cough and collapse of the distal lung; colonic carcinoma may present with disturbed bowel habit and obstruction; brain tumours may cause raised intracranial pressure or focal neurological signs; cancer of the head of the pancreas will cause obstruction of the bile duct leading to jaundice. As the primary tumour gets larger, it may ulcerate and bleed. Haemoptysis is a common symptom of bronchial carcinoma, and chronic blood loss leading to iron deficiency anaemia frequently occurs with carcinoma of the colon. The tumour may infiltrate nerves and bone leading to pain, or pain may arise from stretching of the capsule of an organ – for example, pain over the liver with advanced hepatoma. Nerve entrapment frequently occurs with pelvic tumours such as carcinoma of the cervix. Similarly, carcinoma of the bronchus occurring in the superior sulcus (Pancoast tumour) may be accompanied by intense pain in the arm, due to involvement of the brachial plexus.

Metastatic disease in bone causes pain which is often intense and distressing. Bone pain may occur in the absence of a pathological fracture or vertebral collapse, but it becomes worse when this occurs. In the liver, metastases cause pain by stretching the capsule. Cerebral metastases give rise to raised intracranial pressure, fits, focal signs and symptoms, and mental confusion. Pulmonary spread may

Fig. 9.9 Section of nasopharyngeal tumour. A. Staining with anti-cytokeratin; the epithelium of normal respiratory gland stains strongly but tumour cells are negative. **B.** Staining with antibody to the leucocyte common antigen reveals that the tumour cells are expressing the leucocyte antigen and that the tumour is a lymphoma.

9

cause breathlessness due to large intrapulmonary tumour masses, diffuse lymphatic permeation (lymphangitis carcinomatosa) and massive pleural effusion.

Systemic symptoms

Primary and metastatic cancer may cause a variety of metabolic and other disturbances which are important causes of symptoms. In general, these are produced in one of three ways:

1. as a result of the tumour mass, both primary and metastatic;
2. as a result of secretion of hormones by the tumour (Table 9.4);
3. by ill-understood mechanisms which give rise to specific cutaneous, neurological and other syndromes remote from the tumour and not due to metastasis – *paraneoplastic syndromes* (Table 9.5).

The commonest metabolic disturbance associated with advanced cancer is cachexia. This is a state of profound weight loss, muscle wasting and weakness. Many factors contribute to the state, of which anorexia is perhaps the major cause. Loss of appetite occurs early with tumours of the upper gastrointestinal tract, even before metastases have occurred. For most tumours, loss of appetite is an accompaniment of advanced disease, particularly hepatic metastases. Anorexia may be made worse by treatment with radiation and cytotoxic drugs, by psychological factors such as depression, and by unrelieved pain. The tumour may promote weight loss by direct metabolic effects. For example, there may be excess lactate production by the tumour which is recycled into glucose (a process wasteful of energy), and an increased glucose consumption at a time when carbohydrate intake has declined. Some tumours may cause malabsorption (carcinoma of

pancreas) or intestinal obstruction (colon cancer) which contributes to weight loss. Unlike patients who are starving, many cancer patients have a normal or high metabolic rate but the reason for this is not clear.

Fever may accompany cancer – not always due to infection, although this must always be excluded. Fever is particularly likely to occur with lymphomas, renal carcinoma, sarcomas and any tumours which have metastasised to the liver.

Anaemia may be due to blood loss, malabsorption or dietary deficiency of iron or folate. The most common mechanism is a failure of release of iron (stored in macrophages) into the plasma – the anaemia of 'chronic disease' (p. 1061). This anaemia is unresponsive to iron therapy. Chemotherapy and radiation both depress bone marrow function and contribute to anaemia.

The hormonal syndromes which accompany cancer (Table 9.4) are important because they are a cause of symptoms which are frequently treatable. In many patients, hypercalcaemia is due to bone destruction by metastases, but some cancers produce hypercalcaemia by an ill-understood hormonal mechanism. In these cases, the calcium level falls if the tumour is removed. The mechanism was thought at one time to be production of parathormone by the tumour; but the situation is probably more complex, with production of a parathormone-related peptide and other factors (such as growth factors) which can mobilise bone calcium. Hypercalcaemia associated

Table 9.5 Paraneoplastic syndromes

Syndrome	Associated tumours
Neurological	
Neuropathy (usually sensory)	Small cell lung cancer Cancers of breast and ovary
Cerebellar degeneration	Small cell lung cancer
Eaton-Lambert syndrome	Small cell lung cancer
Musculoskeletal	
Clubbing Hypertrophic pulmonary osteoarthropathy	Carcinoma of the lung (particularly squamous cell)
Dermatomyositis	Lung cancer Oesophageal cancer Other cancers
Polyarthritis	Adenocarcinomas of breast, gut and ovary
Haematological	
Multiple venous thrombosis	Pancreatic cancer Other adenocarcinomas
Erythrocytosis	Renal carcinoma Hepatoma Cerebellar haemangioblastoma Uterine cancer
Disseminated intravascular coagulation	Mucinous adenocarcinomas

Table 9.4 Hormonal syndromes in non-endocrine cancers

Hormonal syndrome	Tumour	Mechanism
Hypercalcaemia	Squamous carcinoma Carcinoma of kidney	? Tumour-derived growth factors ? Other calcium mobilising factors
Hyponatraemia	Small cell lung cancer Lymphoma Pancreatic carcinoma	Ectopic ADH produced by tumour
Cushing's syndrome	Small cell lung cancer Bronchial and thymic carcinoids	Ectopic ACTH produced by tumour
Gynaecomastia	Teratoma Hepatoma Large cell bronchial cancer	? Excess oestrogen activity
Hyperpigmentation	Small cell lung cancer	? Ectopic MSH produced by tumour

with cancer can be very severe, requiring urgent treatment (see Ch. 19 p. 738). Hyponatraemia, due to production of antidiuretic hormone (ADH) by the tumour, is a frequent accompaniment of small cell lung cancer. Malaise, fatigue leading to fits, and coma may result. The condition can be reversed by demeclocycline and water restriction (Ch. 22). Adrenocorticotrophic hormone (ACTH)-like peptides may also be produced by small cell lung cancer. In this disease, the high levels of ectopic ACTH produce profound metabolic disturbances, with proximal muscle weakness, hyperglycaemia and hypokalaemic alkalosis. These symptoms can be reversed by treatment of the tumour.

The paraneoplastic syndromes (Table 9.5) can cause diagnostic difficulty in two ways. Firstly, the syndromes have to be distinguished from other diseases causing a similar clinical picture. For example, the peripheral neuropathy accompanying cancer may be clinically indistinguishable from other causes. Secondly, the underlying carcinoma may not always be clinically apparent. Tumours such as carcinoma of the ovary or pancreas may be associated with multiple migratory venous thromboses at a time when the primary disease is not detectable.

The diversity of symptoms caused by primary and metastatic cancer, together with the hormonal, metabolic and paraneoplastic syndromes which accompany many malignant tumours, mean that a diagnosis of cancer must be considered in any unexplained illness, particularly in a middle-aged or elderly patient.

STAGING AND INVESTIGATION

Once a diagnosis of cancer has been established, further investigation is usually needed to establish the degree of spread of the primary tumour and to determine if metastasis has occurred. It has been known for many years that the prognosis of a patient depends, among other things, on the size of the tumour and the presence of metastases. Our ability to locate the tumour and distant metastases accurately has improved immeasurably in recent years with the introduction of radionuclide and ultrasound scanning, CT scanning and magnetic resonance imaging (MRI). These techniques have shown that, in many patients, the cancer is metastatic at the time of presentation. This realisation has led to a greater emphasis on systemic treatments such as hormone therapy and chemotherapy and, in some cases (e.g. breast cancer), a tendency towards less radical surgical procedures for the primary tumour. The determination of the degree of spread at presentation is generally known as *staging*. The international acceptance of staging systems has meant that, in treatment trials, comparable groups of patients can be treated allowing a comparison between different methods.

TNM classification

A generally accepted system, which is applicable to some (but not all) cancers, is the TNM (*Tumour, Nodes, Meta-*

stases) classification. The *T* component defines certain characteristics of the primary tumour such as its size, site or depth of invasion; the defining criteria will be different with each type of cancer. *N* refers to the presence or absence of involved nodes; the degree of node involvement may be designated as N0 (no involved nodes) and N1, N2, N3, as more nodes are involved. If no metastases are present, the designation is M0, and M1 if they are detected. Clearly, the TNM stage assigned to a tumour will depend on the thoroughness of the clinical and radiological investigation, and this will change as new techniques are invented and perfected.

The TNM stages can be grouped into categories which have prognostic significance. These categories or 'stage groups' have been of great value in the design of treatment trials. The TNM stages and related stage groupings for carcinoma of the kidney are shown in Table 9.6 and the prognosis related to the stage grouping in Figure 9.10.

The TNM system is not applicable to some tumours and is of limited value in others; it is clearly inappropriate,

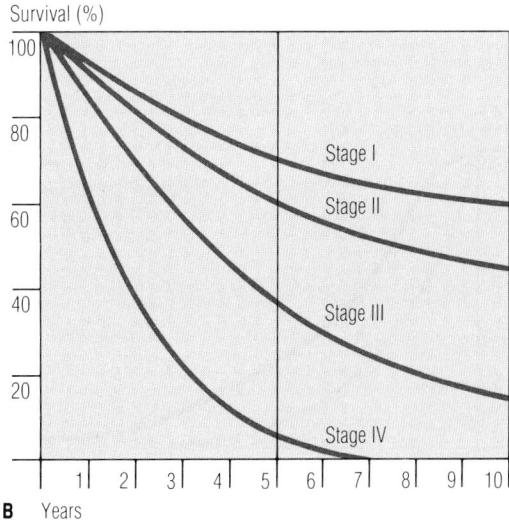

Fig. 9.10 A. Carcinoma of the left kidney. T = degree of local spread; N = involvement of adjacent lymph nodes; M = metastasis to bone or other sites. **B. Prognosis according to stage grouping.**

Table 9.6 Renal carcinoma TNM staging and stage grouping

Stage	Definition
	T stage
T1	Small tumour surrounded by normal kidney
T2	Large tumour with kidney deformity
T3	Perinephric infiltration or renal vein extension
T4	Invasion of local structures (e.g. abdominal wall)
	N stage
N0	No nodes involved
N1	Ipsilateral nodes involved
N2	Contralateral nodes involved
N3	Fixed nodes
	M stage
M0	No distant metastases
M1	Distant metastases

	Stage grouping		
Stage I	T1	N0	M0
Stage II	T2	N0	M0
Stage III	T3	N0–2	M0
Stage IV	T4	N0–3	M1

(The stage grouping refers to the worst prognostic feature of the case: e.g. a T1 N1 tumour would be Stage III)

for example, in acute leukaemias, and prognostic factors in these diseases are based on other criteria (see Ch. 25). Nevertheless, staging classification is possible and useful in diseases such as chronic lymphatic leukaemia and myeloma. The criteria have nothing to do with a TNM system, but are related to tumour mass. In lung cancer, the TNM system is useful and widely used in squamous carcinoma, but is of considerably less value in small cell carcinoma. In this disease, a rough categorisation is made into *limited* disease (confined to one hemithorax) and *exten-*

sive disease (spread beyond one hemithorax including metastases). There is a clear difference in prognosis in these two categories (Fig. 9.11).

Staging investigation

As techniques are developed, the *sensitivity* (ability to detect an abnormality if it is present) and *specificity* (ability to distinguish a metastasis from other pathologies) of the investigations changes. At present, radionuclide bone scanning is the most sensitive method of detection of bone metastases. The new CT scanners are better than, or at least equal to, ultrasound scanning in detection of hepatic metastases, but ultrasound is much cheaper and can be repeated regularly to assess reponse. CT scanning is superior to any other method of detecting pulmonary metastases, and much more sensitive than radionuclide scanning in demonstrating brain secondaries. MRI is superior to CT scanning in detecting deep-seated brain tumours, especially in the brain stem.

CT scanning has proved of value in detecting lymph node enlargement in the thorax and the abdomen. Unfortunately, nodes can be replaced by secondary tumour and yet not be enlarged. Lymphography – in which contrast material is injected into lymphatics in the dorsum of the feet – is of value in showing filling defects in normal size nodes, as well as node enlargement. Unfortunately, the contrast material may not enter grossly enlarged nodes and does not give good visualisation of the upper para-aortic, coeliac, mesenteric or porta hepatis nodes. For those tumours which spread transperitoneally, such as carcinoma of the ovary, laparoscopy (peritoneoscopy) is the most sensitive method of detecting spread of tumour if a laparotomy is not carried out. Although invasive, this procedure can also be used to obtain liver biopsy material under direct vision.

Tumour markers

Tumours may secrete substances into the blood which can be used both diagnostically (to detect the presence of disease) and in therapy, to monitor the effects of treatment. A variety of biochemical disturbances may be induced in the body by a tumour, such as the rise in alkaline phosphatase caused by liver or bone metastases, but these are crude and insensitive guides to the effect of treatment. The markers in common clinical use (Table 9.7) are oncofetal antigens, placental products, isoenzymes, ectopic hormones and some cellular antigens usually derived from the cell membrane.

Ideally, the tumour marker should always be produced by the cancer in question. In choriocarcinoma, human chorionic gonadotrophin (HCG) is produced in over 95% of cases; and 75% of germ cell tumours secrete either alphafetoprotein (AFP), HCG or both. Carcinoembryonic antigen (CEA) is found in the serum in 65% of cases of colorectal cancer. With some markers, e.g. HCG, AFP and placental alkaline phosphatase (PLAP), the serum level of the marker is a reasonably accurate and sensitive reflection

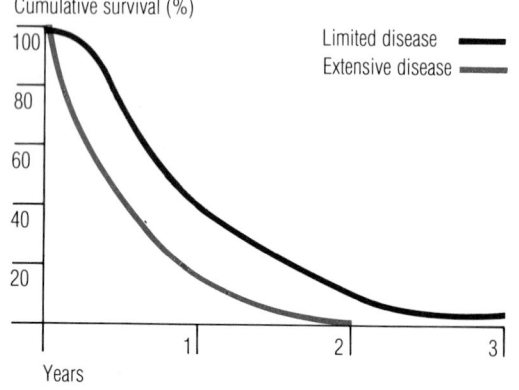

Fig. 9.11 Prognosis of small cell carcinoma of the lung related to the disease extent at presentation. Limited disease = disease confined to one hemithorax. Extensive disease = more widespread local extent or metastasis.

Table 9.7 Tumour markers present in blood

Marker	Tumour
Oncofetal antigens	
Alphafetoprotein	Germ cell tumours of ovary and testis Hepatoma
Carcinoembryonic antigen	Gastrointestinal cancer
Pancreatic oncofetal antigen	Pancreatic carcinoma
Placental products	
Human chorionic gonadotrophin	Choriocarcinoma Teratoma
Placental lactogen	Choriocarcinoma
Placental alkaline phosphatase	Seminoma Ovarian cancer
Isoenzymes	
Alkaline phosphatase	Osteosarcoma
Lactic dehydrogenase	Neuroblastoma
Acid phosphatase	Prostatic carcinoma
Neurone specific enolase	Small cell carcinoma of lung
Ectopic hormones (see Table 9.4)	
Other cellular antigens (defined by antisera)	
Antigens of ovarian carcinoma	
Antigens of cervical carcinoma	

of the tumour mass in an individual patient, and can therefore be used as a guide to therapy. In other cases, e.g. alkaline phosphatase in osteosarcoma, the relationship to tumour response is inconsistent.

The serum marker may be a valuable guide to tumour recurrence and, in most cases of germ cell tumours (such as teratoma of the testis) is a more sensitive indicator of tumour recurrence than any other technique. There is, of course, little value in knowing when relapse is occurring if there is no effective treatment. However, in the case of early stage germ cell tumours, the markers have allowed a policy of observation following initial surgery, since highly

effective chemotherapy is available for relapse. An example of the use of tumour markers is shown in Figure 9.12.

The tumour marker may be produced in other diseases; for example, serum AFP is raised in early pregnancy, and CEA may be present in inflammatory bowel disease. Other markers, such as ADH, are too difficult to measure for routine use.

AFP is produced in the fetal liver, in the malignant yolk-sac cells in teratoma, and in hepatoma. It has a plasma half-life of 5–7 days. HCG is produced by the placenta and by choriocarcinoma, and by the trophoblastic elements in teratoma. The plasma half-life is 30 hours. The beta subunit is measured to avoid cross reactivity with luteinising hormone. CEA is a group of glycoprotein antigens produced by epithelial tumours and by normal colonic mucosa.

Another possible use for tumour markers would be in screening populations for the presence of a tumour. Mass screening programmes are only feasible if the disease has a high incidence and this is not the case for those diseases (such as germ cell tumours) where most tumours produce markers and there are few false positives. However, colorectal cancer is common enough in the elderly for screening to be a practical possibility. Unfortunately, CEA is neither sensitive nor specific enough for it to be used in this way.

PRINCIPLES OF CANCER TREATMENT

Surgery and radiotherapy are the principal methods of treating the primary tumour. For many early-stage cancers – e.g. in cancer of the breast, squamous cancer of the lung, and cancers of the ovary, kidney, testis and gastrointestinal tract – surgery alone has a good chance of cure. Unfortunately, many patients cannot be cured surgically, either because the tumour is so advanced locally as to make resection impossible, or because investigation has revealed metastases.

Advances in radiotherapy technique and the recent developments in combination cytotoxic chemotherapy

Fig. 9.12 Tumour markers in management of testicular cancer. A. Both HCG and AFP markers are elevated before orchidectomy but fall following operation (HCG more rapidly because of its short half-life). **B.** No evidence of recurrence, followed by a rise in marker levels. **C.** Combination chemotherapy for recurrence is followed by a fall in levels to normal (**D**). **E.** A further rise in marker levels is treated more intensively and the patient is disease-free at three years (**F**).

9

have meant that, for many patients, a combined approach to treatment is needed to achieve the best results. This in turn involves close collaboration between surgeon, radiotherapist and medical oncologist. Before treatment begins, it is essential to decide if there is a possibility of cure or whether the intention should be palliative. Many factors will influence this decision, including the degree of spread of the tumour locally, the presence of distant metastases, and the patient's age and state of health. It may be very difficult to decide on the best policy if the chances of cure are relatively small and the toxicity of treatment considerable. In a young patient, the aim of cure would probably overcome doubts about toxicity, but this would not be so in the elderly.

If the clinical evidence makes it quite clear that there is no hope of cure, then it becomes unnecessary and wasteful to undertake elaborate staging investigations since these are unlikely to alter management. Investigation, as previously outlined, will be necessary in all other patients to determine the degree of spread of the disease before deciding on the treatment plan. The principles of surgical management of cancer are beyond the scope of this chapter, but it is important for all physicians to have an understanding of the basis of treatment using radiotherapy, chemotherapy and hormone therapy.

RADIOTHERAPY

Most radiotherapy treatment involves the use of electromagnetic waves with very high energy and short wavelength – gamma rays and X-rays. The therapeutic use of gamma rays started with the discovery of the naturally occurring isotope radium which emits gamma rays as it decays. Some modern radiotherapy machines use ^{60}Co as a source which decays to a more stable form with a half-life of 5.3 years. The process of decay (with loss of a neutron) is accompanied by emission of gamma rays with a high energy (1.2 MeV). X-rays were first produced by Roentgen, who heated an electrode in a sealed vacuum tube. The electrode produced electrons which bombarded a target, resulting in emission of electromagnetic waves which were designated 'X-rays' and whose nature was the same as gamma rays. By increasing the voltage, X-rays of shorter wavelength and higher energy are produced which have greater tissue penetrating power than those produced from low voltage machines (Fig. 9.13). Modern machines accelerate the electrons almost to the speed of light, which results in a high-energy beam. These machines (linear accelerators) have become standard equipment in most departments. They provide a sharper beam than that obtained from ^{60}Co sources and greater depth doses. When the target is moved out of the path of the electrons, the high-energy electron beam can be used for the treatment of superficial tumours.

The tissue penetrating power of high-energy X-rays and gamma rays means that normal tissues will be irradiated as well as the tumour. With lower voltage X-rays, the penetrating power is less and more energy is deposited in superficial tissues, especially bone. With electrons, the

Fig. 9.13 Diagrammatic representation of tissue penetration of different types and energies of radiation.

radiation decays rapidly in tissue, the depth of penetration depending on the energy of the beam (Fig. 9.13).

The important site of radiation damage is nuclear DNA. The damage appears to be induced indirectly. The radiation first produces highly reactive radicals which in turn damage the DNA, impairing the reproductive integrity of the cell. The damaging effects of radiation are less marked in cells which are hypoxic. Some areas of tumour may not be well vascularised and these cells are relatively radioresistant. The mechanism of resistance is not well understood. The amount of cell death following exposure to irradiation is also proportional to the dose administered. At low doses the damage is sublethal. Nevertheless, radiation administered as a few large fractions may not be as effective as multiple fraction regimens using smaller daily doses. This technique may be more effective because it allows the tumour to shrink and become less hypoxic, may be easier to tolerate, and allows normal tissues to recover at a faster rate than the tumour. In treating tumours, multiple fractions are usually employed and the total dose administered depends on what is known of the radiosensitivity of the neoplasm (Table 9.8). The total dose received by the tumour is measured in Gray (1 J/kg) or rad (100 rad = 1 Gray).

The planning of the radiation field is often a highly

Table 9.8 Relative radiosensitivity of tumours

Highly radiosensitive	Relatively resistant
Lymphomas	Squamous cell lung cancer
Ewing's sarcoma	Hypernephroma
Seminoma	Bladder carcinoma
Wilm's tumour	Rectal carcinoma
Myeloma	Soft tissue sarcoma (adults)
	Cervical carcinoma
Moderately radiosensitive	
Breast cancer	**Very resistant**
Small cell lung cancer	
Ovarian cancer	Melanoma
Medulloblastoma	Osteosarcoma
Basal cell carcinoma	Pancreatic carcinoma
Teratoma	

complex procedure that has been greatly facilitated in recent years by the use of CT scanning, which gives a more accurate assessment of the local spread of the tumour, and simulators, which allow the fields to be constructed with precision. In planning the fields, the radiotherapist must therefore consider the localisation of the tumour, its probable inherent radiosensitivity, the tolerance of the normal tissues in the path of the beam, and the necessity to include draining lymph nodes in the treatment. Multiple fields may be necessary to achieve the desired dose in the tumour without damaging normal tissues. The fields may be *open* (or *direct*). Here, the radiation beam is applied directly, usually at right angles to the skin. Alternatively, if several fields are used, the field may be *wedged*. These wedges, inserted into the beam, alter the dose distribution so that the tumour dose is homogeneous and problems of irradiation of normal tissue are minimised where fields overlap. An example of a multiple field is shown in Figure 9.14. The treatment area is immobilised and for some tumours, such as head and neck cancers, moulds and shells are used to ensure accurate and reproducible positioning. The radiation source is mounted in a gantry which moves isocentrically about the patient.

Radiotherapy may also be given by placing a sealed source containing a radioactive isotope inside a body cavity or in tissues. This is known as *brachytherapy*. Examples of such isotopes are ^{137}Cs, which is widely used as an intracavity source of radiation in treating carcinoma of the cervix; and iridium wires, which may be placed in breast tissue to provide interstitial irradiation when radical radiotherapy is used following conservative surgery for breast cancer. Unsealed sources of radioactivity may be taken by mouth, e.g. ^{131}I in the treatment of thyroid cancer, or given intravenously, e.g. ^{32}P in the treatment of polycythaemia rubra vera.

The complications of radiotherapy depend on the radiation sensitivity of normal tissues in the path of the beam, and may be immediate or delayed. A summary of some of these is given in Table 9.9.

SYSTEMIC TREATMENTS

In the last 40 years, there has been a dramatic increase in interest in the use of drugs to kill cancer cells. So many cancers are either disseminated at diagnosis or too advanced locally to resect, that a systemic approach to treatment offers the only chance of remission or cure. The two treatments in general use are *cytotoxic chemotherapy* and *hormone therapy*.

Cytotoxic chemotherapy

Few areas of medicine have undergone a development comparable to the recent advances in the use of cytotoxic drugs. The earliest compounds to be introduced were nitrogen mustards, which were shown to be cytotoxic to lymphoid tissue and then to have activity against lymphomas in humans. In 1948, Farber demonstrated remissions of leukaemia using the antifolate aminopterin,

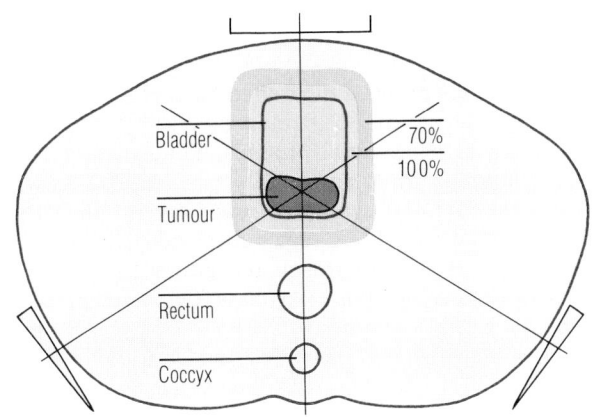

Fig. 9.14 Radiation planning for carcinoma of bladder, showing relationship of the three beams to the tumour and the dose levels (% of maximum) achieved within the tumour and surrounding normal tissue.

Table 9.9 Complications of radiotherapy

TISSUE	COMPLICATION Immediate	Delayed
Skin	Erythema, desquamation	Fibrosis Telangiectasia Squamous carcinoma
Oral cavity	Mucosal ulceration	Loss of saliva
Gut	Nausea, diarrhoea	Fibrosis and stricture
Bone	Bone necrosis	Loss of bone growth in children
Kidney	Acute nephritis	Chronic nephritis Hypertension
CNS	Radiation myelitis and encephalitis	Demyelination Possible alteration of personality and intellect
Eye	Conjunctivitis	Dry eye Cataract formation
Gonads	Sterility	Sterility
Bone marrow	Leucopenia	Suppression of haemopoiesis in area irradiated

and this led to the development of a wide variety of antipurines and antipyrimidines. Anti-tumour antibiotics were first developed in 1940 (actinomycin A) with a significant step forward in 1963 with the isolation of anthracyclines. More recent developments include platinum complexes and epipodophyllotoxins. There are now about 35 cytotoxic drugs of proven value in routine use, and the increasing complexity of medical treatment of cancer has led to the development of medical oncology as an important specialty in cancer management.

151

Cancer Medicine

Mechanisms of action

Cytotoxic drugs produce their effect mainly by damaging the capacity of the cell to divide, and also by interfering with synthesis of essential proteins. For many of these agents, the most important toxicity concerns DNA, with impairment of DNA synthesis, reaction with the DNA helix or damage to DNA repair mechanisms. This and other sites of damage are shown in Figure 9.15.

During cell division there is a phase (G₁) which precedes the phase of DNA synthesis (S). Following the S phase there is a postsynthetic phase (G₂) which is followed by mitosis (M). The daughter cells then either enter into the cycle of division or remain in a non-reproductive stage (G₀). Because of their action on DNA, most cytotoxic drugs exert their maximum effect on replicating rather than resting cells. If, after damage to DNA (e.g. by alkylation), the cell does not divide, there will be time for DNA repair mechanisms to excise the attached alkyl groups and to repair strand breaks. Rapidly proliferating cells are thus more susceptible to cytotoxic damage, but this is not the only determinant of susceptibility since, as with radiation, different tissues and tumours show inherent differences in susceptibility, the biochemical basis of which is poorly understood.

Alkylating agents are very reactive compounds which exert their effect by the linkage of the alkyl group to DNA bases, particularly guanine. If the drug is bifunctional (having two alkyl groups), inter- and intrastrand crosslinks will form. Nitrogen mustard, phenylalanine nitrogen mustard (melphalan), cyclophosphamide, busulphan and chlorambucil are commonly used alkylating agents. Cyclophosphamide itself is inactive but is metabolised by the liver to 4-hydroxycyclophosphamide, which is transported to the tissue and there releases the active alkylating compounds. Nitrosoureas and cisplatin probably act mainly as alkylating agents.

Methotrexate inhibits dihydrofolate reductase, thus preventing the formation of tetrahydrofolate which is necessary for thymidine synthesis. Other antimetabolites include: 5-fluorouracil (5FU), which also blocks thymidine formation; 6-mercaptopurine (6MP), which interferes with purine nucleotide biosynthesis; and 6-thioguanine, which has a similar mechanism of action to 6MP.

Several plant alkaloids have anticancer activity. The vinca alkaloids interfere with the formation of the mitotic spindle by blocking the assembly of tubulin. The epipodophyllotoxins, which have been introduced more recently, appear to damage DNA through an action on topoisomerase II.

Anthracycline antibiotics intercalate between DNA bases, as does actinomycin, which has the additional action of interfering with RNA synthesis. Bleomycin causes DNA strand breaks.

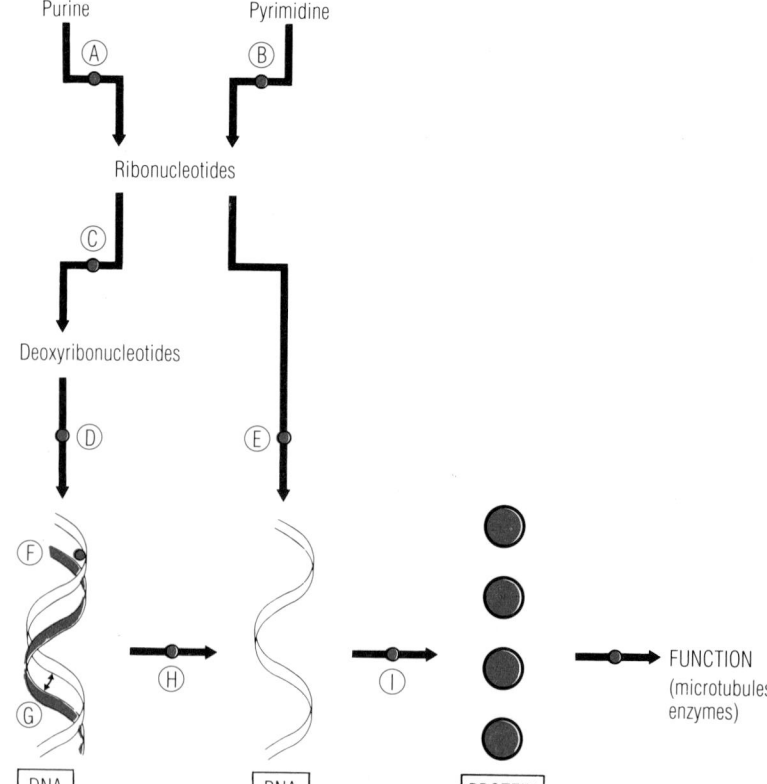

Fig. 9.15 Sites of action of some cytotoxic drugs.
A, B. Blocks to purine (6MP) and pyrimidine metabolism (azaribine).
C. Block of ribonucleotide reductase (hydroxyurea).
D. Inhibition of DNA polymerase (cytosine arabinoside).
E. Alteration of synthesis and function of RNA (5FU, azacytidine).
F. Intercalation with DNA and inhibition of topoisomerase II (anthracyclines, epipodophyllotoxins).
G. Cross-linking of DNA (bifunctional alkylating agents).
H. Impaired synthesis of RNA (actinomycin, anthracyclines).
I. Impaired protein synthesis (asparaginase).
J. Impaired function of proteins (vinca alkaloid blocking of microtubule formation).

Testing a new drug

When a new drug has shown activity in the laboratory, it is tested in patients with cancer. At first, it is given in gradually increasing doses to patients with advanced drug-resistant cancer. These trials are called *Phase I* studies and the aim is to monitor toxicity and to study metabolism and distribution of the drug as well as to note any activity. In *Phase II* studies, patients with a wide range of tumours are then treated in order to determine the spectrum of activity of the drug. Later, *Phase III* studies are performed in which the drug is tested, usually in previously untreated patients, either alone or in combination with other drugs and sometimes as part of a randomised comparison. In practice, there are considerable difficulties with this approach since, in Phase II studies, the patients have usually been previously treated, which decreases the likelihood of response to the new agent. In Phase III, it may not be justified to use the drug alone in previously untreated patients, thus making an evaluation of the activity of the drug very difficult.

Combination chemotherapy

In recent years, it has become standard practice to use cytotoxic drugs in combination. The aim is to produce a variety of different biochemical lesions in the tumour, if possible without increasing toxicity. The first attempts to adopt this approach were in acute leukaemia and lymphomas, and it quickly became apparent that quadruple therapy in, for example, advanced Hodgkin's disease, produced a far higher *complete response rate* (disappearance of all symptoms and signs of the tumour) than single-agent therapy. Furthermore, many of these complete responses were sustained – about 40% of patients being disease free between five and 10 years later. This had not been observed with single-agent therapy. Similar results were reported with non-Hodgkin's lymphoma and, later, with testicular teratoma, Ewing's sarcoma and other childhood tumours. In the common tumours of adults (such as cancer of the breast and small cell lung cancer), an increased response rate is also obtained with drugs in combination; but most of these responses are partial (greater than 50% reduction in size) and not sustained for long.

Most of the regimens used today have been derived empirically by oncologists with knowledge and experience. There are, however, some general principles governing selection of the drugs (Table 9.10). Using these general principles, combination chemotherapy has been introduced into the treatment of many cancers, and forms the mainstay of management in an important minority of uncommon tumours. Unfortunately, most of the common adult cancers are only moderately sensitive to these drugs, and some are very resistant (Table 9.11). Cancer is a disease of the elderly and many patients are not fit enough to risk the toxicity of chemotherapy, especially if the intention is to palliate rather than cure.

Complications of chemotherapy

There are both immediate and long-term complications of chemotherapy (listed in Summary 1).

Immediate

The most troublesome immediate side effects of chemotherapy are nausea and vomiting, mucosal ulceration, bone marrow depression and alopecia. Nausea and vomiting are probably initiated by a centre in the medulla. Intravenous alkylating agents tend to produce nausea at 12–18 hours,

Table 9.10 General principles governing the selection of drugs used in combination therapy

- The drugs are known to be effective when used as single agents.
- Where possible, drugs with differing modes of action are combined.
- The major toxicity of each drug should be as different as possible from that of other agents.
- Pulsed intermittent treatment is used to allow recovery of the gut and bone marrow.
- If possible each drug should be used in its optimum dose and schedule, although in practice some reduction in dose is nearly always necessary.
- There should be no known synergistic toxicity.

Table 9.11 Relative chemosensitivity of tumours

Highly sensitive tumours (which may be cured by chemotherapy)

Teratoma of testis
Hodgkin's disease
High grade non-Hodgkin's lymphoma
Wilm's tumour
Embryonal rhabdomyosarcoma
Choriocarcinoma
Acute lymphoblastic leukaemia in children
Ewing's sarcoma

Moderately sensitive tumours (in which chemotherapy may sometimes contribute to cure and often palliates)

Small cell carcinoma of lung
Breast carcinoma
Low grade non-Hodgkin's lymphoma
Acute myeloid leukaemia
Ovarian cancer
Myeloma

Relatively insensitive tumours (in which chemotherapy may sometimes produce palliation)

Gastric carcinoma
Bladder carcinoma
Squamous carcinoma of head and neck
Soft tissue sarcoma
Cervical carcinoma

Resistant tumours

Melanoma
Squamous carcinoma of lung
Large bowel cancer

9

and cisplatin and doxorubicin typically produce nausea about six hours after administration. Nausea is often accompanied by vomiting and the symptoms usually last 12–24 hours. The patient is often anorexic for the next day or two. These symptoms can be very troublesome but are tolerated by the majority of patients. Skilled and meticulous use of antiemetics is essential. Piperazine phenothiazines (e.g. prochlorperazine) are of some help when given in full dose, but aliphatic phenothiazines (e.g. chlorpromazine) have less antiemetic effect. Metoclopramide is of some value, and its effect may be increased by giving it in high dosage. Benzodiazepines are useful sedatives which enable the patient to sleep during the period of maximum nausea, which is then not remembered clearly. In choosing an antiemetic, a flexible approach is essential. Nurses trained in administration of cytotoxic drugs become adept in knowing which antiemetic suits a particular patient.

Mucosal ulceration in the mouth and gut is a complication of chemotherapy which is particularly likely to occur following methotrexate and anthracyclines. It is dose related, but some individuals are especially susceptible and the dose may then need to be lower than usual. Alopecia is very common with many drugs, especially doxorubicin and cyclophosphamide, and is due to damage to the proliferating cells of the hair follicle. Although the hair regrows when treatment is finally stopped, many patients find this a distressing side effect. With anthracycline, the hair loss can be minimised by scalp cooling during drug administration. The patient must be warned of the likelihood of hair loss, and a wig ordered if desired.

Bone marrow depression results in acute leucopenia and thrombocytopenia and the slower onset of anaemia (because of the greater lifespan of red cells). The nadir of the leucocyte count often comes at 7–9 days after intravenous chemotherapy and it is at this time that the patient is most susceptible to serious infection. Increasingly, oncologists are tending to adjust the dosage in each cycle of very myelosuppressive regimens according to nadir counts, even though this involves an extra blood count between visits. Patients must be forewarned of their susceptibility to infection and bleeding, so that they can report symptoms promptly.

Long-term

The long-term sequels of cancer chemotherapy are now becoming better defined as more children and adults are surviving cancers which were previously incurable. While these complications may be an inevitable risk of regimens that are potentially curative, they are a reminder of the risks attached to increasing the intensity of treatment.

Cytotoxic drugs impair fertility in adults. In men, complete and irreversible loss of fertility occurs with many regimens, particularly those which include an alkylating agent or procarbazine. Prepubertal boys do not become infertile, but Leydig cell function may be impaired and testosterone levels may fall. It is important to inform men of this risk and to arrange sperm storage before chemotherapy begins. Curiously, in Hodgkin's disease, where there is greatest experience of this problem, patients are often subfertile even before chemotherapy begins. For women, the problem is more complex. Amenorrhoea is common during chemotherapy, especially if an alkylating agent is used. Menstruation will usually return when treatment is finished, although subfertility is common. Chemotherapy may, however, induce the onset of menopause and this is more likely to occur in older women who are nearer the natural menopause. In both sexes, patients who are receiving chemotherapy should be advised of possible teratogenic effects and to use a contraceptive during treatment.

Second cancers are increasingly recognised as a long-term consequence of chemotherapy, particularly in ovarian cancer or Hodgkin's disease. In both cases, the risk is especially of acute myelomonocytic leukaemia. In Hodgkin's disease, there is a 40-fold increase in incidence of leukaemia. The risk is greater in patients over 40, and in those treated with both chemotherapy and total nodal irradiation. Second cancers are also more common in patients receiving immunosuppressive therapy with cytotoxic drugs, and in these patients there is an increased incidence of brain lymphoma, cervical carcinoma and skin cancer.

Pulmonary fibrosis is a complication of treatment with busulphan (e.g. for chronic myeloid leukaemia), and acute pneumonitis leading to fibrosis is a dose-related complication of bleomycin. Other cytotoxic agents rarely produce lung damage, although pulmonary fibrosis is a long-term complication of cyclophosphamide and nitrosoureas treatment.

Anthracyclines such as doxorubicin cause a cardiomyopathy, the risk being dose related. Above a total dose of 500 mg/m^2 about 50% of patients will have measurable impairment of cardiac function, but only 5% will develop cardiac symptoms. Established cardiomyopathy leads to cardiac failure which is irreversible on stopping the drug.

Vinca alkaloids cause damage to peripheral and autonomic nerves. The earliest symptoms are of tingling paraesthesiae. There is loss of tendon reflexes and, later, sensory loss and motor weakness. Autonomic neuropathy produces ileus and postural hypotension. Vincristine and vindesine are particularly likely to produce neuropathy, and vinblastine less so. The neuropathy is usually reversible, is total-dose related and more common and severe in the elderly. Cisplatin may cause irreversible loss of hearing, particularly of high frequencies. Renal impairment is also

---

Summary 1	Complications of chemotherapy
Immediate	*Long-term*
Nausea and vomiting	Impairment of fertility
Mucosal ulceration	Secondary cancers
Bone marrow depression	Pulmonary fibrosis
Alopecia	Cardiomyopathy
	Nerve damage
	Loss of hearing
	Renal impairment

Fig. 9.16 Diagrammatic representation of mechanism of action of oestrogen on cell growth. Tamoxifen acts by binding to the oestrogen receptor and blocking its action.

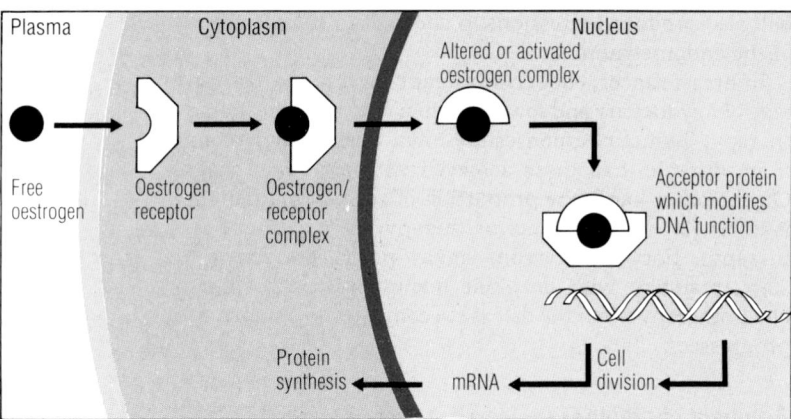

common and irreversible.

These toxic effects are a reminder that the treatment of cancer with cytotoxic drugs is a matter requiring skill and judgement if the benefits are not to be outweighed by the disadvantages. Nevertheless, the improvement in prognosis in some cancers as a result of cytotoxic drug treatment fully justifies the acute and long-term risks involved.

Hormone therapy

The growth of many normal tissues is under hormonal regulation, and the cancers which arise in them often retain sensitivity to changes in the hormone environment. Hormone therapy is an essential part of management of cancers of the prostate, breast, and endometrium. In these cases, the steroid hormone binds to a hormone binding molecule (*receptor*) in the cytoplasm and the receptor/hormone complex is transported to the nucleus where it modifies the activity of DNA. There is an increase in RNA polymerase activity, resulting in increasing production of cytoplasmic proteins followed by cell division (Fig. 9.16). In some cases, the hormone provokes the increased synthesis of receptors for other hormones; oestrogen, for example, increases the synthesis of progesterone receptor in breast epithelium.

It is now possible to measure the cellular concentration of receptors in cancers by measuring the binding of isotopically labelled hormone to homogenised cells. It has been found that the likelihood of response to hormone therapy is strongly associated with the presence of receptors in high concentration. In breast cancer, the presence of oestrogen receptor is associated with a 60% likelihood of response to hormone manipulation, with only a 5% chance of response if the cancer contains very low levels of receptor. The likelihood of response is even more strongly associated with progesterone receptor status.

In breast cancer, it is paradoxical that tumour regression may occasionally be seen both by blocking the effect of oestrogen and by the administration of oestrogen. The cellular basis of these effects is not well understood, but the following general approaches are taken in hormone-sensitive tumours.

Blocking the action of circulating hormones

In breast cancer, the use of tamoxifen has been a major advance. It appears to exert its effect by binding to the oestrogen receptor, thereby preventing the activity of circulating oestradiol. Paradoxically, the drug is effective in postmenopausal women whose tumours are receptor-positive, but in whom circulating levels of oestrogen are likely to be low.

Reduction in concentration of circulating hormones

Until recently, this was the mainstay of hormone therapy and was usually accomplished surgically. In breast cancer, oophorectomy was performed, or a radiation menopause induced in premenopausal women. In those who showed an initial response, but then relapsed, further responses could be obtained by adrenalectomy, which prevented sex hormone synthesis in the adrenal, and by hypophysectomy which produced a similar effect.

The advent of aminoglutethimide has led to a decline in frequency of these operations. This drug blocks the formation of pregnenolone in the adrenal, which diminishes the production of cortisol and androstanedione. Androstanedione is converted in peripheral tissues (and in the breast itself) to oestradiol by enzymes known as aromatases, and aminoglutethimide is a powerful aromatase inhibitor thus preventing oestradiol formation. The drug is widely used in postmenopausal women with breast cancer. Common side effects include transient skin rash, fever and somnolence.

Addition of hormones

The hormonal environment can be altered by administration of hormones which are judged to provide an unfavourable environment for the tumour. Stilboestrol has, for many years, been used to produce regression in carcinoma of the prostate; while androgens, glucocorticoids and progestogens may all slow the growth of the tumour in breast cancer. Progesterone derivatives will also produce regressions in about 20% of carcinomas of the endometrium.

In breast cancer, endocrine therapy has the great advantage of low toxicity and low cost when compared to chemotherapy. Tumour responses are often more complete and more durable than those achieved with cytotoxic drugs. On the other hand, the proportion of responding patients is lower (30% with endocrine therapy, 60% with chemotherapy). For these reasons, many physicians prefer to start treatment with hormone manipulation, moving to chemotherapy when the disease becomes unresponsive and progresses.

Adjuvant chemotherapy and hormone therapy

There are many situations in which a cancer has been removed surgically or treated with radiotherapy, but the risk of local or systemic recurrence is high. Examples include: breast cancer, where there is involvement of axillary nodes or where the tumour is poorly differentiated in a young woman; gastric and other cancers, where the regional nodes are involved; or Ewing's sarcoma of bone, where the tumour is highly sensitive to radiotherapy but the risk of metastasis is very great. In these situations, advances have been made by the use of cytotoxic drugs or hormones in an attempt to delay or prevent recurrence. Even if these treatments are not very effective against advanced cancer (of the stomach or breast), they may be more so when the residual tumour mass is small, when the penetration of the drugs may be better and the degree of cell kill may lead to cure rather than temporary tumour regression.

In recent years, many large-scale trials have been undertaken to assess the value of adjuvant cytotoxic or endocrine therapy. In the best of these studies, the treatment has been compared with an untreated control group. For the results to be accepted with confidence, there must be both sufficient numbers of patients in the study, and prospective randomisation of the allocation of the treatment policy. (The difficulties involved in these trials are discussed below).

In patients with stage II breast cancer, both adjuvant endocrine therapy (using tamoxifen) and cytotoxic therapy (usually using drug combinations such as cyclophosphamide, methotrexate and 5-fluorouracil) have been shown to give a relapse-free survival advantage of about 10–15% at five years. Since previously untreated patients can be treated after relapse, the more important question is whether there will be an overall survival advantage. This seems to be the case for both modalities of treatment (the advantage being 8–10% at five years), but as the toxicity of tamoxifen is far lower, it is a much more acceptable treatment to offer routinely after mastectomy. Breast cancer often has a slow evolution and it is possible that relapse is only delayed rather than prevented by adjuvant therapy. If this is the case, the percentage survival at, say, 10–15 years will be the same, with patients in the treated group relapsing and dying later than those who were not treated (Fig. 9.17).

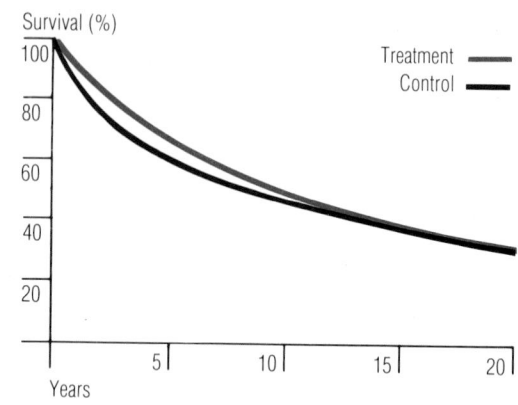

Fig. 9.17 A *possible* long-term result of adjuvant chemotherapy in the treatment of breast cancer. A 5–10% survival advantage might be seen at five years, but not at 15 years.

Adjuvant drug therapy after surgery or irradiation has become an essential part of management in most childhood tumours (rhabdomyosarcoma, Wilm's tumour, osteosarcoma, Ewing's sarcoma), and in a number of adult tumours, such as some stages of breast cancer and ovarian cancer. There are many other tumours (gliomas, gastric carcinoma, colorectal carcinoma, operable lung cancer) in which adjuvant chemotherapy has been shown not to contribute significantly to survival. The situation may of course change with the advent of more active drugs.

SUPPORTIVE CARE IN CANCER TREATMENT

Patients with cancer need supportive care for both the psychological impact of the disease and the physical effects of the tumour and its treatment. Even if there is no prospect of cure, the quality of life of the patient can be greatly improved by the attitude of the medical staff and by meticulous attention to the treatment of pain, anaemia, infection, nausea and anorexia.

Psychological support

The last 20 years have seen an increasing readiness, on the part of doctors, to discuss the diagnosis of cancer with their patients and to explain the principles of treatment. Indeed, the complexities of modern cancer management make it difficult to withhold the facts of the diagnosis, even if it were desirable to do so. Nevertheless, the manner in which the diagnosis is explained and the words used is of great importance, and must be carefully judged in each case. Cancer is the only word which conveys the nature of the complaint accurately, other words used are often misinterpreted by patients as implying a less, or even more, serious condition. The problem is that, in the mind of many patients, cancer is an invariably fatal disease; thus, any explanation of the diagnosis must be accompanied by an unhurried and easily comprehended account of treatment and the possibilities of cure. It is nearly always wrong to offer no hope of either cure or a prolonged period of normal life. Usually, the physician will need to talk to the patient on several occasions, since the patient's understanding of the problems may be incomplete at the beginning. Time taken in unhurried, private conversation is always well spent and greatly appreciated. One of the advantages of having specialised oncology units in hospitals is that all members of the medical team – nurses, doctors, social workers and counsellors – become familiar with the problems that are associated with malignant disease and skilful in dealing with them. It is important that all members of this team know what has been said to the patient in the way of explanation, in order to avoid conflicting advice.

A relapse of the disease or the appearance of a new symptom will often cause a slump in morale and confidence which will require more explanation and reassurance. The emotional demands of this aspect of cancer medicine are considerable and are one reason why some doctors are reluctant to spend time in discussion with their patients.

Pain relief

This is a very important aspect of management, particularly in patients with widespread disease who are terminally ill. No single analgesic will suit all patients all of the time. A patient will need to change from one to another depending on the severity of pain. A brief classification of some of the most useful analgesics is given in Table 9.12. When using opiates, the dosage should be adjusted to the patient's requirements. A wide range of dosage is encountered. Long-acting morphine and oral heroin are

Table 9.12 Useful analgesics

Drugs	Duration of action (hours)
Mild analgesics	
Aspirin	4–6
Paracetamol	2–4
Indole derivatives (e.g. indomethacin)	6–8
Proprionic acid derivatives (e.g. ibuprofen)	4–6
Moderate analgesics	
Codeine (and dihydrocodeine)	4–6
Pentazocine	3–4
Dipipanone	6
Oxycodone	8
Strong analgesics	
Morphine sulphate	4–6 (up to 12 with sustained release forms)
Diamorphine	4–6
Dextromoramide	4–6
Pethidine	3
Methadone	12–30

especially useful and should be given regularly rather than 'as required'. The constipating effects of opiates can be partly relieved by regular laxatives.

If pain is at a particular site, it may be possible to give relief by local measures, such as radiotherapy to a bone metastasis, a nerve block or a coeliac plexus block. The advice of colleagues specialising in these forms of pain relief is often helpful, and the procedures may allow a reduction in dosage of opiate.

Nutritional support

Patients lose weight because of the local effects of the tumour (especially if this is in the alimentary tract), metastases and as a result of treatment. Successful treatment of the primary tumour (e.g. by surgery) will be accompanied by a return of appetite and weight gain. During radical treatment with surgery, radiotherapy and intensive chemotherapy, weight loss is common.

In recent years, it has become possible to administer calories to patients undergoing cancer treatment both in the form of oral supplements and intravenously. However, the value of nutritional support is difficult to demonstrate. It is usual practice to consider total parenteral (intravenous) nutrition in patients undergoing exceptionally intensive treatment, such as high-dose chemotherapy or total-body irradiation with bone marrow transplantation, or during the intensive phases of chemotherapy for acute leukaemia, where there is prolonged hypoplasia. At these times, mucosal ulceration, nausea and diarrhoea make it difficult to feed the patient by mouth, and nasogastric tubes may produce monilial infection or exacerbate acid reflux and oesophagitis. Parenteral nutrition is also used for patients undergoing extensive surgery, particularly gut resection. The aim is to maintain the patient's weight and nutritional status so that recovery is more rapid, allowing further treatment with chemotherapy or irradiation to begin as soon as possible. There is no evidence that additional enteral or parenteral feeding is of value in the treatment of advanced cancer where cure is impossible. It is, however, important to encourage the patient to eat by giving food which appeals (often in the form of smaller more frequent meals), by controlling nausea with drugs such as metoclopramide, and by the careful use of corticosteroids which improve well-being and stimulate the patient's appetite.

Tumour lysis syndrome

In some very sensitive untreated cancers, chemotherapy may produce massive tumour breakdown when treatment is first given. This process may be accompanied by severe metabolic disturbances which constitute the *tumour lysis syndrome*. The syndrome is usually associated with the early phases of treatment of lymphoma and leukaemia in children and, less frequently, in other chemosensitive childhood tumours. In adults, the syndrome is infrequent but may occur with treatment of lymphoma, especially if there is impairment of renal function (such as ureteric

9

obstruction by lymph nodes) which diminishes renal excretion of the tumour products.

The tissue destruction releases large amounts of urate, phosphate and potassium. The urate may be deposited in the renal tubule causing reversible renal failure which, in turn, diminishes further urate excretion. Severe hyperuricaemia and renal failure may necessitate dialysis. This complication of therapy can largely be avoided by using the xanthine oxidase inhibitor allopurinol before and during the early phase of treatment, and by establishing and maintaining a diuresis during the first 24–48 hours. Hyperkalaemia may be severe, particularly if renal failure occurs, and may need treatment with glucose and insulin (see Ch. 20). Hyperphosphataemia can be partly prevented by hydration and diuresis before and during the initial treatment.

NEW APPROACHES TO TREATMENT

Progress in cancer treatment is slow, and results usually improve after many small refinements in treatment rather than by sudden steps forward. The introduction of combination chemotherapy has greatly improved results in drug-sensitive tumours, and CT scanning has greatly helped in staging and in planning local treatment. Since the late 1970s, only modest progress has been made and the search for new drugs and new approaches continues.

High-dose therapy and bone marrow transplantation

Allogeneic (from one individual to another) bone marrow transplantation was introduced for the treatment of acute myeloblastic leukaemia in the early 1970s. The allogeneic marrow was infused after an attempt had been made to eradicate the leukaemia by total-body irradiation and high-dose cyclophosphamide. The results (Ch. 25) showed that the leukaemia might be eradicated. This finding led to the consideration of total-body irradiation in the treatment of other disorders, such as lymphomas and myeloma. More recently, attempts have been made to eradicate leukaemia, lymphoma and some solid tumours with very high-dose chemotherapy (rather than total-body irradiation) using *autologous* (taken from, and re-infused into, the same individual) bone marrow, harvested just before treatment, as a means of preventing life-threatening myelosuppression. These approaches are based on the assumption that increasing doses of chemotherapy will eradicate residual disease when multiple conventional doses will fail. As yet, it is too soon to know whether the approach has any value, and autologous bone marrow transplantation remains an unproven method of treatment in any tumour.

Half-body irradiation

Stimulated by the effects produced by a single fraction of whole-body irradiation in the eradication of leukaemia,

radiotherapists have begun to explore the use of a single fraction of irradiation given first to one half of the body and then the other, allowing time for bone marrow recovery between treatments. Significant responses can be seen in radiosensitive tumours such as lymphoma or myeloma, and palliation of pain from widespread bone metastases can be achieved in diseases such as carcinoma of the prostate. There is much more to be discovered about the use of radiation as a 'systemic' treatment of cancer.

Monoclonal antibodies to cell surface antigens

There is little evidence that human tumours express unique antigens, but many tumours appear to express oncofetal or differentiation antigens not usually found in the normal tissue from which the cancer is derived. An example is the common acute lymphoblastic leukaemia antigen (CALLA) found on the surface of both acute lymphoblastic leukaemia cells and normal lymphatic progenitor cells. The development of somatic cell hybridisation to produce monoclonal antibodies of defined specificity has resulted in the production of monoclonal reagents, which bind preferentially to antigens on the surface of some tumour cells (and to those normal cells which express the antigen). Cytotoxic drugs, cell poisons such as ricin or abrin, and radioactive isotopes can be attached to such antibodies in the hope of selectively destroying the tumour. There are considerable difficulties with this approach – heterogeneity of antigen expression within the tumour; variable uptake and distribution of antibody in normal and malignant tissue; and the production of antibodies by the patient against the foreign (usually mouse) protein. Nevertheless, there are interesting future possibilities for treatment and tumour localisation using this approach.

TRIALS OF TREATMENT

Many cancers have a long and unpredictable natural history: cancer of the breast, for example, is associated with an excess mortality for over 25 years after diagnosis. If survival is the endpoint of treatment then assessment of therapy in this disease will mean prolonged periods of observation. In small cell lung cancer or acute myeloblastic leukaemia, on the other hand, the majority of patients are dead within two years, and relapse in those that survive is less frequent beyond that point. Treatment trials will therefore give answers quickly. In assessment of treatment of a cancer (such as breast cancer), there may be more than one endpoint to be considered: does the treatment give effective local control; does the treatment influence the onset of metastasis; is the proportion of survivors at five and 10 years or longer increased?

Comparison of a treatment with historical controls is very unreliable, since diagnostic and staging criteria are changing constantly and selection of cases is thereby altered. Randomised, prospective studies are now regarded as the only reliable way of making a comparison between two treatments. Such studies must include sufficient numbers of patients to allow the questions to be answered with confidence statistically. The studies require careful documentation and prolonged observation of the patient groups. The treatments being compared must be justifiable ethically and the design of the study capable of giving a clear answer to the central question.

These considerations mean that treatment trials in cancer are complex and usually demand collaboration between many different centres; even, in the case of rare tumours, between different countries. To detect a 5% difference in survival with confidence, may require many hundreds or even thousands of patients in a study. Nevertheless, a 5% difference in long-term survival in breast cancer, if achieved by a non-toxic hormonal means, would mean 1000 lives saved a year in the UK alone – greater than the number of patients with Hodgkin's disease cured. However, a 5% difference achieved by means of toxic chemotherapy might be regarded with less enthusiasm. At present, because progress in cancer treatment is slow and achieved only by small improvements, large-scale clinical trials are the only reliable way of validating new treatments.

CARE OF THE DYING

Many patients with cancer die from their disease, and it is the responsibility of the oncologist to be sure that aggressive treatment of the tumour is not thoughtlessly continued beyond the point at which cure is possible. This does not mean that treatment is discontinued but, rather, that the aim of treatment becomes palliative rather than curative. Palliative treatment can often, if in skilled hands, give the patient a period of happy life free from distressing symptoms. Palliation may require: radiotherapy, e.g. for painful bone metastases or bronchial obstruction; chemotherapy at low dose to suppress constitutional symptoms in lymphoma; aspiration of ascites or pleural effusion; or surgical pinning of a bone weakened by metastasis. There is more to palliative treatment than pain relief. Nevertheless, relief of pain, control of nausea and treatment of depression become increasingly important as the disease progresses.

The most important component of treatment at this stage is the psychological support of the patient and his or her family. Support comes from the nature of the relationship that the patient has established with the medical team throughout the illness. Extra help may be needed from domiciliary nursing teams, which are increasingly providing expert and readily available advice on symptom control to patients in their own homes. Many patients prefer to remain at home in the last few weeks of life, and the family doctor and specialist nurses can often make this possible. Alternatively, the patient's wishes or family circumstances may make admission to a hospital or hospice necessary. The nursing practices and the approach to symptom control that have been developed in hospices are now being incorporated into hospital practice. In some hospitals, nurse specialists have been appointed to advise on these aspects of management.

The gradual awareness of death produces many different reactions. The patient may become angry and direct this at the medical or nursing staff. Feelings of apathy, hopelessness and fatigue are common, and depression may be severe enough to need treatment with antidepressants. The support of relatives and friends is essential.

Meticulous attention to detail and a willingness to take time to talk to the patient are just as important at this stage in treatment as during the early stages when the intention may have been curative. Even though treatment has finally failed, this does not mean it was not worthwhile, nor is it a reflection on the abilities of the medical or nursing staff. The fact of treatment failure leads some doctors to avoid seeing their patients at this stage. This is bad practice and increases the patient's feeling of isolation and helplessness.

Many non-medical agencies are able to help the patient and his or her family. Patients with religious beliefs may gain great comfort from their clergyman and other members of their local religious community. Counselling and support groups have been set up in many towns to provide help during the illness and to the bereaved relatives afterwards.

ALTERNATIVE THERAPY

A multitude of unorthodox approaches to treatment of cancer have been offered to patients over the years. These usually have echoes of current medical practice. Serotherapy was used after antitoxins were introduced for infectious disease; tooth extraction was practised, based on the interwar notions that dental sepsis was responsible for chronic inflammation. Nowadays, psychological ideas are translated into visualisation therapy; and concern over pollution and diet are transmitted into strict vegetarian or fat-free diets. The uncritical assumption that answers will be found in nature has led to a wide range of herbal remedies some of which (e.g. laetrile) are somewhat dangerous. As with many chronic diseases, the practitioners of homeopathy and faith healing offer their remedies.

Most of these approaches share certain recognisable characteristics. These include: a tendency to borrow the jargon of medicine without its science; a belief that all tumours can be treated by the same or similar remedies; a tacit or explicit assumption that there exists a medical conspiracy to conceal the truth about the remedy in question; and a complete failure to adopt any of the proven methods of validation of the results of treatment.

What these approaches offer distressed and anxious patients is a feeling that they can themselves do something to combat their disease, a glimmer of hope that they might be cured, and relief from the side effects of conventional treatment if this is abandoned. These benefits are often a reflection of inadequacy in the relationship of the patient

9

and doctor, rather than a clearly held view by the patient and family. The damaging aspects of these approaches are that they may induce the patient to abandon a worthwhile treatment, weaken the relationship between doctor and patient, and impose unpleasant constraints on the patient's life, such as rigid dietary control. These disadvantages should be discussed with the patient and, if patients are thinking of abandoning a potentially curative treatment, every attempt should be made to persuade them not to do so. Nevertheless, the doctor's role in treatment is to offer help, advice and expertise; the patient has the right to choose what to do. In many cases, no great harm will be done and an experienced doctor will make it clear that the patient is welcome to continue under his or her care in the future.

FURTHER READING

Calabresi P, Schein P S, Rosenberg S A 1985 Medical oncology. Macmillan, New York. *A comprehensive textbook of medical oncology*

Cancer Surveys 1986 Hormones and cancer. Vol 5, No 3. Oxford University Press, Oxford. *One of a series of reviews of cancer topics*

DeVita V T, Hellam S, Rosenberg S 1986 Cancer: principles and practice of oncology. Lippincott, Philadelphia. *A comprehensive cancer textbook*

Easson E C, Pointon R C S 1985 The radiotherapy of malignant disease. Springer-Verlag, Berlin. *A textbook of radiation treatment*

Saunders C M 1985 The management of terminal malignant disease. Edward Arnold, London. *An excellent account*

Souhami R L, Tobias J S 1986 Cancer and its management. Blackwell, Oxford. *A medium-sized text covering most aspects of cancer treatment*

Ageing and Disease

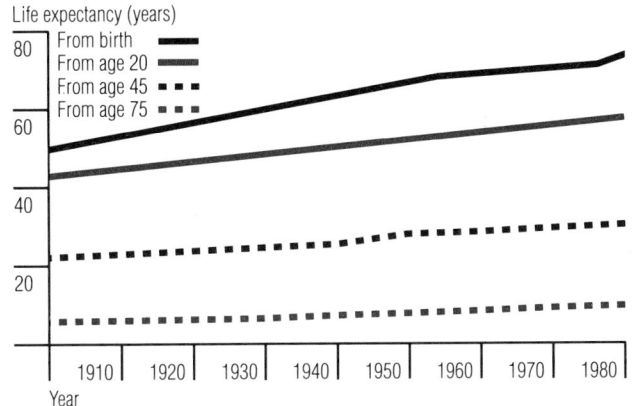

Fig. 10.1   Changes in life expectancy this century. Most of the increase in life expectancy results from reductions in infant mortality rather than an extension of the natural lifespan.

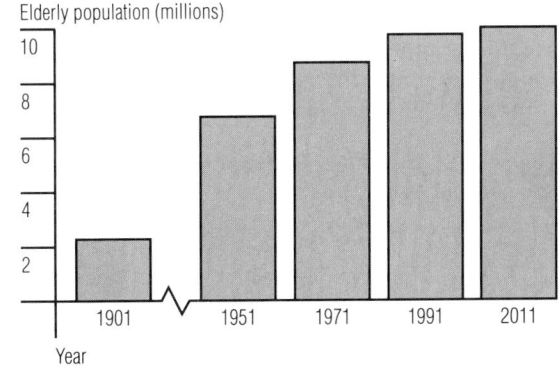

Fig. 10.2   Increases in the elderly population of the United Kingdom since 1901.

Most ill health in developed countries now occurs in elderly persons. Not only are the elderly more prone to illness, but the proportion of elderly people has increased enormously in most societies since the middle of the 20th century.

While ageing is an experience common to all, the response of an individual to growing old depends more upon the previous pattern of life than upon anything in the ageing process itself. Thus, although some generalisations may usefully be made about old age, the elderly should not be regarded as an homogeneous group. Indeed, one of the features of old age is increased differences between individuals.

Life expectancy

Life expectancy is the average observed years of life from birth or from any stated age. Since the beginning of the century, life expectancy at birth in the United Kingdom has increased from 49 to 70 years for men and from 52 to 76 years for women (Fig. 10.1, see also Ch. 1, p. 12). This is mainly the result of reductions in infant mortality from the major infectious diseases: tuberculosis, acute rheumatic fever, smallpox, diphtheria, tetanus and poliomyelitis now account for less than 2% of the ill health they caused in 1900. These changes are largely due to improvements in nutrition and to public health measures which have reduced water- and food-borne diseases. The influence of immunisation and treatment on mortality from infectious

disease is comparatively much smaller. The recent dramatic growth in the number of elderly people in developed countries is due largely to the survival of children born in the latter half of the 19th century (Fig. 10.2).

In 1901, the United Kingdom's 2.4 million elderly (i.e. women over the age of 60 and men over 65) made up 6.3% of the population, yet by 1971, this figure had increased to

16.3%, an elderly population of 8.8 million. By 1991, the numbers of people aged between 65 to 74 will have increased by only 1%; but there will have been a 33% increase in those aged 75 to 84, and a 46% increase in those aged 85 and over (Table 10.1 and Fig. 10.3).

The rate of increase of the elderly population in developed countries will be dwarfed, however, by that in the developing world. Between 1980 and 2000, the percentage increase in the population over 60 years is estimated at 100% for Brazil, Kenya and Nigeria, and 80% for India, compared with less than 2% in the United Kingdom. The level of disability among the middle-aged and elderly is also greater in developing than in the developed countries – due less to strokes and ischaemic heart disease than to polio, leprosy and trachoma. Thus, the problems faced by the health services of the developing countries – already overstretched by common infectious diseases such as TB and malaria – are considerable.

Table 10.1   Projected increase in the World's elderly population (aged 65 and over), 1980–2000

Area	Projected increase in elderly population (in millions)
The world	138
Developing areas	
China	32
India	17
Other	51
Total	100
Developed areas	
USSR	10
USA	7
Other	21
Total	38

THEORIES OF AGEING

No single cause of ageing has been found. Some gerontologists believe that *extrinsic* wear and tear eventually causes malfunction within different tissues, at a rate dependent on each particular individual's genetic background and environment. Others regard the main underlying causes of malfunction as *intrinsic* to the ageing tissue and programmed to occur, like the running down of a biological 'clock'.

Genetic factors

There is general agreement that ageing is, at least in part, genetically determined. Each animal species has a specific lifespan: the maximum recorded longevity of Marion's tortoise, for example, is over 152 years, for man approximately 115 years and for golden hamsters two or three years. In species of *Drosophila*, the F1 hybrid has a greater

longevity than either parental strain. Female sex also generally confers increased longevity, with the male sex shorter-lived in a number of different species; and persons whose parents live to the age of 75 years or more live longer than persons whose parents died before the age of 60. The mean difference in longevity in dizygotic twins is twice that of monozygotes.

Wear and tear

Accumulation of damage may eventually affect the function of single cells, intact organs or the whole individual. In the ageing process, the likely site of such damage is nuclear DNA. Actively dividing cells depend on the accurate transmission of genetic material from parent to daughter cell. Thus, an accumulation of abnormalities in DNA during somatic cell division might lead to cell malfunction and consequent susceptibility to degenerative or oncogenic change.

'Programmed' ageing

It has been proposed that there is a predetermined or 'programmed' alteration in cellular function which contributes to ageing, but there is no agreement as to where such a biological 'clock' might be located. It may be intrinsic to all cells, or it may be that malfunction of a single organ – such as the pituitary gland – may contribute directly through changes in the internal environment. A third possibility is that repair processes which minimise damage from wear and tear are programmed to decline with age.

The concept of cellular ageing is supported by observations that a normal cell undergoes a fixed number of divisions before it dies. This *in vitro* doubling capacity declines with increasing age of the individual. While these observations challenge previously held ideas that ageing occurs at a supra-cellular level in the animal as a whole, it is unlikely that the finite number of cell doublings acts to limit the human lifespan. Indeed, some replicating cell

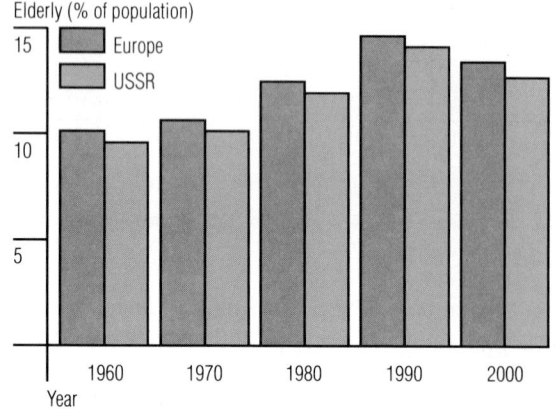

Fig. 10.3   Percentages of people aged over 80 years among those aged over 60 years in Europe and the USSR, 1960–2000 (projected).

populations (such as lymphoid stem cells) are capable of functioning normally for many times the lifespan of the parent organism.

Simmonds' description, in 1914, of senile changes in a patient with severe pituitary deficiency, focussed attention on the pituitary as a possible regulator of ageing. But there is no firm evidence pointing to pituitary hypofunction as a major cause of ageing in normal individuals.

SOCIOLOGICAL ASPECTS

There is no satisfactory definition of what constitutes old age. Ageing is a continuous process that occurs throughout life and there is considerable individual variation. It is a commonplace observation that some persons of 60 years of age look and act a good deal older than a sprightly 80-year-old. In earlier times, 'old' was a term generally applied to persons who had the appropriate physical appearance, such as white hair, wrinkles and a stooped, shuffling gait. This century, however, society has tended increasingly to describe anyone who reaches a pre-selected, arbitrary age as old. The Contributory Pension Act of 1925 was the first attempt in the United Kingdom to establish a retirement pension for most manual workers, based on compulsory contributions made during working life. The chosen retirement age (60 for women and 65 for men) was the result of political, economic and trade union pressures, rather than any biological considerations or the longer life expectancy of women.

An old person might be more appropriately defined as someone in the last 10 years of their life expectancy (i.e. over 70 for men and 75 for women in the United Kingdom). Certainly, the use of health and social services by persons over the age of 75 is very much greater than it is by those between the age of 60 and 75.

Attitudes to the elderly

In Western societies, the elderly do not enjoy a specially favoured position. In part, this reflects a cultural emphasis on the development of new technology rather than the preservation of traditional skills and knowledge. In addition, as a society becomes wealthier and more able to provide institutional care for its elders, the younger are relieved of some of their responsibilities for them and may feel freer to express their own fears of dying in the form of denigratory attitudes towards the elderly.

At the individual level, there is no evidence of any waning of affection or concern for elderly relatives and friends. While it is true that institutionalisation rates for the very old have increased considerably in the last 30 years, this can be explained by the steady decline in the amount of family support available to the elderly. The probability of an elderly person needing to go into residential care is inversely related to the number of his surviving children. With the fall in family size, the number of children available to care for their parents has declined by about 20% since 1948. Families do still care for their elderly relatives and, indeed, provide far more support than is available from health or social services. The belief that families no longer look after their elderly members is simply not true.

It is wrong to regard all old persons as in a state of poor mental and physical health and supported largely by hospitals and residential homes. On the contrary, the great majority of the elderly live in their own homes, and most rate their health as good or fair. It is also often thought that the elderly tend to be bad tempered and feel sorry for themselves, but there is, in fact, little or no sign of a significant decline in happiness or life satisfaction with age.

Retirement

Compulsory retirement means the loss not only of a job but also of a routine, and of comradeship, status and income. In general, retirement is most successful if some thought is given to it in advance. A new routine needs to be worked out, budgets redrawn and part-time work considered. The retiring worker should also sometimes be discouraged from moving to his dream cottage by the sea, because the problems associated with the loss of friends and neighbours, isolation, lack of transport and overstretched health and social services may outweigh the bracing effect of sea breezes.

It is vital to stay physically active, and any sport or pastime that the person enjoys should be encouraged. Those tolerating only the briefest forays from their armchair should be advised to do whatever exercise is necessary to raise their pulse rate to 120 beats per minute for two minutes each day, and to put every joint through a full range of movement. Keeping up morale after retirement is very dependent on mental activity and on finding a new role both within the family and within the larger social circle of friends and acquaintances.

Factors influencing longevity

Claims of large numbers of super-centenarians living in certain geographical regions – such as Vilcabamba in Ecuador, Hunza in Pakistan and Abkhasia in the USSR – have been shown to be exaggerated. The number of people

---

Summary 1 Epidemiology of ageing

- In the UK, the increase in life expectancy at birth this century is largely due to a decrease in infant mortality

- In the UK in 1971, 16.3% of the population were above retirement age

- In the UK by 1991, there will have been a 33% increase in the proportion of elderly between 75 and 84 years of age, and a 46% increase in those aged 85 or over

- In developing countries, the increase in the population over 60 years of age is estimated at over 80%.

Ageing and Disease

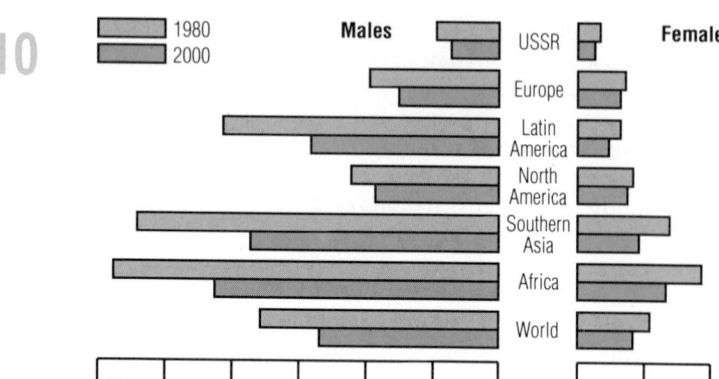

Fig. 10.4 **Percentage of the population aged 65 years and over that is economically active worldwide.** The developed countries have still to find a satisfactory role for their unemployed elderly.

claiming, or claimed to be, centenarians in any one society tends to be inversely proportional to the literacy rate. However, it is true that the inhabitants of each of the above areas are relatively long-lived, and in each case the esteem and merit enjoyed by a person increases with age. There is no retirement age and old persons continue to play an active role in the economic and social life of their communities (Fig. 10.4). The psychological benefit of this should not be underestimated, and industrialised countries must find ways of encouraging the psychological attitudes that lead to a vigorous and happy old age.

SPECIAL FEATURES OF DISEASE IN OLD AGE

Measurement of various physiological functions in healthy young adults give fairly uniform results, with a narrow range between the upper and lower limits of normal. From

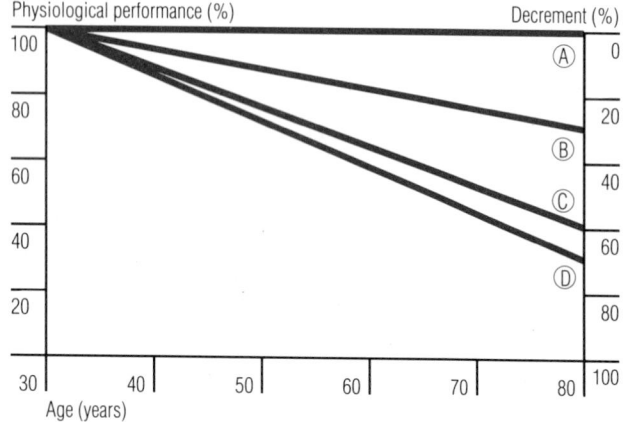

Fig. 10.5 **Age decrements in physiological functions in males. A.** Fasting blood glucose; **B.** Resting cardiac index; **C.** Maximum breathing capacity; **D.** Maximum work rate.

about 30 years of age, a functional decline in performance can be detected in most organs and body systems (Fig. 10.5). However, the organs and systems age differentially so that the variation both within, and between, individuals increases with age. The chronological age of an old person may therefore bear little relation to his functional age (Fig. 10.6), and the response of an old person to the stress of illness – which depends on functional reserve – will be more unpredictable than that of a young adult.

Degenerative changes occur throughout the body with increasing age, but these may become sufficiently marked to constitute a pathological process. The distinction between this and normal physiological ageing is often difficult to make and may at times be merely academic. At other times, however, it can have an important bearing on the management of the patient, as will be seen in the examples that follow.

Most of the data on degenerative changes with age are based on cross-sectional studies, where individuals of different ages are compared. These studies give only a partial indication of what happens to an individual throughout his lifetime. Longitudinal studies usually show a less rapid age-related decline in performance than cross-sectional studies.

The ageing eye

The force required to focus the eye increases considerably at about 40 years of age and, by 45 or 50, accommodation will be so poor that for most persons small print can be read only at arm's length (*presbyopia*). This is a result of both a reduction in elasticity of the lens capsule, and also a thickening of the lens which prevents it adapting its shape to focus near objects. Whether the change is regarded as pathological or physiological is unimportant, since the defect can be readily corrected with spectacles.

The ageing ear

Impaired hearing increases with age and can contribute to poor health, social isolation, depression and (probably) paranoid psychosis. About 30% of the elderly regard themselves as having a hearing impairment but audiometric testing reveals a much higher prevalence (60%) in those aged over 70. *Presbyacusis* is age-related loss of high frequency hearing, but this cannot be reliably distinguished from the effect of ototoxic drugs, diuretics or vascular disorders. It is also likely that some of the hearing loss usually regarded as an inevitable part of old age is due to our noisy environment or hypertension. It is as well to check that the patient does not have wax in his ears before referring him for fitting of a hearing aid.

Osteoporosis

Bone loss from the skeleton begins around 35 years of age and can, when sufficiently advanced, be detected on X-ray by a loss of density of the bone and thinning of the cortex

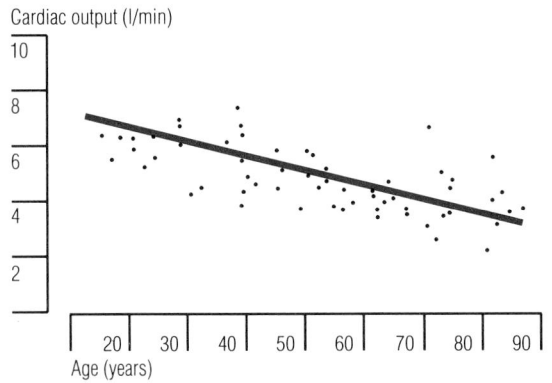

Fig. 10.6   The relation between resting cardiac output and age in men without circulatory disorders. Note that several men over the age of 70 have values similar to men in their 30s.

characteristic pathological findings – neurofibrillary tangles, senile plaques and lipofuscin pigment in the brain – also occur, albeit to a much less extent, in very old persons, it is still unclear whether SDAT is a distinct entity or a mere exaggeration of normal ageing. The early stages of dementia in a patient with SDAT are, however, often difficult to distinguish from the simple forgetfulness of old age.

Impairment of biochemical homeostasis

Most normal old persons can, under resting conditions, maintain their internal environment at levels similar to those in the young. When stressed, however, it is apparent that homeostatic mechanisms in the elderly are impaired. The control of blood glucose, and osmoregulation are two good examples of this.

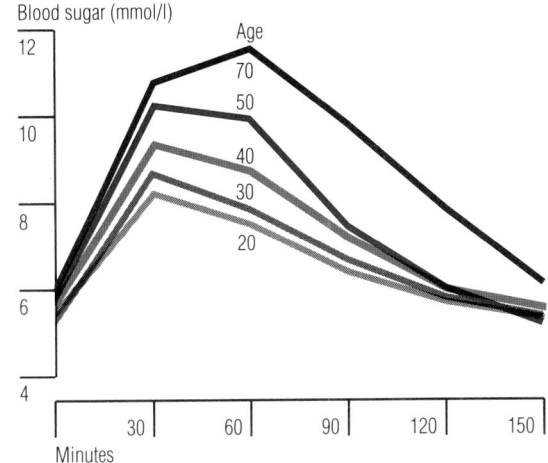

Fig. 10.7   Mean blood sugar levels after a 50 g oral glucose load in a cross-sectional population study. Known diabetics have been excluded.

of the long bones. For the majority of elderly persons, this age-related osteoporosis is asymptomatic, but a minority suffer 'accelerated' osteoporosis and will develop fractures. The causes of this pathological osteoporosis are not well understood but it appears to be related to a number of factors, particularly the skeletal status at maturity, the rapid bone loss occurring after the menopause, hyper-adrenocorticism and immobility. Oestrogen supplements provide partial protection against postmenopausal bone loss; however, because only 25% of women will have suffered one of the common osteoporotic fractures (distal forearm, vertebral compression or femoral neck) by the age of eighty, it is difficult to decide whether or not to treat all women with oestrogens, given the inability to detect at, say, 50 years of age, who will later go on to develop accelerated osteoporosis.

Dementia and normal ageing

Cross-sectional studies have demonstrated a decline in intellectual function with increasing age, as measured by certain tests such as Raven's progressive matrices. However, other tests (e.g. the number of digits that can be remembered and repeated backwards) show no age effect. There is suggestive evidence that individuals who have had better than average intellectual performance throughout life deteriorate more slowly than those with below average performance which, if true, would imply that maintenance of mental activity protects against age related intellectual loss. Thus, the physiological decline in intellectual performance with age may be very small and, where it does occur, we should be looking for pathological processes such as hypertension. Untreated hypertensives do less well in intelligence tests than those free of disease or whose hypertension is medically controlled. There is also a correlation between reduced cerebral oxygenation (as may occur in cardiac failure, for example) and impaired mental performance.

The major cause of intellectual loss in old age is senile dementia of the Alzheimer's type (SDAT). Although its

The control of blood glucose

The average fasting blood glucose level increases only slightly with advancing age. When a glucose load is imposed, however, the rise in maximum blood glucose levels is clearly greater, and the return to resting levels slower, in old persons (Fig. 10.7). The upward drift of blood glucose with age produces diagnostic difficulties since, if criteria used to diagnose diabetes in young populations were applied to the elderly, there would be a considerable increase in the number of those diagnosed as diabetic from the glucose tolerance test. Thus, elderly patients with an impaired glucose tolerance test (i.e. a 2 hour post glucose load of 7–11 mmol/l) should probably not be regarded as diabetic if they are asymptomatic, but they do carry a higher risk of developing frank diabetes.

Osmoregulation

On average, young adults maintain their blood osmolality in the range, 280–295 mmol/kg. Although resting plasma osmolality is unchanged in the elderly, the osmoregulatory response to 24 hour water deprivation is impaired, even in good health. Old subjects develop higher plasma osmolality and sodium concentrations in response to dehydration, and their maximum urine osmolality is lower. Importantly, the elderly also tend to be less thirsty despite higher plasma sodium and osmolality. Particular care is needed in correction of established hypernatraemia with hypotonic fluids in the elderly, because of the risk of cerebral oedema.

Summary 2 Normal vs pathological decrements in physiological performance in old age	
Normal age-related functional decline	*Pathological process*
Impaired sight (presbyopia)	Pathological in extreme cases
Impaired hearing (presbyacusis)	Effects of ototoxic drugs, diuretics or vascular disorders, hypertension
Bone loss	'Accelerated' osteoporosis
Decline in intellectual function	Reduced cerebral oxygenation (e.g. in cardiac failure); SDAT
Impaired glucose tolerance	Diabetes
Impaired balance (increased sway), shorter steps, slower gait	e.g. Parkinson's, Alzheimer's or cerebrovascular disease; dementia; vestibular lesions; cervical spondylosis, visual problems.
Altered sleep pattern	Insomnia due to nocturia (e.g. due to detrusor instability); pain; depression, etc.

AGEING AND THERMOREGULATION

Under normal circumstances, the organs in the body core are kept at a temperature of about 37°C with, under normal comfortable conditions, a skin temperature of 33°C, giving a core/skin temperature gradient of 4°C. The deep body temperature usually remains fairly constant despite wide variation in environmental temperatures, but thermoregulatory responses are impaired in old age due to disordered autonomic function. This usually passes unnoticed; but in times of environmental stress, the old person is less able to maintain a constant deep body temperature. Surveys made during the winter of old persons living at home show that only 0.5% had frank hypothermia (deep body temperature less than 35°C) but 10% had a deep body temperature below 35.5°C. The latter individuals had impaired thermoregulation – as shown by a core/skin temperature gradient only half that of normal individuals – and could therefore be considered 'at risk' (as should anyone with a previous history of hypothermia).

The elderly may also suffer impairment of thermal perception. Young persons can detect temperature differences as small as 0.8°C, but old persons only perceive much greater differences of 2–5°C. Furthermore, the elderly either do not shiver or shiver less efficiently in response to cooling, with little more than half the metabolic heat production seen in young subjects.

Old people are thus not only less able to maintain their deep body temperature when subjected to cold stress, but may also be less aware of cold conditions and therefore fail to take the appropriate steps – putting on extra clothing or increasing heat within the home. This may explain why some old people can tolerate cold living conditions without discomfort. Indeed, a survey in the winter of 1972 (which was slightly warmer than average) showed that 75% of old persons had a living room temperature at or below 18.3°C (the Parker-Morris standard for council housing). Poverty is, of course, another reason for these low levels of heating.

About 80% of the variation in mortality rates throughout the year is associated with changes in temperature (Fig. 10.8). For every degree change in the average winter temperature, the number of annual winter deaths rises or falls by about 8000. Thus, in the mild winter of 1983/4, about 30000 more elderly people died than during the summer months (a 14% increase). Whereas in the cold winter of 1984/5, this figure rose to 46000 (an increase of 20%). The consequence of impaired thermoregulation which attracts most attention in the UK is hypothermia. However, the majority of these 'excess' deaths are due not to hypothermia, but to coronary and cerebral thrombosis resulting from haemoconcentration and hypertension after cold exposure.

The elderly are also less able to cope with excessive heat, and the mortality rate during heat waves rises with increasing age. Heat illness is only rarely recognised as a

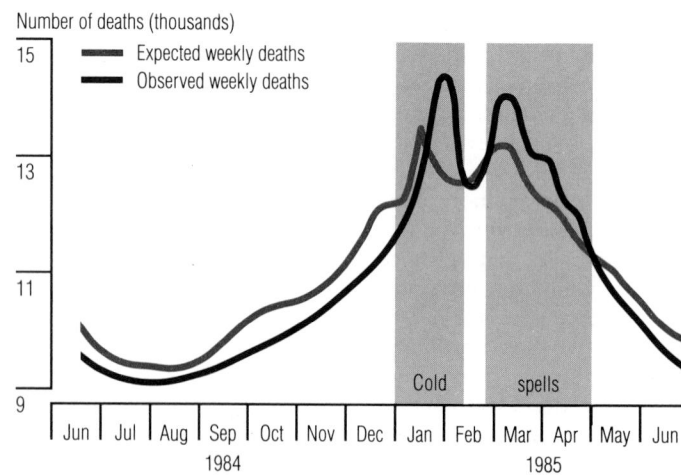

Fig. 10.8 Observed and expected deaths in the UK during the cold winter of 1984/5. Note the rise in death rate during the winter months and the excess deaths during the two exceptionally cold periods in early 1985.

contributory factor, however, and the cause of death is usually recorded as cerebrovascular or ischaemic heart disease.

Hypothermia

Hypothermia is a common problem in the elderly; the diagnosis and treatment of this condition are discussed in Chapter 5.

Autonomic dysfunction and disease

Impaired thermoregulation is only one consequence of autonomic dysfunction. Other important clinical consequences which occur include postural hypotension, bowel and bladder disturbances and impotence.

Diabetes mellitus is the commonest cause of an autonomic neuropathy in the elderly. However, there are also central causes of autonomic dysfunction such as Parkinson's disease, damage to the hypothalamus (commonly due to cerebrovascular disease), the Shy-Drager syndrome and Wernicke's encephalopathy (due to thiamine deficiency associated with alcoholism). Autonomic dysfunction may also be caused by drugs such as phenothiazines, tricyclic antidepressants and haloperidol.

NUTRITION AND AGEING

Even mild obesity may be harmful for certain individuals (e.g. those with hypertension or diabetes), but modern population studies do not support the view that obesity is necessarily bad for everyone. Mortality is generally lowest when the weight is slightly above the ideal weight (see Fig. 10.9).

Nutritional surveys have shown a marked decrease in energy requirements and intakes of nutrients with increasing age (see Table 10.2). However, this is mainly due to physical illness and reduced physical activity which reduce appetite and energy expenditure. With increasing age there

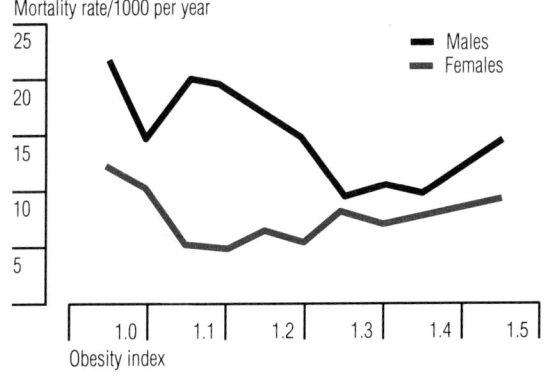

Fig. 10.9 Relation of obesity to mortality found in the Framingham study. The obesity index is the ratio of the subject's weight to a reference weight obtained from height and frame charts compiled by large insurance studies. Note that the lowest mortality occurs at an obesity index rather above 1.0.

Table 10.2 Fall in intake of nutrients in women in their late seventies compared with those in their early seventies (cross-sectional study)

Calories and nutrients	Fall in intake (%)
Calories	19
Protein	24
Fat	30
Carbohydrate	8
Calcium	18
Iron	29
Vitamin C	31

is a gradual decline in metabolism at rest but this is relatively unimportant. For healthy, active persons over 60 years of age, the energy and nutrient requirements are similar to those of a 30-year-old; and longitudinal studies have shown that nutrient intakes are maintained in old people who remain in good health. Housebound elderly women consume 15% less carbohydrate and 46% less vitamin C than active age-matched controls.

Nutritional deficiencies

A survey of old people living at home found that 3% were suffering from malnutrition, including protein-calorie malnutrition, iron deficiency and specific vitamin deficiencies. In most cases, this was the result of some underlying medical problem and was only rarely due primarily to economic or social factors (see Table 10.3). Social factors are, however, likely to be important in cases of subclinical malnutrition. For example, 31% of those living alone had leucocyte ascorbic acid levels below $7.0 \,\mu g/10^8$ wbc; compared with 8% of those living with a spouse. Scurvy remains rare even amongst the most isolated patients.

Megaloblastic anaemia due to a folate-poor diet is rare in old people in the UK. However, low serum folate levels are found in about 8% of elderly hospital patients and are often found in patients with physical disability and dementia.

Osteomalacia may contribute significantly to the skeletal rarefaction seen in old age (although this is more commonly due to osteoporosis). Twenty to forty per cent of elderly patients with proximal femur fractures have histologically proven osteomalacia. There are many causes of this condition, but two of the most important are reduced vitamin D intake and low exposure to sunlight – two factors often present together in the elderly. Housebound old people

Table 10.3 Primary and secondary causes of malnutrition in the elderly

Primary	Secondary
Ignorance	Impaired appetite
Social isolation	Inefficient mastication
Physical disability	Intestinal malabsorption
Mental disorder	Alcoholism
Iatrogenic	Drugs
Poverty	Increased requirements

with poor exposure to sunlight are four times more likely to have a dietary intake of vitamin D less than the recommended level (30 iu/day) than ambulatory women of the same age.

Although nutrient intakes and their serum levels in the elderly are often lower than in younger people there is no correlation between nutrient intakes and mortality in the old. Nutrition thus appears to have little effect on longevity once a person has reached the age of 65.

BALANCE AND FALLS

Normal balance is maintained by keeping the body's centre of gravity within its supporting base. In a normal standing position, the centre of gravity – which lies on average a few centimetres in front of the transverse axis of the ankles – tends to pull the body forwards. This is corrected by active contraction of the calf muscles, so that even during quiet standing the body sways slightly in the anterior-posterior plane. Major displacing forces which cause the centre of gravity to fall outside the support base, are corrected by stepping and hopping reactions or sweeping movements of the arms.

Threats to balance are detected by vision, by proprioceptors in the neck and lower limbs and by vestibular sensors. Coordinated muscular activity is then initiated to move neck, trunk and limbs so that balance is restored. Disease in any part of this system will impair balance, but single lesions are rarely completely disabling because of good overall reserve.

Changes in balance in old age

With increasing age the first change in balance detected in normal persons is increased sway. Sway is measured in the anterio-posterior plane with the person standing still; and is a way of quantifying the Romberg test (see Fig. 10.10). There is also a change in gait with age (Fig. 10.11). Normal, active older people have a shorter step length as compared to the young; the step length is also more variable and they walk more slowly. Elderly persons who have had falls have significantly impaired sway and gait when compared with age-matched controls.

FALLS

The pathological changes underlying the alterations in sway and gait found in normal older people are similar to, but of a lesser degree than, those in patients who fall. Motor nerve conduction time declines with increasing age but, in general, the consequent impairment of the efferent limb of the balance control system is not particularly important. Of much greater relevance is an organic disease such as Parkinson's disease, cerebrovascular disease or Alzheimer's disease. It is not uncommon to find a specific neurological defect such as a mild hemiparesis or Parkinson's disease in patients with repeated falls. Demented

elderly persons are more likely to fall than non-demented and, though mobility appears unimpaired, demented patients also sway more, have a shorter and more variable step length, and slower walking speeds.

Effective balance control depends on both unimpaired sensory input and a stable support base. When the eyes are closed there is generally a slight increase in postural sway, and it appears that peripheral vision in particular is necessary for normal balance. Wearing an artificial limb following an above-knee amputation only affects postural sway when the subject's eyes are closed, indicating that the instability of the base and loss of proprioception is compensated for by increased dependence on vision. Similarly, patients with chronic bilateral impairment of vestibular function walk perfectly normally when their eyes are open. They are unsteady, but can still walk satisfactorily when blindfolded unless they are also on uneven ground (i.e. supporting base unstable), in which

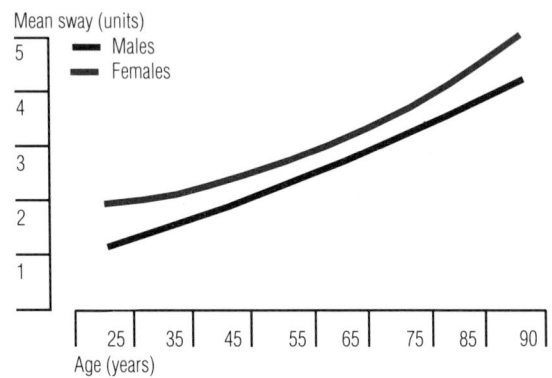

Fig. 10.10 Postural sway (measured as movement in the anterior/posterior plane with the subject standing) increases with age. At all ages, women sway significantly more than men. 1 unit = $3\frac{1}{3}°$ of angular movement.

Ⓐ Young control

Ⓑ Active elderly

Ⓒ Hospitalised elderly faller

	Ⓐ	Ⓑ	Ⓒ
Mean step length	65 cm	46 cm	22 cm
Step width	12 cm	14 cm	14 cm
Frequency (steps/min)	112±10	94±14	95±40
Variability of step length	5%	9%	28%

Fig. 10.11 Changes in gait with age. A step where the heel of the leading foot comes to just beyond the mid point of the trailing foot is about 30 cm. The hospitalised faller walks with a slow, short paced gain: the step length is very variable. This indicates considerable instability and poor confidence.

case they fall over. An important contribution to postural control is provided by the activity of mechanoreceptors in the apophyseal joints of the cervical spine. These exert a reflex influence on the activity of neck and limb muscles, and damage to this mechanism – typically from cervical spondylosis – can cause a feeling of unsteadiness during movements, often worse on turning the head.

In man, the vestibular system plays little part in static posture or in the righting reactions. It is, however, important if the supporting base is uneven (e.g. when walking on a cobbled street) or if the body is unstable.

Balance is usually only seriously impaired if more than one of these sensory systems is affected. Cervical spondylosis, for example, affects nearly everyone over 70 years of age, and probably only becomes important if there are also visual problems or vestibular defects (e.g. Menière's disease). Patients with spontaneous falls (see below) nearly always have multiple defects and their identification allows a rational treatment programme to be planned.

Examination of the patient

The first step in examination of the patient with falls is a good history, since that will allow differentiation between a straightforward trip or accident and a spontaneous fall (Table 10.4). Patients with trips or accidents are generally younger and more active, and their balance and gait no worse than non-fallers of the same age. Their prognosis is good, and no specific measures need to be taken other than advice about maintaining activity and improving home safety.

Patients who suffer spontaneous falls are quite different. They often have difficulty in describing why they fell, and may try to rationalize the fall by saying 'I must have tripped'. Comments such as 'All of a sudden I fell' or 'I came over queer and down I went' are common. Some may say that they felt dizzy (particularly if prompted by the doctor). However, only very rarely does the patient experience true vertigo (a sensation of the patient's surroundings or the inside of his head spinning around). They do not so much feel dizzy, as an unsteadiness when standing or walking, and are frightened that they are going to fall over

Table 10.4 Possible causes of spontaneous falling

Patient generally impaired in one or more of the systems concerned with balance control:
  Vision e.g. poor illumination
  Cervical mechanoreceptor dysfunction e.g. cervical spondylosis
  Vestibular lesions e.g. Meniere's disease
  Impaired central coordination e.g. cerebrovascular disease
  Unstable support base e.g. walking down stairs

Falls may be precipitated by:
  Occult illness e.g. chest infection
  Drugs e.g. hypnotics, anti-Parkinsonians, anti-hypertensives
  Cardiac arrhythmia
  Postural hypotension
  Hypoglycaemia
  Epilepsy

(see Ch. 23, p. 881). Some of these patients suffer drop attacks. These are falls which occur without warning; the patient suddenly crumples to the ground and there are no neurological sequelae. Like other spontaneous falls, their aetiology is multifactorial; but regardless of their precise nature, patients with spontaneous falls tend to have certain characteristics in common. They are usually older and more frail, their gait and balance noticeably impaired, and their general health poor. They are also more likely to be taking drugs such as sedatives and diuretics, and to have incontinence of urine or mental impairment. Their mortality is about five times that of non-fallers.

Points to note in the history are:

1. Whether the patient felt unsteady and fell after turning his head (which suggests cervical spondylosis or vestibular disease).
2. If the fall occurred soon after standing up (raising the possibility of postural hypotension).
3. If there have been repeated falls with loss of consciousness (suggesting that an arrhythmia may be causing cardiac syncope).
4. The patient's drugs will need to be checked. Sedatives or hypnotics frequently slow the patient down and may precipitate a fall. Hypotensive drugs may cause postural hypotension, with the patient complaining of feeling faint when he gets out of bed or stands up from a chair. Drugs used for the treatment of hypertension and anti-Parkinsonian drugs are most commonly involved.
5. Mental state should be assessed if there is a suspicion of dementia or depression.
6. A history of tinnitus, deafness or vertigo should be sought. Tinnitus and deafness indicate a vestibular lesion and suggest a labyrinthine disorder (e.g. Meniere's disease), especially if unilateral or of recent onset.

In the general examination:

1. The lying and standing blood pressure should be measured (a drop in systolic pressure of more than 2.66 kPa (20 mmHg) indicates postural hypotension).
2. The range of neck movements should be assessed.
3. The patient should be observed standing and walking.
4. Normal old persons should not have a positive Romberg test (i.e. closing the eyes when standing should not markedly impair balance).
5. Patients with spontaneous falls will often be unsteady even with eyes open; and their righting reflex may be so poor that they fall following a very light tap with the examiner's finger on their sternum.
6. Such patients walk with short steps (sometimes these are very short, a gait known as a *marche à petits pas*).
7. In severe cases, there will be manifest anxiety and fear of falling, with the patient reluctant to move without clutching onto furniture or onlookers for support.

In addition to routine investigations:

8. A 24-hour ambulatory ECG should be ordered for patients suspected of having Stokes-Adams attacks

(although without a reliable witness at the time of the fall, this is a difficult diagnosis to make). Palpitations before the fall or loss of consciousness are important pointers, but a useful clue is that, despite repeated falls, the patient's gait, balance and confidence are normal.

9. An EEG will be needed for patients suspected of having epilepsy (see Ch. 23, p. 859).

10. The occurrence of early morning falls in patients taking a long acting hypoglycaemic drug (e.g. chlorpropamide) raises the possibility of hypoglycaemia, and blood glucose estimations will need to be checked.

11. Patients suspected of having a vestibular lesion can have this accurately localized only by specialist examinations, which include electronystagmography and caloric tests.

12. The patient's vision, both with and without his usual spectacles, should be noted.

Summary 3 Typical features in patients with spontaneous falls

- Older, frailer and in poorer health than patients with trips or accidents

- Significantly impaired gait and balance (normal in Stokes-Adams patients)

- Difficulty in accounting for how they fell

- Positive Romberg's test; often very unsteady even with eyes open

- Short steps, *marche à petits pas*

- Generally have multiple defects in the sensory systems concerned with balance control – vision, proprioreceptors and the vestibular system

---

Management

Many patients with spontaneous falls have multiple defects and their balance is precarious. Movements such as rising from a chair (even when there is no postural hypotension) or turning suddenly when standing, may place too great a demand on an impaired balance system. Going downstairs in the dark (which involves the additional stress of loss of vision and an unstable base) is also likely to be hazardous. Sometimes a minor illness such as a chest infection, or a newly prescribed sedative drug can simply prove too much for a frail patient. Identification of precipitating factors enables the patient to be appropriately advised. Cervical spondylosis should be treated with neck exercises, not a cervical collar which often makes the patient feel more unsteady. Faulty spectacles should be replaced and everything possible done to improve the patient's vision, including better illumination in the home. Peripheral vestibular lesions may be improved with cinnarizine (15 mg tds) or betahistine (8 mg tds), but these drugs may have troublesome sedative effects. Central vestibular lesions are rarely helped by drugs and the latter therefore should be avoided if this diagnosis is definitely made. Phenothiazines should not be prescribed for vague complaints of dizziness, because of the risk of drug induced Parkinsonism.

The patient's chair should be at the right height (the seat level with the top of his knee) so that getting out of it is not difficult. A walking frame may initially help both mobility and confidence, but should be removed once the patient's walking is better. Balance exercises and measures to improve confidence and well-being are often very helpful. If the falls have been such as to warrant hospital admission, then follow-up for a few weeks in a day hospital is helpful. In case of another fall, the patient should be taught how to get up off the floor, and advised of the various alarm systems he can have installed in his home. An occupational therapist should also visit the home and correct obvious hazards, such as unguarded fires or a broken light bulb over the stairs.

SLEEP AND INSOMNIA

Insomnia is a common complaint in the elderly and there is great pressure on doctors to prescribe hypnotics. The elderly receive more hypnotics than any other age group.

It is often assumed that hypnotics are both harmless and effective, but for the elderly neither assumption is true. Elderly patients taking hypnotics regularly, rate the quality of their sleep as worse than those not on hypnotics; and more than one in ten persons aged 70 or over taking nitrazepam (10 mg) at night, have troublesome daytime sedation. Any patient complaining of insomnia – but particularly an elderly one – needs careful assessment and not just the unthinking prescription of a hypnotic.

Normal sleep

When a person falls asleep he 'descends' rapidly through progressively deeper stages of sleep. Stages three and four are known as *slow wave sleep* because of the characteristic EEG pattern. After about 90 minutes there is the first episode of rapid eye movement (REM) sleep – a time of physiological arousal when dreaming takes place. These REM periods occur at regular intervals and occupy about 20–25% of the night. The pattern of REM sleep remains the same throughout adult life (although it may be reduced in the very old). However, slow wave sleep – instead of occupying about 20% of the night as it does in the young – is reduced to only 5% by 70 years of age, and stage four is almost completely absent.

The elderly wake more frequently and take longer to fall asleep so that, even for the normal old person, sleep becomes increasingly fragmented. Thus, the doctor needs to decide whether the patient's complaint of insomnia is simply – given his age – an unrealistic expectation of what constitutes a good night's sleep. Less physical activity and daytime cat naps will further reduce the ability to sleep well at night.

Causes of insomnia

Insomnia may be age related as discussed above. Nocturia is another common reason for an old person waking up, a

Summary 4   Causes of insomnia

- Age-related changes in sleep pattern
- Nocturia (probably due to detrusor instability)
- Pain
- Anxiety and depression
- Drug induced e.g. alcohol, withdrawal from hypnotics
- Specific problems e.g. sleep apnoea, myoclonus

condition which may be caused by prostatism, renal failure or diabetes but is most likely due to detrusor instability (especially if associated with some urgency). Pain is also an important cause of insomnia, and the akinetic Parkinsonian patient who cannot turn over in bed will find that his sleep is disturbed.

Specific problems such as sleep apnoea, myoclonus and the restless leg syndrome are rare and will usually only be discovered by questioning the bed partner. Anxiety and depression commonly cause sleep disturbances, and are best managed by psychiatric treatment directed at the primary condition.

Insomnia may be drug induced. The most familiar example is alcohol which, if taken in the evening, will quickly induce sleep but results in rebound insomnia with awakening later the same night because of its rapid metabolism. A similar effect can be seen after hypnotics are withdrawn, when the patient complains of anxiety, tension and insomnia. These are essentially withdrawal symptoms and may be related to alterations in REM sleep. In the case of nitrazepam, the symptoms may continue for four or five weeks after treatment is stopped, and are lessened if the hypnotic is gradually tailed off. The patient should be warned of what might happen. If these withdrawal effects are not understood by the doctor then a hypnotic may be needlessly represcribed.

Choosing a hypnotic

Hypnotics should only be used where it is clear that insomnia is impairing the patient's daytime performance. There should be a clear indication, such as a recent bereavement or impending major surgery, and the prescription should be limited to seven or ten days wherever possible.

The drug should have a rapid onset of action, particularly if the patient's main complaint is difficulty in falling asleep. There should be no daytime sedation, although this may occur due to accumulation of long acting hypnotics and their active metabolites, or because of an age-related alteration in sensitivity to the drug.

Benzodiazepines

Diazepam has a half-life in hours approximately equivalent to the person's age, but the constant clearance rate means that the average steady state plasma level of diazepam is unaffected by ageing. However, the half-life of its major active metabolite, desmethyldiazepam, is prolonged due to reduced plasma clearance (Fig. 10.12). The dose necessary

to produce sedation is therefore inversely correlated with age, due partly to an increased sensitivity to the drug in old age and also to accumulation of the active metabolite. Diazepam (2 mg or 5 mg) may be a suitable hypnotic for anxious old people where daytime anxiolitic effect is required. Daytime drowsiness, confusion and falls, however, may be a problem.

Nitrazepam also produces more sedation in the elderly, probably as a result of increased receptor sensitivity (since the pharmacokinetics remain unaltered). The unwanted daytime sedation is largely dose dependent (Fig. 10.13); 2.5 mg is the maximum dose that should be given to an old person.

Temazepam has a half-life of only 5–10 hours in young

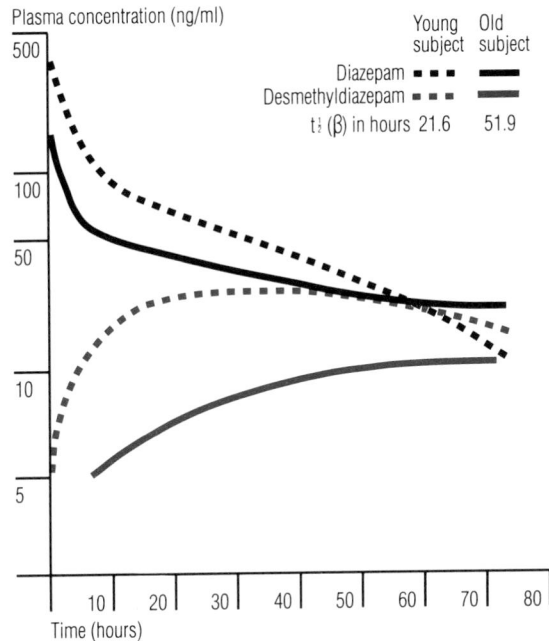

Fig. 10.12 Comparison of plasma concentration/time profiles of diazepam and desmethyldiazepam after intravenous diazepam in a young and an old subject. Significant accumulation will occur on daily dosing with a drug whose half-life exceeds 16 hours.

Fig. 10.13 Relationship of daily dose (5.0–9.9 mg/day and 10.0 or more mg/day) to the frequency of unwanted CNS depression attributed to nitrazepam, with the population stratified according to age.

10

persons but may be as long as 30 hours in the elderly. Accumulation therefore occurs and, after a week of continuous dosing at 20 mg each night, subjects show a significant slowing of reaction times. The effect is likely to be dose related; 10 mg at night rarely causes serious problems.

Lormetazepam has a good pharmacokinetic profile for use in the elderly. Although the elimination half-life of 10 hours (in the young) is prolonged to about 14 hours in elderly subjects, accumulation does not occur and there is no impairment of daytime performance with a nightly dose of either 0.5 mg or 1.0 mg.

Triazolam (a very short acting hypnotic) has a half-life in young persons of 2–3 hours, but its pharmacokinetics have not been adequately studied in the elderly. The half-life is so short that rebound insomnia can occur in the early morning after a bedtime dose; chronic use increases anxiety.

Other hypnotics

Chloral hydrate is usually dispensed as a syrup with an unpleasant taste. The usual dose in the elderly is 1 g and, apart from a gastric irritant effect, it is largely free from side effects although it does potentiate the effect of warfarin. It is particularly useful for treating confused patients, many of whom are made worse by benzodiazepines.

Chlormethiazole is a valuable hypnotic for use in the elderly. Its pharmacokinetics are virtually unaltered by age and its short plasma half-life of 3–4 hours means that accumulation does not occur. It is extensively metabolized by the liver, and should therefore be used with caution in patients with cirrhosis of the liver or in chronic alcoholics. One capsule (192 mg of chlormethiazole base) may be sufficient but two capsules is still a safe dose.

Restless and confused patients are often best sedated by a *phenothiazine* such as thioridazine (25–75 mg nocte) or haloperidol (0.5–3 mg nocte). Both drugs carry a long term risk of extrapyramidal side effects.

SEXUAL FUNCTION

In Western society, sexuality amongst adolescents and young adults is studied and discussed openly. No such liberal attitude exists towards sex in old age and, unfortunately, the stereotype of the sexless old persists. Although sexual activity does decline with advancing age, much of this is due to ill health or the death of the marriage partner. Old age itself causes very little impairment of sexual enjoyment. Twenty per cent or more of men over 80 continue to have intercourse and to masturbate; and, while sexual activity rates among very old women are lower this is often attributable to lack of a partner or their partner's loss of libido. Overall, it would appear that continued sexual activity in old age depends on the frequency and enjoyment it afforded in middle age, the availability of a suitable partner and (particularly in men) continuing good health.

The main physical changes in women result from a lack of oestrogen, which may cause vaginitis with reduced lubrication and painful intercourse. Length of orgasm may be reduced but many postmenopausal women report increased desire and arousability. Male fertility is usually maintained into extreme old age although the volume of prostatic secretions reduces, it takes longer to achieve an erection, orgasm is briefer and the following refractory period is longer.

Many doctors are reluctant to discuss sexual practice with their elderly patients and thereby lose the opportunity for helpful counselling. Vaginitis due to oestrogen deficiency may come to light during the investigation of urinary incontinence and responds readily to dienoestrol cream. Complaints of impotence in the male should prompt a thorough physical examination, including a blood sugar estimation. Many drugs interfere with sexual function and the elderly should be warned about this when they are prescribed. Methyldopa can cause loss of libido and failure of ejaculation, and propranolol and thiazide diuretics may produce impotence. All of the phenothiazines may cause impotence, while thioridazine may also cause lack of ejaculation; haloperidol is free of these problems.

Sexuality – or the lack of it – in old age should not be seen in isolation. The need for affection, tenderness and caressing may be more important than intercourse, and counselling as to what is normal and appropriate may dispel fears of inadequacy or embarrassment. The elderly postcoronary patient (unlike his middle-aged counterpart) does not usually ask when he may resume sexual activity. But, together with advice on diet and exercise, it is often helpful to mention that intercourse can be resumed once the patient can climb a flight of stairs without distress.

ALTERED REACTIONS TO DISEASE

In the elderly, a disease such as bronchopneumonia often causes much less of a temperature rise than would be expected in a young adult. The clinical picture of infection or other diseases may instead be dominated by non-specific presentations, such as confusion, falls and urinary incontinence. Another common age-related change in reaction to disease is a reduced ability to feel pain in illness and trauma.

The usual pattern of disease in the elderly is of multiple disorders, several of which may go unreported.

Confusional states

A toxic confusional state is the ageing brain's response to a number of insults – the stress of a physical illness, a variety of powerful drugs and alterations in the old person's familiar environment. It tends to occur more commonly in persons whose mental state is already impaired (e.g. by senile dementia of the Alzheimer's type) or who has communication difficulties because of defective hearing and

Summary 5   Altered reaction to disease in old age

- Response of an older person to illness is more unpredictable due to differential ageing of organs and systems both within and between individuals.

- In the elderly, there may be less of a temperature rise in response to infection.

- Pain normally expected in illness or trauma may be minimal or absent.

- Disease tends to be manifested through non-specific symptoms e.g. a toxic confusional state, falls or incontinence.

- Tendency to multiple disorders, as reduced reserve renders organs and systems more susceptible to stress. Many may go unreported.

vision. However, confusion can also occur in perfectly normal old persons when they develop a major illness such as pneumonia or cardiac failure.

Falls

Old persons who suddenly start to fall frequently, often have an underlying physical illness as well as an age-related balance impairment (see p. 168). The central control of posture and balance may be affected by reduced cerebral oxygenation due to cerebrovascular disease or cardiac failure or as a result of diuretic induced hyponatraemia. Drug side-effects are another fairly frequent reason for old people starting to fall over; the culprit is frequently long-acting hypnotics or tranquillisers (see p. 171).

Urinary incontinence

A patient may become incontinent due to a confusional state which renders him unable to control bladder function normally, or because he is immobile as a result of physical illness. Thus, an old man living alone may develop broncho-pneumonia and take to his bed, fall several times when in the lavatory because he is too weak to stand properly, give up further attempts and consequently become incontinent in bed. He presents as an immobile, incontinent and confused patient, with the underlying diagnosis not immediately apparent.

Absence of pain

For reasons not clearly understood, pain due to illness or trauma which would be expected in a younger individual, is often minimal or absent in the elderly. Thus, myocardial infarction is commonly pain free, and the patient presents instead with dyspnoea or non-specific illness. Similarly, abdominal pathology such as gastric ulcers or mesenteric thrombosis may be silent; however, acute appendicitis often has a fulminating course in older patients, with the rapid development of gangrene and peritonitis. Even a fracture of the neck of femur may cause the patient only slight discomfort, evidenced by a disinclination to walk.

Multiple pathological processes

The explanation of all symptoms, signs and abnormal investigations by one diagnosis is seldom possible in older patients. The reduced reserve in organs and bodily systems renders them more susceptible to the stress of disease in another part of the body, so that the usual pattern is one of multiple disorders. Thus, a momentary cardiac arrhythmia which may produce only a slight feeling of dizziness or palpitations in a young person may cause loss of consciousness or even a stroke with hemiplegia in an old patient. Similarly, a chest infection may precipitate heart failure because the cardiac reserve is already impaired by ischaemic heart disease. Common conditions such as obesity, osteoarthritis, diverticular disease, hypertension, diabetes, dementia and presbyacusis may all be present in a single individual, and the aim then is to decide which are causing important functional disability.

Unreported illness

Prevention is an important part of geriatric medicine, and the early identification of disease or disordered function allows treatment to be initiated or social support organised before things have gone too far. Studies in general practice show that an elderly person has, on average, at least three disabilities; and for every one known to the general practitioner there is another which is not. Typically, cardiac, chest and neurological disabilities are known to the GP, but incontinence, difficulty in walking, painful feet, dementia and depression often go unreported.

CLINICAL APPROACH

When assessing an elderly patient it is generally more useful to think in terms of functional ability than to lay emphasis on the underlying pathology. The pathological conditions producing ill health in the elderly are often irreversible, whereas some degree of functional improvement is nearly always possible – particularly if the patient is seen early enough. For example, the distinction between rheumatoid and osteoarthritis in a patient with arthritis of the knees may be largely academic. The fact that the patient has poor mobility, and can no longer get out of doors to shop or collect his pension is much more important; and the emphasis is placed on physiotherapy, walking exercises and possibly surgery to improve mobility and independence.

History

A full history remains the primary investigative tool. In a confused patient, it is necessary to get additional information from a relative or community nurse, or someone else who knows the patient well.

The tempo with which the symptoms have developed is particularly important. Forgetfulness which has been gradually increasing over two or three years suggests senile dementia of the Alzheimer's type; whereas a sudden onset of confusion over a day or two indicates a toxic confusional state, and requires a search for underlying physical problems such as an infection or myocardial infarct. A sudden onset of headaches or recent change in bowel habit is never normal in old age; whereas gradually failing hearing and vision may be, but might be remedied by a hearing aid or suitable spectacles.

The history must include: a full list of the patient's medication, including details of dose and frequency; details of the patient's functional ability (to do his own shopping, cooking, cleaning and attend to personal toilet); and social circumstances. The main carer at home should be identified, as well as additional support which might be provided by family, neighbours and social services.

Assessment

It is possible (though not good medicine) to overlook social and psychological problems in a young patient with an acute illness. However, the chances of successfully discharging an elderly, frail person, if his homelessness, anxiety and inadequate personality are ignored, are remote. Such a patient either cannot be discharged at all, or has to be re-admitted within a day or two of discharge, because of an inability to cope. Seeing the patient as a whole is thus not only good for the patient, it is essential if limited health service resources are to be used effectively. An overall view of the patient includes assessment of his medical, functional, social and psychological status, and usually brings together the professional views from several disciplines.

The doctor attends to the physical and mental diagnosis and appropriate treatments. The nurse notes to what extent the patient can wash and feed himself or use the lavatory, and also particular problems such as incontinence, pressure sores or nocturnal confusion. The physiotherapist is concerned with whether the patient can get in and out of bed, rise from a chair, balance and walk; and as the patient improves, the occupational therapist assesses how well the patient can dress, bathe, cook and care for himself. As soon as possible after admission, the social worker inquires into the patient's social background to find out what circumstances are like at home – whether the old person is already receiving support from relatives or neighbours, and whether this support will be continued or need to be increased once the patient returns home.

The aim is to ensure that patients are speedily and effectively treated and returned to their own home in a planned and thoughtful manner, so that the gains resulting from treatment are likely to be maintained. A similar process of assessment can be initiated by GPs using community staff, for patients living at home.

Physical examination

Because of the multiplicity of disorders often found in an elderly patient, it might appear that an extensive and detailed examination of every system is required. This can exhaust a frail patient, and a prolonged neurological examination is liable to frustrate and confuse the doctor. However, the examination can, with practice, be thorough, informative and quick if the doctor concentrates on identifying disabilities and assessing loss of function.

General appearance

The examination should begin with an observation of the patient's general appearance and clothes, noting any signs of self neglect. Facial pallor is frequently present and so is a poor indicator of anaemia. An arcus senilis due to the deposition of lipids at the periphery of the cornea is of no significance in the elderly. Pupil size is often small with reduced response, and upward gaze is often limited. Angular stomatitis – if not due to ill-fitting dentures – suggests multivitamin deficiency or iron deficiency anaemia; but a black hairy tongue or sublingual varicosities are of no significance.

Skin changes

Loose, dry, scaly skin is a common finding, as are senile purpura due to increased capillary fragility on the dorsum of the hands and extensor surface of the arms. Sun-exposed skin should be searched for basal cell carcinomas or actinic keratoses which are potentially malignant. The incidence of both conditions increases with years of exposure to the sun, and are common in the elderly.

Intertrigo – sore, inflamed patches of skin under the breasts or in the abdominal folds of obese patients – is often the result of poor personal hygiene. A keratinised transverse crease across the abdomen is the consequence of long-standing kyphosis, following osteoporotic spinal wedging.

Feet

The ankles and feet should be inspected for signs of oedema and the need for chiropody.

Cardiovascular

Abnormalities of cardiac rhythm are frequently present: occasional ectopic beats occur in about one-sixth of elderly

---

Summary 6 Assessment of an elderly patient

- Main stress is on functional disability, rather than underlying pathology

- Overall view essential:
  Medical status – manner of onset of symptoms is important. Full drug history required.
  Functional ability – washing, cooking, shopping, etc.
  Psychological status – depression, anxiety, confusion, etc.
  Social circumstances – support available at home from family and friends.

- Involves a multidisciplinary team of doctors, nurses, occupational and physiotherapists and social workers.

persons, but any other arrhythmia should be regarded as abnormal and investigated by electrocardiography. Systolic and diastolic blood pressure increases with age although there is little change over the age of 65. There is a wide range of blood pressures in healthy old persons without heart disease; and values up to 160/90 can be regarded as normal. Above this level, the risk of cardiovascular disease increases; but the value of treatment needs to be set against the risk of unwanted drug effects (see p. 169). Systolic murmurs – usually of the ejection type and present at the left sternal edge and aortic area – are found in up to 60% of the elderly. They are commonly associated with significant disease such as cardiac failure, ischaemic heart disease, arrhythmias and hypertension and should not therefore be regarded as necessarily benign.

Breast palpation

The breasts should be examined for lumps.

Bowels and bladder

A rectal examination is essential: carcinoma of the rectum or prostate is common in the elderly, and there may be loading of the rectum with faeces – a common cause of faecal incontinence. The presence of urinary incontinence should be noted and – particularly in bedridden patients – the pressure areas inspected for sores.

Eyesight and hearing

The patient should be asked whether his vision is satisfactory and, if not, should be tested with eye charts. Hearing is probably adequate if the patient can hear a normal conversational voice. Examination of the eardrums for wax should be a routine, particularly where a hearing aid is worn, since the earpiece may compress wax into a hard, impenetrable lump.

Neurological changes

Ankle jerks tend to be absent in about 10% of elderly patients although whether this is a true age-related change, or due to mild peripheral neuropathy, is uncertain. Superficial abdominal reflexes are also often absent, but the presence of extensor plantar responses is best regarded as pathological.

Vibration sense in the lower limbs is reduced, and may be absent at the ankles, in up to a half of patients over 75. However, joint position sense is usually normal. Appreciation of pain, temperature and light touch is very variable, but one or other of these sensations is impaired in about a quarter of the elderly. Both the glabellar tap, and primitive reflexes such as the pout reflex (tap the upper lip and the lips pout), grasp reflex and palmomental reflex (the palm is scratched and the chin wrinkles on the same side), can often be elicited in the elderly, particularly in those who have dementia. Hearing loss of old age (presbyacusis) is a sensory neural loss of high frequencies and affects perhaps 60% of persons over 70.

Gait and balance

Changes in posture and gait with old age follow an essentially extrapyramidal pattern. The stance of an old person is one of general flexion with increased muscle tone, poverty of movement and bradykinesis. These changes are also those seen in Parkinson's disease but, in normal old age, are of a much milder degree. That postural control is impaired is shown by the increased number of falls occurring in the elderly. Although more unsteady when standing than the young, normal elderly people should be able to maintain standing balance with feet together and eyes closed. A tendency to sway and fall when the eyes are closed and the feet approximated (Romberg's sign) is abnormal at any age. The typical gait changes found in the elderly are reduction in speed, shorter step length and greater step length variability.

INVESTIGATION IN THE ELDERLY

One of the more difficult aspects of caring for the elderly is knowing when and how far to investigate. Potentially remediable conditions cannot be ignored simply because the patient is elderly, but it is not good medicine to order invasive, uncomfortable and possibly expensive tests when the potential benefit to the patient is minimal. A middle way must be found, and the following points should be borne in mind.

Overall state of health

Age itself is only a minor consideration when assessing the patient: the overall state of health is much more important. Does the patient have the physical and mental capacity to benefit from a proposed treatment? If surgery is an option, would the patient be fit for operation? If the patient is debilitated and being looked after by his family at home, then the views of these relatives must be included when assessing the benefits and risks of investigation and treatment. For example, an active old person who is having repeated falls associated with transient loss of consciousness should have 24-hour ambulatory ECG monitoring to detect whether the falls are related to a cardiac arrhythmia. If they are, then a pacemaker can be safely inserted – even in the very elderly – with the potential for a considerable improvement in the quality of life.

Will the investigation influence management?

Before ordering an investigation it is necessary to consider whether the result is likely to usefully influence management. For example, a severely demented patient with an abdominal mass and positive faecal occult bloods could have the presumptive diagnosis of carcinoma of the colon confirmed by a barium enema. However, if surgery is not being considered (because of the patient's poor general condition and inability to cope with a colostomy), there is little point in the barium enema. On the other hand, if the same patient is found to be unable to walk following a fall, he should certainly have his hips X-rayed. Repair of a fractured neck of femur will not only relieve the patient's pain, it is also much easier to nurse an ambulant patient than one who is bedridden.

Will the diagnosis affect prognosis?

It is important to consider whether the investigation will establish a diagnosis which significantly affects prognosis. A very frail patient with severe dyspepsia can simply be treated with a full course of an H_2 antagonist. But if symptoms persist – and even if surgery is not being contemplated – it may be important for the patient and his relatives to know if the diagnosis is peptic ulceration or carcinoma of the stomach.

Routine screening

Most patients seen in clinic or admitted to hospital will have a full blood count, ESR (or viscosity), urea and electrolytes, glucose and free T4. Urine should be analysed for protein, glucose and blood. All of these tests can usefully detect treatable disease where the clinical diagnosis is unsuspected or doubtful. This is particularly true of thyroid disease, which is found on screening in about 4% of elderly in-patients. In the elderly the diagnosis can be difficult, because classical symptoms and signs of hypo- or hyperthyroidism may be absent or because the illness may masquerade as depression or confusion. Thyroid function tests can be considerably distorted by systemic illness or drugs: the best screening test is the free T4 with the TSH as a confirmatory test.

A routine chest X-ray is usually taken since about 5% of patients over 65 admitted to hospital are found to have an unexpected lesion on chest X-ray. It is particularly valuable in patients presenting with falls, immobility, incontinence or deteriorating mental function; nearly a quarter of these have cardiopulmonary disease without classical features. The X-ray may also disclose tuberculosis – commonly a disease of the elderly.

An electrocardiogram is not routine, but is required for patients with cardiopulmonary disease, strokes (quite commonly associated with a myocardial infarct) and falls (which might be caused by a cardiac arrhythmia).

Investigation of dementia

The main concern in the investigation of dementia is not to miss a cause for which there is specific treatment. Although rare among elderly patients referred to a geriatrician or general physician, such reversible dementias are relatively common amongst referrals to specialist neurological centres. Conditions which may respond to treatment include:

1. depression and other psychiatric disorders
2. normal pressure (communicating) hydrocephalus
3. resectable tumours
4. subdural haematoma
5. toxic drug effects
6. thyroid disease
7. pernicious anaemia
8. syphilis.

In addition to the routine blood tests, the patient should have the serum B_{12} level checked and a Venereal Disease Reference Laboratory (VDRL) test to exclude syphilis. Although it cannot positively diagnose dementia or Alzheimer's disease, a CT scan is a valuable – though expensive – screening test as it can identify multiple infarctions, space-occupying lesions and hydrocephalus. However, only 2% of all demented patients could expect an improvement in their mental state from treatment following a CT scan. Thus, they are only indicated in patients with mild to moderate dementia of less than one year, who are fit enough for surgery if a remediable lesion is found. Where a CT scan is not available, an isotope scan and EEG can be helpful. Lumbar puncture is indicated if the patient has tuberculosis or positive syphilis serology.

Investigation of gastrointestinal lesions

In the investigation of gastrointestinal lesions, both barium meal and endoscopy give accurate results. However, endoscopy has the advantage of providing a tissue diagnosis where a tumour is suspected, and is also tends to be better tolerated by a frail elderly patient. It is thus probably the investigation of choice when readily available but needs to be preceded by a barium swallow (to check if a blind sac is present) when investigating dysphagia.

When investigating lower bowel disorders, the first steps are usually rectal examination, sigmoidoscopy, stool culture, examination of the stool for occult blood and – finally – barium enema and possibly colonoscopy. Detection and treatment of non-metastatic colonic malignancies gives a good prognosis; vigorous investigation of fit and active elderly patients is therefore justified. In the frailer patient, however, more caution is necessary before ordering a barium enema. Both the preparation (laxatives and soap and water enema) and the barium enema itself are uncomfortable and difficult procedures for elderly patients to undergo. They are also frequently unable to retain the barium so that no useful results are obtained. Thus, if physical examination and stool testing is negative in these patients, only a very suggestive history would justify a barium enema.

Ultrasound scans have the advantages of being non-invasive, quick and relatively cheap, and are particularly useful for investigating jaundice, abdominal masses, pancreatic tumours and possible liver metastases.

Investigation of urogenital system

A routine mid-stream urine (MSU) test in elderly patients admitted to hospital will show significant bacteriuria (bacterial count of more than 100 000 organisms/ml) in 20–30% of women. Over half will be asymptomatic, and antibiotics seem to have only a temporary effect on clearing the urine – eventually another, more resistant organism usually

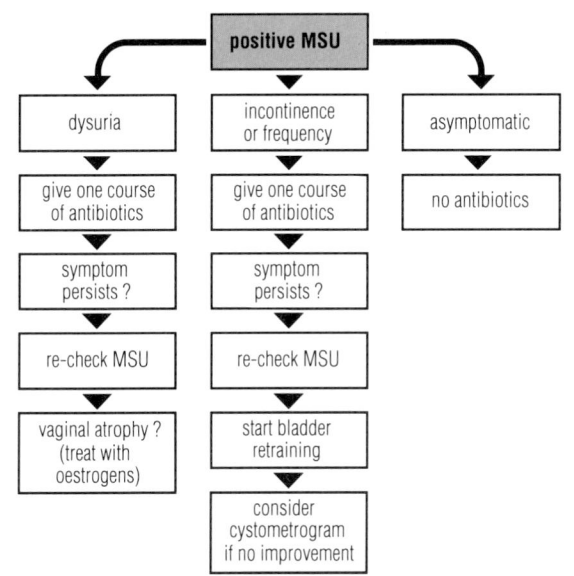

Fig. 10.14 Suggested approach to bacteriuria in elderly women.

appears. Routine MSUs may therefore cause confusion unless there is a clear management policy (Fig. 10.14). Half of patients with bacteriuria have a renal infection rather than cystitis so there is a possibility of renal damage. However, little is known about the natural history of these infections and their recurrence rate with or without antibiotics. To complicate matters further, some incontinent patients have dysuria whether they have a urinary tract infection or not. Many incontinent patients have a significant bacteriuria which is not the cause of the incontinence, but the result of detrusor instability which often leaves a residual urine and thus encourages bacterial growth.

An approach to these problems is as follows. Patients with dysuria should have an MSU taken and be examined for vaginal atrophy (this atrophy also affects the urethra and is treatable with oestrogens). If the MSU shows infection, it should be treated. When the dysuria is accompanied by incontinence, the initial approach is the same; but if the incontinence or dysuria persists – and particularly if there are other symptoms such as urgency and frequency – then the patient should be treated as if she had detrusor instability (p. 837). If the symptoms show no improvement, a cystometrogram is performed. Patients who are incontinent without dysuria and have a positive MSU should have the infection treated on only one occasion before proceeding with bladder retraining (p. 838).

ASSESSMENT OF FITNESS FOR OPERATION

Advanced age is no longer a contraindication to surgery yet the risks are undoubtedly higher. The mortality rate for surgical patients over the age of 65 is about 5%. This doubles to 8–10% in those aged over 75 and rises to 15–20% in those over 85. Such high risks are only justified if surgery offers a reasonable prospect for improving the quality of the patient's life, or of preventing loss of function. Surgery for relief of severe pain or complete bowel obstruction would probably be indicated even in the most severely disabled patient. However, a patient would need to be relatively fit and active before removal of a non-obstructive malignant bowel tumour, repair of an aortic aneurysm or a coronary artery bypass would be considered. The complications of surgery for colorectal carcinoma in the elderly are shown in Table 10.5.

The increased surgical mortality in the elderly is due to several factors:

1. the presence of unsuspected heart disease
2. reduced pulmonary and cardiac reserve (making a postoperative chest infection or myocardial infarct more likely)
3. greater susceptibility to anaesthetic drugs
4. the risk of developing pressure sores or pneumonia during the postoperative period of immobility.

The mortality risk must be weighed against the likely final outcome of surgery. Total hip replacement has transformed the lives of many old people and is now a routine operation. However, if chronic lung disease or an old stroke has reduced the patient's exercise tolerance to a few yards, the operation is unlikely to be worthwhile. Before surgery, heart failure and diabetes should be controlled, dehydration and electrolyte disturbance corrected, and severe anaemia remedied by blood transfusion.

A routine preoperative ECG is worthwhile. Its major use is in detecting a recent myocardial infarct which would mean postponement of surgery for six months (if this is practicable). Many patients will have a minor ECG abnormality which provides a useful baseline measurement for comparing postoperative changes. Preoperative ECG abnormalities do not reliably predict postoperative cardiovascular complications, which can be expected in about one-fifth of elderly patients and consist mainly of heart failure with some cases of myocardial infarction. Car-

Table 10.5 Results of surgery for carcinoma of colon and rectum in 96 patients aged 70 years and over

Postoperative mortality: 8%

Postoperative complications (47/96)

Wound abscess	13	Heart failure	3
Myocardial infarct	6	Embolism	2
Wound dehiscence	5	Atrial flutter	1
Anastomatic leakage	5	Thrombosis	1
Pneumonia	5	Transient ischaemic attack	1
Intra-abdominal abscess	4	Disorientation	1
Urinary tract infection	3		

Age-corrected 5 year survival for whole group: 41%*
10 year survival : 10%

*Age-corrected 5 year survival for patients of all ages with colorectal carcinoma is 43%.
Source: Wobbes T H 1985 Carcinoma of the colon and rectum in geriatric patients. Age and Ageing 14: 321–326.

diovascular disease is the major cause of increased mortality following general surgery in the elderly.

Impaired mental function and poor motivation are also barriers to postoperative rehabilitation. If concentration and short-term memory are poor, the patient may be unable to grasp the physiotherapist's instructions; episodes of mental confusion and agitation may also occur.

PRESCRIBING FOR THE ELDERLY

A general rule of thumb when prescribing drugs for the elderly is 'not too many and not too much'. There is an understandable tendency, when faced with a patient with multiple ailments, to prescribe a treatment for each of them. Thus, while the elderly make up only 18% of the total population, they receive almost one third of all prescriptions issued.

About 75% of persons over the age of 65 and living at home are taking some kind of medication, with 15% receiving four drugs or more. However, multiple prescriptions increase the risk of drug interactions and adverse effects, and compliance is likely to be poor.

Adverse reactions are two or three times more common in the elderly than in those under the age of 60. This is due primarily to slower rates of inactivation and excretion but also, with some drugs, to increased sensitivity of the target organ. Thus, many drugs need to be given in lower dosage.

No new treatment should be prescribed without careful consideration of whether it is truly necessary. Only in exceptional circumstances can the prescription of more than four drugs to an older person be justified.

Altered pharmacokinetics

Drug absorption

Changes in gastrointestinal function with increasing age include: a rise in gastric pH, decreased gastric emptying time, decreased splanchnic blood flow, and loss of small bowel mucosal surface area. Although these changes are theoretically rate-limiting for drug absorption, none appear to be important for passively absorbed drugs.

Distribution

There are a number of theoretically important changes that affect drug distribution in the elderly.

1. A decrease in lean body mass and total body water reduces the distribution of water soluble drugs such as phenazone (Antipyrine) and paracetamol.
2. Increase in body fat results in an increased volume of distribution of lipid soluble drugs such as lignocaine, chlordiazepoxide and diazepam.
3. The small decrease in plasma albumin that occurs in the elderly will reduce drug binding and may thus result in an increased distribution of the drug. Since

it is the unbound fraction that is clinically active, there may be an increased pharmacological effect. In normal elderly people, the reduced plasma protein binding is of little clinical significance; but it may be important in sick or malnourished patients who have a greater reduction in plasma albumin concentration.

4. Conversely, if the drug binds predominantly to α-1 acid glycoprotein (e.g. lignocaine and disopyramide) then protein binding is likely to be normal, or even slightly increased, in the elderly.

Metabolism

There is a decrease in functional liver volume and a reduced rate of hepatic metabolism with increasing age. This reduces presystemic metabolism and causes a marked increase in the bioavailability of drugs metabolised by the liver, such as propranolol, labetalol, lignocaine, chlormethiazole and verapamil. In the case of propranolol, the age differences in plasma concentrations are large, with the mean concentration in the elderly about twice that found in the young. However, because of reduced sensitivity, the dosage need not be lowered. Age-related effects on drug metabolism are variable, so that even some extensively metabolised drugs, e.g. warfarin or diazepam, may show no change in clearance.

Excretion

Advancing age is accompanied by a decline in renal function due to a reduction in both glomerular filtration rate and tubular function. At 60 years of age, renal function is about half that at age 30; and renal function will be further impaired by dehydration, congestive cardiac failure and urinary retention; as well as by specific renal diseases such as diabetic nephropathy. However, normal elderly persons may have significant reductions in glomerular filtration rate and tubular function yet still have a normal blood urea and serum creatinine because of reduced muscle mass.

For those drugs excreted by glomerular filtration, the rate of excretion correlates with glomerular filtration rate. Some of these drugs, e.g. digoxin, gentamicin, lithium, cimetidine and chlorpropamide, have a low therapeutic index and their dosage therefore needs to be carefully chosen in the elderly. In general, a lower dose will be needed than in young patients. Some estimate of the appropriate dosage may be made from reference to standard tables of creatinine clearance and blood urea; but once treatment is started, there is no substitute for checking the drug plasma concentration.

Altered pharmacodynamics

The most clinically important result of altered pharmacodynamics occurs with drugs acting on the central nervous system. Sedatives and tranquillisers are more likely to produce drowsiness and hangover effects in the elderly (Fig. 10.15). Although nitrazepam and diazepam have similar plasma concentrations in young and old,

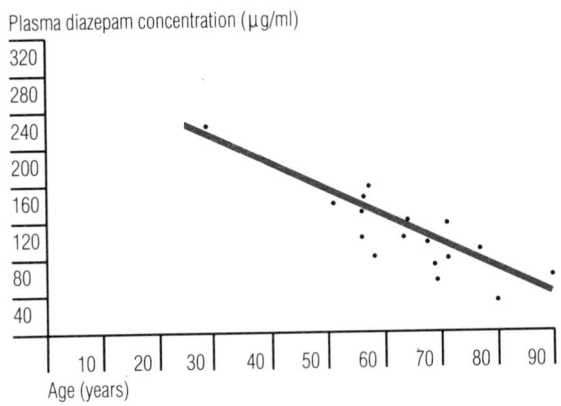

Plasma diazepam concentration (μg/ml)

Age (years)

Fig. 10.15 Relationship between age and the concentration of plasma diazepam required to produce sedation, in patients undergoing cardioversion for cardiac arrhythmias.

psychological testing shows that the elderly make more mistakes and have longer reaction times for 36 hours after a single dose. They also show increased sensitivity to anaesthetic agents such as halothane.

A reduced sensitivity to adrenergic agonists is seen in the elderly heart. The dose of isoprenaline required to raise the heart rate increases with age, indicating a four to six fold decrease in isoprenaline sensitivity. Sensitivity to propranolol also decreases so that – despite the higher plasma propranolol concentrations seen in elderly subjects – the degree of beta blockade is reduced.

The dose of warfarin needed to produce anticoagulation in the elderly is reduced, but this is not due to an age-related rise in plasma warfarin concentration. Warfarin acts by inhibiting the synthesis of vitamin K-dependent clotting factors, and this inhibitory effect is greater in the elderly, resulting in an increased sensitivity.

Adverse reactions

Whenever a reduction in drug elimination or increase in receptor sensitivity occurs, there is the likelihood of an excessive drug effect and hence an adverse reaction. The risk of these adverse reactions increases with age (Fig. 10.16A). About 3% of all admissions to geriatric units in the UK are solely due to unwanted drug effects; and in a further 8% of cases, an adverse reaction is a contributory cause. Two-thirds of all reactions are caused by two groups of drugs.

1. Cardiovascular drugs – diuretics, digoxin and hypotensive drugs.
2. Drugs acting on the central nervous system – anti-Parkinsonian drugs, antidepressants, hypnotics and tranquillisers.

Although more than 70% of patients taking the cardiovascular drugs make a full recovery from the adverse reaction, only 46% recover from the ill effects of anti-Parkinsonian drugs.

The risk of an adverse reaction increases with the number of drugs taken (Fig. 10.16B). Elderly persons are more likely to have multiple diseases than the young, and also tend to visit their doctor more frequently. Since over 50% of all patients' visits to a doctor result in a drug treatment, the likelihood of polypharmacy is therefore high. Not only is the patient apt to be muddled by a large number of drugs and inadvertently take the wrong dose; but drug interactions lead directly to an increased adverse reaction rate. This is particularly likely to occur when drugs with a low therapeutic index, e.g. anticoagulants, antidepressants, anticonvulsants and antihypertensives, are used in combination.

There are a number of important causes of adverse drug reaction in the elderly other than altered pharmacokinetics and pharmacodynamics. Inadequate clinical assessment is perhaps the most common. Dependent leg oedema, for example, is commonly due to immobility rather than congestive cardiac failure, and a diuretic is thus not an appropriate treatment. Similarly, old persons who complain of dizziness are often expressing a sensation of unsteadiness and fear of falling rather than true vertigo. Prochlorperazine – an effective vestibular sedative – is frequently prescribed in this situation but is quite useless and also carries a serious risk of Parkinsonian side effects.

The assumption that there is 'a pill for every ill' sometimes causes the doctor to prescribe excessively. Loneliness and social problems often present as minor aches and pains, unhappiness or insomnia. Although both difficult and

Fig. 10.16 Adverse drug reactions. **A.** The increase in adverse drug reactions with age. **B.** Prevalence of adverse reactions related to number of prescribed drugs. The risk in a patient taking only one drug is about 11% but is 27% if six drugs are taken.

A   Adverse drug reactions (%)

Age (years)

B   Adverse drug reactions (%)

Number of drugs

time-consuming, it is far better to deal with the underlying problems than simply issue a number of drug prescriptions.

Regular reviews of a patient's medication will reduce the risk of adverse reactions. Drugs needed at the time of an acute illness may not be appropriate six months later; and it is often the case that stopping a drug is more beneficial to the patient than writing a new prescription.

Compliance

There is no evidence that the elderly are less compliant than the young, but they do make more medication errors. These errors occur in up to three-quarters of old persons taking drugs, but only about a quarter are potentially serious, usually because of underdosage. Medication errors are more commonly made in patients over the age of 75 who are living alone and are confused. Poor visual acuity often prevents an old person from reading the instructions correctly; and impaired manual dexterity may make it difficult or even impossible for him to unscrew the cap on the bottle (particularly if it is one of the child resistant types). Compliance can be improved, and errors in medication reduced, by careful counselling and an explanation of when and how to take the drug. Written instructions or a calendar pack can be helpful.

REHABILITATION

The aim of the rehabilitation team concerned with the elderly patient is to help restore maximum capability within the limits of the patient's needs and disability.

Principles of rehabilitation

When setting a realistic rehabilitation goal, it is important to consider the patient's needs. For a very elderly and frail amputee, wheel-chair independence may be perfectly satisfactory; but this would not be acceptable for a fit 65-year-old amputee who is a keen golfer.

The principles of rehabilitation in the elderly are essentially the same as for young patients, but some special features of old age should be noted. Multiple pathology is likely to be present, so that the speed with which a stroke patient can be mobilised is often hampered by shortness of breath due to chronic lung or heart disease. The mental barriers to recovery may also be greater, whether due to dementia or to the increased feelings of passivity and dependence sometimes shown by older persons. There may be difficult social problems due to lack of family support or poor housing; and sometimes low expectations, 'I am too old to try this', also reduce the patient's efforts.

Rehabilitation is concerned not with doing things for the patient, but with helping him to learn to do things for himself. It is far better for a stroke patient to spend half an hour trying to feed himself – even if most of the food ends up down his shirt-front or on the floor – than to have a well-meaning relative or nurse spoon it in with speed and efficiency. Patients enjoy exercising their painfully regained skills and it is essential to regain independence before leaving hospital and returning home.

The multidisciplinary team

The most effective approach to rehabilitation is through a multidisciplinary team, with each member contributing their special skills and working together with the patient and his family towards an agreed goal. The team meets regularly to discuss the patient's progress and review future plans. With a good team, the patient is undergoing rehabilitation all the time and not just during the half an hour a day he may spend with the physiotherapist or occupational therapist. Although elderly patients can be successfully rehabilitated on a busy general medical ward, there are definite advantages in grouping them together in one ward. The nurses develop greater expertise, the pace of treatment can be better geared to the patient's needs, and it is easier to create an atmosphere of 24-hour-a-day rehabilitation. Correctly positioning a stroke patient is something all nurses and doctors should be aware of (Fig. 10.17). Whoever helps the patient stand up or transfer to a chair should do it in the correct manner and not haul him up by his paralysed arm.

At some stage before discharge, the occupational therapist will generally take the patient on a home visit to see how well he copes in his own familiar surroundings. This also allows assessment of the need for a specific aid – e.g. a grab handle on the wall next to the lavatory – and the opportunity to have it fitted before the patient arrives home. The social worker has a valuable role to play over and above organising a home help or arranging a place in a residential home. Some old people have severe problems with loneliness, isolation and dependency and the social worker can do a great deal to help the patient and his family adjust to these difficulties.

Fig. 10.17 Positioning the stroke patient. A. Incorrect. **B.** Correct. The forearm on the affected side should be supported and should point straight forwards with wrist and fingers extended and thumb abducted. The arm must not be allowed to hang from the shoulder in internal rotation. Choosing a suitable chair – with unrestricted view and with arm rests – is important. **C.** Transferring the stroke patient to a chair. Note the support given to the affected arm.

COMMUNITY CARE AND LONG-STAY CARE

In the UK in recent years, the emphasis has been to look after elderly persons in their own homes rather than in institutions. This is nearly always what the old person prefers but it is a mistake to regard good community care as a cheap alternative. There may be a saving in capital costs and maintenance, but there is unlikely to be any reduction in the number of health or social service staff required. Keeping an old person at home often means that support is needed for the family looking after that person; otherwise the strain can easily become intolerable and the family can no longer cope.

In addition to the everyday support of home helps and community nurses it may also be necessary to arrange regular relief admissions to the local hospital. This is primarily to relieve the strain on the caring family, but is also a useful opportunity for the hospital staff to improve the patient's mobility and independence.

The geriatric day hospital may be used either to investigate or to treat patients living at home. It sometimes avoids the need to admit a patient to hospital at all or, through close follow-up, allows an early discharge. It should be stressed that the day hospital is a medical, not a social institution. It is staffed by nurses with remedial therapists and doctors in attendance, and is particularly useful for, say, investigating and treating a patient with falls or anaemia, or following up patients who have had a stroke or a proximal femur fracture.

Long-stay care

Many departments of geriatric medicine have found that, as their acute facilities improve, so the number of long-stay beds that they need diminishes. In other words, early intervention and good management reduce long-term disability. Since much effort is put into keeping elderly patients in the community – either in their own homes or in a local authority or private residential home – it follows that only the most severely dependent and frail elderly persons end up in a long-stay hospital bed.

For most patients admitted to a long-stay hospital, this will be their home for the rest of their lives. It should therefore be homely, pleasant and comfortable. As in rehabilitation, the emphasis is on educating patients to do as much for themselves as possible and there is thus still a need for physiotherapy and occupational therapy within long-stay hospitals. It is always a happy day for everyone involved when, after six or twelve months of steady perseverance, a stroke patient improves sufficiently to be discharged.

FURTHER READING

Andrews K 1987 Rehabilitation of the older adult. Edward Arnold, London. *A good mix of practical advice and learned discussion.*

Brocklehurst J C, Allen S C 1987 Geriatric medicine for students. Churchill Livingstone, Edinburgh. *A short introduction; good value for money.*

Harrogate seminar report 7: effective geriatric medicine 1983 Department of Health and Social Security, London. *Discussions on the philosophy and organisation of medical services for the elderly.*

Mandelstam D 1988 Understanding incontinence. Routledge, Chapman and Hall, Andover, Hants. *The best small book on the subject.*

Organic mental impairment in the elderly 1981 Journal of the Royal College of Physicians of London 15: 141–167. *A useful outline of all the major points relating to dementia.*

Seymour D J, Vaz F G 1987 Aspects of surgery in the elderly. British Journal of Hospital Medicine 37: 102–113. *Review article.*

10

Psychological Medicine

Psychiatric disease constitutes a large proportion of disability and illness within society (Fig. 11.1). In their origins psychiatry and medicine were not divided, but from about 1850 onwards they went separate ways. Medicine became dominated by a powerful but increasingly narrow scientific approach; while psychiatry became increasingly isolated, both institutionally, in the mental hospitals, and intellectually set apart from the rest of medical science through its low status and the esoteric nature of its subject matter. Part of the challenge of present-day psychiatry is to bring this division to an end. The large mental hospitals are closing and acute psychiatric illness is now treated in general hospital units alongside the other medical disciplines. Patients and their illnesses are no longer seen by physicians purely as scientific puzzles to be solved; and psychological aspects of physical illness are, through *liaison*

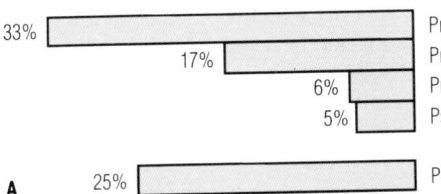

33% Prevalence of psychiatric ill health in the community
17% Prevalence of psychiatric disorder in general practice
6% Prevalence of psychiatric disorder among school-children
5% Psychiatric referral rate from general practice

25% Psychiatric beds as a proportion of all NHS beds

A

Fig. 11.1 **Psychiatric epidemiology. A.**
Prevalence of, and provision for, psychiatric ill health in the community. **B.** Cases per annum of various psychiatric disorders in a general practice population of 2500.

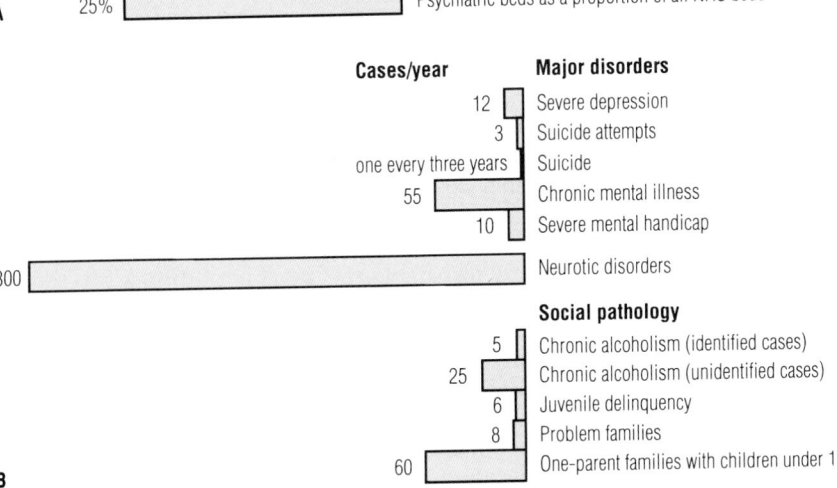

Cases/year	Major disorders
12	Severe depression
3	Suicide attempts
one every three years	Suicide
55	Chronic mental illness
10	Severe mental handicap
300	Neurotic disorders

	Social pathology
5	Chronic alcoholism (identified cases)
25	Chronic alcoholism (unidentified cases)
6	Juvenile delinquency
8	Problem families
60	One-parent families with children under 15

B

psychiatry, now recognised to be of great importance. Medical science is, in turn, making an increasingly important impact on psychiatric knowledge and practice. The basic disciplines underlying psychiatry are psychology, psychoanalysis and sociology; but biochemistry, genetics, immunology and virology are also making some important contributions to the subject.

The central meeting ground for medicine and psychiatry is the *doctor-patient relationship*. All patients, whatever their illness, have feelings and fears which the doctor needs to understand and know how to handle. The meaning to the patient of a particular symptom – chest pain, for example, whether due to angina or anxiety in a 40-year-old man whose father died suddenly of a heart attack in middle age – needs to be understood, in order to appreciate its impact on the patient, as well as diagnosed and investigated. Psychiatry is concerned with meaning as well as explanation, and with methods of communication with the patient, as well as the technology of treatment.

Despite this intimate association with everyday medicine, many doctors find psychiatry difficult and confusing. This is partly because the subject is inherently complex and multifaceted, but also because psychiatry involves the doctor's own feelings and attitudes in a way that can often be avoided in other branches of medicine. In approaching psychiatry, doctors have to learn to deal not just with the patient, but with themselves as well.

CLASSIFICATION

The classification of psychiatric illness is summarised in Table 11.1.

MINDS AND BRAINS

An eminent neurologist once stated that 'psychiatry is neurology without physical signs'. This would be true if psychiatry were simply concerned with the *brain* and its disorders, and the problem of psychiatric diagnosis and classification would, in this case, be no different from that of any other system of the body. A significant part of psychiatry is indeed concerned with diseases of the brain – the organic psychoses such as confusional states for example, or the affective symptoms caused by adrenal disorders. The 19th century discovery that the psychosis known as general paralysis of the insane (GPI) was caused by syphilis, stimulated Emil Kraepelin to search for other physical causes of insanity, with the expectation that all mental illness would soon be found to be caused by diseases of the brain. The attempt has failed, not simply because brain research is difficult, but because psychiatry is concerned with *minds* as well as brains.

Mind has three main properties:

1. the ability to experience emotions
2. intentionality (i.e. having desires and goals)
3. self-awareness.

Table 11.1 Classification of psychiatric illness

Organic syndromes	**Personality disorders**
Delirium	Hysterical
Dementia	Schizoid
Intoxication and withdrawal syndromes	Obsessional
	Psychopathic
Functional psychoses	**Others**
Schizophrenia	Addictions
Manic-depressive psychosis	Alcohol
Paranoid states	Drugs
	Eating disorders
Neuroses	Sexual dysfunction and deviation
Anxiety	
Phobias	
Depression	
Obsessive-compulsive neurosis	
Somatoform disorders	
Conversion	
Somatisation	
Hypochondriasis	

Modern medicine sometimes treats patients as though they were mind-less – assuming they are lacking in feelings, self-consciousness and the capacity to choose. This is bad medicine. The body cannot be treated as if the mind did not exist; the mind cannot be approached as though it were just another part of the body.

Although psychiatric diagnosis approaches the mind as if it were an organ, this is often merely an analogy. When we speak of psychiatric illness we may be speaking about a brain disease, e.g. GPI, Alzheimer's disease or (possibly) some forms of schizophrenia, in the same way we speak of pneumonia as a disease of the lungs. On the other hand, while conditions such as personality disorders or agoraphobia are, in some ways, like illnesses, they also differ in many important respects because they affect the mind.

This important distinction between mind and brain may help to explain the discomfort which some feel when confronted with the essentially rather simple issue of psychiatric diagnosis. The categories of mental illness are few and not difficult to memorise. The main problem is philosophical rather than one of classification.

A number of other difficulties may also be encountered on first approaching psychiatry. Firstly, psychiatric diagnoses tend to be at a rather general level. They are *symptomatic/syndromic* rather than *pathological/specific*. The diagnosis of anxiety neurosis or schizophrenia bears more resemblance to that of heart failure than that of mitral stenosis.

Secondly, with the exception of the organic psychoses, the underlying pathology of psychiatric disorders is usually complex and *multifactorial*. This follows from the nature of mental phenomena. Just as there is usually no simple reason why an individual chooses medicine as a career, so there is rarely a single 'cause' of depression. There may be many explanations for a particular symptom or problem.

A third difficulty encountered in psychiatric diagnosis is that of deciding what is normal or abnormal, sometimes more a political or ethical question than a technical one. The doctor's own standards and feelings are involved in assessing a psychiatric patient. This also leads to two errors commonly made by psychiatric novices: either the student identifies the patient with himself, and so decides there is nothing much wrong; or identifies himself with the patient and worries that he must be psychiatrically ill!

PSYCHOSIS AND NEUROSIS

The distinction between psychosis and neurosis is fundamental to psychiatric classification, although neither is easily defined on its own. The difference turns on four main issues (Table 11.2).

Relationship to reality

The essence of psychosis is that the patient loses contact with everyday reality. This may happen as a result of either hallucinations or delusions, or both.

Delusions and hallucinations are not a feature of neurosis. In contrast to the situation in psychosis, the neurotic patient does not lose touch with reality. His feelings and beliefs about himself may be distorted, but his perception and understanding of the external world remains intact.

Hallucinations

An hallucination is a false perception. The patient undergoes a sensory experience in the absence of an external stimulus, for example hearing a voice when there is nobody there. For this to be diagnostic it should be clear-cut; hearing an 'inner voice' which the person recognises as really part of himself is not an hallucination. Any of the five senses may be involved in the patient's altered perception of reality.

Hearing. Auditory hallucinations are probably the commonest type of hallucination, found especially in paranoid states, in schizophrenia and occasionally in psychotic depression.

Sight. Contrary to popular belief, psychotic patients rarely 'see things'; visual hallucinations occur most commonly in drug and alcohol withdrawal states, temporal lobe epilepsy, and hysterical psychosis.

Smell and taste. Olfactory hallucinations are usually a sign of organic psychosis, e.g. temporal lobe seizures.

Touch. Tactile hallucinations are rare, but can occur in schizophrenia and drug withdrawal.

Hallucinations are not always a sign of pathology. After bereavement, visual or auditory hallucinations of the lost loved one are common.

Delusions

A delusion is a fixed and firmly held false belief. The patient's perceptions are unaltered; but his interpretation of them is, and is at variance with common experience. He sees people chatting at a bus-stop and is convinced they are talking about him, saying he is homosexual or a spy. These beliefs may be well concealed and not evident in superficial conversation.

We normally assume that our thoughts are private, that individuals are autonomous, that the non-human world is indifferent to our existence, that we are not in any special danger, and that we are not of any particular importance or interest to strangers. The deluded patient (e.g. in schizophrenia) has experiences which conflict with these everyday beliefs. He may feel that his thoughts can be interfered with from outside, or that his movements can be controlled by others; he may believe there is some special significance in the number plate of a passing car, that he is in great danger from hostile forces, or that television programmes or public events are caused by, or directed at, himself.

Unusual beliefs about the world may be held by normal members of cultural subgroups (it would, for example, be abnormal for a member of the Flat Earth Society to believe that the world was round!), but the deluded patient is, except in the rare instance of *folie-à-deux*, alone with his false beliefs.

Severity

In general, psychotic disorders are more severe, more disabling and produce greater overall disturbance of mental functioning than neuroses. There are exceptions to this. Obsessional neurosis, in which the individual may spend many hours a day engaged in complicated washing or dressing rituals, can be incapacitating. Conversely, a patient with limited (*encapsulated*) paranoid delusions (e.g. that shopkeepers are plotting against him) may sometimes continue to function relatively normally both at work and at home despite being deluded.

Relationship to normality

In psychosis there is a clear departure from normality. Despite the occasional occurrence of psychotic phenomena in normal people subjected to extreme stress, it is usually possible to make a firm distinction between normal and

Table 11.2 The distinction between psychosis and neurosis

Feature	Psychosis	Neurosis
Relationship to reality	Loss of contact with reality. Delusions and/or hallucinations	Perception of external reality intact. Problem is with the self
Severity	More severe, more global disturbance	Areas of normal function remain
Relationship to normality	Clear distinction between normal and psychotic experience	Represents extremes of normal difficulties
Insight	Usually lacking	Present

psychotic experience. In contrast, minor neurotic symptoms, e.g. depression, anxiety, obsessional symptoms and hysteria, are common in normal people. The neurotic population is best seen as an extreme end of a normal distribution curve in which quantitative, but not qualitative change has taken place.

Insight

It is commonly stated that the difference between neurosis and psychosis is that the psychotic 'lacks insight'. The psychotic patient attributes his symptoms to reality rather than illness, and cannot be persuaded out of his delusions or hallucinations; the neurotic, on the other hand, can usually see that his view of the world might be mistaken. However, while it is undoubtedly true that the psychotic lacks insight, there are several reasons for giving less prominence to insight than is customary. Firstly, if the psychotic is identified on the basis of a loss of touch with reality, then he will, by definition, lack insight. If he knew that his delusions or hallucinations were false, he would not be deluded or hallucinating. Secondly, he often tacitly accepts that he is ill by coming for help despite the apparent illogicality of complaining to a doctor about a delusion. Thirdly, the word 'insight' has two distinct meanings in psychiatry: one, given above, which refers to the patient's relationship to reality and his illness; and another more literal meaning referring to the ability to look into oneself and one's emotions and motives without denial or self-deception. While insight in this second sense may be desirable, it bears no relationship to the presence or absence of illness. It is possible to be perfectly healthy yet lack self-knowledge, or to be profoundly insightful yet mentally ill.

THE PSYCHOSES

Psychoses may be divided by their features and causes into two main groups: *organic* and *functional* (or, more accurately, 'of unknown origin'). In organic psychosis there is established biochemical, infective or structural brain disease. In functional psychosis no such disease process can be demonstrated. Organic psychoses can be divided into acute organic psychoses (also known as acute confusional states, delirium, or 'acute brain syndrome') and chronic organic psychoses (also known as dementia and 'chronic brain syndrome').

Functional psychosis vs acute organic psychosis

It is essential to be able to distinguish functional psychoses from acute confusional states since the former

require psychiatric, the latter medical, treatment. The key difference is the state of consciousness. In functional psychosis consciousness is clear, and patients fully orientated: it is possible to complete a complicated crossword puzzle while suffering from paranoid schizophrenia. In organic psychosis, however, there is almost always some disturbance of consciousness; this is usually variable ('fluctuating level of consciousness') and is often worse at night. The spectrum of altered consciousness is very wide. It ranges from a mild vagueness and inability to concentrate, through disorientation in time and place, to a florid delirium in which the patient is restless, disorientated, grossly deluded and fearful. Some causes of acute organic psychosis are given in Table 11.3.

Table 11.3 Some causes of acute organic psychosis

Cause	Examples
Systemic infection	Malaria, HIV, pneumonia (especially in the elderly)
Metabolic disturbance	Electrolyte imbalance, renal failure, liver failure
Vitamin deficiency	Thiamine deficiency (Wernicke-Korsakoff syndrome in alcoholics, and beri-beri)
Endocrine	Hypoglycaemia, hypothyroidism, steroid administration
Drug intoxication	Anticonvulsants, hypnotics, antidepressants, LSD, amphetamines
Intracerebral	CVA, subarachnoid haemorrhage, tumour, cerebral abscess
Withdrawal syndrome	DTs, benzodiazepine withdrawal

Functional psychosis

One hundred years ago, Kraepelin divided the functional psychoses into two main groups: manic-depressive psychosis, and schizophrenia (or, as he called it, 'dementia praecox'). Manic-depressive psychosis is primarily a disorder of *mood*. The patient becomes psychotically depressed or elated ('unipolar manic-depression') or experiences episodes of both ('bipolar manic-depression'). There are usually periods of normality between episodes of illness. Schizophrenia is primarily a disorder of *thinking* and it produces, on the whole, a more severe and more general disturbance of mental functioning. The prognosis is less good than for manic-depression.

THE NEUROSES

Unlike the situation in psychosis, in neurosis the patient experiences no alteration of external reality. Instead, the patient is troubled by, and tries to avoid, some unacceptable aspect of himself or of his internal reality.

There are four main patterns of neurosis.

Summary 1 Classification of psychosis	
Organic	*Functional*
Acute (delirium)	Manic-depressive psychosis
Chronic (dementia)	Schizophrenia

Anxiety neurosis and phobia

Anxiety is an almost universal feature of all psychiatric illness. It is the psychic equivalent of pain. Anxiety is normally a response to external threat or unpredictability in the environment. In *anxiety neurosis*, the patient is not alerted and mobilised into action by anxiety; he is paralysed or overwhelmed by it. Where anxiety is experienced only in specific situations, the patient is said to suffer from a *phobia*. In phobic disorders the patient attempts to master anxiety by avoidance (e.g. an agoraphobic patient avoids public places).

Depressive neurosis

If anxiety is the psychic equivalent of pain, depression is the equivalent of disability (although anxiety can also of course be disabling, and depression intensely painful). In depression, the patient has lost not a limb or a function but a relationship. It is usually a person who is lost, but the 'lost object' can also be a job or a house, or his own self-esteem. Depression can be seen as an attempt to avoid painful reality by withdrawal.

Hysteria

The basic themes of hysteria are *denial, dissociation, displacement* and *dependency*. The patient denies a painful conflict and thus avoids anxiety or depression, but at a price: she (most hysterical patients are female) dissociates herself from her feelings and displaces the latter into her body instead. Psychic pain is thereby converted into physical symptomatology, and the patient becomes dependent on doctors and others.

Obsessive-compulsive neurosis

Here the patient deals with anxiety – often aroused by fear of his own feelings of aggression, sexuality or wish for power or independence – by an attempt at control. A ritual action or a repetitive thought is performed over and over again in the magical hope that this will keep the patient safe from imagined danger. The patient knows it is absurd (thus he has insight and is not psychotic), tries to resist, but still has, say, to wash in a particular way every morning or he will not feel safe to start the day.

PERSONALITY DISORDER

Individuals are recognisable not just by their appearance but by their personality which, despite ageing and change, remains relatively constant through time.

Personalities can be classified dimensionally or categorically. A dimensional approach is exemplified by Hans Eysenk who, following his intellectual opponent Jung, devised a grid for assessing personalities along the dimensions of *extrovert* (outgoing, gregarious, stimulus-seeking) and *introvert* (inner-directed, shy, stimulus-avoiding).

The problem of differentiating between normal and

Summary 2   Classification of personality

Dimensional approaches
e.g. extrovert/introvert

Categorisation
e.g. schizoid
   obsessional
   hysterical
   sociopathic

---

abnormal personality is even more difficult than for neurosis. There are undoubtedly individuals whose personalities are very unusual, at least in the statistical sense, but they are not necessarily abnormal. An alternative approach to the classification of personality uses psychiatric categories to describe different types of individual. The *schizoid personality*, for example, is withdrawn and aloof, preoccupied with material objects or intellectual pursuits rather than people, lacking in close emotional contact, and is defensive and easily hurt. These features may only be a personality trait, and may even be advantageous: many creative people have schizoid tendencies. However, when taken to extremes they become a personality disorder. Here, the individual is so handicapped by his personality that he seeks, or is brought, for help, e.g. the schizoid personality who suffers from severe social isolation.

Unlike psychosis and neurosis, a personality disorder is not an illness. Its features date back to childhood or adolescence and so there is no premorbid period of normality. However, personality disorder often co-exists with, and may predispose to, neurosis.

Important types of personality disorder (other than schizophrenia) include the following:
Obsessional personality disorder. Here the individual is meticulous, controlled, orderly and rigid; he may find the sloppiness of others unbearable. Such characteristics may be advantageous in certain circumstances, e.g. the armed forces or the operating theatre, but may also bring the individual into conflict with others when flexibility is needed, e.g. under stress and in intimate relationships.
Hysterical personality disorder (p. 201).
Psychopathic personality disorder (p. 208).

'MINOR' PSYCHIATRIC ILLNESS

Patients with minor psychiatic illness are clearly suffering from emotional distress but fit none of the above diagnostic categories. Minor psychiatric illnesses are hard to classify and often go undetected, hiding behind and contributing to physical symptoms. They have been described as *somatoform disorders* (p. 197) in which a somatic 'facade' conceals difficulty in adjustment to social stress ('adjustment disorders'), symptoms of anxiety and/or depression, or personality difficulties. Once these are explored, and the patient reassured, the physical symptoms may be relieved.

In considering patients with somatisation disorders, a

Psychological Medicine

1. *Stress factors*, especially recent losses such as bereavement, unemployment, children leaving home, financial difficulties, divorce and termination of pregnancy.
2. *Social support*, relationship with partner (including sexual relationship), parents, children and friends, housing conditions.
3. *Personality*, how the person has reacted to stress in the past, previous stressful or painful experiences, especially in childhood, and whether the patient is able to respond with appropriate anger or sadness.
4. *Alcoholism, drug abuse and eating disorders*, which frequently present indirectly via physical symptoms.

THE CAUSES OF PSYCHIATRIC ILLNESS

The complexity of the interactions underlying psychiatric illness can be confusing. A causal model of the type 'one pathogen–one disease' rarely applies in psychiatry.

There are three types of causal factor in psychiatric illness: genetic/biochemical; developmental; and social. All play at least some role in most psychiatric disturbance, and part of the art of psychiatry lies in assigning the appropriate weight to each factor and identifying which may be the most important.

Genetic/biochemical ('organic')

Occasionally a single genetic defect can determine a psychiatric illness: the psychiatric manifestations of Huntington's chorea can be explained in this way. However, although genetic inheritance may, as in schizophrenia, be a necessary cause of illness, it is rarely sufficient. Biochemical, viral, immunological and nutritional factors may well be important in a number of psychiatric illnesses; few have so far been convincingly demonstrated as a unique cause. Genetic/biochemical factors can best be seen as creating a 'diathesis' or predisposing condition which can, under certain conditions, lead to illness.

Developmental ('intrapsychic')

Each individual is a product of, and in a sense contains and continues, his past. Psychological development, especially that shaped by early childhood experience and family relationships, plays a crucial part in determining personality and ways of reacting to stress in later life.

Social ('interpersonal')

Many psychiatric illnesses are triggered by recent social events, such as bereavement, divorce or unemployment. The patient's social and family situation can play a major role in both initiating his illness and helping or hindering his capacity to recover. The quality of family relationships is itself influenced by the personality, which is in turn a product of both genetic and developmental factors.

ANXIETY

Anxiety, like pain, is an unpleasant necessity. A person unable to feel anxious would be severely incapacitated. Arousal, which may be experienced subjectively as anxiety, leads to an adaptive response to threat: fight or flight.

AROUSAL AND ANXIETY

There are three main components of the arousal response:

1. psychophysiological
2. psychological
3. interpersonal.

The psychophysiological component

This is mediated by the autonomic nervous system and is accompanied by increased adrenalin, noradrenalin and corticosteroid secretion. These result in: tachycardia, pilo-erection, sweating and pupillary dilatation; and subjective manifestations of autonomic activity including paraesthesiae, giddiness, 'butterflies in the stomach', breathing difficulties, a sensation of painful pressure in the chest, and muscular tension, especially around the head and neck. These symptoms may be mistakenly attributed by both patients and doctors to organic illness.

The psychological component

There is a continuum of arousal responses to threat, running from alertness and readiness, through mild fear, to severe anxiety and incapacitating panic. Effective action depends on an optimal state of arousal; little can be achieved when an individual is either barely aroused or in a state of panic. Examination nerves, if not too great, improve results.

During a panic attack, the patient experiences a sense of threat, or even of impending death. Chronic anxiety states may produce irritability, lack of concentration and a subjective sense of failing memory. Anxious patients fail to habituate to stimuli and so remain chronically over-aroused; this can result in extreme sensitivity to sudden noises or movements. In extreme anxiety, a state of detachment may supervene in which anxiety suddenly disappears, to be replaced by a feeling of being outside of oneself (*depersonalisation*) and cut off from one's surroundings, which appear unreal and distant (*derealisation*). These experiences may be misinterpreted by the patient as signs that he is 'going mad'.

The interpersonal component

A frightened individual clings to those he loves and on whom he depends. This is part of 'attachment behaviour' and, like anxiety, is adaptive: species survival depends on secure bonding. The dependency and excessive demands on others that so often accompany anxiety states (and can be trying to both relatives and doctors) can be understood as part of the attachment response to threat.

ANXIETY SYNDROMES

Anxiety may be a primary diagnosis, or secondary to a psychiatric or physical illness. It is a non-specific symptom which occurs in a wide range of psychiatric syndromes, including benzodiazepine withdrawal, depression, alcoholism and schizophrenia. It can also be an important manifestation of organic illness, particularly thyrotoxicosis, paroxysmal tachycardia, carcinoid syndrome, hypoglycaemic attacks, phaeochromocytoma, and temporal lobe seizures.

Classification

Primary anxiety syndromes may be classified as shown in Table 11.4.

Table 11.4 Classification of anxiety syndromes

Primary anxiety	Secondary anxiety
Generalised	Psychiatric illness
Situational	e.g. depression
Agoraphobia	Organic illness
Social phobia	e.g. thyrotoxicosis
Hypochondriasis	Alcohol-related
Specific (e.g. spiders)	withdrawal symptoms
Panic attacks	Benzodiazepine-related
(hyperventilation syndrome)	withdrawal symptoms

Generalised anxiety

Individuals who experience anxiety symptoms, either chronically or intermittently, without a clear stimulus or an obvious focus of fear suffer so-called 'free-floating' anxiety.

Situational anxiety

In situational anxiety there is an identifiable precipitant to which the anxiety is related. Phobias are closely related to anxiety syndromes because in a phobia the patient avoids the feared situation and is thus restricted by his underlying anxiety. Situational anxiety syndromes include:

1. *Specific phobias*, e.g. snake or spider phobia or fear of heights. These have a good prognosis, are found in otherwise healthy individuals and respond well to behavioural treatment (p. 215).
2. *Agoraphobia*, named after the Greek *agora*, or meeting place. In agoraphobia the patient is frightened to leave home unaccompanied, avoids public places like supermarkets and department stores and cannot travel on public transport, especially underground railways and aeroplanes. (Claustrophobia is usually part of agoraphobia.) The patient is usually female and may be very

Summary 3   Manifestations of anxiety

Physical	*Psychological*
Tachycardia	Irritability
Tightness/pain in chest	Inability to memorise
Difficulty in breathing	Inability to concentrate
Headache	Fear of impending death
Paraesthesia	Fear of madness
Muscular pains	(depersonalisation)
Muscular weakness	
Dizziness	
Difficulty in swallowing	
Abdominal discomfort	
Diarrhoea	
Frequency	

dependent on her mother, daughter or husband. The prognosis is less good than with specific phobias, but behaviour therapy can be helpful. Agoraphobic symptoms may develop as part of a depressive illness (p. 193).

3. *Social phobia*, fear of meeting people in social situations, e.g. parties, canteens. This affects mainly young people and is an extreme form of normal 'shyness'. Patients can be helped by social skills training in groups with fellow-sufferers in which they 'role-play' the feared situations.
4. *Hypochondriasis*, a morbid fear of illness, leading to a frequent need for reassurance by family, friends and doctors.

Panic attacks (hyperventilation syndrome)

These may be part of a specific syndrome, e.g. agoraphobia, or may occur on their own. They frequently present to physicians as medical emergencies and are usually self-limiting. The patient presents in a state of terror, over-breathing, complaining of chest pain and often feeling he is dying. The diagnosis can be established by provoking these symptoms by voluntary overbreathing, which are then relieved by rebreathing from a paper bag. Tetany may be a feature. Organic causes (e.g. hyperthyroidism) must be eliminated and a positive psychiatric history should be established (i.e. a history of recent stress/conflict or background of chronic difficulty).

Aetiology

There is no single cause of anxiety syndrome. Individuals vary in their tendency to become over-aroused: *genetic factors* may play a part in this. Anxiety may also arise from *faulty learning*. A child who senses his mother's tension in social situations may become socially phobic himself. Repeated avoidance of a feared stimulus then exaggerates the threat associated with it, since there is no opportunity for mastery through repeated exposure.

Attachment theory explains how early childhood relationships may predispose to anxiety in later life. A

> **Summary 4   Aetiology of anxiety syndromes**
>
> | Past | Present |
> |------|---------|
> | Genetic factors (predisposition) | External threat |
> | Faulty learning (as a child) | Relationships to attachment |
> | Early childhood relationships | figures |
> | (Attachment theory) | Internal conflict |

developing child must, if he is to survive, bond to an attachment figure (usually the mother). If the mother is consistently present, reliable in her handling and 'good enough' in her emotional responsiveness, then a bond of secure attachment will develop. This enables the child to engage in exploratory behaviour, to deal with new situations without becoming over-anxious, and so gradually to separate, safe in the knowledge that the mother is available if necessary. The child builds up an internal image of a good parent which provides a sense of security. If, on the other hand, the early relationship with the parent is disrupted – by separation or by inconsistent handling, for example – the child may develop a bond of anxious attachment. Rather than being able to explore and become autonomous, the child clings to the mother, at first physically and later emotionally, showing signs of distress when separation is threatened. This childhood experience then acts as a template for separations in later life. Faced with threat, the anxious individual clings to attachment figures – spouse, parent, child or doctor.

The following factors should be considered in cases of anxiety:

1. *The nature of the current external threat.* This may be obvious, such as major illness in the patient himself or a close relative. The 'threat' may, on the other hand, appear as trivial or 'normal' as an adolescent leaving home, or a family holiday. For an anxiously attached individual these can be major hurdles.
2. *The relationship to attachment figures, past and present.* A pattern of anxious attachment in childhood, now repeated in relationship to spouse or children, is often found.
3. *'Internal threat'.* Anxious patients often experience an inner conflict between their need for dependency and their feelings about those on whom they depend. The patient is threatened not so much by external circumstances as by himself. A patient who feels angry, for example with an unfaithful spouse, but is unable to express this because of fear of separation and loss, may develop anxiety symptoms. He fears to bite the hand that feeds. The patient is frightened by his own inner impulses: sexual or aggressive feelings, or the wish for independence and autonomy. Anger in particular often co-exists with anxiety; the angry patient is often a frightened one and vice versa.

Management

Michael Balint, a psychoanalyst who pioneered the use of psychotherapeutic methods in medicine, wrote 'the doctor

is a drug: the question is in what dose, and with what frequency it should be prescribed'. The two drugs most commonly prescribed for anxiety are tranquillisers and 'doctor'. Both can be effective in the short term, but can in the long term produce the complication of dependence, and may even exacerbate the symptoms of anxiety.

Exploratory psychotherapy

Normal individuals who become anxious are usually relieved of their fears by *reassurance*, and the ability to reassure is thus an important part of a doctor's skill. Reassurance in neurotic individuals is often ineffective, however, because it deals only with the surface fear and not with the underlying conflict. A man who develops repeated attacks of pain, in which he is convinced that he is about to die of a heart attack, can be reassured that his ECG is normal and that he is a fit man, and be discharged. Yet a few days later, he may develop another attack and present again to the doctor. The *underlying fear*, and root cause of his anxiety, of which he may be unaware or unconscious, may be that his mother, on whom he is very dependent and who has recently had an illness, will die and that he will be left alone. Only when this fear is exposed and when he has learned to accept the dependent part of himself, will his panic attacks cease.

This kind of exploration is helpful in the evaluation of most cases of anxiety. In some cases, it may need to be followed by longer-term psychotherapy. If the patient can learn to resolve his inner conflicts through his relationship with a doctor or therapist, and so move from a position of anxious attachment to one of secure attachment, he will be relieved of his symptoms.

Behavioural psychotherapy

In exploratory psychotherapy the doctor aims to be understanding, but is non-directive. When the patient feels better about himself, then his symptoms and phobic behaviour will disappear. In behavioural psychotherapy, on the other hand, the doctor aims to change the patient's behaviour directly. A phobic patient *associates* the feared stimulus (e.g. a spider or department store) with unpleasant feelings. The therapy aims to *desensitise* the patient by gradual exposure to the feared stimulus, often in the

> **Summary 5   Management of anxiety syndromes**
>
> | | |
> |---|---|
> | *Exploratory psychotherapy* | Exploration and resolution of underlying conflict. Non-directive. |
> | *Behavioural psychotherapy* | Aims to change patients' behaviour directly, through desensitisation |
> | *Psychotropic drugs* | Antidepressants
Minor tranquillisers
Beta-blockers |

reassuring presence of the therapist. An important feature of behavioural treatment for anxiety is *relaxation training*. Here the patient learns to control his anxiety through muscular relaxation and deep breathing, sometimes with the aid of tape-recorded instructions. Physiological measures of arousal – galvanic skin response and pulse rate – may provide objective evidence of anxiety reduction. When self-administered, this is known as *autogenic training*.

Psychotropic drugs

When anxiety is a manifestation of depressive illness, the treatment of depression with antidepressants (many of which are sedative) also relieves the anxiety. Short-term (up to 10 days) prescription of minor tranquillisers such as benzodiazepines is justified for the relief of stress-related anxiety. Longer-term prescription of tranquillisers should be avoided. Beta-receptor blocking drugs relieve the peripheral symptoms of anxiety and may also occasionally be useful. Side-effects of benzodiazepines include: a hangover syndrome (drowsiness, incoordination, ataxia) from the cumulative effect of long-acting drugs like diazepam; and a withdrawal syndrome characterised by insomnia, anxiety, irritability, muscular pains or twitching, perceptual distortion and depression. Occasionally, withdrawal fits may occur.

DEFENCE MECHANISMS

Life is beset with threat. A variety of social and psychological defence mechanisms exist which keep anxiety within manageable limits. Many of these can be observed on hospital wards, where both patients and staff face the daily threat of illness and death and yet usually manage to remain cheerful and efficient.

Denial

'Everything's wonderful'.

One way of dealing with fear or pain is simply to pretend it does not exist. Men are particularly prone to this in everyday life, but false cheerfulness (sometimes known as *manic denial*) may conceal unvoiced fears or sadness.

Dissociation or conversion

'I'm not worried about anything doctor, it's just that I keep getting this pain ...'.

Akin to denial is dissociation, in which a fear is displaced or converted into a bodily symptom. Patients who have inexplicable and elusive pains, in addition to established physical disease, may well be harbouring unspoken fears and conflicts.

Splitting

'You're wonderful doctor, not like those terrible doctors at the other hospital'.

As the Trojans should fear Greeks bearing gifts, so

Summary 6 Defence mechanisms against anxiety	
● Denial	● Idealisation
● Dissociation or conversion	● Regression
● Splitting	● Obsessional defence
● Projection	● Intellectualisation

doctors should beware the patient who heaps excessive praise (as opposed to expressing genuine gratitude). He may be dealing with anxiety by splitting his world into good and bad, and clinging to the good in the vain hope of absolute security. As with the Trojans, the tables may suddenly turn and *we* may be seen as bad, and *they* good. Patients can sometimes split ward staff in this way; physicians and nurses must learn to take both praise and condemnation with a pinch of salt.

Projection

'It's the psychiatrists who are mad, not me'.

Closely linked to splitting is projection, in which unwanted feelings are attributed instead to a convenient other. The reputation of psychiatrists for being neurotic, mad, waffly and sex-obsessed is no doubt partially justified, but is also an example of the disposal of universal fears of inadequacy and madness by projecting them on to others.

Idealisation

'The doctors here are the best in the world'.

White-coated medical attendants are often viewed through rose-tinted spectacles. After all, who would want to be looked after by a *bad* doctor? The defence of idealisation is closely linked to splitting and projection. It is probably best seen as an example of positive *transference*, in which past childhood feelings towards one's parents are, under the threat of illness, transferred on to present medical attendants.

Regression

'Nurse ... nurse ...'.

The sick, like children, are tucked up in bed, fed, pampered and waited on. This sometimes helps the physiology of recovery, but can also lead to helpless behaviour on the part of the patient, who may deal with the fear associated with illness by becoming more and more child-like, regressed and demanding.

Obsessional defences

'I always have my bowels open at such-and-such o'clock doctor'.

The *'malade-à-petit-papier'*, the patient who presents with a written list of symptoms, is a familiar figure in medical folklore. The obsessional defence is an attempt to deal with fear by *control*. This may produce feelings of irritation and discomfort in the doctor that mirror the way the patient feels. This is an example of how the doctor's subjective response to the patient (technically known as *counter-transference*) can be a useful guide to what the patient himself is feeling.

Intellectualisation

'Just a few more tests should clinch the diagnosis'.

This defence applies more to doctors than their patients. Incurable illness and death are inescapable reminders of the limitations of medicine. The feelings of inadequacy and sadness that this creates may be defended against by preoccupation with diagnostic precision and excessive investigation and treatment.

LOSS, GRIEF AND BEREAVEMENT

Man is not an island, and human beings are inevitably vulnerable to loss. The mourning response – a patterned sequence of psychophysiological reactions to the loss of a loved one – is as deeply embedded in our psyche as are the phases of inflammation in our pathophysiology. Common to both are the experience of pain, immobility and gradual recovery.

MOURNING

The mourning response is divided for convenience into a number of stages, but emotional reality does not conform to any such neat sequence. Grief is characterised by surges and cycles of often confused feelings rather than an orderly progression of recognisable developments.

Denial

The initial reaction, especially to sudden bereavement, may be denial: 'Oh no ...'. This attempt to resist the reality of death may persist long after the bereaved have consciously and rationally accepted their loss; they find themselves talking to their lost loved one, or may 'hear' or 'see' them in one of the hallucinatory experiences that may occur after bereavement.

Numbness

Another early response to bereavement is a complete absence of feeling. The bereaved person may appear to be coping very well because of this emotional shutdown which, like the analgesia of a soldier injured in battle, enables him to get through the initial phase of loss. When this is prolonged, however, it produces chronic impoverishment of emotional life.

Searching

Part of the 'work' of grief involves a mental combing-through of events leading up to the loss of the loved one.

Summary 7 Mourning responses	
● Denial	● Anger
● Numbness	● Detachment
● Searching	● Acceptance
● Guilt	

This phase is often accompanied by intense anxiety and restlessness. Searching, a form of separation anxiety, may lead to apparently aimless wandering or visits to familiar spots associated with the lost one. The bereaved person appears to be struggling to negate the reality of the loss, or to rewrite history with a different, happy ending. Acceptance of loss only occurs when this impossible task has been attempted countless times.

Guilt

Pangs of guilt or self-blame are a very common feature of bereavement. Survivors blame themselves, often quite irrationally, for the loss of their beloved. 'If only', they say, 'I had phoned the doctor earlier/not gone on holiday/been kinder ...'. This response can be seen as an example of *omnipotence*, a relic of childish thinking which attempts to deny human vulnerability to fate and fortune.

Anger

Anger and guilt go together in bereavement. Outbursts of anger towards medical staff or close relatives often occur after a death, and should be met by acknowledgement rather than retaliation.

Detachment

As mourning proceeds, so the grieving individual begins to separate himself from his loss and develop new interests and attachments. Pangs of grief recur, particularly at times of stress and on special dates like birthdays, Christmas, and anniversaries of loss.

Acceptance

When mourning is 'successful' and circumstances favourable, the bereaved individual may come to accept that death and loss are part of life and may even be enriched by the experience. This mature state is rare. More usually, scars remain, and many bereaved people continue to struggle with feelings of meaninglessness and diminished vitality for many years.

Physiological changes

Psychological reactions to loss are accompanied by physiological changes, including disturbance of corticosteroid metabolism and depression of T lymphocyte response.

Death from 'a broken heart' is a reality: mortality rates, mainly from coronary artery disease, are higher in widowers than their non-bereaved counterparts.

DELAYED OR PATHOLOGICAL MOURNING

Return to near-normality after a major loss generally takes from nine to eighteen months. However, chronic states of depression, numbness, anger, anxiety and hopelessness can continue for much longer following a bereavement. The patient becomes stuck in one of the phases of mourning and is unable to progress towards detachment and acceptance. The patient becomes frozen at the moment of loss, still surrounded both emotionally and physically by thoughts of the lost one and his or her 'things' and unable to put them aside.

The likelihood of pathological grief depends on four main factors:

1. *Type of death.* A sudden, untimely (for example of a child) or horrifying death is especially hard to accept.
2. *Nature of the relationship.* An *ambivalent* relationship (one in which love and hate co-exist) is more likely to lead to pathological mourning than a straightforward one. Feelings of guilt (associated perhaps with past fantasy-wishes that the person would die) are more intense in such cases. 'Symbiotic' relationships, such as those involving unmarried daughters living with their mothers, are also often difficult to recover from when they are severed.
3. *Personality of the survivor.* Dependent, insecure or depression-prone individuals are more vulnerable to prolonged grief, as are those with difficulty in expressing feelings. The latter may in part account for the greater vulnerability of men to lasting problems after bereavement.
4. *Social circumstances of the survivor.* The lack of close family, friends, religious beliefs or employment all make recovery from loss more difficult.

Management

About one-third of bereaved persons may be in need of professional support or intervention. Support groups, such as those for widows or for parents whose children have died, can be very helpful. Brief psychotherapy may be necessary in order to recapture and work through buried feelings associated with the loss. Sometimes this is systematised as *guided mourning*, in which the sufferer is encouraged to think about his lost one, talk about the details of his or her death, visit the grave, and so face and accept loss with diminished denial.

DEPRESSION

The complaint of 'depression' can refer to a number of different feelings and reactions – anger, boredom, frus-

tration, anxiety, hopelessness and helplessness – as well as the specific psychophysiological state which psychiatry recognizes as 'depressive illness'.

DEPRESSIVE ILLNESS

Clinical features

Clinical depression can be distinguished from both 'ordinary' depression or sadness (transient depressive moods) and depressive personality by three main features:

1. Depressive illness is a *sustained* depression of mood lasting for weeks or months.
2. The *severity* of the depression is great enough to interfere with normal functioning.
3. The depression has a definite onset with a distinct *change* from normal to depressive thinking.

Depressive illness involves an alteration of many different aspects of mind, body and behaviour. It is nearly twice as common in women as in men. The features of depression may be summarised under four main headings:

1. *Depressed mood.* The patient feels weepy and miserable, 'low-in-spirits', anxious, lacking in concentration and irritable. He can take no pleasure in anything. He feels he has no future and that it is pointless or impossible to make plans. Suicide attempts are common and thoughts of suicide almost invariably present, although the patient may try to resist these by saying 'I would not have the courage'.
2. *Low self-esteem.* The patient feels worthless, inadequate, unwanted and useless. He feels intense guilt and plagues himself with thoughts of past failures and mistakes. He can only see himself in a negative light and emphasises his weaknesses and faults.
3. *Physiological changes.* The most important of these is sleep disturbance (Fig. 11.2). Anorexia, weight loss, loss of libido, constipation, retardation (slowing of thought and movement) or occasional agitation are all important features, especially in severe or psychotic depression.
4. *'Atypical' features.* Sometimes a depressed patient may present atypically, with physical symptoms such as unexplained pain, obsessional thoughts, agoraphobia, criminal behaviour (such as shoplifting) or episodes of anger and violence. These may have been brought to the surface by a depressive illness. In a so-called

---

Summary 8 Features of depressive illness

- Sustained
- Severe
- Definite onset
- Depressed mood
- Low self-esteem
- Physiological changes
- Atypical features brought to the surface by depressive illness

---

Normal

Depressed

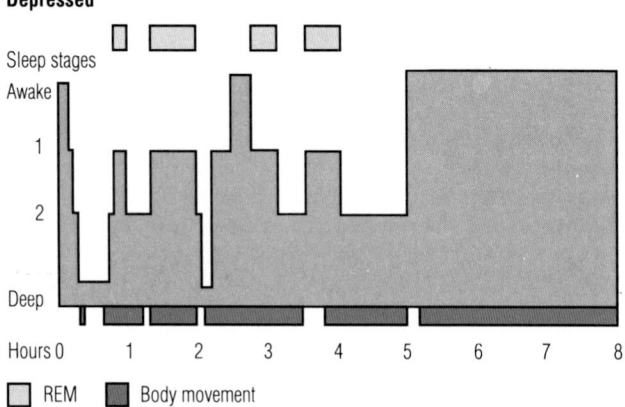

☐ REM   ◼ Body movement

Fig. 11.2 Comparison of sleep patterns in depressed and normal individuals.

Table 11.5 Clinical features of neurotic and psychotic depression

Clinical features	Psychotic	Neurotic
Severity of depression	More severe	Less severe
Delusions/hallucinations	Yes	No
Sleep disturbance	Early morning wakening	Difficulty in getting off to sleep
'Vegetative features' e.g. weight loss, constipation	Yes, prominent	Yes/No
Diurnal mood variation	Worse on wakening and a.m.	No, or worse p.m.
'Reactive', i.e. precipitated by loss	Yes	Yes
Genetic factors e.g. family history of manic-depressive psychosis	Yes	No
Dexamethasone suppression tests	Yes	No
Response to tricyclic antidepressants	Yes	Yes
Response to ECT	Yes	No

'smiling' or 'masked' depression, the patient conceals severe depressive feelings behind a cheerful facade.

Although the presentation of depressive illness can vary greatly, there are two common clinical pictures (Table 11.5).

Neurotic depression

Here the patient, despite depressive feelings, remains in contact with reality: 'I know it is stupid, but I feel *as though* I have let everybody down'. The patient might be a woman in her thirties with several small children, living in poor housing and with a husband who drinks and is having an affair which she has just discovered. She is tearful, has lost weight and cannot fall asleep at night. She feels she is not coping with her job or housework, and no longer enjoys company or television.

Psychotic depression

Depressive psychosis is a part of manic-depressive psychosis, an *affective psychosis*. The depth of the depression is here much greater than in neurotic depression. The ratio of women to men affected is more equal. The patient becomes immobilised both in thought and action. He wakes very early in the morning (Fig. 11.2) and has marked diurnal mood variation, feeling at his worst in the morning and improving slightly towards the evening. He develops depressive delusions, becoming convinced that he has, for example, brought ruin on his family, that he is evil or ugly or radioactive. Depressive hallucinations may occur: he may hear a voice telling him that he is evil, or he may feel that his insides are rotting and complain that he smells. Endocrine disturbance may occur in psychotic depression, with disruption of the pituitary-adrenal axis. The normal diurnal variation of cortisol output is abolished, providing the basis of the *dexamethasone suppression test*. Dexamethasone is administered but fails to reduce urinary steroid levels in many, but not all, cases of severe/psychotic depression.

Differential diagnosis of depression

The differential diagnosis of depression includes:

1. *organic illness*, especially hypothyroidism
2. *drugs*, especially steroids and some antihypertensive drugs
3. *alcohol-induced depression*, where depression is secondary to alcoholism (or drug addiction), and withdrawal of the intoxicant results in lifting of depressive symptoms
4. *anxiety states*, as anxiety is a common feature of depression. When they co-exist, treatment of the depression usually, but not always, removes the anxiety
5. *depressive psychoses*, which must be distinguished from other psychoses, especially schizophrenia.

The causes of depression

Depression is often divided into:

1. *Reactive depression*, whose symptoms correspond with neurotic depression and which is said to be a response to external events
2. *Endogenous depression*, where the symptoms are psychotic in character and where there is no clear environmental precipitant.

The distinction is misleading. Psychotic depression is usually also 'reactive', in the sense that it is triggered by a painful event in the patient's life; and neurotic depression can be 'endogenous', in the sense that genetic and personality factors influence the likelihood of an individual developing depression in response to misfortune.

Loss

Loss plays a central role in the origins of depression, and is the link connecting *grief* with depression. The grieving person is in pain not only because he has lost an external relationship, but because he has lost a part of himself. His internal world as well as his external world has been impoverished. The similarity between the clinical features of grief and those of depression are striking. In grief, an external loss dominates the picture; in depression, it is an internal feeling of loss. In 70% of depressions, there has been a preceding external loss or stress: a bereavement (delayed grief is best seen as a special case of depression), loss of job, break-up of a relationship, child leaving home or a theft, for example. It is when this then leads to a feeling of internal loss – of optimism, vitality and (especially) of self-esteem – that a depression occurs.

Whether or not a particular individual reacts to loss by developing depression depends on a number of inter-

---

> **Summary 9   Factors contributing to depression**
>
> - Loss
> - Genetic
> - Biochemical
>   e.g. neurotransmitter biochemistry
> - Social
>   e.g. lack of close relationships, unemployment, lack of good child-hood experiences to build self-esteem, learned helplessness.

related factors: genetic, social, developmental and psychological.

Genetic/biochemical make-up

Twin studies have shown that genetic factors play an important part in manic-depressive psychosis. Changes in neurotransmitter biochemistry in depression are important: current views emphasise reduction of catecholamine levels at postsynaptic nerve endings. Antidepressant drugs may work through the prevention of breakdown, or reduction in re-uptake, of cerebral amines at central nerve endings (Fig. 11.3).

Current social situation

The presence of a close confiding relationship, usually with a spouse, protects individuals from developing depression after the experience of loss. Employment is another protective factor; the unemployed are thus doubly vulnerable to depression, the loss of a job being a precipitant and lack of a job being a vulnerability factor. Women with three or more children under 15 and long-term social and financial difficulties are more vulnerable to depression following loss.

Fig. 11.3   Cellular mode of action of antidepressants. 1. In normal individuals, there is an adequate quantity of neurotransmitter amine within the presynaptic neurone (A). Some amine is degraded by MAO (B). Amine is then stored in presynaptic vesicles (C) or released from the neurone and taken up by the postsynaptic neurone (D). Some released transmitter is taken up into the presynaptic vesicles (E). **2.** With depression, neurotransmitter amines are reduced, and less are therefore available for release from the presynaptic neurone and subsequent uptake by the postsynaptic neurone. **3.** Treatment with monoamine oxidase inhibitors reduces neurotransmitter breakdown, thereby increasing the amine available for release from the presynaptic neurone. **4.** The tricyclic drugs increase the amine available for uptake by the postsynaptic neurone, by blocking the re-absorption of released amine by the presynaptic neurone.

Early childhood experience

Women who have lost their mothers before the age of 11 – whether through death, separation (for example, due to illness) or divorce – are especially vulnerable to depression in later life. A reservoir of good experiences in childhood is needed for an individual to develop a lasting sense of self-esteem. This provides a child with a good and secure internal world which can withstand the inevitable separations and losses of later life, and enables him to respond to such situations with appropriate sadness rather than by developing depression. If, however, the child has insufficient good experiences with which to balance the bad, he will find it difficult to be self-assertive or to express anger openly for fear of driving away what little support he has. He may turn his anger on himself and become stuck with bad feelings which then form the nucleus of depressive low self-esteem. He is liable to form dependent relationships and is vulnerable to depression.

Psychological factors

Recent studies of depression have focused on the vicious circle of depressive thinking. The depressed individual has developed *learned helplessness* – he feels that nothing he can do will make any difference to his situation. He therefore avoids actions and experiences which *might* make him feel better, and continues to view himself in a negative light. His depression thus becomes a self-fulfilling prophecy.

Management

Mild depression

This is best dealt with by psychotherapy, which may take one of three forms.

Exploratory psychotherapy.   Here, the patient is encouraged to express depressive feelings, to vent his anger and despair and – through the relationship with the therapist (who may be a GP, social worker, psychotherapist or physician) – to experience the containment that was lacking in childhood and so to recognise and recapture some of the good experiences which the depression has blotted out.

Cognitive behaviour therapy.   This counteracts learned helplessness and negative depressive thinking both by challenging the erroneous assumptions on which they are based and by considering positive features of the self. The patient is encouraged to set himself small, easily accomplished tasks and to feel pleased if he succeeds.

Family and marital therapy.   Here, the aim is to improve the marital relationship which can then provide a bulwark against depression in response to loss.

Moderate depression

A combination of antidepressant drugs and psychotherapy can be more effective than either alone in treating moderate depression. Both depressed mood and biological symptoms improve with drugs; low self-esteem and social difficulties improve with psychotherapy. The first-line drugs are the tricyclics such as dothiepin or amitriptyline (75–200 mg/day), which should always be tried when sleeplessness and guilt are prominent features. They take 10–14 days to produce full effect. Side-effects include parasympathomimetic symptoms of dry mouth and urinary retention, constipation, blurred vision and 'muzziness'; and cardiac arrythmias can occur. Tricyclics should be avoided in patients with prostatism or a history of heart disease. Mianserin, a tetracyclic, has fewer side-effects but can produce haematological reactions and is possibly also less effective in its antidepressant action. The mode of action of antidepressant drugs is summarised in Figure 11.3. Monoamine oxidase inhibitors (MAOIs) such as tranylcypromine are still occasionally useful as second-line drugs, especially when phobic symptoms are present; but dietary restrictions (e.g. no cheese or yeast-extract) are needed because of harmful (hypertensive) interactions with tyramine-containing substances.

Severe depression

Depressed patients who are severely ill, psychotic or actively suicidal require hospital admission. Tricyclics, which may have to be given in large doses (up to 250 mg of amitriptyline daily), are the first line of treatment. Despite debate about its mode of action and efficacy, controlled trials of electroconvulsive therapy (ECT) have shown it to be an effective and rapid treatment for depressive delusions and hallucinations; it is also free of side-effects. ECT is a first-line treatment in depressive stupor or where the patient is refusing food and drink. In the United Kingdom it can only be given without the patient's consent after Section 3 of the 1983 Mental Health Act has been applied and a second, independent, psychiatric opinion obtained.

Chronic or recurrent depression

Most depressive illness has a tendency to remit, but relapse is common. Prolonged low-dose treatment with tricyclics may have a prophylactic effect, as may psychotherapy. Relapse of depressive psychosis may in some cases be prevented by prophylactic lithium carbonate. Chronic depressive states are rare but disabling, and prolonged attendance at a supportive day hospital may be required.

MANIA AND HYPOMANIA

Clinical features

In depression, mood is abnormally lowered. In *mania*, or its milder form *hypomania*, it is abnormally elevated. In *unipolar manic-depressive psychosis*, the patient may have recurrent depressive, or recurrent manic episodes. If both manic and depressive episodes occur, the patient has *bipolar manic-depressive psychosis*.

There are three main groups of symptoms in mania and hypomania:

1. *Psychological symptoms*. The patient feels elated, cheerful and expansive, and his thoughts are speeded up. He may develop *grandiose delusions* of wealth, potency and fame. He is full of optimistic (and unrealistic) plans for the future.
2. *Physical symptoms*. He is restless, sleeps little, eats voraciously or not at all, often loses weight, has poor concentration and tries to do several things at once.
3. *Behavioural symptoms*. The patient often spends large amounts of money, dresses flamboyantly and may behave in an outrageous, disinhibited and promiscuous manner. Outbursts of irritability and aggression are common. His speech is rapid, may be incoherent and flits from subject to subject (known as *flight of ideas*). He is often humorous in an irreverent and infectious way.

Hypomania frequently co-exists with depressive symptoms: the patient laughs and cries almost simultaneously. This is known as a *mixed affective state*.

Hypomanic episodes may, like depression, be triggered by a painful rejection or loss. This has led to the concept of *manic defence*, whereby the patient escapes into mania as a way of avoiding unhappy or sad feelings.

Management

A hypomanic patient can cause havoc to both himself and his family. Hospital admission is often indicated but may be hard to achieve voluntarily as the patient denies illness, often indeed claiming he has never felt better, or has discovered the secret of life. Immediate management is with tranquillisers such as chlorpromazine or haloperidol. Subsequent relapses may be prevented by prophylactic lithium carbonate.

SOMATOFORM DISORDERS

Somatoform disorders are conditions in which (a) physical symptoms are present for which no organic or physiological basis can be found, and (b) where there are demonstrable underlying psychological factors or conflicts. In other words, *the physical symptoms may be manifestations of psychological distress*.

Terminology and definitions

There are several terms commonly used to describe physical disorder in which psychological mechanisms may be important.

The outmoded, but still widely used, term *psychosomatic* illness refers to conditions in which there is definite *structural* physical illness (e.g. bowel inflammation in ulcerative colitis) but whose precipitant or maintaining factors are considered to be in part psychological.

The term *functional* is sometimes used to describe symptoms produced by changes in organ *function* in the absence of structural change. Functional illness may or may not be psychological in origin. Functional bowel disease (irritable bowel syndrome, see p. 609), for example, may result from faulty diet or disturbance of the autonomic system (potentially stress-related) or both.

The term *psychogenic* usually implies that the symptoms are entirely psychological in origin. Many of the ill-defined conditions seen in general practice and medical outpatients could be labelled as psychogenic, although this term may obscure the fact that physical factors (e.g. muscular tension) are also important.

The concept of *hysteria* (p. 199) has a long history and has become differentiated from the more non-specific psychogenic symptoms. Hysteria is divided into two types:

1. *Conversion disorders*. These are psychogenic illnesses – often simulating neurological disorders – based on unconscious mechanisms, in which mental conflict is avoided both by converting anxiety into physical symptoms (hence *conversion* hysteria) and by *dissociation* (i.e. a split between the mental self and the physical self).
2. *Somatisation disorders*. These are polysymptomatic disorders in which the patient experiences multiple unexplained symptoms without physical disease and in the context of a disturbed personality.

In psychosomatic illness psychological factors may well aggravate, prolong or cause relapses in an illness whose basis is physical (just as a poor ward atmosphere has been shown to delay postoperative wound healing). Psychogenic symptoms are often based on circular patterns in which, for example, emotional conflict produces muscular tension, which results in pain which leads to greater emotional stress, or anxiety (e.g. fear that the pain may be due to cancer) which results in more muscular tension and so on.

MIND-BODY MODELS

There are two extreme but widely held views on the nature of psychosomatic illness. The first, corresponding to the philosophical position of *materialism*, holds that all phenomena are physical in origin and denies the existence of the mind. For the materialist, there are no psychogenic conditions, only illnesses whose physical cause has yet to be determined. The second, *idealist*, view holds that psychosomatic illness is mental in origin.

There are problems in both these models. The materialist might point to the numbers of patients labelled as hysterical who have subsequently died of carcinoma or multiple sclerosis; but he cannot altogether deny the existence of mind. The idealist, on the other hand, tends to confuse the symbolic *meaning* of an illness with its *cause*, claiming, for example, that a man who developed oesophageal cancer did so because he could not *swallow* his wife's infidelity. A classic error of this type was the pre-1956 theory of Down's syndrome. This held that Down's syndrome was caused by physical or mental trauma in pregnancy, since mothers of Down's syndrome babies regularly reported such traumatic incidents. Only when the chromosomal abnormality responsible was found, was it realised that the trauma theory was a retrospective rationalisation rather than a causal explanation.

In reality, the relationship between mind and body is far more complicated than either the pure materialist or idealist models allow. The interesting questions concern the *interactions* between the mental and the physical, just as the interesting problems in genetics involve interactions between heredity and environment.

Experimental evidence

There is evidence that painful events in a person's life can precipitate physical illness. The link between stress and myocardial infarction, for example, is well documented (Fig. 11.4). Bowel disease, such as ulcerative colitis or even appendicitis, may also be triggered by a preceding painful or stressful life event.

Personality plays an important part in determining the impact of such events. Individuals with 'type A personality' (competitive, driving) are, other factors being equal, more likely to develop coronary artery disease than those with more placid temperaments. Similarly the prognosis of breast cancer may depend in part on personality; women who are emotionally inhibited appear to have, on average, a less good prognosis than those more able to express anger and sadness. The *intervening variables* that link the psychological to the physical are largely unknown. Autonomic and corticosteroid responses to stress play their part, as do changes in the immune system (especially T-lymphocytes); but the precise pathways and links remain to be elucidated. Current evidence does not support the view that psychosomatic diseases are *primarily* psychological in origin; nor that any *specific* relationship exists between personality type and a particular disease or target organ.

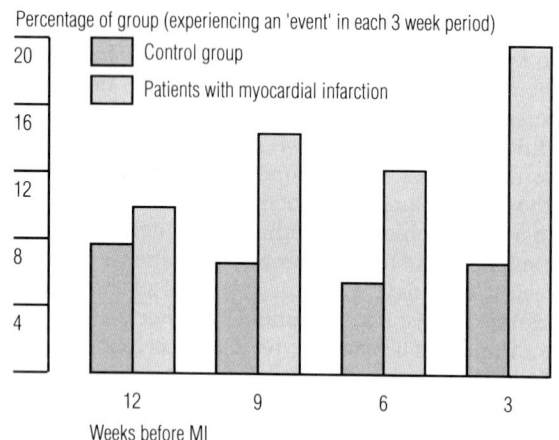

Percentage of group (experiencing an 'event' in each 3 week period)

Control group
Patients with myocardial infarction

Weeks before MI

Fig. 11.4 Experience of potentially stressful life events by myocardial infarction patients in the 12 weeks before MI occurred.

PSYCHOLOGICAL APPROACHES TO SOMATOFORM DISORDERS

The contribution of psychiatry to the understanding of psychosomatic and psychogenic illness can be considered under three headings: the development of the body image; repression and the unconscious; and the language of illness.

Development of the body image

In adult life mind and body are separate realms. The body is experienced as an object among other objects in the world; but is also, for its 'owner', the source of knowledge and sensation, and the means by which contact and communication with others is possible. The mind, though experienced as a separate domain, is indissolubly connected to the body. As Freud pointed out, it only takes a toothache to feel that 'the molar hole contains my soul'.

The adult state in which the self comfortably inhabits both mind and body, experiencing each as separate and yet connected, is a complex product of health, maturity and culture. The infant is born in a state of psychosomatic unity: pain for a young child is both mental and physical. In adult life physical illness may produce *regression* to a child-like state. Childhood experiences may play a crucial part in determining later relationships between mind and body. In early childhood, the parents' love and care for the child and his body sow the seed of healthy self-love in later life. A girl who was 'meant' to be a boy may have to struggle with the effects of her parents' disappointment for years to come. Later, the adolescent has to learn to accept his or her body and sexuality. Self-acceptance is an essential precondition of loving others. When this process is disturbed some individuals may, when anxious, ask their doctor for an examination, complaining that there is something wrong with their body or even asking for it to be changed by plastic surgery. The patient is looking for the acceptance and care he feels he missed from his parents. If external relationships fail, he may turn for interest and gratification to his own body and this too can lead to development of, and preoccupation with, psychogenic physical symptoms.

Repression and the unconscious

Repression is the active removal from consciousness of painful or disturbing thoughts, feelings or memories. The mind's eye is blinded to problems and conflicts. The difficulties and the feelings they evoke remain, however, even though the patient is *unconscious* of them. They may then manifest themselves in physical symptoms, by the process of displacement.

The language of illness

Not all cultures make the firm distinction between mind and body customary in the West. In such societies, emotional distress is habitually expressed via physical symptoms; it is this easy traffic between body and thought that holistic medicine attempts to recapture. Even in the West, words such as 'energy', 'stress', 'pain' and 'weakness' have both psychological and physical connotations, and are often used in both senses simultaneously. The doctor should always listen to the specific language used by the patient to express his distress. A woman who is 'choked' with grief about her mother's death may develop globus hystericus (p. 566). A man who complains of 'weakness' or poor 'performance' at work may really be worried about impotence.

HYSTERIA

The three essential features of hysteria are: physical symptoms, absence of organic pathology and psychological conflict. The modern concept of hysteria can be traced back to ancient Greece, the word deriving from *hysteros* (the womb). Although it is no longer believed that hysteria is due to a wandering or sex-starved womb, emotional conflict is still thought to be a possible element in its origin.

Classification and clinical features

There are three main patterns of hysteria: monosymptomatic, polysymptomatic and epidemic.

Monosymptomatic hysteria (conversion disorder)

Typically there is gross loss of neurological function. This may involve:

1. the limbs, e.g. paralysis, anaesthesia or dystonia
2. the higher functions, e.g. hysterical fits, hysterical blindness, *fugue states* (in which the patient has complete memory loss), or even *hysterical psychosis* (where the patient develops a short-lived and dramatic psychosis in response to external stress).

The pattern of dysfunction follows the patient's 'idea' of how the body works rather than anatomy. Similarly, in hysterical psychosis the patient behaves in the way he thinks a madman ought to behave, rather than demonstrating the specific symptoms of schizophrenia. A neurologist can usually determine the integrity of the nervous system either by subtle physical examination (extensor activity in apparently paralysed limbs) or by investigation (intact visual-evoked potentials in hysterical blindness). The patient may also exhibit the *belle indifférence* described by Janet, i.e. an apparent lack of anxiety in the face of crippling disorder. Psychophysiological measures of arousal show that hysterical patients are in fact often highly aroused despite the absence of manifest anxiety.

Polysymptomatic hysteria (Briquet's syndrome, somatisation disorder)

Polysymptomatic hysterics (usually women in their thirties) develop a wide variety of physical complaints with no organic basis over a number of years. These often involve pain centering around the abdomen, back and pelvis. Such patients have often been extensively investigated by physicians and frequently admitted to hospital. Their medical notes are thick but inconclusive. Unlike patients with monosymptomatic hysteria, their prognosis is poor and is related to general personality difficulties rather than a specific conflict.

They risk developing iatrogenic illness as a result of inappropriate medication or investigation; they may, for example, present with a genuine recurrent 'acute abdomen' due to postoperative adhesions, stemming from exploratory laparotomy for unexplained abdominal pain.

Epidemic hysteria

This rare and self-limiting condition occurs in schools and other situations where young people are in close proximity. Fainting, nausea and paraesthesia brought on by overbreathing are common presentations. The condition is sometimes, wrongly, assumed to have an infective cause.

Diagnosis

Hysteria is not an easy diagnosis to make. It can be made too readily and should never be a substitute for thorough history-taking and examination, or diagnostic acumen. A proportion of patients diagnosed as hysterical turn out to have genuine organic disease: multiple sclerosis or occult cancer, for example. Others may develop another psychiatric condition such as a depressive illness or even schizophrenia. However, it is important to recognise and diagnose hysteria when it does occur, so as to spare the patient unnecessary investigation. Hysteria and organic illness can also, and often do, co-exist; establishing one diagnosis should not prevent searching for another.

Meaning and aetiology

The manifestations of hysteria are often dramatic, and therein lies a clue to its nature. Most people, especially as children, have the capacity to act a role. This involves an internal *splitting*, or *dissociation*, between the actor and his part. The actor is not really Hamlet, yet becomes Hamlet as he acts the role. The hysteric is not paralysed and yet, psychologically, can become so.

According to Freud, the symptoms in hysteria have a *meaning* which can be understood in terms of the patient's

---

Summary 10   Psychological mechanisms in hysteria

- Dissociation
- Denial
- Primary gain – elimination of mental pain
- Secondary gain – attention, care
- Identification
- Illness behaviour
- Unconscious avoidance of conflict

life. Psychological theories of hysteria also highlight several other important aspects of the illness:

1. *Defence.* Hysteria is a defence against the anxiety created by conflict. A young man from an academically minded family was facing exams which he feared he would fail; he became paralysed. A young woman left home to get married, missed her parents desperately but did not want to leave her husband; she developed hysterical fits.

2. *Unconscious behaviour.* Although a conflict is often obvious to others, the patient is *unconscious* of it.

3. *Personal gain.* There are two kinds of gain for patients in being ill. The *primary gain* is the fact that they are unaware of their conflict. The *secondary gain* is the care and attention they get from family, friends and relatives. This is only possible if the family to some extent go along with, or allow the patient to *manipulate* them. Here they may be meeting their own needs, for example, the husband who only feels potent when he has a sick wife to look after. 'Manipulation' is a normal process in childhood, and hysteria always has child-like aspects. The child who does not want to go to school develops a tummy-ache; his mother lets him stay at home with her. A similar process is at work in hysteria. The child is not consciously making himself ill or *malingering* (as, for example, the soldier is, who deliberately shoots himself in the foot to avoid going to battle). There really is a pain, even if it clears up quickly once the danger of having to go to school has passed.

4. *Identification.* A common finding in the histories of hysterical patients is that there has been a close relative who has suffered illness, often serious. The young man who became paralysed because he feared his exams had had a younger brother who had died with cerebral palsy and on whom his parents had lavished all their care and attention. The patient often has such a model of illness and its accompanying behaviour which influences him. Sociologists speak of 'illness behaviour' to describe the socially sanctioned behaviour which accompanies illness and which is not strictly related to the pathophysiology of the disease. Sick people are allowed to retire temporarily from work and spend time in bed; they receive flowers, cards and gifts from relatives and are treated with special consideration; they are allowed to be childish and demanding. Their medical attendants also adopt a particular role, usually one of reassurance, benevolence and quasi-omniscience. One of the rules of illness behaviour seems to be that the patient should recover, or at least attempt to recover. When this does not happen there may be a sudden switch: the previously privileged patient may be seen as manipulative, attention-seeking and deviant, and be shunned or covertly punished by irate relatives and medical attendants. In hysteria this often results in a worsening of the symptoms.

Management

It is tempting to try to argue a hysterical patient out of his illness: to tell him there is 'nothing wrong' with him. Occasionally, this can be helpful; but more often it entrenches the patient more deeply in his symptoms and an escalating battle between doctor and patient may then ensue. There is, moreover, a sense in which the patient is right (it is a useful principle in medicine to assume that the patient, like the customer, is always right). There is something wrong, namely a psychological conflict, albeit one of which he is unconscious.

A more helpful approach is therefore to adopt a *psychosomatic attitude*. This involves explaining to the patient that stress can cause illness, that he may have a psychological conflict, and that there may be a connection between this and his physical problem, both of which are real. The patient who has committed himself to a physical illness should be offered appropriate physical treatments (e.g. physiotherapy, massage) and should not be deprived of it out of spite. And when recovery does take place the temptation to say 'I told you so' should be resisted. Instead, the patient needs a face-saving formula; the paralysed person must be allowed to put his crutch down gradually, inadvertently even, not have it knocked from under him.

The psychological principles of treatment of hysteria may be summarised as follows:

1. *Exploration of conflict.* With allowance for face-saving, this is perhaps the most helpful strategy. If the conflict is removed (e.g. the time for exams past) the symptoms will usually remit.

2. *Behavioural approaches.* These are often useful. They (a) aim to avoid reinforcement of the symptoms, for example by suggesting to ward staff or relatives that they respond positively to any signs of movement in the paralysed patient, but as far as possible ignore (non-punitively) helpless behaviour; (b) are directed towards helping the patient overcome his cognitive responses (e.g. of panic and catastrophe) towards the imagined illness.

3. *Drugs.* Where hysteria is secondary to a depressive illness antidepressants should be prescribed. In general, however, drug treatment should be avoided in hysteria as the patient is often very suggestible and tends to develop dramatic reactions and side-effects. Hysterical amnesia can sometimes be approached by *abreaction*, in which painful experiences are 'relived'

Summary 11   Treatment in hysteria

- 'Psychosomatic' attitude on part of doctor
- Exploration of conflict
- Behavioural approaches
- (Antidepressants)
- Abreaction
- Long-term psychotherapy

with the help of an intravenous injection of a sedative drug such as diazepam.
4. *Psychotherapy.* Some patients will benefit from long-term psychotherapy.

HYSTERICAL PERSONALITY AND RELATED CONDITIONS

There are a number of conditions which are related to hysteria, but take the form of a life-long personality disorder rather than an illness. These conditions share with hysteria the capacity for *dissociation* and the use of illness for *manipulation* of those around them.

HYSTERICAL PERSONALITY

A patient with hysterical personality (usually female) finds it difficult to form close attachments and when she does they are highly dependent. Her emotions are often superficial and rarely satisfying. She may be very alluring and attractive to men, but finds it difficult to enjoy sex herself. She carries with her an atmosphere of drama: her life is often a series of emotional or practical crises. Her feelings are dramatised and exaggerated; her headaches are always 'migraines', her diarrhoea 'dysentery' and her pains invariably 'excruciating'. She uses her crises to coerce those around her (including doctors and nurses) and sometimes has a husband whom she abuses and yet clings to, and who appears to submit willingly to all her demands. As a child she may have felt emotionally neglected and insignificant, helpless and dependent. The anger and manipulation which manifest themselves in adult life can be seen as a continuation of this, an attempt, through the coercive power of illness, to keep attached to her those whom she feels may otherwise ignore or abandon her. Patients with hysterical personality sometimes develop the physical symptoms of hysteria.

MULTIPLE PERSONALITY

The adult personality is made up from a number of elements:

1. Some come from *identifications* based on parents ('he has his father's temper and his mother's charm').
2. Some represent different aspects of the *self*: the caring self, the aggressive self, the childish part of the self and so on.
3. Some can be defined in terms of *relationships*: in a marriage a partner may be expected to be a spouse, lover, parent, colleague and friend.

Eric Berne has summarised these different aspects of the self as 'parent', 'adult' and 'child', all of whom co-exist within one person. In the mature personality, there is a blending together of the different aspects into a coherent whole so that a person is all of a piece, although minor discontinuities and splits in the personality are common.

The fascinating but rare clinical cond[...] sonality, in which several quite s[...] appear to inhabit the same individua[...] works as *Dr Jekyll and Mr Hyde* an[...] *Eve*), is an extreme example of this [...] multiple personality, the different p[...] of their own which are entirely a[...] another; the good self is totally unaware [...] would be horrified by its activities. Th[...] prudish aspect of the self to live alongside the sexual side without being aware of it, thereby avoiding anxiety or guilt. Patients with multiple personality can occasionally be helped towards integration with psychotherapy.

FACTITIOUS ILLNESS

Patients with unexplained symptoms are sometimes found – often after lengthy investigation – to have caused their own illness. A patient with unexplained and extensively investigated 'haemoptysis' was found to be vene-puncturing herself, swallowing blood and then spitting into a sputum pot; a person with unexplained intestinal bleeding may be inserting foreign bodies into the rectum; hypoglycaemic attacks can be produced by insulin injections in non-diabetics; and dermatitis artefacta (p. 1150) is yet another example of such factitious illness. Occasionally, such behaviour is due to psychosis but more often it is a manifestation of a personality disorder. These patients are often very 'nice'; they may be nurses or members of the other caring professions. They are often on good, even intimate, terms with medical staff. They may induce incomprehension, abhorrence and anger once they are discovered. Factitious illness is best seen as an extreme example of hysterical personality disorder. The patient has split off an angry, destructive, defiant part of herself which acts semi-autonomously and of which the 'good' self may be partially unaware. The principles of management of hysteria may be applied in these cases. A full history will reveal underlying conflicts, and the patient can then be told, in as gentle and unconfrontational a way as possible, that these conflicts may be responsible for her symptoms and that she may thus be playing a part in causing her own illness. Although the patient may become angry, the results of such an approach are rarely disastrous. The patient will often be relieved and even begin to accept psychological help.

FICTITIOUS ILLNESS: MUNCHAUSEN SYNDROME

Baron von Munchausen was a 19th century fictional character who travelled extensively and told fantastic stories. His name is now used to describe a group of patients with characteristic features:

1. The patients often experience recurrent unexplained symptoms, especially abdominal or chest pain, which are often thought to be due to renal colic, myocardial infarction or intestinal obstruction. The patient may be given opiates and have had several inconclusive

Summary 12	Conditions related to hysterical personality
Multiple personality	Aspects of the self entirely dissociated from one another, with lives of their own
Factitious illness	Illness, or a symptom suggestive of illness, which is self-inflicted
Fictitious illness (Munchausen syndrome)	Patient travels from hospital to hospital with fictitious illnesses. Pseudologia phantastica

laparotomies which reveal themselves as multiple abdominal scars.

2. These patients travel from hospital to hospital, usually discharging themselves after a brief admission, and using a variety of assumed names.
3. They give dramatic accounts of their lives, for example stories of heroic wartime feats or tragic losses, none of which can be corroborated and none of which quite adds up. These stories are sometimes labelled *pseudologia phantastica*.

Munchausen patients may be seen as the male counterparts of factitious illness patients. They are hard if not impossible to manage or help but awareness of the diagnosis will avoid unnecessary or dangerous investigations. Most doctors have had at least one experience of being hoodwinked in this way and this may be a necessary learning experience. The doctor must be friendly but firm in his refusal to treat these patients as though they are ill. The patient usually disappears, but may occasionally accept social help. Although patients with Munchausen syndrome are not of course immune to real organic illness, obsessional medical preoccupation with 'missing something' and hence unnecessary admission and investigation should be avoided.

EATING DISORDERS

Eating is not just about physiology. Food has great psychological and sociological significance. Morality starts with the child's discovery of what is good and bad to eat and a mother's self-evaluation may continue to depend on how well she feels she feeds her family. Birth, the reaching of adulthood, marriage and death are all marked by a meal. In addition, there are two factors, specific to many highly industrialised Western societies, of especial relevance to eating disorders: the role of the food industry with its large marketing system; and the emphasis on a slim body image as a mark of vitality and attractiveness.

Eating disorders are increasingly common, especially among women (Fig. 11.5). Although the overall incidence of anorexia nervosa is only 1 per 100 000 population, 1% of 16–18 year olds are affected; 2% of women attending a family planning clinic suffer from bulimia nervosa; and the prevalence among dance students is 20%.

ANOREXIA NERVOSA

Aetiology and pathogenesis

No single cause of anorexia nervosa has been found. A number of factors appear to be involved:

1. *Social pressures* towards eating and thinness, though often contradictory, are important.
2. The *fear of losing control* – both of eating and of sexuality – and a feeling of inadequacy and of not being a separate person are characteristic of the anorexic's inner world. Anorexia is an attempt by the individual to remain in complete control by regulating her food intake and her weight, and thereby putting her sexuality into reverse.
3. *Family function* in anorexia is often abnormal. The families (where food is frequently a central theme) tend to be 'enmeshed', i.e. mutually overdependent. This causes little difficulty in early childhood, but with the advent of adolescence the family may be threatened by the possibility of autonomy and separation. There is often a fear that the parents will split up when the children leave home and the anorexic adolescent may thus sometimes be seen as vainly trying to separate herself from the family without leaving home.
4. *Endocrine abnormalities* occur in anorexia nervosa. Hypothalamic function is disturbed with reduced luteinising hormone (LH) and gonadotrophic

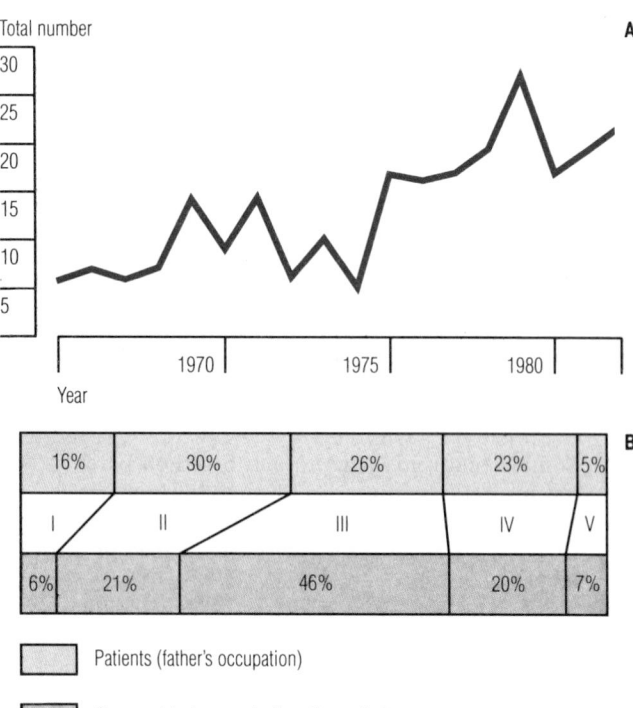

Fig. 11.5 Epidemiology of anorexia nervosa. A. New cases of anorexia nervosa appearing on the Aberdeen Psychiatric Register, 1965–82 (both sexes and all ages). **B.** Social class distribution of anorexic patients (father's occupation) compared with that for general population.

hormone output, but this is more probably a consequence rather than a cause of weight loss. Low levels of plasma thyroxine and plasma TSH are also common. There may be alkalosis if there is surreptitious vomiting.

Summary 13 Features of anorexia nervosa

- Phobic avoidance of normal weight
- Relentless dieting
- Self-induced vomiting, laxatives
- Excessive exercise
- Amenorrhoea
- Lanugo hair
- Hypotension
- Denial, concealment
- Overperception of body image
- Enmeshed families

Clinical features

Four features are characteristic of anorexia nervosa.

1. The most important is *phobic avoidance of normal weight*. The patient is terrified by the idea of her normal weight.
2. With this goes a distortion of body image, known as *overperception*. By asking women to choose a silhouette that they feel represents their shape, it can be shown that it is normal for women aged 15–30 to perceive themselves as up to 50% fatter than they really are. Patients with anorexia nervosa see themselves as at least 100% bigger than they are: an emaciated girl of 35 kg may be disgusted by what she perceives as her gross obesity.
3. The consequence of phobic avoidance and overperception is *relentless dieting*, especially the renunciation of carbohydrates.
4. *Amenorrhoea* is an essential diagnostic feature. In males (10% of all anorexics) there is *disturbance of sexual function*, usually with loss of libido.

Anorexia nervosa usually starts in early or mid-adolescence. There is frequently an initial period of mild overweight, which may appal the girl, who then begins to pursue thinness. Her thoughts are dominated by food and how to avoid it. She absents herself from family meals although she may pride herself on providing food for others, whilst secretly despising and envying those who eat normally, or as she sees it, gluttonously. As long as she is thin she will be happy. To be thin is to be good; fat, bad. She may augment her efforts at dieting by taking laxatives, amphetamines or diuretics, and by self-induced vomiting. Battles about food may develop with her parents. *Denial* of weight loss (p. 191) is an important feature: she may conceal her emaciation within voluminous and floppy clothes. She is physically active or over-active as part of her secret plan for weight loss. Sometimes, deliberately *excessive exercise* may be a major factor in the weight loss. She complains of a feeling of 'fullness' in her stomach which prevents her from eating. She will be emotionally and socially, but not intellectually, less mature than her peer-group.

Physical examination will reveal thinness, scanty secondary sex characteristics, a possible peripheral cyanosis, a soft downy covering of the face and body (*lanugo hair*), hypotension and bradycardia.

Differential diagnosis

The clinical picture may be one of two types:

1. In *typical* anorexia the only obvious psychological abnormality is the difficulty in eating. Here, the main differential diagnoses are organic causes of weight loss in a young woman: malabsorption syndrome, thyrotoxicosis or occult neoplasm. These can usually be excluded by the history but relevant investigations should be carried out.
2. An *atypical* picture also occurs. Here the woman is often older (in her twenties) and her anorexic symptoms co-exist with other psychiatric features, such as depressive symptoms of misery and withdrawal; obsessional symptoms centering, for example, around cleanliness; and personality difficulties.

Summary 14 Factors contributing to anorexia nervosa

- Contradictory social attitudes towards eating and thinness
- Enmeshed, i.e. mutually overdependent, families
- Fear of loss of control of eating and of sexuality
- Fear of separation

Management

A patient weighing less than 35 kg should be admitted to hospital. A behavioural regimen in which the patient agrees on a target weight and is rewarded with privileges (watching television, being allowed visitors) in return for weight gain is usually effective in the short run. Occasionally, a small dose of a phenothiazine (e.g. chlorpromazine 50 mg bd) is helpful. However, the patient will often lose weight again once she is discharged unless psychotherapy is also started. Psychotherapy is the treatment of choice for outpatients. Mild anorexia can respond to simple counselling. In more severe cases, family therapy is the best treatment for those under 17; while for older patients (especially if they have left home) individual psychotherapy is the preferred treatment. In each case, the aims of therapy are:

1. to help both patient and family to move away from the area of food as a focus for all conflicts and difficulties
2. to help the patient accept herself as she is, in terms of both her body and her feelings.

Prognosis

Twenty five per cent of anorexic patients spontaneously recover; 25% make a full recovery with medical intervention; about 25% continue to experience some difficulties with eating but can lead a normal life; 25% remain quite severely handicapped. About 5–10% of anorexics die of the condition. Poor prognosis is associated with later onset, 'atypical features' (see above), marked body image disturbance and self-induced vomiting. Recovery is accompanied by reversal of the hormonal abnormalities and the onset of normal menstruation.

BULIMIA NERVOSA

Bulimia nervosa is a syndrome of 'binge eating' (bulimia: to stuff oneself with food) and self-induced vomiting in the presence of normal weight. There is an overlap here with anorexia nervosa, where binge-vomit cycles can also occur; but in anorexia the patient is always abnormally thin and also amenorrhoeic. The usual age of presentation in bulimia also tends to be older, with patients (usually women) in the 20–30 age range, rather than the teens.

The bulimic is frightened of becoming fat, but can accept her normal weight. She is terrified by her greed and tries to avoid its consequences by making herself sick. She normally feels deeply ashamed about this. She lives in a state of *dietary chaos* in which she is determined to fast, succeeds for a while, then succumbs to hunger and starts eating. She binges, then feels guilty, makes herself sick and then starves; and so the cycle starts again.

The physical consequences of bingeing and vomiting include erosion of dental enamel from exposure to gastric acid, Mallory-Weiss oesophageal tears, and even oesophageal rupture. Repeated vomiting causes hypokalaemia which may in turn produce tetany, paraesthesiae, ileus, cardiac arrhythmias, and epileptic fits.

Bulimic symptoms are common: 20% of women attending a family planning clinic admitted to bingeing, while 2% had the full syndrome. Like anorexia, bulimia may exist either on its own, or as part of a general disturbance of personality and be associated with alcoholism, deliberate self-harm or shoplifting, all of which make the prognosis less good.

Treatment of bulimia nervosa is usually successful and involves helping the woman to re-establish a regular eating pattern, and to feel less guilty. The bulimic often feels a great relief when dietary control is re-established, unlike the anorexic, who feels threatened at the idea of giving up her own control. In addition to a behavioural approach, exploration of the conflicts underlying the bulimia (such as marital difficulties or feelings of anger which the patient is unable to express) is also necessary.

OBESITY

Obesity in itself is not a psychiatric problem, but gross obesity can be experienced as a severe handicap, comparable to amputation or disfigurement. Obese people feel ostracised, and experience self-disgust. They long to be 'normal' and may become depressed by unsuccessful efforts at dieting. There are often marital and family difficulties which are both a cause and a consequence of their obesity. Prognosis for weight loss, either by dieting or surgery (e.g. intestinal by-pass) is not good. Paradoxically, psychotherapy can be a precursor to weight reduction if it

helps the patient to accept herself as she is. The patient may then find it easier to diet as she is less inclined to resort to the comfort of food whenever an emotional upset occurs.

SCHIZOPHRENIA

Just under 1% of the population develop schizophrenia at some point in their lives, a statistic that appears to hold true for all cultures and countries. Chronic major mental illness in people under 65 is mainly due to schizophrenia. Until the move towards community care began, about half of all hospital beds in the United Kingdom were in mental hospitals, and the majority of these (for the under 65s) were occupied by patients with a schizophrenic illness. As the number of hospital beds has fallen, a significant proportion of the vagrants living in large inner-city hostels and prison recidivists have been found to be suffering from schizophrenia.

Aetiology

It may be that schizophrenia is not a single entity, but a group of related conditions. Both genetic and environmental factors are important in the aetiology of schizophrenia.

1. Twin and adoption studies have demonstrated the role of heredity in schizophrenia (Fig. 11.6). The concordance rate for identical twins is about 50%, for non-identical twins around 15%.
2. The efficacy of antipsychotic drugs like chlorpromazine, with its inevitable Parkinsonian side-effects, suggests a disturbance of mid-brain dopaminergic pathways in schizophrenia.
3. A subgroup of patients shows abnormalities on CT scan. These patients lack a family history of the illness, suggesting that non-genetic organic factors, perhaps associated with perinatal brain injury, may be important in some cases.
4. Family and social factors have also been shown to be important. In established schizophrenia, relapse rate is high when the patient is living in an over-involved family where there is a negatively charged emotional atmosphere (high 'expressed emotion').
5. Schizophrenic patients have a high state of psychophysiological arousal, possibly related to family stress. This may reflect limbic system dysfunction and lead to a difficulty in processing sensory stimuli.

Clinical features

Schizophrenia usually starts in young adulthood, (the single exception being *paraphrenia*, a form of paranoid schizophrenia affecting the elderly). There is a slight preponderance of men. The features of the illness can be divided into two parts: the effects on mental processes, and the effects on social functioning.

Mental disturbance

There is a general disturbance of mental functioning in schizophrenia. The normal progression of logical thought is disrupted ('thought disorder'). The privacy of the self is breached. Certain patterns of disorganisation of thinking are characteristic of schizophrenia. These are known as *Schneider's first-rank symptoms*, and consist of:

1. *Passivity feelings*, i.e. the conviction that one's thoughts or actions are not one's own.
2. *Characteristic auditory hallucinations*, which may be in the third person, with voices commenting on one's actions, and thoughts being spoken aloud.
3. *Delusional perception*, a sudden delusional significance of a neutral perceptual stimulus, e.g. traffic lights sending a message.
4. *Disorders of thought possession*, including thought insertion, thought withdrawal, and thought broadcasting.
5. *Hallucinations*, i.e. certain types of 'kinaesthetic' or somatic hallucinations.

Hallucinations

These are usually auditory. Characteristic of schizophrenia are 'third person' hallucinations, in which more than one person is heard discussing the patient and referring to him as 'he', 'she' or 'it'. Voices commenting on a person's actions like a 'running commentary' are also characteristic, as are voices that echo the patient's thoughts. Tactile or 'kinaesthetic' hallucinations, for example electric shock feelings in the limbs, are rare but pathognomonic.

Delusions

In schizophrenia these include the feeling that one's thoughts originate from outside ('thought insertion'), that they are being interfered with, removed ('thought block') or transmitted to outsiders as though on a loudspeaker ('thought broadcasting'). 'Passivity feelings' are the feeling that one's thoughts or actions are 'made' from outside.

Delusional perception

In delusional perception, a natural stimulus (e.g. a car number plate or a traffic light) suddenly acquires special and often frightening significance for the patient.

Social deterioration

The second main feature of schizophrenia is social deterioration. This is known as a *negative feature* of the illness, as opposed to the *positive features* of thought disorder, delusions and hallucinations. The patient may withdraw from social contact, give up his job, shun his friends and family, and spend many hours in isolation. This was once believed to be due to the effects of institutionalisation in a mental hospital, but it now appears that such social deterioration is also a product of the illness itself.

Differential diagnosis

An important subtype of schizophrenia is *paranoid schizophrenia* characterised by paranoid delusions. Here the onset is later (around 30–40 years of age), social deterioration is much less marked, and the personality is relatively well preserved.

Not all madness is schizophrenia. The differential diagnosis includes:

1. organic psychosis, such as acute confusional states and drug- and alcohol-related psychosis;
2. manic or depressive psychosis (in which auditory hallucinations occur but are more often 'second person', in which voices speak directly to the patient)
3. hysteria
4. stress-induced or 'psychogenic' psychosis
5. severe personality disorder.

Prognosis

The course of schizophrenia is very variable. About 30% of patients have only one episode. A good prognosis is more likely if the psychosis has an acute onset, a clear precipitant, florid symptoms, marked mood change in addition to disturbance of thinking, and good previous social adjustment and personality. At the other end of the scale, about 15% remain severely disabled and will still be in hospital after a year ('new long stay' patients). In these patients the

Fig. 11.6 Expectation of schizophrenia in relatives of schizophrenics.

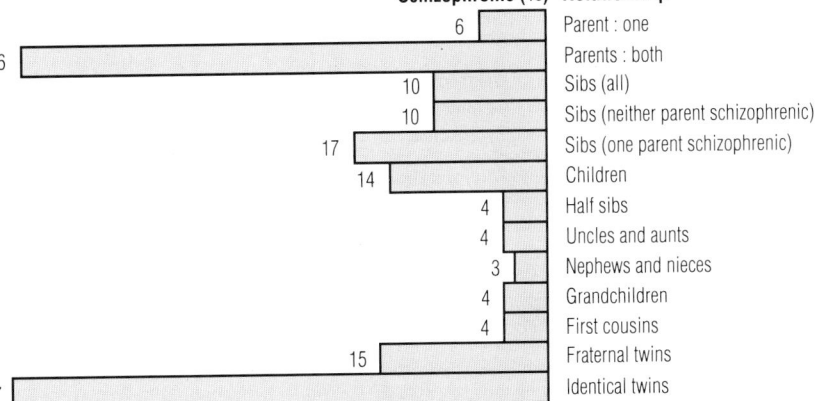

Schizophrenic (%)	Relationship
6	Parent : one
46	Parents : both
10	Sibs (all)
10	Sibs (neither parent schizophrenic)
17	Sibs (one parent schizophrenic)
14	Children
4	Half sibs
4	Uncles and aunts
3	Nephews and nieces
4	Grandchildren
4	First cousins
15	Fraternal twins
47	Identical twins

negative features of schizophrenia (withdrawal and inertia) may predominate. In the middle group, representing the majority of patients, the illness has a fluctuating course but relapse and some residual disability are likely to occur.

Treatment

Acute schizophrenic symptoms respond well to phenothiazines. There is some evidence that prompt treatment is associated with a good prognosis. The patient will normally be admitted to a psychiatric unit and treated initially with 100–1000 mg daily of chlorpromazine or its equivalent.

The longer-term management of schizophrenia is difficult. It involves both prevention of relapse, and management of chronic disability.

Prevention of relapse

Long-term maintenance on phenothiazines (often given in depot form because of problems of compliance) has been shown to prevent relapse. Phenothiazines can, however, have unpleasant and serious side-effects, especially a feeling of tiredness and a Parkinsonian syndrome of stiffness and involuntary movements (Table 11.6). Anti-Parkinsonian drugs should be given to counteract these. Reducing family tension has also been shown to prevent relapse. This can be achieved by family counselling sessions and by physical separation of the patient from an over-involved family through provison of hostel accommodation and/or attendance at a day centre.

Management of chronic disability

Chronic mentally ill patients are severely handicapped. Their prospects of employment are poor; they may have little or no family support; and their capacity to care for and occupy themselves may be very limited. They are sometimes also shunned or made scapegoats by society which tends to fear and despise madness. For at least 150 years these problems were dealt with by removing patients from society and locking them away in mental hospitals, thereby reinforcing the helplessness and isolation produced by the illness. Because of this, and also because mental hospitals are expensive to run and often sited on valuable land, government policy in the UK has now shifted away from the mental hospitals and towards *community care*. Patients are supposed to be cared for within the local community, in a network of hostels, sheltered houses, day hospitals and day centres. These are to be run by a locally based team of professionals, the '*multidisciplinary team*', including community psychiatric nurses, social workers and general practitioners as well as psychiatrists. However, although this pattern of care is indeed desirable for many patients, and already a reality for some, it is not necessarily suitable for all patients and it is not yet clear whether adequate funds and facilities will be made available to replace those previously provided in the mental hospitals.

PARANOID STATES

Paranoia means literally 'to be beside oneself', or 'out of one's mind'. In psychiatry, it refers to a psychosis whose central theme is a feeling of persecution and fear of being attacked. Paranoid states are common in general medical and hospital settings. A postoperative patient may suddenly rip out his intravenous cannula and attack one of the nurses. A patient may refuse all drugs, convinced that the staff are torturers dressed up as doctors and nurses. A patient with cancer may refuse to leave hospital because she is convinced she is in danger of being attacked or raped by marauding gangs outside.

The conditions resulting in paranoid states are as follows:

1. *Organic psychosis.* This is by far the commonest cause in the hospital setting. Paranoid delusions are frequently found in patients with acute confusional states. Any of the causes of organic psychosis (p. 186) may be responsible, with steroid-induced psychosis, alcohol withdrawal syndrome and amphetamine psychosis particularly common. Alcoholism may also produce a chronic paranoid state in which auditory hallucinations predominate (p. 74).
2. *Manic-depressive psychosis.* Feelings of being disliked and shunned are common in depression, and may

Table 11.6 Side-effects and toxic effects of antipsychotic drugs (e.g. chlorpromazine, flupenthixol)

Type of effect	Examples
Autonomic	Blurred vision Dry mouth Constipation Precipitation of glaucoma Postural hypotension Inhibition of ejaculation Urinary hesitancy
Extrapyramidal	Akinesia (Parkinson-like) Acute dystonia Tardive dyskinesia (involuntary repetitive movements) Akathisia (motor-restlessness)
Endocrine effects	Weight gain Galactorrhoea and amenorrhoea Gynaecomastia
Hypersensitivity reactions	Agranulocytosis Cholestatic jaundice Skin rashes
Provocation of epileptic fits	
Hypothermia (especially in the elderly)	
Skin photosensitivity	

assume psychotic proportions if the patient feels he is so wicked that he is deservedly in danger of attack. Paranoid ideas can occur in mania, but elation and over-activity are usually more prominent features.
3. *Paranoid schizophrenia* (see p. 205).
4. *Paranoid psychosis.* Sometimes the patient develops paranoid delusions and hallucinations without the full range of features of schizophrenia. There is often a sexual content to the psychosis. The patient may, for example, become convinced that his spouse is having an affair (morbid jealousy or *Othello syndrome*). The feeling that work-mates or strangers are accusing the patient of homosexuality is often a prominent feature of paranoid psychosis.
5. *Paranoid personality.* The paranoid personality has a tendency to mistrust and blame others and thus frequently becomes involved in complaints and battles with authority. He is often sensitive, isolated, insecure and quick to take offence and misinterpret the behaviour of others as hostile. When his fragile self-esteem is threatened by illness or rejection, he may develop a paranoid psychosis.
6. *Paranoia in the elderly.* Elderly patients may develop a paranoid psychosis (*paraphrenia*) with schizophrenic features. Deafness, social isolation and previous paranoid personality are important predisposing factors.

Common to all the different forms of paranoia are isolation, insecurity, mistrust and misperception. In some cases the defence of *projection* seems to be operating. The above-mentioned cancer patient refuses to leave hospital, because she attributes the hostility felt from the cancer within to the outside world as well. Paranoid states can be treated symptomatically with phenothiazines, but the underlying cause itself should be treated whenever possible.

MENTAL HANDICAP

Mental handicap can be defined as the arrested or incomplete development of the cognitive (i.e. intellectual) part of the mind. Such a broad definition covers a wide range of individuals:

1. *Severely mentally handicapped*, who lack speech, are unable to learn, cannot dress or feed themselves, may be incontinent, and may have stereotyped movements such as rocking or thumb-sucking. The majority are

looked after in institutions.
2. *Moderately mentally handicapped*, who have a considerable handicap (e.g. very restricted speech) but are able to live in sheltered accommodation in the community.
3. *Mildly mentally handicapped*, who have the capacity to learn and to live normal, if somewhat restricted, lives. Their primary problems are social and educational rather than medical. Most can live independently in the community.

Mental illness and mental handicap

It is only recently that mental illness and mental handicap have been properly distinguished. It is now understood that the majority of mentally handicapped people are not psychiatrically ill, and that they should be cared for by the social, rather than medical, services. Nevertheless, the mentally handicapped are particularly vulnerable to mental illness due both to their physical handicap and to emotional and social immaturity. They can develop the full range of mental illness including schizophrenia, manic depression, anxiety states and hysteria. Distress is likely to be expressed behaviourally, for example through withdrawal, temper tantrums, compulsive masturbation or law-breaking (e.g. shoplifting or self-exposure) rather than verbally.

Causes of mental handicap

Moderate and severe mental handicap usually has a distinct cause. This may be:

1. *A single gene disorder*, e.g. untreated phenylketonuria, tuberous sclerosis, mucopolysaccharidoses, untreated galactosaemia and Tay-Sachs disease.
2. *Chromosomal*, e.g. Down's syndrome, fragile-X mental retardation, deletion and duplication syndromes.
3. *Traumatic*, e.g. birth injury or anoxia. Here, the mental handicap is usually associated with spasticity.
4. *Infective*, e.g. maternal toxoplasmosis, cytomegalovirus and rubella; bacterial and viral meningitis. All may cause severe mental handicap.
5. *Other causes* include rhesus incompatibility, lead poisoning, and maternal drugs such as anticonvulsants or alcohol.

Mild mental handicap usually lacks a specific inherited or environmental cause. It is thought to be a result of polygenic inheritance, often coupled with an impoverished environment.

Management

The principles of management of adult mental handicap are shown in Summary 16.

Prevention

Primary prevention is exemplified by rubella innoculation and the provision of lead-free paint. Secondary prevention

> **Summary 16 Principles of management of adult mental handicap**
>
> - Accurate diagnosis
> - Treatment of co-existing mental and physical illness
> - Provision of training facilities, day centres, sheltered workshops and social clubs
> - Residential provision e.g. hostels for those whose relatives cannot cope or are not available
> - Provision of emotional support for carers who, e.g., worry about what will happen when they are no longer able to care for their mentally handicapped dependant

is made possible by genetic counselling and by prenatal diagnosis and screening (see Ch. 6, p. 96). For example, the mental impairment of phenylketonuria can be prevented by low phenylalanine diet in infants identified initially through neonatal screening. Where potential handicap has been identified by amniocentesis, a therapeutic abortion is offered if appropriate.

PSYCHIATRY AND THE LAW

In Samuel Butler's satirical novel *Erewhon*, illness was a punishable crime while criminals underwent medical treatment. Although most criminals are not mentally ill, there are indeed some who are. Mental illness may be associated with crime in one of three ways:

1. *Psychosis.* The most famous example of a crime being the result of a psychosis is the 19th century McNaughten case in which a man who had tried to shoot the American President was acquitted 'by reason of insanity'.
2. *Neurotic disorder.* Depression, for example, may make a criminal act such as shoplifting more likely ('diminished responsibility').
3. *Psychopathic personality.* Crime is associated with this type of disorder.

Psychopathic personality disorder

People with a psychopathic personality disorder may be described as those with persistent social difficulties (often, but not always, involving law-breaking) in the absence of a psychosis or neurosis. Their crimes, if they do occur, may be as trivial as repeatedly breaking shop windows; or they may be serious, such as murder. In the 19th century these individuals were classified as 'morally insane'; they were not deluded or hallucinated, but they appeared not to know right from wrong or to be aware of the consequences of their actions. The term *sociopathic* is now sometimes used in order to avoid the derogatory connotations of 'psychopath'.

The concept of psychopathy implies:

1. a persistent abnormality extending backwards to a childhood which was often disrupted and poor ('depraved because deprived')
2. a major problem of social adjustment.
3. the absence of another psychiatric disorder.

A psychopathic individual has trouble not just in relationship to himself, or his immediate family (although this usually does happen), but also to institutions like the law, school, the armed services, employment and marriage. He is both dependent on institutions, and unable to co-exist peaceably with them. There is usually associated alcohol and/or drug abuse. Since medical settings, and especially hospitals, are institutions, they too may fall prey to the problems created by patients with personality disorders.

The dividing line between normal and abnormal is harder to draw in psychopathy than any other psychiatric category and it is not a diagnosis that should be applied lightly. It is also important not to make such patients scapegoats. Sociopaths sometimes benefit from psychotherapy (providing firm limits are set), and from help with the social consequences of their psychopathy, such as homelessness and unemployment.

THE UNITED KINGDOM MENTAL HEALTH ACT 1983

Psychotic patients lack insight and may, occasionally, be dangerous either to themselves or to others. In the United Kingdom, until the 1930s, nearly all psychiatric inpatients were legally detained in hospital. Today, less than 10% of patients are detained on a 'Section'. While compulsory admission is sometimes necessary for the protection of the patient and the public, this power is open to misuse or even abuse. The United Kingdom Mental Health Act of 1983 aimed to provide safeguards against such abuse, and the Sections of the Act of particular relevance to general physicians are described below. In all cases, it is a duty of the hospital administration to inform the patient of his Section and a statutory right of the patient to appeal against compulsory detention.

Admission for assessment (Section 2)

The patient may be detained for up to 28 days if (a) he is suffering from mental disorder which warrants assessment; or (b) he is a danger to himself or others. The *application* for such assessment must be made by a social worker or the patient's nearest relative. There has also to be a *medical recommendation* from two medical practitioners. One of these must be a doctor officially approved as having special psychiatric experience; the other should if possible have known the patient previously (and is thus usually the patient's GP). In an emergency, the patient may be detained for up to 72 hours (Section 4) on the basis of only one medical recommendation which need not necessarily be by a psychiatrist.

Admission for treatment (Section 3)

The patient may be detained for up to six months. The conditions of the application and recommendation are therefore more stringent, and the rights of appeal greater than under Section 2. The patient must have a defined mental disorder, be thought likely to improve, and be unable to be cared for within the community.

Emergency detention of patients already in hospital (Section 5)

An informal patient may be held in hospital for up to 72 hours on the recommendation of the doctor in charge of his treatment without a Section 2 or 3 being instituted. Under Section 5(4), a psychiatric nurse can detain an informal patient already being treated for mental illness for up to six hours. Under Section 5(2), a patient in a general hospital who is being treated by a non-psychiatrist can be detained, under the report of the doctor in charge of the case, for up to 72 hours. A psychiatrist should see the patient as soon as possible to decide whether further detention is needed. Section 5(2) cannot be renewed.

Powers of the Courts (Sections 36, 37, 38)

Under these sections, mentally ill offenders can be compulsorily admitted to psychiatric units for assessment and treatment, rather than going to prison.

Place of safety order (Section 136)

Police officers have the power to remove to a place of safety any person whom they find in a public place who appears to be suffering from mental disorder, and who is in immediate need of care and control for his own sake, or that of others. Once removed, the patient must be medically examined and assessed. The place of safety is often a police station but may also be a hospital casualty department.

Consent to treatment (Sections 57, 58)

An important feature of the Act is a tightening of the procedure surrounding consent to treatment. Compulsorily detained patients can still be treated without their consent (for example, given ECT or phenothiazine drugs), but a second opinion must first be obtained from a doctor appointed by the Mental Health Commission. Patients may not undergo *psychosurgery* (a brain operation occasionally undertaken in cases of depression or phobic anxiety) if they do not consent to it. Even if they do, a doctor and two non-medical appointees of the Mental Health Commission will scrutinise the case to ensure that consent has been validly given.

People have a right to both liberty and health; and these basic rights may on occasion conflict. By curbing some of the powers of psychiatry the Mental Health Act has introduced important safeguards of the patient's liberty, but this may, occasionally, jeopardise the patient's mental health.

SUICIDE AND PARASUICIDE

Suicide has a long history and is an integral part of human psychology. There are few individuals lucky and happy enough never to have had even a fleeting thought of suicide at some point in their lives.

'Parasuicide', a syndrome of *deliberate self-harm*, appears to be a relatively recent phenomenon, and has reached epidemic proportions over the past 25 years (Fig. 11.7). It is the commonest cause of hospital admission for women under 65, and the second commonest for men. Many cases of deliberate self-harm go unreported; probably only about one third reach hospital.

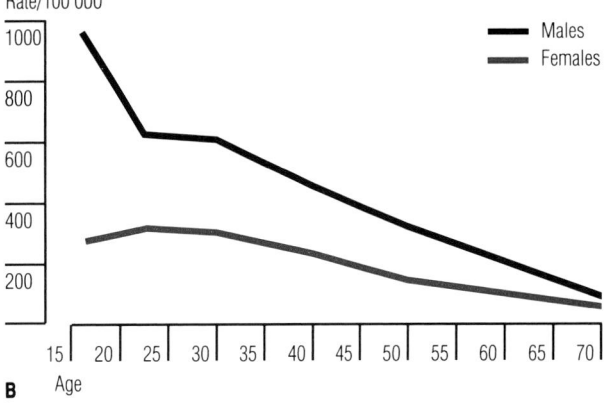

Fig. 11.7 Comparison of suicide and parasuicide rates. A. Suicide rates per 100 000, by age and sex, in England and Wales in 1969–71. **B.** Parasuicide rate per 100 000, by age and sex in Edinburgh in 1973.

Clinical profiles

The clinical profiles of suicide and parasuicide are, on the whole, distinct (Table 11.7). A person who commits suicide could be a middle-aged man with a previous history of depression and alcoholism, recently divorced or made redundant, living alone and with few close friends or relations. He deliberately tells the neighbours and milkman that he is going away for the weekend and then takes a bottle of aspirin or shoots himself. A parasuicidal person

Table 11.7 Clinical profiles of suicide and parasuicide

	Suicide	Parasuicide
Central theme	Despair, depression	Anger, frustration
Epidemiology	Slight decline 1963–83	Fourfold increase 1963–83
Age, sex, class	Commoner over 50; commoner in men than women; no class preference	Commoner in women aged 18–35 and in social classes IV and V
Social circumstances	Isolated e.g. unemployed, retired, divorced, children left home, few friends or religious/social groups	Disturbed but not isolated e.g. teenager unhappy with parents or boyfriend
Method and build-up	Planned. Usually leaves a note; method often violent e.g. hanging, shooting, drowning	Impulsive. Commonest method is swallowing pills. Cutting (usually wrists) a more disturbed subgroup
Alcohol	May play a part – 'Dutch courage'	Attempt very commonly associated with alcohol/drugs i.e. reduced impulse control
Illness	90% of suicide cases are mentally ill, usually with depressive illness. Physical illness also common	Only about 30% are mentally ill. Some have personality disorder. Majority normal or with 'minor affective illness'
Outcome	Not all 'succeed'. Survivors need hospital admission for treatment of mental illness	Not all survive, but most do. About 5% repeat. May benefit from counselling or psychotherapy

might be a woman in her late teens living with her mother and stepfather, and getting on badly with her boyfriend. After a row with him, in which both have been drinking, she goes home, swallows some of her mother's sleeping tablets, and is then noticed to be drowsy. When challenged about what has happened, she immediately 'confesses' and is rushed to hospital.

The central theme of suicide is *despair* and depression; in parasuicide it is *anger* and frustration. Although there are important differences there are also psychological similarities. Both involve a physical attack on self, on the body. In both cases the patient feels a combination of personal inadequacy and anger towards friends and family. This anger is directed inward but there is often a wish to punish or harm those to whom the patient feels close. This is done indirectly via the suicide or suicide attempt.

A second point of contact is the wish to die. It is often said that parasuicide cases 'do not really mean it'. This is only partially true, and can sometimes be used by staff as

justification for adopting a punitive attitude. It is best to assume that both suicide cases and parasuicide cases want *both* to die, *and* not to die. The relative proportion of the two feelings varies greatly but both feel both.

A third point of overlap follows from this. Not all suicide cases succeed, and conversely it is possible in parasuicide to die by mistake. Patients who have made major suicide attempts may recover and, with the help of drugs, psychotherapy and time, regain the will to live. In the majority of parasuicide cases the attempt resolves the difficult social situation which prompted it and so is not repeated. In a minority, about 5%, the attempts are repeated, and a proportion of these will eventually 'succeed'. Parasuicide repeaters are more likely than those who do not repeat to have a personality disorder, be addicted to drugs or alcohol, or to have been in trouble with the law.

Management of failed suicide

The causes of suicide are essentially the causes of depressive illness and the management of attempted suicide is that of prevention, and particularly the early detection of, depression. About one half of successful suicide cases have contacted a helping agency – The Samaritans, a general practitioner, social worker or priest – in the month before they kill themselves. It is important to ask troubled, unhappy or depressed patients about suicidal feelings. Fleeting suicidal thoughts, 'I would like to sleep' or 'I would like to be dead but would never have the courage to do anything', are less worrying than a definite suicide plan. Talking about suicidal thoughts may in itself be a relief. Suicidal patients with symptoms of depressive illness should be admitted to a psychiatric unit. Patients who are managed as outpatients need to be seen frequently while they are in a suicidal state. Antidepressants can be prescribed but only in small amounts, as hoarding of tablets can be a danger.

Although the prevention of suicide remains the ideal this is in practice difficult to achieve. Counselling organisations such as The Samaritans seem not to have had a major impact on overall suicide rates, but the incidence of suicide in the UK has fallen slightly over the past 30 years as compared with the rest of Europe.

Suicide is a reminder of the limitations of psychiatric and social care. When a patient who is receiving treatment commits suicide, it is especially stressful for the doctors and nurses involved, as it always is for the patient's family. Feelings of guilt and anger are inevitable. Suicide, like any death, is a reminder that doctors are not omnipotent. In dealing with suicide or the threat of it, it should be remembered that, ultimately, a person determined or ill enough can always find a way to end his life.

PARASUICIDE

Causes

The causes of attempted suicide cannot be found solely within the individual. The sociologist Émile Durkheim coined the term *anomie* to describe the anonymity and restlessness of urban life, which he saw as a breeding-ground for suicide. Anomie, in his view, explained the higher suicide rates among the Protestant poor, as compared with poor Catholics and Jews among whom mutual support and strong beliefs provided cohesion and a sense of purpose. Social factors which need to be considered in understanding the increase in parasuicide rates include:

1. *Complex family structures* without clear rules or roles, such as unsupported one-parent families; adolescents who want freedom but lack the emotional or financial resources to leave home; families with step-parents.
2. *Drugs* being a socially acceptable means of dealing with *distress*: the commonest tablets taken in parasuicide are mild analgesics and minor tranquillisers.
3. *An epidemic factor.* Deliberate self-harm is often behaviour learned from friends, fellow-patients, relatives or television.

Management

The medical management (Ch. 4) of the parasuicide patient takes initial precedence over the social and psychiatric assessment. Doctors should avoid the temptation to use procedures such as gastric lavage as a means of punishment rather than necessary treatment. Medical staff often feel angry with overdose patients compared with those whose illness is not self-inflicted and, like alcoholics and drug addicts, these patients may become scapegoats. Their irresponsibility affronts the overworked nurses and doctors who are often similar in age and maturity to the patient. In addition, medical staff work in a stressful and hierarchical situation in which they can at times feel angry or frustrated; and these emotions can be displaced into a punitive attitude towards parasuicide patients. This can be avoided if ward procedures give time for discussion of these patients and the feelings they arouse.

History

A careful history must be taken from the overdose patient, who should be kept in hospital until alert and co-operative enough for this to be possible.

The presence of depressive illness and suicidal rather than parasuicidal features must be identified. The risk of repeat has to be assessed (Table 11.8). Social isolation, marked sleep disturbance preceding the attempt, strong feelings of guilt or unworthiness, evidence of pre-planning, inability to look to the future, and previous psychiatric history – especially if there are drug or alcohol problems – all point to serious disturbance and should lead to referral to a psychiatrist.

A detailed account of the attempt itself and of events surrounding it should be taken. It is often unhelpful to ask the patient 'why' he harmed himself. If he knew he might not have had to do so. In attempted suicide one often finds an *acting-out* of feelings rather than the capacity to contain

Table 11.8 Deliberate self-harm: assessment of severity of disturbance. Ideally, all cases should be referred for psychiatric assessment. Psychiatric referral essential if any of the following are present:

Circumstance of the attempt
Evidence of pre-planning (e.g. suicide note, use of car exhaust)
Violent method used (e.g. attempted hanging)

Social circumstances of patient
Alone
Away from home

Personal history of patient
Recent loss (e.g. bereavement, divorce/separation, unemployment)
Physical illness
Previous attempts
Alcohol or drug addiction
History of depressive illness

Family history of patient
Suicide
Depressive illness

Mental state examination
Sleep disturbance, low mood before attempt
Low self-esteem, hopelessness
Psychotic features (e.g. 'I deserve to die')

Future
No relatives or other supports
Unresolved crisis
Continued determined suicidal intent

or verbalise them. The patient will find it much easier to answer questions about 'what happened, and how'. This provides an 'action replay' of the attempt which will contain the clues to the question of 'why'. Most commonly the patient feels *angry* but is unable to express this directly, usually for fear of rejection by a partner, spouse or parent on whom he feels dependent. As in depression, he dare not bite the hand that feeds, so attacks himself instead. It can be useful to ask the patient who he thinks would have been most distressed if he had died. Later, it is often helpful to discuss alternative strategies with the patient, to examine what he could have done in the same situation other than attempt suicide. Follow-up counselling after discharge either as an individual or in a family, by a social worker, psychiatrist or psychotherapist may be offered, although less than half of patients accept such help. However, even without follow-up the prognosis of parasuicide, in the absence of depressive illness or personality disorder, is fairly good.

Preventative measures

Preventative measures for parasuicide are important but difficult to achieve, and probably involve social change beyond the scope of the medical profession. However, doctors can contribute to prevention by placing greater emphasis on counselling for those in distress, and less on indiscriminate prescribing of psychotropic drugs. Guidelines to management are given in Table 11.9.

Table 11.9 Management of deliberate self-harm

Suicide risk	Management
Definite suicide risk (e.g. psychotically depressed; determined to repeat)	Admit to psychiatric unit (Mental Health Act if necessary)
Moderate suicide risk	Consider admission to psychiatric unit *or* Inform GP *and* Arrange attendance at day hospital *and/or* Daily visit by community nurse
Less strong suicide risk	Arrange social work help if necessary (e.g. if homeless) Inform GP Follow-up by psychiatrist, psychotherapist or social worker (N.B. 50% do not attend at follow-up)

MEDICINE AND THE EMOTIONS

There are two basic types of mental activity. One is pictorial, non-rational and emotional, and concerns the biological fundamentals of 'birth, copulation and death' as well as art and creativity; the second is rational, verbal and logical and concerns the achievement of specific goals and solving of particular problems. Freud called these the primary and secondary processes. Non-rational thinking is primary because it precedes rational thinking developmentally: infants and young children think in feelings and pictures. The secondary processes are only gradually acquired. In healthy adult life both co-exist. Much of waking life is dominated by secondary processes, but in dreams, daydreams and instinctual activity the primary processes take over. In mental illness the balance of primary and secondary processes may be disturbed: the psychotic, for example, is dominated by primary processes, while the patient with obsessional neurosis is trying to apply the false logic of secondary processes to his emotions.

Modern medicine is based on scientific rationality. This means that, at times, doctors may find it difficult to comprehend the emotional reactions of the patient to illness, death or sexuality. For the doctor, the patient who needs a routine hernia operation presents a technical problem to be solved; meanwhile, the patient may, at some level, be wondering whether he will survive the operation and, if he does, whether his sex life will continue. Medical training is predominantly a training in rationality, in learning to set feelings aside. In order to understand the 'irrational' anxieties that trouble patients the doctor has to remain in touch with and respect the primary processes. The following sections on sex, and on death and dying, will highlight some of these issues.

SEX AND MEDICINE

Sex matters for three main reasons: identity, attachment and continuity.

Identity

Gender is fundamental. When a baby is born the mother asks 'Is it alright?' then 'Is it a girl or a boy?'. Gender is essential to a sense of identity, and this can be threatened by illness at any of the stages of development. Hypospadism, hirsutism, hernia, delayed puberty, amenorrhoea, infertility, hysterectomy, prostatectomy, diabetes-related impotence – these are just a few of the many medical conditions which may threaten the sense of identity that is rooted in gender and sexual functioning.

Attachment

Human attachment occurs through the body. Even when communication is at a distance, hands are needed to write a letter, a voice to speak on the telephone. Sexual bonding is a powerful and rewarding form of attachment. The adolescent worries whether his or her body is 'good', 'big' or attractive enough to find a partner.

Where sexuality is threatened by illness and disability, the patient fears that the basis of his or her attachment may be undermined: 'who will want me if . . . I have a colostomy . . . a mastectomy . . . am impotent . . . ?'

Psychogenic symptoms such as lower abdominal discomfort, pruritus or back pain may both arise from, and lead to, sexual difficulties. Such symptoms may draw attention to an underlying sexual anxiety, and at the same time provide the patient with the care and attention which he fears he may lose through sexual failure. Occasionally, guilt about masturbation may be based on the misconception that it is 'wrong' or harmful and this too may lead to psychogenic symptoms.

Continuity

Psychologically, sex and reproduction may serve as an insurance against the fear of extinction. The idea of personal death is more acceptable if there is family continuity, or if an individual feels he has contributed something, that children, memories, ideas or objects will live on in the next generation. Threat to this sense of continuity can lead to feelings of anxiety or depression. Nuclear weapons are particularly frightening because they threaten this sense of continuity in mankind itself.

Taking a sexual history

Sex is, at least in theory, no longer a taboo subject, but in practice both doctor and patient are likely to feel anxious about some aspects of their sexuality. It is important that the doctor feels reasonably comfortable when asking about a patient's sexual life. All human beings have a sexual life –

Summary 17   Common anxieties about sex

Adolescence
Masturbation
Homosexuality
Genital inadequacy

Young adults
Impotence
Anorgasmia
Infertility
Lack of libido

Middle-aged
Extramarital affairs
Sex and illness

Any age
Incest
Fetishism
Non-consummation of marriage

General principles of the Masters and Johnson approach include the following:

1. Treatment is in couples. Sexual difficulties are often complementary (e.g. premature ejaculation and anorgasmia) even though one member may present as the person with the problem. The non-presenting partner is given the role of co-therapist.

2. Physical examination and careful history-taking of both partners are required both to rule out organic causes of sexual dysfunction and to reassure the patients that they are 'normal'. Organic problems include autonomic neuropathy, which may cause impotence, vaginal infections, and the side-effects of psychotropic or hypotensive drugs which may produce impotence or delayed ejaculation.

3. There is more to sex than penetration. Sexual arousal depends – especially in women – on a series of steps, and a man may need to learn that foreplay cannot usually be omitted if full sexual arousal in his partner is to occur.

in the sense of thoughts, fantasies and feelings about sex – regardless of whether or not they are celibate. The doctor needs to be sensitive to the common anxieties about sex and to be aware of those that may apply to a particular patient's age and situation (Summary 17).

SEXUAL AND MARITAL DIFFICULTIES

Divorce and family disruption are becoming increasingly common. More than one in three marriages in the UK now ends in divorce, while in the USA the figure is one in two. The effects on developing children are unknown but are likely to be considerable. Partly in response to this there is now great interest in marital and family therapy. Sexual dysfunction may be both a cause and a consequence of marital disharmony. A couple whose sex life improves will get on better; a couple who, through marital counselling, get on better, will have a more enjoyable sex life.

The commonly encountered sexual difficulties are impotence, premature ejaculation and delayed ejaculation for men; and vaginismus and lack of sexual enjoyment (including anorgasmia) for women. Both sexes may suffer diminished libido. Transient difficulties are common; it is only when they are persistent and cause distress that they constitute a problem. Sexual problems may be primary, i.e. present from the onset of sexual life, or secondary, i.e. develop after a period of satisfactory sexual functioning.

The Masters and Johnson approach

Current thinking about sexual dysfunction has been greatly influenced by the work of Masters and Johnson, who studied the physiology of sexual response and introduced a new classification and treatment for sexual difficulties.

4. Anxiety is seen as a central element in sexual dysfunction. Anxiety is antagonistic to sexual arousal and a vicious circle can arise in which the patients fear they will fail (for example, to maintain erection, not to ejaculate prematurely, or to have an orgasm), which makes them 'try' harder, which makes them less able to relax and respond to sexual stimuli and thus more rather than less likely to fail.

5. The aim of treatment is to break this circle. Paradoxically, the couple are initially instructed not to make love, in order to prevent performance anxiety. They are given a series of graded exercises based on sensate focus or stroking, in which they learn to give and receive pleasure. Initially this is non-genital, but later moves on to 'genital sensate focus', i.e. mutual masturbation. It is ironic that whereas masturbation was viewed (wrongly) by 19th century psychiatry as a major cause of insanity, it is now considered important that both sexes are able to masturbate without guilt.

6. Psychological factors in sexual dysfunction may also need treatment, through either individual or marital therapy. Unexpressed anger is a common cause of sexual dysharmony: a couple who cannot row may also not be able to make love. Fear of loss of control, ignorance or guilt may also affect sexual pleasure.

The results of the Masters and Johnson approach are generally good, with 60–70% improvement rates reported in well-motivated couples.

Summary 18   The Masters and Johnson approach

- Treatment in couples
- Physical examination/history taking (to reassure they are 'normal')
- Instruction in sexual arousal
- Instruction initially not to make love (to dispel anxiety)
- Graded exercises based on sensate focus
- Psychotherapy if necessary

DEATH AND DYING

Death is an integral part of medicine, but doctors and other medical staff often feel confused by the psychological and moral questions it poses. Should a terminally ill patient be kept alive as long as possible, or allowed to die in peace? Should every patient with a fatal illness be told of his diagnosis, and if so how should he be told? Can a dying patient be helped to come to terms with death and how can this happen? What are the psychological reactions in the relatives of dying patients, and what support do they need?

These questions are problematic not only because of a lack of training and technique, but also because death is an intrinsically difficult subject which all but the exceptionally compassionate find it hard to face. Patients and doctors alike deny the reality of death in order to carry on with life.

Reactions in the patient

The response of the patient to the knowledge that he has a terminal illness can be compared to a bereavement reaction. The patient enters a state of grief for the loss of his own life. People commonly say they would prefer to die suddenly and without warning, partly to avoid the physical pain and fear of illness, but also, perhaps, to avoid this grief. The initial reaction to discovering that one has a terminal illness is usually one of numbness and shock, a struggle between denial and acceptance. The patient attempts to fight off what is happening; he cannot believe it is true, that it is happening to him. This is often followed by a period of severe anxiety, in which the patient becomes dependent on visitors, family and medical staff, and finds it very hard to be alone. A period of sadness and weeping is inevitable. Anger is also a normal feature of this phase and the patient may become difficult, complaining, ungrateful and demanding. With time, however, the patient gradually becomes calmer, and during this phase the opportunity to talk may be very helpful. This series of reactions may be compressed into a few hours or spread over months, and, as with bereavement, does not follow a neat, orderly course.

Some of the problems posed by dying patients can be seen as exaggerations or arrests in this sequence of feelings. They include:

1. *Manic denial.* The patient becomes inappropriately cheerful, making plans and having hopes quite out of keeping with the reality of his situation.
2. *'Non-attention denial'.* The patient appears to be completely unaware of the diagnosis even though he has been told he has a terminal illness. He carries on as if nothing has happened, but may complain of 'inexplicable' – to him – feelings of exhaustion or depression.
3. *Anxiety states.* This is the opposite of denial. The patient may become excessively tearful, and troubled by minor symptoms unrelated to the illness. He requires far more analgesics than would normally be expected, may panic when left alone and may require frequent 'unnecessary' hospital visits or admissions.
4. *Depressive reactions.* The patient may give up, refusing to talk or see visitors. Often the patient feels angry – with himself, his body, his doctors, nature, fate or

God – and improves if these feelings can be expressed and acknowledged.
5. *Paranoid reactions.* The patient may become very quarrelsome and accusatory or develop psychotic fears of being attacked.

Summary 19 Emotional reactions in terminally ill patients

- Numbness and shock
- Struggle between denial and acceptance
- Severe anxiety
- Sadness and weeping
- Anger
- Eventual calmness

Talking to dying patients

Breaking bad news and talking to dying patients is an art which can be learned through watching others, and through discussion of the feelings and difficulties it arouses. The patient can often be helped if staff and family recognise the subsequent reactions for what they are and then let the patient talk about his anger, panic and sadness. When this has happened the patient may feel better.

The issue of 'to tell or not' is a false alternative. Some patients want to know their diagnosis in great detail; others would rather not know. It is unnecessary and inappropriate to confront all patients with the stark reality of their illness. On the other hand, far more patients than are officially 'told' want to know their diagnosis or know it already. The patient needs space and time in which to discuss his feelings and ask questions. Gentle probing may be needed to help the patient make use of this opportunity: 'I wonder how you felt when we told you we could not remove the whole tumour ...?'. Doctors should be sure that it is not themselves, rather than the patient, whom they are protecting when they withhold information. No one wishes to be the bearer of bad tidings but many patients want, and need, to know the truth.

Reactions in the family

Like the patient, families also go through an anticipatory grief reaction when a loved one is dying. The death of a child or adolescent is especially painful and unsupportable. Sometimes, the family receives help while the patient is almost neglected; but more usually it is the other way round. Spouses of dying patients are particularly vulnerable. They may, for example, feel angry with their husband or wife for being ill, and feel very guilty about having such unvoiced thoughts. The stress of death may lead to tense and angry outbursts, either within the family or outside it at medical staff. Doctors and nurses should be prepared for this. Family counselling can help with these grief reactions and help to make death and bereavement, when they come, more bearable.

TREATMENT IN PSYCHIATRY

The final section of this chapter is aimed at those who claim that there are few effective treatments in psychiatry. In view of both developments in psychopharmacology, and an increasing recognition of the importance of counselling and psychotherapy, this claim can no longer reasonably be made (if, indeed, it ever could). It is true that both psychotherapeutic and drug treatments in psychiatry tend to be broad-spectrum, rather than specific, in their action and that their mechanism of action is not fully understood. But perhaps this matches the syndromic nature of many psychiatric disorders.

Psychotherapy and pharmacotherapy are not incompatible, and many patients, for example those with moderate or severe depression, do better if treated by a combination of drugs and psychotherapy than with either alone.

Physical and drug treatments

A summary of some of the important and effective physical and drug treatments in psychiatry is given in Table 11.10.

Table 11.10 Drug treatment and ECT in psychiatric illness

Class of treatment	Indication	Side-effects
Major tranquillisers e.g. Phenothiazines (chlorpromazine) Butyrophenones (haloperidol)	Functional psychoses, especially florid symptoms. Depot preparations prevent relapse	Parkinsonism including dyskinesia (unwanted movements); dry mouth; idiosyncrasy; jaundice; photosensitive rash; blood dyscrasias
Antidepressants e.g. Tricyclics: (dothiepin, amitriptyline) Tetracyclics (mianserin)	Depressive illness	Parasympathomimetic; cardiac arrhythmias; confusion in elderly
Lithium salts e.g. lithium carbonate	Prevention of relapse in hypomania	Hypothyroidism; nephrogenic diabetes insipidus; tremor; drowsiness (serum concentration should not exceed 1.5 mmol/l)
Beta-blockers e.g. propranolol	Reduction in peripheral symptoms of anxiety	Asthma; bradycardia
ECT	Delusion and hallucinations in severe depressive illness	Those of anaesthesia; short-term memory impairment
Benzodiazepines e.g. temazepam diazepam	Transient stress-related anxiety or insomnia	'Hangover'; addiction; withdrawal syndrome

Psychotherapy

One of Freud's first patients called psychotherapy the 'talking cure'; but perhaps it is better defined as the 'listening cure'. Psychotherapy can be classified either by the nature of the technique used, or by the setting in which it takes place.

Summary 20 Classification of psychotherapy

Psychotherapy can be classified by:

Technique	*Setting*
Directive	Informal
e.g. Behaviour therapy	e.g. Doctor-patient relationship
Exploratory	Formal
e.g. Psychoanalysis	e.g. Individual psychotherapy
Analytic psychotherapy	Group psychotherapy
Psychodynamic psycho-therapy	Marital/family therapy
Counselling	Self-help groups

Techniques

The two basic technical modes of psychotherapy are directive and exploratory.

Directive

Here the patient is given suggestions, tasks and directives. An alcoholic patient might be asked to keep a 'drinking diary', for example; or an agoraphobic patient to go to the corner shop unaccompanied. *Behaviour therapy* is a specialized form of directive psychotherapy, in which a socially phobic patient, for instance, is helped to become *desensitised* to a feared stimulus, first in imagination (imagining a pleasant conversation), then in reality, e.g. by 'practice conversations' in a social skills group with other similar patients.

Exploratory

Here, the aim is to explore the patient's feelings, fears and fantasies. Initially, the role of the therapist is mainly that of a non-judgemental listener; but later he may suggest interpretations of the meaning of the patient's problem or behaviour. He might, for example, suggest that a patient is, deep down, feeling angry and sad about an abortion that was necessary for practical reasons. The aim is always to help the patient understand (gain insight into) her behaviour and feelings, and so to feel less at their mercy.

Psychoanalysis, analytic psychotherapy, psychodynamic psychotherapy and *counselling* are all examples of exploratory therapy. Frequently, exploratory therapy focuses on the nature of the relationship between the therapist and patient, as this often typifies the problem the patient has with relationships generally. The patient who is very deferential and servile with the doctor while, underneath, feeling disappointed and angry, may deal with his boss or wife in a similar way. He may have had a dominant mother who evoked the same feelings and behaviour in him as a child. *Transference* is the term used to describe this transfer on to the therapist or doctor of feelings originally experienced with parents or other significant figures in childhood.

All doctors are involved in counselling and psychotherapy as a matter of course, in the sense that their work is not purely mechanical but necessarily involves communication. The *doctor-patient relationship* contains both directive and exploratory elements. The patient will be directed to take tablets, stop smoking, etc. but he will also, if the doctor is sensitive, have the opportunity to explore his feelings and fears in a safe and trusting atmosphere.

Setting

Psychotherapy can take place in a number of settings. These may be *informal*, as in the normal doctor-patient relationship, or more formal in nature. *Formal psychotherapy* can be further classified as individual psychotherapy (one patient, one therapist), group psychotherapy (usually 6–8 patients, one or two co-therapists) and marital/family therapy (where feelings are explored but directions are also given, e.g. that husband and wife should spend an evening alone together). A self-help group is a psychotherapy group without a formally designated therapist.

FURTHER READING

Beck A, Emery G 1979 Cognitive therapy of depression. Basic Books, New York. *A classical account of an increasingly used mode of therapy.*

Clare A 1980 Psychiatry in dissent, 2nd edn. Tavistock, London. *A stimulating discussion of contemporary issues in psychiatry.*

Gelder M (ed) 1983 Oxford textbook of psychiatry. OUP, Oxford. *Good, standard, medium-size textbook.*

Holmes J, Lindley R 1989 The values of psychotherapy. OUP, Oxford. *A discussion of the uses and abuses of psychotherapy.*

Malan D 1979 Individual psychotherapy and the science of psychodynamics. Butterworth, London. *Very readable account of brief psychotherapy.*

Wolff H, Bateman A, Sturgeon D (eds) 1989 The UCH handbook of psychiatry, 3rd edn. Duckworth, London. *Comprehensive up-to-date textbook with a psychodynamic slant.*

Infectious, Tropical and Parasitic Diseases

The relationship between humans and micro-organisms is usually one of balanced conflicts. In the first months of life encounters with micro-organisms are both a threat and a stimulus to the development of complex immune responses. In many parts of the world micro-organisms appear to have the upper hand, particularly over children. Worldwide, infectious gastroenteritis is the most common cause of death in children below the age of 1 year. This may surprise anyone brought up in a wealthy Western environment where gastroenteritis is regarded as a relatively minor illness. The causative organisms are similar in underdeveloped and Western countries so the statistic reflects more frequent exposure to infection, more severe disease and inadequate treatment. These, in turn, relate to water supplies, methods of food preparation and general standards of hygiene, including disposal of sewage. The outcome of the disease is determined by the extent to which the child becomes dehydrated and, although the type of organism and the severity of the infection are important, the key factor is the child's fluid intake.

Table 12.1 shows how the frequency of some infections varies in different areas of the world. The figures are somewhat inaccurate since most diseases are under-reported, but they illustrate differences which are attributable to climate (malaria), standards of hygiene (typhoid) and immunisation (poliomyelitis, measles and diphtheria). The mortality associated with these diseases is proportionally higher in underdeveloped countries because the victims tend to be in a poor nutritional state at the onset of illness and access to medical facilities is limited.

The pattern of infections is constantly changing, and infectious diseases become less important as a cause of death as the standard of living improves. Examination of historical records show that England in 1860 was much the same as parts of Africa and South-east Asia today with respect to some infectious diseases (Table 12.2). Improvements in standard of living and immunisation account for the change in many of these diseases but sometimes the pathogen itself changes in virulence. Scarlet fever (scarlatina) is no longer the feared disease it was 50 years ago due to erythrogenic toxin-producing streptococci becoming less virulent. Other changes in micro-organisms produce less dramatic changes in the disease but they are no less significant. The type of meningococcus most commonly incriminated in bacterial meningitis in the United Kingdom has been group B for many years, but recently there has been a resurgence of group C infections. Meningococcal vaccine will protect against group A or C infection but group B meningococci are poor immunogens.

Infectious, Tropical and Parasitic Diseases

Table 12.1 Cases of infection reported to WHO from different geographical regions and countries

Region or country	Malaria (1984)	Poliomyelitis (1984)	Measles (1982)	Typhoid (1980/1)	Diphtheria (1982)
Americas (all)	914 000	571	130 977	42 160	3 782
USA*	1 007	8	2 587	390	1
Europe	60 000	238	187 043	7 810	138
E. Mediterranean	305 000	1 959	203 764	75 203	9 930
Africa	5 570 000	1 833	629 345	28 418	1 529
S.E. Asia	2 711 000	15 167	229 873	329 980	20 067
W. Pacific	1 300 000	4 513	664 170	145	17 803
England and Wales†	1 691	3	97 408	177	4

(Data supplied by Communicable Diseases Surveillance Centre, Colindale)   * All figures for USA are for 1984.   †All figures for England and Wales are 1985.

A better-known example of antigenic variation is the constant drift in influenza virus strains. Another change which affects bacteria, including meningococci, is the development of resistance to antibiotics described on p. 222, but this is a change stimulated by exposure to antibiotics.

Most of the changes in the pattern of infections are gradual. New infections (as opposed to the newly discovered cause of an old disease) are extremely rare but can have an enormous impact. Current evidence suggests that human immunodeficiency virus (HIV), the cause of the acquired immunodeficiency syndrome (AIDS), is new in the sense that retrospective studies of stored sera show no evidence of infection in humans before the 1960s. All of the infections encountered in temperate and developed areas of the world will be found in tropical regions. Certain infections are exclusive to the tropics because of climate, and the presence of animal reservoirs and insect vectors.

Table 12.2 Deaths from infection in England in 1860 (all age groups)

Cause	Number
Measles	9 557
Scarlatina (scarlet fever)	9 681
Smallpox	2 749
Diphtheria	5 212
Typhus	13 012
Whooping cough	8 553
Cholera	327
Tuberculosis	58 564

THE RELATIONSHIP BETWEEN MAN AND MICRO-ORGANISMS

Micro-organisms which can cause disease in man are widely distributed in nature and man is colonised by vast numbers of organisms. Whether a particular organism causes disease in man is determined by its natural dis-

tribution, its pathogenicity and the state of the host defence systems.

The more common a pathogen is in the environment, the more likely it is that we will develop immunity to it at an early age. The age at which this first encounter occurs can influence the outcome of infection. At extremes of age the immune system is either immature or in decline and the patient is highly vulnerable. Paradoxically, during childhood many viral infections are silent or mild but the same infection in an adult may be severe and complicated. This may reflect a difference in the vigour with which inflammatory responses are generated.

PATHOGENICITY

Microbial *pathogenicity* – that is, the potential of a micro-organism to cause disease – is determined by its ability to enter the host and colonise, to penetrate tissues, to evade host defences and to damage tissues. The *virulence* of an organism is its degree of pathogenicity. An organism is described as highly virulent if a small number of microbes can cause severe disease.

Skin is an effective barrier to most organisms and they usually enter either through a breach or via more delicate mucosal surfaces such as those of the oropharynx and respiratory tract. Attachment to the cell membrane is essential for viruses, and bacterial colonisation is also often facilitated by a specific attachment mechanism. Examples are *Vibro cholerae* or *Escherichia coli* in the intestine and *E. coli* in the urinary tract. In each case a determinant on the bacterial surface interacts with a specific receptor on epithelial cells.

Some pathogenic organisms cause disease at the site of colonisation by producing toxins (*V. cholerae*) but most traverse the epithelium and their further success depends on their ability to compete with host defences. If this is the first encounter between man and organism innate immunity is man's only defence. In the case of bacteria this centres on phagocytosis and some bacteria are equipped with capsules which confer resistance to phagocytosis. Interferons play a major part in first-line resistance to viruses but viruses differ both in their ability to stimulate interferon production and in their susceptibility to its effects.

The mechanisms of tissue damage by bacteria are very complex but a distinction can be made between damage caused by exotoxins (tetanus or diphtheria toxins, for example) and that resulting from release of bacterial components such as endotoxins. These are lipoprotein-polysaccharide complexes which are major constituents of bacterial cell walls. In addition some bacteria, such as streptococci, secrete enzymes which are destructive to surrounding tissues.

SUSCEPTIBILITY TO INFECTION

The effect of even the most virulent of microbes is curtailed by a healthy individual who has developed an immune response to it. Infectious diseases therefore typically result from a small number of identifiable situations, which are as follows:

1. first encounter with a virulent organism, in sufficient numbers, entering by an appropriate route
2. breach of normal anatomical barriers, e.g. by surgery or injury
3. impairment of innate immune responses
4. impairment of adaptive immune responses.

When anatomical barriers are breached by surgery, tissues which are usually sterile are exposed to the normal microbial flora at the site. Similarly accidental injury often results in exposure to environmental organisms such as *Clostridium tetani* present in the soil.

Impairment of immune responses leads to susceptibility to infection by organisms of low pathogenicity as well as to virulent organisms. Infection by organisms of low pathogenicity is called *opportunistic*. Patients with impaired immunity may therefore present with frequent infections, infection caused by opportunist micro-organisms, unusually severe disease caused by infection, or repeated infection by the same organism.

PRINCIPLES OF DIAGNOSIS AND MANAGEMENT

The principles guiding the clinician in the diagnosis of an infective illness can be considered by asking some simple questions:

1. Is the disease caused by infection and, if so, where is the site of infection?
2. What is the micro-organism responsible?
3. Which drugs can eliminate the organism and will treatment benefit the patient?

This approach will often lead to a simple plan for management of the patient. It is, however, a good principle to establish the source of the infection, since there may be others in the community who are infected and indeed the present patient may still be infectious to others. In some cases the doctor has a legal obligation to notify the disease (see 'Control of infection', p. 227).

Is the disease caused by infection and, if so, where is the site of infection?

A careful history and examination will provide important indicators that the patient is suffering from infection.

History

Three aspects of the history are likely to be helpful:

1. pattern of the illness
2. history of contact with patients with a similar illness or types of behaviour that confer risk of infection
3. history of travel to places where particular infections are known to be common.

Illnesses caused by infection tend to have a form which is reproduced in most individuals and which is characterised by the following features:

1. *incubation period*: time from contact with micro-organisms to onset of symptoms (Fig. 12.1)
2. *prodromal illness*: minor symptoms preceding the definitive illness
3. *overt disease*
4. *resolution (convalescence)*.

This pattern is often influenced by the immune state of the patient and may be altered by drug therapy.

Some symptoms, such as sore throat and fever, are more commonly associated with infection than with other disease processes. Establishing the pattern of fever may be helpful, but caution is necessary since patients are inclined to say that they have had a fever when they have not measured their temperature. They may mean anything from an aching sensation in the limbs to sweatiness or true rigors. The former is not necessarily associated with fever whereas rigor is a good indicator. A *rigor* is a sensation of coldness accompanied by shivering, followed by a hot sensation and marked sweating. These phases correspond with a sudden rise in temperature (during the shivering) followed by a sharp fall.

While there is no symptom which is specifically associated with infection there are many symptom complexes which are highly suggestive of an infective aetiology. For

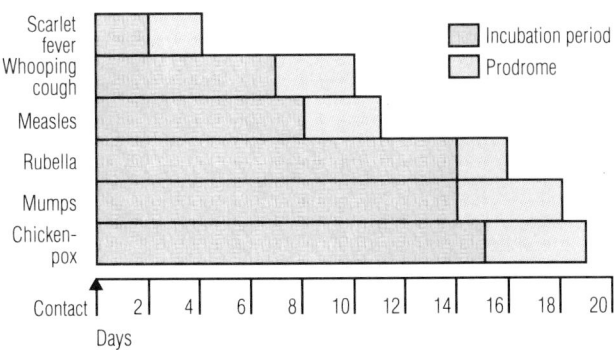

Fig. 12.1 Incubation periods of common infectious diseases.

example, while headache has many causes, the combination of headaches with fever, photophobia and vomiting strongly suggests infection of the meninges (meningitis).

Examination

The findings on examination may be helpful in three ways:

1. Some infections are associated with signs which are specific or which suggest only a short list of differential diagnoses. Examples are the rash of chickenpox or measles, neck stiffness caused by acute meningitis or the characteristic cough of whooping cough.
2. More commonly a combination of signs is highly suggestive of an infection. For example, exudative tonsillitis, generalised lymphadenopathy and splenomegaly together suggest infectious mononucleosis; fever, relative bradycardia, splenomegaly and rose spots suggest typhoid.
3. Physical signs may indicate the site of infection. Consolidation in the lungs suggests pneumonia; loin tenderness is associated with pyelonephritis; inflammation, swelling and fluctuance beneath the skin suggest an abscess.

What is the micro-organism responsible?

Although a careful history and examination will often point to a diagnosis of infection and, in some cases, be specific for infection with a single micro-organism, more frequently infection is strongly suspected but the site and the organism responsible are unknown. Imaging techniques are often helpful in finding the site of infection: for example, ultrasound or CT scanning can demonstrate an abscess in soft tissues. A gallium scan or [111]Indium leucocyte scanning frequently demonstrates a soft tissue abscess. In the latter technique the patient's leucocytes are separated from a whole blood sample, labelled with [111]Indium and re-injected into the patient intravenously (Fig. 12.2). Labelled leucocytes are attracted into sites of acute inflammation such as an abscess, where they are detected by gamma scanning. [111]Indium-labelled leucocytes are also concentrated in surgical wounds and in the bowel wall of patients with inflammatory bowel disease.

Before appropriate treatment can be started the right samples must be collected and sent to the laboratory. Doctors should collect samples and make requests in a way which will allow the laboratory to perform the right tests and to give back the maximum amount of relevant information. The laboratory can give most help if the request is accompanied by a brief summary of the patient's illness so that the tests can be orientated towards detection of likely organisms. The drug history is particularly important since antibiotic in the sample may inhibit growth of bacteria in vitro. There are simple rules for the collection of samples:

1. Avoid contamination of the sample with irrelevant organisms by careful cleaning, e.g. clean skin with iodine before taking blood for culture and wear gloves during venepuncture.
2. When infected fluid is to be cultured (e.g. pus) send a fluid sample in a sterile bottle rather than a swab if the volume of fluid permits. The yield will be higher and a Gram stain can be performed.
3. Think of culture before allowing a tissue specimen to be immersed in fixative such as formalin.
4. Ensure that specimens for culture are transported to the laboratory without delay. Micro-organisms must be nurtured and all too often they die sitting on a shelf waiting for transport or are outgrown by contaminant organisms.

Specimens for viral or fungal culture often require special techniques of collection and the laboratory should be consulted before obtaining the specimen.

A   B

Fig. 12.2 [111]**Indium white cell scan in a paracolic abscess. A.** At 3 hours the scan shows dense accumulation of labelled cells in the right side of the abdomen, with normal uptake of cells in the liver (top left) and spleen (top right). **B.** At 24 hours the activity remains in the original site of localisation, indicating the accumulation represents an enclosed abscess rather than inflamed bowel. (Reproduced by kind permission of Dr Seth Saverymuttu)

Which drugs can eliminate the organism from the infected site and will treatment benefit the patient?

Some guidelines for the choice of antimicrobial drugs are given on page 222. Whether treatment is to be started immediately or after the results of laboratory tests are available depends on the severity of the disease and the likely consequences of delay. There is virtue in waiting until the precise diagnosis is known if the clinical situation permits, and this applies particularly when antibiotics have been given before admission to hospital. Acute meningitis and septicaemia are obvious exceptions because the patient may die before a final result is available but even then it is vital that the correct specimens are obtained before treatment is started. Valuable preliminary information can be obtained by Gram staining and microscopy of specimens such as sputum or pus. As yet direct testing for microbial antigens has made little contribution to rapid diagnosis but with the increasing availability and use of monoclonal antibodies, direct testing is gaining in importance for disease caused by a limited range of organisms such as acute meningitis.

Treatment is not always beneficial to the patient, even when an antimicrobial drug with appropriate activity can be delivered to the site of infection in adequate concentration. Intestinal bacterial infections rarely respond to antibiotics and excretion of salmonellae may be prolonged by treatment.

ANTIMICROBIAL AGENTS

The choice of antimicrobial drugs is central to the management of infection. General measures should not be neglected; these include use of analgesics, attention to nutrition and hydration, and cleaning, debridement or drainage of infected areas.

The term 'antimicrobial agent' can be applied to any substance which is active against micro-organisms. Strictly, an antibiotic is a substance produced by a micro-organism which inhibits the growth of another. The forerunner of antibiotics was penicillin, discovered by Fleming in 1929 and shown to be clinically important in 1940 by Florey and Chain. Sulphonamides (azo dyes) were first synthesised in 1932 and their efficacy in treatment of infections was published in 1935 by Domagk. In this chapter 'antibiotic'

Table 12.3 Common sensitivities of some bacteria to antibiotics

Bacteria	1st choice	2nd choice
Streptococci (except anaerobic)	Penicillin	Erythromycin
Staphylococci	Flucloxacillin	Erythromycin
Neisseria meningitidis	Penicillin	Chloramphenicol
Neisseria gonorrhoeae	Penicillin	Tetracycline
Gram-positive bacilli	Penicillin	
Escherichia coli (urinary tract)	Trimethoprim	Nitrofurantoin
Pseudomonas aeruginosa	Gentamicin and azlocillin (usually requires a combination)	

will be used (inaccurately) to refer to antibacterial drugs, whether synthetic or naturally produced.

Choice of appropriate drugs

Selection of a suitable antimicrobial agent is fairly straightforward when the micro-organism responsible is known (Table 12.3), but often this is not the case and a sensible guess has to be made as to the organisms most likely to cause the clinical condition of the patient. In the case of a urinary tract infection in a previously healthy young woman, for example, faecal organisms such as *E. coli* would be by far the most likely pathogens and initial therapy would be guided by this fact.

The information required to make an appropriate choice of antimicrobial agent can be summarised:

1. probable organism/s
2. probable antimicrobial sensitivities of the organisms
3. ability of the chosen drugs to reach the site of infection
4. history of allergy to drugs
5. interaction of these drugs with any other drugs the patient is taking
6. side-effects of the chosen drug
7. cost of the drug.

An example of the process of decision is shown in Figure 12.3. This logical sequence assumes a considerable knowledge of antibiotics, including the known sensitivity of particular organisms to them. The latter are not constant,

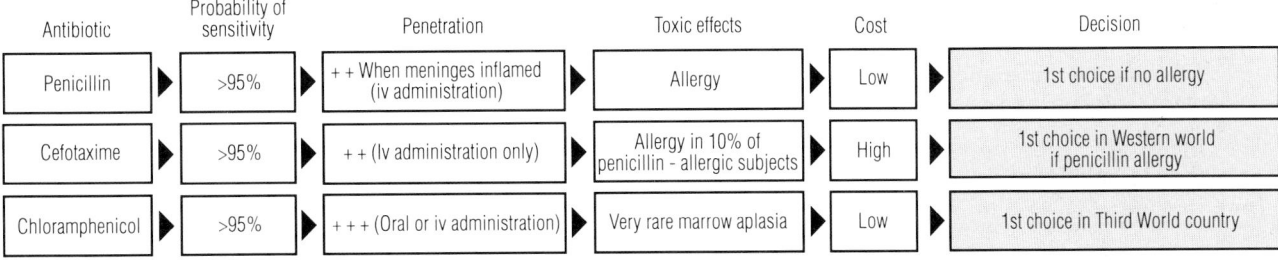

Fig. 12.3 Choice of antibiotic in a patient with acute pneumococcal meningitis.

Infectious, Tropical and Parasitic Diseases

so treatment is often started on the basis of an intelligent guess and modified later according to laboratory results.

In the laboratory, sensitivity of bacteria is tested using discs impregnated with antibiotic and measuring the size of the ring of inhibition on culture plates. This gives a guide to the sensitivity of the organism. In the choice of antibiotic other factors are also important, such as absorption and penetration to the site of infection. Whenever possible the antibiotic chosen should have a spectrum of antibacterial activity limited to a few organisms, since the broader the spectrum, the greater the chance of side-effects due to disturbance of the normal microbial flora. The choice between a bactericidal and a bacteriostatic drug is not usually critical but it may be important when the organisms are fairly inaccessible, as in infective endocarditis, or when host defences are impaired (Table 12.6).

Combinations of antibiotics are used for one of three purposes:

1. to obtain a spectrum of antibacterial activity which could not be achieved with a single agent (e.g. treatment of septicaemia when the causative organism is not known)
2. to take advantage of synergism between drugs (e.g. during the initial treatment of infective endocarditis)
3. to prevent the emergence of resistant organisms (e.g. treatment of tuberculosis).

Route of administration

The ideal drug would give adequate serum levels after oral administration, whatever the state of the patient. However, an ill patient often cannot swallow tablets and absorption from the gut cannot be relied on. Parenteral treatment is preferred and the choice between intravenous (iv) and intramuscular (im) administration is determined by the form in which the drug is available and its pharmacokinetics; the discomfort of intramuscular administration, which varies between drugs and according to the musculature of the patient; and practical issues such as accessibility of veins and other drugs being administered.

Mechanism of action of antibiotics

Antibiotics act in one of the following ways:

1. inhibition of bacterial cell wall synthesis (penicillins and cephalosporins)
2. inhibition of particular aspects of bacterial cell function: *protein synthesis* (aminoglycosides, chloramphenicol, tetracyclines, macrolides, clindamycin); *DNA replication* (rifampicin, 4-quinolones); *microbial enzymes* (sulphonamides, trimethoprim, isoniazid).

Resistance to antibiotics

There are two major ways in which resistance occurs:

1. Production of an enzyme which inactivates the antibiotic. The best-known example is β-lactamase which

Fig. 12.4   Structure of β-lactam ring.

alters the β-lactam ring of penicillins and cephalosporins (Fig. 12.4). Aminoglycosides and chloramphenicol are other drugs broken down by bacterial enzymes.
2. The bacterium itself may alter such that the antibiotic is rendered ineffective. This occurs either by a change in the permeability of the bacterial cell wall or by an alteration at the target site of the antibiotic.

Resistance tends to emerge by natural selection in a population of bacteria exposed to antibiotic – that is to say, those bacteria which have a genetic advantage survive. This advantage may be acquired by mutation but more often it is the result of incorporation of new genetic material into the bacterial nucleus or transfer of genetic material from other organisms in the form of extrachromosomal DNA as plasmids (episomes).

ANTIBACTERIAL ANTIBIOTICS IN COMMON USE

β-lactams

These are the most commonly used antibiotics and have in common the β-lactam ring (Fig. 12.4). There are two major groups, the penicillins and cephalosporins.

Penicillins

Benzyl penicillin or penicillin G is a highly potent bactericidal natural penicillin which was the forerunner of all the other penicillins. Long-acting forms, procaine and benzathine penicillins, allow longer intervals between

222

doses. Its disadvantages are that it can only be given parenterally, it has little activity against Gram-negative organisms, and many staphylococci are resistant to it. Semi-
synthetic and synthetic penicillins have been developed
to circumvent these problems. Doses are now usually
expressed in mg (600 mg = 10^6 units = 1 megaunit).

Phenoxymethyl penicillin is a natural penicillin which is
acid-resistant and can therefore be taken by mouth for
treatment of minor infections with streptococci which are
highly sensitive. Absorption is variable so it should not be
used for more serious infections.

Broad-spectrum penicillins, such as ampicillin, amoxycillin and pivampicillin, have useful activity against Gram-
negative organisms excluding *Pseudomonas* species. They
are well absorbed from the intestine.

β-lactamase-resistant penicillins, such as flucloxacillin
and methicillin, are used mainly to treat penicillinase-
producing staphylococci.

Antipseudomonal penicillins: carbenicillin, ticarcillin and
the ureidopenicillins (azlocillin, mezlocillin and piperacillin) are all distinguished by their activity against *Pseudomonas* species but the ureidopenicillins have a broader
spectrum of activity against Gram-negative organisms.

Cephalosporins

Cephalosporins have a similar structure and mode of action
to penicillins but modifications to their structure have
produced a range of drugs with a broader spectrum of
activity. Examples are cephradine, which has a broad spectrum of activity including some against staphylococci and
can be taken orally; cefotaxime, a parenteral drug with a
very broad spectrum excluding *Pseudomonas*; and ceftazidime, similar to cefotaxime but including *Pseudomonas*
activity. The problem with these drugs is their high cost
and their use should be restricted to situations where there
is no alternative.

Erythromycin

Erythromycin is an extremely useful drug with a macrolide
structure. It can be used in many situations as an alternative
to penicillin when the patient is allergic. In addition it is
active against *Haemophilus influenzae*, *Mycoplasma*,
Legionella, *Bordetella pertussis* and *Campylobacter*.

Chloramphenicol

Chloramphenicol is a cheap drug, well absorbed and distributed, with useful activity against Gram-positive and
negative cocci, *H. influenzae* and *Salmonella typhi*. Its
major drawback is the very rare but usually fatal induction
of marrow aplasia. It is also difficult to use safely in babies.

Tetracyclines

Tetracyclines were widely used to treat exacerbations of
chronic bronchitis until resistance became common. Now
their main use is for treatment of chlamydial infection but

they are also active against *Mycoplasma*, *Brucella*, rick-
ettsiae and *Coxiella*. They should not be used in pregnant
females and children under 9 years old.

Aminoglycosides

Aminoglycosides such as gentamicin, amikacin and tobramycin are used in serious Gram-negative infections. They
are ototoxic and blood levels have to be monitored
carefully, especially when there is renal impairment, since
they are excreted purely by the kidneys. Peak blood levels
are measured 15 minutes after intravenous or 1 hour after
intramuscular administration, and trough levels immediately before the next dose.

Sulphonamides

Sulphonamides were the first synthetic antimicrobial drugs
but their use is now limited by the development of resistance and by the frequency of troublesome side-effects.
Sulphamethoxazole is still widely used in combination with
trimethoprim since they were thought to be synergistic, but
it now seems that trimethoprim alone is just as effective in
the treatment of Gram-negative urinary infection. Trimethoprim can cause thrombocytopenia and megaloblastic
anaemia.

Clindamycin

Clindamycin is a lincosamide with activity against Gram-
positive organisms, including resistant staphylococci, but
also against anaerobic organisms. It achieves good penetration into bone and can be used to treat osteomyelitis.
It went out of favour because of its reported association
with pseudomembranous colitis but it is now clear that it
is no more likely to cause this than other antibiotics.

Metronidazole

Metronidazole is an excellent drug for the treatment of
anaerobic infection. It is cheap when administered orally
or rectally and the more expensive intravenous preparation
is rarely indicated. It is also the first choice in treatment
of *Giardia lamblia*, amoebic disease and *Trichomonas
vaginalis*.

Sodium fusidate

Sodium fusidate is highly bactericidal against staphylococci, including penicillin-resistant ones, but resistance
develops during treatment unless another drug is given
concurrently. It is expensive and is therefore reserved
for treatment of serious infections such as septicaemia
and osteomyelitis.

Vancomycin

Vancomycin is another expensive drug reserved for
serious, penicillin-resistant staphylococcal infection.

4-quinolones

Nalidixic acid has been used exclusively in the treatment of urinary infection by Gram-negative organisms, since adequate levels are only found in the urine. Resistance to this group of drugs is rare since they are not susceptible to plasmid-mediated resistance. A new generation of 4-quinolones has appeared recently, an example of which is ciprofloxacin, which is well absorbed from the intestine and widely distributed. It is the only oral drug active against *Pseudomonas* and may become important for this reason.

Rifampicin

Rifampicin, a synthetic derivative of rifamycin, is central to the treatment of tuberculosis (p. 480) but it is also very active against staphylococci, streptococci and *E. coli*.

ANTIFUNGAL DRUGS

Most fungal infections of the skin are treated with topical preparations but cuticular infection requires prolonged systemic therapy. Visceral infections also require systemic therapy. A limited number of drugs are available for treatment of fungal infections and their use is described in appropriate sections.

Amphotericin B and nystatin

Amphotericin B and nystatin are the best known of the polyene group of antibiotics produced by *Streptomyces* species. They exert a fungistatic effect by binding to sterols in the fungal cell membrane, causing leakage of cell components. Amphotericin B acts synergistically with the unrelated compound flucytosine, probably by increasing permeability to flucytosine.

Neither amphotericin B nor nystatin is absorbed from the intestine but amphotericin B can be administered intravenously, after which there is wide tissue distribution but little penetration to brain and meninges. The plasma half-life is 24 hours and it is excreted very slowly in the urine, 40% of the infused dose appearing in the urine during the following week.

Amphotericin B has a broad spectrum of activity and it is used against the agents of candidiasis, aspergillosis, histoplasmosis, blastomycosis, coccidiomycosis, cryptococcosis and some organisms causing mucormycosis. Minor symptoms following infusion are common and a wide variety of symptoms may be unpleasant enough to require suppression with analgesics, anti-emetics, etc. More serious side-effects occur when there is impairment of renal function which is exacerbated by the resultant rise in plasma drug levels. Renal and haematopoietic toxicity are the main problems. Therapy has to be interrupted to allow a fall in plasma level.

A test dose of 1 mg is given to assess side-effects, followed by 1.0 mg/kg body weight per day infused iv over 6 hours, withdrawing treatment intermittently as required to maintain plasma level at 1–1.5 mg/litre.

Nystatin is not absorbed from the intestine and cannot be given parenterally, but it is useful as a topical or mucosal preparation, particularly for treatment of *Candida* infections. It is available as a suspension or pastilles for oral infection; cream and pessaries for vaginal infections; and cream or ointment for skin infections.

Flucytosine

Flucytosine is a synthetic fluorinated pyrimidine which enters fungal cells and inhibits metabolism by interfering with DNA and RNA synthesis. It is usually given in combination with amphotericin B for treatment of systemic fungal infections and it adds a fungicidal effect to the fungistasis caused by amphotericin. Resistance develops rapidly when it is administered alone.

Flucytosine is well absorbed from the intestine and widely distributed, giving a cerebrospinal fluid concentration 75% of plasma level. Intravenous infusion is difficult and confined to patients unable to take oral medication. Excretion is in the urine, so dosage must be reduced in the presence of renal failure. Side-effects are gastrointestinal disturbance, neutropenia and thrombocytopenia.

Imidazoles

Ketoconazole, miconazole and clotrimazole are examples of drugs in the imidazole group. Most are available only topically and have activity against dermatophytes and *Candida*.

Ketoconazole is an oral preparation which is useful for treatment of severe mucosal infections, such as oesophageal candidiasis which is not responsive to topical treatment. Imidazoles have no place in treatment of systemic fungal infections. The mode of action is not fully understood but imidazoles interfere with synthesis of sterols and other fungal membrane lipids, resulting in defective cell wall synthesis. They may also reduce adherence to mucosal cells and in vitro they enhance killing of *Candida* by leucocytes. Their major toxicity is drug-induced hepatitis, which can progress to irreversible hepatic failure.

Triazoles

Triazoles are a new group of antifungal agents including fluconazole and itraconazole. Early results suggest that they will be useful in treating some systemic mycoses; for example, fluconazole has been used successfully in *Candida* oesophagitis and cryptococcal meningitis. Side-effects appear to be rare.

Griseofulvin

Griseofulvin, produced by *Penicillium griseofulvum*, is absorbed from the gastrointestinal tract and deposited in keratin, where it inhibits growth of dermatophytes. It is relatively non-toxic and can be used in extensive dermatophyte infections which are unresponsive to topical treatment. It is particularly useful for nail and scalp infections (p. 1116).

ANTIVIRAL TREATMENT

Virus metabolism is so closely woven into the metabolism of infected cells that few antiviral agents have been discovered which destroy the virus without also severely damaging host cells. In recent years considerable progress has been made in synthesising agents which specifically inhibit an essential step in virus replication (Table 12.4), without causing host toxicity. This has been achieved in two ways:

1. by using an agent which is activated by the virus, thus localising its action within infected cells
2. by using an agent which inhibits virus metabolism specifically. Usually this is achieved when the agent inhibits a viral enzyme.

Acyclovir, for example, the most widely used agent presently available, produces its specific effects using both of these mechanisms. It is inactive until phosphorylated to a triphosphate by viral thymidine kinase in infected cells. In this form it produces its main antiviral action by inhibiting viral DNA polymerase, essential for synthesis of viral DNA. Acyclovir triphosphate is a more powerful inhibitor of viral than of host DNA polymerases. Although acyclovir seems to be a safe drug it is expensive and its use must therefore be restricted to situations in which it is shown to be clearly beneficial (Table 12.5).

During acute viral infections much of the inflammation is caused by the host response in the later part of the illness and antiviral treatment must be started early to be effective. Antiviral treatment does not affect virus integrated into the host genome and treatment of the primary herpes simplex infection does not influence subsequent viral reactivation. Ganciclovir is an antiviral drug which is licensed for treatment of cytomegalovirus (CMV) infection. It is activated by phosphorylation in a similar way to acyclovir, but ganciclovir depends on human cellular enzymes for this process. Since phosphorylation is not confined to infected cells its toxicity is greater than that of acyclovir and it causes bone marrow suppression. Zidovudine is an inhibitor of human immunodeficiency virus replication which is achieved by inhibition of reverse transcriptase activity.

Table 12.4 Current antiviral treatment

Treatment	Example	Uses	Route
Contact inactivation	Dry ice	Warts	T
Inhibition of virus metabolism			
Uncoating	Amantadine	Influenza A	O
Replication	Acyclovir	HSV, VZV	O,P,T
	Zidovudine	HIV	O
	Ganciclovir	CMV	P
	Vidarabine	HSV, VZV	P,T
	Idoxuridine	HSV, VZV	T
Assembly	Interferons	VZV, HBV	P

HSV = herpes simplex virus; VZV = varicella zoster virus; HIV = human immunodeficiency virus; CMV = cytomegalovirus; HBV = hepatitis B virus
T = topical; O = oral; P = parenteral

Table 12.5 Treatment of herpes virus infections with acyclovir

Virus	Infection	Route
Herpes simplex virus	Encephalitis	IV
	Neonatal infection	IV
	Primary genital infection	O
	Keratoconjunctivitis	T
	Prophylaxis: bone marrow transplantation	O
Varicella zoster	Shingles in immunocompromised patient	IV
	Chickenpox in immunocompromised children	IV
	Chickenpox in neonates	IV

IV = intravenous; O = oral; T = topical

INFECTION IN THE IMMUNOCOMPROMISED PATIENT

An immunocompromised patient is defined as a patient in whom any part of the innate or adaptive immune response is defective. Defects of the immune system are physiological (neonates and the aged), and primary or secondary. Primary immune deficiency diseases are rare and an account is given in Chapter 7. Secondary immune deficiency is more common and of increasing importance (Table 7.5, p. 109). Causes of secondary immune deficiency are:

1. *malignant disease and its treatment*
2. *drug-induced chronic immune suppression*, e.g. in organ transplantation or chronic inflammatory diseases such as systemic lupus erythematosus (SLE)
3. *infection*; the most severe infection is human immunodeficiency virus (p. 250) but many other viruses cause a milder deficiency of cell-mediated immunity (CMI)
4. *splenectomy*
5. *chronic diseases*, e.g. chronic renal failure, malnutrition, protein deficiency, diabetes mellitus.

These conditions cause varying combinations of neutropenia and impairment of humoral and cellular immunity. To some extent organisms likely to cause infection can be predicted from the nature of the underlying disease or the type of treatment. Deficiencies of antibody or neutrophils are associated with infection by encapsulated bacteria, yeasts and fungi. Deficient CMI causes infection by a wider range of pathogens including Gram-positive and *negative* bacteria, viruses, yeasts, fungi, protozoans

Table 12.6 Some micro-organisms causing infection in immuno-compromised patients

Type	Micro-organism	Remarks	Deficiency
Bacteria	Gram-positive e.g. Pneumococcus	Encapsulated	Ab/Neut
	Gram-negative e.g. *H. influenzae*	Encapsulated	CMI
	Mycobacteria e.g. *Avium intracellulare*	Both typical and atypical	CMI
Viruses	Herpes e.g. Herpes simplex virus Varicella zoster virus Cytomegalovirus	Reactivation	CMI
	Echo	Encephalitis	Ab
	Live vaccines e.g. Measles	Virulent	Ab/CMI
Yeasts	*Candida*	Septicaemia/ pneumonia	Ab/Neut
		Mucosal	CMI
Fungi	*Aspergillus*	Systemic	CMI
	Cryptococcus	Meningitis	CMI
Protozoa	*Pneumocystis*	Pneumonia	CMI/Ab
	Toxoplasma	Cerebral	CMI
	Cryptosporidium	Gut	CMI
	Giardia lamblia	Gut	CMI/Ab
Helminths	*Strongyloides*	Systemic	CMI

Ab = antibody; Neut = neutrophil; CMI = cell-mediated immunity

and helminths (Table 12.6). In all these situations immunisation with live viral vaccines is dangerous since the attenuated organism may behave as a pathogen.

The pattern of infection in immunocompromised patients is unusual in several respects. Bacterial infections in splenectomised patients are of sudden onset and rapidly progressive, fulminant pneumococcal septicaemia being the most common. Cellular immune deficiency causes viral infection to be more severe, prolonged and widely disseminated than is usual.

Important examples of particular problems in immunocompromised patients are discussed below.

Fever in the neutropenic patient

During periods of neutropenia hospitals are a hostile environment, since there are many potential pathogens often resistant to antibiotics. The onset of fever should be taken to indicate serious infection unless history and examination reveal an obvious alternative explanation. 'Blind' treatment with antibiotics is started immediately after collection of specimens including blood cultures. Blood cultures are negative in over half of such fever episodes but the choice of antibiotics is guided by positive results in which Gram-negative bacteria, including *Pseudomonas* species, predominate and a combination of a broad-spectrum penicillin with activity against *Pseudomonas* (e.g. piperacillin) and gentamicin is often used (p. 223).

New pulmonary infiltrates on chest radiograph

New pulmonary infiltrates may not be due to infection but the range of possible pathogens is so wide (Table 12.7) that diagnostic specimens often have to be obtained by biopsy. If sputum production is low, bronchoscopy with bronchial lavage and transbronchial or even open lung biopsy may sometimes be helpful, but these investigations are not without risk in a neutropenic and thrombocytopenic patient.

Table 12.7 Organisms causing pneumonia in immunocompromised patients

Bacteria
Gram-positive, e.g. *Strep. pneumoniae*
Gram-negative, e.g. *Haemophilus influenzae*, *Klebsiella pneumoniae*

Viruses
Cytomegalovirus, herpes simplex, varicella zoster
Measles (giant cell pneumonia)

Protozoa
Pneumocystis carinii

Fungi/yeasts
Candida
Aspergillus

Reactivation of herpes viruses

Patients with impaired CMI may suffer severe herpes virus infection. Shingles (varicella zoster) in patients with Hodgkin's disease tends to involve more than one dermatome and there may be dissemination of virus causing widespread chickenpox lesions on the skin and occasionally in viscera. Within affected dermatomes lesions are dense and heal slowly. Reactivation of herpes simplex virus (HSV) may cause extensive perioral ulceration and occasionally visceral dissemination. Cytomegalovirus (CMV) reactivation causes pneumonia in renal transplant recipients.

NOSOCOMIAL INFECTION

Hospitals contain patients who are particularly susceptible to infection and hospital bacteria are often resistant to common antibiotics as a result of previous treatment. Susceptibility to infection is increased in postoperative patients, patients with burns, patients on ventilators, in malnourished patients and in disease states which compromise immunity specifically. Hospital acquired infections are known as 'nosocomial' and are a particular problem on intensive treatment units. The bacteria associated with particular situations can sometimes be predicted; for example, staphylococci and streptococci are common causes of surgical wound infections and *Pseudomonas* frequently infects burns. In ventilated patients difficulties arise in deciding whether bacteria such as *Pseudomonas* are merely colonising the respiratory mucosa or whether they are pathogenic. Antibiotic treatment of colonising organisms is undesirable since the local flora then change to more resistant organisms.

With increasing use of antibiotics in recent years there has been a resurgence of outbreaks of nosocomial infection with methicillin- (and flucloxacillin-) resistant *Staphylococcus aureus* (MRSA). MRSA colonise the skin and nose of normal or diseased subjects but they are particularly persistent in patients with any form of skin lesion. In most cases MRSA do not cause disease but occasionally vulnerable patients can develop septicaemia or local suppuration which necessitates the use of vancomycin. Since MRSA spreads rapidly from patient to patient it is important to isolate infected patients and to screen staff for carriage. Colonised subjects are treated with topical antiseptic preparations and, in the case of staff, removed from work until repeated swabs are clear.

The emergence of bacteria resistant to multiple antibiotics is largely a result of heavy usage of antibiotics and emphasises the need to control their employment both in hospitals and in the community. Most hospitals have antibiotic policies which recommend the antibiotic to be used in a particular situation and restrict administration of some drugs to special situations. The policy is individual to a hospital because it is partly determined by the local microbiological flora.

CONTROL OF INFECTION

Containment of outbreaks of infection is required when susceptible subjects may develop a serious illness if they become infected. It is not always desirable to contain infection. Chickenpox, a mild disease in normal children, is usually severe in adults and so outbreaks among schoolchildren should not be controlled. In a hospital where non-immune patients are liable to develop severe manifestations, however, it is important to prevent cross-infection to non-immune individuals (about 10% of the adult population).

Isolation of patients in single rooms greatly facilitates control of infection. Other measures are determined by the mode of transmission and the degree of infectivity of the organism. Transmission is by:

1. respiratory secretions (e.g. measles, pulmonary tuberculosis)
2. excretions and secretions (e.g. gastroenteritis, hepatitis A, typhoid)
3. skin contact and fomites (e.g. MRSA).

Respiratory transmission can be prevented by having the patient and/or the attendants wear appropriate masks. Organisms transmitted in respiratory secretions usually infect others through the upper or lower respiratory tract, and gowning and hand washing are of minor importance.

When *excretions and secretions* are infectious the most important containment measure is hand washing. When close contact is necessary with a highly infectious patient, such as a patient excreting *Shigella* in the faeces, gowns and gloves are worn. Special arrangements are needed for disposal of excreta, contaminated dressings and contaminated clothing and bedding.

When micro-organisms are found in significant number on the *skin*, in *fomites* and in dust around the patient, as when MRSA colonise patients in hospital, additional precautions must be taken, including the use of overshoes together with gowns and gloves.

In many countries some infections are notifiable (Table 12.8); that is, the medical attendant is obliged by law to report the case to the authority which controls the area in which the patient lives so that steps can be taken to trace contacts. Notification also allows surveillance of the incidence of these infections. Most patients have ceased to be an infectious risk by the time they are discharged from hospital but intestinal pathogens often remain in the stools for several weeks. Carriers of such pathogens are advised to avoid handling food for others, to wash hands regularly and to avoid towel sharing. Following notification stool samples will be checked by the local authority until they are pathogen-free.

Table 12.8 Notifiable diseases (UK, October 1988)

Under the Public Health (Control of Disease) Act 1984	Under the Public Health (Infectious Disease) Regulations 1988
Cholera	Acute encephalitis
Plague	Acute poliomyelitis
Relapsing fever	Anthrax
Smallpox	Diphtheria
Typhus	Dysentery (amoebic or bacillary)
	Leprosy
	Leptospirosis
	Malaria
	Measles
	Meningitis
	Meningococcal septicaemia (without meningitis)
	Mumps
	Ophthalmia neonatorum
	Paratyphoid fever
	Rabies
	Scarlet fever
	Tetanus
	Tuberculosis
	Typhoid fever
	Viral haemorrhagic fever
	Viral hepatitis
	Whooping cough
	Yellow fever

AIDS is not a statutorily notifiable disease but doctors are urged to participate in a voluntary confidential reporting scheme.

IMMUNISATION

Active immunisation

Active immunisation is the administration of antigen to induce a protective immune response in the host. Antigens used include crude preparations of killed organisms, extracellular products of organisms and live, attenuated organ-

Infectious, Tropical and Parasitic Diseases

Table 12.9 UK immunisation schedule (1989)

Age	Immunisation	Type of vaccine	Route
3 months	Diphtheria	Toxoid	IM or SC
	Tetanus	Toxoid	IM or SC
	Pertussis	Killed	IM or SC
	Polio	Live attenuated	O
5 and 8 months	As above	As above	As above
15 months	Measles, mumps, rubella (MMR)*	Live attenuated	IM
5 years	Diphtheria		
	Tetanus }	As above	As above
	Polio		
11–13 years	BCG	Live attenuated	ID
11–13 years (girls only)	Rubella†	Live attenuated	IM
School-leaving	Tetanus }	As above	As above
	Polio		

* MMR introduced into UK in October 1988
† Retained in UK until MMR established
IM = intramuscular; SC = subcutaneous; O = oral; ID = intradermal

isms. The immunisation schedule current in the UK in 1989 is shown in Table 12.9. This schedule is kept under constant review and a judgment has always to be made about whether the benefits of an individual vaccine outweigh its potential hazards. Smallpox vaccination was routine until the disease was eliminated from the world. Mumps vaccine, which had been in use in the USA for many years, was introduced as part of the routine childhood immunisation schedule in October 1988. The policy of immunising only females against rubella has also been changed since there is still a notable incidence of congenital rubella. Immunisation of both sexes in the second year of life has been introduced. BCG (bacille Calmette-Guérin) immunisation for protection against tuberculosis is more important among children of racial groups with a high incidence of the disease, such as Asian immigrants to the UK. In North America the incidence of tuberculosis is not high enough to justify its routine use. In contrast BCG vaccination of neonates is a common practice in the tropics.

Contra-indications to immunisation

1. Live vaccines should not be given to anyone with untreated malignant disease or with any form of immunodeficiency, including those receiving immuno-suppressive therapy, or to pregnant women.
2. A live vaccine dose should not be given within 3 weeks of another injected live vaccine.
3. Coincidental severe febrile illness may limit the response to immunisation. Immunisation should therefore be postponed *but not forgotten*.
4. Significant documented allergy to any component of the vaccine may be a contra-indication to its use.
5. Rubella vaccine should not be given in pregnancy and

pregnancy should be avoided for 1 month after immunisation against rubella.
6. Pertussis immunisation should be discussed with a specialist if a parent or sibling has a history of epilepsy.

Passive immunisation

Passive immunisation is the administration of antibody preparations to prevent or ameliorate infection. Pooled human immunoglobulin is the crudest form which is used commonly to protect travellers against hepatitis A virus infection. More defined preparations of hyperimmune globulin contain high levels of antibodies to particular organisms, usually viruses, which are not present in sufficient concentration in pooled human immunoglobulin to provide protection. Examples are hepatitis B immune globulin given following needle-stick injuries; varicella zoster immune globulin used in neonates born to mothers who have recently developed chickenpox (p. 238), and tetanus immune globulin used for patients at risk of developing tetanus. Most current antibody preparations are derived from human serum, avoiding the problems of administering foreign serum protein. The disadvantages of this form of immunisation are that passively administered antibody has a short half-life, giving protection for only a few weeks, and that the treatment has to be given soon after exposure to be effective.

PREVENTIVE MEASURES FOR OVERSEAS TRAVEL OR RESIDENCE

The individual who is going to travel to the tropics and subtropics can do much to protect himself against the risks of infection with a range of pathogens.

Protection of skin

The skin must be protected against biting insects. This is not only important for the prevention of malaria, but also for protection against viral, rickettsial, protozoal and filarial diseases transmitted by insect vectors.

Exposure to ticks occurs mainly in rural bush areas and so appropriate clothing and footwear is needed to prevent ticks getting on to the skin. Evening and night hours are times for maximum frequency of biting by many insects and at these times the skin should be covered as much as possible and insect repellants applied to exposed areas or as impregnated wrist and ankle bands. Mosquito nets should be used in malarious areas if doors and windows are not screened. It is also useful to spray bedrooms with insecticide last thing at night.

Schistosomiasis is acquired by contact between skin and slow-flowing or still water containing cercariae. Swimming and paddling in fresh water are best avoided in endemic areas.

Protection against malaria

Preventing the bite of the mosquito is very important (see

above). The traveller should be told that there is *no* vaccine against malaria and that none of the vaccines that he receives prior to travel is of any benefit in this regard. Chemoprophylaxis against malaria is the other mainstay of protection (details in Table 12.35, p. 302).

Immunisation for travellers or overseas residents

A range of vaccines is available and the commonly used ones are listed in Table 12.10. *Poliomyelitis* is still common in many areas of the world and so adequate vaccination should be assured in all travellers. *Yellow fever* vaccination is essential for those visiting tropical Africa, the Caribbean and South America. Oral poliomyelitis and yellow fever vaccines should be given either together or separated by an interval of 3 weeks. *Hepatitis B* vaccination is only recommended for those who are likely to be at particular risk, i.e. health care and hospital laboratory workers. *Anti-hepatitis A virus* immunoglobulin is presently the only protection that can be offered to those who are susceptible. Pre-exposure *rabies* vaccination is needed by those who may have any contact with animals. Increasingly tourists undertaking overland travels are having pre-exposure vaccination. The intradermal route allows more economical use of the vaccine.

Tetanus vaccination is needed for any who may be at particular risk of trauma, e.g. military personnel, construction workers, etc. *Typhoid* vaccination is a sensible precaution for many areas but those vaccinated should be told that having the vaccine does not mean that they are 100% protected and can be careless about sources of water and food. Cholera vaccination is not effective.

Table 12.10   Immunisation for travellers to and residents in the tropics and subtropics

Vaccine	Route	Duration of protection	Comments
Poliomyelitis			
Live attenuated	O	Lifelong	Not in pregnancy or immune-suppressed
Killed	SC	Several years	
Yellow fever	SC	10 years	Not in infants or pregnancy
Hepatitis B	IM	Not yet known	For health care workers
Rabies	IM or ID	Not known	For workers with animals
Tetanus	SC	10 years	
Typhoid	SC	3 years	
Meningococcal	SC	3 years	Types A and C only
Passive immunity			
Hepatitis A	IM	4 months	Endemic areas

O = oral; SC = subcutaneous; IM = intramuscular; ID = intradermal

Protection of the gut

Gastrointestinal infection is the most common affliction faced by the traveller. Boiled water used to make tea and coffee or left to cool in a covered, clean container is safe to drink. Bottled drinks are safe. Water from the tap or water used to make ice cubes may not be safe. Tincture of iodine (2%) can be used to sterilise water, adding 0.5 ml per litre and allowing it to stand for 30 minutes. Iodine is more potent than chlorine-based sterilising tablets.

SYNDROMES OF INFECTION

SEPTICAEMIA

Septicaemia is uncontrolled bacterial infection in the blood, causing systemic illness. In contrast to septicaemia, transient bacteraemia is fairly common in normal subjects. Septicaemia is a much more serious condition which is likely to lead to death if untreated.

Aetiology

A wide range of bacteria can cause septicaemia but they can be divided into those which do so as *part of a primary infection* by a single organism acquired in the community, and those which cause septicaemia as a *complication of another process*, such as abdominal sepsis following surgery, when there is often a mixed infection. Community acquired infections are usually recognised as part of a specific illness, as when *Streptococcus pneumoniae* septicaemia complicates pneumonia, meningococcaemia with meningitis, or *E. coli* septicaemia with pyelonephritis. The other kind of septicaemia is usually seen in hospitals, often in a debilitated patient, and the likely bacteria can often be predicted from the clinical situation.

Pathogenesis

Whole bacteria and substances released by bacterial lysis trigger a complex series of events. A major component is endotoxin, the lipopolysaccharide component of Gram-negative bacterial cell walls, of which lipid A is the part responsible for most of the toxic effects. Experimentally, lipid A can activate complement and Hageman factor and it reproduces in animals many of the signs associated with 'Gram-negative' septicaemia in man. Its role in human infection is still controversial, since assays for its presence in serum remain unsatisfactory. Important pathological consequences ensuing from activation of the potent inflammatory pathways are hypotension, increased vascular permeability and consumptive coagulopathy.

Less attention has been paid to the effects of Gram-positive organisms, but activation of inflammatory processes can certainly be triggered by cell membrane components of these organisms. An example is alternate

229

pathway complement activation (Fig. 7.2, p. 101) by teichoic acid found in *Staph. aureus* membranes.

Clinical features and diagnosis

The manifestations of septicaemia depend on the age of the patient, the illness being more featureless and more lethal at extremes of age. On the whole, signs are non-specific but there are signs in the skin suggestive of the diagnosis, such as purpuric lesions associated with meningococcaemia and pustular lesions in staphylococcal septicaemia. Usually there is a rapid deterioration in the patient's condition, including a change in mental state. Fever is often present, with tachycardia and bounding pulse, but as the condition progresses the patient becomes hypothermic with a rapid thready pulse and peripheral vasoconstriction. The latter situation is often considered to be typical of Gram-negative septicaemia, but it also occurs with septicaemia caused by Gram-positive organisms. For this reason the general term 'septicaemic shock' is usually used. Prolonged hypotension leads to acute renal failure and disseminated intravascular coagulation causes bleeding. Adult respiratory distress syndrome (p. 518) frequently complicates hospital acquired septicaemia.

The diagnosis is based on clinical assessment but blood cultures, urine cultures, wound swab and any aspirate from an infected site should be obtained at the time the patient is seen, so that antibiotic treatment can be started without undue delay. The antibiotic regimen can be changed if necessary when culture results are available and the response to treatment has been assessed. Blood cultures should be taken whether the patient is febrile or not.

Treatment

Treatment is urgent because of the high mortality. Antibiotics and circulatory support are the mainstays of management. The use of plasma expanders and selective vaso-active drugs is discussed on page 548.

Antibiotics

The initial choice of antibiotics is based on a logical guess at the bacteria responsible (p. 221). As few antibiotics as possible are given to achieve the necessary cover. As new drugs are developed the following simple guidelines to management will change. The common choice is a combination of a broad-spectrum penicillin such as ampicillin, with an aminoglycoside such as gentamicin. One problem with this approach is that many patients are in incipient renal failure, which enhances the toxicity of gentamicin. Newer drugs, like cefotaxime and piperacillin, are active against Gram-positive and Gram-negative bacteria, and lack the toxicity of gentamicin, but they are more expensive. If anaerobic septicaemia is suspected metronidazole is often used, and for hospital acquired staphylococcal infection a β-lactamase-resistant penicillin, such as flucloxacillin, is added. *Pseudomonas* infections are treated with a combination of drugs: for example, azlocillin and gentamicin.

PYREXIA OF UNKNOWN ORIGIN

When a patient has an elevated body temperature for a period of longer than 3 weeks without a cause being found the diagnostic problem is called pyrexia (or fever) of unknown origin (PUO). This is a challenging clinical problem and it is important to adopt a systematic approach guided by the clinical situation. Regulation of body temperature is discussed on p. 166.

A febrile patient may lose the normal diurnal variation in body temperature or may sometimes have an exaggerated diurnal pattern, with a rise during the night causing drenching night sweats (common in tuberculosis and lymphoma) followed by a rapid fall. Many patterns of fever are described but they are rarely helpful in diagnosis.

Causes of PUO

The most common causes of PUO vary according to the age of the patient, and published incidences vary with the type of institution at which the problem is studied. Infection is usually the most common cause in children, whereas infection and neoplastic disease are equally important in adults. Connective tissue disease can present with fever at any age. Still's disease and SLE are commoner causes in children and young adults, and polymyalgia and giant cell arteritis more frequent in the elderly.

Infection

Most bacterial infections cause an illness which is clinically manifest within 3 weeks, but there are some exceptions. Bacterial endocarditis can cause low-grade illness, particularly in the elderly. Most cases can be diagnosed by blood culture but occasionally blood cultures are repeatedly negative. Infection in the biliary tract may be associated with only minor clinical signs and little abnormality of liver function tests.

Intracellular bacteria, such as *Brucella* and some *Salmonella* species, can cause recurrent septicaemia, but this can usually be diagnosed by blood culture. Deep-seated abscess is a possible cause of PUO and modern imaging techniques are helpful in locating the collection (p. 220).

Summary 1   Causes of pyrexia of unknown origin in UK
Frequency is given in brackets

- Infection   (30%)
- Neoplasia   (25%)
- Connective tissue (autoimmune) disease   (20%)
- Miscellaneous   (12%)
- Undiagnosed   (13%)

Tuberculosis is still a major cause of PUO in developing countries and in some temperate countries such as the UK, especially in Asian patients. Often the granulomatous lesions of tuberculosis are too small to cause pulmonary radiological abnormalities and the site of infection is often outside the lungs.

Viral infections rarely cause PUO (within the definition), with the important exception of human immunodeficiency virus. The history should therefore enquire into sexual practices, intravenous drug abuse and transfusions.

Fungal infections rarely cause PUO without a predisposing cause but they may do so as a complication of immunosuppressive disease or therapy. An exception is histoplasmosis.

Neoplasia

Lymphomas frequently produce a prolonged period of fever before any other manifestation emerges, and it has been shown that they can secrete pyrogens. Leukaemias can also cause PUO but this is sometimes caused by a complicating infection. Many occult solid tumours can present as PUO, among them hypernephroma, pancreatic carcinoma, intestinal tumours, bronchial carcinoma, ovarian tumours and sarcomas. Fever is particularly likely when there are hepatic metastases. Atrial myxoma is a rare benign tumour (p. 428) which occasionally produces an illness similar to bacterial endocarditis.

Connective tissue (autoimmune) disease

Most diseases in the category of connective tissue disease can present with PUO before the characteristic disease pattern emerges. SLE, rheumatoid arthritis and Still's disease (including the adult form), polyarteritis nodosa, temporal arteritis and polymyalgia rheumatica should be considered according to the clinical setting.

Miscellaneous

Granulomatous conditions. Granulomatous conditions include sarcoidosis, granulomatous hepatitis and Wegener's granulomatosis. Sarcoidosis often lacks overt signs in the early phase of the disease and should be considered, particularly in ethnic groups with a high prevalence, such as West Indians.

Factitious. One of the most odd forms of human behaviour is the habitual feigning, or deliberate inducement of, illness. Factitious fever is caused in two ways:

1. In the first the fever disappears when the temperature is measured by someone other than the patient, with the patient under continuous observation: the patient is either saying that fever exists when it does not, or is manipulating the thermometer when the nurse's back is turned.
2. In the other, more serious, form the patient induces true fever by self-injury or self-infection. The methods used are diverse, but faeces are the usual source of

organisms and infection is induced by rubbing or injecting organisms into the skin or blood. Suspicion is aroused when mixed and varying organisms which could be faecal are found in an unexpected site, or when infection persists despite treatment which would normally be effective.

Patients are often nurses or young women associated with medical work and there are sometimes personal problems which suggest that this behaviour is a plea for attention or help. When suspicion grows that fever is factitious it is wise to avoid directly confronting the patient with the possibility. Usually it will be denied and sometimes confrontation can precipitate a psychiatric crisis, even resulting in suicide. It is preferable to attempt to solve the associated problems if they can be identified and to create a situation in which it is difficult for the patient to continue to provoke sepsis, e.g. by removing intravenous catheters or covering inflamed sites. The patient should be made to realise that the manœuvres are understood, if possible without a direct accusation. The best efforts to resolve factitious fever often fail and patients either return intermittently or present themselves to another medical team.

Inflammatory bowel disease. Inflammatory bowel disease is usually associated with incriminating symptoms such as weight loss and diarrhoea, but these may be slow to emerge.

Drug reaction. Once thought of, drug reaction is a straightforward cause of PUO. The possibility that the fever is caused by a drug is tested by withdrawal.

Multiple pulmonary emboli. When frequent small embolic events occur, pyrexia may be the sole manifestation before the pulmonary circulation is greatly compromised.

Other causes. Other occasional causes of PUO are alcoholic hepatitis, familial Mediterranean fever, Whipple's disease and occult haematoma. There are some young women whose normal evening temperature runs above the normal range by up to 0.5°C. This usually comes to light after an infection with slow recovery. Once it is established that there is no underlying pathology the patient can be reassured. Tropical causes are discussed on page 232.

Diagnosis

A careful history and examination of the patient is essential and it is important to return to the patient repeatedly to go over parts of the history and to look for emergent physical signs. Simple screening tests which may need to be repeated at intervals include full blood count and ESR, routine biochemistry of blood and urine, cultures of blood, urine and other relevant samples, and chest radiograph.

Additional investigations are guided by the clinical findings. There are two approaches. One is to perform tests which are more or less specific for particular diseases, e.g. the Kveim test for sarcoid, auto-antibodies in autoimmunity or antibodies to particular pathogens. The other is to investigate a particular site which seems to be generating symptoms or signs. The latter is more often helpful and it is in this area that advances in imaging techniques have changed the methods for diagnosing PUO. *Ultrasound* is particularly useful for abdominal examination, both in detection of solid tissue abnormalities, such as tumours of the kidney or pancreas, lymph node enlargement or infiltration of the liver, and in locating collections of pus (subphrenic, perinephric, intrahepatic, etc.). *CT scanning* is less widely available but it supplements, and is in some situations superior to, ultrasound. A further use of these techniques is to guide the needle during *tissue biopsy*. Conventional *contrast radiology*, such as barium studies of the intestine and intravenous pyelogram still has an important role. The use of ^{111}Indium labelled leucocytes is described on page 220. Even if no localised lesion has been found by imaging techniques, certain biopsy procedures are sometimes rewarding. If the liver enzyme tests are abnormal, percutaneous *liver biopsy* should be considered, since diffuse granulomatous or infiltrative diseases such as sarcoidosis or lymphoma may be detected. *Marrow aspiration and biopsy* may reveal cryptic tuberculosis, or lymphomatous or carcinomatous infiltration. The marrow and liver biopsy should be cultured for *Mycobacterium tuberculosis*.

Patience and persistence are essential in managing PUO. Neoplasia is the only major cause of death among PUO patients, so exclusion of treatable neoplastic disease is a priority. In most studies about one-fifth of cases remain unsolved despite the best efforts.

The approach to the patient with fever in the tropics

Febrile illness is one of the common reasons for seeking medical attention in the tropics, or after travels in the tropics. The range of causes encompasses infectious and non-infectious sources. Among infections, those that have a worldwide distribution, such as pneumonia or urinary tract infection, must be considered, as well as infections which are peculiar to the tropics and subtropics.

Clinical features

A detailed history is again essential in making a diagnosis. This should include accurate recording of the dates of travel, the duration of stay, the countries visited, with information on the places involved (cities, rural areas, beach resorts, etc.), and the reasons for travel. Information about sexual contact during travel is also important. The history should include details about vaccination prior to travel and malaria prophylaxis, with some assessment of the regularity of taking prophylaxis.

In recording the history of the present illness the chronology of events should be recorded, particularly noting the interval between the end of the patient's travels and the onset of illness where this has occurred after return home. This information gives an idea of the incubation period of the disease (Table 12.11). Physical examination should pay attention to the presence of skin lesions, oral lesions, jaundice, adenopathy, hepatosplenomegaly and involvement of the nervous system. After initial assessment it is vital to re-assess the patient at frequent intervals, looking for the appearance of symptoms and signs that may lead to diagnosis and to assess the response to any specific treatment given. *Appendix table 1* (p. 326) gives a differential diagnosis of common syndromes.

Investigations

The investigations done will depend on the clinical diagnosis or the differential diagnosis, but *blood films* should be examined for malaria parasites in any febrile patient who has been to a malarious area. *Blood films* may also be examined for trypanosomes. A *full blood count* is useful for looking for leucocytosis (suggesting bacterial infections), leucopenia (typhoid, viral infections), pancytopenia (visceral leishmaniasis) or eosinophilia (helminthiasis: schistosomiasis, fascioliasis, visceral larva migrans, clonorchiasis,

Table 12.11 Incubation periods for some tropical diseases

Type of organism	Short (less than 2 weeks)	Intermediate (2–6 weeks)	Long (more than 6 weeks)
Viruses	Arbovirus infections Marburg virus disease	Poliomyelitis Hepatitis A virus Arenavirus infection Ebola virus infection Lassa fever virus infection Haemorrhagic fever with renal syndrome	Hepatitis B Non-A, non-B hepatitis Rabies
Rickettsia		Q fever	
Bacteria	Typhoid	Typhoid Brucellosis Leptospirosis Relapsing fever Lymphogranuloma venereum	
Protozoa	*Trypanosoma cruzi* infection	Malaria Toxoplasmosis *Trypanosoma rhodesiense* infection	Visceral leishmaniasis *Trypanosome gambiense* infection
Helminths		Schistosomiasis (Katayama syndrome)	

Bancroftian filariasis). A *Mantoux test* should done early in the course of investigation. *Blood cultures* should be taken and, if brucellosis is a possibility, kept under observation for up to 6 weeks, as this organism grows slowly. *Serological tests* that may be useful include those for syphilis, leptospirosis, rickettsial diseases, brucellosis, amoebiasis, leishmaniasis, trypanosomiasis, toxoplasmosis, filariasis and schistosomiasis. It is not implied that these serological tests should be requested routinely in the febrile patient. They should be used selectively in relation to the clinical presentation. As a routine a serum sample should be obtained from a febrile patient on admission and saved, and a second sample should be obtained 10 days later. This pair of sera can then be used in tests for viral, leptospiral and other infections, looking for a change (usually a rise) in titre. A *chest radiograph* should be obtained. The scanning procedures mentioned above are used as clinically indicated.

When investigations have failed to show a cause additional investigations may be required, including *bone marrow aspiration* and *liver biopsy*. Smears of marrow aspirate should be stained for *Leishmania* and tubercle bacilli and aspirate should be cultured for these organisms and fungi. Liver biopsy material should be cultured for these organisms as well as examined histologically.

Treatment

Ideally treatment will follow from the specific microbiological diagnosis of the cause of fever. Occasionally it may be necessary to treat the patient for a disease suspected clinically but not or not yet proven by laboratory tests. This may be treatment for malaria, or typhoid or rickettsial infection, or tuberculosis in fevers of longer duration.

GASTROENTERITIS

Gastroenteritis is defined as an acute disease with diarrhoea and/or vomiting and a variable degree of systemic illness. 'Food poisoning' is a term used to describe a self-limiting form of gastroenteritis, which is caused by eating contaminated food.

Aetiology

A large variety of micro-organisms can cause gastroenteritis (Table 12.12) but the causative organism cannot be identified in over half of all cases. Salmonellae and *Campylobacter* species are among the most frequent causes. In children the spectrum of organisms is slightly different and rotavirus is the most frequently recognised agent.

Epidemiology

Gastroenteritis is a common infection in all parts of the world, occurring sporadically or in epidemics. Epidemics occur when a common source of food or drink is con-

Table 12.12 Common causes of gastroenteritis

Cause	Clinical presentation
Tissue-damaging bacteria	
Salmonella enteritidis	Diarrhoea, vomiting
Campylobacter jejuni	Diarrhoea predominantly
Shigella species	Dysentery
E. coli	Diarrhoea predominantly
Toxin-producing bacteria	
E. coli (enterotoxigenic)	Secretory diarrhoea
Vibrio cholerae	Secretory diarrhoea
Clostridium difficile	Pseudomembranous colitis
Staphylococcus	Vomiting (short incubation)
Bacillus cereus	Vomiting (short incubation)
Tissue-damaging viruses	
Rotavirus	Infantile diarrhoea
Norwalk virus	Winter vomiting
Adenovirus	Diarrhoea, vomiting
Enterovirus	Diarrhoea, vomiting
Others (tissue-damaging mainly)	
Cryptosporidium	Diarrhoea
Entamoeba histolytica	Dysentery
Giardia lamblia	Chronic diarrhoea (steatorrhoea)

taminated with micro-organisms and when infection spreads from person to person by the faecal–oral route. For example, *Salmonella enteritidis* species frequently colonise the gut of chickens bred in battery conditions and may infect the oviduct and eggs of hens in batteries. During evisceration of the chicken in the factory the meat is contaminated and the salmonellae survive freezing and thawing. If such chickens are not thoroughly cooked, salmonellae are ingested and colonise the intestine.

Some forms of gastroenteritis show striking seasonal variations in frequency but these are usually significant only in temperate areas. Rotavirus is the most common cause of infantile diarrhoea worldwide. In Britain and the USA its peak incidence is in two or three months during the winter, but in tropical climates there is little seasonal variation. Outbreaks of food poisoning caused by *Salmonella*, *Campylobacter* or toxin-producing *Staph. aureus* are more common in summer.

Pathogenesis

Organisms must evade the host defences and colonise the intestine before they can cause disease. Gastric acid is an important defence and patients with a partial gastrectomy are unusually susceptible to intestinal infection. The bacteria adhere to intestinal epithelium and some bacteria have on their surface determinants which bind to epithelial receptors. Examples are *Vibrio cholerae* and some strains of *E. coli*.

The known mechanisms by which micro-organisms cause diarrhoea can be divided into two groups: toxin secretion

12

and mucosal damage. These are not mutually exclusive and the precise mechanism is unknown for many organisms.

Toxin secretion

Cholera is a good example of small intestinal, toxin-mediated, secretory diarrhoea. The toxin is a complex molecule which is released into the enterocyte where it stimulates adenyl cyclase activity (p. 275). Enterotoxigenic strains of *E. coli* secrete a heat-labile enterotoxin which acts in a similar way. In staphylococcal food poisoning enterotoxin-secreting staphylococci multiply in food, and the toxin causes vomiting and diarrhoea within hours of ingestion. Staphylococci are not detected in the stools of patients with this type of food poisoning. *Bacillus cereus*, which contaminates reheated rice, causes vomiting by a similar mechanism.

Mucosal damage

Shigellae invade the colonic mucosa and cause local inflammation, so the faeces contain blood and inflammatory cells. Impairment of water absorption from the colon is the cause of fluid stools. Salmonellae, *Campylobacter* and rotavirus are also invasive and cause tissue damage but the precise mechanisms are not understood. Damage to the brush border of the enterocytes causes temporary disaccharidase deficiency which may prolong the diarrhoea after small intestine infection, even after the pathogen has been eliminated.

Clinical features

Most episodes of gastroenteritis are mild and self-limiting. The incubation period is usually short, ranging from a few hours with staphylococcal food poisoning up to 5 days with *Campylobacter* infection. Vomiting, diarrhoea and cramping abdominal pains are typical features. Large-volume stools suggest a small bowel diarrhoea. The stools are fluid without blood or pus in toxin-mediated disease (e.g. cholera), but when invasion and mucosal damage occurs in *Salmonella*, *Shigella* and *Campylobacter* infections blood and mucus may be seen in the stool. The appearance of the stools is an unreliable guide to the type of organism.

The major consequence of gastroenteritis is dehydration with electrolyte imbalance. Babies are more vulnerable and can rapidly become severely dehydrated. It is essential that the clinician can make a reasonably accurate assessment of the degree of dehydration and Table 12.13 gives some guidelines.

Fever and signs of systemic illness suggest invasive pathogens. Some invasive organisms can cause septicaemia (e.g. *Salmonella typhimurium*), and some shigellae produce neurotoxins which enter the circulation in the absence of septicaemia and, reaching the central nervous system, cause headache and meningism.

The illness is over within 7 days in most infections but symptoms are liable to persist for longer with shigellae and *Campylobacter*. Persisting diarrhoea suggests *Giardia*

Table 12.13 Assessment of degree of dehydration

Degree	Body weight loss	Clinical assessment Symptoms/signs	Degree
Mild	4–5%	Thirst	Present
		Conscious level	Normal
		Skin turgor	Normal
		Mucosae	Moist/dry
		Fontanelle	Normal
		Pulse rate	Normal
		Blood pressure	Normal
		Urine output	Normal
Moderate	6–9%	Thirst	Present
		Conscious level	Irritable, lethargic (infants and young children)
		Skin turgor	Reduced
		Mucosae	Dry
		Fontanelle	Sunken
		Pulse rate	Increased
		Blood pressure	Normal or reduced
		Postural hypotension	Present (older children/adults)
		Urine output	Reduced
Severe	More than 10%	Conscious level	Drowsy/coma
		Skin turgor	Inelastic
		Mucosae	Very dry
		Fontanelle	Sunken
		Pulse rate	Increased (may be impalpable)
		Blood pressure	Reduced (unrecordable)
		Urine output	May be anuric

infection, especially if steatorrhoea is present; persistent diarrhoea and bleeding suggest amoebic dysentery.

Diagnosis

Clinical diagnosis is usually straightforward but problems arise when there is vomiting in the absence of diarrhoea; when abdominal pains are accompanied by localised tenderness, suggesting pelvic inflammatory disease or appendicitis; and when blood in the stools is taken to indicate inflammatory bowel disease. A positive diagnosis is established by identification of the organism in stools by microscopy (electron microscopy or antigen assay for rotavirus) or culture.

Treatment

Rehydration can usually be achieved by administration of oral fluids containing glucose and electrolytes. Oral rehydration therapy is discussed in more detail on page 257. In the home, a simple method of preparation is to add 1 heaped teaspoon of sugar and a pinch of salt to a beaker (250 ml) of water. Fruit squash drinks can exacerbate diarrhoea because of excess sugar (secondary disaccharidase deficiency is common), but a very dilute solution is occasionally helpful when a child finds the salty rehydration fluid unpalatable. In children milk is completely withdrawn in the first 24 hours and is re-introduced as rapidly as possible. Breast-feeding should be maintained, especially in tropical countries.

Intravenous fluid replacement is rarely required but persistent vomiting or severe dehydration with circulatory collapse is an indication for its use.

Antibiotics are normally not required but there are some situations in which their use is justified:

1. septicaemic *Salmonella* infection
2. severe shigellosis
3. severe *Campylobacter* infection
4. infection with *Yersinia, V. cholerae, Entamoeba histolytica* or *Giardia lamblia.*

Problems associated with use of antibiotics are exacerbation of diarrhoea, prolonged carriage of some organisms (e.g. salmonellae) and development of resistance to multiple antibiotics (e.g. shigellae).

ACUTE UPPER RESPIRATORY INFECTION

Common cold and pharyngitis

The common cold is familiar to all since its incidence is 1–4 episodes per person per year. Despite this frequency large gaps remain in our knowledge of pathogenesis although it is clear that many viruses can cause the same clinical entity. There is considerable overlap between organisms causing colds and those causing pharyngitis (Table 12.14). Pharyngitis is more important, since it is often part of a more systemic illness. In the developed world, group A streptococcal pharyngitis is now rarely complicated by rheumatic fever or glomerulonephritis. Since these complications can be prevented by treatment up to a week after onset of pharyngitis and since the majority of episodes of pharyngitis are caused by viruses, antibiotic treatment should be reserved for culture-proven cases of streptococcal pharyngitis. Penicillin, as a single im dose or orally for a minimum of 10 days, is the treatment of choice for streptococcal pharyngitis, with erythromycin for penicillin-allergic subjects. Ampicillin and related drugs should be avoided, since they often cause a rash in patients with infectious mononucleosis.

Upper respiratory infections are frequently complicated by otitis media in children and, less often, by sinusitis in adults or children. These are usually caused by secondary bacterial infection and it is therefore important to recognise them and treat with antibiotics.

Common bacterial causes of otitis media include *Strep. pneumoniae, H. influenzae* (mainly untypable), group A β-haemolytic streptococci and *Branhamella catarrhalis.*

The bacteria which cause acute sinusitis are similar to those incriminated in otitis media but anaerobes, Gram-negatives and *Staph. aureus* should also be considered. Upper respiratory anaerobic bacteria are usually penicillin-sensitive in contrast to those found in the large bowel.

Table 12.14 Causes of upper respiratory infection

Disease	Causative organism
Common cold and pharyngitis	Rhinovirus Coronavirus Influenza virus Para-influenza virus Respiratory syncytial virus Adenovirus Unknown
Pharyngitis/tonsillitis	as above, plus: Epstein-Barr virus β-haemolytic streptococcus group A *Mycoplasma pneumoniae* Mixed anaerobes and spirochaetes* *Corynebacterium diphtheriae** *Neisseria gonorrhoea**
Stomatitis	*Candida albicans* Herpes simplex virus Coxsackie A and other enteroviruses Mixed anaerobic bacteria

* Less common.

Acute stomatitis

In contrast to pharyngitis, the microbial cause of acute stomatitis can often be diagnosed from the appearance of lesions in and around the mouth. *Candida* is a common pathogen, particularly in debilitated patients, patients receiving broad-spectrum antibiotics and patients with human immunodeficiency virus infection. The appearance of white plaques on an erythematous background is characteristic and the wide distribution, including the buccal mucosa, is helpful. Ulcers are usually superficial and not easily confused with primary herpes simplex infection. The latter is often associated with perioral clusters of vesicles. Severely painful ulceration of the mouth and lips in a young immunocompetent patient is usually due either to Stevens-Johnson syndrome or to primary herpes simplex infection. Coxsackie virus infection may cause small, scattered vesicles and ulcers but they are more sparse than those of herpes simplex and less painful. Other, non-infective causes of ulcers must also be considered, such as aphthous ulcers and, rarely, Behçet's disease (p. 1002).

Infections in the subcutaneous tissue spaces of the face and neck often originate from periodontal infection. Ludwig's angina is an anaerobic bacterial infection of the submandibular and sublingual spaces, which causes firm swelling of the tissues below the chin. These may press inwards and compromise the airway. There is accompanying fever and tachycardia and the patient requires urgent antibiotic treatment, usually penicillin and metronidazole.

SEXUALLY TRANSMITTED DISEASES

Sexually transmitted diseases (STD) are infections commonly transferred through sexual contact. Our appreciation of the range of agents capable of being transmitted sexually has increased.

Epidemiology

The prevalence and incidence of sexually transmitted infections varies in different parts of the world. This is due to a variation both in the diseases found and in the methods of reporting such infections. The type of sexual behaviour and the sexual orientation of the person involved also influence the transmission of the infectious agents.

For England and Wales there has been a marked increase in STD in recent years (Fig. 12.5). In the UK there was a fall in incidence of syphilis and gonorrhoea after the introduction of penicillin, but the number of reported infections rose again during the 1960s. Figure 12.6 shows the most commonly found sexually transmitted diseases treated at genito-urinary medicine clinics in England and Wales. This is an underestimate of the problem. Morbidity associated with sexually transmitted disease is more common in women and the agents responsible are more difficult to identify.

Reported STDs are observed mostly in the 20–24-year-old age group, followed by 25–29 and 15–19-year-olds. In the Western world male homosexuals are more likely to

contract hepatitis B, syphilis and HIV infection than their heterosexual counterparts. However, the incidence of newly acquired syphilis and gonorrhoea in homosexual men is falling as trends in sexual behaviour change.

The basis of any STD service is the control of sexually transmitted infections. There are basic requirements:

1. The patient needs ready access to a specialist centre for accurate diagnosis and treatment of any infection. Attendance needs to be voluntary. Treating the index case only partly helps in controlling an infection, therefore sexual partners need to be identified and treated.
2. The patient's co-operation in all these matters is optimum if he/she is assured of absolute confidentiality. The STD service is the most confidential in the present health service and details are generally only released with the patient's consent.
3. Education about sexually transmitted diseases, both for an individual and as part of a general health education, is important in helping to control the spread of infection.
4. The clinics keep a record of the number of patients seen with each infection and these figures form part of a detailed national epidemiological report.

CHRONIC FATIGUE SYNDROME (POSTVIRAL SYNDROME, 'MYALGIC ENCEPHALOMYELITIS')

A common medical problem is a patient, usually teenager or young adult, who experiences a prolonged period of lethargy, usually after an episode of infection reminiscent of a viral illness but sometimes in the absence of an evident acute illness. The problem causes great distress to patient and relatives because an explanation is lacking and because there is prolonged inability to work or play at expected levels, often coupled with an unreasonable need for sleep. Doctors are frustrated by their inability to establish a positive diagnosis or to give any specific treatment and the patient often turns to 'alternative medicine' (with varying financial consequences).

Aetiology

The postviral syndrome is heterogeneous and no single explanation will fit all patients. The term 'myalgic encephalomyelitis' is very misleading since there is no evidence of encephalitis and myalgia may not be present. A number of infections have been associated with this syndrome and they are not all viral. Infectious mononucleosis is the best known and studied but cytomegalovirus infection and toxoplasmosis have been incriminated, and it is likely that many other organisms can act as triggers in susceptible individuals. Enteroviruses, particularly of the Coxsackie group, have also been incriminated but evidence is inconclusive. Often the only evidence for infection at the onset is a history of febrile illness, perhaps with pharyngitis or lymphadenopathy, and a full blood count may have revealed some atypical mononuclear cells.

The relationship of postviral syndrome to depression is

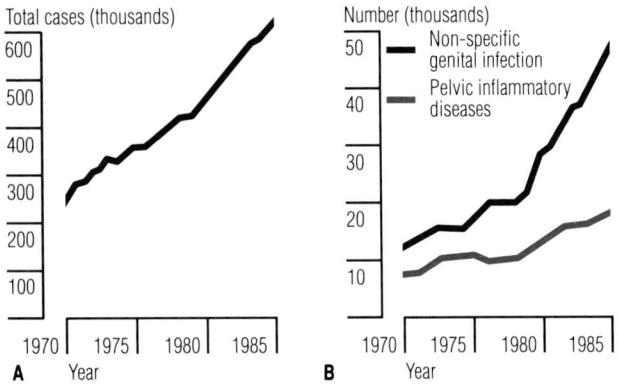

Fig. 12.5 Sexually transmitted diseases. A. Total numbers of cases of sexually transmitted diseases in England and Wales, 1970–1985. **B.** Incidence of non-specific genital infection in women, 1970–1985 (Communicable Diseases Surveillance Centre, Colindale).

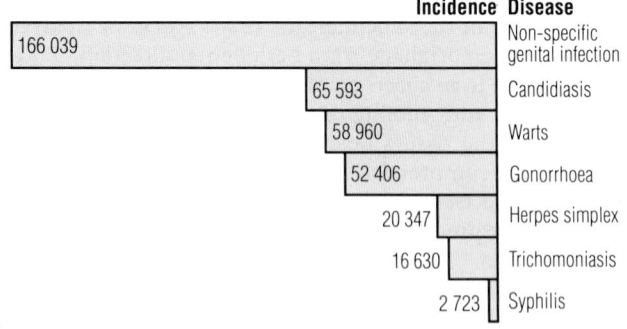

Fig. 12.6 Incidence of sexually transmitted diseases in the UK, 1985 (Communicable Diseases Surveillance Centre, Colindale).

complex. There is no doubt that some patients develop the symptoms and signs of depression and benefit from antidepressant treatment. More commonly the patient becomes depressed as a result of the illness but lacks many of the features of primary depression. In this situation antidepressant therapy is unlikely to be beneficial.

Clinical features

The central symptoms are profound lethargy and easy fatiguability. Often these are accompanied by muscular pains, headaches and symptoms suggestive of fever, such as sweating. This is usually mild, and when the temperature is recorded it is normal or only minimally elevated in the evenings. Exertion exacerbates tiredness and the patient often goes to bed early and wakes late still feeling tired.

Treatment

Patients benefit greatly from having their illness taken seriously and if a precipitating infection can be positively identified this also helps. Sometimes the greatest problem is anxiety about the outcome or about whether there is an underlying disease which has not been diagnosed, so reassurance is important. When patients have restricted their activity it is worth trying to rehabilitate them by a programme of daily exercise, starting with something light like walking or swimming and gradually increasing it in a documented way. The patient is assured that exercise is not harmful and advised to sleep as required.

Most patients recover spontaneously within weeks rather than months, which is another basis for reassurance, but a few continue to suffer for over a year.

VIRUS INFECTIONS

Viruses are usually classified according to their nucleic acid content and morphology. The classification of viruses used in this section is shown in Table 12.15. Arboviruses (*arthropod-borne*) are viruses transmitted by the bite of an insect vector. Most arboviruses are togaviruses, but bunyaviruses and orbiviruses (RNA viruses in the reovirus family) are also included.

Table 12.15a   Classification of viruses: DNA

Morphology	Virus
Enveloped double-stranded	Herpes viruses 　Varicella zoster (VZV) 　Herpes simplex (HSV I, II) 　Epstein-Barr (EBV) 　Cytomegalovirus (CMV) 　Human herpes virus 6 (HHV6) Pox viruses 　Vaccinia 　Variola (smallpox) 　Orf
Enveloped single-stranded	Parvovirus
Non-enveloped double-stranded	Adenoviruses Papovaviruses 　Papilloma 　Polyoma

Table 12.15b   Classification of viruses: RNA

Morphology	Virus
Enveloped single-stranded	Orthomyxoviruses 　Influenza Paramyxoviruses 　Para-influenza 　Respiratory syncytial 　Mumps 　Measles Togaviruses 　Rubella 　Alpha 　Flavi Bunyaviruses 　Rift Valley fever Arenaviruses 　Lassa 　Marburg-Ebola Retroviruses 　Human immunodeficiency (HIV) 1, 2 　HTLV I, II Rhabdoviruses 　Rabies
Non-enveloped double-stranded	Reoviruses 　Rota
Non-enveloped single-stranded	Picornaviruses 　Rhino 　Entero 　　Coxsackie A, B 　　Echo 　　Polio

12 ENVELOPED DOUBLE-STRANDED DNA VIRUSES

HERPES VIRUSES

Six herpes viruses cause disease in man:

1. varicella zoster virus (VZV)
2. *two* herpes simplex viruses (HSV I and II)
3. Epstein-Barr virus (EBV)
4. cytomegalovirus (CMV)
5. human herpes virus 6.

Morphologically, herpes viruses are very similar and indistinguishable by electron microscopy. They are similar in some aspects of their behaviour, notably their ability to establish latent infection with the potential for reactivation. During latency in dorsal root ganglia VZV shows no demonstrable evidence of viral replication for many years. With HSV there is evidence of a low level of replication and reactivation is more frequent. EBV infects B lymphocytes, and EBV and CMV replicate at a low level continuously. CMV can often be detected in the urine of asymptomatic carriers, and herpes simplex in saliva. The mechanisms by which virus replication is suppressed are incompletely understood but cell-mediated immunity probably has an important role, since all the herpes viruses are liable to reactivate in patients with depression of cell-mediated immunity.

Varicella zoster virus infection

Chickenpox (varicella)

Chickenpox is caused by the varicella zoster virus (VZV). The illness is easy to recognise, common and highly infectious. It is a febrile illness with a vesicular rash (Plate 1, p. 251).

During the primary infection there is a viraemic phase when VZV becomes widely disseminated in white cells. In normal subjects it only produces significant lesions in the skin and mucous membranes, but infection of cutaneous sensory nerves leads to infection of dorsal root ganglia and here the virus enters a latent state. Reactivation later causes herpes zoster (shingles). During primary infection VZV is present in nasopharyngeal secretions and is transmitted readily by coughing and sneezing. It is also in vesicle fluid in chickenpox and shingles and this can be a source of transmission.

The incubation period of chickenpox is 15–18 days and the patient is infectious from a few days before the rash erupts until new lesions cease to appear.

The severity of chickenpox is determined by the age and immunological state of the patient. It is most severe in neonates if they have no maternal antibody to VZV, and in patients immunocompromised by disease such as leukaemia or by immunosuppressive therapy. It is usually a mild disease in children but it becomes increasingly severe after puberty.

Clinical features

In children chickenpox starts with the appearance of the rash, which is often sparse and not accompanied by constitutional symptoms. The most troublesome feature of the illness is itching. In adults there is a notable prodromal illness lasting 2–3 days, during which headache, backache, shivering and fever occur, sometimes with sore throat and cough. The more severe the prodromal illness, the more profuse is the rash which follows.

The rash starts on the trunk and spreads to the face and limbs (Plate 1, p. 251). Lesions appear in crops which progress rapidly through the sequence macule, papule, vesicle, pustule, scab. Often the first visible lesions are vesicles containing clear fluid with little surrounding erythema, but the pustular stage is reached within 24 hours. Vesicles on the palate, tonsils and pharynx rapidly burst, leaving superficial ulcers. Crops of skin lesions erupt over 2 or 3 days, but it takes several more days for them all to heal. Constitutional symptoms, if present, lessen with the onset of the rash and disappear within 2 days.

Complications

Secondary infection of the skin lesions, including the scalp, occurs because of scratching, but it usually responds to cleaning and bathing and rarely requires antibiotics. Chickenpox pneumonia occurs in one-fifth of adults and more frequently in immunocompromised patients. It varies in severity from transient dyspnoea to a fulminant pneumonia.

Postinfectious encephalitis is extremely rare and has a variable course, but it is often severe or fatal. Its onset is within a week of the rash and cerebellar involvement is characteristic.

Bleeding into the skin, nose or intestine, also rare, is due either to steroid-responsive thrombocytopenia or to consumptive coagulopathy, when the prognosis is much worse.

Neonatal chickenpox

When a mother develops chickenpox within a few days of having a baby the child is born without the protection of maternal IgG antibodies transferred across the placenta, and it is immediately exposed to the virus. If the child becomes infected during the first 5 days of life disease is severe, with multi-organ involvement, and the mortality is 20%. Fortunately this is rare because most women are immune by the time they reach child-bearing age.

Disease can be prevented or modified to a milder form by administration of varicella immune globulin but this is in short supply.

Congenital chickenpox

VZV can cross the placenta during the first 20 weeks of pregnancy, causing fetal damage or death. This is rare because most mothers are immune.

Diagnosis and treatment

A clinical diagnosis of chickenpox suffices in most cases. Electron microscopy is the quickest way to establish that a herpes virus is present in vesicle fluid but does not establish its type. The virus can be identified by tissue culture inoculation, and antibodies are detected by a complement fixation test.

Treatment with acyclovir (p. 225) is required only in severe cases with complications such as chickenpox pneumonia, in patients with inadequate cell-mediated immunity (such as children with malignant disease), and in neonates without maternal antibody infected in the perinatal period (Table 12.5, p. 225). The virus is sensitive to acyclovir given intravenously.

Shingles (zoster)

When VZV reactivates within a dorsal root ganglion it migrates down the nerve into the skin and causes a crop of lesions identical to those of chickenpox but confined to the dermatome (Plate 2, p. 251). Pain within the dermatome may precede the eruption by a few days and is often severe. One or two adjacent dermatomes on the trunk are most commonly affected but involvement of the ophthalmic division of the fifth cranial nerve is important because the eye can be damaged by the virus or by secondary bacterial infection.

In the elderly it is common for a mild viraemia to occur, causing a few scattered lesions to appear outside the involved dermatome. More serious dissemination with visceral involvement is seen in immunocompromised patients. Patients with Hodgkin's disease are particularly susceptible to shingles, which often starts during chemotherapy.

The skin heals over 2–3 weeks and there is often some residual pain for a few weeks. Rarely, intractable pain continues for years (post-herpetic neuralgia). This is more common following ophthalmic zoster and after severe infections in immunocompromised patients.

Treatment

Most patients do not require admission to hospital and treatment of pain is the main concern. Continuous treatment with simple analgesics such as paracetamol is often effective and should be tried before drugs which have more side-effects.

Topical treatment of the skin with antiviral drugs is of limited benefit, but a small increase in the rate of healing has been demonstrated when high-dose oral acyclovir is used. This benefit must be weighed against the cost of treatment. When the ophthalmic division of the trigeminal nerve is involved, prophylactic topical treatment with an antibiotic such as chloramphenicol and an antiviral drug such as acyclovir is advisable.

Systemic antiviral treatment – for example with intravenous acyclovir – should be given to immunocompromised patients. It reduces pain, shortens the healing time and limits dissemination of the virus.

Herpes simplex virus infection

The two types of herpes simplex virus (HSV I and II) cause patterns of disease which differ clinically and epidemiologically but share some characteristics. Both establish permanent, latent infection within sensory nerve ganglia following primary infection, with reactivation causing episodes of disease in the area supplied by the nerve.

These viruses are indistinguishable morphologically but can be separated by the base composition of their DNA and by differences in antigen expression.

Infection with HSV I is more common. Antibodies are detectable in 80–100% of adults in lower socio-economic groups, and 30–50% in higher socio-economic groups.

Both types of virus are readily transmitted, mainly in vesicle fluid. HSV I is usually acquired during childhood but HSV II infection is mainly transmitted sexually and is most common in sexually promiscuous adults.

Clinical expression of infection with these viruses is strongly influenced by age, nutrition and the immunological state of the patient. An immunologically immature neonate is overwhelmed by disseminated HSV infection acquired during parturition. Infection in older children is often asymptomatic or causes localised disease which is most severe in the presence of malnutrition.

Primary infection with HSV I

Acute herpetic gingivostomatitis in children 2–4 years old presents with fever, sore throat and submental and anterior cervical lymphadenopathy. Clusters of vesicles appear around the lips and in the mouth from gums to pharynx (Plate 3, p. 251). Inside the mouth, lesions rapidly ulcerate, causing pain and dysphagia with consequent drooling of saliva. The child is miserable and may become dehydrated if not encouraged to drink through a straw. The lesions heal over 1–2 weeks.

Primary infection can occur anywhere on the skin and, on the finger, a *herpetic whitlow* can closely mimic a bacterial paronychia. Widespread involvement of the skin can occur in individuals with atopic dermatitis (eczema herpeticum, p. 1126), and particularly in infants, this can be associated with systemic symptoms. In the eye *keratoconjunctivitis* can cause scarring of the cornea and loss of vision.

Herpetic encephalitis in adults presents a characteristic clinical picture due to necrotic lesions in the temporal lobe. This rare manifestation of primary HSV infection is described on page 962.

Primary infection with HSV II

Although HSV I and II can cause identical disease, HSV II is largely associated with genital infection. Primary genital infection is most common in young, sexually active adults and the risk of infection is proportional to the number of sexual partners. After an incubation period of 2–7 days, clusters of vesicles with surrounding erythema appear at the site of virus entry, on the glans or penile shaft in men or on the vulva and vaginal mucosa in women. Homosexual men develop rectal and peri-anal lesions. The lesions are usually painful and there may be systemic illness with headache, myalgia, fever and local lymphadenopathy.

Occasionally paraesthesiae develop in areas supplied by infected nerves and there may be urinary retention or constipation. Skin and mucosal lesions resolve over 2–3 weeks. Virus may be shed for up to 12 days from the lesions.

Infection of neonates can occur during parturition when the mother has genital herpes, particularly if her infection is primary rather than recurrent. The infant develops scattered clusters of vesicles which recur in the same sites subsequently. Alternatively there may be rapid deterioration as the virus disseminates to all the viscera, causing encephalitis, pneumonia and hepatitis with a high mortality. Usually this severe illness starts in the few days after birth but occasionally onset is delayed several weeks.

Reactivation of HSV I and II

The mechanisms involved in maintaining latency are not fully understood but reactivation is well recognised after exposure to ultraviolet light, an episode of infection, such as pneumonia, and trauma to the sensory nerve, though many episodes of reactivation in normal subjects have no identifiable precipitant. Reactivation is more common in some immunocompromised patients, particularly leukaemics undergoing treatment.

The characteristic lesion of reactivated HSV I is a *cold sore*. Patients often experience minor discomfort in the form of tingling or itching up to 24 hours before a lesion appears. This presumably corresponds with migration of the virus from the sensory ganglion into the area of skin supplied by the relevant nerve. Lesions can occur anywhere on the skin or mucous membranes but are commonly adjacent to the lips. A macule rapidly progresses to a papule and then to a cluster of vesicles which involute, ulcerate and scab. The whole process takes 1–2 weeks.

Reactivation of genital HSV causes lesions similar to but milder than those of the primary episode, with more localised lesions occasionally accompanied by shooting pains in the buttocks or legs.

Reactivation in immune deficient patients causes more severe disease which may become disseminated. For example, the virus often reactivates in patients undergoing bone marrow transplantation, causing cold sores which are large and progressive, and dissemination results in pneumonia or hepatitis. Patients with acquired immune deficiency syndrome (AIDS) may develop oesophagitis or proctitis.

Asymptomatic secretion of virus can occur in the mouth (HSV I) or in the vagina (HSV II) but this is rarely a source of transmission.

Treatment of herpes simplex

Herpes simplex viruses are highly sensitive to acyclovir and other DNA polymerase inhibiting drugs. Only serious primary infections with HSV I, such as encephalitis in adults, severe eczema herpeticum or disseminated neonatal infection, warrant treatment with systemic antiviral drugs. Appropriate forms of treatment are shown in Table 12.5. Initial attacks of genital herpes are treated with 5 days of acyclovir, with an antibiotic if secondary infection has occurred. For recurrences attention to local hygiene is all that is required and 5% acyclovir ointment may be helpful for local lesions.

Epstein-Barr virus infection

Epstein-Barr virus (EBV) is a herpes virus which is transmitted by close oral contact. Infection is frequently acquired asymptomatically during early childhood in underdeveloped countries and in crowded living conditions, but infection is delayed in more prosperous environments. Infection in adolescents and adults usually causes infectious mononucleosis (glandular fever).

Other diseases related to EBV infection are nasopharyngeal carcinoma; Burkitt's lymphoma; the very rare syndrome, X-linked recessive progressive combined variable immunodeficiency; and lymphoid interstitial pneumonitis in children with AIDS.

Infectious mononucleosis

Infectious mononucleosis is an acute febrile illness caused by EBV, characterised by severe sore throat and generalised lymphadenopathy.

Pathology and pathogenesis

EBV enters through the pharyngeal epithelium and replicates in B lymphocytes, causing them to proliferate. Fifteen per cent or more of blood mononuclear cells appear 'atypical' during acute infection; these cells are T lymphocytes reacting to the presence of infected B lymphocytes. EBV does not establish a true latent state but maintains a low level of replication throughout life. During infectious mononucleosis, the spleen and lymph nodes are intensely infiltrated with mononuclear cells and the spleen is unusually friable. Haemorrhage may occur into the subcapsular area and rarely this leads to intraperitoneal haemorrhage.

Clinical features

Infectious mononucleosis is most common in adolescents and young adults, but children as young as 5 years old may be affected. The illness is more severe in older patients.

The incubation period is uncertain but is probably 1–2 weeks. There is gradual onset of malaise, general aching and fever. The throat becomes painful and engorged with enlarging lymphoid tissue so that speech is nasal and swallowing is inhibited by pain. The tonsils are large and coated with thick, white exudate (Plate 4, p. 251). Petechiae may be seen on the soft palate. There is generalised lymphadenopathy in most patients and splenomegaly is common. Uncommon features (occurring in less than 15% of patients) are rash, jaundice and tender hepatomegaly. Thrombocytopenia or autoimmune haemolytic anaemia occur rarely. The acute stage of the illness lasts 2–3 weeks and most patients are entirely well within a month. A small proportion of patients, particularly when older, make a slower recovery, continuing to feel lethargic for a variable period (see chronic fatigue syndrome, p. 236).

Differential diagnosis

Other viral causes of sore throat and lymphadenopathy, such as adenovirus, influenza virus and rhinovirus, must be considered (Table 12.14). Streptococcal infection can cause an identical appearance in the throat but the lymphadenopathy is mainly in the anterior cervical region. Streptococci are found on throat swabs in 10% of patients with infectious mononucleosis and their role is unclear.

Many virus infections are associated with atypical lymphocytes on the blood film but these can be distinguished from 'glandular fever cells' by an experienced observer. The latter are also seen in acute cytomegalovirus infection and occasionally in toxoplasmosis. Both of these conditions can cause lymphadenopathy but they rarely produce sore throat.

Laboratory features

Atypical mononuclear cells are usually present in the blood film at some stage of the disease. Simple tests for heterophil antibodies – that is, antibodies to heterologous erythrocytes – are the Paul Bunnell and Monospot tests. Heterophil antibodies are present in 90% of patients by the third week of illness but in only 30% during the first week. Specific IgM antibody measurements are not reliable. Liver function tests are often deranged.

Treatment

No specific treatment is available. Simple analgesic therapy is used to relieve discomfort in the throat and frequently the patient can only take fluids in the early stages. Occasionally the degree of congestion is such as to threaten the airways and a short course of prednisolone starting at 30 mg daily, tailing off over 2 weeks, can produce a rapid reduction in size of the tonsils.

If penicillin therapy is indicated for treatment of concurrent streptococcal infection, ampicillin and amoxycillin should be avoided, since they cause a severe maculopapular rash.

X-linked recessive progressive combined variable immunodeficiency (Duncan's disease)

This rare inherited disease is now recognised as an abnormal response to EBV infection. Patients either die of overwhelming EBV infection in the acute stage or develop a progressive immunodeficiency following infection. Lymphoma may complicate the late stages.

Cytomegalovirus infection

Cytomegalovirus (CMV) is a herpes virus which rarely causes significant disease in immunologically competent subjects. Infection is usually asymptomatic but it may be associated with a mild febrile illness during which atypical mononuclear cells appear in the blood; these cells are similar to those seen in infectious mononucleosis.

Primary infection in the neonate causes serious disease, and primary infection of pregnant women can cause congenital defects in the fetus. As with other herpes viruses, infection is lifelong. CMV behaves like Epstein-Barr virus (EBV) in that it replicates at a low level throughout life, but when immunity is suppressed the rate of replication increases. Patients with kidney or heart transplants are particularly at risk and CMV sometimes causes severe disease in patients with acquired immune deficiency syndrome (AIDS, p. 250).

Transmission

The virus is present in blood during primary infection and can cross the placenta. It can also be transmitted in blood used for transfusion.

Infected organs transplanted from seropositive donors can cause primary infection in the recipient, but most CMV disease in renal transplant patients is caused by reactivation.

The virus is shed from the cervix during active infection and is also present in semen and urine.

Acute infection in normal adults

When infection is symptomatic there is a mild non-specific febrile illness which is recognised as viral infection when atypical mononuclear cells are seen in a blood film. Sore throat, generalised lymphadenopathy and splenomegaly occur in less than one-third of patients. Abnormal liver function tests show that there is usually a mild hepatitis but jaundice is rare. The average age for symptomatic infection is 30 years, about 10 years older than for infectious mononucleosis.

Complications are rare in immunocompetent patients and, when they occur, they are mild. Pneumonitis, myocarditis, meningo-encephalitis, Guillain-Barré syndrome, thrombocytopenia and haemolytic anaemia have all been described.

Infection in immunosuppressed patients

Both primary infection and reactivation can cause disease in immune suppressed patients, but in renal transplant recipients the more severe disease is seen during primary infection. Asymptomatic reactivation is common and is shown by culture of virus from urine. Fever, sometimes with atypical mononucleosis, is the most common presentation of disease, followed by interstitial pneumonitis.

Interstitial pneumonitis presents with insidious onset of fever, non-productive cough and dyspnoea. Chest radiograph shows bilateral diffuse interstitial changes indistinguishable from those of many other opportunistic infections. Diagnosis is usually made by transbronchial biopsy. *Hepatitis* is usually mild but occasionally causes hepatic failure.

CMV may be a harmless passenger in the gastrointestinal tract of patients but a pathological role with the production of *enteritis* is strongly suggested by the coincidence of seroconversion with the occurrence of haemorrhagic lesions anywhere from the stomach to the rectum. These correspond with a severe diarrhoeal disease and blood loss. A response to treatment with antiviral drugs supports the existence of this clinical entity.

Severe *choroidoretinitis* causes progressive loss of sight starting in one eye and then affecting the other. Large white exudates containing haemorrhagic areas occur.

Diagnosis

Virus can be cultured from urine during active replication and IgM antibodies are detectable in serum by an immunofluorescence test. In histological sections 'owl's eye cells' are strongly suggestive of CMV infection.

Treatment

New drugs such as phosphonoformate or ganciclovir are becoming available for treatment of CMV pneumonia, retinitis and enteritis, but unfortunately disease has tended to recur as soon as treatment is stopped. Hyperimmune globulin containing high titre antibody to CMV has been used to treat neonates with CMV pneumonia with possible success.

Human herpes virus 6 infection

Human herpes virus 6 (HHV6) has recently been identified in patients with AIDS and has subsequently been found to be widely distributed. It is the cause of roseola, a common febrile illness of young children characterised by the appearance of a rash when the fever and illness are resolving. Despite having a temperature as high as 104°F, the child is relatively well, but there is often cervical and postauricular lymphadenopathy. When the temperature starts to fall or within 2 days, a maculopapular erythematous eruption appears on the trunk; this lasts for a few days. Blood count reveals neutropenia initially, which may be followed by mild leukocytosis. The illness resolves without complications.

POX VIRUSES

Variola and vaccinia

Variola virus is the cause of smallpox, an infection of low infectivity transmitted between humans by close contact. Edward Jenner introduced vaccination against the disease at the end of the 18th century, using material from the pustules of cowpox (vaccinia). In 1967 the World Health

Organisation (WHO) launched its global campaign for smallpox eradication using the refined vaccine containing vaccinia virus, which is morphologically indistinguishable from variola virus but non-pathogenic. This remarkably successful venture reached its conclusion in 1979, when the eradication of smallpox was announced 2 years after the last naturally occurring case was reported in Somalia. Only accidental laboratory infections have occurred since then. Vaccination against smallpox is no longer justified.

Orf virus infection

Orf virus causes a single nodular lesion at the site of an abrasion which has been in contact with an infected lamb.

Molluscum contagiosum

Molluscum contagiosum is an infection of the skin caused by a pox virus. The incubation period is variable and may be up to 6 months. A typical lesion is a smooth, firm papule, with the vertex of the papule umbilicated and containing a waxy substance.

Lesions commonly appear on the genitalia, suprapubic area and inner thighs but can appear anywhere on the skin surface. They appear to be more common in people who are HIV positive, in whom the face, including the eyelids, may be involved.

Treatment

Spontaneous regression may occur. Therapies include curettage and liquid nitrogen cryotherapy or application of phenol, podophyllin or iodine after disruption of the lesions.

ENVELOPED SINGLE-STRANDED DNA VIRUSES

PARVOVIRUS

The association between infection with human parvovirus and disease has only been recognised in the last decade. The virus was first noticed in sera from normal subjects during screening by electron microscopy (1975), but in 1983 it was reported to be the cause of erythema infectiosum ('slapped cheek disease' or 'fifth disease'). More seriously, it was reported from the West Indies that the virus can cause aplastic crises in patients with sickle cell disease. The delay between finding the virus and associating it with a disease was partly because asymptomatic viraemia precedes the disease, but viraemia is no longer present during the illness.

Clinical features

Parvovirus infection is probably transmitted from human to human by nasopharyngeal secretions and causes a range of illness ranging from asymptomatic to a febrile systemic illness with a rash. After a mild prodromal illness consisting of fever, headache, upper respiratory symptoms and myalgia lasting 2–4 days, a rash appears on the arms and chest, spreading peripherally, even to the palms and soles. The classic 'slapped cheek' appearance of erythema infectiosum is seen in less than half of infected patients. Elsewhere the rash is maculopapular and fluctuates in intensity, increasing on exercise, for example. It often develops a lacy reticular pattern on the limbs and leaves a short-lived pale brown pigmentation as it fades over a week, although occasionally it can be much more long-lasting. The rash is frequently pruritic. Other features during the rash are generally mild but include fever, malaise, headache and sometimes arthralgia, lymphadenopathy and splenomegaly.

Complications

Complications are rare. Adult women may develop symmetrical peripheral polyarthritis, which can be the sole manifestation of infection. Although it usually resolves within 3 months it may continue for several years.

Aplastic crises are not a feature of infection in patients who are otherwise normal haematologically, but when the red cell life is reduced, as in sickle cell disease or hereditary spherocytosis, arrest of erythropoiesis for 5–10 days causes a significant fall in haemoglobin level.

Diagnosis and treatment

IgM serum antibodies detected by enzyme-linked immunosorbent assay (ELISA) or radioimmunoassay (RIA) are diagnostic of recent infection and persist for about 2 months. A change in titre of IgG antibodies also indicates recent infection. Virus isolation is not feasible and detection of viral protein is reserved for research purposes.

There is no specific treatment at present.

NON-ENVELOPED DOUBLE-STRANDED DNA VIRUSES

ADENOVIRUSES

Adenoviruses are a common cause of upper respiratory infection in children, and cause a variety of other illnesses depending on the serotype of virus and the age of the patient. Over 40 serotypes have been isolated from man and many of these are known to have pathogenic potential. Virus can frequently be isolated from the posterior pharyngeal lymphoid tissue of asymptomatic subjects, suggesting that it can remain latent for long periods.

Upper respiratory infection. Common cold and pharyngitis occur in all age groups and serotypes 1–6 are the usual cause.

Lower respiratory infection. Tracheobronchitis and pneumonia are rare in children but young adults may be affected. This is one of the differential diagnoses of atypical pneumonia. Types 4 and 7 are the most common causes.

Pharyngo-conjunctival fever. An acute infection spreads among young children in close contact, often caused by adenovirus type 3.

Epidemic keratoconjunctivitis. Epidemic keratoconjunctivitis is a more severe form of eye infection which affects adults and often follows minor trauma to the eye. Type 8 is the usual pathogen.

Haemorrhagic cystitis. Caused by types 11 and 21, haemorrhagic cystitis is a childhood infection.

Adenoviruses are also uncommonly associated with diarrhoeal disease, intussusception and meningitis or encephalitis.

There is as yet no effective antiviral treatment for adenoviruses.

PAPOVAVIRUSES

The important members of the papovavirus group are *papilloma* or wart viruses and *polyoma* viruses, one of which, the JC virus, causes progressive multifocal leucoencephalopathy, a rare neurological disease (p. 964).

Palmar and plantar warts are benign infections, common in childhood, which often spontaneously regress with increasing age. They are caused by viruses which are distinct from the anogenital warts viruses; the latter are sexually transmitted (p. 1119) and are regarded as important in view of increasing evidence associating them with cervical cancer.

Genital warts

In men warts can appear on any part of the genitalia but especially the frenum, coronal sulcus and the inner surface of the foreskin. They are called condylomata accuminata. They may involve the male urethra and appear as bright red lumps at the meatus.

In women the vulva, vagina, cervix and perineal area can be involved. Cervical condylomata may be flat and identifiable only by colposcopy. They may be associated with dyskaryosis and koilocytosis and with cervical cancer.

Treatment

Local application of cytotoxic agents such as podophyllin and 5-fluorouracil, or destructive agents or methods such as trichloracetic acid, cautery, diathermy or cryosurgery, are still the main therapeutic approaches. Ablation of cervical warts by laser therapy is effective.

ENVELOPED SINGLE-STRANDED RNA VIRUSES

ORTHOMYXOVIRUSES

Influenza type A and type B are the main viruses in this family. Influenza is described in Chapter 14.

12

PARAMYXOVIRUSES

Para-influenza virus infection

There are four types of para-influenza virus and the organisms are a common cause of mild upper respiratory infection in children under 2 years of age (Ch. 14). Types 1–3 occasionally cause more severe lower respiratory tract disease, such as croup and bronchiolitis. Although there is little antigenic variation in para-influenza viruses, immunity is poor and reinfection causing mild disease is common.

Respiratory syncytial virus infection

Respiratory syncytial virus (RSV) is the most important cause of lower respiratory tract infection in young children. Outbreaks occur annually, usually in late winter or spring, and about half of primary infections result in pneumonia, bronchiolitis or tracheobronchitis. Upper respiratory involvement is also common and otitis media is a frequent complication. Children over the age of 3 usually suffer milder disease and adults are occasionally infected. RSV is highly infectious and is commonly transmitted to other patients in hospital. Respiratory isolation procedures should be applied (but rarely are). Successful therapy for RSV has been described using ribavirin administered as an aerosol, but in practice this is difficult to apply. Vaccines which induce a good immune response have been prepared but they do not protect and indeed appear to exacerbate the disease.

Mumps

Mumps is a systemic paramyxovirus infection which commonly causes inflammation of salivary glands. It is transmitted by droplets from the mouth. Infection in childhood is common but infectivity is low and many people reach adulthood without becoming infected.

Clinical features

The incubation period is about 18 days (Fig. 12.1, p. 219). Mumps is a mild disease in childhood and about one-third of children infected have no symptoms. In its mildest form there is fever with discomfort and swelling in the parotid glands, which lasts a week or less. In more severe forms there is considerable malaise, the glands are painful and there may be trismus. Other salivary glands are often inflamed and glands are sometimes involved sequentially. Swollen parotid glands can be distinguished from lymphadenopathy because the angle of the mandible is obliterated by the former. The mouth is dry and there may be redness around the orifices of the parotid ducts, but there is no purulent discharge.

About 20% of adult males develop *orchitis* in the course of mumps but *oophoritis* is rare. Usually orchitis starts a few days after the onset of parotitis, but it may be earlier and it may occur in the absence of parotitis. The swollen inflamed testicle is exquisitely tender and remains so for 3–4 days before gradually recovering. Orchitis is accompanied by fever and malaise and the latter often persists for some weeks.

Orchitis is bilateral in 15–30% of cases but even in these patients sterility is extremely rare. Although some shrinkage of involved testicles may be detected shortly after the illness, this does not imply complete loss of function and it is important to reassure patients on this point.

Mumps virus is highly neurotropic and involvement of the central nervous system is the most common complication of this infection. Although this is often referred to as meningo-encephalitis, there are in fact two distinct entities, *meningitis* and *encephalitis*.

Lymphocytic meningitis occurs in about 5% of patients with mumps parotitis, but this figure underestimates its prevalence since it also occurs in the absence of parotitis. There is some seasonal variation in the clinical manifestations, meningitis with parotitis being more common in spring whereas meningitis alone is seen more in summer. The time of onset of meningitis varies but it usually becomes apparent a few days after parotitis. The cerebrospinal fluid shows a lymphocytic pleocytosis and virus can be isolated from it. The course is invariably benign.

Encephalitis is rare. It either occurs during parotitis as a result of direct viral invasion of the brain, or its onset is 7–10 days after that of parotitis, when it represents a postinfectious encephalitis. Most patients recover completely but there is a mortality of 1–2%.

Pancreatitis is rarely severe but may account for some of the abdominal symptoms in mumps. Some degree of abdominal pain is not infrequent and may be accompanied by vomiting. In severe cases there is marked abdominal tenderness and the serum amylase level is elevated.

Diagnosis

A clinical diagnosis usually presents little difficulty, but if necessary the virus can be isolated from saliva and throat washings or from CSF in cases of meningitis. Complement-fixing antibody detection can be used to make a retrospective diagnosis.

Treatment

There is no specific treatment, but oral hygiene is important both for comfort and to prevent secondary infection. Orchitis requires testicular support and adequate analgesia. There is little evidence that corticosteroid treatment is beneficial in orchitis.

Prevention

Vaccination with a live attenuated vaccine was adopted as part of the routine programme in the UK from 1988. It is given in combination with measles and rubella in the second year of life.

Measles

Measles is an easily recognised, highly infectious disease

of childhood caused by measles virus, an RNA virus of the paramyxovirus group.

Epidemiology

Infection is spread by droplets coughed on to mucosal surfaces of the conjunctiva and nasopharynx, and since cough is a feature of the illness from the onset it is not surprising that infection spreads rapidly between non-immune subjects. The rapidity of spread and the completeness of immunity after measles are illustrated by the experience of measles on virgin soil. In 1846 measles was introduced to the Faroe Islands by a Danish traveller and the disease spread to affect 6000 of the 8000 inhabitants. The majority of those infected were less than 65 years old and the previous epidemic of measles had been 65 years before. There are many similar examples and one of the interesting features of the disease in older epidemics was the high mortality rate. It is not clear whether measles virus has changed to a more benign form or whether environmental factors are responsible, but the latter is more likely since the disease is still severe in Africa. The size of the pool of non-immune humans determines whether there is an epidemic of measles; in the past epidemics have occurred in Britain every 2 years or so, but immunisation has made this pattern less apparent.

Pathogenesis

Measles virus can infect many different cell types and during the incubation period, which is 8–11 days from infection to the onset of prodromal symptoms (Fig. 12.1, p. 219), the virus multiplies and becomes widely disseminated. It reaches most tissues, including skin, mucous membranes, lungs, gut, brain and lymphoreticular tissue.

The lesions of measles, containing mononuclear and giant cells, are caused by a combination of viral cytopathic effect and non-specific and specific inflammatory reactions. The role of immune mechanisms is demonstrated by the modified or absent skin rash in immunodeficient subjects, who may nevertheless die from a giant cell pneumonia. Antibody is detectable in serum 24–48 hours after the onset of rash and virus is rapidly cleared during this period.

Clinical features

In Britain measles is most common at the age of 3–5 years but the age is lower in underdeveloped countries. In the period 2–4 days before eruption of the rash the features are similar to many upper respiratory infections. The patient feels unwell and has a fever, red eyes, swollen eyelids, congested streaming nose, diffuse redness in the mouth and a hacking cough. Koplik's spots, 1–2 mm white spots like a grain of salt on a red background, may be seen on the buccal mucosa (Plate 5, p. 251). Their number varies from a few to hundreds and they often persist after the rash appears.

The worst of the illness is the first few days after eruption of the rash, when there is a spiking fever and the child is irritable and miserable. Spots appear first behind the ears and on the forehead, and then spread to the rest of the face, on to the trunk and out to the limbs over 24–72 hours (Plate 6, p. 251). This pattern of spread is characteristic but the rash of rubella (German measles) spreads in the same direction. Measles spots are red macules and maculopapules initially a few millimetres in diameter, which enlarge and coalesce to form irregular blotches, the most striking of which are on the cheeks. As the rash fades and the patient starts to feel better there is transient brown staining of the skin and sometimes fine desquamation.

At the height of the eruptive stage the mucous membranes and eardrums are red, and there is generalised lymphadenopathy, a barking cough and widespread crackles in the chest.

Complications

Major complications are rare in Britain today.

All complications are more common in malnourished children, and severe skin desquamation with secondary bacterial infection, diarrhoea, appendicitis, laryngitis, stomatitis and major weight loss all occur frequently in Africa. Measles sometimes precipitates the onset of kwashiorkor. Secondary bacterial infection usually manifests itself 3–4 days after the rash and prolongs the illness. The timing is an important clue, as renewed fever heralds a third phase of illness. Bronchopneumonia and otitis media are examples. Giant cell pneumonia is rare and usually affects immunocompromised children, such as leukaemics.

As far as the central nervous system is concerned, febrile convulsions may occur as the temperature rises in the incubation period or at the beginning of the eruptive phase. Encephalitis is rare and varies in severity. It occurs in the convalescent phase and in fatal cases virus is not recovered from the brain, so encephalitis may be caused by an immune reaction to viral antigen in neural tissue. Subacute sclerosing panencephalitis (SSPE) is a progressive fatal form of encephalitis affecting older children who had measles many years before. High titres of measles antibodies and recovery of a measles-like virus from the brain suggest that it is related to measles.

Diagnosis

Clinical diagnosis of measles is usually straightforward. The rash of rubella has a similar distribution, but lesions are smaller and they tend to remain discrete. Rubella is a milder illness with a characteristic distribution of lymphadenopathy (occipital and posterior cervical). Laboratory confirmation of measles is rarely necessary, but measles virus can be cultured from nasopharyngeal specimens during the prodrome and for about 2 days into the eruptive phase. Blood count normally shows leukopenia and the finding of neutrophilia suggests secondary bacterial infection. Antibody titres are measured by a complement fixation test.

Infectious, Tropical and Parasitic Diseases

12

Treatment

Most children with measles are looked after at home but if hospital admission is required for social reasons, or because of complications, the patient should be nursed in isolation. Antiviral treatment is not available at present and management is directed at providing comfort and maintaining hydration. Prophylactic antibiotics have no place but appropriate antibiotics must be given for secondary bacterial infection. Important organisms in respiratory infection and otitis media are *Streptococcus pneumoniae*, *Haemophilus influenzae* and, less commonly, *Staphylococcus aureus*. Therefore the usual first choice of antibiotic is a broad-spectrum penicillin (e.g. amoxycillin) or erythromycin.

Management of encephalitis is described on page 962. Passive immunisation with 500 mg normal human immunoglobin intramuscularly (250 mg for children less than 1 year old) attenuates or prevents clinical manifestations if it is given within 6 days of contact. This is useful in children under 18 months and in those whom immunosuppression makes susceptible to severe forms of measles. Protection lasts for about 3 weeks.

Active immunisation

Live attenuated measles virus vaccine is given in the second year of life in Britain. In parts of the world where the disease is common in younger children immunisation is recommended at an earlier age. A single subcutaneous or intramuscular dose gives prolonged protection.

Contra-indications are immune deficiency disease (primary or secondary), immunosuppressive therapy, and severe egg allergy. Atopy and febrile convulsions do not preclude use of the vaccine.

The uptake rate for measles immunisation is disappointingly low in Britain: approximately 65%. If it were

Table 12.16 Effect of measles immunisation in the USA, compared with the UK (Communicable Diseases Surveillance Centre, Colindale)

Year	Cases/year	Incidence per 100 000
USA		
Before introduction of immunisation (1963)	500 000	211
1980	13 506	
1981	3 125	
1982	1 714	
1983	1 497	
1984	2 587	
1985	2 813	1.2
UK/England		
1860 (England)	(4767 deaths)	
1985 (UK)	104 127 (11 deaths)	184

to be increased measles could become a rare disease, as it has in the United States (Table 12.16).

TOGAVIRUSES

The togavirus group comprises the rubella virus, alphaviruses and flaviviruses. *Rubella* is the commonest togavirus infection in the Western world. *Alphaviruses* are the cause of Eastern, Western and Venezuelan equine encephalitis. *Flaviviruses* cause dengue and yellow fever.

Rubella

Postnatal rubella (German measles) is a mild illness occasionally complicated by arthritis or encephalitis. By contrast, infection in utero can have devastating effects on the fetus.

Pathogenesis

Rubella virus infects nasopharyngeal secretions, where it is found during subclinical as well as overt infection. During the viraemic phase it is disseminated widely and, as for measles, the clinical illness corresponds in time with the development of immunity. The incubation period for rubella is 14–16 days.

Clinical features

The derivation of the name German measles is unknown but it may have come from 'germane' (Latin *germanus*), implying a similarity to measles. The similarities are that both are associated with fever, lymphadenopathy, rash and conjunctival suffusion. The distinguishing features of rubella are that it is a mild, short-lived illness which may be asymptomatic. Severity increases with age but at worst it is no more severe than a bad cold. The lymphadenopathy of rubella is characteristically suboccipital, postauricular and posterior cervical. It may persist long after the rash has faded. Although, as in measles, the rash starts on the face and behind the ears, spreading downwards and outwards over the trunk and limbs, the spots are paler red, circular macules which remain discrete and do not coalesce into bright irregular blotches (Plate 7, p. 251). The rash varies from hour to hour, fading and re-appearing for up to 4 days. It is common to find petechiae on the soft palate (Forscheimer spots) but these are not diagnostic, unlike the enanthem of measles.

Complications

Arthritis is the only common complication of rubella. It usually affects young women, who develop polyarthritis of small joints, especially those of the fingers and wrists, although larger joints may be affected. It is easily confused with acute rheumatoid arthritis, especially in the absence of rash. It usually subsides within a few days but can last up to 3 months. Encephalitis and thrombocytopenic purpura are very rare complications.

246

Congenital rubella

The relationship between maternal rubella and congenital defects was first described in 1941, when Gregg observed a high incidence of unusual cataracts following a rubella epidemic in Australia.

Both the risk and the severity of damage to the fetus are closely related to the time of infection. Following infection during the first month of pregnancy, over half of fetuses are affected, whereas by the fourth month only 5% have defects, although this is still twice the frequency in control groups. Minor damage can result from later infection.

During the viraemic phase of the maternal illness rubella virus invades the placenta, damaging chorionic blood vessels and causing villous placentitis. Entering the fetal circulation, the virus becomes widely disseminated but the degree of damage is variable, even in twins infected at the same time.

The common major abnormalities resulting from infection in the first trimester are cataracts, patent ductus arteriosus with or without pulmonary stenosis, and deafness. Rubella virus can be isolated from the baby's pharynx for several months, a much longer period than in acquired rubella. The virus is present in all other secretions and these babies can readily infect nurses handling them.

Diagnosis

Serology is the mainstay of diagnosis in both congenital and acquired rubella. The haemagglutination inhibition (HAI) test, which is used extensively, exploits the ability of rubella virus to agglutinate chick red cells. Serum antibodies inhibit this agglutination. IgM antibodies are detected by separating an IgM fraction from the serum and testing this fraction for rubella antibodies by HAI or by an immunofluorescence test. A rise in total antibody titre or the presence of specific IgM antibodies indicates recent infection.

In acquired infection antibody is detectable by HAI 14–16 days after infection and reaches a peak 6–12 days later. The fetus starts to produce IgM antibody at about the twentieth week of life, and since only IgG antibody can cross the placenta, the presence of IgM antibodies to rubella virus in the fetus or infant implies active infection. Rubella virus can be cultured from clinical specimens but this is rarely used for diagnosis.

Immunisation

Live attenuated virus vaccine is given routinely as part of measles/mumps/rubella (MMR) vaccination to boys and girls aged 15 months. This was introduced in 1988 and replaces the policy of immunising girls aged between 11 and 13 years. Vaccine virus can cross the placenta so it should not be given during pregnancy, and pregnancy should be avoided for 2 months after immunisation.

Exposure to rubella during pregnancy

Definite exposure to rubella of a non-immune, pregnant woman during the first trimester is an indication for termination of pregnancy. If the woman does not know whether she is immune to rubella, the following course of action is recommended:

1. If possible, establish by serology the diagnosis of rubella in the patient with whom the pregnant woman was in contact. Often it may not have been rubella at all. Find out whether contact was close enough to allow transmission of virus.
2. Test the pregnant patient for rubella antibodies:
   If positive by HAI within 14 days of exposure to rubella, the patient was immune previously and she can be reassured.
   If negative by HAI then test further sample 2–3 weeks from contact. If the second serum is positive or if IgM antibodies are detected, discuss risks and offer termination. Some women prefer to continue with the pregnancy despite the risk to the fetus. In this case intramuscular rubella immunoglobulin should be given as soon as possible after exposure.

ARBOVIRUSES

Arboviral infections (*Appendix table 2*, p. 327) are a group of virus infections of man that are transmitted by the bite of an arthropod vector. There are two main diseases: dengue and yellow fever.

Dengue

Dengue is an acute febrile illness with severe bone pains, rash and lymphadenopathy. It is due to a flavivirus. The vectors are *Aedes* mosquitoes. The dengue virus is a 50 nm RNA-containing flavivirus. Four serotypes are recognised, and these can be differentiated in a range of standard serological tests. The serotypes are closely related antigenically but cross-protection between serotypes is lacking. The dengue shock syndrome and haemorrhagic fever occur in patients experiencing re-infection with a different serotype.

Distribution and incidence

Dengue occurs throughout tropical and subtropical areas of the world closely related to the distribution of the *Aedes* mosquito vector.

Transmission and epidemiology

The most common vector is *Aedes aegypti* but other species have more limited roles in transmission. Eight to eleven days after ingesting dengue virus in a human blood meal the mosquito is infective to a receptive host by biting; it remains infective for the rest of its life.

Both sexes and all age groups are susceptible to dengue provided they have not been infected before with that serotype. Dengue haemorrhagic fever is predominantly a disease of children.

Pathology and pathogenesis

After inoculation virus replicates in cells in local lymph nodes. Viraemia follows and reticulo-endothelial cells in skin and other tissues become infected. Local inflammatory changes occur around small vessels in the skin. The pathogenesis of dengue haemorrhagic fever is poorly understood. It is characterised by hypovolaemia, due to increased vascular permeability, and coagulation defects.

Clinical features

The incubation period is about 7 days prior to the onset of high fever, headache, eye pains, backache and chills. Limb pain is often severe in dengue and this gives rise to its common name, 'breakbone fever'. A blanching, erythematous, macular rash may appear on the third or fourth day of the illness. Lymphadenopathy may be present. Leukopenia is usual in the peripheral blood.

In dengue haemorrhagic fever the patient is more ill, and the peripheral blood shows thrombocytopenia and increased haematocrit. There may be spontaneous bleeding into the skin and at other sites. The loss of circulating blood volume causes shock with low blood pressure, rapid pulse, restlessness and abdominal pain (the dengue shock syndrome), which can have a mortality of 50% untreated. This occurs most often in children but occasional cases are reported in adults.

Diagnosis

Virus can be isolated from blood using *Aedes* or mammalian cell lines. A rising antibody titre in paired sera obtained 10–14 days apart is diagnostic, although the serological response may not be so clear-cut in areas where populations are exposed to other flaviviruses.

Treatment

Patients with uncomplicated dengue require simple supportive measures, such as attention to nutrition and hydration and relief of pain. Paracetamol should be used in preference to aspirin. Dengue haemorrhagic fever and dengue shock syndrome require early intensive therapy with intravenous fluids. This much reduces mortality.

Control

Vaccines are not yet available. Vector control comprises removal of breeding sites, which are often collections of water in tins, tyres, tubs and water storage vessels around homes, and larviciding.

Yellow fever

Yellow fever is an acute arboviral infection caused by the yellow fever virus, a flavivirus. The illness is characterised by high fever, jaundice and encephalopathy in its severe form. The disease occurs in focal outbreaks in Africa, the Caribbean and Central and South America.

Distribution and incidence

Sub-Saharan tropical Africa (especially West Africa), the Caribbean islands (most recently Trinidad) and South America (Brazil, Peru, Bolivia, Ecuador, Venezuela and Colombia) are the areas affected by yellow fever. Relatively small numbers of cases occur every year in these areas, although cases in isolated areas may go unreported.

Transmission and epidemiology

Transmission is shown in Figure 12.7. In South America, and Central and East Africa, a jungle cycle involves monkey–mosquito–monkey and maintains the virus in the mosquito reservoir. *Haemagogus* mosquitoes are the vector. The epidemiology in savannah and forest-savannah areas involves other *Aedes* species with man and monkeys. The insect vector passes infection to the next generation of mosquitoes by transovarial transmission.

Non-immune persons of all races, all ages and both sexes are susceptible to infection. Prior exposure to other flaviviruses produces some degree of cross-protection. Men are at particular risk of infection because of occupations which take them into forests.

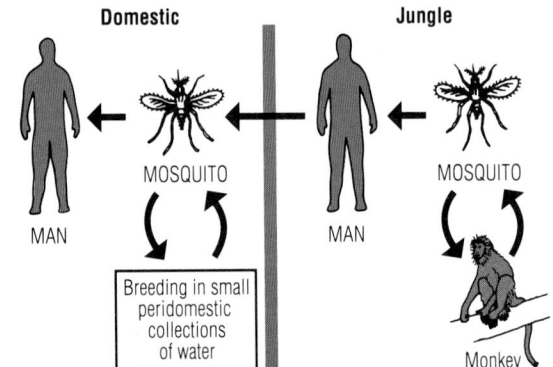

Fig. 12.7 Cycle of transmission of yellow fever virus. Infected humans bring the virus from the jungle. Mosquitoes can breed peridomestically in small collections of water such as puddles and water pots.

Pathology and pathogenesis

The liver is the main organ involved and shows midzonal necrosis of hepatocytes. Councilman bodies result from the degeneration of hepatocytes. The kidneys show acute tubular necrosis which may relate to shock and hypovolaemia. There may be haemorrhage into mucous membranes and the skin, associated with the bleeding tendency that is common in yellow fever. The underlying pathogenic mechanisms are poorly understood.

Clinical features

There is a range of severity of disease from mild to severe, life-threatening illness. The latter constitutes a minority of all those infected. The incubation period is about 6 days before the onset of headache and fever. More severe illness is associated with marked limb pains. Proteinuria is usual. High fever, headache, severe limb and back pain and chills associated with fetor oris, haemorrhages in the gums, and nosebleeds are early features in severe cases. There may then be a short period of remission of symptoms for up to 24 hours before the recurrence of fever with vomiting and jaundice. Bleeding into the gut, skin and other sites is usual in severe cases. Occasional cases are seen with the brunt of organ damage limited to heart or kidneys, causing cardiac or renal failure. Bleeding and renal failure are the main causes of the high mortality (up to 50%) in severe cases. Resolution in severe cases can take from 3 days to 6 weeks.

Diagnosis

The clinical features in severe cases suggest the diagnosis but in milder cases without evidence of organ dysfunction the diagnosis may not be made. Virus can be isolated most often from blood taken in the first 4 days of clinical illness. Rising antibody titres in paired sera may also give the diagnosis, but serological tests may not be easy to interpret in people exposed to related viruses.

Differential diagnosis

In mild cases the range of febrile illnesses to be considered is extensive and includes malaria, typhoid, the prodromal phase of viral hepatitis, leptospirosis and rickettsial diseases. The presence of jaundice with fever prompts consideration of leptospirosis, malaria, East African trypanosomiasis, typhoid, biliary tract sepsis and Marburg virus diseases. Ebola virus disease and Lassa fever are other causes of haemorrhagic fever, although marked jaundice is not usual.

Laboratory features

Anaemia, leukopenia and thrombocytopenia are usual features in more severe cases. Conjugated bilirubin levels and transaminases are high in jaundiced cases. Coagulation abnormalities comprise prolonged prothrombin time, reduced fibrinogen levels and detectable fibrin degradation products. Renal failure with proteinuria, oliguria and raised creatinine and urea may occur.

Treatment

More severe cases are likely to come to medical attention. Paracetamol may be helpful symptomatically and in relief of fever. Severe cases require intensive care but this is rarely available in the endemic areas.

Prevention and control

All travellers to endemic areas, apart from pregnant females, infants under 1 year and immunosuppressed patients, should receive the attenuated 17D yellow fever vaccine. Patients with yellow fever should be nursed under mosquito nets to prevent mosquitoes becoming infected.

Other arboviral infections

There are a considerable number of arboviruses which affect man (Appendix table 2). In these infections the main clinical manifestations are fever, chills, joint pains and a maculopapular rash. Mild forms of the diseases are frequent. Vaccines are not available.

VIRAL HAEMORRHAGIC FEVERS

The viruses causing viral haemorrhagic fevers, a group of clinically similar infections, mainly comprise togaviridae and arenaviridae (Table 12.17). The diseases have a wide geographic distribution. They are characterised, in the clinically severe cases, by a bleeding tendency evident by purpura and ecchymoses in the skin, bleeding from the gums and rapidly falling haemoglobin level, often associated with bleeding into the lungs, gut and other internal organs. Haemorrhagic fever with renal syndrome was first described from Korea in the 1950s but cases have been reported from Finland, Sweden and Belgium. In this infection progressive renal failure occurs with a rapidly declining haemoglobin, often due to bleeding into the lungs. It should be noted that not all patients infected with these viruses develop severe disease; many have a febrile illness which resolves spontaneously. Treatment in severe cases is mainly supportive, comprising restoration of blood volume, transfusion, platelet support, and dialysis where there is renal failure.

Table 12.17 Causes of viral haemorrhagic fever

Type of virus	Disease	Frequency and distribution
Togaviridae	Dengue haemorrhagic fever Yellow fever	Relatively common
Arenaviridae	Lassa fever Argentine haemorrhagic fever	Epidemics/endemic
Marburg-Ebola group	Marburg virus disease Ebola virus disease	Rare, focal epidemics

Lassa fever

Lassa fever is an acute febrile illness first described from the region of Lassa in north-eastern Nigeria in 1969. It is an arenavirus (RNA) infection characterised by high sustained fever, ulcerative pharyngitis and swelling of the neck and face in typical cases.

Transmission and epidemiology

The multimammate rat, *Mastomys natalensis*, is the peridomestic reservoir and persistently excretes virus in its

Infectious, Tropical and Parasitic Diseases

12

urine. Man is infected by ingesting food contaminated with urine containing virus.

Person-to-person spread can occur through contact with vomit, urine, faeces, blood and serum. The virus may enter the body through cuts, abrasions or mucous membranes. Studies in endemic areas indicate that mild infections commonly occur, with a low mortality. The disease may be milder in children than adults. Virus replication occurs in many organs with cell death and necrosis.

Clinical features

The incubation period can be up to 17 days. Gradual onset of fever with anorexia, lethargy and headache is usual followed by prostration and ulcerative pharyngitis. Cervical lymphadenopathy and swelling of the neck and face may appear. Bradycardia is often present. Vomiting, diarrhoea, cough and chest pain are common features. A maculopapular rash on face, trunk and upper limbs is seen in the second week of the illness. Bleeding from gums and other mucosal sites occurs in more severe cases. The blood pressure is low. Recovery occurs during the third week of the illness but convalescence may be protracted. Nerve deafness is a common sequel. Fatal cases usually show declining renal function and oliguria, declining conscious level and secondary bacterial infection. Laboratory investigations show leukopenia, low albumin, raised blood urea and elevated transaminases. Platelet counts are normal but function is impaired.

Diagnosis

In the endemic areas this will be based on the clinical features plus the exclusion of important treatable causes of fever. The specific laboratory diagnosis is made by finding the virus in blood, urine or throat washings, using electron microscopy or culture, or by detecting antibodies or antigen in serum.

Treatment

Hydration and nutrition should be maintained. Oral toilet and analgesics such as paracetamol may be helpful. Volume replacement is necessary in shocked patients. Ribavirin given intravenously or orally reduces mortality from the disease.

Diagnosed cases of Lassa fever in Europe and North America are managed in secure isolation facilities to give maximum protection to the attendant nursing and medical team, although standard barrier nursing precautions are adequate.

Marburg and Ebola virus disease

Marburg and Ebola virus disease are African diseases caused by morphologically identical arenaviruses; they are distinguished from each other serologically. The course of Marburg virus disease is similar to that of Lassa, with sudden onset of fever, headache and general systemic upset, progressing to prostration with watery diarrhoea and dehydration. The diarrhoea may last for a week and be associated with cramping abdominal pain. Haemorrhagic manifestations may be seen at the end of the first week of the illness with bleeding from mucosal surfaces. A maculopapular rash also occurs. Recovery occurs after 2–3 weeks in those surviving.

Management is supportive and symptomatic, with fresh blood transfusions for significant haemorrhage.

RETROVIRUSES

The acquired immunodeficiency syndrome (AIDS) and human immunodeficiency virus (HIV) infections

The acquired immunodeficiency syndrome (AIDS) was first described in the USA in 1981. Homosexual men were reported as having opportunistic infections, such as *Pneumocystis carinii* pneumonia, and Kaposi's sarcoma. It was known that such illnesses occurred in people undergoing renal transplants and receiving immunosuppressive therapy, and therefore an underlying immune deficiency in these men was assumed. The spread of the condition resembled that of hepatitis B. The causal agent, called human immunodeficiency virus (HIV; previously HTLV III) was isolated in 1983.

Epidemiology

The epidemic is now traced in two ways: the number of people showing antibodies to HIV, and those with clinically defined AIDS (Fig. 12.8). Many homosexual and bisexual men have opted not to be tested for HIV anti-

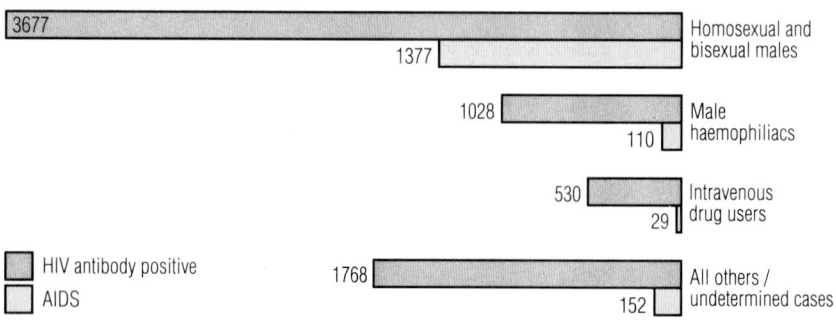

Fig. 12.8 Totals of HIV antibody positive persons and AIDS cases reported in the UK July 1988 (Communicable Diseases Surveillance Centre, Colindale).

1 Vesicles and pustules in a patient with chickenpox.

2 Dermatomal distribution of varicella zoster lesions.

3 Gingivo-stomatitis caused by primary herpes simplex I.

4 Acute tonsillo-pharyngitis caused by primary Epstein-Barr virus infection.

5 Koplik's spots in measles.

6 Measles rash.

7 Rubella rash.

8 Scarlet fever rash.

9 Necrotic haemorrhagic lesions in meningococcal septicaemia.

251

bodies and the overall prevalence of HIV infection will not be known until anonymous surveys have been conducted.

In Europe and the USA the majority of AIDS cases are in homosexual men, injecting drug users and haemophiliacs. Metropolitan areas have the greatest numbers. The first case of AIDS in haemophiliacs was reported in the USA in 1982. The lyophilised clotting factor concentrates made from cryoprecipitates pooled from a large number of donors contained HIV and these pooled blood products from the USA were used in the UK.

HIV and AIDS have now been reported in heterosexual men and women and in babies. In the Western world sexual intercourse with an injecting drug user, or a past user, is still the major risk factor for heterosexuals contracting HIV. In Africa, however, the epidemic is spread heterosexually. It is hypothesised that the high prevalence of other sexually transmitted diseases, particularly those causing genital ulceration (Table 12.18), is a factor in the spread of HIV. In some areas of Africa up to 10% of women of childbearing age are infected.

HIV is not transmitted by saliva, although the virus has been cultured from saliva and tears as well as from blood and semen. Breast milk may rarely transmit infection. HIV is *not* transmitted by normal household contact and only very rarely by needle-stick injury.

Table 12.18 Causes of genital ulceration

- Genital herpes
- Trauma
- Syphilis
- Chancroid
- Lymphogranuloma venereum

Human immunodeficiency virus

HIV has a lipid envelope and is about 100 nm in diameter. It has a dense cylindrical nucleoid containing core protein, genomic RNA, and the reverse transcriptase enzyme which classifies HIV as a retrovirus. HIV is closely related to a group of viruses called the lentiviruses; this includes the visna virus, which is capable of causing chronic neuro-degradation in sheep. There are also similarities with lymphotropic retroviruses HTLV I and II. There are many minor variations between human immunodeficiency viruses but only two major variants, HIV 1 and 2, have been identified. HIV 2 was first found in West Africa and it exists both as a single infection and as a co-infection with HIV 1. It is much less common than HIV 1 and it may be less pathogenic.

The main action of HIV is to cause depletion of the T4 helper or inducer lymphocytes. The CD4 molecule appears to be the HIV receptor. After HIV enters the cell, the genomic RNA is transcribed into DNA by the reverse transcriptase. The DNA is then integrated into the host genome. HIV replication remains at this stage till the infected cell is activated. It may be that other infections can act as the triggering mechanism. After activation, tran-

scription occurs, followed by protein synthesis, and the T4 cell dies. The virus spreads to infect other cells. As well as T4 lymphocytes, other cells of the immune system can be infected by HIV. The monocytes and macrophages are vulnerable. The monocytes may carry HIV to the central nervous system. B cell abnormalities are also seen as an effect of HIV infection. There is polyclonal activation, with high immunoglobulin levels, but a poor antibody response to newly acquired antigens, leading to susceptibility to bacterial infections which are common in HIV-infected individuals.

Clinical features

HIV infection is asymptomatic and produces no abnormal physical signs in over half of affected subjects. The remainder are often described as having persistent generalised lymphadenopathy (PGL), AIDS-related complex (ARC) or AIDS. Their relationship is shown diagrammatically in Figure 12.9. The time from infection to development of AIDS is a few months to more than 5 years (mean 8–10 years).

AIDS is defined as a reliably diagnosed disease that is indicative of cellular immunodeficiency, such as an opportunistic infection or Kaposi's sarcoma (in a patient aged less than 60) in a patient who has serum antibodies to HIV and no other cause of deficient CMI. This definition does not embrace the neurological manifestations or recognise the bad prognosis of ARC. The groups shown in Summary 2 are more useful in this respect, and group IV contains patients with AIDS and ARC.

Fig. 12.9 Usual evolution of HIV infection to AIDS. Individual stages may be bypassed in some patients; for example, an asymptomatic carrier may present with AIDS without going through the intermediate stage.

Summary 2 Classification system for HIV-infected patients (Centers for Disease Control, Atlanta)

Group I   Acute seroconversion illness

Group II   Asymptomatic infection

Group III   Persistent generalised lymphadenopathy

Group IV   Other disease (including ARC and AIDS)
  Subgroup A   Constitutional disease (ARC)
  Subgroup B   Neurological disease
  Subgroup C   Opportunistic infection
  Subgroup D   Secondary cancers
  Subgroup E   Other conditions

Group I: acute seroconversion illness

Some people infected with HIV develop a febrile illness about 6 weeks after infection. With the fever they have oral ulcers, rash, lymphadenopathy and arthralgia. After 2 weeks the majority become asymptomatic (group II) but a few have persistent generalised lymphadenopathy (group III).

Group II: asymptomatic infection

The majority of people, for at least the first 2 years after infection, are completely well. They are seropositive and can transmit infection.

Group III: persistent generalised lymphadenopathy

Persistent generalised lymphadenopathy (PGL) is diagnosed when lymph nodes in extra-inguinal sites remain enlarged for more than 3 months. Commonly the posterior cervical, anterior cervical, submandibular, posterior occipital and axillary nodes are involved. The nodes may swell up and cause pain intermittently. Biopsy of the nodes usually shows reactive hyperplasia. A large single node or rapidly enlarging nodes are an indication for biopsy to exclude opportunistic infection or tumour. About one-third of patients with PGL develop AIDS within 5 years.

Group IV A: constitutional disease or AIDS-related complex

AIDS-related complex (ARC) is a collection of symptoms and signs including chronic fatigue, unexplained weight loss, night sweats and recurrent fever, a variety of cutaneous manifestations including recurrent herpes simplex infections, oral candida, chronic tinea infection, seborrhoeic dermatitis, molluscum contagiosum (p. 1120), intermittent diarrhoea, and myalgia.

Many of these infections are treatable but there is an inevitable progression to AIDS.

Group IV B: HIV-related neurological disease

Psychoneurological defects are associated with HIV infection for which HIV itself may be responsible. Peripheral neuropathy and subacute encephalitis (AIDS encephalopathy or dementia complex) occur. Clinically, subacute encephalitis is characterised by poor memory, inability to concentrate, apathy and psychomotor retardation. There may also be focal motor abnormalities and behavioural changes. For the majority of patients, before the use of zidovudine, dementia rapidly followed subacute encephalitis.

Group IV C: opportunistic infection

Table 12.19 shows part of the spectrum of opportunistic infections in patients with AIDS. The incidence of these infections varies considerably in different parts of the

Table 12.19 Opportunistic infection in AIDS

Syndrome	Organism
Pneumonia	*Pneumocystis carinii*
	Mycobacterium tuberculosis
	Cytomegalovirus*
Stomatitis	*Candida*
	Herpes simplex
Oesophagitis	*Candida*
	Herpes simplex
	Cytomegalovirus
Enterocolitis	*Cytomegalovirus*
	Cryptosporidium
	Isospora belli
Proctitis	*Herpes simplex*
Retinitis	*Cytomegalovirus*
CNS disease	
Meningitis	*Cryptococcus neoformans*
Encephalitis	*Cytomegalovirus*
	JC virus and SV40
Mass lesion	*Toxoplasma*
Septicaemia	*Salmonella typhimurium*
	Mycobacterium avium intracellulare

* This is a questionable cause of pneumonia.

world. *Pneumocystis carinii pneumonia* (PCP) is the most common presentation of AIDS in the UK and other Western countries. There is a history of slowly increasing dyspnoea and fever, sometimes accompanied by dry cough. The patient is often hypoxaemic and chest X-ray changes lag behind the clinical signs. In a developed pneumonia the radiological changes are classically a bilateral ground glass appearance.

Diagnosis is made by identifying trophozoites in bronchial lavage fluid or in sputum induced by inhalation of nebulised hypertonic saline. The organisms can be seen with a silver stain or by immunofluorescent staining using a monoclonal antibody.

Therapy consists of high-dose co-trimoxazole (20 mg trimethoprim per kg body weight per day) for 3 weeks. There is a high incidence of skin rashes during treatment and alternative treatment with trimethoprim plus dapsone is sometimes used. Addition of corticosteroids has been advocated for severe unresponsive cases (p. 296).

Many other organisms can cause pneumonia in AIDS but tuberculosis caused by *Mycobacterium tuberculosis* is a common initial presentation in poor countries. Whereas PCP and Kaposi's sarcoma predominate in the Western world, tuberculosis and weight loss are the main features in Africa, with candida providing a common thread.

Intestinal infection is common, particularly in African patients, in whom weight loss is so striking that AIDS is sometimes referred to as 'slim disease'. HIV infects gut epithelial cells and it may be this or an as yet unidentified secondary infection which causes malabsorption and weight loss. Profuse watery diarrhoea occurs with several

Infectious, Tropical and Parasitic Diseases

12

unusual protozoal infections such as *Cryptosporidium* or *Isospora belli.*

Central nervous system opportunistic infection presents major problems because of inaccessibility to diagnosis. *Toxoplasma* is the most common cause of a mass lesion within the brain and when CT scanning is available, the main differential diagnosis is from a cerebral lymphoma. This distinction may require a stereotactically directed brain biopsy. Meningeal infection is most often caused by the yeast *Cryptococcus neoformans.*

Retinitis is the most frequent manifestation of cytomegalovirus infection in AIDS, and this can be bilateral, resulting in loss of sight.

Blood and bone marrow are affected by septicaemia, which is caused by conventional bacteria, particularly in children, but *Candida* or atypical mycobacteria may be responsible. *Mycobacterium avium intracellulare* also infects bone marrow and causes a pancytopenia. This is usually a late complication.

Group IV D: secondary cancers

Kaposi's sarcoma (KS), the most common secondary cancer, shows initially as a purple nodule or plaque on the skin or mucous membranes. Unlike KS seen in the past in elderly men, KS found in AIDS may spread to other parts of the body and eventually the patient may have hundreds of lesions.

In the early stages, patients with KS alone are relatively well, but later there may be rapid spread to lymph nodes, gut and lung associated with constitutional symptoms. In the UK and the USA, KS is almost confined to gay men. Diagnosis is by biopsy and histological examination. The lesion consists of a mixture of spindle cells and vascular spaces which are infiltrated by plasma cells. The cell of origin is thought to be endothelial.

Therapy is unsatisfactory at present. Skin cream can be used to camouflage unsightly lesions and local radiotherapy will shrink large nodules. In the later stages treatment is with cytotoxic agents such as vinblastine or etoposide, or drugs acting on the immune system like alpha interferon.

Group IV E: other conditions

This heterogenous subgroup contains other symptomatic conditions which have not been classified elsewhere. *Lymphoid interstitial pneumonitis* is a descriptive term for a common pneumonia of unknown aetiology in children with AIDS. It has a variable course, sometimes responding to corticosteroid therapy.

Thrombocytopenia may occur during an asymptomatic or a symptomatic phase of infection. When it is early it often remits without having any apparent influence on the subsequent prognosis.

Other patients are included in this group when they have infections, tumours or other conditions which do not fit into one of the other subgroups. An example would be an HIV positive drug addict with frequent bacterial (i.e. not opportunistic) chest infection.

Diagnosis

The diagnosis of AIDS rests on the demonstration of infections or tumours associated with immunodeficiency.

The presence of HIV is usually determined by demonstration of antibody to the HIV envelope or core proteins. HIV antigen can be measured and HIV itself can be grown in culture, but these tests are not routinely available.

Identification of a patient as having HIV-related disease usually requires the demonstration of HIV antibody or antigen, followed by the measurement of T4 helper cell numbers, and clinical examination and follow-up looking for symptoms or signs of ARC or AIDS. By regular examination of known HIV antibody positive patients and appropriate medical intervention, patients may be kept well for many years.

Paediatric HIV infection

About a quarter of babies born to HIV positive mothers are infected; the baby is usually infected in utero but can also be infected from contact with the mother's blood at birth. HIV antibody passively acquired from the mother can be demonstrated in the baby's blood for several months after birth. The presence of HIV antigen confirms active infection but its absence does not exclude infection. If the antigen is present the baby is likely to show signs of HIV infection within the first year of life. Signs of HIV infection in a baby include failure to thrive, loss of weight, psychomotor retardation, interstitial pneumonitis, skin rashes and many of the infections seen in adult AIDS.

Treatment

There is no curative therapy for AIDS or HIV infection. Patients are told to lead a healthy life and have all associated infections, such as candida, treated promptly. Zidovudine, an antiviral drug, is effective against HIV. It is a thymidine analogue which inhibits reverse transcriptase, which in turn terminates the viral DNA-chain elongation. It has been shown to increase life expectancy and to reduce the incidence of opportunistic infections, particularly PCP in patients with AIDS or ARC. The main side-effects of zidovudine are megaloblastic anaemia unrelated to vitamin B_{12} or folate deficiency and neutropenia. Regular full blood count measurements are necessary.

Counselling

A substantial amount of distress is experienced by patients with HIV infection. Trained counsellors have an important input at several stages of the disease. Counselling prior to antibody testing is important so that people are aware of what they are being tested for and to discuss the health education aspects of HIV disease. Counsellors can also help people who are HIV positive or have AIDS to cope with the many problems caused by having a new and commonly fatal infection.

HTLV infection

See page 1087.

RHABDOVIRUSES

Rabies

Rabies is an acute encephalomyelitic illness, caused by an RNA-containing rhabdovirus. It is characterised by paroxysms of muscle spasm, particularly of muscle groups associated with inspiration and swallowing, in response to attempts to drink water as well as at the sight, sound or mention of water. It is almost invariably fatal.

Aetiology

The rabies virus is an RNA rhabdovirus which, with five related viruses, comprise the *Lyssavirus* genus. The rabies virus is shaped like a bullet and measures 180×75 nm. It is pathogenic for all mammals. The virus can be grown in cell culture.

Distribution and incidence

Antarctica and Australasia are the only continents free of rabies. It is endemic in the rest of the world, with the exception of the United Kingdom, the Scandinavian countries, Japan and Taiwan. The incidence of human rabies is difficult to estimate. Occasional cases occur in Europe and North America. Rabies is much more common in the tropics, although accurate figures are not available. It is a considerable health problem in Asia, Africa and Central and South America.

Transmission and epidemiology

Rabies virus cannot penetrate the intact skin and so must be inoculated in saliva by the bite of a rabid animal; this is most often a dog, less often a cat (Fig. 12.10). Licking of abraded or cut skin can transmit infection. Virus can penetrate the mucous membranes of mouth and eye.

All mammals can become infected but transmission to man is mainly caused by biting animals, most often stray dogs in the tropics. Wolves, jackals, mongooses, bats (fruit-eating, insectivorous and vampire), monkeys and ungulates (sheep, cattle and deer) can all become infected and to a greater or lesser extent transmit the infection. Apart from bats, all infected species die from the disease. In Europe the red fox is the reservoir of infection. Vampire bats infect cattle in the countries of South America, causing considerable economic losses through cattle rabies. These bats painlessly incise veins around the lower legs of cattle and lap the blood. Human rabies has been acquired from vampire bats.

Pathology

Virus first penetrates skeletal muscle cells where it remains for some time. It then enters nerves through the fibres supplying muscle spindles and travels centripetally to the neuraxis to infect nerve cell bodies. Virus replication occurs and cell rupture releases new virions to infect other neurones. At post-mortem examinations the neuropathological changes are not gross. Collections of inflammatory cells around small vessels, dead neurones and phagocytosis of degenerating neurones are seen, especially in the medulla and midbrain. Viraemia is not thought to contribute to dissemination of virus. There is centrifugal spread of virus via autonomic nerve fibres to cornea, skin and salivary glands.

Clinical features

The incubation period is 20–60 days on average, with a range of up to 1 year.

Initial symptoms are non-specific, with headache, fever, anorexia, insomnia and paraesthesia or altered sensation at the site of biting or some peripheral site. After 2–3 days the patient may become markedly agitated, hyperexcitable, anxious, confused and lucid in turn. The earliest hint of fear of water may be evident at this stage; this rapidly progresses to typical hydrophobia, with involuntary contraction of main and accessory inspiratory muscles in a sustained spasm, brought on by attempts to drink water, the sight of water, the sound of water or even the mention of water. Variations in mood persist. Saliva may continuously be spat out as it cannot be swallowed. The spasms may be provoked by fanning air across the face. Cranial nerve palsies, paralysis and bizarre patterns of breathing follow. Ascending paralysis without hydrophobia occurs in a few patients and this may pose problems in diagnosis. Death occurs within 7–14 days, due to respiratory failure or cardiac arrhythmias. There is no effective treatment for established disease.

Differential diagnosis

Tetanus, other causes of ascending paralysis and encephalitis, and rabies hysteria form the main differential diagnosis.

Laboratory features

Virus particles may be grown from saliva, nasal washings, cerebrospinal fluid or urine. Viral antigen can be identified

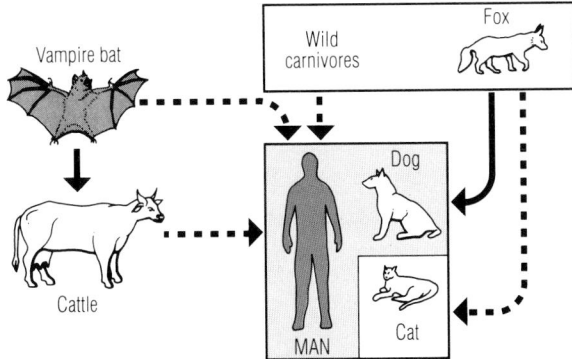

Fig. 12.10 Cycle of transmission of rabies. The commonest routes of spread are shown in solid lines. Man is usually infected by dog bites.

in skin biopsies, or less easily, in corneal impression smears using direct fluorescent antibody techniques. Rising titres of antibody to rabies virus in blood or cerebrospinal fluid also confirm the diagnosis.

Prevention, control and treatment

Correct management at the time of biting prevents rabies. First aid treatment consists of thorough washing of the wound with soap and water for 5 minutes, followed by washing with clean water. This is followed by application of 40–70% alcohol, povidone iodine or 0.01% aqueous iodine. Extensive areas of necrotic tissue should be excised. An occlusive dressing should not be applied and the wound should not be sutured, as this may inoculate virus into skeletal muscle. Delayed suture may be appropriate. Tetanus prophylaxis should be started. Antibiotics are given as needed.

When exposure takes place in an endemic area rabies vaccination must be considered. When the animal concerned was a cat or dog, the attack was unprovoked, and the exposure comprised licks of the skin or minor bites of the extremities of trunk through clothing, the vaccine is given. If the animal remains healthy through 5 days of observation or the animal's brain contains no rabies virus by direct immunofluorescence, vaccination is stopped. If the animal becomes rabid or the virus is detected, vaccination is continued and antirabies immunoglobulin (ARIG) is given. When the attack is by a wild animal or a dog or cat not available for observation, both serum and vaccine are given. When there are major bites, i.e. extensive or involving the head and neck, or licks of the mucosa, give serum and vaccine. Vaccination is stopped if the dog or cat remains healthy at 5 days or animal brain examined by immunofluorescence shows no virus.

Antirabies immunoglobulin is obtained from two sources, equine and human. Reactions to horse and mule serum are common and so a test dose should be given first. The vaccine of first choice comprises killed virus grown in human diploid cells (HDCV).

The problem of controlling reservoirs of infection remains. The capturing and killing of stray dogs in endemic areas has reduced an important source of human rabies.

Vaccination of household dogs and cats is a helpful measure but does not exclude the possibility of the animal contracting rabies. The spread of rabies in Europe has been uncontrolled so far. Attempts are being made to vaccinate foxes through vaccine-contaminated bait.

NON-ENVELOPED SINGLE-STRANDED RNA VIRUSES

PICORNAVIRUSES

Rhinovirus infection

Rhinoviruses are the most common cause of colds (p. 470). There are over 90 serotypes and reinfection with the same serotype can occur. Infection is usually confined to the nasal mucosa, but complications such as sinusitis and otitis media can occur as a result of mucosal swelling and obstruction to drainage of secretions. Rhinoviruses can also cause exacerbations of chronic bronchitis but the mechanism for this is not clear.

Enterovirus infection

Coxsackie A, Coxsackie B and *Echoviruses*, of which there are 24, 6 and 34 types respectively, cause a wide variety of clinical infections, but overall the majority are asymptomatic. A febrile illness with upper respiratory symptoms is another common manifestation of infection with many different serotypes. More specific disease associations are shown in Table 12.20. *Polioviruses* types 1, 2 and 3 cause poliomyelitis, which is described on page 963.

Acute meningitis

Enteroviruses are a common cause of lymphocytic meningitis (more than 70% of cases), which is a benign disease. Enteroviral meningitis is common in young children and rare over the age of 40. The clinical features are described on page 962.

Table 12.20 Enterovirus types and their disease associations

Disease	Virus types most commonly associated		
	Coxsackie A types	Coxsackie B types	Echo types
Acute meningitis	Most	All	Most
Encephalitis	One-fifth	Most	One-third
Herpangina (pharyngitis)	2–6, 8, 10, 22	None	None
Hand, foot and mouth disease	5, 7, 9, 10, 16	None	None
Pleurodynia (Bornholm disease)	None	1–5	None
Pericarditis/myocarditis	None	1–5	None
Chronic meningo-encephalitis in hypogammaglobulinaemics	None	None	One-third

Other neurological disease

Encephalitis is a rare manifestation of enteroviral infection which may occur with or without meningitis. Flaccid motor paralysis is only seen with any frequency in poliomyelitis.

Fever and exanthem

A variety of skin rashes are associated with enteroviral infections. Maculopapular eruptions associated with fever are more common with Echo than Coxsackie viruses. In some forms the exanthem follows a febrile illness in a sequence resembling roseola. Petechial or purpuric eruptions are uncommon.

The most distinctive exanthem is the vesicular eruption of hand, foot and mouth disease caused by Coxsackie virus A16 (and occasionally others). Lesions are found in the mouth consistently and on the palms, soles and extensor sufaces of the hands and feet in 75% of cases. Vesicles are sometimes surrounded by a ring of erythema and lesions may be slightly tender. The child feels unwell for one or two days and has a fever but recovers completely. Virus can be isolated from vesicles, throat washings or stools.

Respiratory tract infection

Most enteroviruses can cause non-specific upper respiratory infection but group A Coxsackie viruses are the common cause of herpangina, an acute painful vesicular eruption on the fauces and soft palate, associated with fever, malaise and myalgia and lasting up to 10 days.

Pleurodynia

Pleurodynia (sometimes known as Bornholm disease) is an acute febrile illness characterised by 'pleuritic' chest pain; it is usually caused by group B Coxsackie viruses. The pain is due to infection of muscle and there is no pleural inflammation. About half of patients have pain in an area of the thorax but upper abdominal pain occurs in others, especially children, and this may mimic an abdominal emergency. Tenderness over involved muscles is the characteristic sign.

The illness is usually over in 5 days but it may last up to 3 weeks and it sometimes recurs.

Myopericarditis

Enteroviruses, mainly group B Coxsackie, are an important cause of acute myocarditis and pericarditis in young adults. Usually the two conditions occur simultaneously but one predominates in the clinical presentation. The clinical features are described on page 416.

Epidemic haemorrhagic conjunctivitis

This epidemic form of acute conjunctivitis, which is associated with pain, subconjunctival bleeding and oedema of the eyelids, lasts about 1 week and is usually caused by enterovirus 70, one of the recently recognised enteroviruses.

The disease was first noticed in 1969 and appears to have been new. The virus is highly infectious and is spread by contact and fomites rather than by droplet.

NON-ENVELOPED DOUBLE-STRANDED RNA VIRUSES

REOVIRUSES

Rotavirus diarrhoea

Rotavirus diarrhoea is an acute dehydrating diarrhoeal disease caused by a 70 nm RNA-containing virus. This organism is the commonest cause of diarrhoea in children up to 2 years old in the tropics.

Transmission

Rotavirus diarrhoea is spread by the faecal–oral route but the occurrence of upper respiratory tract symptoms at the onset of the illness has raised the possibility of droplet transmission. The infection occurs in both endemic and epidemic forms worldwide.

Clinical features

After an incubation period of up to 5 days (most often 2 days) anorexia, vomiting, diarrhoea and fever begin suddenly. There may also be a blocked nose and sore throat. The stools are watery and non-dysenteric. The illness is self-limiting, terminating in about 5 days in most cases. Moderate dehydration is the usual consequence of the illness but a number of fatalities from severe dehydration have occurred. The organism may be found in faeces by immune electron microscopy and viral antigen detection using an enzyme-linked immunosorbent assay.

Treatment

Management comprises assessment of the degree of dehydration (Table 12.13, p. 234) and replacement of that volume of fluid in the first 4–6 hours after presentation. Continuing fluid losses must also be replaced until diarrhoea ceases.

Oral rehydration solution (ORS) can be used for rehydration. The standard WHO/UNICEF formulation comprises glucose 20 g (or sucrose 40 g), sodium chloride 3.5 g, sodium bicarbonate 2.5 g (or sodium citrate 2.9 g) and potassium chloride 1.5 g made up to a volume of 1 litre with clean water. Additional water, not ORS, must be allowed for insensible losses and obligatory urinary losses. When there is shock, intravenous rehydration is necessary. As soon as the child wishes to start eating again he should be allowed to do so.

12   CHLAMYDIAL, MYCOPLASMA AND RICKETTSIAL INFECTIONS

CHLAMYDIA

Chlamydia are bacteria which contain both DNA and RNA (unlike viruses) but are unable to replicate extracellularly (Table 12.21). They are Gram-negative and have a lipopolysaccharide endotoxin.

Chlamydia psittaci is a common pathogen of birds and animals which can infect man, causing psittacosis (ornithosis). *Chl. trachomatis* is transmitted between humans by sexual contact or from a mother's infected genital tract to her newborn infant, causing conjunctivitis or occasionally pneumonia. Different serotypes of *Chl. trachomatis* cause lymphogranuloma venereum (LGV) and trachoma.

Psittacosis

Although ornithosis is a commonly used name for infection with this organism, this is a misnomer because a wide range of animals other than birds are infected by *Chl. psittaci*.

Epidemiology

Psittacosis is worldwide and occurs sporadically but it is most frequent in people closely associated with birds through work or hobbies. Infected animals and birds usually have an overt illness but they continue to shed organisms in excreta and feathers for months after recovery if they do not die. Humans are infected by inhalation.

Clinical features

After an incubation period of about 2 weeks the patient experiences fever, malaise, headaches, myalgia and sometimes arthralgia. Dry cough is notable and there is variable dyspnoea with confusion and clouding of consciousness if severe hypoxia develops. As with other atypical pneumonias (e.g. mycoplasma) there are few abnormal signs on examination of the chest, although there may be fine crackles in the lower zones. The chest radiograph shows unilateral or bilateral patchy infiltrates; there are more in the lower zones, but occasionally there is the appearance of lobar consolidation. Gastrointestinal symptoms occur uncommonly. Rarely the disease is complicated by aortic or mitral valve endocarditis. Abortion in pregnant women has been reported.

Diagnosis and treatment

Diagnosis is suspected from the history and evidence for atypical pneumonia, and confirmed by testing for serum antibodies by immunofluorescent or complement fixation tests. Tetracyclines given for at least 10 days are the most effective treatment.

Non-specific genital infection (NSGI)

Urethritis, cervicitis and proctitis are most commonly caused by organisms that are not identifiable by routine staining of the exudate. Among the relevant organisms are *Chlamydia*, mycoplasmas and *Ureaplasma*. Chlamydial infection appears to account for more than 50% of NSGI in the UK.

Chlamydia trachomatis is an obligatory intracellular parasite whose replication results in the death of the infected cell. During its life cycle the infectious particle, the elementary body, changes to an actively dividing form – the reticulate or initial body. These later re-organise into the infectious form which is released on cell lysis.

Clinical features

Men usually have a urethral discharge and dysuria about 10 days after exposure to infection. In women the infection is usually silent. If uncomplicated rectal infection occurs there may be anal discharge, peri-anal dampness, irritation and tenesmus.

Complications are more common in women than in men. In women they include bartholinitis, salpingitis and peri-

Table 12.21 Chlamydial infections

Type	Transmission	Disease	Clinical features
Chlamydia psittaci	Zoonosis	Psittacosis	Pneumonia
Chlamydia trachomatis			
Types A, B, C	Fingers, flies, fomites	Trachoma	Keratoconjunctivitis
Types D–K	Sexual	Non-gonoccol urethritis, salpingitis	Urethritis, pelvic inflammatory disease, Reiter's syndrome, perihepatitis (rare)
	Mother-to-infant		Conjunctivitis, pneumonia (rare)
Types L_1, L_2, L_3	Sexual	Lymphogranuloma venereum	Suppurative inguinal lymphadenitis

hepatitis (Fitz-Hugh-Curtis syndrome); in men epididymo-orchitis, prostatitis and sexually acquired reactive arthropathy (Reiter's syndrome, p. 1000).

Diagnosis

In men a urethral smear, Gram-stained, shows excess of polymorphonuclear leucocytes but no gonococci. In men and women chlamydial infection is diagnosed by identifying antigen at the site of infection or serum antibody.

Treatment

Most NSGI responds to tetracycline therapy. The commonest therapy in the UK is oxytetracycline (250 mg four times daily) or doxycycline (100 mg daily) for at least 10 days. Erythromycin (500 mg twice daily) may be used as an alternative and is the first choice in pregnancy and tetracycline allergy.

Relapse or recurrent infection is common in both sexes. There may be symptoms of a postinfective urethritis with no signs of infection. Sexual partners of both sexes should always be examined and treated. The management of anxiety may have a role in therapy.

Congenital Chlamydia trachomatis infection

Chl. trachomatis infection is now frequently seen as a cause of ophthalmia neonatorum. The infected baby will develop a conjunctivitis about 10 days after birth. Investigation of ophthalmia neonatorum should include culture of or monoclonal antibody test for *Chl. trachomatis*. In addition, it may be a cause of pneumonia in the neonate.

Treatment is with erythromycin syrup. The baby's parents should always be examined for *Chlamydia* or other infections.

Trachoma

Trachoma is a chronic infection of the conjunctiva of the globe and eyelids caused by *Chlamydia trachomatis* serotypes A, B, Ba and C. The inflammatory responses in the eyelids may eventually cause fibrosis, scarring and deformity of the eyelids, which in turn cause entropion, continuing corneal trauma and blindness due to corneal scarring.

Distribution and incidence

Trachoma is widespread throughout the tropics and subtropics, and is primarily a disease related to poor personal and public hygiene. It is one of the commonest causes of blindness in the world, with 500 million affected, 2 million blind and 100 million with severe visual impairment.

Transmission and epidemiology

The organisms present in ocular secretions infect other people by direct contagion on contaminated fingers or clothes. Absence of water for washing means that infected secretions are wiped on to hands and clothes. Flies may also carry the organisms from one person to another. Infection occurs early in life and subsequently there are episodes of reinfection and secondary bacterial infection.

Pathology and pathogenesis

Acute inflammation is present in the conjunctiva. This progresses to a chronic state, with lymphoid aggregates around infected conjunctival cells. It is likely that damage due to trachoma is exacerbated by repeated bacterial infections. The tarsal plates fold inwards due to fibrosis (entropion) and the cornea is continually damaged by the inverted eyelashes, resulting in corneal opacity from scarring.

Clinical features

The earlier features are hypertrophic follicles on the upper tarsal conjunctiva and at the corneo-scleral junction superiorly. With time and repeated reinfections, this inflammatory response leads to fibrosis. The scarring disorganises the arrangement of Meibomian glands, and their orifices are pulled away from the lid margin. The eyelid is inverted and sites of eyelash trauma on the cornea are seen. New vessels grow into the cornea (pannus formation) and corneal scarring follows.

Diagnosis

Diagnosis is made on the appearances described above. Giemsa staining of scrapings from the affected conjunctiva shows intracytoplasmic inclusion bodies. Antigen can be detected by enzyme-linked immuno-assay.

Treatment

Tetracycline (2.0 g per day in divided doses) is given for 3 weeks to all patients apart from pregnant women and children under 8 years. Erythromycin is an effective alternative (250 mg or 4 mg/kg four times daily for 3 weeks). Topical 1% tetracycline eye ointment, applied 2–4 times daily for 3 weeks and repeated at 1-month intervals up to 6 times, is effective.

Continued trauma to the cornea must be prevented. Removal of offending eyelashes helps. Surgical reconstruction of the eyelid may be needed.

Prevention and control

Education concerning the importance of washing with soap and water is an important measure in preventing transmission. This depends on the availability of an adequate water supply sufficient for all domestic needs. The use of antibiotics in infected persons reduces the inflammation in their eyes and prevents progression of the disease, while eradicating sources of infection for others.

Lymphogranuloma venereum

Lymphogranuloma venereum (LGV) is caused by L_1, L_2, or L_3 serotypes of *Chlamydia trachomatis*. It is most prevalent in parts of Africa, Asia and South America.

Clinical features

The most common primary lesion of LGV is a shallow ulcer appearing on the genitals of men or women 3–10 days after exposure to infection.

In men there may be an associated lymphangitis of the dorsal penis. More commonly in men there may be an inflammation and swelling of the inguinal lymph nodes. This sign may appear 10 days to 6 months after infection. The inguinal bubo is unilateral in about 60% of cases. The bubo may enlarge, causing pain, and may rupture. About 20% also have involvement of femoral lymph nodes. This creates a groove over the inguinal ligament, the characteristic 'groove sign'.

LGV may also cause a rectal infection. After the initial inflammation of the rectal mucosa a chronic inflammatory process may follow; this invades the bowel wall, with noncaseous granulomas and crypt abscesses forming. A partial or complete stricture of the rectum may develop.

Diagnosis and treatment

Diagnosis is based on a positive complement-fixation or micro-immunofluorescent (micro-IF) test. Doxycycline (100 mg daily for 2–4 weeks) is the therapy of choice.

MYCOPLASMAS

Mycoplasmas are the smallest organisms able to grow in cell-free media, wherein they differ from viruses. They differ from bacteria in lacking a cell wall. *Mycoplasma pneumoniae* is an important cause of atypical pneumonia and a number of other clinical syndromes described in Chapter 14. *M. hominis* and *Ureaplasma urealyticum* can cause non-gonococcal urethritis, prostatitis, pelvic inflammatory disease and postpartum fever. They are sensitive to tetracycline, the treatment of choice (p. 223).

RICKETTSIA

Rickettsial infections comprise a group of acute infectious diseases caused by small bacteria. They cause the typhus group of infections, the spotted fever group of infections, scrub typhus, Q fever (*Coxiella burnetii*) and trench fever (*Rochalimaea quintana*). These organisms produce diseases with a range of severity from mild to severe and life-threatening (*Appendix table 3*, p. 327).

Apart from *Rochalimaea* all are obligate intracellular parasites and can only be grown in cells in vitro. *Rochalimaea quintana* grows in acellular cultures. They are Gram-negative organisms and, like Gram-negative bacteria, produce endotoxin which may contribute to the pathogenesis.

Q fever

Q fever is an acute illness caused by *Coxiella burnetii*; it is transmitted between animals by ticks and to humans from domestic animals by close contact, particularly with aborted placentas or with infected carcasses in abattoirs or, more often, by inhalation of the endospores.

The main clinical features of acute infection are high fever with severe headache and myalgia, after an incubation period of about 20 days. Hepatosplenomegaly is common, with biochemical evidence of hepatitis. Pneumonia is less common but may be severe and bilateral. Q fever may present as pyrexia of unknown origin (p. 230).

The natural history of the disease is to resolve spontaneously within 2 weeks in most patients, but a slower recovery with progression to chronic disease may occur. The main feature of chronic Q fever is endocarditis, which is usually fatal if left untreated (p. 420).

Diagnosis

Diagnosis is usually made by serology, since laboratory handling of the organisms is dangerous. Tetracycline is the treatment of choice but it is not known whether it prevents progression. Endocarditis is very difficult to eradicate and surgery is often required.

Typhus

Distribution and incidence

Typhus group

Louse-borne typhus (*Rickettsia prowazekii*) occurs in louse-infested populations. These are usually relatively poor people living at high altitude, who wear as much clothing as they can to keep warm, and do not change or wash their clothing. Mountainous areas of South America, the Himalayas and highland regions of Ethiopia are endemic areas. Louse-borne typhus is less common than it used to be. Brill-Zinsser disease represents a recrudescence of latent *R. prowazekii* infection some time, possibly years, after initial infection. Murine typhus (*R. mooseri*) is widely distributed where rat and man live close together.

Spotted fever group

Rocky Mountain spotted fever (*R. rickettsii*) occurs most often in the hills and mountains of the eastern seaboard of the United States. Countries of South America are also affected.

African tick typhus affects the countries of North Africa, where *fièvre boutonneuse* is well recognised, and eastern, central and southern Africa, where tick-bite fever is well known. The incidence is unknown. African tick typhus is the commonest imported rickettsial infection in the United

Kingdom. Rickettsial pox infections occur in Asia, Asian regions of the USSR and Korea.

Scrub typhus

Scrub typhus (*R. tsutsugamushi*) occurs throughout Asia and is probably one of the commonest causes of fever there. Studies in Malaysia showed that it accounted for 23% of patients with febrile illnesses presenting at rural hospitals.

Trench fever

Trench fever is not common now. It is thought to have a focal distribution in Africa and Central America.

Transmission and epidemiology

Typhus group

Louse-borne typhus is transmitted by *Pediculus humanus*. The louse defecates after taking a blood meal, and *R. prowazekii* in the faeces of an infected louse is scratched into the bite site or abrasions in the skin. Man is the reservoir for *R. prowazekii* and infection passes from one person to another.

Epidemic disease occurs when infection is introduced into a large group of people not previously exposed. Refugee camps present an ideal situation for such epidemics.

Spotted fever group

The spotted fever group of infections are also zoonoses transmitted by the bite of infected ticks which are also the reservoir of infection. Occupational and leisure exposure, such as walking, camping, farming, lumber work and hunting, are activities that take man into tick-infested areas in North America. Tourism, tending animals and gathering wood are activities that take people into similar areas in Africa.

Scrub typhus

Scrub typhus is a zoonosis transmitted by chiggers, larvae of leptotrombiculid mites. Occupational exposure in rural areas – farming, animal tending, rubber plantation work, etc. – is the usual means of infection.

Trench fever

Trench fever is transmitted by rubbing infective louse faeces into the bite or a skin abrasion. Man is the reservoir of this infection and conditions which favour human lousiness will favour the occurrence of trench fever. Its name goes back to the First World War, when it occurred among men during trench warfare. Epidemics occurred in the Second World War.

Pathology and pathogenesis

These organisms replicate within vascular endothelial cells of small vessels in many tissues. The vasculitic responses and blood vessel damage underlie the pathogenesis. *R. rickettsii* infection is more invasive than the other organisms, and causes more severe illness due to full-thickness vessel wall damage.

The effect of blood vessel damage is a rash that may become purpuric and haemorrhagic, even ecchymotic in louse-borne typhus and *R. rickettsii* infection. Leakage of protein-rich fluid from the vascular compartment into the interstitium causes hypovolaemia, hypotension and reduced tissue perfusion. Thrombotic lesions occur in a variety of organs, including the brain. Renal and liver damage from vasculitis occur in severe cases.

Clinical features

Typhus group

The incubation period is usually about 12 days with a range of 10–14 days. Headache and mild fever are usual initial symptoms, followed after 48 hours by a sharp rise in temperature to 40°C, which is sustained. Conjunctival suffusion is seen. Meningism and photophobia also occur. The rash occurs at about the sixth day and begins as red macular lesions on the axillary folds and trunk, spreading on to the limbs, with palms, soles and face affected in the most severe cases. The rash may evolve through purpuric stages to form ecchymoses. Initial bradycardia progresses to tachycardia in hypotensive patients. Haemorrhagic manifestations and hypotension lead to renal involvement, with rising blood urea and falling urine output. Mild cases get better in the second week of the disease but untreated severe cases may go into the third week before recovery begins. Death from shock, cerebral involvement or renal failure occurs in the second or third week.

Brill-Zinsser disease is a mild form of louse-borne typhus due to recrudescence of latent infection. Recovery is the rule.

Spotted fever group

The incubation period is about 7 days for Rocky Mountain spotted fever (RMSF) and African tick typhus, and rather longer – around 13 days – in rickettsial pox. Fever and headache with generalised limb pains are usual features early in the course. The clinical features are similar to typhus. There is early deterioration in those with severe RMSF. Death may occur between 3 and 6 days of onset.

African tick typhus is generally mild and self-limiting. Fever, systemic upset and headache are the usual presenting features. Rash may occur, causing macular lesions which have a widespread distribution on trunk and limbs. Palms and soles may be affected. A black, ulcerated eschar is usually found marking the site of the tick bite.

Scrub typhus

The incubation period is about 10 days (range 6–18). Fever, headache, chills and general body pains are usual symptoms. Conjunctival suffusion, macular skin rash, pneumonitis and hepatosplenomegaly may occur.

12

Trench fever

The incubation period may be as long as 22 days or as short as 4 days. Fever, headache and chills are usual symptoms, appearing and usually settling over about 5 days. Relapses may occur.

Diagnosis

The clinical features usually lead to suspicion of a rickettsial infection. This can be confirmed by serological tests using group-specific rickettsial antigens. The main differential diagnosis in RMSF is meningococcal septicaemia, which also requires urgent treatment.

Laboratory features

Severely affected patients with all forms of rickettsial disease will show generalised derangement of coagulation and evidence of liver and renal dysfunction. Platelet counts are low, in association with prolongation of the pro-thrombin time, reduced fibrinogen levels and elevated levels of fibrin degradation products. Anaemia is usual. Plasma albumin levels fall. Declining urine output indicates renal failure.

Treatment

Typhus group

Tetracycline (500 mg 6-hourly for 7 days) is very effective (30 mg/kg/day). Pregnant women and children under 8 years should receive chloramphenicol (50 mg/kg per day in divided doses for 7 days; 25 mg/kg per day in divided doses for infants under 1 month). Doxycycline, 100 mg (single dose) for adults or 50 mg for children, is the ideal treatment for louse-borne typhus.

Spotted fever group

Tetracycline or chloramphenicol as above are effective and must be started promptly.

Scrub typhus

As for louse-borne typhus.

Trench fever

There is little experience with chemotherapy. In vitro sensitivities suggest a good response to tetracyclines.

Supportive measures

Prompt administration of antibiotics is essential. Management comprises restoring blood volume with infusions of plasma and fluids, and restoring coagulation mechanisms by fresh blood transfusions or fresh frozen plasma.

Prevention and control

Delousing is the main way to control louse-borne typhus. Thorough and regular washing of clothes in hot water with detergent kills lice and their eggs. DDT 10% or malathion 1% can be applied to clothed people with good effect. Appropriate clothing should be worn to prevent ticks getting to the skin. In tick-infested areas the skin should be carefully inspected at the end of the day. Any that are found should be removed by gentle pulling to keep the tick intact.

BACTERIAL INFECTIONS

Table 12.22 Classification of bacteria

Gram-positive cocci	Gram-positive bacilli
Streptococci	Bacilli
Strep. pneumoniae	*B. anthracis*
Strep. pyogenes	*B. cereus*
Strep. viridans group	*Corynebacterium diphtheriae*
Anaerobic	*Listeria monocytogenes*
Staphylococci	Clostridia (anaerobic)
Staph. aureus	*Cl. tetani*
Staph. epidermidis	*Cl. botulinum*
	Cl. perfringens
	Cl. difficile
	Cl. septicum

Gram-negative cocci	Gram-negative bacilli
Neisseria	Enterobacteria
N. meningitidis (meningococcus)	*Escherichia coli*
N. gonorrhoeae (gonococcus)	*Klebsiella*
	Proteus
	Salmonella
	Shigella
	Parvobacteria
	Haemophilus
	Bordetella
	Brucella
	Yersinia
	Pseudomonas
	P. aeruginosa
	P. pseudomallei
	Francisella tularensis
	Bartonella bacilliformis
	Cat-scratch bacillus
	Vibrios
	V. cholerae
	Campylobacter jejuni
	Anaerobic bacteria
	Bacteroides
	Fusobacteria

Mycobacteria

Spirochaetes
Treponema
  T. pallidum
  T. pertenue
  T. carateum
Borrelia
Leptospira icterohaemorrhagiae

A classification of bacteria is given in Table 12.22.

GRAM-POSITIVE COCCI

STREPTOCOCCI

β-haemolytic streptococci are classified by the Lancefield grouping system which detects polysaccharide antigens on their surface by a panel of antisera. Table 12.23 shows these and other streptococci which are α-haemolytic or non-haemolytic. Not all group D streptococci are β-haemolytic. Cutaneous streptococcal infections are described in Chapter 26.

Table 12.23 Streptococci

Group and name	Characteristics	Disease/syndromes
Group A		
S. pyogenes	β-haemolytic	Pharyngitis
	Secrete enzymes,	Scarlet fever
	e.g. hyaluronidase,	Otitis media
	and toxins,	Sinusitis
	e.g. erythrogenic	Erysipelas/impetigo
		Lymphangitis
		Puerperal sepsis
Group B		
S. agalactiae	β-haemolytic	Neonatal infection
	Common vaginal	(puerperal sepsis)
	commensal	
Group D		
Enterococci,	β- or non-haemolytic	Urinary tract infection
e.g. *S. faecalis*	Anaerobic	Septicaemia
	Normal bowel flora	Endocarditis
	Antibiotic resistance	
S. pneumoniae	α-haemolytic	Pneumonia
(pneumococcus)	Common throat	Acute meningitis
	commensal	Otitis media/
	More than 80 serotypes	mastoiditis
S. viridans group,	α- or non-haemolytic	Endocarditis
e.g. *S. milleri, mitior,*	Dental commensals	Cerebral abscess and
mutans, salivarius,		empyema
sanguis		(*S. milleri*)

Scarlet fever

Scarlet fever is a febrile illness with a characteristic rash caused by infection with an erythrogenic toxin-producing strain of *Streptococcus pyogenes*. Infection is usually in the throat, but the skin or genital tract may be the primary site.

It is now a much milder disease than it was 50 years ago. The severity of disease is probably determined by variations in the micro-organism but host factors also play a part. The same bacterium may be a harmless passenger in one subject, or produce a sore throat or scarlet fever. Host antibodies are largely responsible for these differences. Antibodies to the erythrogenic toxin prevent the rash of scarlet fever but not tonsillitis.

Clinical features

Infection is spread by droplets, and after an incubation period of 2–4 days there is abrupt onset of sore throat, pain on swallowing and fever. There is tender cervical lymphadenopathy. The tonsils are enlarged, congested and often covered with exudate. The tongue is coated and initially red papillae are visible through the fur, but later the fur is lost, leaving the classical 'strawberry tongue' appearance. The rash (Plate 8, p. 251) appears within 2 days on the face, where it consists of a diffuse erythema often with peri-oral pallor (not specific for this condition). On the trunk the rash is a punctate erythema which is less brightly coloured. Superficial peeling of the skin starts on about the fourth day. The overt illness resolves within a week, although the patient may continue to feel unwell for several more days.

Complications

Complications are now rare. Septic complications include otitis media. Late complications are rheumatic fever (p. 426) or acute glomerulonephritis (p. 816), which may develop 2–3 weeks after the infection.

Diagnosis and treatment

Strep. pyogenes can be cultured readily from a throat swab, and the presence of neutrophilia helps to distinguish from infectious mononucleosis, which can cause an identical appearance. Retrospective diagnosis can be made by measuring antistreptolysin O antibodies. Treatment with oral penicillin is commonly used, and although this may not eliminate streptococci from the throat unless given in high dose for 10 days, the importance of eradicating the organism has diminished since complications have become so uncommon. Erythromycin is an alternative agent for penicillin-allergic patients.

STAPHYLOCOCCI

Staphylococcus aureus and *Staph. epidermidis* are the clinically important staphylococci. Both are common skin commensals but *Staph. aureus* is more virulent and is commonly associated with disease.

Staphylococcus aureus infection

There are two distinct mechanisms by which *Staph. aureus* can cause disease. Most often it is by *direct invasion of tissues* (Table 12.24), when some of the enzymes produced by *Staph. aureus* may be important in pathogenesis, e.g. catalase, coagulase, hyaluronidase. Less often, the major disease manifestations are the result of *toxin secretion* (Table 12.25).

Staph. aureus often produces β-lactamase, particularly in hospital acquired infections, so treatment is usually started with a β-lactamase-resistant antibiotic such as flucloxacillin. Methicillin-resistant *Staph. aureus* (MRSA) has re-appeared recently in European hospitals. The cutaneous syndromes of staphylococcal infection are described on page 1113. The management of septicaemia is discussed on page 230. Lung abscess is described on page 481.

Table 12.24 Invasive disease due to Staphylococcus aureus

Site of infection	Disease
Skin	Impetigo
	Boils and carbuncles
	Surgical wound infections
Blood	Septicaemia
Lungs	Pneumonia with abscesses
Liver, bone and other	Abscess
Heart	Acute endocarditis

Staphylococcus epidermidis infection

Staph. epidermidis is a skin commensal which was thought to be a contaminant when it appeared in cultures; now, however, it is apparent that it causes serious infections in patients who are immunocompromised and in patients with intravenous cannulae, prosthetic heart valves, pacemaker

Table 12.25 Staphylococcus aureus toxin-mediated diseases

Disease	Manifestations	Organism	Pathological effect	Site of infection
Staphylococcal scalded skin syndrome	Skin erythema; may progress to bullae, exudate, crusting, positive Nikolsky sign	*S. aureus* phage group II, often phage type 71 (produce epidermolytic exotoxins)	Split skin at stratum granulosum	Skin
Toxic shock syndrome	Diarrhoea and vomiting. Hypovolaemia. Erythema of mucosae and skin leading to peripheral desquamation. Fever and myalgia	*S. aureus* phage group I, often phage types 29 and 52 (Produce enterotoxin F, identical to exotoxin C)	Uncertain	Vagina, skin or other (occurs mainly young women using tampons)
Food poisoning	Vomiting and diarrhoea	*S. aureus* phage group III (produce enterotoxins A, B, C, D, E)	Uncertain	Food (toxin ingested)

wires, CSF shunts and other foreign materials in place for long periods. *Staph. epidermidis* produces β-lactamase and is usually resistant to a wide range of antibiotics including methicillin. Resistance to methicillin is mediated by alteration to penicillin-binding proteins. The mainstay of treatment is vancomycin.

GRAM-NEGATIVE COCCI

NEISSERIA

Neisseria meningitidis (meningococcus) infection

There are three types of meningococcus – groups A, B and C – which are the most common cause of acute bacterial meningitis (p. 955). They also cause septicaemia with or without meningitis (Plate 9, p. 251). Disease occurs sporadically or in epidemics and the epidemiology is poorly understood.

Neisseria gonorrhoea (gonococcus) infection

Gonorrhoea is an important sexually transmitted disease causing urethritis, endocervicitis or proctitis. The annual incidence of cases reported by clinics in the UK declined after the introduction of penicillin treatment but soon rose again (Fig. 12.11). The different reported incidence for females is largely artefactual, since 70% or more of female cases are asymptomatic. The incubation period is between 2 and 7 days.

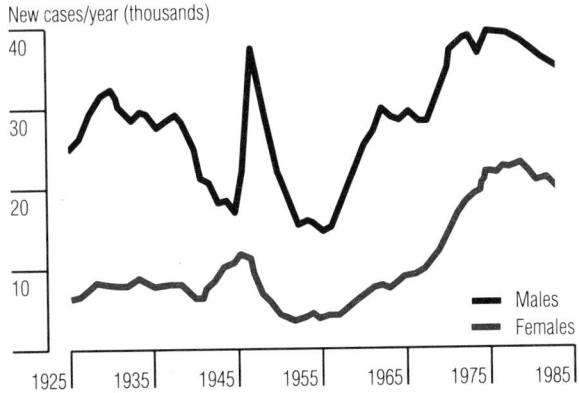

Fig. 12.11 Annual incidence of gonorrhoea in England and Wales, 1925–1983 (Communicable Diseases Surveillance Centre, Colindale).

Clinical features

In men there is urethritis, with creamy discharge, dysuria and frequency. Homosexual men also develop proctitis, with pruritus, tenesmus and rectal discharge often containing blood.

In women the infection is usually asymptomatic (discovered by contact tracing) or causes vaginal discharge, dysuria, frequency and lower abdominal pain. Pharyngeal infection follows oral sex but is usually asymptomatic.

Complications

Ascending infection causes pelvic inflammatory disease, with salpingitis, peritonitis or abscess formation in 10–20% of infected women. Less commonly septicaemia occurs, with a rash on the extremities. Gonococcus is an important cause of acute septic arthritis (p. 1004). Perihepatitis (Fitz-Hugh Curtis syndrome) is rare. Disseminated gonococcal infection is commoner in women than in men. Signs include fever, pustular rash and arthritis.

Infection in pregnancy may cause abortion or premature labour and is associated with high perinatal mortality. The baby is infected in utero, at birth or postnatally, and at worst develops disseminated infection. Ophthalmia neonatorum is a sign of infection.

Diagnosis

Microscopy of Gram-stained smears shows pus cells and both intra- and extracellular Gram-negative diplococci. Specimens should be taken from the endocervix in women; a high vaginal swab is inadequate. Culture is essential since β-lactamase-producing gonococci are becoming more common. Serology is not helpful in diagnosis.

Treatment

Treatment is with amoxycillin (3 g) plus probenecid (1 g orally), or procaine penicillin (2.4 g im) with probenecid (2 g orally). These combinations allow single dose treatment, probenecid delaying excretion of the penicillin. If the patient is allergic to penicillin, kanamycin (2 g im) or co-trimoxazole (4 tablets twice daily for 2 days) is an alternative. Neither of these preparations has any antitreponemal activity.

β-lactamase-producing strains of gonococcus comprise about 2% of isolates in the UK at present. If a resistant strain is cultured, appropriate drugs are spectinomycin (2 g im) or cefuroxime (1.5 g im). Follow-up is essential, since 50% of patients have concurrent non-specific urethritis. This is suspected if symptoms persist a week after treatment of gonococcal infection. Contacts should be traced, examined and treated.

GRAM-POSITIVE BACILLI

BACILLI

Bacillus anthracis: anthrax

Few cases of anthrax are seen in Western countries but about 100 000 cases occur in the world each year. The Gram-positive rods of *B. anthracis* give rise to spores in conditions unfavourable for replication, and spores survive for many years. The spores can contaminate the hides, hooves, hair, horns and bones of herded animals, particularly goats, and contact with these can cause cutaneous anthrax both in the endemic areas and in industrialised countries to which these animal materials are taken for processing. Bacilli are found in the tissues of animals dying of systemic infections. Transmission to man is by skin contact with infected material such as hides or meat, by inhalation of spores or by ingestion of infected meat, causing skin, respiratory and gastrointestinal disease respectively. Disease onset is within 5 days in all forms and usually about 2 days.

Cutaneous anthrax

Cutaneous anthrax is the most common form of the disease and the most benign. A red macule or papule develops at the contact site, e.g. the neck of a meat carrier in a slaughterhouse. A pruritic vesicle develops, satellite lesions appear, and the whole evolves into an ulcer, then a black eschar. There is usually some surrounding oedema, but occasionally there is a severe local reaction with gross oedema, and general toxaemia ensues.

Inhalation anthrax

At first there are mild general symptoms and non-productive cough. Improvement over a few days is followed by abrupt decline into severe respiratory distress. Rapidly the patient becomes very ill, with cough, fever, tachypnoea, cyanosis, tachycardia, vomiting and chills. Diffuse crackles are heard over the affected lung fields. The spleen may enlarge. There is massive enlargement and oedema of the neck and chest wall. Untreated, the patient often dies within 24 hours.

Gastrointestinal anthrax

Following ingestion, lesions can occur anywhere in the gastrointestinal tract, including the throat. There is severe gastroenteritis with haemorrhage, and mortality is high.

Haematogenous dissemination of organisms can sometimes cause meningitis with bloody CSF.

Diagnosis

Many cases may go undiagnosed in the tropics and subtropics. The cutaneous form is probably most often diagnosed on the clinical appearances. Occupational exposure may be suspected from the nature of the patient's job. The severity of a pneumonic illness may prompt consideration of pulmonary anthrax.

The organisms are readily found in Gram-stained smears from skin lesions and grow well in blood culture samples.

Treatment

The cutaneous form may resolve without treatment. Benzyl penicillin is very effective and is given for 7–10 days. For mild cutaneous disease 2 g/day is given; 4–6 g/day are required for more severe infection. When the patient is allergic to penicillin, tetracycline or chloramphenicol can be used. The latter is given to children and pregnant females. Pulmonary or intestinal cases will require considerable supportive care, with maintenance of oxygenation and infusions to maintain blood volume and hydration.

Prevention is by elimination of the infection from animals. Immunisation is available when there is danger of occupational exposure.

Bacillus cereus infection

Bacillus cereus is one of the causes of food poisoning (see Gastroenteritis, p. 233). Two illnesses are associated with different incubation periods. Short incubation (1–6 hours), vomiting and abdominal pain caused by heat-stable enterotoxin are often related to ingestion of reheated rice. Longer incubation (8–16 hours), diarrhoea and abdominal pain are caused by a heat-stable toxin formed in the infected intestine. The treatment is directed at maintaining the patient's hydration. There is no specific therapy.

CORYNEBACTERIUM DIPHTHERIAE INFECTION

Corynebacterium diphtheriae is the cause of diphtheria, a toxin-mediated disease which is rare in countries with an effective immunisation programme. Transmission is mainly person-to-person by nasopharyngeal droplets, but skin infection is also important in tropical countries.

Pathogenesis

C. diphtheriae infects the throat and causes minor local disease, but its major effects result from production of a protein toxin of MW 62 000. The toxin is elaborated only by *C. diphtheriae* strains infected by a bacteriophage. Its main effects are on the myocardium and nervous tissue.

Clinical features

After an incubation period of 2–6 days there is slow onset of malaise and fever, sometimes with mild sore throat. At an early stage the predominant findings are profound weakness, restlessness and irritability, with fever, pallor and a rapid thready pulse. Examination of the throat reveals the characteristic membrane which is adherent, attempts to scrape it off resulting in bleeding. In laryngeal diphtheria, the membrane involves the larynx and trachea, causing respiratory obstruction which may require tracheostomy. The primary infection may also involve the nose, larynx or bronchi. ECG abnormalities suggesting myocarditis appear in the first week (flattening or inversion of T waves most commonly) and acute circulatory collapse may occur. Neurological complications start later, with paralysis of the palate, followed by the ocular muscles, then the pharynx, larynx and respiratory muscles, and lastly the limbs.

Treatment and outcome

Since the most dangerous effects of diphtheria are caused by the toxin, administration of antitoxin is essential. Intensive nursing is necessary and the patient must be isolated, with respiratory precautions to avoid spread of infection. Penicillin or erythromycin will eradicate the organism from the primary infection site. Contacts must be traced, treated if infected, and immunised. If the patient survives the acute illness, recovery from complications such as paralysis is complete.

LISTERIA MONOCYTOGENES INFECTION

Listeria monocytogenes is a Gram-positive bacillus which is commonly dismissed as a diphtheroid contaminant on examination of CSF specimens. Microbiologists are now aware of its significance as a cause of serious disease, particularly in immunocompromised patients, pregnant women and neonates. The bacillus is a common contaminant of soft cheeses, especially if these are unpasteurised. It causes septicaemia, often associated with meningo-encephalitis. Ampicillin or penicillin is the drug of first choice, with erythromycin in reserve for penicillin-allergic patients.

CLOSTRIDIA

Clostridia are a group of obligate anaerobic bacteria; they cause illness largely through toxins which act locally or enter the circulation. Clostridia are frequent wound contaminants without necessarily causing disease; when disease occurs, however, it is severe.

Tetanus

Tetanus is a potentially fatal disease dominated by muscle spasm caused by an exotoxin, tetanospasmin, produced by *Clostridium tetani*.

Epidemiology and pathogenesis

Cl. tetani is found in the faeces of man and animals, and its spores abound in soil. It is anaerobic and proliferates in ischaemic or necrotic tissue. In Western countries the usual situation is a wound which is not properly tended in an unimmunised individual. In rural areas farm workers or gardeners are infected, but in cities the disease has been observed in drug addicts. Since immunisation against tetanus toxin is standard in Western countries, and immunised patients with susceptible wounds normally receive prophylaxis, tetanus is rare (12 cases notified in England and Wales during 1985). In poorer countries immunisation is variable.

Tetanospasmin is a neurotoxin which acts in several different ways. It inhibits the release of acetylcholine from nerve endings in muscle but, more importantly, it interferes with synaptic reflexes in the spinal cord, causing disinhibition which results in muscle spasms.

Clinical features

The incubation period can be up to 3 weeks, depending on inoculation dose and site. A short incubation and rapid onset of first spasm indicate a severe infection. Symptoms are most severe at either extreme of age.

The first (and sometimes sole) sign of tetanus is often spasm of muscles local to the wound. In the majority the central nervous system is involved and trismus (lockjaw) heralds the onset of generalised tetanus. The patient notices difficulty in opening the mouth and in swallowing, followed by stiffness in the neck and back. Examination reveals the initial site of infection and 'risus sardonicus', the facial expression caused by trismus and contraction of facial muscles. Muscles of the back and abdomen become stiff, and painful spasms, provoked by sudden movement or noise, occur in the back muscles, causing opisthotonos. Autonomic involvement causes sweating and cardiovascular instability. Death is from exhaustion, aspiration or secondary infection.

Treatment

Further toxin production is prevented by local débridement of wounds and parenteral treatment with benzylpenicillin (tetracycline in penicillin-allergic patients). Human immune globulin containing antibodies to tetanus toxin in high titre is given to neutralise free toxin. If surgery is indicated, it should be delayed for an hour after administration of antibody.

The patient is nursed in a quiet room to avoid stimuli likely to provoke spasms. Neuromuscular block is indicated when spasms become generalised, and then the patient is ventilated. Since prolonged ventilation is usual, tracheostomy is performed early. In countries where intensive care is not available, anticonvulsant drugs such as diazepam are used as an alternative to paralysis. Nutrition is maintained enterally or parenterally.

An attack of tetanus does not render the patient immune and a full course of immunisation should be given after recovery.

Prevention

Immunisation with tetanus toxoid is the only way to prevent the disease altogether. A full course of toxoid confers immunity for at least 5 years. Neonatal tetanus can be prevented by immunising the mother during pregnancy.

Patients with wounds susceptible to *Cl. tetani* infection are managed according to their state of immunity. All patients require local wound toilet. Fully immunised patients receive a booster dose of toxoid. Unimmunised patients with a wound considered susceptible to *Cl. tetani* receive human tetanus immune globulin and, simultaneously, active immunisation with adsorbed tetanus toxoid is started. Injection of long-acting penicillin, followed by a course of oral penicillin, is also indicated in these cases.

12

Botulism

Botulism is a virulent form of food poisoning caused by enterotoxins of *Cl. botulinum*. The toxins cause disease when produced in contaminated food, usually tins of meat. These highly potent poisons interrupt cholinergic neurotransmission. The initial illness is an afebrile gastroenteritis developing within 12–36 hours of ingestion in one-third of patients, but the remainder have only malaise and dizziness (with postural hypotension), progressing to extreme dryness caused by autonomic paralysis. Other neurological symptoms appear during the next 3 days: diplopia followed by bulbar signs, then symmetrical weakness of the limbs – usually in that order. Bulbar and respiratory muscle weakness may lead to inhalation pneumonia. Treatment is supportive and recovery is very slow, taking several weeks. Polyvalent horse antitoxin is available but it is poorly tolerated by many patients and of uncertain value.

Other clostridial syndromes

Gas gangrene

Cl. perfringens (welchii) is one of a number of gas-producing clostridia which contaminate wounds containing necrotic, anoxic material. *Cl. perfringens* produces 12 toxins, alphatoxin being the one associated with gas gangrene. It proliferates rapidly, producing myonecrosis. Gas infiltrates neighbouring tissues, causing crepitus. Toxins entering the circulation cause profound toxaemia with a high mortality.

Skin and soft tissue infections

Local infections, often involving muscle, occur in amputated stumps, diabetic ulcers of the foot, decubitus ulcers, perirectal abscesses and in abscesses at injection sites of drug addicts. Such infections frequently contain multiple organisms, including clostridia.

Gut infections

Pseudomembranous colitis is caused by toxin-producing strains of *Cl. difficile* which colonise the large intestine after antibiotic therapy. Although the early association was with clindamycin therapy, most antibiotics have caused this disease. Watery diarrhoea (without blood) and abdominal pain are associated with severe systemic toxicity. Treatment is with oral metronidazole or vancomycin.

Suppurative intra-abdominal infection caused by clostridia is particularly associated with carcinoma of the colon or pancreas. Neutropenic patients may develop severe *enterocolitis* caused by *Cl. septicum*.

GRAM-NEGATIVE BACILLI

ENTEROBACTERIA

The enterobacteria group comprises *Escherichia coli* (*E. coli*), *Klebsiella*, *Proteus*, *Salmonella* and *Shigella*.

E. coli causes a wide variety of diseases, usually as a result of auto-infection. Urinary tract infection is the most common, but systemic infection is a major problem in hospitals. Septicaemia arises from the bowel when there is a bowel disease or surgery has been carried out, or from the urinary tract as a complication of infection or surgery there. In neonates, *E. coli* is a common cause of septicaemia and meningitis. Several strains of *E. coli* cause gastroenteritis by a number of mechanisms; they are referred to as enteropathogenic, entero-invasive, enterohaemorrhagic, entero-adherent and enterotoxigenic. The latter produce toxins, one of which acts in a similar way to cholera toxin.

Klebsiella causes urinary tract infection, septicaemia and pneumonia. *Klebsiella pneumoniae* causes an acute, severe, cavitating pneumonia most frequently seen in alcoholics (p. 474).

Proteus is mainly associated with urinary tract infection.

Salmonella is found in several hundred strains. Salmonellae other than *S. typhi* and *S. paratyphi* are amongst the most common causes of gastroenteritis related to food poisoning (see Gastroenteritis, p. 233). They cause disease by direct invasion of the intestinal mucosa, and some strains, e.g. *S. typhimurium*, cause septicaemia, but usually disease remains localised. Typhoid (enteric fever) is caused by *S. typhi*, and is described below.

Shigella is also related to gastroenteritis. Four strains of shigella are the cause of bacillary dysentery, a form of acute diarrhoeal disease characterised by severe, bloody, purulent diarrhoea and abdominal pain. Bacillary dysentery describes the type of diarrhoeal disease caused by *Shigella* bacilli.

Shigella dysentery

Shigella sonnei and *S. flexneri* are the common organisms in the UK, the incidence of *S. flexneri* infection having increased in recent years; the other species are *S. dysenteriae* and *S. boydii*. Shigella infections occur worldwide, and epidemics are common where conditions are crowded and hygiene poor. Faecal–oral transmission results from lack of hand washing, and the organism is highly infectious, ingestion of less than 200 organisms causing disease in healthy adults.

The infection localises in the colon, where the epithelium is invaded and becomes inflamed. There is an acute inflammatory exudate which produces diarrhoea containing large numbers of leucocytes. Enterotoxin production contributes to the intestinal damage and the organisms may also produce a neurotoxin which may influence the clinical presentation.

Clinical features

After an incubation period of 2–3 days there is rapid onset of vomiting, abdominal colic and diarrhoea, which is usually bloody and purulent. Severity ranges from mild to fulminant. The most severe illness is caused by *S. dysenteriae*. Although the main illness is usually over within 1–2 weeks, diarrhoea and abdominal discomfort may persist for several weeks. Fever is common in the first few days and dehydration can occur rapidly, especially in children.

Postinfective aseptic arthritis and Reiter's syndrome (conjunctivitis, urethritis and arthritis) are complications which vary in frequency in different epidemics but are more common in HLA-B27-positive individuals.

The diagnosis is made when organisms are cultured from faeces.

Treatment

Patients are managed as for any severe form of gastroenteritis, rehydration being the key factor. Antibiotics are usually given to severely ill patients, although plasmid-mediated resistance is common and transfers rapidly. Ampicillin or co-trimoxazole is usually effective.

Typhoid

Typhoid (enteric fever) is a serious, prolonged, systemic infection with the Gram-negative bacillus *Salmonella typhi*.

Epidemiology

Typhoid is endemic in many poor countries, and although uncommon in Britain (about 200 cases reported per year), it is an important cause of fever in returning travellers. Humans are the reservoir of infection and spread of infection is by contamination of water or food by human faeces. Epidemics usually occur when a common water supply is contaminated. Small outbreaks sometimes result when a chronic excreter of the organism works as a food handler.

Pathogenesis

Ingested organisms invade the small intestinal mucosa. In the absence of specific immunity, organisms phagocytosed by macrophages survive and proliferate. After an incubation period varying from 1–3 weeks (usually 10–14 days), determined by the infecting dose, septicaemia develops and foci of infection may be established in any organ.

The gall bladder is an important site, since it is the source of chronic excretion when this occurs. Focal inflammation of Peyer's patches may be so vigorous as to cause intestinal perforation or haemorrhage.

Clinical features

In Britain typhoid usually presents as a pyrexia of insidious onset in a patient returning from abroad, often travelling from the Indian subcontinent.

The classic stepwise rise in temperature is rarely seen but the untreated illness has a remorseless progression. Headache and dry cough are common in the first week, and the patient is often vague and withdrawn. Constipation is usual. In the second week the spleen is often palpable and the elusive rash consisting of rose spots is seen in less than half of patients. The rash is sparse, less than a dozen spots in all, and consists of 1–2 mm pale red macules, which are hard to discern on a pigmented skin. By the third week diarrhoea may develop and the patient, now extremely ill, may lapse into coma.

The overall mortality in untreated typhoid is about 10%, but with appropriate antibiotic therapy it is less than 5%. Spontaneous remission is often followed by relapse within 2 weeks.

Typhoid in children

Typhoid is even more featureless in children than in adults and presents as an abrupt severe septicaemic illness. The mental state is striking, the child initially being irritable but later frankly delirious. Febrile convulsions may be the presenting feature and some degree of meningism is not uncommon. Diarrhoea is perhaps more frequent than in adults with typhoid, although intestinal infection with other organisms complicates the issue.

Complications

The most serious complications in the acute phase are intestinal haemorrhage or perforation. In severe cases there may be myocarditis or bone marrow suppression. Later complications are relapse, even after correct antibiotic treatment, in 15% of cases, and local sepsis in any organ as a result of septicaemia. Osteomyelitis is slow to cause symptoms.

Chronic carriage

Faecal excretion of *S. typhi* often continues several weeks after resolution of the illness and, rarely, patients excrete the organism for years. The organism is not detected in faeces during antibiotic treatment but re-appears after therapy is stopped. The source of organisms in long-term carriers is probably the gall-bladder, and gallstones readily become infected. Chronic excretion has obvious epidemiological consequences and some well-known outbreaks have been traced to a single chronic excreter.

Diagnosis

The diagnosis is usually made by blood culture. The organism is not present in stools initially but can be isolated in the second to third week. It may also be cultured from urine in 30% of patients. Serology is rarely helpful in diagnosis and the Widal test for agglutinating antibody is not often performed now. The blood count is helpful since neutropenia is common.

Treatment

Patients with typhoid must be barrier nursed, preferably in an isolation unit. Person-to-person transmission is not common. As with other prolonged febrile illnesses attention must be paid to management of fluid balance, oral hygiene and prevention of bed sores. Chloramphenicol, co-trimoxazole, trimethoprim alone and amoxycillin have all been used successfully. Promising results have been obtained with ciprofloxacin. Although duration and severity of symptoms, as well as mortality, are reduced by treatment, the response to treatment is not immediate. Treatment is continued for a week after resolution of fever and in any case for at least 2 weeks. Relapse can be treated with the original antibiotic, provided the organism was sensitive. Prolonged carriage is difficult to treat but success has been reported with high-dose amoxycillin and with ciprofloxacin. Cholecystectomy may be necessary.

Perforation of the intestine is dangerous and carries a high mortality. Opinions have changed with regard to the place of surgery in its management. Good results have been achieved by laparotomy and perfusion of the peritoneum and intestinal lumen with chloramphenicol.

Summary 3 Antibiotics for typhoid in adults

Minimum 2 weeks

Chloramphenicol 500 mg 4-hourly initially, then 500 mg 6-hourly

Co-trimoxazole 2 tablets (trimethoprim 80 mg, sulphamethoxazole 400 mg each) 12-hourly

Amoxycillin 500 mg 6-hourly

Ciprofloxacin 500 mg 12-hourly

Prevention

A monovalent vaccine to protect against *S. typhi* is more effective and has fewer side-effects than the old TAB vaccine, which included *S. paratyphi A* and *B* antigens.

Salmonella paratyphi infection

S. paratyphi B (*S. schottmuelleri*) is the most common paratyphoid infection in Britain. Other strains are called *S. paratyphi A* and *C* (*S. hirschfeldii*). Paratyphoid has a shorter incubation period than typhoid and is a milder disease with fewer complications. Diarrhoea tends to occur early, in contrast to typhoid. Treatment is with co-trimoxazole.

PARVOBACTERIA

Haemophilus infection

Haemophilus organisms are normal colonisers of the upper respiratory tract. *H. influenzae* is a major human pathogen; other *Haemophilus* species rarely cause disease, although *H. para-influenzae* can cause problems similar to *H. influenzae*.

Table 12.26 Diseases caused by Haemophilus influenzae

Type	Disease	Age
Type b	Acute meningitis	
	Epiglottis	
	Septic arthritis	Up to 5 years
	Orbital cellulitis	
	Pneumonia	
Non-encapsulated	Exacerbations of chronic bronchitis	
	Otitis media and sinusitis	Any age
	Conjunctivitis	
Other encapsulated types	Rarely pathogenic	

A small proportion of *H. influenzae* isolated from humans are encapsulated and six antigenic types are recognised. The most important is type b, which can cause septicaemia and several clinical syndromes in children under 5 years old (Table 12.26). Older children acquire immunity to the capsular antigens. Untypable (non-encapsulated) *H. influenzae* are potential pathogens in the lower respiratory tract.

Strains of *H. influenzae* have become increasingly resistant to antibiotics in recent years: 5–15% of strains are resistant to amoxycillin. This is particularly relevant to children with life-threatening diseases like acute meningitis, in which a delay in treatment with the right antibiotic could be fatal. Resistance is mediated by β-lactamases.

Vaccines have been prepared to the polysaccharide capsular antigens but so far their protective value has been limited and they are not used routinely.

Whooping cough (pertussis)

Whooping cough is a prolonged lower respiratory tract infection caused by the Gram-negative coccobacillus *Bordetella pertussis*. It is highly infectious and is transmitted by droplet.

Epidemiology

Spread of infection is entirely human-to-human and the disease is endemic, cases occurring continuously. Every few years the number of susceptible children is high enough for an epidemic to start, and this has tended to happen about every 4 years in the UK (Fig. 12.12). Since reports of a possible association between pertussis immunisation and encephalopathy in 1973 the rate of immunisation has fallen off and epidemics have been larger. In regions where uptake was less than 60% the reported incidence was 112 per 100 000 population, but where uptake was above 70% the incidence was only 58 per 100 000.

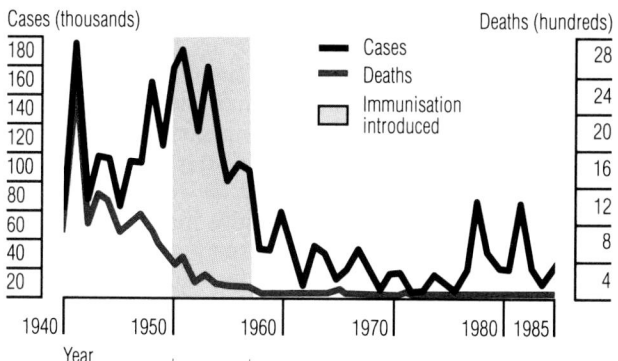

Fig. 12.12 Incidence of whooping cough in England and Wales, 1940–1985. Note the effect of immunisation on incidence. The death rate was falling before immunisation was introduced (Communicable Diseases Surveillance Centre, Colindale).

The disease may affect any age group, but it is most common in children under 5 years and most severe in those below 1 year.

Pathogenesis

The infection is concentrated in the bronchial walls, producing damage to the epithelium and accumulation of viscid mucus. Toxins produced by *B. pertussis* probably have a role in the tissue damage. Collapse of segments of lung distal to obstructed bronchioles is common.

Clinical features

After an incubation period of 7–10 days there is sometimes a prodromal illness resembling a cold and lasting 2–3 days (catarrhal stage). This is followed by onset of the characteristic cough, with long spasms of coughing interrupted by inspiration. At the end of a spasm there is a rapid inspiration which sometimes produces a whooping sound. This is often followed by vomiting.

During a spasm of coughing the child becomes pink and then blue, and small babies may become apnoeic after a spasm. Between spasms the child looks and feels deceptively well.

Whooping cough lasts about 2 months on average and in the later stages the cough is mainly at night. It is distressing to watch small children rendered helpless by the spasmodic cough, and anxiety and disruption of sleep cause a major disturbance to family life.

Complications

Secondary bacterial infection causing pneumonia or mucus plugging with segmental collapse are the most common serious complications. Cerebral hypoxia during prolonged coughing spasms may cause convulsions. Minor complications are subconjunctival haemorrhages, peri-orbital bruising and frenal ulcer, all of which result from prolonged spasms of coughing.

Diagnosis

Clinical diagnosis rests on recognition of the pattern of cough and is fairly simple when whooping is heard. In the early stages it is often difficult to distinguish from other causes of cough and babies frequently fail to whoop. The disease occurs in non-immune adults and again the whoop may not be obvious.

Laboratory support comes from the profound lymphocytosis in the blood and culture of *B. pertussis* from a pernasal swab; the latter is taken by passing a special swab through the nostril to the nasopharynx.

Treatment

Attentive nursing is the most important aspect of treatment and parents need help and reassurance to learn to manage coughing spasms. Babies frequently feed poorly and lose weight, necessitating feeding through a nasogastric tube.

The organism is sensitive to erythromycin and early treatment may be beneficial, although the effect is seldom pronounced. Antibiotic treatment of secondary bacterial pneumonia is along conventional lines.

Prevention

Pertussis vaccine is a crude preparation of killed organisms, but it is 80% effective in preventing whooping cough and often ameliorates the disease, if not wholly preventing it. There is a small risk of convulsions after immunisation (1 in 6000 doses) and a minute incidence (1 in 100 000 doses) of encephalitis with lasting consequences. Since there is severe morbidity and a small mortality in whooping cough epidemics the vaccine is strongly recommended. Work is in progress to develop more refined vaccines, but the ravages of the disease continue in the mean time.

Disappointingly, prophylactic erythromycin treatment of close contacts has proved ineffective.

Brucellosis

Brucellosis (undulant fever) is a septicaemic infection caused by *Brucella abortus*, *Br. melitensis* or *Br. suis*. *Br. abortus* is acquired from cattle, *Br. melitensis* from sheep or goats (Malta fever), and *Br. suis* from swine. Most northern European infection is by *Br. abortus* acquired during occupational exposure of vets, farm workers and slaughterhouse employees, by ingestion of raw milk or by accidental infection in the laboratory. As the name implies, *Br. abortus* causes abortion in cattle and the abortus is highly infectious. Most herds in the UK are brucella-free and pasteurisation is an additional insurance against infection of milk. As a result of control measures the disease is now very rare in the UK but it remains a major problem in parts of Europe, the Middle East, Central and South America and perhaps elsewhere.

Brucellae are Gram-negative coccobacilli which proliferate intracellularly. The incubation period of the disease is about 3 weeks.

Clinical features

A proportion of patients are infected asymptomatically but the common presentation is an acute illness with swinging fever and profuse sweats, which is otherwise fairly featureless. Back pain is more prominent than in other febrile illnesses. There are no specific physical signs but 40% of patients have hepatosplenomegaly, 20% have splenomegaly only, and 20% have arthritis in one large joint. Less common manifestations are epididymo-orchitis, spondylitis, an erythematous papular eruption on the extremities, and neurological involvement with meningitis, encephalitis or radiculitis.

If no treatment is given, fever may persist for weeks or months, although it gradually declines, only to relapse again in many cases. A prolonged debilitating illness can be associated with depression and the question is sometimes asked if a depressed patient with moderate brucella antibody titres has chronic brucellosis. This is rarely the true explanation in the absence of a preceding history suggestive of acute brucellosis.

Diagnosis

There is neutropenia and lymphocytosis in the acute phase, and brucellae can be cultured from blood in 50–60% of cases and also from bone marrow. Complement fixing and agglutinating antibodies can be detected in rising titre following acute infection.

Treatment

Inadequate treatment is associated with a high rate of relapse within 3 months, and some relapses occur despite the best known therapy. Tetracycline combined with rifampicin or streptomycin gives the lowest relapse rates. Co-trimoxazole has also been used but should not be given alone.

Preventive measures are concentrated on elimination of brucellae from domestic animals and avoiding contact with infected materials. In the United States the cost of prevention runs to 100 million dollars per annum.

Yersinia infection

Yersinial infections are zoonoses. The important human pathogens are *Y. enterocolitica* and *Y. pseudotuberculosis* which are enteric pathogens, and *Y. pestis*, the cause of plague.

Y. pseudotuberculosis and Y. enterocolitica

Infection with *Y. pseudotuberculosis* and *Y. enterocolitica* (see also p. 608) is less common in the UK than in some other European countries, notably Scandinavia and Belgium; Belgium has the highest rate of *Y. enterocolitica* infection. The latter is probably the result of the habit of eating raw pork, which is started at an early age. The organism is a common commensal in the pharynx and tonsillar tissue of pigs, which are included in ground pig meat. Other foods, including milk and seafoods, have been incriminated in human outbreaks.

Y. enterocolitica causes febrile enterocolitis in young children (less than 5 years old), but in adolescents an illness which is difficult to distinguish from acute appendicitis is caused by mesenteric adenitis. The latter is also the most common manifestation of *Y. pseudotuberculosis* infection. The presence of exudative pharyngitis may give a clue in *Y. enterocolitica* infection. Many laparotomies have been carried out for these self-limited infections, which may be partially responsive to gentamicin therapy (often given as blind treatment or prophylaxis for surgery).

Reactive polyarthritis and erythema nodosum are well-recognised complications which are more common with *Y. enterocolitica*.

Plague

An acute severe infection caused by *Y. pestis* manifests by either lymphadenitis with suppuration, bubonic plague or necrotising pneumonitis (pneumonic plague). It is a zoonosis.

Aetiology

The organism is a Gram-negative aerobic bacillus in the parvobacteria family. It grows well at 28°C. At 37°C it produces an antigen which inhibits phagocytosis. It has a lipopolysaccharide capsular endotoxin.

Distribution and incidence

Asia, Africa, the Middle East and the Americas (South America and the southern states of the USA) are endemic areas with comparatively small numbers of reported cases each year. The disease is probably under-reported.

Transmission and epidemiology

The infection is transmitted to man by the bite of the rat flea (Fig. 12.13). The natural hosts are rodents and the vector is the rat flea, *Xenopsylla cheopis*, which takes blood meals from its rodent hosts. Infected rats die and the fleas leave the dead rats for other hosts. The organisms produce a coagulant which prevents the flea taking a full blood meal. The flea bites the host repeatedly, encouraging transmission. The coagulant is inactive above 28°C and transmission diminishes.

Pathology

Necrosis and haemorrhage are the main features, together with marked inflammatory changes. An eschar at the bite site is occasionally found. Buboes are grossly enlarged inflamed lymph nodes draining the site of the flea bite. The normal lymph node architecture is destroyed and necrotic, with large numbers of bacilli. The pathological changes in pneumonic plague are very similar, with haemorrhagic necrosis of lung tissue.

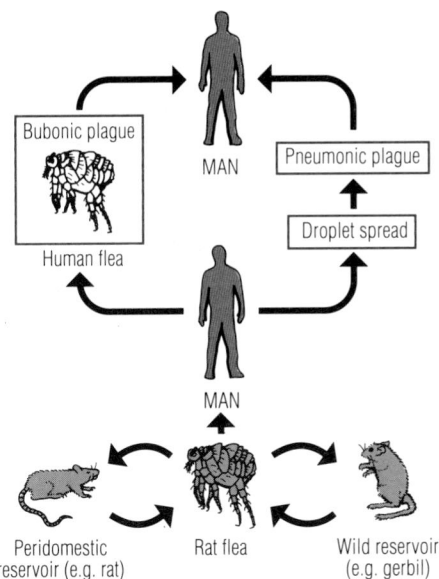

Fig. 12.13 Cycle of transmission of plague.

Clinical features

The incubation period is 2–8 days before the onset of systemic upset, fever, chills and headache. Within 24 hours of this, the patient finds a bubo which is exquisitely tender. Any group of lymph glands can be involved. Tachycardia and high fever are usual, with hypotension and shock in severely affected patients. Purpuric skin lesions are occasionally found.

Pneumonic plague results from haematogenous spread of organisms to the lungs. Cough, chest pain and haemoptysis in a severely ill patient are usual features. Patchy shadowing is seen on the chest X-ray. Aerosol spread of plague can occur from patients with pneumonic plague. Septicaemic plague has a high mortality.

Laboratory features comprise a neutrophil leucocytosis which may be very high. Some degree of disseminated intravascular coagulation is common, although spontaneous bleeding is uncommon.

Diagnosis

The organism may be found in material aspirated from the necrotic centre of buboes and in blood films. Smears made on slides can be stained with Giemsa stain, which shows the Gram-negative coccobacilli. The organism grows readily on standard media.

Treatment

The high mortality in untreated plague (over 50%) has been altered by antibiotics. Streptomycin (15 mg/kg twice daily im) for 10 days is the treatment of choice. Defervescence occurs by the third or fourth day. Tetracycline and chloramphenicol are alternative choices. Supportive treatment is needed in those with low blood pressure and shock, with volume replacement using saline or plasma. Buboes should be aspirated.

Prevention and control

A vaccine is available for those working with plague in the laboratory or in the field. Proven cases are not infectious unless there is pneumonic involvement, when isolation of cases, with respiratory precautions to avoid aerosol spread, is necessary. Antibiotics rapidly reduce infectivity. Vector control with insecticides and rat control will minimise transmission in towns and cities.

PSEUDOMONAS

Pseudomonas aeruginosa infection

Pseudomonas aeruginosa is an opportunist organism which rarely causes disease in immunocompetent subjects. It causes serious infection in patients with deficient immunity and in patients who have had surgery. Septicaemia, osteomyelitis, infection of burns and pneumonia are examples. Skin changes due to *P. aeruginosa* are described in Chapter 26. Patients in intensive care units may become colonised superficially and treatment with antibiotics is often counterproductive, since resistance develops rapidly. Antibiotic treatment of serious infection requires combinations of agents such as gentamicin and azlocillin.

Melioidosis

Pseudomonas pseudomallei is a Gram-negative, aerobic bacillus that is found contaminating surface water. The south-east Asian countries and northern Australia are endemic areas. Infection occurs by ingestion or inhalation of contaminated water, or by contact of infected water with abraded skin. The outcome of infection is determined to a great extent by the health of the infected person. If his health is good, then there may be subclinical infection shown by seroconversion without systemic upset. Debilitating illness from many causes enhances susceptibility, and some degree of immunosuppression may be needed to allow clinical infection, which can be acute or chronic.

Acute disease has an incubation period measured in days before the onset of fever, with myalgia, vomiting, confusion or delirium. Diarrhoea may also occur, as may shock with features of endotoxic shock. Pustular skin lesions may be found. The lungs may be involved in acute disease, with consolidation, cavitation and pus formation. Chronic and relapsing sepsis may occur, with abscess formation affecting lymph glands, lungs, skin, liver, genito-urinary tract and bones.

The organism is a dangerous pathogen which may be grown from pus, lymph gland biopsies, liver biopsy material and bone marrow aspirate. Serological responses using indirect haemagglutination (IHA) or complement-fixing antibody techniques are available.

Treatment is with ceftazidime (30 mg/kg given intra-

12

venously 8-hourly) and co-trimoxazole (5 mg trimethoprim/kg; 25 mg sulphamethoxazole/kg) 12-hourly, given for 4 weeks.

TULARAEMIA

Francisella tularensis is a Gram-negative bacillus that infects a wide range of wild animals; man is occasionally infected in rural areas of the northern hemisphere (North America, Sweden, Norway, northern Europe, Russia and Japan). Infection occurs in several ways:

1. by the bite of an infected insect
2. by mucosal or skin contact with an infected animal
3. by inhalation of material contaminated with bacilli
4. by eating inadequately cooked meat.

The effects in man may be localised cutaneous pustular disease with regional adenopathy, a pneumonic illness, or a systemic illness sometimes with diarrhoea. Inapparent (subclinical) infections occur.

The North America rabbit strain produces severe disease, with a mortality of up to 10% without treatment. Mortality with the other strains is negligible, even without treatment.

The diagnosis is made by finding the organisms in material from infected tissues. Direct immunofluorescence may be used. Serological tests may also be used to detect antibodies to the organism by ELISA and agglutination techniques. Great caution is needed in handling specimens to avoid the risk of laboratory infection.

Streptomycin (10 mg/kg twice daily for 14 days) is very effective. Tetracycline and chloramphenicol are effective. Patients need to be isolated until they have been on treatment for 48 hours to minimise the risk of cross-infection.

BARTONELLOSIS

Bartonella bacilliformis is a Gram-negative aerobic bacillus transmitted by the bite of the female sandfly, *Lutzomyia verrucarum*. The disease is limited to the valleys of the western Andes, mainly in Peru, Colombia and Ecuador, between 2500 and 8000 feet above sea level. Man is the reservoir of infection. There are two manifestations of the disease: *haematological* and *cutaneous*.

After a 21-day incubation period there is sudden onset of systemic upset. The onset of fever is often followed by acute severe intravascular haemolysis which may last up to 4 weeks before resolution. Several weeks to several months later the eruptive phase of the disease appears, with nodular lesions of various sizes over the body in the miliary form, or fewer nodular, deep lesions particularly concentrated on the extensor aspects of the limbs. Mucous membranes of the mouth and gut, and serous cavities can be affected.

The organisms can be grown in blood cultures taken in the first week of the illness and can be readily found in Giemsa-stained thick and thin blood films, or in material obtained from skin lesions.

Treatment with antibiotics kills the organisms and produces rapid defervescence and clearance of organisms from the blood. Penicillin, streptomycin and chloramphenicol are effective; the latter is recommended in view of the reported association between systemic salmonellosis and bartonellosis.

CAT-SCRATCH DISEASE

Cat-scratch disease (CSD) is a benign lymphadenopathy in a site determined by an area scratched by a cat, most often in the neck or axilla.

Aetiology and pathogenesis

Histology of affected lymph nodes reveals scanty small pleomorphic rod-shaped bacilli which stain erratically with Gram stain. The other histological features are micro-abscesses and sometimes necrotic granulomas. The histological picture suggests a hypersensitivity reaction and skin tests with cat-scratch disease antigen confirm this.

The infection is transmitted by scratching or licking by a cat which does not itself appear ill. The cat is probably infectious for only about 3 weeks. It is not clear how cats transmit the infection, since bacilli have not been found in their saliva or on their claws, but they are present in lymph nodes.

Clinical features

Most cases occur in children or young adults. The main feature of the disease is gross enlargement of a single group of lymph nodes, which are usually tender. Lymphadenopathy develops about 2 weeks after the scratch and usually lasts for 2–4 months, but it may persist for up to a year. A papule may occur at the site of the scratch; it appears about a week after the scratch and persists for 1–3 weeks. Although most patients remain well, one-third have a low-grade fever for a few days and may experience malaise, headache and sore throat. Rare manifestations are conjunctivitis and pre-auricular lymphadenopathy (oculoglandular syndrome), encephalopathy, thrombocytopenic purpura, osteomyelitis and pneumonia.

Diagnosis

The diagnosis is usually based on the histology of excised lymph node with negative cultures for bacteria and mycobacteria. The Warthin-Starry silver impregnation stain may reveal the CSD bacilli but they are present in small numbers. The CSD antigen for skin testing is not widely available.

There may be a mild neutrophil leukocytosis but other tests are unhelpful. Antibody tests are being developed.

Treatment

Since the disease resolves spontaneously the only treatment usually required is analgesia if the lymph nodes are painful, and reassurance. Antibiotics do not help.

VIBRIOS

Cholera

Cholera stems from infection with the Gram-negative bacillus *Vibrio cholerae*, which causes acute secretory diarrhoea with death due to dehydration.

Aetiology

Vibrio cholerae is a curved Gram-negative motile bacillus. Two biotypes are recognised, the *classical biotype* and the *El Tor biotype*. The organism is present in vast numbers in the faeces of infected patients. The El Tor biotype tends to cause more asymptomatic and mild infections which resolve spontaneously and leave the patient excreting vibrios to infect others. The organism is sensitive to desiccation but survives in saline waters.

Distribution and incidence

Distribution and incidence are shown in Figure 12.14. South America remains free of the disease. Cholera has been imported into European countries but no outbreaks have resulted, apart from that in Naples in 1974.

Fig. 12.14 World distribution of cholera 1961–1986 (WHO).

Transmission and epidemiology

Organisms are ingested in contaminated food and water. In India, Bangladesh and Pakistan, where cholera is endemic, it is predominantly a paediatric disease. All ages are affected in epidemic cholera. Individual susceptibility is governed by the infecting dose and by the gastric acid barrier.

Pathogenesis

Vibrio cholerae secretes an exotoxin which binds to the GM1 ganglioside, a glycolipid on the surface membrane of jejunal enterocytes (Fig. 12.15). The effects of cholera toxin are mediated by direct effect on epithelial cell adenylate cyclase, causing accumulation of cyclic adenosine

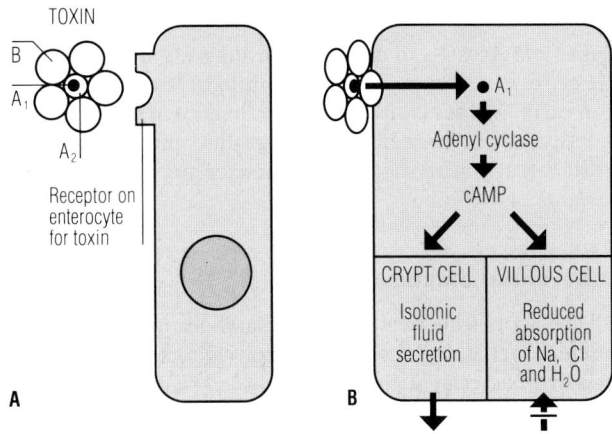

Fig. 12.15 Mechanism of action of cholera toxin on intestinal cells.
A. Attachment of cholera toxin to receptor on enterocyte. **B.** Activation of cAMP – note different effects on villous and crypt cells.

monophosphate in the cell. Local neurohumoral stimuli also contribute to the diarrhoea.

The outcome is that the upper small intestine becomes a site of net secretion with accumulation of isotonic fluid containing Na^+, Cl^-, HCO^-_3 and water. This fluid passes down the intestine and in the colon K^+ exchanges for Na^+ under the influence of aldosterone. Stooling rates of 500 ml/hour are common and up to 1 l/hour may be produced. The effect of cholera toxin lasts for the duration of the life of the enterocyte, which is 3–4 days; during this time the cell migrates from the crypt to villous tip, where it is desquamated into the gut lumen.

Vibrio cholerae and its exotoxin cause no histological changes in the affected mucosa. Cholera is a secretory diarrhoea with no mucosal inflammation. Secondary changes in a range of tissues, e.g. kidney, occur as a result of hypovolaemia and shock.

Clinical features

The incubation period is about 2 days. Diarrhoea begins suddenly, with vomiting during the first 24 hours of illness. Faecal residues are present in the stool at first but these are soon washed out of the gut, and opalescent, rice-water stools are passed. There are no pus cells in faecal smears. The abdomen may be distended and bowel sounds are increased. Stool losses are maximal within the first 48 hours of the illness and decline thereafter spontaneously, but death can occur from dehydration within 24 hours in the most severe cases.

The clinical features of cholera relate to isotonic volume depletion reducing the circulating blood volume and organ perfusion (Table 12.13, p. 234). Haematocrit and plasma specific gravity rise with haemoconcentration. Hypoglycaemia may occur in young children and may be associated with convulsions. Loss of bicarbonate causes acidosis. There is pre-renal uraemia.

There is a considerable range in the severity of diarrhoea in cholera, particularly the El Tor biotype.

12

Diagnosis

Rapid progression to dehydration suggests that cholera is the cause in severe cases that are brought to medical attention early. Milder cases will not be diagnosed unless a stool is cultured, or immediate dark ground microscopy of a fresh faecal smear shows the characteristic motility of *V. cholerae*.

Differential diagnosis

All the acute infective causes of diarrhoea need to be considered, including ingestion of staphylococcal enterotoxin, invasive bacteria, such as *Salmonella*, *Shigella* and *Campylobacter*, and enterotoxigenic strains of *Escherichia coli*. Rotavirus infection may also be difficult to distinguish from cholera.

Treatment

Mild to moderate dehydration can be managed with oral rehydration solution (ORS) (p. 257), while those with severe dehydration need intravenous infusions, e.g. Ringer's lactate, to restore blood volume. The aims of rehydration are:

1. to replace estimated fluid losses in the first 6 hours after presentation
2. to replace continuing intestinal fluid losses with equal volumes until diarrhoea stops.

ORS can be drunk from a cup, given using a spoon or syringed down a nasogastric tube. Frequent small amounts of ORS are better tolerated than less frequent large volumes, especially if the patient is vomiting. Additional fluid, such as water, fruit juice, tea or breast milk but *not* ORS, should be given to allow for insensible losses and obligatory urinary losses. The glucose in ORS is not sufficient to counter hypoglycaemia and so extra sugar should be given orally.

Antidiarrhoeal and antisecretory drugs have no part to play in the management of dehydrating diarrhoeal disease. Tetracycline reduces the duration of diarrhoea and reduces the duration of faecal excretion of *V. cholerae*. Tetracycline (250 mg for 4 days) can be given to adults and non-pregnant females. Pregnant women and children under 8 years can be given furazolidone. Co-trimoxazole is also effective.

Prevention and control

Adequate clean water supplies and safe disposal of faecal wastes would do much to prevent the occurrence of cholera. Concurrent education of the population about the relationship of infective diarrhoeal disease to personal and general sanitation practices is essential. The widespread use of ORS early in the course of all diarrhoeal illness reduces mortality.

Vaccination with the present killed vaccine is of no benefit, either for prophylaxis in the traveller or for the control of epidemics.

CAMPYLOBACTER

Campylobacter are morphologically similar to *Vibrios* but are now regarded as a separate genus since they have different biochemical characteristics. There are six species, of which *C. jejuni* and *C. fetus* are important human pathogens.

C. jejuni is a major cause of prolonged, severe enterocolitis, frequently associated with bloody stools and abdominal pain and tenderness suggestive of peritonitis. Infection may be acquired from food or drinks but there is often a relationship with domestic animals, many of which are normally colonised (e.g. dogs and cattle).

C. fetus rarely infects normal subjects but can cause septicaemia in debilitated patients. Like many gastrointestinal pathogens *Campylobacter* may cause a reactive arthritis.

C. jejuni is sensitive to erythromycin in vitro, and oral treatment renders stool specimens culture-negative, but its effect on the rate of resolution of disease is disappointing. Nevertheless it is sometimes used in ill patients.

ANAEROBIC BACTERIA

Bacteroides fragilis is the most commonly encountered pathogenic anaerobe but many other anaerobes are found among the normal flora of the gastrointestinal tract and genital tract; these include other *bacteroides*, *fusobacteria* and some *anaerobic cocci* such as peptostreptococci and micro-aerophilic streptococci. Anaerobic organisms often cause wound infection, abscesses and septicaemia in patients who have had abdominal surgery or intestinal perforation. Antibiotic sensitivity is restricted; metronidazole is a key drug, since it is well absorbed after oral or rectal administration and *B. fragilis* is usually sensitive to it. Clindamycin is another useful agent against anaerobes.

Mixed infections

When infection arises as a result of contamination from an endogenous source, particularly the colon, it may involve several different bacteria including anaerobes. Abscesses associated with the bowel or vagina are examples and, less obviously, cerebral abscess. Some tissue infections also contain multiple pathogens but these usually occur in debilitated patients. Severe stomatitis, one form of which is known as *Vincent's angina*, commonly occurs in malnourished patients with poor dental hygiene. The pathogens responsible are members of the normal mouth flora, including anaerobes and spirochaetes which are sensitive to penicillin. Metronidazole is an alternative drug which is better absorbed after oral administration.

Necrotising fasciitis is a rapidly spreading subcutaneous infection; it results in extensive necrosis, which may involve any part of the body but most often involves the periphery, particularly in diabetic patients, and the perineum. Scrotal infection is called *Fournier's gangrene*. The organisms involved are mixed anaerobic bacteria, mainly *Bacteroides* or peptostreptococci. Treatment is by a combination of aggressive surgery and antibiotics aimed mainly at anaerobes.

MYCOBACTERIA

Mycobacteria are classified as a group because they contain mycolic acids. They are bacilli which are mostly slow-growing and able to survive within macrophages. On staining by the Ziehl-Neelsen method they are acid- and alcohol-fast. The most important pathogens within the group are *Mycobacterium tuberculosis* and *M. leprae*.

Tuberculosis is now uncommon in the Western world but still a major problem in less developed countries. The disease is discussed fully on page 477. *M. bovis* is rarely incriminated now but can cause similar disease. Other mycobacteria, sometimes called atypical, such as *M. kansasii*, are less pathogenic than *M. tuberculosis* but can cause disease. *M. avium intracellulare* has become more familiar in recent years because it is one of the infections which afflict patients with AIDS. It causes pulmonary disease or septicaemia with disseminated infection. Mycobacteria other than *M. tuberculosis* are often resistant to standard antituberculous drugs, so their treatment presents difficult problems in immunocompromised patients.

LEPROSY

Leprosy is a chronic infection of skin and cutaneous nerves caused by *Mycobacterium leprae*. The manifestations in the patient may be localised or generalised, and are determined largely by the host response to the infecting organism.

Aetiology

M. leprae was the first pathogenic bacterium recognised in man (Hansen 1873). It is an acid-fast bacillus. It cannot be cultured in vitro. Ziehl-Neelsen staining of smears of the organism differentiates viable (solid staining) from granular (non-viable) organisms. In man the cooler superficial regions of the body are the preferred sites for bacterial proliferation. The generation time is about 13 days.

Distribution and incidence

Leprosy is mainly a disease of the tropics and subtropics (Fig. 12.16). It is relatively common in Africa and Asia, with a prevalence of 2–9 per 1000 in most areas and higher rates in a few countries. Lepromin skin test positivity rates in endemic areas are much higher than rates of clinical cases, suggesting that host factors do much to influence the outcome of the disease. The disease has almost completely disappeared from Europe.

Transmission and epidemiology

There is little evidence to support skin-to-skin contact as the route of infection. Leprosy bacilli injected into the skin

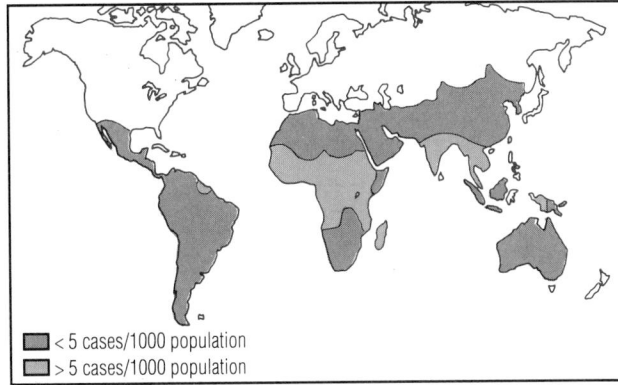

< 5 cases/1000 population
> 5 cases/1000 population

Fig. 12.16 Geographical distribution of leprosy.

do not cause infection. Aerosol spread from the upper respiratory tract of patients with multibacillary (lepromatous) leprosy may be a source of infection.

There is considerable variation in the course of infection from person to person, and the majority of those infected develop no clinical disease.

Among those developing clinical disease there appears to be a racial variation in the type of leprosy occurring: up to 50% of cases in Asia have lepromatous disease, compared with 10% in Africa. The male-to-female ratio is 2:1 in adults and unity in children.

Pathogenesis and pathology

The host's cellular immune responses determine the outcome of infection. If macrophages are able to kill the infecting organisms there is either no clinical disease or the lesions of indeterminate leprosy at most (Fig. 12.17). Those in whom the infection progresses further develop one of the forms of disease described in Table 12.27 and classified as one of the following:

1. tuberculoid (TT)
2. borderline tuberculoid (BT)
3. borderline (BB)
4. borderline lepromatous (BL)
5. lepromatous (LL).

Few bacilli are found in the tuberculoid forms (*paucibacillary*) while vast numbers are found in patients with lepromatous leprosy (*multibacillary*). Host cellular responses to mycobacterial antigens determine the form of disease that develops, with delayed type *hypersensitivity* at the tuberculoid end of the spectrum and *anergy* at the lepromatous end. The borderline forms are immunologically unstable and without treatment will deteriorate to the lepromatous end of the spectrum.

The earliest lesions in leprosy begin in cutaneous nerves, where bacilli are phagocytosed by Schwann cells. The most severe damage to nerves is seen in TT leprosy. At the lepromatous end of the spectrum the involved nerves are

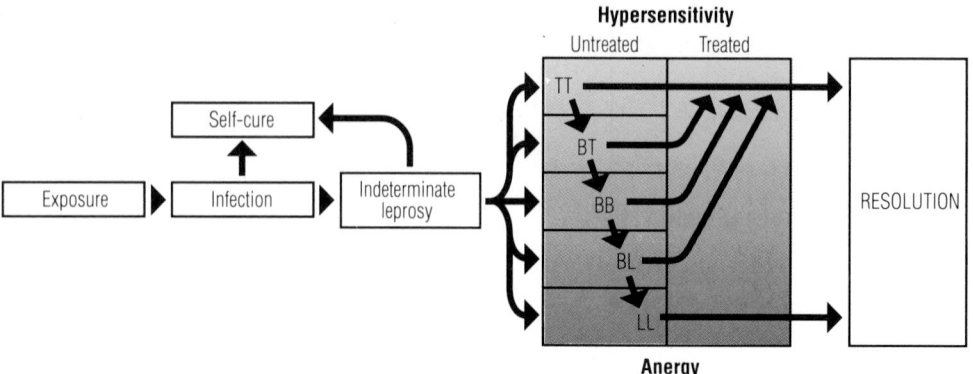

Fig. 12.17 Evolution of leprosy lesions with and without treatment. (TT = tuberculoid; BT = borderline tuberculoid; BB = borderline; BL = borderline lepromatous; LL = lepromatous) (After Ridley D S 1977 Skin Biopsy in Leprosy. Ciba-Geigy, Basle.)

not so large. The auriculo-temporal, ulnar, median, radial cutaneous, lateral popliteal and sural nerves are pre-ferentially involved at sites where the nerve trunks are close to the skin and therefore cooler, e.g. the ulnar nerve behind the medial epicondyle at the elbow.

The bacterial load and the morphology of the organisms need to be assessed, initially for classification purposes and subsequently to determine the response to treatment. Slit skin smears are obtained from the edges of lesions, the ear lobes, elbows and knees. Numbers of bacilli and their viability can be graded. Lepromin is a skin test antigen obtained from *M. leprae*. The antigen is injected intra-dermally, and the test is read at 3 weeks, when a nodule at the site of injection indicates a positive response supporting a classification at the tuberculoid end of the spectrum.

Two types of acute reaction are recognised in leprosy:

1. *Erythema nodosum leprosum* (ENL) is an immune-complex-mediated vasculitis occurring in LL patients and, less often, in BL, either while on treatment or in the untreated patient. The histological features are those of acute inflammation with oedema and a promi-nent infiltrate of neutrophils.
2. A *reversal reaction* indicates a change in cellular responsiveness to the infecting organism, either increasing or decreasing responsiveness. Skin lesions and affected nerves become more inflamed. The swollen lesion resolves completely in time, becoming smaller in 'upgrading' and bigger with 'downgrading'.

Clinical features

Indeterminate leprosy

Indeterminate leprosy is manifest as a hypopigmented macule on a dark skin, and as a slightly reddened macule on a light skin, with either normal or mildly reduced sensation. These lesions may regress spontaneously or progress to one of the stages described below.

Tuberculoid leprosy

Tuberculoid leprosy (TT) is characterised by a hairless, hypopigmented, anaesthetic lesion with a flat centre and a well-defined, raised edge with minimal inflammation. The skin of the lesion does not sweat. Single lesions are usual but up to three may be found. Common sites are the extensor aspect of the arm, around the elbow and the knee. A thickened cutaneous nerve supplying the affected area may be felt. To detect a thickened nerve the examiner should run his finger over the nerve trunk, at sites of subcutaneous nerves, in a direction at right angles to that of the nerve trunk. Neural TT leprosy occurs with a single thickened nerve as the only physical sign.

Borderline tuberculoid leprosy

Borderline tuberculoid (BT) lesions are similar to those of TT but more numerous and asymmetrically distributed. The edges of the lesions are inflamed and irregular. The

Table 12.27 Major features in leprosy

Feature	Tuberculoid leprosy (TT)	Borderline leprosy (BB)	Lepromatous leprosy (LL)
Lesions	Few (1–3)	More numerous	Large numbers
Nerve involvement	Local	Present in nerves of predilection	Diffuse, symmetrical late in disease
Numbers of bacilli	Fragmented only	Viable bacilli present in lesions	Vast numbers of viable bacilli
Lepromin test	+++	–	–
Reactions upgrading/downgrading	–	+++	–
Erythema nodosum leprosum (ENL)	–	–	+++

nerves preferentially involved in leprosy are usually thickened and damaged, causing anaesthesia, loss of function and deformity to a variable extent in hands and feet. Penetrating ulcers in the soles of the feet, burns and skin sepsis are often present. There may be osteomyelitis of the bones of the feet due to an infected penetrating ulcer.

Borderline leprosy

Borderline leprosy (BB) produces multiple lesions that vary in form, size and shape. Papules, plaques and lesions with elevated wide outer rims and depressed, well-defined, anaesthetic centres are seen. The lesions may be hypopigmented or hyperpigmented. There is diffuse involvement of the peripheral nerves.

Borderline lepromatous leprosy

Borderline lepromatous leprosy (BL) causes numerous, asymmetrically distributed, inflamed or hyperpigmented lesions which may be papules, nodules or plaques. Sensation over the lesions may be normal. Vague macules that vary in size are present in some patients. Peripheral nerves may only show slight enlargement.

Lepromatous leprosy

Lepromatous leprosy (LL) is associated with numerous symmetrically distributed skin lesions. At the very earliest stage of the disease numerous slightly reddened hypopigmented macules and nodules are seen. These evolve into papules and plaques without treatment. The eyebrows are lost and the skin of the face and ears become diffusely thickened (leonine facies). Involvement of the nasal mucosae may block the nose and cause a bloodstained nasal discharge. *M. leprae* is found in nasal scrapings but the diagnosis of leprosy must *not* be made by finding acid-fast bacilli in this site only, as saprophytic acid-fast bacilli (not *M. leprae*) may be found on the nasal mucosa of healthy persons. Destruction of the nasal cartilage may occur later. Iritis and keratitis are often present. The voice may alter because of inflammation and thickening of the laryngeal mucosa. Testicular atrophy and gynaecomastia occur because of testicular damage. Bilateral oedema of the legs is often present. Nerve involvement occurs late in the course of the disease. Renal failure due to glomerulonephritis and amyloid disease are late complications in LL.

Reactional states

The skin lesions and involved nerves become more inflamed and swollen in *reversal reactions*. These reactions may also be accompanied by swelling of face, hands and feet. Involved nerves become very tender, often with further deterioration in function. This type of reaction may persist for 2–3 months before subsiding.

Erythema nodosum leprosum produces acute inflammation of existing skin lesions in BL. The lesions become swollen and painful and slowly evolve through a livid appearance to residual hyperpigmentation of the affected skin. Bullae form over some lesions and these ulcerate and are slow to heal. New papules appear in LL cases, typically on the extensor aspects of the limbs. They may evolve over 2–3 days, through a bullous stage, to indolent ulcers which are slow to heal. Uveitis, lymphadenitis, orchitis and neuritis are also features of ENL.

Diagnosis

Diagnosis is based on the clinical features, characteristic histology, a positive lepromin test (at the tuberculoid end of the spectrum) and acid-fast bacilli in slit skin smears taken from the edge of lesions and other sites, the ear lobes, elbows and knees (BB to LL). Most patients are diagnosed from these features. In pure neural leprosy the diagnosis can be made from a biopsy of a few fascicles of an affected distal cutaneous nerve with no motor functions, such as the radial cutaneous nerve at the wrist, or sural nerve.

Treatment

Multidrug therapy is now the rule and the current World Health Organization recommendations are set out in Table 12.28. These drugs are generally well tolerated. Dapsone

Table 12.28 Treatment of leprosy

Type	Classification	Drugs	Duration
Paucibacillary	Tuberculoid (TT) and borderline tuberculoid (BT)	Rifampicin, 660 mg monthly, supervised + dapsone, 100 mg daily, unsupervised	6 months
Multibacillary	Borderline (BB), borderline lepromatous (BL), lepromatous (LL)	Rifampicin, 600 mg monthly, supervised + dapsone, 100 mg daily, unsupervised + clofazimine, 300 mg monthly, supervised + clofazimine, 50 mg daily, unsupervised Ethionamide or prothionamide may also be added	2 years from time of diagnosis and thereafter until slit skin smears contain no bacilli

12

occasionally causes haemolysis. Clofazimine may stain the skin a rather reddish hue. Ethionamide and prothionamide may cause hepatitis.

Mild upgrading reactions may be controlled with aspirin or non-steroidal anti-inflammatory drugs. More severe reactions that threaten nerve function require oral steroids. Erythema nodosum leprosum may be controlled by steroids but sometimes thalidomide is needed. This drug is only available for the treatment of ENL in the United Kingdom through designated specialist physicians.

The patient needs careful instruction regarding the care of hands and feet, prevention of cracking and infection of the skin of the feet and appropriate footwear. Where the cornea is exposed as a result of facial nerve palsy, early lateral tarsorrhaphy is essential to prevent corneal damage. Tendon transplants may help in managing foot and hand deformities.

Prevention and control

There is still a considerable stigma attached to leprosy; this is based on ignorance. Education of the public regarding the disease and the efficacy of treatment is being attempted. BCG vaccination reduces the incidence of leprosy. Currently there are efforts to define protective antigens which may result in a genetically engineered vaccine. Until then control depends on detection and effective treatment of cases, particularly LL. Public education creates a climate in which patients may seek medical attention earlier.

MYCOBACTERIUM ULCERANS

Mycobacterium ulcerans causes chronic ulceration, usually on an exposed area of the body, often the lower limbs. The condition has a wide distribution in the tropics and is often called *Buruli ulcer*. The lesion may begin as a subcutaneous nodule which ulcerates through the skin. Lateral, subcutaneous extension produces an ulcer with markedly undermined edges. The organisms (acid-fast bacilli) are numerous and can be grown in Löwenstein-Jensen medium at 30–33°C.

Prior to ulceration rifampicin is of help. Local heat will encourage healing, as the bacteria are killed by temperatures over 33°C. When the lesion affects a region near to a joint, active and passive movement of the joint must be encouraged to prevent contractures.

SPIROCHAETES

SYPHILIS

Syphilis is caused by *Treponema pallidum* (TP), one of a small group of treponemes. TP is a bacterium 6–15 microns in length, and is narrow, with regular tight spirals and mobile in all axes. Transmission is usually by sexual contact although transplacental infection may occur. Exposure to moist mucosal or cutaneous surfaces is

required; transmission is commonly during the first 1–4 years of infection.

The incidence of syphilis in England and Wales fell after the introduction of antibiotic therapy but there was a resurgence during the 1970s in males (Fig. 12.18). These cases were mainly in homosexual men with numerous sexual partners. More recently there has been a decline in the incidence of syphilis.

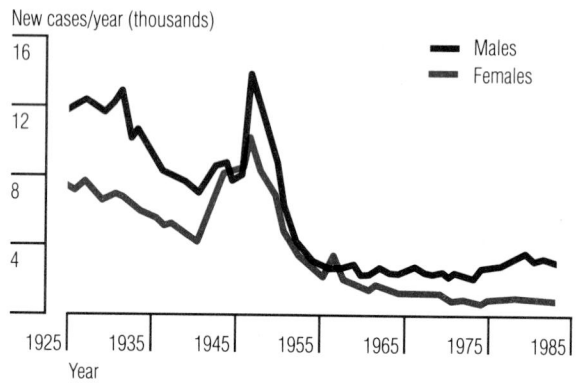

Fig. 12.18   Incidence of syphilis in England and Wales, 1925–1983.

Clinical features

There may be signs of active infection, or the disease may be latent. Clinically, syphilis may be divided into four stages: primary, secondary, tertiary and quaternary.

Primary

The primary lesion is a chancre, which starts as a painless pink papule and may develop into an ulcer. The ulcer has a button-like feel on palpation. The base is initially pink and shiny, becoming grey later. Painless inguinal lymphadenopathy is common and may be unilateral. On occasions the chancres may be multiple and painful. A chancre usually appears about 3 weeks after exposure to infection (range 10–90 days), and heals. Men, especially homosexual men, are infected more often than women.

In the male the common genital sites of infection are coronal sulcus, glans penis and prepuce. In the female chancres may be found in the vagina, and on the labia, fourchette and cervix.

In both sexes infections can occur in the pharynx and anus. In the anal area a chancre resembles a fissure and may be painful. Rarely other parts of the body, such as the finger, mouth, tongue or axillae, may be infected. Chancres, because they can be small and painless, are often missed.

Secondary

The secondary stage may take 3 months or more to appear after infection (average 6 weeks). At this stage there is a bacteraemia. Systemic upset is common, including low grade fever, malaise, headache, generalised lymph-

Summary 4   Sites of involvement in secondary syphilis
The proportion of cases is given in brackets

Skin   (90%)
Lymph glands   (50%)
Mouth and throat   (35%)
CNS
   symptomatic   (20%)
   asymptomatic   (2%)
Kidneys   (Rare)
Gastrointestinal tract and liver   (Rare)
Bones and joints   (Rare)

adenopathy including epitrochlear glands, and rarely hepatosplenomegaly and transient proteinuria. Arthralgia, acute meningitis and cranial nerve palsies are rare features (Summary 4).

The skin is most frequently involved in secondary syphilis. A non-pruritic rash is common. The lesions are usually papules or plaques and in early secondary syphilis tend to be symmetrical and widespread. The palms, soles and face are often involved. Scaling is common and the lesions can resemble psoriasis. In late secondary syphilis lesions tend to be fewer and asymmetrical. Patchy and partial hair loss can occur, giving a moth-eaten appearance. Other signs of secondary syphilis include patchy alopecia, erosive lesions of the mucous membranes (mucous patches) common in the mouth, and soft, flat-topped and highly infectious warts found in the peri-anal area and known as condylomata lata. At this stage all tests for syphilis are positive. The veneral disease research laboratory slide test (VDRL, see below) shows a very high titre.

Latent period

Syphilis, if untreated, will go into a latent phase, when clinical symptoms and signs are absent, approximately 2 years after the initial infection. Before this, there may be periods of infectivity; over 90% occur in the first year. These relapses may be characterised by rashes and lymphadenopathy. During the latent phase, sexual transmission is rare, although feto-maternal transmission may occur. Transplacental passage becomes unlikely in late latent syphilis. The VDRL will be negative or have a very low titre, e.g. 1:8. The *T. pallidum* haemagglutination assay (TPHA) and fluorescent treponemal antibody absorption test (FTA-Abs) – see below – are always positive.

Late (tertiary) syphilis

Tertiary syphilis is now rare, since effective treatment prevents progression.

The characteristic pathological lesion at this stage is a gumma, which is a destructive granuloma sometimes associated with vasculitis. Treponemes are very scanty and not usually seen under the microscope. Gummas can involve any organ. In the skin they cause punched-out ulcers, and in the nose the nasal septum is destroyed.

Lesions in bones and joints are common, and lead to fractures and joint destruction. Liver involvement causes fever and local tenderness. Gummas respond remarkably rapidly to treatment.

Quaternary

Quaternary syphilis is either neurosyphilis (described on p. 964) or cardiovascular syphilis, which is due to endarteritis obliterans of the vasa vasorum of the aorta. This causes aneurysm, most commonly of the ascending aorta (p. 445).

Congenital syphilis

T. pallidum crosses the placenta after the third month of pregnancy, usually when the mother has early disease. If she is not treated, infection of the fetus may cause abortion, stillbirth or the birth of a child with congenital syphilis. The child may have signs of infection at birth, similar to those of secondary syphilis in adults, or he may be asymptomatic but develop signs of late congenital syphilis, equivalent to adult tertiary, after the age of 2 years. The predominant signs in early presentation are snuffles and rash which may vesiculate (not seen in adults).

Possible late signs are facial abnormalities including frontal bosses, saddle nose, protruding mandible, Hutchinson's incisors (peg-shaped, splayed), interstitial keratitis, eighth nerve deafness, periostitis and Clutton's joints, juvenile neurosyphilis, and paroxysmal cold haemoglobinuria.

As in adult syphilis diagnosis depends on serology in the later stages.

Diagnosis

Primary syphilis is diagnosed by identifying the *Treponema pallidum* by using dark ground microscopy. *T. pallidum* can be identified in serous exudate from the surface of the chancre, which is placed in a drop of saline and examined using an oil immersion lens. A negative result does not exclude the diagnosis, as topical (e.g. antibiotic ointments) or systemic therapy may alter the findings. The FTA-Abs is positive in approximately 70% of cases at this stage.

Later stages require serological testing for confirmation of the diagnosis. Serological examination of the CSF is necessary if neurosyphilis is suspected.

Antibodies to treponemal antigens are present, i.e. positive TPHA and FTA-Abs, in 80% of cases of primary syphilis.

Two types of antibody tests are employed (Table 12.29):

1. *Non-treponemal tests* (e.g. venereal disease research laboratory slide test or VDRL; rapid plasma reagin card test or RPR). These tests detect cardiolipin antibodies in serum. A high titre indicates an active infection. They become negative after therapy or during the latent phase of untreated syphilis. False positive results may be found in acute febrile illness, autoimmune diseases and after immunisations.

12

2. Treponemal tests (e.g. fluorescent treponemal antibody absorption test or FTA-Abs; *Treponema pallidum* haemagglutination assay or TPHA). These detect antibodies against the treponemal antigen. They are positive earlier in the infection, but remain positive after therapy and in latent syphilis.

Table 12.29 Serological tests for syphilis

Disease/stage	VDRL or RPR*	Test TPHA†	FTA-Abs†
Primary syphilis	Negative	Positive/ negative	Positive
Secondary syphilis	>1:64	Positive	Positive
Latent (over 2 yrs) syphilis	<1:16	Positive	Positive
Latent (over 2 yrs) late syphilis	Negative/ <1:2	Positive	Positive
Yaws	Negative/ <1:2	Positive	Positive
Treated syphilis	Negative/ <1:2	Positive	Positive

* Tests for cardiolipin antibodies: VDRL = Venereal Disease Research Laboratory slide test; RPR = rapid plasma reagin card test.
†Tests specific for treponemal antibodies: FTA-Abs = fluorescent treponemal antibody absorption test; TPHA = *T. pallidum* haemagglutination assay

Yaws, another treponemal disease caused by *T. pertenue* (see below), gives a serological picture similar to that of untreated syphilis. Careful history is necessary to differentiate the cause, and if doubt about the diagnosis persists, treatment for syphilis is given.

Treatment

Table 12.30 shows acceptable treatment regimens.

Benzathine penicillin does not effectively cross the blood–brain barrier. Patients may, but do not commonly, experience Jarisch-Herxheimer reaction 1–2 hours after the first dose of penicillin. This reaction is more commonly seen in secondary syphilis.

In cardiovascular syphilis the inflammatory response to antibiotic therapy may result in small vessel occlusion in the coronary ostia; to prevent this, prednisolone is given in decreasing doses for 24 hours before and up to 48 hours after commencing therapy. The success of therapy is ensured by repeating serological examinations for at least 1 year after treatment. This is of especial value in primary and secondary syphilis.

It is always important to examine the sexual partners of people with syphilis; tracing their partners should therefore be regarded as an integral part of treatment.

If the erythromycin regime is used for a pregnant patient, it is always advisable to treat the baby at birth with procaine penicillin (30 mg/kg daily for 10 days). Since erythromycin is not a fully reliable treatment, the mother should be treated with doxycycline after delivery; doxycycline is, of course, contra-indicated during breast-feeding.

YAWS

Yaws is a chronic infection due to *Treponema pertenue*; it is characterised by a primary site of skin infection, with later dissemination to other cutaneous sites and periosteum. Unlike syphilis, cardiovascular and nervous systems are not affected and congenital infection does not occur.

Distribution and incidence

Following mass eradication campaigns yaws became very uncommon, but there has been a resurgence of cases in South America, West and Central Africa, Indonesia and the Pacific region.

Transmission and epidemiology

The organism must be introduced into the skin by contact between an infective lesion and an abrasion in the skin of the recipient.

Clinical features

The primary papillomatous lesion or 'mother yaw' develops at the site of infection. This lesion is highly infectious. Other forms are a localised area of dry papules or a localised maculopapular rash. Regional lymph nodes are often enlarged. Secondary infectious lesions appear within a few weeks, either before or after the primary lesion has

Table 12.30 Treatment of syphilis

Stage	Drug*	Dose and route†	Duration (days)
Early (incl. latent for under 1 year)	Procaine penicillin	600–1200 mg/day, IM	14
Late (incl. latent for over 1 year)	Procaine penicillin	600–1200 mg/day, IM	21
Congenital	Procaine penicillin	30 mg/kg per day, IM	10
Penicillin-allergic patients			
Early	Oxytetracycline	500 mg 4 times/day, O	15
Late	Oxytetracycline	500 mg 4 times/day, O	30

* Probenicid is usually added for treatment of neurosyphilis and cardiovascular syphilis.
† 1 megaunit penicillin = 600 mg; IM = intramuscular; O = oral

healed. Rashes continue to appear over the next 5 years and take various forms. Condylomata form at moist sites, e.g. peri-anal and perineal areas, and are highly infectious. Later periostitis may occur, affecting fingers, tibia (causing sabre tibia) and nose (a destructive lesion called gangosa). Painful, deep fissures in the soles of the feet also occur, so-called crab yaws.

Diagnosis

The organisms are readily found in serous material from the primary and secondary lesions examined by dark ground microscopy. Serological tests for syphilis are positive.

Treatment

Penicillin aluminium monostearate (PAM) is very effective given once only in a single dose of 1.5 g, or 0.75 g for children under 10 years. Tetracycline (2.0 g per day in divided doses for 14 days) can be used in those allergic to penicillin, apart from pregnant women and children under 8 years, who should receive erythromycin for 2 weeks.

Prevention and control

Chemotherapy is very effective in controlling yaws, with surveillance to detect resurgence of infection.

ENDEMIC SYPHILIS (BEJEL)

Endemic syphilis is due to non-venereal infection with an organism that is intermediate between *T. pallidum* and *T. pertenue*. It is present in the desert regions of North Africa and the Middle East. Infection probably occurs by person-to-person spread among children and older females who look after children.

The first lesions are mucous patches in the mouth. Later, moist raised lesions of various sizes in axillae, groins, perineum and between the buttocks are seen. Hyperkeratotic lesions like those of yaws affect palms and soles. Bone involvement (periostitis) is associated with pain in the knees and shins. Destructive lesions of the nose, similar to gangosa in yaws, may occur. Congenital transmission does not occur, and late disease affecting the cardiovascular and nervous systems is very rare. Treatment with pencillin aluminium monostearate, as in yaws, is effective.

PINTA

Pinta is a treponemal infection caused by *Treponema carateum*. Geographically it is localised to the drier regions of Central and South America. Transmission occurs by direct contagion from infectious skin lesions, and breaks in the skin may be a route of entry for the organism.

The primary skin lesion is a papule sited on the extremities, around which smaller, similar lesions appear. Spirochaetes may be found in serous material expressed from the erythematous and violaceous lesions. Serological tests for syphilis are positive. Treatment is with a single dose of benzathine penicillin (1.5 g intramuscularly, or 0.75 g for children under 10 years).

RELAPSING FEVER

Relapsing fever is an acute infectious illness caused by spirochaetes of the genus *Borrelia*. *Borrelia recurrentis* is the cause of louse-borne relapsing fever, while a range of other species cause the tick-borne variety. The disease is characterised by febrile episodes lasting several days, followed by afebrile periods and then relapse of fever. Febrile periods correspond to recurrence of spirochaetaemia.

Aetiology

Borrelia are spiral organisms which can be identified in peripheral blood smears using Giemsa and Leishman stains; they can also be readily identified using dark ground microscopy and cultured on artificial media.

Louse-borne relapsing fever

Man is the reservoir of infection; the human body louse, *Pediculus humanus*, is the vector. War, famine and natural disasters that cause sudden migrations of large numbers of people grouped together in adverse conditions encourage the spread of lice and louse-borne diseases, relapsing fever and typhus.

Tick-borne relapsing fever

Tick-borne relapsing fever is a sporadic zoonosis in man when he enters an area where there is a cycle of transmission between ticks and wild rodents. The disease has a worldwide distribution, except for Australia and the Pacific region.

Pathogenesis and pathology

During the incubation period spirochaetes divide intravenously. Platelets are sequestered intravascularly and this, together with intravascular coagulation, produces a bleeding tendency manifest as a purpuric rash. After 4–5 days of symptoms there is a crisis associated with massive phagocytosis of *Borrelia* helped by opsonising antibody. Following the crisis there is an afebrile period, during which numbers of organisms expressing a different surface antigen build up and symptoms recur. This can occur up to five times.

The spleen, liver, heart and brain are the main sites of pathological lesions, which consist of macrophages surrounding and ingesting large numbers of organisms.

Clinical features

After an incubation period that varies from 4–18 days the illness begins suddenly with rigors and a fever which rises rapidly to 40°C. Headache, joint pains, anorexia, malaise, nausea and vomiting are usual features, with mental confusion frequently present. Hepatosplenomegaly is common, with jaundice present in some patients. A petechial rash, most prominent on the trunk, is seen. Bleeding from the nose, the respiratory tract or the gut may occur, as may focal neurological signs.

The first febrile period lasts about 5 days before spontaneous defervescence. This follows a severe febrile paroxysm with cold extremities, a rising pulse rate, a rising blood pressure and tachypnoea. An afebrile period lasting about 7 days recurs before the first relapse. Tick-borne disease is milder than louse-borne disease described above. In both types death can occur during the initial rigor or during defervescence.

Diagnosis

Organisms can be found in peripheral blood smears stained with Giemsa stain. Dark ground microscopy can be used to demonstrate the motile spirochaetes in a fresh blood smear.

Treatment

Antibiotics kill spirochaetes readily. Tetracycline can be used in patients over 8 years old, apart from pregnant females. Erythromycin can be used in pregnant women and young children.

Louse-borne relapsing fever requires a single dose of 500 mg of either drug. Tick-borne relapsing fever requires treatment for 10 days.

Supportive care is needed, particularly in patients with louse-borne disease, as they can develop severe reactions after being treated. Central venous pressure monitoring is essential if facilities are available. Hypoxia is corrected by giving oxygen continuously. Vitamin K is given if the prothrombin time is prolonged.

Prevention

Delousing by washing with soap and water, followed by dusting with 10% DDT, is effective. Clothes should be washed with soap in water at 55°C to kill lice and nits (lice eggs) which are found in the seams of clothes. Lice cannot survive on a person who has two sets of clothes which he wears on alternate weeks.

LYME DISEASE

Lyme disease is due to infection with *Borrelia burgdorferi*, transmitted by the tick *Ixodes dammini*. It is described on page 1007.

LEPTOSPIRAL INFECTION

Infection with *Leptospira icterohaemorrhagiae* is discussed on page 660.

ACTINOMYCOSES

Actinomyces species, despite their name, are bacteria which are often confused with fungi because of their filamentous appearance and their propensity to produce chronic suppurative infection with sinuses discharging purulent material. Most human disease is caused by *Actinomyces israelii*, an oral commensal, and occurs in the presence of chronic lack of dental hygiene. The characteristic pathological feature is that tissue boundaries are crossed and bone is infected. There is a fibrotic reaction around suppurating areas, which accounts for the induration detected in palpable lesions. Three major forms of disease occur: cervicofacial, thoracic and disseminated actinomycosis.

Cervicofacial actinomycosis

The characteristic lesion is a painless swelling below the border of the mandible, bluish, fluctuant and slowly enlarging. Sometimes the abscess is painful and usually it is apparent long before there is any spontaneous discharge.

Thoracic actinomycosis

Thoracic actinomycosis may result from aspiration of oral debris, or may occur after thoracic surgery; it is easily confused with carcinoma. Chest radiograph shows unilateral consolidation with evidence of chest wall involvement. Nowadays the disease is usually diagnosed before discharging sinuses develop.

Disseminated actinomycosis

Lesions may occur at almost any site following rare haematogenous dissemination; the abdomen is the most common site, however, and within the abdomen, ileocaecal disease heads the list. Because of the chronic course and difficulty in diagnosis, sinus or fistula formation is still seen in abdominal actinomycosis.

Diagnosis and treatment

Microscopy of tissues reveals the Gram-positive organisms, with surrounding acute or chronic inflammatory reaction and foamy macrophages. The organism can be cultured from tissues and rarely from blood.

Penicillin is the drug of choice and *prolonged* treatment is necessary, with intravenous treatment for 4–6 weeks, followed by oral treatment for at least 6 months. Tetracycline, erythromycin and choramphenicol are alternatives in penicillin-allergic subjects.

MADUROMYCOSES

Maduromycosis is a descriptive term for a group of chronic infections of the subcutaneous tissues and bone of the limbs. Two groups of organisms cause this condition:

1. *actinomycetes*, causing 60% of cases, which are bacteria and respond to antibiotics
2. *true fungi* such as *Madurella mycetomatis* which are almost totally unresponsive to antifungal drugs.

These two groups of organisms are found in the soil and enter the skin by penetrating injuries.

Pathology

The main features are chronic inflammation with micro-abscesses and granulomatous reactions around collections of the organisms. Sinuses form and organisms are extruded. There may be localised erosion of bone. Infection spreads along fascial tissue planes. Progressive destruction of affected tissue occurs.

Clinical features

Chronic indurated swelling of the affected area, with healed or open sinuses, are usual features.

Investigations

The most important investigation is an adequate surgical biopsy of diseased tissue. This specimen is divided to give samples for histology and culture for the two groups of organisms.

Treatment

Actinomycetoma responds well to prolonged courses of antibiotics. Co-trimoxazole for 9 months, plus streptomycin for the first 2 months, is effective. Fungi respond poorly to antifungal drugs, even though there may be in vitro sensitivity. Wide local excision with grafting may be effective in early lesions, but amputation is necessary in more advanced cases.

NOCARDIOSES

Nocardiosis is a systemic infection due to species of *Nocardia* (*N. asteroides* and, less often, *N. brasiliensis* and *N. caviae*). *Nocardia brasiliensis* is the common cause of actinomycetoma in the tropics and subtropics. *Nocardia* are higher bacteria which exist in a filamentous and coccobacillary form, depending on culture conditions.

Aetiology, pathogenesis and epidemiology

Nocardia are aerobic, filamentous, branching Gram-positive bacteria and grow well on standard culture media. The organisms are found in rotting vegetation, and infection is acquired by inhalation in most instances, although inoculation of organisms in the skin occurs. Initial pulmonary lesions may lead to dissemination of infection by the bloodstream. Necrosis and suppuration are the typical pathological changes.

Adults are most often affected, with cases in males exceeding those in females. Infection mainly occurs in immunosuppressed individuals.

Clinical features

Acute and sometimes fulminant or chronic suppurative pulmonary disease occurs in nocardiosis. Fever, cough with viscid sputum, night sweats and weight loss are usual features. Signs of lobar pneumonia may be found. Pleural thickening and empyema may develop, and the affected lung may cavitate. Haematogenous dissemination to cause brain abscess, kidney lesions, bone lesions and subcutaneous sepsis is reported.

Actinomycetoma due to *Nocardia* presents with long-standing swelling of the extremity, most often foot or ankle, and sinuses discharging on to the skin.

Diagnosis

Diagnosis depends on finding the organism in discharges, exudates, bronchial washing or biopsy sections. *Nocardia* grow well on media used for growing tubercle bacilli and on Sabouraud's medium. Serological tests are of help in diagnosis and can give useful information about the response to treatment, although they are only available in a few centres. When a case of Madura foot is being investigated, the importance of taking an adequate, deep biopsy cannot be overemphasised, as an adequate biopsy will give the best chance of isolating the organism concerned.

Treatment

Chemotherapy usually involves the use of a sulphonamide given in combination with trimethoprim (co-trimoxazole) or with ampicillin or erythromycin. Prolonged treatment (6–12 months) is needed, continuing for 6 weeks after apparent resolution of the condition.

SYSTEMIC MYCOSES

Mycoses are infections caused by organisms which are classified by morphology as yeasts or filamentous fungi. Yeasts are round or oval and reproduce by budding. Filamentous fungi grow by branching and longitudinal extension of hyphae. This is not a simple distinction, since several organisms can grow in either form, depending on conditions.

CANDIDA INFECTIONS

The range of disease caused by *Candida albicans* is very broad. It is a common commensal of the oral and vaginal mucosae at one extreme. At the other it can cause pneumonia, endocarditis, septicaemia and death.

Candida can become a pathogen on damaged skin, in severely ill patients, in patients who have specific immune deficiency, and in patients receiving broad-spectrum antibiotics when the local microbial ecology is disturbed. Both cell-mediated and humoral immunity participate in control of *Candida*, since specific inherited deficiency of T cell function causes severe but localised disease, whereas in mixed inherited deficiency the infection becomes disseminated. In practice, severely ill patients under intensive care frequently have a mixed immune deficiency and are also receiving antibiotics which predispose to *Candida* infection. Disseminated infections are also seen in intravenous drug abusers. Cutaneous and mucosal surface candidiasis is described in Chapter 26.

Diagnosis of systemic Candida infection

Often candida septicaemia is a terminal event and over half of patients are diagnosed at post-mortem. Clinical signs are usually minimal, but there may be *endophthalmitis* with fluffy yellow/white retinal spots resembling cotton-wool spots, or small *abscesses* may be detected elsewhere, such as in the liver, where ultrasound-guided biopsy or aspiration can clinch the diagnosis. *Pulmonary infiltrates* may occur on chest X-ray, with *Candida* in bronchial washings. Isolation of *Candida* from a single site on one occasion does not necessarily indicate serious infection, even when it comes from a blood culture. Measurements of *Candida* antigen and antibody levels in serum have shown too many false negatives to be valuable in diagnosis, so the judgment that *Candida* is responsible for disease manifestations remains clinical. In view of the difficulty in diagnosis, treatment is given for disseminated candida infection if *Candida* is cultured from more than one site in a severely ill patient in whom there is new evidence of infection (e.g. fever) but bacterial infection is judged to be unlikely.

Treatment

The only effective treatment for disseminated candidiasis is amphotericin B administered intravenously. In view of the possibility that it will cause acute toxicity with hypotension and collapse, an initial test dose is infused. If this is tolerated the full dose is instituted by slow intravenous infusion. If the blood urea level rises, treatment is withheld temporarily. Oral flucytosine is synergistic with amphotericin.

ASPERGILLUS

Aspergillus is a less common fungal pathogen which can cause disseminated disease in terminally ill patients. However, its more common manifestations are a range of respiratory diseases, the nature of which is determined by the immune response of the host (Ch. 14).

CRYPTOCOCCOSIS

Cryptococcosis (torulosis) is a systemic infection with the yeast-like fungus *Cryptococcus neoformans*. The organism is commonly found in soil contaminated by bird droppings, notably those of pigeons. Disease occurs following inhalation of the organism, but it is unusual in immunocompetent people and currently is seen most often in patients with acquired immunodeficiency syndrome (AIDS).

Clinical features

CNS infection causes chronic meningitis with very low-grade symptoms at presentation. Cranial nerve palsies may cause visual abnormalities, loss of acuity or diplopia, or facial weakness and numbness. The course is slow or rapidly progressive, depending on the patient's immune status. Corticosteroid therapy accelerates progression.

Respiratory infection usually occurs in the absence of CNS involvement. It is more chronic and may regress spontaneously.

Skin lesions are found in 10% of patients. The face and scalp are the most common sites of the painless lesions, which are variable nodules, sometimes ulcerating.

Diagnosis

It is important to think of the possibility of cryptococcosis, since routine culture is often negative. In the CSF little abnormality is found, apart from a few cells, mainly lymphocytes, mildly reduced glucose compared to the blood, and slightly raised protein. The organisms may be stained with India ink but the most sensitive method of diagnosis is by detection of antigen in CSF and sometimes in blood.

Treatment

Amphotericin B is the drug most likely to eliminate infection. In view of its toxicity it is encouraging that preliminary reports are appearing of successful treatment with some of the new triazoles such as fluconazole.

HISTOPLASMOSIS

Histoplasma capsulatum is a common environmental fungus found in the soil in a filamentous form, but it behaves as a yeast when it infects humans. It multiplies rapidly in soil containing the droppings of birds and bats, and humans are usually infected by inhalation of spores in infected dust. Infection has been shown to be common by skin test surveys in the eastern central part of the United States, but there are also scattered areas of infection in both temperate and tropical areas of the world. *H. capsulatum var. duboisii* is a variant found in central Africa.

H. capsulatum infects macrophages and the pathogenesis of disease is similar to that of tuberculosis. Delayed hypersensitivity skin tests show that the majority of infected individuals are asymptomatic.

Clinical features of H. capsulatum

Acute pulmonary infection in normal hosts causes a febrile illness with headache, often accompanied by cough and chest pain, with malaise, myalgia and weight loss. Erythema nodosum or multiforme may occur. Symptoms usually last less than a week, but occasionally severe infection is seen following a high inoculation dose and it may even be fatal. Radiological changes occur in only 25% of acute infection, with scattered pulmonary infiltrates and hilar and mediastinal lymphadenopathy. The histoplasmin skin test is not helpful in diagnosis but a complement fixation antibody test may be useful. Treatment is not usually required, as spontaneous resolution is the rule, but in severe cases amphotericin B is given intravenously for 2 or 3 weeks. Imidazoles such as ketoconazole have been used successfully.

Chronic pulmonary histoplasmosis affects normal individuals with structural defects of the lung. Infection of emphysematous lesions causes chronic destructive disease in the lung apices, similar to tuberculosis. Fever may be accompanied by night sweats and one-third of patients have chest pain. Diagnosis requires repeated sputum cultures. Antibody and skin tests are usually unhelpful.

Treatment is problematic, since it is impractical to give long courses of amphotericin B intravenously, but imidazoles have now been shown to be of value. The need for treatment is judged on the basis of clinical severity.

Disseminated histoplasmosis is a rare and often fatal manifestation of infection in immunocompromised hosts. It may be acute, subacute or chronic, depending on the age of the patient (acute is more frequent in infants) and the degree of parasitisation of macrophages (more severe parasitisation causing more acute disease). Fever, hepatosplenomegaly, anaemia, leucopenia, thrombocytopenia and interstitial pneumonia are most common in the acute disseminated form. Intestinal ulceration, Addison's disease, meningitis and endocarditis in the subacute form, and oropharyngeal ulcers occur in the chronic disseminated disease. Diagnosis is by histology and culture of relevant tissues and treatment is as for the other forms of the disease but with a poorer prognosis.

Histoplasma capsulatum var. duboisii

Histoplasma capsulatum var. duboisii infection occurs in Africa. The route of infection is poorly understood; asymptomatic pulmonary infection, with later spread to the skin and bones or inoculation into the skin, is a possibility. Skin, subcutaneous tissues and underlying bone can be affected causing:

1. superficial, cutaneous granuloma
2. subcutaneous granuloma and abscess
3. cutaneous lesions secondary to underlying osteomyelitis.

The cutaneous granulomas present as raised papules, which may later ulcerate. The subcutaneous granulomas present with localised areas of tender induration which can progress to abscess formation and discharge through the skin. Osteomyelitis of flat bones produces discharging sinuses on the skin which may heal spontaneously. Involved skin over affected bone-marrow-containing bone, e.g. sternum, produces vigorous granulomatous responses. Smears from exudate or discharges show numerous large yeast cells. Histological sections of infected tissue show giant cell granulomas with the large yeast cells. Treatment with amphotericin B may be needed in those lesions which show no signs of regression.

COCCIDIOIDOMYCOSIS

Coccidioidomycosis is a fungal infection caused by *Coccidioides immitis*. Its distribution is confined to arid areas of the western hemisphere, including the south-west USA, Central America and some countries of South America. Dust contaminated with fungal spores is the source of infection. Granulomatous responses occur around fungal spherules, while suppurative lesions with leucocytes characterise the tissue response to endospores.

The host response to the organism determines the outcome of disease. Asymptomatic infection occurs in about three-fifths of patients and is detected by skin testing. A smaller number of those infected present with respiratory symptoms, cough, fever and chest pain, with malaise, muscle pains, night sweats and chills. A macular erythematous rash, erythema nodosum and erythema multiforme also may be seen (pp. 1128 and 1129). Radiograph appearances include pneumonitis, hilar adenopathy and pleural effusion. In most of these patients the disease resolves spontaneously. The diagnosis is made by finding the endospore of the organism in material from affected lung. There is a considerable risk of laboratory infection with this organism. Serological tests are an aid to diagnosis. Antigen detection may develop as a routine method of diagnosis. In some patients pulmonary infiltrates and systemic symptoms persist, sometimes with cavitation.

Dissemination of infection from an initial site of pulmonary disease may occur. Pregnant females show increased incidence of dissemination. All tissues and organs of the body may be affected. Meningitis is one of the most severe manifestations of disseminated infection.

Amphotericin B is used in treatment. The main difficulty lies in deciding which patients will benefit from treatment. Persistent, symptomatic pulmonary infection and disseminated infection require chemotherapy.

PARACOCCIDIOIDOMYCOSIS

Paracoccidioidomycosis, or South American blastomycosis, is unrelated to coccidioidomycosis. It is caused by *Paracoccidioides brasiliensis* and occurs exclusively in the area between Mexico and Argentina. The natural environment of the pathogen is uncertain, as is its mode of acquisition by humans, though inhalation is likely.

Clinical features, diagnosis and treatment

Adults usually present with progressive respiratory symptoms, sometimes accompanied by ulcers in the mouth and nose, dysphagia, voice changes, skin lesions and cervical lymphadenopathy.

Diagnosis is usually made by culture or histology, and treatment is with imidazoles (particularly itraconazole), sulphonamides or amphotericin B.

BLASTOMYCOSIS

Blastomycosis is a primarily pulmonary disease caused by the dimorphic fungus *Blastomyces dermatitidis*. It is much less common than histoplasmosis, and it occurs mainly in the eastern United States. The organism has been isolated from soil, and infection may be by inhalation of dust.

Clinical features

Primary infection may be asymptomatic, or it may lead to an acute pneumonia which either resolves spontaneously or progresses to chronic pulmonary disease which may be confused with tuberculosis. Extrapulmonary manifestations are caused by haematogenous spread from the lungs, and the most common is skin disease with verrucous or ulcerative lesions.

Diagnosis is by demonstration of the yeasts in sputum or other specimens, or by culture of the organism. Amphotericin B is the mainstay of therapy but imidazoles have been used successfully.

SPOROTRICHOSIS

Sporothrix schenckii is a dimorphic fungus found in soil, on plants and on plant debris. Infection is uncommon and is seen in the Americas and Africa. Disease usually results from traumatic inoculation into the skin, and the common form is a red painless papule at the site which enlarges and forms a granulomatous plaque that commonly ulcerates. Further lesions often appear proximally along the course of the lymphatics, and regional lymph nodes can be involved. Disseminated disease is rare and usually only occurs in immunosuppressed patients.

Diagnosis is by culture of the organism from skin lesions. Cutaneous lesions are treated with oral potassium iodide, and extracutaneous disease with amphotericin B.

MUCORMYCOSIS

Mucormycoses are a group of similar diseases caused by members of the order Mucorales. The organisms are common in the environment, often growing on fruit or bread. They cause disease almost exclusively in immunosuppressed patients.

Clinical features

In rhinocerebral disease in an uncontrolled diabetic, the fungus invades the palatal, nasal and paranasal sinus mucous membranes, and destructive lesions spread directly back towards the brain. Black necrotic lesions are visible, and from these a variety of secondary bacterial pathogens are often isolated. Pulmonary, cutaneous and intestinal disease may occur.

Diagnosis and treatment

Diagnosis is made by examination of scrapings, and biopsies and cultures are often negative. Successful treatment depends on management of the underlying cause. Amphotericin B is the only useful drug in treatment, but the response is often poor.

Protozoa are single-cell organisms, and man's protozoan parasites have adapted to a range of ecological niches in the human host (Table 12.31). They are a major cause of human disease, especially in Third World countries.

Table 12.31 Classification of protozoa

Gut protozoa
Giardia lamblia
Cryptosporidium
Entamoeba histolytica
Balantidium coli
Isospora belli
Sarcocystis

Genital tract protozoa
Trichomonas vaginalis

Free-living protozoa causing human disease
Naegleria fowleri
Acanthamoeba

Non-pathogenic gut protozoa
Entamoeba coli
Entamoeba hartmanni
Endolimax nana
Iodamoeba beutschlii
Chilomastix mesnili

Tissue and blood protozoa
Toxoplasma gondii
Pneumocystis carinii
Plasmodium species
Babesia species
Trypanosoma gambiense, rhodesiense and *cruzi*
Leishmania species

Fig. 12.19 Scanning electron micrograph of *Giardia lamblia*. (Reproduced by kind permission of Dr David Warhurst.)

PROTOZOAL INFECTION OF THE GUT

GIARDIASIS

Infection with the flagellate protozoan *Giardia lamblia* can cause asymptomatic infection or diarrhoeal disease, of variable severity from mild to severe, with malabsorption.

Aetiology

The parasite is a flagellate, pear-shaped protozoan (Fig. 12.19), which is found in the lumen of the upper small intestine; under influences that are not understood some trophozoites encyst to be passed in the faeces. The cyst is infective for others and can survive for 2 months at 8°C in water. It is resistant to normal levels of chlorination, and sand filtration is used to clear municipal water supplies of this and other parasites. The parasite can now be grown in culture.

Distribution and incidence

The distribution is worldwide, although it is more common in the tropics. It is endemic in the countries of Eastern Europe. Epidemics have occurred at day care nurseries, on cruise ships and in towns in the USA. Giardiasis is fairly common in children in some inner-city populations in Britain, and has caused diarrhoea in the elderly. It is the commonest protozoan parasite reported by microbiology laboratories in England and Wales.

Transmisson and epidemiology

Spread is by the faecal–oral route. As few as 10 cysts will cause infection, while 1000 cysts consistently cause infection. Contaminated food and water are vehicles of infection. Person-to-person spread is common in childhood, particularly when children are not toilet-trained. Mothers are often infected by changing nappies of an infected child. Any circumstances in which standards of personal and public hygiene (such as water treatment) are low lead to transmission.

In the tropics children are most often infected, although both indigenous and visiting adults in endemic areas can develop symptomatic disease. Male homosexuals and retarded children are often infected. Hypogammaglobulinaemia and reduced gastric acid secretion are host factors that increase susceptibility.

Pathology and pathogenesis

The main abnormalities relate to the function and morphology of the upper small intestine. Markedly symptomatic patients have impaired absorption of fat, d-xylose and vitamin B$_{12}$, and lactose maldigestion. The jejunal mucosa is abnormal, with a ridged or convoluted mucosa on dissecting microscopy and reduced villous height with increased crypt depth, and an increased infiltrate of plasma cells in the lamina propria. The changes are moderate. Subtotal villous atrophy may occur with giardiasis but is uncommon. Patients with mild or no symptoms have normal jejunal morphology and function. Lactose maldigestion may be present.

The pathogenesis is not well understood but there is a growing body of evidence to suggest that the parasite itself may damage the enterocyte surface membrane to impair function and cause increased rates of cell loss from the jejunal mucosa. Jejunal colonisation with bacteria may also contribute to some of the mucosal dysfunction. It seems likely that parasite numbers in the gut lumen are controlled by antigiardia IgA secreted from the mucosa and in bile. This antibody may bind to trophozoites and immobilise them, allowing them to be washed away down the gut.

Clinical features

The incubation period is usually about 10–14 days, although it can be much longer. Many patients with giardiasis are asymptomatic or have minimal bowel upset. Acute giardiasis is characterised by the sudden onset of anorexia, nausea, abdominal distension, discomfort and diarrhoea with frequent yellow, offensive, frothy stools by day and night. Lethargy is often severe and weight loss is usual. There is no systemic upset. After about 3 weeks there may be the beginnings of spontaneous improvement. This may progress to complete resolution over a month. Some people remain mildly symptomatic, often because of continuing lactose intolerance.

Some patients remain markedly symptomatic, and fail to regain lost weight or continue to lose weight. Examination in this group shows evidence of weight loss with loss of muscle bulk. The abdomen is distended and bowel sounds are prominent. The stools are yellow and offensive. These people have malabsorption clinically and objective testing confirms this. Children are occasionally brought to medical attention because of failure to thrive. Giardiasis has been reported as a cause of chronic diarrhoea in elderly persons in the United Kingdom.

Diagnosis

Diagnosis depends on finding the parasite. Stool microscopy shows cysts in most patients, although examination of several samples may be necessary. Trophozoites may be found in diarrhoeal stools. When the parasite is not found and symptoms are marked, investigation of intestinal morphology and function is indicated. Jejunal juice and jejunal mucus obtained at the time of biopsy can be examined for trophozoites. Giardia may be seen in the intervillous spaces of the sections of the biopsy. Giardia antigens can be detected in stools by immunological techniques. This type of test may become routine in parasitological diagnosis in the future.

Differential diagnosis

A range of viral and bacterial pathogens cause acute diarrhoea. Cryptosporidiosis causes self-limiting diarrhoea in healthy persons (see below). *Campylobacter* species can cause a small bowel type of diarrhoea but usually cause systemic upset. Among causes of chronic diarrhoea with weight loss, tropical sprue, intestinal tuberculosis and chronic calcific pancreatitis are conditions that must be considered in the tropical areas. In temperate areas of the world coeliac disease, jejunal diverticulosis, intestinal strictures and other anatomical lesions need to be considered.

Laboratory features

Laboratory investigations show malabsorption of fat, d-xylose and vitamin B$_{12}$ in severely affected patients. D-xylose malabsorption and lactose maldigestion may be present in those with mild symptoms. Occasional patients are seen who have marked malabsorption and folate deficiency. Barium follow-through examinations show non-specific changes, with dilatation of small bowel loops and thickened mucosal folds in patients with malabsorption.

Treatment

Metronidazole is the drug of first choice, given either as a low dose (200 mg 3 times a day) for 10–14 days, or as a high dose (2 g daily) for 3 days. Tinidazole is more expensive but can be given as a single dose of 2 g (50 mg/kg in children). Both drugs cause nausea in high dose and have a disulfiram-like interaction with alcohol. Asymptomatic giardiasis in pregnancy need not be treated. When there is symptomatic disease in pregnancy associated with weight loss or failure to gain weight, then metronidazole (200 mg 3 times a day for 10 days) may be given. Symptoms due to giardiasis improve rapidly after treatment. Dietary measures are sometimes helpful for continuing gut symptoms. Avoidance of alcohol, spicy foods and lactose is often helpful. Repeat stool microscopy 6–8 weeks after treatment provides a test of cure. Abnormalities in intestinal structure and function disappear over 6–12 weeks after treatment.

Prevention and control

Travellers in areas where the tap water is not safe to drink should avoid salads, uncooked foods, unpeeled fruits and ice cubes in drinks. Sterilising drinking water with 2% tincture of iodine (0.5 ml/l of water and allow to stand for 30 minutes) may be necessary. Treatment of asymptomatic cyst excreters is worthwhile, particularly in a non-endemic area, as it reduces the risk of transmission to others.

CRYPTOSPORIDIOSIS

Cryptosporidiosis is an infection of the gastrointestinal tract with the sporozoan parasite *Cryptosporidium*. It causes enteritis in man and a range of other animals. It is a zoonosis with a worldwide distribution.

Its life cycle is complex, with asexual and sexual cycles. Infection is by the faecal–oral route. Ingested oocysts are disrupted in the intestinal lumen, liberating four sporozoites which enter the apical regions of intestinal cells within a membrane-bounded vacuole. Trophozoites develop from the sporozoites and undergo asexual reproduction. Merozoites liberated by schizogony can undergo further asexual cycles, or become gametocytes which fuse to form oocysts which are passed in the faeces.

Transmission and epidemiology

Early reports recognised this organism as a gut pathogen causing persisting watery diarrhoea in immunosuppressed patients, especially those with AIDS. Later studies showed that cryptospiridiosis was associated with diarrhoea in 4–9% of otherwise healthy children and adults. Children at nursery school may transmit infection person-to-person. Susceptible animals include calves, lambs, goats and birds, although a history of contact with animals is often absent.

Clinical features

An acute watery diarrhoeal illness, often with offensive stools, is the usual history. There may be fever and vomiting. The disease is self-limiting, with a median duration of about 12 days, but prolonged diarrhoea with weight loss occurs in patients with humoral and cellular immunodeficiency states, especially AIDS.

Diagnosis

Faecal smears stained by the modified Ziehl-Neelsen technique show the pinkish-red-staining oocysts. Other forms of the parasite are seen at the luminal surface of enterocytes in intestinal biopsies.

Treatment

In most patients the disease is self-limiting and symptoms resolve spontaneously in 10–12 days. There have been reports of successful treatment of symptomatic immunosuppressed persons with oral spiramycin (3.0 g per day in divided doses) but relapses do occur.

Prevention and control

Hand washing is the most important factor in limiting the spread of infection by the person-to-person route.

AMOEBIASIS

Amoebiasis is infection with *Entamoeba histolytica*. The infection may be:

1. non-invasive and confined to the lumen of the colon
2. invasive, causing colonic ulceration (amoebic dysentery)
3. invasive, causing amoeboma
4. invasive, with spread to the liver to cause amoebic liver abscess.

Aetiology

Entamoeba histolytica has two forms, a motile trophozoite (Fig. 12.20) and an encysted trophozoite. The motile trophozoite is found in the stools of a person with amoebic dysentery and contains ingested red cells. The cyst is the infective form. It is resistant to the chlorine in potable domestic water supplies. Sand filtration is the best method of removing cysts from water.

Fig. 12.20 *Scanning electron micrograph of* Entamoeba histolytica. (Reproduced by kind permission of Dr David Warhurst.)

Distribution and incidence

Amoebiasis has a worldwide distribution. It is common in those areas of the world where standards of sanitation are low. Most instances of invasive disease occur either in endemic areas or in travellers who have recently been exposed. Occasional cases are seen in people who returned from endemic areas years before, or who have never left a country such as Britain.

Transmission and epidemiology

Faecal-oral spread by ingestion of amoebic cysts in contaminated food and water or on fingers or other direct personal contact is the route of infection. Asymptomatic amoebiasis is not uncommon in male homosexuals in Britain with transmission by person-to-person spread, and this route of infection also occurs in the mentally retarded.

Amoebiasis is more common in adults than children. Men tend to be affected by amoebic liver abscess more often than women but dysenteric disease occurs in both sexes. Invasive amoebiasis can be more severe in pregnancy.

Pathology and pathogenesis

There are no pathological changes in those persons who are asymptomatic cyst excreters. Their amoebae live on the colonic mucosa but do not invade. Not all organisms are capable of causing invasive disease, but the reasons for this are not well understood. Trophozoites invade the colonic epithelium in amoebic dysentery and lyse host cells on contact. Necrosis is the main feature of invasive amoebiasis. Areas of the mucosa are excavated and the overlying epithelium disintegrates, leaving multiple flask-shaped ulcers. Amoebae are found in the slough and in the advancing edge of the lesions. The rectum and caecum are commonly affected areas, but the extent can vary from localised proctitis to a pancolitis with a diffusely inflamed ulcerated mucosa.

Amoeboma is an uncommon late complication occurring after amoebic dysentery has resolved. The lesion consists of a mass of granulation tissue containing few amoebae. The caecum is a usual site but any part can be involved and lesions may be multiple.

Amoebic liver abscess (ALA) results from the haematogenous spread of amoebae from the colonic mucosa via the portal vein. Amoebae reach the liver, and liver cells are lysed on contact with amoebae. The affected area enlarges progressively and the necrotic cells liquefy in the abscess cavity, which may be unilocular or multilocular. A single abscess in the right lobe is usual. Multiple abscesses are unusual, as is involvement of the left lobe of the liver. The contents of the abscess are bacteriologically sterile on culture and contain few pus cells. The pus is typically odourless and pinkish-brown, but cream or yellow-coloured pus may be found.

Clinical features

No symptoms are attributable to the commensal amoeba. In the patient with amoebic dysentery symptoms vary according to the extent and site of colonic involvement. The usual symptoms are abdominal discomfort and increased frequency of bowel action, with softer stools. Blood may be noticed in the stools, especially when the rectum is involved. Physical signs usually consist of mild colonic tenderness. Sigmoidoscopy may show the typical appearance: scattered ulcers are surrounded by mucosal erythema with normal mucosa intervening, but the mucosa may be diffusely inflamed and ulcerated. With increasing extent of colonic disease, symptoms and signs are more marked.

Dehydration, anaemia and septicaemia may occur in severe disease, and perforation, toxic dilatation and significant haemorrhage may complicate the clinical course. Rarely the superficial part of the mucosa may be sloughed over a variable length of colon and passed per rectum. Late complications of amoebic dysentery are colonic stricture

and amoeboma, where a mass of granulation tissue forms in response to the presence of relatively few amoebae. Localised pain and blood in the stools are usual symptoms and one or more masses may be felt in the abdomen or rectally.

Symptoms and signs in ALA

Symptoms and signs in ALA relate to the site and size of the abscess. There may be no history to suggest past or present intestinal amoebiasis and many patients do not have amoebic cysts in their stools. Fever, sweats, lethargy and anorexia are usual early symptoms and examination may reveal no abnormal physical signs, or only tenderness on springing the right lower rib cage. With larger abscesses pain becomes a more prominent feature related to the site of the abscess. This pain may be continuous when the abscess is sited in the lower part of the right lobe. Abscesses sited laterally or superiorly cause chest pain which may be pleuritic, or referred pain in the right shoulder or scapular region indicating diaphragmatic irritation. Rigors occur with multiple large abscesses.

The liver may be palpably enlarged and tender, with a localised tender mass on the surface. Physical signs at the base of the right lung are found with superiorly sited abscesses, causing dullness to percussion and impaired movement. Absence of breath sounds indicates an effusion or collapse of lung. Palpation with the fingertip in the intercostal spaces may reveal a point of localised tenderness. Left lobe abscesses may present with symptoms and signs related to the epigastrium or left hypochondrium.

Complications

The main complication in ALA is extension outside the liver (Fig. 12.21). Spread to the brain occasionally occurs, where a necrotising abscess-like lesion is produced. Rarely

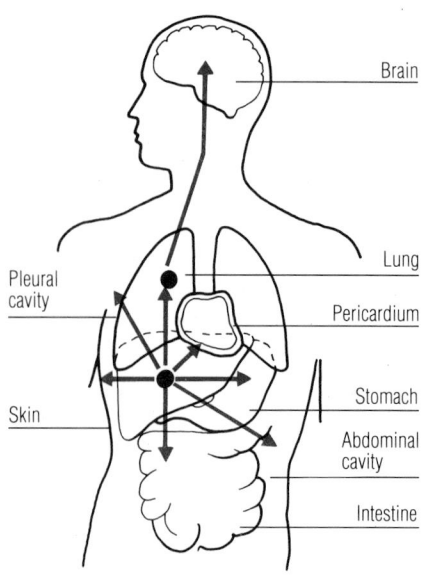

Fig. 12.21 Sites of spread of amoebic liver abscess.

the skin of the peri-anal region is ulcerated by local extension of amoebic proctitis, and the skin of the chest or abdominal wall is involved after percutaneous rupture of ALA.

Diagnosis

Cyst passer

Amoebiasis is usually diagnosed when stool microscopy is carried out during screening after overseas travel or residence, investigation of diarrhoea due to some other microbial pathogen, or examination of other groups at risk of infection, e.g. male homosexuals or the mentally retarded. Serological tests for amoebiasis are negative.

Amoebic dysentery

Amoebic dysentery is diagnosed by finding motile trophozoites with ingested red cells in faecal smears or scrapes from ulcerated colonic mucosa. Amoebae can be seen in the edges of ulcers in rectal biopsies. Serological tests for amoebiasis (e.g. indirect fluorescent antibody test, or IFA) are positive in 60% of cases. Diagnosis depends on finding the parasite.

Amoeboma

Amoebic cysts may be found in the stools. Colonoscopy allows the lesion to be visualised and biopsied. Serology for amoebiasis is positive in over 90% of cases and is a reliable test in this situation.

Amoebic liver abscess

Diagnosis of amoebic liver abscess depends on the clinical features suggesting an intrahepatic lesion and strongly positive amoebic serology (found in over 95% of cases). Cases seen early in the course of disease occasionally have a negative IFA but have a definitely positive test 7 days later.

Additional investigations

Intestinal disease

With increasing extent of colonic involvement there is increasing exudation of protein-rich fluid into the gut. Plasma albumin levels fall; normochromic, normocytic anaemia and a raised sedimentation rate develop. These investigations are normal in more localised disease. Barium enema studies show non-specific features with ulceration in dysentery. Amoeboma appears as one or more mass lesions, causing narrowing of the colon, simulating colon cancer.

Amoebic liver abscess

There is neutrophil leucocytosis, a normochromic, normocytic anaemia and raised ESR. Bilirubin levels are usually normal, while aminotransferase levels are slightly raised; alkaline phosphatase levels are raised and plasma albumin levels are low.

Imaging techniques allow accurate localisation. A chest X-ray will show elevation of the diaphragm above an abscess in the right lobe superiorly, and sometimes basal linear atelectasis or consolidation or pleural effusion. Isotope liver scanning with technetium shows a 'cold' area at the site. Ultrasound scanning and computerised tomography scanning give more accurate information about the abscess, and its precise site and size. Ultrasound scanning is particularly useful. It can be repeated frequently to assess changes and it can be used to guide insertion of a needle for percutaneous aspiration.

Differential diagnosis

Intestinal disease

All causes of infective colitides enter the differential diagnosis: *Shigella*, *Salmonella*, *Campylobacter* and *Yersinia* infections all may cause colitis. Non-specific inflammatory bowel disease, Crohn's colitis and ulcerative colitis must be considered. If amoebic infection may be a cause of disease in a patient, this should be rigorously excluded before treatment for non-specific inflammatory bowel disease is started, as steroids may promote rapid progression of invasive amoebiasis with perforation and death. Carcinoma of the colon, tuberculosis of the ileocaecal region or colon, and schistosomiasis are possible causes of a colonic mass.

Amoebic liver abscess

Subphrenic and intrahepatic pyogenic abscesses cause similar symptoms and signs. Often the history is more acute and the patient more toxic with chills and rigors, but their presence does not exclude amoebic infection. Abscess in these sites is often secondary to intra-abdominal sepsis and surgery, although primary pyogenic liver abscess does occur. Primary hepatoma and bacterial infection of a hydatid cyst often present like ALA.

Treatment

The drug treatment of amoebiasis is set out in Table 12.32. Symptoms and signs improve rapidly within 48 hours. Surgical treatment of amoebic dysentery is rarely needed, except where large areas of mucosa are sloughed; in this case resection of the affected colon can be life-saving.

When amoebic liver abscesses are very large, or are pointing or are likely to rupture, percutaneous aspiration is needed. This is done using a large-bore needle inserted under local anaesthetic, if possible under ultrasound guidance. Variable amounts of fluid can be removed. Amoebae are sometimes found in the material aspirated from the edge of the abscess. Aspiration has a low morbidity. Rupture of ALA dramatically increases the mortality, which is low in uncomplicated cases.

12

Table 12.32 Drug treatment of amoebiasis

Clinical situation	Drug
Cyst passer	Diloxanide furoate 500 mg 3 times a day (8 mg/kg 3 times a day)
Amoebic dysentery Amoeboma Amoebic liver abscess	Metronidazole 800 mg 3 times a day for 5–10 days (40 mg/kg per day in 3 divided doses) or Tinidazole 750 mg twice a day for 5–10 days (12.5 mg/kg twice a day) followed by Diloxanide furoate 500 mg 3 times a day (8 mg/kg 3 times a day)

Prevention and control

The provision of clean water and safe disposal of faecal wastes would do much to prevent transmission. Patients with invasive amoebiasis should always receive diloxanide furoate as well as metronidazole to eradicate any pathogenic amoebae remaining in the gut lumen. Where water supplies are not treated, boiling and filtering drinking water is advised. Tincture of iodine (2%) is effective in killing amoebae used as above. Salads, unpeeled fruits and ice cubes are possible sources of infection with amoebae and other gut pathogens and should be avoided in endemic areas.

BALANTIDIUM COLI INFECTION

The ciliate *Balantidium coli* is the largest of man's protozoan parasites. It can be seen with the naked eye in cultures. It is a parasite of pigs, and humans who have close contact with pigs become infected. It causes no disease in most infected humans. Occasional cases of enteritis affecting small and large intestine due to *B. coli* are reported. Death occurs as a result of bacterial peritonitis after ulceration and perforation of the gut. Metronidazole is effective in symptomatic cases.

ISOSPORA BELLI INFECTION

Isospora belli is a sporozoan parasite of the gastrointestinal tract in man. It has a worldwide distribution and man is the only reservoir of infection. The life cycle has asexual and sexual phases. Infection occurs by ingestion of oocysts containing sporozoites which are released in the small intestine and invade epithelial cells; there they undergo asexual reproduction, or schizogony. The host cell ruptures, releasing merozoites which invade other epithelial cells and which reproduce asexually to form oocysts. These are released into the gut lumen by the normal des-

quamation of epithelial cells and passed in the faeces. Infection occurs by ingesting oocysts in contaminated food and water.

Most infections cause no symptoms. Some cause a diarrhoeal illness, with weight loss, pale stools, lethargy and low-grade fever. Patients with immunodeficiency syndromes including AIDS exhibit chronic diarrhoea with more marked symptoms.

The diagnosis is made by finding oocysts in stools, jejunal juice and in stained sections of jejunal biopsies.

Co-trimoxazole appears to be effective in treatment, giving 2 tablets twice daily for 10 days. Longer courses of treatment may be needed in patients with immunodeficiency.

SARCOCYSTOSIS

Two species of sarcocystis are recognised parasites of man; they are *Sarcocystis bovihominis* and *Sarcocystis suihominis*, which have cattle and pigs as their intermediate hosts respectively. The parasites have a worldwide distribution, with infection rates of up to 100% in cattle and pigs. However, the infection is not common in man. The parasites have a complex life cycle involving both asexual and sexual reproduction.

Volunteer infections have shown abdominal discomfort, distension, nausea and diarrhoea within hours of infection, and sporocysts were found in the stools 14–18 days later. A small series of cases has been reported from Thailand, but it may be that these parasites cause more gastrointestinal disease than we presently appreciate. Diagnosis requires zinc sulphate flotation to concentrate the small numbers of cysts shed in the faeces.

Treatment with pyrimethamine and sulphadiazine or nitrofurantoin has been successful in patients with chronic symptoms. Freezing meat reduces the infectivity of muscle cysts, and thorough cooking of meat prevents infection.

GENITAL TRACT PROTOZOA

TRICHOMONIASIS

Trichomonas vaginalis (TV) is a pear-shaped, flagellate protozoan. It causes vaginal discharge and urethritis in women and urethritis in men. It is a sexually transmitted infection.

Clinical features

Most women with TV have an offensive vaginal discharge associated with vulvovaginal pruritus, and occasionally dysuria and dyspareunia. Clinically the vulva is erythematous and excoriated; the vaginal discharge may be seen at the introitus. The discharge is grey, yellow or green and may be frothy. Vaginal erythema and punctate haemorrhages of the cervix may be seen.

In men TV is a rare cause of non-specific urethritis.

Diagnosis

Examination of the discharge on a wet mount is essential. The trichomonads are easily seen.

Treatment

Metronidazole (200 mg 3 times a day for 7 days; or 400 mg twice daily for 5 days) is effective but recurrences are common. Sexual partners should be treated. Single doses of tinidazole (2.0 g, or 50 mg/kg) are very effective.

FREE-LIVING PROTOZOA CAUSING HUMAN DISEASE

NAEGLERIA FOWLERI INFECTION

Naegleria fowleri is a free-living amoebo-flagellate which causes primary amoebic meningo-encephalitis. It is found in water from hot springs as well as in ponds and pools, and has a worldwide distribution. Amoebae in fresh water are carried into the nasal passages by activities like swimming. They adhere to areas of the nasal mucosae bearing terminal filaments of the olfactory nerves, and then migrate through the cribriform plate along the nerve fibres. The amoebae replicate asexually and spread through the subarachnoid space.

Pathology

The olfactory bulbs show massive invasion with amoebae and necrotic changes. There is a superfical encephalitis of the affected areas. In the meninges there is a prominent fibrinous and purulent reaction that is most marked over the infero-medial regions, with particular involvement of the basal subarachnoid cisterns. The amoebae, which are circular and 6–9 μ in diameter, have a fine cell membrane.

Clinical features

The patients are often children or young adults. Fever, headache, nausea, vomiting and lethargy are usual early features, followed by deterioration of conscious level. Neck stiffness is usual. Papilloedema may be present.

Lumbar puncture in these patients shows features suggesting acute pyogenic meningitis. The cerebrospinal fluid (CSF) is turbid, with a very high cell count, predominantly neutrophils. Protein levels are very high and sugar levels are reduced or normal. The amoebae are readily seen on phase contrast microscopy if a direct smear of CSF is examined. They stain well with iron haemotoxylin and can be grown in special culture media.

Treatment

Amphotericin B is effective in treatment, possibly in combination with miconazole. The high mortality in this condition is probably related to delay in diagnosis and initial trials of antibiotics, as for pyogenic meningitis.

ACANTHAMOEBA INFECTION

Acanthamoebae are free-living amoebae. Infection may occur by ingestion or inhalation of cysts, which are very light and may be distributed on the wind.

A considerable range of clinical features has been reported for this infection. Cerebral abscess, meningitis and involvement of the scalp, orbit and middle ear have occurred. Acanthamoeba have been identified in corneal ulcers. Lung involvement has also been reported. Amoebae may be identified in smears from cerebrospinal fluid or from corneal ulcers, or in stained tissue sections. Amphotericin B is used in systemic infections, and 5-flurocytosine and clotrimazole can be used topically on corneal ulcers.

NON-PATHOGENIC GUT PROTOZOA

There are a number of protozoa which infect man but cause no disease. These are listed in Table 12.31. When they are found in patients with abdominal symptoms, the symptoms should not be ascribed to these parasites and further investigations should be undertaken.

TISSUE AND BLOOD PROTOZOA

TOXOPLASMOSIS

Toxoplasmosis is caused by *Toxoplasma gondii*. It is a zoonosis, the definitive host in the life cycle being cats. Primary human infection is acquired by ingestion of oocysts derived from animal excreta or from undercooked meats such as pork or mutton, the pig or sheep having acted as an intermediate host (Fig. 12.22). Infection is common, 20–40% of adults in Britain having antibodies. The most serious effects are seen after congenital infection or in immunocompromised patients.

Pathology and pathogenesis

Trophozoites released at the site of entry multiply and

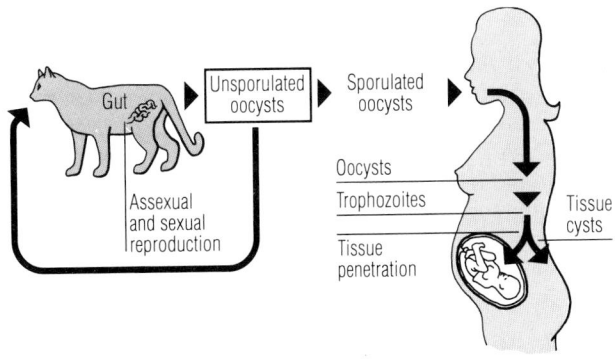

Fig. 12.22 Transmission of toxoplasmosis. Infection can occur in either sex and at any age. Reactivation causes disease in immunosuppressed patients.

spread via blood and lymphatics to all tissues. They can invade any cells, and intracellular proliferation leads to cell death. Development of immunity results in restriction of proliferation and the organism is eliminated, or forms tissue cysts. Cysts 10–200 mm in diameter, containing several thousand organisms, may remain in the tissues for life. Depression of cell-mediated immunity results in reactivation.

Clinical features

Congenital infection

Congenital infection usually follows primary asymptomatic infection of the mother during the third trimester of pregnancy. The effect on the fetus may be spontaneous abortion, stillbirth, premature birth or normal birth with subsequent illness. The latter outcome is most frequent and results in disease of the eye, usually bilateral choroidoretinitis, or of the brain, with hydrocephalus, microcephaly, cerebral calcification or convulsions. Fever, lymphadenopathy, hepatosplenomegaly and rash may also occur.

Acquired infection

Asymptomatic infection is common in adults, but there may be a mild chronic febrile illness with lymphadenopathy. Often a group of enlarged lymph nodes in a single area is the only finding, although more diffuse adenopathy may occur with splenomegaly. Sore throat does not occur. Choroidoretinitis is a rare manifestation of acquired infection.

Reactivation in the immunosuppressed patient

Most toxoplasmal disease in patients with deficient immunity is caused by reactivation of latent cysts. The most common manifestation is necrotising lesions in the brain, often presenting as intracerebral mass lesions; these have been a major problem in patients with acquired immunodeficiency syndrome (AIDS). Myocarditis and possibly pneumonitis have also occurred.

Diagnosis

Serology is the mainstay of diagnosis. The Sabin-Feldman dye test, indirect haemagglutination or fluorescent antibody tests (FAT) are used to measure IgG antibodies, and an FAT is also available for measurement of IgM antibodies. Histology of affected lymph nodes shows reactive changes which are not specific for toxoplasmosis. The organisms are rarely seen in tissue sections. Diagnosis of cerebral lesions is helped by computerised tomography.

Treatment

Acquired infection in normal adults rarely requires treatment and there is no evidence that specific treatment affects the prolonged lethargy which sometimes follows such disease. Severe infections are treated with a combination of pyrimethamine and sulphadimidine (e.g. Sulphatriad), which are synergistic in their action against trophozoites. Pyrimethamine is a folic acid antagonist and causes bone marrow suppression, which can be prevented by concurrent administration of folinic acid.

There is no treatment for tissue cysts.

PNEUMOCYSTIS CARINII INFECTION

Pneumocystis carinii is a common organism that is found worldwide. Although currently classified as a protozoan, recent evidence suggests that it may be fungal in nature. It infects the lungs and causes no problems in normal human hosts. The organism is found in autopsy material from healthy people in up to 4% of cases and serological studies in Europe have shown up to 75% seropositivity in healthy children. The reservoirs of infection and the mode of transmission are poorly defined, but it seems likely that human-to-human droplet infection occurs.

It causes interstitial pneumonitis in premature and young infants, in children with protein-energy malnutrition, in immunosuppressed patients during treatment for haematological malignancies, and in patients with AIDS.

In normal lung the organisms are found singly or in clusters on the alveolar septal wall, with no surrounding host response. When there is pneumonitis large numbers of parasites are found in the alveoli, with desquamation of alveolar cells and accumulation of proteinaceous material in the alveolar spaces.

Clinical features and diagnosis

The clinical features of *Pn. carinii* pneumonia are progressive dyspnoea, cough, fever and weight loss. Chest examination is often normal; chest radiographs may be normal initially but progress fairly rapidly to show extensive interstitial shadowing. The diagnosis should be suspected in any immunosuppressed patients, especially those with AIDS, and confirmation is obtained from examination of bronchial washings obtained at bronchoscopy or in sputum induced using nebulised hypertonic saline.

Treatment

The treatment is adequate oxygenation and ventilatory support when necessary, and chemotherapy with either high-dose co-trimoxazole (4 tablets 4 times a day) or pentamidine given by intramuscular injection or slow intravenous infusion in 250 ml of normal saline or 5% dextrose over 1–2 hours. Nebulised pentamidine is effective in treatment and prophylaxis in AIDS patients. Studies in children with malignancies and adults with AIDS have shown no difference in outcome with either drug. Fever, rash and leucopenia have been seen in patients with AIDS after about 7–10 days on co-trimoxazole, and a change to pentamidine may be necessary, as treatment for at least 21 days is required. Pentamidine side-effects include renal and hepatic failure and prolonged hypoglycaemia. There is a 20% mortality in AIDS patients in their first episode of *Pn. carinii*, irrespective of treatment. Prophylaxis with co-trimoxazole for this infection has been effective in patients with acute leukaemia. Prophylaxis in AIDS patients with drugs combining an antifolate with a sulphonamide/sulphone may be of value, and nebulised pentamidine has also been used successfully.

MALARIA

Malaria is an acute febrile illness characterised clinically by paroxysms of fever; these are the consequence of asexual reproduction by species of *Plasmodium* within red cells (schizogony). *Plasmodium vivax*, *P. ovale* and *P. malariae* are associated with morbidity but no major mortality, while *P. falciparum* causes both morbidity and considerable mortality. The infection is transmitted by the bite of the female anopheline mosquito.

Distribution and incidence

Malaria occurs widely throughout the tropical areas of the world, in the Americas, Africa, Asia and the Pacific area (Fig. 12.23). *Falciparum* malaria is particularly common in tropical Africa, where it causes about 1 000 000 deaths per

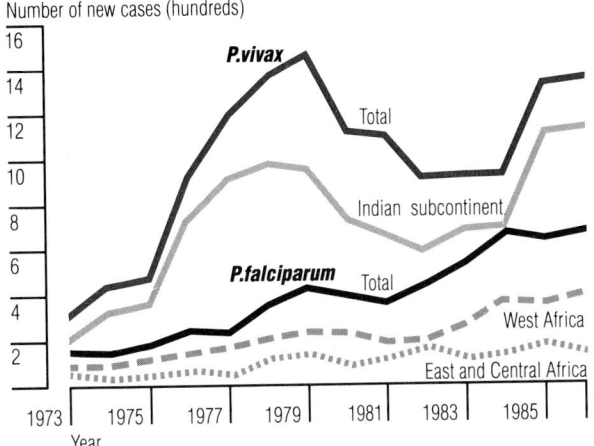

Number of new cases (hundreds)

Fig. 12.24 Incidence and sources of malaria in the UK, 1973–1986 (Communicable Diseases Surveillance Centre, Colindale).

A

B

Fig. 12.23 Malaria. **A.** World distribution of malaria, 1986. **B.** World distribution of chloroquine-resistant malaria (Both WHO).

year, mainly in children. The resurgence of malaria in the Indian subcontinent was led by a rising incidence of *vivax* malaria in the 1970s, and now *falciparum* infection is more widespread in the region. *Ovale* malaria is predominantly an East African disease. *Malariae* malaria is the least common form.

Malaria is imported into temperate regions by tourists, people employed overseas, business travellers and immigrants. The numbers of cases have progressively risen over the past 20 years (Fig. 12.24).

Transmission and epidemiology

Life cycle

The life cycle is shown in Figure 12.25. *Vivax* and *ovale* life cycles are similar, with primary exo-erythrocytic schizogony (EES) in hepatocytes leading to infection of the peripheral blood with merozoites. These enter red blood cells (rbcs) and undergo erythrocytic schizogony (ES) every 48 hours; this is benign tertian and *ovale* tertian malaria. Some of the sporozoites produce latent forms, the hypnozoites, within liver cells, and these produce EES and then ES up to 2 or 3 years after infection, i.e. relapsing malaria.

Falciparum malaria has no hypnozoite form, and so the infection is cured when parasites are cleared from the blood by treatment. Erythrocytic schizogony has a periodicity of less than 48 hours and 'subtertian malaria' is one of the names for this type of malaria. *Malariae* parasites lack the hypnozoite stage but can cause re-appearance of parasitaemia (parasites in peripheral rbcs) up to 20 or more years after infection, i.e. recrudescence. Small numbers of parasites persist in rbcs to cause this. The periodicity of ES is 72 hours (quartan malaria).

Vivax, *ovale* and *malariae* parasites invade 1–2% of rbcs at most. *Falciparum* parasites invade any proportion of RBCs and this accounts for the severity of disease and high mortality.

297

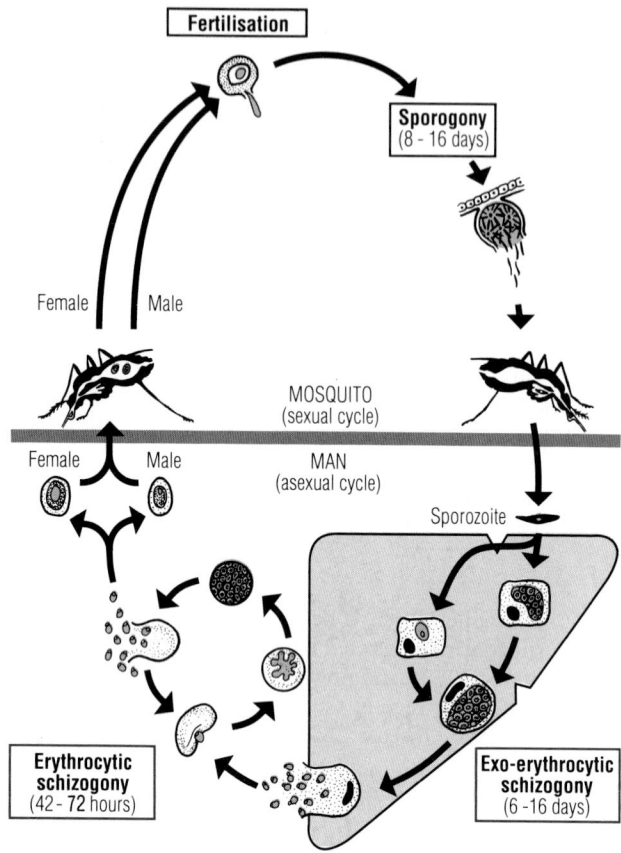

Fig. 12.25 Life cycle of malaria.

Host

A baby born of an indigenous mother in an endemic *falciparum* area will be protected against infection during the first year of life by maternal antimalaria IgG crossing the placenta in the last trimester of pregnancy. This passive immunity wanes during the first year, leaving the child fully susceptible. Without chemoprophylaxis the child experiences repeated attacks of malaria, and by the age of 4 or 5 years will have acquired protective immunity; this persists while he remains in the endemic area. Parasites are often found in the peripheral blood of an asymptomatic child. The immunity declines if an individual leaves the endemic area. Maternal immunity declines during pregnancy, particularly in primapara, with transplacental transfer of IgG. Anaemia, fever and intense parasitisation of placenta make miscarriage, premature labour and low birth weight common, especially in areas such as West Africa where there is heavy, seasonal transmission with a high risk of infection. Where transmission is not so intense, effective immunity is not built up and all ages in the exposed population are at risk.

Any individual, of any age, from a malaria-free area may contract severe malaria. Sickle cell trait protects against severe malaria, and the heterozygous state for glucose-6-phosphate dehydrogenase (G6PD) deficiency is also protective.

Vector

Climatic factors have a profound influence on the transmission of malaria through effects on survival and reproduction of the mosquito population, and on the development of the parasite in the vector. Mosquitoes survive up to several months and their lifespan is not affected by malaria parasites. Ambient temperatures in the range 20–30°C, with a relative humidity of 60% or more, are ideal. Sporogony will not occur below 16° or above 33°C. The vector species vary considerably in different localities. *Anopheles gambiae* is one of the most effective vectors.

Additional routes

Additional routes for transmission of malaria are:

1. *transplacental*, which is uncommon
2. *transfusion-associated*, which is uncommon in Europe and North America but common in endemic areas
3. *syringe-transmitted*, among intravenous drug abusers who share syringes.

Pathogenesis and pathology

The pathogenesis of malaria is complex and incompletely understood. Most attention has been directed to *falciparum* infections. The initial steps are concerned with adhesion of the merozoite to the erythrocyte membrane. Glycophorin A is the major glycoprotein on erythrocyte membranes and is a receptor for binding specific surface proteins of the merozoites. Red cells deficient in glycophorin A are resistant to invasion. The Duffy blood group antigen is a specific receptor for invasion by *P. vivax* merozoites.

The parasitised red cell is less flexible than normal and develops small projections on the erythrocyte surface membrane. These result in sequestration of rbcs containing *mature* trophozoites in the postcapillary venules. (Mature trophozoites are not seen in peripheral blood films.) Maximum numbers of adherent rbcs are found in venules in brain, liver, spleen, kidney and lung. The trophozoite matures into the schizont and at schizogony the red cell membrane bursts, releasing merozoites, malaria antigen, malaria pigment and red cell cytoplasmic constituents. This may damage the endothelium further locally and possibly more generally. The cycle continues, progressively building up the numbers of parasitised red cells.

How these changes lead to altered consciousness in cerebral malaria is not clear. Computerised tomography of the brain in patients with cerebral malaria has not shown oedema. Diffuse irreversible vascular obstruction is also an unlikely cause, in view of normal cerebral flow and complete recovery without neurological deficit in those surviving. Cerebrospinal fluid lactate levels are increased in cerebral malaria and this may indicate some degree of anaerobic cerebral glycolysis.

Renal damage occurs because of pre-renal and renal factors. Acute tubular necrosis is the usual effect of severe malaria on the kidney. This may occur both with and without severe intravascular haemolysis. Vessels in the heart are parasitised but cardiac function is well preserved. Reduced peripheral vascular resistance, dehydration from sweating, vomiting and reduced fluid intake may contribute to hypotension.

In cerebral malaria the brain shows swelling with small haemorrhages throughout the white matter. The spleen is enlarged and has a slate-grey hue over the normal red colour. Centrilobular necrosis is seen in the liver with the accumulation of malaria pigment in Küpffer cells. The pulmonary venules contain large numbers of parasitised red cells. Pulmonary oedema may occur but the cause is not understood. The placenta is usually heavily parasitised. The above are seen at post-mortem.

The anaemia of malaria has several causes which include rupture of parasitised red cells in schizogony, sequestration of red cells in tissue venules, destruction of parasitised red cells in the reticulo-endothelial system (especially the spleen), haemolysis due to the presence of malaria antigen, antibodies and complement on rbcs and marrow suppression. Abnormalities of coagulation are usual with low platelet counts due to peripheral consumption and consumption of clotting factors. Disseminated intravascular coagulation does occur in a few patients with severe malaria but is probably not a major factor in pathogenesis.

Clinical features

Vivax and ovale

After an incubation period of about 13 days (*vivax*) or 18 days (*ovale*), prodromal symptoms – headache, fever, shivering without rigors, and general aches – begin. These last for up to 3 days before the first paroxysm of coldness, then extreme heat, then defervescence with a profuse sweat. Forty-eight hours later the full paroxysm occurs, with a feeling of extreme coldness and a rigor beginning in the late afternoon. Headache, nausea and vomiting are usually present. The temperature is high, the pulse rapid and of low volume, and the skin is cold. This phase lasts for 45 minutes to 1 hour. The patient will cover himself with anything available to try to get warm. When the rigor ceases, peripheral dilatation occurs; the patient feels very hot and thirsty and is unable to relieve the sensation of hotness. The pulse is rapid and of full volume. The skin is hot and dry. This lasts about 1 hour and defervescence follows, with a profuse sweat. The symptoms settle completely and the patient will usually sleep. The following day there may be a little weakness. One day later the malaria paroxysm recurs. Daily paroxysms occur when parasite broods are undergoing schizogony on successive days. Untreated, the paroxysms continue for 6 weeks and die out spontaneously, only to recur 2–3 months later. By the time symptoms have been present for a week the spleen is usually palpable and there may be mild anaemia. Rupture of the enlarged spleen is reported in *vivax* malaria.

Malariae malaria

The incubation period is usually about 28 days. Non-specific prodromal symptoms last for 2–3 days before the onset of the first paroxysm, which is accompanied by a rigor. The periodicity of symptoms is every 72 hours. The spleen is enlarged when symptoms have been present for 7–10 days.

Falciparum malaria

The incubation period is about 12 days. Headache, anorexia, nausea, vomiting, weakness and fever are prominent symptoms. The periodicity of symptoms is less than 48 hours, but periodicity is an unreliable clinical feature, present in only 30% of cases. The patient feels ill all the time, with exacerbation of symptoms at the time of paroxysms, which are similar to those described above but usually more severe. Convulsions may occur in children. Vomiting and diarrhoea are sometimes prominent features in the history. Herpes simplex vesicles may appear on the lips during the illness.

Complications

Complicated malaria occurs in falciparum infections (Summary 5). Altered consciousness in the presence of *falciparum* malaria must be taken as a clinical indication of cerebral malaria. Neck rigidity is not a feature, although mild neck stiffness may be present. Raised intracranial pressure is not a feature, and focal neurological signs are uncommon. Generalised convulsions occur in children and adults. Hypoglycaemia occurs in children, pregnant women with severe malaria and, less often, in adults with severe infection.

Jaundice may be a prominent physical sign in some patients with severe malaria. Haemolysis can cause this, but tender hepatomegaly and abnormalities of liver function suggest liver involvement. Some degree of uraemia is common but this resolves after treatment. Uraemia with

Summary 5	Organ involvement in complicated falciparum malaria
Brain	Impaired consciousness: drowsiness, progressing to coma
	Convulsions
Kidney	Oliguria
	Blood urea raised, K^+ raised, pH lowered
Liver	Upper abdominal tenderness from enlarged liver
	Marked jaundice
	Bilirubin and aminotransferases elevated
Lungs	Dyspnoea
	Tachypnoea
	Cyanosis
	Scattered bilateral crackles
Intravascular haemolysis	Haemoglobinuria
	Tachycardia
	Blood pressure lowered
	Jaundice
	Oliguria (= blackwater fever)

12

oliguria indicates renal involvement. Pulmonary oedema can result from overhydration, but can also occur in the patient whose infection is coming under control. Blackwater fever due to acute massive intravascular haemolysis is an uncommon complication. It became less common after chloroquine replaced quinine in the prophylaxis and treatment of malaria, suggesting that quinine itself contributed to pathogenesis; blackwater fever does, however, occur in people who have not taken quinine. The urine is black in colour, the haemoglobin falls rapidly and jaundice appears. Hypotension and tachycardia are usual, and renal failure may follow. Gram-negative septicaemia has been reported in patients with severe malaria and may be responsible for hypotension.

Late complications

Tropical splenomegaly syndrome (TSS) occurs in areas of endemic *falciparum* malaria. It is characterised clinically by considerable splenomegaly, a lesser degree of hepatomegaly, anaemia and pancytopenia. There is polyclonal elevation of serum IgM levels, and malaria antibody titres are high.

Quartan nephrotic syndrome is related to *P. malariae* infections, and presents with gross oedema and proteinuria in children aged 4–6 years. The histological features are segmental endothelial proliferation with obliteration of capillary loops by periodic acid-Schiff (PAS) positive material. There is segmental thickening of the basement membrane. Progression of the glomerular lesion leads to diffuse glomerulosclerosis. Immunoglobulins and complement are deposited in the glomerulus, and *P. malariae* antigen is detectable in 25% of biopsies. The prognosis is poor, with progressive deterioration in renal function. Treatment of malaria and chemoprophylaxis do not influence the course of established disease.

Diagnosis

The clinical diagnosis of malaria is based on the history of a febrile illness after exposure in an endemic region. Differential diagnosis is shown in Table 12.33. Cases in non-endemic areas present most often in the first 3 months after leaving the endemic area. *Ovale* and *vivax* infections may present later, and the latency in *malariae* malaria may be prolonged. The diagnosis is confirmed by the finding of parasites in stained blood films. If *falciparum* malaria is diagnosed, the percentage of red cells parasitised should be determined and the film should be carefully examined for schizonts which are seen in blood film from patients with severe malaria. Severe malaria is defined parasitologically as over 5% of red cells parasitised, although complicated malaria can occur with only 1% of red cells parasitised; clinical assessment is therefore very important. The blood film is positive on the first occasion in most cases.

A blood film should be made and examined as soon as the diagnosis of malaria is considered. It is not necessary to wait for fever to occur. An antimalarial drug taken before blood films are obtained may clear the blood of parasites. If necessary further blood films should be made and examined once or twice daily until the febrile illness either is diagnosed or resolves. During a period of observation in hospital prophylactic antimalarial drugs should be stopped to give the best chance of demonstrating parasites. It may be necessary to start treatment for malaria after taking blood films but before they have been examined.

Laboratory features

Laboratory investigations are normal or mildly abnormal in *vivax*, *ovale* and *malariae* malaria, but consistently abnormal to some degree in *falciparum* malaria. Haemoglobin levels may be normal or slightly reduced at presentation but they fall thereafter. Reticulocyte counts may be low both before and after treatment, suggesting a period of marrow suppression, followed by recovery and reticulocytosis. White cell counts are normal but leucocytosis occurs in severe malaria. Platelet counts are reduced, often below 100 000/mm³. The prothrombin time and other measures of blood coagulation may be abnormal, particularly in *falciparum* infections, but gross clotting abnormalities are not usual.

Biochemical tests are often abnormal. Plasma sodium levels are low in *falciparum* malaria and urea may be raised. Abnormalities in liver function tests are frequent, and there may be a minor elevation in both total and unconjugated bilirubin in mild infections or greater elevation in more severe *falciparum*. Serological tests for malaria have no place in diagnosis of individual cases but may be helpful in assessing previous exposure.

Treatment

Drug treatment

The prime aim of treatment is to stop further ES cycles (Table 12.34). There is usually a prompt response in *vivax*, *ovale* and *malariae* malaria. The fever in *falciparum* infections may take 2–4 days to settle. Where radical cure of relapsing malaria is required, glucose-6-phosphate dehydrogenase levels should be checked and, if normal, primaquine is given. When there is severe deficiency of G6PD, primaquine should not be given, because of the risk of severe haemolysis; chemoprophylaxis can be given

Table 12.33 Differential diagnosis of malaria

Fever alone	Fever and renal failure
Any cause of pyrexia of unknown origin (see Summary 1, p. 230)	Septic shock
	Leptospirosis
Fever and jaundice	Viral haemorrhagic fevers
Yellow fever	**Fever and impaired consciousness**
Typhus	Meningitis
Leptospirosis	Encephalitis
Biliary sepsis	
Septicaemia	

Table 12.34   Treatment of malaria

Type of malaria	Drug	Dose	Additional treatment
Vivax and ovale	Chloroquine base	600 mg (10 mg/kg) stat, then 300 mg (5 mg/kg) 6 hours later, then 300 mg (5 mg/kg) daily for 2 days given orally	Primaquine, 7.5 mg twice a day for 14 days (children 250 µg/kg per day)
Malariae	Chloroquine base	As above	Nil
Falciparum Chloroquine-sensitive			
Mild	Chloroquine base	As above	
Severe	Chloroquine base	300 mg (5 mg/kg) given by iv infusion in 250–500 ml fluid, repeated 12-hourly. Change to oral chloroquine as soon as the patient's condition permits	Nil
Chloroquine-resistant or sensitivity unknown			
Mild	Quinine base	500 mg max (10 mg/kg) 3 times a day for 7 days orally	Fansidar, 3 tablets as a single dose for adults; reduced doses for children
Severe	Quinine base	500 mg max (10 mg/kg) by iv infusion in 250–500 ml fluid over 4 hours given 12-hourly until the patient can take oral quinine, giving a total of 7 days' treatment	Fansidar as above

to prevent relapse, e.g pyrimethamine (25 mg weekly). Primaquine is not recommended in pregnancy and a chemoprophylactic should be given.

Plasmodium falciparum malaria is a serious infection demanding urgent treatment. Chloroquine resistance in *P. falciparum* parasites has added to the difficulties in treatment. The distribution of chloroquine-resistant strains is shown in Figure 12.23 and the areas affected will increase with time. Quinine is the drug of first choice for treatment of chloroquine-resistant or potentially resistant strains. The route of administration must be chosen carefully. A patient who is vomiting will need parenteral treatment. Intravenous treatment is needed when there is severe *falciparum* malaria – judged either on the clinical condition of the patient or on the presence of complications (Summary 5) – or high parasitaemia (2% or more of the red cells parasitised) or schizonts in the peripheral blood. The dosage regimens used are set out in Table 12.34. Impairment of renal or hepatic function will prolong the half-life of the two main schizonticidal drugs, and so the dosage regimen will need to be modified, reducing the amount given and, if necessary, the frequency of administration. As soon as the patient's condition has improved sufficiently, oral treatment should be given. Tinnitus, deafness and headache are common side-effects of quinine and if they are very troublesome, the frequency of administration of the drug can be reduced.

Quinine alone will not cure *falciparum* malaria and another drug is needed. Fansidar, a combination of pyrimethamine with the long-acting sulphonamide, sulphadoxine, has been effective but Fansidar resistance is becoming more common. Mefloquine is being used with very good results.

Chloroquine is generally well tolerated by mouth; nausea and blurring of vision are transitory side-effects. Upper abdominal discomfort may occur after taking the drug. Pruritus is common in Africans taking chloroquine. This is not associated with a rash and is not a manifestation of allergy. Chloroquine can be used in pregnancy. The route of administration of the drug is determined by the severity of the illness, judged by the criteria detailed above.

Additional measures

Patients with severe or complicated malaria should be managed in an intensive care unit. Convulsions should be controlled with diazepam. Apart from effective treatment of the malaria and the usual care of the unconscious patient, no additional treatment is needed in cerebral malaria. Hypoglycaemia has been reported in severe cases, particularly in young children and pregnant women. This appears to be an effect of quinine on insulin release and metabolism. Blood sugar should be monitored regularly and 50% glucose injections given as needed. Dialysis is needed when there is renal failure. Attention to fluid balance is essential to prevent fluid overload. Pulmonary oedema can occur because of fluid overload, but can also occur without evidence of heart failure. Mechanical ventilation may be needed when pulmonary oedema occurs. Transfusion is indicated when there is acute intravascular haemolysis and when the haemoglobin falls below 7.0 g/dl. Fresh frozen plasma and platelet transfusions are given when there are major clotting defects. Whole blood exchange transfusion appears to be effective in severely ill patients, and is indicated when more than 10% of rbcs are parasitised and when complications are present.

Management of other complications

Quartan nephrotic syndrome has a poor prognosis, with progressive deterioration of renal function to end-stage

301

12

renal failure. Fluid restriction, diuretics and albumin infusions may be of help in relieving the oedema and fluid retention.

The idiopathic *tropical splenomegaly syndrome* is treated with maintenance antimalarial chemoprophylaxis. On this treatment the splenomegaly regresses, haematological indices improve, and abnormal serological findings return towards normal. Cessation of chemoprophylaxis may cause relapse.

Prevention and control

Everything possible must be done to prevent mosquito bites (p. 228). With the increasing problems posed by drug-resistant malaria, these measures occupy a central place in prophylaxis and their importance must be stressed to travellers and residents in endemic areas. This applies particularly to infants, children and pregnant women. The drugs currently used are listed in Table 12.35 but up-to-date information should be obtained by those advising travellers to endemic areas.

Eradication is no longer perceived as an achievable goal and control is the current aim. Insecticide resistance among mosquitoes, particularly to the cheapest compound, DDT, and chloroquine resistance among *falciparum* parasites, have contributed to the problems of controlling malaria. The main methods used are:

1. reduction of vector breeding sites
2. larviciding pools that cannot be drained
3. spraying insecticides inside houses and on other sites where mosquitoes rest
4. treating cases in man.

BABESIASIS

Babesia is a genus of intracellular protozoa that invade, divide asexually within, and finally rupture host erythrocytes. There are 70 species in the genus, affecting a wide range of vertebrates including cattle (*Babesia divergens*) and rodents (*B. microti*). The parasites are transmitted by the bite of hard-bodied (ixodid) ticks. Transovarial transmission of the parasite occurs in the tick. Babesia are widely distributed geographically, with reports of cases in humans from many countries including Scotland and the United States.

The incubation period is up to 4 weeks, less in patients who have had a splenectomy. There is a considerable range in the severity of infection, from mild to severe. Asymptomatic infections also occur. Prodromal features include headache, malaise and gastrointestinal upset prior to the onset of fevers and rigors, with jaundice, haemoglobinuria and renal impairment in *B. divergens* infections. *B. microti* produces a more prolonged but less severe illness. Increasing age is associated with more severe clinical illness.

The laboratory diagnosis is made by finding organisms similar to malaria parasites in Giemsa-stained peripheral blood films.

There is no single treatment of proven value in the management of babesiasis. Survival in the rapidly progressive *B. divergens* infections depends largely on sup-

Table 12.35 Malaria prophylaxis

General measures
Protection against mosquito bites (insect repellants, nets, clothing)

Chemoprophylaxis
Low risk of malaria – chloroquine-sensitive
  Chloroquine or proguanil
High risk of malaria – chloroquine resistant
  Chloroquine and proguanil
High risk of malaria – multiple drug resistance
  Chloroquine and proguanil
  or mefloquine (visits of ≤3 weeks only)

Points to note
- Where the risk of drug-resistant malaria is high, severe malaria may occur despite regular prophylaxis, but this is *not* a reason to omit prophylaxis.
- Prophylaxis should be started 1 week before entering the area, and continued for 4 weeks after leaving.
- Mefloquine is a new drug and there is limited experience of its use for prophylaxis
- Useful UK telephone numbers:
  Dept of Communicable and Tropical Diseases, East Birmingham, Hospital: 021–766 6611; Hospital for Tropical Diseases Travel Clinic, London: 01–388 9600/8989; Liverpool School of Tropical Medicine: 051–708 9393.

portive measures such as renal dialysis according to the usual criteria, with transfusion and/or exchange transfusion. Treatment with intravenous quinine in standard doses appears to be effective. *B. microti* infection is usually self-limiting and requires only symptomatic treatment.

TRYPANOSOMIASES

African trypanosomiasis (sleeping sickness)

Infection with species of *Trypanosoma gambiense* causes an initial febrile illness which progresses slowly to a chronic phase dominated by infection of the central nervous system, causing neuronal death and a variety of organic neurological syndromes. Neurological involvement occurs early in *Trypanosoma rhodesiense* infections within weeks of inoculation of parasites and, untreated, there is rapid deterioration and death. The two species cannot be distinguished on morphological grounds. Various species of tsetse fly, *Glossina*, are the vectors.

Distribution and incidence

The specific names of these parasites suggest a West African (*T. gambiense*) or East African (*T. rhodesiense*) origin for the infections, but there is a considerable overlap of the distribution of the two species in Central Africa (Fig. 12.26). Numerically the total numbers of cases are far fewer than malaria, but *rhodesiense* infections have a considerable economic impact as valuable farming and grazing lands cannot be used because of the high risk of infection.

Transmission and epidemiology

Tsetse flies become infected by ingesting trypanosomes in

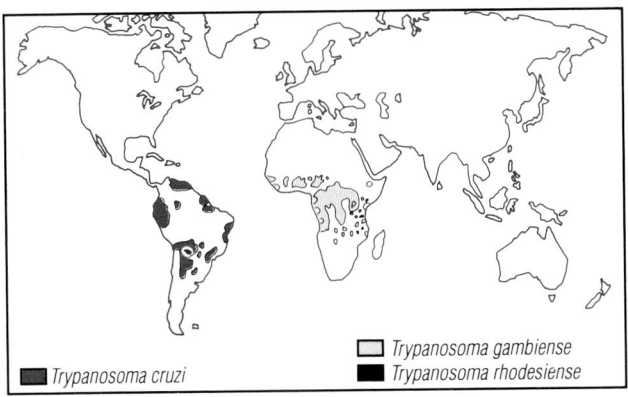

Fig. 12.26 World distribution of trypanosomiases.

a blood meal. Once infected, a fly remains infective for life. About 1% of flies in an area are infected. Man is the reservoir in *gambiense* infections, while a variety of wild mammals, including bush buck and hartebeest, are the reservoir of *rhodesiense* infection and man is an incidental host. Transmission of *gambiense* trypanosomiasis occurs in wooded areas around rivers and streams that are water sources for local populations. Blood transfusion and transplacental transmission are also possible routes of infection.

Pathology and pathogenesis

Following infection there is an early marked inflammatory response at the site of inoculation and in the lymphoid tissues of the body, lymph glands, liver and spleen. Trypanosomes may be seen in tissue sections. *Rhodesiense* infections progress rapidly to involve the heart and brain. Myocarditis and pericarditis are common. An obliterative endarteritis with vascular occlusion is found in the central nervous system, causing the degenerative changes. The neuropathological features include thickening of the meninges, which are infiltrated by lymphocytes and plasma cells. This infiltrate extends into brain substance in a perivascular distribution.

The pathogenesis is poorly understood. The parasites continuously shed surface antigens which evoke antibody responses in the host, but the antigens change in sequence – a possible mechanism of evading host immune responses. Auto-antibodies to brain and heart may cause tissue damage. Disseminated intravascular coagulation can occur in *rhodesiense* infections.

Clinical features

With both species, fever, chills and weakness are usual initial symptoms, beginning about 10 days after the bite. An inflamed lump is present at the bite site and there is regional adenopathy. On white skins it is possible to see transient irregular areas of erythema in both types of disease. Posterior auricular and posterior cervical adenopathy develops after 1–2 months of infection in *gambiense*

infections. Unpleasant dysaesthesia follows squeezing of the calf muscles. Hepatosplenomegaly is often present in both infections early on. Jaundice occurs in *rhodesiense* infections. Purpuric rashes on the extremities are occasionally seen in severe *rhodesiense* infections.

Neurological involvement appears within weeks of infection in *rhodesiense* infections, but it may be months or years later with *T. gambiense*. Indifference, lassitude, personality change and altered behaviour are early features. Sleep rhythm is reversed. The basal ganglia, cerebellum and brain stem regions are most affected, producing tremor, incoordination, and problems with speech, balance and walking. Parkinsonian features may be prominent. Epilepsy occurs. In the terminal stage the patient is scarcely rousable, unable to swallow and cannot feed himself. Bronchopneumonia is a common cause of death.

Diagnosis

Diagnosis depends on finding trypanosomes. Early in the course of infection with either species parasites may be found in peripheral blood films. There are usually many more parasites in *rhodesiense* than *gambiense* infections. *Gambiense* parasites may be seen in bone marrow smears. Smaller numbers of parasites can be detected in smears of the buffy coat. When there is cervical adenopathy material aspirated from a gland by syringe and needle can be smeared on a slide and stained. Repeated examinations must be made to detect the low levels of parasitaemia in *gambiense* infection.

Cerebrospinal fluid (CSF) must also be examined. The cell count is determined and the stained deposit is examined for trypanosomes. An increased white cell count (over $5/mm^3$) and/or an increased CSF protein (over 250 mg/l) indicates CNS infection in a patient with parasites in his blood or tissues. Serum immunoglobulin concentrations are increased, with IgM levels very high. Increased CSF IgM indicates nervous system involvement. Serological tests are available but do not have diagnostic value for individual patients.

Treatment

Suramin is used to kill parasites in blood and lymphoid nodes, and cures patients early in the disease. It does not cross the blood–brain barrier and so is ineffective when the CNS is involved. Pentamidine is a second-line alternative to suramin.

The arsenical compound, melarsoprol (Mel B), is used when there is CNS involvement. It will also kill blood forms but its high toxicity prohibits its use as a first-line drug.

Examination of blood films, IgM levels, CSF and the condition of the patient is helpful in assessing the response to treatment. Improvement in the condition of the patient and resolution of the abnormalities indicate a good response. Relapse is indicated by a rise in the CSF protein or cell count and further treatment should be given.

When patients are treated early, complete recovery is

12

the rule. In more advanced cases treatment arrests progression of the disease.

Prevention and control

Wearing appropriate clothing in endemic areas is a basic preventive method to minimise the area exposed to biting, although tsetses can bite through thin material. Pentamidine has been used as a prophylactic agent against *gambiense* infections in those heavily exposed. Improvement of facilities for diagnosis and treatment is also important. Efforts to control vectors by destruction of habitats may be helpful.

American trypanosomiasis (Chagas disease)

American trypanosomiasis is an infection caused by *Trypanosoma cruzi*. It can cause an acute febrile illness with myocardial damage and sudden death in some cases. Chronic infection can be associated with cardiomyopathy and the 'mega-syndrome' of the oesophagus and colon particularly. Reduviid bugs are the insect vector.

Aetiology

The parasite exists in several forms during its life cycle. The trypomastigote is found in the blood and has similar appearances to the African trypanosome. Amastigotes are found within host cells. Human blood forms are ingested by the bug when it takes a blood meal. The bug defaecates infective faeces on the skin after taking a blood meal, and the metacyclic forms enter the host through the bite or other skin abrasion, or through the conjunctiva if the faeces are carried to the eye on fingers.

Distribution and incidence

American trypanosomiasis is most common in the countries of South America among people living in poorly constructed housing, as the bugs live in roof thatch and cracked mud walls. Infection occurs most often in the home. Many people are infected in South America, with about 6 000 000 cases in Brazil, although not all those infected develop disease (Fig. 12.26).

Transmission and epidemiology

Contact with infected bugs, transplacental infection and blood transfusion are the routes of infection (Fig. 12.27). Infected bugs are the most important source. Infection in bugs is maintained from a reservoir of *T. cruzi* in dogs. Infection of children in the first decade of life is common.

Pathology and pathogenesis

Trypanosomes invade cells, including myocardial and gut smooth muscle cells. Rupture of the cell releases trypomastigotes and evokes inflammatory responses in the surrounding tissues. The trypomastigotes circulate, invade

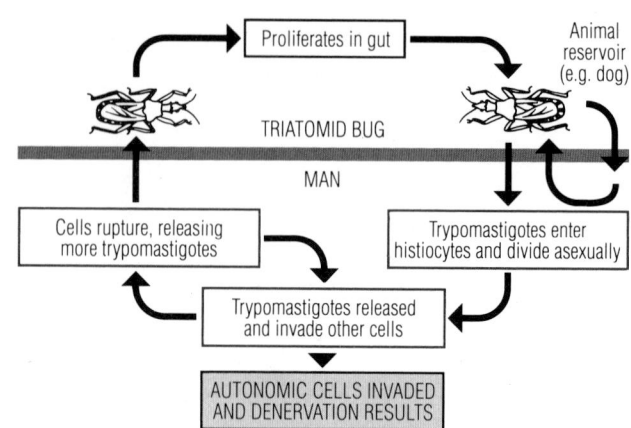

Fig. 12.27 Life cycle of *Trypanosoma cruzi.*

other cells and replicate as amastigotes. Phagocytic cells in any tissue, as well as heart muscle, skeletal and smooth muscle, and central nervous system, are among the tissues involved. Pericarditis and cardiomegaly are often present.

The heart and the gut are the organs severely affected in chronic Chagas disease. The heart is enlarged, with apical ventricular aneurysm commonly present. Thrombus is often present in the atrial appendage and in the ventricles. There is diffuse myocardial cell necrosis, with fibrosis and involvement of the conducting system. Parasympathetic plexuses of the gut are destroyed, causing dilatation of the intestine, frequently the oesophagus or colon (the mega-syndrome).

The pathogenesis of the disease is complex. There are several different strains of *T. cruzi*, some of which cause the cardiac and mega-syndromes. Other strains cause lifelong infection but no disease. Autoimmune mechanisms are probably involved in damaging tissues.

Clinical features

Acute infection may be inapparent in young children, but in older children and adults there may be an acute febrile illness. The patient may find a lump in the skin marking the site of the infected bite and initial parasite replication (the chagoma). Unilateral peri-orbital oedema indicates a conjunctival route of infection. Local adenopathy and hepatosplenomegaly are found. Cardiomegaly, heart failure, arrhythmia and conduction defects indicate myocarditis in the acute illness. This may cause sudden death. Meningo-encephalitis may also be present. The local signs at the bite site, hepatosplenomegaly and fever subside in 6 weeks.

Chronic Chagas disease presents with heart and gut disease. Cardiac failure is common, with right and left heart failure. There may be signs suggesting pulmonary or systemic embolisation from thrombus in the cardiac chambers. Conduction abnormalities are often present and may cause Stokes-Adams attacks and sudden death. Mega-oesophagus causes dysphagia and aspiration pneumonia in the most severely affected. Megacolon causes constipation and faecal impaction. Volvulus of sigmoid megacolon may occur.

Diagnosis

Acute infections can be diagnosed by finding parasites in the peripheral blood film. Trypanosomes may also be found on microscopy and culture of CSF, even when evidence of CNS involvement is lacking. Serological tests are usually positive in both acute and chronic cases by indirect immunofluorescence, indirect haemagglutination and complement fixation techniques.

Treatment

Treatment is unsatisfactory. Two drugs are available, nifurtimox and benzonidazole. Both will clear the blood of parasites in the acute phase but prolonged follow-up suggests that neither gives a radical cure. Control of arrhythmias and heart failure is all that can be done for cardiac disease in the chronic phase. Relief of obstruction at the oesophagogastric junction by dilatation or surgery may help the patient with mega-oesophagus. A dilatated segment of small or large intestine can be excised.

Prevention and control

Improvements to housing would do much to prevent this disease. Residual spraying with gamma benzene hexachloride is a useful method of vector control.

LEISHMANIASIS

The *Leishmania* are obligate intracellular protozoan parasites that infect man and other mammals, including dogs, foxes, gerbils and rats. Infection is transmitted by the bite

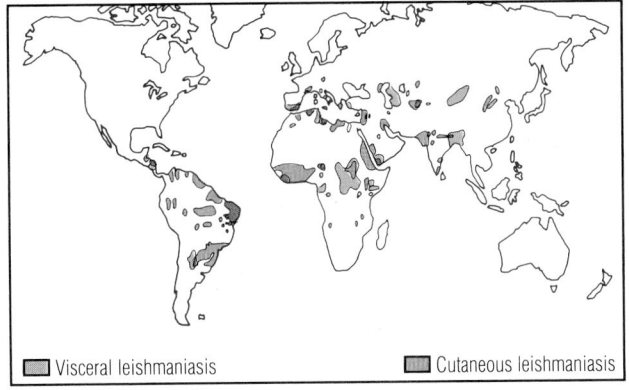

Visceral leishmaniasis ▨ Cutaneous leishmaniasis

Fig. 12.29 World distribution of leishmaniasis.

of infected sandflies. The generalised life cycle is shown in Fig. 12.28. These organisms parasitise cells of the reticulo-endothelial system and evoke granulomatous responses in infected tissue. Genetic factors controlling the host-cell-mediated responses determine the outcome of infection, with only a proportion of those infected developing clinically apparent disease.

The geographical distribution is shown in Figure 12.29. Two forms of disease are recognised. *Cutaneous leishmaniasis* denotes infection with species of *Leishmania* that affect primarily reticulo-endothelial cells in the skin, while *visceral leishmaniasis* denotes infection with a species that primarily infects reticulo-endothelial cells of deeper tissues (Table 12.36). The species causing cutaneous disease are geographically distinct between the Old and New World. Speciation of leishmania depends on iso-enzyme typing, as species cannot be distinguished by morphological criteria.

Cutaneous leishmaniasis

Cutaneous leishmaniasis is a granulomatous infection of the skin caused by various species of *Leishmania*, which results in one or more chronic ulcerating skin lesions. In time, the ulcers usually heal with scarring.

Aetiology

The organisms causing cutaneous leishmaniasis are listed in Table 12.36. Morphologically they are all identical.

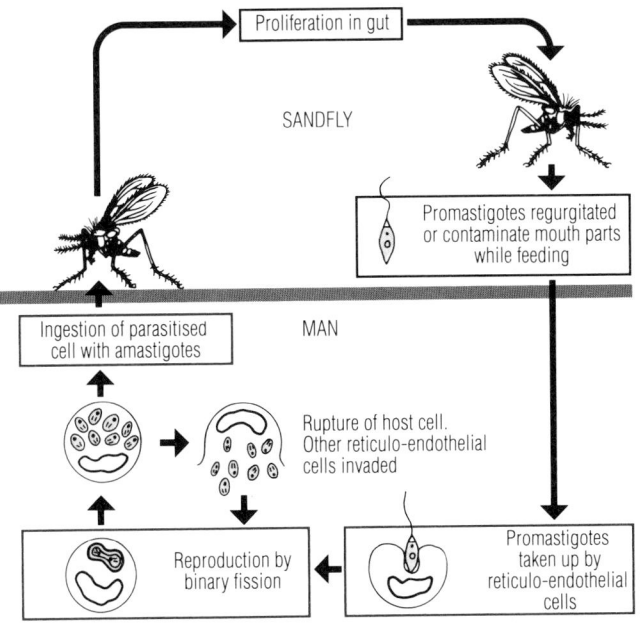

Fig. 12.28 Generalised life cycle of *Leishmania*.

Table 12.36 Forms of Leishmania infection

Location	Cutaneous leishmaniasis	Visceral leishmaniasis
Old World	Leishmania tropica Leishmania major Leishmania aethiopica Leishmania infantum	Leishmania donovani Leishmania infantum
New World	Leishmania mexicana complex Leishmania braziliensis complex Leishmania peruviana	Leishmania donovani

305

Distribution and incidence

The incidence is difficult to estimate, as many self-healing cases never come to medical attention. World Health Organization figures put the incidence at 100 cases per 10 000 of the population in endemic areas (Fig. 12.29).

Transmission and epidemiology

Female sandflies of the genera *Phlebotomus* (Old World) and *Lutzomyia* (New World) transmit these infections by their bite. Apart from *Leishmania tropica* (transmitted in towns and cities with man as the reservoir), these are zoonotic infections; humans are infected when they move into areas where there is a mammal–sandfly cycle. Urban infections tend to be more common among children.

Pathology and pathogenesis

Promastigotes change to amastigotes after inoculation into the skin, and the amastigotes are very rapidly phagocytosed by macrophages where they replicate (Fig. 12.28). The local granulomatous reactions produce a subcutaneous nodule and then the overlying skin ulcerates. The lesion persists as long as amastigotes proliferate within macrophages. This occurs despite the presence of sensitised T lymphocytes, shown by a positive delayed hypersensitivity reaction to a leishmanin skin test antigen. Healing occurs spontaneously in time in most infections.

Recidivans leishmaniasis is a relapsing form of the disease due to *L. tropica*, which can persist over many years despite good cell-mediated responses. Mucocutaneous leishmaniasis (espundia) due to *L. braziliensis braziliensis* is a late manifestation of a primary cutaneous infection up to 30 years before. Total lack of host response to the parasite characterises the lesions in diffuse cutaneous leishmaniasis (DCL), caused by *L. aethiopica* in Africa and the *L. mexicana* complex in Central and South America. Leishmanin tests are negative and there is a paucity of lymphocytes in the lesions, but many parasitised macrophages.

Clinical features

Persisting cutaneous ulceration on an exposed part of the body continuing for more than a month is the usual feature. The ulcer is painless and may crust over, only for the crust to separate again. Regional adenopathy is not seen unless there is secondary infection. Around the main ulcer, which has well-defined indurated margins, a number of smaller nodular lesions may be present. These infections will heal spontaneously in 2–8 months, leaving a residual scar. Recidivans leishmaniasis caused by *L. tropica* infection is characterised by a chronic relapsing course. In contrast, diffuse cutaneous leishmaniasis causes numerous nodular or plaque-like lesions which tend not to ulcerate. These patients represent a kind of 'lepromatous' cutaneous leishmaniasis (p. 277). The South American species cause lesions similar to those of *L. major*. *Leishmania braziliensis braziliensis* causes an initial ulcerating skin lesion which heals, but may subsequently produce a recurrence of disease with destruction of tissues at a mucocutaneous junction.

Diagnosis

Parasites can usually be found in Giemsa-stained smears of material from slit skin smears, material aspirated from the edge of the lesion or touch impression smears from the surface of a biopsy. Material from the biopsy can also be cultured in Novy-McNeal-Nicolle (NNN) medium. Serological tests for leishmaniasis are positive at low titre in most forms of cutaneous leishmaniasis.

Differential diagnosis

A variety of infective disorders can cause indolent ulceration. Among these are yaws, tertiary syphilis, lupus vulgaris, *Histoplasma duboisii*, diphtheritic ulcers (desert sore) and blastomycosis. Malignant ulcers and tropical ulcer should also be considered. Diffuse cutaneous leishmanias can be mistaken clinically for lepromatous leprosy unless the causative organism is demonstrated in skin smears.

Treatment

The treatment of cutaneous leishmaniasis is unsatisfactory, not least because the commonly used drug, sodium antimony gluconate, has to be given by daily intravenous injection for 20–30 days. Intralesional antimonials, emetine and γ-interferon have been used successfully. Self-cure is a feature of infection with *L. tropica* and *L. major*, and so a single lesion caused by these parasites in a site that will not produce disfiguring scarring or be particularly exposed to secondary bacterial infection may be left to heal spontaneously. Patients with multiple lesions, large lesions or lesions in exposed places should receive treatment. Patients in areas where diffuse cutaneous leishmaniasis or mucocutaneous leishmaniasis occurs must be treated.

Sodium antimony gluconate (Pentostam) is the first choice of drug for both Old and New World leishmaniasis, and usually results in healing in most types of disease. Diffuse cutaneous leishmaniasis is often resistant and pentamidine is the alternative drug.

Prevention and control

Among Old World cutaneous leishmaniasis, cure is usually associated with immunity to re-infection with the same strain, but vaccination is not yet available. Destruction of burrows of rodent vectors can be successful in removing reservoirs. Removal of sandfly breeding sites around houses and spraying with insecticides will help to control peridomestic transmission. Protection against the bites of sandflies may be helpful, e.g. mosquito nets and insect repellants, although the insects will bite through a shirt.

Visceral leishmaniasis (kala-azar)

Visceral leishmaniasis, an infection due to *Leishmania donovani*, is spread by the bite of an infected female sandfly and causes a prolonged febrile illness with wasting, hepatosplenomegaly and lymphadenopathy.

Distribution and incidence

The areas affected are shown in Figure 12.29. This condition is endemic in some countries of southern Europe and Mediterranean islands that are regularly visited by tourists. Infections acquired in these areas are seen in the United Kingdom. Children are commonly affected in the endemic areas. Subclinical cases probably exceed clinical cases by 5 to 1. Endemic, epidemic and sporadic forms of the disease occur. All ages and both sexes are susceptible to infection.

Transmission and epidemiology

The dog seems to be an important reservoir throughout the endemic areas. Man is the reservoir in north-eastern and eastern India.

The vectors are female sandflies of the genus *Phlebotomus* in the Old World and *Lutzomyia* in the New. These insects, guided by scent plumes, bite at night-time.

Pathology and pathogenesis

Amastigotes (Fig. 12.28) replicate asexually within macrophages and are carried to lymph nodes draining the site of the bite; they then disseminate to macrophages in other tissues, particularly the liver, spleen, nodes and marrow. There is progressive enlargement of liver and spleen. Hypersplenism results, with anaemia, leucopenia and thrombocytopenia. There is also marrow suppression. Wasting of the muscles and low plasma albumin are metabolic responses to the infection. The malnutrition will impair immune responses to the parasite and to other diseases such as tuberculosis or pneumococcal pneumonia, which may complicate the patient's illness. Leishmanin tests (a delayed hypersensitivity skin test) are negative before treatment and become positive after cure.

Clinical features

The incubation period is very variable, from 2 weeks to 2 years or more. Early symptoms consist of lethargy, sweats, and fever with a pattern that typically has two peaks in a day. Within weeks of onset the liver and spleen are palpable and progressively enlarge. Body weight falls. Lymphadenopathy may be found. Emaciation is obvious in more long-standing cases. Darkening of the skin of hands, feet, face and abdomen is common in eastern India ('kala-azar' means 'black sickness'). Lymph glands may be enlarged. Poorly nourished patients should be carefully examined for co-existing tuberculosis or other infection such as pneumonia. Leishmaniasis has been recognised as one of the infections that may complicate the course of AIDS.

Investigation shows anaemia and pancytopenia, low plasma albumin and high globulin (e.g. 50 g/l) with polyclonal elevation of IgG. Serological tests for leishmaniasis are positive in most cases.

Diagnosis

The clinical features, together with exposure in an endemic area, suggest visceral leishmaniasis. The parasites are usually found on examination of Giemsa-stained smears of bone marrow aspirate, which should also be put into NNN culture medium. Percutaneous splenic aspiration has a high yield of positive results (95%); it can be done safely in a co-operative patient whose prothrombin time is not more than 5 seconds greater than the control, and whose platelet count is 40 000/μm^3 or more. Again, material should be cultured and used for making smears.

Treatment

Sodium antimony gluconate (Pentostam) is the drug of first choice, given by daily intravenous injection for about 30 days depending on the response. Fever settles quickly and there is progressive improvement in the clinical and laboratory findings. Relapse occasionally occurs and the options are to give more sodium antimony gluconate continuing for longer periods, or to give a second-line drug, e.g. pentamidine or amphotericin B. One of these is certainly needed if there is no response to a second course of sodium antimony gluconate.

Prevention and control

Prevention is difficult. Where man is the reservoir, finding and treating cases and insecticiding homes may help in control. Control of canine reservoirs can be of help. Vaccines are under study but not in clinical use yet.

HELMINTH INFECTIONS

A large number of helminthic parasites affect man. Man is the definitive host in most instances and the sexual phase of the life cycle takes place in the human host. A classification is given in Table 12.37. Less commonly man is an inadvertent intermediate host infected either with larvae that do not develop any further because they are in the wrong host, e.g. *Toxocara canis*, or with larvae that are unlikely ever to be consumed by the definitive host, e.g. hydatid disease.

The life cycles of these parasites differ markedly; faecal-oral transmission or percutaneous infection by infective larvae is characteristic of the soil-associated gut nematodes. In contrast the filariases have blood-sucking insect vectors in which there is development to infecting larvae that will infect man when later blood meals are taken. The life cycles of the trematode platyhelminths are more complex, involving more than one intermediate host in many instances.

The climatic conditions favouring transmission are warmth and humidity. These factors promote the survival of the soil-transmitted helminths and the insect vector of the filarial parasites. Local traditions in food preparation and consumption are important in transmission of a number of parasites: eating meat raw or very lightly cooked (*Trichinella spiralis, Taenia saginata*), or eating fish or crabs raw (*Clonorchis sinensis, Paragonimus westermani*). Among sheep- and goat-herding communities where dogs are used, definitive and intermediate hosts of *Echinococcus granulosus* are brought together, and it is common for sheep and goat offal containing hydatid cysts to be fed to dogs. Dogs become heavily infected and, because they live close to man, there is a considerable risk of human infection from dog faeces which contaminate the environment around houses.

The effect of helminthic infections on the health of communities is difficult to assess. *Ascaris lumbricoides* is one of the most common helminthic infections. It undoubtedly causes disease (for example, through a mass of tangled worms obstructing the small intestine), but these events probably do not happen very often among the 290 million people infected worldwide. In contrast, *Onchocerca volvulus* in the savannah belt of West Africa causes significant morbidity through the ocular complication, sclerosing keratitis, which can progress to blindness.

The chemotherapy of helminthic infections has become progressively simpler. The benzimidazoles – thiabendazole, mebendazole and albendazole – are broad-spectrum antihelminthics active against the soil-transmitted helminths. The incidence of side-effects decreases in the order given; albendazole, the newest, has much better absorption from the gut than mebendazole, but lacks the nausea and vomiting associated with thiabendazole. Praziquantel has actions in a range of cestode and trematode infections, with a low incidence of side-effects. It is the first drug to be effective in cysticercosis.

NEMATODES

HUMAN INTESTINAL NEMATODE INFECTION

Ascariasis

Ascariasis is infection of the gut lumen with the nematode parasite, *Ascaris lumbricoides*.

Aetiology

The adult female worm measures up to 400 mm long by 6 mm wide at its thickest. The male is up to 300 mm long by 2–4 mm. They live for about 1 year. Both are a greyish-white colour. The female lays up to 200 000 eggs per day. The worms do not attach themselves to the gut mucosa but maintain their position by actively moving against the flow of intestinal contents. The eggs survive well in warm moist soil but are killed by heating to 50°C. The adult parasite survives for about 1 year.

Distribution and incidence

Ascariasis is common in the tropics and subtropics, and up to 90% of people may be infected. Poor or absent sanitation and frequent faecal contamination of the environment with vast numbers of ascaris eggs lead to a high frequency of infection, often with large worm loads in children.

Table 12.37 Classification of helminth infections

Nematodes (round worms)

Human intestinal	Filarial	Animal intestinal
Ascaris	*Onchocerca*	*Trichinella*
Ancylostoma	*Wuchereria*	*Toxocara*
Necator	*Brugia*	
Strongyloides	*Loa loa*	
Enterobius		
Trichuris		

Trematodes (flukes)

Schistosoma
Clonorchis
Opisthorcis
Fasciola
Fasciolopsis
Paragonimus

Cestodes (tapeworms)

Human intestinal	Larval tissue cestodes
Taenia species	*Taenia solium* (cysticercosis)
Diphyllobothrium	Hydatid (*Echinococcus*)
Hymenolepis	

Transmission and epidemiology

Eggs are ingested in food or water or from fingers, and the larvae are released in the small intestine. They enter the mucosa and then blood vessels to reach the lungs, where they leave blood vessels and enter air spaces. Here they undergo two further moults and then ascend the bronchial tree to the pharynx. They migrate down the oesophagus and through the stomach to reach the small intestine.

Pathology

No intestinal mucosal lesions are attributable to the adult worms. Pulmonary infiltrates with eosinophils are found during the larval migratory phase of the life cycle.

Clinical features

Symptoms due to the migrating phase of ascariasis are very uncommon. Pulmonary infiltrates on X-ray, eosinophilia and restrictive pulmonary function defects might be expected. There are also few symptoms attributable to established infection.

Worms may be vomited, or passed with the stools, or may even emerge from a nostril. Bolus obstruction of the small intestine occurs, particularly in children with very heavy infections. An adult worm in the bile duct causes pain and obstructive jaundice with ascending cholangitis. Pancreatitis may result from ascaris obstruction of the pancreatic duct. Ascarids can also migrate through intestinal suture lines to cause leakage from an anastomosis.

Diagnosis

Diagnosis is made by finding eggs in faecal samples. The complications of ascariasis are usually diagnosed at surgical exploration or endoscopic examination. Eosinophilia is uncommon, apart from at the stage of tissue migration.

Treatment

Mebendazole (100 mg twice daily for 3 days) or albendazole (400 mg as a single dose) is effective. Both drugs are relatively expensive.

Piperazine hydrate elixir (750 mg of hydrate per 5 ml) is effective. The dose depends on age and weight. Where a mixed infection of ascaris and hookworm is being treated with piperazine and tetrachlorethylene (TCE) for hookworm, it is usual to treat the ascaris first, as TCE may stimulate ascaris migration into biliary or pancreatic ducts.

Prevention and control

The use of latrines would prevent infection. Faecal contamination of the environment and the use of human faeces as fertiliser on crops encourage transmission. Before use as fertiliser, faeces can be treated with sodium nitrate or calcium superphosphate to kill the eggs of gut parasites.

Education of the community about the control efforts, and its active co-operation, are essential to the success of control programmes.

Hookworm

This is infection of the gut with either *Ancylostoma duodenale* or *Necator americanus*. Both grip the wall of the mucosa with their mouth parts and take a small amount of blood from the host each day. A relatively small number of people develop disease related to hookworm infection.

Aetiology

The worms are small, about 9 mm long. The female *Ancylostoma* produces 30 000 eggs per day and *Necator* 9000 eggs per day. Eggs must be passed into warm, moist soil for the ovum to develop into the larval stage. The life cycle is shown in Figure 12.30. Larvae of *Necator* grow in the lungs. *Ancylostoma* larvae can be ingested with food and develop in the gut lumen without tissue migration.

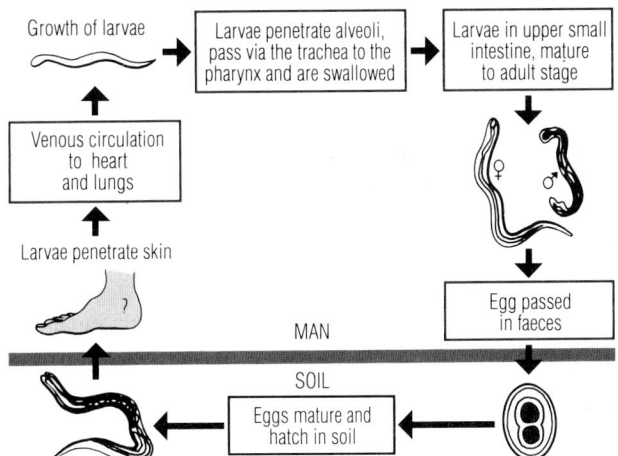

Fig. 12.30 Life cycle of hookworm.

Epidemiology

Both species occur worldwide where temperature and soil conditions are suitable. *Ancylostoma* eggs are capable of resisting desiccation to some extent. Infection rates of 80–90% are common in endemic rural areas. The use of untreated faeces as fertiliser on crops accounts for the high infection of farm workers.

Pathogenesis and pathology

Each worm takes a small amount of blood from the host. Nutrients are removed by the parasite and the residue passes into the gut, where it can be digested and absorbed. Iron deficiency anaemia occurs when iron losses exceed intake and iron stores are depleted. Anaemia may be severe, with haemoglobin levels of less than 5.0 g/dl. Hypoalbuminaemia is usual at this stage. There is no evidence to support an association between hookworm infection and malabsorption.

Clinical features

No symptoms are attributed to hookworm infection. Hookworm anaemia appears to cause few symptoms until oedema due to hypoproteinaemia develops. Salt retention and water retention exacerbate the oedema. Dyspnoea and some degree of exertional dyspnoea are usual. The findings are those of severe iron deficiency anaemia, with mucosal pallor and koilonychia. Some patients present with high-output congestive cardiac failure.

Diagnosis

Diagnosis is confirmed by finding eggs in the faeces. Worm burden can be assessed from 24-hour faecal egg outputs.

Laboratory features

The haematological features of hypochromic microcytic anaemia are evident on blood films and in red cell indices in hookworm anaemia. It is important to distinguish between iron deficiency and β-thalassaemia trait. Eosinophil counts may be normal or increased. Plasma albumin levels are low in hookworm anaemia.

Treatment

Mebendazole (100 mg twice daily for 3 days) or albendazole (200 mg twice daily for 2 days) is effective. Bephenium hydroxynaphthoate granules (5.0 g) are given on an empty stomach. The cheapest treatment is tetrachlorethylene (TCE), giving 0.5 ml/kg to a maximum single dose of 5.0 ml.

Eradication of the worms is not the priority in hookworm anaemia. Packed cell transfusion after giving diuretics may be needed. Where there is heart failure diuretics and cautious blood transfusion with packed cells are needed. Exchange transfusion is another way of correcting anaemia without risking adverse effects of fluid overload. Later iron stores will need replacing by oral or parenteral iron preparations.

Prevention and control

Safe disposal of faeces would prevent transmission. Where night soil must be used to fertilise crops, prior chemical treatment kills ova (see ascariasis above). Wearing shoes or sandals would also prevent infection. Where possible, vegetables with a high content of ferrous iron, e.g. soya beans, should be introduced into the diet.

Cutaneous larva migrans

The hookworm parasite of dogs and cats, *Ancylostoma braziliense*, produces eggs which are passed in the animal faeces; they hatch in warm, moist soil conditions to release larvae which mature to the infective stage and can penetrate the skin of humans. The larvae cannot follow their usual migration in man and instead meander around in the subcutaneous tissues close to the site of entry until they die. The feet are the most common site for this condition, but any part in contact with contaminated soil or sand can be affected.

The appearances are readily recognised. A red papule marks the tip of the track produced by the migrating worm. The papule is in fact a little way behind the migrating worm. A raised, red, serpiginous track, about 3 mm across, stretches out behind. The affected skin is itchy and may be blistered. Secondary bacterial infection can occur. The lesion can be active for several months.

The diagnosis is made on the appearances. Treatment is with thiabendazole, either orally, or topically as a cream. Following effective treatment the migration of the worm ceases and the track will slowly disappear. Secondary bacterial infection requires treatment with antibiotics.

Strongyloidiasis

Strongyloidiasis is an infection of the small intestine with the nematode parasite *Strongyloides stercoralis*. Most people are asymptomatic. A small number have cutaneous manifestations and immunosuppressed patients may develop massive systemic invasion with filariform larvae.

Aetiology

Strongyloides stercoralis adult females are small, 2 mm long, and are found in the intestinal lumen, where they insinuate their anterior ends between the villi. The life cycle is described in Figure 12.31.

A variation of the life cycle involves rhabditiform larvae developing into filariform larvae during transit down the gut. These larvae penetrate the rectal or anal mucosa or the peri-anal skin, and then enter the usual migratory tissue phase.

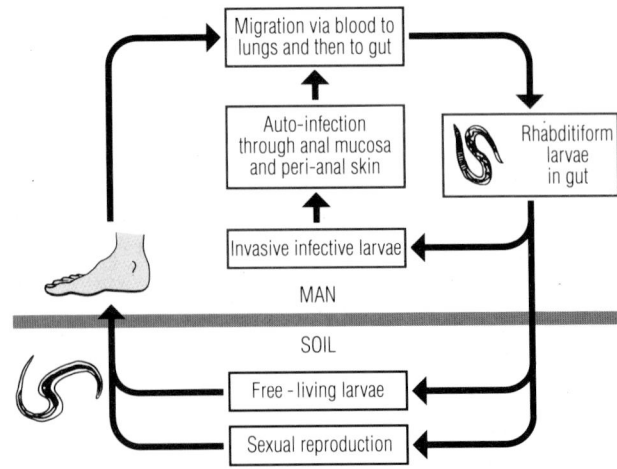

Fig. 12.31 Life cycle of *Strongyloides stercoralis*.

Transmission and epidemiology

Transmission and epidemiology are broadly the same as those of hookworm but tend to be focal depending on soil conditions. The occurrence of auto-infection in strongyloidiasis allows infection to persist for 30 years or more, successive generations of adults maintaining infection.

Pathology

The migrating larvae in lung evoke some degree of eosinophilic pneumonitis. Where adults lie in between the villi there is some local cellular response, but this is mild. Strongyloidiasis has been associated with a malabsorption syndrome. Diarrhoea, hypoproteinaemia and oedema of the small bowel wall have been found in children with *Strongyloides fulleborni* infection. The mechanism is not understood.

Massive auto-infection with filariform larvae can occur in immunosuppressed patients, with dissemination of larvae to gut, lungs and CNS.

Clinical features

Most patients are asymptomatic and the diagnosis is made by stool microscopy or in the investigation of eosinophilia. Some patients present with a transient, linear or serpiginous urticaria that comes and goes within 40–60 minutes. This is caused by subcutaneous migration of infective filariform larvae. The massive auto-infection syndrome occurs most often in people on steroids or immunosuppressive drugs. Fever, abdominal distension, diarrhoea, vomiting and ileus are common presenting symptoms. There may be signs of meningitis. Dyspnoea, cyanosis and pulmonary infiltrates indicate pulmonary involvement. Septicaemia with organisms from the colonic microflora is common. The prognosis is poor.

Diagnosis

Diagnosis is usually made by finding rhabditiform larvae in stools or juice obtained from the duodenum by intubation. Eosinophilia is usual in normal persons but absent in patients with massive auto-infection. Larvae are readily found in sputum, jejunal aspirate or faeces in patients with massive auto-infection.

Treatment

Thiabendazole (25 mg/kg to a maximum single dose of 1.5 g) is given twice daily for 3 days. Albendazole (400 mg twice daily for 3 days) is also effective; it causes fewer side-effects and may become the drug of first choice. Treatment is continued for 7 days in massive auto-infection. Intensive care is also needed for these patients.

Prevention

Safe disposal of faeces would prevent *S. stercoralis* infection. Sandals would help to prevent skin/soil contacts.

Treatment with cytotoxic or immunosuppressive drugs for leukaemia, lymphoma and other malignancies, reactional states in leprosy or organ transplantation should be preceded by thiabendazole treatment in patients from or in the tropics.

Threadworms

Infection with the intestinal nematode, *Enterobius vermicularis*, causes pruritus ani. Children are most often affected but adults can also become infected. The life cycle is described in Figure 12.32. The full cycle can take 14 days.

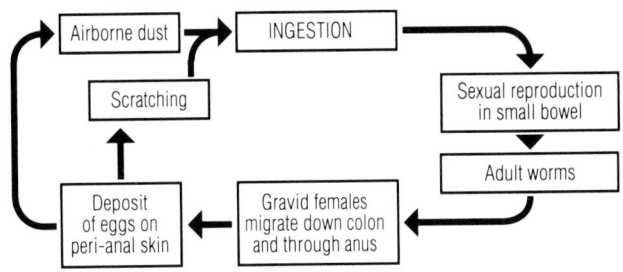

Fig. 12.32 Life cycle of threadworm.

Transmission

Auto-infection maintains the parasite in the host. Person-to-person spread is the likely route of infection in children and other family members, or by handling pyjamas, sheets or towels with adherent eggs.

Clinical features

Intense pruritus ani is the usual symptom of this infection. The pruritus often disrupts sleep. When symptoms are present the worms may be seen on the peri-anal skin. In females vulvo-vaginitis and vaginal discharge may occur.

Diagnosis

Diagnosis is made either by identifying a female obtained from the peri-anal skin or from the faeces, or by finding eggs. To give the best chance of finding eggs the peri-anal skin should not be washed before the swab is taken. Eosinophilia is not found in this infection.

Treatment

A number of drugs are available and it is usual to treat the whole family. Mebendazole (100 mg as a single dose, followed by a second dose 2 weeks later) is effective. Piperazine citrate (65 mg/kg to a maximum dose of 2.0 g/day for 6 days, repeated after 3 weeks) can be used. Pyrvinium pamoate (5 mg of base/kg as a single dose) is also used.

In addition to chemotherapy it is helpful to prevent finger sucking and nail biting. The importance of hand washing after going to the lavatory and before eating should be stressed. Occasionally one child is chronically afflicted by enterobiasis, and this causes both child and family great distress. This may occur in families that are particularly careful about washing, cleanliness, and so on. Reassurance that this is not uncommon and that enterobiasis is occasionally difficult to treat is necessary.

Trichuriasis

Trichuriasis is infection of the intestinal lumen with the nematode, *Trichuris trichiuria*. Most patients are asymptomatic. Malnourished children suffer heavy infections with this parasite, causing symptomatic disease. Eggs are swallowed and larvae hatch. They mature during their transit down the small intestine, and adults are found in the terminal ileum and colon. The eggs mature in soil and are ingested. The adult worm has a long, thin anterior end and a short, thick posterior end. This appearance is described by the common name of the parasite, the whipworm. The thick posterior end grips the colonic mucosa.

Clinical features

Most people are asymptomatic and eggs are found on faecal microscopy. Malnourished children may become infected with large numbers of these worms, and diarrhoea with blood in the stool may result. By proctoscopy large numbers of worms can be seen adhering to the rectal mucosa. Rectal prolapse is sometimes seen in these malnourished children. It is difficult to know if the worm burden is the cause or the result of malnutrition.

Diagnosis

Diagnosis is made by finding eggs in faecal smears or concentrates.

Treatment

Mebendazole (100 mg twice daily for 3 days) is effective.

FILARIAL INFECTION

The filariae are a group of helminthic parasites whose adult and larval forms are found in man, the sole reservoir of infection for all but one species. Transmission occurs by the bite of blood-sucking insects. The larvae, referred to as microfilariae, develop into infective stages by two further moults. The infective microfilariae migrate out from the insect's mouth parts on to the skin when the insect is taking a blood meal, and then enter the skin through the puncture site. Development from the infective larval form to the adult then takes about 6 months.

The adult worms are very long-lived; shedding of microfilariae begins about 6 months after infection and lasts for many years. The severity of disease relates to the burden of adult worms in the host.

Onchocerciasis

Infection with the filarial parasite *Onchocerca volvulus* causes chronic intense pruritus with a papular eruption. This is caused by the death of microfilariae in the skin. Death of microfilariae in the cornea over a prolonged period results in scarring of the cornea and unilateral or bilateral blindness.

Aetiology and transmission

Infective larvae escape on to the skin from the proboscis of an infected *Simulium* blackfly, when it takes a blood meal, and enter the skin through the bite site (Fig. 12.33). The infection is maintained in the vectors when adult blackflies ingest microfilariae in blood meals. These develop into infective larvae over about 9 days. In humans the larvae develop into adults over 6 months. Adult worms survive for up to 15 years and may shed microfilariae for most of that time.

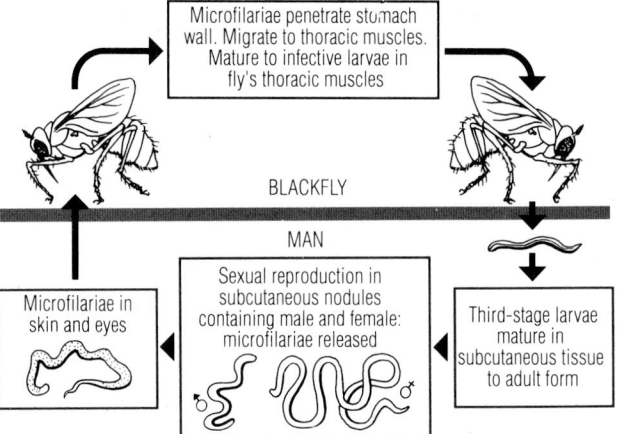

Fig. 12.33 Life cycle of *Onchocerca*.

Distribution

Tropical Africa and Central America are the main endemic areas, with foci of disease in Yemen, Colombia, Venezuela and the northern Amazonian region of Brazil. In Africa two distinct areas are affected: the savannah area throughout West Africa where ocular involvement is common, and the tropical rain forest area where ocular involvement is less common (Fig. 12.34).

Epidemiology

The distribution of the disease relates closely to the ecology of the *Simulium* vector, which requires fast-flowing, freshwater streams and rivers for breeding. Most human cases occur in people who live close to these water sources and visit the stream or river to collect water, wash clothes or, in the case of children, play.

Pathology and pathogenesis

The changes in the skin and eyes are caused by the death

of microfilariae. Following an acute response to the worm there is granuloma formation and fibrosis. Enlargement of regional lymph nodes is often present. Over a number of years the result is destruction of elastic fibres, fibrosis and thickening in the affected skin. Microfilariae die in the cornea, leading to irreversible corneal scarring. Worms also may die in the iris and ciliary body, causing uveitis with secondary glaucoma as a further complication.

A range of immune responsiveness has been suggested to account for the observation that some heavily infected patients have no symptoms, while others have marked symptoms and signs. Antibody and eosinophils are the principal effectors in killing microfilariae.

Clinical features

The earliest symptom is pruritus. The itch may be made worse by a hot bath. Examination shows a papular eruption with excoriation. When the arm or leg is affected, the limb may be obviously swollen in the early phase of the infection. Regional glands are often enlarged and non-tender. The lateral corneo-scleral junction should be examined with a slit-lamp for keratitis, which appears first as small diffuse white spots. Slit-lamp examination may show microfilariae in the anterior chamber. The posterior segment of the eye should be examined for retinal lesions.

The papular rash is less apparent in chronic cases where fibrosis has produced inelastic thickened skin. There may be patchy destruction of the pigment layer in a black skin, giving a 'leopard skin' appearance. Destruction of the elastic fibres of skin in the inguinal region creates pouches containing enlarged inguinal glands, 'hanging groins', and the same process predisposes to inguinal hernia. Onchocercal nodules may be seen and felt over bone prominences.

Diagnosis

The parasitological diagnosis is confirmed by examining skin shavings from affected areas for microfilariae. Eosinophilia and a positive serological test for filariasis are usually found in the peripheral blood but are not diagnostic for onchocerciasis.

Differential diagnosis

Scabies and lichen planus are common or relatively common itching skin diseases in the tropics and should be considered. Nodules and ocular disease are not found, and the appearance and distribution of lesions in both conditions is different. Loa loa infection (p. 315) causes transient soft tissue swelling that produces short-lived pruritus. The lymphatic filarial infections cause unilateral limb swelling with regional adenopathy but no pruritus or papular rash.

Treatment

Diethylcarbamazine (DEC) has been the mainstay of treatment for many years. The starting dose is 25–50 mg,

increasing on alternate days to a maximum of 200 mg 3 times a day, maintained for 21 days. The disadvantage of this drug is that it causes gross exacerbation of the symptoms and signs of the disease, even at the lowest doses. When this is severe, doses should be increased more slowly. When ocular disease is exacerbated, topical or systemic steroids may be needed. Malnourished patients or those with intercurrent infections should have these problems corrected *before* DEC is given, as reactions on treatment may be fatal in malnourished or infected persons. Without re-infection about 50% of patients relapse by 1 year after treatment. This does not indicate parasite resistance, as DEC kills microfilariae effectively but does not kill adults.

Suramin (Antrypol) is effective against adult worms and microfilariae but is used mainly for its ability to kill adult worms when ocular involvement is present. Anaphylaxis to the drug can occur and the drug is nephrotoxic. Mebendazole (1.0 g twice daily for 4 weeks) has been used in onchocerciasis with good effect and no exacerbation of the symptoms and signs of the disease. This regimen is very expensive, and can cause liver and bone marrow toxicity. Ivermectin has been tried in onchocerciasis with good microfilaricidal activity and much less exacerbation of the disease. Excision of onchocercal nodules is recommended, particularly those on the head and shoulders.

Prevention and control

The Onchocerciasis Control Programme in West Africa has been very successful in reducing transmission of the disease by application of insecticides to vector habitats and by treating cases. The success is evidenced by a striking reduction in infection rates among children. The costs involved are considerable. Insecticide resistance may become a serious handicap to further progress.

Lymphatic filariasis

Lymphatic filariasis is a group of filarial infections in which adult worms, found in major abdominal lymphatic vessels, shed microfilariae which are carried to the bloodstream. In contrast to onchocerciasis, it is the adults that cause the pathological changes resulting in lymphoedema. This occurs in a relatively small proportion of those infected. The three species involved are *Wuchereria bancrofti*, *Brugia malayi* and *B. timori*. Geographical distribution of *W. bancrofti* is shown in Fig. 12.34.

Aetiology and transmission

Wuchereria bancrofti (Fig. 12.35) females measure 80–100 mm long by 0.3 mm. The males are smaller, 40–50 mm long. The adults live in lymphatic channels and the female sheds about 50 000 sheathed microfilariae per day; these are carried to the bloodstream in lymph. They circulate in the blood and are taken up by mosquito vectors of the genera *Culex*, *Anopheles* and *Aedes*. The infective larvae moult twice after they enter a human host when the insect bites. *Wuchereria bancrofti* exhibits periodicity of micro-

Fig. 12.34 World distribution of filariasis. Onchocerciasis distribution is very focal and not uniform over the areas shown.

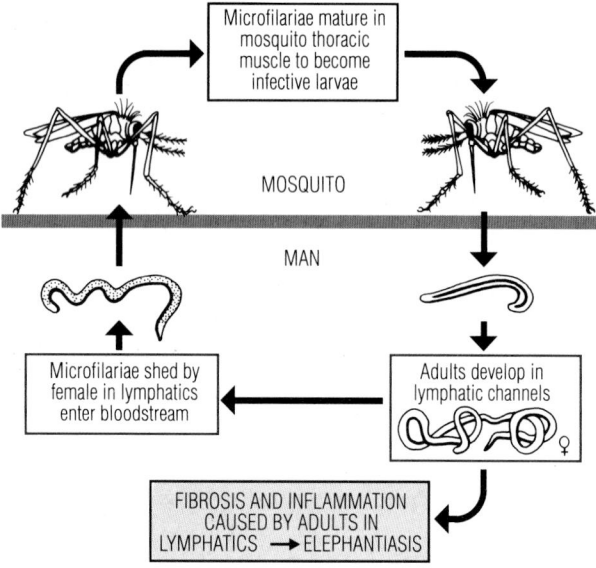

Fig. 12.35 Life cycle of lymphatic filariasis.

filaraemia throughout most of its geographic distribution, releasing microfilariae during the night hours; maximal counts are at about 1 a.m., in close relation to the nocturnal feeding habits of the mosquito vectors. Subperiodic strains release microfilariae throughout the 24-hour period.

Brugia malayi and *B. timori* have similar adult morphology and a similar life cycle.

Distribution and incidence

Bancroftian filariasis has the widest geographical distribution, covering tropical Africa, Asia east of Pakistan as far as eastern China, Indonesia, the Philippines, Papua New Guinea, the Caribbean and the north-eastern regions of South America (all periodic forms). Subperiodic forms are widely distributed in S.E. Asia and the Pacific.

Current estimates indicate that about 905 million people live in endemic areas, of whom about 10% are infected. Of these, 90% have *W. bancrofti*. Two-thirds of all those infected live in China, India and Indonesia.

Pathology and pathogenesis

Obstructive lymphoedema of arm, breast, genitalia or legs is the main outcome of inflammatory changes in main lymphatic channels elicited by the presence of adult worms. Swelling of the affected area, often the leg, may appear within months of infection. Adult worms may be found in lymphatics or lymph nodes. Distal to this obstruction the lymphatics are dilated. Inflammatory changes in the epididymis can be an early manifestation of the host response to *W. bancrofti*. Similar histological features occur in infection with *Brugia* species but these most often affect the legs. In established infections, episodic non-bacterial lymphangitis and lymphadenitis occur, evoked by allergy to filarial antigens. Eosinophils, giant cells, dead adult worms and fibroblasts are seen in the affected lymphatics and glands.

In the chronic phase lymphatic channels are obstructed by fibrosis with distal lymphoedema. There is fibrosis in the lymphoedematous tissue.

Clinical features

Many infected people have no symptoms related to the disease, and so there is likely to be an element of idiosyncrasy in the responses of those that develop disease. The earliest feature is often generalised painless swelling of the leg. There is no rash and inguinal glands may be normal. The swelling is worst in the evening and declines while the patient is recumbent overnight. This occurs within months of infection before microfilariae are shed, which indicates a response to adult worms. Without treatment this swelling may progress to the chronic lymphoedema of filariasis. Recurrent lymphangitis is another presentation of filariasis. Lymphatics are red and tender, and inguinal glands are swollen and painful. The lymphangitis may spread distally in a limb, which is the opposite of spread in bacterial lymphangitis. Epididymitis which may or may not relapse is another manifestation of the same process.

The end stage is non-pitting lymphoedema with thickened, lichenified skin. The penis, scrotum or labia may be involved. The breast is sometimes involved. Infection with *Brugia* species tends only to affect the lower limbs. Filarial abscesses can develop along the line of lymphatic channels, more often proximally in the limb. These rupture and discharge, and the ulcerated area heals well.

W. bancrofti infection may cause intermittent chyluria, in which anastomoses between intestinal and renal lymphatic channels are open; these are due to more proximal obstruction in main lymphatics leading to the cisterna chylae and thoracic duct.

Diagnosis

Diagnosis is usually made on the history, physical signs

and marked peripheral blood eosinophila when patients are seen at the early lymphoedema stage. Later, when there is relapsing lymphangitis or epididymitis microfilariae are found in the blood, maximally at 1 a.m. in the periodic forms, and by day and by night in the subperiodic forms. When there are many microfilariae they are readily found in stained blood smears; alternatively, filtration of blood through a millipore filter to retain the microfilariae may be needed to demonstrate parasites in lighter infections. The parasitic infection may have died out in patients with end-stage disease, and so parasites cannot be found. Serological tests are not specific for filarial infections and cross-reactions with *Strongyloides* are common, so that a positive test should stimulate a further search for parasites.

Differential diagnosis

Tuberculosis, malignancy and chronic bacterial lymphangitis may all cause lymphoedema in the tropics.

Treatment

Diethylcarbamazine (DEC) is used, as for onchocerciasis (p. 313). Reactions due to death of worms do occur. Lymphoedema is best controlled by elevation of the affected limbs at night and pressure bandaging. Surgery is not satisfactory and is only a final resort. Prophylactic penicillin (penicillin V, 250 mg twice daily) is helpful in patients who have had repeated attacks of bacterial lymphangitis.

Prevention and control

Traditionally these have depended on vector control and treating cases. Recent work in Indonesia and Kenya has shown that low-dose DEC can be used to control the infections.

Loa loa

Loa loa is a filarial infection characterised clinically by transient soft tissue swellings at sites of adult worm death. *Chrysops* flies are the vectors.

Aetiology

Loa loa adults measure about 60 mm by 0.5 mm (female) and 30 mm by 0.4 mm (male). They migrate freely in subcutaneous tissues. Six months after infection adults have developed, and fertilised females start to shed microfilariae which are found in peripheral blood during the daytime. *Chrysops* flies ingest microfilariae in blood meals. Development to adult worms takes place in subcutaneous tissues, and shedding of microfilariae begins by 90 days after infection. Adults live for up to 15 years.

Epidemiology

The endemic areas are shown in Figure 12.34, and these cover the tropical rain forest regions of West and Central Africa, extending as far east as the southern Sudan and Uganda.

The vectors live in the forest canopy and descend to lower levels to feed. The prevalence in some populations is 100%. Animal reservoirs do not play a part in the cycle of transmission.

Clinical features

Transient itchy soft tissue swellings up to 7 cm across, on the limbs or less often the face, are a common presentation; these are called 'Calabar swellings'. Occasionally an adult worm migrates across the globe of the eye beneath the conjunctiva, causing local irritation, a feeling of movement and some alarm. Occasionally a worm dies immediately beneath the skin, producing a linear swelling in the skin.

Problems can arise in patients who have large numbers of microfilariae in the peripheral blood (over 25–50/mm^3), beginning a short time after starting treatment with diethylcarbamazine (DEC). Encephalitis or encephalomyelitis can occur, probably due to death of microfilariae occluding vessels of the brain and spinal cord. Cerebral oedema and granulomatous reactions around microfilariae are found in fatal cases.

Diagnosis

The diagnosis is confirmed by finding typical sheathed microfilariae in peripheral blood samples taken during the day. When there are few microfilariae, millipore filtration of blood may show parasites (see above). Eosinophilia in the peripheral blood is usual and a positive serological test, e.g. filaria indirect fluorescent antibody test, provides only indirect evidence of infection.

Treatment

Diethylcarbamazine is the most active drug in the treatment of loiasis. It kills microfilariae very well and adults more slowly. While the patient is on DEC, Calabar swellings may appear. Also, worms dying close to the skin may be seen. When microfilariae counts are above 25–50/mm^3 DEC cannot be given alone because of the danger of precipitating cerebral complications. Removal of microfilariae from circulation is recommended. Whole blood exchange transfusion or leucapheresis using a blood separator can be used to remove large numbers of microfilariae. This makes it safe to give DEC in the usual way. Steroids may be given before DEC.

Prevention and control

Measures for control of loiasis have not been successful. Vector control is difficult. Mass chemotherapy is not appropriate because of the need for individual supervision of treatment in people with heavy infections, and because of the co-existence of onchocerciasis in the same endemic areas. Other measures include protection from biting by clothing and the use of insect repellants.

Tropical pulmonary eosinophilia (TPE)

Tropical pulmonary eosinophilia is a condition that has been seen most often in India but can occur wherever there is transmission of Bancroftian filariasis. It is thought to represent pulmonary hypersensitivity to the microfilariae of *W. bancrofti*.

The patients present with a range of nocturnal respiratory symptoms, including unproductive cough, dyspnoea waking the patient from sleep, and wheezing (not common). The severity of symptoms ranges from mild to severe. The physical signs may be minimal, with pulmonary crackles or minimal wheeze. Radiological changes are prominent, with linear and nodular shadowing that may alter with time. Pulmonary function tests show a predominantly restrictive defect.

Gross eosinophilia is usual, with absolute counts often in the range of 2000 to 10 000 per mm³. Serological tests for filariasis are strongly positive. Studies in TPE patients using species-specific antigens showed the highest titres to *W. bancrofti* antigens. Blood samples contain no microfilariae. It is thought that these hypersensitive patients sequester the microfilariae in the pulmonary circulation, clearing the blood before it passes to the left heart. Post-mortem studies have shown microfilariae in lung with surrounding inflammatory responses in lung vessels.

Treatment with DEC is effective but there may be initial exacerbation of pulmonary symptoms. If these are particularly bad, oral prednisolone may be given. Symptoms and signs regress and radiological changes return to normal. The eosinophil count returns to normal.

ANIMAL INTESTINAL NEMATODE INFECTION

Trichinosis

Aetiology

Trichinella spiralis is a nematode parasite with very low host specificity. It will infect over 100 species of animals, particularly carnivores. Infection of man occurs by eating undercooked meat containing encysted larvae (Fig. 12.36). These hatch in the human gut and mature to the adult stage. Fertilised females shed viviparous larvae for up to 14 weeks until the adults are expelled. The larvae penetrate the gut mucosa to reach the circulation and are disseminated to all the tissues, where they excite inflammatory responses. Larvae encyst and survive in skeletal muscles.

Distribution and incidence

T. spiralis is widely distributed in nature through the Americas, Asia, Africa and the Arctic. Sporadic cases and epidemics occur. Outbreaks occur in Europe.

Transmission and epidemiology

All ages and both sexes are susceptible but children seem

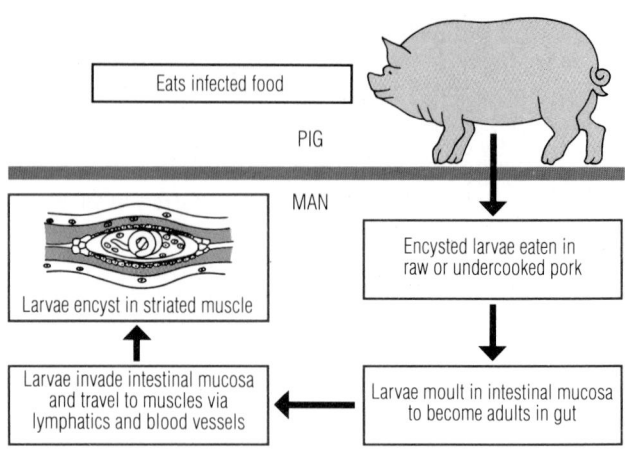

Fig. 12.36 Life cycle of *Trichinella spiralis*.

to have milder attacks, probably related to a lower infecting dose of larvae in their smaller meals. Exposure to infection is more likely among those nationalities whose cuisine involves eating raw or lightly cooked meats.

Pathology

Granulomata form around worms dying in the tissues. Focal interstitial myocarditis is found in the heart, with a marked infiltrate of eosinophils. A non-suppurative meningitis with granulomata and capillary thromboses is seen in fatal cases. Invasion of the eye muscles may contribute to the peri-orbital oedema. Skeletal muscles show encysted larvae, myositis with marked eosinophil infiltrate, and patchy degeneration of muscle fibres. Calcification may occur in the capsule of the cyst or in the larvae by 6 months after invasion, but larvae can remain viable in muscle for 10–15 years.

Clinical features

Four main features of the disease are fever, orbital oedema, myalgia and eosinophilia. Bowel upset is variable. Vomiting occurs, and the alteration in bowel habit may be diarrhoea or constipation. In the phase of muscle invasion the affected muscles are tender on movement. Fever, urticaria, splinter haemorrhages in fingers and toes, difficulty with swallowing and difficulty with breathing may all be present. Invasion of the nervous system can cause a meningitis-like picture. Fits, paralysis, disturbed conscious level, difficulty with balance and personality disorders may occur. Heart failure can result from severe cardiac involvement. Symptoms due to reactions to larvae in the tissues start to resolve gradually from about 14 days onwards in milder cases, but can take several months to settle completely.

Diagnosis

Trichinosis is suspected clinically and confirmed by examination of muscle biopsy for encysted larvae. Muscle biopsies can be obtained under local anaesthetic using a Trucut needle and are examined immediately, squashed between microscope slides. Eosinophil counts are very high, over 2.00×10^9/l, and muscle enzymes are raised. Trichinella serology is strongly positive. Differential diagnosis includes polyarteritis and other causes of eosinophilia.

Treatment

Thiabendazole is used in doses of 25 mg/kg, up to a maximum single dose of 1.5 g, twice daily for 5 days. Mebendazole is recommended (200 mg twice daily for a similar time). It eradicates adult worms from the gut lumen but does not affect larvae. Steroids should be given to those who have marked systemic upset and muscle tenderness.

Prevention and control

Thorough cooking or freezing ($-15°C$ for 20 days) of meat will prevent trichinosis. Public health measures include boiling pig swill and inspecting meat.

Toxocariasis

Toxocariasis is caused by infection with larvae forms of *Toxocara canis* or *Toxocara cati*.

Aetiology

Toxocara are primarily parasites of dog and cat, where the adult worms are found in the gut lumen. Eggs are shed in the faeces. Humans are infected by ingesting eggs, and the larvae released burrow into the gut wall to enter vessels and disseminate. Larvae mature outside the host over 14 days and then are infective to the definitive host or to man.

Distribution and incidence

The distribution is worldwide in dogs and cats, although there is considerable variation in the frequency of animal infection and contamination of the environment. Studies in Britain showed that 17% of soil samples were contaminated with toxocara eggs. Moist soil conditions are more suitable for transmission than hot, dry conditions.

Transmission and epidemiology

Children are most often infected. Infection is likely to occur when fingers contaminated with soil or sand containing eggs during play are put in the mouth. Dog faeces deposited in public parks, especially around playgrounds, represent a potential source of infection. Dog breeders and people who work in kennels are at risk of infection. Toxocariasis due to *T. cati* is much less common.

Pathology and pathogenesis

Disease in man relates to the number of infecting larvae and the host response. Clinical manifestations are due to dying and dead larvae, which evoke granuloma formation with eosinophils, macrophages and lymphocytes. The eye, brain, liver, spleen and lungs may be involved in toxocariasis, but granuloma formation may occur in any organ of the body.

Clinical features

Ocular toxocariasis and visceral larva migrans (VLM) are two clinical presentations of this disease, which is often a subclinical infection. Unilateral visual impairment is the usual symptom in ocular toxocariasis. Lesions directly on the visual axis will cause severe impairment. A child may develop a squint. The granuloma can form in relation to the lens and ciliary body, or on the retina itself. A cataract may develop secondary to a granuloma affecting the ciliary body. Visceral larva migrans is due to a heavy infection with larvae. Fever, anorexia, chills, night sweats and weight loss are usual features. Examination shows hepatosplenomegaly as the main physical sign. Pneumonitis may be present as well.

There is usually a marked eosinophilia in the peripheral blood in VLM, but eosinophilia is less common with ocular disease. Serological testing is valuable, the ELISA technique using a toxocara secretory antigen being a sensitive and specific test.

Differential diagnosis

Toxoplasmosis usually causes bilateral choroidoretinitis with destruction of the retina. Lymphoma, tuberculosis and sarcoidosis are usually considered in the differential diagnosis of VLM, although the gross eosinophilia is against the former conditions and supports a helminthic infection. The toxocara antibody test is strongly positive.

Treatment

Diethylcarbamazine is the usual treatment, giving initial doses of 50 mg and doubling the dose on alternate days till the maximum dose (10 mg/kg per day in 3 doses for 21 days) is reached. Ocular disease is not specifically affected by DEC because the worm is dead. There may be some spontaneous improvement as inflammation and granuloma size reduce. The DEC is given in these cases to kill any worms that are still migrating.

Prevention and control

Regular deworming of dogs, particularly pregnant bitches and puppies, reduces the numbers of eggs contaminating the environment. Dog owners should try to ensure that their dogs defaecate in a place where the faeces will not contaminate open spaces, playgrounds and parks.

Dracunculiasis

Dracunculus medinensis, the Guinea worm, is a tissue nematode widely distributed through Africa and Asia. Man is infected by drinking water containing minute crustaceans of the *Cyclops* genus infected with Guinea worm larvae. The larvae penetrate gut tissues and migrate through host tissues, maturing to the adult stage. The female is fertilised by the male, which dies, and the gravid female migrates out into a limb, producing a painful, fluid-filled blister about 3 cm across. The blister bursts and about 5 cm of the female protrudes. Vast numbers of larvae are released from the worm. Patients often put the affected limb into cold water to relieve the pain; this stimulates discharge of larvae to provide the opportunity for larvae to continue the life cycle by infecting other cyclops. The diagnosis is made on the clinical appearances. Treatment comprises:

1. relief of pain
2. treatment of secondary bacterial infection with antibiotics
3. administration of thiabendazole.

This does not have any direct effect on the worm, but reduces inflammation around the worm, allowing it to be gently wound out of the subcutaneous tissues on a stick.

TREMATODES

Schistosomiasis

Infection with digenetic flukes of the genus *Schistosoma* affects the bladder and urinary tract (*S. haematobium*), or intestine (*S. mansoni, S. japonicum*). These worms cause disease because of the host's response to eggs retained in the tissues. The severity of disease relates to the number of eggs in the tissues, which is proportional to the worm burden.

Aetiology

Eggs are passed in stools or urine; those deposited in still or slow-flowing fresh water hatch to release the ciliate miracidium, which can survive for up to 48 hours before it dies (Fig. 12.37). During this time it must find an aquatic snail of the appropriate genus, *Bulinus* for *S. mansoni*, *Biomphalaria* for *S. haematobium*, and *Oncomelania* for *S. japonicum*. Cercariae are released from the snail and these penetrate the skin of a suitable host, almost always man, becoming schistosomules during penetration. These migrate via the blood vessels to the pulmonary vasculature, where some traverse the pulmonary circulation to enter the systemic circulation. Schistosomules of *mansoni* and *japonicum* mature in the hepatic branches of the portal vein, and by 6 weeks after infection they are mature. They migrate out of the liver against the flow of blood in the portal vein to small veins around the colon and small intestine. The colon is mainly involved in *mansoni* infections, and both colon and small intestine are involved in *japonicum* infections. The life cycle of *S. haematobium* is similar, but maturation takes place in pelvic veins; the worm pairs migrate into small branches of the internal iliac vein around the bladder principally, although other pelvic structures – the prostate and seminal vesicles in men, and the uterus and adnexal structures in women – may be involved. Adult worms survive for about 7 years on average, but survival of over 30 years has been reported.

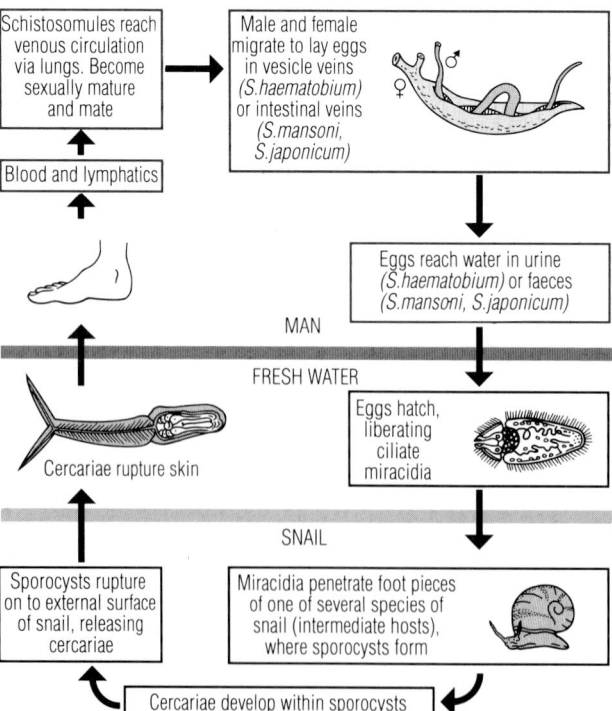

Fig. 12.37 Life cycle of schistosome parasites.

Distribution and incidence

The extent of the distribution is shown in Figure 12.38. There is considerable overlap in the endemic areas for *haematobium* and *mansoni*, but *japonicum* has a distinct, Asian distribution. The prevalence and incidence of infection vary considerably, with rates up to 70% or more in the endemic areas. Infection rates tend to be highest in children and decline with increasing age.

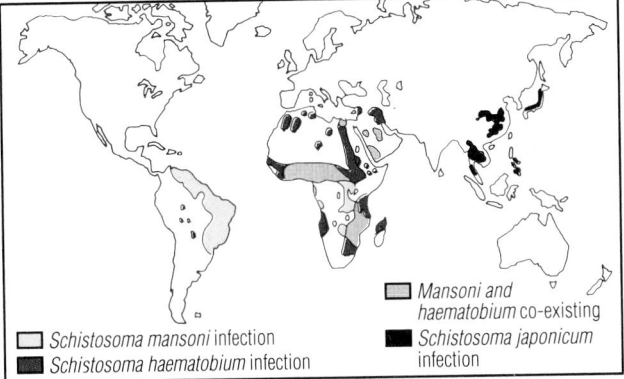

Key:
□ Schistosoma mansoni infection
■ Schistosoma haematobium infection
▨ Mansoni and haematobium co-existing
■ Schistosoma japonicum infection

Fig. 12.38 World distribution of schistosomiasis.

Transmission and epidemiology

Freshwater contact is the major factor in becoming infected and maintaining transmission. Children are infected early in life by playing in infected water. They are also likely to urinate and defaecate in and around pools and streams, further enhancing the local intensity of transmission. The highest rates and intensities of infection are found in the second and third decades of life.

Pathology and pathogenesis

The pathological changes relate to the presence of eggs in the tissues. Eggs laid in the small branches of veins may:

1. pass through the wall of the viscus to reach the exterior in faeces or urine
2. be retained in the tissues
3. embolise through vessels to lodge in presinusoidal branches of the portal vein in *mansoni* and *japonicum* infections, or in pulmonary arterioles in *haematobium* infections.

The egg excites a granulomatous response. Macrophages, lymphocytes, plasma cells and eosinophils constitute the granuloma. Granuloma formation is important for the transition of the egg through the mucosa to the lumen of the viscus. The chronic inflammation they may cause in the epithelium may be a factor in carcinogenesis in the bladder (*haematobium*) and the colon (*japonicum*).

Eggs retained in the tissues within granulomata gradually break down until all that may remain is remnants of the egg case. The granuloma heals by fibrosis. Early in the course of infection exuberant granuloma formation in the colon can cause polyps in *mansoni* and *japonicum* infections; in *haematobium* infection it can cause bladder polyps. These polyps resolve after treatment and may also resolve spontaneously.

Fibrotic polyps and strictures are not often seen in *mansoni* infection, although they are more common in *japonicum* infection. *Haematobium* infection causes fibrosis of the bladder, which is often shrunken with a thick wall. Bladder stones may form and cystitis is common. Unilateral or, less commonly, bilateral ureteric strictures cause obstructive uropathy. Stones may form in the dilated ureters. Distortion of the ureterovesical junction may allow vesico-ureteric reflux of urine with associated recurrent pyelonephritis.

Squamous cell carcinoma of the bladder is common in highly endemic *S. haematobium* areas. It is suggested that schistosomiasis acts with dietary factors to produce malignancy. Reports from China have associated colonic cancer with *S. japonicum* infections. Chronic schistosomal colitis causing epithelial cell dysplasia, a premalignant stage, and later carcinoma is the suggested sequence of events. This has not been found in *S. mansoni* infection.

Mansoni and *japonicum* eggs embolise to the liver. The granulomas add to the volume of the liver and increase its size, and obstruct the flow of blood through the portal circulation in the liver, causing congestive hepatosplenomegaly in those with heavy worm burdens. Over a period of years periportal fibrosis results, causing irreversible portal hypertension. The anatomy and architecture of the hepatic lobules are not altered and there are *no* regenerating nodules, therefore cirrhosis is not caused. In the lungs granulomatous reactions in the vessels cause fibrosis and pulmonary hypertension.

Involvement of the central nervous system occurs in *S. japonicum*, *S. mansoni* and *S. haematobium*, in descending order of frequency. Granulomas form around eggs that have embolised to the brain or spinal cord.

Clinical features

Cercarial invasion of the skin may cause a local, irritant, papular eruption but this is uncommon. Marked rashes develop when avian schistosome cercariae invade the skin. Most patients have no symptoms related to the phase of migration and maturation. Occasionally non-immune people develop the *Katayama syndrome* with the phase of worm migration. Those mildly affected may have malaise and lethargy, while fever, profuse sweats, muscle pain, abdominal pain, joint aches, unproductive cough, urticaria, swollen eyelids and hepatosplenomegaly occur in more severely affected patients. These symptoms begin 3–4 weeks after exposure and persist for up to 3 months with reducing severity.

Chest X-rays may show coin lesions due to worms dying in vessels and evoking local inflammatory reactions. Marked eosinophilia is common. Eggs are not found until 3–6 weeks after infection.

S. mansoni and S. japonicum

The onset of egg laying in *S. mansoni* infection is inapparent in most patients. Diarrhoea with blood in the stool occurs occasionally in those heavily infected.

Many infected patients go through life without any symptoms related to this infection. Rectal examination is normal; sigmoidoscopy is normal or shows scattered mucosal haemorrhages. Occasional patients present with anaemia and oedema because of bleeding and protein loss from schistosomal polyps. The most common physical sign in infected patients in endemic areas is hepatomegaly, which correlates with the intensity of infection in the first two decades but not in older age groups. Similar findings are noted in *S. japonicum* infection. Abdominal pain and subacute intestinal obstruction occasionally occur in the rare patients who develop fibrotic strictures in the colon or, less often, the small intestine. Hepatosplenomegaly with congestive splenomegaly suggests end-stage schistosomal hepatofibrosis. These patients often present with haematemesis and ascites. Porto-systemic encephalopathy is not a usual feature after variceal bleeding in schistosomiasis. Severe pain over a grossly enlarged spleen may indicate splenic infarction.

S. haematobium

Dysuria, frequency and haematuria occur in some patients at the start of egg laying. More commonly, the presenting symptom is terminal haematuria. The last drops of urine passed are blood-stained. Physical examination is usually normal. Most persons have light infections and suffer no long-term adverse effects. Reversible granulomatous polyps and obstructive uropathy occur in the early stages of heavier infection. This appears to be spontaneously reversible and it is certainly reversible after treatment. Those with heavy infections develop fibrotic and obstructive complications which can cause recurrent urinary tract infections, stone formation and finally renal failure. In these patients the infection is associated with an increased risk of bladder cancer. Excretion urography often shows bladder polyps and obstructive uropathy, either unilateral or bilateral, in older children and teenagers.

Chronic infection causes 'sandy' patches on the trigone as a typical cystoscopic finding. Calcification in retained eggs is seen in the bladder wall as a rim of calcium in the pelvis on a plain abdominal X-ray. Tramline calcification in the ureter may also be seen.

Other manifestations

Pulmonary involvement may be subclinical up to the stage when significant pulmonary hypertension develops. Right heart failure develops and this is difficult to treat. Cutaneous involvement is indicated by a collection of subcutaneous papules. The skin of the scrotum and perineum may be affected in *haematobium* infection.

Symptomatic involvement of the central nervous system is uncommon. Intracranial disease occurs with *S. japonicum* infections, with a frequency of 2–4% among those infected. It is much less common in *mansoni* and *haematobium* infections. Focal signs and Jacksonian epilepsy may occur with involvement of the cerebral hemispheres, while posterior fossa lesions are associated with raised intracranial pressure, cerebellar signs and brain stem compression.

Lesions of the spinal cord may present with features suggesting cord compression, transverse myelitis or spinal artery occlusion. Granulomas may also form around the cauda equina. The occurrence of focal signs in the neuraxis in a patient in or from an area endemic for schistosomiasis should prompt a search for schistosome eggs in stools and urine that would indicate active infection. Eosinophils in the cerebrospinal fluid suggest the possibility of schistosomiasis affecting the central nervous system. The use of antischistosomal drugs also needs to be considered.

Diagnosis

Diagnosis is made by finding schistosome eggs. Eggs of *S. mansoni* and *S. japonicum* are found in concentrates of faecal samples. Eggs of *S. haematobium* are found in the centrifuged deposit of terminal urine samples. Eggs of all three species may be found in rectal snips. Squash preparations can also be made from fragments of bladder mucosa obtained at cystoscopy.

Eosinophilia is a common finding in the peripheral blood but occurs in several helminthic infections. Serological tests can be helpful. An enzyme-linked immunosorbent assay (ELISA) for antibodies to schistosome egg antigens is useful because it indicates that infection has progressed to the stage of oviposition. The test takes 18 months to revert to negative after treatment and so is not helpful in assessing cure.

Excretion urography, isotopic renography, ultrasound scanning and computerised axial tomography give anatomical and functional detail of the urinary tract in chronic schistosomiasis. Colonoscopy and barium enema can be used to examine the colon in more detail. Ultrasound scanning of the liver demonstrates the presence of periportal fibrosis. Chest radiographs show dilatation of the pulmonary arteries and right ventricular hypertrophy in pulmonary hypertension. Myelography and computerised tomography allow localisation of schistosomal lesions of the neuraxis. Eosinophilia in the cerebrospinal fluid supports the diagnosis of CNS involvement in schistosomiasis.

Treatment

Three safe, effective drugs are available for use in schistosomiasis (Table 12.38). Their safety has not been confirmed in pregnancy and so treatment should be delayed until after delivery unless there are urgent indications for prompt treatment. All cases should be treated, even the advanced cases, as further oviposition causes further urinary tract, intestinal, liver or pulmonary damage. Ideally stools and rectal snips should be examined for viable ova 3 months after treatment.

Table 12.38 Drug treatment of schistosomiasis

Drug	Active against	Dose	Side-effects/contra-indications
Oxamniquine*	Schistosoma mansoni	West Africa and South America 15 mg/kg × 1 (adult) 20 mg/kg × 1 (child) Elsewhere 20 mg/kg per day ×3	Occasional febrile episode 5 days post-treatment
Metrifonate*	S. haematobium	7.5 mg/kg ×3 (2 weeks between doses)	Anticholinesterase actions may prolong neuromuscular blockade after surgery. Avoid elective surgery for 3 days post-treatment and provide ventilatory support after emergency surgery within 48 hours of administration
Praziquantel*	S. mansoni S. haematobium S. japonicum	40 mg/kg × 1 20 mg/kg ×3 (4 hours between doses)	Dizziness, nausea and occasional vomiting beginning 1 hour after dosing, lasting up to 4 hours

* The safety of these drugs has not been confirmed in pregnancy; treatment should be delayed until after delivery unless there are urgent indications for prompt treatment.

Prevention and control

Control measures are expensive and require a change in the behaviour pattern of the exposed population. Education regarding the reasons for the measures is essential. Dams and irrigation projects for the improvement of the economy of an area may create new habitats for snail hosts of schistosome parasites. Molluscicides can be used, but are expensive and may have detrimental effects on other water creatures. Biological methods of snail control are an attractive concept but are not yet effective.

Clonorchiasis

Clonorchis sinensis is a hermaphroditic trematode parasite of the biliary tract in man.

Aetiology

The adult fluke is 10–25 mm long by 3–5 mm wide. The life cycle is shown in Figure 12.39.

Transmission and incidence

Fish-ponds into which human faeces are poured as fish feed are an important source of infection as eggs, snails and fish are conveniently found together. The disease occurs in Asian countries. Dogs and cats are also important hosts.

Pathology

The worms obstruct small branches of the biliary tree, and bile accumulates in cysts proximal to the obstruction. Hypertrophy of the bile epithelium with adenomatous proliferation occurs. Later there is cellular infiltrate of the bile duct wall with chronic inflammatory cells. Pigment stones and biliary mud form. Flukes obstructing the pancreatic ducts can cause pancreatitis. Long-standing heavy infections are associated with malignant change in the adenomatous hyperplasia, leading to cholangiocarcinoma.

Clinical features

Clinical features relate to the worm burden. Mild infections cause no symptoms. Upper abdominal discomfort, diarrhoea and weakness occur with heavier infections; with the heaviest worm burdens upper abdominal pain, diarrhoea, weight loss, obstructive jaundice, hepatomegaly, cholangitis and Gram-negative septicaemia occur.

Diagnosis

The eggs are found in faeces or in duodenal aspirate. Eosinophilia is usual in the peripheral blood. Endoscopic retrograde cholangiopancreatography or percutaneous transhepatic cholangiography shows dilated branches of the biliary tree, and the worms appear as filling defects.

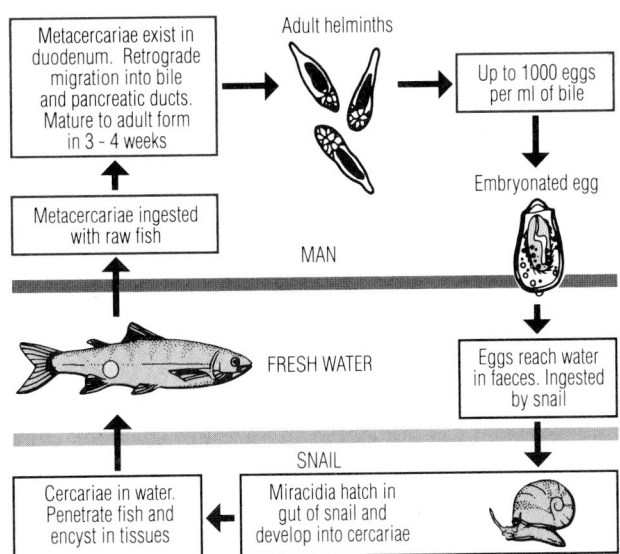

Fig. 12.39 Life cycle of *Clonorchis* and *Opisthorcis*.

Treatment

Praziquantel is the treatment of choice, giving 25 mg/kg on 3 occasions 4 hours apart on 1 day. When there is obstructive jaundice with cholangitis and septicaemia, relief of biliary obstruction, vigorous treatment of the bacterial infection and circulatory support for the patient are needed.

Prevention and control

Transmission can be interrupted by safe disposal of faecal wastes. Usually this involves a major change in social habits, which is difficult to achieve. Thorough cooking of fish before it is eaten prevents infection, as does freezing fish, $-10°C$ for 5 days, and salting in 10% saline.

Opisthorciasis

Opisthorcis viverrini and *O. felineus* have similar life cycles to that of *C. sinensis*, and in man they parasitise the intra- and extrahepatic branches of the biliary tree (Fig. 12.39). Raw, pickled, smoked and undercooked fish are the sources of infection. The pathological change and consequences are those of chronic irritation and obstruction of the biliary tree with ascending cholangitis in severely affected patients. Cholangiocarcinoma occurs in *O. viverrini* patients.

The diagnosis is made by finding eggs of the parasite in stools or duodenal aspirate. Praziquantel is used for treatment as for *clonorchiasis*.

Fascioliasis

Fascioliasis is an infection of the biliary tree with the hermaphroditic trematode, *Fasciola hepatica*. It is primarily an infection of sheep. The life cycle is similar to that of *Clonorchis* (Fig. 12.39).

Aetiology and distribution

The parasite measures 3 cm by 1.5 cm. Eggs are released in the biliary passages and pass to the exterior in the faeces. The miracidium hatches in fresh water and penetrates the tissues of a freshwater snail (*Lymnaea* species). After a cycle lasting 4 months in the snail, cercariae are released. These encyst on the leaves of watercress and other types of aquatic vegetation. Man is infected by eating watercress with encysted metacercariae. Maturation to the adult stage in bile ducts takes about 4 months until egg laying starts. Sheep are the normal hosts of this infection, and human infections are likely wherever sheep are herded in wet pasturelands.

Pathology

There is hepatic parenchymal necrosis in the phase of migration through the liver. The liver tissue regenerates. The worm burden determines the severity of disease. In the bile ducts there is chronic inflammation with regenerative hyperplasia of the epithelium and some degree of duct obstruction.

Clinical features

Pain in the liver area, fever, chills, tender hepatomegaly and marked eosinophilia are usual features during the tissue migration phase. Upper abdominal discomfort and hepatomegaly are present in mild to moderate infections, while heavy infections may cause obstructive jaundice and cholangitis in addition to pain and hepatomegaly.

Diagnosis

Eggs of the parasite are found in stools or duodenal aspirate. Eosinophilia is usual and serological tests for this infection are usually positive.

Treatment

Bithionol is effective (40 mg/kg in two divided doses after food on alternate days for 15 dosage days).

Prevention and control

Watercress production must be separate from sheep pastures. Wild watercress should not be sold for human consumption.

Fasciolopsiasis

Fasciolopsis buski is the largest trematode parasite, measuring up to 7.5 cm long by 3.0 cm wide. It has a wide geographic distribution through eastern Asia with a reservoir of infection in pigs. The metacercariae are found on bamboo shoots or water chestnuts, and infection occurs when these are eaten uncooked. After about 3 months the adult has matured in the small intestine; egg production begins and lasts for most of the 6-month lifespan of the adult. Upper abdominal discomfort, diarrhoea, preprandial upper abdominal pain relieved by food, and symptoms and signs of intestinal obstruction may occur, more marked symptoms being found with heavier infections. Eggs are found in the faeces. Tetrachlorethylene is effective in treatment. Praziquantel may prove to be effective.

Paragonimiasis

Paragonimus westermani is a hermaphrodite fluke that is usually found in the lungs but occasionally in other sites, e.g. central nervous system. It has a wide distribution in South America, West Africa, South-east Asia and the Pacific. Human infection occurs when raw or undercooked freshwater crustacea with metacercariae encysted in their muscles are eaten. The development cycle outside the host involves a freshwater snail: from the snail the cercaria is released and this finds a suitable crustacean host.

In man the metacercaria excysts and penetrates the full

thickness of the gut wall to enter the peritoneal cavity. The phase of tissue migration continues with the parasites reaching and crossing the diaphragm to enter the lungs. Where the worm finally comes to rest in lung tissue it elicits first a cellular response and then fibrosis, so that the worm is enclosed but for a connection to an airway. Dead worms calcify.

Radiological appearances comprise pleural thickening, infiltrates at the site of recent invasion, nodular lesions (encysted adults), fibrosis and finally calcification.

Eggs released by the worms are coughed up or swallowed. Cough productive of sputum, dyspnoea and chest discomfort are usual features. Bacterial infection of the affected area causes fever, systemic upset, purulent sputum and haemoptysis on occasions. Abdominal organs and brain are affected less often.

Diagnosis

Eggs are found in the sputum in most cases. Serological tests are available.

Treatment

Praziquantel is effective in doses of 25 mg/kg given three time daily for 3 days.

CESTODES

HUMAN INTESTINAL CESTODE INFECTION

Taenia saginata

Human infection with *T. saginata* is common in Africa, the Middle East, Asia and South America. The infective stage is the cysticercus in beef, and man is infected by eating rare or undercooked beef (Fig. 12.40). The cyst is released in the gut and the scolex everts from the cyst. It adheres to the gut wall and proglottids start to develop. Each segment has testis and ovaries, and is self-fertile. The worm may be 5–10 m long. The distal segments are full of eggs. Lengths of worm are passed in the stools, and when defaecation occurs in pasture, cattle may eat the gravid segments and develop cysticercosis bovis.

The infection causes no symptoms in man, although often a variety of vague abdominal symptoms have been attributed to it. Occasionally a patient will present with pruritus ani and find segments in his underwear. The motile segments have wriggled out of the anus.

The diagnosis is confirmed by examining segments. *Taenia saginata* segments have 15–20 lateral branches to the uterus. The eggs are occasionally found in the stools or on the peri-anal skin, but are identical in *saginata* and *solium* infections (see below).

Treatment with praziquantel (10 mg/kg as a single dose) is effective in 96% of patients. Niclosamide is also effective. Both praziquantel and niclosamide destroy the scolex and

Fig. 12.40 Life cycle of *Taenia* species.

so it is no use looking for it in the expelled worm remnants. If segments have not been passed by 4 months after treatment the infection is cured.

Thorough cooking of meat and freezing meat to −10°C for 10 days kills cysticerci. Meat inspection is also an effective control measure.

Taenia solium

The life cycle is the same as that of *T. saginata*, except that the pig is the intermediate host (Fig. 12.40). Infections with *T. solium* adults cause no symptoms. The segments are distinguished from those of *T. saginata* by the small number of lateral branches of the uterus, 7–13. Treatment is the same as for *T. saginata*, with the addition of an antiemetic prior to dosing and giving a purge 2 hours after dosing. Thorough cooking of pork or freezing to −10°C for 10 days prevents infection. Cysticercosis is discussed below in the section on larval cestodes.

Diphyllobothrium latum

The fish tapeworm has a more complex life cycle than the other intestinal cestodes: coracidia released from eggs infect water fleas (copepods). Further development takes place in fish that eat the copepods and in bigger fish that eat plerocercoid-infected fish. Mammals are infected by eating the plerocercoid-infected fish. Digestion releases the plerocercoid, which adheres to the gut wall and starts to produce proglottids. Proglottids break up, releasing eggs which are passed in the stools. Man is infected by eating uncooked fish.

A variety of abdominal and general symptoms are attributed to this infection, including abdominal discomfort, fatigue, weakness, sensations of hunger and diarrhoea. It is associated with deficiency of vitamin B_{12} and, less commonly, with overt megaloblastic anaemia. When the worm is sited in the upper part of the gastrointestinal tract, it can take up both free and intrinsic factor-bound vitamin B_{12}. Features of vitamin B_{12} deficiency appear when body stores are exhausted.

The diagnosis is made by finding eggs or, less often, typical segments in faecal samples. Purging may provide a sample of segments. Praziquantel gives a high cure rate. Niclosamide is also effective. Thorough cooking of fish and freezing fish to $-10°C$ for 48 hours kills plerocercoids.

Hymenolepiasis

Hymenolepis nana and *H. diminuta* are two species of small tapeworm. *H. nana* is predominantly a parasite of man with person-to-person transmission, while *H. diminuta* is predominantly a rodent parasite with man as an occasional host.

Children are most often infected with *H. nana*. Heavy infection causes abdominal pain, anorexia, diarrhoea, irritability, pruritus ani and urticaria. Eosinophilia is found in heavy infections. Treatment with praziquantel (15 mg/kg as a single dose) is effective.

H. diminuta has a more complex life cycle involving an insect intermediate host which ingests eggs with rodent faeces. Most infections cause no symptoms and are diagnosed when eggs are found in faeces. Treatment with niclosamide is effective.

LARVAL CESTODE INFECTION

Cysticercosis

Infection with the intermediate stage of the *T. solium* parasite (see above) can occur in two ways:

1. by ingesting eggs of the worm, which hatch in the gut to release the cysticercus
2. by regurgitation of gravid segments into the stomach to initiate the process of egg digestion and release of cysticerci.

The cysticerci released by either route of infection then invade host tissues. The first route is more common.

The development of subcutaneous lumps is a common presentation. Uni-ocular disturbances of vision occur with cysticerci in the eye. The most serious consequences occur in cerebral cysticercosis, causing epilepsy, raised intracranial pressure and localising signs related to space occupation. Frequently numerous cysts are found in the brain. The diagnosis is based on the geographic history, a positive serological test for cysticercosis on serum, and the finding of cystic lesions on computerised tomography (CT) of the brain. In the endemic areas where CT is not available, the diagnosis would be made on the clinical picture plus a high index of suspicion. Antibodies to cysticerci can be detected in cerebrospinal fluid, which contains increased amounts of protein, a normal glucose and normal or increased cell count. Skeletal muscles are often involved in cysticercosis. Usually this causes no symptoms and calcified cysticerci are seen on X-rays. There may be muscle pain at the time of invasion. If cysticerci are found at any site in the body a CT brain scan should be done to detect cerebral involvement.

Praziquantel is effective in cysticercosis. The dose is 50 mg/kg per day in three equal doses for 14 days. Dexamethasone is also given in doses of 4 mg three times daily prior to the start of treatment and tailed off after treatment. Follow-up shows that two-thirds of cerebral cysts will disappear, and symptoms and signs will improve. This treatment should be given in centres where neurological expertise is available.

Hydatid disease

Aetiology and distribution

Echinococcus granulosus is a tapeworm of dogs. The life cycle is shown in Figure 12.41. The ingested eggs release the onchosphere, which penetrates the gut mucosa and spreads by vascular or lymphatic channels to other organs, most often the liver, with lung, spleen, brain, eye, bone and other tissues infected less often. Cyprus, Turkey, Middle Eastern countries, the Turkana area of Kenya, and South America are among the endemic areas.

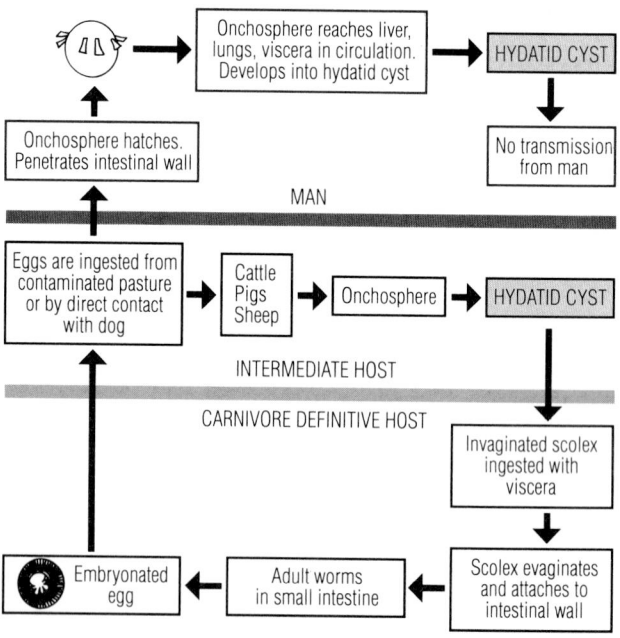

Fig. 12.41 Life cycle of *Echinococcus granulosus*.

Clinical features

The clinical presentation is very variable. Unexplained painless hepatomegaly is fairly common, but an expanding cyst can cause right upper quadrant abdominal discomfort.

Rupture of the cyst may produce pleuritic discomfort, abdominal pain and tenderness, and allergic manifestations such as urticaria and anaphylaxis. Rupture of hydatid cysts is infrequent, although the consequences of release of daughter cysts to seed the peritoneal cavity are serious.

Pulmonary hydatids may be symptomless and may be found on chest X-rays. They may rupture spontaneously. Hydatid material, membranes and scolices with hooklets may be coughed up and disseminate endobronchially to seed the lungs bilaterally, causing numerous small cysts in both lung fields. Bone and joint hydatids cause pain, swelling and sinuses discharging hydatid material. The latter may follow surgical exploration. The cyst wall may calcify.

Diagnosis

There may be blood eosinophilia and positive serological tests. Ultrasound and CT scanning allow accurate localisation and measurement of hydatid cysts in internal organs. Bone hydatid produces areas of lucency surrounded by sclerosis. Joints are destroyed.

Treatment

Management is difficult. Mebendazole in high doses has been successful in occasional cases where cysts are young and newly formed. Albendazole, which is much better absorbed, is currently being evaluated and may prove effective. Surgical treatment is difficult. Solitary pulmonary hydatids can often be excised with the relevant segments or lobe. Excision of hepatic hydatids is more difficult. Surgery for hydatids of the central nervous system requires great care to avoid rupture.

Complications

Secondary bacterial infection of a hydatid cyst is not un-common. Amoebic abscess, pyogenic abscess and perihepatic sepsis must be considered in the differential diagnosis when liver cysts are concerned. Gallium scanning may help to indicate bacterial infection and blood cultures should be taken. Amoebic serology is strongly positive in amoebic liver abscess. When infected hydatid cyst is probable, vigorous antibiotic treatment is first needed, followed by safe surgical drainage of the cysts.

Prevention and control

Regular deworming of dogs, killing of stray dogs, and safe disposal or boiling of offal are important control measures. These measures, plus effective communication of the dangers of hydatid disease among populations in Iceland and New Zealand, have controlled the disease.

FURTHER READING

Adler M W (ed.) 1984 ABC of sexually transmitted diseases. British Medical Association, London. *The only book a medical student needs on STD: summarises the important facts*
Adler M W (ed.) 1988 ABC of AIDS. British Medical Association, London. *This BMA booklet gives a clear summary, with good pictures, of all aspects of HIV disease*
Lambert H P, Farrar W E 1982 Infectious diseases illustrated. W B Saunders, London. *Illustrations of a wide variety of infections*
Lambert H P, O'Grady F 1990 Antibiotic and chemotherapy, 6th edn. Churchill Livingstone, Edinburgh. *A comprehensive guide to antimicrobials and their use*
Mandell G L, Douglas R G, Bennet J E 1989 Principles and practice of infectious diseases, 3rd edn. Churchill Livingstone, New York. *A major reference work*
Strickland G T (ed.) 1984 Hunter's tropical medicine, 6th edn. W B Saunders, London. *A major reference work*
Wilcox R R, Wilcox J R (eds) 1982 Venerological medicine. Grant McIntyre (now Blackwell, Oxford). *A major reference work*

Appendix table 1 Some clinical presentations, with fever, and their causes in the tropics and subtropics

Syndrome	Virus	Bacterium	Protozoon	Fungus	Helminth
Fever	Prodrome of viral hepatitis Arboviruses Influenza Lassa/Marburg/Ebola virus infections	Typhoid Brucellosis Leptospirosis *Borrelia* spp. Rickettsial disease	Malaria Toxoplasmosis Amoebic liver abscess Trypanosomiasis Babesiosis		
Fever + splenomegaly/ hepatomegaly/ hepatosplenomegaly	Epstein-Barr virus Cytomegalovirus	Typhoid Brucellosis Q fever Typhus Tuberculosis	Malaria Toxoplasmosis Amoebic liver abscess Visceral leishmaniasis Trypanosomiasis Babesiosis	*Paracoccidioides brasiliensis* Candida Histoplasmosis	Schistosomiasis (Katayama fever; also with *S. typhi*) Toxocariasis Infected hydatid cyst
Fever + jaundice	Fulminant viral Hepatitis Epstein-Barr virus, cytomegalovirus (both rarely) Yellow fever	Leptospirosis Typhoid Septicaemia	Malaria Trypanosomiasis		Worm obstruction of the biliary tree: *Ascaris* *Fasciola* *Clonorchis* *Opisthorcis*
Fever + adenopathy	Epstein-Barr virus Cytomegalovirus Herpes zoster virus	Tuberculosis Brucellosis Leprosy Melioidosis Syphilis	Toxoplasmosis Visceral leishmaniasis Trypanosomiasis		
Fever + rash	Dengue Coxsackie Enterovirus Epstein-Barr virus Cytomegalovirus Lassa/Marburg/Ebola virus infections Measles Rubella Varicella	Typhoid Rickettsial disease Meningococcal disease Leprosy Brucellosis (rare) Disseminated gonococcal infection	Trypanosomiasis Toxoplasmosis	*P. brasiliensis*	Bancroftian filariasis Schistosomiasis (Katayama fever) Trichinosis
Fever + neurological features	Mosquito-borne viral encephalitis Tick-borne viral encephalitis Rabies Encephalitis type of poliomyelitis	Leptospirosis Rickettsial disease Tuberculosis Brucellosis (uncommon)	Malaria Trypanosomiasis (Africa/S. America) Toxoplasmosis (in immunosuppressed hosts)		Strongyloides stercoralis (massive auto-infection)

Appendix table 2   Arbovirus infections

Genus*	Virus	Distribution	Clinical illness†
Alphaviruses	Chikungunya	E. Africa, India	2, 3
	O'nyong nyong	E. and W. Africa, Zimbabwe	2
	Eastern encephalitis	N. and C. America, Trinidad, Guyana, Brazil	4
	Venezuelan encephalitis	C. and S. America	1, much less often 4
	Western encephalitis	N. America, Mexico, Brazil, Argentina	4
	Ross river	Australia	1, with arthritis
Flaviviruses	Yellow fever	Africa, Caribbean, C. and S. America	See text
	Dengue	S.E. Asia, Pacific Islands, Papua New Guinea, Caribbean	1, 2, 3
	St Louis encephalitis	USA, Jamaica, C. and S. America	1, 4
	Murray Valley encephalitis	Australia, New Guinea	4
	Japanese encephalitis	Coastal region of E. Asia	4
	West Nile fever	Egypt, C. and S. Africa, Israel, Cyprus, France	2, 4
Phleboviruses	Naples virus ⎫ Sicilian virus ⎭	Mediterranean, Middle East, Africa, Asia	1

* All mosquito-borne, except phlebotomus group, which are transmitted by sandfly.
†Clinical features: 1 = febrile illness; 2 = febrile illness with rash; 3 = haemorrhagic fever; 4 = encephalitis.

Appendix table 3   Rickettsial infections

Organism	Disease	Usual host	Vector	Transmission	Distribution
Coxiella burnetti	Q fever	Domestic animals	Nil	Inhalation or ingestion	W. Europe, Australasia
Typhus group					
R. prowazekii	Louse-borne typhus	Man	Human body louse (*Pediculus humanus*)	Infective louse faeces rubbed into bite site or skin abrasion	Colder areas of the world: Himalayas, highlands of Ethiopia
R. mooseri	Murine typhus	Rats, other rodents	Rat flea (*Xenopsylla cheopsis*)	Infective flea faeces rubbed into bite site or skin abrasion	Tropical areas: especially around warehouses, grain stores, houses
Spotted fever group					
R. rickettsii	Rocky Mountain spotted fever (RMSF)	Small wild mammals	Ixodid ticks (= reservoir of infection)	Tick bite not seen	USA (Atlantic seaboard), S. America
R. conori	Tick typhus	Small wild mammals	Ixodid ticks (= reservoir of infection)	Tick bite usually present	N., E. and S. Africa, countries of Mediterranean littoral
R. akari	Rickettsial pox	Rodents	Mites (= reservoir of infection)	Infective mite faeces rubbed into bite site or skin abrasion	N. America, USSR, Korea
Scrub typhus					
R. tsutsugamushi	Scrub typhus	Small wild mammals	Larvae of leptotrombiculid mites, chiggers (= reservoir of infection)	Chigger bite not usually seen	Asia, S.E. Asia, Pacific area

Cardiovascular Disease

A

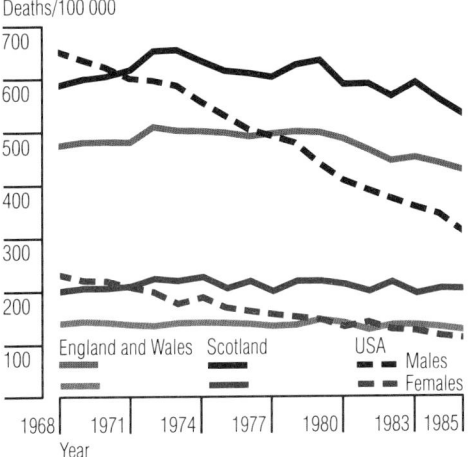

B

Fig. 13.1 Mortality from cardiovascular disease. A. Causes of death from cardiac disease (England and Wales, 1987). **B.** Deaths due to coronary artery disease in Scotland, England and Wales, and the USA in the years 1968–1985. Note the steep decline in mortality in males and females in the USA. (Source: WHO)

THE SCOPE OF MODERN CARDIOLOGY

More than 40% of patients admitted to medical wards in the United Kingdom have some form of heart disease. Hypertension, coronary artery disease, heart failure, and cardiac arrhythmias are among the commonest causes of emergency hospital admission. Ischaemic heart disease is the most important cause of death in the Western World, causing more than a million deaths per year in the USA and about 160 000 deaths annually in the United Kingdom (Fig. 13.1). Ischaemic heart disease accounts for 40–50% of all deaths in the developed world and is the main reason for men not reaching their seventh decade.

A recent concerted effort to change life-styles with respect to smoking, diet, and exercise, as well as better control of hypertension, appears to have led to a decline in coronary heart disease deaths in the USA and the more affluent Northern European countries, but has yet to make a major impact in the United Kingdom. Coronary artery surgery, although extremely effective, may be making only a small contribution to decreasing mortality.

Rheumatic heart disease has declined rapidly in importance in the West over the last 30–40 years (p. 426). It now accounts for less than half the cases of heart valve disease coming to surgery and, with only a small number of new cases presenting, its importance will probably decline much further. However, it is still a major cause of morbidity and mortality in the developing world – those countries least able to afford heart surgery.

Congenital heart disease is one of the principal causes of neonatal death and is likely to remain a significant cause of morbidity and mortality in childhood. However, more cases are now treatable by cardiac surgery in childhood, and major cardiac defects can now be detected during pregnancy, raising the possibility of neonatal, or even antepartum, cardiac surgery.

Some types of cardiac disease, for example cardiomyopathy, are increasing in frequency. The reasons for this are unknown and, until recently, treatment had not improved the generally poor prognosis.

The development of sophisticated methods of investigation in cardiology now allows great precision in diagnosis, enabling full advantage to be taken of the advances in cardiac surgery and catheter-based treatments. Diagnostic methods have expanded from simple ECG and X-ray, to include an ever-widening range of techniques, using ultrasound (both imaging and Doppler), isotope imaging, angiography, intracardiac electrophysiology and 24-hour ECG recording, pressure measurement and magnetic resonance imaging. Therapeutic options have also increased, to include complex cardiac surgery possible at all ages, pacemaker therapy and non-surgical interventions such as angioplasty. The efforts of cardiac surgeons and bioengineers have produced a generation of patients with prosthetic heart valves, implanted pacemakers, modified congenital heart disease and, now, heart transplants; these present a new spectrum of pathology and altered natural history.

NORMAL AND DISORDERED PHYSIOLOGY

CONTRACTION

Cardiac muscle is striated and shares with skeletal muscle the same basic contractile unit, the *sarcomere*. The components of the sarcomere are the myosin thick filaments, and the thin filaments composed of actin, troponin and tropomyosin. A local increase in calcium concentration allows an interaction to occur between the heads of myosin molecules and the thin filaments which produces crossbridges between the filaments. During contraction, a conformational change between the globular head of the myosin molecule and its rod-like tail causes a tension in the cross-bridge, making the filaments slide past each other (Fig. 13.2). This shape-change is brought about by the

Fig. 13.2 Diagrammatic representation of sarcomere contraction. A. In the relaxed state (diastole) tropomyosin inhibitory subunits prevent the interaction of the myosin heads with actin. **B.** In the presence of calcium, this interaction can take place enabling contraction (systole) to occur.

hydrolysis of adenosine triphosphate (ATP) by myosin ATP-ase to produce adenosine diphosphate (ADP) and inorganic phosphate (Pi).

Energy for contraction

Adenosine triphosphate is only present in small amounts in heart muscle, so that its production must occur at a rate equal to its consumption. The metabolism of fats and glucose by oxidative phosphorylation, in the mitochondria, yields ATP. Free fatty acids (FFA) are the major source of myocardial energy, yielding 2.5 times more ATP per gram weight than glucose. Breakdown of glucose can occur in the absence of oxygen, but, under these circumstances, only two molecules of ATP are produced per molecule of glucose metabolised to pyruvate (instead of the 36 obtained by aerobic metabolism of glucose to carbon dioxide and water). The normal heart consumes lactate, which, by the action of lactate dehydrogenase, yields pyruvate.

The action potential

Rhythmic contraction and relaxation of myocardial cells is achieved by the sequential release of calcium near the myofibrils and its subsequent removal. This cyclical change in cytosolic calcium concentration is due to release of calcium from the sarcoplasmic reticulum, initiated by the depolarisation of the cell membrane (sarcolemma) during the action potential. The sequence of events is outlined in Figure 13.3.

Fig. 13.6   The relationship of LV volume to pressure in a normal cardiac cycle (A-B-C-D). At (A) systole begins. The pressure rises isovolumically until at (B) the aortic valve opens. The ventricle ejects to (C) and then isovolumic relaxation occurs until (D), at which point filling occurs. With acute elevations in aortic diastolic pressure (red line), pressure in the ventricle rises to (E) before the aortic valve opens. Ejection occurs to (F). The pressure volume relationship at the end of systole is defined by the black line (E $_{max}$) passing through (C) and (F). The beat A-E-F-G has a low stroke volume (A minus G). For this to be restored to the original volume (A minus D), the line E$_{max}$ must shift to the left (dotted line); i.e. a positive inotropic effect is required, where a given end-systolic pressure is associated with a lower volume and more complete ejection.

dilated ventricle with an increased diameter can only generate the same pressure with an increased wall tension. This increased wall tension can only be produced by an increase in oxygen consumption, and this may outrun the supply, leading to further ischaemia and dilatation.

Ventricular hypertrophy

Usually a response to an abnormal pressure load, hypertrophy is characterised at the ultrastructural level by a parallel increase in sarcomere numbers. Hypertrophy may also cause increased myocardial oxygen demand, a burden that the coronary circulation may not be able to maintain, particularly for the less well-supplied subendocardial layer of muscle. The thick walled hypertrophied myocardium has abnormal properties in diastole: compliance is reduced so that filling may be impaired and diastolic pressure higher for any given filling volume. At the extremes, this also tends to impair adequate perfusion of deep myocardial layers.

SYMPTOMS AND SIGNS OF CARDIAC DISEASE

The major cardiac symptoms are chest pain, shortness of breath, palpitations, syncope and presyncope, oedema and fatigue. These symptoms are similar to those of other conditions. Thus, a careful history is essential and may show that the patient's symptoms are more likely to arise from the heart than from, say, a combination of indigestion and bronchitis. It also provides an opportunity for the patient to indicate the degree of disability and intrusion into

normal life. An inquiry into the extent to which the patient has had to change how and what he does is most instructive. Some patients avoid symptoms by grossly restricting their activities; others take their symptoms as a matter of course without realising their significance. It can also be very useful to ask for a history of heart disease in the family or a close acquaintance, since cardiac symptoms may follow dramatic cardiac events in close relatives or contacts (but are not always functional in origin). Some diseases, such as hypercholesterolaemia, are familial.

Chest pain

There are several types of chest pain arising from the heart and great vessels. The pain may be from cardiac ischaemia, pericarditis, aortic dissection, massive pulmonary embolism or, in introspective patients, from ectopic beats, in which case the patient will complain of occasional, apical, stabbing pain.

Cardiac ischaemic pain

The typical pain of angina pectoris or myocardial ischaemia is a squeezing, gripping pain, usually felt in the praecordium but often felt in the throat (hence the term *angina* or sore throat). It may radiate down the arms, usually the left, up into the jaw and lower teeth, or even through to the back. The pain is reproducible in its location and distribution, except that mild attacks may not gain the full distribution of more severe attacks. For example, an anginal attack may always start in the praecordium and only go through to the back if it becomes more severe.

The discomfort may be very severe and be associated with frightening feelings of impending death, an inability to get enough air and sweating. It can also be a mild discomfort or ache in the chest which may be thought trivial and ignored. Some patients have difficulty in describing their angina as a pain, and feel it as a faint constriction in the chest. Many attacks of cardiac ischaemia are unaccompanied by any pain (*silent ischaemia*).

Angina usually disappears fairly rapidly if the patient rests, or takes glyceryl trinitrate (GTN). Angina builds up over a few seconds and is usually not greatly influenced by posture; whereas muscular skeletal chest pain, which may occur with exertion, comes on very suddenly and is often greatly influenced by posture. Although similar in nature and radiation, the pain of myocardial infarction lasts much longer than angina. It is more intense and does not pass off with rest or GTN. In an attack, a patient with cardiac ischaemia usually looks pale and sweaty, unlike someone with an attack of indigestion, who often appears flushed.

Other causes of chest pain

Pericardial pain is described more fully on page 433. It is very similar to anginal pain but is often influenced by posture, sometimes being relieved by leaning forwards, and aggravated by swallowing. It is more often described as a burning pain, and is less likely to be associated with breathlessness than is cardiac ischaemia.

The pain of *dissection of the ascending aorta* is described as a very severe, tearing pain, often starting suddenly, usually felt retrosternally at first and then going through to the back if the dissection extends to the arch and descending aorta.

Massive pulmonary embolism can also produce a retrosternal constricting discomfort (p. 505). The pain of oesophageal rupture can be confused with myocardial infarction. *Oesophageal spasm* due to reflux can also produce a severe retrosternal pain which may be confused with that of myocardial ischaemia. *Jabbing precordial pains* are common in highly strung patients. They may have a muscular origin, but, on occasion, coincide with the accentuated post-ectopic contraction of the heart which is perceived by the patient as a stabbing pain.

Dyspnoea or shortness of breath

Everyone breathes more heavily on exertion, but they do not necessarily feel 'short of breath'. This symptom is a feeling of laboured, or unnaturally difficult, breathing. In heart failure, it is due to decrease in compliance of the lungs owing to the congestion that occurs with a rise in pulmonary venous pressure, and the patient's limited cardiac output. The reduced cardiac output limits the oxygen-carrying capacity of the circulation, so that, during mild activity, anaerobic metabolism occurs with the muscles producing lactic acid. The acidosis causes increased ventilation which persists for longer than normal after exertion. Thus, even minor exertion produces disproportionate and prolonged dyspnoea. Finally, in severe left heart failure with pulmonary oedema, the dyspnoea may be caused by arterial oxygen desaturation.

The degree of exertion that produces dyspnoea (or angina) can be categorised using the New York Heart Association scale (Table 13.1). Severe forms of left heart failure are associated with dyspnoea at rest, closely related to posture. This degree of pulmonary venous hypertension is commonly accompanied by a dry, non-productive cough. The dyspnoea may prevent sleep, and the severity can be graded on the basis of the height of the pillows required to enable the patient to sleep (*orthopnoea*). It is common for patients with left heart failure to be woken from their sleep by severe dyspnoea resulting from pulmonary congestion.

This passes off after a few minutes of sitting up, or even walking about slowly, and is known as *paroxysmal nocturnal dyspnoea*. This may be the first symptom of left heart failure, and may be difficult to distinguish from nocturnal asthma, as some patients with left heart failure develop a considerable degree of wheeze with bronchospasm.

Palpitations

The term 'palpitation' is used by patients to describe a wide variety of disorders in which there is an awareness of the heart beat. A careful interpretation of what the patient means is therefore essential. It may be simply an awareness of the normal heart beat, which may be more forceful or faster than usual because of anxiety; it may, however, be indicative of a serious cardiac arrhythmia. It is useful to ask the patient to tap on the table to indicate the rate and rhythm during the attack. Many patients can do this remarkably accurately, especially if they have had a true paroxysmal tachycardia. It is helpful to determine if the attacks stop suddenly or gradually, whether they were preceded or stopped by a forceful thump in the chest (ectopic beat) and whether there were symptoms of cardiac insufficiency, such as faintness and dyspnoea (suggesting low cardiac output and blood pressure, and pulmonary venous hypertension respectively). Irregular thumping suggests ectopics or atrial fibrillation; the occurrence of angina implies a very fast and potentially dangerous heart rate; and true syncope indicates an urgent need for investigation, as the arrhythmia is potentially fatal. Polyuria sometimes occurs in supraventricular tachycardias, but is not usually described by the patient unless a leading question is asked. Patients sometimes claim to have palpitations which, on closer questioning, are twitching of superficial muscles over the left breast. The term palpitations can also be used to describe a fluttering feeling over the praecordium from ectopics, or a marked pulsation in the neck from a tachycardia.

Syncope and presyncope (dizziness)

Exertional syncope

Sudden collapse with loss of consciousness *during* exertion, such as running for a bus, almost always has a cardiac cause. It is due either to an obstruction to outflow from the left or right ventricle which prevents an adequate increase in cardiac output on exertion, or to a cardiac arrhythmia, such as heart block, induced by the exertion. Both may result in a sudden fall in blood pressure and cerebral perfusion.

Syncope *after* exertion is not uncommon and may simply be due to blood pooling in the legs and a poor venous return. However, syncope under other circumstances may be cardiac, and an eye-witness account is invaluable. Cardiogenic syncope usually occurs without warning; the collapsed patient is vasoconstricted and grey and the pulse is either absent or very slow. In a classical 'Stokes-Adams' attack, the unconscious patient blushes dramatically with

Table 13.1   New York Heart Association grading of dyspnoea or angina

Grade	Criteria
1	Symptoms only occur on severe exertion. Almost normal life style possible.
2	Symptoms occur on moderate exertion. Patient has to avoid certain situations, such as carrying shopping up several flights of stairs.
3	Symptoms occur on mild exertion. Activity is markedly restricted.
4	Symptoms occur frequently, even at rest.

the return of circulation and subsequent return of consciousness.

A degree of mental confusion after cerebral anoxia is almost invariable. A prolonged period of unconsciousness is unlikely to be cardiogenic since (unless the patient is concussed) cardiac asystole or a malignant cardiac arrhythmia sufficiently rapid to cause unconsciousness is unlikely to last long without proving fatal.

Other forms of syncope

'Common' syncope. The common faint, often triggered by pain or an unpleasant sight, gastrointestinal upset, haemorrhage or pyrexial illness, is a vagal phenomenon, and a syncopal episode followed by profuse cold sweat, a feeling of sickness or actual vomiting, and bradycardia is very rarely 'cardiogenic'.

Micturition syncope and *cough syncope* are rarely cardiogenic, but are probably triggered by a Valsalva manœuvre, the first when initiating micturition with a full bladder (and usually in a vasodilated state) and the latter after repeated bouts of coughing, which inhibit venous return.

Presyncope or *dizziness* is a common and much less defined symptom, and has a variety of causes other than heart disease. It may result from a cardiac arrhythmia, but, even then, is much more common in elderly patients with associated cerebrovascular disease.

Oedema

Right heart failure causes pitting oedema of the feet and legs. It is usually worse at the end of the day and is relieved by rest and keeping the legs up. Unlike other causes of oedema (such as hypoalbuminaemia), it may be associated with other symptoms of heart failure, such as dyspnoea and fatigue. The oedema may spread to the thighs and even to the abdominal wall and skin of the sacrum and back. There is then often some ascites and hepatic congestion, so the patient also complains of abdominal distension. Occasionally, the hepatic congestion is aggravated by exertion and the patient complains of pain over the liver (usually epigastric) during exercise and for several minutes after. This symptom of right heart failure can be confused with true angina.

The differential diagnosis of cardiac oedema includes fluid retention from other causes, such as nephrotic syndrome and cirrhosis of the liver, oedema of one or both legs from venous insufficiency or lymphatic insufficiency.

Fatigue

Fatigue is such a non-specific symptom, and is so often a feature of depression or an anxiety state, that it tends to be neglected in the history. It is, however, a very real feature of heart disease, a result of the reduced effort tolerance and lactic acidosis produced by anaerobic muscle metabolism and changes in the skeletal muscle. It is a prominent feature of low cardiac output.

EXAMINATION OF THE CARDIOVASCULAR SYSTEM

Examination of the cardiovascular system is part of the general examination of the patient.

Position

The patient must be stripped to the waist and lying on a couch or bed with the head and thorax supported at about 45 degrees to the horizontal. There should be a strong light for examining the hands, and a side light for looking at the jugular venous pressure. For auscultation, there should be a minimum of competing noise.

General examination

Dyspnoea. Observation will reveal whether the patient is unduly breathless at lying down (orthopnoea) or on undressing. There may be a degree of intercostal recession in left heart failure from stiffening of the lungs and decreased lung compliance.

Cardiac cachexia. Although acute weight gain is common with development of oedema, in the long term, the cardiac patient usually loses fat and muscle bulk with prolonged heart failure and low cardiac output.

'Mitral' facies. The pulmonary hypertensive patient with a long-standing low cardiac output may develop a loss of subcutaneous fat from the face and the appearance of dilated cyanosed blood vessels over the cheek-bones. This characteristic appearance is seen in patients with long-standing mitral valve disease, but is not pathognomonic. It indicates a prolonged period of low cardiac output.

Peripheral cyanosis. A low cardiac output results in poor perfusion of the skin, particularly of the peripheries, such as the hands and nose, which become cyanosed and cold.

Central cyanosis. An intracardiac right-to-left shunt of blood causes central cyanosis, with a blue tongue as well as blue peripheries. In this situation, the peripheral circulation may be adequate with warm extremities and there will usually be clubbing of the fingers and toes. In cardiac failure, central cyanosis is not associated with clubbing and the extremities are cold and cyanosed.

Pallor. A low cardiac output causing vasoconstriction can lead to generalised pallor, including the mucous membranes, fingernails, and skin.

Oedema. There may be obvious pitting oedema of the legs extending to the scrotum (in males) and trunk. In a patient who has been in bed, oedema is often found over the sacrum. Pitting oedema is demonstrated by firm finger pressure for 5–10 seconds. Other signs of salt and water retention which may be present are abdominal distension from ascites and greatly engorged and pulsatile neck veins.

Hands

Clubbing is an incidental finding in most cardiac patients unless they have central cyanosis from congenital heart disease or infective endocarditis.

Cardiovascular Disease

13

Splinter haemorrhages are only seen in a good light and consist of small dark subungual petechiae. They are not specific to infective endocarditis but can be found after trauma and in other medical conditions, such as polyarteritis nodosa. Recurrent crops of splinter haemorrhages are a sign of continuing infection in infective endocarditis.

Blood pressure

Good technique is essential for accurate registration of the blood pressure. Although usually recorded early in the examination, it may be worth repeating when the patient is more relaxed and hypertension due to anxiety is likely to have settled. Hostility or anxiety in the patient causes a rise in blood pressure. Blood pressure readings tend to fall with successive visits, as the patient becomes more used to the same observer.

The interpretation of the Korotkoff sounds and a detailed description of blood pressure measurement are given on page 436.

Radial pulse

Rhythm

A regular pulse has almost equal pulse volume with each beat, so that the examiner can predict when the next beat is coming, e.g. by counting or tapping the foot. There may be slight variation in rate with respiration, particularly in young patients (*sinus arrhythmia*).

An irregularity of the heart rhythm may occur infrequently, or regularly after a number of normal beats; both are likely to be caused by ectopics. If the heart rate is totally irregular and the pulse volume changing all the time, the patient is likely to be in atrial fibrillation or having a large number of ectopics arising from different parts of the heart. If the pulse is irregular, the heart rate is best counted by auscultation, as observers vary considerably in their ability to feel weak beats.

Apex/radial deficit

The difference between the heart rate at the apex (by auscultation) and radial pulse rate at the same time is called the apex/radial deficit. This sign is of limited diagnostic value, as there is always a deficit if the apex rate is fast and irregular but a negligible one if the apex rate is slow.

Pulse types

The arterial pulse consists of a percussion wave and tidal wave separated by the dicrotic notch (Fig. 13.7). Usually, the tidal wave cannot be felt unless the patient has a high fever or is markedly vasodilated, when the pulse is called *dicrotic*. The time interval from the upstroke to the dicrotic notch is the ejection time of the left ventricle; this increases with stroke volume, and decreases with inotropic drive.

The characteristic pulse waveforms for aortic disease are best appreciated in the carotid pulse. *Pulsus alternans*

(alternating pulse volume with a regular pulse) is a feature of left ventricular dysfunction; *pulsus paradoxus* (exaggerated dimunution of pulse pressure and volume with respiration) is found when ventricular filling is embarrassed by pericardial constriction, tamponade or a cardiomyopathy; *pulsus bigeminy* and *trigeminy* are found with regular ventricular ectopics (Fig. 13.7).

Pulse volume

The pulse volume at the wrist depends on the stroke volume, which varies with cardiac output and pulse interval. It also depends on the state of the arterial tree proximal to the radial pulse and the state of vasodilatation of the skin of the hands. A patient will therefore have a smaller radial pulse volume when cold than when warm.

Carotid pulse

The pulse contour of a peripheral pulse is influenced by the state of vasodilation of the peripheral vascular bed. However, the carotid pulse supplies a vascular bed with a less variable blood supply, and is therefore more constant in its pulse contour.

The carotid pulse is most easily examined with the patient reclining at about 45 degrees, with the head fully supported and the chin central. The left thumb can be used to feel the right carotid and the right thumb, the left. The pulse is most easily felt half-way up the sternomastoid muscle at the level of the major skin crease.

The carotid pulse is used to time the first heart sound, which immediately precedes the upstroke. It gives an indication of the pulse volume and ejection time, and abnormalities of the waveform indicative of aortic valve disease can also be detected. A thrill may be present, caused by turbulence in the flow.

Pulse types

The characteristic types of carotid pulse are shown in Figure 13.7.

Collapsing pulse

The collapsing pulse is a sign of aortic regurgitation but may be found in any patient with a low impedance to aortic outflow in diastole (e.g. persistent ductus arteriosus, arterial venous fistula or immediately after exercise). The pulse has a very large volume with an abrupt fall following the upstroke. There is a large pulse pressure in the blood pressure measurement, with a low diastolic reading, and the carotid pulse may be visible in the neck (Corrigan's sign). A collapsing pulse may be so dramatic that the whole body shakes in time with the pulse.

Bisferiens pulse

There is a double peak to the bisferiens pulse (Fig. 13.7), which is characteristic of aortic regurgitation accompanied by some stenosis of the valve. However, it may also be

336

Normal carotid

Collapsing

Bisferiens

Anacrotic or plateau pulse of aortic stenosis

Pulsus alternans

Pulsus bigeminy

Pulsus paradoxus

Fig. 13.7 Carotid pressure tracing showing various pulse waveforms.

found in aortic regurgitation without a measurable aortic valve gradient.

Plateau (slow rising, or anacrotic) pulse

The characteristic pulse of aortic stenosis is a small volume sustained pulse which rises slowly to its peak displacement, often with a palpable thrill (Fig. 13.7).

'Jerky' pulse

The 'jerky' pulse is a pulse waveform found with shortened left ventricular ejection. It occurs with severe mitral regurgitation, hypertrophic obstructive cardiomyopathy (which may produce a type of bisferiens pulse if the tidal wave is palpable), and in heart failure. In the latter, the small pulse pressure and tachycardia may make it difficult to appreciate.

If the carotid pulse cannot be examined, any large artery such as the femoral, subclavian or brachial may give similar information, but, being more remote from the heart, they are less reliable as indicators of aortic valve disease.

Jugular venous pulse

The jugular venous pulse (JVP) is visible in the majority of patients if a little time and care are devoted to the examination. The height of the JVP is dependent on central venous pressure; it is therefore low in states of fluid depletion and haemorrhage, and raised in right heart failure and fluid overload. The waveform of the jugular venous pulse can be a useful diagnostic aid in heart disease.

The patient should be reclining on a bed or couch with the head supported at about 45 degrees. Jugular pulsation is often better seen with side-lighting than direct illumination, and is often better appreciated from the foot of the bed, when widening of the neck can be seen in time with the JVP. Turning the head may make the external jugular visible, but the internal jugular is more freely pulsatile and is the vessel that best repays inspection.

The JVP falls on inspiration and rises on expiration. Patients with increased airway resistance may be difficult to assess, especially if they are using external muscles of respiration, but should be requested to stop breathing with their mouths open for a few seconds while the height of the JVP is assessed.

If the JVP cannot be seen, the patient can be positioned more horizontally, when the pulse usually becomes visible. Alternatively, abdominal compression can be used to see whether the patient has a low JVP which then becomes visible. *Gentle* pressure anywhere on the abdominal wall, or over the liver, temporarily increases the venous return (hepato-jugular reflux). The normal right ventricle increases its stroke volume within two or three seconds, so there is a transient (if any) increase in venous pressure. The failing right ventricle, however, cannot increase its stroke volume, so that pressure produces a sustained rise in the venous pressure.

Discrimination of arterial from venous pulsation

Venous pulsation has a sinuous quality due to the low pulse-wave velocity and the fact that it varies with respiration. Arterial pulsation is always palpable, whereas venous pulsation is only palpable when there is tricuspid regurgitation.

Height of the JVP

The height of the JVP is measured vertically from the sternal angle and is normally less than 3 cm above it. It can be increased slightly in pregnancy and in patients on beta-blocking drugs.

Jugular venous waveform

The jugular vein's waveform is influenced by right heart events and arrhythmias. The principal components and classical waveforms are shown in Figure 13.8. The *a* wave is generated by atrial systole (there is no valve between the atrium and the jugular vein); it is absent in atrial fibrillation and exaggerated in right ventricular disease with a raised right ventricular filling pressure. The *v* wave coincides with ventricular systole, which causes a pressure pulse in the right atrium as the tricuspid valve bulges into the atrium.

Extra-large *a* or cannon *a* waves are seen when the atrium contracts against a closed tricuspid valve (Fig. 13.8) as in complete atrioventricular block, ventricular ectopics and nodal rhythm. Regurgitation through the tricuspid valve causes a giant *v* wave (sometimes called an *s* wave) with a very rapid *y* descent. A slow *y* descent is characteristic of tricuspid stenosis.

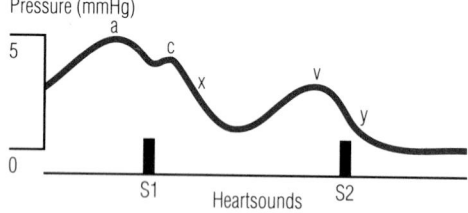

Fig. 13.8 Relationship of venous waveform to heart sounds. The a wave of atrial contraction is followed by the x descent. The c wave is not usually visible. The v wave coincides with ventricular systole.

The precordium

On inspection, there may be thoracic deformity. This sometimes indicates congenital heart disease, as the thorax remains plastic until ossification is complete. The apex beat may be visible.

Palpation is performed to detect cardiac hypertrophy and the presence of palpable heart sounds and thrills. Palpation over the lower end of the sternum, with the heel of the hand and light pressure applied, may reveal evidence of right ventricular hypertrophy or a very dynamic left

atrium, as in severe mitral regurgitation. Palpation at the apex is used to locate the position of the apex beat, which is defined as the furthest laterally and caudally that the pulsation can be felt. The cardiac apex is normally in the fifth space in the midclavicular line, but can be displaced by cardiac hypertrophy or mediastinal shift.

The *character* of the apex beat is often best appreciated with the patient tipped to the left, but the *position* of the apex must be judged with the patient lying on his or her back. The left ventricle usually makes up the apex, but in severe right ventricular enlargement it may be pushed posteriorly and the apex can be right ventricular. Left ventricular hypertrophy produces an apex beat which displaces the palpating fingers. The impulse may be generated by a pressure-loaded left ventricle (e.g. aortic stenosis or hypertension), in which case the apex impulse feels very muscular and thrusting but is not markedly displaced; alternatively, it may be generated by a volume-loaded left ventricle (e.g. mitral or aortic regurgitation), in which case the left ventricle feels very dynamic and the apex beat may be displaced considerably.

Left ventricular aneurysm may produce a rocking feeling at the apex, from a double or dyskinetic impulse. A grossly dilated damaged heart may have a very diffuse impulse with a presystolic thrust from a prominent *a* wave. In dextrocardia, the impulse will be on the right. Abnormal praecordial pulsation due to other types of heart disease is described in the relevant section below. Aortic aneurysm can produce pulsation retrosternally and 'tracheal tug'.

Auscultation

Hearing abnormal heart sounds and murmurs depends on training faculties of perception, particularly the ability to concentrate on listening for one short period of the cardiac cycle and perceiving a noise which is much quieter than that immediately preceding or following it. A quiet environment and well-fitting earpieces on the stethoscope are essential.

The diaphragm of the stethoscope is used for mid-range and high frequency sounds – normal valve closures, heart sounds, systolic murmurs and early diastolic murmurs. The bell favours low frequencies and should only be applied gently to the chest wall (or else the skin becomes a diaphragm). It is used for atrial and third heart sounds and the low-pitched, mid-diastolic murmurs of mitral stenosis, tricuspid stenosis and atrial septal defects.

Heart sounds

The timing of the heart sounds is shown in Figure 13.9.

First and second

The first heart sound, S1, signals the onset of systole and is produced by a variety of events, principally the closure of the atrioventricular valves and the tensioning of the wall of the left ventricle. It is identified by palpating the carotid pulse. The upstroke of the carotid pulse follows closely

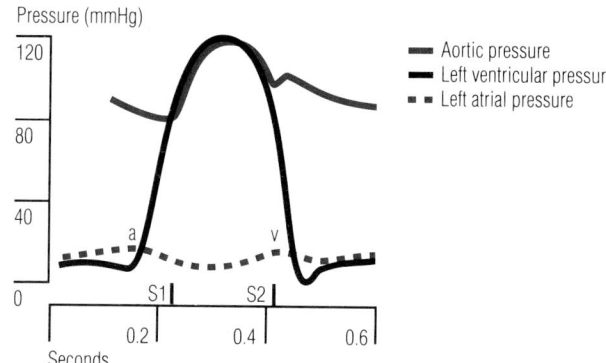

Fig. 13.9 Relationship between pressures in the aorta, left ventricle and left atrium. The timing of the heart sounds (S1 and S2) are shown.

after S1. The second heart sound, S2, separates systole and diastole and is due to the closure of the aortic and pulmonary valves and the sudden tensioning of their leaflets, like a sail flapping.

The normal sequence is S1 (mitral before tricuspid) and S2 (aortic before pulmonary). Splitting of S1 into its components is not usually very obvious, but splitting of S2 increases with inspiration so that S2 may become two distinct sounds which resynchronise with expiration. This is called normal splitting of S2 (Fig. 13.10). As the pulmonary valve closure sound (P2) is usually much softer than the aortic valve closure sound (A2) this normal splitting is most easily heard over the pulmonary area.

Third and fourth

The third and fourth heart sounds, S3 and S4, are low-pitched and not usually heard. However, they may be audible in fit young patients with bradycardia, such as athletes, and they become audible in patients with heart failure or a high ventricular filling pressure. They may arise from either side of the heart, but more usually from the left. S3 coincides with rapid ventricular filling and occurs in early to mid-diastole. Various mechanisms, such as tensioning of the chordae tendinae or ventricular wall, have been proposed. A loud S3 is common in a dilated left ventricle with rapid diastolic filling, such as severe mitral regurgitation. A much higher-pitched S3 is heard in pericardial constriction and restrictive cardiomyopathy, as ventricular filling is suddenly truncated in early diastole.

The fourth heart sound, S4 or atrial sound, coincides with atrial systole in patients with a high ventricular filling pressure. It is absent where there is no atrial systole and in mitral stenosis. In sinus rhythm, it immediately precedes the first heart sound and may be heard (and sometimes felt) at the apex of the heart. Typically, it is heard in hypertension and heart failure.

Gallop (triple) rhythm. If either the third or fourth heart sounds are very loud, a triple rhythm or gallop results, which almost invariably accompanies heart failure. With an associated tachycardia, the third and fourth heart sounds

come together in a *summation gallop*. This is particularly common in hypertensive heart disease with left heart failure.

Added sounds

Ejection clicks are heard in young patients with aortic and pulmonary stenosis, where there is 'doming' of a mobile stenotic valve.

Mid-systolic click is heard in mitral valve prolapse, where the redundant chordal length allows mid-systolic prolapse of a mitral valve cusp. This may be single or multiple.

Opening snap. Normally an inaudible event, the opening snap becomes audible and, indeed, as loud as a heart sound, in mitral stenosis (and tricuspid stenosis) where the tethered valve cusps cannot separate adequately and the raised atrial pressure forces the valve to open to its full extent with sudden development of tension.

Other added sounds include pericardial rub and pericardial clicks, which may be found in pneumothorax.

Heart murmurs

Murmurs are generated along the path of turbulent flow and are convected in the same direction. They change their character slightly as they 'radiate' downstream, tending to acquire a harsher character as the low-frequency components become more prominent. A murmur is therefore often best heard 'downstream' from the lesion producing it, and the same murmur may sound different at different sites on the precordium. A *thrill* is a murmur radiating to the chest wall with sufficient low-frequency components to be palpable. The classical valve 'areas' (mitral, aortic, tricuspid and pulmonary) for auscultation were defined in the 19th century, and reflected the findings in rheumatic and infective cardiac disease (Fig. 13.10B). They are not always the best sites for auscultation of all murmurs arising from those particular valves.

Causes of murmurs

Murmurs may be generated by a high velocity jet, such as a stenotic or regurgitant jet, passing from a high-pressure to a lower-pressure chamber or vessel. They may occur with increased flow velocity in a normal vessel or with flow into a dilated or distorted vessel, such as the aorta in hypertension or the pulmonary artery in sternal depression. Murmurs therefore do not always indicate valve pathology. They may indicate a high flow, such as in pregnancy, or a minor anatomical distortion not amounting to true pathology, so-called *innocent murmurs*.

Description of murmurs

Murmurs are described in terms of their timing, precordial location, radiation, relative intensity and, if warranted, the influence of respiration and posture (Fig. 13.10). It is possible to grade the *loudness* of murmurs from 1/6 (almost inaudible) to 6/6 (a murmur which can be heard in a

Cardiovascular Disease

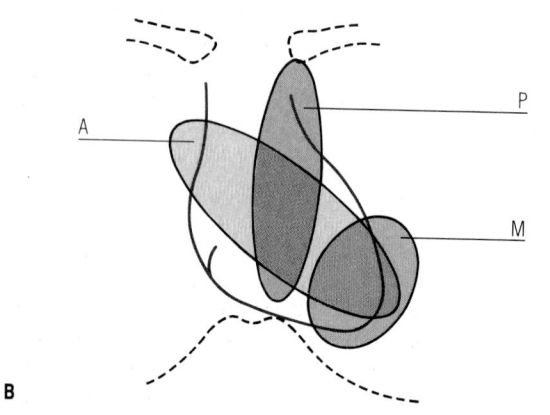

Fig. 13.10 Heart murmurs. A. Diagrammatic representation of murmurs. S1 and S2 = first and second heart sounds; A2 = Aortic valve closure sound; P2 = pulmonary valve closure sound; OS = opening snap. **B.** The precordial areas where murmurs are usually heard maximally. A = aortic; P = pulmonary; M = mitral.

quiet room without using a stethoscope). These grades are, however, of limited value, as they are highly subjective and the loudness of a murmur varies considerably depending on circumstances. The *length* of a diastolic murmur can be expressed on a scale of quarters, 1/4 being very short, and 3/4 an almost full-length diastolic murmur.

Systolic murmurs

Ejection murmurs are crescendo-decrescendo (diamond-shaped) and are characteristic of flow across a stenotic aortic or pulmonary valve, or flow into a dilated aorta or pulmonary artery. They may also occur with increased flow across these valves.

Pansystolic murmurs are generated by jets passing from a high-pressure chamber to a low-pressure chamber throughout systole, including the normally isovolumic phases of contraction and relaxation. The best example is mitral regurgitation, but tricuspid regurgitation and ventricular septal defects produce similar murmurs. The murmur obscures both the first and second heart sounds and is of almost even intensity throughout systole. The long ejection murmur of pulmonary stenosis, in which the prolonged right ventricular ejection can go through the aortic second sound, can be mistaken for a pansystolic murmur.

Late systolic murmurs. Mitral valve prolapse gives rise to a high-pitched murmur of even intensity starting halfway through systole, often preceded by a mid-systolic click. Papillary muscle dysfunction can give rise to a mitral pansystolic murmur which appears to get louder in late systole.

Diastolic murmurs

Diastolic murmurs are always pathological, but are often much harder to detect than systolic murmurs.

Mitral and tricuspid mid-diastolic murmurs. The mitral (and tricuspid) stenotic jets strike the apex of the ventricle and induce a low-frequency, largely subsonic vibration. These are heard as low-pitched, rumbling murmurs starting after the opening snap, best heard with the bell. They are often missed by the inexperienced, who are expecting to hear a much higher-pitched sound. The mitral diastolic murmur is accentuated by the patient lying on the left, and often resembles a low-frequency vibration of an underground train shaking the ground. If short, it can be confused with a third heart sound.

Early diastolic murmurs start immediately after the second heart sound. They are high-pitched noises, which can be very short or persist throughout diastole. Aortic diastolic murmurs are often faint and are best heard with the patient leaning forwards in expiration. A soft aortic diastolic murmur is missed by up to 50% of doctors who examine the patient.

Other types of murmur

Musical or mewing murmurs may occur in systole or diastole if a valve cusp adjacent to a jet vibrates at a characteristic frequency. These murmurs can be very loud, but the jet causing them may be small. A mewing murmur is characteristic of a small hole in an aortic valve cusp as a complication of endocarditis.

'Innocent' murmurs

Many mid-systolic and ejection systolic murmurs are unaccompanied by any signs or features of heart disease. These murmurs are common in children and pregnancy. They are maximal in the pulmonary area, but may also be heard along the left sternal edge and at the apex, and often have a low-pitched vibratory quality. They are usually of low intensity. If there is doubt as to their 'innocent' nature, an echocardiograph and, particularly, a Doppler study can be performed to rule out a small ventricular septal defect, pulmonary stenosis or unsuspected trivial mitral regurgitation. If no pathology is found, the murmurs can be considered innocent and do not require endocarditis prophylaxis unless residual doubt remains.

Bringing out a murmur

It is not uncommon to see a patient in whom valvular disease is suspected, but in whom a murmur cannot be heard, or who has been referred because of a murmur which is not evident. Murmurs can be accentuated by exercise; this increases cardiac output and is best accomplished by asking the patient (if well enough) to lie on the couch and do, say, 20 cycles of toe-touching and then resting back. Murmurs in mitral valve prolapse and hypertrophic cardiomyopathy commonly come and go, and are best assessed both with patient in the usual auscultatory position and when standing and squatting. If the patient has severe emphysema, heart sounds and murmurs can be so faint as to be inaudible. The location and characteristics of murmurs and other methods of accentuating them are described in more detail below, in the sections dealing with the clinical conditions giving rise to them.

Concluding a cardiac examination

Cardiac examination is incomplete without examination of the lung bases for signs of cardiac failure, the sacrum and ankles for oedema, and assessment of the peripheral pulses.

Lungs

The lungs are examined not only for signs of failure, but also because chronic lung disease can complicate and add to the symptoms and signs generated by heart disease.

Peripheral pulses

A patient with angina may well have atheromatous peripheral vascular disease, shown by loss of pulses in the legs. Examination of the carotid arteries for signs of atheromatous carotid stenosis may reveal loss of a carotid pulsation, a carotid bruit or loud systolic murmur. Atrial fibrillation may have caused embolic loss of some pulses. If the patient is hypertensive with a systolic murmur, radial and femoral pulses should be felt to detect any delay and weakness of the femoral pulse indicating coarctation. Possible aortic aneurysm should lead to careful assessment of the pulses and the blood pressure in both arms.

Abdomen

Tricuspid regurgitation is confirmed by finding a pulsatile liver. If the patient has hypertension, the abdomen is examined for renal enlargement or bruits. A patient in right heart failure may well have ascites and considerable liver enlargement.

Neck

Mediastinal shift may be detected by a deviated trachea. Atrial fibrillation or tachycardia may be caused by thyrotoxicosis, so the thyroid is examined for goitre and other signs of thyroid overactivity looked for.

Optic fundi

If the patient is hypertensive, the optic fundi are examined for hypertensive retinopathy. They should be examined regularly in patients suspected of having endocarditis.

CARDIAC INVESTIGATION

THE ELECTROCARDIOGRAM

The electrocardiogram (ECG) is a record of the electrical activity of the heart and thus gives only indirect information on the mechanical activity and health of the heart. A 'normal ECG' at rest can be reassuring but also misleading, as it can be found even with life-threatening coronary disease; in the absence of symptoms, a routine ECG is thus of limited value and a relatively poor screening test. The main value of a routine ECG is for use at the time of subsequent events to see if there has been any change.

Technical background and recording an ECG

The lead and electrode positions are shown in Figure 13.11. Correct calibration is essential. Accurate positioning of the V leads in women can be difficult; if possible the electrodes should be positioned underneath the breast rather than on the surface. The electrical resistance is minimised if the electrodes are clean and the electrode jelly is massaged into the skin.

Three bipolar limb leads (I, II and III), three augmented unipolar limb leads (aVR, aVL and aVF) and six unipolar ventricular leads (V1 to V6) are routinely used. The six limb leads provide an electrical 'view' around the heart in the frontal plane, while the six ventricular leads view the heart from the complementary horizontal plane (Fig. 13.11). By convention, the lead connections have been made to show a positive deflection as a wave of depolarising electrical activity travels towards the electrode (Fig. 13.12). The final shape of the electrocardiogram is determined by the lead being sampled and by the angle (vector) at which it 'views' the activity in the heart; the magnitude of the recorded deflection is affected by the mass of tissue undergoing electrical activation. Understanding the electrocardiogram thus requires that the anatomy of the heart, the route taken by electrical activation and the viewpoint of the electrode are known. Differences in anatomy and minor variations in lead positions can account for some of

341

13

A

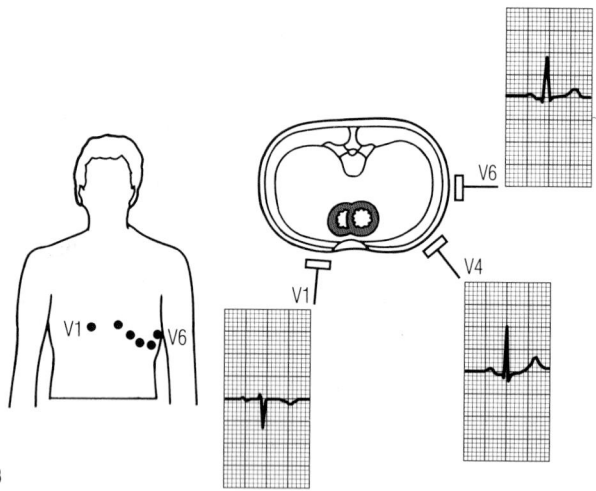

B

Fig. 13.11   Positions of leads and electrodes in the ECG. A. Frontal plane. **B.** Horizontal plane.

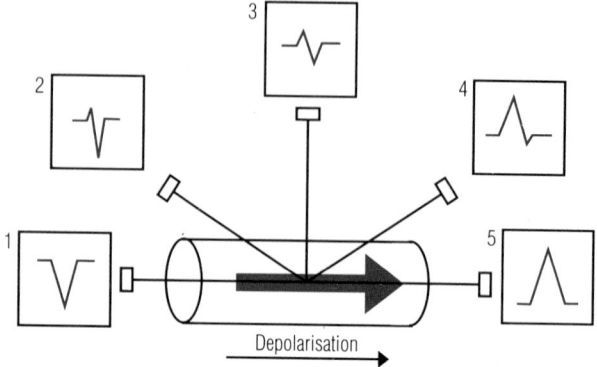

Fig. 13.12   Vectorial effect on QRS size and polarity. Panel 1 shows a negative deflection as depolarisation moves away. Panel 3 shows a small equiphasic deflection because it is perpendicular to the direction of depolarisation.

first and arrives at the left atrium fractionally later. The wave front moves in a general direction towards + 60°. The surface ECG records a P wave which is positive and best seen in leads II, V1 and I. Right atrial hypertrophy produces a tall (over 2.5 mm) peaked P wave, sometimes called the *P pulmonale* from its association with the pulmonary hypertension of pulmonary disease. Left atrial hypertrophy (*P mitrale*) produces a broad notched P wave (more than 0.12 s duration) in lead II or III, with a negative secondary deflection in V1 which exceeds the right atrial positive deflection in that lead (Fig. 13.13). P waves that

Fig. 13.13   Normal and abnormal P waves. On the left is shown the direction of atrial activation ➡ that produces the normal P waves shown in lead II. In P pulmonale (PP) the P wave is abnormally tall and peaked. When activation is retrograde (nodal rhythm shown by dashed line), the P wave is inverted. In left atrial hypertrophy (e.g. in mitral stenosis) a broad bifid P wave is seen in lead II and a prominent negative deflection in lead V1; this is P mitrale (PM).

the variability in clinical electrocardiograms; pathological processes account for the rest.

Standard gain settings (1 cm/mV deflection) and paper speed (25 mm/s) complete the electrocardiogram recording.

Atrial activity and the P wave

In the normal heart, the dominant pacemaker is to be found in the high right atrium at the sino-atrial node. The depolarising wave front moves through the right atrium are inverted in lead II are caused by an abnormal direction of the depolarising wave front, and may be seen when atrial activation is initiated at the atrioventricular (AV) node low in the right atrium. Other ectopic atrial rhythms may produce P waves of varying shapes.

The PR interval

Between atrial and ventricular depolarisation, the ECG signal records a flat isoelectric line for 0.12–0.20 seconds (Fig. 13.14). This is the delay encountered by the depolarising wave front in the AV node before rapid propagation to the ventricular myocardium. The PR interval will diminish at increased heart rates and under the influence of adrenaline. It increases in diseased atrioventricular nodes, with certain drugs and, occasionally, in normal people.

The QRS complex and ventricular activation

Normal QRS

The normal QRS parameters are shown in Figure 13.14. Normal ventricular activation is orderly and rapid, being complete within 0.12 s with virtually simultaneous activation of the left and right ventricles. This is achieved by a system of specialised rapidly conducting muscle cells, which form the bundle of His and the Purkinje network. Activation of the interventricular septum begins first from left-to-right and accounts for the small q wave (duration less than 0.04 seconds and depth less than 25% of R wave height) seen in leads V5, V6 and, usually, V4. This wave is matched by the r wave in V1 and V2. Since the left ventricular muscle mass is greater than that of the right ventricle, it is the left ventricular forces which dominate the chest leads, with rS waves in leads V1 and V2 and qR waves in leads V5 and V6, with an intermediate transition zone to be found between leads V3 and V4.

The mean QRS axis

The mean frontal plane vector, obtained from the six limb leads, describes the direction of the dominant electrical forces. It can be determined for all the major electrocardiogram deflections (P wave, QRS complex and T wave) but is mainly used to summarise ventricular depolarisation as the *mean QRS axis*. This parameter is roughly estimated by determining the lead with the smallest equiphasic deflection, and assuming the vector is at right angles to this lead. The limb lead on this vectorial line, which shows a positive deflection, indicates the direction of the axis. The units are degrees, with values above the equator (0°) being prefixed negative (Fig. 13.15).

The mean frontal plane vector is normally about +60°. Left axis deviation is variously defined, but a shift further than −30° is definitely abnormal; right axis deviation is definite at greater than 120°. The latter can be due to right ventricular hypertrophy or, less commonly, to abnormal patterns of activation caused by interruption of the posterior fascicle of the left bundle branch, in left posterior

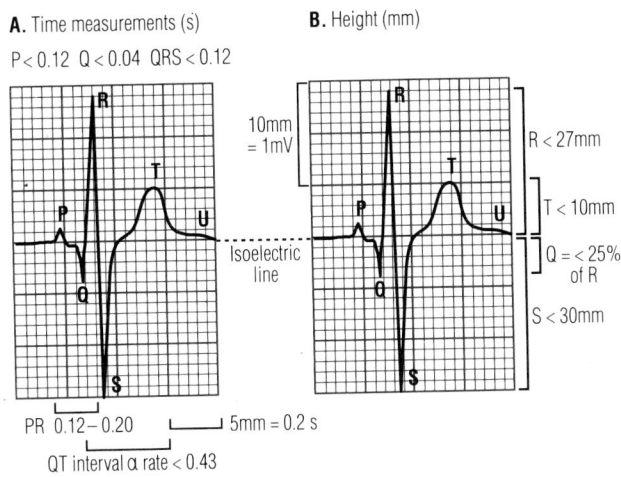

A. Time measurements (s)   **B.** Height (mm)

P < 0.12   Q < 0.04   QRS < 0.12

10mm = 1mV

Isoelectric line

R < 27mm
T < 10mm
Q = < 25% of R
S < 30mm

PR 0.12–0.20   5mm = 0.2 s

QT interval α rate < 0.43

Fig. 13.14   Normal PQRST parameters.   **A.** Duration.   **B.** Height.

hemiblock. Left axis deviation is an 'electrical' phenomenon, caused by interruption of the anterior fascicle of the left bundle branch. It is associated with the loss of the normal septal depolarisation and hence the loss of q waves in V5 and V6. This is called left anterior hemiblock; in these conditions, the QRS duration remains less than 0.12 s.

Bundle branch block

Interruption of the right or left bundle branches produces a bundle branch block pattern characterised by broad QRS complexes of greater than 0.12 s duration. With *right bundle branch block*, an rSR or 'M'-shaped pattern is seen in the right facing chest leads V1, V2 ± V3, as right ventricular forces occur late and unopposed by left ventricular contraction (Fig. 13.16); this is also manifested by late deep slurred S waves appearing in V4 to V6. *Left bundle branch block* causes a delay in left ventricular activation, which occurs from right to left, causing a marked axis shift (greater than −60°) and loss of q waves in V5 and V6. Lead V1 shows only a qS wave and the lateral leads (V5 and V6) the characteristic slurred RsR or 'M' pattern (Fig. 13.16).

Left bundle branch block is virtually always pathological, the single commonest cause being ischaemic heart disease. Right bundle branch block may be a normal finding, but the change from normal conduction to one or other of these patterns implies heart disease.

Rate-dependent bundle branch block

Occasionally, normal QRS morphology is present at low heart rates, but a bundle branch block pattern appears at faster rates. This is usually right bundle branch block, as its refractory period is generally longer than that of the left bundle branch. Rate-dependent bundle branch block may be a particular problem if it occurs with a supraventricular tachycardia, where the broad QRS complexes may wrongly suggest the diagnosis of ventricular tachycardia.

A

B

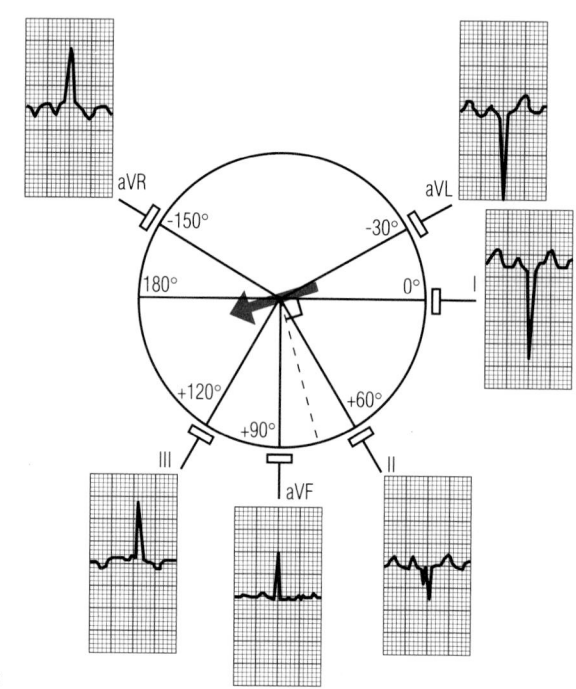

C

Fig. 13.15 Determining the mean frontal plane axis. In **A.**, lead aVL has the smallest biphasic signal. The axis is perpendicular to this and its direction given by the upward deflection produced in lead II. The axis, shown by the arrow, is therefore +60°. In **B.**, the axis is −90° (perpendicular to I and away from aVF). This is left axis deviation. In **C.**, the smallest and most biphasic complex lies between II and aVF and the axis is therefore greater than 120° (severe right axis deviation).

Ventricular hypertrophy

The tallest R wave should not exceed 27 mm nor the deepest S wave 30 mm, and the sum of the tallest R wave and deepest S wave should not exceed 40 mm (Fig. 13.14). Left ventricular hypertrophy (LVH) is diagnosed when these criteria are exceeded, with a normal total QRS duration of less than 0.12 s. The intrinsic deflection is delayed by more than 0.04 s in the left-facing leads, this measurement being taken from the onset of the QRS deflection to the point at which the R wave swings abruptly downwards.

Associated ST segment depression and T inversion occur in the left-facing limb and praecordial leads, particularly with pressure-overloaded ventricles, and is said to represent ventricular 'strain'.

Right ventricular hypertrophy is suspected when there is a dominant R wave in V1, associated with a rightward QRS axis shift (more than +90°) in a QRS complex of less than 0.12 s duration. There is also ST segment depression and T inversion in the right precordial leads, and often also by clockwise rotation of the ventricular leads with the normal transition zone (V3–V4) moving towards V5–V6.

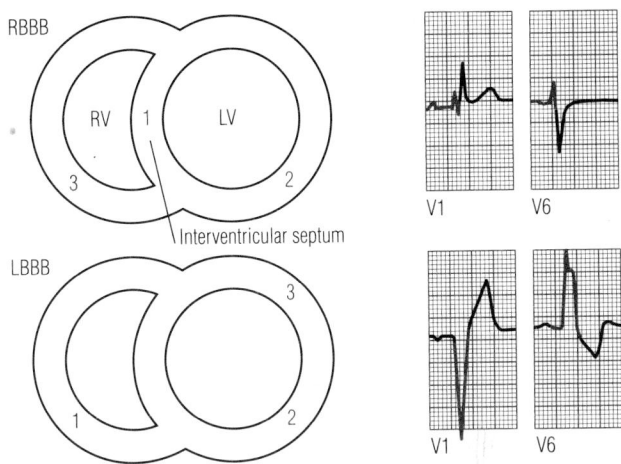

Fig. 13.16 The production of the QRS complex in right (R) and left (L) bundle branch block (BBB). The order of activation is shown by numbers 1–3. In RBBB, the interventricular septum and left ventricle depolarise normally (red tracing) and the right ventricle is delayed (black tracing). In LBBB, the left ventricular depolarisation is delayed and prolonged.

The ST segment

The ST segment begins where the QRS ends, and is normally on the isoelectric line gently curving upwards into the T wave (the J or *junction point*). There may be 1–2 mm of elevation in the high anterior chest leads (V1 and V2), but greater elevation is seen with myocardial infarction, the so-called current of injury (p. 407, Fig. 13.62) and pericarditis (p. 434, Fig. 13.65). A normal variant – particularly common in young black men – exists, in which there is marked anterior ST elevation. The clinical context is usually sufficient to differentiate this appearance from acute infarction.

Depression of the ST segment (p. 401, Fig. 13.58) is the hallmark of cardiac ischaemia; this can vary from subtle loss of the normal slight upward curvature and acute angulation with the T wave origin, to more marked depression, sloping downwards before abruptly changing direction with the T wave onset. The degree of depression of the ST segment is a rough indication of the severity of the myocardial injury. The duration of the ST segment is encompassed within the QT interval. This shortens with increasing heart rate, but may be prolonged (more than 0.40 s or more than 50% of previous R-R interval) by hypocalcaemia or hypomagnesaemia.

The T wave: myocardial repolarisation

There is more variability in T wave amplitude and orientation than in other parts of the ECG, so that criteria for normality have to be more flexible. The T wave may be flat or abnormal in non-cardiac disease and in some normal patients. It is asymmetrical in shape, with a slower upstroke than downstroke and a smooth rounded peak. Symmetrical, peaked T waves may indicate ischaemia, whereas

notching may be a feature of pericarditis. T wave height should not exceed 10 mm in the precordial leads, and larger examples occurring without LVH suggest acute myocardial infarction (Fig. 13.64) or hyperkalaemia. T wave orientation is normally upright in leads with R waves over 5 mm in height, so that, in the normal adult, T waves are upright in I, II and V3 to V6, are always inverted in aVR and may be inverted in aVL, aVF, III, V1 and V2. The evolution of acute infarction (p. 407) involves T inversion in leads affected by the injury, and these changes may persist.

The U wave

The U wave follows the T wave (Fig. 13.14), is of small amplitude and shares the T wave orientation. It is best seen in lead V3 and is enlarged in hypokalaemia. Its genesis is uncertain, but it coincides with the period of supra-normal excitability in the ventricles.

Exercise testing

The normal 12-lead resting ECG often shows no abnormalities in patients who develop symptoms on exercise. The exercise test may be performed for the following reasons:

1. to reproduce the symptoms of which the patient is complaining, so that he can describe them as they happen under standardised exercise conditions
2. to assess the patient's 'functional capacity', i.e. the amount of work he can perform before he becomes limited by symptoms, and also how rapidly he recovers from exercise
3. to ascertain whether the symptoms are accompanied by any objective evidence of myocardial ischaemia, cardiac arrhythmia, hypertension or other events which would make unsupervised exercise hazardous
4. to monitor treatment with serial studies
5. to assess prognosis in patients with known cardiac disease.

Modern exercise testing regimes consist of an incremental load on either a treadmill or a cycle ergometer, in which the exercise load is started at an easily managed level, kept stable for 1.5–3 minutes at each load, and then serially increased with the aim of 'exhausting' the subject within 15 minutes (although, in submaximal tests, exhaustion is not usually the end point).

The patient is connected to an ECG monitor and, ideally, all 12 leads are recorded at frequent intervals to demonstrate ischaemia or arrhythmia and monitor the heart rate. The blood pressure is also recorded. The exercise test is stopped when the patient is incapable of continuing, or has achieved the target heart rate (calculated as 220 minus the patient's age). It is also stopped if there is significant objective evidence of ischaemia on ECG, or if the patient has a significant arrhythmia, such as salvos of ventricular ectopics, or atrial fibrillation. A defibrillator should be available.

Sensitivity and specificity

The exercise test is conclusively positive if the patient develops classical anginal pain and severe downsloping (greater than 2 mm) ST segment depression is shown on the ECG (p. 401, Fig. 13.58). Minor degrees of ST segment depression are common, particularly in anxious individuals and especially young women, but are usually upsloping. T wave inversion is not necessarily ischaemic in origin. A commonly used criterion is 1 mm ST depression more than 0.08 s after the previous QRS complex. Severe ischaemia is shown by widespread ST depression in several leads which takes several minutes to return to normal. There may be a sudden drop in blood pressure during exercise; this may be unaccompanied by ECG changes but is diagnostic of severe ischaemia and an absolute indication to terminate the test.

CHEST X-RAY

Because of the almost uniform density of its components, the cardiac shadow on a PA chest film is a silhouette of a three-dimensional structure displayed on a two-dimensional film. The size and visibility of the component parts of the heart as seen on the chest X-ray is therefore dependent not only on any magnification, but also on any rotation of the heart and masking of one structure by another (Fig. 13.17).

Examination of a cardiac X-ray requires a logical approach, and includes the following:

1. a check of the technical quality of the film, and the position of the thoracic skeleton
2. an assessment of heart size (and changes from previous films if available)
3. a search for evidence of specific chamber enlargement and abnormalities of cardiac anatomy
4. an examination of the lung fields and vessels
5. identification of valve or other calcification.

The film should be well centred with no gross rotation of the patient, who should have taken a full inspiration. An A-P film is usually marked as such, and is only of value in assessing the lung fields or gross changes in heart size. There may be evidence of thoracotomy, rib resection, scoliosis or severe kyphosis which may result in an abnormal appearance of the heart. Lateral films may show a depressed sternum or abnormal sternal segmentation. There may be rib notching, suggesting coarctation.

Heart size and cardiothoracic ratio

Minor variations in heart size can be technical in origin. It is usual to measure the *cardiothoracic ratio* – the maximum transverse diameter of the heart compared with that of the ribcage – which is 0.5 or less in normals. This commonly

Fig. 13.17 **Composition of the normal cardiac silhouette on chest X-rays. A.** PA view. RV and LV = right and left ventricles; RA = right atrium; SVC = superior vena cava. **B.** Lateral view.

accepted criterion is, however, rather rigid and needs to be modified with athletes and people of African descent, many of whose hearts exceed this limit, but are by other criteria physiologically normal. When comparing successive chest X-rays, an increase in transverse diameter of the heart of more than 1.5 cm is regarded as significant. There is obviously some variation depending on whether the film was taken in systole or diastole, and on the heart rate (bradycardia being associated with a larger heart).

Anatomy and specific chamber enlargement

The border-forming structures of the cardiac silhouette in the PA and lateral views are shown in Figure 13.17. The approximate positions of the heart valves are also shown.

Left atrium

Left atrial enlargement may produce splaying of the angle of bifurcation of the trachea into the main bronchi (carina) with lifting of the left main bronchus. The increased density of an enlarged left atrium (LA) may make it visible within the right heart border, or it may protrude beyond it. On the left side, the left atrial appendage makes up part of the normal border, and enlargement of the LA can cause straightening, and even bulging, of the left heart border.

On lateral chest X-ray (Fig. 13.17B), left atrial enlargement produces posterior displacement of the upper posterior cardiac border.

Left ventricle

The left ventricle (LV) makes up the cardiac apex and part of the left heart border on PA X-rays, and much of the posterior heart border on lateral views. Left ventricular enlargement usually displaces the apex of the heart downwards and laterally on the PA view, while on the lateral view, the LV produces a prominent convexity of the lower half of the posterior border of the heart.

Aorta

In young adults, the upper right cardiac border may not include the ascending aorta, but, with ageing, the aorta elongates and becomes more prominent on chest X-ray. In elderly patients, the aorta becomes tortuous. Prominence of the ascending aorta may thus be due to age as well as hypertension, post-stenotic dilatation or aortic dilatation from aortic valve disease, aneurysm or dissection. Computerised tomography, ultrasound or angiography may be needed to define the cause of a prominent aorta. The aortic arch may also be prominent in any of these conditions. Calcification of the ascending aorta is almost pathognomic of syphilis, but is very common in the arch and descending aorta in normal individuals.

Right atrium

Enlargement of the right atrium (RA) is seen as prominence of the lower half of the right heart border, and is usually accompanied by superior vena cava (SVC) prominence. The SVC forms the highest part of the right border of the cardiac silhouette and is prominent in right heart failure, SVC obstruction or displacement of the SVC by the aorta.

Right ventricle

The right ventricle (RV) is an 'internal' structure on the PA X-ray unless there is massive RV dilatation with the left ventricle rotated posteriorly. Right ventricular dilatation results in a more globular appearance to the heart on PA film, with the cardiac apex being more elevated.

Pulmonary conus and trunk

The pulmonary trunk is more prominent in young subjects than later in life. A dilated pulmonary trunk may indicate a post-stenotic dilatation, pulmonary hypertension, increased pulmonary flow or can be idiopathic. It therefore needs to be interpreted along with the appearance of the lung fields.

Lung fields and vessels

Assessment of pulmonary vascularity is difficult. It tends to be subjective and demands a good quality film. Normal pulmonary vascularity will show larger vessels in the lower zones, with symmetry between the two lungs. There is a steady diminution in vessel size peripherally.

A number of diagnoses can be made from the pulmonary vascularity.

Pulmonary venous hypertension

If the pressure in the pulmonary veins rises above about 15 mmHg, the upper lobe vessels dilate and become of greater size than the lower lobe vessels, which constrict with perivascular cuffing. There is redistribution of flow to the upper lobes (p. 355). If the venous pressure rises higher than about 20–25 mmHg, the pulmonary lymphatics become engorged, and appearances of interstitial oedema are seen on the chest X-ray. These are the appearance of *Kerley B lines* (horizontal septal lines best seen at the costophrenic angles) and increased haziness of the perihilar regions, sometimes resulting in the classical but uncommon 'bat's wing' appearance of the chest X-ray, often with small effusions (Fig. 13.18). Further rise in pressure above 30 mmHg results in alveolar oedema with dense opacification of the lung from fluid collection.

Increased lung blood flow

With increased blood flow to the lungs (as in a left to right shunt), the lungs look very vascular, with quite large vessels running right to the periphery of the lungs. This can be distinguished from left heart failure by the lower lobe vessels remaining larger than the upper lobe vessels.

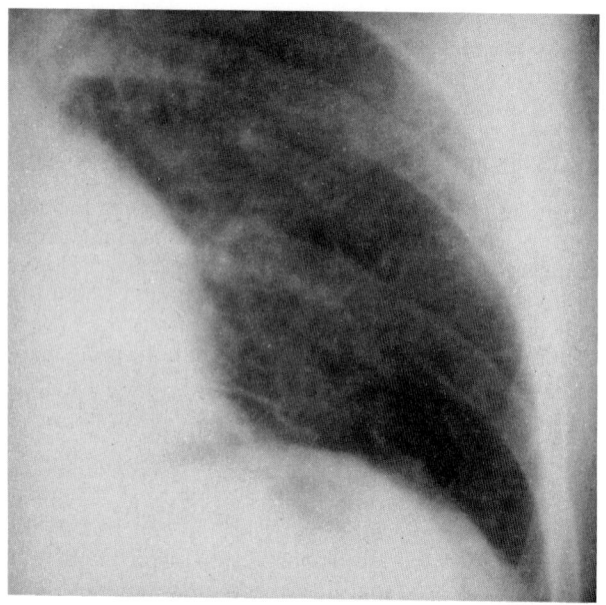

Fig. 13.18 Radiological features of left heart failure. A. PA chest X-ray showing bilateral shadowing spreading from the hila typical of acute pulmonary oedema. **B.** Detail of the left costophrenic lung field showing horizontal lines (Kerley B lines).

Pulmonary oligaemia

Pulmonary oligaemia (as in severe pulmonary stenosis) is associated with an avascular appearance of the lung fields but normal size central pulmonary arteries (although the pulmonary trunk may be dilated as a post-stenotic dilatation in pulmonary stenosis).

Pulmonary arterial hypertension

The presence of pulmonary arterial hypertension gives rise to large central pulmonary arteries which are rapidly pruned peripherally with relatively avascular-looking lung fields.

Calcification

Calcification may be found in any cardiac structure. It is usually best seen on penetrated PA and lateral films, as much of the calcification seen within the heart overlies the spine on PA films. The mitral and aortic valve may both calcify; on lateral film, the latter is usually lying above a line joining the tracheal bifurcation and the costophrenic angle, whilst the mitral is predominantly below the line (Fig. 13.19). Calcification is also sometimes seen in the great vessels, the wall of a rheumatic left atrium, the pericardium (p. 435) and, sometimes, within the LV in thrombus in an LV aneurysm. It is commonly seen in severely diseased coronary arteries.

ULTRASOUND TECHNIQUES

Echocardiography

If a beam of ultrasound is directed into the thorax through a suitable 'acoustic window' it travels through the soft tissues and blood at an almost uniform velocity of 1340 m/s. The various tissue interfaces in the line of the beam of ultrasound reflect some of the sound back towards the transmitting transducer, and the red blood cells in its path scatter the ultrasound. The reflected ultrasound takes varying times to get back to the transducer, depending on the depth of the interface from which the reflection occurs. As the velocity of the ultrasound is constant, the time of the returning echoes is an indication of their depth, while their strength is an indication of the change in acoustic impedance producing the echo. The beam of ultrasound can be pulsed, using the same transducer as transmitter and receiver, to give a map of the tissue interfaces in one or various beam direction(s).

M mode echocardiography

The technique of M mode electrocardiography is illustrated in Figure 13.20. If the beam is maintained in a single direction, an M mode display is produced, where the line of echoes of varying strength at different depths is shown as a vertical line of varying intensity on a cathode ray tube, this line being swept across the tube with time. Signals of differing depth and intensity are therefore displayed against time with centimetre and second calibration markers. Hard copy of the display can be produced simultaneously.

Since both the fronts and backs of tissue interfaces reflect the ultrasound, M mode echocardiography can be used to display the cardiac chambers, the valves and the wall thickness of the left ventricle throughout the cardiac cycle. Their size and thickness can be measured with a resolution of about 2 mm (depending on the ultrasound frequency). An ECG is used for timing.

Two-dimensional or sector echocardiography

If the beam of ultrasound is swung through an arc, a two-

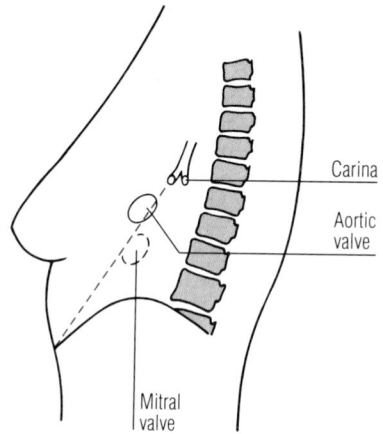

Fig. 13.19 Calcification in the heart. A. PA chest X-ray showing abnormal calcification in pericardium (due to previous pericarditis) and normal calcification in the aortic knuckle. **B.** Lateral chest X-ray showing sites at which valve calcification may be found.

Fig. 13.20 M mode echocardiography. The diagram shows the position of the transducer and directions of the ultrasonic beam. In **A** the beam traverses the left ventricle (LV) below the mitral valve. Systole (S) and diastole (D) are indicated. In **B** the beam is aimed to demonstrate the mitral valve (MV). In **C** the aortic valve (Av) and aorta (Ao) are shown.

dimensional 'sector scan' is produced; this can be recorded as a moving image on videotape, or stored and recorded as hard copy in frozen images (Fig. 13.21). The frame rate is limited by the speed of ultrasound, as the echoes have to return from the deepest structures to the transducer before it can be moved to record another scan line. Two-dimensional (2D) echocardiography is therefore useful for 'real time' dynamic records, but does not give as high a resolution as M mode.

Echocardiography is particularly useful for demonstrating valve thickening, calcification and vegetations, as well as chamber size and wall thickness and LV function.

It is the method of choice for demonstrating pericardial effusion. Under good conditions, 2D echocardiography can demonstrate the presence of thrombus in the heart and can also be used with injected saline contrast to demonstrate intracardiac shunting.

Doppler ultrasound

The technique of Doppler ultrasound makes use of the change in frequency of the backscattered ultrasound energy from the red blood cells. This change of frequency is proportional to the blood velocity; thus, if the beam of

349

Cardiovascular Disease

13

Fig. 13.21 **Two-dimensional echocardiography.** Parasternal long axis views of the heart in systole and diastole are shown. (The direction of the beam is equivalent to that shown by line B in Figure 13.20). The opening and closure of the aortic and mitral valves are clearly shown.

ultrasound is aligned with the jet of blood within the heart, accurate measurements of blood velocity can be made and the gradient across the valve calculated (Fig. 13.22). The relation between the pressure gradient across the valve (P measured in mmHg) and the increase in velocity (V expressed in metres per second) is $P = 4V^2$. In most cases, the peak jet velocity is used as the flow velocity upstream of the jet is usually trivial compared with the jet velocity. The predicted pressure gradient from Doppler measurements is the instantaneous pressure gradient, whereas cardiac catheterisation often measures only the peak-to-peak pull-back gradient (Fig. 13.24).

Doppler ultrasound is used predominantly for measuring pressure gradients and can also be used to dem-

onstrate the presence and severity of valvular regurgitation. It is extremely sensitive in detecting minor degrees of regurgitation, which are often unexpected. The combined techniques of echocardiography and Doppler ultrasound save many patients, particularly children, from invasive studies, as in many cases the complete pathology can be demonstrated with ultrasound. These techniques cannot, however, measure chamber pressures, such as the left ventricular end diastolic pressure, or show the coronary arterial anatomy.

Colour Doppler

Colour Doppler is a form of pulsed Doppler in which the blood velocity is colour-coded and superimposed on a 2D sector echo image. The colour code demonstrates whether the mean velocity of the sample is towards or away from the transducer, and the hue can be changed depending on the velocity. Its main use so far is in providing a non-invasive type of colour angiogram which makes the rest of Doppler technology easier to use and appreciate.

Limitation on use

All ultrasound techniques are limited by the size of the acoustic windows, which have to avoid bone and lung. These are large in babies and young children (almost infinite in the fetus) and can be supplemented, if justified, by a transoesophageal approach. The windows become smaller with age and can become particularly limited in people with lung disease, denying the benefits of these techniques to many who would be helped by a non-invasive diagnosis. The usual windows are parasternal, apical, subxiphoid, and suprasternal.

NUCLEAR IMAGING

The development of gamma cameras and relatively short-lived nuclear isotopes (most commonly ^{99m}Tc) with suitable emission characteristics has led to a rapid increase in the diagnostic and imaging capability of isotopic techniques.

A

B

C

Fig. 13.22 **Two-dimensional echocardiogram and Doppler ultrasound. A.** Apical four chamber view of the heart. **B.** Diagrammatic representation of A, the transducer position and beam direction of Doppler signal (dotted line) are shown. **C.** The continuous wave Doppler signal that is obtained from position B shows a diastolic jet (upwards towards the transducer). An abnormal systolic jet away from the transducer, due to mitral regurgitation, is also shown. The velocity trace indicates peak velocities of 2 m/s and 5 m/s respectively (corresponding to peak gradients of 16 and 100 mmHg).

350

Nuclear angiography

Nuclear angiography uses intravenously injected radio-nuclides in the cardiac blood pool; this provides a non-invasive assessment of ventricular wall motion and ejection fraction and demonstrates valvular regurgitation and shunts. In the *first pass technique*, a discrete bolus of labelled blood is followed through the heart, and data collected by an externally placed gamma camera for 30–50 s. A fresh injection is required for each view, and allowance made for the background activity of the first and subsequent injections. This technique can be facilitated by the use of short-lived isotopes such as ^{195}Au, whose half-life of 30 s enables rest and exercise studies to be performed with relatively low cumulative exposure to the patient and little residual background emission in serial studies.

In an *equilibrium study* the whole of the circulating blood is labelled and data collection can take much longer, with serial views obtained at leisure. Both first-pass and equilibrium techniques are constrained by the need to limit patient exposure to radiation. In order to increase resolution of the gamma camera image from the low level of emission, a large number of images are acquired over several cardiac cycles and the images from different phases of the cardiac cycle are averaged. This process is accomplished by 'gating' with reference to the ECG as a time marker and dividing the cardiac cycle into a series of time intervals each of, for example, 30–50 ms (Fig. 13.23).

Fig. 13.23 Radionuclide ventriculography: the multiple uptake gated acquisition (MUGA) scan. The blood pool is labelled and counts over the left ventricle are related to defined proportions of the cardiac cycle (1–15 in the diagram). These are summated to give an average radioactivity for end systole (B) and end diastole (A) from which the ejection fraction can be calculated.

Derived images and measurements

The prolonged data acquisition and storage of the data in a computer, although limiting the immediacy of the results, enables the individual counts to be handled in a variety of ways to give a variety of measures.

End diastolic and end systolic volumes. Ejection fraction and stroke volume (and thus cardiac output) can be cal-culated. The ejection fraction is normally above 50%, and should rise with exercise by at least 5%.

Regional wall motion abnormalities are shown by quantitative colour-coding of emission over the heart. This identifies areas showing little change in counts compared with the rest, or showing decreasing counts when the rest of the ventricle is increasing.

Limitations of nuclear angiography

In severe right heart failure, a peripheral venous injection of isotope is dissipated through a large mixing volume before it reaches the heart. Tricuspid regurgitation aggravates the problem, leading to greatly degraded imaging. An injection into the pulmonary artery by means of a transvenous catheter overcomes this problem, but changes a non-invasive technique into one requiring cardiac catheterisation.

Time-gating over many cycles is not usually possible in patients with atrial fibrillation or other significant arrhythmias. More than a minor degree of movement of the thorax relative to the gamma camera also tends to limit studies during exertion.

Thallium (^{201}Tl) perfusion scan (myocardial scintigraphy)

The technique of myocardial scintigraphy depends upon thallium (^{201}Tl) being taken up by viable myocardium which is normally perfused. These tests are more difficult to perform than nuclear angiography, and the isotope not as easily available as ^{99m}Tc. Generally, exercise is incorporated in the protocol. Areas of viable myocardium which are not perfused during exercise appear as cold spots which 'fill in' during the rest scan. Cold spots on the scan that do not perfuse after exercise represent infarcted myocardium.

MAGNETIC RESONANCE IMAGING (MRI)

Magnetic resonance imaging (MRI) – a new development in non-invasive technology – relies on the use of extremely powerful magnets to generate changes in the resonant frequency of atoms; these can then be detected by radiofrequency receivers and used to generate a sectional map of the tissues within the magnetic field. The technology promises much but is, at present, limited by data acquisition time, the cost of the equipment and the prerequisite that the patient be in a regular cardiac rhythm. However, it is proving invaluable in paediatric cardiology for complex congenital abnormalities and can now be used for studying flow velocity patterns as well as structure.

CARDIAC CATHETERISATION

Cardiac catheterisation is a diagnostic procedure in which a flexible tube is passed, under local anaesthetic, from a superficial vein into the right side of the heart, or from the brachial or femoral arteries to the left side of the heart. In children, the procedure may require a general anaesthetic.

13

In *right heart catheterisation* the catheter tip can be passed to all the right heart chambers. Using an end-hole catheter, an indirect left atrial pressure can be obtained by wedging the catheter in a small pulmonary artery. *Left heart catheterisation* from a peripheral artery is restricted to the aorta and left ventricle, by passing the catheter retrogradely through the aortic valve.

Uses of cardiac catheterisation

Catheterisation allows pressure measurements to be made and cine angiograms performed by the injection of contrast agents. Selective catheterisation of the *coronary arteries* can provide high-quality angiographic views of the coronary tree to demonstrate its anatomy. This has become the major use of cardiac catheterisation, since non-invasive techniques have become very accurate and can be used for diagnosis in most patients with valvular and congenital heart disease.

In valvular heart disease, the objectives of cardiac catheterisation are as follows:

1. *To measure pressures in the chambers of the heart*, and so establish the presence of valve stenosis or ventricular disease (Fig. 13.24).
2. *To measure valve pressure gradients.* Although the gradient across a normal valve is trivial and cannot be measured with conventional fluid-filled catheters, pathological pressure gradients are very much larger. An aortic valve pressure gradient is considered surgically significant when it reaches about 50 mmHg if the cardiac output is normal. A mitral valve gradient of less than 5 mmHg is considered trivial.
3. *To enable radio-opaque contrast to be injected selectively* in the different chambers of the heart and thus demonstrate by cine *angiography* the presence of valvular regurgitation, intracardiac shunts and abnormal morphology or contractility of the ventricles.
4. *Measurement of oxygen content for demonstration of shunts* (Fig. 13.25). Sampling in the different chambers

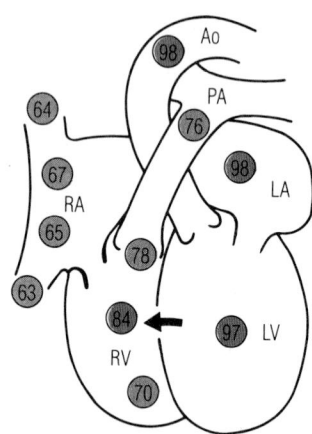

Fig. 13.25 Oxygen saturation in the cardiac chambers and great vessels in ventricular septal defect. A step up in saturation occurs in the right ventricle. Ao = aorta; PA = pulmonary artery.

of the right side of the heart can be used to demonstrate the presence and size of a left-to-right shunt by the rise in oxygen content (saturation) of the blood. Persistent arterial desaturation, despite the patient breathing 100% oxygen, demonstrates the presence of a right-to-left shunt. Measurement of pulmonary artery and systemic arterial blood oxygen content, together with measurement of oxygen uptake by timed expired air gas collection (or, in many centres, estimated oxygen uptake from normograms of patient's surface area), are used to calculate cardiac output.

Complications of cardiac catheterisation

The complications of cardiac catheterisation are shown in Table 13.2. The risks are small (below 0.1%), and are minimised by current techniques. They are increased if the patient has small vessels, is in heart failure, or has very severe coronary artery or valvular disease.

Table 13.2 Complications of cardiac catheterisation

- Peripheral arterial damage (dissection, haematoma)
- Cardiac arrhythmia (SVT, VT, VF)
- Cardiac tamponade
- Dissection of a coronary artery
- Heart failure due to hyperosmolar contrast agents
- Thromboembolism, due to clot on catheter, air embolism, dislodged atheroma

HEART FAILURE

Heart failure is a poorly defined clinical entity in which the heart ceases to respond normally to the demands made on it. Inadequate perfusion of the tissues leads to a variety of

Fig. 13.24 Cardiac catheter pressure tracing in aortic stenosis. As the catheter is withdrawn from the left ventricle into the aorta, there is an abrupt drop in pressure demonstrating a gradient across the aortic valve of 140 mmHg. Lower tracing is the ECG.

symptoms, of which fatigue, oedema and breathlessness are the most important. It is now appreciated that some of the symptoms are not easily explained, and that secondary changes occur in skeletal muscle which limit exercise tolerance, and may give rise to feelings of fatigue and breathlessness.

Diuretic treatment may lead to improvement in the clinical manifestations of heart failure related to salt and water retention, but without much improvement in cardiac output or other haemodynamic indices. Definitions of heart failure thus become difficult and *haemodynamic* definitions of heart failure should, perhaps, be avoided. The condition may be best regarded as the end of a spectrum which starts with trivial heart disease or overload without any symptoms or signs; progresses to more severe heart disease or overload with limitation of exercise performance; and finally passes to severe cardiac damage, hypertrophy or overload, with symptoms at rest, limitation of activity and severe fluid retention. The precise point at which the heart is said to 'fail' is thus arbitrary. Heart failure in a high-output state, such as severe anaemia, may differ in many ways from heart failure in constrictive pericarditis or massive myocardial infarction.

PATHOPHYSIOLOGY OF HEART FAILURE

The clinical syndrome of heart failure affects more than 1% of the population and accounts for a very large number of hospital admissions. The condition includes a complex interplay of factors: impaired cardiac performance (from many causes), impaired pulmonary gaseous exchange, activation of neurohumoral systems causing alterations in sodium and water homeostasis, and changes in skeletal muscle function. Early on in heart failure, when cardiac output falls and the venous pressure rises, activation of the sympathetic nervous system and salt and water retention can be regarded as adaptive responses maintaining perfusion pressure by vasoconstriction and increasing circulating volume. However, as the condition develops, these compensatory mechanisms contribute to the signs and symptoms of heart failure.

Impaired myocardial function

In many conditions, a change in cardiac myocyte function has been demonstrated, but it is not always clear if the observed changes are the cause of, or secondary to, the heart failure. Change in myocyte calcium handling, abnormal ATPase isoenzymes, energy metabolism and cellular buffering capacity have been described. These observations have not yet led to a single unifying hypothesis of the nature of contractile malfunction in heart failure.

Systolic muscle performance can be improved by the use of inotropic agents (Table 13.3), of which digoxin is the most established. Long-term inotropic therapy does not, however, appear to improve prognosis and, with some agents, may even be harmful due to the increased oxygen demand that may be caused. Indirect improvements in systolic performance may accompany the use of vaso-

Table 13.3 Commonly used inotropic agents

Drug	Mechanisms/comments
POSITIVELY INOTROPIC	
Digitalis glycosides, e.g. digitalis, digitoxin, ouabain	Sodium pump inhibition Parasympathetic stimulation
Adrenergic agonists	
Adrenaline and noradrenaline	Mixed beta and mixed alpha stimulation
Isoprenaline	Mixed beta stimulation
Dobutamine	Beta-1 stimulation
Dopamine	Low dose: release of noradrenaline Medium dose: beta-1 stimulation High dose: alpha stimulation
Phosphodiesterase inhibitors	
Aminophylline (also enoximone, Amrinone, Milrinone)	Increase intracellular cAMP
NEGATIVELY INOTROPIC	
Beta-adrenoceptor agents	
Propranolol Atenolol Metoprolol	All may cause deterioration in LV function
Calcium antagonists	
Verapamil	
Diltiazem	
Other drugs used in arrhythmias	
Bretylium	
Amiodarone	Safe if given slowly iv
Disopyramide	
Mexiletine	(with toxic doses)
Flecainide	
Lignocaine	(only with toxic doses)

dilating drugs that primarily affect afterload (p. 358). Many drugs used in heart disease have a direct myocardial depressant effect, especially those used in treatment of arrhythmias (Table 13.3).

Neurohumoral factors

Sympathetic neural stimulation and increased levels of circulating catecholamines are found in heart failure, but these compensatory mechanisms may become counterproductive.

Sympathetic stimulation arises from afferent stretch receptors in the baroreceptors of the aorta which respond to diminished stroke volume, while stretch receptors on the atria and pulmonary veins respond to the rise in venous pressure (Fig. 13.26). These vagal afferent signals cause sympathetic stimulation via the vasomotor centre of the brain stem. In the heart, beta-1 receptors are responsible for an increased heart rate, aided by simultaneous vagal inhibition. Contractility of ventricular muscle cells is also enhanced by beta-1 stimulation with a possible contribution from alpha-1 receptor activation.

The peripheral circulation is also the source of powerful afferent signals when perfusion is diminished due to failing

13

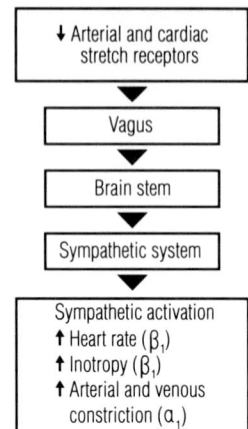

Fig. 13.26 Pathway of response to cardiac and arterial stretch receptors.

pump performance. Vasomotor centre activity increases pre-capillary arterial tone, thereby increasing peripheral vascular resistance and maintaining pressure. Similarly, constriction of the capacitance veins occurs, increasing venous return to the heart.

Renin-angiotensin-aldosterone system

Activation of the renin-angiotensin-aldosterone system causes salt and water retention and vasoconstriction, thus contributing to the clinical picture of heart failure. Reduced perfusion pressure of the afferent glomerular arteriole of the kidney, and a diminished sodium load at the macula densa, are the stimuli to activation of renin release (Fig. 13.27). Sympathetic activation via beta-1 receptors in the afferent arteriole also stimulates renin

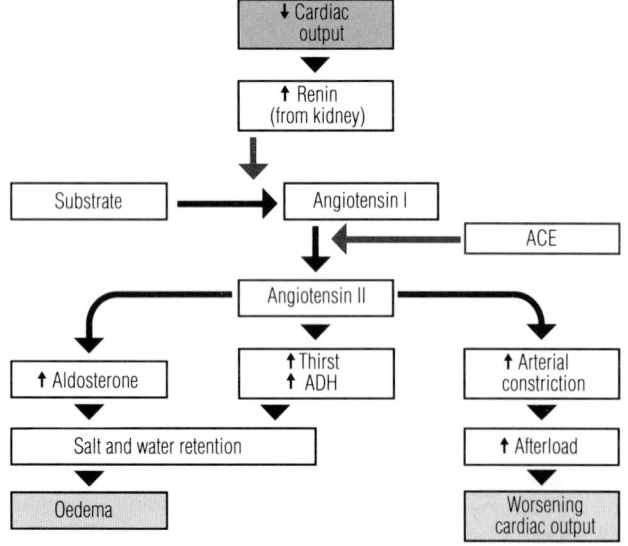

Fig. 13.27 The renin-angiotensin-aldosterone system in cardiac failure. Activation of the renin-angiotensin system by falling cardiac output leads to salt and water retention and worsening cardiac output (ACE = angiotensin-converting enzyme).

release. The action of renin on circulating renin substrate produces angiotensin I which is converted to the active form, angiotensin II, by angiotensin-converting enyme (ACE). Angiotensin II is a powerful vasoconstrictor and stimulator of aldosterone secretion.

Modern treatment of patients in heart failure with severe degrees of pump impairment now includes drugs which inhibit ACE (p. 444). Peripheral vascular resistance is thus diminished, reducing the afterload on the ventricles, and inhibition of aldosterone secretion counteracts the tendency to retain sodium and water.

Other humoral factors in heart failure

The secretion of antidiuretic hormone (ADH) is probably increased to some degree, but its importance in the pathophysiology of heart failure is not clear. Atrial natriuretic peptide or factor (ANP or ANF) is produced in the atria and secreted in response to atrial wall distension. Its role has not yet been precisely defined, but it may counteract some of the salt- and water-retaining mechanisms that are activated by diminished stroke volume. Prostaglandins act as vasodilatory hormones within the kidneys; thus, drugs which interfere with prostaglandin synthesis (such as indomethacin), may precipitate a rise in vascular resistance which can severely impair renal function and lead to a rise in blood pressure.

CLINICAL ASPECTS OF HEART FAILURE

In more severe forms of heart failure, the output of the heart at rest is insufficient for adequate tissue perfusion. Before this stage is reached, the heart may only give an adequate resting output at the expense of a raised filling pressure, and be incapable of increasing output sufficiently during even moderate degrees of exertion; the latter thus occurs anaerobically, rather than aerobically. The end result of the raised filling pressure and reduced output, together with the compensatory mechanisms that come into action, is retention of salt and water, so that the lungs and/or the systemic circulation become overloaded with excess fluid.

Terminological confusion arises since the heart is really two pumps in series separated by the lungs and the systemic circulation. Either side may fail independently – either the left, when the lungs become congested, or the right, in which case the dependent parts of the body become oedematous. Alternatively, there may be failure of both sides at the same time, or, more frequently, left heart failure leading to right, producing both pulmonary congestion and peripheral oedema. *Congestive cardiac failure*, to most clinicians, means combined right and left heart failure; others, however, also use the term to refer to pure right heart failure. The term is probably best avoided.

Blood flow to the kidneys, abdominal viscera and the skin is reduced, and the patient looks pale with pale conjunctivae. A normal flow to the brain is maintained at first; in severe cases, however, poor cerebral perfusion probably adds to the feeling of lethargy and fatigue and, in some

Summary 1	Symptoms and signs of heart failure

Symptoms
- Fatigue
- Shortness of breath
  on exertion
  on lying flat
- Paroxysmal nocturnal
  dyspnoea
- Haemoptysis
- Weight gain
- Swollen ankles
- Abdominal distension
- Abdominal pain

Signs
- Pallor
- Peripheral cyanosis
- Pulsus alternans
- Cardiomegaly
- Gallop rhythm
- Positive hepatojugular reflex
- Basal crackles
- Pitting oedema
- Raised JVP
- Ascites
- Hepatomegaly

cases, mental confusion. The main symptoms and signs of heart failure are listed in Summary 1.

LEFT HEART FAILURE

Left heat failure is usually left *ventricular* failure, resulting from damage to, or chronic overload of, the left ventricle. The overload may be from either a pressure overload, as in hypertension, or a volume load, as in aortic regurgitation. There may be inadequate filling of the ventricle, due to an arrhythmia or disease, such as mitral stenosis or atrial myxoma proximal to the ventricle; in this case, left *heart* failure is the more accurate term, as the left ventricle is blameless.

The principal causes of left heart failure are shown in Table 13.4. The left ventricle may have failure of *systolic* function, such that it cannot efficiently eject a normal stroke volume and has a reduced ejection fraction (normally over 60%). Alternatively, there may be failure of *diastolic* function, so that it cannot relax and fill adequately in diastole, without an increase in its filling pressure (normally below 15 mmHg).

When the filling pressure of the left heart rises sufficiently, the pulmonary venous and capillary pressures exceed the level at which the pulmonary lymphatics can cope with the additional filtration of fluid out of the lung capillaries. As a result, the lung parenchyma becomes congested, and there is an increase in lung blood volume and lung water. When the capillary pressure exceeds about 35 mmHg, the fluid starts to accumulate in the alveoli, and

Table 13.4 Principal causes of left heart failure

Increased load	Myocardial damage

• Systemic hypertension	• Ischaemic heart disease
	  Infarction
	  LV aneurysm
	  LV fibrosis

• Mitral and aortic valve disease	
• Cardiac arrhythmias	• Myocarditis

• High output states,
  e.g.: anaemia
  thyrotoxicosis
	• Cardiomyopathy

• Overtransfusion	• Cardiac depressant drugs

pulmonary oedema develops, with fluid frothing in the airways.

Clinical features

Symptoms

The typical symptoms are related to the congested lungs and include unnatural shortness of breath on exertion, paroxysmal nocturnal dyspnoea (waking up at night severely breathless) and dyspnoea and cough on lying down (orthopnoea). The congested bronchial mucosae may produce wheeze ('cardiac asthma'), and bronchial veins may bleed, causing haemoptysis – a feature of severe mitral stenosis. Severe left heart failure results in pulmonary oedema, with the patient 'drowning' in the alveolar transudate. In extreme cases, the symptoms of this often terminal condition are profound air-hunger and respiratory distress, a feeling of suffocation, panic and impending death, and frothing sputum, which eventually becomes blood-stained, pouring out of the mouth.

Chronic left heart failure produces a dramatically reduced effort tolerance, lethargy and chronic fatigue.

Signs

Signs vary with the cause of the failure, which may be evident, such as severe hypertension or severe valve disease. Left ventricular failure is commonly accompanied by a tachycardia, a short ejection resulting in a small volume pulse and small pulse pressure, a dilated left ventricle with presystolic atrial thrust, and an audible gallop rhythm from third and fourth heart sounds which may coincide in a summation gallop (p. 339). There may be pulsus alternans, and a jugular venous pulse with a prominent A wave. Often, there are basal crackles in the lungs, but these may not develop until later in the condition and are not necessary for the diagnosis. Inspiratory and expiratory wheeze, which not uncommonly occurs in patients with left heart failure, especially the elderly, may lead the doctor mistakenly to diagnose respiratory disease. Another source of confusion is the profound vasoconstriction that occurs with heart failure; this often results in a slight increase in blood pressure which is diagnosed falsely as the 'cause'. The pallor of heart failure may lead to a mistaken clinical diagnosis of anaemia.

Investigation

A chest X-ray is helpful; this shows the engorged lymphatics as Kerley B lines at the lung bases (Fig. 13.18). The upper zone veins become dilated because of splinting of the lower zone veins by congested lymphatics. In pulmonary oedema, the hilae become hazy and a full 'bat's wing' shadowing can develop. Small basal effusions are common at the costophrenic angles. Large pleural effusions are more typical of right heart failure, pulmonary embolism or other aetiologies.

The ECG may indicate infarction or left ventricular

hypertrophy, but is not very useful in diagnosing heart failure except by indicating left atrial hypertrophy (Fig. 13.13). It may be almost normal in severe heart failure, but, if left ventricular hypertrophy or strain is indicated, it is imperative to exclude 'silent' aortic stenosis as a remediable cause.

RIGHT HEART FAILURE

Right heart failure is usually secondary to pulmonary hypertension, although there are some processes which damage the right ventricle (Table 13.5). Lung disease is a common cause (described on page 502), and massive pulmonary thromboembolism can cause acute right heart failure (p. 502). Right-sided valve disease is a common cause in congenital heart disease. Myocardial infarction, cardiomyopathy and myocarditis usually involve both sides of the heart. When faced with a considerably increased load, the right ventricle dilates. This causes a rise in the filling pressure, which increases the systemic venous pressure. The capillary pressure of the lower body rises, and fluid transudates from the capillaries into the tissues. Cardiac output falls, increasing salt- and water-retention by the kidneys (Fig. 13.27) and expanding the extracellular volume. The systemic capillary pressure increases, causing further oedema.

Table 13.5 Principal causes of right heart failure

- Pulmonary hypertension
  Secondary to left heart failure
  Secondary to lung disease
  From increased lung blood flow (left to right shunt)
  Pulmonary embolism
- Right ventricular infarction
- Right-sided involvement in cardiomyopathy and myocarditis
- Pulmonary and tricuspid valve disease

Clinical features

Symptoms

The earliest symptom of right heart failure is pitting oedema of the lower body – the ankles and feet in those who are mobile, and the sacral area and legs of those in bed. The oedema can spread upwards to involve the groin and the abdominal wall, and ascites can cause abdominal distension. Pleural effusion may contribute to breathlessness. Liver engorgement and distension of the capsule can cause abdominal pain, particularly on exercise, (*hepatic angina*).

Signs

The jugular venous pressure is raised and, if the right ventricle is very dilated, there may be tricuspid regurgitation, with a large V wave and pulsatile liver. After an initial gain in weight through oedema, long-standing

failure is associated with a fall in lean body mass. If the oedema is treated, the patient loses weight and eventually becomes cachectic. The cachexia is not fully understood, but is probably due to loss of appetite and a degree of malabsorption due to venous congestion of the gut.

'Consequential' right heart failure

Breathlessness due to left heart failure may be relieved when the right heart starts to fail. This occurs because the pulmonary arterial tree appears to be sensitive to a rise in left atrial pressure. Not only is there a passive rise in pulmonary artery pressure sufficient to maintain normal flow through the lungs, but there may also be an active constriction of the pulmonary arteries. This lessens pulmonary vascular congestion, but, by increasing the resistance to flow, puts an increased load on the right ventricle, which then fails.

Diagnosis

Severe fluid retention from any cause can mimic right heart failure. The characteristic findings, apart from the oedema (which can have a variety of causes), are a raised jugular venous pressure, cardiomegaly, a gallop rhythm and an enlarged heart on chest X-ray. The severely oedematous patient may have a raised jugular venous pressure, increased heart size, proteinuria and reduced plasma albumin. A patient with severe right heart failure may also have deranged liver function tests, and be jaundiced from hepatic congestion complicated by hepatic cirrhosis. Establishing the differential diagnosis of hepatic cirrhosis, nephrotic syndrome or severe right heart failure may therefore take a little time. The albuminuria of heart failure is not gross and, although the liver may be considerably enlarged and tender, splenomegaly is relatively uncommon in right heart failure and usually only occurs in very long-standing cases.

MANAGEMENT OF HEART FAILURE

The management of heart failure has several objectives. Relief of symptoms is paramount, but it is also essential that the cause of the heart failure be established. The treatment should aim to improve the survival and quality of life for those patients who have, on average, a poor life expectancy.

Acute left heart failure

In an emergency, acute left heart failure is best managed in the following sequence (Summary 2):

Posture

The patient is sat up, so that the oedema settles to the lung bases. An oxygen mask giving a high concentration of oxygen may improve central saturation. Patients start to feel better in a few minutes.

Depress respiration and allay anxiety

Diamorphine (or morphine) is given intravenously or by deep intramuscular injection to depress the exaggerated respiratory effort (which is itself using a large proportion of the limited cardiac output), reduce the patient's distress and redistribute some of the increased central blood volume to the periphery. Patients usually start to feel better in about 10 minutes.

Promote diuresis

An intravenous diuretic is given, such as frusemide (20 mg). Larger doses are appropriate if the patient is already on diuretics. The diuresis takes about 30 minutes or more and the patient does not feel better until then.

Venesection

If a patient is moribund and not responding to intravenous diuretics, the most direct way of reducing left atrial pressure is by *venesection*, which requires about 500 ml of blood to be removed. A brisk diuresis may then follow. Unfortunately, venesection is usually attempted too late. It is preferable to the technique of cuffs blown up to between systolic and diastolic blood pressure on the limbs, which is tedious and has little effect.

More intensive treatment

A more aggressive approach is needed in left heart failure which is not responding to initial measures. This is particularly appropriate in endocarditis or severe valve disease, where young patients may have an excellent prognosis with surgery if they can be maintained until then. Positive pressure ventilation, the use of intravenous nitrates for preload reduction, inotropic agents to improve blood pressure and renal perfusion, and afterload reduction with nitroprusside, may be needed. Use of these techniques can be extremely hazardous if left atrial pressure and cardiac output are not monitored.

Treat cause

The cause is identified and treated if possible. Malignant hypertension should be treated (p. 444) but mild hypertension may be secondary and should not be treated unless it is sustained for more than 24 hours after initial therapy. Disease of native or prosthetic valves must be excluded. A severe tachycardia should also be treated, but sinus tachycardia is secondary to the increased sympathetic drive.

Chronic heart failure

Right heart failure, chronic left heart failure and biventricular failure are all managed in a similar fashion. The cause (valvular disease, rhythm disturbance, hypertension)

Summary 2 Principles of management of heart failure

Acute left heart failure	
Posture	Sit patient up. Give oxygen
Depress respiration and allay anxiety	Give morphine or diamorphine (with anti-emetic)
Reduce left atrial pressure, promote diuresis	Give iv diuretic
Treat cause	e.g. serious arrhythmia, severe hypertension
Other treatments	Venesection. Ventilation (see text for details)
Chronic heart failure	
Rest	Bedrest. Small meals
Salt restriction	No added salt
Combat fluid and salt retention	Diuretics plus potassium ACE-inhibitors Spironolactone
Preload reduction	Nitrates
Afterload reduction	Vasodilators ACE-inhibitors
Inotropic agents	Digoxin. Sympathomimetics
Prevent venous thrombosis	Anticoagulants Stockings, leg exercise
Treat cause wherever possible	

---

is treated wherever possible. The main principles of symptomatic treatment are shown in Summary 2.

Bedrest

Bedrest is important. In the previously ambulant patient, it will produce diuresis, as it allows an increased proportion of cardiac output to perfuse the kidneys. Early mobilisation, when the oedema has gone, does not allow the heart time to reduce in size as much as with further rest. Bedrest also, of course, potentiates the risk of venous thrombosis and thromboembolism.

Salt restriction

Nowadays, severe salt restriction is not advised, but salty food should not be eaten nor salt added to food.

Fluid restriction

Fluid restriction is occasionally necessary as a secondary measure where diuretics and other measures have failed. It becomes particularly important where there is evidence of hyponatraemia.

Diuretics and potassium

Diuretics help to eliminate the excess salt and water, thus reducing the oedema and, by removing fluid from the circulation, helping to reduce the preload. Mild failure responds well to thiazide diuretics, which have a sustained action and are given once a day in the morning. Loop diuretics, such as frusemide and bumetanide, have a more powerful and shorter action. They may be given morning and at lunchtime, and, in resistant heart failure, may be effective when given intravenously, even when ineffective orally. All of these diuretics encourage loss of sodium, water and potassium; potassium supplementation therefore becomes necessary, particularly as a patient in heart failure already has a low total body potassium, and marked diuresis can produce hypokalaemia (p. 850).

Some potassium supplementation is possible with fruit juices or a high fruit diet. Larger amounts require potassium given as an effervescent tablet or in a slow-release preparation. Certain diuretics conserve potassium, the most commonly used being amiloride and spironolactone. The latter is an aldosterone antagonist which has diuretic and hypotensive effects as well as maintaining serum potassium levels. Although spironolactone has the undesirable effect of producing gynaecomastia in men, it has a valuable potentiating effect when given with loop diuretics. It can cause nausea, but is less likely to do so when given with food.

Afterload and preload reduction

Angiotensin-converting enzyme inhibitors are now being given earlier in the management of heart failure, on the grounds that they help to break the vicious cycle induced by the renin-angiotensin-aldosterone effects of salt retention and vasoconstriction (Fig. 13.27). ACE inhibitors are extremely potent vasodilators, and their main effect often appears to be reduction of afterload, rather than a major impact on diuresis. They are usually used in resistant heart failure, but, in some trials, gave better survival than conventional treatment, even in milder heart failure. They are used in combination with loop diuretics.

Other afterload reducers include hydralazine, intravenous nitroprusside and nifedipine. Nitrates are agents which reduce *preload* by increasing venous capacitance. They have a useful complementary role to diuretics and often improve effort tolerance.

Ancillary treatment

Anticoagulation. A large heart and sluggish circulation with oedematous legs and prolonged bedrest predispose to venous thrombosis and thromboembolism. Clot may also form in the heart, giving pulmonary or systemic emboli. In patients at risk, prophylactic anticoagulation with heparin, and then warfarin, is therefore advisable, but may require special care in patients with congested livers, who may need very small doses of warfarin.

Anti-arrhythmics. Heart failure may be complicated by arrhythmias. Ventricular arrhythmias may settle as the heart becomes smaller, and all cardio-depressant anti-arrhythmic drugs, such as beta-blockers and verapamil, must be used with great caution in the presence of heart failure, as it may be severely exacerbated by their use.

Atrial fibrillation is conventionally treated with digoxin or alternative digitalis glycosides. However, the inotropic effect of these drugs is questionable, and they are becoming less used for this effect alone. Slow sinus rhythm, or slow atrial fibrillation, can be treated with oral salbutamol, which increases the heart rate and has a vasodilator effect.

Inotropic agents may initiate a diuresis and shrinkage in heart size in resistant heart failure, but their place in long-term survival is still controversial. They are most widely used in cardiogenic shock after infarction, or after cardiac bypass (p. 389).

RHYTHM DISTURBANCES

INVESTIGATIVE TECHNIQUES

The principal tool for analysing disorders of cardiac rhythm is the 12-lead ECG. The correct interpretation of the ECG may depend on comparison with previously acquired recordings. A systematic approach is essential.

24-hour ECG (Holter monitor)

Recorders able to monitor two channels of an ECG in ambulant patients over a continuous 24-hour period (Fig. 13.28) have helped enormously in investigating patients with paroxysmal symptoms. However, since some rhythm disturbances may occur very infrequently, this type of recorder may not always be the most helpful. Alternatives are available. One small recorder can be applied by the patient directly to the chest during symptoms and records 30 seconds of ECG in a solid state memory. This can be replayed subsequently through an ECG machine, or transmitted by telephone to a central station, where a doctor can advise on the nature of the event. For those patients who receive no warning of impending rhythm disturbance, there are newer automatic solid state

1920 hours

Fig. 13.28   24-hour continuous ambulatory ECG monitoring. At 19.20 hours, the sinus rhythm is interrupted by ventricular ectopic beats and a short run of ventricular tachycardia.

recorders that continually sample the ECG over long periods but only memorise significant events.

Intracardiac electrophysiological testing (EP testing)

The techniques of cardiac catheterisation enable localised intracardiac ECGs to be recorded, using catheters similar to pacing catheters with electrodes mounted near their tips. Thus, the activity of the atria, atrioventricular node, bundle of His and ventricles can be recorded independently. By combining recording with artificial stimulation from intracardiac pacemakers, a detailed analysis of intracardiac conduction can be made. This has proved useful in studying patients with tachycardia, in whom the abnormal rhythm may be induced and its origin (ventricular or supraventricular) confirmed. The site, number and potential danger from accessory atrioventricular bypass tracts (e.g. in Wolff-Parkinson-White syndrome), is ideally assessed in this way. The effectiveness of drug regimens and the potential for using anti-tachycardia pacemakers are also tested using EP studies.

Exercise ECG

The exercise test is more commonly used to assess ischaemic heart disease, but also has a role in managing certain patients with arrhythmia. Those with recurrent ventricular tachycardia, or Wolf-Parkinson-White syndrome, may undergo exercise testing to check the efficacy of their drug treatment. However, not all these patients have exercise-induced arrhythmia, and may instead require more sophisticated EP studies (see above).

NORMAL SINUS RHYTHM

Each ventricular (QRS) complex is preceded by a P wave with a normal P wave axis (i.e. from the sinus node, P wave axis = 0° to +90°) and normal PR interval (0.11–0.20 s). In some circumstances, sinus rhythm may control the atrial, but not the ventricular, activity; this is most commonly encountered in complete heart block (p. 361 and Fig. 13.32).

Sinus arrhythmia is the quickening of the heart rate which occurs cyclically with each inspiration. It is most marked in those individuals (often young) who have high vagal tone.

ECTOPIC OR EXTRASYSTOLIC BEATS

Beats which occur prematurely, before the next sinus beat, may arise in the atria, the atrioventricular node and bundle of His or from the ventricles.

Atrial ectopics

Atrial ectopics or atrial premature beats (Fig. 13.29) are usually preceded by a P wave of different shape, different PR interval and, frequently, a different axis to the sinus P wave. The following QRS complex is normal. Atrial

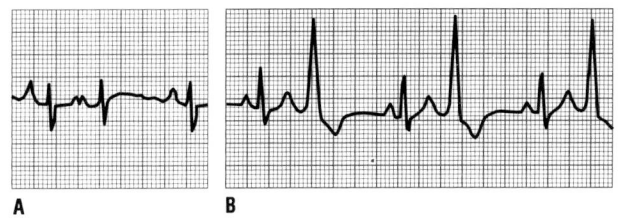

Fig. 13.29 ECGs showing ectopic beats. A. An atrial ectopic beat, demonstrated by the varying shape of the P wave. **B.** Coupled ventricular ectopics (bigeminy).

ectopics are common even in normal hearts, although, like all extrasystoles, they may be felt as uncomfortable fluttering, palpitation or 'skipped beats' in the chest. Stimulants, such as alcohol or caffeine-containing drinks and cigarettes, may be precipitants. Other predisposing factors include anti-arrhythmic drugs, especially digoxin, and electrolyte disturbance. High vagal tone suppressing sinus activity may allow atrial 'escape' beats to occur. Atrial distension may precipitate ectopic beats or tachycardias.

Junctional extrasystoles

Junctional extrasystoles may arise from the atrioventricular node or proximal bundle of His, although this differentiation cannot normally be made, hence the less specific term 'junctional' rather than the older 'nodal beat'. Atrial activation occurs retrogradely so that the P wave axis is towards aVR and produces negative P waves in II, III and aVF. The delay between ectopic activation and ventricular activity depends on its site of origin and will vary the timing of the P wave. This can precede, be buried in, or follow the QRS complex, which has a configuration identical to that in sinus rhythm (Fig. 13.29).

Blocked atrial premature beats occur when the premature atrial contraction encounters a fully refractory AV node and the impulse fails to conduct to the ventricles. Lesser degrees of P wave prematurity may encounter relative refractoriness in the AV node and be associated with longer PR intervals than the sinus beats.

Ventricular ectopics

Ventricular ectopic (VE) beats, by definition, are not preceded by a P wave and have a broad QRS configuration (Fig. 13.29). There is no prognostic significance attached to whether the ectopic beat has a left or right bundle branch block pattern. However, when frequent or multiform ventricular ectopics are found in association with underlying ischaemic heart disease or cardiomyopathy, then there is an increased risk of sudden death. Control of ventricular ectopics with drugs may improve symptoms, but does not improve the prognosis for the patient. This is probably because the severity of the underlying heart disease is a more important influence on survival. In addition, the drugs used to suppress VE may themselves precipitate serious ventricular arrhythmias.

BRADYCARDIA AND HEART BLOCK

Bradycardia

Defined as a heart rate less than 60 bpm, bradycardia may be seen as a manifestation of vagal tone in trained athletes or, more commonly, as an unwanted effect of beta adrenoreceptor blocking drugs. It generally requires no treatment, unless severe and producing symptoms. In an emergency (such as when severe bradycardia complicates a myocardial infarction), intravenous atropine (600 mcg iv to a maximum of 2.4 mg in 2 hours), or adrenaline (2–10 ml of 1/10 000 iv) may be used; if persistent, a temporary artificial pacemaker should be implanted. Chronic bradycardia may be a manifestation of the sick sinus syndrome (p. 371) and may benefit from pacemaker implantation.

Sinus node block and sinus arrest

Both sinus node block and sinus arrest are associated with a pause in the normal train of sinus rhythm, leading to a delay in the appearance of the P wave. In *sinus node block*, the resultant pause between P waves is approximately double the preceding sinus (P-P) interval. This implies that a normal discharge of the SA node pacemaker cells failed to be transmitted to the atria (and cannot be seen on the ECG). The essential pacemaker rate, however, remains constant. In *sinus arrest*, the pause is not a simple multiple of the sinus interval, from which it is inferred that a transient change in pacemaker automaticity has led to the loss of P wave.

First degree heart block

In first degree heart block (Fig. 13.30), the PR interval is prolonged (greater than 0.20 s). This may occur in otherwise normal patients and is caused by delayed propagation within the atrioventricular (AV) node. Increased vagal tone decreases both sinoatrial (SA) node firing rate and AV node conduction, so that a modestly prolonged PR interval may accompany vagally-induced bradycardia. However, long PR intervals in the presence of normal or fast heart rates imply an intrinsic defect in the AV node. This is generally benign. The development of first degree heart block in the context of infective endocarditis usually means aortic root abscess formation; the prognosis is bad unless rapidly dealt with surgically. Similarly, widespread conducting tissue disease is suggested by the combination of first degree block, left axis deviation and bundle branch block

Fig. 13.30 ECG showing first degree heart block. Note prolonged PR interval (0.28 s).

(Fig. 13.16). First degree block may also occur following a myocardial infarction (p. 413).

Second degree heart block

Second degree heart block (Fig. 13.31) is defined as intermittent failure to conduct an impulse from the atria to the ventricles, and may be temporary or permanent. It occurs in two major forms which have different anatomical sites for the block and somewhat different implications for the patient.

A

B

Fig. 13.31 ECGs showing second degree heart block. A. Mobitz type I showing progressive lengthening of the PR interval until the P wave is not conducted to the ventricles (arrow). **B.** Mobitz type II. Four sinus beats are followed by cessation of conduction following the P wave (arrowed).

The Wenckebach phenomenon or Mobitz type I block

The Mobitz type I block (Wenckebach phenomenon) produces successively increasing PR intervals until a P wave is not conducted; the cycle then repeats itself. There are usually 3–5 beats in a cycle. This block occurs *within* the AV node, and is probably relatively benign. It may complicate acute inferior myocardial infarction and generally does not require specific treatment. It may also be seen in patients with generalised conducting tissue disease and as part of the sick-sinus syndrome (p. 371).

Mobitz type II block

In the Mobitz type II block, an unheralded failure to conduct a P wave occurs. The site of the block is *below* the AV node in the proximal bundle of His. This condition has a tendency to progress unpredictably to complete block, which may cause Stokes-Adams' attacks or even death. This conduction disturbance is much less common than type I block and, because of its implications, usually requires treatment with an artificial pacemaker.

Other special forms of second degree block

During atrial tachycardia (e.g. atrial flutter), there may often be conduction of alternate beats to the ventricles in a ratio of 2 P waves:1 QRS complex. When a tachycardia is present, this block constitutes the normal physiological function of the AV node, and block can often be increased further (to 3:1 or 4:1 or more) by manœuvres, such as carotid sinus massage, which stimulate vagal activity. In the absence of an atrial tachycardia, established 2:1 conduction represents a form of second degree block. High grade block is present when the ratio of P waves to QRS is 3:1 or greater. In either case, artificial permanent pacemaker implantation is the treatment of choice when the arrhythmia persists.

Complete or third degree heart block

In complete or third degree block (Fig. 13.32), the atrial impulses fail to be conducted to the ventricles. The block may be within the atrioventricular node, when the escape ventricular rhythm will be within the lower regions of the node or bundle of His, giving narrow, normal configuration QRS complexes and heart rates of about 40 bpm. Complete heart block may also occur at the level of the bundle of His, so that ventricular or distal bundle pacemakers control the heart rate, producing a much slower pulse (about 30 bpm) and wide, bundle branch block QRS complexes.

A

B

C

Fig. 13.32 Three rhythm strips demonstrating complete heart block. A. Atrioventricular dissociation with a relatively rapid ventricular rate and narrow QRS complex (with acute inferior infarction). **B.** A slow idioventricular rate with broad QRS complexes. **C.** The unusual combination of complete heart block and atrial fibrillation (no P waves).

Clinical features

Symptoms

First degree heart block is asymptomatic, as are many cases of second degree heart block, but patients may be aware of

the dropped beat and the stronger post-pause beat in Mobitz types I and II. In complete heart block, the most dramatic symptoms are related to recurrent asystole or the common ventricular arrhythmias that complicate severe bradycardia. However, complete heart block may present: without any symptoms, despite a marked bradycardia; with heart failure secondary to a low cardiac output; and, often, as a confusional state secondary to poor cerebral perfusion and multiple syncopal episodes.

Stokes-Adams' attack

The Stokes-Adams' attack is the classical syndrome of transient asystole (but can, equally, be the result of a transient burst of ventricular fibrillation or flutter). The attacks are usually unheralded. The patient may first be aware of lying on the ground or falling. Recovery is usually rapid and complete. Unlike epilepsy, there is no subsequent headache or confusion, unless a head injury or a prolonged period of anoxia complicate the picture. Skin pallor may be followed by flushing. If the anoxia lasts more than a few seconds, a convulsion may occur and, on occasion, incontinence. Incomplete attacks are common, presenting with transient giddiness (without true vertigo) or near fainting (pre-syncope).

Attacks are sporadic and random. There may be months to years between symptoms in some patients with intermittent block, so that 24-hour ambulatory electrocardiographic recordings (p. 358) may have to be made repeatedly for the diagnosis to be made. Occasionally, treatment with a pacemaker is warranted on the basis of the history alone, although intracardiac electrophysiological studies (p. 359) may help in these difficult patients.

Signs

There are few clinical signs in heart block. The first heart sound is quiet in first degree block, and intermittent dropped beats will be felt at the pulse in second degree block. In complete heart block, a slow pulse and intermittent cannon waves will be seen in the jugular venous pulse, due to occasional simultaneous contraction of the atria and ventricles. The large stroke volume and collapsing pulse with a systolic murmur may mimic aortic valve disease.

Management

In congenital complete heart block, there is a surprising degree of tolerance to the slow heart rate, which may show some modest rate responsiveness with exercise. Nevertheless, it is possible that adults with this condition risk sudden death, and that permanent pacemaker implantation is helpful.

In acute inferior myocardial infarction, complete heart block is due to transient ischaemia of the SA and AV nodes, and may not need a temporary pacemaker unless symptoms or heart failure occur (p. 365). In extensive anterior myocardial infarction, complete heart block is related to

13

extensive muscle damage and carries such a poor prognosis that many consider temporary pacemaker implantation unnecessary; however, this view may change with increasing salvage of damaged myocardium.

Drug treatment of complete heart block with isoprenaline slow-release capsules is now hardly ever justified, and permanent pacemakers should be offered to virtually all patients.

THE PERMANENT ARTIFICIAL PACEMAKER

Artificial cardiac pacemakers that can be implanted permanently have been one of the success stories of modern medicine. The basic pacemaker consists of a small battery container which can be implanted under the skin and connected by an insulated electrode to the heart. Small electrical impulses can be transmitted through the electrode to stimulate the heart to contract. Since the first permanent pacemakers were used to treat heart block in 1960, there has been a great increase in their use, so that between 0.75 and 1 million people worldwide now live with an implanted pacemaker. The initial sole indication for pacing was the treatment of chronic complete heart block, but now a major indication is the treatment of the sick sinus syndrome (p. 371). More recently, units able to treat tachycardias and administer internal DC cardioversion have been developed, although these are not yet widely used.

Early implantable pacemakers were fixed rate, i.e. they provided a constant stimulus irrespective of the patient's cardiac activity, and had battery lives of 12–18 months. Modern pacemakers, however, are almost exclusively demand (or standby) units, providing a pulse only when the heart rate falls below certain predetermined limits, and have battery lives of 8–15 years. They may offer considerable adjustment and analysis via transcutaneous telemetry. The complexity of cardiac pacemakers has increased for a number of reasons:

1. To increase battery life by reducing unnecessary pacing and by reducing the electrical output from the generator to the lowest safe limit.
2. To allow fine control of the pacing heart rate, and, with dual chamber devices, to restore the atrial contribution to filling, which may be very important to individuals with impaired ventricular function.
3. To enable detection of when the patient will need an increase in heart rate (e.g. with exercise), and increase the pacing rate accordingly.
4. To detect tachycardias and abort them by programmed bursts of pacing (anti-tachycardia).

A letter coding system, used internationally (e.g. VVI = a ventricular pacemaker in demand mode), describes the type of pacemaker used. In some pacemakers, a facility (hysteresis) allows the interval between the last natural beat and the paced beat to be longer than the pacing interval. Thus, only when a pause corresponding to a very low heart rate is exceeded will the pacemaker step in and gradually accelerate to its programmed paced rate. This stops the pacemaker inserting beats for trivial slowing of the heart (e.g. during sleep).

Dual-chamber pacemakers

Dual-chamber pacemakers have been developed to achieve a more physiological situation than is possible with ventricular pacing alone. These require implantation of electrodes in the right atrium as well as the right ventricle, adding slightly to the complexity of the implantation procedure. They also use more complex, and therefore more expensive, generators. In addition, the capacity to 'fine-tune' the multiplicity of programmable functions to each individual patient requires both time, and the availability of skilled pacemaker technicians or doctors in special clinics within pacing clinics. Nevertheless, these units are justified in certain groups of patients:

1. Patients with AV block but normal SA activity, in whom a true physiological situation can be achieved, with normal rate increase with activity, and maintained atrioventricular sequential contraction. This is usually reserved for young, or very active, patients.
2. Patients with poor ventricular function or valve disease where the atrial contribution to filling is of prime importance.
3. Patients with the 'pacemaker syndrome'; a small number of patients develop severe symptomatic hypotension with pacing of the right ventricle alone.

Dual-chamber pacemakers should be avoided in patients with unstable SA activity or atrial fibrillation.

Pacemaker implantation and complications

Permanent pacemakers are almost always inserted by a cardiologist using local anaesthesia and full surgical sterile technique. Like temporary pacemakers (p. 413), the pacing electrode is passed down a central vein to the right heart; usually, the cephalic or subclavian veins are used. The electrode and generator box are then buried subcutaneously, above pectoralis major on the high anterior chest wall. Complications of implantation are similar to those of temporary pacemakers. Infection is rare, but when it occurs, it requires major revision of the entire system and accounts for considerable morbidity and a small mortality. Lead displacement and lead fracture are very rare with modern pacing systems.

Specific pacemaker malfunction is now very rare. With current telemetry, the pacemaker (and lead) function can be assessed transcutaneously, so that premature battery failure can be predicted, problems with lead impedance (electrical resistance), current leak and failure to sense can often be diagnosed, and the unit reprogrammed to compensate for problems until replacement is required. Failure to sense the patient's electrical activity and intermittent failure to capture may sometimes cause problems. Dual-chamber pacemakers, although potentially much closer to normal physiology, carry their own problems, the most serious being is the capacity to generate pacemaker-induced arrhythmia. Fortunately, these problems are rare.

Interference with pacemaker function by external sources of high magnetic and electromagnetic fields is less of a problem than might be expected; few problems arise in the normal environment of most patients. However, magnetic resonance imaging is contraindicated, and cautery during surgery has to be performed with care, avoiding placing the ground electrode near the generator.

THE TACHYCARDIAS: INTRODUCTION

Tachycardias are defined as a heart rate above 100 bpm, and are divided according to the origin of the pacemaker impulse. A classification is given in Table 13.6, and a guide to the use of anti-arrhythmic agents in Table 13.7. A decision tree to aid in diagnosis is shown in Figure 13.33.

Mechanisms of production of tachycardias

Three basic mechanisms have been established: abnormalities of automaticity; early after-depolarisations and triggered activity; and abnormal impulse conduction and re-entry.

Abnormalities of automaticity

Under normal circumstances, only sino-atrial and atrio-ventricular node cells display automaticity. Abnormal automaticity may be displayed by diseased atrial and ventricular muscle. Stretch, alkalosis, increases in temperature and hypoxia all increase the rate of repolarisation and reduce the maximum diastolic (resting) potential (Vm), thereby accentuating the tendency to abnormal automaticity. Cardioactive drugs also influence heart rate and rhythm via these mechanisms. Therapeutic doses of some anti-arrhythmics achieve their beneficial effects by decreasing the rate of depolarisation (Table 13.9). Toxic doses may cause atrial and ventricular tachyarrhythmia by increasing the diastolic depolarisation slope and lowering Vm.

Early after depolarisations and triggered activity

Following an action potential, there may be a further spontaneous depolarisation which can occur early during repolarisation or late. Single 'after-depolarisations' can precipitate further spontaneous beats, to produce a rapid cycle of spontaneous activity. Factors which encourage their occurrence include hypoxia, hypercapnia, high circulating catecholamines, non-specific muscle injury and stretch. There is evidence that this activity occurs frequently and is important in producing tachycardia, particularly in the long QT syndrome (p. 372) and with drugs of the Vaughan-Williams classes IA and III.

Table 13.6 Features and classification of tachycardias

Type	Rate (bpm)	ECG P-waves	QRS complex	Response to carotid sinus pressure	Clinical Symptoms and signs
Supraventricular					
Sinus	>100	Normal	Normal	Transient minor slowing	Palpitation or none
Atrial Paroxysmal atrial tachycardia	120–250	Abnormal shape	Regular and normal unless aberrant conduction produces broad QRS of RBBB or, less commonly, LBBB type. Broad QRS also if BBB already present.	May terminate tachycardia	Palpitation, dizziness, breathlessness, chest pain may occur. Diuresis on cessation
Atrial fibrillation	>140	Absent	Irregular	Transient slowing	As above
Atrial flutter	150	Flutter waves; sawtooth pattern in lead V1	Very regular QRS complexes	Conduction may decrease from usual 2:1 to 4:1 or less	As above
AV NRT	180–240	None seen (buried in QRS)	Normal and regular	None, or abrupt cessation	As above
AV RT	180–240	Inverted P waves after QRS	Normal and regular	None, or abrupt cessation	As above
Ventricular					
Ventricular tachyardia	150–250	Dissociated P waves diagnostic, but can be difficult to see	Regular broad QRS >120 ms sometimes ≥140 ms. QRS look similar V1–V6 – 'concordance'	No response	May cause collapse; sometimes well-tolerated
Ventricular fibrillation Ventricular flutter	150–300	None seen	Loss of regular discernible QRS features	Inappropriate	Collapse with rapid loss of consciousness

Heart rate >100

Regular — No → Atrial fibrillation

Yes

QRS complexes

Broad > 0.12 s

Narrow < 0.12 s

> 0.14 s

0.12–0.14 s

P wave visible ◄ No ◄ Delta wave in resting ECG

Heart rate >180

QRS similar to previous ECG at resting rate ◄ Yes ◄ Pre-existing BBB

No

No   Yes   Don't know

No   Yes

Yes

Yes

Consider SVT

Rate-dependent BBB or VT

AVNRT Nodal tachycardia

WPW

Re-entry likely

Concordance V1–V6

Dissociated P waves present

Fusion beats present

Before QRS

No

Yes

AVRT Nodal tachycardia

Abnormal P wave

Normal P wave and PR interval

Yes

No

Yes

Yes

VT likely

SVT more likely than VT

Paroxysmal atrial tachycardia Nodal tachycardia Atrial flutter

Sinus tachycardia

Fig. 13.33   Decision tree for diagnosis of tachycardia.

Table 13.7 Guide to use of anti-arrhythmic drugs

Vaughan-Williams classification	Electrophysiological action		Indications	Toxic effects
	On action potential	On ECG		
Class I: Membrane stabilising drugs				
IA Quinidine	Increase threshold for activation. Slow rate of rise of action potential ?(Inhibit fast sodium channel)	QRS and QT prolongation, especially quinidine	Toxicity now limits use. Effective in VT, and may convert AF or A flutter to sinus rhythm.	GI disturbance. Pro-arrhythmogenic. Interacts with digoxin and numerous other drugs
Procainamide			Not used long-term, due to side-effects. Acute iv for ventricular and supraventricular arrhythmia	Lupus syndrome. Other autoimmune disorders.
Disopyramide			Ventricular and supraventricular arrhythmia. Prophylaxis in paroxysmal AF	Negative inotropy Anticholinergic side-effects
IB Lignocaine Mexiletine Phenytoin	Inhibit fast sodium channel. Shorten action potential	Usually none	Ventricular arrhythmia during and after myocardial infarction. Phenytoin useful for digoxin toxicity arrhythmia	CNS side-effects
IC Flecainide Propanfenone	Inhibit fast sodium channel. Inhibit His-Purkinje network with QRS widening	QRS duration prolongation and QT lengthening	Mainly ventricular arrhythmia.	Major pro-arrhythmic potential with flecainide. Use only in potentially lethal conditions.
Class II: Beta-adrenoreceptor blockers				
e.g. Propanolol Atenolol	Slow diastolic depolarisation	Bradycardia	SVT. Exercise-induced VT. Rate control of AF, as adjunct to digoxin	Hypotension, wheeze
Class III:				
Amiodarone	Prolong action potential	QT prolongation	Extremely wide-spectrum against SVT, VT and VF. For life-threatening arrhythmia	Pneumonitis Pro-arrhythmogenic potential. Interference with thyroid function
Bretylium tosylate	Prolong action potential	QT prolongation	iv for resistant VF	Profound hypotension
Sotalol	Additional beta-blocking effects	QT prolongation	SVT and VT	Beta blocker side-effects
Class IV: Calcium antagonists				
e.g. Verapamil Diltiazem	Inhibit slow calcium channel	None	SVT, except acute AF	Hypotension Profound AV nodal block

Abnormal impulse conduction and re-entry

A wave of depolarisation may sometimes circle endlessly around a loop of cardiac tissue. The necessary conditions for re-entry (arrhythmias) are a closed loop conduction path, a local region within the loop with unidirectional block and a conduction time around the loop longer than the longest refractory period in the area proximal to the block (Fig. 13.34).

The loops of myocardial tissue may be found as a combination of alterations in anatomy (congenital or acquired), and abnormal function of parts of the heart. The best-known and documented form of this arrhythmia is that due to the presence of anomalous pathways connecting the atria with ventricular myocardium. This is the basis of the *pre-excitation syndromes*, so-called due to the tendency of the aberrant pathways to excite areas of adjacent ventricle and produce the *delta* wave on the ECG (Fig. 13.35). The clinical syndrome that results is the Wolff-Parkinson-White (WPW) syndrome (p. 372). Slow conduction in the anomalous pathways is the basis for the arrhythmia in

Fig. 13.34 Mechanism of re-entry tachycardias. A. Normal conduction. **B.** An area of abnormal conduction affects one limb of the circuit. This interrupts the antegrade conduction (large red arrow) but is able to conduct retrogradely some moments later (black dashed line). This combination allows re-entry of the impulse (black arrow) and a tachycardia ensues.

WPW, while, in ischaemia, segments of diseased ventricular muscle with slow conduction or unidirectional block is the cause. Surgical or catheter ablation of the anomalous pathways interrupts the circuit in WPW to provide a treatment for the tachycardias; treatment may be difficult when localised segments of diseased myocardium are the source of re-entry circuits within the ventricles.

Fig. 13.35 ECG characteristics of the Wolff-Parkinson-White syndrome. Note the short PR interval and pre-excitation of the ventricle producing the slurred upstroke of the R wave (delta wave, arrowed in V4).

SUPRAVENTRICULAR TACHYCARDIAS

Supraventricular tachycardias (SVT) arise in the atria or atrioventricular node. They are characteristically associated with *narrow* QRS complexes, but there are certain important exceptions:

1. when there is pre-existing bundle branch block – a situation impossible to diagnose with certainty unless there are ECGs available in normal sinus rhythm – before or after the arrhythmia
2. when there is rate-dependent bundle branch block (p. 343, Fig. 13.16).
3. in the pre-excitation syndromes (although the delta waves often do not show during tachycardia, as the anterograde conduction may be normal).

Clinical features

The symptoms of SVTs are commonly those of an unpleasant awareness of rapid heart beats or palpitations in the chest. Associated cardiac disease may dominate the picture when the combination of arrhythmias and underlying disease is sufficiently severe to lower cardiac output or produce chest pain. The patient will then complain

of breathlessness, dizziness, fatigue or chest pain. The tachycardia may precipitate acute left ventricular failure. Patients who suffer paroxysmal SVT, particularly those with structurally normal hearts, may notice polyuria during, or after, the attack.

Diagnosis

Differentiating between the many forms of SVT may, occasionally, be difficult. The ECG is the basic diagnostic tool, although aspects of the history and, occasionally, physical examination can give clues to the diagnosis. Very fast heart rates may produce ST and T wave changes on the ECG which persist for some hours after cessation of the arrhythmia.

Sinus tachycardia

Sinus tachycardia is a persistent sinus rate over 100 bpm. It can be regarded as pathological when inappropriate and chronic, e.g. with diseases such as thyrotoxicosis, or when secondary to heart failure. Under these circumstances, treatment consists of control of the underlying disorder. A number of uncommon diseases of sinus node function produce a chronic sinus tachycardia, and the latter may also complicate the dysautonomia of diabetes, extrapyramidal disease of the Shy-Drager syndrome and cardiac infiltration with amyloid.

Atrial tachycardia

In atrial tachycardia (Fig. 13.36), the ECG shows abnormal P waves at rates from 120 to 250 bpm. The mechanism of the arrhythmia is usually enhanced, or abnormal, automaticity in the sino-atrial node. The normal AV node may not conduct at rates much greater than 200 bpm, so that very fast atrial rates may be associated with intermittent failure of contraction. This may lead to an atrial tachycardia with 2:1 conduction or higher degrees of block. Conduction through the AV node may be further impaired by disease, or by drugs, such as digoxin. Indeed, one of the manifestations of digoxin toxicity is atrial tachycardia (at a relatively slow rate) with block. Other causes include ischaemic heart disease, cardiomyopathy, rheumatic heart disease and the sick sinus syndrome.

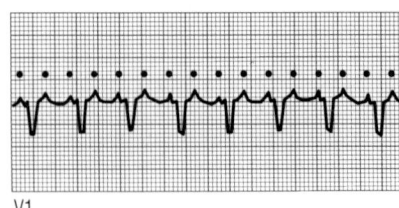

Fig. 13.36 ECG showing atrial tachycardia with 2:1 conduction. Dots indicate position of P waves. (Atrial rate is 300/s.)

Treatment

Withdrawal of digoxin is important if toxicity is suspected.

Otherwise, measures to control ventricular rate include intravenous verapamil (slow bolus of 5 mg repeated to a maximum of 10–20 mg in 20 minutes), when there has been no prior beta-blocker therapy, and intravenous digoxin when glycoside toxicity is not the cause. Patients who have received beta-blocker therapy should be given verapamil with great caution, for fear of precipitating severe bradycardia or high-grade atrioventricular block. Intravenous beta blockade may also terminate the tachycardia, as will DC cardioversion or atrial overdrive pacing.

Atrial fibrillation

Atrial fibrillation (AF) is probably the commonest of the arrhythmias, and one which may be permanent in many patients. It is characterised by a chaotic, rapid and low-amplitude waveform on the ECG (Fig. 13.37). The ventricular response is characteristically completely irregular in rhythm, and usually shows a narrow QRS complex unless there is pre-existing disease, or rate-dependent bundle branch block. Despite an atrial activity of 350–600 impulses/min, the AV node conducts only intermittently and randomly. The nodal rate is usually less than 200 impulses/min, or even less in the presence of AV nodal disease or drugs suppressing nodal activity (e.g. digoxin). An exception to the rule of irregular ventricular activity in atrial fibrillation is when it co-exists with complete heart block, when a subnodal pacemaker provides a slow, regular ventricular complex (Fig. 13.37).

The rhythm is believed to be caused by localised re-entry

Table 13.8 Causes of atrial fibrillation

With structural heart disease	Without structural heart disease
● Rheumatic mitral valve disease	● Alcohol
● Hypertension	● Thyrotoxicosis
● Cardiomyopathy Dilated Hypertrophic	● Acute pericarditis
	● Constrictive pericarditis
● Atrial septal defect	● Pulmonary embolism
● Ischaemic heart disease	● Sick sinus syndrome
	● Myocarditis

circuits within the atria, and is a frequent consequence of chronic atrial distension from any cause. The causes of atrial fibrillation are shown in Table 13.8. The commonest underlying condition is probably hypertension. Some patients develop the rhythm for no discernible reason and are said to be suffering *lone atrial fibrillation*; they appear to have a normal prognosis. For other patients, the immediate consequence of the arrhythmia and its long-term prognosis are determined by the underlying condition.

Atrial fibrillation may be paroxysmal or permanent. Even when structural heart disease is absent, paroxysms of AF can sometimes be symptomatically disabling and, although drug therapy to control the ventricular rate during an attack is reasonably effective, there may be considerable difficulty in providing adequate prophylactic therapy.

The loss of a mechanical atrial systole can be very important in patients with severe heart disease, and, in some, is sufficient to precipitate heart failure. The loss of atrial contraction predisposes to stasis of blood in the atria, particularly in the atrial appendages; this encourages the formation of thrombi, which pose the threat of systemic embolisation. This tendency is accentuated where there is associated rheumatic mitral valve disease, especially mitral stenosis. Stroke due to embolism is nearly five times commoner in patients with AF than in those in sinus rhythm, and this relative risk rises to seventeen-fold if there is associated mitral valve disease.

Clinical features

Clinically, the symptoms are determined by the rate of the arrhythmia and the underlying cardiac state, but they do not differ significantly from those of any SVT (p. 366). The pulse is of variable rhythm and volume. Very early beats, especially with fast AF, may not produce sufficient stroke volume to produce a pulse at the wrist, producing an apex to radial pulse deficit in 'uncontrolled' AF. The venous pulse shows only a single waveform, corresponding to ventricular systole (the V wave).

Treatment

The aim of treatment is control of the ventricular rate; ideally, this is achieved by re-establishing sinus rhythm.

Fig. 13.37 Rhythm strips showing atrial fibrillation and flutter. A. Atrial fibrillation. Note the irregular ventricular rate. **B.** Atrial flutter with typical saw-tooth P waves and a regular ventricular response (4:1). **C.** Atrial flutter with a variable ventricular response.

Many patients are, however, likely to remain in atrial fibrillation permanently, and the goal is then to control the ventricular rate both at rest and during exercise. In individuals with paroxysmal AF, prevention of recurrences is attempted.

Acute

Ventricular rate control is achieved by digoxin. In the acute situation, with fast AF causing symptoms or cardiac decompensation, intravenous digoxin is the drug of choice, as it uniquely combines bradycardic actions and positive inotropy. Intravenous loading is achieved by slow bolus injection of digoxin (0.5 mg over 30–60 min, to a total of 0.75–1.0 mg in 24 hours). Other drugs which may be used acutely include verapamil (5–10 mg iv, bolus or slow infusion) and amiodarone (up to 5 mg/kg over 20–30 min, diluted and infused through a central venous catheter). Where fast AF has caused severe haemodynamic disturbance, DC cardioversion can be used successfully. Its danger in previously digitalised patients has often been overstated. There is an increased risk of inducing malignant ventricular arrhythmia when there is digitalis intoxication, but this risk is small in patients without digoxin toxicity who have normal serum potassium.

In less urgent situations, digitalisation can be achieved moderately rapidly by a combination of intravenous injection (0.5 mg) followed by oral digoxin (0.25 mg) once or twice in the next 24 hours. The commonest maintenance dose is digoxin 0.25 mg by mouth daily. Renal function is the most important determinant of digoxin dosage, which also has to be adjusted (downwards) in the elderly, even if a normal plasma creatinine is present. Verapamil by mouth (80–120 mg) can achieve rapid rate response (within 2 hours), but it has negative inotropic effects.

Chronic

Chronic treatment of AF aims to reduce the resting rate to about 90 bpm, with a modest increase in rate with exertion. Digoxin alone, although effectively controlling the resting heart rate, is insufficient to control the rate response to exercise in a large proportion of patients. A combination of digoxin with verapamil (or digoxin with a beta-blocker) is superior to digoxin alone in these circumstances.

Anticoagulation with warfarin reduces the risk of emboli considerably and is essential when rheumatic valve disease is present, or if the heart, particularly the left atrium, is enlarged. It is probably indicated in patients with a previous history of systemic emboli, and where the cause is thyrotoxicosis. If AF has been present for more than one week, anticoagulation for at least three weeks should precede attempts to restore sinus rhythm.

Paroxysmal AF can be disabling. Digoxin is less effective at preventing attacks, but disopyramide, quinidine and amiodarone used alone, or in combination with digoxin, have some effectiveness against relapses in paroxysmal AF. In some patients, although satisfactory prevention of paroxysmal AF is not achieved with drugs, the symptoms may be blunted by drugs such as verapamil, which lowers the peak heart rate during a paroxysm of AF. Ablation of the AV node and pacemaker implantation have been used with some success.

Atrial flutter

Closely allied to atrial fibrillation but much less common, atrial flutter is an arrhythmia due to multiple re-entry circuits producing atrial contraction at 300 ± 50 bpm. Conduction block at the AV node (most commonly 2:1) is almost always present, producing a steady pulse of 150 bpm. This pulse rate should always lead to the clinical suspicion of atrial flutter. Vagal slowing of AV conduction produced by carotid sinus massage will temporarily increase the degree of AV block, and the sudden halving or more of the ventricular rate can easily be detected at the bedside. On the ECG monitor, P waves previously concealed within T waves become visible as a saw-tooth pattern, thus establishing the diagnosis (Fig. 13.37). Physical examination may show flutter waves in the neck. The causes of atrial flutter are the same as those of atrial fibrillation (Table 13.8), but, unlike the latter, flutter is rarely permanent. Drugs are less effective in flutter compared to fibrillation and, since this rhythm is very responsive to DC cardioversion, this is usually the therapy of choice. Energies of 25–50 J are frequently sufficient to achieve successful cardioversion to sinus rhythm. Intravenous verapamil will successfully convert many patients to sinus rhythm, as will pacing the atria at, or below, the tachycardia rate (underdrive pacing) or rapidly for a few minutes (overdrive pacing).

Chaotic atrial tachycardia and wandering atrial pacemaker

Chaotic atrial tachycardia is characterised by multiple P wave shapes and PR intervals. It is quite common in elderly patients while, in younger patients, it is usually associated with severe respiratory disorders. It requires no specific intervention, except for control of any associated illness and withdrawal of digoxin if this has previously been prescribed. Conversely, a sustained rhythm may be slowed by digoxin or verapamil.

The wandering atrial pacemaker is a slower arrhythmia often associated with variations in vagal tone, allowing various subsidiary atrial pacemakers to become established. It requires no special treatment.

JUNCTIONAL TACHYCARDIAS

Atrioventricular nodal re-entry (AVNRT) or paroxysmal supraventricular tachycardia

As the name suggests, the mechanism involved in AV nodal re-entry tachycardia (AVNRT) is re-entry through a functionally distinct area of the AV node or tissues surrounding it. This is a common arrhythmia, particularly in (young) patients with structurally normal hearts. There is a 1:1 relationship between atrial and ventricular activity. P waves generally cannot be identified; if they can be seen, they will be buried within the QRS or immediately follow it (Fig. 13.38). The onset is abrupt, usually precipitated by an atrial extrasystole, and an equally abrupt cessation is the rule, although the latter may not be appreciated by the patient since a sinus tachycardia may follow the arrhythmia. The usual rates are about 180–240 bpm, with narrow QRS complexes, except if there is pre-existing, or rate-dependent, bundle branch block. If manœuvres or drugs induce a lower degree of conduction than 1:1, AVNRT is excluded and a paroxysmal atrial tachycardia or flutter is the more likely diagnosis.

Rhythm strip

Fig. 13.38 AV nodal re-entry tachycardia. Note rapid narrow QRS complex tachycardia (rate 185 bpm).

Treatment

Treatment may not be necessary if the attacks are transient and infrequent. For sustained episodes, restoration to sinus rhythm may be achieved by altering AV nodal conduction to a degree that is able to interrupt the re-entrant cycle. Several vagotonic manœuvres may be helpful (Table 13.9), all of which can be taught to the patient who suffers paroxysmal attacks. Failing these simple approaches, drug therapy is usually successful. Intravenous verapamil is the drug of choice, although intravenous injections of beta-blocker, disopyramide, amiodarone and adenosine may also prove useful. Atrial and ventricular pacing may also be used, the former following a similar procedure to that used to convert atrial flutter (p. 368). A more elegant

Table 13.9 Simple procedures to terminate paroxysmal SVT

- Carotid sinus message. If effective, the rhythm is abruptly stopped; occasionally only moderate slowing occurs.
- Cold water splash on face (to mimic the diving reflex). This may be effective, but is often difficult to administer.
- Performance of Valsalva's manœuvre (often effective).
- Swallowing cold drinks.

approach is to interrupt the re-entry circuit with critically-timed ventricular or atrial ectopic impulses using chronically implanted anti-tachycardia pacemakers.

Long-term prevention can often be achieved with beta-blockers, disopyramide, digoxin or amiodarone. Failing this, anti-tachycardia pacemakers have been used for disabling symptoms. Finally, disruption by transcatheter ablation of accessory pathways or the AV node can be undertaken. These latter techniques are rarely required, and need a prior definitive intracardiac electrophysiological study (p. 359).

Atrioventricular re-entry tachycardia

The hallmark of atrioventricular re-entry tachycardia (AVRT) – a less common rhythm than AVNRT – is the occurrence of retrograde P waves immediately after the QRS complex.

Non-paroxysmal AV nodal or junctional tachycardia

Non-paroxysmal AV nodal tachycardia is a narrow complex tachycardia associated with inverted P waves in II, III and aVF. Characteristically, it is caused by ischaemia and digoxin toxicity, although junctional rhythms may be precipitated by most forms of heart disease; the mechanism is enhanced automaticity. Since the atria and ventricles are stimulated virtually simultaneously, the P waves may precede the QRS complexes with a short PR interval. Alternatively, they may be buried within the QRS complex or follow after it. The onset of the tachycardia is gradual and the established rates, between 60 and 130 bpm, considerably slower than the paroxysmal forms of tachycardia. Therapy is along the same lines as for AVRT, although lignocaine may also be useful. Withdrawal of digoxin may be all that is required when toxicity is implicated.

BROAD-COMPLEX TACHYCARDIAS

The hallmark of ventricular rhythm is the broad QRS complex. Ventricular fibrillation and flutter do not cause diagnostic difficulties, but ventricular tachycardia (VT) is often wrongly diagnosed as SVT with rate-related aberration, or with pre-existing bundle branch block. There is often a reluctance to diagnose VT, particularly on the part of less experienced physicians, probably because the implications for the patient are so much worse for VT than for SVT. Guidelines for their differentiation are given in Table 13.10. In the context of acute infarction, or when there is severe underlying myocardial disease, the observation of a broad complex tachycardia should always be assumed to be ventricular in origin until proved otherwise.

Ventricular tachycardia

Ventricular tachycardia (Fig. 13.39) is defined as the appearance of three or more ventricular ectopic beats in a sequence. When sustained, the rate is between 150 and 250 bpm and regular. Unsustained VT can be seen in

Table 13.10 Differentiation of VT from SVT with aberration or bundle branch block (BBB)

Feature	Value in differentiation
Broad QRS complex (>120 ms),	Very broad (more than 160 ms) – almost always VT. Broader than 140 ms favours VT, but may be due to pre-existing BBB.
Bizarre QRS morphology, similar in V1–V6 and not resembling any BBB pattern	Characteristic of VT when present.
Independent P wave activity	Diagnostic of VT, when found
QRS between sinus and tachycardia morphology in VT, fusion beat.	Diagnostic of VT, when found.
Variability of rate from 10 ms to 20 ms; except for fusion/capture beats	Not good
Hypotension, shock and collapse	No value
When V-A conduction occurs with 2:1 block	When ventricular rate is shown to be greater than atrial, the rhythm is VT.

people with normal hearts, but organic heart disease is suspected if the rhythm is sustained or produces symptoms. Causes are ischaemic heart disease, cardiomyopathy or myocarditis. Ventricular tachycardia carries the risk of sudden death, usually due to degeneration of the rhythm to ventricular fibrillation (VF).

Even with the guidelines to diagnosis given in Table 13.10, VT can, in some circumstances, be difficult to diagnose, and prolonged examination of the ECG or the use of an oesophageal ECG lead may be necessary. In about one-half of patients, the sinus node continues to fire independently, so that atrial P waves dissociated from ventricular activity can sometimes be observed, if not buried within the QRS complex. In a few patients, retrograde activation of the atria occurs; this may be recognised by

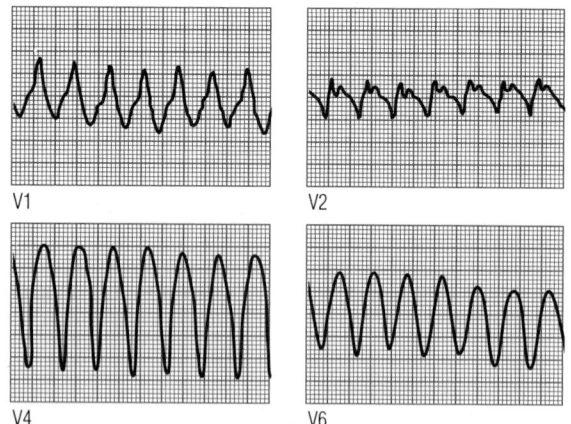

Fig. 13.39 Ventricular tachycardia. A rapid, broad QRS complex tachycardia illustrating the similarity of appearance in complexes from V1 to V6 (concordance).

finding inverted P waves.

In paroxysmal VT (150–250 bpm) the onset is abrupt, usually following a critically-timed ectopic beat. A slower form of VT, *accelerated idioventricular rhythm* (rate 60–130 bpm), occurs as an enhanced automatic rhythm during periods of suppressed sino-atrial activity. It is usually seen in acute infarction and its prognosis – unlike that of paroxysmal VT – is generally good.

Treatment

Acute

In the presence of acute haemodynamic disturbance or acute myocardial infarction, immediate DC cardioversion with a synchronised shock is the treatment of choice; this is followed by an intravenous lignocaine bolus dose of 100 mg (or 1 mg/kg), followed by an infusion, starting at 4 mg/min for 30 minutes, reducing to 2 mg/min for two hours and continued at 1 mg/min thereafter, for approximately 24 hours. This approach is generally successful, particularly in acute infarction, when there is rarely any indication to continue to chronic oral anti-arrhythmic therapy. In resistant or recurrent cases, an alternative therapy is amiodarone. Mexilitene, flecainide or bretylium may be required in certain instances, although the acute use of many different anti-arrhythmic drugs should be avoided. The serum potassium must be maintained at, or above, 4.5 mmol, and acidosis and hypoxaemia reversed.

Chronic

Episodic or paroxysmal VT complicating organic heart disease (e.g. hypertrophic cardiomyopathy, chronic ischaemic heart disease and cardiomyopathy), requires prophylactic therapy. In choosing the drug, information on its efficacy in the individual patient should be taken into account. This may be difficult to judge in some patients, but the response to exercise testing and monitoring the effectiveness of therapy with Holter 24-hour ECG recordings is helpful. In those patients in whom VT is inducible by exercise, beta-blocking drugs may be useful; sotalol, with its class III effects (Table 13.7), may be the rational first choice. Patients with poor ventricular function are probably most at risk from VT. The choice of drug for these patients is very limited, due to the negative inotropy of most anti-arrhythmic agents. Amiodarone or mexilitene are the most useful in these patients.

A new form of therapy is being developed for those patients in whom drug therapy fails. This involves the use of small implantable automatic defibrillators which detect the arrhythmia (VT or VF) and, after an appropriate pause, deliver a DC shock. At present, their use is limited by their high cost and a number of difficulties in arrhythmia recognition.

Surgery

Certain patients have an anatomical basis for their ventricular arrhythmia, either a ventricular aneurysm or localised area of ischaemically injured myocardium. After suitable electrophysiological testing, including endocardial electrical mapping during surgery, the excision of the aneurysm or electrically abnormal tissue can sometimes be curative.

Ventricular fibrillation and ventricular flutter

Ventricular fibrillation (VF) is characterised by rapid, irregular and uncoordinated electrical activity in the ventricles, probably due to re-entry circuits within localised areas of myocardium. The ECG shows more or less coarse, irregular waveforms, without discernible P, QRS or T waves (Fig. 13.40). In ventricular flutter, the entire tracing appears as a rough saw-tooth with a rate of 160–250 bpm, without normal QRS morphology. If either rhythm occurs, effective contraction and cardiac output cease, leading to unconsciousness within seconds. These rhythms do not usually revert spontaneously and are often precipitated by an ectopic beat or runs of VT, particularly when they complicate acute myocardial infarction. Ventricular fibrillation is probably the arrhythmia responsible for most cases of sudden death in the community (pp. 405–6). In the context of acute myocardial infarction, when VF occurs early, within 24–48 hours of onset of the illness (*primary VF*) and is successfully treated, the prognosis for the patient is not adversely affected. However, VF occurring late in the course of acute infarction (*secondary VF*), often follows extensive muscle damage and carries a grave prognosis unless adequate prophylactic treatment is given.

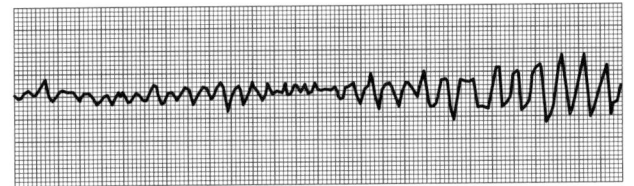

Fig. 13.40 Rhythm strip showing ventricular fibrillation.

Treatment of VF

Witnessed collapse due to VF (usually an event seen only in coronary care units), requires immediate action, and a precordial chest thump (p. 374) may convert up to 15% of cases without the need for electrical defibrillation. In all other circumstances, basic cardiopulmonary resuscitation should begin until the treatment of choice is available, namely defibrillation by application of an external DC

shock (p. 374). Correction of acidosis, hypoxaemia and electrolyte imbalance improves the likelihood of conversion to a stable rhythm. Drug treatment and long-term prophylactic therapy follow the same lines as for ventricular tachycardia. Primary VF does not generally require subsequent prophylactic therapy.

Torsade de pointes ventricular tachycardia

Torsade de pointes VT is an uncommon but important arrhythmia, characterised by a ventricular tachycardia, often of modest rate but associated with an undulating QRS height due to a slow but continual variation in the QRS axis (Fig. 13.41). Its importance is due to its precipitation by anti-arrhythmic drugs, particularly if electrolyte disturbances coexist. It is associated with prolongation of the QT interval, whether it is acquired due to drug therapy (Class IA and III anti-arrhythmic drugs, tricyclic antidepressants and phenothiazines) or electrolyte imbalance (low K^+, Ca^{2+} or Mg^{2+}), or present as a congenital abnormality (Romano-Ward, Jewell and Lange-Nielsen syndromes).

Treatment

Treatment of the acquired forms means withdrawal of the offending agent and correction of electrolyte abnormalities. In less stable situations, infusion of isoprenaline, or increasing the heart rate with a temporary pacemaker, are the appropriate remedies. The congenital syndromes may be caused by abnormalities in sympathetic supply to the heart, and are best treated with beta-blocking agents.

OTHER ARRHYTHMIC SYNDROMES

Sick sinus syndrome

The sick sinus syndrome (SSS) is a relatively common condition, characterised by episodic arrhythmias combining episodes of profound bradycardia and heart block with episodes of tachycardia (it is sometimes called the tachycardia-bradycardia syndrome). The bradycardias may be paroxysmal or sustained sinus bradycardia, episodes of sinus arrest, or sino-atrial block producing long pauses in pulse rate and pauses after atrial ectopics. Immediately following a tachycardia there may be a prolonged pause or very slow sinus rhythm sufficient to cause dizziness or a Stokes-Adams' attack. The tachycardias are mostly supraventricular, with atrial fibrillation, flutter,

Fig. 13.41 Rhythm strip illustrating torsade de pointes, a broad complex ventricular tachycardia. Note the fluctuation in size of the complexes.

chaotic atrial rhythm and atrial tachycardia being the most common, although ventricular tachycardia (especially torsades de pointes) is occasionally seen. Chronic atrial fibrillation with a slow ventricular rate due to associated atrioventricular node disease is sometimes included in SSS.

The pathology is probably degeneration and fibrosis in the sinus node and conducting tissues. The AV node is often involved in the degenerative process. Ischaemic heart disease and amyloid infiltration of the heart may be the cause in some patients and SSS has also been associated with many other pathologies, from cardiomyopathy to Friedreich's ataxia. It is important to exclude as causes digoxin, beta adrenoreceptor blockers or quinidine, since all of these may mimic SSS.

Apart from discomfort and Stokes-Adams' episodes, the condition carries a risk of systemic embolisation and is the cause of episodic heart failure.

Treatment and prognosis

Treatment is with anti-arrhythmic drugs and pacemaker implantation. The prognosis is generally good but mainly dependent on any underlying condition; it is not greatly influenced by pacemaker implantation.

Wolff-Parkinson-White syndrome

The ECG abnormality of short PR interval (less than 0.12 s) with abnormal QRS widening due to delta-wave (Fig. 13.35) is relatively common. The clinical syndrome, Wolff-Parkinson-White syndrome (WPW), with paroxysmal tachycardias is much less common, although the precise incidence of arrhythmia in individuals with the ECG abnormality is not clearly established. The syndrome generally occurs in an otherwise normal heart, although it may complicate Ebstein's anomaly (p. 393) or mitral valve prolapse (p. 381). The abnormality is due to an accessory pathway between the atrium and ventricle allowing a re-entry or reciprocating tachycardia to develop (p. 365). The tachycardia produces narrow QRS complexes without the delta-wave, because conduction is anterograde through the AV node. Thus, the diagnosis of WPW may not be made until an ECG in sinus rhythm is obtained. There is an increased incidence of atrial fibrillation. In a small proportion of patients who have a short refractory period in the accessory pathway, AF may conduct very rapidly (1:1) to the ventricles; this may degenerate to ventricular fibrillation and is the usual cause of sudden death in these patients.

Investigation and treatment

Investigation of symptomatic patients includes electrophysiological studies to establish the site, number and refractory period of the accessory pathway or pathways. Treatment may include anti-arrhythmic drugs, but sometimes requires ablation of localised accessory bundles; catheter techniques are generally used, although surgical interruption of these tissues may sometimes be required.

Lown-Ganong-Levine syndrome

Patients with Lown-Ganong-Levine syndrome (LGL) have short bypass tracts that connect the atria to various portions of the proximal bundle of His or distal AV node. The ECG manifestation is of a short PR interval (less than 0.12 s) without pre-excitation (no delta-waves). Such patients are subject to paroxysmal tachycardias, but are less commonly threatened by rapidly conducted AF.

Long QT syndrome

Several congenital disorders are described characterised by a long (more than 0.45 s) QT interval and associated with ventricular tachycardia, syncope and sudden death. Children respond to treatment with beta-blocking agents. In adults, amiodarone and quinidine may prolong the QT interval.

SYNOPSIS OF DRUG TREATMENT OF ARRHYTHMIAS

A decision tree for the diagnosis of tachycardias is shown in Figure 13.33. Summaries of the treatment of and drug doses used in arrhythmias are given in Tables 13.11 and 13.12.

Table 13.11 Emergency drug treatment of common arrhythmias

Arrhythmia	First line therapy	Second line therapy
Atrial fibrillation	Digoxin iv, then oral. DC cardioversion if blood pressure very low	Verapamil DC cardioversion
Atrial flutter	DC cardioversion (50–100 J)	Verapamil Vagotonic manœuvres Atrial pacing
Atrial tachycardia and junctional tachycardia	Vagotonic manœuvres Verapamil	DC cardioversion Digoxin (if not digoxin toxicity)
SVT of AVNRT or AVRT type	Vagotonic manœuvres Verapamil	Beta-blocker Disopyramide Flecainide Amiodarone DC cardioversion
SVT in WPW with narrow QRS	Verapamil	DC cardioversion
SVT in WPW with broad (δ-wave) QRS	Amiodarone Flecainide (Adenosine/ATP)	DC cardioversion
VT and VF	DC cardioversion Lignocaine	Flecainide Mexiletine Amiodarone
Bradycardia	Atropine Isoprenaline	–
Complete heart block	Pacemaker Isoprenaline	–

Table 13.12 Doses and methods of administration of drugs commonly used in acute arrhythmia

Drug	First dose	Method	Maintenance	Side-effects
Amiodarone	2–5 mg/kg	iv slow bolus	Usually required. 600–1200 mg/day iv infusion	↓ BP Need central venous access
Atropine	0.6–1.2 mg	iv bolus	Not used	Anticholinergic side-effects
Beta-blockers Atenolol Metoprolol Propranolol	5–10 mg 5–15 mg 0.1 mg/kg	iv bolus iv bolus iv bolus	Usual. 50–100 mg oral/day 100–400 mg oral/day 120–360 mg oral/day	↓ Heart rate; ↓ BP; bronchospasm
Bretylium	5–10 mg/kg	iv rapid in emergency	Optional. 1–2 mg/min (iv infusion)	↓↓ BP; nausea
Digoxin	0.5 mg	iv slow bolus	Optional. 0.75–1.0 mg for first 24 h, then 0.25 mg/day (oral)	Toxicity: lower dose in renal impairment and in elderly
Flecainide	1–2 mg/kg	iv bolus over 10 min	Optional. 0.15–0.25 mg/kg/h (iv infusion)	↓ BP; cardiac failure
Isoprenaline	50 μg	iv rapid in emergency	Optional. 0.02.0.18 μg/kg/min	↑↑ Heart rate
Lignocaine	100 mg	iv bolus	Essential. 4 mg/min reducing to 1 mg/min in 24 h (iv infusion)	CNS toxicity
Verapamil	5 mg, repeat with 10 mg after 10 min	iv slow bolus	Optional. 0.005 mg/kg/min for 1 h (iv) or 80–120 mg/8-hourly (oral)	↓ BP; ↓ Heart rate

RESUSCITATION

Within 20 seconds of cardiac inactivity the victim falls unconscious, breathing soon ceases and the pupils dilate. Sudden death affects about 50 000 people a year in the UK. One-half of these are not previously known to have coronary artery disease.

About 60% of deaths due to myocardial infarction occur within an hour of the first symptom (Fig. 13.61), the majority occurring outside hospitals. The commonest rhythm disturbance (over 60% of cases) is ventricular fibrillation (VF).

Cardiopulmonary resuscitation (CPR) may involve:

1. *basic life support*, requiring training but no special equipment
2. *advanced life support*, which requires equipment and specialised skills.

Many cities in the UK and other industrialised countries are involved in training the public in basic life support skills, and provide specialised ambulances with very rapid response times and facilities for advanced life support and DC cardioversion. Examples are Belfast and Brighton in the UK, and Seattle in the USA. With basic life support available to the victims of cardiac arrest, about 20% of victims may reach hospital and 11% live to be discharged. These numbers are halved when basic life support is not

available. Survival is worse in older patients, and when arrest occurs at home or in the street. In hospital, when cardiac arrest due to VF occurs within 4 hours of symptoms and is successfully treated, 80% of patients are alive three years later.

BASIC LIFE SUPPORT

The basic cardiac arrest procedures are given in Table 13.13. Initial assessment is rapidly followed by establishing a clear open airway. This is done by head tilt with chin lift and jaw thrust. In the absence of airway obstruction, rescue breathing begins with the mouth-to-mouth technique. Recommendations vary, but in the UK, four quick breaths are advocated. In the USA, two slow breaths (1–1.5 s each) have been suggested, in order to diminish the likelihood of gastric distension with air, and subsequent vomiting (risking inhalation of vomit into the unprotected airway). Protective masks and airway equipment should be provided for personnel most often exposed (ambulance and paramedical staff), even though the risk of infection (such as from hepatitis B or HIV) is likely to be very small. Bag mask techniques are taught to nursing and medical staff, but are frequently more difficult to use and less effective in inexperienced hands than is mouth-to-mouth ventilation.

Closed cardiac compression follows at a rate of 60–80 compressions/min. Training in the technique is essential. Mid-sternal compression is carried out with the heel of one

Table 13.13   Basic cardiac arrest procedures

A	**Assessment**	Assess whether patient is unconscious or asleep: call for help if unconscious.
		Determine whether or not airway is clear: clear it, pull chin up.
B	**Breathing**	If patient is breathing: turn to recovery position.
		If patient is not breathing, but is choking: blow to back, Heimlich manœuvre
		If patient is not breathing, but is not choking: start artificial ventilation call for assistance
C	**Circulation**	If no pulse: start external cardiac massage
		call for assistance
		continue ventilation

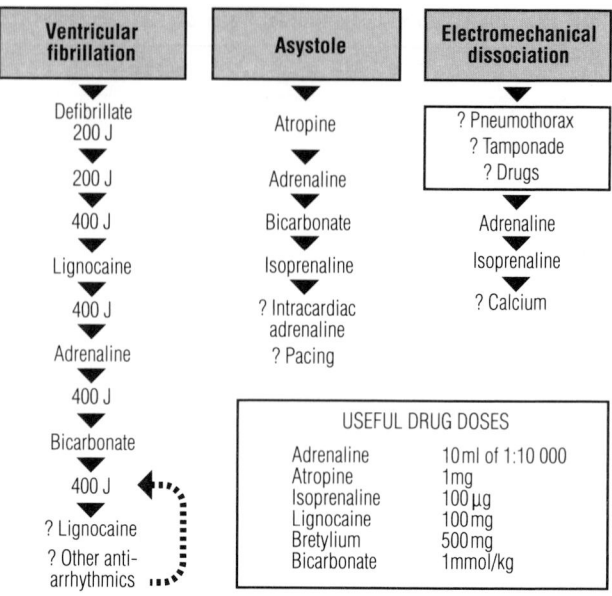

Fig. 13.42   Flow diagram of resuscitation procedures. (Based on recommendations of the UK Resuscitation Council.)

hand to depress the sternum by 2–4 cm. The patient should be on a rigid, flat surface with the resuscitator kneeling alongside. The arms are kept straight, and compression produced primarily by body weight movement. Closed chest compression achieves a cardiac output by virtue of cyclical changes in intrathoracic pressure, rather than by squeezing the heart.

A single-handed resuscitator should provide 15 chest compressions for every two mouth-to-mouth breaths. If two people are available, the ratio should be 4:1. Cardio-pulmonary resuscitation must be continuous, and pauses to reassess the situation or allow for advanced life support techniques should not be greater than 10 seconds.

The first response to a *witnessed* arrest should be a force-ful precordial thump. This may be sufficient to convert VF or VT to a more stable rhythm by localised myocardial depolarisation, or even to initiate a rhythm in cases of acute asystole.

ADVANCED LIFE SUPPORT

Advanced life support (summarised in Figure 13.42) con-sists of defibrillation with DC shock, endotracheal intu-bation, the use of drugs and pacemakers.

DC defibrillation

When cardiac arrest is due to VF, the earlier DC shock is given, the more successful the outcome. When defib-rillators are immediately available, such as in coronary care units, the first procedure following the precordial thump should be defibrillation at 200 J. This will be sufficient to revert 85% of cases to a more stable rhythm. In 9% of patients, a further 200 J shock is required and is successful. If these approaches are unsuccessful, life support must be begun immediately. Outside coronary care units, basic life support must be begun and interrupted only when the defibrillator is ready to produce the first shock of 200 J. If no monitor is available, major pulses are checked and, if absent after 3 seconds, 15 chest compressions are given with the appropriate mouth-to-mouth breaths. A second

shock follows the same pattern of events and, if VF persists, intravenous lignocaine (100 mg iv bolus) is given before the third shock at 400 J. Adrenaline may be given before the fourth shock at the highest energy and, if an acidosis is demonstrated by arterial gases, an infusion of bicarbonate (1 mmol/kg) is given before the fifth high-energy shock (Fig. 13.42).

The technique of DC shock administration can be taught to nursing and paramedical personnel. Early defibrillation administered out of hospital by ambulance crews has been shown to improve survival from VF. Defibrillation paddles are placed on the chest with firm pressure, one under the right clavicle and one just lateral to the usual cardiac apex. Skin impedance is reduced with conducting gel or pads, and the administrator of the shock ensures that no-one is touching the patient before the shock is delivered. Com-plications are remarkably few, although very high-energy shocks or many repeated shocks carry the risk of some myocardial damage; both ECG changes and cardiac enzyme release have been shown in experimental studies.

Endotracheal intubation

If there is no recovery after a few minutes of basic life support, endotracheal intubation is necessary. This is a skilled technique which can be mastered by medical and paramedical staff alike, but which requires frequent prac-tice. In hospital, anaesthetists form part of the cardiac arrest team. After the cardiac arrest, it may be necessary to continue ventilation, via a mechanical ventilator, of seri-ously ill patients, those with damaged ribcage from cardiac massage and those who sustain cerebral damage.

Drugs in advanced life support

There is controversy over the value of many drugs used during advanced life support. The number of drugs of proven benefit is small, despite the large number of drugs available to treat ventricular arrhythmia.

Adrenaline

Adrenaline is the inotropic and chronotropic agent of choice. It is given intravenously in a dose of 1 mg (1 ml of 1/1000) or 2 mg via the endotracheal tube. Its benefit comes from beta stimulation with minor alpha effects, causing peripheral constriction which maintains systemic pressure. Its risks include arrhythmia induction and the possibility of increasing myocardial oxygen demand.

Lignocaine

Lignocaine is routinely given after VF and during the attempts to treat VF. A bolus of 1 mg/kg (or 100 mg) is followed by an infusion (4 mg/min reducing to 2 mg/min over 24 hours). A second half-dose bolus can be given 10–20 minutes after the first. Despite its widespread use, there is surprisingly little evidence of its effectiveness in prophylaxis after VF.

Sodium bicarbonate

Sodium bicarbonate can no longer be recommended for routine administration in cardiac arrests. It causes tissue damage if accidentally extravasated, may produce an untreatable alkalotic state and gives a large sodium load. Bicarbonate infusion is used in established acidosis, an average dose being 1 mmol/kg of 4.2% sodium bicarbonate solution. As metabolic acidosis following a cardiac arrest is a relatively late event, current management includes frequent estimations of blood gases and pH by arterial blood sampling during the arrest.

Calcium chloride

Trials have shown that routine administration of calcium chloride does not aid resuscitation. Calcium may also exacerbate cerebral vasospasm. Consequently, it is no longer recommended, but continues to be useful in specific circumstances, such as resuscitation after cardiopulmonary bypass and in calcium antagonist overdose. The usual dose is 10 ml of 10% calcium chloride. This must not be given in the same infusion set as bicarbonate, or precipitation will occur; nowadays, this would in any case seem an unlikely combination of therapies.

Other drugs

The treatment of resistant VF or ventricular tachyarrhythmias may require the use of one or other of the alternative drugs available (p. 370). None, however, has a proven role as 'standard' therapy in CPR, and their indications have to be determined individually at the time of the resuscitation attempt.

Special techniques

Cardiac pacing

Cardiac pacing can be used to treat bradycardia, heart block and, sometimes, asystole. The various methods by which this can be achieved are shown on p. 372, Table 13.11. During a cardiac arrest, access to the central and antecubital veins may be difficult. The femoral vein may then provide a suitable venous approach. Asystole, unless it has been caused by drugs, rarely responds to cardiac pacing.

Intracardiac injection

Intracardiac injection has been used to administer calcium or adrenaline during cardiac arrest with asystole. However, this is seldom necessary, since, with adequate basic life support and central venous cannulation, delivery of drugs to the heart can be achieved with much less hazard to the patient.

Intra-aortic balloon counterpulsation

Highly specialised techniques such as intra-aortic balloon counterpulsation have a very limited role in specialised centres, where they can be used to support the circulation until a definitive procedure can be performed. One such circumstance might be a cardiac arrest during cardiac catheterisation or angioplasty. Arterial support can be given whilst preparations are made to perform cardipulmonary bypass and revascularise the heart.

When to stop

Rigid rules as to when to stop resuscitation cannot be given, but guidelines are possible. Resuscitation is almost never successful in patients who have a cardiac arrest complicating another serious illness, such as pneumonia or malignancy. It is important, therefore, that the staff likely to be first to witness a collapse should have had clear guidance concerning the desirability of resuscitation in individual patients.

In general, the outlook for a useful neurological recovery is poor if the arrest occurred out of hospital and was not witnessed, or if more than four minutes passed without even basic life support being attempted. If no spontaneous respiration or cardiac output is achieved after 30 minutes of adequate advanced life support, and there is no evidence to implicate drug overdose or drowning, then further attempts at resuscitation are questionable. The state of the pupils, whether widely dilated and reacting or not, is unreliable with respect to outcome. Age should not be used as the sole determinant of policy on resuscitation.

RESUSCITATION FROM NEAR-DROWNING

Resuscitation from near-drowning is discussed on page 81.

13

RESUSCITATION FROM CHOKING

Collapse due to acute airway obstruction is often due to a lump of food. In the UK, it is still recommended that active coughing with gravity drainage be encouraged whilst the subject is still conscious. This is supplemented by back blows and, finally, the abdominal thrusts known as the Heimlich manoeuvre. The latter depends upon gripping the subject from behind and, with clenched fist, producing a rapid, powerful upward thrust in the upper abdomen. This produces rapid airflow which may be sufficient to dislodge the offending obstruction.

ACQUIRED VALVULAR DISEASE OF THE HEART

AETIOLOGY AND NATURAL HISTORY

In Western countries, rheumatic heart disease was, until recently, the commonest cause of valve disease, and this is still the case in most developing countries. Various forms of degenerative valvular disease are now seen increasingly, some based on congenital abnormalities of the valve, others apparently arising in middle-age or later.

It is difficult to predict the progression of what initially may seem a trivial lesion of no consequence, to one that is life-threatening 30 or more years later. A child in India may have rheumatic fever at five years of age, and develop severe triple valve disease within another five years; on the other hand, one occasionally sees patients in their seventies presenting with mitral stenosis 60 years after their rheumatic fever. The situation is similar with a congenital bicuspid aortic valve. Some progress to severe stenosis, others to mixed stenosis and regurgitation, while others never cause problems. In the last 20 years, more exact diagnostic criteria have been developed that will enable longitudinal studies to be performed to indicate the natural history of valve lesions.

What dictates progression of the valve lesion? Mechanical forces must be involved; pressure and shear forces on the valve probably make it thicken and even calcify. The patient may also have myocardial disease which, combined with the valve disease, leads to symptoms. Even if it were possible to predict the progression of the valve lesion in terms of gradual reduction of valve area or increasing regurgitation, the tolerance of the myocardium to increasing work load would remain unpredictable.

THE EFFECTS OF STENOSIS AND REGURGITATION

Heart valve disease can occur either due to a narrowing of the valve (*stenosis*), causing obstruction to blood flow through the valve, or when the valve leaks, when the lesion is termed *regurgitant*, *incompetent* or *insufficient*. A *combined* or *mixed* lesion is common.

Valve stenosis

Mild degrees of stenosis may produce an audible murmur and produce a risk of endocarditis, but place an insignificant physiological burden on the heart. For significant symptoms to result, stenosis has to progress until the valve is narrowed to less than 30% of its normal area. Flow through the valve is maintained at close to normal levels by a compensatory increase in pressure in the chamber of the heart upstream of the stenotic valve. This chamber therefore hypertrophies.

The severity of the stenosis is quantified by the pressure drop across the valve. In a normal valve, this pressure drop is not measurable by conventional techniques. However, in severe aortic stenosis, the left ventricular pressure may rise to as much as 200 mmHg more than the aortic pressure, and the valve area may be less than 25% of normal. In mitral stenosis, the left atrial pressure cannot rise above 40 mmHg because the pulmonary capillaries are unable to withstand a higher pressure. Thus, the mitral valve gradient is usually much less than the aortic valve gradient in significant stenosis, and the residual valve area accordingly greater.

It follows that there are three ways of assessing the severity of a valve stenosis:

1. *The pressure gradient across the valve.* This indicates the additional work required to push blood through the valve. However, this is flow-dependent (no flow, no gradient); if there is heart failure, with low flow, the valve gradient is smaller.
2. *The valve area.* Formerly, this could only be calculated from cardiac catheterisation data (p.352), but direct measurement is now possible from ultrasound. There is, however, controversy over the accuracy of the measurements, because of the beam spread and lateral resolution of the ultrasound.
3. *The peak blood velocity across the valve.* Measured by Doppler ultrasound, this bears a very simple relationship to the pressure gradient (p. 350).

Valvular regurgitation

Normal human valves are highly efficient. The aortic valve closes without any significant reverse flow other than the swept volume of the valve cusps. They start closing as the flow decelerates, and are fully closed with about 97% efficiency. However, severe mitral or aortic valve regurgitation can be associated with up to 80% regurgitation (efficiency 20%). The forward flow then has to be five times greater than normal to allow for this leakage, and the chamber supplying the blood dilates accordingly. In aortic regurgitation, the left ventricle enlarges; in mitral regurgitation, the left atrium and left ventricle both enlarge dramatically.

Acute regurgitation (such as mitral valve chordal rupture or aortic regurgitation from acute endocarditis), are badly tolerated, since the left ventricle and left atrium require time to increase in volume. The rapid increase in left ventricular diastolic pressure or left atrial pressure, has severe consequences for left ventricular perfusion and pulmonary capillary pressure.

Combined valve lesions

The combined effect of even mild stenosis with regurgitation is potentially catastrophic. Since the forward flow of as little as 50% regurgitation is twice normal, even a 50% stenosis becomes highly significant. This may be explained using the concept of blood velocity. If peak aortic velocity is normally 1 m/s, a 50% stenosis of the aortic valve produces a peak velocity of 2 m/s, or a pressure gradient of 16 mmHg. This is an insignificant additional load on the left ventricle. However, if there is associated 50% regurgitation, the compensatory increase in forward flow produces a peak velocity of 4 m/s. This gives a pressure gradient of 64 mmHg, a significant valve gradient which will rise much higher on even mild exercise as flow increases further (Table 13.14). Thus, with a combined lesion, the regurgitation greatly potentiates the effect of the stenosis. This is particularly true of the mitral valve, where pressures need to rise much less before producing symptoms.

Table 13.14 Relationship between valve area, blood velocity and pressure gradient

Condition of valve	Area (cm^2)	Velocity (m/s)	Pressure gradient (mmHg)
Stenosis alone			
Normal	3	1	4
Mild stenosis	1.5	2	16
Severe stenosis	0.6	5	100
Stenosis and regurgitation			
Normal area, no regurgitation	3	1	4
Normal area, 50% regurgitation	3	2	16
Mild stenosis, 50% regurgitation	1.5	4	64
Mild stenosis, 66% regurgitation	1.5	6	144

The Bernouilh equation ($P = 4V^2$), relating blood flow velocity (V) to pressure gradient (P) across a valve, shows the effects of regurgitation on the pressure gradient if the forward stroke volume is maintained. The figures are chosen for simplicity. With 50% regurgitation, the forward stroke volume and (theoretically) the flow velocity doubles; with 66% regurgitation, they increase three-fold. In practice, the flow time also increases.

MITRAL STENOSIS

Aetiology

Mitral stenosis is almost always a consequence of rheumatic heart disease, and is the commonest valvular manifestation of the disease. A rare congenital form exists. The two valve cusps become adherent along their commissures, producing progressive stenosis with a 'fish mouth' orifice. Initially the cusps remain fairly pliable, but they become increasingly rigid with time and eventually calcify. The increasing degree of stenosis produces a rise in left atrial pressure and left atrial dilatation. The raised pulmonary venous pressure leads to left heart failure and can lead to progressive pulmonary hypertension.

Clinical features

Mitral stenosis may remain asymptomatic for many years with the patient unaware that she has a limited exercise tolerance. However, an additional load on the heart such as pregnancy, exertion, emotional stress or intercurrent chest infection (which is more common in patients with mitral valve disease because of the pulmonary vascular congestion), may produce the first symptoms of left heart failure. The onset of fast atrial fibrillation in middle-age is a common presentation, often leading to left heart failure, and thrombus formation with the risk of embolism. Right heart failure eventually develops as a consequence of pulmonary hypertension.

Symptoms

Of left heart failure

The symptoms of left heart failure (not to be confused with left *ventricular* failure) are shortness of breath on exertion, orthopnoea, paroxysmal nocturnal dyspnoea, pulmonary oedema, and haemoptysis of fresh blood occurring from rupture of a congested bronchial or pulmonary vein (uncommon with other causes of left heart failure). Haemoptysis may be due to pulmonary infarction, which is more common in mitral valve disease.

Summary 3 Symptoms and signs of mitral stenosis

Symptoms	
Of left heart failure	Shortness of breath, orthopnoea, paroxysmal nocturnal dyspnoea, haemoptysis
Of atrial fibrillation	Palpitations and syncope (at onset); May precipitate left heart failure Systemic embolism, to CNS, limbs, gut, kidneys
Of pulmonary hypertension	Weight loss and cachexia Right heart failure
Signs	
Uncomplicated (auscultatory only)	Opening snap Mitral diastolic murmur Presystolic murmur
With atrial fibrillation	Irregular pulse
With pulmonary hypertension	Parasternal lift (RVH) Loud P2 Tapping apex
If very severe	Mitral facies Cardiac cachexia

Due to atrial fibrillation

The raised left atrial pressure may lead to atrial fibrillation, sometimes paroxysmal at first, but then stable. The onset of atrial fibrillation can change an asymptomatic patient into one severely disabled by breathlessness. The loss of atrial filling and the shortened diastolic filling period may convert a quiescent, slowly progressive, stenosis into a life threatening condition.

Systemic embolism. The atrial fibrillation and raised left atrial pressure lead to left atrial enlargement, more marked in patients who have suffered myocardial damage from the rheumatic fever. Thrombus can form in the left atrium and give rise to systemic emboli. A hemiplegia is a not uncommon presentation of mitral valve disease, and embolism to other sites is frequent. The patient in sinus rhythm is also at risk from embolism but to a lesser extent. The greatest risk is in the patient who, having been in atrial fibrillation, reverts to sinus rhythm, as the return of coordinated atrial contraction can dislodge clot.

Due to an enlarged left atrium

Massive enlargement of the left atrium can lead to hoarseness from pressure on the recurrent laryngeal nerve, dysphagia from oesophageal compression, and bronchiectasis from distortion of the left main bronchus. Long-standing raised left atrial, and thus raised pulmonary capillary, pressure often leads to constriction of pulmonary arterioles and thickening of the capillary basement membranes. There is increased resistance to flow through the lungs and, thus, pulmonary hypertension.

Right ventricular hypertrophy compensates for the increased load on the right ventricle. When pulmonary hypertension is severe, right ventricular failure follows, usually, but not always, associated with left heart failure. The typical facial appearance of a patient with mitral valve disease – ruddy complexion, with red or vaguely cyanosed cheeks – is secondary to pulmonary hypertension (*mitral facies*).

Signs

The main signs of mitral stenosis are illustrated in Figure 13.43. Pure mitral stenosis in sinus rhythm without pulmonary hypertension is relatively uncommon. The signs are then purely auscultatory, as cardiac output is maintained and there is no significant right ventricular hypertrophy. The auscultatory signs are:

1. *An opening snap*, best heard halfway between the apex and the left sternal edge. It occurs close to the aortic second sound in severe stenosis, but is more separated from it in mild stenosis.
2. *A rumbling diastolic murmur*. This commences with the opening snap and fades rapidly in mild stenosis, but is full length and runs into the presystolic murmur in severe stenosis.
3. The *presystolic murmur* coincides with atrial systolic flow through the valve. It is of the same character as the mid-diastolic murmur and is sometimes heard when the latter cannot be heard. It is absent in atrial fibrillation.

A

B

Fig. 13.43 Features of mitral stenosis. A. Chest X-ray showing cardiomegaly with gross left atrial enlargement. **B.** Diagrammatic illustration of the pressures in left atrium (red) and left ventricle (black), showing a diastolic pressure gradient (shaded pink). The timing of an opening snap (OS) and diastolic murmur is shown. S1 and S2 = first and second heart sounds. **C.** Typical M mode. The mitral valve (arrowed) movement is abnormal (compare with Fig. 13.20B). **D.** 2D echocardiographic appearance in mitral stenosis. Thickened mitral valve (MV), dilated left atrium (LA) and the LV cavity (LV) are shown.

C

D

4. A *loud first heart sound*. In the mobile stenotic valve, the cusps are still fully open as systole starts, so they close with a louder sound than normal. This is an unreliable sign.

Atrial fibrillation and pulmonary hypertension of some degree are found in most middle-aged patients. These patients also have signs of a low cardiac output, mitral facies, small stroke volume with small volume pulse, a raised jugular venous pressure, right ventricular hypertrophy, and a mid-diastolic murmur following the opening snap. The severe pulmonary hypertensive patient may have a very low cardiac output and the mitral murmur may then be virtually inaudible, especially if the patient is in heart failure – so-called *silent mitral stenosis*. The symptoms and signs of mitral stenosis are listed in Summary 3.

Investigation

The most useful investigations in mitral stenosis are echocardiography and Doppler ultrasound. In sinus rhythm, the ECG may show P mitrale. Severe pulmonary hypertension may produce right ventricular hypertrophy or 'strain', but this aspect of the ECG is often unhelpful.

Chest X-ray. The chest X-ray may show enlargement of the left atrium (Fig. 13.43), redistribution of flow to the upper zones, left heart failure and enlargement of the right side of the heart if there is coincident pulmonary hypertension. A penetrated lateral X-ray will show a calcified valve in the majority of patients over the age of 50.

Echocardiography. The echocardiogram shows thickening of the cusps (Fig. 13.43), which are fused together so that the posterior cusp moves anteriorly in diastole with the anterior cusp. The severity of the stenosis is assessed by the rate of ventricular filling, direct assessment of the valve area from 2D echo, and Doppler ultrasound measurement of the mitral jet velocity. The echo is extremely useful for examining the size of the left atrium and, thus, the risk of thrombus formation and embolism. Occasionally, clot can be demonstrated in the left atrium with 2D echo.

Doppler ultrasound demonstrates the blood velocity and, by calculation, can give a fair approximation of the pressure gradient across the valve non-invasively. It can also detect mitral regurgitation which may well be missed by echocardiography. Where there is doubt as to whether a patient's symptoms are from mitral valve disease or left ventricular disease and trivial mitral stenosis, cardiac catheterisation is still used to measure the valve gradient and left ventricular function, and to examine the state of the coronary circulation.

Management

Management of mitral stenosis consists of three phases:

1. *Monitoring* the asymptomatic patient with mild disease who does not require any treatment, with eventual decision on anticoagulation.
2. *Medical* management of the symptomatic patient with a decision on surgery.

3. *Surgical* management of the patient with more severe disease.

Medical

In the asymptomatic patient in sinus rhythm, no treatment is necessary; but the patient should be advised about prophylaxis against infective endocarditis (p. 425) and carefully assessed during pregnancy (p. 429). The onset of atrial fibrillation may lead to the development of symptoms. Even asymptomatic patients in sinus rhythm with moderate stenosis are at risk from thrombo-embolism from the left atrium, so the relative risks of anticoagulation have to be weighed against the benefits in each individual case. The indications for anticoagulation in mitral stenosis are listed in Summary 4.

In the symptomatic patient, the aim of medical management should be to control the symptoms of left heart failure with diuretics. In atrial fibrillation, the ventricular rate should be controlled with digoxin, either alone or in combination with (or substituted by) a beta-blocker or verapamil (p. 368). The risk of thrombo-embolic episodes should be reduced by anticoagulation.

Summary 4   Indications for anticoagulation in mitral stenosis

- Moderate or severe stenosis
- Enlarged left atrium
- Atrial fibrillation
- Sinus rhythm with recurrent palpitations
- Any symptoms suggestive of arterial embolism

Surgical

Closed valvotomy

Closed mitral valvotomy – first attempted as a treatment for mitral stenosis in the 1920's – is an extremely effective operation. The aim is to separate the valve cusps where they are adherent along the commissures, without tearing the cusps and rendering the valve regurgitant. The closed valvotomy is performed through an apical subcostal incision; it does not require cardiac bypass and can even be performed during the second trimester of pregnancy without much hazard to the fetus. A limited thoracotomy allows the atrium to be opened through the atrial appendage (which is usually amputated as it is the seat of clot formation), and enables a mechanical dilator to be passed through a stab incision at the apex of the left ventricle to the mitral orifice, where it is opened and splits the valve. This operation is most suitable for young patients with non-calcified valves. It produces an unobtrusive scar which is often hidden under the left breast.

Open valvotomy

Nowadays, open valvotomy through a midline sternal

incision, with the patient on cardiac bypass, is more popular. It allows direct inspection of the valve, and, should regurgitation result from splitting the valve, it can be replaced or even repaired. Valve replacement is essential if there is significant regurgitation or if the valve is heavily calcified.

Prognosis

Mitral valvotomy can dramatically improve the symptoms of the patient with mitral stenosis. With time, however, the valve tends to become more rigid and calcify, effectively becoming restenotic even if there is no fusion of the commissures. Often, a degree of regurgitation develops and, occasionally, other heart valves affected by rheumatic heart disease start to cause problems. For example, a valvotomy at 25 years of age may well be followed by a further, less successful, valvotomy at 35, a mitral valve replacement at 45 and an aortic valve replacement at the age of 60, with tricuspid valve plication.

MITRAL REGURGITATION

Aetiology

Until recently, most cases of mitral regurgitation were thought to be rheumatic in origin, but the percentage of valves coming to surgery which are rheumatic is now below 50% in many series. The mitral valve apparatus is complex and regurgitation can result from:

1. dilatation of the valve ring
2. damage, retraction or perforation of the valve cusps
3. damage to the subvalvular apparatus (chordae, papillary muscle, or the ventricular muscle to which the papillary muscles attach).

There are therefore many causes of mitral regurgitation.

Heart failure

Heart failure with dilatation of the left ventricle will produce 'functional mitral regurgitation' due to dilatation of the valve ring and a shift in the attachments of the chordae tendinae. This may disappear as the ventricle shrinks with treatment, but may become a permanent feature in the end stages of a congestive cardiomyopathy.

Myocardial infarction

Papillary muscle *dysfunction* can arise due to inferior myocardial infarction, producing a characteristic type of mitral regurgitation which is usually not severe. In contrast, infarction complicated by rupture of the papillary muscle produces catastrophic regurgitation and is usually fatal.

Degenerative changes

Degenerative changes are often seen in mitral valves at surgery. The pathogenesis is not fully understood, as degenerative changes can occur in rheumatic valves or others which are known to be mildly incompetent for a long period.

Rupture of the smaller chordae tendinae can occur slowly and progressively in an atretic valve, causing increasing mitral regurgitation. Acute chordal rupture of a major trunk causes sudden severe mitral regurgitation, and may present with a sudden sharp pain in the chest followed by pulmonary oedema.

Other causes

The *click-murmur syndrome* (*floppy mitral valve* or *Barlow's syndrome*) is due to prolapse of a mitral valve cusp late in systole, often from a degree of 'redundancy' in the length of the chordae tendinae. Elderly patients often develop a minor degree of mitral regurgitation from *calcification of the valve ring*. This produces a characteristic wheezy systolic murmur. *Endocarditis* may make even a trivial degree of regurgitation more severe, and acute endocarditis can rapidly destroy a normal valve. There is a degree of mitral regurgitation in most cases of *hypertrophic obstructive cardiomyopathy* (p. 418).

Congenital forms of mitral regurgitation include cleft cusps in atrioventricular canal defects and endocardial cushion defects in association with ostium primum atrial septal defects (p. 395). It may also be found in Marfan's syndrome, and osteogenesis imperfecta.

Sharp (stabbing) and blunt (steering wheel injury) trauma to the precordium, acromegaly and Libman-Sacks endocarditis in systemic lupus erythematosus, are other rare causes.

Clinical features

Symptoms and pathophysiology

Chronic

The symptoms of chronic mitral regurgitation are essentially the same as those of mitral stenosis, but severe pulmonary hypertension is less common with pure mitral regurgitation. The slowly progressive regurgitation is accommodated by gradual increase in size of the left ventricle, which ejects the blood into a slowly enlarging and compliant left atrium and pulmonary venous vasculature. Up to 80% of the left ventricular stroke volume may be regurgitant in severe cases, and the left ventricular stroke volume can exceed 250 ml. Symptoms in chronic mitral regurgitation usually develop when the left ventricle dilates sufficiently for there to be a significant rise in its filling pressure. Usually, systolic function and ejection fraction are well-maintained, because the left ventricle is ejecting largely into a low impedance outflow. The symptoms of left heart failure, atrial fibrillation, and pulmonary hypertension are the same as for mitral stenosis (p. 377).

Acute

In acute mitral regurgitation, e.g. due to rupture of chordae tendinae, a small left ventricle is regurgitating into a small uncompliant left atrium (high impedance), with a resultant very high pressure pulse or *v* wave in the left atrium which may reach 60 mmHg. Left atrial pressure rapidly exceeds pulmonary oedema levels, especially if the low forward output precipitates a tachycardia – during which the heart spends a disproportionate amount of time in systole, which makes the regurgitation worse. Acute mitral regurgitation thus usually presents with severe left heart failure or pulmonary oedema.

Signs

Uncomplicated pure mitral regurgitation, if trivial, has only auscultatory signs (Fig. 13.44). However, if the regurgitation is more severe, the left ventricular volume load becomes clinically evident by a hyperactive left ventricle with displacement of the cardiac apex down and laterally. Enlargement of the left atrium in systole may be felt as a parasternal heave. In severe regurgitation, the pulse may become small and rather jerky from a shortened ejection time. Severe regurgitation is evident on auscultation by the presence of a third heart sound and short mid-diastolic murmur, produced by the greatly enhanced forward flow through the mitral valve during diastole.

The pansystolic murmur of rheumatic mitral regurgitation, or other types of regurgitation with a central jet, is best heard at the apex of the heart and may be louder with the patient tipped to the left. The murmur of mitral regurgitation may be well heard posteriorly over the lungs.

Many other types of mitral regurgitation – including the late systolic murmur of the floppy valve syndrome – are best heard at the left sternal edge, and a number of others are also not pansystolic in character. Differential diagnosis from trivial aortic stenosis and ventricular septal defect can therefore be difficult, and requires non-invasive tests such as echocardiography and Doppler ultrasound or even cardiac catheterisation.

Mitral valve prolapse

Mitral valve prolapse (also known as floppy mitral valve, or Barlow's syndrome), spans an enormous range of severity, from a trivial abnormality picked up on echocardiography which has little or no consequence to the patient, to severe mitral regurgitation and heart failure. At the mild end of the spectrum is a group of patients with the auscultatory features of single or multiple systolic clicks audible in the mitral area, which may be associated with a late systolic murmur of mild mitral regurgitation. There may be a tendency to supraventricular arrhythmia and atypical chest pain and associated mild skeletal abnormalities, commonly a straight back (loss of thoracic kyphosis).

The underlying abnormality consists of redundancy in the chordae tendinae allowing posterior prolapse of one or other mitral cusp in late systole. More severe degeneration of the sub-valvular apparatus is seen in certain patients, particularly those with Marfan's syndrome (Ch. 6, p. 93), although severely floppy mitral valves may occur in isolation. Isolated mitral regurgitation, even if severe, can

Fig. 13.44 Features of mitral regurgitation. A. Illustrates diversion of blood into the left atrium. **B.** Shows the pressures in the left ventricle and left atrium in both mild and severe cases and the accompanying murmurs. PSM = pansystolic murmur; MDM = mid-diastolic murmur. **C.** M mode echocardiogram through the left ventricle (LV) in a case of severe mitral regurgitation due to valvular disease. The ventricle is dilated and hyperkinetic. **D.** M mode echocardiogram at the same level in a patient with mitral regurgitation due to poor LV function. The LV is dilated and hypokinetic. IVS = interventricular septum; PW = posterior wall.

be tolerated for long periods if its development is gradual. It is uncertain whether patients with the mild 'click-murmur' syndrome suffer a significant number of complications, but systemic embolisation, arrhythmia and endocarditis are potential risks. Treatment of severe regurgitation is surgical.

Investigation

ECG. The ECG is of little value in indicating the severity of the regurgitation. There may be P mitrale and left ventricular hypertrophy, but very severe regurgitation can exist in the presence of an almost normal ECG. Severe left ventricular hypertrophy would suggest another cause.

Chest X-ray may show enlargement of the left ventricle as well as the left atrium. Sudden increase in size of the left ventricle precedes left heart failure. There may be evidence of raised pulmonary venous pressure.

M mode echocardiography is useful in demonstrating the volume load on the left ventricle and the size of the left atrium. It is seldom capable of showing the presence of, or the cause of, mitral regurgitation, but will show a rheumatic thickened mitral valve, mitral valve prolapse or flail cusp. Two-dimensional echocardiography will often show lack of co-aptation of the mitral valve cusps in rheumatic mitral regurgitation.

Doppler ultrasound is an excellent technique for demonstrating mitral regurgitation, differentiating it from aortic stenosis or a ventricular septal defect.

Cardiac catheterisation will give a direct measurement of the left ventricular filling pressure and the left atrial pressure, which helps to distinguish left ventricular muscle pump failure from severe valvular regurgitation. *Angiography* shows the severity of the leak and often its mechanism.

Management

Trivial regurgitation is very well-tolerated and requires only endocarditis prophylaxis (p. 425). Moderately severe mitral regurgitation can be well-tolerated for years, but the patient may slowly come to accept a diminishing exercise tolerance and the role of a cardiac invalid, while at the same time denying symptoms. Eventually, heart failure will require treatment, and a decision will be required concerning valve replacement or, exceptionally, repair. Severe regurgitation and acute regurgitation merit early valve replacement.

MITRAL REGURGITATION WITH STENOSIS

The combination of mitral regurgitation with stenosis is almost invariably a result of rheumatic heart disease but occasionally arises in other conditions, such as Libman-Sacks endocarditis in SLE. Mixed mitral valve disease presents later than pure stenosis, and is very common after mitral valvotomy.

The physical signs are shown in Figures 13.43 and 13.44. Atrial fibrillation is more likely here than with pure stenosis, and severe pulmonary hypertension is less likely. Even a mild degree of regurgitation makes the effective degree of mitral stenosis much greater (p. 377). The predominant lesion can be difficult to assess in the presence of hypertension or aortic valve disease, which will also produce left ventricular hypertrophy. A pansystolic murmur alone may arise from coincident tricuspid regurgitation with pure mitral stenosis. The degree of mitral regurgitation can vary with the heart rate and the degree of left ventricular dilatation. What may appear to be severe regurgitation when the patient is in heart failure, may settle considerably as the patient improves. Management is as for mitral stenosis alone (p. 379).

Assessment of the mitral valve with Doppler ultrasound shows that minor degrees of mitral regurgitation are extremely common even when these cannot be detected clinically.

AORTIC STENOSIS

Aetiology

Outflow obstruction to the left ventricle can be at the valve itself (valvular), above it (supravalvular), or below (subvalvular). About 1% of cases of 'aortic stenosis' are supra- or subvalvular. Supravalvular stenosis is a congenital form of atresia of the ascending aorta, and is associated with a characteristic 'elfin' facies. Subvalvular stenosis is either a congenital ring lesion (which is amenable to surgery) or is a variable muscular obstruction produced by hypertrophic obstructive cardiomyopathy (p. 418).

Valvular aortic stenosis can result from a number of conditions:

1. *Congenital* aortic stenosis, presenting in childhood, the valve having one, two or three cusps.
2. *Bicuspid aortic valve* presenting in adulthood. About 1% of the population are born with two, instead of three, cusps. About one third of these develop calcific aortic stenosis, one third mixed aortic valve disease, and one third have no significant valvular abnormality. The valve itself seems to be mechanically unsatisfactory and suffers mechanical stresses which lead to progressive damage. Heavy work may hasten the onset of the stenosis, so that a heavy manual labourer can present in his forties and a desk-worker in his or her sixties.
3. *Rheumatic heart disease*. This involves the aortic valve in about 50% of cases of rheumatic valvular disease, most frequently producing aortic regurgitation, often a mixed lesion but sometimes pure stenosis. As with mitral valve disease, stenosis with rheumatic heart disease seems more common in women, and regurgitation in men.
4. *Senile aortic calcification*. Although calcification of the valve ring is commonly benign, it can invade the cusps and produce a calcified tricuspid valve as it renders the cusps immobile. This aetiology is more common over the age of 70. The valve cusps are not fused.

Pathophysiology

Outflow obstruction to the left ventricle leads to:

1. *Concentric left ventricular hypertrophy*. The walls may thicken from 1 to 2 cm without the heart appearing enlarged on chest X-ray.
2. *Compensatory enlargement of the coronary arterial circulation* as the metabolic demands of the hypertrophied left ventricle with its large pressure load are increased.

3. *A relatively fixed cardiac output.* A resting pressure gradient of 100 mmHg would have to become 400 mmHg for the flow velocity through the valve to double. The heart is incapable of generating such a pressure, and the heart is therefore near its limit at rest.

Clinical features

Symptoms

Aortic stenosis may remain asymptomatic until it is very severe and is then life-threatening. The symptoms (Summary 5) are those of:

1. *Left ventricular failure.* The thickened ventricle has an increased filling pressure which rises dramatically should the ventricle dilate. Shortness of breath on exertion may precede paroxysmal nocturnal dyspnoea and orthopnoea, or the patient may present with acute pulmonary oedema.
2. *Myocardial ischaemia.* Left ventricular work is greatly increased and, with the grossly thickened ventricular wall, subendocardial ischaemia is common. The thickened myocardium is perfused by a lower than normal perfusion gradient due to low aortic diastolic pressure and a high LV end diastolic pressure. For these reasons, angina can occur without any coronary atheroma. In the older age group, aortic stenosis may well coexist with coronary artery disease.
3. *Syncope on exertion.* This is a sinister symptom which indicates a fixed cardiac output and presages sudden death. The mechanisms may be: skeletal muscle vasodilatation, causing a drop in blood pressure since no rise in cardiac output is possible; a sudden rise in ventricular pressure which activates ventricular baroreceptors, producing reflex bradycardia and vasodilation; myocardial ischaemia triggering ventricular arrhythmia.
4. *Sudden death,* probably resulting from myocardial ischaemia and ventricular irritability, leading to a fatal arrhythmia. This may be provoked by exertion and is the main reason why tight aortic stenosis is an urgent indication for valve-replacement, even in the asymptomatic patient.
5. *Right heart failure.* Progressive myocardial ischaemia can lead to a 'myopathic heart', in which the most prominent symptom is oedema from right heart failure supervening on left.
6. *Emboli from a heavily calcified valve.* These are usually fairly small and cause small strokes or visual disturbances. The calcific embolus can occasionally be seen on fundoscopy.

Signs

The signs of pure aortic stenosis are shown in Figure 13.45. Although the systolic ejection murmur is the feature that attracts attention to the possible diagnosis, the most important physical sign is the slow-rising (Fig. 13.7), poor volume pulse, best felt at the carotid where a systolic thrill may also be evident. The heart is not enlarged unless the patient has been in failure, but the left ventricular apex beat is powerful and 'pressure loaded'. Differential diagnosis from a 'flow murmur' is based on the single second sound (in calcific aortic stenosis), the pulse, and the presence of left ventricular hypertrophy. The loudness of the murmur is a poor index of severity and the murmur may

Fig. 13.45 Features of aortic stenosis. A. Pressures in the left ventricle (black) and aorta (red) showing a systolic pressure gradient due to aortic stenosis. The ejection systolic murmur is illustrated. **B.** 2D echocardiogram showing severe aortic valve (AV) thickening. Ao = aorta; LV = left ventricle; LA = left atrium; RV = right ventricle. **C.** Position of probe and direction of Doppler beam. **D.** Continuous wave Doppler record showing high velocity signals. Peak = 4.5 m/s (dotted line), predicting a gradient of 82 mmHg.

Summary 5 Symptoms of aortic stenosis

- Left ventricular failure – dyspnoea, orthopnoea, pulmonary oedema
- Angina
- Exertional syncope
- Sudden death
- Right heart failure
- Small cerebral emboli

even be absent in heart failure. In congenital aortic stenosis, there may be an ejection click as the valve cusps tent as they tension.

Investigation

Electrocardiography

An ECG is very useful. A normal ECG virtually rules out significant aortic stenosis, except in congenital disease when the trace may remain remarkably normal despite a large gradient. However, severe left ventricular hypertrophy in any patient with a systolic murmur, or in any patient presenting in heart failure who is not hypertensive, should suggest aortic stenosis as a possible diagnosis.

A number of ECG changes are seen in aortic stenosis:

1. *Left ventricular hypertrophy*. Often widening of QRS and T wave changes of 'strain' predominate over voltage change. T wave inversion over LV leads may be the only feature. Loss of anterior R waves may mimic a picture of old anterior infarct.
2. *Left axis deviation* and, eventually, *left bundle branch block* may occur either from severe hypertrophy or invasion of conduction system by calcium from the valve.
3. *Complete heart block*.
4. *Left atrial hypertrophy* or '*P mitrale*'. A large negative component to the P wave in V1 indicates raised LV filling pressure.

Chest X-ray

The chest X-ray can be normal but may show a post-stenotic dilatation of the ascending aorta, prominence of the left ventricle, and a calcified aortic valve on lateral chest X-ray. The latter is of great significance in suggesting tight stenosis in any patient under the age of 55; above this age, the valve may calcify even with an insignificant gradient. Significant enlargement of the left ventricle occurs with heart failure or coincident aortic regurgitation.

M mode echocardiography

M mode echocardiography can display thickening and calcification of the valve cusps, but is less useful in congenital stenosis. The compensatory hypertrophy of the left ventricular wall is well shown. Two-dimensional echocardiography may give a good view of the aortic valve orifice from the apex, but resolution of the ultrasound picture is not sufficiently good to predict the gradient.

Doppler ultrasound

Doppler ultrasound is used to measure the jet velocity and predict the valve gradient. If the probe can be aligned with the jet, velocities as high as 6 m/s can be recorded – equivalent to 150 mmHg. A high blood velocity (more than 4 m/s) indicates a surgically significant gradient but, since

jet velocities can be underestimated, a negative or low jet velocity record is of less significance than a high one.

Cardiac catheterisation

Measurement of the valve gradient by cardiac catheterisation is not essential if the diagnosis is well established. Catheterisation is indicated where there is doubt about the site of the stenosis and when it is important to check on left ventricular function or associated mitral valve disease. It is usually performed before surgery to obtain coronary angiograms.

Management

Surgical

Tight aortic stenosis has such a poor prognosis that surgery should be offered to everyone with this diagnosis. Valvuloplasty in elderly patients was considered attractive in the past, and can still be used as a temporary 'holding' procedure, but it provides only partial relief of the obstruction for a few months and has as high a mortality as surgery. Valvuloplasty or valvotomy in children may gain sufficient time for them to reach a reasonable size before having aortic valve replacement. For adults, valve replacement is the only long-term treatment. If the ventricle has already been badly damaged the results are poor, but in the asymptomatic patient with a good ventricle, the left ventricular hypertrophy regresses fairly rapidly.

Lesser degrees of stenosis, with valve gradients of less than 50 mmHg (or equivalent valve area), need serial follow-up, as the stenosis may become more significant with time. The patient with aortic stenosis and coronary disease would require both valve replacement and coronary grafts.

Medical

Treatment of heart failure is along conventional lines (p. 357). Vasodilator agents are contra-indicated, as reduction of systemic resistance can lead to a severe drop in blood pressure.

AORTIC REGURGITATION

Aetiology

The aortic valve cusps normally overlap on closure to the extent of about 25% of the cusp area. Aortic regurgitation can arise from:

1. dilatation of the valve ring so that the cusps no longer meet adequately to prevent leakage
2. damage to the cusps themselves
3. in some diseases, a combination of these factors.

Dilatation of the valve ring occurs classically in syphilitic aortic regurgitation, but can also occur with hypertension and aortic dissection; less common causes include cystic medial necrosis in Marfan's syndrome, and osteogenesis imperfecta.

Damage to the valve cusps is a feature of rheumatic aortic regurgitation, infective endocarditis, and also less common conditions, such as Libman-Sacks endocarditis, mucopolysaccharidoses, and pseudoxanthoma elasticum. The seronegative arthritides, ankylosing spondylitis, Reiter's disease and psoriatic arthritis can be associated with an aortitis and cusp damage, leading to aortic regurgitation; rarely, rheumatoid arthritis is associated with a nodular cusp damage leading to aortic regurgitation.

Bicuspid aortic valve (found in 1% of the population) can lead to predominant aortic regurgitation (p. 382). There are other congenital forms of aortic regurgitation, e.g. that associated with a supracristal ventricular septal defect.

Clinical features

The clinical features of aortic regurgitation are listed in Summary 6.

Symptoms and pathophysiology

Aortic regurgitation can be well-tolerated for years if it develops slowly. Up to 80% regurgitation can be found in severe chronic aortic regurgitation, but acute regurgitation (such as follows aortic dissection or acute infective endocarditis) is poorly tolerated. The patient with chronic aortic regurgitation has a very low peripheral resistance and this contributes to the physical signs (see below). These are not so apparent if the patient develops heart failure, when there is peripheral vasoconstriction and the 'collapsing pulse' and other peripheral signs disappear.

The severity of the regurgitation is normally indicated by a low diastolic blood pressure and wide pulse pressure, both of which may appear more normal in heart failure as the stroke volume falls and the end diastolic pressure of the left ventricle rises. As aortic regurgitation progresses, the increasing leakage requires a larger and larger forward flow. This is usually achieved not by a tachycardia but by the left ventricular end diastolic size increasing with an increased stroke volume. Initially, the ejection fraction of the left ventricle is well-maintained and exercise tolerance is excellent; however, after an unpredictable time, there is steady or sudden deterioration in left ventricular function, often with a dramatic increase in heart size and the development of symptoms of left ventricular failure. Eventually, right heart failure follows with the development of pulmonary hypertension. Paradoxically, patients with severe aortic regurgitation may have symptoms of paroxysmal nocturnal dyspnoea yet retain a reasonable exercise tolerance, since exercise reduces the aortic impedance with respect to the left ventricle. The development of heart failure indicates serious dilatation of the left ventricle and need for urgent consideration of valve surgery. Unlike mitral valve disease – where some delay in surgery even in the presence of heart failure does not greatly affect the prognosis – heart failure in aortic regurgitation is associated with rapidly worsening left ventricular function which may never recover.

Angina can develop because the dilated left ventricle has increased oxygen requirements (as in congestive cardiomyopathy), but it is usually associated with coronary artery disease. Atrial fibrillation occurs in about 15% of cases, usually those with long-standing failure. The presence of atrial fibrillation means that associated mitral valve disease should be suspected.

Physical signs

The physical signs of aortic regurgitation (Fig. 13.46) are related to the large stroke volume, the peripheral vasodilatation and the compensatory increase in size of the left ventricle. The pulse may be collapsing or bisferiens, or feel normal if there is heart failure. The blood pressure indicates the large pulse pressure and low diastolic pressure. If the diastolic pressure is well-maintained in the presence of severe aortic regurgitation, coincident hypertension should be suspected. The left ventricle is very active and, in severe cases, the apex beat is displaced.

The increased forward flow is often accompanied by a systolic flow murmur which, of itself, does not indicate coincident stenosis. The early diastolic murmur is notoriously difficult to hear, and the non-cardiologist should therefore entertain the diagnosis if the other physical signs are present. The lack of a murmur is often a defect in the observer rather than the patient. The murmur is best heard with the diaphragm of the stethoscope, with the patient sitting forward having breathed out. It may be best heard at the left sternal edge, nearer the apex or the aortic area depending on the direction of the jet. Typically, valve ring dilatation regurgitation is better heard in the third right interspace rather than the third left.

An *Austin Flint murmur* may be associated with aortic regurgitation. This is an apical diastolic murmur, similar to that of mitral stenosis, arising from the anterior cusp of the mitral valve which vibrates in the jet of aortic regurgitation. Because aortic regurgitation may be both difficult to hear and is a frequent lesion in infective endocarditis, a

---

Summary 6 Clinical features of aortic regurgitation

Symptoms
Left heart failure: breathlessness
Myocardial ischaemia, angina
Atrial fibrillation (less frequently)

Physical signs
Large stroke volume with vasodilatation
  Collapsing pulse
  Wide pulse pressure
  Head nodding, capillary pulsation
Enlarged left ventricle with dynamic displaced apex
Auscultatory
  Forward flow systolic murmur
  High-pitched early diastolic murmur
  Premature first heart sound (in severe cases)

patient with a fever and steadily widening pulse pressure is regarded as having aortic regurgitation and endocarditis until proved otherwise.

Investigation

ECG shows left ventricular hypertrophy of the diastolic overload type, in that, initially at least, voltage changes with prominent Q waves over the lateral leads predominate over T wave changes. Later, the T waves invert and this has been taken by some as an indication for surgery (see below).

Chest X-ray shows increasing size of the left ventricle and often some dilatation of the proximal aorta. Generalised cardiac enlargement may follow and, eventually, changes of raised pulmonary venous pressure.

Echocardiography. M mode shows the dilated LV and its wall thickness. Calculation can be made of the stroke volume and ejection fraction, which are useful for following progress. In many cases, vibration of the anterior cusp of the mitral valve or the septum can be seen, confirming the

Fig. 13.46 Features of aortic regurgitation. A. Pressures in the aorta (red) and left ventricle (black) are illustrated with the accompanying murmurs (3 = third sound). **B.** Direction of regurgitant flow (arrow) and orientation of M mode and Doppler beams (dotted lines). **C.** Continuous wave Doppler signal showing a regurgitant jet throughout diastole with a maximal velocity of 4 m/s (upwards signal). The small downward signal excludes aortic stenosis. **D.** M mode echocardiogram showing flutter of the anterior mitral valve leaf (arrowed), which may close prematurely in severe aortic regurgitation causing early first heart sound.

diagnosis. *Doppler ultrasound* will confirm the diagnosis but cannot yet quantify the lesion, although attempts have been made by examining ascending aortic flow velocity.

Cardiac catheterisation can be used to examine left ventricular function, severity of the aortic regurgitation and its anatomy, as well as looking for other pathology, such as mitral regurgitation and coronary artery disease.

Management

Most patients are asymptomatic and require no therapy.

Surgery

Those in heart failure have been left too late to get the best results from surgery, since a dilated 'myopathic' heart never returns to normal and is associated with a high risk of sudden death. Cardiologists have therefore tried to find criteria to predict the best time to operate before heart failure develops. The currently used criteria are based on echocardiographic dimensions; others are now being developed based on the use of isotope left ventricular angiography. A fall in the ejection fraction of the left ventricle on exercise has been suggested as a criterion for surgery, since the ejection fraction is normally well-maintained or even increases. Acute aortic regurgitation requires very close attention and urgent valve replacement at the first sign of heart failure. Delay can result in catastrophic heart failure and death of the patient, as the degree of regurgitation and size of the heart rapidly increase.

Medical

Medical management of chronic regurgitation consists of treatment of heart failure and control of other problems, such as arrhythmias and endocarditis prophylaxis (p. 425).

MIXED AORTIC VALVE DISEASE

About one-third of patients with aortic valve disease have a combined lesion with significant regurgitation and stenosis. As previously described, regurgitation makes a dramatic difference to the valve gradient (p. 377), and a stenotic valve with a gradient of 16 mmHg in systole would have a gradient of over 60 mmHg if twice the flow is accommodated, because of 50% regurgitation. The physical signs of the combined lesion are distinctive, with a large volume sustained or bisferiens pulse (Fig. 13.7), a markedly hypertrophied left ventricle which is both pressure and volume loaded, and both systolic ejection and early diastolic murmurs. The aortic second sound is single. Combined regurgitation and stenosis can only arise in valves that would stenose. A combined lesion cannot be caused by syphilis or other pathologies that primarily dilate the aortic root.

Investigation and management

Assessment of combined lesions has been greatly helped by

Doppler ultrasound and echocardiography. The gradient measured by Doppler ultrasound may appear much greater than the pull-back pressure gradient measured at cardiac catheterisation.

Surgery for combined lesions is based on the same criteria as for single lesions; onset of symptoms means that there is severe left ventricular hypertrophy and probably fibrosis, with consequent poor left ventricular function. Surgery is therefore ideally timed to anticipate symptoms and allow the left ventricular hypertrophy to regress. Opinions as to how this is judged differ, but a gradient of over 50 mmHg, the development of a left ventricular strain pattern on ECG, left ventricular dilatation and any evidence of heart failure are all considered indications for aortic valve replacement.

COMBINED MITRAL AND AORTIC VALVE DISEASE

Over 50% of patients with rheumatic mitral valve disease will eventually develop evidence of aortic valve disease, most commonly aortic regurgitation, but sometimes stenosis as well. The presence of disease of both valves makes assessment of the severity of the individual lesions more difficult. Mitral valve disease, in particular, tends to reduce cardiac output and stroke volume, which may make the physical signs of aortic valve disease, such as the carotid pulse, far less evident. Aortic regurgitation and mitral regurgitation both cause a volume load on the left ventricle, so the contribution of each lesion to this is difficult to assess. The auscultatory signs may also be far more difficult to elicit, particularly if the patient is in heart failure.

Investigation and management

The presence of aortic valve disease should be suspected in every patient with rheumatic mitral valve disease, particularly if they have ECG evidence of left ventricular hypertrophy, or a slightly sustained carotid pulse. Fortunately, echocardiography and, in particular, Doppler ultrasound enable the valves to be individually examined for evidence of stenosis and regurgitation; this is far more accurate than inspection of the valves at surgery. If a patient is being considered for mitral valve replacement in the presence of aortic valve disease, it is unwise for the surgeon to leave anything but trivial aortic valve disease, as the patient may otherwise require a further valve replacement within a few years. What may seem a trivial degree of aortic regurgitation or stenosis at presentation, may become clinically important with replacement of the mitral valve.

TRICUSPID REGURGITATION

Tricuspid regurgitation most commonly arises as a result of dilatation of the valve ring secondary to right heart failure with pulmonary hypertension. Less common causes are actual rheumatic involvement of the tricuspid valve leaflets producing 'organic tricuspid disease', and right-sided endocarditis, which is rare in anyone other than intravenous drug addicts. Floppy tricuspid valve may be associated with floppy mitral valve, and some congenital heart disease is associated with tricuspid regurgitation either as a primary phenomenon or secondary to right heart enlargement (e.g. atrial septal defect). Endomyocardial fibrosis, a disease occurring in the tropics, especially Africa, causes mitral and tricuspid regurgitation.

Doppler ultrasound has shown that a right-sided cardiac enlargement in rheumatic heart disease is almost invariably associated with a regurgitant jet through the tricuspid valve, very often in the absence of any physical signs. Similarly, it may be the cause of an 'innocent systolic murmur'.

Clinical features

Pathophysiology and symptoms

The leakage of a small percentage of the right ventricular stroke volume is easily accommodated by the right atrium. However, as the volume of regurgitation increases, there is increasing enlargement of the right atrium and right ventricle, and the movement of the interventricular septum becomes dominated by the right ventricle and so 'paradoxical'. The large systolic pressure pulse in the right atrium leads to stagnation and, eventually, reversal of flow of the blood in the great veins; the liver becomes distended and pulsatile (Fig. 13.47). The high hepatic venous pressure leads to cardiac cirrhosis and this may occasionally lead to secondary portal hypertension and splenomegaly.

The poor venous return, high venous pressures and poor hepatic function are associated, in most patients, with a degree of cardiac cachexia, poor wound-healing and difficulties with haemostasis.

Organic tricuspid regurgitation is much better tolerated, as the regurgitation is at a much lower pressure than when it is secondary to pulmonary hypertension. An extreme example of this is when the tricuspid valve has been totally resected in some cases of endocarditis. The patient can tolerate this situation for some weeks without any serious consequences, until a prosthetic valve is inserted.

The principal symptoms are those of right heart failure, with low cardiac output, fatigue, oedema, and pain from hepatic congestion which may arise on exercise – so-called 'hepatic angina', i.e. epigastric or right-sided subcostal pain arising on exercise and gradually (more gradually than 'true' angina) disappearing with cessation of exercise.

Signs

The patient may be in atrial fibrillation and is often slightly jaundiced. In moderate to severe cases, there is a highly pulsatile jugular vein with a big v wave and rapid y descent. The height of the v wave peak may be as much as 15 cm above the sternal angle and, in these circumstances, the jugular vein is palpably pulsatile and can be confused by the novice with an arterial pulse. The right ventricle is very active and gives rise to a right parasternal impulse. There is a pansystolic murmur heard at the left sternal edge, or

Fig. 13.47 Features of tricuspid regurgitation. A. Illustration of regurgitant flow and direction of Doppler beam (dotted line). PA = pulmonary artery; SVC and IVC = superior and inferior vena cava. **B.** and **C.** Continuous wave Doppler signals, both showing tricuspid regurgitation (downwards signal). In **B**, there is severe (organic) regurgitation with normal pulmonary artery pressure and increased triscuspid forward flow. In **C** there is pulmonary hypertension with a high velocity regurgitant jet through the triscuspid valve.

even at the cardiac apex, which may be formed by the right ventricle under these circumstances. The murmur is often of lower pitch than a mitral murmur, possibly because of the lower blood velocity. There can be a right ventricular third heart sound.

Abdominal examination reveals a pulsatile liver which is often visible, but is best felt bimanually with the hands hinged at the wrists.

Investigation

ECG may be unhelpful and is usually dominated by other factors associated with the underlying cardiac disease.

Chest X-ray shows right-sided cardiac enlargement, and there may be a fullness in the region of the distended superior vena cava.

Echocardiography shows an enlarged right ventricle with paradoxical movement of the interventricular septum suggesting 'volume load' of the right ventricle. The tricuspid valve leaflets are more easily seen with an enlarged right heart.

Doppler ultrasound will confirm a regurgitant jet through the tricuspid valve. The jet velocity will give an indication of the gradient across the valve, and hence the right ventricular pressure and the severity of the pulmonary hypertension (if any).

Management

As tricuspid regurgitation is most frequently functional, the treatment is frequently that of the associated condition. Bedrest and diuretics will have a dramatic effect in many cases, with the murmur and pulsatile jugular veins disappearing. Intravenous diuretics may be required, as the oral drugs may be poorly absorbed in these patients. Organic tricuspid valve disease may require surgical treatment at the same time as other cardiac surgery. Tricuspid valve replacement is unsatisfactory, as all prosthetic valves

are functionally stenotic. However, an annuloplasty of the tricuspid valve may reduce the amount of regurgitation, or even cure it.

TRICUSPID STENOSIS

Tricuspid stenosis is a very uncommon manifestation of rheumatic heart disease. It mimics mitral stenosis, but produces right heart failure rather than left. It almost always complicates rheumatic involvement of the mitral and aortic valves, and should be suspected if there is a high venous pressure with a slow *y* descent in the jugular venous pulse. The diastolic murmur is reputedly enhanced on inspiration and is heard best at the left sternal edge. There can be a tricuspid opening snap. Often, there is coincident tricuspid regurgitation.

Investigation and treatment

The diagnosis can be confirmed by echocardiogram which will show the thickened cusps. Doppler ultrasound can be used to measure the jet velocity and thus calculate the diastolic gradient. Cardiac catheterisation with a double lumen catheter is needed to measure the rather small valve gradient.

Treatment is by valve replacement.

PULMONARY REGURGITATION

Pulmonary regurgitation is usually caused by dilatation of the pulmonary valve ring in pulmonary hypertension. It may also follow pulmonary valvotomy or valvuloplasty. In severe cases, the right ventricle is hyperactive from volume loading, and the murmur is difficult to distinguish from that of aortic regurgitation, being an early diastolic murmur at the left sternal edge starting immediately after the pulmonary component of the second sound. It may have a slightly lower pitch and be more obvious on inspiration, but the two can easily be confused. The Graham Steell murmur of pulmonary regurgitation in mitral valve disease is far more frequently due to aortic regurgitation than was formerly believed.

Pulmonary regurgitation is usually well-tolerated but can be one reason why the heart size remains enlarged after surgical correction of Fallot's tetralogy.

PULMONARY STENOSIS

Pulmonary stenosis is the second most common form of congenital heart disease in adults; it is commoner in women. Mild cases, with gradients of less than 50 mmHg are common. Stenosis may occur at valvular or subvalvular level, or even in the pulmonary arteries. There is a raised pressure in the right ventricle and, in severe cases, reduced lung blood flow and poor effort tolerance.

Clinical features

Most cases are asymptomatic, but with gradients of over 80 mmHg, the most common symptom (surprisingly) is dyspnoea on exertion. In very severe stenosis, symptoms of exertional syncope and angina become prominent, similar to those associated with aortic stenosis. In children and young adults, pulmonary stenosis may present with severe right heart failure.

The physical signs are of a small volume pulse, a large *a* wave in the jugular venous pressure, a right ventricular substernal heave and a harsh systolic murmur in the pulmonary area; the latter appears very long and drowns the heart sounds in severe cases of infundibular stenosis, but can be a short ejection murmur in mild cases. The timing of pulmonary valve closure, which is delayed in severe cases, is a useful indication of severity.

Investigation and treatment

ECG shows right ventricular hypertrophy. The chest X-ray shows oligaemic lung fields; and a large post-stenotic dilatation with dilatation of the pulmonary conus is common in valvular stenosis, but not infundibular. The right ventricle is not significantly enlarged unless it has failed.

Doppler ultrasound assessment of the valve gradient has become invaluable. Echocardiography will show the hypertrophy of the right ventricle and the site of the obstruction, as well as showing other anomalies.

Surgical valvotomy has been largely replaced as a treatment of pulmonary stenosis by balloon valvuloplasty, in which a balloon catheter is inserted and dilated at the site of the obstruction.

SURGICAL MANAGEMENT OF ACQUIRED HEART VALVE DISEASE

The choices in surgical management of heart valve disease have recently become more complex, with closed valv-otomy, open valvotomy and balloon valvuloplasty all being possible approaches.

Cardiac bypass

The technique of cardiac bypass involves valve replacement performed with the circulation arrested and with extracorporeal circulation from a roller pump and external oxygenator. Since the brain is perfused at relatively low pressure, and the oxygenator and perfusion system produce progressive damage to blood constituents and introduce microemboli into the arterial circulation, there is a significant morbidity associated with cardiac bypass which increases considerably with the length of time on bypass. Most of the morbidity seems to be reversible (e.g. intellectual impairment) but patients with cerebrovascular disease, such as carotid stenosis, are at particularly high risk from cerebral infarction. Occasionally, carotid artery surgery may have to precede cardiac bypass.

Balloon valvuloplasty

The advent of balloon angioplasty to dilate coronary and other vessels has triggered an interest in the application of similar techniques to stenosed valves. In balloon valvuloplasty, a balloon catheter is inserted through the valve orifice and then dilated to split open the valve. This technique has been shown to work in both congenital aortic stenosis and pulmonary stenosis and has now been applied to the mitral valve. Balloon valvuloplasty is still being developed, but it has been disappointing in adult aortic stenosis, providing only temporary palliation. If torrential regurgitataion is produced, valve replacement is essential.

Valve repair and replacement

Nowadays, a badly leaking valve is almost invariably replaced. The other options are: a delicate plastic surgical repair of the valve, sometimes with pericardial or other tissue to repair defects in the valve cusps; or suturing of the valve ring to a prosthetic former to correct a grossly dilated valve ring. The latter operation is commonly performed in severe tricuspid regurgitation. Owing to the time-consuming nature of plastic surgical procedures, and the technical demands and variable results, many surgeons never attempt plastic surgery but invariably replace the valve.

Prosthetic and biological valves

The type of valve used in valve replacement depends very often on local preference and expertise. The original prosthetic Starr-Edwards valve – essentially a ball in a cage – was built for durability, but formed thrombus on its struts and was also rather noisy. Numerous attempts have been made to improve on this valve, with disc valves of lower profile and greater orifice area, but many of these have developed mechanical problems.

In order to avoid the anticoagulation essential with

13

mechanical valves, various attempts have been made to use biological valves. Fresh human homografts have been used very successfully in the aortic position, but the chances of a fresh homograft of the right size becoming available at the right time is small; furthermore, it is impossible to transplant the mitral valve, which therefore has to receive an aortic valve mounted in a stent. The most widely used biological valves are pig xenografts which have been treated with denaturing agents to preserve them and render them less likely to provoke biological rejection. They are usually mounted on a ring or stent and have the advantages of not requiring long-term anticoagulation, nor producing the loud prosthetic clicks of mechanical valves. Their disadvantages are that they have an unpredictable lifespan and can calcify and become stenosed very rapidly in young patients. However, most of them last at least five years and can therefore be used in women of child-bearing age who wish to have a family without the risks of long-term anticoagulation. Such patients must be prepared to face the subsequent re-operation for valve replacement when the biological valve fails. Under current legislation in the UK, a heavy goods or public service vehicle licence holder cannot drive if he is on anticoagulants, so these patients may have to opt for biological valves if they wish to maintain their occupation.

CONGENITAL HEART DISEASE: INTRODUCTION

Congenital heart disease has a different spectrum in the neonate from that in adult life. Many complex forms of congenital heart disease are incompatible with survival to adulthood, as they depend on the persistence of the fetal circulation (Fig. 13.48). As the ductus arteriosus closes, babies with some of these anomalies are at risk and the neonatal paediatric cardiologist (and surgeon) may have to intervene within a few days of birth.

With the dramatic advances in cardiac surgery over the last 20 years, more babies are having severe abnormalities corrected and are surviving into adolescence (if not yet adult life) with modified congenital heart disease. The physician may therefore see patients who have congenital heart disease presenting for the first time in adult life, or who have had their congenital lesions modified or corrected by surgery in infancy or childhood.

Congenital heart disease can therefore be present at any age, but the relative frequency of different lesions changes dramatically depending on the compatibility of the lesion with longevity. Atrial septal defect, for example, can present in the patient's seventies, but congenital aortic stenosis or co-arctation of the aorta presents much earlier, either to the physician or as a cause of sudden death.

INCIDENCE

The overall incidence of congenital heart disease is about 8 per 1000 live births. (This does not include the congenital bicuspid aortic valve which accounts for about 50% of cases of adult aortic stenosis.) The actual incidence of congenital heart disease and the relative preponderance of different lesions depends, to some extent, on whether minor degrees of pulmonary stenosis are included, and also on the age at which the assessments are made, since some ventricular septal defects close early. Almost every premature baby has a 'patent ductus arteriosus' which can really only be considered abnormal if it persists beyond 40 weeks from conception and becomes a *persistent* ductus arteriosus.

Fig. 13.48 Diagram of the fetal circulation. SVC and IVC = superior and inferior vena cava.

Table 13.15 Relative frequency of types of congenital heart disease

Congenital defect	Frequency (%)
Live births	
Atrial septal defect	30
Pulmonary stenosis	25
Tetralogy of Fallot	10
Ventricular septal defect	9
Eisenmenger syndrome	7
Patent ductus arteriosus	7
Coarctation of the aorta	5
Other	7
Stillbirths	
Ventricular septal defect	35
Univentricular heart (with tricuspid and mitral atresia)	13
Atrial septal defect	10
Coarctation of the aorta	9
Complete transposition	9
Atrioventricular septal defects	9
Hypoplastic left heart	6
Tetralogy of Fallot	3
Other	6

Similarly, some adult heart disease, such as aortic stenosis, develops on a congenitally abnormal valve (in this case bicuspid), and mitral valve prolapse may also, in many cases, be congenital rather than acquired. If these lesions were included, the rate of 8 per 1000 live births would be much higher.

The commonest forms of congenital heart disease seen after birth are shown in Table 13.15. Note the difference between these lesions and those found in stillbirths. Congenital defects may occur in combination and, even when not occurring as part of complex syndromes, there are often associated minor thoracic abnormalities, such as anomalous sternal segmentation.

AETIOLOGY

The causes of congenital heart disease are listed in Table 13.16. Most cases of congenital heart disease remain unexplained. The morphogenesis of the heart involves complex embryological processes of flexing, twisting and formation of septa and the formation and closure of foramina; it is

Table 13.16   Causes of congenital heart disease

Cause	Defect
Rubella	Patent ductus, atrial septal defect, pulmonary stenosis
Drugs	
Alcohol	Ventricular septal defect
Lithium	Ebstein's anomaly
	Tricuspid atresia
Thalidomide	Multiple defects
Inherited disease	
Connective tissue disorders	
Marfan's	Aortic dilatation and incompetence; mitral incompetence
Ehler-Danlos	Mitral regurgitation; arterial dilatation
Inborn metabolic errors	
Mucopolysaccharidoses	Valve disease, cardiomyopathy
Homocystinuria	Aortic and pulmonary dilatation
Pompe's disease	Glycogen deposition in myocardium
Chromosomal abnormalities	
Down's syndrome	Atrial and ventricular septal defect; Fallot's tetralogy; endocardial cushion defect
Trisomy 13	Ventricular septal defect; right ventricular anomalies
Turner's syndrome	Coarctation of aorta, bicuspid aortic valve; pulmonary stenosis
Other inherited syndromes	
Di George	Fallot's tetralogy; aortic arch anomalies
Friedreich's ataxia	Cardiomyopathy
Holt-Oram	Atrial septal defect
Kartagener	Dextrocardia
Tuberous sclerosis	Cardiomyopathy

thus not difficult to conceive of minor 'mistakes' in this process leading to the congenital defect. Most of these lesions develop in the first trimester of pregnancy, many at about the seventh week; other defects are related to delivery. The formation of a *patent ductus arteriosus* (more correctly a *persistent* patent ductus arteriosus) and coarctation of the aorta, appear to be due to physiological mechanisms that go wrong after birth.

Environmental factors

In some cases a maternal *viral infection* in early pregnancy, typically rubella, appears to be the cause of the congenital heart defect. Rubella produces a characteristic association of defects, including deafness, cataract and often persistent ductus arteriosus, although other lesions may occur. Although rubella is the best documented viral agent, mumps and influenza epidemics have been shown to increase the risk of congenital defects if the mother has the illness early in pregnancy. Other agents, such as cytomegalovirus, herpes and coxsackie, have also been implicated. About 5% of cases of congenital heart disease can be explained by viral illness.

Maternal illness has been suggested as an agent for congenital atrioventricular block. In one series, 30% of the mothers had evidence of collagen disease, most commonly SLE. *Drugs* taken by the mother can be teratogenic, and drugs now associated with congenital heart disease include alcohol, lithium, amphetamines, phenytoin, oestrogen/progesterone and trimethadione.

Chromosomal abnormalities and counselling

Chromosomal abnormalities can be accompanied by congenital heart disease. Down's syndrome (Mongolism or trisomy 21, see Ch. 6, p. 89) is associated with endocardial cushion or atrioventricular canal defects (ASD mitral and tricuspid regurgitation), but ventricular septal defects and pulmonary stenosis also have an increased incidence. Turner's syndrome (XO) – characterised by stunted growth, web neck, female sexual stunting and cubitus valgus – has a greatly increased incidence of coarctation of the aorta and pulmonary stenosis. Spontaneously aborted fetuses have a much higher incidence of severe congenital heart disease than do normal term infants (Table 13.15), and this natural mechanism prevents a higher neonatal death rate from congenital heart disease incompatible with an independent existence.

A mother who has congenital heart disease herself, or who has one affected child, can usually be counselled that subsequent pregnancy carries a low risk (1–5%) of congenital heart disease. Occasionally, there are families who have a dominant Mendelian inheritance for heart disease (e.g. hypertrophic cardiomyopathy). Concordance rates for identical twins are between 15 and 20%, and for non-identical twins between 3 and 5%, suggesting environmental as well as genetic factor(s) in the development of congenital heart disease.

Cardiovascular Disease

CYANOTIC CONGENITAL HEART DISEASE

Central cyanosis occurs when venous blood in sufficient quantity passes across to the arterial side of the heart without passing through the lungs. A degree of shunting through the ductus arteriosus occurs for several hours, or even days, after birth and this may persist; more commonly, however, right-to-left shunting occurs through persisting embryonic defects or through the foramen ovale (Fig. 13.49). The persistence of central cyanosis after birth, or its onset later on, only occurs if such a 'hole-in-the-heart' is present, and if the resistance to outflow from the right heart is higher than that of the left.

High resistance to outflow of the right heart is usually caused by congenital pulmonary stenosis (valvular or muscular) or by the development of pulmonary hypertension from constriction of the pulmonary resistance vessels. Acquired pulmonary hypertension occurs with high flow through the lungs, so a left-to-right shunt can eventually reverse and become right-to-left with cyanosis (the *Eisenmenger reaction*).

Cyanotic heart disease produces a characteristic appearance with central cyanosis which may vary with activity, clubbing, impaired growth and intellectual development (if severe) and marked polycythaemia after the first year of life. Complications of the right-to-left shunt include cerebral abscess and paradoxical emboli, in which embolism from clot in peripheral veins gains access to the systemic circulation through the shunt. The severe polycythaemia can lead to thrombosis and infarction. Pulmonary hypertension can be complicated by recurrent haemoptysis, with severe haemorrhage. The high pulmonary artery pressure may lead to calcification of the pulmonary arteries.

FALLOT'S TETRALOGY

Fallot's tetralogy is the commonest form of cyanotic congenital heart disease seen after the age of one year. The four main features of this abnormality (Fig. 13.50) are:

1. *a ventricular septal defect* (through which the shunting occurs)
2. *pulmonary stenosis*, which may be muscular or valvular and acts as the obstruction which leads to the right to left flow

3. *an over-riding aorta.* The aorta is positioned above the ventricular septal defect
4. *right ventricular hypertrophy*, due to the pressure and volume load to which the RV is subjected.

Incomplete forms of the condition exist in which not all the features are present and the child may be acyanotic.

Clinical features

The child is deeply cyanosed and subject to cyanotic and exertional syncopal episodes which appear to be related to changes in the degree of muscular pulmonary stenosis and, thus, shunting. The physical signs are cyanosis, clubbing, right ventricular hypertrophy, a harsh systolic murmur at the upper left sternal edge (often with a thrill) and a single second heart sound.

Investigation

The characteristic features of Fallot's tetralogy on investigation are illustrated in Figure 13.50. Chest X-ray shows a characteristic cardiac silhouette of severe right ventricular hypertrophy which lifts the cardiac apex (*coeur en sabot*) and oligaemic lung fields. ECG shows right ventricular hypertrophy. Echocardiogram shows the over-riding aorta and ventricular septal defect and, with Doppler, can demonstrate the pulmonary stenosis, the right ventricular pressure and, sometimes, the flow through the ventricular septal defect. Cardiac catheterisation can be used to measure the pressures and show the severity of the outflow tract obstruction.

Treatment

Total surgical correction is now often attempted at an early age, but a holding or palliative operation to increase the lung blood flow is often performed. A subclavian artery is anastomosed to a pulmonary artery (the Blalock-Taussig anastomosis), and this provides sufficient flow for the baby to grow before the full correction is attempted.

LESS COMMON FORMS OF CYANOTIC CONGENITAL HEART DISEASE

Some of the less common forms of cyanotic congenital heart disease are important causes of neonatal and infant

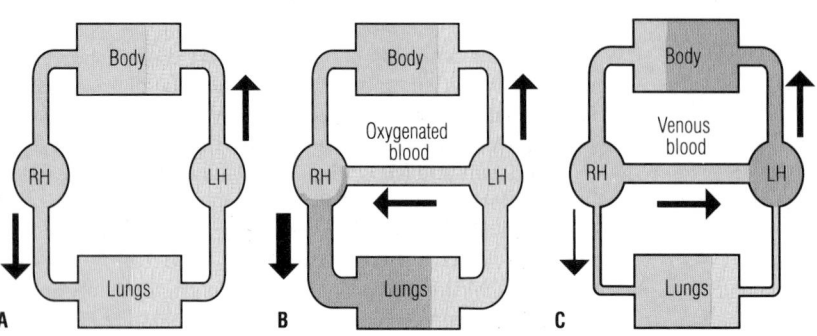

Fig. 13.49 Diagrammatic representation of blood flow in the systemic and pulmonary circulation. **A.** Normal. **B.** Left-to-right shunt. **C.** Right-to-left shunt; the pulmonary blood flow is reduced as a result of development of high resistance. RH = right heart. LH = left heart.

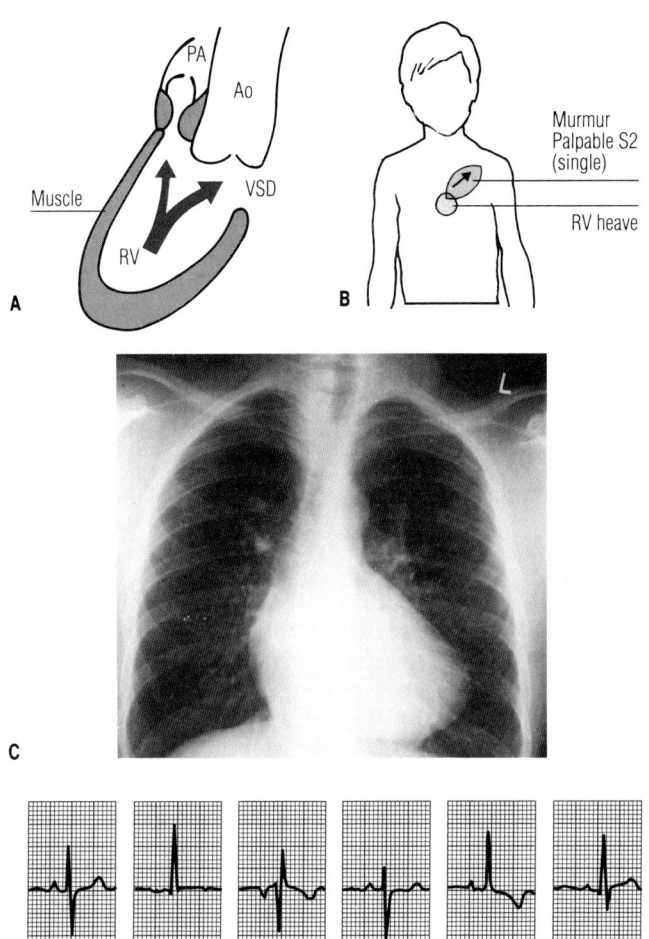

Fig. 13.50 Features of Fallot's tetralogy. A. Diagram of abnormality. VSD = ventricular septal defect; PA = pulmonary artery; Ao = aorta. **B.** Physical signs. **C.** Chest X-ray showing right ventricular hypertrophy, typical 'coeur en sabot'. **D.** ECG showing right atrial and ventricular hypertrophy and right axis deviation.

death; however, they may be diagnosed accurately with modern imaging techniques and can then be treated surgically. Even in neonates, cardiac transplantation and heart lung transplantation may make some formerly inoperable conditions amenable to surgery.

Transposition of the great arteries

Transposition of the great arteries (TGA) comprises some 4% of congenital heart disease at birth. The aorta and pulmonary arteries are connected to the 'wrong ventricles'. The RV gives rise to an anterior aorta, and the LV to a posterior pulmonary artery. This results in two separate circulations joined usually by an atrial connection, often a persistent ductus arteriosus and, in 30% of cases, a ventricular septal defect. This is termed *d-transposition* after the embryonic origin of the defect. In corrected transposition (*l-transposition*), the malpositioned aorta and pulmonary artery are connected to similarly malpositioned left and right ventricles. This results in a 'corrected circulation' which may be asymptomatic, but which is often associated with other cardiac anomalies. Various degrees of transposition (or malrotation) are possible, giving rise to other conditions; these include double outlet right ventricle (DORV), in which both great vessels arise from the right ventricle, and (less common still) double outlet left ventricle. The clinical features are dyspnoea and cyanosis from birth, leading to cardiac failure.

These anomalies may complicate many other types of congenital heart disease. TGA is treated by atrial septostomy when diagnosed and, eventually, by full surgical correction using the 'Mustard' technique, in which an intra-atrial baffle (membrane) redirects the blood flow.

Total anomalous pulmonary venous drainage

Total anomalous pulmonary venous drainage occurs when the pulmonary veins enter the right atrium and there is an interatrial connection. There is a large range of associated congenital lesions and a wide range of types of anomaly of the venous system. Partial anomalous venous drainage also occurs. Infants present with dyspnoea, cyanosis and right heart failure. Treatment is by surgical correction.

Truncus arteriosus

In truncus arteriosus, a single major vessel arises from both ventricles. There is a large VSD and, often, an incompetent valve with from two to four leaflets. There may be a single coronary artery. Survival is only possible with successful repair, but even then the long-term prognosis is poor.

Tricuspid atresia

Tricuspid atresia is often present as a complex and variable malformation which includes an absent tricuspid orifice and an interatrial communication. There may be a hypoplastic right ventricle associated with a VSD and various degrees of pulmonary stenosis and transposition of great arteries. The infant is cyanotic and survival is unusual without surgical intervention. Shunting operations are performed, with 20-year survivals of up to 40%.

Ebstein's anomaly of the tricuspid valve

In Ebstein's anomaly of the tricuspid valve, the septal and posterior leaflets of the tricuspid valve are attached to the right ventricular wall so that a large part of the right ventricle becomes atrialised. The right ventricle is small, but the right atrium becomes enormous. There is often some tricuspid regurgitation, and occasionally the abnormal valve obstructs filling, or even emptying, of the right ventricle. There is a high incidence of patent foramen ovale or atrial septal defect, and supraventricular arrhythmias are

393

very common and often produce the presenting symptoms. The condition often presents in adult life. It may remain asymptomatic for years and present with an abnormal chest X-ray or ECG. The patient may, on the other hand, present with right heart failure, dyspnoea on exertion and, sometimes, mild cyanosis and clubbing. Occasionally, there are other associated congenital defects.

Clinically, the heart is large and inactive. There is often a murmur of tricuspid regurgitation and a cV wave in the neck. ECG shows small voltages, right atrial hypertrophy and right bundle branch block. A Wolff-Parkinson-White configuration (p. 367) is common. Chest X-ray shows a globular or flask-shaped heart with a prominent convex right atrial border. Echocardiogram and cardiac catheterisation findings are quite characteristic.

ACYANOTIC CONGENITAL HEART DISEASE

Left-to-right shunting commonly occurs through atrial septal defects, ventricular septal defects and through persistent ductus arteriosus.

ATRIAL SEPTAL DEFECT

Atrial septal defects (ASD) can be of three types – secundum, primum or sinus venosus defect (Fig. 13.51). In adult cardiology, they occur in the above order of decreasing frequency, and the foramen ovale only acts as an ASD if right-sided pressures exceed left; such as may occur with massive pulmonary embolism.

Pathogenesis

The defect in the atrial septum allows blood from the left atrium to join the venous blood passing into the right ventricle and lungs. Because the lungs have a low impedance to flow, shunting is considerable and is increased further by any associated lesion of the left side of the heart that raises the left atrial pressure. The patient has a limited exercise capacity, as a maximal systemic cardiac output cannot be achieved on exercise. The right ventricle hypertrophies and the lung blood flow is increased, which seems to increase the likelihood of pulmonary infections. Symptoms are usually not prominent until middle-age and include dyspnoea, fatigue (low exercise cardiac output) and, quite frequently, palpitations which are caused by atrial arrhythmias. Heart failure, when it occurs, is usually both right and left-sided, since any rise in atrial pressure on one side of the septum will shunt the blood to the other side.

After middle-age, the pulmonary vascular resistance may rise, with the development of massive pulmonary arteries (visible on chest X-ray) and, occasionally, reversal of the shunt.

Secundum atrial septal defect

Clinical features

Secundum ASD (Fig. 13.52) is usually uncomplicated. The physical signs are the result of right ventricular hypertrophy and increased flow through the right side of the heart; this causes pulmonary and tricuspid flow murmurs and delayed closure of the pulmonary valve. The associated signs are wide, fixed splitting of the second sound and pulmonary systolic murmur; a tricuspid diastolic murmur is usually heard if shunting is significant.

Investigation and treatment

Chest X-ray (Fig. 13.52) shows enlargement of the heart commensurate with the size of the shunt, prominent pulmonary arteries, pulmonary plethora and, usually, a small aortic knuckle. ECG shows right bundle branch block in most cases, with right axis deviation. Echocardiography shows dilated RV with a 'volume load' of the RV which dominates the septal movement; the latter therefore appears 'paradoxical', i.e. it moves away from the free wall of the left ventricle in systole towards the free wall of the right ventricle. The shunt can be demonstrated by contrast

Fig. 13.51 **Sites of atrial septal defect. A.** Ostium secundum. **B.** Ostium primum (or atrioventricular canal defect). The septal leaflet of the mitral valve is often involved, allowing a communication between the left ventricle (LV) and both atria. **C.** Sinus venosus defect, where the abnormality involves anomalous pulmonary venous drainage. SVC and IVC = superior and inferior vena cava. PV = pulmonary vein.

A

B V1 V6

ECG

Phono

C S1 A2 P2

RV

IVS

LV

PW

D

Fig. 13.52 Features of atrial septal defect. A. Chest X-ray showing enlarged pulmonary arteries, pulmonary plethora and relatively small aortic knuckle. **B.** ECG showing a vertical axis (normal) and partial RBBB. **C.** Phonocardiogram demonstrating wide splitting of second heart sound. **D.** M mode echocardiogram at the ventricular level, shows a volume overload RV with paradoxical movement of the interventricular septum (IVS) which is out of phase with the posterior wall of the left ventricle (PW).

injection of saline or with colour Doppler.

Cardiac catheterisation was traditionally used to demonstrate the size of the shunt. Blood samples taken in the different cardiac chambers show a step-up in oxygen content of the blood occurring at the lower right atrium. The shunt size can be calculated from the oxygen content of the pulmonary artery blood and left-sided samples. Angiography demonstrates the type of ASD and any associated mitral regurgitation.

Surgical closure is usually advised if the defect is associated with a shunt which gives a pulmonary flow greater than 1.5 times systemic flow.

Primum atrial septal defect

Primum ASD is a much less common form and accounts for 10% of ASDs but is relatively common in Down's syndrome. Apart from a different anatomical site, there are often also associated abnormalities of the mitral valve and the structures forming the atrio-ventricular valve region.

Clinical features, investigation and treatment

The clinical features are similar to those of secundum ASD, but there may be associated mitral regurgitation

and the ECG usually shows a left axis deviation. Left ventricular angiography shows a 'swan neck deformity' of the LV and any associated mitral regurgitation.

Surgical correction is more complex than for a secundum defect, and may involve mitral valve repair or replacement.

Sinus venosus defect

Sinus venous defect is a high right atrial defect near the junction with the superior vena cava. It is often associated with anomalous pulmonary venous drainage into the right atrium.

VENTRICULAR SEPTAL DEFECT

Ventricular septal defects may occur as isolated lesions or be associated with other congenital defects of the heart. They are relatively common (Table 13.15), but many close spontaneously during childhood. They may occur as muscular, membranous, infundibular or posterior (AV) defects and may be multiple. The left ventricular pressure exceeds the right throughout most of the cardiac cycle, so there is considerable shunting of blood from left to right unless a rise in pulmonary outflow resistance occurs. This tends to happen in pulmonary hypertension if there is a very large pulmonary flow. In extreme cases, the flow reverses causing cyanosis and the Eisenmenger syndrome.

Small ventricular septal defects

Small VSDs are common and are asymptomatic. There is a loud systolic murmur with a thrill at the left sternal edge (Maladie de Roger), with no associated cardiomegaly and minimal, if any, changes of pulmonary plethora on chest X-ray. Differential diagnosis is from mitral regurgitation and is simply accomplished with Doppler ultrasound. Echocardiography may not show a small defect and the ECG is usually normal.

The only complication of a small VSD is the risk of *endocarditis*, and endocarditis prophylaxis is essential. Although the surgical mortality and morbidity for closure of small defects is low, surgery is not usually necessary.

Moderate and large-sized ventricular septal defects

With larger VSDs, systemic cardiac output is limited on exercise and can produce symptoms of fatigue and dyspnoea. As they are both volume loaded, both ventricles enlarge with displacement of the cardiac apex. The pansystolic murmur and thrill of Maladie de Roger may be softer in these patients, as the jet velocity of the VSD and the pressure gradient between the ventricles becomes smaller the larger the defect. As pulmonary hypertension becomes prominent, the murmur may almost disappear as the pressures in the two ventricles balance.

Investigation and treatment

The features of VSDs on investigation are illustrated in Figure 13.53. ECG shows biventricular hypertrophy, and there is increasing right ventricular hypertrophy with pulmonary hypertension. Chest X-ray shows pulmonary plethora, and cardiomegaly with both right and left ventricular hypertrophy. As pulmonary hypertension develops, the central pulmonary arteries increase in size and the peripheral vessels become pruned.

Echocardiography and Doppler ultrasound can show the location of the VSD, and can be used to calculate RV pressure from the VSD jet velocity (the derived pressure gradient; see p. 350) and the systolic blood pressure.

Surgical closure is advised unless pulmonary artery pressure has risen too high.

COARCTATION OF THE AORTA

Coarctation of the aorta is a narrowing, or even complete interruption, of the aorta distal to the aortic arch, with blood flow to the lower body augmented by flow carried through collateral vessels. Coarctation represents about 5% of adult congenital heart disease, and is seen in males three times as frequently as females. The condition leads to upper body hypertension and also an increased risk of aortic dissection. There is frequently a bicuspid aortic

Fig. 13.53 Features of ventricular septal defect. A. The characteristic systolic murmur associated with a widely split second heart sound with a premature aortic second sound (A2) and maintained mobility of P2 with respiration (dashed line on inspiration). **B.** Doppler ultrasound showing high velocity jet (6 m/s). **C** and **D.** 2D echocardiogram showing the septal defect (VSD). IVS = interventricular septum.

valve, which can become stenotic (or is congenitally stenosed). Other congenital defects are sometimes associated. There is also an associated risk of subarachnoid haemorrhage from berry aneurysm of the circle of Willis. These occur with greater frequency than in essential hypertension, and are presumed to be an associated congenital anomaly.

The coarctation is nearly always at the aortic isthmus distal to the left subclavian artery, but can, rarely, occur proximal to it. The mechanism is thought to be related to ductal tissue in the wall of the aorta leading to progressive stenosis of the aorta by the same mechanism as results in ductal closure. The degree of stenosis becomes comparatively more severe as the child grows, so that a baby with minimal signs may grow into an adult with features of severe coarctation. The coarctation is followed by a post-stenotic dilatation in most cases; however if there is complete interruption of the aorta, there may be some atresia of the descending aorta.

Clinical features

Hypertension with a systolic murmur and delayed or absent femoral pulse are the hallmarks of the condition, and these should be sought in any young hypertensive.

Presenting complaints include left ventricular failure, subarachnoid haemorrhage and aortic dissection; however, most cases should be identified in childhood. The coarctation itself may become the site of an endocarditis, as may the bicuspid valve.

The physical signs are hypertension, a large volume

pulse in the arms and carotids, and weak, delayed, femoral pulses; occasionally, the left subclavian is involved in the coarctation, producing weak left arm pulses. There is often palpable left ventricular hypertrophy, a systolic murmur over the precordium and in the back, and palpable collateral arteries running over the medial aspects of the scapulae.

Investigation

Diagnosis is confirmed by demonstrating a lower systolic blood pressure in the ankles than in the brachial artery with Doppler ultrasound. The chest X-ray often shows the characteristic '3' sign over the aortic knuckle, with the upper half being the left subclavian artery and the lower half the post-stenotic dilatation of the aorta. Rib-notching is seen in most adults with coarctation, and is caused by the collateral arteries.

Visualisation of the coarctation is sometimes possible from the suprasternal notch using 2D echocardiography, and the jet can often be located with Doppler ultrasound from the same site. Angiography of the aorta is not always needed, but cardiac catheterisation is often performed to look for associated lesions and to confirm the length of the narrow segment.

Treatment and prognosis

Significant coarctation should always be treated surgically in children. If the diagnosis is made in adulthood, the surgical management is more difficult and carries a high morbidity and mortality, as the patient then has established hypertension with changes in the aortic wall. In addition, reversal of hypertension does not occur. The associated aortic valve lesions may progress and complicate matters, as may subarachnoid haemorrhage.

PERSISTENT DUCTUS ARTERIOSUS

Persistent ductus arteriosus (PDA) is a congenital abnormality caused by failure of the ductus arteriosus to close and form the ligamentum arteriosum. The result is a shunt of blood from the aorta into the pulmonary circulation. The shunt is from the aorta just distal to the left subclavian artery, and so an increased flow occurs through the left heart and pulmonary circulation but not the right heart.

The ductus arteriosus remains patent for a variable time after birth, and failure to close can be associated with congenital abnormalities other than PDA. The isolated lesion is usually diagnosed in childhood from the presence of a continuous or 'machinery murmur' at the upper left sternal edge.

Clinical features

Overload of the left heart can lead to heart failure in older patients. The increased lung blood flow in infants can present with the consequences of increased pulmonary vascular resistance; extremely rarely, reversal of the flow

through the ductus with cyanotic blood passing to the distal aorta occurs, and clubbing of the toes but not the fingers. Rarely, the ductus may be the site of endocarditis.

Investigation and treatment

Diagnosis is based on the physical findings of the characteristic murmur, a collapsing pulse and a chest X-ray which usually shows a prominent pulmonary conus and increased lung blood flow.

Echocardiography and Doppler ultrasound are extremely useful in demonstrating both the lesion and the volume load on the left ventricle. Cardiac catheterisation with aortography is not usually necessary in the uncomplicated case, but it may be useful in differentiating the much less common aorto-pulmonary window, which requires much more complex surgery.

The simple case requires ligation and transection of the PDA.

COR TRIATRIATUM

In cor triatriatum the left atrium is divided by a diaphragm above the mitral valve which gives rise to obstruction to pulmonary venous return to the left heart. There is a variable size orifice (or none at all) which is easily opened surgically. The condition is thus eminently treatable.

DEXTROCARDIA

Dextrocardia – in which there is a mirror image of the normal heart – is usually quite benign if associated with situs inversus (stomach bubble also on the right); however, it may be associated with other congenital abnormalities and can be confused with dextroversion, in which the heart is rotated rather than being a mirror image.

ISCHAEMIC HEART DISEASE

Although ischaemia may be produced whenever there is an imbalance between tissue demand for blood supply and its delivery, ischaemic heart disease (IHD) can be considered virtually synonymous with coronary artery disease, and hence with a failure in supply. Atheromatous disease outweighs all other causes, but coronary arteritis and embolism can cause ischaemia. Demand exceeds supply in very hypertrophied ventricles, especially in aortic valve disease.

THE CORONARY CIRCULATION

Flow in normal and abnormal coronary arteries

Flow through the coronary arteries is regulated, with mean flow maintained through wide changes in mean arterial pressure (Fig. 13.54). However, coronary vascular resistance is greatly affected by extrinsic compression during

13

Fig. 13.54   Coronary arterial flow. A. Aortic pressure. **B.** Flow in the left and right coronary arteries. Note the abrupt fall in left coronary flow with the onset of systole.

Fig. 13.55   Effect of mean coronary arterial pressure on flow (solid line). Coronary occlusion affects flow as shown by red circles. The limits of coronary autoregulation are shown by the arrows.

cardiac muscle contraction. Compression of the intra-myocardial vessels during systole means that flow occurs in diastole. This is particularly marked for the left coronary artery. Myocardial vessels are innervated and respond to neural, humoral and local metabolites.

The heart has little capacity for anaerobic metabolism, nor for the build-up of an oxygen debt. It is therefore dependent on increased perfusion to cope with an increased oxygen demand if irreversible damage is to be avoided. The major determinant of oxygen consumption is contractile activity, and this can be related to myocardial tension production (more accurately, the index of tension and time). Myocardial oxygen extraction is not increased with increasing demand during exercise, so that an increase in demand must be met by increased coronary flow following coronary vasodilatation. The coronary vascular resistance will fall to 20–25% of its basal state in response to maximal demand during exercise. This ability to lower the resistance to flow explains why it is possible to maintain normal flow at rest, even when there is an 80% reduction in the diameter of a large coronary artery. The relationship between changes in the luminal diameter in coronary arteries and flow is shown in Figure 13.55.

Coronary anatomy

The anatomy of the coronary circulation is shown in Figure 13.56. Three major coronary arteries provide the heart with its blood supply. The major anatomical features are remarkably constant for the three main epicardial vessels. The main stems of the left coronary artery (LCA) and the right coronary artery (RCA) arise from the aorta at the sinuses of Valsalva. The main stem of the left coronary is a relatively short vessel. It divides into the left anterior descending artery (LAD) – which is responsible for the blood supply to the major part of the left ventricle and the

interventricular septum – and the circumflex artery (Cx, usually the smaller branch of the left main stem), which supplies the posterior and variable amounts of the inferior walls of the left ventricle. The right coronary artery supplies the right ventricle and inferior left ventricle. In some individuals, variable amounts of the left ventricular apex, septum and posterior wall may be supplied by the RCA. This artery usually provides the sino-atrial and atrio-ventricular nodes with their blood supply.

Major anatomical variations exist, but are rare. Individual differences in supply usually relate to the relative importance of the RCA and Cx, with occasional individuals where the LAD appears to be of relatively minor importance. The myocardium has a very rich capillary network which appears to be regulated by precapillary resistance vessels; these form the anatomical substrate for autoregulation. In addition, there is sometimes (but not always) a network of collateral vessels connecting coronary arterial networks to each other. If present, these collaterals become important in coronary artery disease.

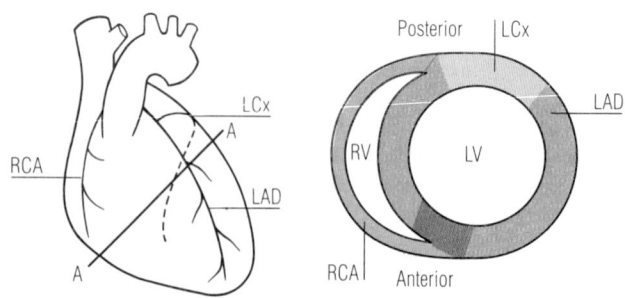

Fig. 13.56   Anatomy of the coronary circulation. LAD = left anterior descending, LCx = left circumflex, (dotted line represents position of LCx at the back of the heart), RCA = right coronary artery. Section across heart (A-A) shows the approximate distribution of blood supply.

ATHEROMATOUS DISEASE OF THE CORONARY ARTERIES

The commonest cause of changes in the luminal diameter of the epicardial coronary arteries is the presence of atheromatous plaques. These are complex lesions which are not uniform in structure even within one vessel. The lesions may encircle an artery or be eccentric; they may be discrete and localised or involve the greater length of the vessel. The eccentricity of some plaques may be important when vasospasm is the cause of angina; the normal arterial wall opposite the plaque (Fig. 13.57) maintains its ability to contract, producing a very marked reduction in cross-sectional area even if the smooth muscle contraction is modest in degree and the atheromatous plaque small. Other acute changes in the plaques may account for unstable angina, myocardial infarction and sudden death. There is evidence from post-mortem studies, and direct visualisation of affected arteries, that an acute fissure develops, breaching the thin endothelium which covers a lipid-rich plaque. Haemorrhage occurs into the plaque, acutely increasing the stenosis. Additionally, the endothelial breach may precipitate the rapid development of a clot, with total or subtotal occlusion of the vessel. These events appear to account for many instances of the more acute forms of coronary disease, and have renewed interest in the role of thrombosis in acute cardiac ischaemia. This has led to the successful use of fibrinolytic agents and aspirin in the treatment of infarction (p. 410).

As well as becoming more severe, there is now reason to believe that under some circumstances atheromatous plaques may regress. This has been achieved by drugs which lower LDL cholesterol and triglyceride and increase HDL cholesterol.

Clinical features

Ischaemic heart disease is a condition with characteristic symptoms but few physical signs until its complications become severe.

Symptoms

The cardinal symptom is angina. This is a chest discomfort precipitated by exertion and relieved by rest. It is often described as a pressing or constricting feeling and, less often, as a pain. It remains remarkably constant within each individual, even though its precipitants may vary significantly from day to day. The patient may often accompany the description with a clenched fist held in front of the sternum indicating the squeezing nature of the pain, and he may describe radiating discomfort in the arm (left more often than right), the jaw or even a choking sensation in the throat. Dyspnoea frequently accompanies angina. There is usually rapid relief of the symptom with sublingual, or spray, glyceryl trinitrate.

The pain of myocardial infarction may be similar in many ways, but generally begins at rest, does not respond so well to nitrates, lasts longer than 20 minutes and is often associated with feelings of impending death, nausea, sweating and collapse.

Unfortunately, in a large proportion of patients with ischaemic heart disease, the first manifestation of the disease may be sudden death. Prevention of atheroma will be necessary to reduce this, although out-of-hospital resuscitation may improve the survival of the few fortunate enough to collapse within reach of a person competent in basic life support.

Signs

Some individuals undoubtedly have significant ischaemic episodes without symptoms. This may be discovered by routine ECG, when pathological Q waves may be found with no history of any antecedent chest pains. Investigations of patients with ambulatory recorders have also shown some individuals to have changes in the ST segments usually associated with ischaemia, despite a total lack of symptoms. Even patients with known angina may have episodes of ST segment change which appear to be clinically silent. Patients with known coronary disease who have silent ischaemia fare worse than those without this finding.

There are few physical findings in uncomplicated ischaemic heart disease. There may be evidence of hypertension or hyperlipidaemia. Cardiac dilatation, hypertrophy and failure are all late features and are non-specific.

Other anginal syndromes

The above is a description of the typical stable atheromatous coronary artery disease. Several other anginal syndromes occur which are less common but which often have implications for management.

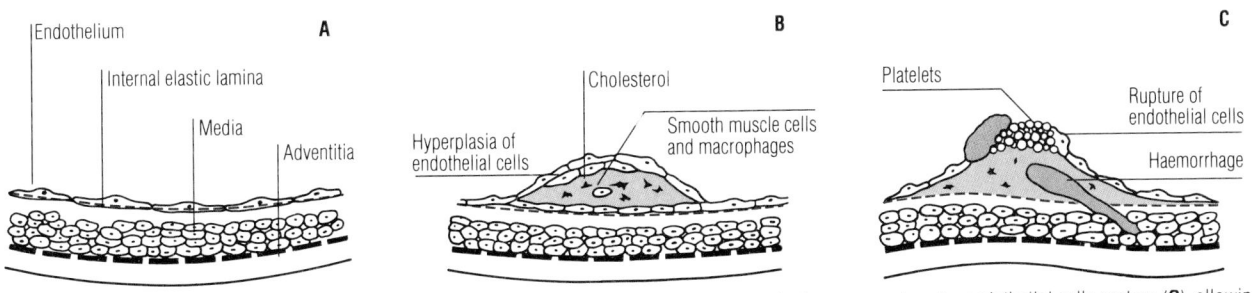

Fig. 13.57 Progression of atheromatous lesion. A. Normal endothelium. **B.** Acute expansion of the lesion occurs when the endothelial cells rupture (**C**), allowing haemorrhage into the plaque and platelet aggregation on the endothelial surface.

Crescendo angina and unstable angina

Both crescendo and unstable angina may represent states of pre-infarction, when atheromatous plaques have fissured and the degree of coronary stenosis is waxing and waning. In *crescendo angina*, a history of increasingly frequent attacks of angina with ever-diminishing levels of exertion is obtained. *Unstable angina* includes situations where episodes of pain are frequent, may occur without obvious cause and at rest, and where acute infarction has been excluded. *Decubitus angina* is angina occurring at rest in bed.

Vasospastic angina

It is now recognised that abnormalities other than fixed stenotic lesions are important in angina. Some degree of arterial spasm is probably present in most episodes of angina, but spasm occurring in an otherwise normal coronary artery has also been observed. It can be severe enough to cause infarction, but is very rare. In *Prinzmetal's syndrome*, rest pain is frequent and is associated with acute ST segment elevation which resolves to normal with cessation of pain. This condition is rare and almost certainly involves coronary vasospasm.

Differential diagnosis

Recently, the management of acute myocardial infarction and chest pain due to unstable angina has become much more active; it has thus become even more important to diagnose correctly the condition even before confirmatory changes on ECG and in biochemical tests are available. In particular, the use of thrombolysis in the earliest phases of infarction means that certain possible alternative causes of chest pain should be excluded before treatment is begun. Confusion may also arise due to the coexistence of two relatively common conditions in the same patient. Angina is a common symptom in aortic stenosis (p. 383) and aortic regurgitation (p. 385), particularly when the valve lesions are severe or acute. In cases of aortic regurgitation due to syphilis, chest pains may be due to severe aortic reflux, but coronary ostial stenosis may also occur. In hypertrophic cardiomyopathy, hypertrophy may lead to angina.

Acute pericarditis. Chest pain may be severe with acute pericarditis and is exacerbated by movement, deep respiration or coughing. It is often relieved by sitting forward and by non-steroidal anti-inflammatory drugs (NSAIDs). The clinical sign of pericardial friction rub may come and go, much to the consternation of GPs.

Oesophageal spasm. The pain of oesophageal spasm may be severe and, since it occurs at rest and can be associated with T wave changes on the ECG, it may cause considerable confusion and be diagnosed as unstable angina in some patients. Just how commonly this condition is missed is disputed; interestingly, the calcium antagonist drugs may be effective therapy. Oesophageal manometry has been used to study the condition, but is not often resorted to (by cardiologists) in routine practice.

Hiatus hernia with oesophagitis can cause chest pain. This can be demonstrated by infusions of mild acidic mixtures into the oesophagus of affected individuals. Radiological and endoscopic methods will demonstrate the abnormalities, but these are common conditions and ischaemic heart disease may coexist in the same individual.

Acute cholecystitis and peptic ulceration can produce severe pains in the lower chest and xiphisternal areas and may, infrequently, be mistaken for acute myocardial infarction. Non-specific T wave changes on the ECG have been observed during these acute illnesses.

Da Costa's syndrome (also known by several other names, e.g. neurocirculatory asthenia) has a long history and is characterised by sharp transient chest pains which occur with relaxation, may disappear with exertion and are associated with easy fatigue.

Mitral valve prolapse. Atypical (for IHD) chest pains may occur in patients with mitral valve prolapse of mild degree. This condition can be very troublesome and difficult to treat.

Hyperventilation. Patients who hyperventilate may produce symptoms indistinguishable from angina, and may have an abnormal resting and exercise ECG to accompany their symptoms.

So-called *Syndrome X* is characterised by typical angina in association with radiologically normal coronary arteries.

Finally, *Tietze's syndrome* (p. 499) may cause diagnostic confusion until the painful costal cartilage is palpated.

Investigation

The aim of investigations is to confirm that the clinical history is due to significant coronary artery disease, and to determine at how much risk of infarction or progression the patient may be, and whether any remediable risk factors may be present. Once coronary artery disease has been confirmed using non-invasive tests, an assessment of ventricular function may be necessary and, finally, coronary angiography performed if surgery or angioplasty are being considered. (Investigation of myocardial infarction is considered on pages 407–9.)

ECG

The resting ECG may be normal in ischaemic heart disease, even when it is severe. Signs of ischaemia characteristically involve the ST segments, with depression in the leads corresponding to the myocardial territory involved (Fig. 13.58). The associated T waves may be flattened or biphasic. These electrocardiographic signs are not specific, however; they may be found in some normal individuals and may be produced by hyperventilation or change in posture.

Exercise test

The exercise test has been described on page 345. Exercise will induce ischaemia with coronary stenoses of 70% or more (Fig. 13.58). Its uses and its sensitivity and specificity depend upon the clinical context of the test. Thus, if a

Fig. 13.58 Exercise ECG showing typical and severe down-sloping ST segment depression.

population of asymptomatic individuals is subjected to an exercise test there will be a higher incidence of false positive tests (10–20%) than if it is being used in a group of patients with suspected angina (less than 8%) It is therefore not a very good screening test for coronary artery disease in the population, although it is routinely used in late middle-aged aviators.

The exercise ECG has several uses:

1. to detect ischaemic heart disease in patients with suspicious symptoms
2. to gauge severity and the site of the coronary artery disease, although accurate anatomical localisation is not possible
3. to identify patients at high risk of further infarction or death early after myocardial infarction
4. to assess functional capacity.

Although changes in the ST segment are the most characteristic features of a positive exercise test (Fig. 13.58), the development of angina and the workload performed up to the development of symptoms or ECG change are additional variables which aid interpretation. A normal blood pressure response consists of a rise in systolic pressure by at least 20 mmHg. Diastolic pressure falls with exercise, but is so difficult to measure under these circumstances that it is not routinely taken. The gravest prognostic indicator in exercise testing is a failure of systolic pressure to rise, or even a fall. The appearance of multiple ventricular ectopic beats is also associated with severe disease.

Radionuclide studies

Radionuclide techniques (discussed on page 350) are complementary to the other non-invasive methods used in assessing ischaemic heart disease. Information on ventricular wall motion abnormalities (MUGA scan) and regional perfusion (^{201}Tl scan) can be obtained, which is not available from the resting and exercise ECG.

Echocardiography and Doppler ultrasound

Echocardiography (p. 348) may be useful to assess ventricular function and wall motion abnormalities, while Doppler ultrasound (p. 349) can show valvular regurgitation and intracardiac shunting, such as acute septal rupture.

Ambulatory ECG (Holter) monitoring

Ambulatory ECG monitoring (p. 358) is generally used to detect arrhythmias, but these recordings may also detect episodes of ST segment change during normal activities. Some of these episodes may not be accompanied by symptoms of angina (silent ischaemia). In the patient with known coronary disease, frequent episodes of silent ischaemia are associated with a high risk of infarction. In the patient with few or no symptoms the implications of this finding are not at all clear. The role of routine 24-hour ECG recording for ST segment analysis in IHD is not established, since it remains to be proven that the information gained is any more useful than the exercise test, which is rather easier to perform and currently more widely available.

Magnetic resonance imaging

The non-invasive technique of magnetic resonance imaging (p. 351) may yet be used for the assessment of ventricular function in ischaemic heart disease. However, the equipment is large, costly and as yet unable to image the coronary arteries. Magnetic resonance spectroscopy is a non-invasive technique enabling quantification of the amount of high energy phosphate within working muscle cells.

Left ventricular and coronary angiography

Left ventricular and coronary angiography (p. 351) are the standards by which all other techniques used in the assessment of ischaemic heart disease are judged. The aim of the investigation is to establish the functional state of the left ventricle, to exclude valve lesions which might account for the symptoms (such as occult aortic stenosis), and to obtain detailed pictures of the coronary arteries.

A global LV ejection fraction (EF) of 60–70% is normal, and end diastolic pressure is usually below 12 mmHg. Subjective assessment is often sufficient to describe LV wall motion abnormalities without recourse to the numerical estimation of EF.

The coronary arteries are selectively intubated and cineangiograms taken in several projections. A 70% reduction in the diameter of an artery is generally considered to be a clinically significant stenosis.

Cardiac catheterisation provides unambiguous information on the location of coronary artery stenoses. However, the clinical significance of stenoses is sometimes difficult to judge, so that the exercise test and thallium scan may provide complementary information. Cardiac catheterisation is indicated in all patients in whom treatment of angina by coronary angioplasty or coronary bypass surgery is being contemplated. In some patients with troublesome symptoms and a low likelihood of IHD, this examination is performed in order to finally exclude the possibility of coronary artery disease. This group may comprise between 10 and 20% of all patients undergoing cardiac catheterisation.

The invasive nature of catheterisation is necessarily associated with a morbidity (less than 1.0%) and mortality

Cardiovascular Disease

(less than 0.1%). This means that angiography cannot assume the role of a screening test for coronary disease.

Special catheterisation techniques in IHD

Intracoronary infusion of thrombolytic agents in acute myocardial infarction was designed to deliver high doses of thrombolytic agents to the site of the thrombus in acute infarction. However, because the financial and organisational requirements allow only a tiny minority of acute myocardial infarction patients to receive this treatment, the approach will not be adopted.

Coronary angioplasty has developed rapidly since its introduction in 1977. Its use is described on page 405.

MANAGEMENT OF CHRONIC STABLE ANGINA

Once the diagnosis is established, treatment should be aimed at restoring a normal exercise capacity. Investigations should establish the individual's risk, and contributory risk factors reduced as far as possible. A flow diagram of the management of angina is shown in Figure 13.59.

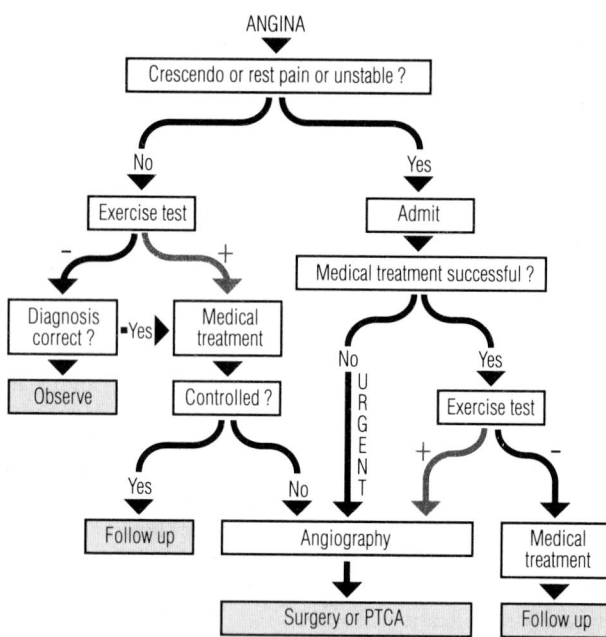

Fig. 13.59 Flow diagram of management of angina. PTCA = percutaneous transarterial coronary angioplasty.

General measures

All patients should be advised to cease smoking, achieve their ideal weight and have raised blood pressure controlled. Lipid measurements should be made in young patients (below 50 years of age), and those with severe abnormalities (total cholesterol greater than 7.1 mmol/l; HDL/LDL less than 20%; triglyceride greater than 2.0 mmol/l) should be given an appropriate diet (p. 136) until repeat estimations are within the normal ranges. Family members and children of young patients with IHD

should have their lipid levels measured. The benefit of these measures in those over 50 years of age is questionable. There is disagreement amongst doctors, particularly in the UK, regarding the importance of dietary fat in coronary heart disease and its management.

The patient with angina of effort, and a normal resting ECG and chest X-ray, and whose symptoms are well-controlled on simple treatment, can probably be managed adequately without further investigation. The prognosis in ischaemic heart disease is dependent on the severity of the stenoses, the number of coronary arteries involved and on left ventricular function. This information can only be obtained accurately at cardiac catheterisation. This investigation should be offered to young patients with angina (below 40 years of age), whose risk is highest. The risk of death may be approximately 4% per year in other patients, but it increases to between 7 and 9% if there are associated abnormalities in the resting ECG. In many (up to 33%), angina may spontaneously resolve. Thus, although a resting ECG may be sufficient investigation for many patients, further determination of the risk to the individual is obtained by non-invasive tests, especially the exercise test. Catheterisation may then be required for those with a positive test at low workloads, or those in whom medical treatment is not being successful.

Drug treatment

The drugs commonly used in the treatment of angina are listed in Table 13.17.

Nitrates

Therapy begins with sublingual or aerosol spray nitrates. These are used to treat an anginal episode and can be successfully used in prophylaxis by patients with predictable symptoms. The aerosol spray has the advantage of a long storage life compared to glyceryl trinitrate tablets, which deteriorate rapidly in their container. The onset of action is very rapid (within 1–2 minutes) and its duration is under 10 minutes. With all nitrates, troublesome headache can prevent their use in certain susceptible individuals, although this side-effect usually stops after a few days of treatment.

Longer-acting nitrate preparations include glyceryl trinitrate given via the skin, using small sustained-release plasters or patches. Isosorbide dinitrate is absorbed from the gut and metabolised by the liver to the active mononitrates. The duration of action is longer, but 6–8-hourly doses are needed to maintain blood levels. Mononitrates are absorbed in the gut and do not require hepatic conversion; thus, some variability in effectiveness due to liver metabolism is avoided. Their duration of action is longer, so two or three daily doses are adequate.

Tolerance

Tolerance to nitrates develops as sulphydryl (SH) groups on the vessel walls become oxidised by constant exposure

Table 13.17 Drugs commonly used in the treatment of angina

Drug	Route	Dose	Frequency
Nitrates			
Glyceril trinitrate (GTN)			
Tablets	Sublingual	0.3–0.6 mg	PRN and prophylaxis
Spray	Oral	0.4 mg/puff	PRN and prophylaxis
Ointment	Skin	1–5 cm	3–4-hourly
Patches	Skin	5–10 mg/cm^2	Daily
Isosorbide dinitrate (ISDN)	Various types oral sustained release	20–80 mg	12-hourly
Isosorbide mononitrate	Oral	20 mg	12-hourly
Parenteral preparations			
GTN	iv	0.6–12 mg/h	infusion
ISDN	iv	1.25–5 mg/h	infusion
Beta-blockers. Many alternatives, including:			
Atenolol (beta-1 selective)	Oral	50–100 mg/day	Daily
Propranolol (non-selective)	Oral	30–360 mg/day	6-hourly
Calcium antagonists			
Nifedipine	Oral	10–20 mg	8-hourly (12-hourly for sustained release form)
Diltiazem	Oral	60–120 mg	8-hourly
Verapamil	Oral	80–120 mg	8-hourly (12-hourly for sustained release form)

to nitrates; this prevents the stimulation of guanidylate cyclase, which is believed to be fundamental to the smooth muscle relaxation produced by these drugs. A nitrate-free period is sufficient to allow recovery of SH groups. Thus, the very rapidly-acting sublingual or spray glyceryl trinitrate is not associated with tolerance, whereas longer-acting preparations may be. Prolonged administration of the longer-acting nitrates may therefore be associated with a lessening in their efficacy which may respond to a change in dosing to produce a nitrate-free period (about 8 hours). A reduction in efficacy can also be due to a worsening of the underlying ischaemic heart disease.

Beta-blocking drugs

Beta-adrenoreceptor blockade has become established as a cornerstone in the treatment of angina. Although many beta-blocking drugs with varying pharmacological properties are available, there is no overwhelming evidence to suggest one drug is any better than the others. They are specifically contra-indicated in patients with obstructive airways disease and severe ventricular dysfunction, and relatively contra-indicated in diabetes and in those with peripheral vascular disease, bradycardia or heart block. Some patients find they are unpleasant due to a mild 'sedative' action and an interference with exercise capacity.

In angina, these drugs achieve their benefit by a reduction in myocardial oxygen demand consequent upon the fall in heart rate, blood pressure and myocardial contractility that is produced. In coronary vasospasm and variant (or Prinzmetal's) angina, beta-blockers may worsen symptoms, due to the unmasking of alpha-adrenoreceptor-mediated vasospasm. A reduction in mortality has not been shown in angina patients, nor does there appear to be any marked cardiac protective action in treated hypertensives, especially those who continue to smoke. Table 13.17 shows some commonly prescribed regimens.

Calcium antagonists

Nifedipine, diltiazem and verapamil are the first generation calcium antagonists; they vary in their pharmacological properties so that their indications may be different. Calcium antagonists are certainly effective in angina, achieving their effect by smooth muscle relaxation in the coronary arteries and the peripheral circulation, increasing myocardial supply and reducing myocardial work. The manner in which this is achieved varies with the three drugs, all of which inhibit cellular calcium entry, but differ in their tissue specificity. Nifedipine acts primarily by arteriolar vasodilatation with minimal effects on the SA node and the myocardium. It may cause a reflex tachycardia, so is often used in combination with a beta-blocker. The action of diltiazem is more marked on the SA and AV nodes, producing a mild bradycardia but less negative inotropy than verapamil.

Other compounds

Amiodarone is an effective anti-anginal preparation but has such potentially toxic side-effects (Table 13.7) that its use is limited to the treatment of potentially lethal arrhythmia.

13

Perhexilene alters the metabolism of cardiac muscle from free fatty acids to glucose and can be effective in refractory angina. However, it can have serious side-effects, including hepatotoxicity and peripheral neuropathy. *Trimetazidine* is a compound currently being investigated, which also alters myocardial metabolism and potentially diminishes the effects of ischaemia.

Drug combinations in angina

There is a progression in therapy before medical treatment can really be said to have failed. Most patients begin treatment with nitrates and a beta-blocker or a calcium antagonist. Elderly patients may well be adequately controlled with nitrates and a reduction in activity, and many find that beta-blockers induce unpleasant lethargy; whereas younger patients may not wish to reduce their activity, and find the prophylactic action of beta-blockers or calcium antagonists a considerable advantage. Verapamil and diltiazem may produce profound bradycardia or heart block when used with a beta-blocker, so these combinations should be avoided. Patients with severe disease commonly require 'triple therapy' to control their symptoms. Compliance with treatment appears to be less of a problem with treatment of angina, compared to the treatment of asymptomatic conditions such as hypertension.

Surgical treatment of angina

Effective surgical treatment has had a marked effect on the management of ischaemic heart disease in the developed world. Coronary artery bypass grafting can now be performed with an overall operative mortality of approximately 2–3%. Symptoms can be eradicated in 80–90% of patients and improved considerably in a further 5–10%. A small number are no better or, indeed, worse following surgery. It might therefore be asked why this form of therapy, which aims to 'revascularise' the heart, is not offered to all patients with angina. Several factors are responsible, including:

1. deterioration of grafts
2. a distinct survival advantage for surgical treatment has been proven for only certain subgroups of patients.

Deterioration of grafts

Saphenous vein bypass grafts have an appreciable rate of deterioration; 85–90% are patent immediately after surgery, but then occlude at a rate of approximately 2% of grafts per year between 5–10 years and at 4% per year thereafter. About 60% of grafts are patent ten years after operation. This implies surgery is not a permanent cure, merely another method of symptom control in these patients.

Improvements in early vein-patency rates have been achieved by the use of antithrombotic agents, such as aspirin and dipyridamol. Even more significant has been the use of the internal mammary artery (or internal thoracic artery) as a graft. The use of this vessel is slightly more demanding technically, but has been shown to provide greater than 90% patency rates at 10 years. Unfortunately, complete cardiac revascularisation is not often possible even when both internal mammary arteries are used.

Survival advantage

A distinct survival advantage for surgical treatment over medical treatment has only been clearly demonstrated by randomised trials for certain subgroups of patients (Table 13.18). Survival is improved by surgery in those with left main stem disease and those with three vessel coronary disease and impaired left ventricular function. It is very likely to improve survival in patients with severe angina, three vessel coronary disease and normal ventricular function. The situation is less clear for patients with less marked symptoms and those with little in the way of symptoms but with a positive exercise test, although evidence is mounting that this group of patients also benefit from surgery.

From the point of view of improvement in symptoms, exercise tolerance and diminution in the numbers of medicines required, surgery appears to be a more effective treatment for patients with continued symptoms not controlled by drugs. There is a diminution in fatal heart attacks, but probably not in non-fatal events. Randomised studies have failed to show any differences between medical and surgical treatment in the numbers of patients who return to work, nor in the amount of recreational activity they take up. However, the sociological measures may not reflect the changes in perceived quality of life in the two groups of patients.

Thus, in general, patients are considered for coronary artery surgery if medical therapy fails to adequately control their symptoms, or if they fall into the high-risk groups who do considerably better with surgical rather than medical treatment. These broad guidelines conceal a large number of patients in a rather grey area, in whom individual assessments must be made to gauge the relative merits of one approach over the other. These might include young patients with severe stenoses causing highly positive exercise tests, in whom the consequences of occlusion might be a disabling infarction and in whom an internal mammary graft might be expected to be highly successful treatment.

Table 13.18 Indications for coronary artery surgery in angina

Indication	Comment
Left main-stem stenosis	Proven survival benefit of surgery
Symptoms uncontrolled despite maximal medical treatment	Improved survival with surgery in some subgroups of patients
Three vessel coronary artery disease with impaired LV function	Improved survival with surgery
Proximal stenosis in left anterior descending coronary artery *with* positive exercise test at low workload	Likely improved survival with surgery (but debatable)

Patients with extensive left ventricular aneurysm may often improve, in terms of heart failure control and anginal symptoms, with resection of the aneurysmal area.

Percutaneous transarterial coronary angioplasty

The indications for percutaneous transarterial coronary angioplasty (PTCA), first introduced in 1977, are changing with experience (Table 13.19). In general, the patients treated are the same as those that would be selected for surgery. In most centres, one or two stenoses are tackled by angioplasty, and patients with severe three-vessel coronary disease are not generally considered. Patients with left main stem disease and very poor ventricular function are also not considered for PTCA, unless surgery is impossible for technical reasons or due to coincidental disease.

The technique of PTCA is illustrated in Figure 13.60. Problems that remain to be solved are a high recurrence rate and the prevention of complications.

Recurrence rate. This varies from 15–30% of successful dilatations. Virtually all recurrences occur within 3 months of the first dilatation. The vast majority of these can be redilated, and 70–80% remain patent. The cause of recurrence is unknown, but most patients are given antithrombotic treatment with aspirin or dipyridamole, and antivasospastic medication with calcium antagonists and/or nitrates.

Immediate complications. Occlusion of the vessel being dilated may occur, causing myocardial infarction in 3–4% of patients, and precipitating urgent coronary artery surgery in 3–4% and death in 1–3%. The difficulty lies in predicting which patients are going to have problems. Some complications are related to the experience of the operator, but occur even in the most experienced centres. Most operators use nitrates, aspirin, calcium antagonists and anticoagulation but it is not clear which of these, if any, is able to prevent complications.

Fig. 13.60 Technique of coronary angioplasty. A. The catheter is introduced into the coronary ostium. **B.** A steerable guide wire is advanced across the lesion. **C.** The balloon catheter is advanced from the guiding catheter over the guide wire and positioned so that the balloon straddles the narrowing. **D.** Balloon inflation splits and compresses the atheromatous plaque. **E.** After deflation, the balloon and wire are removed and the arterial wall shows only mild irregularity at the site of the narrowing.

MYOCARDIAL INFARCTION

About 200 000 people suffer a myocardial infarction each year in the United Kingdom. Half die from the infarction, and of these, half do so before they reach hospital (Fig. 13.61). Most of this group suffer an arrhythmia and death occurs instantaneously or within one hour of the first symptom. These victims of 'sudden death' form a distinct subgroup, whose pathology and management is different from survivors of acute infarction. Clearly, these deaths will only be avoided by measures which prevent the development of coronary disease, although pre-hospital

Table 13.19 Indications for coronary angioplasty

Indication	Comment
All indications for surgery (except left main stem stenosis) where coronary lesions suitable*	Single and double vessel PTCA. Low risk, high efficacy
Symptomatic single vessel coronary disease	?Treatment of choice before surgery. Remains to be proven if PTCA is as good or safe as surgery in these patients
Coronary disease where surgery impossible ('salvage PTCA')	Uncommon, but a suitable approach in the very elderly or infirm
Severe stenoses after thrombolysis or after non-Q wave infarction	Remains to be proven whether a survival advantage will be demonstrated over medical treatment

*Suitable coronary lesions: Proximal, discrete, not involving major branches, recent onset, non-calcified, circumferential lesions.

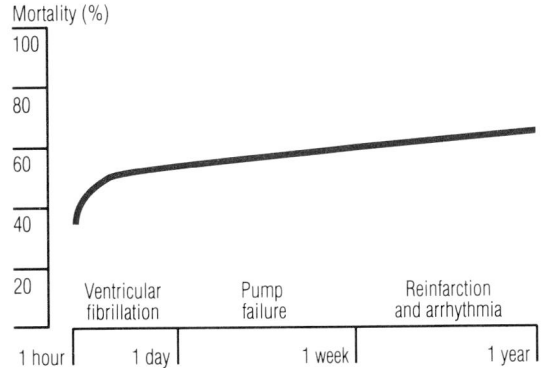

Fig. 13.61 Mortality following onset of acute myocardial infarction. A high proportion of patients die of ventricular fibrillation within one hour of onset.

13

and community resuscitation schemes can make an impact.

Hospital admissions for infarction total 70–80 000 per year in the UK, with an overall in-hospital mortality approaching 10% and a 10% mortality in the first year.

Within the overall figure of 10% hospital mortality, the prognosis varies widely, from 3–6% for the patient with an uncomplicated infarction injuring only a limited amount of myocardium, to 80% for the victim of massive myocardial necrosis and shock (Table 13.20). The amount of muscle damaged determines both early and late outcomes from infarction, so that the current major impetus in acute management is to reduce the size of the infarct.

In hospital, the patient should be cared for in a specific coronary care unit (CCU). The rationale behind this development was the observation that many of the early deaths in myocardial infarction were due to arrhythmia and, in the 1960's, it was demonstrated that external cardiac massage and external DC countershock could save some of the victims of infarction. This led to CCUs with nurses trained to recognise arrhythmia and to deliver DC countershock rapidly. Soon after their introduction, the mortality fell from 20–25% to 15–20% for patients admitted to CCUs rather than to general wards. This trend has continued, particularly in countries with active CCU policies such as New Zealand. Here, mortality has fallen from over 20 to 10% from 1966–67 to 1981–84. It has been estimated that 20% of the fall in ischaemic heart disease deaths could be attributed to better coronary care. Although this view has not gone unchallenged, the trials which appeared to show no benefit were limited in scope and size and there is now considerable doubt that they had the statistical power to reliably detect any differences in outcome between hospital and home care. With the current emphasis and recent successes in infarction limitation by early treatment, the vast majority of heart attack victims will continue to be dealt with in CCUs within hospitals.

Table 13.20 Mortality from acute myocardial infarction

Class	Definition	Admissions (%)	Mortality (%)
I	Uncomplicated, without clinical signs of LV failure	33	6
II	Generally asymptomatic, but manifesting a ventricular third sound, basal crackles or raised venous pressure	38	17
III	Clinical evidence of pulmonary oedema	10	38
IV	Cardiogenic shock indicated by a systolic BP below 90 mmHg and at least one of: oliguria (<20 ml/h) low skin temperature mental confusion	19	81

Data from: Killip and Kimball 1969 A M J Cardiol 20:457–467.

Some elderly patients, and those seen very late after the event, may be managed at home.

DIAGNOSIS OF MYOCARDIAL INFARCTION

Strictly, the diagnosis of myocardial infarction is a pathological diagnosis depending on the demonstration of irreversible myocardial necrosis. The clinical syndrome is rather less precise, but, for most purposes, a working diagnosis includes two of the following:

1. a typical history
2. the evolution of characteristic ECG change ending with Q wave formation
3. a significant elevation and subsequent fall in creatine phosphokinase (CPK), preferably the MB isoenzyme fraction (CPK-MB), aspartate transaminase (AST) or hydroxybutyrate dehydrogenase (HBD).

CLINICAL FEATURES

History

A squeezing or tight chest, or epigastric pain with its onset at rest is reported by 80% of patients, a large proportion (40%) of whom may have an antecedent history of angina. The pain lasts longer than angina, typically more than 20 minutes, and is resistant to treatment with sublingual or buccal nitrates. Associated symptoms are sweating, nausea, vomiting, breathlessness and collapse. Like angina, the pain may radiate to the arms, throat and jaw. At the onset of symptoms, many patients believe they are suffering from indigestion and consume antacids; belching may be associated with their discomfort, confusing in their minds the likely cause of the pain. With the advent of thrombolytic therapy, with its emphasis on early treatment, it has become even more important to be aware of possible differential diagnoses in the patient with acute chest pain (p. 400).

Examination

There are no specific features that accompany myocardial infarction. During the acute phase, patients vary a great deal in their appearance, and the physical signs are largely those associated with pain and fear and are initially dominated by autonomic nervous activity. With *acute anterior infarction*, there is a tendency for sympathetic activity to dominate, with a tachycardia, cool pale periphery and a normal, or even slightly raised, blood pressure in the early minutes. This contrasts with *acute inferior infarction*, which is commonly associated with massive vagal discharge, stimulated by the Bezold-Jarisch reflex producing a cold sweaty periphery, bradycardia, hypotension, nausea and vomiting.

Even in the absence of cardiogenic shock, the blood pressure tends to fall to lower than normal levels for the patient within a few hours of infarction. The venous pressure is generally normal in the early stages unless there has been extensive right ventricular involvement, which may occur with an inferior or posterior infarction. In left ventricular infarction, heart failure may develop and the venous pressure will rise signifying severe myocardial damage. Auscultation commonly reveals a fourth heart sound and a third sound over the apex in those patients in incipient left ventricular failure. The left ventricular impulse may be anterior and dyskinetic when a large segment of left ventricular wall is moving paradoxically; this is particularly marked later in those individuals who develop an aneurysm. Orthopnoea and basal crackles are present in patients developing pulmonary oedema.

A pyrexia develops within 12 hours in patients who suffer significant myocardial injury; it may persist for up to a week and is associated with a polymorphonuclear leucocytosis. Pericardial friction rubs are occasionally encountered soon after infarction, and signify a large loss of myocardium extending to the epicardium. This finding is distinct from the pericarditis and pneumonitis of Dressler's syndrome which usually, but not always, occurs during the first six weeks after a myocardial infarction and has an immunological basis (p. 416).

Other physical signs in myocardial infarction are due to the mechanical complications of the condition and are discussed individually below.

INVESTIGATION

ECG changes in acute infarction

The ECG changes of acute infarction may take some hours to develop and, occasionally, are absent completely. Treatment of acute infarction must often begin before there is any objective evidence confirming the diagnosis (a rise in plasma enzyme levels also takes some hours to occur).

ST segment elevation

The most characteristic feature of infarction on the ECG is the development of ST segment elevation, with a convex upward pattern in the leads facing the area of ventricle infarcted. The diastolic iso-electric line is depressed, so accentuating the ST elevation that follows it (Fig. 13.62). Reciprocal ST depression is often seen in leads opposite the infarction; this is usually indicative of severe multiple vessel coronary disease, but may on occasion represent a purely electrical phenomenon.

ST elevation (the *current of injury*), is produced by ischaemia, and can occur in the absence of infarcted tissue. Thus, such ST changes can be associated with anginal pain due to coronary vasospasm (Prinzmetal's angina) and resolve rapidly and completely when spasm is relieved and ischaemia reversed. ST elevation during acute infarction lasts for some days but may persist longer. If it is still present some weeks after infarction, left ventricular aneurysm or extensive dyskinesia is likely.

T wave inversion

The terminal portion of the T wave begins to invert within hours of infarction and produces symmetrical inversion after a few days (Fig. 13.64). This appearance persists for

Fig. 13.62 Evolution of ECG change in an acute inferior infarction. Initially, there is marked ST segment elevation in II, III, aVF and reciprocal depression in V2–V4. At 12 hours, a Q wave is developing in II, III and aVF and the ST segment has returned to the baseline. At 48 hours the Q wave has deepened and broadened and there is T wave inversion.

weeks or months and, occasionally, is a permanent feature of the ECG. In some patients at the very earliest stage of infarction, the only ECG change may be in the T waves, which become very prominent, peaked and symmetrical. This appearance is sometimes called the *hyperacute pattern* of infarction. Symmetrical T inversion alone, without Q wave formation, may indicate a limited infarction in some patients (see non-Q wave infarction, p. 408) and this has important implications for their management.

Q wave formation

Q waves are often the latest change to be seen on ECG. They are often permanent and are sometimes considered the definitive ECG change of infarction. They must have a depth of at least 25% of the succeeding R wave height (or greater than 3 mV) and last longer than 40 ms (one small square at 25 mm/s). They may appear within 24 hours of infarction and are associated with loss in R wave height of the corresponding leads.

Alternative patterns

Ideally, electrocardiographic proof of infarction should include successive traces showing the presence and resolution of ST segment elevation, T wave inversion and pathological Q wave formation (Fig. 13.62). Often, such a classical progression is missing and the diagnosis may rest upon a slightly deeper than normal Q wave in V4, loss of R wave height or the absence of the small *q* waves of initial septal depolarisation in I, aVL, V5 and V6; this may occur in septal infarction, but is also produced by incomplete left bundle branch block.

In the presence of bundle branch block, the ECG changes due to infarction may be difficult to detect or be absent. With right bundle branch block septal depolarisation occurs normally. Changes in ST segments and T waves may appear, but the ECG diagnosis of infarction often cannot be made with certainty. Bundle branch block patterns may precede infarction or be a consequence of it.

The posterior infarction (see below) may cause difficulty.

Localisation of infarction from the ECG

Although myocardial infarction can be endocardial, epicardial or involve the whole thickness of the ventricular wall, these distinctions cannot reliably be made by ECG. Localisation to an approximate region of the left ventricle is possible, however. The precordial leads give most information in this respect. If they have been correctly positioned: leads V1 and V2 face the right ventricle, although an extra lead (V4R, at the level of V4 on the right of the sternum below V1) is better; V3 faces the interventricular septum; V4 the anterior and lateral borders; and V6 the postero-lateral wall of the left ventricle (this is because the apex faces backwards).

Inferior infarction

In inferior infarction, changes are seen in leads III, aVF and II, with reciprocal change in I, aVL and the anterior leads. Infero-lateral infarction extends to involve lead V6. The right coronary and its posterior descending branch account for the majority of these cases (Fig. 13.62).

Anterior infarction

Anterior infarction is extensive when leads V2 to V6 are involved with changes in I, aVL and II. There may be reciprocal changes in the inferior leads III and avF. Anterior infarction implies involvement of the left anterior descending coronary artery. Infarction may be antero-septal when the ECG changes are limited to leads V3 and V2. Antero-lateral infarction may present with changes in I, aVL, V5 with some involvement in V4 and V6 (Fig. 13.63).

Posterior infarction

The true posterior infarction is usually caused by occlusion in the circumflex coronary artery, and its hallmark on the ECG is a tall R wave in V1. There is often associated ST depression in leads V3 and V4, but little else on the electrocardiogram (Fig. 13.64).

Non-Q wave infarction

Non-Q wave infarction is a rather imprecise term used to identify patients who have suffered a relatively minor infarction. The interest in identifying these patients is that they appear to have a very high (40–60%) chance of developing a full-thickness, or Q wave, infarction in the weeks and months following their presentation. Their mortality is also 20–30% higher than that for hospital survivors of infarction, presumably because a proportion of these patients suffer sudden death as the next manifestation of their ischaemic heart disease. Previously, the term subendocardial infarction was used for these patients, but this implies a rather more accurate anatomical localisation than is warranted from the ECG and other clinical findings.

The features of non-Q wave infarction are a typical history with or without a modest enzyme rise, and often with T wave changes alone on the ECG. Management is along the lines followed for all high-risk post-infarction patients (p. 409).

Laboratory tests

Infarction causes the release of intracellular enzymes into the circulation; these can be assayed in the laboratory to confirm the diagnosis and may be used to estimate the size of the infarction. The most specific enzyme available is an isoenzyme of creatine phosphokinase (CPK) called the MB fraction (hence, CPK-MB). It is a better indicator than creatine phosphokinase itself, which is released into the blood with any skeletal muscle trauma. Creatine phosphokinase and the MB fraction rise within hours of infarction, but the concentration falls within 24–48 hours after the event. Although the absolute peak of CPK or CPK-MB that is measured gives a crude estimate of the size of infarction, a more reliable approach is to assess the area under the concentration-time curve.

Lactate dehydrogenase – or its more cardiac-specific isoenzyme LDH_1 – is assayed as hydroxybutyrate dehydrogenase (HBD); it appears in blood within 12–24 hours after infarction and may remain elevated for some days. Aspartate aminotransferase (AST) is relatively non-specific,

Fig. 13.63 ECG of acute anterior infarction. ST segment elevation in V1–V6 and Q waves in V2–V4 are shown.

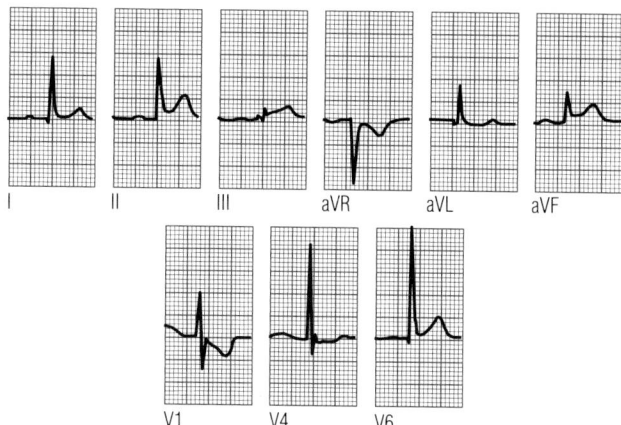

Fig. 13.64 ECG of acute posterior infarction. Inferior ST elevation (in II, III, aVF) and a tall R wave in V1 (mirror of the Q wave) are shown.

but rises with an intermediate temporal position to CPK and HBD.

A raised polymorphonuclear leucocyte count, and an elevated ESR are non-specific accompaniments of acute infarction. A very high ESR in the early stages of infarction raises the possibility of infarction being secondary to a giant cell arteritis or immunological disease such as polyarteritis nodosa.

Imaging techniques

Hot-spot scanning with technetium labelled pyrophosphate has been used to confirm infarction, but now a more common use of radionuclide studies is to establish ventricular function (MUGA scan; see page 351) or document areas of potentially reversible ischaemia (^{201}Tl scan; see page 351). The echocardiogram can be used to assess ventricular function and localise areas of infarction and dyskinesia.

DIFFERENTIAL DIAGNOSIS

Acute chest pain syndromes can pose diagnostic difficulties in acute myocardial infarction (p. 400), particularly as there are no specific physical signs in acute infarction and the diagnostic tests may be normal in the initial hours of the attack. With the advent of thrombolysis and acute beta-adrenoreceptor blockade used early in the management of acute infarction, diagnostic accuracy has become even more important.

The symptoms of *aortic dissection* (p. 445) may be very similar. Pain indistinguishable from acute cardiac ischaemia can be produced by the sudden increase in right ventricular work associated with an *acute massive pulmonary embolism*. Syncope is often the first manifestation of the embolism, and the marked dyspnoea, tachypnoea and cyanosis accompanying *acute pericarditis* (p. 433) produces chest pain, often accompanied by a fever and a friction rub.

MANAGEMENT OF ACUTE INFARCTION

The aims of management of acute infarction have altered over the years from the provision of pain relief alone, through the treatment of arrhythmic and mechanical complications, to the current era of infarct limitation. Having helped (or watched) a patient survive, management should be directed to defining the relatively small proportion of patients at a greater than normal risk in the post-infarction period, and to rehabilitation and secondary prevention.

Analgesia and oxygen

In addition to the discomfort of chest pain, many of the patients are afraid for their lives, exacerbating some of the unwanted ill effects of sympathetic hyperactivity. Analgesia and sedation is achieved with opiates, preferably diamorphine (2.5–5.0 mg iv) or morphine sulphate (4–8 mg im). These drugs combine sedation with an advantageous vasodilatory action which improves haemodynamics. Respiratory depression is rare in the setting of acute infarction. The relief of pain itself may help raise blood pressure and reduce the heart rate. Associated nausea is treated using cyclizine (50 mg iv) or prochlorperazine (12.5–25 mg im). An inhaled mixture of nitrous oxide and oxygen (Entonox) is widely and successfully used in continental Europe to provide pain relief prior to arrival in hospital.

Oxygen by mask is frequently given to patients with acute infarction to counteract the hypoxaemic effects of pulmonary oedema. However, many patients are not hypoxaemic and in these, oxygen delivery to the tissues will not be improved by this treatment.

Acute beta-adrenoreceptor blockade

Acute intravenous beta blockade can be given safely to many acute infarction patients. Large-scale trials have shown a reduction in early deaths caused by reinfarction and cardiac rupture. An additional effect is a reduction in pain. It has been calculated that acute intravenous beta blockade would have to be given to 200 patients to prevent one death, one reinfarction and one cardiac arrest; chronic therapy after infarction saves two lives for every 100 patients treated for one year.

Limitation of infarct size

The essential feature of measures aimed at infarct size limitation is that they must either restore blood supply to the affected myocardium or very significantly reduce oxygen requirements very early in the condition, before permanent damage has occurred. Six hours appears to be the usual limit before which there is maximum likelihood that a restored blood supply will salvage ischaemic muscle. If collateral channels are poor, this time limit may be considerably less.

Thrombolysis

In approximately 80% of patients, a myocardial infarction is caused by thrombotic occlusion of a vessel. This is almost always superimposed on an atherosclerotic plaque. Early trials of the intravenous fibrinolytic agents, streptokinase and urokinase, were negative, probably because the therapy was given too late and the trials were too small.

Intravenous infusion of streptokinase ($1. \times 10^6$ units over 1 hour) has been shown to be nearly as effective as intra-coronary treatment infusion, with a 60–70% restoration of patency. A large-scale trial has shown a reduction in acute mortality for patients treated with a single injection of streptokinase within 24 hours.

Unfortunately, fibrinolysis is not limited to the site of the thrombosis, and haemorrhagic complications occur – though sufficiently rarely not to interfere with the overall beneficial effect of therapy. Patients with clotting disorders, a previous history of stroke or peptic ulceration, and those with severe hypertension or any injuries are excluded from this treatment. It is important to exclude aortic dissection, as fibrinolytic treatment would prove catastrophic. This may sometimes be difficult (p. 446). Other relative contra-indications are a known hyper-sensitivity to the drug, recent streptococcal infection, sur-vivors from cardiac arrest who have had cardiac massage and those with heart block who may need a temporary pacemaker.

Unresolved problems with this undoubtedly effective treatment include managing the 15% or so of patients who suffer a reocclusion of the artery within a few days of treatment. Newer agents with less immunological side-effects, and a tendency to be more clot-specific, include tissue plasminogen activator, now manufactured using recombinant DNA technology.

Benefit from thrombolysis is increased if it is given within 6 hours, and preferably 3 hours, of the first symptom. This has led to a suggestion that newer fibrin-olytic agents be produced which can be administered at the site of the presenting symptoms either by the ambu-lance crew or the family general practitioners. These will probably have to be given by intramuscular injection.

Aspirin and heparin

The use of aspirin has been extended from angina to infarc-tion. The ISIS trial has shown a reduction in acute mor-tality of about 13%, and, with streptokinase, a combined reduction in acute mortality of 25%. Heparin by sub-cutaneous injection prevents pulmonary embolism in patients on bedrest. However, myocardial infarction patients now rarely spend more than 24–48 hours in bed, unless complications such as severe heart failure develop. Continuous infusion of heparin after thrombolysis and after coronary angioplasty is routine in many centres, but formal proof that it keeps vessels patent or improves the prognosis in infarction is not yet available. A suitable man-agement plan might therefore include 150 mg of oral aspirin once the patient is able to eat and drink, with heparin by constant infusion for those that cannot. Sub-cutaneous heparin can be given to patients with congestive cardiac failure who are confined to bed for more than 24 hours.

Angioplasty and surgery

Early revascularisation during acute infarction is possible. However, the logistics and cost of providing a 24-hour service for these complex, labour-intensive techniques are similar to those required for intracoronary streptokinase treatment. At present, none of these treatment options can realistically be expected to be adopted. Individual cases will continue to be so treated in centres where angioplasty or surgical suites are closely linked to the acute admission wards.

Nitrates and calcium antagonist drugs

Nitrates by intravenous infusion (2–10 mg/h for isosorbide, 5–10 μg/min for nitroglycerin) are frequently used in the acute phase of infarction, where persistent pain is a prob-lem. They can be used with relative ease, and have the advantage of causing reduction in preload and afterload, which may have an haemodynamic advantage in some patients. Hypotension can be a problem, particularly in patients who are dependent on a high right heart filling pressure to maintain stroke volume, such as patients with right ventricular infarction. Nitrates can also be given by skin using ointment applied over a sufficient area to reduce blood presure by 10%. Cutaneous therapy is best reserved for the less acute stages of infarction, when converting patients from intravenous infusion to maintenance therapy. Calcium antagonist drugs are effective in improving ischaemic cardiac pain, but their use has not been associ-ated with any improvement in infarction mortality. Nitrates and calcium antagonists are particularly useful if coronary vasospasm is contributing to the production of pain, such as in Prinzmetal's angina.

In general, nitrate infusion should be reserved for patients unable to tolerate beta blockade, for those in whom the latter is insufficient to control symptoms, or for those in acute pulmonary oedema. Calcium antagonists can be used when there are contra-indications to beta-blockade, or when adjunctive treatment is necessary.

Bedrest, mobilisation and rehabilitation

Prolonged bedrest is unnecessary and, indeed, harmful in myocardial infarction. Mobilisation can begin within 24 hours in uncomplicated infarction. Patients can generally be discharged on the tenth day, having demonstrated their ability to walk and manage a flight of stairs before returning home. Mobilisation should be slowed if there is a return of chest discomfort, a heart rate below 50 bpm or above 120 bpm, the return of ischaemic ST elevation on the ECG or an increase of more than 15 mmHg in systolic pressure with gentle ambulation.

Individual advice is required when patients are

discharged. Many centres now issue booklets with advice on activity, work, diet and risk factor modification. Many patients, however, benefit from a more formal approach with a structured and supervised course of rehabilitation following a pre-discharge exercise test. This exercise test serves the purpose of identifying high-risk patients to the physician, and can be reassuring to the patient, illustrating the degree of exertion which can be undertaken with safety at home; this is often much more than he would have imagined.

Rehabilitation programmes

Rehabilitation programmes with supervised exercise training, and usually associated relaxation therapy, counselling and educational sessions, have been taken up with variable enthusiasm. The results suggest a benefit in survival of between 25 and 35%, with an additional decrease in other coronary events. The risks in exercising post-myocardial infarction patients are small. Out of 51 303 patients who exercised for a total of 2.3 million hours, there were 21 cardiac arrests, 18 of which were successfully resuscitated. This compares with the reported incidence of sudden death in 'healthy' joggers (1 per 396 000 person-hours). Indices of general well-being and psychological status have been shown to improve, but it appears that the return to work is not always hastened by exercise programmes.

There is some evidence that ventricular function and, possibly, myocardial perfusion improve with prolonged exercise training. Most centres encourage the continued use of beta-blockers throughout exercise programmes. The amount and duration of exercise training that is required to produce benefit is 20 minutes of exercise at 75–80% of the maximal safe heart rate achieved on exercise testing, 2–3 days per week. Training effects may be seen after 6–12 weeks of this degree of effort. Compliance and continuation with unsupervised exercise, as well as cessation of smoking and improvements in the diet, are more likely to occur in patients who have been monitored for a prolonged period.

Drug therapy in myocardial infarction survivors

Beta-blockers

The most successful agents in secondary prevention of further coronary events following myocardial infarction are the beta-blocking drugs. Despite differences in the pharmacology of different agents, it is likely that this effect is common to the whole class of drugs, the only exceptions being those with high intrinsic sympathomimetic activity such as oxprenolol. Sudden death and reinfarction appear to be the events that are successfully prevented. As noted elsewhere, pooled data from all the randomised trials suggest a 25% reduction in mortality. Most events occur within the first 6–12 weeks of infarction. Treatment with beta-blockers is therefore recommended for at least three months, and, in high-risk individuals, for years if not indefinitely, although conclusive data regarding the benefit

of this is not available. Patients at very low risk of reinfarction or death may not require this form of treatment.

Antithrombotics

The second most important class of drugs in secondary prevention is the antithrombotic drugs, *aspirin* in particular. Aspirin is safe, economical and well-tolerated in the absence of peptic ulcer disease. Its effectiveness is now beyond doubt in unstable angina, but its role after infarction is not so well-established, and the precise dosage is contentious. In theory, a very small dose of 75 mg every day, or even alternate days, may have advantages over larger doses, since the desired antiplatelet activity is then achieved without the unwanted inhibition of endothelial wall prostacyclin activity. At present, trial information is available only for relatively large doses of from 300 mg to 2 g daily. Until further information becomes available, an enteric coated or soluble aspirin at a dose of 300 mg per day would be appropriate therapy. Two other antiplatelet drugs, *sulphinpyrazone* and *dipyridamole*, have no demonstrated advantage over aspirin alone. Dipyridamole and aspirin together probably have a specific role in the management of patients after saphenous vein bypass grafting, where improvement in graft patency with this combined therapy has been demonstrated.

Anticoagulants

Anticoagulation with *warfarin* following myocardial infarction has been a topic for controversy for many years. Although a small benefit in survival is apparent, particularly for a small subgroup of compliant elderly patients, there are considerable problems associated with its safe usage over many years. Where warfarin has been compared to aspirin, the benefits are equivalent and side-effects are equally common, although different. However, aspirin therapy requires much less supervision, and hence is preferable for the patients and physicians alike.

Patients with extensive anterior infarction, with demonstrable intraventricular clot (shown by echocardiography) and with evidence of systemic embolisation, can have the risk of further emboli reduced by warfarin anticoagulation. The risks of emboli are highest in the first few weeks; hence, treatment may only be required for 3–4 months.

COMPLICATIONS OF MYOCARDIAL INFARCTION

ARRHYTHMIAS

Arrhythmias are a common complication of myocardial infarction.

Tachycardias

Sinus tachycardia

Sinus tachycardia (heart rate greater than 100 bpm) is associated with a poor prognosis if it persists, despite control of pain, anxiety and cardiac failure. It requires no specific therapy in most instances. Beta-blockers will reduce its incidence but cannot be given to patients with severe impairment of ventricular function.

Ventricular fibrillation

Ventricular fibrillation (VF) is a lethal arrhythmia which can complicate acute myocardial infarction from the moment of coronary occlusion. It is the cause of most cases of sudden death due to ischaemic heart disease. Its peak incidence is in the first few hours of the attack when it is termed primary VF and, if successfully dealt with in an otherwise uncomplicated infarction, has a good prognosis. Secondary VF occurs several days or weeks after infarction, usually in patients who have suffered extensive muscle damage and heart failure. Its prognosis is then very poor. There is only one treatment that is effective in VF – direct current (DC) defibrillation. The earlier it is used, the more likely is a successful outcome. The procedure itself and the sequence with which it should be given is described fully in the section on resuscitation (p. 374).

Lignocaine is also given after successful defibrillation to prevent further episodes. Limitations on the use of lignocaine include its narrow therapeutic margin, with central nervous system side-effects being the most common. Doses have to be reduced in the elderly and in those with poor hepatic function. The use of lignocaine to prevent VF is controversial.

Warning arrhythmia

Many episodes of VF are preceded by multiple or frequent ventricular ectopic beats or early ectopics falling on the vulnerable period of the ECG – the *R on T phenomenon.* Although it was hoped that recognition and treatment of these 'warning' arrhythmias might reduce the incidence of VF, this promise has not been fulfilled, since warning arrhythmias gave frequent false positive and false negative associations.

Ventricular ectopic beats

At an early stage (6–72 hours) in an acute myocardial infarction, frequent ventricular ectopic (VE) beats (more than 10 VE/h) are seen in 70% of patients. Ectopy then diminishes so that only 10% of patients have frequent VEs at the time of discharge. Frequent VEs at the time of discharge from hospital carries an increased (two- to three-fold) risk of death in the first year. This association appears to be independent of ventricular function. Although drugs to effectively inhibit ectopic activity are available, controlled trials have not shown any benefit on survival associated with treatment of frequent or complex VE. The reasons are unknown, but include inadequate trial sizes and possible pro-arrhythmogenic effects of treatment.

Treatment of frequent VEs is indicated if their occurrence causes an effective bradycardia and diminished output.

Ventricular tachycardia

The risks of dying after an infarction are greatly increased if ventricular tachycardia (VT) is present on the ECG at the time of discharge. Haemodynamic disturbance and degeneration to VF is common with sustained VT in acute infarction. Direct current shock therapy is indicated in almost all cases, to be followed by intravenous or oral therapy (p. 370). Lignocaine is usually used in the acute situation, followed by other Vaughan-Williams class I drugs and amiodarone. Unfortunately, although drug therapy may suppress the arrhythmia the survival of patients has not always been improved.

Patients with non-sustained VT should probably be monitored carefully, receive a pre-discharge exercise test and oral anti-arrhythmic therapy for the first few weeks after infarction.

Accelerated idioventricular rhythm

On occasion, a ventricular rhythm at a rate of 60–90 bpm can arise. It generally has broad complexes, but they may be narrow if the origin is high in the bundle of His. This rhythm rarely requires specific treatment, but may be an indication of profound sinus and AV nodal suppression which may respond to atropine (0.6–1.2 mg).

Supraventricular tachycardia

Atrial fibrillation (AF) is the commonest supraventricular tachycardia (SVT) seen in acute infarction, atrial flutter being relatively uncommon. Tachycardias causing severe haemodynamic disturbance are usually best dealt with by DC cardioversion. In *atrial flutter* (AF), this is generally the treatment of choice, as low energies are often required to convert to sinus rhythm. In AF, intravenous digoxin is given followed by oral treatment (p. 368). Maintenance digoxin is usually only required for a few days, since there is some evidence that chronic digoxin treatment after infarction may increase mortality. Control of AF rate may require the concurrent administration of another drug (p. 368). Beta-blockers are often used, and verapamil or diltiazem are also effective.

Paroxysmal atrial tachycardia may complicate acute infarction; if hypotension is severe, DC cardioversion is the therapy of first choice. Intravenous verapamil is effective in terminating many of these episodes, and intravenous beta blockade (atenolol 5 mg or metoprolol 5–15 mg) may be an alternative. If the first-choice drug fails to produce a satisfactory slowing of the rhythm or conversion to sinus rhythm, it is best to use DC cardioversion to avoid additive negative inotropic effects of anti-arrhythmic drugs.

An alternative therapy for atrial flutter and atrial tachycardia is overdrive pacing; this has the advantage of avoiding negatively inotropic drugs, but requires a temporary transvenous pacemaker placed in the right atrium.

Bradycardia

Many instances of bradycardia are transient and require

no treatment. However, in any circumstance where the bradycardia produces symptoms or significantly impairs the haemodynamics, then treatment with a pacemaker or drugs is required.

Sinus bradycardia

Up to 80% of patients with acute inferior infarction develop a heart rate less than 60 bpm in the very early stages of the condition. This usually responds to atropine (0.5–1.0 mg iv), but if symptomatic bradycardia persists a temporary pacemaker is required. This is preferable to infusions of isoprenaline, which may produce dangerous arrhythmia.

Heart block

First degree heart block

The lengthening of the PR interval may be seen during the evolution of an infarction, particularly inferior infarction. When pre-existing it requires no action. However, lengthening PR intervals deserve observation, as this implies interference with AV node function, and progression to higher grades of block may occur.

Second degree heart block

The differentiation of second degree heart block into a more benign Mobitz type I block (Wenckebach block), due to intranodal malfunction, and a more sinister Mobitz type II block, due to subnodal conduction disturbance, is an oversimplification. Both require very careful observation. Progression to complete heart block and sudden death is uncommon with inferior infarction, where Mobitz type I is a frequent, though transient, complication (about 15% of cases). In anterior infarction with extensive involvement of the interventricular septum, Mobitz type II block may be seen and carries a poor prognosis (80% mortality), which owes more to the associated large mass of muscle loss than to conduction disturbance itself.

Temporary pacemakers should be used in all cases where second degree block produces symptoms (e.g. syncope), or haemodynamic disturbance, or when anti-arrhythmic drugs are to be given. A permanent pacemaker should be considered for survivors of anterior infarction with persistent block.

Third degree or complete heart block

Complete heart block is a common complication of inferior infarction (about 10% of cases), when treatment is along the same lines as for second degree block. It needs no specific treatment if well-tolerated, but temporary cardiac pacing should be employed if heart failure, or rates less than 50 bpm, occur. In anterior infarction, complete block (incidence approximately 5% of cases) may occur suddenly or be preceded by bifascicular block (see below). It generally occurs in the context of large infarctions involving the septal tissue where the conducting tissue is concentrated, and always requires treatment with a pacemaker. This may not always improve survival but management is eased considerably.

Complete heart block rarely persists, but if it does persist beyond 7–14 days after infarction a permanent pacemaker is required.

Bifascicular and trifascicular heart block

Interruption of conduction through the right bundle and either fascicle of the left bundle constitutes bifascicular block. When the anterior fascicle is involved (*left anterior hemiblock*, LAH) the QRS axis is greater than $-30°$ with small r waves in II, III and aVF and absent initial q waves in V5 and V6. Posterior fascicular block (*left posterior hemiblock*, LPH) produces a rightward axis shift (greater than $+100°$) with an S wave in I and Q in III. Trifascicular block is any combination of bifascicular block associated with a long PR interval.

The association of right bundle branch block with LPH in anterior infarction indicates considerable ischaemic damage, and its appearance is an indication for prophylactic use of a temporary pacemaker, since progression to complete block may be sudden. Right bundle branch block with left anterior hemiblock does not carry such a poor prognosis, and is a slightly less powerful indication for pacing. There was a vogue for recommending permanent pacemaker implantation in survivors of infarction with bifascicular block. However, this was not shown to improve long-term survival and is rarely required.

Temporary transvenous cardiac pacemakers

The indications for implanting a pacemaker in acute infarction are summarised in Table 13.21. There are various methods by which pacing can be achieved but, in general, transvenous routes are the most stable and can be maintained for the few days that are required. The methods require the insertion of a bipolar electrode into the right ventricular apex, usually under radiological control. Pacing thresholds of under 1 volt at 2 ms pulse width duration should be established, since the threshold tends to rise after implantation. To achieve this, it may be necessary to try various positions in the right ventricular apex. The pacemaker is an external box which is always set in the demand mode; this ensures the patient's ventricular activity is sensed and pacing only begun when the intrinsic heart rate falls below a pre-set rate (usually between 70 and 90 bpm). A stable position of the temporary electrode is confirmed by establishing pacing at an output of 1 volt, and ensuring ventricular capture is not lost during maximal inspiration, coughing or sniffing. There should be sufficient slack in the electrode to accommodate these movements of the thorax without displacing the tip of the electrode. Once the electrode position is finalised it is secured to the skin under a sterile dressing. Except in an emergency, it is rarely justified to manipulate a temporary pacemaker after it has been inserted for some time, since sterility cannot be

Table 13.21 Indications for temporary pacemaker in acute myocardial infarction

A. Indicated regardless of MI site	B. Indicated in anterior MI	C. Not indicated
Symptomatic and drug-resistant bradycardia due to:	All indications in **A**	First degree heart block alone
Sinus bradycardia, sinus arrest, S-A block	RBBB + LPHB	Asymptomatic Mobitz type I
Second degree heart block	RBBB + LAHB	Asymptomatic bradycardia or junctional
Third degree heart block	Trifascicular block:	rhythm
Sick sinus syndrome with bradycardia-tachycardia	Long PR + LBBB	LAHB
Drug-resistant tachycardia	Long PR, RBBB + LPHB or LAHB	LBBB in
DC shock-resistant tachycardia	Second degree heart block, especially if	RBBB isolation
Ventricular standstill	Mobitz type II	LPHB
Alternating LBBB with RBBB		

ensured. If displacement has occurred, a replacement pacemaker will be required. Threshold measurements should be checked daily or more frequently if the patient is pacemaker-dependent. The pacemaker settings are adjusted to provide a voltage output of at least 3–4 times threshold. A threshold of over 1–2 volts is an indication to replace the electrode.

Atrial and dual-chamber pacing

Although pacing via a ventricular electrode is sufficient in the vast majority of instances, there are circumstances where atrial pacing or dual-chamber pacing are required. The former can be used to treat atrial flutter or bradycardia-dependent rhythms when AV nodal conduction is intact. Electrode positioning is more difficult and stability can be a problem.

In dual-chamber or physiological pacing, sequential pacing of first the atria followed, after a suitable pause, by the ventricles, offers a near physiological system maintaining the atrial contribution to cardiac filling. This can be very important in severe ventricular impairment, right ventricular infarction or when there is associated valvular disease, such as aortic stenosis. The technique requires suitable dual chamber pacemakers and the expertise to implant atrial as well as ventricular electrodes; availability is thus likely to be limited to specialised cardiac centres.

CARDIAC FAILURE

Dyspnoea, basal crepitations and the radiographic signs associated with pulmonary oedema (p. 355), are frequently encountered in the early stages of infarction.

Treatment

Prompt treatment with intravenous loop diuretics (frusemide 20–60 mg iv or bumetanide 1–2 mg) is the mainstay of treatment, which usually results in a brisk diuresis and resolution of signs, although the chest X-ray may remain abnormal for some time thereafter. Larger initial doses are often given, but these are rarely necessary and may produce hypotension worsening the patient's overall condition. Opiates are also helpful, and oxygen, given by a close-fitting, low dead-space mask (e.g. MC mask at 4 l/min)

is indicated. Pulmonary oedema that persists or worsens despite diuretic treatment requires the addition of vasodilatation to the treatment. This is best achieved using intravenous nitrates, which reduce preload as well as afterload and are thus preferred to sodium nitroprusside in ischaemic heart disease. Ideally, these drugs are used in combination with arterial and indirect left atrial pressure measurement. The latter is obtained with a Swan-Ganz catheter placed in a pulmonary arterial branch (see below). The aim of treatment should be to decrease the indirect left atrial pressure (or pulmonary capillary wedge pressure) to less than 20 mmHg, whilst maintaining systolic blood pressure above 100 mmHg and diastolic pressure over 60 mmHg. Facilities for invasive pressure monitoring may not be available in some hospitals and under these circumstances, the patient's blood pressure, heart rate and clinical condition will have to be monitored with care and the doses administered titrated against these observations.

CARDIOGENIC SHOCK

Cardiogenic shock in myocardial infarction is defined as hypotension with a systolic pressure under 100 mmHg; it is invariably accompanied by ventricular failure, peripheral vasoconstriction and oliguria (less than 20 ml/h of urine) and usually arterial hypoxaemia, mental confusion and metabolic acidosis. Remediable causes, such as uncontrolled pain, arrhythmia or excesses of negatively inotropic drugs (e.g. beta-adrenoreceptor blockers or calcium antagonists, such as verapamil), should be excluded and treated specifically. Shock is caused by damage affecting 30–40% of ventricular muscle mass and, if untreated, carries an 80–95% acute mortality. Treatment may reduce early mortality but it remains high (approximately 70% at one month), because of the amount of muscle damage.

Right ventricular infarction may produce cardiogenic shock, as defined above, but carries a very much better prognosis. The findings are a lower than expected indirect left atrial pressure and a relatively high right atrial pressure. The ECG shows changes of inferior or posterior infarction, and lead V4R may reveal the infarction clearly. Treatment consists of maintenance of a high right-sided filling pressure which may have been inadvertently lowered by diuretics given to treat the seemingly high venous pressure. The cardiac output and systemic pressure may respond to infusion with colloid. Inotropes and diuretics may be avoided altogether in these patients.

Treatment

Pressure monitoring, including indirect left atrial pressure, systemic arterial pressure and a facility for measuring cardiac output, are the minimum requirements for managing patients with shock. Therapy consists of inotropic agents, diuretics and, very rarely, mechanical support of respiration by ventilation and of the circulation with intra-aortic balloon counterpulsation (see below).

Inotropic agents are required to maintain the systolic pressure to perfuse the tissues, but these have the disadvantage of increasing oxygen requirement unless the doses are kept at the minimum required level. Diuretics are used to relieve pulmonary oedema, but adequate ventricular filling pressures must be maintained or else cardiac output falls. The inotropic agents of choice are dopamine and dobutamine.

Dopamine

Dopamine has three important actions which appear at increasing dose ranges. Low-dose dopamine infusion (0.5–2.5 μg/kg/min) primarily produces renal and mesenteric vessel dilatation, and is frequently used at this dose as a renal protector during times of systemic hypotension. Medium-dose dopamine infusion (5.0–10 μg/kg/min) has a direct myocardial inotropic action and at high doses (more than 10 μg/kg/min), the drug produces peripheral vasoconstriction (alpha-adrenoreceptor-mediated) so raising systemic pressure at the cost of vasoconstriction in tissue beds, including renal. The drug must be infused through a large central vein and, at medium to high infusion rates, may precipitate cardiac arrhythmias.

Dobutamine

Dobutamine is a synthetic dopamine analogue which directly stimulates beta$_1$ receptors; unlike dopamine, it does not release noradrenaline, and hence is less affected by the reduction in cardiac stores of this hormone in chronic heart failure. Dobutamine can be used via a peripheral vein and the dose is usually between 2.5 and 10 μg/kg per min. Its action is primarily inotropic, and hence improves cardiac output whilst at the same time reducing ventricular filling pressures.

Combination therapy

Dopamine in low dose to promote renal bed vasodilatation, and dobutamine in doses to achieve an improved cardiac output are often used in combination in cardiogenic shock; thus, lower doses of each can be used. Filling pressures (measured via a Swan-Ganz catheter) are titrated against systemic pressure, and the drug dosages adjusted every 10 minutes to achieve an optimal cardiac output and sufficient perfusion pressure to maintain renal, cerebral and myo-cardial function, whilst avoiding excessive heart rates and pulmonary oedema. Ideally, therefore, the dose of dobutamine is adjusted each 10 minutes until the cardiac output reaches a plateau. Dopamine is adjusted to achieve a reasonable urinary output (more than 60 ml/h); this may require support with intermittent bolus doses of loop diuretics. Left atrial pressure is maintained between 15 and 20 mmHg; this is below the threshold to produce pulmonary oedema and above the level which begins to impair cardiac output. The right atrial pressure is maintained at a level high enough to support the cardiac output and left atrial pressure. The heart rate is kept between 100 and 120 bpm and systolic blood pressure between 110 and 120 mmHg with a diastolic pressure near 80 mmHg. The patient should be comfortable in this state, with near normal arterial oxygen saturation and no acidosis.

Mechanical support

Mechanical support of the circulation can be achieved using intra-aortic balloon pump counterpulsation (see below). Mechanical ventilation of patients in cardiogenic shock is rarely justified, since it prolongs survival for a period but does little for the overall outlook of these seriously ill patients.

ACUTE VENTRICULAR SEPTAL RUPTURE AND RUPTURED PAPILLARY MUSCLE

Acute ventricular septal rupture and ruptured papillary muscle are uncommon and very severe complications of acute myocardial infarction. They tend to occur 2–10 days after the acute event and produce sudden deterioration with acute heart failure, shock and the development of a new systolic murmur. It can be impossible to differentiate the two conditions clinically, although echocardiography and Doppler ultrasound can do so in most cases.

Treatment is early surgery in both instances, although mortality remains high. There may be an advantage to allow tissues to 'heal' before closure of a VSD, but, unfortunately, most patients will succumb before sufficient time elapses. There are some conspicuous successes with early surgery and, when possible, circulatory support prior to operation may be life-saving. This is one of the only indications for intra-aortic balloon counterpulsation outside that of post-surgical shock.

CARDIAC RUPTURE

Cardiac rupture is a much commoner cause of sudden death in hospital than has previously been recognised, and is responsible for 10–20% of in-hospital deaths. It typically occurs several days after the acute infarction and appears to be commoner in men, in those with higher blood pressures and in those who suffer anterior infarction. Acute beta blockade protects from this complication which is manifested clinically by the sudden onset of severe pain followed rapidly by cardiovascular collapse. Resuscitation from this event is unusual.

13

VENTRICULAR ANEURYSM

Ventricular aneurysm is a late complication of myocardial infarction in 10–15% of patients. *True aneurysms* cause thinning and paradoxical motion of portions of ventricular wall. They interfere with cardiac mechanical function by directing some of the stroke volume into the aneurysm sac. Recurrent arrhythmia, refractory heart failure, embolisation and early rupture are the complications associated with true aneurysms, which are manifest clinically by paradoxical precordial pulsation, persistent ST elevation on the ECG and an abnormal LV border contour on the chest X-ray. *False aneurysms* are limited cardiac ruptures whose structure has become organised and stabilised; the main complications include those of true aneurysms as well as a significant tendency for late and fatal rupture.

Surgery is the treatment of choice for aneurysms once angiography has established the anatomy in detail. Antiarrhythmia therapy may be necessary and anticoagulation for true aneurysms with clot in the sac (60–70% of cases).

DRESSLER'S OR POST-MYOCARDIAL INFARCTION SYNDROME

Dressler's syndrome is an immunological syndrome of pleuro-pericarditis which may occur in 1–4% of patients, 2–12 weeks following infarction (or open heart surgery). Antiheart antibodies directed against the sarcolemma and subsarcolemma of myocytes may be found. The clinical syndrome is similar to acute pericarditis (p. 433), with pain, fever, leucocytosis, a high ESR and a 'pericarditic' ECG in half the cases. It must be differentiated from extension of myocardial infarction, pulmonary embolism or pneumonia.

Treatment usually consists of non-steroidal anti-inflammatory agents, although steroids may be required for severe and recurrent episodes. The prognosis is good.

DISEASES OF HEART MUSCLE

MYOCARDITIS

The causes of myocarditis are shown in Table 13.22. In the Western World the commonest causes are viral, of which the most important are Coxsackie B and echovirus infections. Toxoplasmosis affects the myocardium in the neonate. *Trypanosoma cruzi* is the major cause of infective heart muscle disease in South America and is discussed on page 302.

Acute viral myocarditis may complicate many severe viral infections and has been described with almost all common viral diseases. Clinically important myocarditis is uncommon, but ECG changes possibly due to myocarditis are more frequent.

Table 13.22   Causes of myocarditis

Cause	Example
Viral	Coxsackie B, but a wide range including echoviruses, adenoviruses, polio, influenza
Rickettsiae	Chlamydia and Coxiella (Q fever)
Toxoplasma	Infants and immune-compromised adults
Trypanosomiasis	*T. Cruzi* (Chagas' disease of S. America)
Bacteria	Often toxin-mediated, e.g. diphtheria
Physical	Radiation, severe hypothermia
Drugs and poisons	Emetine, carbon monoxide

Clinical features

A febrile illness accompanied by acute unexplained heart failure, cardiac arrhythmias and chest pain are the main presenting features of myocarditis. Chest pain usually results from a myopericarditis. An arrhythmia, such as frequent ventricular ectopic beats, is probably the most frequent manifestation of a mild attack of myocarditis, and is often seen after an attack of influenza.

The physical signs may include gallop rhythm and heart failure with cardiac enlargement.

Diagnosis and investigation

Diagnosis is made on the basis of the history and an ECG which may show a variety of arrhythmias, conduction defects, and myocardial injury with ST and T wave abnormalities. An echocardiogram is helpful in diagnosis and shows reduced ventricular contractility. Endomyocardial biopsy is occasionally necessary to make the diagnosis. This technique is used to obtain a small piece of myocardium for histological examination. In acute myocarditis, there is a marked lymphocytic and inflammatory cell infiltrate. Necrosis of myocytes is seen and, often, interstitial fibrosis. Later in the disease, the histological appearances become less marked and merge into those of congestive (dilated) cardiomyopathy (p. 417). The main differential diagnosis is then from other causes of congestive cardiomyopathy.

Treatment

Rest is advised until symptoms and signs and ECG abnormalities have resolved. Strenuous exercise is prohibited during this period. Cardiac arrhythmias are treated. Although the majority of patients make an apparently full recovery, about 15% have a poor prognosis with continuing evidence of cardiac enlargement and, in some cases, of progressive heart failure. It seems likely that some patients will progress to a dilated cardiomyopathy. Immunosuppressive therapy is now being advocated in the more severe cases.

CARDIOMYOPATHIES

An increasing number of patients are found to suffer from heart muscle disease. In most cases, the causes are not known, and the term *cardiomyopathy* is usually only used when hypertension and coronary artery disease have been excluded. Cardiomyopathy is more frequent in people of African origin – not only in Africa and the Caribbean, but also in the UK. The reasons for this are still unknown. There is a higher incidence of hypertension in people of African descent which causes disproportionate hypertrophy, but many have congestive cardiomyopathy with no obvious cause.

Cardiomyopathies are now classified into three main groups, shown in Table 13.23.

Congestive (dilated) cardiomyopathy

Congestive cardiomyopathies comprise half or more of patients diagnosed with cardiomyopathy. The aetiology is usually not identifiable since an identical clinical histological and pathological picture can arise after damage to the heart from many causes, including toxins (such as cobalt), drugs (such as adriamycin), or following an attack of acute myocarditis. Chronic alcoholism is associated with congestive cardiomyopathy, and, since alcohol has a direct suppressant effect on the heart, it is thought to be an aetiological agent in many cases. The precise mechanism has not, however, been clarified. Other known causes are given in Table 13.23.

Clinical features

Presymptomatic congestive cardiomyopathy may be present for several years without coming to the notice of a doctor unless there is a routine chest X-ray. There may, at this stage, be some diminution in maximum effort tolerance (should it be measured), but unless the subject concerned is an athlete, this usually goes unnoticed or is ascribed to normal ageing.

Later on, symptoms are dominated by heart failure in severe cases, with both left- and right-sided failure being eventually intractable. Atrial fibrillation and thromboembolism are frequent complications and some 10% of patients have recurrent chest pain or angina on effort, despite normal coronary arteries.

The clinical picture is of a dilated heart that contracts very poorly, with a markedly reduced ejection fraction and a high filling pressure. Physical examination usually reveals cardiomegaly, with a gallop rhythm and, often, secondary atrioventricular valve regurgitation. Both mitral and tricuspid regurgitation are common when the patient presents in heart failure, and are secondary to the ventricular dilatation.

Investigation

Chest X-ray reveals the cardiomegaly, which often involves all the chambers of the heart. The ECG is non-specific, and may show features of ventricular hypertrophy, Q waves, and widespread T wave inversion.

Echocardiography is the most important diagnostic aid, especially in the differential diagnosis of the enlarged cardiac silhouette. It can be used to exclude a pericardial effusion and haemodynamically significant valve disease. In congestive cardiomyopathy, the left ventricle is dilated and contracts very poorly. In severe mitral regurgitation, however, although the left ventricle will be dilated, it will contract vigorously with a normal or better than normal ejection fraction.

Management and prognosis

When these patients present with heart failure, the prognosis is poor, with a 50% mortality in the following two years. Treatable causes of heart failure such as heart valve

Table 13.23 Types of cardiomyopathy*

Type	Features	Causes
Congestive (dilated) cardiomyopathy (CCM)	Large cavity, poor contraction. AV valve regurgitation. Low ejection fraction	High percentage unknown (idiopathic) Following myocarditis Alcohol, cobalt, adriamycin, daunorubicin Systemic illness: amyloid; sarcoid; haemochromatosis; glycogen storage diseases; neuromuscular, e.g. Friedreich's ataxia; collagen diseases
Hypertrophic (obstructive) cardiomyopathy (HCM or HOCM)	Idiopathic ventricular wall thickening, often asymmetric. Small cavity. High ejection fraction	Usually familial or sporadic, but also associated with some left-sided lesions, e.g. aortic valve disease
Restrictive cardiomyopathy	Thick-walled ventricle or fibrosed endocardium restricts filling, but systolic function (ejection fraction) maintained. Much less common.	Endomyocardial fibrosis and Löffler's endocarditis. Amyloid; sarcoid; haemochromatosis (some cases)

*Some patients may have features of more than one type of cardiomyopathy, e.g. congestive and restrictive, and individual diseases, such as haemochromatosis, may commonly have features of both.

disease must be excluded, and endomyocardial biopsy may be necessary in the young patient to exclude an active myocarditis. Heart failure is treated conventionally with diuretics and bedrest. Anticoagulation is often advised because of the high risk of thrombo-embolism.

Inotropic agents may give a temporary improvement in symptoms but do not seem to improve prognosis. Angiotensin-converting enzyme (ACE) inhibitors are being used increasingly, and there is some early evidence that quality of life and possibly also survival are improved. Cardiac arrhythmias are treated conventionally but, as most antiarrhythmic agents are myocardial depressant, they have to be used very carefully in the presence of heart failure.

Hypertrophic cardiomyopathy

Hypertrophic cardiomyopathy is characterised by marked left ventricular wall-thickening with a small left ventricular cavity. Usually, the wall-thickening is asymmetric and predominantly affects the interventricular septum; this is known as *asymmetrical septal hypertrophy* (ASH). The hypertrophy can lead to left ventricular outflow obstruction with abnormal systolic anterior motion (SAM) of the mitral valve; when this occurs, there is almost always a variable degree of mitral regurgitation. The condition is then known as *hypertrophic obstructive cardiomyopathy* (HOCM). Similar processes can occur, but less frequently, on the right side of the heart, and sometimes both sides of the heart are involved.

Aetiology and pathology

There is a familial incidence of hypertrophic cardiomyopathy. It is sometimes inherited as an autosomal dominant, but sporadic examples account for most cases. The condition may be mild and show only on echocardiographic examination. Some cases have associated 'triggers' for left ventricular hypertrophy, such as hypertension or aortic valve disease, but there is usually no obvious cause.

On microscopy, the muscle fibres are thickened and appear to be arranged haphazardly. The appearances are not specific and other causes of left ventricular hypertrophy, such as aortic valve disease and hypertension, must be excluded. One theory suggests that the geometrical arrangement of the fibres is such that they pull antagonistically during systole, and that this results in myofibrillar hypertrophy and disruption.

Clinical features

Syncope and palpitations from a variety of arrhythmias are common and sudden death may occur. Angina can develop without coronary artery disease. The thickened myocardium can produce an inflow obstruction and lead to heart failure from a raised filling pressure. In later stages, there is an enlarged heart and a risk of systemic embolism.

The physical signs depend on whether there is outflow obstruction. In its absence, there may only be third or fourth heart sounds and a rather muscular feel to the left ventricular impulse. In the presence of outflow obstruction, systolic ejection is shortened, there is a jerky carotid pulse (compared with a sustained and weak pulse in aortic stenosis) and the apex beat has a characteristic presystolic lift. Outflow obstruction produces a harsh late systolic murmur which may be masked by a pansystolic murmur of coincidental mitral regurgitation.

The presence of exertional angina, exertional syncope and a systolic murmur with left ventricular hypertrophy can easily lead to a mistaken diagnosis of aortic stenosis. Although the physical signs differ from those of true aortic stenosis, echocardiography has proved invaluable in establishing the correct diagnoses.

Investigation

Chest X-ray is often unremarkable in the absence of heart failure. The ECG is non-specific, showing left ventricular hypertrophy and, occasionally, Q waves. Echocardiography demonstrates the left ventricular wall thickening, particularly ASH, and, with obstruction, shows SAM of the mitral valve (see above). Two-dimensional echocardiography shows that the septal hypertrophy can be a localised bulge, and also the high ejection fraction. Doppler ultrasound will demonstrate the mitral regurgitation, as well as the high velocity jet in late systole that develops in the outflow tract of the left ventricle in the presence of obstruction.

Cardiac catheterisation and angiography carry some risks because of the high incidence of arrhythmias and the very small left ventricular cavity. It is sometimes necessary to perform these investigations where there is coincident aortic valve disease or suspicion of significant coronary artery disease.

Treatment

Sudden death is a continuing hazard even with anti-arrhythmic therapy, and various agents are used to control symptoms of palpitations without apparently preventing sudden death. Beta-blockers can abolish outflow obstruction, and may help in the management of heart failure. Calcium antagonists, such as verapamil, have been used to reduce ventricular hypertrophy with variable results. Both types of drug slow the heart rate and aid diastolic function.

Surgical intervention has been used quite extensively, with mitral valve replacement and outflow tract myomectomy being used to abolish outflow tract obstruction. There is a high surgical mortality and, unless the myomectomy is radical, outflow tract obstruction can recur. The role of surgery therefore remains controversial.

Screening of siblings of those affected reveals a high incidence of mild degrees of asymptomatic asymmetrical hypertrophy. Investigation and monitoring of these subjects may eventually enable the mortality and morbidity of this condition to be reduced, but may also cause great anxiety in an asymptomatic individual.

Restrictive cardiomyopathies

There is a small subgroup of heart muscle disorders characterised by a very high filling pressure to the ventricles resulting from rigidity of the walls due to infiltration with abnormal tissue. Reasonable systolic function is usually maintained. Clinically, such restrictive cardiomyopathies present with very similar features to constrictive pericarditis, with evidence of severe heart failure and a relatively small heart. Unlike the case with the other cardiomyopathies, a distinct disease entity can often be identified, the commonest being amyloid, endomyocardial fibrosis, haemochromatosis, glycogen deposition, fibroelastosis and eosinophilia.

Cardiac amyloid

Cardiac amyloid is the commonest cause of death in primary amyloidosis – the form which develops in patients who do not have pre-existing long-standing systemic disease, such as myeloma. The gastrointestinal tract and tongue are often also involved, as are the nerves and skin. Presentation is either with heart failure secondary to poor systolic function (like a congestive cardiomyopathy) or with severe right heart failure secondary to a restrictive pattern.

There may be evidence of tricuspid and mitral regurgitation with a loud gallop rhythm, and echocardiography shows thickening of the ventricular walls with a small LV cavity. Characteristically, the ventricular walls, infiltrated by amyloid, have a very bright echo appearance, and there may be conduction abnormalities which may require a pacemaker. The diagnosis may be confirmed by rectal or gingival biopsy or, sometimes, by cardiac biopsy. There is no specific treatment for these patients, who fortunately present late in life.

Haemochromatosis and transfusion haemosiderosis

Overload of the body with iron can damage the heart. Haemochromatosis is a genetic disease in which iron overload occurs (Ch. 17, p. 649). The gene is situated on the short arm of chromosome 6, and the disease is inherited as an autosomal recessive character with a carrier frequency of 8% in Caucasian populations. The disease is due to excessive intestinal iron absorption. Cardiac iron overload also occurs in transfusion haemosiderosis, in which repeated blood transfusion (usually more than 100 units) for chronic anaemias, such as thalassaemia, causes similar tissue loading with iron. The iron damages the liver, heart, gonads and pancreas causing hepatomegaly, heart failure, testicular dysfunction and diabetes. There is a characteristic dusky skin pigmentation.

Cardiac manifestations are found in about 30% of patients. But cardiac involvement does not necessarily parallel other organ involvement, although cardiac failure is always associated with high levels of iron in the heart. There is usually myocardial thickening and dilatation, so the patient presents with features of both a dilated and restrictive cardiomyopathy. The diagnosis is based on demonstration of excessive iron in the body with the serum ferritin being particularly high.

Cardiac findings are of heart failure and arrhythmias – both supraventricular and ventricular – with disorders of conduction. There may be a low voltage ECG.

The heart failure is often refractory to treatment. The main aim of management should be to reduce body iron levels by chelation or, in the case of haemochromatosis, by repeated venesection.

Cardiac carcinoid

In the carcinoid syndrome, where a carcinoid tumour (usually ileal) has metastasised widely, over 50% of the patients have cardiac involvement which consists of endocardial plaques of fibrous tissue. This is almost always on the right side of the heart and involves the tricuspid and pulmonary valves, the vena cava and the coronary sinus, producing distortion and valvular stenosis. Serotonin and kinin peptides produced by the tumour are normally inactivated in the liver and lung; thus the left side of the heart is protected.

Clinically, the patient has the systemic manifestations of carcinoid syndrome – flushing, diarrhoea and, sometimes, bronchoconstriction. In addition, there are symptoms and signs of right heart failure, often with pulmonary stenosis and tricuspid regurgitation. The circulating vasodilators may also produce a hyperkinetic circulation with high output heart failure.

Sarcoidosis

Between 20% and 30% of autopsied cases of generalised sarcoid show cardiac involvement, although clinical manifestations are present in only about 5% of patients. Presentation may be with a cardiomyopathic picture of either the congestive or restrictive type, although it can also present with conduction abnormalities, heart block and sudden death. Heart block in a young patient may be the first manifestation of sarcoid.

Diagnosis and treatment

In the presence of the classical pulmonary findings, diagnosis does not require myocardial biopsy, but where there is doubt a biopsy can be extremely helpful. Isotope and magnetic resonance imaging may show infiltration.

Treatment is on the whole unsatisfactory. Pacing may reduce the risk of sudden death in patients with conduction system damage, and large doses of corticosteroids are usually advocated in an attempt to prevent progressive myocardial infiltration.

Endomyocardial fibrosis

Endomyocardial fibrosis is relatively common in regions of Africa, particulary Nigeria and Uganda, where it accounts for more than 20% of cardiac deaths. It is also found in other tropical areas and, occasionally, in Europeans who have been resident in endemic areas. Pathologically, there is gross fibrous thickening of the endocardium of one or both ventricles, usually associated with severe atrioventricular valve regurgitation. It commonly presents in young people of both sexes, often from low income groups.

Clinical features

The clinical presentation of endomyocardial fibrosis depends on whether one or both ventricles are involved. The disease may be heralded by fever, but usually presents with severe heart failure and sometimes arrhythmias. The heart is not usually markedly enlarged, although pericardial effusion is not uncommon. Clinical signs of the valvular regurgitation and heart failure predominate. Systemic and pulmonary emboli may complicate the clinical course. Echocardiography, particularly 2D scanning, may demonstrate the thickened endocardium, which can obliterate parts of the ventricular cavity. Intraventricular clot may also be shown.

Surgical excision of the thickened endocardium with tricuspid and mitral valve replacement has given some encouraging results in a disease that appears to have, for most, a relentless progression.

Endocardial fibroelastosis

Endocardial fibroelastosis is a condition of infancy in which there is gross thickening of the endocardium with subsequent heart failure. It may present as a primary condition or follow aortic stenosis, other left-sided heart conditions or cardiac surgery in which endocardial perfusion may have been at risk.

Löffler's endocarditis

Löffler's endocarditis – a syndrome of prolonged eosinophilia with associated localised or widespread eosinophilic infiltrates – involves the heart in over 90% of cases. The hypereosinophilic syndrome is most commonly idiopathic, but may occur with eosinophilic leukaemia or secondarily with Hodgkin's disease, polyarteritis nodosa, tumours and parasitic infestation.

The clinical picture is of a severe progressive cardiomyopathy with a restrictive picture, often with systemic embolism, in a patient with a wasting disease and marked eosinophilia.

The disease process starts as an eosinophilic myocarditis, and progresses with the formation of multiple endocardial thrombi. In the third stage, there is fibrosis and a hyaline membrane forms over the endocardium. The disease thus has some similarities to endomyocardial fibrosis, but the difference in the aetiology and clinical presentation separates the two conditions.

The clinical course of the disease can be from a few months to 12 years.

INFECTIVE ENDOCARDITIS

Infective endocarditis is a multisystem disease due to infection of the heart valves or adjacent endocardium. It is characterised by prolonged fever, weight loss, embolic phenomena and renal failure.

Classification

Until recently, it was usual to divide the disease into two groups:

1. subacute bacterial endocarditis
2. acute bacterial endocarditis.

Subacute bacterial endocarditis (SBE) affected relatively young patients with an identifiable pre-existing cardiac abnormality, usually rheumatic valvular heart disease or a congenital abnormality of the heart associated with a jet lesion. These patients had normal immune mechanisms, but the heart valves became infected with an organism of normally low virulence which slowly formed vegetations on the damaged valve and produced progressive valvular regurgitation. This was accompanied by intracardiac abscesses, embolic episodes and a slow, wasting fever, often associated with evidence of formation of immune complexes leading to glomerulonephritis.

Acute bacterial endocarditis was a disease occurring in immune compromised patients or those suffering from a staphylococcal septicaemia. Apparently normal mitral or aortic valves were rapidly destroyed in the course of 24–48 hours, resulting in torrential regurgitation and death from heart failure. This usually occurred in someone with a pre-existing severe disease.

Over the last two or three decades, the clinical spectrum of infective endocarditis has changed greatly. This is due to the gradual decline in the numbers of patients with rheumatic heart disease, an increase in the number of patients who have had cardiac surgery, increasingly sophisticated investigative techniques being used in elderly patients, and the epidemic of intravenous drug abuse.

Nowadays, infective endocarditis occurs quite frequently in elderly patients with degenerative disease of the heart valves and in whom there is no evidence of either rheumatic or congenital heart disease. Furthermore, infective endocarditis is not easily divided into the subacute and acute forms. There are a wide range of infective agents of different virulence, and the same organism, such as *Staphylococcus aureus*, can behave quite differently on different occasions depending on the patient's host defences and the particular strain of organism.

The intravenous drug abuser may develop infective endocarditis with a variety of unusual organisms, sometimes on apparently normal valves and quite commonly on the tricuspid valve. Bacteria are not the only causes of infective endocarditis. Fungal and rickettsial infections, as well as viral infective endocarditis, can occur. For these reasons, the more general term *infective endocarditis* is preferred to the earlier classification.

Pathogenesis

Pre-existing cardiac lesions

It is still the case that endocarditis most commonly develops in congenitally abnormal or rheumatic hearts in which there is a 'jet' lesion. Experimental work has shown that normal 'laminar' flow results in particulate matter, such as bacteria, in the bloodstream being insulated from the endocardium by a sleeve of plasma. However, if a turbulent jet of blood is present, the bacteria may impinge directly on the endocardial surface. Damage to the endothelium (for example as a result of rheumatic heart disease) may be followed by platelet aggregation and the formation of fibrin, to form non-bacterial, thrombotic endocarditis, which is easily colonised by bacteria present in the bloodstream. For this to occur, the bacteria in the bloodstream have to stick to the endocardial lesion and multiply before it has time to heal. A chronic lesion, such as one produced by a jet of blood impinging on the endocardium, would remain susceptible. However, transient lesions, such as those produced by passing a cardiac catheter or cannula through the heart valves for as little as 15 minutes, heal rapidly and, as a result, rarely become infected.

Bacteraemia

Transient bacteraemia is common with trauma to the mouth and teeth; the organism most commonly present, *Streptococcus viridans*, is also very likely to stick to an endocardial lesion and colonise it. Gram-negative bacilli, which can be grown from the blood in Gram-negative infections and at the time of urogenital manipulation and surgery, are less likely to cause endocarditis and stick less readily to endocardial lesions.

In practice, any surgical procedure that involves manipulation of any organ or part of the body that is not normally bacteria-free, should be regarded as a potential cause of bacteraemia. Bacteraemia is usually transient, but repeated episodes may induce antibody production and it has been demonstrated that antibodies to the circulating organism make them clump, and so stick more readily to the endocardial lesion.

Infective endocarditis may occur following a chest or urinary infection or septicaemia. It can also occur following a variety of operative and investigative procedures, but the risk of these procedures producing a bacteraemia is variable. Minor medical procedures which may provoke bacteraemia include the following:

1. *Dental extraction and manipulation.* Transient bacteraemia with streptococci and some enterococci lasts from 15 minutes to several hours. Chewing can cause bacteraemia even in edentulous individuals.
2. *Oropharynx.* Tonsillectomy, rigid bronchoscopy, orotracheal intubation and nasopharyngeal suction.
3. *Gastrointestinal tract.* Barium enema, sigmoidoscopy, and colonoscopy.
4. *Urogenital tract.* Urinary catheterisation, prostatectomy and prostatic massage have all been found to produce a bacteraemia, but normal vaginal parturition only does so occasionally.
5. *Intravenous cannulae.* These are a potential source of bacteraemia and should not be used unnecessarily in patients at risk.

Growth of the vegetation

The vegetation grows not simply as a mass of bacteria, but as a concretion of bacteria and the reaction of the blood to their presence. The bacteria become covered in platelets and layers of fibrin. The exuberance of the vegetation depends on the organism. Fungal infections with Candida produce large vegetations which can even occlude the orifice of prosthetic valves. Other organisms may provoke so little reaction that the vegetations are too small to be demonstrated by echocardiography (which has a maximum resolution of a few millimetres).

Vegetations remains the classical pathological manifestation of endocarditis, but infection can perforate the valve cusps, and track into the adjacent myocardium and valve ring, causing abscesses and a variety of complications depending on the site. These include fistula formation, bundle branch block, complete heart block, infective pericarditis and papillary muscle and chordal rupture.

Embolism and immune complex manifestations

Embolism of fragments of infective vegetation can produce embolic abscesses in the spleen, kidneys, brain and elsewhere, with 'mycotic' aneurysm of the arterial wall which may result in rupture and sudden haemorrhage. Embolic episodes result in cerebral and peripheral ischaemic attacks, transient haematuria, splenic infarcts and coronary occlusion.

Long-standing infection leads to the formation of immune complexes which may themselves complicate the presentation and course of the disease. These complexes are probably responsible for the glomerulonephritis which may accompany infective endocarditis, and for the skin lesions.

Valve involvement

As in rheumatic heart disease, the frequency of involvement of the four cardiac valves is in direct relationship to the mechanical loading on the valves, i.e. mitral, aortic, tricuspid and pulmonary in descending order of frequency. This is related to the much higher jet velocities usually found on the left side of the heart, although the very low incidence of involvement of the pulmonary valve in pulmonary stenosis remains unexplained. Untreated infective endocarditis of the aortic valve may rapidly lead to infection of the mitral valve, as the regurgitant jet of blood through the aortic valve most commonly strikes the anterior cusp of the mitral valve. Tricuspid valve endocarditis leads to a picture of recurrent lung 'pneumonitis' of a patchy nature due to embolism of vegetation and organisms into the lung.

Infecting organisms

Streptococci

At present, about 50% of cases of infective endocarditis are caused by alpha haemolytic streptococci from the mouth and oropharynx, formerly classified as *Streptococcus viridans* but now subdivided into many organisms, for example, *Strep. mitior* and *Strep. sanguis*. These organisms are most likely to reach the bloodstream after dental extraction or manipulation, bronchoscopy and tonsillectomy and adenoidectomy.

The *Enterococci* of Group D streptococci have become more frequent causes and can be found in the gastrointestinal tract, the genitourinary tract and the periodontal tissue. Accurate identification is sometimes difficult, and the prognosis is worse than for *Strep. viridans* infection. *Strep. bovis*, a non-enterococcal organism from Group D, is an increasingly common finding in infective endocarditis, and the disease in these cases is very similar to that caused by *Strep. viridans*.

Strep. pneumoniae is a less common agent but still causes some cases of acute infective endocarditis; the infection may be complicated by meningitis.

Anaerobic streptococci, organisms which are initially difficult to grow, are found increasingly frequently but necessitate anaerobic cultures. The discovery of *Strep. faecalis* should lead to investigation of the gut, since colonic carcinoma may be an underlying cause.

Staphylococci

A staphylococcal septicaemia with *Staph. aureus* often involves the heart valves; if several positive cultures are obtained, a prolonged course of anti-staphylococcal therapy is indicated even without definite evidence of cardiac pathology. Acute endocarditis can damage apparently normal valves very quickly. The same organism can produce a subacute picture. It is a frequent finding in intravenous drug abusers and diabetics with endocarditis.

Staph. epidermidis (albus) may be grown as a contaminant of blood cultures, but repeated positive cultures are significant since it is a common cause of infective endocarditis both in patients with prosthetic valves and in intravenous drug abusers. It is occasionally found in patients with indwelling subcutaneous intravenous lines.

Other organisms

Neisseria gonorrhoea and Gram-negative bacilli are relatively uncommon causes of infective endocarditis, but *Pseudomonas* is becoming more frequent.

Q fever endocarditis is uncommon and is diagnosed by finding a rising titre of antibodies in the blood. *Fungal* endocarditis occurs with prosthetic valves and in patients who have had prolonged periods of antibiotic or corticosteroids, or who are intravenous drug abusers.

Clinical features

The clinical features of infective endocarditis can be divided into several categories (Summary 7).

Features of chronic infection

The features of chronic infection include a remittent pyrexia, myalgia, arthralgia and general fatigue. These symptoms are accompanied by anaemia, anorexia and weight loss. Splenomegaly may be present but is usually not marked. Splenic infarction can lead to pain and a friction rub over the spleen. A splenic abscess can delay resolution of the fever. In long-standing cases, cachexia and mild finger-clubbing may occur.

Cardiac manifestations

Heart murmurs are present in over 85% of cases but may easily be missed by the inexperienced, especially in the presence of heart failure. Early diastolic murmurs are notoriously difficult to hear, and a wide pulse pressure is often the first clue that aortic regurgitation is present. Changing heart murmurs are uncommon but, when present, are very suggestive of the diagnosis. Cardiac arrhythmias and conduction abnormalities may follow the spread of infection from the valve ring to form myocardial abscesses.

Heart failure can be a presenting symptom. Its presence

Summary 7 Clinical features of infective endocarditis	
Infection	Fever, anorexia, weight loss, splenomegaly, cachexia, clubbing. Also arthralgia, bone pain.
Cardiac	(History of cardiac murmur, bacteraemic procedure.) Heart murmur, increasing valvular regurgitation, conduction disorders.
Systemic embolism (about 50%) Arterial Pulmonary	CVA, mesenteric, renal. Recurrent pneumonitis. (Infective emboli cause abscesses and arterial rupture.)
Immunological Renal Skin	Glomerulonephritis leading to renal failure. Subungual: splinter haemorrhages Skin and buccal mucous membranes – petechiae Finger and toe tips – Osler nodes Thenar and hypothenar eminences – Osler nodes and Janeway lesions Retina – Roth spots and boat-shaped haemorrhages

signifies a poor prognosis and is an indication for early surgery. Sudden heart failure can occur with rupture of a valve cusp or chordae tendinae, or sinus of Valsalva aneurysm.

Systemic embolism

Embolism is a prominent feature of infective endocarditis and the presentation may be with a cerebrovascular event (such as a dense hemiplegia), an ischaemic limb, mesenteric embolus or haematuria from renal infarction. Over 50% of cases exhibit embolic phenomena; fungal endocarditis with large friable vegetations is notorious for producing large emboli. Right-sided endocarditis most commonly presents with recurrent patchy consolidation (pneumonitis).

Immunological phenomena

Renal

A diffuse glomerulonephritis is present in many patients and is due to the deposition of immune complexes. The renal disease is shown by proteinuria and microscopic haematuria. In untreated endocarditis the blood urea begins to rise, but renal failure develops in less than 10% of cases. Even when advanced, renal failure recovers with adequate treatment of the infective endocarditis.

Skin and mucous membranes

Typical skin manifestations of infective endocarditis were much more common in the pre-antibiotic era, but are now seen in only $20-40\%$ of cases. Thorough examination of the patient's skin, mucosae of the oropharynx, conjunctivae and retinae should be repeated during the course of the disease, to check for new lesions.

Petechial haemorrhages. Examination of the soft palate, pharynx, conjunctivae, hands, feet and anterior body wall may reveal *petechial haemorrhages*, often with a pale centre.

Subungual or '*splinter haemorrhages*' are usually seen as a faint dark line away from the nail margin in the fingers and, occasionally, toes. They may also be seen in patients who are debilitated for other reasons, or after trauma. When present, they occur in 'bursts' and indicate activity of the disease.

Osler nodes are painful, nodular, red to purple lesions that form most commonly on the fingertips but can also occur on the backs of the toes, soles of the feet, the thenar and hypothenar eminences and, occasionally, elsewhere. Formerly common, they are now seen in less than a fifth of cases. The lesions can last a few hours to a few days.

Janeway lesions are painless, 1–4 mm erythematous macules which are most common on the thenar and hypothenar eminences and the soles of the feet, and blanch on pressure.

Retinal lesions. The Roth spot is a 'cotton-wool exudate' consisting of a perivascular collection of lymphocytes. It is not specific to infective endocarditis. Boat-shaped haemorrhages with a pale centre and white spots have also been described, but, like the Roth spot, are less common than formerly.

All of these retinal and cutaneous lesions have been ascribed to 'septic emboli', but are now thought to be immunological manifestations of the disease.

Diagnosis

Infective endocarditis is a possible diagnosis in any patient with a fever and a heart murmur, and is established by taking blood cultures. The cardinal diagnostic criteria are:

1. fever
2. evidence of chronic infection
3. a heart murmur suggestive of a jet lesion
4. positive blood culture on more than one occasion
5. presence of vegetations on echocardiography.

In many cases, a patient with a heart murmur may have an intercurrent viral infection or some other cause for fever; but where the source of the fever is not manifest, it is essential for such a patient to have blood cultures taken before being started on an antibiotic, should that be considered necessary. This is especially important when a patient at risk of endocarditis develops a fever following a procedure such as dental extraction that has not been covered with antibiotic prophylaxis.

Any febrile patient who has had open heart surgery (other than coronary bypass grafting), should be considered at risk fom infective endocarditis, even if no murmur is evident. This may be the result of infection at the time of surgery or at any time later. In the elderly patient, endocarditis can exist without significant fever. Other signs of chronic infection, such as unexplained anaemia and high ESR in a patient with a heart murmur should arouse suspicion and lead to blood cultures being taken.

Blood cultures

Blood cultures should be taken on 6–8 occasions, over the first 48 hours; it is not necessary to wait for peaks of fever. The blood should be inoculated into several bottles with a large inoculum. Special culture conditions may be needed, such as anaerobic. The organisms may not grow for several days. Although a higher percentage of positive cultures has been claimed for arterial blood culture (and even bone marrow culture) over venous blood culture, the safety and ease of venous sampling dictates that multiple venous samples are usually obtained and incubated under various culture conditions before the other more difficult techniques are used.

The laboratory must be told of the suspicion of endocarditis and whether there is a prosthetic valve, so that *any* organism that grows is kept in subcultures and not discarded. Appropriate culture techniques can then be instituted for poorly-growing organisms.

Where the clinical evidence of the disease is overwhelming, especially if there is evidence of deteriorating valve function, antibiotic therapy may be started as soon

13

as 4–6 cultures have been taken and before positive cultures are reported by the laboratory. There is, however, an inevitable risk that this may interfere with identification of the organism if the initial cultures are negative.

Where infective endocarditis is a high probability, and particularly if *Strep. viridans* is grown from blood culture, a dental opinion on possible septic foci in the mouth should be obtained. It is then possible to time any dental extraction or other dental work to follow by one hour or so the initiation of antibiotic therapy. This then removes the possibility of septic foci in the mouth harbouring antibiotic resistant organisms, which can then superinfect the heart after the initial organisms have been eradicated.

Culture-negative endocarditis

In over 20% of cases, no organisms are grown despite many other features of the disease being present. This may occur because the patient has been treated with an antibiotic (which may render cultures negative for days or weeks after stopping treatment), because the organism involved is present in very small numbers, or because it is difficult to culture. Even in average cases of endocarditis, there may be only 100 organisms per ml of blood and, particularly in long-standing cases with renal failure the patient's antibodies may render the blood almost sterile, despite the presence of organisms in large vegetations. Repeated blood culture samples of 10 ml should be inoculated into 100 ml of culture broth and incubated both aerobically and anaerobically. The organisms may require special nutrients and may not grow for several days, or, in a few cases, for several weeks. If repeated cultures are negative, or the patient's condition is deteriorating, it may be necessary to embark on treatment without positive cultures of an organism.

This course of action must only be followed after close consultation with a microbiologist, who may suggest unusual sampling techniques (occasionally bone marrow or urine are positive when blood is not), and after blood has been taken for fungal and rickettsial antibodies.

Treatment

Successful treatment of infective endocarditis should involve close cooperation between admitting physician, cardiologist and microbiologist. In the uncomplicated case, 4–6 weeks of bactericidal antibiotic therapy is required with serum levels of antibiotic sufficient to penetrate the vegetations and abscesses and eradicate the organism. Bacteriostatic antibiotics and bacteriostatic levels of bactericidal antibiotics are not sufficient, even with the host's natural defences to eradicate the organism.

Antibiotic therapy

Although oral antibiotic therapy can be used for sensitive *Strep. viridans* infection, the intravenous rate is preferred for initiating therapy, and while awaiting 'back titrations'. Suitable antibiotic regimens are shown in Table 13.24.

Table 13.24 Representative antibiotic regimens for infective endocarditis (see cautionary remarks in text)

Indication	Antibiotic regimen
PROPHYLAXIS (Note: the first dose is given 1 to 2 hours pre-operatively)	
Dental (local anaesthetic)	
No history of penicillin hypersensitivity	Oral ampicillin or amoxycillin, 3 g 1 hour pre-dental work, repeat 3 hours later
Penicillin allergy	Oral erythromycin 1.5 g, repeat 500 mg 6-hourly × 2
Dental (general anaesthetic)	Triplopen im (benzathine, procaine, and benzyl penicillins) or erythromycin iv, 1 g and then 500 mg 6-hourly × 2 or Vancomycin iv, 1 g
Non-dental gastro-intestinal and urogenital tract and prosthetic valves	
No history of penicillin allergy	Triplopen im 1 vial and gentamycin 80 mg iv, then gentamycin 80 mg iv 8 hourly × 2
Penicillin allergy	Vancomycin im 1 g instead of triplopen
INITIAL ANTIBIOTIC TREATMENT: (Drug regimens are adjusted on the basis of laboratory results of organism sensitivity and blood levels of antibiotic)	
***Strep. viridans* species**	Penicillin 3 g iv 6-hourly, plus gentamycin 80 mg iv 8-hourly. If organism is very sensitive to penicillin, continue penicillin alone either iv or im.
Culture-negative endocarditis and *Strep. faecalis*	As for *Strep. viridans*, but dual therapy continued.
Staph. aureus	Flucloxacillin 2–4 g iv 6-hourly Gentamycin 80 mg iv 8-hourly Fusidic acid iv 500 mg 6-hourly
Staph. epidemidis (albus)	As for *Staph. aureus*, although benzyl penicillin may be used instead of flucloxacillin if organism sensitive. Vancomycin may be necessary.
Gram-negative endocarditis	Ampicillin iv 2–4 g 6-hourly Gentamycin iv 80 mg 8-hourly Metronidazole iv 500 mg 8-hourly may be added if needed, but may be well-absorbed orally.
Fungal endocarditis (Monilia)	Systemic antifungal therapy and surgery
Q fever endocarditis	Has to be treated with bacteriostatic drug tetracycline, usually followed by valve replacement.

For intravenous therapy, a central venous catheter may overcome the problems of superficial venous cannulae. These may require repeated change of drip site. All cannulae must be inserted under strict aseptic conditions and kept scrupulously clean to prevent the risk of super-infection with fungi.

After culture and identification of the organism, its antibiotic sensitivity must be urgently assessed. The bacteriology laboratory assists by monitoring the patient's blood levels of antibiotic and titrating to determine what serum dilutions are bactericidal to the organism in culture. A level of 1 in 8 is considered satisfactory, but lower levels may be acceptable if the serum levels of antibiotic are sufficiently high to raise the possibility of renal or oto-toxicity should they be increased.

It is essential that the antibiotic regime for an acute septicaemic endocarditis includes anti-staphylococcal antibiotics. Where a subacute infection is being treated, it is usual to use wide-spectrum antibiotics, such as gentamycin and ampicillin. The response to treatment is then monitored and the treatment changed or continued, depending on whether it appears to be controlling the infection. Culture-negative endocarditis, particularly with large vegetations or other indication of severe valvular involvement, may be an additional criterion for early surgical intervention, particularly if potentially hazardous antibiotics are being used.

Monitoring treatment

Successful antibiotic treatment ideally results in disappearance of the fever within a few days, a fall in the ESR, rise in the haemoglobin and an increase in the patient's weight and wellbeing. Measurement of C-reactive protein may give a more reliable guide to response than the ESR. Evidence of micro-emboli, such as fresh splinter haemorrhages and microscopic haematuria, take longer to go, and large vegetations take several weeks to regress. Occasionally, the fever and high ESR do not settle although repeated blood cultures remain negative. If other causes for persistent fever (e.g. splenic abscess or superinfection) are eliminated, then the fever may be antibiotic-induced and disappear with cessation of antibiotic treatment.

Surgery

Severe valve failure and uncontrolled infection may require emergency valve replacement. If the patient presents with heart failure, early surgery is essential as, even with rapid successful antibiotic treatment of endocarditis, damaged valves shrink and fibrose with progressive increase in the degree of valve regurgitation and the heart failure may become irreversible. Prosthetic valve endocarditis almost invariably requires valve replacement for the infection to be eliminated.

A few days of antibiotic therapy prior to surgery reduces the risk of valve dehiscence from sewing the new valve into an infected valve ring, and reduces the risk of prosthetic valve endocarditis. A heavily infected valve with large veg-

etations may be electively replaced where there is risk of major embolism, or where the patient cannot be given effective bactericidal therapy. Tricuspid valve endocarditis with large vegetations can be treated by excision of the tricuspid valve without replacement, while the course of antibiotics is given. The prosthetic valve can then be sewn into a sterile ring.

Apart from valve replacement, surgical closure of intra-cardiac fistulae, such as aortic-to-right-atrial shunts and limited thoracotomy for epicardial pacing for heart block, are occasionally required.

Prophylaxis

The recommended regimens for endocarditis prophylaxis vary slightly, but all are based on the use of a bactericidal antibiotic to cover a procedure likely to produce bacteraemia. If a general anaesthetic is involved, the antibiotic is given intravenously or intramuscularly. If no general anaesthetic is involved, oral preparations are given if possible. It is usual to give a single-day, large-dose regimen. Prophylaxis is given one hour before the procedure if oral, and 30–60 minutes before if given systemically. Regimens are shown in Table 13.24.

A safe general rule is that prophylaxis should be given for all dental work where the teeth are manipulated, all pelvic, colonic and bladder instrumentation and surgery. Normal parturition does not need routine cover but if the bladder is catheterised or forceps used, this should be covered.

SYPHILITIC ENDOCARDITIS

Pathogenesis

Syphilis is much less common as a cause of heart diseae than formerly. The cardiac involvement is a manifestation of the tertiary stage of the disease, which often follows a prolonged quiescent period. An endarteritis obliterans of the vasa vasorum of the aorta weakens the media, which undergoes a slow necrosis and causes thickening and scar formation in the intima. The changes are irregular, and complicated by fibrosis and calcification. Dilatation of the aorta occurs and can be localised, giving a fusiform or saccular aneurysm; it often also involves the valve ring, causing progressive, and often severe, aortic regurgitation. There may be damage to the aortic valve cusps leading to retraction, but never stenosis. The intimal scarring of the aorta can lead to coronary ostial stenosis. The changes do not always lead to overt heart disease. There is a higher percentage of cases of aortic regurgitation and aortic aneurysms in manual labourers with aortitis, compared with sedentary men and women with necropsy evidence of aortitis. Thus, it may be that physical activity produces additional loads on the aorta which induce these changes.

Clinical features

The patient is usually a man (there is a 3:1 sex ratio for

uncomplicated aortitis, but this rises to 10:1 for aortic aneurysm) in late middle-age.

Aortic regurgitation

The presentation may be with pure aortic regurgitation with evidence (best shown echocardiographically) of a dilated aortic valve ring, and serological proof of previous *Treponema pallidum* infection. If untreated, the regurgitation tends to be progressive and severe; indeed, the classical 19th century physical signs described for aortic regurgitation are almost all based on patients with severe syphilitic aortic regurgitation (water hammer pulse, head rocking etc.). With a dilated aortic root, the early diastolic murmur is louder in the third right interspace than the third left interspace. If there is coronary ostial stenosis, severe angina is usually present, often leading to status anginosus (continuous pain), heart failure and death unless there is early surgical intervention.

Aortic aneurysm

Aortic aneurysm (p. 445) is much less common than regurgitation. It usually occurs in the ascending aorta or arch rather than the descending aorta, where aneurysms are much more likely to be arteriosclerotic. The clinical features depend on the position of the aneurysm. Classically, the ascending aortic aneurysm produces signs of aortic regurgitation, the arch aneurysm symptoms, such as dysphagia, cough, pain, dyspnoea, and the descending aneurysm pain from erosion of the spine.

Diagnosis and investigation

Serological proof of previous spirochaetal infection is usually followed by CSF examination, because of the close association with neurosyphilis. Positive serology cannot be taken as proof of syphilitic infection in patients with yaws scars, who often have persistent positive serology even after treatment. However, the combination of aortic dilatation and positive serology would be taken as confirmatory. Arteriosclerotic aneurysms, cystic medial necrosis of the aorta and aortic dissection are now common differential diagnoses.

Aortic regurgitation is investigated with particular emphasis on excluding coronary ostial stenosis. Aortic aneurysm is now often investigated by computerised tomography. There is often laminated clot in the aneurysm, and classically, in aortitis, there is calcium seen in the ascending aorta. The treatment of syphilis is described on p. 282. The Herxheimer reaction is particularly dangerous in aortic regurgitation with coronary ostial stenosis. The regurgitation may progress after effective penicillin treatment, due to further fibrosis. Surgical treatment is as for other causes of aortic regurgitation or aortic aneurysm, after effective chemotherapy.

NON-INFECTIVE ENDOCARDITIS

RHEUMATIC FEVER AND RHEUMATIC HEART DISEASE

Rheumatic heart disease is now uncommon in Western Europe and North America, but is an important historical cause of what was once the bulk of valvular heart disease. It is still important in the Third World as a disease of childhood and a major cause of heart disease. Its decline in Western countries started before the widespread use of antibiotics, and probably reflects increased standards of nutrition and hygiene and, possibly, a decline in the virulence and prevalence of Lancefield Group A haemolytic streptococci.

Rheumatic fever and chorea are the exclusive causes of chronic rheumatic heart disease, in which there is interstitial muscle fibrosis as well as the heart valve disease. However, some 50% of patients with chronic rheumatic heart disease give no history of either condition.

Rheumatic fever develops in about 3% of young people exposed to an epidemic strain of beta haemolytic Lancefield Group A streptococcus. These patients most commonly have pharyngitis, but may have scarlet fever. After apparent recovery, they develop fever, sweats, skin rashes, arthritis and, sometimes, cardiac involvement from what appears to be an autoimmune disease starting 2–4 weeks after the initial sore throat and lasting 6–8 weeks, but occasionally as much as 26 weeks. Some patients give no definite history of an antecedent sore throat.

Following the attack of rheumatic fever, some 70% of the patients will eventually have evidence of rheumatic valvular heart disease, although the time-interval can be as long as 50 years. On the other hand, the valve disease may become manifest during the attack of rheumatic fever, especially where regurgitation develops. Rheumatic fever may be recurrent, and the chances of valve disease increase with the number of attacks.

Pathology

Although rheumatic fever follows a streptococcal infection, no bacteria are found in the lesions, however, they may still be present in the pharynx. There is an acute inflammatory reaction, with oedema in the affected tissues, and then granulomatous lesions develop in the myocardium (Aschoff nodules). Oedema of the valve cusps is followed by verrucous fibrin deposits developing along the lines of apposition of the valve cusps, which eventually adhere at the commissures. In the acute illness, there is an acute non-bacterial synovitis in the joints, and granulomata may develop subcutaneously on extensor surfaces of the limbs and over the Achilles tendons (rheumatic nodules). There is usually a high anti-streptolysin O titre, and other anti-streptococcal titres may also be high. It is thought that cross-reactivity between the streptococcal antigens and host tissue antigens leads to an autoimmune inflammatory process.

Clinical features and diagnosis

The diagnosis of rheumatic fever depends on criteria proposed by Duckett-Jones (Table 13.25); two major criteria, or one major and two minor criteria establish a high probability for the diagnosis.

The patient is almost always between the ages of 3 and 30 years (usually 5–15 years); he suffers drenching sweats and a prolonged feverish illness with extremely painful arthritis that moves from joint to joint – usually involving large joints such as the knee and elbow – which become hot, red, swollen and extremely painful for a few days and then recover fully. The flitting arthritis is characteristic, as is the classical skin rash, erythema marginatum. Subcutaneous nodules may develop after several weeks, usually over the elbows.

Carditis may be pericarditis, myocarditis or, more importantly for the eventual appearance of valve disease, endocarditis. All may occur at once as *pancarditis*. The pericarditis is similar to any acute pericarditis (p. 433), with precordial pain, ECG changes (raised ST segments) and often an increase in cardiac silhouette on chest X-ray. Myocarditis is manifest by a tachycardia disproportionate for the degree of pyrexia, gallop rhythm, heart failure; there are also ECG changes, such as prolonged PR interval or greater degrees of AV block and T wave flattening or inversion, and raised serum creatine phosphokinse AV. Death occasionally occurs from myocarditis.

Endocarditis is indicated by transient or changing murmurs. The classical murmur, which is specific for the condition, is the Carey-Coombs murmur; this is a short rumbling diastolic murmur indicating mitral valvulitis.

Table 13.25 Criteria for the diagnosis of rheumatic fever

Major criteria	Minor criteria
● Polyarthritis	● Fever
● Carditis	● Arthralgia
● Subcutaneous nodules	● Prolonged PR interval on ECG
● Chorea	● Raised ESR
● Erythema marginatum	● Raised white blood count or C-reactive protein
	● Preceding beta-haemolytic streptococcus infection
	● Previous rheumatic fever or inactive heart disease

Sydenham's chorea

Sydenham's chorea (St Vitus' dance) is usually a separate disease entity but, like rheumatic fever, appears to be related to recent beta haemolytic streptococcal infection and an autoimmune process; occasionally, it accompanies the rheumatic fever, although it may follow some weeks later. It is characterised by sudden, jerky, purposeless movements of the face and limbs such that the child is thought to be clumsy and grimacing. Pure chorea, even when unaccompanied by other evidence of rheumatic fever, is followed by a high incidence of rheumatic valve disease, indistinguishable from that following conventional rheumatic fever.

Investigation

Laboratory investigations show a raised ESR, C-reactive protein and anti-streptolysin O titre. Blood cultures are negative. Throat swab may be positive for beta haemolytic streptococcus, if the preceding pharyngitis has not been treated with antibiotic.

Differential diagnosis

Since there is no absolute diagnostic test, it is extremely common to find patients who have been diagnosed as having rheumatic fever on weak evidence, such as a childhood fever with a few aches and pains and the presence of a systolic murmur. In one study, some 50% of patients with mild congenital heart disease claimed to have had rheumatic fever, suggesting that a child with a heart murmur alone is very likely to be diagnosed as having rheumatic fever during the course of a febrile illness.

Treatment

Aspirin is traditionally used to control the arthritis and fever; it is used in maximum doses (p. 993). Where the patient is extremely ill, corticosteroids are commonly used, but there is no evidence that these reduce the incidence of endocarditis or subsequent development of rheumatic valvular disease.

Prophylaxis

Anyone who has had acute rheumatic fever is at risk from a recurrence and is usually maintained on phenoxymethylpenicillin (250 mg orally daily or an im depot preparation of benzathine penicillin) or, if allergic to penicillin, oral sulphonamide, either until the age of 21 or for 5 years after the last attack of rheumatic fever, whichever comes later.

LIBMAN-SACKS ENDOCARDITIS

Systemic lupus erythematosus (p. 1015) may lead to heart failure from hypertension and a myopathic process affecting the left ventricle. In some post-mortem series, involvement of the heart valves by a verrucous endocarditis is described as involving a significant proportion of post-mortem specimens; however, valve disease is a clinical problem in only a small proportion of long-standing cases of SLE. The warty outgrowths occur at, and away from, the free edges of the valve cusps and over the mural endocardium. They involve the mitral valve in particular, and may lead to thickening of the chordae and subvalvular apparatus. Mitral regurgitation and aortic regurgitation are said to be the commonest lesions, but mixed valve lesions occur. Aortic stenosis has also been described in SLE. Libman-Sacks endocarditis may become the site of infective endocarditis and, if clinically important, is treated by prosthetic valve replacement. This cannot be undertaken lightly, however, because of the risks of coincident use of anticoagulants, corticosteroids and other anti-inflammatory drugs.

RHEUMATOID ARTHRITIS

A small percentage of patients with very active rheumatoid arthritis develop mitral and aortic valve disease, with exuberant nodular granulomatous lesions on the valve cusps but also at other sites throughout the body. These lesions only occasionally cause significant valve disease but, very occasionally, may cause significant stenosis or regurgitation in a patient who has very exuberant and severe rheumatoid arthritis.

REITER'S DISEASE AND ANKYLOSING SPONDYLITIS

Reiter's disease and ankylosing spondylitis (p. 997) can produce a degree of aortitis and aortic root dilatation and cusp retraction similar to that seen in syphilitic aortitis. There may be associated conduction abnormalities as well as aortic regurgitation, and, occasionally, these patients require aortic valve replacement and cardiac pacemakers.

CARDIAC TUMOURS

Cardiac tumours are extremely uncommon. They can present a variety of clinical features and mimic a large number of other cardiac and systemic diseases. A classification is shown in Table 13.26. Benign tumours comprise 75% of primary cardiac tumours.

Table 13.26 Most frequent cardiac tumours

Tumour	Frequency (%)	Prognosis
Myxoma	30	Benign
Lipoma	10	Benign
Papillary fibro-elastoma	10	Benign
Rhabdomyoma	8.5	Benign
Angiosarcoma	9	Malignant
Rhabdomyosarcoma	6	Malignant
Other (including secondary)	26.5	–

MYXOMAS

The origin of myxomas is controversial. They appear as a gelatinous pedunculated mass usually arising from the fossa ovalis in the atria; three out of four are on the left side, but occasionally the tumour invades both atria. About 75% are found in women. There is a slight familial tendency, and current theory suggests that myxomas arise from embryonic cells in the septum. Clinical presentation is in late middle-age, when they reach sufficient size. The clinical features are haemodynamic obstruction, embolisation and constitutional symptoms.

Left atrial myxoma

In left atrial myxoma, the large gelatinous mass obstructs the mitral valve and simulates mitral stenosis, producing left heart failure. A ball-valve mechanism can produce recurrent pulmonary oedema or syncope, which can lead to sudden death. Pulmonary hypertension with subsequent right heart failure mimics mitral valve disease. In one-third of patients, there are systemic emboli, with the brain the most frequent site. Systemic symptoms are found in 90% of patients and mimic those of a collagen disease or infective endocarditis, with fever, anorexia, weight loss, myalgia, arthritis, Raynaud's phenomenon, petechiae and finger-clubbing. These features are thought to result from immunological reactions to necrosing tumour.

Physical signs can mimic those of mitral stenosis, with a diastolic murmur in about 20% of patients. More common is a systolic murmur of mitral regurgitation and, classically, there is a 'tumour plop' instead of the opening snap of mitral stenosis. However, the tumour can be silent or give only intermittent auscultatory findings.

Right atrial myxoma

Right atrial myxomas are less common than those on the left side; they can cause severe right heart failure with oedema, hepatomegaly, ascites and pleural effusion. Syncope and sudden death are also recorded, and recurrent emboli can lead to severe pulmonary hypertension and a paradoxical path to the left side through a patent foramen ovale. Constitutional symptoms are as common as on the left. Physical signs are more frequent than on the left side, with systolic and diastolic murmurs being audible in over 80%, and endocardial friction rub audible in 20%.

Myxomas may arise in the ventricles, but these are less common. As with atrial myxomas, they are likely to embolise and cause obstruction.

Investigation

Electrocardiography may show atrial hypertrophy from obstruction. Chest X-ray may show left atrial or right atrial enlargement, pulmonary hypertension or other secondary effects of the tumour. Occasionally, a slow-growing myxoma calcifies and can be seen on plain film or, better, on screening.

Echocardiography has revolutionised the diagnosis of myxoma, initially using M mode, but now with 2D echo. The tumour can often be visualised popping backwards and forwards through the valve orifice. However, the tumour can be missed by the inexperienced operator in M mode if inappropriate gain settings are used, and a 2D study from several windows may be needed to show small tumours and, particularly, right atrial myxomas.

Formerly, left atrial myxoma was visualised angiographically by injecting dye into the pulmonary artery and following it to the left atrium and ventricle. Occasionally, tumour was visualised with left ventricular injection. If satisfactory echo pictures are available, there is now nothing to be gained from cardiac catheterisation, which runs the risk of dislodging tumour and causing systemic emboli.

Laboratory tests are frequently abnormal, especially in patients presenting with systemic symptoms. Haemoglobin is low (with normochromic normocytic film), but may, occasionally, be high with right atrial myxoma, severe pulmonary hypertension and right-to-left shunting through a patent foramen ovale. A neutrophil leucocytosis occurs. The ESR is often raised, with an increase in plasma gamma globulins.

Treatment

Surgical excision of the tumour is essential but carries some risk of tumour embolisation and recurrence, both from the site of excision, if incomplete, and from other sites in the heart. The tumour is therefore excised with its atrial attachment, and the atrial septum then patched. Many surgeons now inspect all four cardiac chambers, because of the high incidence of local recurrence and the occasional multiple tumour.

Atrial myxomas are relatively easily treated and should be suspected wherever there is unexplained systemic embolism, particularly if there are features of a 'collagen disease', if a case of 'infective endocarditis' is persistently culture negative, and if features of mitral valve disease are accompanied by syncopal episodes. Right atrial myxoma should be suspected in unexplained right heart failure and recurrent pulmonary emboli.

CARDIAC DISEASE AND PREGNANCY

Pregnancy places a sustained load on the heart which increases throughout the pregnancy and then peaks with labour. There is a considerable increase in cardiac output (30–50%), blood volume (40–50%) and extracellular volume (about 7 litres), with an increase in heart rate of about 10 beats per minute and a slight fall in mean blood pressure.

The circulation of the pregnant woman is as if she were vasodilated, with warm peripheries and an increase of up to 30% in resting oxygen uptake. The increase in cardiac output is accomplished by an increase in heart rate, stroke volume and ejection fraction. Venous pressure of the upper body increases marginally, if at all, whereas there can be an increase in lower body venous pressure when supine or standing, due in part to pressure of the gravid uterus on the inferior vena cava. This pressure increase, and the increase of up to 8.5 litres in total body water, often leads to oedema of the ankles. The increase in plasma volume occurs earlier than a compensatory increase in total red blood cell volume, so that an apparent anaemia ensues.

Diagnosis

Pregnancy makes the diagnosis of heart disease more difficult. The pregnancy may produce symptoms of fatigue, shortness of breath, ankle oedema and syncope (from pressure of the gravid uterus on the inferior vena cava). Physical examination may reveal flow murmurs, a mammary souffle, venous hum, a third heart sound, a raised *a* wave in the jugular venous pulse, displacement of the cardiac apex (by the elevated diaphragm) and basal rales (which clear on coughing) for the same reason, all of which may be taken to indicate heart disease.

The above confounding symptoms and signs are unfortunate because of the increased risk posed by heart disease to both the mother and the fetus. Another reason for establishing if heart disease is present, even if it appears to be asymptomatic, is the small risk of puerperal endocarditis. The murmur of pregnancy (*Still's murmur*) is a low-pitched, often vibratory murmur heard at the left sternal edge but usually loudest in the pulmonary area. It is extremely common, is mid-systolic and is unaccompanied by any other signs of heart disease. High-pitched systolic murmurs, and all diastolic murmurs, indicate heart disease. The use of echocardiography and Doppler ultrasound will often be of great value in these cases. Chest X-ray is relatively contra-indicated. If essential, the fetus can be shielded. The risk to the fetus late in pregancy is much smaller than first thought.

The ECG is usually normal but the axis may shift to the left, with T wave inversion in lead 3, a small Q wave and sometimes even ST and T wave inversion in the limb and precordial leads; these ECG changes revert to normal at the end of pregnancy and recur in later pregnancies.

Management

If the pregnant mother is known to have heart disease and is in functional class 3 or worse of the New York Heart Association classification (p. 334, Table 13.1), it is hazardous for the pregnancy to continue; certain types of heart disease, such as coarctation of the aorta, severe hypertension, severe aortic or mitral stenosis or cardiomyopathy, present particular hazards.

Surgery during pregnancy may offer a solution to the mother who is anxious to continue with the pregnancy; closed mitral valvotomy, or open valvotomy and valve replacement under cardiac bypass, have been performed with a low maternal mortality and acceptable fetal risk.

If valvular disease or a jet lesion (ventricular septal defect, etc) is diagnosed, appropriate antibiotic cover is given at the time of labour – particularly if instrumentation (e.g. urinary catheterisation) is used at the time of delivery.

Anticoagulants

A particular problem may be the need for anticoagulants. Discontinuation of anticoagulants is dangerous for a mother with a prosthetic heart valve, and possibly also for a mother who has had a pulmonary embolus. Warfarin is avoided if at all possible during the first trimester, because of an increased risk of fetal abnormality. It may be given in a later stage of pregnancy, but is discontinued towards term. For a planned pregnancy, heparin can be given during the first trimester and is given near term. However, if continued for long, it may accentuate calcium loss from the mother.

Peripartum cardiomyopathy

Pregnancy and labour may make occult heart disease manifest. Occasionally, catastrophic heart failure supervenes and appears to be associated with a progressive cardiomyopathy.

Hypertension

Hypertension in pregnancy and pre-eclamptic toxaemia and eclampsia are discussed on page 438.

SECONDARY HEART DISEASE

A wide variety of pathological conditions may also increase cardiac output and produce heart failure. These include thyrotoxicosis, anaemia, cor pulmonale, beriberi, arteriovenous fistulae, generalised Paget's disease of bone and exfoliative dermatitis.

Thyrotoxicosis

Thyrotoxicosis dramatically increases metabolic rate, but the thyroid hormones also have a stimulant effect on the autonomic nervous system and the heart itself. There is usually a sinus tachycardia which is indicative of the severity of the disease, but in 15% of cases, thyrotoxicosis triggers a supraventricular arrhythmia, most frequently atrial fibrillation. Pulse pressure and blood pressure rise slightly and the heart contracts more vigorously in thyrotoxicosis. Heart failure does not usually occur in the absence of other heart disease.

Anaemia

Severe anaemia makes a two-fold demand on the heart. In order to supply the oxygen requirements of the body, the heart has to pump an increased cardiac output, but it has to do so while itself being perfused with anaemic blood. Small degrees of anaemia are of marginal importance, but life-threatening anaemia may lead to cardiac dilatation and severe heart failure, with pathological changes in the myocardium of 'fatty heart'. As the myocardium extracts vir-

tually all the oxygen from the blood in the coronary circulation, autoregulation of flow demands a dramatic increase in coronary flow to compensate for the extra myocardial work of severe anaemia. This cannot be accommodated if there is coronary disease of any severity, and continuous angina and heart failure may result.

Beriberi

Beriberi is uncommon outside Asia, but minor forms may occur in some alcoholics and food faddists. Severe thiamine deficiency (classically due to subsistence on polished rice) results in autonomic and other nervous system damage, with profound vasodilatation and a high cardiac output. In its fulminant form, the patient may die from pulmonary oedema within 48 hours of the onset of symptoms. Response to conventional heart failure therapy without thiamine is poor. Thiamine is given as soon as the diagnosis is suspected, and should be given to alcoholics in heart failure (in case there is a degree of thiamine deficiency), and in all cases of resistant heart failure where the nutritional background of the patient is doubtful.

Arteriovenous fistulae, Paget's disease of bone, exfoliative dermatitis

If they are severe enough, arteriovenous fistulae, Paget's disease of bone and exfoliative dermatitis may all cause a considerable reduction in peripheral resistance leading to a large increase in resting cardiac output. The patient has a bounding pulse and hyperkinetic circulation, often with a third heart sound and systolic murmur. Heart failure may supervene if the heart is already damaged or if the stress is severe enough. Treatment of the condition will alleviate the strain on the heart.

Inborn errors of metabolism and connective tissue disorders

Heart disease may complicate or be part of many other medical conditions. Table 13.27 shows the cardiac lesions associated with inherited connective tissue disorders; Table 13.28 lists some inborn errors of metabolism associated with cardiac disease; Table 13.29 gives the main chromosomal abnormalities in which there are cardiac abnormalities; and Table 13.30 gives the main skeletal syndromes associated with heart disease.

Athlete's heart

Endurance athletes often have hearts which exceed 50% of the transverse diameter of the chest on chest X-ray, and they may have clinical cardiac enlargement as well. Associated with the cardiac enlargement is a slow resting heart rate and an increased stroke volume. The degree of enlargement seems to vary with the extent of the resting bradycardia which can be as low as 35 bpm in extreme cases, but is more usually between 45 and 60 bpm. Exercise

Table 13.27 Inherited connective tissue diseases and the heart

Condition	Cardiac condition	General features
Cutis laxa	Peripheral pulmonary stenosis	General skin laxity, disrupted elastic fibres
Ehlers-Danlos	Mitral regurgitation Arterial rupture	Hypermobile joints Hyperelastic skin
Marfan's	Aortic dilatation, dissection, aortic and mitral regurgitation	Gracile habitus arachnodactyly, lens subluxation, sternal abnormalities
Osteogenesis imperfecta	Aortic regurgitation	Fragile bones, blue sclera
Pseudoxanthoma elasticum	Peripheral and coronary artery disease	Degeneration of elastin fibres leading to yellow pseudoxanthomas of skin, retinal angioid streaks, hypertension

Table 13.28 Inborn errors of metabolism and the heart

Condition	Cardiac condition
Pompe's disease	Glycogen storage disease involving the heart muscle
Homocystinuria	Aortic and pulmonary artery dilatation
Mucopolysaccharidoses: Hurler's and Hunter's syndromes (mental deficiency)	Multivalvular disease, coronary artery disease and cardiomyopathy
Morquio's disease	Aortic regurgitation

Table 13.29 Chromosomal abnormalities and the heart

Chromosomal defect	Cardiac abnormality
Trisomy 21 (Down's syndrome)	Endocardial cushion defects, ASD, VSD, pulmonary stenosis
Trisomy 13	VSD, double-outlet right ventricle
Trisomy 18	VSD, persistant ductus arteriosus, pulmonary stenosis
Cri du chat (short arm deletion 5)	VSD
XO (Turner's syndrome)	Coarctation
XXXY and XXXXX	Persistant ductus arteriosus

ASD = atrial septal defect; VSD = ventricular septal defect

Table 13.30 Skeletal syndromes and the heart

Syndrome	Cardiac abnormality	Skeletal syndrome
Ellis von Crevold	Single atrium or ASD	Chondrodystrophic dwarfism
TAR	ASD or tetralogy of Fallot	Absent radius, thrombocytopenia
Holt Oram	ASD (and others)	Upper limb deformity, hypoplasia of clavicles
Laurence Moon-Biedl Bardet	Variable	Polydactyly, obesity
Noonan	Pulmonary valve dysplasia	Pectus excavatum
Tuberous sclerosis	Cardiomyopathy	Bone lesions
Leopard	Pulmonary stenosis	Broad facies, ribs abnormal
Cockayne	Accelerated atherosclerosis	Cachectic dwarfism
Progeria	Accelerated atherosclerosis	Skeletal hypoplasia
Apert	VSD	Craniosynostosis syndactyly

ASD = atrial septal defect; VSD = ventricular septal defect

rate and endurance performance. A variety of ECG changes have been described in young athletes, some resulting from marked vagal tone, others from both right and left ventricular hypertrophy. The increased stroke volume can result in a soft systolic murmur, and third and fourth heart sounds are sometimes faintly audible with subjects who have marked bradycardia.

Diagnosis

Extreme examples of this condition can easily be confused with cardiomyopathy, and it is essential not to arrive at an erroneous pathological diagnosis. Fortunately invasive investigation is not usually required. The assessment is based on exercise testing and echocardiography (unless there have been symptoms or are signs suggestive of ischaemic heart disease), which usually show superior performance of the heart.

Where an athlete has symptoms suggestive of heart disease, he should be rapidly investigated. Athletes are not immune from heart disease, and superior athletic performance is compatible with a number of forms of cardiac pathology, some of which are potentially lethal. However, an athlete who is in strict training can lose form very rapidly if prevented from training. It is unfortunate for both the athlete and the credibility of the doctor concerned, if training is interrupted for investigation of a suspected abnormality which is only part of the 'athletic heart syndrome'.

training appears to promote the bradycardia, which has both a vagal component and a component which appears to arise from desensitisation of the heart to chronotropic sympathetic drive. Elite endurance athletes with extremely slow resting heart rates and a large stroke volume can generate very high cardiac outputs, since their maximum exercising heart rate is the same as the normal (180–210 bpm). The high cardiac output enables them to maintain a superior oxygen uptake, and thus a superior work

Sternal depression and straight back syndrome

Abnormalities of the shape of the thorax are a common cause of systolic murmurs; they may also give rise to musculoskeletal chest pains, an abnormal X-ray appearance of the heart and, in severe cases, ECG changes. Sternal depression and an abnormally vertical dorsal spine (straight back syndrome) both allow very little room for the heart in the anterior-posterior axis; this is well shown on the lateral chest X-ray. There is often a systolic murmur arising from the distorted great vessels; respiratory function may be impaired because of restricted chest wall expansion on inspiration, giving rise to a poor effort tolerance; and there may be associated mitral valve prolapse as a congenital anomaly. The ECG commonly shows right bundle branch block, and there may be anterior T wave inversion in the V leads in the most severe cases.

Assessment includes careful clinical examination to exclude primary cardiac pathology, and echocardiography and Doppler ultrasound where doubt exists as to whether there is more than a 'flow murmur'. Mild forms of this condition are commonly seen in pregnancy, when the patients are referred because of the murmur. Reassurance often helps the chest pains, which usually have a musculoskeletal basis and become worse when the possibility of heart disease is raised. Simple back exercises may also help.

CARDIAC TRANSPLANTATION

Since the first human heart transplant in December 1967, the technique has become an accepted form of treatment for the patient who is dying from heart failure, and for whom no other form of therapy offers any help. In the period 1968–81, the mortality from surgery and graft rejection steadily decreased.

Indications

The British Cardiac Society reported on the indications for cardiac transplantation in 1983. The main indications proposed were:

1. dilated cardiomyopathy with congestive failure
2. advanced ischaemic myocardial damage with severely damaged left ventricle.

Less common indications were:

3. hypertrophic cardiomyopathy with intractable heart failure
4. rare causes of intractable congenital heart disease, unassociated with a raised pulmonary vascular resistance in the lungs
5. severe myocardial damage related to previous cardiac surgery for valve disease.

Patients were only considered for transplantation if they had reached end-stage heart failure and were considered to have a life expectancy measured in weeks.

The British Cardiac Society also assessed the number of potential patients who would be considered suitable for transplantation in the United Kingdom. They calculated that there could be 150 patients with congestive cardiomyopathy under 50 years of age, 150 cases a year of ischaemic left ventricular damage, 30 cases of hypertrophic cardiomyopathy and 50 cases of congenital heart disease. This gives a total of 450 to 500 patients under 50 years of age considered, on medical and psychological grounds, to be suitable for transplantation. Subsequent experience and improvements in surgery have increased these numbers considerably.

Donor hearts

The main limitation on cardiac transplantation, apart from access to surgical teams skilled in the technique, is the availability of donor hearts. These must be from young adults free from heart disease, so that donor hearts only become available after severe head injury or cerebral catastrophe in the donor. These hearts can now be removed remote from the recipient and kept in a cold 'cardioplegic' solution for long enough to survive a journey of several hundred miles; this removes the necessity for the brain-dead donor to be brought to an adjacent operating theatre. ABO blood group compatibility with the recipient is essential; HLA compatability has not been shown to influence graft rejection, but a negative lymphocyte cross-match between recipient and donor cells has been found necessary, and the donor and recipient have to be of similar size.

Technique

The recipient heart is excised leaving as much aorta and pulmonary artery as possible, and leaving the posterior walls of the atria with their venous connections. The donor heart is anastomosed by the atria to the recipient atria with preservation of the donor sino-atrial node; the aorta and pulmonary artery are also anastomosed. Two temporary pacemaker electrodes are attached to the right atrium for pacing and recognition of early graft rejection; this shows on the ECG recorded from the atrial surface (the right atrial electrogram).

The surgical technique itself is relatively simple. The principal problems apart from the preservation of the donor heart in transit are rejection and infection.

Rejection and immunosuppression

Rejection occurs early and can be recognised from the ECG by loss of R wave voltage, and by serial percutaneous endomyocardial biopsy which is carried out at frequent intervals. Rejection is prevented and controlled by prophylactic immunosuppression which is increased if evidence of rejection is found. Regimens vary, but consist of combinations of azathioprine, methylprednisolone, antithymocyte globulin and cyclosporin A.

Because of their therapy, transplant patients are at risk

from infection and, as late complications, may develop accelerated arteriosclerosis in the donor hearts, an increased incidence of malignancies and lymphomas. However, life expectancy and quality of life have greatly improved with the evolution of better techniques of donor heart preservation, surgery and immunosuppression. The Stanford series produced by Shumway showed survival of nearly 40% at 5 years and, for younger patients under 40, 55% at 3 years.

PERICARDIAL DISEASE

The pericardium is a fibrous bag which supports and invests the heart. Like the pleura, it may be the site of inflammation, neoplastic infiltration and calcification, and may also be the site of fluid collection with or without inflammation.

Aetiology

The causes of pericardial disease are shown in Table 13.31. All of these conditions can produce the clinical features of pericarditis with effusion. Heart failure can also cause a pericardial effusion, but these are small asymptomatic effusions, often discovered at routine echocardiography.

Acute viral pericarditis

The commonest viral causes are Coxsackie virus A or B, varicella, herpes simplex, influenza virus and echovirus (type 8). Frequently, a definite viral cause cannot be established. Typically, it occurs in young adults one or two weeks after an upper respiratory infection. The patient then develops fever, pericardial pain and malaise which may persist for a few weeks. Unfortunately, recurrences occur in about 25% of cases possibly from an autoimmune mechanism. Tamponade is unusual.

Acute pyogenic pericarditis

Acute pyogenic pericarditis can follow pneumonia or a septicaemia and is treated with the appropriate antibiotics and repeated drainage, which may require surgical intervention. Staphylococcus and Haemophilus are the most common organisms involved. It may also occur in immunosuppressed patients and following cardiac surgery.

Tuberculous pericarditis

Tuberculous pericarditis may be asymptomatic until it presents as pericardial constriction (see below). It may present as a large pericardial effusion with enlargement of the cardiac silhouette on chest X-ray, or as a low-grade fever with weight loss, fatigue and features of pericarditis. Pericardial aspiration may reveal the organisms but occasionally (as with pleural effusions), culture of the fluid or pericardial biopsy may be required before the diagnosis is established.

Table 13.31 Causes of pericardial disease

Infections	Autoimmune
Viral, e.g. Coxsackie, influenza	Collagen disease, rheumatoid
Bacterial; pyogenic and tuberculosis	arthritis, SLE
Fungal	Post-pericardiotomy and post-
	infarction (Dressler's) syndromes
Metabolic	Serum sickness and drug reactions
Uraemia	Idiopathic (benign recurrent viral)
Hypothyroidism	relapsing pericarditis
	Rheumatic fever
Neoplastic	
Carcinoma of the bronchus	**Haemopericardium**
Lymphomas	Cardiac rupture
	Aortic dissection
Myocardial infarction	Trauma and surgery
Radiotherapy	

Malignant pericarditis

Pericardial effusion fluid should always be sent for cytology, as malignancy may present with a pericardial effusion. The clinical features are similar to other types of pericarditis, but may be complicated by direct tumour extension into the pericardium with a degree of constriction. Lung cancer is the commonest cause.

Uraemic pericarditis

Uraemic pericarditis develops with severe untreated uraemia and disappears with dialysis. It appears to be directly related to the blood urea level.

Other types

In most other types of pericarditis, such as in autoimmune disease, pericardial involvement is an incidental finding, but occasionally may lead to constrictive pericarditis.

Clinical features

The principal symptoms of pericarditis are pericardial pain, breathlessness (if the effusion becomes large enough) and, eventually, tamponade. There may be systemic symptoms related to infection, such as fever, rigors, weight loss and symptoms of the underlying cause (lung cancer, tuberculosis etc).

Pericardial pain

Pericardial pain is a mediastinal pain that can be very similar to that of myocardial ischaemia, but differs in that it is more commonly referred to the shoulder and back and is often influenced by posture and mediastinal movements, such as coughing, sneezing and, particularly, swallowing. It is often relieved by leaning forwards. The diagnosis may be difficult because of the occurrence of pericardial pain following myocardial infarction. There can also be a pleural element to the pain.

Pericardial rub

Pericardial rub – the main physical sign of pericarditis – is very variable and often absent. It is a rough scratching sound which seems nearer to the observer than the stethoscope headpiece. Typically, it has three components – systolic, diastolic and atrial-systolic. However, the atrial-systolic and diastolic components may not be present, and a purely systolic scratchy murmur may have other causes. The noise can sometimes be accentuated by leaning the patient forward or, if conditions allow, by putting the patient in the knee-elbow position. The sound comes and goes and does not necessarily disappear with the formation of an effusion; indeed, it may be found in up to 70% of patients with pericarditis and effusion.

Pericardial effusion

Pericardial effusion does not usually cause symptoms unless it is large, when there may be some breathlessness and, eventually, features of tamponade (see below). The clinical signs of an effusion without tamponade – soft heart sounds, increased cardiac dullness etc. – are not as helpful as chest X-ray and ultrasound.

Cardiac tamponade

If the pericardial cavity fills with blood or pericardial fluid, the pericardial pressure may rise sufficiently to embarrass filling of the heart and lead to a form of cardiogenic shock (*cardiac* or *pericardial tamponade*) with very low cardiac output, cerebral confusion, and severe hypotension proceeding to death, if the pericardium continues to fill.

The pericardium is visco-elastic and can therefore stretch slowly to accept as much as two litres of fluid over a period of time without the development of tamponade, but much smaller amounts of fluid can be fatal if they accumulate quickly.

Aetiology

Tamponade is usually caused by bleeding or effusion into the pericardial space. It can complicate aortic dissection and myocardial infarction with rupture into the pericardium. Bleeding can also follow surgery or trauma to the heart and mediastinum, and may follow perforation of the heart at cardiac catheterisation, or injury after pericardial aspiration. Malignant disease is a common cause, but tamponade is an uncommon complication of other causes of pericardial effusion.

Clinical features

Severe hypotension with impalpable peripheral or very weak peripheral pulses may be present. Classically, careful palpation of the arterial pulses reveals *pulsus paradoxus*, in which the pulse pressure drops considerably on inspiration and the pulse may even become impalpable. The paradox is not that the pulse volume diminishes with inspiration (which happens normally to a small extent), but that the stroke volume of the left ventricle declines markedly whilst – paradoxically – the heart seems to be beating normally. The mechanism of pulsus paradoxus is related to the pericardial tamponade dictating a small fixed volume to the heart. Normally, right ventricular filling is aided by inspiration but with tamponade (or pericardial constriction), this right-sided mechanism inhibits filling of the constricted left ventricle, whose stroke volume falls.

The jugular venous pressure is usually markedly raised, may show a marked systolic drop and, sometimes, rises with inspiration (*Kussmaul's sign*). Chronic tamponade can mimic constriction, with hepatic enlargement and oedema. The heart sounds may be faint and there can be a pericardial rub.

Investigation of pericarditis

The ECG changes of acute pericarditis are shown in Fig. 13.65. The ST elevation remains concave upwards and is followed later by widespread T wave inversion, probably indicating a degree of epicardial myocarditis. A large effusion can produce a diminution of ECG voltages; in extremely large effusions, there can be 'electrical alternans', with the voltage being influenced by the heart swinging backwards and forwards in the effusion.

Chest X-ray (if there is an effusion) shows increased cardiac silhouette, with a globular appearance to the heart but no evidence of raised pulmonary venous pressure. This appearance is not specific.

Echocardiogram is the technique of choice in demonstrating a pericardial effusion, preferably with a 2D scan. A small effusion can be localised, and may be missed unless the operator is experienced. With a large effusion, echocardiography will show the heart surrounded by a large bag of fluid which is seen as an 'echo-free' space.

Pericardial aspiration is described below. The fluid should be sent for bacteriological and cytological examination.

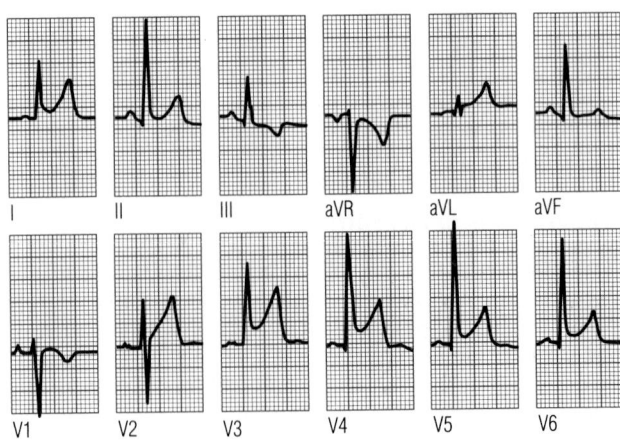

Fig. 13.65 ECG of acute pericarditis illustrating widespread concave ST segment elevation.

Treatment

Pericardial pain often responds to anti-inflammatory agents. Infective pericarditis demands prompt diagnostic aspiration and identification of the infective agent, with appropriate chemotherapy. In viral pericarditis anti-inflammatories alone are used, but where there is an auto-immune element, such as in post-infarction syndrome and recurrent 'viral' pericarditis, corticosteroids may help. A large effusion is drained as described below. If the patient suffers repeated attacks, a pericardial window can be made into the pleural space at operation.

Pericardial aspiration

Pericardial aspiration can be both diagnostic and therapeutic. In an emergency – for example after a road traffic accident with trauma to the chest – if a patient is moribund with features suggesting tamponade (i.e. very high venous pressure), then aspiration from the apex of the heart with a needle of adequate length should not be delayed. Removal of even 50–100 ml of blood from the pericardium may reverse the state of shock.

Elective aspiration is best performed in a coronary care unit with ECG monitoring and a cardiac defibrillator available. After local analgesia of the chest wall, the pericardium is punctured either at the cardiac apex (which is free of major coronary vessels) or by a subxiphoid approach. The ECG monitor shows ventricular ectopics if the ventricles are touched. Ideally, a cannula, rather than a needle, is left in the pericardium, and aspiration or drainage follows. If the fluid looks like blood, pericardial blood from a haemopericardium can be distinguished from ventricular blood by the fact that it is defibrinated and will not clot. It also has a lower haemoglobin and haematocrit than venous blood, since it is almost always diluted with serous pericardial fluid.

Aspiration at the cardiac apex is possibly safer than the subxiphoid approach, since the aspiration needle is likely to puncture the thick-walled left ventricle rather than the thin-walled right ventricle, which is more likely to tear.

Diagnostic aspiration of a large effusion without subsequent drainage can lead to pericardial fluid draining into the pleural cavity. Drainage of a large effusion can take several hours, and recurrent effusion (for example in malignant disease) may require fenestration of the pericardium or insertion of a pericardioperitoneal drain by a cardiothoracic surgeon.

CONSTRICTIVE PERICARDITIS

Constrictive pericarditis results from thickening and fibrosis of the pericardium with, in some cases, extensive calcification.

Aetiology

There may be an antecedent history of acute pericarditis or radiotherapy. Tuberculous pericarditis is now rare in Western countries, but is the classic cause of calcific constrictive pericarditis.

Pathogenesis

The heart is effectively encased in a rigid box, which eventually prevents the heart from filling. Haemodynamically, the diastolic pressures or filling pressures of the two sides of the heart become the same as the intrapericardial pressure; as this rises, the patient goes into bilateral heart failure, in which features of right-sided failure predominate. Sometimes the constriction is selective so that the left or the right side, inflow or even outflow can be compromised most.

Clinical features

Symptoms

The major symptom is of severe oedema, often with ascites, liver engorgement and, often, progressive weight loss secondary to the hepatic engorgement and a low cardiac output. Patients with long-standing disease look cachectic, and with the liver enlargement and a degree of jaundice are easily thought to have carcinomatosis or cirrhosis of the liver. The absence of significant left-sided heart failure symptoms is characteristic. The patient can often lie flat without problems and does not have a history of paroxysmal nocturnal dyspnoea, but he will always have a limited exercise tolerance and dyspnoea on exertion. Constriction may arise with no previous history of pericarditis. A previous history of pericarditis is a valuable clue to the diagnosis.

Signs

A very high venous pressure is invariable, as the end diastolic pressure in both ventricles is about 25 mmHg. The high venous pressure is interrupted by a rapid *x* descent or *systolic collapse* of the venous pressure. This is the result of sudden filling of the right atrium as the two ventricles contract and so allow a greater expansion of the squeezed atria. The pulse exhibits pulsus paradoxus, but this sign is not invariable and the presence of atrial fibrillation in about 30% of cases makes the sign difficult to elicit. The pulse will, in any case, be of small volume. The heart is not clinically enlarged and the rigid pericardium may impede palpation of the cardiac impulse. The heart sounds may be faint with a loud additional sound, the *pericardial knock*. This is a loud early third heart sound, resulting from the rapid filling of the ventricles being suddenly impeded by the rigid pericardium. Murmurs are uncommon unless the constriction is selective.

Investigation

The ECG is non-specific, showing low voltages and, usually, T wave inversion; other changes may reflect epicardial myocardial damage resulting from pericardial impingement on the epicardial coronary arteries.

Chest X-ray shows a normal-sized or slightly enlarged heart, often with an abnormal contour due to flattening of the atria. Calcification may be seen in the A-V groove on a lateral film (Fig. 13.19). Depending on the sites of constriction, there may be signs of left atrial or right atrial hypertension. Pleural effusions are common. Screening of the heart reveals a typical 'diastolic shock', with lack of pulsatility of the atria.

Echocardiography may demonstrate thickening of the pericardium. The ventricles fill rapidly in early diastole, but the differential diagnosis from constrictive cardio-myopathy is not easy.

Treatment

The only effective treatment is surgical decompression of the heart by removing enough of the pericardium to allow the heart to fill effectively. This means removing the adherent pericardium from around the great veins and atria, which are extremely thin-walled. Where the pericardium is adherent to the ventricles the coronary arteries are easily damaged, so considerable surgical skill and patience are required.

SYSTEMIC BLOOD PRESSURE AND HYPERTENSION

Cardiac output and vascular resistance form part of an integrated system which controls arterial pressure and also blood flow to the tissues. Despite our knowledge of many of the component mechanisms of pressure and flow control, many aspects of the system remain unclear, both in health and disease.

CONTROL OF BLOOD PRESSURE

Neurosympathetic blood pressure control

Activation of pre-ganglionic sympathetic neurones to the heart produces an increased heart rate and increased strength of contraction. Vasomotor sympathetic outflow constricts vascular smooth muscle, producing arterial vaso-constriction. The supply to the veins is richer and more sensitive than to the arterial system.

Increased vagal activity reduces the heart rate, but, with the exception of the coronary and salivary gland vascular beds, there is no parasympathetic control of the blood vessels.

Moment-to-moment reflex control of the circulation is via the arterial baroreceptors in the wall of the aorta and in the carotid arteries. These are excited by stretch and activation leads, by the withdrawal of sympathetic tone, by vasodilatation in the peripheral circulation and by a diminished heart rate and strength of cardiac contraction. The speed of this pressure-controlling mechanism is illustrated by its important role in maintaining systemic pressure during abrupt changes in posture.

Neurosympathetic influences on blood pressure and the circulation are rapid but tend to be transient; this is partly due to a tendency for the reflexes themselves to undergo accommodation, and partly because peripheral auto-regulatory mechanisms may overcome neural constrictor effects.

Renin and angiotensin

The renin-angiotensin-aldosterone system (Fig. 13.27) plays a major part in the control of blood pressure, regional blood flow and blood volume, via its control of sodium balance. Renin secretion from the granules in the juxta-glomerular apparatus is stimulated by a fall in plasma volume, a drop in blood pressure and sodium depletion. The consequent rise in angiotensin II production and aldo-sterone secretion leads to sodium and water retention, and hence to restoration of sodium balance and plasma volume. Under conditions of plasma volume reduction and sodium depletion (less than 50 mmol Na^+/day), angiotensin II contributes to the maintenance of blood pressure by both vasoconstriction and interaction with the sympathetic nervous system. In the kidney, angiotensin II has a preferential constrictor effect on efferent (post-glomerular) arterioles, and thus maintains glomerular filtration pressure at times when the overall arterial pressure is diminished.

The renin-angiotensin system plays a crucial role in the increased blood pressure seen with renal arterial constriction; the latter causes a rapid release of renin and angiotensin II and hence a rise in blood pressure. Angiotensin II causes changes in intrarenal flow patterns and stimulates aldosterone release. The combination of haemodynamic and direct effects on the renal tubules increases sodium reabsorption.

The juxtaglomerular apparatus is not the sole source of renin, which is found in the vessel walls of many tissues including the brain. Angiotensin-converting enzyme (ACE) activity is also widespread, but the exact contribution of these facilities for local production of angiotensin II to the control of blood pressure and tissue perfusion is not clearly understood.

BLOOD PRESSURE MEASUREMENT

The routine bedside assessment of systemic blood pressure was first performed by noting the pressure required to occlude the radial pulse with upper arm or forearm constriction. Korotkoff defined the auscultatory features (Korotkoff sounds) over the brachial pulse as pressure was released from an inflatable cuff. Systolic pressure correlates with the first sound (K_1) and diastolic pressure is usually within a few mmHg of sound muffling (K_4). Sound disappearance (K_5) is used to define diastolic pressure in many major trials of blood pressure treatment. In some individuals, K_5 cannot be defined when peripheral vascular resistance is low, as sounds carry on to zero cuff pressure. The anauscultatory gap (K_2–K_3) is particularly prominent in the elderly; this is important, as mistaken identification of K_3 as K_1 might lead to a serious underestimation of systolic pressure – by up to 15–20 mmHg in some cases. Its presence is accentuated by venous distension distal to the cuff.

Accurate blood pressure measurement requires a cuff of adequate size; a small cuff will seriously overestimate pressures. The subject should be seated with the manometer reservoir at the level of the sternal angle. The cuff bladder is arranged medially to overlap comfortably the medial aspect of the upper arm. Pressure in the cuff is inflated rapidly to 20–30 mmHg above that required to occlude the brachial or radial pulse. Pressure is then reduced slowly from the cuff whilst listening with a stethoscope over the previously located brachial pulse. The rate of pressure drop should not exceed 5 mmHg per second, and the line of sight should be such as to avoid parallax errors when reading the falling column of mercury.

SYSTEMIC HYPERTENSION

Definitions

Blood pressure varies considerably in any one individual, depending on the demands of the circulation. Blood pressure rises during exertion, and is subject to a circadian variation which may not be completely activity-related. Ambient temperature and the degree of emotional or physical arousal will also affect systemic pressure levels. In addition, systolic blood pressure rises with age in developed countries (Fig. 13.66). Diastolic pressure does not appear to rise to such a degree. Within a community, blood pressure (systolic and diastolic) has a normal or Gaussian distribution, a factor which becomes very important when definitions of abnormalities of blood pressure are considered (Fig. 13.66).

Insurance companies were amongst the first to note that a reduced lifespan was associated with recordings of elevated blood pressure. It was clear from their data that no cut-off pressure level could be identified at which no increased risk of premature death was present. The absence of an easily identifiable abnormal group of patients with the disease 'hypertension' has led to different strategies designed to isolate those individuals most at risk, those in whom pressure reduction will diminish risk and those in whom treatment would make little difference to their outlook. Hypertension could therefore be defined as a blood pressure above a particular value, for example 160/90 mmHg.

A more flexible definition – able to take into account new information derived from the results of therapeutic trials – might be preferable, for example, 'the level of blood pressure above which investigation and treatment do more good than harm.' Figure 13.67 illustrates how successive treatment trials (the Veterans Administration in 1965, compared to the Medical Research Council in 1985) have lowered the blood pressure at which treatment has been shown to have benefits.

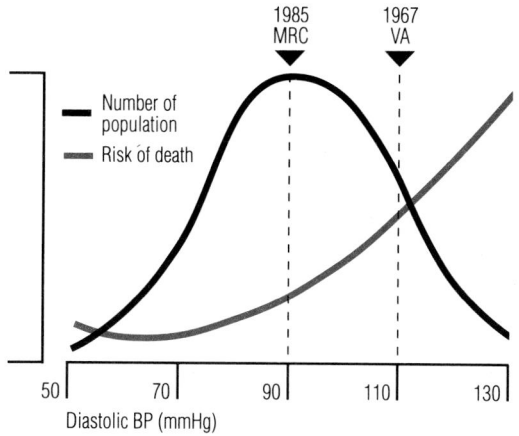

Fig. 13.67   **Distribution of diastolic blood pressure in a Western population (black line).** Risk of death is shown by the red line. The diastolic blood pressure levels are indicated at which treatment reduced mortality in two large trials (see text). VA = Veterans Administration; MRC = Medical Research Council.

Risk stratification

A small number of individuals have very high blood pressure and are at very high risk of complications of the disease, and death. At lower levels, the risk attributable to blood pressure is relatively less for the individual, but that low risk is shared by so many people that the associated complications and premature mortality pose a significant burden on the community.

Blood pressure is not the only risk factor in these calculations. Since drug treatment of great numbers of the population tends to carry unwanted financial and medical

Fig. 13.66   **Changes of blood pressure with age in three different communities: Londoners, urban Zulu and Kalahari Bushmen.**

consequences (due to the requirement for lifelong therapy), it is very important to pay attention to other contributing risk factors as well.

Hypertension in special groups in the community

There is a tendency to a high systolic blood pressure in old age and this carries with it the risks associated with hypertension at any age. Therapy is possible in older patients, and has been shown to reduce the risk of stroke and myocardial infarction.

Urban black populations have a higher incidence of hypertension than their white neighbours. Both environmental and genetic factors are likely to be responsible. Hypertension is rare in some rural African communities but a very major problem in others. Stroke is the most common complication amongst black hypertensives, and myocardial infarction is relatively rare; the opposite is the case for white hypertensives. The effectiveness of treatment is similar amongst blacks and whites; however, there are minor differences in the response to certain drugs, with a slight resistance to the effects of beta-adrenoreceptor blocking drugs being shown by black patients.

PRIMARY HYPERTENSION

Borderline and labile hypertension

About one-third of patients found to have an abnormal blood pressure at their first visit to the doctor will have lower blood pressure on subsequent visits. This borderline group may subsequently develop established hypertension. Some individuals appear to have wide swings in blood pressure, and have been called *labile hypertensives*. It seems likely that they do not form a pathologically distinct group, but manifest an accentuation of normal variability. As a group, they have a higher mortality than consistently normotensive individuals.

Isolated systolic hypertension

Due to arteriosclerotic changes in the major vessels of the elderly, the pulse pressure widens, with a greater rise in systolic compared to diastolic pressure. Thus, isolated systolic hypertension may be observed. Even in isolation, systolic hypertension is associated with an excess risk of morbidity through stroke, myocardial infarction and congestive cardiac failure. Unequivocal evidence of benefit of treatment in such cases is not yet available, but it seems reasonable to aim for a systolic pressure reduction to 140–160 mmHg, as long as treatment is well-tolerated.

Benign or essential hypertension

Hypertension is never 'essential' and rarely benign; nevertheless these terms have the justification of common usage. This is the disease which affects the vast majority of those suffering from high blood pressure – possibly as much as 20% of the middle-aged population of the UK. The diagnosis depends on an established elevated systemic pressure in the absence of changes in the ocular fundi and of proteinuria, and where no identifiable cause of pressure elevation has been demonstrated. Essential hypertension can affect any age group and can, when untreated, lead to many complications, including malignant and accelerated phase hypertension.

Malignant and accelerated-phase hypertension

Malignant or accelerated-phase hypertension is associated with vascular fibrinoid necrosis and loss of pre-capillary arteriolar autoregulation. The consequence is capillary vessel rupture and tissue necrosis through haemorrhage and ischaemia. The brunt of the damage is borne by renal, adrenal, cerebral, retinal, pancreatic and mesenteric vessels, for reasons that remain unclear. The clinical findings are elevated levels of blood pressure (which may be severe), associated with haemorrhages and exudates visible on the retina. Proteinuria due to similar vascular changes in the kidney is usual. Papilloedema (when present) reflects cerebral oedema and was previously used to differentiate malignant hypertension, where it was present, from accelerated phase hypertension, where it was not. This differentiation has no clinical or prognostic value as the conditions are identical, with an untreated mortality of over 80%. Patients may have a past history of hypertension but, in most, this is the first manifestation of their disease. It is one of the few occasions that hypertension is associated with symptoms, which include visual disturbance, headache and breathlessness due to pulmonary oedema; with severe degrees of cerebral oedema, blunting of consciousness, coma and epileptic seizures also occur. It is usually easy to treat and therapy is undoubtedly life-saving.

Many factors have been implicated in the genesis of malignant hypertension. The rate of rise of pressure may be more important than absolute levels of hypertension and there may be associations with other factors which damage blood vessels, such as cigarette smoking.

Hypertension in pregnancy

During pregnancy cardiac output rises, but blood pressure normally falls due to a fall in vascular resistance. Obstetricians regard as abnormal a blood pressure greater than 140/90 (measured using Korotkoff 4 for diastolic pressure) in the first half of pregnancy, and by this criterion nearly one-quarter of the pregnant population will be hypertensive. About 2% will have a blood pressure greater than 160/105. *Pre-eclampsia* and *eclampsia* are distinct clinical syndromes, which are limited to the duration of pregnancy, and of which elevated blood pressure is just one manifestation. Pre-eclampsia was previously defined as hypertension with proteinuria (more than 0.5 g/l per 24 hours) and oedema. However, the latter is a frequent finding in normal pregnancies and often absent in pre-eclampsia, so that it is no longer included as a diagnostic criterion. Proteinuria is a late manifestation of pre-eclamptic renal impairment. Impaired uric acid clearance, which occurs much earlier in the disease process, is more useful diagnostically. Evidence of disseminated intravascular coagulation occurs late in the disease. Eclampsia is defined as the development of convulsions in the above setting.

The diagnosis of pre-eclampsia thus depends on the observations of an abnormal rise in blood pressure between the first and second halves of pregnancy of, or greater than, 30/20 mmHg, associated with abnormal urate levels (more than 0.35 mmol/l at 32 weeks or more than 0.4 mmol/l thereafter); proteinuria, impaired renal function and clotting disorders confirm the diagnosis, but occur very late in the disease.

The consequences of pre-eclampsia are placental ischaemia and infarction and, in severe cases, maternal cerebral haemorrhage. Treatment is elective delivery, which confirms the diagnosis by effecting a rapid and complete cure. Medical management may reduce blood pressure but has not been shown to ameliorate other features of pre-eclampsia, which continues until delivery is effected.

Pre-existing hypertension, low social class and the first pregnancy with a particular partner are risk factors for pre-eclampsia; interestingly, it appears to be less common in smokers.

SECONDARY HYPERTENSION

The causes of secondary hypertension are given in Table 13.32. As a general rule, the younger the patient with hypertension, the greater is the likelihood that a cause will be found. In an adult hypertensive population, less than 5% of patients will have a discernible cause for their elevated blood pressure.

Renal disease

The precise cause of high blood pressure in chronic renal failure is not clear. Adequate management of hypertension is important to prevent vascular complication due to hypertension and prevent further deterioration of renal function. There is no justification for surgical removal of kidneys in unilateral renal disease, since medical treatment of hypertension is now likely to be more effective.

Renal arterial stenosis activates the renin-angiotensin system, and restoration of the normal vascular supply may potentially cure the associated hypertension. Atheromatous disease is the commonest form of renovascular disease; it mainly affects middle-aged male smokers, and is often part of a generalised degenerative disease of the arteries. Angioplasty (p. 405) may be useful, but the disease present in smaller arteries limits the overall prognosis. In fibromuscular dysplasia (a disease of younger age-groups), surgical reconstruction of renal arteries may be very effective.

The importance of diagnosing renovascular hypertension has increased in recent years with the introduction of angiotensin-converting enzyme inhibitor drugs (ACE inhibitors). The latter are to be avoided in renovascular hypertensives, as these drugs have a drastic effect on renal function due to the importance of angiotensin II in main-

Table 13.32 Causes of secondary hypertension

Type of cause	Examples
Renal	
Parenchymal disease	Chronic renal failure of any cause
	Acute and chronic glomerulonephritis
	Polycystic disease
	Pyelonephritis
	Tumours, e.g. haemangiopericytoma,
	Wilm's tumour
	Diabetes
Arterial disease	Arteriosclerotic disease
	Fibromuscular dysplasia
	Embolism
	Polyarteritis nodosa
Endocrine disease	
Adrenal cortical overactivity	Cushing's syndrome
	Conn's syndrome, adrenal hyperplasia
	Enzyme defects, e.g. congenital adrenal hyperplasia
Adrenal medullary overactivity	Phaeochromocytoma
Drug-induced	Contraceptive pill
	Liquorice-containing compounds
	Steroids
	Withdrawal of antihypertensives, esp. clonidine
	Cheese ingestion in patients taking monoamine oxidase inhibitors
	Sympathomimetic decongestant nasal sprays/appetite suppressants
Coarctation of the aorta	
Miscellaneous	Porphyria (during acute attacks)
	Lead poisoning (during acute phase)
	Raised intracranial pressure

taining intrarenal haemodynamics in the underperfused kidney.

Endocrine disease

Hypertension, which may be severe, usually accompanies Cushing's syndrome (p. 708).

Hyperaldosteronism

Over-production of aldosterone may be due to single or multiple autonomous adrenal adenomas (Conn's syndrome) or bilateral micronodular hyperplasia of the zona glomerulosa. Clinical suspicion of primary hyperaldosteronism is raised when untreated hypertension is associated with hypokalaemia (K^+ less than 3.5 mmol/l), alkalosis (HCO_3 greater than 30 mmol/l), and a serum sodium which is high or at the upper limit of normality (Na^+ of, or greater than, 145 mmol/l).

Investigation of *primary hyperaldosteronism* is aimed at differentiating adenomas from adrenal hyperplasia, as the former may be removed surgically. Radionucleotide adrenal scanning with labelled cholesterol, CT scanning and adrenal vein catheterisation to measure the production of aldosterone, offer the best methods of diagnosis. Explorative surgery may be necessary in some instances. Hyperplasia is treated successfully with anti-aldosterone drugs, such as spironolactone or amiloride.

Phaeochromocytomas

Phaeochromocytomas are tumours, usually found in the adrenal, which secrete a mixture of catecholamines. They are responsible for clinical syndromes where hypertension may be episodic and alternate with episodes of postural hypotension. Paroxysms of hypertension are often associated with a constellation of symptoms, including headache, sweating, palpitations, feelings of apprehension and tremor. These symptoms are more sensitive in making the diagnosis than are most biochemical tests. The majority (90%) of the tumours are benign, and 10% arise outside the adrenals, most commonly at the bifurcation of the abdominal aorta. There are associated phaeochromocytomas in Sipple's syndrome (often a familial disorder with the combination of medullary carcinoma of thyroid and parathyroid adenoma) and in neurofibromatosis or von Recklinghausen's disease (p. 1140).

Investigation and treatment

Confirmation of the diagnosis is made by the detection of increased amounts of catecholamines and their breakdown products – normetadrenaline, metadrenaline and vanylmandelic acid (VMA) – in urine or plasma. Localisation of the tumours is by CT scanning and radionucleotide scans with MIBG (^{131}I meta-iodobenzylguanidine).

Treatment is surgical when possible, but can be hazardous due to surges of catecholamine secretion during tumour manipulation. Preliminary treatment with alpha- and beta-blockade is essential, as are agents to raise blood pressure and prevent vascular collapse when the levels of these hormones fall rapidly as the tumour is removed.

Drug-induced hypertension

Mineralocorticoid-induced hypertension with hypokalaemia and alkalosis accompany the use of steroids, and may occur with carbenoxolone and excessive liquorice consumption. Hypertension induced by the contraceptive pill is generally mild and reversible on cessation of therapy, although this may take several months.

Coarctation of the aorta

In coarctation of the aorta, children or young adults present with asymptomatic upper limb hypertension and are noted on physical examination to have characteristically late and low-volume femoral pulses compared to the radial pulses (*radio-femoral delay*).

Hypertension may be difficult to treat medically and, if left until the patient is a teenager, is often only partially helped by surgical repairs of the narrowed aortic segment. Those operated on late (after 20 years of age) frequently suffer the complications of uncontrolled hypertension, and about 12% may die in their thirties of cerebral haemorrhage or ruptured aortic aneurysm. Surgery is now recommended before the age of six, but, more recently, balloon angioplasty has been successfully used in this condition and may be used more frequently in the future if initial good results are maintained.

The hypertension of coarctation is not fully explained, but renal hypoperfusion, aortic baroreceptor activity and mechanical effects of aortic obstruction may all play a part.

CLINICAL FEATURES OF HYPERTENSION

Until complications appear, essential hypertension is a condition without symptoms which, by definition, has no associated physical signs save for the elevated blood pressure. Headaches – once widely regarded as indicators of hypertension – are no more common in hypertension than in the general population, although very severe hypertension, associated with cerebral oedema, does produce headache. Breathlessness may be present, due to elevated left ventricular and end-diastolic pressure and pulmonary venous congestion produced by left ventricular hypertrophy.

Once the complications of essential hypertension are present, they are reflected in the symptoms and physical signs. Ventricular hypertrophy may lead to breathlessness, orthopnoea and frank cardiac failure; coronary disease to angina pectoris or myocardial infarction; cerebrovascular disease to stroke and dementia; and renal disease to all its associated symptoms.

The presence of some symptoms (for example those associated with phaeochromocytoma) will suggest a secondary cause. Symptoms of renal impairment (such as nocturia and polyuria) may reflect the consequence of long-standing hypertension rather than its cause.

Certain points in the examination of the hypertensive deserve emphasis, and require careful observation at diagnosis and during follow-up.

Pulse

Rate and rhythm. Atrial fibrillation is a late consequence of hypertension. A resting tachycardia might imply cardiac decompensation or a secondary cause, such as phaeochromocytoma or hyperthyroidism.

Arterial wall. If thickened arteries are palpated in an under 50-year-old, aggressive treatment of blood pressure and other risk factors would be justifiable.

Peripheral pulses. Radio-femoral delay is a sign of aortic coarctation, which may be a cause of hypertension in young patients. In older patients, atherosclerotic disease may cause peripheral vascular bruits and absent distal pulses.

Apex beat

A displaced and thrusting apex beat indicates left ventricular hypertrophy (LVH) and therefore hypertension worthy of aggressive treatment. The absence of this sign does not exclude LVH.

Abdomen

Palpable kidneys might be found with polycystic renal disease. A systolic and diastolic abdominal or flank bruit raises the possibility of renal arterial stenosis.

Optic fundus

Haemorrhage, exudates and papilloedema are all signs of accelerated or malignant hypertension. Early signs of arterial wall-thickening are narrowing of the arterial lumen (grade 1, which is difficult to identify) and arteriovenous nipping (grade 2).

General aspects

Other important general signs include:

1. signs of risk factors for vascular disease (xanthomata), which might tip the balance in favour of treatment because of the increase in vascular risk
2. signs suggesting Cushing's syndrome or neurofibromatosis (associated with phaeochromocytoma)
3. indications of congestive cardiac failure.

INVESTIGATION

The extent to which patients with elevated blood pressure are investigated depends upon the outcome of the history and clinical examination. Biochemical, radiological and cardiac investigations have two aims:

1. to determine the effect that elevated blood pressure has already had on various organ systems, in particular the kidneys and the heart
2. to identify a cause of the hypertension.

Numerically, the latter is far less rewarding since only about 5% of all cases of hypertension have an identifiable cause. This proportion is higher in young adults, all of whom should be investigated accordingly.

Urine testing

Even though the yield of abnormal results by dip-stick testing is not high, this simple test is essential in all cases. Persistent proteinuria requires detailed testing of renal function (p. 791). The discovery of haematuria should be followed by tests for inflammatory and neoplastic disease of the kidney.

A 24-hour collection of urine is required to quantitate protein excretion; this may be helpful in hyperaldosteronism, Cushing's disease and phaeochromocytoma.

Blood tests

Routine haematological and biochemical tests are seldom

rewarding. However, it is usual to obtain a full blood count and biochemical profile, which may occasionally provide useful information, for example:

1. an indication of renal function (urea and creatinine)
2. electrolyte disturbances (low K^+, raised HCO_3^- and Na^+) that might indicate hyperaldosteronism
3. other associated risk factors, such as hyperuricaemia or hyperlipidaemia
4. anaemia due to chronic renal disease, or polycythaemia secondary to renal disease.

ECG

An initial ECG may be helpful as a baseline for future changes, or as an additional help in deciding whether to offer treatment. Features to be documented are signs of left atrial enlargement ('P mitrale', p. 342) and, with more severe levels of hypertension, evidence of left ventricular hypertrophy (Fig. 13.68) possibly associated with abnormalities in the ST segments and T waves that denote the 'strain' pattern. With effective blood pressure reduction these changes usually resolve.

Fig. 13.68 Typical ECG in severe hypertension showing left ventricular hypertrophy.

Chest X-ray

The chest X-ray is helpful in establishing cardiac size and may reveal cardiac failure. In most Caucasian patients it is normal, but cardiac enlargement is common in hypertensives of African descent. In young hypertensives, signs of a coarctation (p. 396) may be found.

Ultrasound techniques

The echocardiogram can accurately measure ventricular hypertrophy and estimate function, while the abdominal examination shows kidney size, ureteric anatomy and some information on the renal substance. Both tests should be reserved for patients whose initial investigations reveal a problem requiring further definition.

Nuclear medicine techniques

Nuclear medicine techniques are used to measure dynamic aspects of kidney and cardiac function. These specialised methods should be reserved for those in whom a specific problem has been identified.

Intravenous urography

Intravenous urography may be helpful in assessing renal size and function and to exclude obstruction in patients with probable renal disease.

COMPLICATIONS OF HYPERTENSION

The development of left ventricular hypertrophy in hypertension is an adaptive response, but the effects on diastolic function may give rise to pulmonary venous congestion and, with increasing hypertrophy, inner layers of myocardium become ischaemic. The associated acceleration of atheromatous coronary disease contributes to the progression to left ventricular dysfunction and cardiac failure.

Atheroma deposition is accelerated by hypertension, and causes the most numerous of the complications of coronary artery disease; it also is responsible for most of the cases of stroke. Aortic dissection is a consequence of vessel wall degeneration and cystic medial necrosis.

A pathologically distinct process affects smaller vessels particularly of the renal and cerebral circulations; this consists of medial and intimal proliferation. Renal impairment may follow, although renal failure is usually a complication of the fibrinoid necrosis of the resistance vessels, which characterises malignant or accelerated phase hypertension.

SUITABILITY FOR TREATMENT

At the highest levels of blood pressure (diastolic pressure greater than 115 mmHg) the risks to the individual patient are so high that treatment is mandatory. However, confirming that it is beneficial to treat patients with diastolic pressures between 90 and 114 mmHg has been more difficult. The combined results of randomised trials suggest that treatment has decreased the odds of stroke significantly, by about 40%. Treatment only managed to reduce the risk of heart attack by 10%. These large trials have provided no evidence to favour any one particular drug regimen over any other.

Patients with diastolic blood pressures above 105 mmHg are recommended for treatment, particularly if they demonstrate any ventricular hypertrophy, or renal impairment. For the 10–15% of the middle-aged population with diastolic pressures between 90 and 104 mmHg, a more complex strategy is necessary. This is because halving the annual risk of a stroke, from 0.1 to 0.05%, in an asymptomatic middle-aged man may not be worthwhile, particularly when set against the requirement for lifelong treatment.

However if the individual has already suffered a complication, such as a transient ischaemic attack, halving the annual stroke risk from 20 to 10% is a worthwhile goal.

A strategy for patients with diastolic blood pressure between 90 and 104 mmHg should aim to identify those individuals with the highest risk of complications. Treatment begins with measures to reduce associated risk factors, such as smoking, high blood lipids and obesity. Drug therapy of mild hypertension should therefore be reserved for those in whom all other measures have failed and those who carry the greatest risk of progression to severer forms of blood pressure or cardiovascular complications.

Systolic hypertension

Although epidemiological studies have shown that systolic blood pressure is at least as good a predictor of subsequent complications as diastolic pressure, there is less information on the levels of systolic pressure which should be treated. In most cases, systolic and diastolic pressures follow each other closely. However, difficulties arise in elderly patients, where isolated systolic hypertension is more common. Precise guidelines are not available, but the fears that treatment might reduce cerebral blood flow and worsen cerebrovascular risks have not been borne out. Reduction of high systolic pressures (greater than 180 mmHg) might therefore be expected to accrue benefits by reducing the stroke rate, and this indeed has been the finding in the few studies of elderly hypertensive patients.

METHODS OF TREATMENT

The importance of attention to associated risk factors, such as smoking and hyperlipidaemia, has already been emphasised, and is an important part of all treatment strategies. Blood-pressure-lowering drugs may not be needed if other methods are successful.

Non-pharmacological methods

Drug withdrawal. Withdrawal of drugs which may contribute to hypertension, such as non-steroidal anti-inflammatory agents, steroids and oestrogen-containing compounds such as the oral contraceptive pill, should be considered where possible.

Dietary measures. For each kilogram loss of weight, blood pressure can be expected to fall by 2.5–3.0 mmHg systolic and 1.5–2.3 mmHg diastolic. In general, salt restriction has not been found to be an effective treatment for hypertension at the levels of intake achievable with a tolerable Western diet. However, high salt intakes can negate the effectiveness of the thiazide diuretics used in treatment, so that it is important to ensure patients moderate their intake.

Relaxation. Teaching patients to relax – using formal programmes which can be administered by non-medical personnel in general practices and continued at home by the patient – has been shown to produce a modest sustained blood pressure reduction.

Exercise. Aerobic exercise maintained for some 15–20 minutes will lower subsequent blood pressure readings by 5–10 mmHg for about 12 hours. Exercise may also improve associated cardiac risk factors, including obesity.

Drug treatment of essential hypertension

Principles of drug treatment of hypertension are theoretically simple. Therapy with a single drug given once a day is the ideal, but combination treatment is frequently necessary. A step-by-step approach is frequently used, starting with a first line preparation alone, then in combination with another, before third and fourth line drugs are used (Table 13.33).

Diuretics

The long-acting thiazide diuretics such as chlorothiazide and bendrofluazide are effective, although symptomatic side-effects such as impotence and gout are not uncommon. They are less powerful in renal failure, when loop diuretics such as frusemide and bumetanide have an advantage, but they appear to be particularly effective in black hypertensive subjects and in those with more severe elevation of blood pressure.

Thiazide diuretics cause biochemical changes which have given concern about their long-term safety. In particular, mild hypokalaemia is commonly produced, and this may be associated with a risk of cardiac arrhythmias. Hyperuricaemia may produce symptomatic gout and, in conjunction with glucose intolerance and increases in cholesterol and triglyceride concentration, an overall worsening of the cardiovascular 'risk factor profile' is produced by these drugs. It is not at all clear whether these concerns are justified, although the lack of improvement in the incidence of myocardial infarction in the vast majority of hypertension treatment trials has been attributed in part to these unwanted biochemical effects of the thiazide diuretics.

Table 13.33 Indications for specific antihypertensive drugs and their common side-effects

Type of drug	Indication	Advantages	Symptomatic side-effects	Other side-effects
Diuretics				
Long-acting thiazides	First line or adjunct to beta-blockers or Ca-antagonists	Effective, cheap, usually once-daily treatment	Gout, impotence	Hypokalaemia Glucose intolerance ↑ Lipids
Spironolactone Amiloride	First line in Conn's or adrenal hyperplasia	Potassium-sparing	Gastrointestinal upset	Hyperkalaemia in renal impairment
Loop	In renal disease	Powerful diuretics	–	As for thiazides ? lipid effect
Beta-adrenoreceptor blockers	First line	Anti-anginal and anti-arrhythmic	Asthma in some subjects, tiredness, claudication and cold hands/feet	↑ LDL ↓ HDL
Calcium antagonists	First or second line	Anti-anginal and anti-arrhythmic	Flushing, oedema, gastrointestinal upset	Heart block and negative inotropy with some examples
Angiotensin-converting enzyme inhibitors	Second line ? First line in renal disease	Well-tolerated and very powerful; useful in heart failure	Rash, dysgeusia, postural hypotension	Profound hypotension Renal impairment in renovascular disease
Others				
Methyldopa/clonidine	Second/third line Methyldopa in pregnancy ? First line	Can be used alone effectively	Sedation, impotence	Haemolytic anaemia
Hydralazine	Third line	Largely superseded by Ca-antagonists and ACE-inhibitors	Headache	SLE-type reactions
Prazocin/indoramin	Third line	Largely superseded by Ca-antagonists and ACE-inhibitors	Postural hypotension	–
Diazoxide	Third line	Largely superseded by Ca-antagonists and ACE-inhibitors	Oedema	Glucose intolerance
Minoxidil	Third and fourth line	Extremely powerful vasodilator	Hirsutism, oedema	Fluid retention
Bethanidine/guanethidine	Fourth line	Rarely indicated	Postural hypotension/impotence	Hypotensive infarction

Beta-adrenoreceptor blockers

Chance clinical observations led to the recognition that the beta-adrenoreceptor blockers are effective antihypertensives. These drugs are specifically contra-indicated in obstructive airways disease, due to the production of asthma even by drugs with supposed cardiac selectivity. Other troublesome side-effects are related to the beta-receptor blocking action, with bradycardia, tiredness, claudication and cold limbs being prominent. The demonstration of their protective effect following myocardial infarction, as well as their anti-arrhythmic and anti-anginal actions, make beta-blockers a rational choice when ischaemic heart disease complicates hypertension. They have to be used with great caution, if at all, in heart failure. Plasma lipids are altered with beta-blockade, potentially worsening the cardiovascular risk. However whether these alterations are deleterious in the long term has not been clarified.

Beta-blockers with diuretics have become established as the mainstays of the management of hypertension. There are many examples of these drugs. In the UK, atenolol, metoprolol, propranolol, nadolol and pindolol are commonly used examples.

Calcium antagonists

The antihypertensive effectiveness of calcium antagonists is related to the fall in peripheral vascular resistance that follows resistance vessel vasodilatation. Side-effects of nifedipine can be attributed to its vasodilator activity and include flushing, headache and oedema; in contrast, verapamil has more gastrointestinal side-effects, and ought not to be combined with beta-blockade due to its propensity to produce heart block and impair ventricular contractility. Diltiazem fills an intermediate position with fewer peripheral effects and more cardiac effects than nifedipine, but less myocardial effects than verapamil. Although these drugs have not been subjected to close analysis in large trials, there is no doubt of their efficacy and popularity, even as a first line therapy.

Angiotensin-converting enzyme (ACE) inhibitors

The ACE inhibitors were specifically manufactured to inhibit the renin-angiotensin system, by blocking the conversion of angiotensin I to its active form, angiotensin II. These drugs are subjectively very well tolerated, and their associated efficacy, in all but the groups of patients with renal arterial stenoses, has led to their adoption as the first of the second line treatments to be used in the severer degrees of hypertension. Side-effects have included severe neutropenia, rashes and taste disturbance with captopril, and renal impairment and hypotension with both captopril and enalapril. Their hypotensive effect may be severe in relatively hypovolaemic patients and in those with hyponatraemia (which might occur in those taking diuretics). ACE inhibitors will cause a deterioration in function or renal failure in renal arterial stenosis.

Methyldopa

In pregnancy, methyldopa still maintains a place in the treatment of hypertension, but the associated CNS side-effects have made it less popular now that less sedative preparations are available.

Sympathetic ganglion blocking drugs

In the past, the sympathetic ganglion blocking drugs (guanethidine and bethanidine) were important as early effective treatments, but their use is now limited by their troublesome postural hypotensive effects, lack of supine blood pressure control and the sexual dysfunction that they produce in men.

Drug treatment of hypertension in pregnancy

Pre-eclampsia

The treatment of pre-eclampsia (p. 438) requires the delivery of the fetus. Nevertheless, drugs may be needed to control the blood pressure before delivery can be achieved. Methyldopa (250–500 mg, 6-hourly by mouth) is used and, if necessary, can be given parenterally. It has the advantage of being effective and harmless to the fetus, although its sedative side-effects can confuse neurological assessment and its onset of action is slow (1 hour). Hydralazine, orally (less than 300 mg daily), by intramuscular injection (10–20 mg, 3–6-hourly) and by constant infusion (5–10 mg/h) is a suitable alternative, although flushing, tachycardia and vomiting may be side-effects at the higher doses. Given intravenously, it has a rapid onset of action which can be maintained by a constant infusion. Beta-adrenoreceptor blockers and calcium antagonists have been found to be effective in the acute situation, although experience with these drugs and follow-up of the delivered neonates has been shorter than for methyldopa and hydralazine. Diuretics are used only when cardiac failure complicates the picture.

Chronic hypertension in pregnancy

Due to its known lack of effects on the fetus, methyldopa is the drug of choice; hydralazine as the usual alternative, although beta-adrenoreceptor blockers are being used increasingly without undue hazard. Mothers who are known moderate hypertensives may be advised to cease treatment at the time of conception, although no teratogenicity has been associated with any of the commonly used antihypertensive drugs.

Drug treatment of hypertensive emergencies

Accelerated or malignant phase hypertension

This previously rapidly fatal condition is now managed by bedrest with admission to hospital and oral treatment. Parenteral treatment is avoided unless coma, fits or severe heart failure are present. Under these circumstances, an effective treatment is an intravenous infusion of labetalol starting at 25 mg/h and increasing to 120 mg/h with additional diuretic treatment for pulmonary oedema. Hydralazine given intramuscularly has been a popular treatment, but the 20 minute delay in onset of action may lead to additional doses or drugs being given, resulting in hypotension some hours later. Methyldopa, even when given intravenously, is also too slow to be used effectively. For cases due to phaeochromocytoma, phentolamine (2.5–10 mg iv bolus or 1 mg/min by iv infusion) produces a rapid pressure reduction by alpha-adrenoreceptor blockade, but such a response is not limited to this disease.

Oral treatment is optimal in most cases of malignant and accelerated hypertension, and any of the usual antihypertensive drugs can be used successfully. Recent observations show that sublingual nifedipine (10–20 mg) produces a smooth blood pressure reduction beginning within 10 minutes, although the reflex tachycardia it produces may require treatment with a beta-adrenoreceptor blocker. Additional diuretic treatment is often given.

The degree and rapidity of blood pressure reduction is important. In chronic hypertensives, cerebral autoregulation is lost at mean blood pressures above 150–175 mmHg and below 90–120 mmHg. Treatment should reduce mean blood pressure to 100–120 mmHg and no lower. This should be achieved over a 12–36 hour period to allow time for the relatively slow process of re-establishing normal cerebral autoregulation.

Aortic dissection

Aortic dissection is an emergency requiring prompt reduction of mean blood pressure to 100–110 mmHg; this is usually achieved with an infusion of sodium nitroprusside, starting at 12.5 mg/min and titrating the dose against blood pressure every 2–3 minutes. Infusion should not continue beyond 24 hours, but the resulting thiocyanate accumulation can be diminished by concomitant use of hydroxycobalamine by injection. There may be an advantage in reducing the systolic rate of change in aortic pressure as well as mean pressure. This can be achieved with beta-adrenoreceptor blockade, so that labetalol infusion with its mixed, though predominantly beta-receptor effects, has been advocated for use in dissection.

Hypertension in chronic renal failure

A proportion of patients with chronic renal failure have hypertension; in these, blood pressure may be controlled by dietary sodium restriction and fluid removal at haemodialysis. Drug treatment is necessary in some cases, and the excretory metabolism must be taken into account when dosages are calculated. Treatment is generally similar to that in essential hypertension.

Hypertension in phaeochromocytoma

Hypertensive crises in phaeochromocytoma may be treated conventionally, but it is important to avoid beta adrenoreceptor blockade before full alpha-adrenoreceptor blockade has been achieved, in order to avoid unopposed alpha effects exacerbating hypertension. Parenteral phentolamine can be used acutely, and longer term control gained with phenoxybenazamine (10–30 mg tds) with the later addition of small doses of a beta-blocker, such as propranolol (40 mg tds). If a surgical cure cannot be effected, long-term treatment with alpha-methyl-tyrosine can be used, although side-effects are frequently troublesome.

Adrenocortical hyperplasia and Conn's syndrome

Surgical removal of the adenomas in Conn's syndrome may not always cure the electrolyte disturbances and hypertension. In these circumstances, as in idiopathic hyperplasia, treatment with amiloride (20–70 mg daily) or spironolactone (200–400 mg daily) is effective.

VASCULAR DISEASE

DISSECTING AORTIC ANEURYSM

Dissection occurs when there is haemorrhage into the wall of the aorta causing the media to separate from the other layers (Fig. 13.69). The majority of dissections are seen in middle-aged or elderly men with arteriosclerosis and hypertension. More than 50% of patients who present with dissection die within 24 hours. It is a particular complication of Marfan's syndrome, where cystic medial necrosis is common.

Dissections can be clinically classified according to the

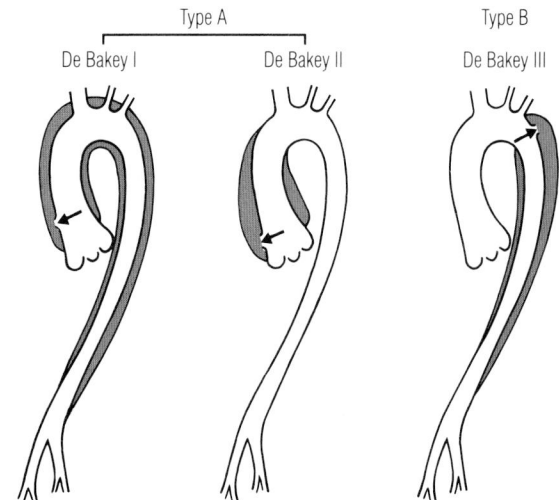

Fig. 13.69 Sites of dissection in aortic aneurysm.

part of the aorta that is affected. When the ascending aorta is involved, it is termed a *type A* dissection (De Bakey types I and II), whereas those where only the aorta beyond the left subclavian origin is involved, are called *type B* dissections (De Bakey type III).

Clinical features

The most prominent symptom is a very sudden onset of excruciating pain, often described as tearing in nature. Unlike infarction pain, the pain is often totally unheralded and at its worst initially, but may uncommonly develop to a pulsating discomfort that persists. The pain may radiate through to the back and, in type B dissection, to the left shoulder. Typical myocardial infarction pain may also coexist if the coronary arteries are involved by the dissection.

Diagnosis and investigation

The diagnosis can be difficult, and its importance has considerably increased with the emphasis on the early acute treatment of myocardial infarction with thrombolytic drugs. Clearly, these have terrible consequences in dissection. The patients are frequently hypertensive or have a history of hypertension, which may or may not have been treated. Patients with Marfan's syndrome are usually easy to identify but these form only a small proportion of cases. In about 10% of patients, a difference in blood pressure (20 mmHg or more) in the two arms may be found and, in some, a prominent pulsation is visible at the root of the neck. Auscultation may reveal aortic regurgitation in type A dissection, which is typically more obvious at the right sternal edge.

The ECG may be normal except in those cases with associated coronary artery involvement. In some individuals, the chest X-ray provides the first clue to the diagnosis, with mediastinal widening, left-sided pleural effusions and expansion of the aortic knuckle border beyond a calcified rim of endothelium. The diagnosis is confirmed at catheterisation by contrast aortography; at present, this is performed by intra-arterial injection, although the development of digital subtraction angiography may well allow venous contrast injection to suffice in the future. Computerised tomography is helpful and is less invasive, often being performed prior to catheterisation but rarely supplanting it totally. Echocardiography by the standard methods may demonstrate a proximal ascending aortic dissection, but transoesophageal echocardiography is the only ultrasound method able to adequately demonstrate the descending thoracic aorta. Transoesophageal colour Doppler is particularly useful, as the flow patterns make the intimal tear more obvious.

Complications

Complications of the dissection include occlusion of arterial branches, including the coronary arteries, head and neck vessels and indeed all distal arterial branches.

Stretching of the aortic annulus in type A dissection is responsible for aortic regurgitation, which may be severe and lead to left ventricular failure and shock. Progressive dilatation of the aorta may obstruct the airways or oesophagus. Finally, rupture of the aortic wall may occur, to produce pericardial or pleural effusion and, occasionally, intrabronchial haemorrhage. This complication frequently, but not always, causes death.

Treatment

Treatment is usually surgical for type A dissection and for many cases of type B. However, acute management includes blood pressure reduction by parenteral treatment, preferably with drugs reducing the inotropic force of the heart, such as labetalol by infusion (p. 455). Pain control and sedation are also very important in this very distressing condition, where the outlook is often very poor.

ARTERITIS

Arteritis is an inflammatory process involving the artery wall. It can occur in vessels of various sizes. If these are small, the condition is called necrotising vasculitis and is found in a large number of 'autoimmune' conditions (discussed in Chapter 24, p. 1022). Involvement of large arteries is much less common and occurs principally in Kawasaki's disease, Takayasu's (or pulseless) disease and giant cell (or temporal) arteritis.

KAWASAKI'S DISEASE

Kawasaki's disease is a disease of children described originally in Japan but now reported from other parts of the world. The aetiological agent is unknown, but, as the disease occurs in cyclical epidemics, an infective agent is suspected. It was originally called 'muco-cutaneous lymph node syndrome' because of the prolonged fever, skin rash and marked cervical lymphadenopathy. Later it was realised that there is a high incidence of coronary artery aneurysms, occlusions and myocardial infarction, which, because many of the patients are infants, were originally missed. Diagnosis of these lesions can often be made non-invasively by ECG and 2D echocardiography. Management is based on the use of antithrombotic agents and steroids, but aspirin alone has been found to result in a lower incidence of coronary artery complications than some other regimens.

TAKAYASU'S ARTERITIS

Takayasu's arteritis – a disease which predominantly affects Oriental women – was first described by an ophthalmologist whose first case was a young woman with cataracts and unusual arteriovenous anastomoses around the optic papillae. It was later realised that similar ophthalmic findings were seen in patients with absent radial pulses, hence its alternative name, 'pulseless disease'.

The disease can be classified into three types:

1. Type I involves the aortic arch and its branches, producing diminished or absent pulses over the upper body (so-called 'reversed coarctation').
2. Type II involves the descending aorta, particularly the renal arteries and vessels supplying the abdominal viscera.
3. Type III is a combination of I and II.

Takayasu's arteritis has also been implicated in the development of primary pulmonary hypertension.

The aetiology is unknown but the disease commonly starts in female teenagers, with a sex ratio of 8:1.

Clinical features

There is often a systemic illness with fever, arthralgia and fatigue. There may be pain and tenderness over the affected arteries. This systemic phase passes and is followed by a latent period. Some time later, these patients, and others who had no systemic prodrome, present with the typical features of weak or absent pulses, low or unrecordable upper body blood pressure, hypertension, heart failure and ocular damage.

The hypertension is produced by an increased aortic impedance secondary to major vessel occlusion or narrowing, and also from renal artery stenoses causing renal hypertension. Bruits over affected vessels are common.

Heart failure is usually secondary to hypertension, but coronary artery ostial stenoses can occur, causing angina; aortic regurgitation has also been described.

Treatment and prognosis

The acute systemic illness is alleviated by corticosteroids, which may reduce the incidence of sequelae. Anti-platelet agents, such as aspirin and dipyridamole, and warfarin have been used to reduce the frequency of cerebral transient ischaemic attacks and possibly retard the progression of arterial lesions.

Morbidity is chiefly from heart failure and cerebrovascular events. Surgical treatment of severe vascular stenoses may become necessary.

GIANT CELL (TEMPORAL) ARTERITIS

Although predominantly affecting the cranial arteries, giant cell arteritis can, like Takayasu's arteritis, involve the aorta and its proximal branches. The disease is described more fully in Chapter 24, page 1024. Where major vessel arteritis occurs, it may complicate the more common presentation with cranial arteritis and polymyalgia rheumatica, or may occur alone. Symptoms are similar to Takayasu's arteritis, including angina, and exercise-related ischaemia of upper and lower limbs. Aortic regurgitation, aneurysm and dissection can complicate giant cell arteritis of the aorta. Treatment, as for the commoner forms of the disease, is with corticosteroids.

ARTERIAL DISEASE

Thoracic outlet syndromes

In the past, the thoracic outlet syndromes were thought to be principally due to arterial compression of the subclavian artery, but it is now appreciated that many of the symptoms are due to compression of the brachial plexus as well. This is from an anomalous fibrous band stretching from a cervical rib to the first rib and, in doing so, compressing the neurovascular bundle. The patient has symptoms in the hand, which appear promptly when the arm is abducted to 90 degrees and externally rotated. A bruit can then be found over the supraclavicular fossa. These features disappear when the arm is returned to a relaxed position.

Aneurysm of, and embolism from, the subclavian artery is a comparatively rare complication of this condition, which can lead to digital gangrene.

Peripheral arterial disease and arteriosclerosis

Arteriosclerotic arterial disease can be from atheroma, focal calcific sclerosis (Monckeberg's arteriosclerosis) or arteriosclerosis. Monckeberg's sclerosis leads to calcification of the media without any narrowing of the vessels, but is often associated with arteriosclerosis and luminal narrowing.

Most symptomatic disease is due to atheromatous plaque formation, with subsequent stenosis, occlusion or embolisation of the vessel. Haemorrhage into an atheromatous plaque may precipitate a sudden vessel occlusion. Emboli may arise from atheromatous plaques (as occurs frequently from the carotid); however, major emboli are more frequently from the heart, in such conditions as mitral valve disease, LV aneurysm, mural thrombus following myocardial infarction, left atrial myxoma, endocarditis and from any enlarged heart, particularly if there is atrial fibrillation.

The sites of predilection for the atheroma are not fully explained, and any one patient may have principally coronary, cerebrovascular or peripheral vascular symptoms, with very similar risk factors to another patient whose symptoms are quite different. Atheroma tends to develop in the abdominal aorta and at the origins of major branches. These may be sites of mechanical stress or low shear.

Intermittent claudication

Ischaemia of the lower limbs is most commonly accompanied by effort-related cramp in the calves, thighs and buttocks, which disappears with rest. The site of claudication indicates the probable site of stenosis or occlusion – the higher the claudication the higher the atheroma is likely to be found. The walking distance on the flat is usually remarkably repeatable. Claudication is often accompanied by profound weakness as well as cramp in the affected muscles, which have become acidotic from anaerobic exercise.

The combination of hip and thigh claudication with impotence in males (the *Leriche syndrome*) is due to severe atheromatous occlusion of the lower end of the aorta.

More severe ischaemia produces a continuous pain at rest, particularly in bed. The pain is most frequently in the toes or foot, with some paraesthesia. The foot is often hung over the edge of the bed and may be subject to ulceration and gangrene.

In diabetics with peripheral neuropathy, there may be no pain but only ulceration and gangrene.

Diagnosis and investigation

Peripheral vascular disease is assessed by a careful history and clinical examination for signs of ischaemia, absent pulses, audible bruits over the proximal arteries, poor skin nutrition, low skin temperature and loss of hair, and then by blood pressure measurement. This is most commonly done using Doppler ultrasound on the ankle arteries with a proximal cuff.

The normal ankle systolic pressure is usually higher than brachial (by about 20%) and should be maintained after exercise. The ischaemic leg often has an ankle pressure of about 50% of brachial at rest, and this becomes unrecordable after exercise when the blood is diverted to areas of vasodilatation elsewhere. The severity of the hypotension is related to the degree of arterial disease.

Treatment

Most patients with claudication benefit from medical measures such as weight reduction, complete cessation of smoking and an energetic training regime which increases the claudication distance. Vasodilators and viscosity-reducing drugs have a limited role. Surgical intervention after angiography now includes angioplasty, as well as endarterectomy and bypass grafting. It is reserved for more severe cases.

Gangrene

Sudden ischaemia of a limb – from trauma, arterial thrombosis or embolism – leads to pain, pallor, coldness, and then numbness of the limb distal to the occlusion. If the perfusion is not restored, sensation is severely diminished in an hour, and within six hours ischaemic contracture of the muscles has started. This is followed by subcutaneous haemorrhage and focal gangrene. Fixed staining of the skin indicates death of the underlying tissues. Persistent pain and numbness without loss of sensation indicate a collateral flow.

Treatment

Treatment is an emergency and is surgical, by embolectomy, emergency bypass grafting or eventual amputation. Embolectomy under local anaesthetic can often

save a limb. Heparin is used to prevent further clotting, particularly if there is an obvious embolic source.

Buerger's disease

Buerger's disease was previously thought to be a distinct disease, but is now considered to be an accelerated form of atheroma affecting young men of 20–40 years of age who smoke (or chew) tobacco heavily. It affects the small arteries of the hands and feet, with an intense inflammatory response, and often involves the veins as well. Hand and instep claudication may occur, with loss of ankle and wrist pulses and gangrene of the toes and fingers. There is often an associated Raynaud's phenomenon (see below) and a migratory nodular phlebitis. Cessation of smoking or chewing tobacco is imperative.

Prognosis

For patients with symptoms of limb ischaemia, the rate of limb loss is about 2% per year for non-diabetics and 7% per year for diabetics.

Raynaud's syndrome and phenomenon

Raynaud's syndrome and phenomenon are vasospastic conditions affecting mainly the hands; they are often precipitated by cold and sometimes by motion, although random spontaneous attacks are common. The attacks are characterised by episodes of arteriolar spasm; these produce cold pale fingers and hands, progressing over minutes or hours to cyanosis and ending finally with a red flushing phase. When the condition is not associated with any underlying disorders, it is termed Raynaud's syndrome and skin changes are not seen. This is commoner in young women. Raynaud's phenomenon occurs secondary to underlying systemic conditions, the most common being scleroderma. Other collagen diseases may be associated with Raynaud's phenomenon, as may thoracic outlet compression, arteriosclerotic vascular disease, vibration trauma in pneumatic drill users and serum protein abnormalities.

Mesenteric ischaemia

Mesenteric ischaemia is described in Chapter 16, page 591.

VENOUS DISEASE

Varicose veins are the commonest vascular disorder affecting the legs, and venous thrombosis is a frequent complication of many medical and surgical conditions.

Varicose veins

Varicose veins are dilated and tortuous veins, varying in size from large palpable bunches to mere discoloured superficial spider bursts on the skin. They arise either through primary abnormalities in the venous wall leading to dilatation and incompetence of the valves, or secondarily after damage caused by previous thrombosis. In either case, factors which impede venous flow or increase venous pressure in the legs contribute to their development, as does the prolonged standing required in certain occupations.

Many patients suffer no symptoms but they can be responsible for discomfort, usually described as heaviness or pulling. Oedema may occur and, in chronic severe disease, pigmentation of the skin, a disfiguring dermatitis, ulceration or, at its severest, gangrene may follow. These complications are more prominent in the areas subject to the highest venous pressures, where skin nutrition is consequently poorest, namely in the lower third of the leg, often more marked medially.

Treatment

Elastic stocking support, injection of sclerosants and surgical removal (or stripping) of the veins are used to treat the varicose veins. Relief of exacerbating factors, such as obesity, ascites and right heart failure, is also important. Ulcers often heal slowly, and must be kept clean and uninfected. Elevation of the limb aids healing.

Venous thrombosis

Occlusion of veins by thrombus is very common. It leads to considerable morbidity and, when the deep veins of the leg and pelvis are involved, to the risk of serious illness or death through pulmonary embolism.

Superficial venous thrombosis

Superficial venous thrombosis causes pain and swelling over the affected vessel, which is often palpable as a tender cord or small nodule. Unless complicated by progression to deep vein thrombosis, superficial venous thromboses are essentially benign and require only symptomatic treatment. Non-steroidal anti-inflammatory agents, such as indomethacin or aspirin, plus local applied heat, are of help.

Deep venous thrombosis

Deep venous thrombosis (DVT) is a frequent complication of the post-operative patient. The factors predisposing to thrombus formation within the veins are abnormalities in the vein wall, venous stasis and hypercoagulability of the blood. Certain operations are more frequently associated with DVT than others. These include orthopaedic procedures, particularly on the hip, and prostate surgery, although any condition leading to immobility is a potential cause of DVT. Congestive cardiac failure, malignant disease, pelvic masses and marked obesity are also recognised as conditions where DVT may occur. In the majority

of instances, it is the deep veins of the calf, thigh and pelvis which are involved and are the source of potentially lethal pulmonary emboli (PE). Deep vein thrombosis of the axillary vein is much less common and rarely gives rise to significant PE.

Clinical features and diagnosis

The diagnosis of DVT is often difficult. The main features are pain and swelling of the affected limb. The symptoms vary with the extent and type of vein involved and may frequently be absent. Dorsiflexion of the foot may produce calf tenderness (Homan's sign) in the extended leg, but this sign is often not very helpful. The diagnostic test of most usefulness is the venogram, which, when technically adequate, will usually establish the presence and extent of any thrombus. Doppler ultrasound velocity profiles can be useful, although only for DVT affecting the veins above the knee.

The major conditions which may mimic DVT include muscle trauma, rupture of a popliteal (Baker's) cyst (which resembles calf vein DVT) and sciatic nerve irritation.

Complications

The most serious complication in DVT is pulmonary embolism (Ch. 14, p. 502). This is usually a complication of thrombus above the knee, but can sometimes occur with calf vein thrombosis. Other complications include vein wall and valve damage leading to long-term venous insufficiency.

Treatment

Treatment of DVT is by intravenous heparin, bolus (5000 U iv) followed by a constant infusion (24 000–48 000 U/24 h) sufficient to maintain a partial thromboplastin time 2–3 times the normal. Oral anticoagulation with warfarin is then instituted after several days, with the heparin being discontinued once a prothrombin ratio of 2.5–3.0 is achieved. Oral anticoagulation is continued for some months unless recurrent DVT is a problem, when lifelong anticoagulation may be considered. Massive venous thrombosis (e.g. common iliac vein) is often treated by fibrinolysis in order to reduce the ensuing morbidity.

It has become clear that prophylactic treatment with relatively low doses of anticoagulants (heparin by subcutaneous or intramuscular injection: 5000 U 8-hourly) can prevent DVT, and hence PE, in patients at risk, such as those on prolonged bedrest after major surgery.

FURTHER READING

Bennett D H 1985 Cardiac arrhythmias: practical notes on interpretation and treatment. Wright, Bristol. *An excellent discussion with good examples.*
Braunwald E (ed) 1983 Heart disease: a textbook of cardiovascular medicine. W B Saunders, London. *The outstanding reference work in cardiology.*

13

Fiegenbaum 1986 Echocardiography, 4th edn. Lea & Febiger, Philadelphia. *Still one of the best books on the topic, with exhaustive discussion and reasonably good examples.*

Opie L H et al 1987 Drugs for the heart, edn. Grune and Stratton, New York. *A small and excellent book with a comprehensive discussion of all aspects of therapy in cardiac disease. An excellent buy.*

Roberts W C 1986 Adult congenital heart disease. Davis, Phildelphia.

The best reference text concerning this increasingly important field of cardiology.

Schamroth L 1982 An introduction to electrocardiography. Blackwell Scientific, Oxford. *Still the best introduction to understanding ECGs.*

Swanton R H 1984 Pocket consultant in cardiology. Blackwell Scientific, Oxford. *Comprehensive manual small enough to be carried in the white-coat pocket. An excellent buy.*

Respiratory Disease

Respiratory diseases are responsible for a large proportion of premature mortality and serious morbidity among the population, and at the same time, for a large amount of minor illness. In 1985 in England and Wales respiratory diseases (including lung cancer) accounted for 21% of all male deaths (60 325 deaths) and 14% of all female deaths (40 481 deaths). They are the second most common cause of death after cardiovascular disease.

STRUCTURE AND FUNCTION OF THE RESPIRATORY SYSTEM

Respiration can be defined as those processes concerned with gas exchange between an organism and its environment. In man respiration begins with the uptake of O_2 and ends with the elimination of CO_2. The adequacy of gas exchange by the lungs depends on four closely integrated processes:

1. ventilation
2. diffusion of gases
3. pulmonary capillary blood flow
4. the carriage of gases by the blood.

In addition, breathing is regulated in accordance with the constantly changing metabolic needs of the body by an intricate control system.

The anatomical organisation of the human lung is eminently suited to its role as an exchanger of O_2 and CO_2. A series of branching airways conduct air into and out of the alveolar spaces. Similarly, the pulmonary circulation delivers blood to and drains blood from the pulmonary capillaries. Ninety per cent of the alveolar surface ($80 \, m^2$ in an adult lung) is covered with capillaries, providing a thin but large film of blood for exposure to the gases in the alveolar spaces.

The lung has other functions besides gas exchange:

1. It provides O_2 and substrates for its own metabolic needs.
2. Its blood vessels serve as a reservoir for the left side of the heart.
3. It modifies the pharmacological properties of a variety of drugs.
4. It provides an elaborate defence mechanism that protects the body against inhaled pathogenic micro-organisms and toxic chemicals.
5. The upper airways filter and humidify inspired air.

Ventilation

Ventilation is the cyclical movement of ambient air into and out of the lungs, and the distribution and mixing of that air within the lungs. This cycle is accomplished by contraction and relaxation of the respiratory muscles and the elastic recoil of the lungs. During normal quiet breathing, about two-thirds of the inspired gas reaches perfused alveoli; this fraction is known as alveolar ventilation (V_A). The rest of the inspired gas fills the conducting airways and alveoli that may not be well perfused and is known as physiological dead space (V_D) or 'wasted ventilation'. Therefore, total ventilation (usually in l/min) $= V_A + V_D$.

14

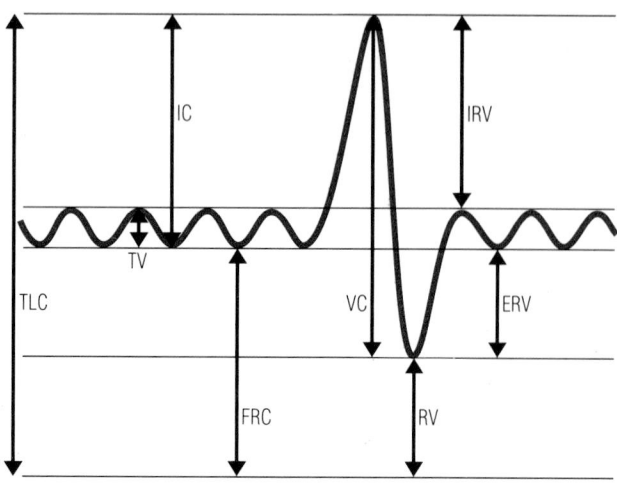

	Vital capacity (l)	Residual volume (l)	Total lung capacity (l)
Age 20 – 39			
Male	3.4 – 5.9	1.1 – 2.3	4.8 – 7.9
Female	2.4 – 4.3	1.0 – 2.0	3.6 – 6.1
Age 40 – 59			
Male	2.7 – 5.3	1.4 – 2.6	4.5 – 7.6
Female	2.0 – 4.0	1.1 – 2.2	3.4 – 6.0
Age 60+			
Male	2.4 – 4.7	1.7 – 2.7	4.3 – 7.3
Female	1.9 – 3.6	1.3 – 2.4	3.3 – 5.8

Fig. 14.1 The subdivisions of lung volume. Functional residual capacity (FRC) is the resting expiratory level. (TLC =total lung capacity; TV =tidal volume; IC =inspiratory capacity; VC =vital capacity; RV =residual volume; IRV =inspiratory reserve volume; ERV =expiratory reserve volume.)

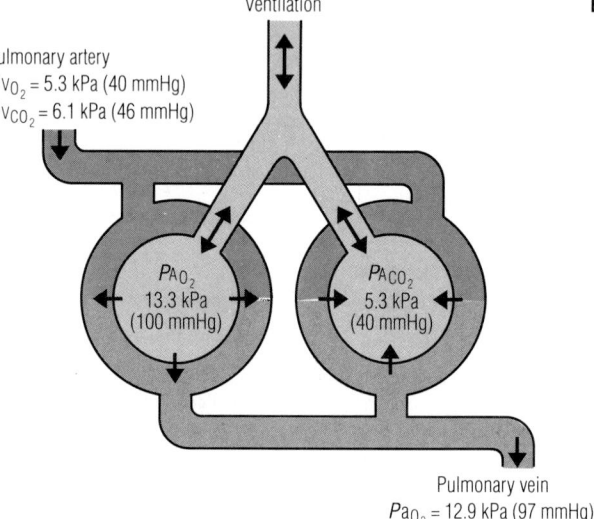

Fig. 14.2 The terminal respiratory unit. In the terminal respiratory unit (**A**) blood from the pulmonary artery is in close proximity to alveolar gas, facilitating gas exchange (**B**) and thus the uptake of oxygen and the elimination of carbon dioxide.

The commonly measured static lung volumes are shown in Figure 14.1. The static volumes depend upon the distensibility (i.e. compliance) of both the lung and chest wall. The distensibility or compliance of the lung is affected by the elastic recoil from the connective tissue elements in the parenchyma and from the surface tension of the surfactant that lines the alveolar surface. Thus the compliance of the lung is increased in emphysema and decreased in both diffuse pulmonary fibrosis (tissue changes) and neonatal respiratory distress syndrome (reduced surfactant).

Diffusion of gases

The term 'diffusion' describes the passive movement of O_2 and CO_2 between alveolar gas and pulmonary capillary blood (Fig. 14.2). It depends on three major factors:

1. the matching of ventilation and blood flow (V/Q)
2. the diffusion of gas from the alveolus to the red blood cell
3. the availability of haemoglobin and the chemical reactions within the red blood cell.

Although O_2 is the physiological gas that is most likely to be affected by abnormalities of diffusion, the diffusion capacity of the lung is usually measured with a non-physiological gas, carbon monoxide (TLCO or transfer factor). If the haemoglobin concentration is normal, a decreased transfer factor means either a change in the alveolar–capillary surface available for diffusion (thickening or loss of membrane), or obstruction or destruction of capillaries (decrease in capillary blood volume).

Pulmonary capillary blood flow

The adequacy of pulmonary capillary blood flow depends upon the volume and distribution of right ventricular output. Because distribution is gravity-dependent, in the upright position there is more blood flow to the bases than to the apices of the lung; in addition local mechanisms exist to divert blood from poorly ventilated regions of the lung.

Carriage of gases by the blood

Oxygen is transported in the blood mainly in combination with haemoglobin; a small amount is present in solution.

The relationship between the per cent saturation of haemoglobin and the partial pressure (or tensions) of O_2 (P_{O_2}) in the blood is shown in Figure 14.3. The shape of the curve is important: blood is nearly fully saturated when the P_{O_2} is greater than 8 kPa (60 mmHg), as it usually is in arterial blood; furthermore, when the prevailing P_{O_2} is low, 5.3 kPa (40 mmHg), as it is in the tissues, haemoglobin readily gives up its O_2, which is then available for metabolic activities. The position of the curve is not fixed, and shifts occur to the right (decreased affinity) and left (increased affinity) in many common clinical conditions. Shifts of the curve to the right, resulting from an increase in P_{CO_2}, H^+ concentration, temperature and organic phosphates (particularly 2,3-diphosphoglycerate) are beneficial because they facilitate O_2 transfer to the tissues and thus serve to maintain tissue oxygenation. (See also p. 1041.)

Carbon dioxide is transported in the blood as HCO_3^- in solution, or in combination with haemoglobin. The chemical reactions are reversed as blood flows through pulmonary capillaries, thus allowing CO_2 to evolve into alveolar gas. Carbon dioxide forms carbonic acid in the blood by the reaction:

$$CO_2 + H_2O \rightarrow H_2CO_3$$

catalysed by carbonic anhydrase, and the carbonic acid then dissociates by the reaction:

$$H_2CO_3 \rightleftharpoons H^+ + HCO_3^-$$

Accordingly, a rise in arterial P_{CO_2} tends to increase H^+ and decrease pH; this mechanism is of fundamental importance in acid–base balance and the regulation of ventilation (p. 854).

Oxyhaemoglobin saturation (%)

■ Arterial
● Venous
■ Oxygen in solution

Oxygen pressure (kPa)

Fig. 14.3 Oxygen dissociation curve. In normal subjects a large fall in arterial oxygen tension causes a small reduction in oxyhaemoglobin saturation (and oxygen carriage). In a hypoxic patient (for example, with a P_{aO_2} of 6 kPa/45 mmHg) a small fall in oxygen tension causes marked desaturation.

Control of ventilation

The rhythmic pattern of breathing is driven by the spontaneous discharge of neurons chiefly located in the medulla.

The activity of these cells is modulated by signals from the pons, hypothalamus and cortex, and from central chemoreceptors and receptors in the lung. Although the physiological mechanisms involved are largely unknown, there is a remarkable matching of metabolic activities and ventilation.

Synthetic and metabolic functions of the lung

Among the important biochemical substances that are modified during a single passage through the pulmonary circulation are:

1. acetylcholine (rapidly inactivated)
2. 5-hydroxytryptamine (almost completely removed)
3. noradrenaline (40% removed)
4. bradykinin (up to 80% inactivated)
5. angiotensin I (converted to angiotensin II)
6. prostaglandins E and F (almost completely removed).

Many of these processes take place on or very close to the luminal surface of the pulmonary capillary endothelial cells.

PATHOPHYSIOLOGY

It is convenient to consider generalised lung disorders under the headings:

1. airflow obstruction
2. restrictive lung disease
3. abnormalities of diffusion
4. abnormalities of pulmonary blood vessels.

These functional categories often show considerable overlap and, of course, do not account for localised abnormalities such as those caused by tumours, pneumonia or pulmonary infarction.

Airflow obstruction

The all-embracing terms 'chronic obstructive lung disease' or 'chronic airflow limitation' are often used as diagnoses for patients who have chronic bronchitis, emphysema, asthma or even bronchiectasis. The disorders are grouped together because they share the common physiological abnormality of expiratory airflow limitation, because some of the symptoms and signs are similar, and because the disorders frequently co-exist.

Determinants of bronchial calibre

The cross-sectional area of the tracheobronchial tree progressively increases as each generation of airways branches because the sum of diameters of the daughter branches exceeds that of the parent branch. Therefore, resistance to airflow, which depends on cross-sectional area, is greatest in the large or central airways and least in the small or peripheral airways. Airway calibre is influenced by the tone of bronchial smooth muscle, which, in turn, is regulated by a variety of neurohumoral mechanisms. Normally, there is a small amount of resting tone because parasympathetic-bronchoconstrictor impulses predominate over sympathetic-bronchodilator impulses. In addition to bronchoconstriction, airway calibre may be decreased by mucosal oedema, muscle hyperplasia, bronchial secretions and loss of elastic recoil.

Tests of airflow obstruction

There are simple tests to assess the severity of airflow obstruction that can be performed at the bedside, doctor's surgery or in the laboratory. Most commonly used are the *forced expiratory volume in 1 second* (FEV$_1$) (Fig. 14.4A) and the *peak expiratory flow rate* (PEFR). Both depend on patient co-operation and effort and predominantly reflect the function of larger airways. Additional useful information can be obtained by recording flow against volume during a forced expiratory manoeuvre, producing a maximal expiratory flow-volume curve (Fig. 14.4B). The earliest changes of several important diseases (e.g. chronic bronchitis and asthma) are in airways less than 2 mm in diameter, and because these airways contribute only 15–20% of total airways resistance, simple tests of airways obstruction are not sensitive enough to detect early disease. Hyperinflation of the lung, an important feature of airways obstruction, can be demonstrated in the laboratory as an increase in residual volume and an increase in the ratio of residual volume to total lung capacity (Fig. 14.5).

In all patients with airways obstruction, reversibility in response to an inhaled β_2 agonist should be assessed. Rapid improvement after inhalation of bronchodilators is characteristic of asthma and may occur to a lesser degree in some patients with chronic bronchitis, emphysema and bronchiectasis.

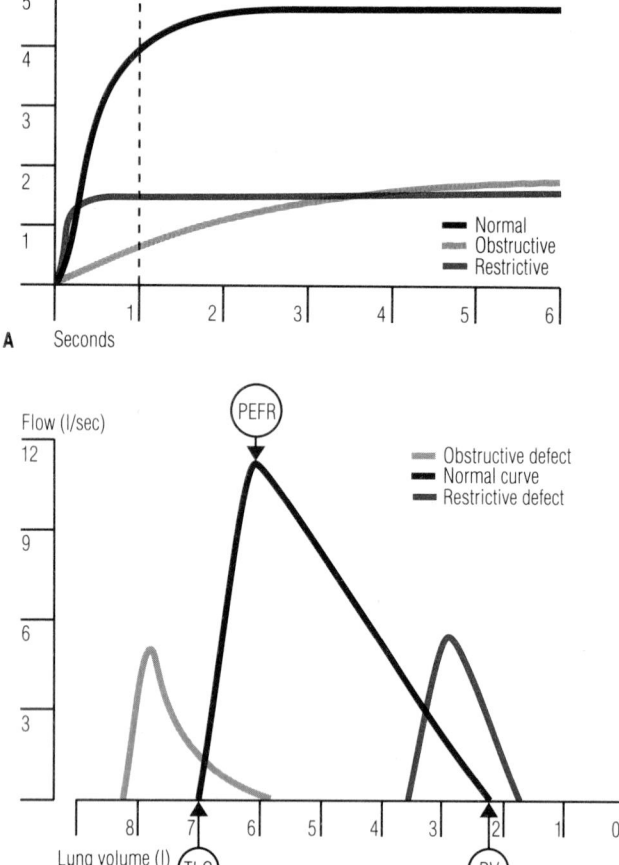

A Seconds

B Lung volume (l)

Fig. 14.4 A. Forced expiratory spirogram. Starting from a full inspiration, the volume expired during a forced expiration (forced vital capacity, FVC) is reduced in both obstructive and restrictive pulmonary disease. However, the volume expired in 1 second (FEV$_1$) is disproportionately reduced in patients with airways obstruction, but not in those with restriction.
B. Expiratory flow–volume curves. In patients with airways obstruction expiratory flow is strikingly reduced as residual volume is approached. In restrictive disorders the shape of the flow–volume curve (although not the magnitude) is normal. (TLC = total lung capacity; RV = residual volume; PEFR = peak respiratory flow rate.)

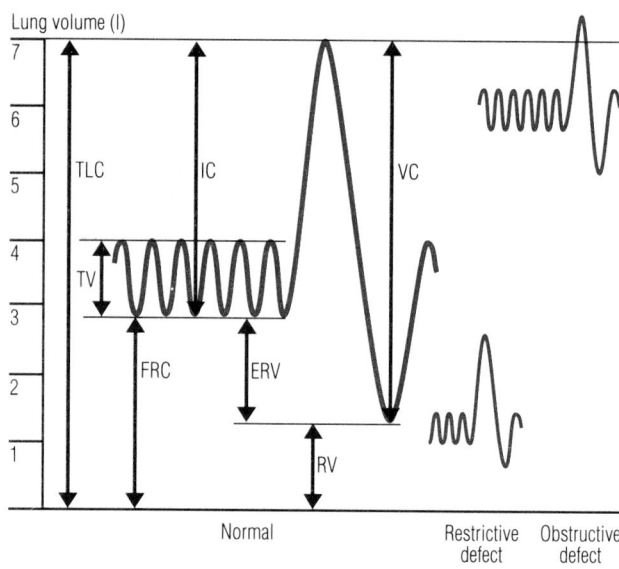

Fig. 14.5 The effect of obstructive and restrictive disorders on lung volumes. Both obstruction and restriction reduce vital capacity (VC). With obstruction, residual volume (RV) and functional residual capacity (FRC) increase and the patient becomes 'hyperinflated'. With restrictive disorders total lung capacity (TLC) and FRC are reduced. (TV = tidal volume; IC = inspiratory capacity; ERV = expiratory reserve volume.)

Upper airways obstruction

This may be caused, for example, by tumours of the larynx or trachea, by post-tracheostomy strictures or by inhaled foreign bodies. Clinically, it can be difficult to distinguish upper airway obstruction from other causes of airflow limitation. The flow volume loop is characteristic (Fig. 14.6). In patients with asthma or chronic bronchitis expiratory flow is most limited; when upper airway obstruction is present, inspiratory flow may also be markedly reduced.

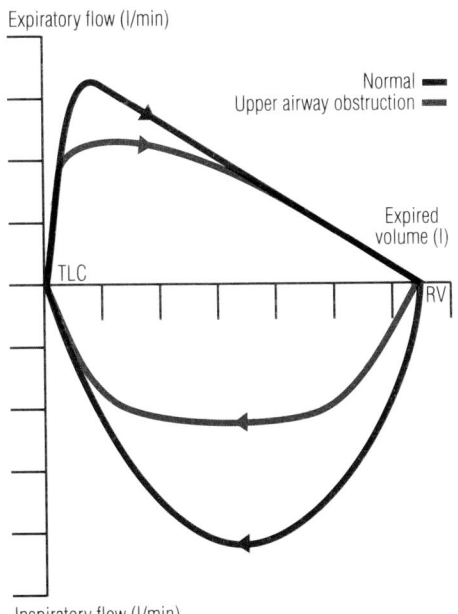

Expiratory flow (l/min)

Normal ■
Upper airway obstruction ■

Expired volume (l)

TLC

RV

Inspiratory flow (l/min)

Fig. 14.6 Flow-volume curves with upper airways obstruction. With obstruction of the upper airways (e.g. tracheal tumour) maximal flow rates are reduced, resulting in the characteristic shape of the flow–volume curve. When breathing out from full inspiration (total lung capacity: TLC), peak expiratory flow rate (PEFR) is reduced. Typically PEFR is reduced to a greater extent than the forced expiratory volume during the first second (FEV$_1$). (RV = residual volume.)

Restrictive lung disease

Limitation of expansion of the lung can result from diseases of the bony rib cage, respiratory muscles, pleura or lung parenchyma. A restrictive defect is therefore a feature of disorders as diverse as kyphoscoliosis, the pneumoconioses and polyneuritis. Pleural thickening or effusion also limits expansion of the lungs. The most common causes of restrictive lung disease, however, are diffuse infiltrative processes within the lung, such as pulmonary fibrosis or extensive sarcoidosis. Regardless of the underlying cause, pulmonary function tests show small lung volumes (Figs. 14.4 and 14.5) and, if there is destruction of the pulmonary capillary bed, a reduced transfer factor. Airways resistance is not increased and the ratio of FEV$_1$ to vital capacity (VC) is not reduced. As would be expected, lung compliance is reduced in diffuse pulmonary fibrosis.

Abnormalities of diffusion

Abnormality of any of the parameters that determine diffusion will reduce TLCO. Tests of diffusing capacity are sensitive to the concentration of haemoglobin; thus TLCO is low in patients with anaemia and high in those with polycythaemia. When corrected for changes in haemoglobin concentration, decreased TLCO values are found in patients with destruction or obliteration of pulmonary capillaries (emphysema, pulmonary vascular disease, interstitial infiltrative diseases). Increased TLCO

values are not common but are found in patients with left-to-right intracardiac shunts, polycythaemia, early left heart failure, pulmonary haemorrhage and asthma. Transfer factor may be expressed as the carbon monoxide transfer coefficient (KCO), which is the TLCO per litre of alveolar volume. When lung volume is reduced (e.g. pneumonectomy) but the remaining lung is normal, TLCO is therefore reduced but KCO is normal.

Abnormalities of pulmonary blood vessels

The function of the pulmonary vascular system is to expose mixed venous blood to adequately ventilated alveoli. Local mechanisms divert blood flow from poorly ventilated to better-ventilated regions. Conversely, if blood flow to part of the lung is compromised, ventilation of that region is reduced. Both these compensatory mechanisms tend to preserve the normal balance between blood flow and ventilation that is essential for efficient gas exchange.

The most common disorder of the pulmonary circulation is pulmonary embolism. This is usually diagnosed by ventilation and perfusion lung scanning or pulmonary angiography (p. 503). Chronic obliterative disease of pulmonary arteries may cause severe dyspnoea on exertion but is difficult to diagnose at an early stage because physical examination, chest X-rays and spirometry show no abnormalities. In such disorders, gas transfer is reduced and hypoxaemia intensifies, or may only be apparent, on exercise.

Abnormalities of arterial blood gases and pH

Arterial blood gases and pH are also discussed in Chapter 22. The prime function of the lung is to add O$_2$ and remove CO$_2$ from blood. Thus the ultimate test of the adequacy of ventilation, diffusion, pulmonary capillary blood flow, and control of ventilation is measurement of P_{O_2}, P_{CO_2} and pH of arterial blood.

Arterial P_{O_2}

Arterial oxygen tension ($P_{a_{O_2}}$) is normally between 11.3 and 13.3 kPa (85 and 100 mmHg) in healthy adults. Arterial hypoxaemia is a decrease in circulating O$_2$ (O$_2$ content), which depends on the amount of haemoglobin available for combining with O$_2$, as well as $P_{a_{O_2}}$. The causes of arterial hypoxia are listed in Summary 1. A low inspired P_{O_2} is usually due to high altitude; of the remaining causes, abnormalities of diffusion seldom cause hypoxia at rest but may be important during exercise. Hypoventilation can be recognised by an increase in arterial P_{CO_2}, and ventilation–perfusion abnormalities and right-to-left shunts can be differentiated by having the patient breathe 100% O$_2$ for 10–20 minutes; 100% O$_2$ substantially 'corrects' a ventilation–perfusion abnormality, but the effects of a right-to-left shunt are still readily apparent. Ventilation–perfusion mismatching usually occurs in patients with diseases that cause obstruction of airways; in contrast, right-to-left shunts occur in patients with disorders associated with

Respiratory Disease

14

> **Summary 1 Causes of hypoxia**
>
> *Arterial hypoxia*
> Ventilation–perfusion abnormalities
> Hypoventilation
> Impaired diffusion
> Right-to-left shunts
> Reduced PO_2 in inspired air
>
> *Anaemic hypoxia*
> Insufficient haemoglobin for O_2 carriage
>
> *Stagnant hypoxia*
> Poor tissue perfusion
>
> *Histotoxic hypoxia*
> Respiratory chain enzyme abnormalities, poisoning of tissue enzymes, e.g. by cyanide.

alveolar closure or filling: for example, pneumonia ('physiological' shunt) or congenital heart disease ('anatomical' shunt).

Patients may have significant arterial hypoxia without symptoms. Central cyanosis only occurs when the saturation of arterial blood is less than 85%. Thus the clinical signs and symptoms of mild to moderate, but nevertheless important, arterial hypoxia are unreliable, and the diagnosis must be made by analysis of arterial blood gases. With chronic hypoxia patients develop secondary polycythaemia and pulmonary hypertension.

Arterial P_{CO_2}

The arterial CO_2 tension (Pa_{CO_2}) at rest is 4.6–6.0 kPa (35–45 mmHg). Regulation of arterial P_{CO_2} is determined according to the equation:

$$\text{Arterial } P_{CO_2} = K \times \frac{CO_2 \text{ production}}{\text{Alveolar ventilation}}$$

Only two variables, CO_2 production and alveolar ventilation, are involved. Deviation from normal values of arterial P_{CO_2} can be viewed as a failure of alveolar ventilation to increase or decrease in accordance with metabolic changes. Hyperventilation, an increase in ventilation in excess of metabolism so that arterial P_{CO_2} decreases, occurs in patients with a variety of common lung diseases (asthma, pneumonia, pulmonary embolism), presumably from reflexes arising from the chest wall or within the diseased lung. Hyperventilation also results from stimulation of the central nervous system by drugs (aspirin), irritative lesions (cerebral tumours, infections) or anxiety. A 'primary' hyperventilation syndrome is not uncommon, and is sometimes, but not always, associated with anxiety. Hypoventilation can result from disorders that involve the airways (chronic bronchitis), lung parenchyma (advanced diffused interstitial fibrosis), chest wall (kyphoscoliosis), respiratory muscles (myasthenia gravis) or central nervous system (sedative drugs).

Like arterial hypoxia, mild to moderate changes in arterial P_{CO_2} produce no or few signs and symptoms. Thus,

analysis of arterial blood gases is required to determine the presence and severity of disturbances in P_{CO_2}.

Arterial pH

The arterial pH (Fig. 14.7) at rest is 7.38. It can also be expressed as H^+ content, and the normal value for this is 35–45 nmol/l. The arterial pH value represents the net effects of both respiratory and non-respiratory factors that regulate P_{CO_2} and HCO_3^- (and other buffers). When ventilation increases acutely, P_{CO_2} decreases and pH increases; conversely, when ventilation decreases acutely, P_{CO_2} increases and pH decreases. If the ventilatory changes persist, pH gradually returns towards normal values as the kidney makes appropriate adjustments in concentration of HCO_3^- in blood. Thus the pH value depends on both the magnitude of the change in P_{CO_2} and whether or not compensation has had time to occur.

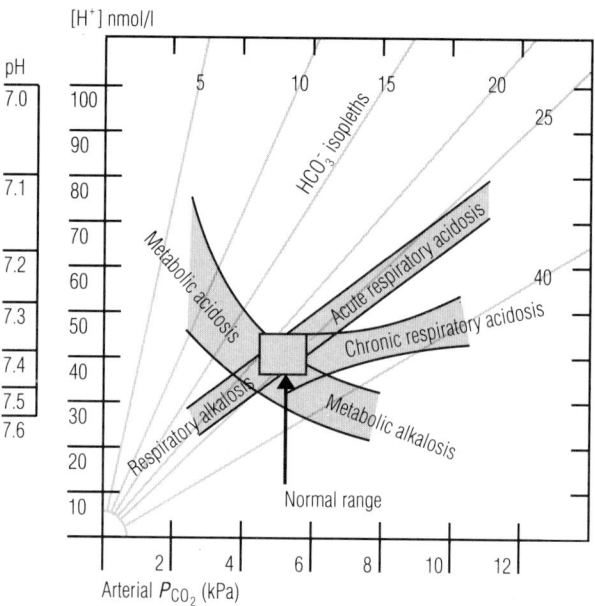

Fig. 14.7 Acid–base diagram. The relationship of arterial pH [H^+] P_{CO_2} and bicarbonate with disturbances of acid–base balance. For example, acute ventilatory failure leads to a raised arterial P_{CO_2} and a reduction in pH; compensatory renal mechanisms then increase bicarbonate and restore pH to normal. (Modified from Flenley D C 1971 Another non-logarithmic acid–base diagram? Lancet 1961.)

Lung function testing

Patterns of lung function abnormality are easily identified (Table 14.1). Airflow limitation without reversibility and with a normal TLCO is compatible with chronic obstructive bronchitis; if emphysema is present, however, TLCO and KCO will be reduced. A more than 15% improvement in FEV_1 or peak flow after inhaled bronchodilator is suggestive of asthma. Restrictive lung disease due to pulmonary fibrosis will show low lung volumes with a normal or high FEV_1/VC ratio and a reduced TLCO, whereas if the restriction is due to chest wall disease the TLCO may be normal or slightly reduced, and the KCO raised.

456

Table 14.1 Patterns of abnormality in lung function tests

Feature	Asthma	Chronic bronchitis	Emphysema	Pulmonary fibrosis	Chest wall abnormalities
Airflow obstruction	Yes	Yes	Yes	No	No
Reversibility	Yes	Slight	Slight	No	No
Hyperinflation	Yes	Yes	Yes	No	No
Reduction of lung volumes	No	No	No	Yes	Yes
TLCO	Normal or increased	Normal	Reduced	Reduced	Normal or reduced
Compliance	Normal	Normal	Increased	Reduced	Normal or reduced

SYMPTOMS AND SIGNS OF RESPIRATORY DISEASE

The most important symptoms of respiratory disease are:

1. cough
2. sputum
3. haemoptysis
4. breathlessness
5. wheeze
6. chest pain.

Cough

Cough is initiated when irritant receptors in the mucous membrane of the respiratory tract are stimulated. Although these receptors are present down to the small bronchi, most of them are in the pharynx, larynx, trachea and major airways. Cough is by far the most common respiratory symptom, and is characteristic in heavy smokers. Frequently, cough is triggered by the presence of sputum in the respiratory tract, and is useful in helping to clear infection from the bronchial tree. In such cases the suppression of cough by drugs is harmful. A wide variety of inhaled irritants other than cigarette smoke (for example, noxious gases or cold air) may stimulate coughing, and this is more likely if the airways are already irritable because of inflammation as a consequence of infection. Similarly the irritant receptors in the bronchial tree may be stimulated by tumours, inhaled foreign bodies, allergens and the asthmatic response, pulmonary oedema and external compression by lymph nodes. With neurological disease laryngeal function may be impaired or oesophageal motility abnormal (e.g. achalasia), and cough may be due to repeated aspiration. In some patients cough is worse at night, particularly in asthma or pulmonary oedema. Prolonged coughing reduces venous return, causes a transient fall in cardiac output and cerebral oxygenation, and leads to cough syncope. Damage to the recurrent laryngeal nerve, commonly at the left hilum due to bronchial carcinoma, leads to vocal cord paralysis and an inability to produce a normal explosive cough, which becomes 'bovine'.

Sputum

In healthy subjects the bronchial tree produces approximately 100 ml of mucus each day; this is carried upwards by ciliary action and is then swallowed. This ciliary mucus escalator is a normal part of the mechanism for clearing debris and pathogens from the bronchial tree. In disease processes causing the production of excess mucus, irritant receptors are stimulated and sputum is coughed up.

Sputum is not reliably described by patients and it is always best to inspect it. Sputum may be clear, white or mucoid, as in chronic bronchitis, or purulent, in which case pus is mixed with mucus and the sputum is yellow or green. Sputum may contain blood, which may be bright red (e.g. pulmonary infarction), a rusty colour (acute pneumonia) or pink (pulmonary oedema due to left heart failure). In asthma, the sputum may contain mucus plugs. Microscopically, sputum may contain bacteria, pus cells, eosinophils (as in asthma and pulmonary eosinophilia) or malignant cells. It is helpful to know the volume of sputum produced each day, and this can be particularly large: greater than 20 ml in bronchiectasis, cystic fibrosis, and lung abscess when there is a bronchopulmonary fistula. Clinical progress can be monitored by documentation of sputum volume. Occasionally patients with asthma or alveolar cell carcinoma produce very large volumes of clear watery sputum (bronchorrhoea). Anaerobic infection results in foul-smelling sputum.

Haemoptysis

Patients may have difficulty in being sure that blood has been coughed rather than vomited. Coughed blood may be from a lesion of the nose, nasopharynx and vocal cords. When infection causes haemoptysis, blood will be mixed with purulent sputum, whereas in non-infective causes (for example, pulmonary infarction) there is usually frank blood and no sputum. In patients with chronic bronchitis it is common for the sputum to contain occasional specks of blood but more substantial haemoptysis is unusual (Table 14.2).

A cause for haemoptysis should be carefully sought in

Table 14.2 Important causes of haemoptysis

Pulmonary infections	Pulmonary haemorrhage
Bronchiectasis (particularly upper lobe bronchiectasis from past pulmonary tuberculosis)	Idiopathic pulmonary haemosiderosis
Lung abscesses	Goodpasture's syndrome
Pneumonias	Systemic lupus erythematosus
Tuberculosis	Pulmonary vasculitis
Aspergilloma	
	Trauma
Pulmonary infarction	Pulmonary contusion
	Needle biopsy
Tumours	Transbronchial biopsy
Carcinoma	
Adenoma	**Vascular abnormalities**
(Haemoptysis is unusual with pulmonary metastases)	Arterio-venous malformation
	Hereditary haemorrhagic telangiectasia
Pulmonary oedema	**Bleeding disorders**
Particularly due to mitral stenosis	Usually severe thrombocytopenia from any cause

Disorders of the upper airways
Epistaxis
Tumours

Table 14.3 Time course for the development of breathlessness

Immediate	Weeks
Pneumothorax	Pleural effusion
Pulmonary oedema due to cardiac arrhythmias	Anaemia
	Muscle weakness
Pulmonary embolism	
Inhalation of foreign body	**Months**
	Tumours
Hours	Pulmonary fibrosis
Asthma	Thyrotoxicosis
Left heart failure	Muscle weakness
Pneumonia	
Laryngeal oedema	**Years**
	Muscle weakness
Days	Chronic airways obstruction
Pneumonia	Pulmonary fibrosis
Adult respiratory distress syndrome	Primary pulmonary hypertension
Left heart failure	Chest wall disorders

all cases, but a definite diagnosis is only achieved in 60–70%. All patients require a chest X-ray, including a lateral film. Pulmonary infarction can be confirmed by isotopic lung scan; lung tumour can usually be confirmed by bronchoscopy. In some series, up to 10% of patients with haemoptysis subsequently found to be due to bronchial carcinoma had normal chest X-rays at the time of presentation. Occasionally haemoptysis can be severe and life-threatening, causing drowning and hypoxia rather than exsanguination. This occurs most frequently in cavitating tuberculosis and bronchial carcinoma. In those patients in whom no definite cause for haemoptysis is found, careful follow-up is necessary, with repeated chest X-rays.

Breathlessness

Breathlessness is an unpleasant awareness of the effort of breathing. The history should document severity: How far can the patient walk on the flat? How many steps can he climb without stopping? Breathlessness may have characteristic features: in left heart failure breathlessness is worse when lying flat; in asthma it is frequently episodic, worse at night. With psychogenic breathlessness the patient complains of difficulty in taking air in, difficulty in fully filling the lungs with air and an inability to take a deep breath. These patients are often breathless at rest but not on exercise. The time period over which breathlessness has developed is of great importance (Table 14.3).

Most causes of breathlessness are relatively easily diagnosed by history, physical examination, chest X-ray and lung function tests. In difficult cases observation of the patient during an exercise test may be helpful.

Although orthopnoea and paroxysmal nocturnal dyspnoea suggest left heart failure, many patients with asthma are worse at night and many patients with severe airways obstruction are more comfortable sleeping with many pillows. Diaphragm weakness can cause profound orthopnoea.

Wheeze

Patients with airways obstruction frequently complain of wheeze which is predominantly expiratory in asthma, chronic bronchitis and emphysema. In some patients with asthma, wheeze may only be present at night, on waking in the morning, following exercise, or on exposure to allergens. Patients may notice that a wheeze is inspiratory, indicating narrowing of the larynx, trachea or main bronchi, and occasionally they will remark that the wheezing sound is from only one side of the chest, as when a tumour narrows a major bronchus. Diffuse expiratory wheezes can occur in left heart failure and frequently are most obvious at night.

Chest pain

The many causes of chest pain can usually be distinguished by careful history-taking, paying particular attention to the duration of the pain, its site and radiation, and the relationship to movement, breathing and exercise. The quality of pain is also diagnostically important, especially if it is pleuritic in nature. Diseases within the lung are usually painless since there are no pain receptors within lung tissue.

Pleural pain

This usually indicates involvement of the parietal pleura by inflammation or malignancy but is also a feature of pneumothorax. Inflammation of pleura can be caused by:

1. pneumonia
2. pulmonary infarction
3. lung abscess
4. tuberculosis
5. rheumatoid arthritis

6. systemic lupus erythematosus
7. uraemia.

Pleural pain is sharp, often well localised, worse on breathing, particularly deep inspiration, and causes the patient to catch his breath. Pain from inflammation of the central diaphragm is referred to the shoulder; pain from inflammation of the lateral diaphragm is referred to the lower lateral chest wall and upper abdomen.

Mediastinal pain

Central chest pain may occur with primary carcinoma of the lung, particularly when there is involvement of mediastinal structures including lymph nodes. Adenopathy due to other disorders, such as sarcoidosis, can cause pain. Usually the pain is poorly localised and dull, but can be sharp, especially with sarcoidosis. The differential diagnosis will include angina, oesophagitis and bone pain. Severe sudden central chest pain can occur with pulmonary embolism (p. 505).

Chest wall pain

With rib fractures there is local pain and tenderness. Occasionally coughing leads to fracture, particularly of the middle ribs posteriolaterally. Osteoporotic ribs and those involved by tumour fracture easily. Perichondritis causes pain and swelling of the costochondral junction, often of the second ribs bilaterally (Tietze's syndrome). Pain within the distribution of thoracic nerves occurs with herpes zoster, the pain frequently preceding the vesicular rash. Nerve root pain, often described as burning, also occurs with an intervertebral disc or malignant and inflammatory diseases of the spine. Local pain and tenderness of the muscles of the chest wall is caused by coxsackie B viral infections (Bornholm's disease) which may sometimes involve the diaphragm. Localised muscle pain without any important underlying pathological process is common in breathless, coughing patients.

EXAMINATION OF THE RESPIRATORY SYSTEM

In thoracic medicine the *history, physical examination, chest X-ray* and *pulmonary function tests* all contribute to diagnosis and assessment in a complementary manner. The chest X-ray gives accurate information on thoracic anatomy, whereas clinical examination is much more useful in assessing pathophysiology and frequently reveals severe disease despite a normal or near-normal chest X-ray.

Before the clinical examination, many relevant observations will have been made while talking to the patient concerning breathlessness, pain, cough and general appearance. In addition, the history will have served to focus attention on particular diagnostic probabilities and possibilities which subsequent examination will confirm or refute. If already available, the information from the chest X-ray will similarly direct the physician's examination of the patient.

Examination of the hands

Examination of the hands may give valuable information:

1. *Finger and toe clubbing* (Fig. 14.8) is an important physical sign. The four criteria for documenting finger clubbing are: increased sponginess of the nail bed; loss of the usual acute angle between the nail and the nail bed; increased nail curvature; and increased bulk of the soft tissues over the terminal phalanges. The majority of patients with clubbing have pulmonary disease (Table 14.4). Clubbing is occasionally familial in otherwise normal subjects. It can develop very rapidly, within a few weeks (e.g. with an empyema), but its onset is usually gradual. The mechanism of clubbing is not understood. The bones of the fingers and toes are normal. If the underlying cause is successfully treated clubbing usually resolves.
2. *Hypertrophic pulmonary osteo-arthropathy (HPOA)*. Virtually all patients with this unusual condition have clubbing, but only a few patients with clubbing have HPOA. There is arthralgia and joint swelling affecting particularly the wrists and ankles. X-rays show subperiosteal new bone formation in the long bones of the lower limbs and forearm, the bone scan demonstrates increased activity, and often the serum alkaline phos-

Fig. 14.8 Finger clubbing.

Table 14.4 Important causes of clubbing

Bronchial carcinoma (particularly squamous cell)	Cyanotic congenital heart disease
Mesothelioma	Bacterial endocarditis
Benign intrathoracic tumours	Atrial myxoma
Pulmonary arteriovenous fistula	
Lung abscess	Cirrhosis
Empyema	
Bronchiectasis	Ulcerative colitis
Fibrosing alveolitis	Crohn's disease
Asbestosis	
Advanced pulmonary fibrosis of any cause	

phatase is raised. Ninety per cent of cases are associated with bronchogenic carcinoma, particularly peripheral squamous cell tumours.

3. *Examination of the nails.* This may show that some or all of them are thickened and yellow or greenish in appearance. This occurs in the *yellow nail syndrome* which is associated with lymphoedema, exudative pleural effusions, bronchiectasis and sinusitis.

4. *Carbon dioxide retention.* When there is carbon dioxide retention, peripheral vascular dilatation greatly enhances blood flow and the hands are strikingly warm. With severe and acute carbon dioxide retention, there may also be an irregular flapping tremor of the outstretched hands. The fingers may be blue (peripheral cyanosis), and if the limb is warm this is likely to reflect central cyanosis rather than poor peripheral perfusion.

Cyanosis

In patients with a normal haemoglobin concentration, oxygen saturation must fall to 85%, corresponding to an arterial oxygen tension of 7–8 kPa (approximately 55–60 mmHg), before cyanosis can be clinically detected. As a consequence of the sigmoid shape of the oxygen dissociation curve (Fig. 14.3), further small falls in oxygen tension then produce large, dangerous falls in saturation. In anaemia, severe hypoxia is required to produce the quantity of reduced haemoglobin (about 1.5 g/dl) necessary to cause cyanosis, whereas patients with polycythaemia become cyanosed at higher arterial oxygen tensions.

The bluish colour of central cyanosis is best appreciated by examination of the tongue in adequate daylight. Cyanosis is a difficult physical sign, and estimates of severity are so unreliable that measurement of the arterial oxygen tension is the next logical step. Cyanosis can not be reliably detected in many black and Asian patients in whom severe hypoxaemia may go undetected.

In most cases central cyanosis is due to lung disease. Right-to-left shunts within the heart or within the lungs (arteriovenous malformation) cause central cyanosis, as do pulmonary shunts in advanced cirrhosis. In patients with lung disease and circulatory failure, severe venous hypoxaemia following increased peripheral oxygen extraction contributes to central cyanosis. Rarely patients appear cyanosed due to methaemoglobinaemia or sulphaemoglobinaemia, most commonly caused by drugs.

Pulsus paradoxus

The curious term 'pulsus paradoxus' is used to describe a greater than normal fall in blood pressure during inspiration. In normal subjects the systolic blood pressure falls by a few mmHg during inspiration. This fall is greater (not paradoxical) when venous return to the right heart is impaired: for example, in patients with hypovolaemia, cardiac tamponade or massive pulmonary embolism. In respiratory disorders pulsus paradoxus is seen when there

are large pressure swings within the thorax during the respiratory cycle. This is particularly likely to occur in severe acute asthma, when systolic blood pressure may fall by 40 mmHg on inspiration (Fig. 14.33). The degree of paradox is best documented using a sphygmomanometer: as the pressure of the cuff is reduced, the systolic sound is noted to be audible, initially only on expiration but with a further reduction in cuff pressure the systolic sound becomes audible throughout inspiration too. The pressure difference between the measurement taken when the systolic sound is first detected and the measurement taken when it is present throughout the breathing cycle is termed the *degree of paradox*; this is then recorded in mmHg. In asthma paradox is dependent on respiratory muscle contraction and is reduced with exhaustion as well as with improvement in airways obstruction.

Jugular venous pressure

The jugular venous pressure is raised in right heart failure, which is itself frequently due to pulmonary disorders such as chronic bronchitis. The venous pressure is also elevated if the resting pressure in the thorax is raised, as with a tension pneumothorax, or the hyperinflation of severe asthma. When there is severe airways obstruction the pressure swings within the thorax are large; intrathoracic pressure is positive during expiration, elevating the jugular venous pressure, which then falls during inspiration. Thus, interpretation of the jugular venous pressure in the tachypnoeic patient, particularly with severe airways obstruction, is difficult.

The jugular venous pressure is raised and not pulsatile in superior vena cava obstruction, most commonly due to malignant nodes or a tumour mass compressing the vein. The most common cause is an extending bronchial carcinoma but lymphoma, thymic tumours and metastases can all cause compression. Very rarely non-malignant lesions are responsible, for example, mediastinal fibrosis or aortic root aneurysm or dissection. Partial obstruction may cause venous thrombosis and subsequent complete obliteration. Superior vena caval obstruction produces drowsiness, a sense of fullness in the head, swelling and cyanosis of the face, neck and arms, and sometimes papilloedema. The chest X-ray most frequently demonstrates a bronchial carcinoma or nodes situated in the right paratracheal region.

Peripheral oedema

Peripheral oedema associated with severe pulmonary disease (cor pulmonale) is common, and is most often seen with chronic bronchitis in which there is hypercapnia as well as hypoxia. Patients with hypoxic normocapnic respiratory failure seldom have oedema. In some patients with oedema the jugular venous pressure is not elevated, the cardiac output is normal and fluid accumulation is related to factors other than right heart failure, perhaps mediated through the action of hypercapnia on renal function.

Examination of the chest

Examination of the chest (Table 14.5) may reveal that the chest wall shows an abnormality of shape (kyphoscoliosis, a barrel chest or pectus deformity) or an abnormality of symmetry (a reduction in the volume of one hemithorax reflecting underlying chronic fibrosis, or perhaps an increase in volume reflecting a pneumothorax). Much can be learned about respiratory function by observing the patients' breathing pattern. An increase in respiratory rate is a sensitive index of cardiorespiratory disorders and is not sustained above 14–20 breaths per minute in normal adults. Disorders that cause widespread functional impairment, such as asthma, pulmonary fibrosis and pulmonary oedema, invariably increase respiratory rate. Conversely, respiratory rate is reduced by central nervous system injury or central depressant drugs. Respiratory rate must be measured without the patient's awareness of the rate being counted.

Visible or palpable contraction of the accessory muscles is abnormal. Sternomastoid activity is particularly obvious in severely hyperinflated patients, whereas in patients who are not over-inflated, accessory muscle activity is an indication of a greatly increased respiratory effort. In severely breathless patients abdominal muscle activity is increased both to assist expiration and aid diaphragm function during inspiration.

Chest wall movements

Both sides of the thorax should be seen to expand equally during tidal and full inspiration. Hands placed flat on either side of the sternum can appreciate the predominantly forward movement of the sternum and upper ribs, whereas hands placed around the lower thorax can best detect the normal outward and upward movements of the mid- and lower ribs.

Overall movement of the ribcage is reduced by hyperinflation (e.g. emphysema), reduced pulmonary compliance (e.g. fibrosis), reduced chest wall compliance (e.g. ankylosing spondylitis) and weak inspiratory muscles (e.g.

myasthenia gravis). Local chest wall movement is reduced in pleural effusion, pleural thickening, pulmonary collapse, and to a lesser degree in consolidation and pneumothorax. With reduced compliance of one lung or pleura (i.e. fibrosis), movement is also delayed compared with the normal hemithorax.

The pattern of breathing is altered by disease. For example, patients with stiff lungs, a poorly compliant ribcage or weak respiratory muscles breathe rapidly and shallowly. It must be stressed that clinical assessment of the depth of respiration is notoriously inaccurate. Patients with airflow obstruction have a prolonged expiratory phase and patients with left heart failure may have marked periodic respiration. With severe weakness or paralysis of the diaphragm the anterior abdominal wall moves paradoxically inwards during inspiration when supine (Fig. 14.72).

Trachea and apex beat

The trachea is an important anatomical landmark indicating the position of the upper mediastinum. It is best palpated by one finger gently placed in the suprasternal notch. Loss of volume in one hemithorax, as with pulmonary fibrosis, pulls the trachea to the same side. Expansion of a hemithorax (as with tension pneumothorax) or local masses (for example, an enlarged thyroid) pushes the trachea towards the opposite side. When examining the trachea, the distance between the suprasternal notch and the cricoid cartilage is noted and is normally 3–4 fingers, and a reduction in this distance is a reliable sign of hyperinflation. Assessment of tracheal shift is difficult in patients with hyperinflation. A shift of the lower mediastinum displaces the cardiac apex. However, a displaced apex must be interpreted with caution because ventricular enlargement also moves the apex beat. In many patients the apex beat is not palpable, usually due to obesity or hyperinflation of the lungs. Less commonly the apex is difficult to palpate because of pericardial disease or poor left ventricular function, and the apex will be located on the right side with dextrocardia. Palpation at the left sternal edge may elicit the heave of right ventricular hypertrophy, common in

Table 14.5 Signs in respiratory disease

	Mediastinal shift	Chest wall movement	Percussion note	Tactile fremitus; vocal resonance	Breath sounds	Added sounds
Collapse	Yes (towards collapse)	Reduced	Reduced	Reduced	Reduced	No
Effusion	Yes (away from effusion)	Reduced	Reduced	Reduced	Reduced	Occasional (rub)
Consolidation	No	Normal or reduced	Reduced	Increased	Increased (bronchial)	Crackles
Pneumothorax	Yes (with tension)	Reduced	Increased	Reduced	Reduced	Occasional (click)
Pleural thickening	No	Reduced	Reduced	Reduced	Reduced	No

patients with severe pulmonary disease causing pulmonary hypertension. In patients with hyperinflation heart sounds are much reduced at the apex, but well heard over the lower sternum in the midline.

Percussion

When percussing the chest comparison should be made between identical areas on both sides in an attempt to detect differences in percussion note. There are no generally applicable standards for 'resonance' or 'dullness' for comparing one patient with another. The percussion note is resonant over aerated lung, and hyper-resonant with emphysema, large bullae or pneumothorax. Percussion is dull over solid organs such as the liver and heart (except with hyperinflation when the aerated lung covers the heart). In the normal subject the upper level of liver dullness when supine is at the sixth rib in the mid-clavicular line.

The percussion note becomes dull when there is fluid in the pleural space, when there is collapse of a lobe or lung and when there is extensive consolidation. Less marked dullness occurs with pulmonary fibrosis, pleural thickening and large peripheral tumours. Basal dullness as a consequence of diaphragm elevation is easily confused with pleural fluid. If the diaphragm is not paralysed, the level of dullness will fall on inspiration.

Tactile fremitus and vocal resonance are both crude physical signs which are increased with pulmonary consolidation and decreased by pleural fluid.

Auscultation

Listening to the chest is of the greatest clinical importance. At the bedside the breathing of patients with airways obstruction is noisy, and this correlates well with the degree of obstruction documented by pulmonary function tests. This noisy breathing is particularly prominent in chronic bronchitis and asthma, but is less marked in emphysema. On auscultation breath sounds are noted to be generally reduced in patients with airways obstruction, particularly emphysema, and there may be local areas of greatly reduced breath sounds over bullae, a pneumothorax, pleural effusions and when a lobe or lung are poorly ventilated, as when there is substantial bronchial obstruction due to tumour. Expiratory breath sounds are prolonged with airways obstruction whereas expiration is rapid in patients with severe restrictive disease. Bronchial breathing is when the breath sounds become harsh and high-pitched due to enhanced transmission of sound through the abnormal lung. Whispered sounds are then easily heard as high-pitched 'whispering pectoriloquy'. Bronchial breathing is most commonly heard over areas of consolidated lung or over large peripheral cavities.

In addition to alteration of the normal ('vesicular') breath sounds the stethoscope may detect additional sounds:

1. crackles
2. wheezes
3. a pleural rub.

Summary 2   Common causes of crackles

- Bronchiectasis
- Pneumonias
- Alveolitis
- Left heart failure
- Adult respiratory distress syndrome
- Pulmonary fibrosis
- Chronic bronchitis and emphysema
- Bronchiolitis

Crackles

Crackles (crepitations or rales – see Summary 2) are short explosive sounds thought to represent the equalisation of intraluminal pressure as collapsed small airways open during inspiration. Crackles therefore occur in disease processes causing small airway closure whether due to airway damage (chronic bronchitis) or increased interstitial volume (pulmonary oedema, pulmonary fibrosis). With diffuse disease the effect of gravity makes crackles more prominent in dependent parts of the lungs. The crackles of chronic bronchitis and emphysema are characteristically early in inspiration, and are transmitted to the patient's mouth where they can be easily heard by the unaided ear. In bronchiectasis the crackles are maximum in mid-inspiration; in pulmonary fibrosis or oedema they occur during mid- and late inspiration; and in both circumstances the crackles are not transmitted to the mouth.

Wheezes

Wheezes are musical sounds reflecting airway narrowing such that the airway oscillates between being open and closed like the reed of an oboe. In asthma, chronic bronchitis and emphysema multiple polyphonic wheezes are heard in expiration. A localised area of narrowing due to tumour or foreign body produces a single monophonic wheeze. Narrowing of the upper airway (larynx and trachea) causes a wheeze in inspiration as well as expiration, which may be audible at the bedside and is then described as stridor. The causes of wheeze are listed in Summary 3.

Summary 3   Causes of wheeze

Generalised	Localised
Asthma	Tumour
Chronic bronchitis	Extrinsic compression
Emphysema	Foreign body
Pulmonary oedema	Bronchial secretions

Pleural rub

Pleural rub is the sound produced when the two layers of pleura move over one another in a jerking motion, generating a creaking sound similar to that produced by bending stiff leather.

IMAGING THE THORAX

THE CHEST X-RAY

In thoracic medicine, the chest X-ray is of fundamental importance in demonstrating anatomy and is a direct extension of the physical examination of the chest. The examination of chest X-rays is an exercise in problem-solving, and it is much more likely to be successful if the concentration of the radiologist is focused by clinical details and questions.

Chest X-rays should be of good quality and correct exposure. Under-exposure of films is a much greater problem than over-exposure because it cannot be compensated for by any viewing conditions. When viewing an abnormal chest X-ray all available films should be studied in the sequence in which they were taken; past films are frequently the most important in understanding the patient's clinical problems. The chest X-ray should be taken with the patient properly centred, with the medial end of the clavicles equidistant from the spinus processes, and the film should be taken in full inspiration, in which case the dome of the diaphragm will normally be at the level of the sixth rib anteriorly and the tenth rib posteriorly.

Viewing the chest X-ray

The chest X-ray is illustrated in Figure 14.9. Points to consider are listed in Summary 4.

Trachea

The translucent tracheal air column is readily seen in the neck and superior mediastinum; it is placed centrally or slightly to the right. The trachea is an anterior structure and slight rotation of the patient produces substantial lateral displacement of the trachea on the chest X-ray. The tracheal air column may be narrowed by intraluminal disease (e.g. tumour), external compression (e.g. enlarged thyroid) or displaced to the right or left (e.g. upper lobe collapse or fibrosis). The paratracheal regions of the superior mediastinum are common sites of pathology (e.g. lymphadenopathy, apical pulmonary tumours).

Diaphragm

Downward displacement of the diaphragm indicates large-volume lungs (e.g. emphysema); upward displacement suggests small-volume lungs (e.g. pulmonary fibrosis) or diaphragm dysfunction – commonly unilateral, or abdominal pathology. Both hemidiaphragms have a curved shape and a clear edge, and can be seen throughout their length. The right hemidiaphragm is 2 cm higher than the left. The level of the left hemidiaphragm, however, is influenced by the volume of gas in the bowel beneath it. The diaphragm becomes flattened by hyperinflation, best appreciated on the lateral chest X-ray. Failure clearly to visualise the diaphragm indicates abnormality of the adjacent pleura or lung.

Fig. 14.9 Normal chest X-ray. Careful inspection will include: 1. Trachea; 2. Diaphragm; 3. Costophrenic angle; 4. Cardiophrenic angle; 5. Subdiaphragmatic region; 6. Cardiac silhouette; 7. Behind the heart; 8. Hilar shadows; 9. Horizontal (minor) fissure; 10. Vessels; 11. Lung fields; 12. Clavicle and lung apex; 13. Ribcage (Fig. 14.62); 14. Soft tissues (Fig. 14.62).

Summary 4   Viewing the chest X-ray

Points to consider

- Trachea
- Diaphragm
- Costophrenic angle
- Cardiophrenic angle
- Subdiaphragmatic region
- Cardiac silhouette
- Behind the heart
- Hilar shadows

- Horizontal (minor) fissure
- Vessels
- Lymphatics
- The lung fields
- Clavicle and lung apex
- Pleura
- Ribcage
- Soft tissues

Costophrenic angle

This sharp angle is obliterated and the lateral aspect of the diaphragm obscured by small pleural effusions. Chronic pleural abnormalities (e.g. from past infection) also blunts the costophrenic angle.

Cardiophrenic angle

This area of the chest X-ray requires careful inspection

and pathology is easily missed. The angle is blunted by pleural effusion or thickening and also obscured by pericardial fat pads.

Subdiaphragmatic region

Posteriorly, the lung extends below the level of the diaphragm as viewed on the PA film, and pathology in this recess is easily missed; inspection of this area is best on the lateral chest X-ray. On the left, gas in the stomach is commonly seen immediately below the diaphragm and provides some indication of the position of the diaphragm even when it is obscured by pleural or pulmonary pathology. Perforation of an abdominal viscus causes free gas below the diaphragm.

Cardiac silhouette

The mediastinum requires careful inspection to confirm that it is centrally placed and that the cardiac silhouette is of normal configuration and size (Fig. 13.17, p. 346). The heart may be displaced by pleural effusions, collapse of a lung or lobe, extensive fibrosis or pneumothorax. The heart is displaced to the left (which may be misinterpreted as cardiac enlargement) by a depressed sternum. Many disorders alter the configuration of the heart and mediastinum (e.g. cardiac disease, aortic disease, mediastinal tumour and lymphadenopathy) and the cardiac silhouette may be enlarged due to a pericardial effusion as well as dilatation of cardiac chambers. The cardiac diameter is usually less than 50% of the transthoracic diameter, but this is a crude measure and absolute measurements are more valuable; the cardiac diameter is less than 14.5 cm in females and less than 15.5 cm in males, and a change in diameter of greater than 1.5 cm between two X-rays is significant. Emergency chest X-rays taken in the anteroposterior plane magnify the cardiac silhouette.

Behind the heart

This is a notorious blind spot on the PA chest X-ray, particularly if the film is underpenetrated. The retrocardiac space is well seen on the lateral chest X-ray. Pleural or pulmonary shadowing adjacent to the medial aspect of the left hemidiaphragm will obscure it. Occasionally this occurs because of massive cardiac enlargement. A retrocardiac shadow can be caused by a hiatus hernia (Fig. 2.2, p. 23), which may contain a fluid level.

Hilar shadows

The left hilum is always higher than the right. The hilar shadows are vascular and the midpoint (the 'hilar point') is where the upper lobe veins cross the basal pulmonary artery. The lateral border of the hilum is concave. Both hila are of similar size, shape and density. Adenopathy (e.g. tumour) is a common cause of hilar enlargement, with increased density and convexity of the lateral border. Volume loss in the lung – for example, fibrotic shrinkage – distorts the hilum and moves the hilar point towards the loss of volume. Any rotation of the chest X-ray will make the hila asymmetrical.

Horizontal (minor) fissure

This fissure is visible in 60% of normal chest X-rays, running from the centre of the right hilum, laterally and horizontally, to meet the sixth rib in the mid-axilla. The fissure is more easily visible when there is increased pleural fluid (e.g. cardiac failure), and encysted pleural fluid, within any fissure, can mimic a mass lesion. Localised volume loss in the right lung (e.g. collapse of the right upper lobe) moves the fissure from its normal position and the position of the fissure is therefore an important landmark when assessing the chest X-ray for possible obstructing lesions in the right bronchial tree.

Vessels

On the X-ray of normal lungs virtually all pulmonary shadows, apart from a few central bronchi, are vascular. Arteries can be traced back to the hilum but this is more difficult with pulmonary veins. As expected, vessels branch asymmetrically and taper towards the periphery. In the erect posture blood flow to the base of the lungs is greater than to the upper zones, and vessels at the bases are therefore larger. Vessels in the second intercostal space are usually less than 3 mm in diameter. The right basal artery measures approximately 15 mm. If vessels are enlarged, this implies that either pressure (e.g. in pulmonary hypertension secondary to chronic bronchitis or distended upper lobe veins due to left heart failure) or flow (e.g. in left-to-right cardiac shunts) is increased. In left heart failure, the arterial flow to the base of the lungs is reduced and the vessels appear narrower than usual; there is therefore a combination of increased size of upper lobe vessels and reduced size of lower lobe vessels.

Loss of vascularity (e.g. in emphysema) makes the affected area of lung abnormally transradiant. Following lobar collapse the remaining lobes of the lung enlarge, the vessels per unit volume of lung are reduced, and the chest X-ray shows increased transradiancy. The vascular pattern of the lung is therefore an excellent index of localised volume loss. It is not possible to see any vessels in a large bulla, cyst or pneumothorax.

Lymphatics

These are not normally visible on the chest X-ray but when distended by fluid and surrounded by oedema (left heart failure) or infiltrated by tumour (lymphangitis carcinomatosa, see Fig. 14.61) they are seen as linear shadows. In left heart failure the distended lymphatics are seen as 1–2 cm horizontal shadows extending inwards from the pleura, best seen just above the costophrenic angle (termed Kerley B lines or septal lines).

The lung fields

Pathological processes within the lung increase its density (with the exception of pulmonary embolism, emphysema and bullous disease). The abnormality may be localised (e.g. tumour mass, pneumonic consolidation) or generalised (e.g. diffuse fibrosis, pulmonary oedema). Abnormal shadowing is often characteristic of a particular condition or group of disorders, e.g. the bilateral apical shadowing with cavitation characteristic of pulmonary tuberculosis. Two particularly important radiological signs arise from increased pulmonary shadowing: the air bronchogram and the silhouette sign.

1. *Air bronchogram.* An air bronchogram (Fig. 14.10) is visible when alveoli are filled with exudate, transudate or other substance and the bronchi remain patent and filled with air. Important causes of an air bronchogram are pneumonia, cardiogenic pulmonary oedema, adult respiratory distress syndrome and alveolar cell carcinoma.

2. *The silhouette sign.* The outline of many structures on the chest X-ray is visible because of an interface between opaque tissue (heart or diaphragm) and air in the lung (Fig. 14.11). If the lung adjacent to such structures also becomes opaque the 'silhouette' is lost. Thus, collapse of the left lower lobe obscures the left hemidiaphragm and collapse of the lingula or right middle lobe obscures the left and right heart borders.

Clavicle and lung apex

The lung behind the clavicle is a blind spot on the chest X-ray and requires careful scrutiny. It is an important site for pulmonary tumours and tuberculosis. If necessary, an apical view should be taken.

Pleura

Pleural effusions usually obliterate the costophrenic angle, but loculated effusions and pleural thickening (e.g. mesothelioma, Fig. 14.71) are easily missed unless care is taken to look all around the inner aspect of the thoracic cage. In some cases the pleura may calcify (asbestos plaques, tuberculosis, past empyema). With pneumothorax the line of the visceral pleura is seen, although small pneumothoraces are only visible at the apex. The differentiation of a loculated pneumothorax from bullous disease can be difficult.

Ribcage

The ribcage should be symmetrical. Each rib, as well as visible parts of the clavicles, scapulae and spine, should be inspected, particularly looking for fractures and destructive processes. Destruction of ribs in the axillary line is easily missed unless care is taken to follow the curve of each bone, the 'skyline', down the outer aspect of both sides of the thoracic cage.

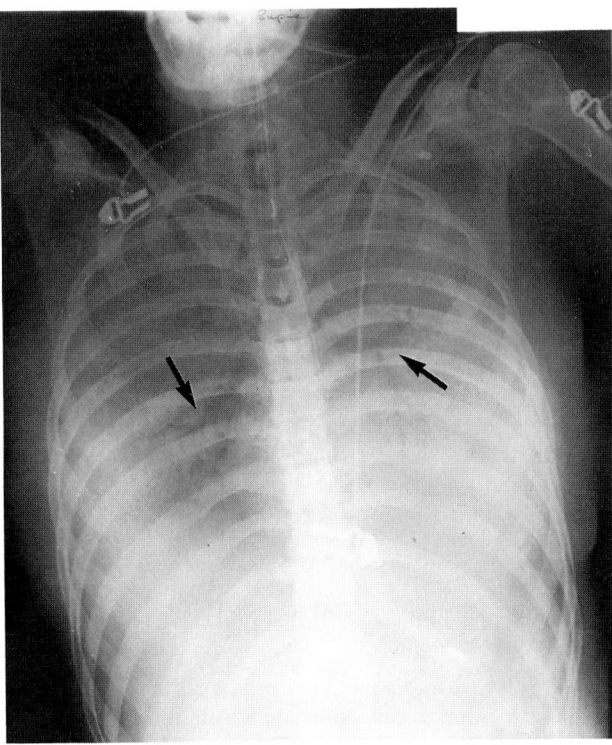

Fig. 14.10 Air bronchogram. The chest X-ray shows bilateral air-space consolidation in a patient with pneumocystis pneumonia and the adult respiratory distress syndrome. Note that the major airways (arrowed) are seen as an 'air bronchogram' against the background pulmonary shadowing.

Fig. 14.11 Silhouette sign. On the normal chest X-ray (Fig. 14.9) there is a clear silhouette of the structures making up the left mediastinum. Collapse of the left upper lobe (including the lingular division) causes an opacity adjacent to the mediastinum and the silhouette is lost. Note the shift to the left of the trachea.

14

Soft tissues

Inspection of the soft tissues not uncommonly provides valuable information which is helpful to the interpretation of lung field abnormalities. Thus, a mastectomy may be noted in a patient with a pleural effusion (Fig. 14.68). When supraclavicular nodes are enlarged, the soft tissue companion shadow, running parallel with the upper border of the clavicle, is lost (Fig. 14.62).

The lateral chest X-ray

A lateral chest X-ray is necessary in all patients with cardiorespiratory problems in whom a comprehensive assessment of thoracic structure is required. On the lateral film some areas are better seen than on the PA view, and three-dimensional localisation of pathology is possible (Fig. 14.12).

Retrosternal area

This area is transradiant and should be of the same density as the retrocardiac area. With hyperinflation (e.g. emphysema) there is an increase in the size and transradiancy of the retrosternal space. Conversely, there is increased retrosternal shadowing with anterior mediastinal masses (e.g. enlarged lymph nodes, ascending aorta, tumour, thymus or thyroid – see Figure 14.67).

Retrocardiac area

Careful inspection of this area, which should be transradiant, is useful because much of the retrocardiac space is not visible on the PA chest X-ray.

Vertebral bodies

Superimposed structures make it difficult to visualise the upper thoracic vertebral bodies but they are progressively more clearly seen towards the lower thoracic spine. If the vertebral bodies are not progressively more easily viewed this suggests that there is pathology (e.g. consolidation or tumour) overlying the spine.

Fig. 14.12   Lateral chest X-ray.
1. Retrosternal area
2. Retrocardiac area
3. Vertebral bodies
4. Diaphragm
5. Greater (oblique) fissure
6. Trachea
7. Cardiac silhouette.

Diaphragm

Both hemidiaphragms should be visible. The gastric gas bubble is beneath the left hemidiaphragm.

Greater (oblique) fissure

The greater fissure passes from where the anterior quarter of the diaphragm meets the posterior three-quarters, through the hilum, and up to the level of the fourth thoracic vertebral body. Displacement of the fissure is an important sign of volume changes within the lobes of the lungs.

Horizontal fissure

The horizontal fissure between the right upper and middle lobes passes anteriorly and horizontally from the level of the hilum. Its position is altered by volume loss, particularly of the right upper and middle lobes.

Trachea

The tracheal air column is frequently better visualised on the lateral chest X-ray than on the PA film.

Cardiac silhouette

Intracardiac, aortic and pericardial calcification is best seen on the lateral chest X-ray.

Summary 5   Viewing the lateral chest X-ray

Points to consider

- Retrosternal area
- Retrocardiac area
- Vertebral bodies
- Diaphragm
- Greater (oblique) fissure
- Horizontal fissure
- Trachea
- Cardiac silhouette

Supplementary radiological examination of the chest

Films taken in expiration are useful for demonstrating small pneumothoraces not easily visible on the PA film at full inspiration.

It is frequently necessary to take chest X-rays with the patient in a supine position (e.g. in the intensive care unit). When the patient is supine, pulmonary blood volume is increased, and there is also a relative redistribution towards the upper zones. These changes result in the vasculature looking more prominent on the chest X-ray, and can be misinterpreted as left heart failure. However, the definition of the vessels remains normal, with no blurring as occurs with interstitial oedema or bronchopneumonia. Cardiac diameter and mediastinal width are both increased when supine.

For the differential diagnosis of pleural effusion from pleural thickening it can be useful to request a chest X-ray taken in the lateral decubitus position, in which free fluid will run along the lateral wall of the thorax. This investigation can detect much smaller effusions (100 ml) than a conventional erect chest X-ray (300 ml).

Tomograms

Conventional tomograms visualise a slice of the thorax to the exclusion of structures both in front of and behind the selected depth. Tomography is particularly useful for more precisely defining masses, demonstrating cavities, examining hilar structure (Fig. 14.13), detecting calcification, and visualising the lumen of the trachea and larger bronchi.

Fig. 14.13 Tomography. Conventional tomogram of hilar structures demonstrating marked right-sided adenopathy due to sarcoidosis (arrow).

Fig. 14.14 Computed tomogram (CT scan) of the thorax. A. CT scan of the normal thorax. B. Scan demonstrating the normal pulmonary vascular pattern. C. CT scan in alpha-1-antitrypsin deficiency. Bullous air spaces occupy most of the left lung and much of the right posteriorly: the peripheral vascular markings are lost.

Computerised tomographic scanning

The vast majority of patients with cardiorespiratory disorders can be satisfactorily investigated with routine radiological techniques. However, when indicated, computerised tomographic (CT) scans of the thorax can provide remarkably detailed information of thoracic anatomy (Fig. 14.14). CT scanning is particularly useful for imaging the mediastinum and demonstrating pleural

467

and chest wall disease. For many patients with bronchogenic carcinoma CT scanning is necessary to stage the disease adequately, particularly when surgery is being considered. Scanning is also valuable in the diagnosis and assessment of emphysema, bullous disease, bronchiectasis, alveolar proteinosis and pulmonary fibrosis.

Magnetic resonance scans provide excellent anatomical visualisation of the thorax and are particularly good for lesions of bone and for detecting lymphadenopathy.

Ultrasound

Ultrasound is not a suitable technique for visualising the lung but it is a good method for imaging pleural disease, both pleural fluid and pleural thickening, and subdiaphragmatic regions (particularly when investigating a subphrenic abscess).

BRONCHOSCOPY AND LUNG BIOPSY

Fibre-optic bronchoscopy

Fibre-optic bronchoscopy is an invaluable technique for diagnosis, assessment and therapy in thoracic medicine. For most patients the procedure is undertaken using local anaesthesia and on a day-case basis. As skills in the technique have increased, so the risks have become small and the indications for fibre-optic bronchoscopy have widened (Table 14.6).

Fibre-optic bronchoscopy is of great value in many patients with seemingly inexplicable respiratory problems. Haemoptysis, for example, may be shown to be due to a tumour above or involving the vocal cords; 'wheeze' may be due to tracheal narrowing; sputum retention may be due to collapse of bronchi during coughing in emphysema; increased breathlessness may be due to endobronchial disease in sarcoidosis; bleeding may be due to telangiectasia of the bronchial tree.

Table 14.6 Major indications for fibre-optic bronchoscopy

Investigation of symptoms, signs or radiological appearances suggesting pulmonary tumour (e.g. haemoptysis, hoarseness; mass, persistent consolidation, or volume loss on chest X-ray)

Diagnosis of pneumonias, tuberculosis and pulmonary shadowing in the immunocompromised host

Removal of mucus, pus and aspirated material from the bronchial tree (frequently on the intensive care unit)

Diagnosis and assessment of activity in diffuse interstitial lung disease (e.g. sarcoidosis, fibrosing alveolitis)

Demonstration of bronchiectasis

Bronchogenic carcinoma

Bronchogenic carcinoma is commonly visible as an obvious endobronchial tumour mass, in which case bronchial biopsy will confirm the diagnosis in 90% of cases. The flushing of saline over the surface of tumours and the subsequent aspiration of this fluid, or the brushing of the surface of tumours, provide cells for cytological examination, and these investigations have a diagnostic yield of 60–80% for visible endobronchial disease.

A small number of patients have positive sputum cytology but no evidence of tumour on chest X-ray. Most commonly, the cause is a centrally placed, squamous cell bronchogenic carcinoma, easily diagnosed at bronchoscopy although the malignant changes may be relatively early and the tumour mass small.

In assessing the extent of malignant disease, fibre-optic bronchoscopy is of great importance, allowing visualisation of the proximal spread of the tumour which determines the feasibility and likely extent of any surgical resection.

In selected patients endobronchial tumour can be destroyed by a laser, transmitted through a fibre passed down the biopsy channel of a fibre-optic bronchoscope. In patients with large central tumours causing breathlessness or haemoptysis that have not responded to radiotherapy, such palliative therapy can be of substantial benefit.

Haemoptysis

All patients with haemoptysis who are at risk of carcinoma of the bronchus should be bronchoscoped; approximately 10% of patients with a chest X-ray which does not obviously suggest tumour will nevertheless have malignancy. When bleeding is not due to tumour, for example, in bronchiectasis, bronchoscopy is useful to determine the site of bleeding, which is important should bleeding become a serious problem and bronchial arterial embolisation or thoracic surgery be considered.

Interstitial lung disease

Sarcoidosis is the most common cause of interstitial lung disease and in the majority of cases the diagnosis is easily confirmed by bronchoscopy. Overall, a bronchoscopic transbronchial biopsy has a positive yield of 90% (p. 508). With the technique of transbronchial biopsy (TBB) a small fragment of lung tissue is obtained when the forceps remove the bronchial wall of the carina of two small peripheral bronchi (Fig. 14.15). In pulmonary fibrosis, including cryptogenic fibrosing alveolitis (p. 516), transbronchial biopsy is less helpful. The small samples obtained are often not representative and if histological confirmation of the diagnosis is required, an open lung biopsy is preferable. Transbronchial biopsy can be diagnostic in the uncommon conditions of alveolar proteinosis, histiocytosis X and pulmonary disease due to inorganic dusts.

Broncho-alveolar lavage

At fibre-optic bronchoscopy saline is instilled into the periphery of the lung, with the tip of the bronchoscope wedged in the segmental or subsegmental bronchus, and the fluid

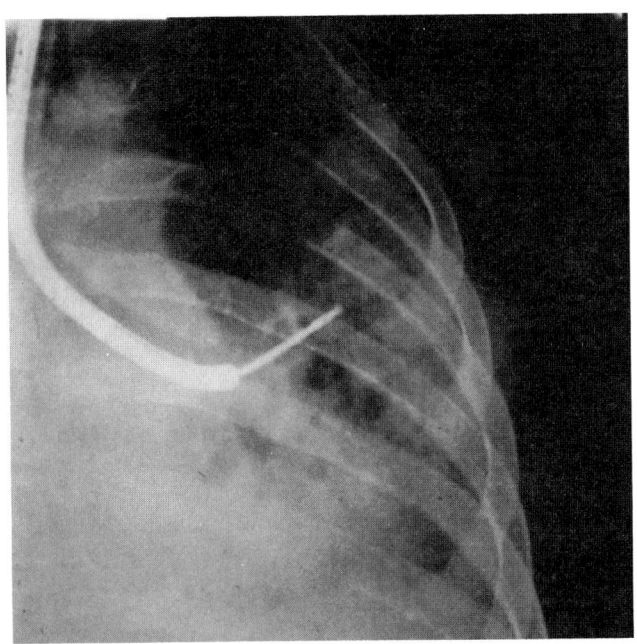

Fig. 14.15 Bronchoscopy. Using the flexible fibre-optic bronchoscope biopsy forceps can be passed into peripheral bronchi and samples of lung obtained by transbronchial biopsy.

is subsequently gently aspirated. The lavage fluid contains millions of cells (macrophages, lymphocytes, neutrophils and eosinophils), the numbers of which, and their differential count, give information on the nature of the interstitial lung disease. In occasional circumstances, bronchoalveolar lavage (BAL) can be diagnostic, as in alveolar proteinosis, pulmonary haemosiderosis and histiocytosis X.

Pulmonary infections

Some patients with pneumonia fail to show an adequate response to chemotherapy, yet do not have sputum for microbiological analysis. In such patients, bronchoalveolar lavage provides helpful information, although when patients are already receiving antibiotics bacterial culture is frequently negative and staining techniques give the most valuable information.

Similarly, patients with pulmonary tuberculosis do not always have sputum and in these cases bronchoscopy and lavage of the affected lobes is an efficient technique for confirming the diagnosis. In miliary tuberculosis, BAL is commonly positive and transbronchial biopsy will confirm the diagnosis in virtually all cases.

Bronchoscopy with BAL and TBB is of great value in the investigation of pulmonary shadowing in the immunocompromised host (p. 475). The importance of these techniques has become greater since the advent of AIDS (p. 476). For most infections, as opposed to other causes of pulmonary infiltration, BAL is virtually as effective as transbronchial biopsy or open lung biopsy in providing diagnostic information but carries less risk to the patient.

Bronchiectasis

With a fibre-optic bronchoscope it is possible to produce high-quality selective bronchograms; the technique is generally well tolerated by patients with bronchiectasis (p. 482).

Bronchoscopy on the intensive care unit

Many patients on the intensive care unit, as well as other ill patients often in the immediate postoperative period, develop sputum retention, basal atelectasis or pulmonary collapse. Bronchoscopy and bronchial lavage are effective at removing impacted secretions. Bronchial lavage is frequently superior to conventional catheter suction in the diagnosis of intensive care unit pneumonias. Bronchoscopy is also valuable for the inspection of the bronchial tree, particularly the trachea, for catheter or endotracheal tube trauma, or stenosis.

Rigid bronchoscopy

As a diagnostic technique rigid bronchoscopy, which requires a general anaesthetic, has been largely superseded by fibre-optic bronchoscopy. Immediately prior to thoracic surgery for bronchogenic carcinoma, rigid bronchoscopy is routinely undertaken. The range of vision of the rigid instrument is less than with the fibre-optic bronchoscope but it is a simple matter to pass a fibre-optic bronchoscope through the rigid instrument. Rigid bronchoscopy remains of great value in the following situations:

1. in the bronchoscopy of smaller children
2. in patients who have a foreign body impacted in the bronchial tree
3. for the biopsy of vascular tumours, particularly adenomas
4. for obtaining a large biopsy sample to confirm submucosal malignancy not demonstrated by the small superficial biopsies that can be taken using the fibre-optic bronchoscope.

Transthoracic needle biopsy

Several techniques are available to biopsy the lung and diagnose pathological processes, most commonly tumours, within it. Cutting needles provide good tissue samples for histological analysis, but except for sampling extensive pleural disease or pulmonary tumour masses invading the pleura, the technique is unacceptably dangerous. The technique of choice is fine needle aspiration biopsy under radiological control. The tissue so obtained is suitable for cytological and microbiological, but not histological, analysis. If it is performed using local anaesthesia, patients seldom experience pain and major complications are rare. A small pneumothorax is common (30%), particularly in patients with emphysema, and a few patients will require tube drainage (5%). The overall mortality is very low and the technique is now extensively used in the investigation of pulmonary disease. In practice, the most common indication is to provide confirmation of malignancy for peripheral tumours not seen at fibre-optic bronchoscopy. With experience and expert cytological support a yield of 90% or more is obtained in malignant disease. A further important use of the technique is in the investigation of pulmonary infections not diagnosed by more conventional techniques, particularly fungal, protozoal and mycobacterial infections in the immunocompromised host.

Open lung biopsy

Open lung biopsy is most commonly undertaken for diffuse interstitial lung disease, atypical tumours, and occasionally, serious pulmonary infections. A limited submammary thoracotomy allows biopsy of the anterior segments of all lobes as well as inspection of the pleura and mediastinum. Complications (approximately 5%) include infection and chronic pneumothorax and there is a small mortality (less than 4%) reflecting for the most part the serious nature of the underlying illness in many of the patients.

Mediastinoscopy and mediastinotomy

These techniques are mainly used to diagnose and to stage bronchogenic carcinoma but occasionally are required to confirm other malignancies (for example, lymphoma) or causes of adenopathy (for example, sarcoidosis or tuberculosis). At *mediastinoscopy* an incision is made above the suprasternal notch, the tissues anterior to the trachea are dissected and the mediastinoscope inserted. Hilar, subcarinal and paratracheal nodes can be inspected, biopsied or removed. The involvement of mediastinal nodes in bronchogenic carcinoma is common (40% of all cases) and a positive diagnosis is achieved in sarcoidosis in more than 80% of cases.

Mediastinotomy is occasionally required to evaluate areas of the mediastinum not accessible at mediastinoscopy, particularly the subaortic fossa on the left side, and most commonly the surgeon gains access through the second left costal cartilage.

The development of CT scanning has reduced the need for mediastinoscopy and mediastinotomy. In carcinoma of the bronchus a CT scan which demonstrates a normal mediastinum obviates the need for surgical evaluation prior to thoracotomy. However, if the CT scan demonstrates adenopathy, such an evaluation may be still required to confirm that the nodes are involved by tumour and are not enlarged due to reactive hyperplasia.

RESPIRATORY INFECTIONS

UPPER RESPIRATORY TRACT INFECTIONS

Most upper respiratory tract infections (URTIs) are viral and the majority of these are the results of infection with picornaviruses of the rhinovirus group. However, adenoviruses, coronaviruses, coxsackie viruses, echoviruses, influenza viruses, para-influenza viruses and the respiratory syncytial virus (RSV) can all cause upper respiratory tract infections. URTIs represent the most common of all illnesses and are responsible for approximately half of all time lost from work.

In addition to URTI the influenza viruses, para-influenza viruses I and II, adenoviruses and RSV can cause acute infection of the larynx, trachea and major bronchi, and are causes of croup. URTIs are most common in the late winter months and early spring. The most frequent manifestation of these viral infections is the *common cold* (acute coryza), which may be complicated by secondary bacterial infection and subsequently by sinusitis, otitis media, obstruction to the Eustachian tubes and infection of the lower respiratory tract. *Viral laryngotracheobronchitis*, particularly in children, may be complicated by severe laryngeal oedema and life-threatening *croup*. Croup is also a feature of acute *epiglottitis* in children and occasionally adults, which is most commonly due to *Haemophilus influenzae* type B infection. The swelling of the epiglottis and surrounding soft tissues can rapidly produce respiratory distress. Unlike laryngitis, the voice is not hoarse. The epiglottis is hugely swollen and attempts to examine the throat can precipitate total upper airway obstruction.

In most patients with URTI the illness is self-limiting and symptoms subside after a few days. Antibiotics are not generally required unless there is acute epiglottitis due to *Haemophilus influenzae*. However, in patients in whom secondary bacterial infection is both likely and potentially serious – for example, in chronic bronchitis and emphysema – immediate treatment with antibiotics is justified. The development of stridor requires careful observation in hospital with anaesthetic support for possible emergency intubation. Patients with stridor, particularly children with croup, adopt the posture that facilitates adequate ventilation and they should be allowed to do so. Inhalation of warm, humidified air is helpful. The value of steroids to reduce oedema is unproven.

Sinusitis

Sinusitis (infection of the paranasal sinuses) is a common complication of upper respiratory tract infection and the bacteria most frequently involved are *Haemophilus influenzae* and *Streptococcus pneumoniae*. Facial pain and tenderness, headache, nasal discharge and a postnasal drip are the usual features. Radiology may demonstrate fluid levels within the maxillary sinuses or show sinus mucosal thickening. Sinusitis may complicate the nasal obstruction of allergic rhinitis, in which case topical steroid therapy is useful, in addition to antibiotics. Persistent or recurrent sinusitis may require surgical drainage. Sinusitis is a common feature of patients with bronchiectasis (occasionally, both are manifestations of the immotile cilia syndromes) and it is equally important to control infection at both sites.

LOWER RESPIRATORY TRACT INFECTIONS

Acute bronchitis

Acute bronchitis is common in smokers and in patients with chronic bronchitis and emphysema. However, it also occurs in otherwise healthy individuals and in both groups the bacteria most often incriminated are *Streptococcus pneumoniae* or *Haemophilus influenzae*. These infections cause an acute inflammation of the trachea and major airways, and as a consequence of this there is chest pain, commonly experienced as a raw feeling maximal on deep inspiration, as well as chest tightness. The patients may wheeze. In patients with pre-existing, chronic airflow limitation the development of acute bronchitis can cause severe breathlessness. Acute bronchitis causes an irritating, persistent, dry cough although after one or two days patients produce small amounts of mucoid thick sputum which subsequently becomes more plentiful and purulent. Appropriate antibiotic therapy is amoxycillin, tetracycline or co-trimoxazole. In patients with chronic airflow limitation, aggressive therapy with bronchodilators is important since acute bronchitis can precipitate a worsening of respiratory failure and necessitate hospital admission.

PNEUMONIA

Pneumonia remains an important clinical problem, causing many more deaths than any other infectious disease in the UK, both in the community and in hospitals. In recent years the aetiology of the pneumonias has changed with, for example, an increased incidence of legionella infection and opportunistic pneumonias in the immunocompromised host, particularly patients with HIV infection.

Although pneumonia is the most common cause of fever ditions must be considered in the differential diagnosis (Table 14.7).

Having arrived at a clinical diagnosis of pneumonia, the next decision is what therapy to institute. For the adult patient, the clinical background of the pneumonia serves to reduce the range of possible pathogens. The most useful

Table 14.7 Differential diagnosis of a presumed pneumonia

Pulmonary infarction

Pulmonary eosinophilia

Allergic alveolitis

Pulmonary drug reaction

Radiation injury

Pulmonary vasculitis or haemorrhage

Alveolar cell carcinoma

Leukaemia, lymphoma, Kaposi's sarcoma and other pulmonary tumours

Empyema

Bronchial obstruction with distal collapse/consolidation

classification of the pneumonias is therefore a clinical one (Summary 6).

Summary 6 Classification of pneumonia

- Community acquired pneumonia
- Hospital acquired (nosocomial) pneumonia
- Recurrent pneumonia
- Aspiration pneumonia
- Pneumonia in the immunocompromised host
- Unusual pneumonias

Community acquired pneumonia

Community acquired pneumonia is commonly due to a limited and predictable group of pathogens (Table 14.8).

Patients with pneumonia commonly have fever, cough, breathlessness, abnormal chest signs and X-ray shadowing. However, specific pneumonias may have additional features. *Mycobacterium tuberculosis* remains an important pathogen and tuberculosis must be considered in the differential diagnosis of many pneumonias: in most cases tuberculosis has characteristic clinical features (p. 479).

Table 14.8 Important causes of community acquired pneumonia

Streptococcus pneumoniae

Mycoplasma pneumoniae

Haemophilus influenzae

Staphylococcus aureus

Legionella pneumophilia

Viruses

Mycobacterium tuberculosis

Pneumococcal pneumonia

Pneumoccal pneumonia is more common in the winter months and upper respiratory tract viral infections are a predisposing factor. Following the penetration of the organism into the lower respiratory tract there is intense inflammatory oedema, and rapid multiplication and spread of organisms proceeding to hepatisation, in which the lung becomes solid and airless. There is substantial ventilation–perfusion mismatch and associated hypoxaemia. The stiff lung produces a rapid, shallow breathing pattern. Fever is often very high and there may be rigors. Pleurisy is common and the cough, which is initially dry and painful, subsequently becomes productive of rusty sputum. Altered blood from the congested lung tissue gives the sputum its characteristic colour. Labial herpes simplex is common (30% of cases). In some cases the onset of symptoms in pneumococcal pneumonia can be very rapid and patients may be critically ill within a few hours. In the usual case clinical examination demonstrates crackles more than classical signs of consolidation, and a pleural rub is common. The chest X-ray shows hazy shadowing, often with an air bronchogram (Fig. 14.10), in any lobe, although lower lobes are the most frequently involved. In the majority of cases the consolidation does not involve the whole lobe.

Mildly or moderately ill patients can be managed adequately at home and are satisfactorily treated with oral amoxycillin, erythromycin or co-trimoxazole. Severely ill patients should be transferred to hospital for the adequate treatment of pain, dehydration and hypoxaemia which may cause the patient to become confused. A Gram stain of the sputum will show typical Gram-positive diplococci and blood cultures will be positive in 25–40% of untreated cases. Pneumococcal antigen can be demonstrated in both blood and sputum. If the specific diagnosis is established benzylpenicillin is the treatment of choice, but patients also do well with amoxycillin.

Recovery from pneumococcal pneumonia is usually rapid, although the X-ray may take several weeks to return to normal, as is the case with most pneumonias. In those patients who are more severely ill, and who are bacteraemic, mortality may be as high as 25%. Of all pneumonias, pleural effusion is most common in association with pneumococcal infection. Empyema complicating the pleural effusion is now relatively rare and occurs in 3% of cases with positive blood cultures. In such blood culture-positive patients pneumococcal pneumonia can be complicated by pericarditis, endocarditis, septic arthritis, peritonitis, cellulitis and, on rare occasions, meningitis.

Haemophilus influenzae pneumonia

It is unusual for *Haemophilus influenzae* to cause pneumonia in previously fit individuals. However, it is probably the most common cause of infection in patients with pre-existing lung disease, particularly in those with chronic bronchitis and emphysema. It is the organism most often responsible for the exacerbations that occur in chronic bronchitis, sometimes complicating an initial viral infection. The chest X-ray distinguishes haemophilus bronchopneumonia from simple infective bronchitis by showing shadowing, usually as nodules 0.5–3.0 cm in diameter, at both bases, and on examination there may be bronchial breathing. The same picture of bronchopneumonia is sometimes seen with staphylococcal and pneumococcal infection.

Bronchopneumonia is very common. Patients are often wheezy and progressively more breathless. There is usually fever but in elderly and debilitated patients the temperature can be normal. Cough and purulent sputum are prominent features. As a consequence of diffuse airway inflammation and intraluminal sputum, patients with chronic bronchitis are frequently precipitated into respiratory failure and cor pulmonale. The first-line treatment of *Haemophilus influenzae* bronchopneumonia is amoxy-

cillin, and where appropriate hospitalisation will be necessary to deal with sputum retention, airways obstruction and respiratory failure.

Staphylococcal pneumonia

Staphylococcal infection causes more necrosis than other organisms responsible for pneumonia and there is a high incidence of abscess formation. In the community staphylococcal pneumonia is not common (about 1% of cases), but it is an important and serious complication of viral influenza and is therefore more common during influenza epidemics and during the winter months. Staphylococcal lobar pneumonia can be fulminant and rapidly fatal. In most cases, the clinical picture is similar to pneumococcal pneumonia, but haemoptysis is more common. Cavitation is unusual in community acquired pneumonias, with the exception of staphylococcal or particularly virulent serotype 3 pneumococcal infections. The chest X-ray typically shows bilateral consolidation, usually basal, with abscesses that are thin-walled and cyst-like. Staphylococcal lung abscesses may rupture into the pleural cavity, resulting in pneumothorax or pyopneumothorax.

In the community, the development of pneumonia as a complication of influenza should be treated with flucloxacillin in addition to amoxycillin. Following admission to hospital, Gram stain of the sputum is helpful in confirming the diagnosis and blood cultures are frequently positive. With a definite diagnosis treatment should be with flucloxacillin and fucidic acid. Although the majority of patients make a good recovery from staphylococcal pneumonia, the combination of influenza A infection and staphylococcal pneumonia still carries an appreciable mortality. Important complications include the haematogenous spread of infection to brain, bone and other organs and occasionally patients can develop acute bacterial endocarditis.

Legionella pneumonia

Legionella pneumonia was first recognised in 1976 after an outbreak of pneumonia with a high mortality at a Legionnaires conference in Philadelphia. The pathogen is now known as *Legionella pneumophilia*, a small Gram-negative coccobacilliary organism. Infection is acquired from contaminated water, usually in air-conditioning systems and showers in hotels and hospitals, and transmission does not occur from person to person. Most cases have been in middle-aged or elderly males and have occurred in the summer months. Legionella is a cause of opportunistic chest infection in immunocompromised patients. Clinically, legionella pneumonia resembles viral or mycoplasma infection. There is a cough but little sputum, and this is mucoid, not purulent. Patients are frequently severely ill with high fever, rigors, confusion, myalgia, abdominal pain, vomiting and diarrhoea. Hyponatraemia, hypo-albuminaemia and haematuria (50% of cases) are common. The white cell count may be normal or modestly elevated but seldom above $15\,000 \times 10^6/l$. Gram stain of the mucoid sputum reveals no organisms. The chest X-ray most commonly shows patchy shadowing which can be bilateral and which progresses to lobar consolidation.

Diagnosis is usually retrospective and based on a greater than fourfold increase in the indirect fluorescent antibody titre. The organism can be isolated from lung tissue, pleural fluid and blood. Treatment is with erythromycin (500 mg six-hourly) for a period of 3 weeks. In patients who fail to respond, rifampicin should be added. Ciprofloxacin may also be effective. The overall mortality is 15%, some patients dying despite appropriate antibiotic therapy.

Viral and viral-like pneumonia

Viral and viral-like pneumonias (Table 14.9) are characterised by fever, systemic symptoms (e.g. myalgia, headache) and a normal or near-normal white cell count.

Respiratory syncytial virus infection is important in children. Influenza and measles are frequently complicated by serious bacterial infection, particularly staphylococcal. Cytomegalovirus is a cause of pneumonia in the immunocompromised host (p. 476). Of the remaining causes, *Mycoplasma pneumoniae*, *Chlamydia psittaci* and *Coxiella burneti* are the most important.

Table 14.9 Organisms causing viral and viral-like pneumonias

Mycoplasma pneumoniae

Respiratory syncytial virus

Influenza

Measles

Cytomegalovirus

Adenoviruses

Para-influenza virus

Rhinovirus

Varicella (chickenpox)

Coxiella burneti (Q fever)

Chlamydial pneumonias (psittacosis, ornithosis)

Mycoplasma pneumonia

Mycoplasma pneumoniae is the most important agent causing the so-called 'atypical' pneumonias. In the past, this organism was the cause of major outbreaks of pneumonias in the armed forces; many cases still occur in clusters, and epidemics typically occur every 3 or 4 years. Infection is caused by an organism of the mycoplasmata group, the smallest known free-living organism. Most cases are aged between 15 and 30 years. After an incubation period of between 1 and 3 weeks the patient develops symptoms suggestive of viral pneumonia with systemic upset, arthralgia and myalgia being particularly common. Typically, the white cell count is not raised. The appearances on chest X-ray are very variable and although seg-

mental and subsegmental shadows are most common, a lobar pattern can also be seen.

In mycoplasma pneumonia cold agglutinins are present in approximately 50% of cases and serological investigations demonstrate antibodies to mycoplasma in most instances. Mycoplasma titres may be raised for several years following infection.

The most effective therapy for mycoplasma infection is erythromycin or tetracycline. Complications can include a haemolytic anaemia and renal failure, due to the presence of cold agglutinins, as well as meningism, central nervous system involvement and myocarditis. For most patients the prognosis is excellent.

Psittacosis and ornithosis

Chlamydial infection is transmitted from parrots to man (psittacosis) or from other birds to man (ornithosis). The organism (intermediate between a virus and a rickettsial organism) is in the dust derived from excreta and feathers. The birds do not always appear to be ill. There is usually a history of close contact with birds (e.g. pigeon racers). The ensuing illness is rather like influenza. There is a cough, mucoid sputum and sometimes haemoptysis. The chest X-ray shows patchy consolidation. A complicating bacterial pneumonia is common. Diagnosis is best made by a rising titre for chlamydia antibodies and effective treatment is tetracycline or erythromycin.

Rickettsial pneumonia (Q fever)

The rickettsial organism (*Coxiella burneti*) is transmitted from animals (most commonly cattle and sheep) to man by dust inhalation. Slaughterhouse workers are most often infected. There is an abrupt onset of a viral-like illness with headache and meningism. Respiratory symptoms are less prominent. The chest X-ray shows patchy consolidation. Diagnosis is confirmed by a rising antibody titre. A prolonged course of tetracycline (or erythromycin) is effective, as is chloramphenicol. Rickettsia can cause endocarditis (p. 420).

Treatment of community acquired pneumonia

Because of the likely pathogens, most patients respond well to amoxycillin. For patients with features of an 'atypical' pneumonia, or legionella, erythromycin should be added, and in patients with a recent influenza-like illness, flucloxacillin.

Hospital acquired (nosocomial) pneumonia

Up to 5% of patients admitted to hospital for other causes subsequently develop a pneumonia; the mechanisms of infection are depicted in Figure 14.16. Particularly important predisposing factors are cigarette-smoking, chronic lung disease, obesity, the effects of anaesthesia and surgery, and prior use of broad-spectrum antibiotics.

Table 14.10   Organisms responsible for hospital acquired pneumonia

Organism	% of cases
Gram-negative bacteria (especially Klebsiella spp. and Pseudomonas spp.)	50
Staphylococcus aureus	15
Anaerobes	9
Streptococcus pneumoniae	6
Others (legionella, fungi, etc.)	20

The causative organisms for hospital acquired pneumonias are different from those responsible for community acquired pneumonia and, in particular, Gram-negative organisms are responsible for 50% of cases. Anaerobic infections are also important (Table 14.10).

The prior use of broad-spectrum antibiotics and the consequent colonisation of the oropharynx with Gram-negative bacilli reduces the value of sputum culture and makes it difficult to find the cause of hospital acquired pneumonia. The management of these pneumonias involves close collaboration between clinical staff and microbiologist. Gram stain of the sputum may be more useful than culture. Blood cultures will be positive in up to 25% of cases. For potentially serious pneumonias clinical management is helped by a precise diagnosis and invasive techniques are appropriate. Transtracheal aspiration and bronchoscopy can yield useful information. The wide range of potential pathogens demands the use of broad-spectrum antibiotics, including good Gram-negative cover, in the initial therapy of hospital acquired pneumonia. An amoxycillin/ceftazidine or ureido penicillin/aminoglycoside combination is usually effective.

A knowledge of the factors concerned in the pathogenesis of hospital acquired pneumonia (Fig. 14.16) indicates ways

in which such infections can be reduced. Careful use of antibiotics is of particular importance.

Recurrent pneumonia

Prior to making a diagnosis of recurrent pneumonia, the possibility of a non-infective cause of recurrent pulmonary problems should be considered. Alternative diagnoses will include pulmonary infarction, pulmonary eosinophilia (including bronchopulmonary aspergillosis) and asthma. Recurrent pneumonia is unusual without a predisposing factor (Table 14.11).

Table 14.11   Important causes of recurrent pneumonia

Diffuse bronchopulmonary disease	Local bronchial obstruction
Bronchiectasis	Tumour
Cystic fibrosis	Adenopathy
Chronic bronchitis, emphysema and chronic asthma	Foreign body
Immotile cilia syndrome	**Local bronchopulmonary disease**
Immune deficiency states	Bronchiectasis
HIV infection	Congenital abnormalities (sequestration)
Hypogammaglobulinaemia	
Myeloma	

Any cause of obstruction to a bronchus can result in recurrent or persistent pneumonia, but tumours are most important (p. 522). The clinical situation is usually that of a pneumonia which is slow to resolve or has recurred in a patient who is a cigarette smoker and who may also have haemoptysis. Haemoptysis occurs with many pneumonias but is much more common with tumours. Volume loss on chest X-ray suggests central airway obstruction.

Aspiration pneumonia

Many patients with aspiration pneumonia have dental sepsis, a predisposition to aspiration, or both (Table 14.12). Infection is usually with anaerobic organisms derived from the upper respiratory tract. Aspiration pneumonia may be acute, extensive and progressive or it may run a more subacute course and progress to lung abscess formation.

When cavitating anaerobic pneumonias communicate with the bronchial tree the sputum is both copious and foul-smelling. The site of the pneumonia or lung abscess will depend on the position of the patient at the time of aspiration. Aspirated material enters the right lung more easily than the left, and will enter the lower lobes when the subject is standing and the apical segment of the lower lobes or the posterior segment of the upper lobes when supine.

An important cause of anaerobic pneumonias and lung abscess is bronchial obstruction (e.g. with bronchogenic carcinoma), and if the diagnosis of aspiration is in doubt bronchoscopy is indicated. Barium swallow will frequently be a rewarding investigation. Anaerobic infection causes

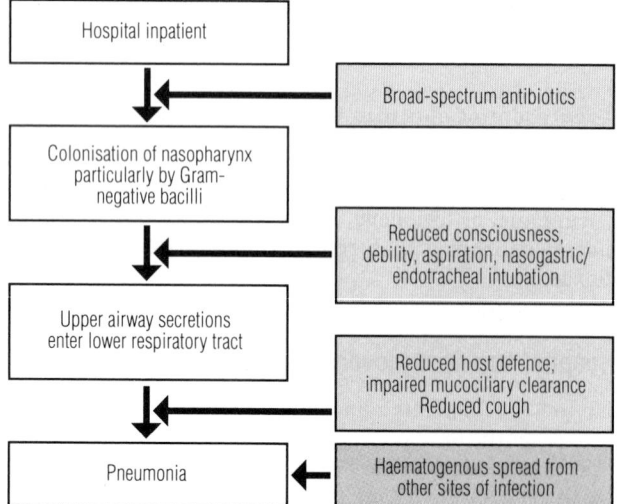

Fig. 14.16   Factors predisposing to hospital acquired pneumonia.

Table 14.12   Factors predisposing to aspiration pneumonia

Altered consciousness	**Neurological disorders**
Drug overdose	Pseudobulbar palsy
Anaesthesia	Myasthenia gravis, etc.
Epilepsy	
Cerebrovascular accident	**Nasogastric tubes**
Alcoholism	**Severe dental and upper airways sepsis**
Dysphagia and oesophageal disease	**Terminal illness**
Stricture	
Achalasia	
Oesophageal pouch	
Fistula	
Hiatus hernia	
Reflux	

considerable tissue destruction with abscess formation, and empyema and metastatic abscesses can also occur. Prompt treatment avoids such problems. Most anaerobes are sensitive to penicillin. Early aspiration pneumonias are adequately treated with amoxycillin but more severe infections and lung abscesses require parenteral penicillin plus metronidazole for penicillin-resistant organisms. Postural drainage is important and antibiotic therapy should be continued for 6 weeks or more to minimise lung destruction.

Inhalation pneumonias

Aspiration pneumonia is the term used to denote aspiration of organisms into the lower respiratory tract (usually anaerobes); inhalational pneumonias refer to the consequences of inhaling non-infected particulate matter, fluids and irritant gases.

The inhalation of gastric contents during anaesthesia or other causes of reduced consciousness, or childbirth (Mendelson's syndrome) produces a chemical pneumonitis and respiratory distress. When severe, the features are of the adult respiratory distress syndrome (p. 518). Management includes antibiotics, and metronidazole provides good cover for anaerobic organisms, but corticosteroids are not helpful.

Inhalation of food produces the clinical picture of a chronic, often recurrent pneumonia. The inflammatory infiltrate in the lung may progress to fibrosis.

Lipoid pneumonia follows the aspiration of liquid paraffin laxatives, oily nosedrops or oily seawater. The lung pathology shows a foreign body giant cell reaction and fibrosis. Chronic pneumonias due to inhalation may mimic lung tumours and the diagnosis may only become evident following surgical resection. Repeated inhalation may eventually produce bilateral fibrosis and bronchiectasis. Hot smoke inhalation causes respiratory burns. There is oedema of the upper airways and bronchial tree, causing

wheeze and croup. Severe injury is unlikely if there is no blistering of the mouth. Several hours or days after inhalation, pulmonary oedema may develop. Early corticosteroid therapy may be beneficial. Patients may progress to develop the adult respiratory distress syndrome (p. 518).

Pneumonia in the immunocompromised host

The increased use of immunosuppressive agents and the emergence of HIV infection has greatly increased the prevalence of pneumonia in the immunocompromised host, so-called 'opportunistic' infections. These infections are particularly common in certain well-recognised groups (Table 14.13).

Table 14.13   Groups at risk of opportunistic pneumonias

Primary immunodeficiency	**Secondary immunodeficiency**
B cell deficiency (agammaglobulinaemia)	HIV infection (AIDS)
	Leukaemias and lymphomas
T cell deficiency (Di George syndrome)	Corticosteroid therapy
T cell and B cell deficiency (combined immunodeficiency)	Cytotoxic agents (particularly following organ transplantation and the treatment of haematological malignancies)
	Malnutrition, general debility, uraemia, liver failure, etc.

In patients who are immunosuppressed, particularly following organ transplantation or cytotoxic therapy for malignancy, the development of fever and pulmonary infiltrates is not always due to infection (Table 14.14).

Occasionally bleeding into the lung occurs in patients who are thrombocytopenic. Radiation pneumonitis is most intense between 4 and 6 weeks after treatment. In a small number of patients a non-specific pneumonitis develops for which no cause is found, even when these patients are submitted to open lung biopsy.

Infection can be due to a wide variety of agents. Immunodeficiency facilitates infection with organisms seldom

Table 14.14   Fever and pulmonary infiltrates in immunocompromised patients

Infection

Pulmonary oedema

Pulmonary haemorrhage

Drug-induced pneumonitis

Radiation pneumonitis

Malignant infiltration (e.g. leukaemia, Kaposi's sarcoma)

Pulmonary emboli

Non-specific pneumonitis

encountered in immunocompetent individuals and the clinical picture is often of a rapid, extensive and life-threatening pneumonia (Table 14.15).

Table 14.15 Important causes of pneumonia in the immunocompromised patient

Bacterial	Viral
Gram-negative organisms as well as Gram-positive	Cytomegalovirus
Nocardia	Herpes simplex
Mycobacteria	**Fungal**
Legionella	Candida
Mycoplasma	Aspergillus
Chlamydia	Cryptococcus
	Protozoal
	Pneumocystis

Management of pneumonia in the immunocompromised patient

Pneumonia in the immunocompromised host is a medical emergency requiring immediate investigation and treatment. All patients should have blood cultures and appropriate serological investigations for likely pathogens. The chest X-ray is of limited value, with the exception of pneumocystis pneumonia in patients with HIV infection. Any pleural fluid should be sampled for diagnostic purposes. Localised shadows are more common in bacterial infection; diffuse infiltration suggests an opportunistic organism. In all patients the likely value (and the risks) of invasive techniques to establish a definite cause for pneumonia must be considered.

Most patients with diffuse pulmonary infiltration do not have sputum and invasive investigations are therefore required to demonstrate the infective agent. Transtracheal aspiration, percutaneous needle aspiration biopsy, bronchoscopy and open lung biopsy can all yield useful information. Bronchoscopy is the most widely available technique. Broncho-alveolar lavage is a valuable technique for diagnosing pneumocystis and cytomegalovirus infection and is safe in patients with thrombocytopenia and bleeding diatheses. Transbronchial biopsy, although an effective investigation, can produce dangerous haemorrhage in patients with bleeding problems (uraemic patients are particularly prone to haemorrhage) and pneumothorax is a complication, particularly hazardous in patients receiving positive pressure ventilation.

Specific pneumonias in immunocompromised patients

Gram-negative pneumonias

Bacterial pneumonias, particularly Gram-negative infections, are common in neutropenic patients (e.g. following bone marrow transplantation or chemotherapy for leukaemia) and may be associated with life-threatening sep-

ticaemia. The chest X-ray usually shows localised shadowing, rather than diffuse infiltration. Following blood cultures empirical therapy should be started immediately. Common organisms are *Pseudomonas aeruginosa, Klebsiella, Enterobacter, Escherichia coli, Serratia*. The use of broad-spectrum antibiotics favours the emergence of resistant organisms and also the development of fungal infections. Treatment of Gram-negative infections commonly requires aminoglycosides, cephalosporins and antipseudomonal pencillins.

Klebsiella pneumonia

The most common clinical setting for this Gram-negative pneumonia is in the elderly male patient, often with chronic lung disease, whose 'immunosuppression' is due to general debility, associated with chronic illnesses such as diabetes and alcoholism. The illness can be severe (mortality 20–50%) with high fever, rigors and pleuritic pain, and haemoptysis occurs more often than in most bacterial pneumonias. The upper lobes are commonly involved with considerable necrosis and cavitation, often bilateral and with bulging of the fissure adjacent to the consolidated lung. There may be diagnostic confusion with tuberculosis.

Patients with Klebsiella pneumonia can develop empyema. Treatment is most effective with gentamicin plus cefuroxime but resolution is often slow and substantial residual pulmonary damage is not uncommon.

Pneumocystis carinii pneumonia (PCP)

It is probable that the sporozoan *Pneumocystis carinii* is inhaled in early life and lies dormant in the lung where it can be reactivated following suppression of the immune system. Pneumocystis pneumonia occurs in patients receiving steroids and other immunosuppressive agents, and is particularly common in AIDS. Simultaneous infection with cytomegalovirus occurs. The clinical picture is of fever, a dry cough and progressive breathlessness. On auscultation the lungs often sound remarkably normal. The chest X-ray is often clear when symptoms first develop, but there is progressive bilateral pulmonary infiltration, commencing in the perihilar regions, without effusions (Fig. 14.17). Untreated, all patients become incapacitated by dyspnoea and die of hypoxaemia. In patients with AIDS pneumocystis pneumonia characteristically evolves over several weeks, whereas in other patients at risk, the time course is more rapid. In AIDS, pneumocystis is the most common cause of diffuse pulmonary shadowing; up to 85% of AIDS cases will have at least one episode of pneumocystis. Since pneumocystis pneumonia is so common in this group it is appropriate in some circumstances to initiate empirical therapy. Whenever there is doubt about the correct diagnosis, or if response to treatment for presumed pneumocystis infection is slow, a definite diagnosis is required; for this, bronchoscopy with broncho-alveolar lavage and, if lavage is negative, transbronchial biopsy, have a very high diagnostic yield. The diagnosis can also be achieved by inducing sputum production by nebulising

Fig. 14.17 Pneumocystis pneumonia (PCP). Note that the diffuse hazy consolidation is bilateral and maximal in the mid- and lower zones. Normal vascular markings are lost. There is relative sparing of the costophrenic angles. In patients with HIV and PCP the lung adjacent to the right heart border is frequently the first area to appear abnormal. PCP is not associated with effusions or adenopathy.

hypertonic saline.

When treated early, pneumocystis pneumonia responds well to therapy with high dose co-trimoxazole given for 3 weeks. Trimethoprim and dapsone is an effective combination, whereas pentamidine, although effective, is a more toxic drug. Unfortunately, recurrence is common. Prophylactic co-trimoxazole is effective in patients undergoing therapy for malignant disease, although in patients with AIDS prolonged administration frequently causes side-effects. The inhalation of pentamidine also provides effective prophylaxis. In AIDS patients with severe pneumocystis pneumonia and respiratory failure steroids may improve survival.

Aspergillus pneumonia

Aspergillus fumigatus is a rare cause of pneumonia and patients usually have severe granulocytopenia or are on corticosteroid therapy, and have frequently received broad-spectrum antibiotics. Patients receiving therapy for leukaemia are particularly at risk. The clinical picture is of fever, dyspnoea, pulmonary infiltrates that resemble pulmonary infarction, sometimes with cavitation, and pleural involvement. There is frequently evidence of aspergillus infection at other sites, notably the brain, bones and endocardium. Diagnosis is most reliably achieved by open lung biopsy or transbronchial biopsy. Broncho-alveolar lavage in immunosuppressed patients frequently demonstrates aspergillus, but biopsy material is required to confirm invasive pulmonary infection. Treatment is with

intravenous amphotericin B but mortality is high.

Candida albicans is an unusual cause of pneumonia, occurring in the same high-risk patient group as those who develop aspergillus pneumonia and presenting a similar clinical picture. Blood cultures are more frequently positive. Treatment is with amphotericin B and flucytosine.

Nocardia pneumonia

Nocardia asteroides can rarely cause a chronic suppurative pneumonia in otherwise normal individuals but more commonly it is a cause of an acute pneumonia in the immunocompromised host. In addition to lung involvement, in which there may be a single lesion or extensive consolidation with cavitation, pleural disease, empyema and metastatic spread also occur. The sputum shows Gram-positive hyphae which are acid-fast and grow rapidly on aerobic culture. The treatment of choice is a sulphonamide.

Unusual pneumonias

A number of unusual infections (bacterial, viral, fungal and protozoal) can cause pneumonia and are particularly important in certain parts of the world (Table 14.16). They are described in Chapter 12.

Table 14.16 Unusual causes of pneumonia

Bacterial	**Rickettsial**
Salmonella typhi and *paratyphi* (typhoid)	Typhus
Brucella abortus and *melitensis* (brucellosis)	**Protozoal, yeast and fungal**
Pasteurella pestis (plague)	*Actinomyces israelii* (actinomycosis)
Pasteurella tularensis (tularaemia)	*Coccidioides immitis* (coccidioidomycosis)
Bacillus anthracis (anthrax)	*Histoplasma capsulatum* (histoplasmosis)
Leptospira icterohaemorrhagicae (leptospirosis)	
Viral	
Varicella (chickenpox)	
Herpes zoster	
Epstein-Barr virus (infectious mononucleosis)	

TUBERCULOSIS

Epidemiology

In 19th-century England 1 person in 5 died of *Mycobacterium tuberculosis* infection. The dramatic decline in notifications (Fig. 14.18) and deaths (Fig. 1.6, p. 12) reflects one of the great medical advances of the century. However, tuberculosis remains a common cause of death in the developing world, in which there are approximately 10 000 000 infectious cases. There are well-recognised 'at risk' population groups in the UK and these include the elderly, immigrants from the Indian subcontinent and Far East, those of poor social circumstances, alcoholics, immu-

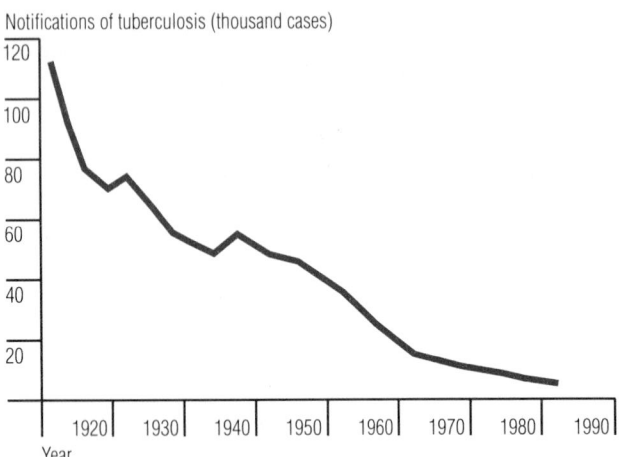

Notifications of tuberculosis (thousand cases)

Fig. 14.18   The decline in tuberculosis in England and Wales.

Primary infection

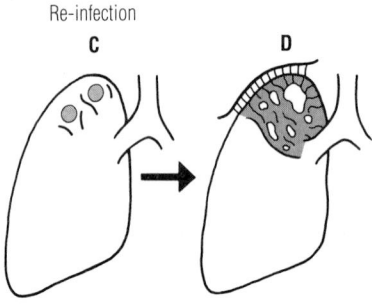

Re-infection

nosuppressed patients and hospital employees. Tuberculosis is a common complication of HIV infection, and as a consequence, the incidence of TB has substantially increased in some areas of the world.

Mycobacterium bovis was once a common cause of human infection but has now been eradicated in developed countries by inoculation of cattle and pasteurisation of milk.

Other 'atypical' or 'anonymous' mycobacteria may occasionally infect man. The organisms are not transmitted between humans (Table 14.17).

Fig. 14.19   Primary and postprimary (re-infection) tuberculosis.   In primary tuberculosis there is pneumonic consolidation (Ghon focus) which is usually subpleural and affects the mid- or lower zones (**A**). Subsequently, infection involves the draining hilar nodes (**B**), which may cause bronchial compression. Re-infection tuberculosis (**C**) is usually apical and progresses to cavitation, fibrosis, volume loss and pleural thickening (**D**).

Table 14.17   Atypical mycobacteria

Group		Example	Clinical feature
I	Photochromogenic	*M. kansasii*	Pulmonary disease
I	Scotochromogenic	*M. scrofulaceum*	Cervical lymphadenitis in children
III	Non-chromogenic	*M. intracellulare*	Pulmonary, lymph node and disseminated disease
		M. avium	Pulmonary disease
		M. xenopi	Pulmonary disease
IV	Rapid growers	*M. fortuitum*	Pulmonary disease

Infectivity, immunology and pathology

The response to a primary infection is shown in Figure 14.19. The usual end result of this is a small subpleural lesion which heals with fibrosis; the glandular lesion also heals, and within about 18 months both may calcify. However, some lesions, especially in children, may erode a blood vessel (Fig. 14.20) and progress to 'miliary' tuberculosis, so named because of the 'millet'-sized lesions on chest X-ray. Alternatively the lung lesion may progress, and cavitate or involve the pleura causing a pleural effusion. Finally the lymph node involvement may progress, especially in Asians and negroes, and occasionally

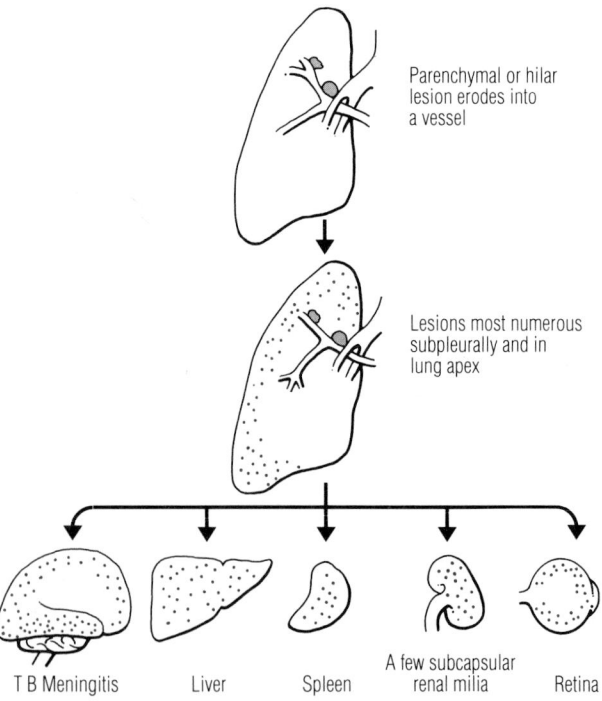

Parenchymal or hilar lesion erodes into a vessel

Lesions most numerous subpleurally and in lung apex

TB Meningitis   Liver   Spleen   A few subcapsular renal milia   Retina

Fig. 14.20   Miliary tuberculosis.   In miliary tuberculosis multiple organs are involved. The diagnosis is most commonly suggested by the chest X-ray. Meningitis is relatively common.

compress, obstruct or erode a bronchus, particularly that of the right middle lobe. Of those that heal, some develop postprimary tuberculosis (Fig. 14.19), sometimes referred to as re-infection adult tuberculosis. Whether the patients become re-infected exogenously or whether their existing lesions become active again is often not clear. Postprimary tuberculosis is usually apical and may have a variety of sequelae, including bronchiectasis and, most seriously, tuberculosis bronchopneumonia.

Clinical features

Some patients are asymptomatic, their disease being noted on routine chest X-ray. Tuberculin testing either with the Mantoux technique or the multiple puncture Heaf or Tine tests is useful in assessing contacts and in children before BCG vaccination. A positive Mantoux should show 5 mm of induration using up to 10 tuberculin units. When performed correctly, a negative tuberculin test almost excludes active tuberculosis infection except in the very ill or in the presence of tuberculin anergy.

Tuberculosis may present insidiously in the elderly.

Investigation

A normal chest X-ray is rare in active pulmonary tuberculosis. Characteristic appearances include:

1. primary tuberculosis with hilar gland enlargement
2. miliary tuberculosis (Fig. 14.21)
3. postprimary (re-infection) tuberculosis with cavitation (Fig. 14.22)
4. tuberculosis bronchopneumonia.

Fluorescent techniques are usually used to screen sputum, and the Ziehl-Neelsen stain to confirm that bacilli are present. Culture of the organism takes 4–8 weeks, and is

Fig. 14.22 Postprimary (re-infection) tuberculosis. The widespread tuberculous consolidation is predominantly involving the upper and mid-zones. The translucent areas in the upper zones are cavities. There is calcification in the right upper zone and the right hemidiaphragm, suggesting that the patient has re-activation of old disease.

important for excluding atypical mycobacteria and determining drug sensitivities. If the patient has no sputum, fibre-optic bronchoscopy with bronchial lavage is a useful diagnostic tool. In adults gastric washings or laryngeal swabs are seldom necessary when bronchoscopy is available. The sedimentation rate is usually raised, and in advanced disease there may be an anaemia with a raised white cell count, occasionally with a lymphocytosis. Liver function tests may be abnormal.

Extrapulmonary tuberculosis can involve most organ systems (Table 14.18).

Table 14.18 Diagnosis of extrapulmonary tuberculosis*

Three early morning urine specimens

Liver biopsy

Lymph node biopsy

Bone marrow aspiration and trephine biopsy

Lumbar puncture

Laparoscopy and biopsy

Joint aspiration

Bone biopsy

Stool specimens in immunosuppressed patients

* All specimens should be cultured.

Fig. 14.21 Miliary tuberculosis. Thousands of small nodules, 'millet-size', all of similar size and distributed throughout the lungs. (This patient was too ill for bronchoscopy and diagnosis was confirmed by bone marrow trephine biopsy.)

Differential diagnosis

In any febrile illness it may be relevant to consider tuberculosis, particularly if there is chest X-ray shadowing or lymph gland enlargement. It must be distinguished from simple pneumonia, and in such cases the usual clinical feature which raises suspicion of tuberculosis is the indolent nature of the illness.

Complications

These may be due to dissemination of the disease, extensive lung damage or non-specific metabolic disturbances. Complications are:

1. *Dissemination (Extrapulmonary tuberculosis).* Tuberculosis may involve lymph nodes, pleura, bones, joints, kidneys, adrenals, liver, peritoneum, bowel, epididymis, meninges and brain.
2. *Extensive lung damage.* This may result in massive haemoptysis, bronchiectasis, breathlessness and eventually respiratory failure with cor pulmonale.
3. *Associated metabolic conditions.* These can include hypokalaemia, hyponatraemia, hypercalcaemia and hypo-albuminaemia.

Treatment

Organisms in the walls of pulmonary cavities, exposed to a high oxygen tension, tend to replicate rapidly, whereas those in caseous areas or within macrophages, in which the pH is low, divide relatively slowly. There are therefore three populations of organisms to be treated:

1. the rapidly dividing extracellular organisms
2. the slowly dividing extracellular organisms
3. the slowly dividing intracellular organisms.

The immediate target for chemotherapy is to kill the large numbers of organisms in the 'rapidly dividing' group and to prevent survival of 'mutant' strains. The slow-growing intracellular and extracellular organisms will be completely eliminated only by a prolonged course of effective drugs, and if there are 'persisters' from these two groups they will cause late relapse of the disease.

Antituberculous drugs and treatment regimes

The four most commonly used drugs in developed countries are listed in Table 14.19. Cure can be achieved by the combination of isoniazid plus streptomycin, but the isoniazid must be continued for 18 months if relapse due to persisters is to be prevented.

With the use of isoniazid and rifampicin, both of which have activity against intracellular organisms, tuberculous lesions should be sterilised much more quickly. Effective chemotherapy of pulmonary tuberculosis is 9 months' isoniazid and rifampicin, with either pyrazinamide or ethambutol given in addition for the first 2 months. Treatment can be shortened to 6 months if, in addition to rifampicin and isoniazid, either streptomycin and pyrazinamide or ethambutol and pyrazinamide are given for the first two months.

In patients with liver disease, standard therapy with rifampicin, isoniazid and pyrazinamide can be given but liver function should be closely monitored. In renal failure treatment of tuberculosis is with rifampicin, isoniazid and pyrazinamide but if ethambutol or streptomycin is used, the dosage should be reduced and drug levels monitored. Dialysis can greatly affect drug clearance. Rifampicin, isoniazid, pyrazinamide and ethambutol are safe in pregnancy but streptomycin should be avoided. Rifampicin reduces the effectiveness of the combined oral contraceptive.

Treatment in special circumstances

There are four major problems that undermine the suc-

Table 14.19 'First-line' drugs for tuberculosis

Drug	Daily dose	Bactericidal (C) or bacteriostatic (S)	Actively multiplying organisms	Slow multiplying organisms Acid pH	Neutral pH	Side-effects
Rifampicin	10 mg/kg usually 450–600 mg	C	Effective	Effective	Effective	Hepatitis, nausea, vomiting, fevers, thrombocytopenia, renal failure (on intermittent therapy), drug interactions (e.g. oestrogens)
Isoniazid (prescribed with pyridoxine 10 mg daily)	Children 6 mg/kg Adults usually 300 mg	C	Effective	Some effect	Effective	Peripheral neuropathy, hepatotoxicity, hypersensitivity reactions
Pyrazinamide	20–30 mg/kg usually 1–2 g	C	Little effect	Effective	Little effect	Hepatotoxicity, hyperuricaemia, arthralgia
Ethambutol	15–25 mg/kg	S	Some effect	Some effect	Little effect	Optic neuritis, rashes

cessful treatment of tuberculosis:

1. drug resistance
2. drug side-effects
3. cost
4. patient non-compliance with treatment.

Drug resistance

Resistance to antituberculous drugs is either primary natural resistance of the organism or due to infection with an organism from an ineffectively treated patient. Resistance to rifampicin and pyrazinamide is rare, but in the Far East and Africa initial resistance to isoniazid or streptomycin, or both, is high. In patients with resistant strains the use of 'second-line' drugs (e.g. streptomycin, capreomycin, cycloserine, prothionamide), particularly in the first 2–4 months of treatment, may be necessary. Four or even five drugs may be required in this initial period and to achieve cure a more prolonged, 18–24-month, regime is necessary.

Drug side-effects

Short-course regimes are relatively non-toxic (Table 14.19) and side-effects are unusual in patients under 35 years.

Cost

Rifampicin is an expensive drug and pyrazinamide is also costly. Cost limits their use in developing countries.

Patient non-compliance with treatment

The treatment of tuberculosis requires disciplined drug-taking, usually on a daily basis, for 6–9 months in most drug regimes. This may be difficult to achieve, particularly in the rural populations of developing countries and in the vagrant populations of the inner cities of Western countries. For this reason supervised twice-weekly regimes, ultra-short courses which accept less than 100% cure, or even supervision in a residential hostel, may have to be considered. Supervision can include direct observations of pill-taking, urine tests for isoniazid and urine inspection for the red discoloration of rifampicin. The advantage of combination tablets of rifampicin and isoniazid is that red urine or a positive urine test for isoniazid confirms that both drugs are being taken.

Treatment of extrapulmonary tuberculosis

Treatment of renal, bone and joint, liver, peritoneum and bowel tuberculosis is in general similar to that of pulmonary tuberculosis. The treatment of tuberculous meningitis deserves special mention, since treatment failure may be lethal. Treatment should include isoniazid, pyrazinamide and rifampicin in conventional doses. A fourth drug is controversial, but streptomycin is considered useful by some physicians. Intrathecal drugs are rarely given. Treatment should be given for 12 months.

The use of corticosteroids in tuberculosis

The administration of corticosteroids, in addition to antituberculous drugs, may sometimes be beneficial. Their use should be considered in the very wasted patient, tuberculous meningitis, intracerebral tuberculomata, as well as pleural and pericardial effusions. Where a patient develops a hypersensitivity to a drug that is essential and irreplaceable in a treatment regime, steroids may allow drug therapy to continue.

Prevention

The dramatic decline in tuberculosis in developed countries is due to several factors. Of great importance is the control of infection from human sources by effective chemotherapy. Isolation of infectious patients (those with smear-positive sputum) for a few days is helpful, although prolonged periods of barrier nursing, disposable cutlery and so on are not essential. Often, the simplest method is to get the patient to wear a face-mask when people come into the room. Contact tracing is crucial and immediate contacts, especially children, should have a tuberculin test and chest X-ray. Host defences are improved by better housing and social conditions and the use of Bacille Calmette Guérin (BCG) vaccination. This vaccine, using an attenuated strain of tubercle bacillus, gives a harmless primary infection and therefore a large measure of immunity. It is given to teenage children in developed countries and to infants elsewhere. However, with the decline in the incidence of the disease, routine use of the BCG in Caucasian children who are not otherwise at risk is questionable.

Chemoprophylaxis with isoniazid is used in children with a positive skin test and a normal chest X-ray.

LUNG ABSCESS

Lung abscess can be defined as an infected, cavitated lesion within the lung parenchyma (Table 14.20). Abscesses can occur as a result of primary infection, or secondary to other conditions. The two factors critical to the pathogenesis of lung abscesses are necrotic tissue and infection. Apart from septic emboli, infection is via the tracheobronchial tree and seeds in an area of necrotic lung tissue. This leads to further breakdown of lung tissue and communication with a bronchus.

The presentation will vary with the cause: patients with acute lung abscesses secondary to bacterial pneumonia (e.g. *Klebsiella*), are acutely unwell, febrile and coughing foul, blood-stained sputum, whereas the presentation of a tuberculous abscess will be much more indolent. The patient's breath and sputum may smell faeculent in the presence of anaerobes. There may be finger clubbing.

14

Table 14.20 Causes of lung abscess

Necrotising infection	Pulmonary infarction
Pyogenic bacteria (*Staphylococcus aureus*, *Klebsiella*, anaerobes, *Pseudomonas aeruginosa*)	Pulmonary thrombo-embolism Pulmonary foreign body embolism (e.g. iv drug abusers) Septic pulmonary embolism
Mycobacteria (*M. tuberculosis* or atypical mycobacteria)	**Cavitation in malignant tumour**
Fungi (*Histoplasma capsulatum*, *Coccidioides immitis*)	Bronchogenic carcinoma (esp. squamous cell)
Parasites (*Entamoeba histolytica*, *Paragonium westermani*)	Metastases Lymphoma
Secondary to bronchial occlusion	**Others**
Bronchial carcinoma or adenoma	Wegener's granulomatosis
Foreign body aspiration	Infected cysts, bullae, sequestrations
Bronchial stenosis	Pneumoconiosis (silica, coal)

Lung abscesses are more common in alcoholics and elderly debilitated patients, who are prone to aspiration, and in intravenous drug abusers. Lung abscess may follow the aspiration of infected material in patients with dental sepsis and sinusitis, and may complicate bronchiectasis.

The chest X-ray initially shows a rounded homogeneous opacity, and only when bronchial drainage is established does an air–fluid level appear (Fig. 14.23). Sputum should be sent for Gram stain, culture and sensitivity and examined for acid-fast bacilli. Fibre-optic bronchoscopy will provide useful information both for bacteriology (especially the isolation of anaerobes) and in identifying neoplasms and foreign bodies.

Patients with staphylococcal or *Klebsiella* pneumonias

Fig. 14.23 Cavitating lung abscess. The abscess is in the lingular segment of the left upper lobe. The patient had a cough productive of large volumes of purulent sputum from the abscess cavity; note the fluid level.

tend to develop abscesses. The commonest radiological appearances with staphylococcus are of multiple, thin-walled, cystic spaces with little fluid. Anaerobic abscesses due to *Entamoeba histolytica* usually involve the liver as well as the lung. The patients may have haemoptysis or cough up 'anchovy paste' or 'chocolate sauce' sputum. Lung abscess is a relatively common sequelae of aspiration pneumonia (p. 474).

The treatment of lung abscess depends on the cause. Foreign bodies and some cavitating tumours can be surgically removed. Bronchoscopic removal of long-embedded foreign bodies is possible, but prophylactic antibiotics, and perhaps steroids, are indicated. When there is no surgically resectable lesion, treatment centres on frequent physiotherapy and appropriate antibiotics, guided by the bacteriology of sputum, blood and bronchial washings, and given for 6 weeks or more. Needle aspiration to obtain samples of pus for microbiology may be helpful. Surgical resection is occasionally necessary.

BRONCHIECTASIS

Bronchiectasis may be defined as chronic dilatation of bronchi, usually associated with deficient local clearance mechanisms. The disease may be localised to a lobe or segment or may be generalised throughout the bronchial tree. Clinically, bronchiectasis presents with intermittent or constant cough and sputum with or without haemoptysis.

Aetiology

Congenital factors

1. *Cystic fibrosis* (p. 484). This multisystem disorder is associated with bronchial obstruction due to inspissated mucus and thus recurrent infection, the consequence of which is bronchiectasis.
2. *Immune deficiency syndromes.* Bronchiectasis is particularly frequent in hypogammaglobulinaemia.
3. *Kartagener's syndrome.* This is the triad of dextrocardia, sinusitis and bronchiectasis. The sinusitis and bronchiectasis are due to disorders of ciliary function. The *Chandra-Khetarpal syndrome* is similar, but with laevocardia and no demonstrable ciliary abnormality.
4. *Pulmonary sequestration.* Bronchiectasis frequently occurs in congenitally sequestrated lung tissue.

Inflammatory factors

A variety of *infective* processes in the lung may produce bronchiectasis. These include infection with necrotising organisms such as *Klebsiella pneumoniae*, staphylococci, *Pseudomonas aeruginosa* and tuberculosis. The damage caused to the bronchial wall by these organisms may lead to dilatation and permanent ciliary damage. Some viral infections, particularly adenovirus and influenza virus, may predispose to bronchiectasis, as may an episode of bronchiolitis or whooping cough in childhood. MacLeod's syndrome is a unilateral emphysema-like condition which follows early childhood infections and may be associated with bronchiectasis.

The other major inflammatory process predisposing to bronchiectasis is *immunological*, the classical example being allergic bronchopulmonary aspergillosis (p. 492). It is likely that antigen/antibody complexes in the bronchial wall fix complement, causing an inflammatory reaction, tissue damage and bronchiectasis, characteristically in proximal large airways.

Bronchial obstruction and retraction

Proximal obstruction of an airway by foreign bodies, tumours, enlarged lymph glands or mucus plugs causes secretions to accumulate distally; these then become infected, causing bronchial wall damage. The result of this process is often an area of bronchiectasis localised to a segment or lobe, which may be amenable to surgical resection.

Retraction of lung tissue can occur with healing of tuberculosis or with extensive pulmonary fibrosis, causing distortion and widening of adjacent bronchi.

Idiopathic

Probably the largest single group of patients are those in whom a cause is never found. They usually have bilateral lower lobe disease.

Clinical features

The usual presentation is with cough and sputum. In the advanced stage of the disease patients may produce up to 40–50 ml of sputum per day, most of it in the morning. Haemoptysis is common, usually as blood-streaking of the sputum. Massive haemoptysis does occur, often in association with a recurrence of infection, and is occasionally fatal. With widespread disease the patient is breathless, with malaise, weight loss and recurrent fevers.

The physical signs depend on the extent and stage of the disease. In the patient with severe, widespread bronchiectasis general health may be poor, finger clubbing is common, there are coarse crackles and wheezes and there may be central cyanosis and cor pulmonale. Complications of bronchiectasis include pneumonia, lung abscess, pleural effusion, empyema, brain abscess and amyloidosis. With effective antibiotic therapy these complications are unusual.

Investigation

The chest X-ray may be normal. However, the more characteristic radiographic changes (Fig. 14.24) include ring, line, and parallel ('tramline') shadows – the appearances of thickened bronchial walls seen end on or laterally. CT scanning is a sensitive technique for demonstrating

Fig. 14.24 Extensive saccular bronchiectasis. There are ring shadows in the left lower zone (due to thickened bronchi viewed end on), and behind the heart can be seen grossly dilated bronchi, filled with fluid.

Fig. 14.25 Bronchiectasis: CT scan. There is extensive disease, with bronchial wall thickening and airway dilatation, easily seen in the left lower lobe (arrow).

dilated bronchi (Fig. 14.25). For the detection of minor changes the best technique is bronchography, which also demonstrates the precise anatomical distribution (Fig. 14.26). If the disease is largely peripheral it usually has a cystic appearance, whereas when the major bronchi are affected the bronchi take on a fusiform or saccular appearance. Bronchography is only indicated for the diag-

Fig. 14.26 Cystic bronchiectasis. Bronchogram demonstrating severe cystic bronchiectasis of the lingula.

nosis of minor disease not demonstrated by other techniques, or when surgery is being considered.

The most common infecting organism is *Haemophilus influenzae*, but pneumococcus is also a frequent pathogen. Colonisation with *Pseudomonas aeruginosa* is not uncommon.

Lung function tests reflect the extent and severity of disease. As the condition worsens a mixed obstructive/restrictive defect develops, with variable response to bronchodilators. Younger bronchiectatic patients require a sweat test to exclude cystic fibrosis and all patients should have a routine estimation of their serum immunoglobulins. When clinically appropriate, neutrophil function should be investigated. A blood eosinophilia is common in allergic bronchopulmonary aspergillus. Ciliary function may require investigation, including a nasal mucosal biopsy with motility studies.

Treatment

The long-term treatment of bronchiectasis includes regular, effective physiotherapy. The patients and their relatives are taught postural drainage. In the majority of patients continuous long-term antibiotics are not appropriate and predispose to colonisation with *Pseudomonas aeruginosa*. Prompt treatment of intercurrent and symptomatic infection with appropriate antibiotics is essential. Regular inhaled antibiotics may be helpful, especially in patients with cystic fibrosis.

Inhaled β agonists are useful in those patients with airways obstruction. Oral steroids are required in bron-

chopulmonary aspergillosis and can be helpful in some other bronchiectatic patients in whom bronchial damage is immunologically mediated. In severe cases patients eventually develop cor pulmonale and require diuretic and domiciliary oxygen therapy. A small number of patients with cystic fibrosis have been successfully treated by heart-lung transplantation.

Surgical resection for bronchiectasis is indicated in only a small number of cases, usually for localised disease caused by previous bronchial occlusion or lobar pneumonia. It may also be necessary to resect bronchiectatic lung for massive haemoptysis. Haemoptysis can sometimes be successfully treated by embolisation of a branch of the bronchial artery with foam.

With the exception of patients with generalised disorders, such as cystic fibrosis or immune deficiency, the long-term outlook for the majority of patients with bronchiectasis is good.

CYSTIC FIBROSIS

Cystic fibrosis (formerly called mucoviscidosis or fibrocystic disease of the pancreas) is the most common potentially lethal genetic disease in Caucasians. It is an autosomal recessive gene which is carried by 1 in 20 of the Caucasian population and its incidence is about 1 in 2000 live births. The incidence amongst Caucasians varies a little from country to country, but it is rare in Asians and negroes.

Mucus in cystic fibrosis patients is no more viscid than in chronic bronchitis; however, mucus-secreting glands throughout the body show morphological changes, and the ducts of mucus glands are obstructed. Pathological changes are seen in the lung, pancreas, bowel, liver and genital tract. The genetic defect is on chromosome 7 and is related to a regulation protein which controls ion and water flux across cell membranes, causing high sodium and chloride levels in the sweat ducts, a high transepithelial potential difference in the respiratory tract and elevated chloride and low water content in pancreatic secretions. The epithelial cells of the respiratory tract and sweat ducts are relatively impermeable to chloride ions with a secondary increase in sodium transport; chloride transport in other cells, such as erythrocytes, is normal. The ion transport abnormality leads to impaired local defence mechanisms in the respiratory tract and abnormal pancreatic secretions. The defect in the lung causes bacterial colonisation, damage to the bronchial wall and bronchiectasis. The defective pancreatic secretions cause a malabsorption syndrome and blockage of the ducts with autodigestion of the pancreas results in diabetes mellitus in 10–20% of adult patients (p. 750).

Clinical features and diagnosis

The clinical presentation differs between neonates, and older children and young adults (Table 14.21). Clinical

Table 14.21 Clinical consequences of cystic fibrosis

Neonates	Older children and young adults
Meconium ileus	Bronchiectasis
Rectal prolapse	Malabsorption
Failure to thrive	Meconium ileus equivalent
Recurrent bronchopulmonary	Infertility
infections	Cirrhosis and portal hypertension

examination of adolescents and adults usually shows finger clubbing secondary to chronic respiratory infection, retarded growth and development and a hyperinflated chest with coarse crackles and wheezes. Gynaecomastia is occasionally seen and there may be hepatosplenomegaly and other signs of chronic liver disease.

The chest X-ray (Fig. 14.27) shows hyperinflated lungs with parallel line and ring shadows, and with multiple nodular opacities, mainly in the mid- and upper zones. Lung function testing shows a progressive obstructive defect. The single most important diagnostic test is the sweat sodium which is consistently greater than 70 mmol/l in children with the disease and greater than 90 mmol/l in affected adults, although the results in adults are less reliable. Sputum bacteriology will often yield *Staphylococcus aureus*, and later in life *Pseudomonas aeruginosa* becomes a major problem. Haemophilus may be an

important pathogen and patients occasionally develop tuberculosis.

Prenatal diagnosis can be achieved by the measurement of elevated levels of enzymes such as alkaline phosphatase in the amniotic fluid or by DNA analysis of chorionic villus biopsies; these techniques are only of value for 'at risk' pregnancies. Neonatal screening for immunoreactive trypsin in the blood is simple and inexpensive.

The differential diagnosis includes hypogammaglobulinaemia, immobile cilia syndromes, asthma, coeliac disease and Shwackman's syndrome (pancreatic insufficiency, neutropenia, metaphyseal chondrodysplasia, growth retardation and frequent infections).

Treatment

The corner-stone of treatment of respiratory disease is regular chest physiotherapy, particularly postural drainage. In the first year of life prophylactic antistaphylococcal drugs may be helpful. Severe infective exacerbations require intravenous antibiotics, usually antipseudomonal agents (e.g. gentamicin, ceftazidime, piperacillin). Bronchodilators and occasionally oral corticosteroids may be useful in patients with airflow obstruction. Pneumothoraces are not uncommon and should be treated conservatively whenever possible. Malabsorption is treated by oral pancreatic enzymes supplements. Abdominal emergencies occur, including adult meconium ileus equivalent, intussusception, acute pancreatitis and bleeding from oesophageal varices. Diabetes is common. Adult patients will need counselling about fertility since 98% of the males are infertile (due to maldevelopment of the vas deferens) and for females pregnancy can be hazardous. Patients and their family need constant moral, psychological and practical support. Genetic counselling of the parents of children with cystic fibrosis and of the patients themselves is essential.

ASTHMA

Understanding of the pathogenesis of asthma has increased over the past two decades and consequent improvements in therapy have reduced the morbidity from this common condition.

Definition

The American Thoracic Society defines asthma as 'a disease characterized by increased responsiveness of the bronchi to various stimuli, manifested by widespread narrowing of the airways that changes in severity either spontaneously or as a result of treatment'. Asthmatics may be said to have 'hyperactive' or 'twitchy' airways, and it is an essential feature of the resulting bronchoconstriction that it is usually reversible with administration of inhaled bronchodilators. Most asthmatics can be classified as either *'extrinsic'* or *'intrinsic'* (Table 14.22). There are a number

Fig. 14.27 Cystic fibrosis. Diffuse changes of bronchiectasis typical of severe disease. There are multiple ring and line shadows from thickened bronchial walls viewed end on or tangentially. The hila are prominent and the lungs are of large volume.

14

Table 14.22   The classification of extrinsic and intrinsic asthma

Extrinsic	Intrinsic
History of allergy (e.g. hay fever, eczema)	No allergic history
Skin tests positive	Skin tests negative
Early onset	Late onset
Family history of atopy	Family history of asthma only
Intermittent attacks, often seasonal	Persisting asthma, perennial
Elevated IgE	Normal IgE
Marked blood and sputum eosinophilia	Variable eosinophilia
Not aspirin-sensitive, occasional polyps	Aspirin-sensitive, nasal polyps
Good response to beta agonists	Variable response to beta agonists
Good response to disodium cromoglycate	Poor response to disodium cromoglycate

of non-specific trigger factors that can start an attack (Table 14.23).

Some late-onset asthmatics who have smoked may also have chronic bronchitis and are therefore difficult to classify, falling into the untidy category of '*asthmatic bronchitis*'.

Asthma caused by sensitising chemicals and industrial agents is increasingly recognised (Table 14.24).

Table 14.23   Non-specific 'trigger' factors in asthma

Upper respiratory tract infection

Exercise

Cold air

Laughter

Irritants: smoke, paint or chemical fumes

Drugs, e.g. beta-blockers

Industrial causes

Table 14.24   Sensitising chemicals and industrial agents as a cause of asthma

Material	Industry
Toluene di-isocyonate (TDI)	Polyurethane industry
Soldering flux	Electrical, engineering industry
Cotton dust (byssinosis)	Textiles
Urine, serum, danders of animals	Veterinary, agricultural and laboratory workers
Flour, grain	Bakers, millers
Wood dust	Carpenters
Sulphur dioxide, ozone, chloride	Chemical industry

Epidemiology

Asthma is common, affecting up to 5% of children and 2% of adults in the UK. The peak age of onset is under 5 years, and in this age group it is more common in boys by a ratio of 3 to 2; above 5 years there is an equal sex ratio. There is an allergic component in one-third to one-half of all cases. About 2000 patients die from asthma in the UK each year, and it is likely that many of these deaths are preventable.

Pathogenesis

Bronchial 'hyper-reactivity' appears to be the key to the asthmatic reaction. It is the unique property of asthmatic airways to react, by bronchoconstriction, inflammation and mucus production, to stimuli that would not elicit this reaction in normal airways. Possible mechanisms for bronchial hyper-reactivity are listed in Table 14.25.

Table 14.25   Mechanisms of bronchial hyper-reactivity

Inflammation, immunological liberation of bronchoconstrictor mediators

Alterations in autonomic nervous control

Abnormalities of Ca^{2+} flux

Damage to epithelial 'tight junction'

There can be little doubt that immunological mechanisms (Ch. 7) play an important part in the asthmatic reaction. Both immediate and delayed responses are involved and these can be demonstrated by the technique of bronchial provocation challenge testing. This is a method of provoking an asthmatic reaction in susceptible subjects by inhalation of antigens or chemicals. The immediate hypersensitivity reaction is mediated by degranulation of mast cells (Fig. 14.28). The mast cell degranulation is produced by the union of antigen with IgE antibody which is bound to the mast cell surface. Degranulation liberates a variety of substances including preformed mediators and newly formed metabolites of

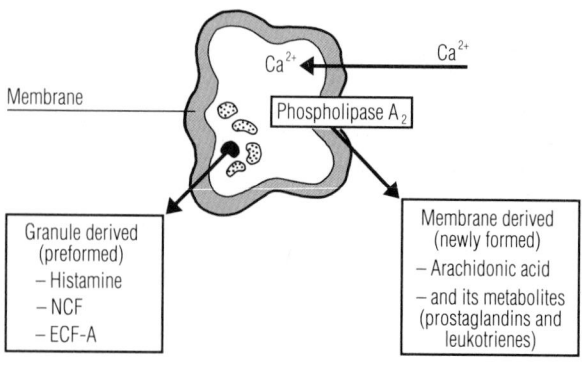

Fig. 14.28   Mast cell mediators. The release of preformed and newly formed mediators from mast cells involves calcium flux across the cell membrane, and in the case of the newly formed mediators, phospholipase A_2 activation.

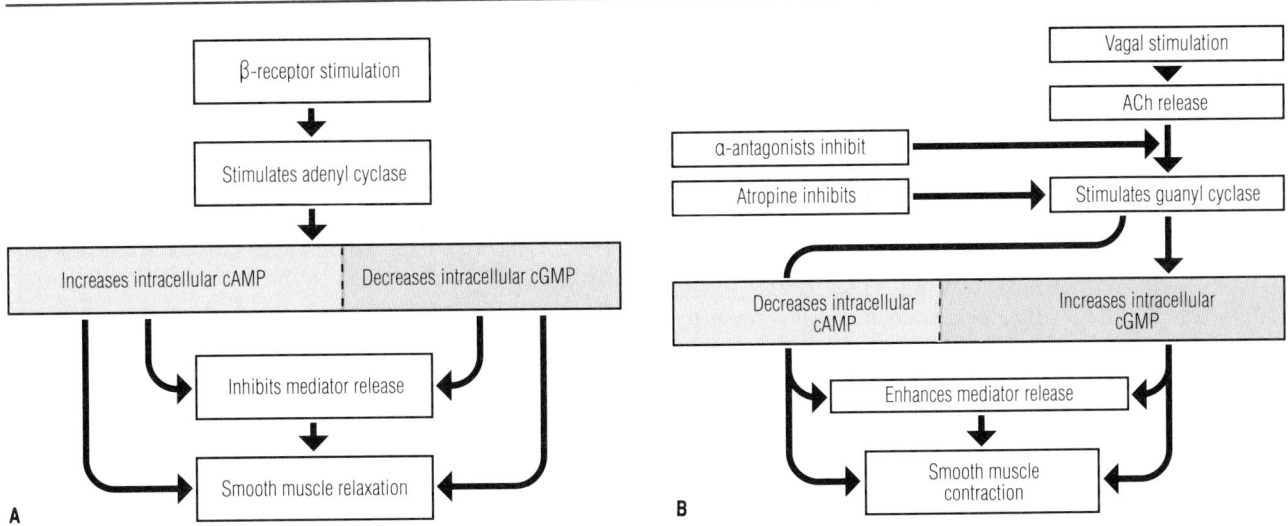

Fig. 14.29 The control of airway calibre. The balance of bronchodilatation from sympathomimetic β-receptor stimulation (**A**), and bronchoconstriction from parasympathetic vagal activity (**B**), is an important determinant of airway calibre.

arachidonic acid from the cell membrane (prostaglandins, leukotrienes, etc. – see below.

The preformed mediators, histamine in particular, have long been known to have a bronchoconstrictor action. Eosinophil chemotactic factor of anaphylaxis (ECF-A) may play an important part in the inflammatory component of the asthmatic reaction. Much interest has been centred recently on the newly formed, membrane-derived mediators which are the metabolites of arachidonic acid. This fatty acid is metabolised via two pathways: the cyclo-oxygenase pathway and the lipoxygenase pathway. Metabolism via cyclo-oxygenase generates prostaglandins and thromboxanes. Their effects on the airway vary: prostaglandin F_2 is a powerful bronchoconstrictor whereas prostaglandin E_2 is a bronchodilator. The metabolites of the lipoxygenase pathway are known as 'leukotrienes'. Leukotriene B_4 has potent chemotactic properties and may play a part in airways inflammation in asthma. Leukotrienes C_4, D_4 and E_4 are now known collectively to be what was originally called 'slow reacting substance of anaphylaxis (SRS-A)': they are amongst the most powerful naturally occurring bronchoconstrictors and there is considerable speculation about their role in clinical asthma. Non-mast-cell-derived mediators such as platelet activating factor (PAF) may also play a part in causing airways inflammation and narrowing; inhaled PAF has been shown to induce prolonged airway hyper-reactivity in man which may be of importance in asthma.

Bronchial smooth muscle and secretions are regulated by neural mechanisms (Fig. 14.29). The balance of autonomic nervous control is important. The cholinergic vagal impulses have bronchoconstrictor and secretory actions. These effects are opposed by β_2 adrenergic receptors which are bronchodilator and antisecretory. The β adrenergic mechanism is supported by circulating catecholamines. In patients with asthma, vagal reflexes may play an important part in bronchial hyper-reactivity, particularly to stimuli such as cold air and exercise.

Other mechanisms may play a part in bronchial hyper-reactivity. Calcium flux across cell membranes is important for smooth muscle contraction and for mast cell degranulation, and agents which block this flux may prove to be useful in treatment. Finally, there is some evidence that the 'tight junction' between epithelial cells on the surface of the bronchial epithelium may be abnormally 'leaky', allowing antigen readier access to the mast cells underneath.

It is therefore clear that no single mediator or mechanism is responsible for the asthmatic reaction, and research continues to elucidate this highly complex process.

Pathology and pathophysiology

The pathogenic mechanisms involved in asthma result in the histological changes shown in Figure 14.30. These changes can be acute or chronic. The sputum of asthmatics is often yellow and tenacious and contains many eosinophils, epithelial cells and bronchiolar casts ('plugs'). At post-mortem in patients who die of acute asthma, many plugs are found in large and small airways.

Fig. 14.30 The pathology of asthma. Intense inflammation, with oedema and intralumenal mucous plugs, is the striking pathology of asthma.

Clinical features

Asthma is episodic. Between attacks, patients, especially younger ones, may be asymptomatic and have no abnormal physical signs. The common symptoms of an asthma attack are cough, wheeze and breathlessness. Cough may be the only symptom, especially in children. Almost all asthmatics are worse at night and most will feel 'tight' in the morning. The fall in peak flow rate in the early hours of the morning is referred to as 'morning dipping' (Fig. 14.31). Acute asthma and sudden asthma deaths occur most frequently in the early hours of the morning. There is a personal or family history of allergy (rhinitis, conjunctivitis, eczema or urticaria) in up to 50% of patients.

In chronic asthma, particularly that which has persisted from childhood, there may be chest wall deformity. When asthma is severe the patient is distressed and vigorously contracting the accessory muscles of respiration. When the condition progresses despite active treatment, the patient is then said to have 'acute severe asthma' (p. 490).

A number of clinical conditions are associated with asthma (Table 14.26). *Allergic bronchopulmonary aspergillosis* occurs mainly in temperate climates. It is due to hypersensitivity to the ubiquitous fungus *Aspergillus fumi-*

Peak expiratory flow rate (l/min)

Days

Fig. 14.31 Peak expiratory flow rate (PEFR) in asthma. The measurement of peak flow is essential for the management of asthma. PEFR is variable in asthmatics; it is lower in the early hours of the morning and on wakening ('morning dipping') and increases with β_2 agonists (e.g. salbutamol). The chart is typical of a patient recovering from an episode of moderately severe asthma.

Table 14.26 Clinical syndromes associated with asthma

Eosinophilic syndromes
  Allergic bronchopulmonary aspergillosis
  Idiopathic pulmonary eosinophilia
  Tropical eosinophilia
  Churg-Strauss syndrome

Aspirin sensitivity and nasal polyposis

Pericarditis

Carcinoid syndrome

gatus. The presenting features, usually in a patient with pre-existing asthma, include intermittent cough productive of green rubbery 'plugs' in the sputum, fever, chest X-ray shadows, blood and sputum eosinophilia, a positive aspergillus skin test, and serum precipitins for *Aspergillus fumigatus.* Other pulmonary eosinophilic syndromes include idiopathic pulmonary eosinophilia and tropical eosinophilia. In some patients with late-onset asthma and nasal polyps, aspirin can induce bronchoconstriction, perhaps through a mechanism involving the arachadonic acid metabolic pathway. Asthma is a feature of the Churg-Strauss syndrome and, rarely, of polyarteritis nodosa.

Investigation

X-ray findings

Most asthmatics have normal or hyperinflated lungs on chest X-ray. Mucus plugs can cause focal or segmental atelectasis, and sometimes collapse of a lobe or lung. Transient infiltrates are seen in association with eosinophilia. Spontaneous pneumothorax can complicate asthma in the acute phase.

Other investigations

Blood eosinophilia is common; it is usually greater in atopic asthma. Skin prick tests to common allergens may occasionally reveal an unsuspected source of allergy.

Lung function tests may be normal between attacks. During episodes of asthma the peak expiratory flow rate (PEFR), FEV_1 and FEV_1/VC ratio will be reduced and airways resistance increased.

In addition to airflow obstruction the patient with acute or chronic asthma will have laboratory evidence of *hyperinflation* with increased total lung capacity, residual volume, and ratio of residual volume to total lung capacity. The *transfer factor* (diffusing capacity) for carbon monoxide is normal or increased in uncomplicated asthma. Hypoxaemia is common.

Diagnosis and management

The four principles of diagnosis and management of asthma are:

1. recognition
2. supervision
3. education
4. treatment.

Recognition of asthma is not always straightforward. It is often not recognised in children who present with episodes of cough, wheeze and dyspnoea. Such 'wheezy bronchitis' in childhood is almost always asthma. The differential diagnosis of chronic asthma includes: 'asthmatic' bronchitis, left heart failure, centrally obstructing tumour or foreign body and recurrent pulmonary emboli. It may be difficult or impossible to distinguish late-onset asthma from chronic obstructive bronchitis in the elderly smoker. Many of them respond well to bronchodilators and have a better prognosis than patients with fixed airways obstruction.

Supervision of chronic asthma is as important as in any serious chronic condition. Some hospitals run a very effective 'open door' policy for asthmatics, allowing them to obtain immediate specialist advice whenever their asthma is severe.

Education about the nature of the disease, the use of drugs and delivery systems, the avoidance of allergens and the recognition of deteriorating asthma are all important. Asthma can seldom be 'cured'. Long-term therapy is usually required, for prophylaxis or control, and it is critically important that this simple truth is appreciated by both the patient and the physician.

Treatment

Treatment regimes (Table 14.27) can be broadly classified as *long-term prophylactic treatment* and *treatment of exacerbations and acute severe asthma*.

Hyposensitisation therapy (desensitisation immunotherapy) is discouraged in the UK but widely practised throughout the world despite little evidence of efficacy.

Table 14.27 Treatment of asthma

Proven benefit	Dubious benefit	Potential benefit
Sympathomimetics	Antihistamines	Calcium antagonists
Theophylline, aminophylline	Expectorants	Prostaglandin analogues/antagonists
Anticholinergics	Cough suppressants	Leukotriene antagonists
Disodium cromoglycate	Mucolytics	
Corticosteroids	Hyposensitisation	

Drugs of proven benefit

Sympathomimetics

Beta agonists exert their action by stimulating the enzyme adenyl cyclase which catalyses the formation of cyclic-AMP within the bronchial smooth muscle cell. The original beta stimulants, adrenaline, noradrenaline and isoprenaline, have almost equal effects on the cardiac β_1 receptors as on the β_2 receptors in the bronchi. Structural alterations in the β agonist molecule have produced much more β_2-specific drugs. All available β_2 agonists can be given by inhalation, which is the preferred route, and some by oral, iv and subcutaneous administration. Salbutamol and terbutaline are the two most commonly prescribed. Salbutamol is available in a metered dose inhaler ($100\,\mu g$ per dose), as a dry powder for inhalation ('Rotacap') for patients whose co-ordination is poor or for children, and as tablets, slow-release tablets, iv injection, a nebuliser solution and a syrup. Terbutaline is available in similar forms. Inhaler spacer devices can improve drug inhalation efficiency in patients unable to manage a conventional

inhaler. With both drugs muscle tremor and tachycardia commonly occur, but tend to settle with prolonged usage.

Methyl xanthine derivatives (aminophylline and theophylline)

Oral use is preferred in routine treatment and intravenous use for acute asthma; theophylline and its compounds are not effective by the inhaled route.

When used in a daily dose of 10 mg/kg body weight, divided doses of slow-release theophyllines are effective and safe bronchodilators. These sustained release formulations are particularly useful when given at night for the prevention of nocturnal asthma and 'morning tightness'. Ideally, blood levels of the drug should be measured, aiming to achieve a therapeutic serum concentration of 10–20 mg/l. If excessive doses are given, or occasionally even when blood levels are in the therapeutic range, side-effects may occur. These include nausea, abdominal pain, headache, tremor, insomnia and palpitations, convulsions and cardiac arrhythmia. The dose administered should be reduced in elderly patients, those with liver disease, and those taking other drugs that increase theophylline blood levels (e.g. erythromycin).

Anticholinergics

Anticholinergic agents have proved to be of some value, particularly in older patients with late-onset asthma or 'asthmatic bronchitis'. Atropine can be delivered by inhalation in its methonitrate form from a nebuliser, although it is more convenient to administer the newer anticholinergic, ipratropium bromide, as a metered-dose aerosol. For patients optimally treated with inhaled β_2 agonists the additional benefit of anticholinergic drugs is seldom important.

Disodium cromoglycate

It has been suggested (but it is by no means certain) that cromoglycate acts by 'stabilising' the mast cell and preventing mediator release. It is only effective when used on a regular prophylactic basis and it has no intrinsic bronchodilator activity. Younger extrinsic asthmatics tend to benefit most from its regular use and it can also be used to 'block' exercise-induced asthma when administered about 20 minutes before planned exertion. It is administered in the form of 'spincaps' which deliver a dry powder for inhalation, and a metered-dose inhaler is also available. Useful nasal and ophthalmic preparations are available for the treatment of hay fever. The drug has no serious side-effects.

Corticosteroids

Corticosteroids, probably by their anti-inflammatory action, are the most powerful drugs available for the treatment of asthma. Attitudes towards, and use of, corticocosteroids for the long-term management of asthma have been dramatically changed by the introduction of powerful, topically active fluorinated corticosteroids for use by the inhaled route. Beclomethasone diproprionate and budesonide are most often prescribed. They enable asthmatics to be treated with low-dose inhaled corticosteroids, which are not absorbed in sufficient quantities to cause adrenal suppression or iatrogenic Cushing's syndrome, and are highly effective when used on a regular basis in the prophylaxis of asthma. In some patients inhaled steroids predispose to oral candida infection but this can usually be easily controlled.

If long-term oral corticosteroids are essential for the control of asthma, patients should also be on maximum doses of inhaled steroids, thereby permitting the oral prednisolone dosage to be reduced by as much as 10 mg daily.

Nebuliser therapy

Nebulisers can deliver large doses of β_2 agonists and anticholinergic drugs. They are increasingly used at home by patients with chronic airflow obstruction, but, in view of the large doses of drug used (particularly β agonists), such treatment requires careful assessment and supervision. It is important to document that nebulised bronchodilators confer a genuine advantage over *maximal* treatment with metered dose inhalers.

Summary of routine treatment of asthma

Figure 14.32 illustrates the treatment strategy for asthma. Drugs are added to therapy, not substituted. Oral steroids are prescribed only when maximum therapy with all other drugs fails to control the disease.

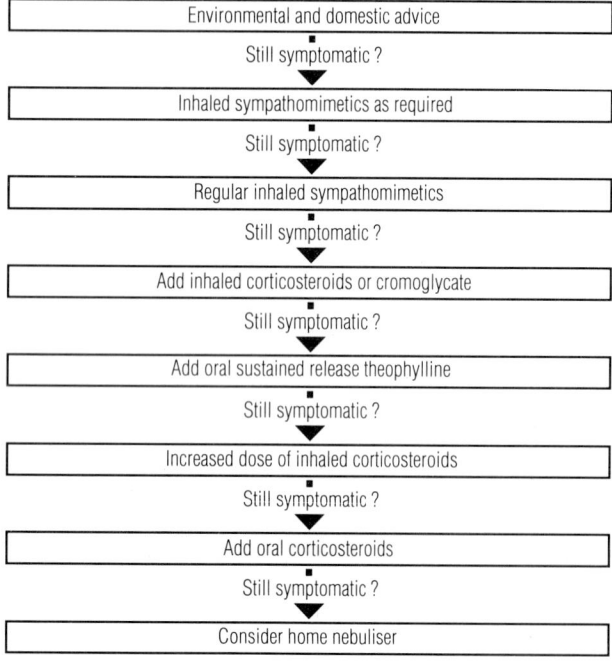

Fig. 14.32 Treatment strategy in asthma. Note the central importance of inhaled steroids in the treatment of moderate or severe asthma. Treatments are usually added, not substituted, as disease severity increases.

Treatment of acute severe asthma

Acute severe asthma is diagnosed when a patient has had severe progressive asthmatic symptoms over a number of hours or days, despite apparently adequate treatment with inhaled sympathomimetics. The patient with acute severe asthma is distressed, dyspnoeic and using accessory respiratory muscles; there are widespread inspiratory and expiratory wheezes and the chest is hyperinflated. When airways obstruction and bronchial plugging is severe and widespread, the flow of air through bronchi is greatly decreased, and wheezing becomes less obvious, eventually resulting in the ominous 'silent chest' of advanced acute severe asthma. As the condition progresses cyanosis, dehydration, exhaustion and ventilatory failure ensue. Indices of the severity of acute asthma are listed in Table 14.28. The patient's condition is best assessed by the repeated measurement of these indices. In the accident and emergency department PEFR, heart rate and pulsus paradoxus should be documented with particular care, and without these measurements the severity of asthma will not be appreciated (Fig. 14.33). Arterial blood gas tensions should be measured in all patients whose asthma is sufficiently severe to require hospital assessment.

Acute asthma requires immediate evaluation and treatment. Oxygen is necessary, and in almost all circumstances can be liberally administered without fear of CO_2 narcosis. Salbutamol solution in a dose of 2.5–5.0 mg can be given via a nebuliser and is usually very effective. This can be repeated 3–6-hourly as required. Alternatively (or in very severe episodes, in addition), aminophylline is given in a dose of 5 mg/kg body weight intravenously over 20 minutes, to be followed by an infusion of 0.5 mg/kg per hr. In patients already taking theophyllines an infusion of aminophylline (0.5 mg/kg per hr) can be started and the blood theophylline level checked. The dose of aminophylline is reduced if the patient is more than 55 years old, or if there is evidence of liver disease or cardiac failure. A theophylline blood level should be measured 18 hours after starting the infusion and the dose adjusted to remain within the therapeutic range of 10–20 mg/l. If there are problems with venous access, subcutaneous terbutaline (0.25–0.5 mg) is helpful.

Systemic corticosteroids must be given to all patients

Table 14.28 Indications of severe asthma

Low PEFR (< 150 l/min, poor bronchodilator response)

Associated with (one or more of)
  Disturbances of consciousness
  Central cyanosis
  Vigorous accessory muscle activity
  Heart rate greater than 130
  Pulsus paradoxus
  Arterial P_{O_2} less than 8 kPa (60 mmHg)
  Arterial P_{CO_2} greater than 5.5 kPa (41 mmHg)
  Gross over-inflation (X-ray)
  ECG abnormalities
  Pneumothorax/pneumomediastinum

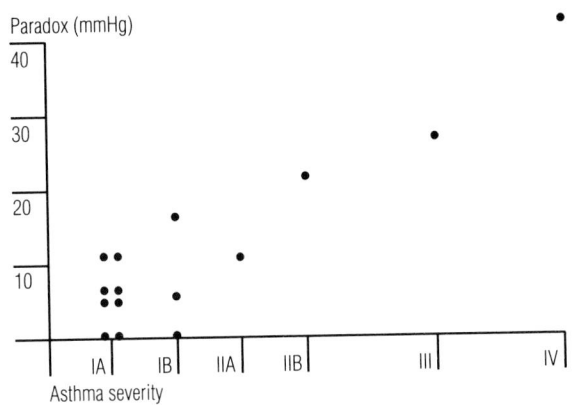

Paradox (mmHg)

Fig. 14.33 Pulsus paradoxus and asthma severity. Asthma can be clinically graded:

IA   Some difficulty with everyday tasks. Sleep sometimes disturbed
IB   Great difficulty with everyday tasks. Sleep often disturbed
IIA   Patient largely confined to chair, but mobile with moderate difficulty. Disturbed sleep, with little improvement with inhaled β_2 agonist
IIB   Patient only able to mobilise with extreme difficulty. Unable to sleep. Pulse greater than 120 per minute
III   Patient confined to chair or bed. Unable to sleep. Inhaler ineffective. Pulse greater than 120 per minute
IV   Patient totally immobilised and approaching exhaustion.

The clinical severity of asthma is closely reflected by pulsus paradoxus, heart rate and peak expiratory flow rate (PEFR). (Modified from Sherwood Jones 1971 The intensive therapy of asthma. Proc. R. Soc. Med. 64: 1151, and Knowles G K and Clark T J H 1975 Pulsus paradoxus as a valuable sign indicating severity of asthma. Lancet ii: 1356–9.

whose asthma is of sufficient severity to warrant hospital admission, and also many less severe cases satisfactorily controlled in the emergency department. It is probably immaterial how corticosteroids are given; it may be as an iv bolus of hydrocortisone 3–6 mg/kg body weight followed by an infusion of 3–6 mg/kg 6-hourly, or alternatively 60 mg of oral prednisolone for the average-sized adult.

Supportive measures are also important. Patients with acute asthma become dehydrated. Physiotherapy is not helpful. Reassurance helps, but the best reassurance is improvement of the asthma. Sedatives should *never* be used unless intubation and mechanical ventilation are being contemplated. Antibiotics are prescribed if there is evidence of bacterial infection.

Some patients fail to respond to treatment and become progressively more hypoxic. At the onset of an asthma attack patients hyperventilate and therefore have an acute respiratory alkalosis. As airways obstruction increases, exhaustion supervenes, ventilatory pump failure occurs, alveolar ventilation diminishes, CO_2 rises and pH falls, leading to an acute respiratory acidosis. At this point the patient requires intubation and mechanical ventilation.

Small tidal volumes should be used, and most asthmatics who need mechanical ventilation will need at least 48 hours on the ventilator to allow their asthma to respond to therapy. Bronchodilator and steroid therapy should be continued while the patient is being ventilated.

Prognosis

About 50% of children 'grow out of' their asthma in early adult life. Late-onset asthma is almost always chronic, tends to be more severe, and usually needs more aggressive treatment. About 30% of asthma deaths occur within 2 hours of the onset of the acute attack and these may be difficult to prevent. However, many of the remaining 70% of the 2000 deaths that occur in the UK should be preventable, by appropriate long-term therapy and the early recognition of deteriorating asthma.

ALLERGIC RHINITIS

Allergic rhinitis (commonly known as 'hay fever', although it is not related to hay and there is no fever) is a condition characterised by rhinorrhoea, nasal obstruction, sneezing, conjunctivitis, lacrimation, and nasal and pharyngeal itching. It is usually seasonal, with tree pollens being the allergen in the spring months and grass pollen in the summer. This causes considerable problems for young people who may be taking important examinations at those times of year. A perennial form occurs in those patients sensitive to allergens such as house dust, which are in the air all year round. Food allergy is an often quoted but clinically rare cause of rhinitis.

Pathologically the mucosa of the nose is oedematous and inflamed, and the secretions are rich in eosinophils. Nasal polyps and sinus infection may be present, especially in the perennial type. The conjunctivae are congested and oedematous. The diagnosis is made by taking a careful history. Skin prick testing for a battery of common allergens is helpful. Serum IgE is usually elevated, and occasionally a radio-allergo-immunosorbent test will help to define the allergen. The major differential diagnosis is from vasomotor rhinitis, which is a similar syndrome but with no documented allergic basis. Other conditions which may present in a similar fashion include exposure to irritants and repeated upper respiratory tract infections.

Treatment

Although the symptoms of allergic rhinitis tend to get better as the subjects get older, they can, when active, be severe. Most of the relevant allergens are ubiquitous and therefore unavoidable. The first line of treatment is topical; nasal sprays or drops containing corticosteroids such as beclomethasone or budesonide, or disodium cromoglycate, are useful when used on a regular basis. Disodium cromoglycate eye drops are also helpful for the conjunctivitis. These drugs can be supplemented by a non-sedating antihistamine by mouth, such as terfenadine or astemizole. The place of hyposensitisation is debatable, and is usually reserved for isolated grass pollen allergy. Occasionally a small dose of oral corticosteroids, e.g. prednisolone (10–15 mg/day), or 1 or 2 injections of a depot corticosteroid during the season may be necessary.

PULMONARY EOSINOPHILIA

Pulmonary eosinophilia may be defined as transient pulmonary infiltrates associated with an elevated blood eosinophil count. A cause can only be identified in some cases (Table 14.29). The blood eosinophil count is elevated above its normal upper level of $400/mm^3$ and may in some circumstances be as high as $50\,000/mm^3$. The serum IgE level is usually elevated in those conditions with an identifiable cause, especially in the allergic mycoses. Asthma is almost always present in cases of allergic bronchopulmonary aspergillosis, occurs in about half the patients with cryptogenic pulmonary eosinophilia, and is unusual with helminth infections apart from filariasis.

Table 14.29 Classification of pulmonary eosinophilia

Known causes	Helminthic infections
Fungal allergy	*Ascaris lumbricoides*
Aspergillus fumigatus	(Loeffler's syndrome)
Candida albicans	*Strongyloides*
Stemphylium canugenosum	*Filaria* ('tropical pulmonary
Dresclera lawaiiensis	eosinophilia')
Curvularia lunata	*Ankylostoma*
Helminosporium	
Drugs and toxins	
Sulphonamides (including sulpha-	
salazine)	
Nitrofurantoin	
Sodium aminosalicylate	
Penicillin	
Tetracycline	
Chlorpropamide	
'Spanish toxic oil' syndrome	

Unknown causes
Cryptogenic pulmonary eosinophilia
Allergic argiitis and granulomatosis (Churg-Strauss syndrome)

Pathogenesis

The eosinophil has cytotoxic and anti-inflammatory properties. The cytotoxic properties act against parasites but may also damage host tissues. The pathological response to the various identifiable causes of pulmonary eosinophilia depends on the route by which they reach the lungs; if inhaled (e.g. allergic mycoses) the response is in the airways (bronchocentric), whereas if delivered to the lung via the pulmonary circulation the response is in the blood vessels (angiocentric).

Allergic bronchopulmonary mycoses

By far the commonest cause is allergic bronchopulmonary aspergillosis (ABPA). This is due to sensitivity to the ubiquitous fungus *Aspergillus fumigatus*. This fungus thrives in warm, wet conditions, and symptoms therefore tend to occur in the autumn. The bronchial tree provides

an ideal environment for colonisation. When the fungus is inhaled there is an immediate hypersensitivity reaction with eosinophils drawn into the area. There may be several responses thereafter:

1. a simple asthmatic reaction with an eosinophilia but no radiological change
2. pulmonary eosinophilic infiltrates with consolidation and chest X-ray shadowing
3. mucus impaction with distal collapse and progressive airway damage due to the release of tissue-damaging factors; this in time may lead to a characteristic proximal bronchiectasis and upper zone fibrosis, sometimes making it difficult to differentiate ABPA from old tuberculosis.

Clinically, ABPA presents, often in early adult life, as worsening asthma. The patient may complain of coughing up rubbery brown or green plugs, and exacerbations of asthma are often accompanied by fever and fleeting pulmonary infiltrates. Almost all patients have a positive immediate-type hypersensitivity to *Aspergillus fumigatus* on skin prick testing and about 90% have precipitating antibody.

Treatment with oral prednisolone (30–40 mg/day) leads to rapid symptomatic and radiological improvement; whether or not it affects the long-term outcome is uncertain. Physiotherapy and occasionally bronchoscopy help to remove troublesome plugs, and the asthma responds to conventional treatment. Many patients require a small maintenance dose of oral prednisolone to prevent relapse.

Drugs and toxins

There are a wide variety of drugs and toxins which can cause a pulmonary eosinophilic syndrome (Table 14.30). The drug reaches the lung via the pulmonary circulation and sets up an allergic reaction in the vessel wall. There is frequently an associated skin reaction. Patients may present with a pneumonia-like illness, with dyspnoea, cough, fever and pleuritic pain, or as a pulmonary vasculitis. Rarely, if the subject is exposed over a prolonged period, a type of fibrosing alveolitis develops. Whatever the progression, fleeting chest X-ray shadows and blood eosinophilia will be present. Almost all cases improve if the offending agent is stopped and oral corticosteroids help speed recovery.

Table 14.30 Some causes of eosinophilia due to drugs and toxins

Nitrofurantoin	Chlorpropamide
Sulphonamides	Inorganic chemicals, e.g. nickel
Penicillin	Lymphangiography
Tetracycline	Blood transfusions

Helminthic infections

Some helminths (*Ascaris*, *Strongyloides*, *Toxocara*) are

borne to the lungs via the circulation, where they are attacked by eosinophils. During this phase the patient may be febrile and have pulmonary infiltrates, and the dying parasite may initiate an allergic response and thus an asthmatic attack. Filarial infection (due to infection with *Wuchereria bancrofti*) may cause asthma and patients can also develop diffuse fibrosis and pulmonary hypertension. The chest X-ray in helminthic infections shows widespread nodular infiltrates which are at first transient but may become persistent. The diagnosis is confirmed by appropriate complement fixation tests and by finding ova in the stools. (See also Ch. 12.)

Unknown causes

There is a spectrum of conditions of unknown aetiology which cause fleeting eosinophilic infiltrates in the lung and a blood eosinophilia. Pathologically, these range from a localised or generalised pulmonary eosinophilia to eosinophilic syndromes with vasculitis and granuloma formation. Classification is difficult; the most important distinction is between the clinical syndrome of cryptogenic pulmonary eosinophilia and those syndromes associated with vasculitis and granuloma formation.

Cryptogenic pulmonary eosinophilia (eosinophilic pneumonia)

Cryptogenic pulmonary eosinophilia is a syndrome of fever, weight loss, cough and breathlessness with widespread, mainly peripheral, pulmonary infiltrates (Fig. 14.34) and a marked blood eosinophilia. The patients

Fig. 14.34 Pulmonary eosinophilia. Extensive, ill-defined peripheral consolidation in the left upper zone and less marked consolidation in the left lower and right mid-zone, in a patient with cryptogenic pulmonary eosinophilia. Characteristically, new shadows appear and previous ones spontaneously resolve.

are usually non-atopic but 10% have previous asthma. No cause can be identified. Some patients progress to the vasculitic/granulomatous type of disease. There is a rapid response to oral corticosteroids; treatment should be carefully tailed off as recurrences are common, and usually corticosteroid treatment for up to 2 years is required.

Allergic angiitis and granulomatosis

This is a rare group of conditions in which asthmatic patients present with symptoms similar to cryptogenic pulmonary eosinophilia. Radiologically, they may show extensive transient pulmonary infiltrates, nodules, cavities and occasionally pleural and pericardial effusions. There is a blood eosinophilia and a raised erythrocyte sedimentation rate (ESR). Lung biopsy shows a vasculitis and if there is an allergic granulomatous reaction this is known as the *Churg-Strauss syndrome*, although there is probably a broad spectrum of pathological overlap in these syndromes. In many ways the syndrome is similar to polyarteritis nodosa, although lung involvement in typical polyarteritis nodosa is rare. Other organs such as liver, spleen, heart, skin and central nervous system may be affected by the vasculitis but, unlike polyarteritis nodosa, renal involvement is uncommon. Treatment with prednisolone in high doses, with or without azathioprine or cyclophosphamide, significantly reduces mortality although infective or cardiac complications may still be fatal.

CHRONIC BRONCHITIS AND EMPHYSEMA

Chronic bronchitis

Chronic bronchitis is a clinical diagnosis in which there is cough productive of sputum on most days for 3 months of the year for 2 or more years, which is not due to a specific respiratory disease such as bronchiectasis. The disorder is characterised by excess mucus secretion. Pathologically there is hyperplasia and hypertrophy of the tracheal and bronchial mucus glands and an increase in the glandular elements of the bronchial wall. The increase in intraluminal mucus and thickening of the bronchial wall produces airways narrowing and increased airways resistance, the FEV_1 correlating with the mucous membrane thickness.

Emphysema

Emphysema is defined by its pathology and is characterised by destruction of respiratory tissue and permanent enlargement of the unit of the lung distal to the terminal bronchiole (the acinus). Lung destruction causes loss of alveolar capillary bed and elastic recoil. Centrilobular emphysema involves the proximal part of the acinus, is frequently associated with cigarette smoking and chronic bronchitis, and affects predominantly the upper zones of the lungs. Panacinar emphysema affects the whole acinus, is maximal in the lower zones and is characteristic of alpha$_1$-antitrypsin deficiency. However, many patients with panacinar emphysema are heavy smokers who also have chronic bronchitis.

In the past much importance has been placed on the distinction between chronic bronchitis and emphysema. In the majority of patients both conditions co-exist, usually in heavy cigarette smokers, and the physician therefore makes a clinical diagnosis of chronic bronchitis *and* emphysema.

Aetiology and prevalence

Chronic bronchitis and emphysema are responsible for the personal disability and misery of tens of thousands of patients and impose a huge social and economic burden on society. Respiratory disorders are an important cause of death in the United Kingdom and of these chronic bronchitis and emphysema constitute a large proportion (p. 13). As a consequence of the gradual development of chronic bronchitis and emphysema mortality is greatest in the elderly, but many younger people are affected and these diseases cause massive loss of working days each year. In the UK 10% of absence from work is caused by chronic bronchitis and emphysema and approximately 10% of occupancy of acute general medical hospital beds is the result of these diseases.

Atmospheric pollution and occupational dust exposure are minor aetiological factors in chronic bronchitis and the dominant causal agent is cigarette smoke. Smoking also causes emphysema, probably damaging the lung by the release of proteolytic enzymes. Smoke-affected pulmonary alveolar macrophages, present in greater numbers than usual, release neutrophil chemotactic factor and the attracted neutrophils are damaged by smoke and release proteolytic enzymes, especially elastase, capable of lysing elastin, collagen and basement membranes. The effectiveness of alpha$_1$-antitrypsin is impaired by smoking and the unchecked proteolysis results in centrilobular emphysema. This process is particularly rapid in patients who are deficient in alpha$_1$-antitrypsin.

Alpha$_1$-antitrypsin deficiency

This genetic disorder affects 1 in 5000 people, is equally common in men and women, and predisposes to the early development of emphysema often before the age of 40. The emphysema is panlobular and basal (Fig. 14.14) and lung destruction is accelerated by cigarette smoke. Non-smoking heterozygotes do not have emphysema but it is possible that smoking heterozygotes develop emphysema more readily than smoking normals. The feasibility and clinical value of alpha$_1$-antitrypsin replacement therapy is under investigation.

Mechanism of airflow obstruction

In chronic bronchitis and emphysema the fundamental cause of reduced ventilatory capacity and breathlessness is the limitation of expiratory airflow. Secondary to expiratory airflow limitation, residual volume is increased, the thorax is hyperinflated and inspiratory capacity is markedly impaired, in part due to the compromised function of the inspiratory muscles. In chronic bronchitis airways resistance is increased and expiratory airflow reduced by the thickening of the bronchial wall and excessive intraluminal mucus. In emphysema a more important mechanism is the narrowing and collapse of airways during expiration as a consequence of loss of the lung elastic recoil which normally keeps airways open. In health the upper airways and trachea contribute most to airways resistance and therefore narrowing of the distal smaller airways has to be substantial before total airways resistance is greatly affected. For this reason the available laboratory tests of airflow limitation are not sensitive at detecting early disease of smaller airways. By the time that increased airways resistance can be demonstrated, the pathological changes of chronic bronchitis and emphysema are substantial.

Clinical features

Chronic bronchitis and emphysema develop over many years and patients are rarely symptomatic before middle age. Symptoms are initially minor, perhaps a morning cough productive of a little sputum. In some patients chronic bronchitis can remain a trivial problem but in many, smoking-related airways obstruction co-exists and the patients then develop breathlessness. Initially breathlessness is on exertion but exercise capacity progressively and slowly deteriorates and eventually patients become respiratory cripples distressed by dyspnoea even at rest. Patients with predominant bronchitis are prone to periodic infections. Often the infective process remains confined to the bronchial tree but sometimes infection involves the surrounding lung with consequent pneumonia; thus, although some patients may have radiological changes of pneumonia in association with an infective exacerbation, the majority show no change on chest X-ray. Eventually patients with chronic bronchitis develop severe hypoxaemia, hypercapnia and peripheral oedema–cor pulmonale (the so-called '*blue bloater*'). Patients with substantial emphysema tend to be very breathless, ventilating sufficiently to maintain normal arterial carbon dioxide and near-normal oxygen tensions. The development of cor pulmonale is a late and terminal event in these '*pink puffers*'. These two clinical extremes overlap; many patients with a normal arterial carbon dioxide tension eventually become cyanosed, but the broad clinical distinction between the 'pink puffer' and the 'blue bloater' is useful. Oxygen therapy is much more difficult in the hypercapnic blue and bloated patient, sedation is more hazardous, and general anaesthesia poses greater risks due to postoperative sputum retention and difficulty in weaning such patients from assisted ventilation.

Patients with chronic bronchitis frequently complain of morning tightness in the chest which usually resolves when they are up and about and is helped by clearing the bronchial secretions that have collected during the night. Unfortunately the bronchial irritation and cough produced by the first cigarette of the day is helpful for expectoration and some patients are reluctant to stop smoking for this reason. Some patients have bronchial hyper-reactivity and exposure to cold air, acute temperature changes, dusts and cigarette smoke causes increasing breathlessness, respiratory distress and wheeze.

The development of cor pulmonale indicates a poor prognosis with a 30% 5-year survival. In association with severe hypoxia and hypercapnia, pulmonary arterial hypertension develops and some patients also have an elevated jugular venous pressure. However, in many patients cor pulmonale is not simple cardiac failure since cardiac output is frequently normal and there can be peripheral oedema without elevation of the jugular venous pressure. The mechanism of cor pulmonale remains obscure but in part it reflects an increase in blood volume perhaps due to hypercapnia causing sodium retention by the kidney. Cor pulmonale is unusual in the absence of hypercapnia. There is evidence that optimum therapy and careful follow-up of patients with cor pulmonale can produce good results.

Physical signs

In the early stages of chronic bronchitis and emphysema physical signs are minimal except perhaps nicotine staining of the fingers and scattered expiratory wheezes. In predominantly emphysematous patients, inspiratory airways resistance is not increased and inspiration is therefore quiet, whereas patients with predominantly chronic bronchitis have noisy breathing. As the diseases progress the physical signs may eventually include those of severe airways obstruction, hypoxia, hypercapnia and cor pulmonale. Patients with chronic airflow limitation often have early inspiratory crackles which can be heard at the patient's mouth by the examining physician. Weight loss is common with advanced emphysema.

Patients with emphysema have translucent lungs on the chest X-ray with few vascular markings, and bullae may also be present (Fig. 14.35). Patients with predominantly chronic bronchitis may show bronchial wall thickening. Hyperinflation is more severe in emphysema. Commonly, radiological abnormality is most striking in the upper zones but in alpha$_1$-antitrypsin deficiency disease is predominantly basal.

Respiratory function

In patients with chronic bronchitis and emphysema the FEV$_1$ is reduced and the FEV$_1$/VC% is low, indicating expiratory flow limitation (p. 454). Vital capacity for a relaxed manœuvre is usually greater than for a forced effort. The peak expiratory flow rate, although low, is a less sensitive measure of the severity of airways obstruction. Hyperinflation is confirmed by the increase in residual volume and total lung capacity. Gas transfer is more dramatically reduced in the 'pink puffer' with a substantial element of emphysema. In the 'blue bloater' there is severe hypoxaemia, hypercapnia and secondary polycythaemia.

Fig. 14.35 Bullous emphysema. The large bullae (right upper zone, right lower zone peripherally) display no vascular markings. Elsewhere the lung markings appear obvious, partly due to increased blood flow through relatively normal lung and partly because bullae compress adjacent lung tissue.

Management

Restoration of normal function is not possible in chronic bronchitis and emphysema. The aim of therapy must therefore be to reduce disability by tackling the inter-related problems of airways obstruction, recurrent infections, breathlessness, hypoxia and poor exercise tolerance. Factors aggravating chronic bronchitis, particularly cigarette smoking, must be withdrawn.

Airways obstruction

In chronic bronchitis and emphysema the increased resistance to gas flow within the bronchial tree increases the work of breathing and overall oxygen consumption. As a consequence of airways obstruction there is excess gas trapping in the lungs, hyperinflation and disordered rib-cage geometry, and these changes shorten the inspiratory muscles and make the diaphragm less curved, thereby greatly reducing ventilatory capacity. Airways obstruction therefore increases ventilatory work at the same time as reducing ventilatory capacity.

Conventionally the airways obstruction of chronic bronchitis and emphysema is regarded as being irreversible. However, the majority of patients show some improvement in lung function with therapy directed at relaxing bronchial

14

smooth muscle and, although small, this improvement can have an important impact on the disability of these patients. Prognosis in patients who respond well to bronchodilators is considerably better than for those with completely fixed obstruction. The most important bronchodilator agents are the selective β_2 adrenergic agonists (e.g. salbutamol and terbutaline), which are best administered as an aerosol.

Inhaled atropine analogues (ipratropium bromide) can be helpful, but provided optimum doses of β_2 agonists are administered, ipratropium bromide confers little additional benefit.

Oral theophyllines available in slow-release formulation are of marginal usefulness in chronic bronchitis and emphysema. It has been claimed that theophylline improves respiratory muscle contractility but recent studies have not confirmed this effect.

Patients with severe airways obstruction should have a therapeutic trial of steroids – for example, oral prednisolone (30 mg daily) for a period of 2–3 weeks – provided there are no contra-indications. Long-term oral steroids will not be indicated in most patients, but when prescribed require regular assessment and dosage should seldom exceed 7.5–10 mg daily, thereby avoiding drug complications. Mucolytic agents (e.g. bromhexine) are of unproven value in chronic bronchitis, but occasional patients report substantial benefits, and when sputum retention is a major problem, a therapeutic trial is justified.

Infection

In acute exacerbations of chronic bronchitis an infective viral or bacterial pathogen is isolated in less than 50% of cases. Viral infections are frequently complicated by bacterial overgrowth and the majority of patients develop purulent sputum. Severe exacerbations have a mortality of up to 25%, and prompt antibacterial therapy is of the greatest importance. Common infective organisms are *Streptococcus pneumoniae* and *Haemophilus influenzae*, and suitable antibiotics are amoxycillin, erythromycin, co-trimoxazole and the cephalosporins. For most patients long-term chemoprophylaxis is not helpful but if intermittent treatment fails, a trial of continuous antibiotic therapy is appropriate.

Oxygen therapy

During acute exacerbation of chronic bronchitis and emphysema, oxygen therapy is necessary to avoid death from hypoxia. In patients with hypercapnia oxygen must be given at low and controlled concentrations (usually 24% or 28% O_2). A more contentious question is the value of long-term domiciliary oxygen therapy. Studies suggest that long-term controlled oxygen therapy can benefit patients with severe airways obstruction who have severe hypoxia and who refrain from smoking cigarettes. It is necessary to administer oxygen virtually continuously, including during sleep (Fig. 14.36).

The administration of continuous oxygen presents considerable practical and financial difficulties. Oxygen may

Fig. 14.36 Long-term domiciliary oxygen therapy. Effect of therapy on survival in patients with severe respiratory failure, due to chronic bronchitis and emphysema (MRC = Medical Research Council; NIH = National Institutes of Health, USA).

be supplied in cylinders or, preferably, generated by an oxygen concentrator. This therapy should be reserved for patients with severe disease who are well motivated. Oxygen therapy requires careful pretreatment assessment and long-term supervision.

In practice much oxygen used by patients in their homes is for a few minutes only and the main purpose is to relieve breathlessness. Oxygen is also available in small portable cylinders and some patients find this helpful in reducing breathlessness on exercise, improving exercise capacity, and permitting excursions from the home.

Patients with severe chronic bronchitis and associated hypoxia, hypercapnia, pulmonary hypertension and cor pulmonale have profound nocturnal hypoxaemia (Fig. 14.37). This hypoxaemia is much more a feature of the 'blue bloater' than the 'pink puffer'. 'Pink puffers' do have nocturnal hypoxaemia but the oxygen desaturation is much greater in the already hypoxic chronic bronchitic. Much of the hypoxia is caused by hypoventilation and irregular breathing patterns during rapid eye movement (REM) sleep and is not due to obstructive sleep apnoea (p. 498). Oxygen therapy during the night (2 l/min by nasal cannulae) can alleviate hypoxaemia and make hypoxic periods less severe.

The return of normal breathing patterns following REM sleep is impaired by sedatives and these should therefore be avoided in patients with chronic bronchitis. Respiratory stimulants may have a place in reducing nocturnal hypoxaemia, but their clinical role is still under evaluation.

Drug therapy for breathlessness

In patients with airways obstruction it is the 'pink puffers' with normal CO_2 values and mild or moderate hypoxia who are most breathless. However, 'blue bloaters' may be equally incapacitated by dyspnoea, which may also be disabling in patients with pulmonary fibrosis. In some

Fig. 14.37 Oxygen saturation during sleep in severe chronic bronchitis. Patients who are already hypoxic can markedly desaturate during sleep, particularly REM sleep (vertical bars).

patients, reducing ventilation with diazepam, promethazine and dihydrocodeine can reduce breathlessness and in patients without carbon dioxide retention a careful trial of such therapy is justified when symptoms are severe. For the devastating dyspnoea which is frequently a feature of terminal respiratory failure diamorphine is helpful.

Secondary polycythaemia

Polycythaemia produces symptoms attributable to hyperviscosity, including somnolence, lethargy, poor concentration and headache. Venesection reduces these symptoms but does not affect lung function or blood gases. Venesection also improves cerebral blood flow, pulmonary hypertension and exercise tolerance. Patients with a haematocrit of 0.60 or greater should benefit and the haematocrit should be reduced to 0.50. This can be achieved either by simple venesection, exchange transfusion with dextran or plasma, or erytropharesis. Continuous oxygen therapy for 6 weeks will also reduce the haematocrit. Whenever possible the first-line therapy for secondary polycythaemia is to improve lung function.

Chest physiotherapy

There have been few scientific studies of the long-term effect of chest physiotherapy techniques aimed at improving breathing patterns in patients with chronic bronchitis and emphysema; no benefit has been proven.

Postural drainage is of undoubted benefit in patients with excessive bronchial secretions. Its effectiveness is increased by coughing or forced expiratory manœuvres ('huffs'). Postural drainage has little place if patients do not have sputum. In asthma vigorous physiotherapy, especially forced expiratory manœuvres, can increase bronchoconstriction.

During acute exacerbations of bronchitis and pneumonia several studies have, rather surprisingly, shown no benefit in physiotherapy. In the absence of excessive secretions physiotherapy is not justified in these patients. Mucociliary clearance is decreased and basal collapse is more common following general anaesthesia and surgery, particularly of the upper abdomen. The case for routine pre-operative physiotherapy in chronic bronchitis patients is, however, not proven except for very high risk patients.

Assisted ventilation in chronic bronchitis

Patients with severe progressive chronic bronchitis and emphysema eventually die of intractable ventilatory failure, having been breathless at rest and confined to their homes in the months before death. The poor quality of life precludes such patients from being treated with mechanical ventilation to delay the inevitable outcome. Difficult decisions are posed by the less severely disabled, who require mechanical ventilation if they are not to die during an acute exacerbation of bronchitis. Many of these patients are difficult to wean from ventilation, particularly those with pre-existing hypercapnia and blunted ventilatory response to CO_2. Before embarking on mechanical ventilation, every effort must be made to establish the background severity of respiratory disability, exercise tolerance and quality of life.

Cessation of cigarette smoking

Tobacco smoke damages the bronchial tree and produces airflow limitation by a number of different actions. Smoke impairs mucociliary clearance and causes bronchial smooth muscle to contract by stimulating receptors and provoking the release of inflammatory mediators. In addition, smoke increases mucus production and causes mucous gland hypertrophy. Smokers are predisposed to bronchial infection and consequent inflammation; the increase in elastase and the impairment of alpha$_1$-antitrypsin, as well as impaired surfactant production, contribute to emphysema. It is therefore not surprising that chronic bronchitis and emphysema are found in 15% of middle-aged males who smoke moderately or heavily but are rare in non-smokers, and that deaths from bronchitis increase with the amount smoked.

If patients with chronic bronchitis and emphysema stop smoking, the rate of decline in pulmonary function is reduced to that of non-smokers (Fig. 14.38). Indeed, if patients stop smoking early in their disease there is improvement in pulmonary function. However severe the disease, stopping smoking will reduce cough.

Patients with chronic bronchitis and emphysema have smoked for many years and have great difficulty in abstaining. Stopping smoking is particularly difficult if a spouse or cohabitant smokes. In patients who are determined to stop smoking, nicotine chewing gum is helpful, but in

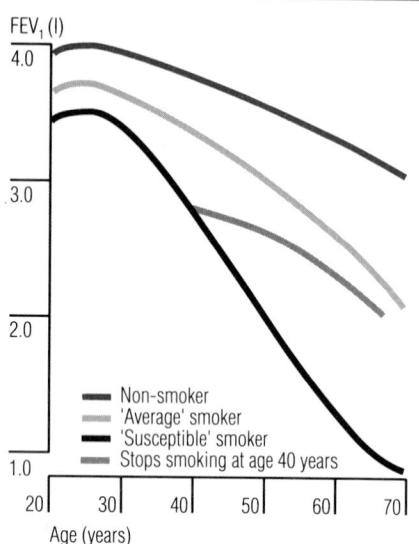

Fig. 14.38 Airflow limitation and smoking. FEV₁ (the maximum volume that can be expired in 1 second) declines with age. In smokers this decline is more marked, particularly in 'susceptible' smokers. Such patients, therefore, become breathless in middle or old age. When smokers stop the habit, the rate of decline in FEV₁ is markedly slowed. (From Burrows B 1986 The natural history of asthma, chronic bronchitis and emphysema. Medicine International 35: 1422–1425.)

Graph legend:
- Non-smoker
- 'Average' smoker
- 'Susceptible' smoker
- Stops smoking at age 40 years

general the firm advice of the patient's physician (and other medical staff) is as effective as any other measure and is most likely to work when the patient is unwell. Cigarette smokers who change to smoking a pipe or cigars inhale the smoke and this change is therefore not helpful. If patients are unable to stop smoking completely, they should smoke as few cigarettes as possible, move to low-tar brands, reduce the number of puffs, and smoke less of each cigarette they do smoke.

RESPIRATION DURING SLEEP

SLEEP APNOEA SYNDROMES

Apnoea is defined as no gas flow at the nose or mouth for 10 seconds, and a sleep apnoea syndrome is diagnosed if more than 30 such episodes occur during the night. Apnoea may be central, when there is no airflow and no chest wall movement; obstructive, when there is no airflow despite chest wall movement because of upper airways obstruction; or the apnoea may result from both mechanisms.

Obstructive sleep apnoea

Obstructive sleep apnoea is more common than central apnoea, perhaps occurring to some degree in up to 1% of the adult male population. The typical features (Summary 7) are hypersomnolence by day and upper airways obstruction during sleep. Many, but not all, patients are obese and

Summary 7 Features of obstructive sleep apnoea	
Snoring	Intellectual deterioration
Disturbed sleep	Systemic hypertension
Witnessed apnoeas	Pulmonary hypertension
Cardiac arrhythmias	Right heart failure
Excessive daytime sleepiness	Obesity
Morning headache	Small oropharynx

hypertension is common. In severe cases there is chronic alveolar hypoventilation at night, daytime hypoxia, secondary polycythaemia and cor pulmonale. Patients often have loud, persistent snoring, and the frequent arousals from apnoeic episodes greatly disturb sleep (although the patient may be unaware of this). Patients fall asleep by day and may have road and other accidents. There is difficulty in concentrating, particularly in the morning, intellectual impairment, personality change and irritability. Abnormal limb and body movements during arousals following apnoea (thrashing around in bed), sexual dysfunction and morning headaches are important features. During apnoea there are cardiovascular disturbances, particularly bradycardia.

In some patients the upper airway is abnormally narrow (e.g. hypertrophy of tonsils and adenoids), but in many cases no anatomical abnormality is found. However, during obstruction the posterior and lateral walls of the pharynx collapse, occluding the oropharynx. The condition is more common in obese patients. The collapse of the upper airway is probably due to a failure to activate the upper airway musculature sufficiently during inspiration, and the negative pressures generated in the upper airway by the contraction of the respiratory muscles suck in the soft tissues of the oropharynx (Fig. 14.39). This negative pressure will be greater if the upper airway is narrowed, and nasal obstruction can be a contributory factor.

Central sleep apnoea

Central apnoea is less common than obstructive apnoea. The patients snore less, are seldom obese, and complain of night-time wakening. The central drive to breathing is abnormal and inspiration may fail to be initiated. The syndrome occurs as a consequence of primary alveolar hypoventilation and of hypoventilation following brain stem surgery and bulbar poliomyelitis.

To document sleep apnoea, to determine whether it is central or obstructive and to assess the severity of nocturnal hypoxaemia, a formal sleep study in a specialist laboratory is required (Fig. 14.40).

Sleep in other respiratory disorders

Patients with airways obstruction and hypercapnia may become profoundly hypoxic at night as a result of hypo-

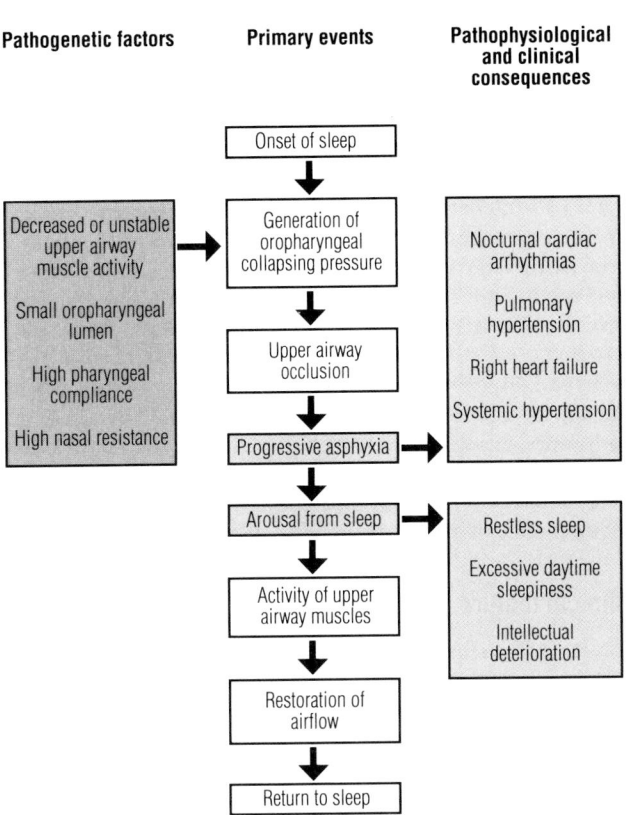

Fig. 14.39 The mechanism of obstructive sleep apnoea (OSA). In severe cases, since sleep stops ventilation, sleep is grossly disturbed and daytime somnolence is very striking. (From Stradling J R and Phillipson E A 1986 Breathing disorders during sleep. Q J Med (New Series) 58:3–18.

Fig. 14.40 Sleep study in obstructive sleep apnoea. The record shows a period when ventilation is obstructed and there is no airflow (V). At this time the diaphragm continues to contract (EMG_{di}); oesophageal (P_{es}) and gastric (P_{ga}) pressure swings occur, and there is ribcage and abdominal movement (RC and AB). As obstruction continues arterial oxygen saturation (So_2) falls. Eventually the activity of the upper airway muscles, including genioglossus (EMG_{ge}), increases, the upper airway becomes patent, and airflow is restored. Patients can have hundreds of similar episodes during the night. (From Onal et al. 1982 Am Rev Respir Dis. 125: 167–74.)

ventilation (Fig. 14.37) (p. 497). Nocturnal hypoxaemia is also a clinical problem in patients with advanced kyphoscoliosis or severe respiratory muscle weakness (p. 538).

Treatment of apnoea syndromes

In the management of obstructive sleep apnoea weight reduction is helpful but difficult to achieve. Tracheostomy is effective but presents management difficulties, and many patients are resistant to this line of therapy. Nasal airway positive pressure (NAPP) is very effective and remarkably well tolerated, although the technique is rather cumbersome. Palatopharyngoplasty (PPP), surgical reconstruction of the pharynx, can also be effective, but the site of obstruction may not be relieved in some patients and the long-term effects of surgery are not yet known. Drugs may sometimes be helpful, particularly protriptyline (a non-sedative tricyclic antidepressant); this reduces rapid eye movement sleep, during which, as a consequence of reduced activity of upper airways musculature, obstruction is most likely. For many patients, weight reduction and perhaps protriptyline are worthy of trial before considering NAPP or PPP.

RESPIRATORY FAILURE

Definition

There is no acceptable clinical definition of respiratory failure; the diagnosis rests on the interpretation of arterial blood gas measurements. A patient can be said to be in respiratory failure if the arterial oxygen tension (Pao_2) falls below 8.0 kPa/60 mmHg (normal range 11.3–13.3 kPa or 85–100 mmHg) or if the arterial carbon dioxide tension (Pa_{CO_2}) rises above 6.6 kPa/50 mmHg (normal range 4.6–6.0 kPa or 35–45 mmHg), when the subject is at sea level, awake and breathing air. The condition may be acute or chronic; if the patient has arterial hypoxaemia with a normal or low Pa_{CO_2} then he is said to have *type I* respiratory failure; and if the Pa_{CO_2} is elevated, *type II* respiratory failure. Arterial hypoxaemia does not always imply respiratory failure: a low inspired O_2 at altitude or an anatomical right-to-left shunt, as in congenital heart disease or arteriovenous malformation, can cause hypoxaemia despite normal lung function. The causes of types I and II respiratory failure are shown in Table 14.31. Chronic respiratory failure in the UK is most commonly due to chronic bronchitis and emphysema (p. 493).

Measurement of the alveolar-arterial (A–a) gradient is useful in hypoxic patients, and may help to decide, for instance, whether the patient's hypoxaemia is secondary to central hypoventilation or to intrinsic lung disease. The A–a gradient indicates the contribution of venous admixture (i.e. true shunt or $\dot{V}/\dot{Q}$ abnormality) to hypoxaemia. It can be calculated by using the concept of 'ideal alveolar air' (Pao_2):

$$Pao_2 = FiO_2 - \frac{Pa_{CO_2}}{0.8}$$

where FiO_2 = inspired Po_2 (20 kPa on room air) and 0.8 = respiratory exchange ratio. Thus the normal alveolar air tension is approximately 14 kPa, the normal arterial oxygen tension approximately 12.5 kPa, and the normal A–a gradient is therefore 1–2 kPa.

In the management of the hypoxic patient it should be remembered that tissue O_2 delivery depends not just on Pao_2 but also on the haemoglobin concentration and cardiac output. The most useful index of tissue oxygenation is the mixed venous (pulmonary arterial)/arterial O_2 content difference. The normal oxygen combining capacity is 1.4 ml O_2/gm haemoglobin (approximately

0.06 mmol/g). The oxygen content of blood is the oxygen combining capacity × haemoglobin concentration × saturation (plus a small amount of dissolved oxygen in plasma, which is negligible at normal atmospheric pressure). Assuming the haemoglobin concentration is 15 g/100 ml, and the oxygen content of arterial blood is $1.4 \times 15 \times 0.95 = 20.58$ ml/100 ml, and the oxygen content of mixed venous blood is $1.4 \times 15 \times 0.75 = 15.75$, the arterial/mixed venous oxygen content difference is 4.83 ml/100 ml. If oxygen delivery is reduced (e.g. reduced cardiac output) the arterial/venous content difference widens.

Type II hypercapnic ventilatory failure represents inadequacy of the respiratory muscle 'pump'. The concept of 'pump' failure leading to hypercapnia is a useful one, focusing attention on the importance of CNS output, neuromuscular function and chest wall movement in the maintenance of adequate ventilation (p. 538).

Clinical features

Acute hypoxaemia or hypercapnia is less well tolerated than chronic gradual alteration in blood gases. Virtually all patients with respiratory failure, with the exception of some patients with CNS dysfunction (for example, drug overdose), are breathless. Acute hypoxaemia causes restlessness, confusion and sweating, with a tachycardia, poor peripheral perfusion and central cyanosis. Cyanosis can be deceptive, particularly if the patient is polycythaemic, so measurement of arterial blood gases is crucial.

Patients with acute severe hypercapnic ventilatory failure are breathless and cyanosed, and in addition may have confusion, flapping tremor of the hands, warm peripheries, bounding pulse and occasionally papilloedema. The mental state is probably the best clinical index to follow, since increasing confusion and restlessness often parallel a rising Pa_{CO_2}. When patients (for instance, those with advanced chronic bronchitis) progress to severe chronic respiratory failure, with a compensated respiratory acidosis, symptoms may also include sleep disturbance with early morning headache and personality change. Such patients develop polycythaemia, pulmonary hypertension and cor pulmonale.

Chronic hypercapnic respiratory failure can occur despite normal lung function. Sleep apnoea syndromes, for example (p. 498), may be severe enough to produce pulmonary hypertension and cor pulmonale. Patients with neuromuscular disorders (for example, myasthenia gravis or the Guillain-Barré syndrome) may also have life-threatening ventilatory failure despite normal lungs (p. 538).

Treatment

The general principles for the treatment of acute respiratory failure are those of any other respiratory emergency. The airway should be cleared of sputum and protected. Oxygen should be given in sufficient concentration to ensure a Pao_2 of 8 kPa (60 mmHg). This can be delivered via a Venturi mask which will give an inspired

---

Table 14.31 Causes of types I and II respiratory failure

Type I (hypoxaemic)
Acute asthma
Pulmonary oedema
Pneumonia
Pulmonary fibrosis
Chronic bronchitis
Emphysema
Pulmonary vascular disease
Miscellaneous: lymphangitis, radiation pneumonitis, etc.

Type II (ventilatory)

CNS	Thoracic cage and pleura
Trauma	Crushed chest
Cerebral tumour	Kyphoscoliosis
Raised intracranial pressure	Extensive thoracic surgery
Drugs	(thoracoplasty)
Hypoventilation syndromes	Ankylosing spondylitis (rare)
Neuromuscular	Lung and airways
Cervical cord lesion	Severe acute asthma, pneumonia
Guillain-Barré syndrome	Upper airway obstruction
Motor neurone disease	Chronic airflow limitation: chronic
Poliomyelitis	bronchitis, emphysema,
Muscular dystrophies and	bronchiectasis
myopathies	
Botulism	
Myasthenia gravis	
Muscle relaxant drugs	
Organophosphorus poisoning	
Status epilepticus	

oxygen concentration of 24–35%, or a Hudson or MC mask which will deliver variable, but higher, inspired oxygen concentrations. If identifiable, the underlying cause should be treated: for example, antibiotics for acute bacterial pneumonias, or bronchodilators and corticosteroids for acute asthma. If the patient's condition is worsening, with deepening cyanosis, disturbance of consciousness and a rising Pa_{CO_2}, then a decision to intubate and employ assisted mechanical ventilation must be made. This decision is based on a number of considerations, including the previous exercise capacity, the possibility of treating the underlying cause, the overall clinical state of the patient and serial arterial blood gas measurements.

Patients with chronic respiratory disease who develop additional acute problems require a rather different pattern of management. Patients with longstanding hypoxaemia and hypercapnia are dependent on hypoxaemia to maintain ventilatory drive. High concentrations of inspired oxygen reduce respiratory drive and ventilation, resulting in a rise in Pa_{CO_2} and a worsening respiratory acidosis. Oxygen must therefore be given in a controlled fashion, starting with an inspired concentration of 24% and with repeated monitoring of arterial blood gases. It should be emphasised that it is not necessary to raise the Pa_{O_2} into the physiological range; a Pa_{O_2} of more than 6 kPa (45 mmHg) is usually sufficient to maintain the patient in a reasonable clinical state. Although it is correct to exercise caution when administering oxygen to hypercapnic patients, it should be remembered that severe hypoxaemia, less than 5 kPa (38 mmHg), is life-threatening and must be relieved, and hypoxaemic patients without CO_2 retention (a common situation in fibrotic lung disease, for example) can receive high inspired oxygen concentrations without developing hypercapnia.

If, with the proper use of oxygen supplements, the Pa_{CO_2} continues to rise, a respiratory stimulant, such as doxapram, may, in the short term, be helpful. This may allow the use of a higher inspired oxygen concentration without precipitating a rise in Pa_{CO_2}. However, some patients will continue to deteriorate and the point may come when a decision will have to be made about whether to offer assisted mechanical ventilation. In this group of patients, above all, their background in terms of respiratory function, exercise tolerance, and when they were last reasonably well, must be taken into consideration. Discussions should involve the patient's family and, very often, the patient himself.

PULMONARY HYPERTENSION

The normal resting pulmonary artery pressure is approximately 25/8 mmHg; values greater than 30/15 mmHg indicate pulmonary hypertension (Table 14.32).

More than one factor may operate in any particular patient; for example, patients with ventricular septal defects eventually develop secondary obstructive and obliterative changes.

Table 14.32 Classification of pulmonary hypertension

Passive pulmonary hypertension	Increased pulmonary vascular resistance
Left heart failure	Vasoconstrictive
Mitral stenosis	e.g. response to hypoxia
LVF	
Hyperkinetic pulmonary hypertension	Obstructive
	Pulmonary emboli
Increased pulmonary blood flow	Veno-occlusive disease
ASD	
VSD	Obliterative
Patent ductus	Polyarteritis nodosa
	Systemic lupus erythematosus
	Systemic sclerosis
	Schistosomiasis
	Chronic bronchitis and emphysema
	Primary pulmonary hypertension

Clinical features

Pulmonary hypertension eventually leads to low cardiac output, right ventricular hypertrophy and failure, syncope, fatigue and breathlessness. Physical signs include a prominent 'a' wave in the jugular venous pulse, right ventricular hypertrophy and a loud pulmonary sound. The ECG confirms right atrial and right ventricular hypertrophy. The chest X-ray shows large central pulmonary arteries. Patients also have signs of the particular underlying cause of pulmonary hypertension (for example, airways obstruction, Fig. 14.41).

Fig. 14.41 Severe chronic bronchitis with marked hypoxaemia and pulmonary hypertension. In keeping with airways obstruction the lungs are of large volume. The main pulmonary artery (see below the aortic knuckle) is massively enlarged, as are the branches of the left and right pulmonary arteries.

> **Summary 8   Important causes of pulmonary hypertension**
>
> - Parenchymal lung disease
> - Recurrent pulmonary embolism (p. 506)
> - Chest wall abnormalities (p. 541)
> - Sleep apnoea syndromes (p. 498)
> - Mitral stenosis and congenital heart disease
> - Primary pulmonary hypertension (Ch. 13)

The most important causes of pulmonary hypertension are listed in Summary 8.

Pulmonary hypertension due to parenchymal lung disease

Chronic bronchitis is by far the commonest cause of pulmonary hypertension, but it also occurs in severe tuberculosis, bronchiectasis, cystic fibrosis, cryptogenic fibrosing alveolitis and other respiratory diseases causing widespread lung destruction and hypoxaemia. Pulmonary hypertension is due to destruction of the capillary bed, a secondary arteritis, and also hypoxic vasoconstriction. In patients with airways obstruction continuous oxygen therapy can reduce pulmonary arterial hypertension and improve prognosis.

Primary pulmonary hypertension

This diagnosis includes classical primary pulmonary hypertension in which the pulmonary arteries are diseased, and also a disorder localised to the pulmonary veins, pulmonary veno-occlusive disease. Both conditions are rare. In the differential diagnosis it is important to consider silent recurrent thrombo-embolic disease, systemic lupus erythematosus and lupus-like syndromes.

Classical primary pulmonary hypertension is of unknown cause and is much more often seen in females, usually young adults. Pulmonary function shows hypoxia due to ventilation–perfusion mismatch, and reduced gas transfer. Patients become increasingly breathless, have syncopal episodes, develop right ventricular hypertrophy and eventually right ventricular failure. There is peripheral cyanosis with a small-volume peripheral pulse and cold, blue hands. Central cyanosis is a late development. The jugular venous pulse has a giant 'a' wave and on auscultation there is a right atrial gallop, tricuspid regurgitant murmur, a pulmonary systolic ejection click, closely split second sound with a loud pulmonary component and a murmur (Graham Steell) of pulmonary regurgitation. The chest X-ray shows a dilated pulmonary artery. The signs are similar in pulmonary veno-occlusive disease, with the important difference that there is pulmonary oedema and therefore more severe hypoxia as well as shadowing on the chest X-ray. The diagnosis of primary pulmonary hypertension is by exclusion of other causes of pulmonary hypertension and the diagnosis of veno-occlusive disease

requires a lung biopsy. In primary pulmonary hypertension, no therapy has been demonstrated to be particularly effective, although pulmonary vasodilators (for example, hydralazine and prostacycline) may be of some value. In veno-occlusive disease anticoagulants and possibly azathioprine may be helpful. A number of patients with primary pulmonary hypertension have been successfully treated by heart–lung transplantation.

PULMONARY THROMBO-EMBOLISM

Tumour, fat, amniotic fluid, parasites, air and injected material can all embolise to the lung but the great majority of emboli are from venous thrombosis, particularly in the lower limbs and pelvis. Although massive pulmonary embolism is an important cause of death, few patients with such large emboli survive to reach hospital. Most commonly, the clinical picture is of less serious pulmonary emboli and pulmonary infarction. There is often a recent history of illness, trauma, anaesthesia or other factors known to predispose to deep venous thrombosis.

PULMONARY EMBOLISM AND INFARCTION

Pulmonary infarction follows embolisation to the peripheral branches of the pulmonary arteries. Emboli are frequently multiple, involving the lower zones more frequently than the upper part of the lungs and only some cause infarction. In many instances of pulmonary embolism without infarction the distal lung remains viable because of adequate oxygenation via the bronchial arterial blood supply and the airways. Pulmonary infarction is much more likely to occur when there is disease of the airways or bronchial circulation. Pathologically, the lesions of pulmonary infarction are markedly haemorrhagic and involve the visceral pleural surface.

Clinical features

The characteristic symptom of pulmonary embolism is the sudden onset of breathlessness. Indeed, relatively few processes cause such a sudden dyspnoea (p. 458). Lateral, usually basal, pleuritic chest pain and haemoptysis develop some time after the onset of breathlessness and are only clinical features if infarction has occurred. The haemoptysis consists of frank red blood without sputum. In addition to respiratory symptoms, there may be pain or swelling of a leg suggesting deep vein thrombosis, or a history indicating an increased risk of thrombosis. A past history of pulmonary emboli is important since such patients are at increased risk of recurrent episodes.

On examination, there may be signs of deep vein thrombosis. The respiratory rate is usually raised and if infarction has taken place, there may be a pleural rub and a small pleural effusion. If embolisation has been extensive there will be cyanosis and signs of cardiovascular stress. The most important cardiovascular sign is a tachycardia. With extensive embolism, patients may have signs of pulmonary hypertension and occasionally a systolic murmur can be heard over the lung fields, as a consequence of turbulent pulmonary blood flow past partial pulmonary arterial occlusion. Within a few hours of pulmonary infarction fever is the rule.

Arterial blood gas analysis demonstrates variable hypoxaemia and hypocapnia, reflecting the ventilation–perfusion mismatch consequent on pulmonary vascular occlusion. However, not all patients are hypoxaemic and hypoxaemia is in itself a very non-specific abnormality. Patients with pulmonary embolic disease are frequently anxious as well as breathless and their hypocapnia is not uncommonly taken to reflect anxiety. However, anxiety hyperventilation syndromes produce hyperoxaemia. Immediately following embolisation, there is often bronchoconstriction, there may even be wheeze, and later, a reduction in surfactant in the affected lung is a contributory factor to atelectasis.

Diagnosis

The clinical diagnosis (Fig. 14.42) of pulmonary embolism is difficult and clinical criteria alone are seldom sufficient. Accurate diagnosis is important, since without specific therapy there may be further, fatal, embolisation. Furthermore, the institution of anticoagulation therapy has important consequences for the patient and is not justifiable without sound evidence. Important clinical factors in the diagnosis are a history of predisposing factors, a

clinically obvious deep vein thrombosis and a pleural rub.

The chest X-ray in pulmonary embolic disease is frequently normal. When pulmonary infarction occurs, radiological changes develop over the following 24 hours and may include peripheral shadows adjacent to the pleura, most often basal and frequently multiple, an elevated hemidiaphragm, some segmental or lobar volume loss, and small pleural effusions (Fig. 14.43A). If pleural fluid is aspirated it is found to be an exudate and is frequently haemorrhagic. With resolution, the linear shadows of pulmonary infarction are characteristic and usually have a pleural component (Fig. 14.43B).

The ECG is rarely helpful, except in the diagnosis of

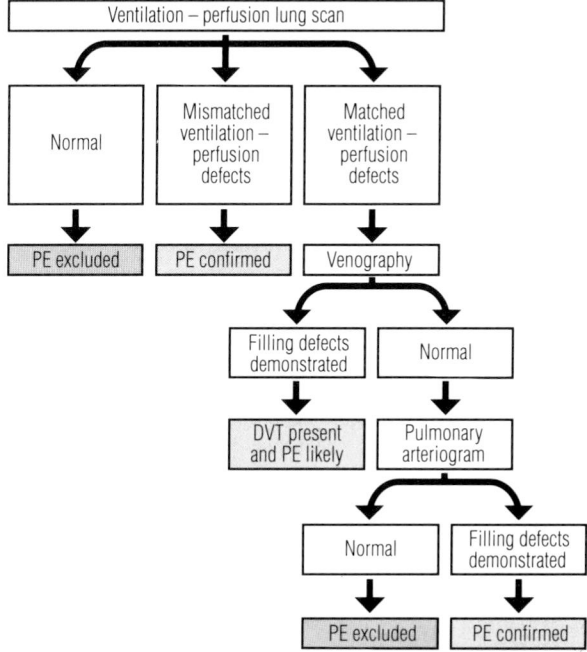

Fig. 14.42 **Strategy for the diagnosis of pulmonary emboli (PE).** The indication for venography to investigate patients with a matched ventilation–perfusion defect will depend on the degree of clinical suspicion of embolic disease. The same argument applies to a subsequent pulmonary arteriogram when venography is normal.

Fig. 14.43 **Pulmonary infarction: chest X-rays. A.** Early changes. There is consolidation at both bases, particularly the left. The left hemidiaphragm is elevated. The patient has made a poor inspiratory effort due to pleuritic pain. **B.** Resolving infarction. Linear basal shadows are characteristic of resolving pulmonary infarction.

myocardial infarction or pericarditis, which may require consideration in the differential diagnosis of pulmonary embolic disease. Occasionally, the ECG changes are suggestive of pulmonary embolism in that they demonstrate right axis deviation, right bundle branch block or the SI, QIII, TIII pattern. However, non-specific abnormalities, particularly T wave changes, are much more common. Severe or recurrent pulmonary emboli may be associated with pulmonary hypertension and the ECG changes of right ventricular and right atrial hypertrophy. Substantial pulmonary embolism is unusual without an associated tachycardia.

Isotope lung scans are the investigation of choice in most patients with pulmonary embolic disease, with the exception of a few patients with massive pulmonary embolism, in whom it may be more appropriate to proceed directly to pulmonary angiography. A normal perfusion lung scan excludes pulmonary embolic disease but an abnormal scan is non-specific. Although an abnormal scan in conjunction with a normal chest X-ray may be taken to suggest pulmonary embolism, perfusion scans may be markedly abnormal in some pulmonary disorders associated with a clear radiograph, as, for example, in asthma. Furthermore, pulmonary angiography demonstrates emboli in only 50% of patients with an abnormal perfusion lung scan and a normal chest X-ray. Thus, for many patients the confirmation of pulmonary emboli, rather than the exclusion of this diagnosis, necessitates a ventilation as well as a perfusion lung scan. Characteristically, the perfusion scan demonstrates the vascular obstruction, whereas ventilation to the affected area is relatively normal (Fig. 14.44). In doubtful cases, particularly patients with airways obstruction in whom ventilation–perfusion mismatching can mimic pulmonary embolic disease, serial scans, during which the perfusion defects of pulmonary emboli resolve, are diagnostically helpful.

Large or multiple ventilation–perfusion mismatched areas are highly likely to be due to pulmonary emboli (80–90% of cases). In a minority of patients, perhaps up to 20% of cases, matched defects can be due to pulmonary embolism confirmed angiographically. For patients with a matched defect and a normal chest X-ray the diagnosis of pulmonary embolism can only be confidently excluded by pulmonary arteriography. The importance of achieving a definite diagnosis in equivocal cases rests on the fact that, untreated, about 50% will have recurrent, sometimes fatal thrombo-embolism.

Venography is often helpful in the management of patients with suspected pulmonary embolic disease. In patients documented to have pulmonary emboli angiographically, 70% will have deep vein thrombosis and therefore the demonstration or exclusion of deep vein thrombosis, by venography, plethysmography or isotopic techniques, is helpful in determining the likelihood of pulmonary emboli. However, a negative venogram occurs in up to 30% of patients with documented pulmonary emboli.

Because of its invasive nature arteriography is only performed in selected cases. However, with imaging techniques such as subtraction digital angiography, that require small volumes of contrast, it is likely that more cases of possible pulmonary embolism causing diagnostic difficulties will be investigated by arteriography in the future.

If treatment is initiated for deep venous thrombosis without a precise diagnosis for the pulmonary pathology, careful follow-up is required to ensure correct treatment of non-embolic disorders such as pneumonia.

Treatment

The purpose of therapy in pulmonary thrombo-embolic disease is to halt the propagation of peripheral thrombus and avoid further pulmonary embolism, and thereby allow time for natural thrombolysis. The treatment of acute pulmonary embolism is intravenous heparin. Massive pulmonary embolism may require additional therapy (p. 505). The most effective heparin treatment regime is probably a continuous infusion such that the partial thromboplastin time is prolonged to 1.5–2.0 times normal, commonly requiring 30 000 to 40 000 units of heparin daily. Heparin requirements tend to fall after 2 or 3 days. If heparin treatment is complicated by bleeding, the action of heparin is rapidly reversed by the administration of

Fig. 14.44 Pulmonary embolic disease: ventilation and perfusion lung scans. Posterior scans demonstrate normal ventilation (**A**), and numerous, mainly peripheral, defects of perfusion (**B**), characteristic of multiple pulmonary emboli. Such changes usually resolve over a period of several weeks.

A   B

protamine sulphate. Heparin therapy should be undertaken for 7–10 days. Thrombolytic therapy, most commonly used with massive pulmonary embolism (see below), is occasionally necessary when heparin treatment is inadequate, including cases with severe or extensive venous thrombosis, particularly when involving the inferior vena cava. Long-term anticoagulant therapy with warfarin is initiated 3–4 days before heparin therapy is stopped; warfarin treatment is continued for 3–6 months unless a chronic predisposing factor for deep venous thrombosis – for example, chronic venous insufficiency of the legs – indicates the need for prolonged therapy. If bleeding complicates warfarin therapy, treatment is with vitamin K_1. In pregnancy, and in patients in whom intravenous heparin therapy is particularly hazardous, subcutaneous heparin administered 12-hourly is the treatment of choice.

The resolution of pulmonary emboli is rapid, usually within 2–4 weeks. Heparin therapy is highly effective in preventing further thrombo-embolism.

MASSIVE PULMONARY EMBOLISM

Massive pulmonary embolism is a relatively rare hospital emergency since most patients with fatal pulmonary emboli die within 2 hours, frequently before reaching medical help. For those who survive beyond 2 hours, the outlook is good in most cases, provided they receive appropriate medical treatment. Surgical intervention is only rarely required.

Clinical features

The clinical features of massive pulmonary embolism reflect the haemodynamic consequences of obstruction to a large proportion of the pulmonary arterial tree; more than 60% obstruction is necessary to produce serious consequences in a previously healthy individual. Less extensive embolism will be life-threatening in patients with severe pre-existing cardiorespiratory disease. Following embolism, some of the increase in pulmonary vascular resistance may be due to vasoconstriction, secondary to the release of agents such as serotonin from thrombus. The dominant symptom of massive embolism is severe breathlessness. In some patients, there is central chest pain due to myocardial ischaemia, reflecting the combination of a massive increase in right ventricular oxygen requirements and reduction in coronary artery blood flow. Hypotension may cause syncope. Examination shows tachypnoea, tachycardia, hypotension and poor peripheral perfusion. Signs of pulmonary hypertension and right ventricular strain are not always present. The ECG is frequently unhelpful, with the most common abnormality, other than a tachycardia, being T wave changes. The main importance of the ECG is in the differential diagnosis from massive myocardial infarction. The chest X-ray is frequently normal or non-specifically abnormal. Oligaemia of the lung fields is helpful when present but can seldom be appreciated on emergency supine chest X-ray films.

Diagnosis and treatment

Therapy is urgent and potentially life-saving. If the diagnosis of massive pulmonary embolism is probable and the ECG does not suggest myocardial infarction, urgent investigations are required but immediate treatment with intravenous heparin (15 000 units) is reasonable. When hypotension is severe, inotropic support to the right ventricle is needed. In patients who have collapsed with massive pulmonary embolism, external cardiac massage can move clot peripherally and restore part of the pulmonary circulation. Patients have and require high right heart filling pressures, and treatment with diuretics and vasodilators, including morphine, is deleterious. If the patient is capable of co-operation and facilities are immediately available a ventilation–perfusion scan is performed. Indeed, a perfusion scan alone will be grossly abnormal and strongly support the diagnosis, provided the chest X-ray is clear. Patients who, for whatever reason, are unable to have isotope lung scans, require a pulmonary arteriogram, as do all patients for whom surgery is being considered. Pulmonary arteriograms normally demonstrate large central filling defects (Fig. 14.45).

Most patients who survive long enough to reach hospital, and who are then treated with intravenous heparin and inotropic support, rapidly improve. Following the confirmation of the diagnosis some are best treated with thrombolytic agents. Thrombolytic therapy achieves more rapid, and possibly more complete, resolution than intravenous heparin. Bleeding complications are, however, twice as likely than with heparin and thrombolytics should not be

Fig. 14.45 Massive pulmonary embolism. The pulmonary arteriogram shows a large filling defect in the right pulmonary artery, with almost no perfusion of the right lung, and little perfusion of the left lower lobe peripherally.

given if patients have active haemorrhage, a history of a recent cerebrovascular accident, recent surgery, recent organ biopsy or childbirth. Streptokinase is the thrombolytic agent most commonly used, but is antigenic. Urokinase is less antigenic but more costly. Thrombolytic agents are usually infused directly into the pulmonary artery.

A small number of patients with severe haemodynamic disturbance fail to improve on medical therapy and require embolectomy. Surgery is performed with the patients on cardiac bypass. It is critically important that the definitive diagnosis of massive pulmonary embolism has been substantiated prior to surgery and if so, the operative results are good (75% survival).

RECURRENT PULMONARY EMBOLISM

With adequate anticoagulation therapy recurrent pulmonary emboli are uncommon. Rarely anticoagulants are absolutely contra-indicated and in such patients, and also those with recurrent emboli despite full anticoagulant therapy, inferior vena caval sieves can be used. Such surgical procedures are not always effective, the inserted devices may become dislodged or blocked and indeed, may become a source of future emboli.

Repeated, often silent, pulmonary emboli can gradually obstruct a large proportion of the pulmonary vasculature and lead to pulmonary hypertension. Such patients may have a chronic low cardiac output state and intractable right heart failure. They have severe breathlessness, the cause for which is frequently not appreciated at first presentation. Any possibility of recurrent pulmonary emboli warrants comprehensive investigations including angiography. Anticoagulant therapy can prevent progression of the disease. When angiography demonstrates central filling defects, some cardiothoracic centres have produced benefit to patients by surgical removal of organised clot.

Prevention of venous thrombo-embolism

The prevention of pulmonary embolism is possible if high-risk patients for the development of deep vein thrombosis and therefore pulmonary emboli are recognised and suitable prophylaxis undertaken. The predisposing factors to thrombosis are stasis, vessel wall abnormalities, and increased coagulability of blood. Rarely, a haematological clotting abnormality predisposes to thrombosis, for example, hereditary antithrombin III deficiency. Patients at high risk include the elderly, patients with a past medical history of thrombosis, cardiac failure, immobility, malignancy, varicose veins, obesity, pregnancy (particularly post-partum) and lower limb orthopaedic surgery. Low-dose subcutaneous heparin (5000 units 12-hourly) is effective prophylaxis and has few complications unless patients are actively bleeding. In addition to older patients undergoing surgery, prophylaxis should be considered in any ill medical patients confined to bed, including patients recovering from myocardial infarction.

SARCOIDOSIS

First described by Hutchinson more than a century ago, sarcoidosis is a disease of unknown aetiology characterised by the involvement of more than one organ or tissue by non-caseating epithelioid cell granulomas which proceed either to resolution or to fibrosis. A more satisfactory definition of this disorder will only become possible when its cause is known.

Prevalence and distribution

Sarcoidosis is now recognised to be a worldwide disease which may present to all specialties and is relatively common. Worldwide, the prevalence is approximately 20 in 100 000. It is more common in temperate climates, American negroes, and West Indian and Irish immigrants to the UK, and is less common in Chinese and peoples of the Indian subcontinent. However, differences in incidence may reflect a difference in the awareness of the disease and the availability of diagnostic facilities, particularly radiology, and in many parts of the world the disorder has been frequently misdiagnosed as tuberculosis. Sarcoidosis is unusual in children and in the elderly and is most common between the ages of 20 and 40, with a slight female preponderance. In general, the disease is more florid in blacks than Caucasians.

Aetiology

The cause of sarcoidosis is not known. It is postulated that an as yet unidentified agent interacts with the host and produces a disease in which immunological factors are important (Fig. 14.46).

Many agents, including viruses, mycobacteria, fungi and pine pollen, have been considered as the cause of sarcoidosis but none has been substantiated. Inhalation is the most likely route for the causal agent and the sequence of events is probably one of alveolar injury and an influx of immune effector cells, followed by an inflammatory alveolitis. The alveolitis of sarcoidosis is predominantly lymphocytic (as shown by examination of lung tissue and broncho-alveolar lavage fluid), mostly activated T lymphocytes, with a reduction in circulating blood T lymphocytes. The increased lymphocytes in the lung are mostly T helper cells which are relatively depleted in peripheral blood. These changes may be responsible for the alveolitis, and partly explain the peripheral anergy of delayed type hypersensitivity of sarcoidosis.

Activated T lymphocytes secrete monocyte chemotactic factor, recruiting circulating monocytes and macrophages into the alveolitis, and lead to granuloma formation. Lymphocytes also activate macrophages to form the epithelioid and giant cells of granulomata. The metabolic activity of macrophages is associated with increased levels of angiotensin converting enzyme (ACE) in lung tissue, broncho-alveolar lavage fluid and serum. Whether the granulomata resolve or progress to fibrosis may be determined by the

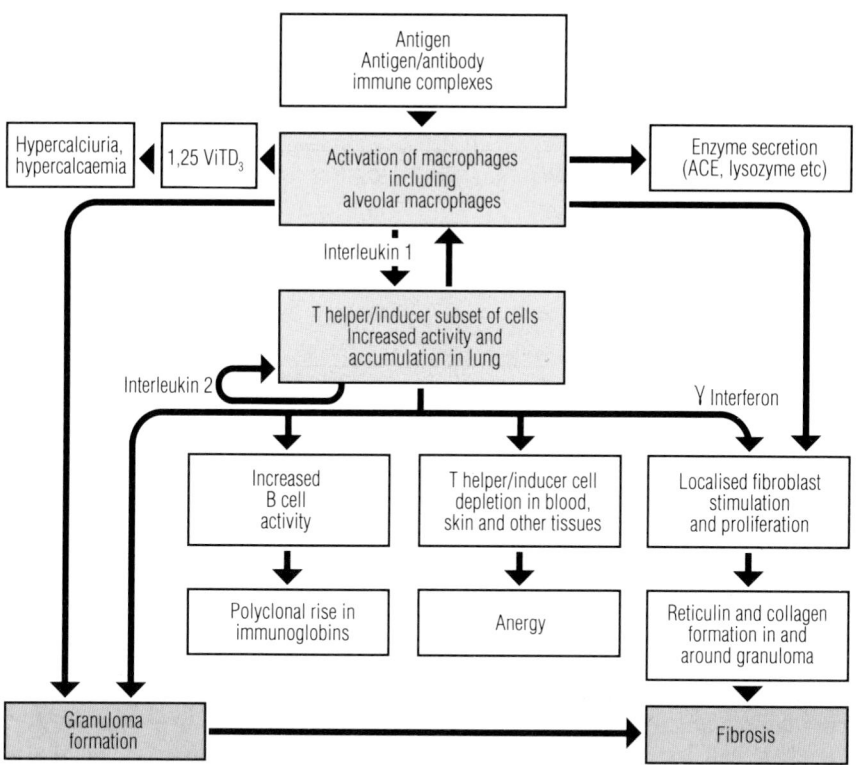

Fig. 14.46 Pathogenesis of sarcoidosis.

intensity of the alveolitis.

The increase in T cell activity stimulates B lymphocytes, which results in raised serum immunoglobulins, circulating antibodies, and immune complexes. Heredity may play a part in the predisposition to sarcoidosis and the condition is more common with some HLA groups.

The characteristic pathological finding of sarcoidosis is therefore granulomata that consist of collections of large histiocytes (epithelioid cells) with occasional multi-nucleated giant cells, and, more peripherally, lymphocytes (T8-suppressor cells). There is no central necrosis, a point of contrast to tuberculosis, and the reticulin between the histiocytes is, therefore, intact. In the lung the granulomata are in the interstitium but can be peribronchial. Non-caseating granulomata are not specific for sarcoidosis and can occur in other disorders (Table 14.33). Sarcoid granulomata are dynamic entities developing, ageing and resolving. In chronic cases the granulomata are replaced by hyalinisation and fibrosis.

Clinical features

Since sarcoidosis can affect virtually all organs and tissues of the body, with the probable exception of the adrenal glands, the clinical features of this disorder are varied (Table 14.34). The lungs, eye and skin are most frequently involved, with more than 85% having some degree of pulmonary involvement, and many cases are diagnosed following a routine chest X-ray. Eye involvement can cause blindness, and important causes of death (2% of all cases) are respiratory, cardiac and renal failure.

Table 14.33 Causes of non-caseating granulomata

Sarcoidosis	Berylliosis
Tuberculosis	Foreign body reactions
Primary biliary cirrhosis	Cat scratch disease
Leprosy	Hypersensitivity pneumonitis
Tertiary syphilis	Granulomatous arteritides
Brucellosis	Lymphomas
Hypogammaglobulinaemia	Carcinoma (regional lymph node)
Fungal infection	Crohn's disease

Table 14.34 Clinical spectrum of sarcoidosis in the United Kingdom

Clinical feature	% of cases
Liver biopsy positive with bilateral hilar adenopathy	80–90
Abnormal chest X-ray (lung involvement ± hilar or mediastinal adenopathy)	>85
Erythema nodosum	20–30
Lymphadenopathy	10–15
Palpable splenomegaly	6
Eye involvement	15–25
Skin sarcoid	5–20
Enlargement of parotid/lachrymal/other salivary glands	5–20
Symptomatic nervous system involvement	5
Bone cysts	3–8
Symptomatic heart disease	<5
Symptomatic myopathy	<1

Table 14.35 Classification of thoracic sarcoid

Stage	Description of chest X-ray	Stage at presentation (%)	Elevated ACE levels (%)	Positive transbronchial lung biopsy (%)	Positive Kveim test (%)	Positive liver biopsy (%)
0	Normal	8	30	–	50	–
I	Hilar adenopathy	51	56	65–80	70	85
II	Hilar adenopathy plus parenchymal infiltrate	29	71	75–100	80	65
III	Parenchymal infiltrate ±fibrosis	12	56	75–85	40	60

Thoracic sarcoidosis

The chest X-ray is abnormal in more than 85% of cases of sarcoidosis and the radiological appearances form the basis for the classification of thoracic sarcoid (Table 14.35).

Stage I

Hilar adenopathy is usually bilateral and symmetrical, but can be unilateral. Adenopathy is the commonest manifestation of thoracic sarcoidosis and more than half of patients have no symptoms. In addition to enlargement of hilar glands, the right paratracheal gland is frequently enlarged (Fig. 14.47). Bilateral hilar adenopathy can also occur in other disorders (Table 14.36).

In up to 40% of stage I cases there is also erythema nodosum, and in the UK 80% of cases of erythema nodosum in young adults are due to sarcoidosis. In association with bilateral hilar adenopathy and erythema nodosum there is commonly low-grade fever, poly-

Table 14.36 Differential diagnosis of bilateral hilar adenopathy

Sarcoidosis*	Beryllium disease
Tuberculosis	Hypogammaglobulinaemia
Lymphoma	Histoplasmosis
Leukaemia	Coccidioidomycosis
Metastatic malignant disease	Enlargement of pulmonary arteries

* Compared with sarcoidosis, all other causes of bilateral hilar adenopathy are uncommon.

arthralgia and a raised erythrocyte sedimentation rate (ESR).

Although few patients have severe symptoms with stage I sarcoidosis a minority have cough and chest pain due to adenopathy. Bilateral hilar adenopathy, with and without erythema nodosum, is usually benign, with 80% of cases resolving in less than 12 months and 90% by 2 years. In 10% of cases, glandular enlargement persists and eggshell calcification may develop, or patients may develop pulmonary opacities. Patients with bilateral hilar lymphadenopathy without erythema nodosum probably do rather less well, with up to 20% developing a pulmonary infiltrate.

Stage II

Pulmonary infiltrates co-exist with adenopathy in about 30% of patients (Fig. 14.48).

More severely affected patients have a restrictive ventilatory defect with exertional breathlessness and a reduction in gas transfer. The chest X-ray appearances correlate poorly with physiological disturbances, the patient being frequently asymptomatic, despite widespread pulmonary shadowing. The prognosis for stage II sarcoidosis is less good than for stage I. Although 50% resolve spontaneously within 2 years, some take longer, 30–40% require steroid therapy and in 10–15% long-term steroid therapy is required, despite which a small number develop progressive pulmonary fibrosis. The differential diagnosis of stage II and stage III sarcoidosis is shown in Table 14.37.

Fig. 14.47 Stage I sarcoidosis. There is bilateral hilar lymphadenopathy (BHL) and also enlargement of the right paratracheal nodes, characteristic of sarcoidosis.

Fig. 14.48 Stage II sarcoidosis. The X-ray shows florid stage II sarcoidosis, with bilateral hilar lymphadenopathy (BHL) and extensive pulmonary infiltrates.

Table 14.37 Differential diagnosis of stage II and stage III sarcoidosis

Cryptogenic fibrosing alveolitis	Bronchopulmonary aspergillosis
Pulmonary tuberculosis	Ankylosing spondylitis
Extrinsic allergic alveolitis	Berylliosis
Carcinoma	Histiocytosis X
Pneumoconiosis	

Stage III

With the development of pulmonary fibrosis, patients become breathless, hypoxic and ultimately develop cor pulmonale. Pulmonary function tests demonstrate a severe restrictive ventilatory defect. In addition to fibrosis, which is characteristically most marked in the mid- and upper zones, the chest X-ray may also show cavitation and bullae formation. As would be expected, the prognosis for stage III sarcoidosis is less good, with about 30% showing significant improvement with steroid therapy.

Extrathoracic sarcoidosis

Skin

Erythema nodosum is the most common skin abnormality, and is associated with acute, usually stage I, sarcoidosis. When there is erythema nodosum and bilateral hilar lymphadenopathy in a young adult, a clinical diagnosis of sarcoidosis can be firmly made without resort to tissue biopsy. Erythema nodosum is an immunological response associated with sarcoidosis and skin biopsy demonstrates a characteristic histology, which is the same as for other causes of erythema nodosum (p. 1129). Sarcoid tissue itself can also infiltrate the skin, and biopsy shows typical non-caseating granulomata. Small papules, plaques and subcutaneous nodules are common, and the skin of the nose may be involved (lupus pernio), as are scars and keloid tissue. When there is lupus pernio the upper respiratory tract is frequently involved by the disease and nasal mucosal biopsy is positive. Skin sarcoid more commonly affects females and is more common, extensive and florid in blacks.

Eyes

Eye involvement is both common (up to 25% of cases) and potentially serious. Early eye involvement may be asymptomatic and all patients should be examined by an ophthalmologist. Uveitis, conjunctivitis and retinal involvement can all occur. Dry eyes (keratoconjunctivitis sicca) occurs in a Sjögren-like syndrome when the salivary glands are involved. The lachrymal, salivary and parotid glands may be enlarged. Eye involvement is an indication for steroid therapy, usually systemic.

Hypercalciuria

Hypercalciuria has, in the past, been reported in up to 60% of patients with sarcoidosis, of which as many as 11% have been reported to have hypercalcaemia. However, more recent series have suggested that these disorders of calcium metabolism are less common. The dangers of hypercalciuria and hypercalcaemia are nephrocalcinosis, with renal failure, and renal stones. The abnormality in calcium homeostasis is enhanced calcium absorption from the gut due to increased calcitriol production by the sarcoid granulomas. There is a hypersensitivity to vitamin D and hypercalcaemia may be revealed as a problem in some patients only when they spend time in sunny climates. Occasionally, hypercalcaemia may be sufficiently chronic to produce corneal calcification. Hypercalcaemia responds rapidly to oral steroids.

Lymphadenopathy

Enlarged lymph nodes are present in 10–15% of patients and splenomegaly occurs in 6%, both abnormalities being more common in blacks. Occasionally, the spleen is very large and associated with anaemia, neutropenia and thrombocytopenia, which may improve following splenectomy.

Cardiac sarcoid

Involvement of the myocardium by granulomatous infiltration may be relatively common, up to 25%, but is usually localised and asymptomatic. More extensive involvement causes conduction defects, arrhythmias and cardiac failure. A 24-hour ECG tape can be a particularly useful investigation. Early cardiac involvement responds well to steroids but the prognosis for extensive involvement is poor. In some patients the heart may be the only organ clinically affected and a careful search is necessary to establish evidence for sarcoidosis of other organs and tissues.

Nervous system

Sarcoid tissue within the nervous system occurs in approximately 5% of patients and can give rise to meningitis, encephalitis, hydrocephalus, pituitary involvement, space-occupying lesions, cranial nerve palsies and a peripheral neuropathy. Facial nerve palsy is the most common neurological manifestation and sometimes resolves with steroid treatment. With the less common neurological problems there may be little evidence of sarcoidosis elsewhere and diagnosis is difficult. CT and magnetic resonance imaging (MRI) may help. Neurological sarcoidosis is often chronic, and has a poor prognosis, despite steroid therapy. Involvement of the hypothalamus and the posterior pituitary can, rarely, cause diabetes insipidus, hypothyroidism and other hypothalamic syndromes.

Bone sarcoidosis

Arthritis, acute and transient, is common with bilateral hilar lymphadenopathy and erythema nodosum, but chronic skeletal problems are unusual (3%), characteristically affecting hands and feet in patients with skin sarcoidosis. Bone cysts, especially of the terminal phalanges, are most typical. Steroids have little effect and bone lesions are usually confined to cases of chronic sarcoidosis. Sarcoid involvement of muscle is usually asymptomatic but occasionally patients have myopathic symptoms.

Diagnosis

Chest X-ray and transbronchial lung biopsy give the diagnosis in the majority of patients. Biopsy of any clinically involved tissue will confirm the diagnosis and a liver biopsy will be positive in 85% of patients. Frequently, the most important differential diagnosis is between sarcoidosis and tuberculosis and tissue should, therefore, be stained for acid-fast bacilli and cultured for mycobacterium tuberculosis. In cases where biopsy is relatively difficult (e.g. hilar adenopathy) or negative, a diagnosis of sarcoidosis can be substantiated by the Kveim test. A suspension of particulate human sarcoid tissue is injected intradermally and in patients with active sarcoidosis epithelioid cell granulomata gradually develop and can be demonstrated following skin biopsy of the purplish red nodule at 4 weeks. A positive Kveim test strongly suggests a diagnosis of sarcoidosis (false positives 1–2%). However, the Kveim test is not always positive in sarcoidosis and there is a relatively high false negative rate in chronic fibrotic disease.

Depression of delayed type hypersensitivity in sarcoidosis reduces tuberculin reactivity. Two-thirds of patients do not react to 100 tuberculin units and more than 90% fail to react to 10 tuberculin units. A depressed tuberculin reaction persists for many years, long after clinical resolution of sarcoidosis. In the differential diagnosis of sarcoidosis and tuberculosis, the tuberculin test is of great value; indeed, a positive tuberculin reaction in a patient with sarcoidosis previously demonstrated to be tuberculin negative strongly suggests the additional development of tuberculosis.

Management

Assessment of the severity and activity of disease

Following the diagnosis of sarcoidosis, patient management, particularly the decision of whether to treat with steroids, will depend on an assessment of the severity of the illness and its activity. Although the symptoms and signs are the main guide to management, further investigations are necessary and helpful in decision-making.

Radiology

Chest X-rays provide a crude index of the extent of thoracic sarcoidosis and the correlation between radiological findings and functional impairment is poor. However, serial chest X-rays over months and years remain indispensable for documenting qualitative changes that occur either spontaneously or in response to therapy.

Serum angiotensin converting enzyme

Serum angiotensin converting enzyme (SACE) levels are high with acute granulomatous disease and correlate with chest X-ray abnormalities. However, not all patients with sarcoidosis have raised SACE levels and conversely, some patients without sarcoid (perhaps up to 20%) can have high levels. SACE is a pointer towards the diagnosis of sarcoidosis, but not an absolute test. Although the correlation of SACE with the extent of alveolitis on lung biopsy or the T lymphocyte count of broncho-alveolar lavage is not particularly good, SACE is nevertheless useful in monitoring granulomatous activity and the response to steroid therapy.

Broncho-alveolar lavage

In normal subjects, broncho-alveolar lavage (BAL) usually shows less than 10% lymphocytes, whereas in sarcoidosis, average figures for lymphocyte counts are 30% with up to 50–60% in florid, acute disease. However, there is an overlap of the cell count in sarcoidosis with those in normal subjects, particularly smokers, as well as in patients with extrinsic allergic alveolitis, lymphomas and cryptogenic fibrosing alveolitis. The findings of an increased number of lymphocytes therefore favours, rather than proves, a diagnosis of sarcoidosis. Serial examination of BAL fluid can provide useful information on the intensity of the alveolitis and the response to treatment. In advanced fibrotic disease lymphocytosis is not a feature and there may be an increased number of polymorphonuclear leukocytes.

Gallium scanning

Gallium is taken up by activated macrophages and gallium scans have been used to delineate the sites involved in sarcoidosis and to assess disease activity. Uptake is increased in a variety of interstitial lung diseases as well as pulmonary tumours. Gallium uptake is increased in 65–70% of all patients with sarcoidosis and appears to reflect the intensity of the alveolitis. The correlation of gallium uptake with symptoms, radiological changes and pulmonary function abnormalities is poor. The definitive role of gallium scanning in the management of sarcoidosis awaits further study.

Lung function tests

The correlation between chest X-ray appearances and pulmonary function is poor. Pulmonary sarcoidosis leads to a restrictive ventilatory defect with a reduction in lung volumes, pulmonary compliance and gas transfer. The most sensitive index of impaired pulmonary function is abnormal gas transfer, which may be reduced even in stage I disease. Some patients with sarcoidosis have an obstructive defect due to endobronchial disease (confirmed by bronchoscopy and bronchial biopsy and improved by steroid therapy) or to airway distortion from fibrosis. With moderate or severe disease, patients may be hypoxic at rest and in mild disease there is hypoxia on exertion. Pulmonary function testing is essential in the assessment of sarcoidosis and repeated measurements are of great value in long-term management.

Treatment

The known effects of steroids on immunological mechanisms suggest that these drugs would be helpful in suppressing the immunologically mediated alveolitis of sarcoidosis and, indeed, patients with acute florid disease appear to respond rapidly. However, given the natural history towards resolution in most patients with sarcoidosis it has proved difficult to demonstrate the long-term value of these drugs. Since most physicians would not be prepared to leave severely symptomatic patients without oral steroids, a prospective controlled trial is not possible. In most patients the short-term effect of steroids is to improve symptoms, suppress inflammation and granuloma production and lower SACE levels. Prednisolone at a dosage of 30–40 mg daily, with a gradual reduction towards the minimum dose that controls disease activity, frequently 7.5–10.0 mg daily, is normally prescribed. Treatment with steroids is indicated whenever vital organs are severely involved or when there is substantial systemic disturbance (Table 14.38).

Alternative immunosuppressive agents (i.e. methotrexate, azathioprine or cyclosporin) may be used for chronic disease, particularly chronic skin infiltration, but there is no evidence that these agents are superior to oral steroids.

Prognosis

Approximately 60% of all patients with thoracic sarcoidosis resolve spontaneously, and have a normal chest X-ray, mostly within 2 years. A further 20% will resolve with steroid therapy which can then be discontinued.

Table 14.38 Indications for steroid treatment in sarcoidosis

Eye involvement

Severe chest X-ray changes (stage II and stage III disease) associated with a high serum angiotensin converting enzyme

Intense alveolitis on broncho-alveolar lavage

Breathlessness

Hypercalcaemia and hypercalciuria

Severe skin infiltration

Severe involvement of the upper respiratory tract

Cardiac involvement

Nervous system involvement

Salivary gland involvement

These patients have an acute or subacute type of the disease, clearly associated with a good prognosis. For the minority 10–20% with chronic disease, resolution, even with steroid therapy, is less likely, with radiographic clearing in about 50% who have stage II and 20% who have stage III disease. Patients with chronic pulmonary sarcoidosis may eventually develop pulmonary fibrosis and respiratory failure. Although only a small percentage of patients with sarcoidosis die of the condition, most of these deaths are from pulmonary fibrosis and respiratory failure. Chronic extrathoracic sarcoidosis often responds poorly to treatment. Central nervous system involvement is particularly chronic and poorly responsive to steroid therapy.

CONNECTIVE TISSUE DISEASES AND THE LUNG

Systemic lupus erythematosus (SLE)

Pleurisy is common in systemic lupus erythematosus, affecting 50% of patients, with effusions in approximately 30%. An acute pulmonary vasculitis can cause widespread pneumonitis in about 10% of cases, sometimes leaving a residual basal atelectasis. Interstitial fibrosis is unusual. Not uncommonly patients develop small-volume lungs, the cause of which is unknown. In patients with the SLE-like syndrome characterised by the presence of anti-cardiolipin antibodies, thrombotic obliteration of the pulmonary vasculature can lead to pulmonary hypertension and severe breathlessness.

Mixed connective tissue disease

Mixed connective tissue disease (MCTD) is a syndrome composed of features of SLE, polymyositis, rheumatoid arthritis and scleroderma; it is not infrequently complicated by pulmonary involvement including pleurisy, pulmonary fibrosis and pulmonary hypertension secondary to vascular involvement.

Rheumatoid arthritis

The most common pulmonary manifestation of rheumatoid arthritis is a *pleural effusion* (p. 530) which at some stage affects up to 30% of patients, most frequently middle-aged or elderly males. Although patients with pleurisy usually have active nodular disease and a high serum rheumatoid factor titre, pleural involvement can predate arthritis. Effusions are usually small. The aspirated pleural fluid has a low glucose content (p. 533). Treatment for rheumatoid effusions is seldom necessary, but if so, steroids frequently lead to resolution. *Pulmonary fibrosis* associated with rheumatoid arthritis is clinically indistinguishable from cryptogenic fibrosing alveolitis (p. 516) and may progress to disabling breathlessness. In large series of patients with fibrosing alveolitis, evidence of rheumatoid arthritis is not uncommon (10%), but in patients with rheumatoid arthritis the complication of fibrosing lung disease is unusual (1–2%). Diffuse pulmonary disease has also been reported as a complication of the treatment of rheumatoid arthritis with penicillamine, gold and immunosuppressive agents. Rheumatoid *pulmonary nodules* may be single or multiple and can occasionally cavitate. Patients usually also have subcutaneous nodules and the histology of both is the same. In patients with pneumoconiosis and rheumatoid arthritis, large diffuse nodules combined with fibrosis can develop (Caplan's syndrome). Occasionally a rheumatoid nodule is difficult to distinguish from a pulmonary tumour. Needle aspiration biopsy can confirm malignancy but a definitive diagnosis of a rheumatoid nodule may require excision biopsy at thoracotomy. Patients with rheumatoid arthritis can develop a vasculitis affecting the pulmonary vasculature and, rarely, an obliterative bronchiolitis.

Systemic sclerosis

The most common pulmonary manifestation of systemic sclerosis is pulmonary fibrosis, and pleurisy is unusual. Occasionally, pulmonary vascular disease occurs in the absence of parenchymal abnormalities, leading to pulmonary hypertension. Aspiration, with consequent pneumonitis, infection and bronchiectasis, is not uncommon in systemic sclerosis.

Pneumonitis and fibrosing alveolitis can occur in Sjögren's syndrome and dermatomyositis. In dermatomyositis muscle weakness can be a major factor contributing to breathlessness.

VASCULITIDES AND THE LUNG

Wegener's granulomatosis

In Wegener's granulomatosis, described by Wegener in 1936, the characteristic pathology is a necrotising granulomatous arteritis of the upper and lower respiratory tract and also of the kidney, where it causes a focal and segmental glomerulonephritis. Upper respiratory tract mani-

Fig. 14.49 Wegener's granulomatosis. There are large, irregular, central nodular shadows in both mid-zones, rather characteristic of Wegener's. Lesions commonly cavitate.

festations, particularly sinusitis and ulceration of the nasal mucosa, is a common presentation, but unlike midline granulomatous disease there is no facial ulceration. In Wegener's, middle-aged males are most frequently affected. Increasing breathlessness, haemoptysis and pleurisy occur with pulmonary involvement, which is present in 95% of cases. In most cases, there is a low-grade pyrexia. In contrast to polyarteritis nodosa, hypertension is unusual. Wegener's granulomatosis is a multisystem disease and the widespread vasculitis may affect eyes, skin, joints, heart and the nervous system. In most instances it is the renal involvement, present in 85% of cases, that is critical. The chest X-ray shows nodules which are commonly bilateral (Fig. 14.49), and which may be large and cavitate. Mediastinal or hilar adenopathy is rare. Endobronchial disease may be visible at bronchoscopy.

In Wegener's, the ESR is greatly raised and the platelet count may also be elevated. Eosinophilia is not a feature. The diagnosis is a clinical one (suggested by disease of the upper as well as the lower respiratory tract and by renal involvement), supported by tissue biopsy demonstrating characteristic histology. Open lung biopsy gives the highest diagnostic yield but the diagnosis is often possible by biopsy of more accessible structures such as the skin or upper airway mucosa. Renal biopsy confirms kidney involvement but the tissue obtained is commonly not diagnostic of Wegener's. A positive antineutrophil cytoplasmic antibody test (ANCA) strongly supports the diagnosis. Without treatment 80% of patients die within one year, the advancing renal disease being the major determinant of survival. Treatment with cyclophosphamide (1–2 mg/kg per day), initially combined with steroids (prednisolone, 60 mg daily), is often remarkably effective. Long-term remission is achieved by such therapy in up to 90% of patients, and in some cases with severe chronic renal impairment successful renal transplantation has been undertaken.

Midline granuloma

This is a rare disease, now thought to be a T cell lymphoma, in which there is destruction of the tissues of the nose and upper respiratory tract. The characteristic pathology is of granulomata; patients are most often middle-aged females. Nasal involvement is the most striking feature, with the development of septal perforation and saddle nose deformity. The disease is localised (unlike Wegener's) and there is no arteritis. Without treatment the disease is fatal. The treatment of choice is local radiotherapy and steroids are not helpful.

Polyarteritis nodosum

Pulmonary involvement in classical polyarteritis nodosa is unusual, but is a feature of the variant of polyarteritis known as allergic granulomatosis or the Churg-Strauss syndrome (p. 493), characterised by a necrotising vasculitis, granuloma formation, eosinophilia and asthma. Treatment is with high-dose steroids, and cyclophosphamide if necessary.

Pulmonary involvement occurs in many other systemic vasculitides including giant cell arteritis, Behçet's, Henoch-Schönlein purpura, hypersensitivity vasculitis (usually drug-induced) and lymphatoid granulomatosis.

PULMONARY FIBROSIS AND DIFFUSE INTERSTITIAL LUNG DISEASE

Fibrosis of the lung parenchyma can be:

1. *replacement fibrosis*, following infective processes such as lung abscesses, bronchiectasis, tuberculosis or occasionally from infarction
2. *focal fibrosis*, which is the hallmark of lung disease due to inhaled inorganic dusts (pneumoconioses)
3. *interstitial fibrosis*, as a consequence of interstitial lung diseases such as extrinsic allergic alveolitis, cryptogenic fibrosing alveolitis, sarcoidosis, histiocytosis X, chronic pulmonary oedema and iatrogenic lung disease.

Focal and interstitial fibrosis are characteristic of a number of specific pulmonary disorders (Table 14.39).

Clinical features of pulmonary fibrosis

The conditions which cause diffuse pulmonary fibrosis share many clinical, radiological and pathophysiological features. The common presenting symptom is dyspnoea, which is mild at first but can progress to total incapacity. Very often a persistent dry cough, particularly at night, is a

Table 14.39 Causes of pulmonary fibrosis

Inhalation of dust or chemicals
Organic dusts (e.g. avian proteins, moulds)
Mineral dusts (e.g. asbestos, silica, coal dust)
Chemicals (e.g. nitrogen dioxide, chlorine)

Unknown causes
Cryptogenic fibrosing alveolitis (syn. diffuse pulmonary fibrosis, idiopathic pulmonary fibrosis, usual or organising interstitial pneumonia)
Sarcoidosis
Idiopathic haemosiderosis
Histiocytosis X (Letterer-Siwe disease, Hand-Schuller-Christian disease, eosinophilic granuloma)

Iatrogenic and poisoning
Drugs (e.g. bleomycin, hydralazine, busulphan)
Paraquat
Radiation pneumonitis
Oxygen toxicity

Pulmonary involvement in systemic disease
Rheumatoid arthritis
Ankylosing spondylitis
Systemic sclerosis
Sjögren's syndrome
Dermatomyositis

Congenital
Niemann-Pick disease
Gaucher's disease
Tuberous sclerosis
Neurofibromatosis

feature. There may be symptoms of an associated systemic syndrome, including fever and weight loss during the acute phase. On examination, the patient may have few physical signs outside the chest. However, when fibrosis is widespread there may be tachypnoea, cyanosis and, at a late stage, cor pulmonale. There may be finger clubbing, especially in patients with cryptogenic fibrosing alveolitis and asbestosis. Auscultation of the chest usually reveals predominantly basal inspiratory crackles but there are exceptions (see below). The chest X-ray in the early stages shows a hazy, nodular infiltrate. As the lungs become more fibrotic, cystic spaces become evident and a 'honeycomb' pattern, sometimes with large bullae, develops.

Lung function tests show a restrictive ventilatory defect (p. 455), reduced transfer factor and hypoxaemia.

OCCUPATIONAL LUNG DISEASE

The lung can be injured by the inhalation of dusts, fumes or other noxious substances at work in certain specific occupations. There are strict criteria for the diagnosis of these conditions and for determining the level of compensation.

Pulmonary damage can occur in several ways:

1. *mechanical effects of dust retention*
2. *fibrogenesis* (e.g. coal dust, silica)
3. *granulomatous reactions* (e.g. berylliosis)
4. *toxicity* (e.g. mercury vapour)

5. *irritation of air passages* (e.g. chlorine)
6. *promotion of bronchial hyper-reactivity* (e.g. occupational asthma in laboratory workers who become hypersensitive to animal fur or urine).

Important occupational lung diseases include those due to *inorganic dusts* (e.g. silica, talc, asbestos, tin, iron); those due to *organic dusts* (e.g. cotton dust, maple bark dust) and those due to *gases and fumes* (e.g. chlorine, ammonia). Occupational exposure can also cause asthma, and lung and pleural malignancy.

Pneumoconioses due to inorganic dust inhalation

The common pneumoconioses are listed in Table 14.40.

Table 14.40   The common pneumoconioses

Disease	Occupation	Cause	Pathology
Coal miners' pneumoconiosis	Coal mining	Coal dust	Nodular and progressive massive fibrosis
Silicosis	Mining, quarrying, metal grinding, stone dressing, etc.	Silica	Focal fibrosis, centrilobular emphysema, progressive massive fibrosis, associated tuberculosis
Asbestosis	Demolition workers, shipbreaking, lagging and brake lining manufacture, etc.	Asbestos	Focal fibrosis, pleural calcification, bronchial carcinoma, pleural mesothelioma
Berylliosis	Electronics, atomic energy reactors, aero-engines	Beryllium	Granulomata and interstitial fibrosis
Talcosis	Rubber industry	Magnesium silicate	Focal fibrosis
Stannosis	Smelting	Tin oxide	Mineral deposition
Siderosis	Arc welding	Iron oxide	Mineral deposition

Coal miners' pneumoconiosis

Inhalation of coal dust over a prolonged period damages the lung. The incidence varies with the type of coal being mined, occurring in about 12% of all miners but up to 50% in those who have mined anthracite for more than 20 years. For certification for compensation the diagnosis is radiological, not clinical. In the disease's early form, these radiological changes consist of small nodules less than 1.5 mm in diameter; this early form is termed *simple*

Fig. 14.50   Pneumoconiosis. There are widespread nodular changes of coal worker's pneumoconiosis plus the large lesions of progressive massive fibrosis (PMF).

pneumoconiosis. In a proportion of cases the nodules grow up to 10 mm in size, are irregular, and form large masses which may cavitate, commonly in the upper lobes: this is referred to as *complicated pneumoconiosis* or *progressive massive fibrosis* (Fig. 14.50).

About 15% of patients have positive antinuclear factor and in a small number, active rheumatoid arthritis is present. This is *Caplan's syndrome* and the chest X-ray shows rounded peripheral nodules in the lung fields 0.5–5.0 cm in diameter. First described in coal miners, the same appearances have since been seen in other forms of pneumoconiosis.

Silicosis

Although now less common as a result of protective measures, silicosis is still a major occupational hazard because of the ubiquitous distribution of free silica. Silicosis results from the inhalation of fine particles of silicon dioxide crystals or quartz particles. Those involved in mining, quarrying, metal casting, sandblasting and the pottery industry are at risk. Inhalation can cause an acute febrile illness with rapidly progressive dyspnoea and cyanosis which can occur after a short exposure and lead to death in a few weeks. This acute syndrome is rare. The more common chronic form of the disease is due to the highly fibrogenic potential of silica and presents as slowly progressive dyspnoea and cough, occasionally with haemoptysis. Co-existing tuberculosis is not uncommon. The disease may progress even after exposure ceases. The radiological appearances are of upper zone fibrosis with characteristic hilar 'eggshell' calcification.

Asbestos-related disease

Asbestos is the generic name for several silicates including chrysolite (90% of all world asbestos), crocidolite (blue asbestos), osmosite and anthopyllate. Fibres persist in the lung long after inhalation and cause characteristic pathological changes. Those at high risk include demolition workers, pipe laggers, brake lining industry workers and boiler makers. The respiratory effects of asbestos are a progressive pulmonary fibrosis (asbestosis), pleural plaques, and malignancy of the lung and pleura.

Asbestosis presents as progressive dyspnoea and cough, with finger clubbing and basal crackles. Like the other pneumoconioses it may progress to respiratory failure. Asbestos fibres are inhaled and phagocytosed, causing damage to cell membranes and the release of lysosomal enzymes. Radiologically there may be basal linear and irregular shadows which in the later stages spread to 'honeycombing' throughout the lung fields with an indistinct heart border (Fig. 14.51). Lung function testing shows a restrictive defect with reduced transfer factor. There are usually 'asbestos bodies' in the sputum or bronchial washings.

Pleural plaques are an indication of previous exposure to asbestos. They do not indicate lung disease or any increased risk over similarly exposed subjects of developing a tumour. They are usually basal or diaphragmatic and frequently calcify. CT scanning of the thorax is very useful in picking up early lesions, demonstrating the extent of pleural involvement, and distinguishing pleural from parenchymal disease.

Fig. 14.51 Asbestosis. Bilateral pulmonary fibrosis of asbestosis. There is also pleural thickening, best seen adjacent to the lateral chest wall on the left and diaphragmatic pleural calcification on the right.

Bronchogenic carcinoma is the most common tumour caused by asbestos exposure; cigarette smoking in asbestos workers greatly increases the risk, exerting a multiplicative rather than an additive effect. The tumours are usually adeno- or squamous cell carcinomas. Mesotheliomas of pleura and peritoneum are associated with asbestos exposure. Eighty per cent of patients with mesothelioma will have had some (although not necessarily much) asbestos exposure 20–30 years before the tumour appears, crocidolite asbestos being the most dangerous (p. 537).

Berylliosis

Berylliosis differs from other pneumoconioses in that the initial pathological response to inhaling beryllium is a granulomatous one, which progresses to fibrosis. Histologically it may be difficult to distinguish from sarcoidosis. It can occasionally cause an acute pneumonic type of illness. Those at risk include workers in the atomic power and aero-engine industry.

Other inorganic dusts

Other inorganic dusts vary in their ability to generate fibrosis; iron and iron oxides in arc welding and silver finishing (siderosis), and tin oxide in smelting (stannosis) are relatively non-fibrogenic, whereas magnesium silicate in the rubber industry (talcosis) can be a potent cause of fibrosis. Other dusts cause mucus hypersecretion and airway irritation with or without pneumonitis, e.g. cement, graphite, cadmium and many others.

EXTRINSIC ALLERGIC ALVEOLITIS

This group of conditions is caused by the inhalation of *organic* dusts (Table 14.41). Chronic exposure to dusts which contain antigen sensitises the individual, a precipitating antibody is produced, and granulomata appear in the lung. These granulomata heal by fibrosis.

Clinically, the patient may present with an acute illness 6–8 hours after heavy antigen exposure, with fever, "flu-like' symptoms, cough, dyspnoea and crackles. These resolve spontaneously in 24–48 hours if there is no further antigen exposure. The clinical features reflect the pathogenic mechanism, which is primarily an IgG-mediated 'late' type III hypersensitivity or Arthus' reaction to the antigen, although there is probably also a cell-mediated response. The result of repeated exposure is granuloma formation and eventually extensive fibrosis. More commonly the presentation is with established fibrosis, with dyspnoea and dry cough. Finger clubbing is uncommon, in marked contrast with cryptogenic fibrosing alveolitis. Inspiratory crackles and squeaks are characteristic. Radiologically, the changes are predominantly upper zone, with nodular and linear shadows (Fig. 14.52) and volume loss. Lung function tests show reduction in lung volumes and transfer factor. Precipitating antibodies are present in the blood and intradermal skin tests, read at 6 hours, are avail-

14

Table 14.41 Some causes of extrinisic allergic alveolitis

Type	Disease	Source	Antigen
From fungi	Farmer's lung	Mouldy hay	Micropolyspora faeni Thermoactino- mycetes vulgaris Thermoactino- mycetes sacherii
	Mushroom worker's lung	Mushroom compost	
	Bagassosis	Mouldy bagasse	
	Ventilator pneumonitis	Air conditioning and hot air systems	
	Malt worker's lung	Mouldy barley	Aspergillus clavatus
	Maple bark stripper's lung	Mouldy maple bark	Cryptostroma (coniosporium corticale)
From birds	Bird fancier's lung	Pigeon/budgerigar/ hen/parrot droppings	Avian serum proteins in droppings
From mammals	Pituitary snuff taker's lung	Porcine pituitary powder	Serum protein/pituitary antigens
	Rat handler's lung	Rat droppings	Rat serum protein

able for some of the causes and are especially useful in the diagnosis of bird fancier's lung. Bronchial challenge tests, with measurement of temperature, lung volumes and gas transfer, are occasionally valuable.

The treatment of these conditions is firstly to stop exposure to the antigen. For the acute type of allergic alveolitis this is usually sufficient. However, when chronic exposure has led to granulomatous change in the lung, treatment with corticosteroids is required. In advanced fibrotic disease, as with all end-stage fibrotic lung diseases, there is little that can be done apart from considering heart–lung transplantation.

CRYPTOGENIC FIBROSING ALVEOLITIS

Cryptogenic fibrosing alveolitis (CFA), of unknown aetiology, is characterised pathologically by migration of large mononuclear cells into the alveolar spaces with later thickening of alveolar walls, with fibrosis. The mononuclear cellular response is associated with acute symptoms, whereas the alveolar thickening and fibrosis is responsible for the more chronic clinical picture.

The pathogenesis of the condition is poorly understood. It is considered to be an altered state of host-responsiveness to an as yet unknown stimulus. An alteration of cell-mediated immunity has been proposed, since stimulated T lymphocytes increase fibroblastic activity. Activation of complement with consequent leucocyte aggregation may play a part. The pathological picture that emerges is, at first, an intra-alveolar inflammatory response, with many mononuclear cells and an increase in reticulin, collagen and elastin. As the disease progresses, there is fibrosis and destruction of lung architecture, with formation of cystic spaces.

Characteristically, CFA is a disease of late middle age, which affects males twice as frequently as females. The acute variant of the disease may present with rapidly progressive dyspnoea and cough, widespread crackles, and progressive respiratory failure within a few months. The chronic (and much more common) form presents with dyspnoea and dry cough, and in approximately 20% of cases, polyarthralgia. About two-thirds of the patients have finger clubbing and almost all have basal crackles. The

Fig. 14.52 Extrinsic allergic alveolitis. Chest X-ray in acute alveolitis, demonstrating widespread nodular opacities. The patient had acute symptoms associated with exposure to racing pigeons; when he was separated from the birds, the X-ray returned to normal. Chronic exposure produces pulmonary fibrosis, predominantly of the upper lobes.

Fig. 14.53 Cryptogenic fibrosing alveolitis (CFA). Diffuse pulmonary fibrosis, with linear and nodular opacities throughout both lungs. In some areas the retracted, enlarged air spaces give a 'honeycomb' appearance. In less severe CFA the radiological abnormalities are commonly maximal at the bases, with differential volume loss of the lower lobes.

condition may be associated with a variety of systemic diseases: rheumatoid arthritis, Sjögren's syndrome and systemic sclerosis. Other known causes of pulmonary fibrosis, such as the pneumoconioses or sarcoidosis, should be excluded, but with end-stage pulmonary fibrosis it is often difficult, even at post-mortem, to determine the aetiology.

The chest X-ray shows fine nodular and irregular shadowing (Fig. 14.53) and eventually 'honeycombing'. Lung function tests show a restrictive pattern with reduced transfer factor. Antinuclear antibodies are present in 45% of patients and rheumatoid factor in 20–25%. Broncho-alveolar lavage usually yields a predominantly poly-morphonuclear leucocyte pattern. To make a definitive diagnosis an open lung biopsy may be necessary. Patients who have a very active cellular histology respond better to treatment than those with established fibrosis.

Treatment

The usual treatment is with oral corticosteroids and the response is variable, with only 10% improving substan-tially. Treatment may need to be continued over several years. Cyclophosphamide or azathioprine may be used as steroid sparing agents. It is unlikely that treatment substantially affects the long-term prognosis. The pro-gression of CFA is variable; some patients with very acute, severe disease (the 'Hamman-Rich' syndrome) may die within months. Overall approximately 50% survive for 5 years and 25% for 10 years. There is a tenfold increase in the incidence of bronchogenic carcinoma. In a few patients fibrosing alveolitis has been successfully treated by heart–lung transplantation.

Honeycomb lung

This is a radiological description of a group of conditions that cause widespread cystic or 'honeycomb' appearances on chest X-ray. A 'honeycomb' appearance can be seen as the end stage of pulmonary fibrosis of any cause. Rare causes include Letterer-Siwe disease, tuberous sclerosis, Hand-Schuller-Christian disease, neurofibromatosis and eosinophilic granuloma. Patients with honeycomb lung tend to develop pneumothoraces. The long-term prognosis is poor, with respiratory and cardiac failure supervening.

Idiopathic pulmonary haemosiderosis

Idiopathic pulmonary haemosiderosis is a rare condition of unknown aetiology, characterised by recurrent episodes of intrapulmonary haemorrhage, pyrexia, haemoptysis and a secondary iron deficiency anaemia. Most cases occur in childhood; patients may die during an acute episode, but more commonly recurrent episodes eventually cause severe pulmonary fibrosis and respiratory failure. Some auth-orities consider that there is an association with Good-pasture's syndrome (p. 822). During acute episodes there may be crackles at the lung bases and occasionally hepatosplenomegaly. Chest X-ray during episodes of haemoptysis may show patchy, usually bilateral, shadowing in the middle zones. Management consists of treatment of the iron deficiency and corticosteroids and/or azathioprine during acute episodes, although their value is as yet unpro-ven. At 3 years from diagnosis one-third of patients will have died, one-third will have active symptomatic disease and one third will be symptom-free.

IATROGENIC LUNG DISEASE

There are a wide variety of drugs and physical agents, including oxygen and ionising radiation, which can cause temporary or permanent lung damage. The drugs most commonly responsible are cytotoxic agents (Table 14.42).

Bleomycin toxicity is commonest, occurring in 3–6% of patients treated with the drug; it is dose-dependent and there is increased toxicity in the elderly and in those who have received thoracic radiotherapy or combination chemotherapy. Likewise, the pulmonary side-effects of the *nitrosoureas* are more common in the elderly. The changes in the lung induced by *methotrexate* may resolve despite continuing treatment with the drug. *Cyclophosphamide* causes a pneumonitis and fibrosis that can respond remarkably well to corticosteroid therapy. Treatment with corticosteroids may be useful in *mitomycin* pulmonary toxicity. The pneumonitis caused by *procarbazine* may have a direct toxic or allergic basis, and may recur on re-introduction of the drug.

There are also a large number of non-cytotoxic drugs which can cause pulmonary toxicity (Table 14.43). The largest single group is antibiotics and the most common of these is nitrofurantoin. The reaction to nitrofurantoin is either an acute hypersensitivity pneumonitis or, in a small number of patients, an interstitial pneumonitis which can progress to pulmonary fibrosis. Other antibiotics (e.g. penicillin, erythromycin, etc.) can cause acute asthma. Pulmonary eosinophilia is associated with drugs such as isoniazid and sulphonamides.

Radiation injury

Patients who receive radiation treatment to the thorax may sustain long-term lung injury. The acute injury is characterised pathologically by pulmonary vascular congestion, alveolar oedema and the formation of hyaline membranes. This may progress, over a period of 6–12 months, to pulmonary fibrosis. Clinically, these processes cause a dry cough, chest wall pain and, depending on the extent of the damage, breathlessness. Radiation injury occurs most frequently in patients receiving treatment for carcinoma of the breast, lymphomas and carcinoma of the bronchus. The chest X-ray in the acute pneumonitis shows localised infiltration of the lung in the path of the radiation beam; when fibrosis has developed there is dense shadowing and volume loss. Symptoms and radiological appearances are poorly correlated; some patients with minor infiltrates may be severely dyspnoeic whilst others with widespread X-ray changes may be asymptomatic. Treatment with corticosteroids may be useful in the acute phase, but once fibrosis is established no treatment is effective.

Oxygen toxicity

The use of high levels of inspired oxygen is now known to cause lung injury indistinguishable from the adult respiratory distress syndrome (ARDS). The injury is related to both the inspired oxygen fraction (FiO_2) and the duration of exposure; a safe level has not yet been established but an FiO_2 of more than 0.7 over a period of more than several days may be associated with X-ray infiltrates and histological change. Toxic O_2 radicals (in particular superoxide anion, O_2^-) are thought to be important in oxygen-induced lung injury.

THE ADULT RESPIRATORY DISTRESS SYNDROME

The term adult respiratory distress syndrome (ARDS) is used to describe a pulmonary condition characterised by progressive hypoxaemia, chest X-ray infiltrates and reduced lung compliance in the presence of a normal left atrial pressure. In many respects the clinical presentation resembles the respiratory distress syndrome of the newborn, hence the name, but in view of its pathogenesis, 'non-cardiogenic pulmonary oedema' might be a more accurate and descriptive title. The condition occurs in response to a wide and seemingly unrelated variety of initiating events (Table 14.44).

The pathogenic mechanisms which produce the syndrome (Fig. 14.54) are due to diffuse damage to the pulmonary capillary endothelium, which results in increased 'leakiness' across the endothelial/epithelial barrier, result-

Table 14.42 Cytotoxic drugs causing pulmonary toxicity

Drug	Toxic effects
Bleomycin	Interstitial pneumonitis Pulmonary fibrosis
Nitrosoureas	Interstitital fibrosis
Mitomycin	Pneumonitis and fibrosis
Busulphan	Diffuse pulmonary fibrosis
Methotrexate	Pneumonitis Blood eosinophilia
Cyclophosphamide	Interstitial fibrosis
Procarbazine	Pneumonitis Pleural effusion Blood eosinophilia
Chlorambucil	Pulmonary fibrosis
Melphalan	Pneumonitis Pulmonary fibrosis

Table 14.43 Non-cytotoxic drugs which cause pulmonary toxicity

Nitrofurantoin	Neomycin
Penicillin	Ethionamide
Erythromycin	Isoniazid
Tetracycline	Sulphonamides
Streptomycin	

Table 14.44 Conditions associated with the adult respiratory distress syndrome

Shock (traumatic, septic, etc.)

Infection
  Pneumonias (viral, bacterial, pneumocystis carinii)
  Gram-negative sepsis

Trauma (fat emboli, head injuries, lung contusion)

Aspiration (gastric contents, fresh or salt water)

Drug overdose (narcotics, barbiturates)

Metabolic disorders (pancreatitis, uraemia)

Inhaled toxins (O_2, smoke, corrosives)

Blood disorders (disseminated intravascular coagulation, massive blood transfusion)

Miscellaneous
  Paraquat ingestion
  Radiation
  Eclampsia
  Raised intracranial pressure
  Seizures
  High altitude

Table 14.45 Clinical features of the adult respiratory distress syndrome

Initiating event	'Stiff lungs'
Dyspnoea and cough	Normal left heart pressures
Crackles over lung fields	With progression
Progressive hypoxaemia	sepsis
Chest X-ray infiltrates	failure of other organs (kidneys, liver, etc.)

cal, neural and vascular responses, all combining to produce the clinical syndrome.

The clinical features are outlined in Table 14.45. A typical radiographic progression is shown in Figure 14.55.

Management

In many situations early diagnosis and efficient treatment of the underlying predisposing disorder may prevent the syndrome. There are, as yet, no definite predictors as to which patients with the conditions listed in Table 14.46 will develop ARDS. However, the warning signs are *deteriorating gas exchange, worsening chest X-ray*, and, if the patient is being mechanically ventilated, *increasing inflation pressures* as the lungs become more 'stiff'. Early diagnosis and effective treatment can shorten the course, minimise the long-term sequelae, and improve the prognosis of ARDS. Unfortunately, early treatment cannot salvage all patients, many of whom die despite vigorous therapy.

The initial clinical assessment should include a detailed history to determine possible aetiological factors. Vital signs should be carefully documented to provide the baseline for future examinations. Cardiogenic pulmonary oedema should be excluded.

As measurements of pulmonary artery pressure, pulmonary artery wedge pressure and mixed venous O_2 content are critical, a Swan-Ganz catheter should be passed into the pulmonary artery (p. 545). For the diagnosis of ARDS to be secure, the clinical features of the disorder are combined with a normal pulmonary artery wedge pressure (normal PAWP = 8–12 cmH$_2$O).

Once the diagnosis of ARDS has been made the patient is usually so hypoxic that endotracheal intubation and mechanical ventilation is required.

The following aspects of the patient's therapy should be considered:

1. fluid balance
2. oxygenation
3. drug therapy.

Fluid balance

Fluid balance is illustrated in Figure 14.56. The physician treating the patient with ARDS is faced with a dilemma. Excessive fluid administration may increase the pulmonary capillary hydrostatic pressure and thus cause further leakage of fluid into the lung interstitium and alveolar

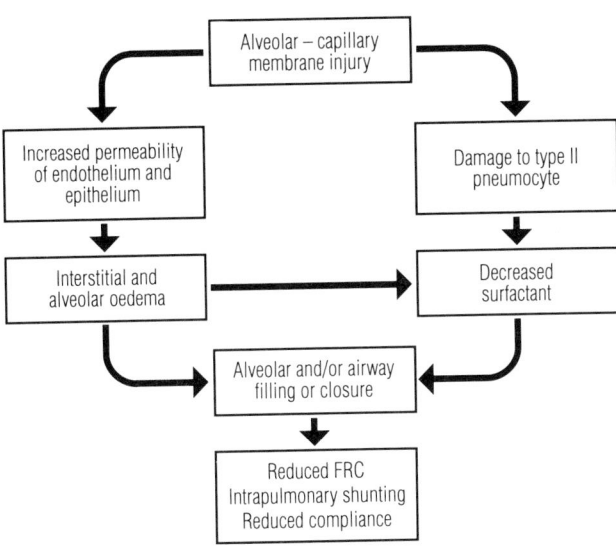

Fig. 14.54 Pathogenesis of the adult respiratory distress syndrome (ARDS). The many causes of ARDS have in common the damage of the alveolar–capillary membrane. The pathological changes that follow cause profound hypoxaemia. (FRC = functional residual capacity.)

ing in the passage of plasma and red blood cells into the interstitial space, and thence into the alveoli, causing alveolar flooding. The mechanisms responsible for the capillary endothelial damage are poorly understood. Activation of complement with leucocytosis and release of lysosomal enzymes, and interactions between mediators such as leukotrienes, prostaglandins, neuropeptides and superoxides are all considered to contribute. Damage is therefore due to a complex series of events involving cellular, chemi-

Fig. 14.55 **Adult respiratory distress syndrome.** The X-rays are of a young man who had sustained severe trauma and blood loss in a road traffic accident; the films cover a period of 5 days from a relatively normal X-ray (**A**), to bilateral infiltrates (**B**), to bilateral 'white-out' (**C**), accompanied by severe hypoxaemia. A Swan-Ganz catheter for measurement of pulmonary artery 'wedge' pressure (as a reflection of left atrial pressure) can be seen *in situ* on X-ray C. The patient died shortly after the last film.

Fig. 14.56 **The relationship of pulmonary extravascular water and pulmonary capillary pressure.** In normal circumstances an increase in pulmonary extravascular water (and pulmonary oedema) does not occur until pulmonary artery 'wedge' pressure exceeds 3.3 kPa (25 mmHg). However, increased permeability (as in ARDS), and hypoalbuminaemia (common in intensive care unit (ICU) patients) can cause pulmonary oedema at normal wedge pressures. (From Hopewell P C and Murray J F 1976 The adult respiratory distress syndrome. Annual Review of Medicine 27: 243–356.)

spaces; if the patient is allowed to become fluid-depleted, however, systemic and pulmonary perfusion may suffer, causing renal and other organ damage. There is no completely correct solution to this, but the best compromise is to administer sufficient fluid to maintain a pulmonary artery wedge pressure of approximately 6–8 cmH$_2$O, and if further circulatory support is required, to administer an inotropic agent such as dobutamine or isoprenaline. Fluid can be given in the form of 5% dextrose solution, or as a crystalloid, and if the patient is severely hypoalbuminaemic, intravenous salt-free albumin should be administered.

Oxygenation

The first step in improving arterial hypoxaemia is to add supplementary O$_2$. Very high concentrations of O$_2$ may be employed initially (up to 100%) but these levels should not be sustained, as they may of themselves cause pulmonary damage. Steps must also be taken to minimise atelectasis, including:

1. efficient removal of secretions by endotracheal suction and physical therapy
2. the use of high tidal volumes on the ventilator (15 ml/kg body weight)
3. occasional hyperinflation with 'sighs', which may be of some value
4. positive end expiratory pressure (PEEP).

PEEP has gained widespread acceptance as an effective method of ventilating patients with ARDS. Positive pressure (usually 5–15 cm H$_2$O) is applied at the end of expiration, thus preventing airway closure, limiting areas of atelectasis and reducing right-to-left shunting of blood through underventilated areas of lung. Patients with

ARDS breathe at a low functional residual capacity, at which, due to the pressure–volume relationships of the lung, compliance is reduced. Application of PEEP increases functional residual capacity (FRC) and therefore reduces lung 'stiffness'. The net result of PEEP is usually an increase in PaO_2 without increasing the inspired O_2 concentration. However, PEEP is not without problems. By increasing intrathoracic pressure it may reduce venous return to the heart and impair cardiac output. Inotropic support may be necessary, as is careful maintenance and monitoring of intravascular fluid volume. The higher the level of PEEP administered, the greater the risk of inducing pneumothorax. The optimum level of PEEP for individual patients can be determined by starting at low levels, say 5 cm H_2O, and working upwards in small increments, measuring at each level the effect of PEEP on gas exchange, lung compliance, cardiac output and mixed venous–arterial oxygen content difference.

The efficiency of oxygenation must not be based on the interpretation of the PaO_2 alone. The PaO_2 must be related to the concentration of O_2 in the inspired air and with this knowledge (using the alveolar air equation), the alveolar–arterial O_2 gradient can be calculated (p. 500). The alveolar–arterial O_2 gradient in normal young adults is about 1 kPa (7.5 mmHg). Tissue oxygenation is also determined by haemoglobin concentration, the characteristics of the oxygen dissociation curve, and cardiac output. The most useful index of tissue oxygenation in patients with ARDS is the mixed venous (i.e. pulmonary arterial)/arterial O_2 content difference (p. 500). This is normally about 5 ml/100 ml blood, and will increase if, for whatever reason, the systemic O_2 transport diminishes.

Drug therapy

Sepsis is now the commonest cause of death in patients with ARDS. Pulmonary and abdominal sepsis is particularly common. Steroids have little role in the treatment of ARDS and in some instances, particularly in septicaemic patients, they may be harmful.

Extracorporeal membrane oxygenation (ECMO) is a technique by which blood is continuously removed from the circulation, passed through a membrane oxygenator, and then returned. The results of controlled studies to date of ECMO in ARDS are discouraging and further technical advances are necessary before this can be considered a realistic option for treatment, except in a small number of selected patients.

The outlook for patients with ARDS remains poor. There is a 50–70% mortality, and if failure of an organ in addition to the lungs (e.g. the kidneys) supervenes, almost 100% of patients die. Effective ventilatory support has meant that most patients die now, not from respiratory failure, but from overwhelming sepsis. However, of those who survive, most recover normal lung function; and only a small proportion, usually those who have required ventilatory support for many weeks, develop bronchiectasis or pulmonary fibrosis.

LUNG TUMOURS

Carcinoma of the bronchus is one of the major causes of death in Western countries. In addition the lungs and mediastinum are common sites for metastatic malignant disease, with about 30% of cancer patients developing lung secondaries, in half of whom metastases are limited to the lungs. By far the commonest primary lung tumour is bronchial carcinoma (Table 14.46).

Table 14.46 Relative frequency of primary pulmonary tumours

Tumour	%
Bronchial carcinoma	95
Alveolar carcinoma	1–2
Bronchial adenoma	1–2
Hamartoma	1
Other tumours	1

BRONCHIAL CARCINOMA

In the 19th century bronchial carcinoma was unusual; by the mid-20th century, associated with the widespread habit of cigarette smoking, it reached epidemic proportions. In the United Kingdom, carcinoma of the bronchus is the commonest malignancy in males and is approaching the importance of breast cancer in females; in all, 35 000 patients die each year from this disease (p. 140).

The UK has a higher death rate from bronchial carcinoma than any other country in the world (p. 139). In America the incidence of the disease has reached a plateau; in the UK a plateau has been reached for males, but the number of female cases continues to rise.

Aetiology

Atmospheric pollution and industrial exposure to dusts, particularly asbestos, increase the incidence of lung cancer, but the dominant causative agent is tobacco smoke. The disease is unusual in non-smokers and the increased incidence in smokers is related to the number of cigarettes consumed (Table 1.1, p. 4). The incidence in ex-smokers rapidly falls towards that of non-smokers. If smoking was completely eliminated the incidence of bronchial carcinoma would be a few hundred cases annually.

Pathology

Bronchial carcinomas are conventionally classified into four main histological groups (Table 14.47).

Squamous cell carcinoma

Squamous cell carcinomas are most common. The neo-

Table 14.47 Natural history of untreated lung cancer*

Histology	%	Doubling time (days)	Earliest diagnosis (1 cm)	Usual diagnosis (3 cm)	Death (10 cm)
Squamous	35	88	7.2	8.4	9.6
Adenocarcinoma	21	161	13.2	15.4	17.6
Large cell undifferentiated	19	86	7.1	8.2	9.4
Small (oat) cell	25	29	2.4	2.8	3.2

* From Geddes D M 1979 The natural history of lung cancer: a review based on rates of tumour growth. Br. J. Dis. Chest. 73: 1–17.

plastic epithelial cells produce keratin and frequently arise from major bronchi. The tumours are thought to originate in areas of squamous metaplasia which progress to carcinoma in situ and then to invasive carcinoma. Squamous tumours frequently cavitate; when peripheral they often invade the chest wall.

Adenocarcinomas

Adenocarcinomas arise both centrally and peripherally, from the bronchial epithelium or submucosal glands. They do not cavitate and their histology is characterised by tubules and gland-like structures, often producing mucin. Adenocarcinomas are related to cigarette consumption but also occur in non-smokers. There can be diagnostic difficulty since an apparent primary tumour may prove to be a metastasis from a tumour of the gastro-intestinal tract, kidney, ovary, pancreas, thyroid or breast.

Small cell carcinoma

Small cell carcinomas (oat cell) show differentiation into cells with amine-precursor uptake and decarboxylation (APUD) characteristics. Electron microscopy frequently shows neurosecretory granules. The malignant cells are small with little cytoplasm and dark, often oval nuclei. The tumours are usually central, highly invasive and disseminate rapidly. They secrete a wide range of hormones, particularly ADH and ACTH.

Large cell (undifferentiated) carcinoma

Large cell undifferentiated tumours constitute a heterogeneous group including giant-cell and clear-cell carcinomas, the cells of which show no evidence of maturation. They frequently arise centrally, invade the mediastinum and disseminate widely.

Studies of the natural history of bronchial carcinoma and analysis of the time taken for tumours to double in size suggest that by the time a tumour can be diagnosed it may have been present for many years, and has frequently metastasised (Table 14.47).

Clinical features

Symptoms of local disease

Bronchial carcinomas frequently arise in major bronchi, and therefore common problems include cough, haemoptysis, breathlessness, wheeze and stridor. Some patients have diffuse, poorly localised chest pain, and many have chest infections. Of these symptoms, haemoptysis, progressive breathlessness and persistent respiratory infection are the most important.

Haemoptysis

There are many causes of haemoptysis (Table 14.2, p. 458), but in a middle-aged or elderly smoker, carcinoma must always be excluded. A normal chest X-ray is unusual in bronchial carcinoma, but does not exclude a tumour.

Breathlessness

This is common in smokers who have developed generalised airways obstruction but progression is usually gradual and accelerated breathlessness commonly occurs as a tumour narrows a major airway. Such narrowing may produce a localised wheeze and occasionally stridor if the trachea or major bronchi are affected. Breathlessness may also be due to the accumulation of a malignant pleural effusion or the development of lymphangitis.

Chest infections

These are not uncommon in chronic heavy smokers and usually resolve quickly when treated with antibiotics. When infection occurs distal to a tumour, however, it frequently persists or relapses. For this reason failure of a pneumonia to resolve is a common presentation of bronchial carcinoma.

Symptoms due to intrathoracic infiltration

The common sites of local infiltration are shown in Figure 14.57. The tumour may extend to involve the chest wall, destroying ribs and vertebral bodies and causing severe pain. In the apex of the lung the tumour may infiltrate the brachial plexus, causing pain in the arm (Pancoast tumour). The pleura is frequently involved and a pleural effusion is common. The tumour may infiltrate the mediastinum, causing recurrent laryngeal or phrenic nerve palsy, central chest pain and superior vena cava obstruction.

Extrathoracic metastasis

In bronchial carcinoma general symptoms such as lethargy, anorexia and weight loss frequently signify disseminated disease. The most important sites of secondary spread are liver, bone and brain, but virtually all parts of the body can be affected. In small cell carcinoma the bone marrow is involved in 10–20% of patients presenting with advanced

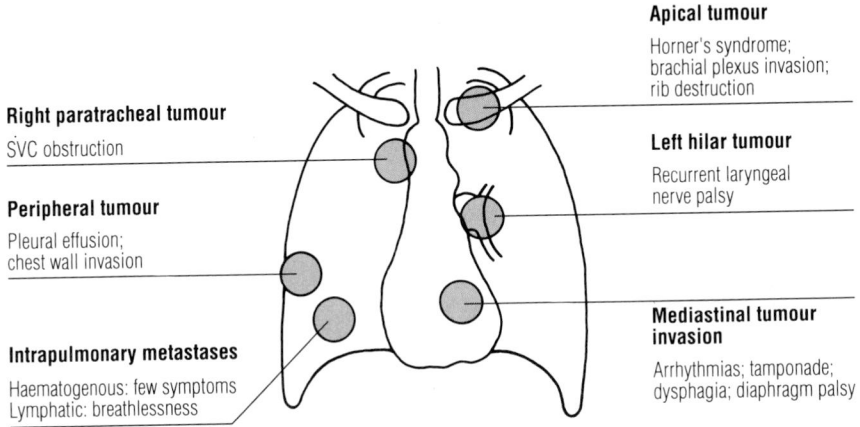

Right paratracheal tumour

SVC obstruction

Peripheral tumour

Pleural effusion;
chest wall invasion

Intrapulmonary metastases

Haematogenous: few symptoms
Lymphatic: breathlessness

Apical tumour

Horner's syndrome;
brachial plexus invasion;
rib destruction

Left hilar tumour

Recurrent laryngeal
nerve palsy

**Mediastinal tumour
invasion**

Arrhythmias; tamponade;
dysphagia; diaphragm palsy

Fig. 14.57 Symptoms and signs of intrathoracic tumour invasion and metastases.

disease and can produce a leuco-erythroblastic anaemia, but in most patients any anaemia is due to the non-specific effects of malignancy (Fig. 25.16, p. 1061).

Non-metastatic manifestations

Endocrine and metabolic changes occur in 10–15% of cases but cause symptoms much less frequently.

Hypercalcaemia

Hypercalcaemia occurs in 6–7% of tumours. In some cases of squamous carcinoma this is due to the production of parathyroid hormone-related peptide elaborated by the tumour. In most patients hypercalcaemia is due to extensive bone metastases. Hypercalcaemia can cause polyuria, polydipsia, constipation, lassitude, depression and confusion (p. 737), and control of hypercalcaemia is an important aspect of management.

Hyponatraemia

The secretion of ADH-like peptides is nearly always associated with small cell cancer, and is a feature in 10% of such tumours. It results in a dilutional hyponatraemia, low blood osmolality and raised urine osmolality. The serum sodium may be very low, less than 120 mmol/l, and the patient may then become confused.

Cushing's syndrome

The ectopic production of ACTH-like peptides by small cell tumours is common but only occasionally causes symptoms (1% of all cases). The main manifestations are hypokalaemia, hyperglycaemia and skin pigmentation. There is usually insufficient time for the other features of Cushing's syndrome to develop.

Clubbing

Clubbing (Fig. 14.8, p. 459) is most frequently seen with squamous cell carcinoma (more than 50%) and is unusual in small cell tumours. Occasionally clubbed patients have hypertrophic pulmonary osteoarthropathy (HPOA).

Neurological manifestations

Neurological manifestations are also described on page 970. These are not common (less then 2%) and most frequently complicate small cell carcinoma. Manifestations include cerebellar degeneration, sensory neuropathy, motor neuropathy, polyneuritis, progressive dementia, myopathy (usually proximal), the Lambert-Eaton syndrome, dermatomyositis and autonomic dysfunction. Neurological manifestations can predate any obvious tumour. They may remit spontaneously but usually progress and, except for rare cases, are little affected by treatment of the associated tumour.

Diagnosis

Carcinoma of the bronchus is so common and has such a variety of symptoms and signs that it should be considered in most heavy smokers presenting to a general physician. Diagnosis is usually straightforward and the first important investigation is a chest X-ray. Indeed, 5% of cases are discovered when a chest X-ray has been taken for unrelated reasons. In a smoker clubbing, haemoptysis, persistent chest infection or weight loss demand an immediate X-ray of the chest.

The most common radiological abnormalities are listed in Summary 9.

Summary 9   Common radiological abnormalities in bronchial carcinoma

- Unilateral hilar enlargement
- Peripheral solid tumour mass
- Peripheral cavitating tumour mass
- Volume loss
- Abnormal mediastinum
- Lymphatic invasion
- Apical (Pancoast) tumour
- Pleural effusion

Fig. 14.58 Carcinoma of the bronchus. The left hilum is enlarged and more dense than the right. There are strands radiating from the hilum and this spiculated appearance is typical of tumour.

Fig. 14.59 Carcinoma of the bronchus: peripheral (squamous cell) carcinoma. Most pulmonary mass lesions more than 4 cm diameter are malignant tumours.

Unilateral hilar enlargement

Unilateral hilar enlargement (Fig. 14.58) is due to tumour and, frequently, involved lymph nodes. Tomography may be helpful in doubtful cases. The hilum appears more dense than the opposite side, and the outer border of the hilum is frequently convex. Phrenic nerve invasion produces unilateral elevation of the diaphragm, and left recurrent laryngeal nerve involvement produces vocal cord paralysis with hoarseness.

Peripheral solid tumour mass

The tumour may be seen as a nodule, a large rounded mass or an irregular density (Fig. 14.59). Streaky shadows often extend into the surrounding lung, particularly towards the hilum, which may be abnormally bulky due to lymphadenopathy.

Peripheral cavitating tumour mass

A peripheral cavitating tumour mass is characteristic of squamous cell carcinomas. The cavitation is due to necrosis within the tumour and the cavity wall is irregular and thick. However, a certain diagnosis is not possible on radiological criteria alone, and the differential diagnosis can include tuberculosis, lung abscess (Fig. 14.23), pulmonary infarction, vasculitic lesions and a rheumatoid nodule. Sometimes cavitation occurs in the consolidated lung distal to an obstructing tumour.

Volume loss

Bronchial carcinoma frequently arises in a major bronchus and gradually narrows the airway, leading to volume loss in a lung or lobe on the chest X-ray. Volume loss is therefore a critically important radiological sign, particularly if progressive. Eventually the tumour causes collapse of a lobe or lung, producing an opacity on the chest X-ray.

Abnormal mediastinum

Bronchial carcinoma frequently involves the mediastinum, and tumour infiltration as well as lymph node enlargement makes the mediastinal outline abnormal (Fig. 14.60). This is common in small cell tumours. Abnormalities of the mediastinum are well demonstrated by a CT scan.

Lymphatic invasion

The widespread involvement of the pulmonary lymphatics by tumour produces lymphangitis carcinomatosa (Fig. 14.61). This also occurs in malignant tumours of the stomach, pancreas and breast. Patients are characteristically very breathless. The differential diagnosis may include left heart failure, in which orthopnoea and crackles are more striking features.

Fig. 14.60 Carcinoma of the bronchus. Central (small cell) carcinoma, lateral and inferior to the aortic knuckle. The usual configuration of the hilar structures is lost. There is a secondary deposit in the left mid-zone.

Fig. 14.61 Carcinoma of the bronchus: lymphangitis carcinomatosa. There are widespread linear and nodular opacities due to lymphatic infiltration. The basal septal lines are radiologically similar to those seen in left heart failure. Patients with lymphangitis usually have severe breathlessness.

Apical (Pancoast) tumour

Apical tumours frequently invade the ribs, sympathetic chain (Horner's syndrome, p. 866), brachial plexus and chest wall (Fig. 14.62). Apical tumours are well seen on a CT scan.

Pleural effusion

A common radiological manifestation of bronchial carcinoma at presentation is a pleural effusion, usually of large volume, which rapidly re-accumulates following aspiration, is blood-stained and contains malignant cells.

Confirmation of diagnosis

In addition to confirming the diagnosis, a knowledge of tumour cell type affects treatment; chemotherapy is frequently appropriate in small cell cancer but seldom useful in non-small cell disease.

Sputum cytology

This simple, non-invasive technique can produce a positive result in up to 40% of patients. Sometimes the inves-

Fig. 14.62 Carcinoma of the bronchus: apical (Pancoast) tumour. The left first rib has been destroyed and there is a soft tissue mass, due to metastatic nodes, in the supra-clavicular fossa. The companion shadow normally visible above the clavicle is lost.

14

tigation confirms malignancy, but fails to determine the specific nature of the tumour.

Bronchoscopy

Fibre-optic bronchoscopy (p. 468) with local anaesthesia has become the most important technique for confirming a diagnosis of bronchial carcinoma (as well as documenting the location of the tumour). A tumour is visible in about 70% of cases, and a definite diagnosis from cytology of bronchial aspirate and tumour brushings and histology of biopsy material is possible in more than 90% of these patients. Submucosal tumour that can be seen to distort the bronchial anatomy may not be sampled by the very small bronchial biopsies, and in such cases rigid bronchoscopy may be necessary to allow large biopsies to be taken.

Needle aspiration lung biopsy

Percutaneous needle aspiration biopsy (p. 469), with X-ray screening to localise the tumour, is particularly effective for peripheral lesions not seen at bronchoscopy. A positive cytological diagnosis is achieved in 75–90% of patients with tumours.

Surgical biopsy

In a small number of patients, surgical biopsy is necessary to establish a diagnosis. Mediastinoscopy and mediastinotomy allow biopsy of tumour within the mediastinum (see p. 470), and thoracotomy gives access for lung and pleural biopsy. The pleura can also be inspected and tumour biopsied under direct vision using a thoracoscope.

Staging notation for lung cancer

Following diagnosis, patients can be staged according to the extent of their disease (Table 9.6, p. 148). In general, only patients with stage I disease are suitable for surgery.

The tumour, node, metastasis (TNM) system is surgically based and is useful for non-small cell lung cancer. In small cell carcinoma a categorisation into 'limited' disease (disease confined to one hemithorax) and extensive disease is made.

Treatment of lung cancer

Surgery

The overall results of surgery are not good, with a 5-year survival of about 25%, but surgery represents almost the only possibility of cure in non-small cell lung cancer. The critical question to be asked for each new patient with bronchial carcinoma is, 'Can this patient be cured by surgery?' The final answer to this question depends in turn on the answer to several intermediate questions:

1. Is the patient's general health good?
   Coronary artery disease is common.
   Patients over 70 seldom do well.

2. Is pulmonary function adequate to cope with major surgery and pulmonary resection?
   Most patients have airways obstruction.
   An FEV_1 of less than 1.5 litres usually precludes pneumonectomy.
   How much 'useful' lung is to be resected?
3. What is the site of the tumour: is surgery technically feasible?
4. What is the tumour histology?
   Small cell carcinoma is usually disseminated.
   Most favourable histology is well differentiated squamous cell carcinoma.
5. Is there evidence of local spread of tumour within the thorax?
6. Is there evidence of distant metastases?

Patients with pulmonary hypertension, hypoxia and hypercapnia should not be operated upon, and those with excessive sputum production often develop post-operative chest infections. Static lung function can be misleading and information on exercise tolerance is helpful. For most cases this information is as easily obtained by the physician walking up the stairs with his patient as by formal exercise testing.

In addition to pulmonary function tests the contribution of the lung that will be resected can be obtained by perfusion and ventilation lung scans, and the postoperative FEV_1 and VC can be predicted from such information.

Recurrent laryngeal nerve invasion, malignant pleural effusion, chest wall involvement, superior vena caval obstruction, pericardial involvement, mediastinal lymph node spread and metastasis to the contralateral lung all preclude surgery. In considering surgery, assessment for mediastinal spread is critical. CT scanning can be helpful; a negative scan usually indicates that the mediastinum is clear, but a positive scan may demonstrate enlarged nodes that are subsequently found to be due to reactive hyperplasia rather than tumour. These cases may require surgical assessment of the mediastinum.

The relatively poor results for surgery in bronchial carcinoma reflect the widespread and early metastases so common in this disease. Prior to surgery biochemical tests may reveal abnormal liver function, and liver secondaries can be confirmed by ultrasound or CT scan. A raised alkaline phosphatase may reflect bone secondaries which can be confirmed by bone scan. CNS symptoms or signs indicate the need for a CT brain scan to exclude cerebral metastases.

Results of surgical therapy

Extent of disease, size of tumour, cell type, age of patient and the operation performed all affect the results from surgery (Fig. 14.63). Although the overall survival rates with surgery of 25% at 5 years and 17% at 10 years are poor, some patient groups do relatively well. Young, fit patients who have a lobectomy for stage I squamous cell carcinoma have a 5-year survival of 55–60%.

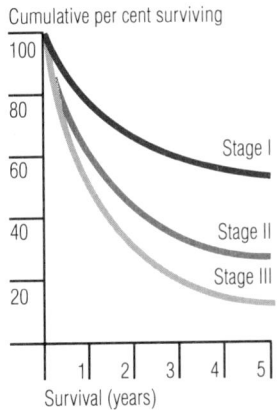

Cumulative per cent surviving

Stage I

Stage II

Stage III

Survival (years)

Fig. 14.63 Survival following surgical resection for non-small cell carcinoma of the bronchus.

Chemotherapy

The results of chemotherapy for non-small cell tumours not suitable for surgery are very poor and chemotherapy is largely reserved for the treatment of small cell lung cancer. Small cell tumours can respond dramatically to multiple drug chemotherapy. The drugs in common use include ifosfamide, cyclophosphamide, vincristine, adriamycin and etoposide.

Treatment is given at 3–4 weekly intervals over a period of several months. A complete response to therapy with a return to normal of the chest X-ray and disappearance of tumour at bronchoscopy can be achieved in 25–50% of patients. Small cell tumours are rarely completely eradicated, however, and the tumours rapidly relapse. Chemotherapy increases the overall median survival from approximately 4 months without drug therapy, to 11 months with treatment (Fig. 9.11, p. 148). Approximately 10% of those patients with limited disease will continue symptom- and disease- free for 2 or 3 years. In general patients with least tumour bulk and good general health have the best prognosis. The great reduction of tumour mass following treatment can produce dramatic symptomatic improvement, often following only two or three courses of drugs. Therapy can relieve breathlessness due to airways obstruction by tumour, bone pain due to metastatic disease, superior vena caval obstruction and haemoptysis.

Chemotherapy is well tolerated by most patients, but avoiding the problems of nausea and infection due to marrow suppression requires careful attention to detail. A few more patients may achieve long-term survival if radiotherapy is combined with chemotherapy. However, the outlook for small cell carcinoma remains poor and is unlikely to be substantially improved until better chemotherapeutic agents become available.

Radiotherapy

In bronchial carcinoma the principal purpose of radiotherapy is to produce symptomatic relief. Radiotherapy is particularly good at controlling bone pain, haemoptysis, superior vena caval obstruction and breathlessness due to narrowing of major airways. Following complete collapse of a lobe or lung, radiotherapy is less effective. Cerebral metastases often respond, albeit temporarily, to radiotherapy, with concomitant steroid therapy to control cerebral oedema. In carefully selected patients, radiotherapy can produce impressive results. For small, localised, well differentiated, particularly squamous cell, tumours in generally fit patients who are frequently not suitable for surgery because of poor lung function, it is possible to achieve a 5-year survival of up to 17% following radical high-dose radiotherapy. Survival in localised small cell carcinoma is not greatly extended by radiotherapy alone, but tumour bulk can be dramatically reduced with consequent excellent control of symptoms. In patients with small cell carcinoma who respond well to chemotherapy, prophylactic cranial irradiation can largely prevent the distressing development of symptomatic cerebral metastases.

Advanced bronchogenic carcinoma

As with all malignant disease, patients with advanced bronchogenic carcinoma which is no longer responding to treatment require much medical nursing and social support during their last months of life. Support and understanding of the patient's family is also important. The large number of patients dying of lung cancer represents an important challenge to hospitals, general practice, community terminal care teams and hospices. Pain is a particularly troublesome symptom and radiotherapy may be required for its control. Pain may also require regular analgesics, particularly oral morphine. For intractable pain peripheral nerve blockade may be necessary. Morphine helps reduce the sensation of breathlessness. Poor appetite and lethargy can temporarily be alleviated by steroids, which may also improve the symptoms from cerebral secondaries for a few weeks or months. Weakness, immobility, poor food intake and analgesics all contribute to constipation. In the last weeks of life pain, constipation, anxiety, breathlessness and weakness can greatly reduce the quality of life. Frequent assessment of the patient's needs is necessary. In this respect the family doctor's contribution is of great importance and the domiciliary terminal care team are able to provide a regular assessment in the patient's home.

ALVEOLAR CARCINOMA

This is an unusual tumour with distinctive pathological and clinical features. It constitutes 1–2% of primary pulmonary tumours. The sexes are equally affected and the tumour occurs in all races. Alveolar carcinoma is most common in patients above the age of 50, and is not related to smoking tobacco.

Pathology

Alveolar carcinoma often arises within a damaged area of lung. Histologically the characteristic feature is malignant

527

cells growing along the alveolar walls. On light microscopy it may be difficult to distinguish alveolar cell from primary or secondary adenocarcinoma. The good prognosis for resection of early single nodule disease suggests that in most cases multinodular disease represents spread of tumour rather than simultaneous multiple foci.

Clinical features

The presenting symptoms of alveolar carcinoma are similar to other tumours although, because the tumour is not endobronchial, haemoptysis, bronchial obstruction and distal infection are less common. When the tumour mass is large or affecting both lungs, patients become very breathless. In a few cases patients produce large volumes of clear, watery sputum (bronchorrhoea). The chest X-ray usually shows a single, irregular peripheral shadow sometimes resembling pneumonic consolidation, frequently with an air bronchogram within the tumour opacity. Cavitation is uncommon, but effusions occur. Obstruction of airways with consequent volume loss is uncommon. Multiple tumour opacities develop, initially within one, and then within both lungs (Fig. 14.64).

Fig. 14.64 Alveolar cell carcinoma of the lung. The appearances of 'consolidation' (note the obvious left upper lobe air bronchogram) are common with this carcinoma. Bilateral disease is also common.

Diagnosis

Malignant cells can be detected in the sputum in some cases, but the distinction from adenocarcinoma is frequently not possible. Bronchoscopy and bronchial biopsy are usually negative although transbronchial biopsy can provide a diagnosis. Diagnosis can be achieved by needle aspiration biopsy or more frequently by surgical biopsy at thoracotomy. Diffuse and multiple lesions are often initially thought to be infective but failure to respond to antibiotic therapy raises suspicion of the true diagnosis.

Treatment

Alveolar carcinoma is often relatively slow growing, and disseminated metastatic disease is less common than in other pulmonary tumours. Surgical resection is therefore the treatment of choice whenever possible, and good results can be achieved with a 5-year survival of 50% for localised disease. More extensive disease has a poor prognosis and is difficult to treat, the tumour being resistant to chemotherapy and radiotherapy.

BRONCHIAL ADENOMA

The term 'adenoma' covers a variety of tumours, approximately 90% of which are carcinoid tumours arising from cells of the APUD series. The diagnosis is often made in young adults and the sexes are equally affected. These tumours are endobronchial, usually arising in larger airways, and they therefore cause airway narrowing, volume loss, collapse and distal infection. Common clinical features are cough, haemoptysis, breathlessness, unilateral wheeze and recurrent infections. Most tumours are of low-grade malignancy and symptoms may be present for a long period before a diagnosis is made. Wheezing dyspnoea may lead to a mistaken diagnosis of asthma. Some tumours become malignant and occasionally (2% of cases) the patients develop the carcinoid syndrome (p. 593). It is important to note that tumour is not usually visible on the chest X-ray and the most common radiological abnormality is volume loss or lobar collapse. Diagnosis is frequently made at bronchoscopy, where 90% of these tumours are visible. The tumour is vascular and bleeds easily and profusely. The best treatment whenever possible is surgical resection, and the prognosis for these tumours is good unless there has been malignant change.

HAMARTOMA

Hamartomas are tumour-like malformations of disorganised tissue; in some the predominant tissue is cartilage, and in others smooth muscle. Unlike carcinoid tumours, hamartomas usually present over the age of 50. Males are three times more likely to be affected than females. Hamartomas are usually peripheral within the lung parenchyma and seldom within the bronchus. They grow slowly and are benign. Most hamartomas are asymptomatic and are incidental findings on chest X-ray. The mass of the hamartoma is usually small, less than 4 cm in diameter, rounded, well defined and occasionally calcified (Fig. 14.65). Cavitation is rare. In most cases in the absence of typical calcification, and without the benefit of past chest X-rays, a malignant bronchial carcinoma will be part of the differential diagnosis and the correct treatment will be surgical excision. At surgery the ha-

Fig. 14.65 Pulmonary hamartoma. Tomogram of a hamartoma in the left lower lobe; note the rounded appearance and the presence of calcification.

martoma is felt to be hard, can be removed without resecting lung, and the prognosis is excellent.

THE SOLITARY PULMONARY NODULE

A common diagnostic and management problem arises when the chest X-ray, frequently a 'routine' investigation, shows a solitary pulmonary nodule (Table 14.48 and Fig. 14.66). The larger the lesion, the more likely it is to be malignant; nodules less than 8 mm are usually benign.

Management

Resection of a single small malignant nodule results in surgical cure for more than 60% of patients. Because 40% of all nodules are malignant, surgery should be considered in all patients who are fit for tumour resection, unless there is compelling evidence that the nodule is non-malignant. Nodules that have not grown in size for 2 years or which show calcification (especially central, diffuse or speckled) within the nodule are likely to be benign. Solitary nodules in patients below the age of 35, especially non-smokers, are likely to be benign. The search for past X-rays is often the most rewarding investigation in these patients. Tomography may show calcification more easily. A CT

Fig. 14.66 The 'solitary pulmonary nodule'. A. Small peripheral 'solitary pulmonary nodule' in the right lower lobe. **B.** When there is doubt, calcification is best demonstrated by CT scan.

Table 14.48 Causes of a solitary pulmonary nodule

Malignant (40%)		Benign (60%)	
Bronchogenic carcinoma	(25%)	Infectious granuloma	(50%)
Alveolar carcinoma	(3%)	Non-infective granuloma	(2%)
Bronchial adenoma	(2%)	Benign tumour	(2%)
Metastasis	(10%)	Other rare causes	(6%)

scan may demonstrate multiple pulmonary metastases. Fibre-optic bronchoscopy is seldom helpful because the lesion cannot be seen endoscopically. Needle aspiration biopsy is much more useful, confirming malignancy in 75–90% of tumours, and a reliable diagnosis that the lesion is benign in up to 40%. However, for some tumours and most benign lesions, the precise diagnosis is only revealed by surgical removal.

MEDIASTINAL TUMOURS

Mediastinal tumours are illustrated in Figure 14.67. *Metastatic malignant disease* is the most common cause of a mediastinal mass, most frequently at the hilum. Lymphoma and sarcoidosis are common, with anterior mediastinal adenopathy favouring the former. In addition to the lateral chest X-ray, CT scanning is helpful in elucidating the nature of mediastinal masses; contrast studies demonstrate vascular lesions, and cystic lesions (usually benign) can be identified. Thyroid isotope scans demonstrate a retrosternal goitre. Solid, non-vascular lesions usually require biopsy for diagnosis (for example, the differential diagnosis of carcinoma, lymphoma and sarcoidosis) by needle aspiration biopsy, mediastinoscopy, mediastinotomy, or thoracotomy.

Neurogenic tumours are the most common cause of a posterior mediastinal mass. Symptoms arise from compression of local structures, a small proportion are malignant and treatment is surgical. Occasionally, a neurofibroma is associated with Von Recklinghausen's disease. *Dermoid cysts* arise from ectodermal tissue, whereas *teratomas* are germ cell tumours that contain ectodermal, mesodermal and endodermal tissue. These teratodermoid tumours arise in the anterior mediastinum, commonly of young adults. Dermoids are usually cystic and benign whereas teratomas are commonly solid and frequently malignant. Treatment of these tumours is surgery to remove all or as much as possible of the tissue. In malignant cases, radiotherapy and chemotherapy may be necessary. *Thymomas* can be benign or malignant (about 25% of cases). Whereas many patients with thymoma have myasthenia gravis, only a minority of patients with myasthenia have a thymic tumour. Treatment of all thymomas is surgical excision and, for malignant cases, postoperative radiotherapy.

PLEURAL DISEASE

The visceral pleura, composed of a layer of mesothelial cells supported on connective tissue rich in lymphatics and blood vessels, covers the lung. The parietal pleura lines the thoracic cavity, covers the diaphragm and meets the visceral pleura at the hilum. The visceral pleura has no pain fibres, whereas irritation of the parietal pleura induces the pain characteristic of pleurisy. Normally, the two pleural layers are adjacent to one another, separated by a thin film of fluid, continually formed at the parietal and drained at the visceral pleural surface. As a consequence of the elastic property of the lung, the pressure within the pleural space is negative, approximately -5 cm H_2O at resting end-expiration.

PLEURAL EFFUSION

Water and electrolytes from the pleural space are taken up by the visceral pleura and cleared by the pulmonary and

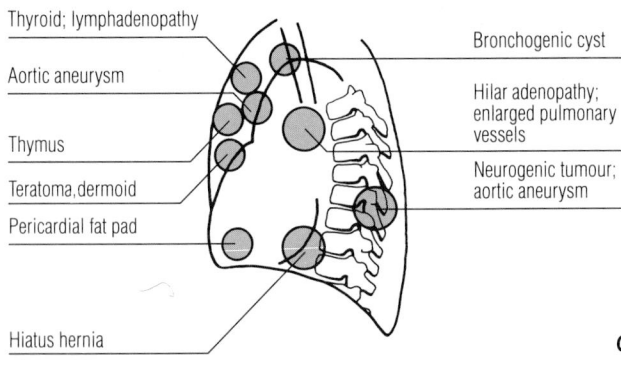

Fig. 14.67 Mediastinal mass lesions. A. The chest X-ray demonstrates a mediastinal mass: the preservation of the silhouette of the descending aorta suggests that the mass is placed anteriorly. **B**. This is confirmed by the lateral chest X-ray: the retrosternal space is opaque. The mass was a malignant thymoma. **C**. Location of the more common mediastinal masses.

systemic (bronchial) circulation, whereas the proteins of pleural fluid are mainly cleared via the lower mediastinal lymphatics. Excess fluid accumulates within the pleural space when visceral or parietal pleural capillary pressure is raised (e.g. left or right heart failure); when capillary permeability is increased (e.g. infection); and when lymphatic drainage is decreased (e.g. lymphatic invasion by tumour). The turnover of pleural water and electrolytes is rapid, even when a large effusion is present, hence the rapid response to diuretics of effusions due to cardiac failure. Protein turnover is less rapid, contributing to the slow clearance of effusions with high protein content. The accumulation of pleural fluid reduces the volume of the underlying lung, causing a restrictive ventilatory defect. There may or may not be pleural pain; if it is present, it contributes to the 'reduction in lung volumes. Large effusions will cause breathlessness, particularly if they develop rapidly, and, when unilateral, mediastinal shift. The collection of fluid, combined with the reduction in volume of the underlying lung and therefore reduced elastic recoil, raises intrathoracic pressure, increases the overall volume of the ipsilateral hemithorax and eventually causes elevation of the jugular venous pressure.

Radiology

The history and particularly the clinical examination may suggest pleural fluid but the most helpful, simple investigation is a chest X-ray (Fig. 14.68). Radiology may suggest fluid but cannot determine the nature of the fluid (e.g. a clear transudate, pus or blood). When there is doubt about pleural fluid a film taken in the lateral decubitus position will demonstrate pleural fluid adjacent to the lateral chest wall. Very small effusions are clearly seen on CT scanning. On occasions, pleural fluid becomes loculated and ultrasound is a simple technique for confirming that fluid is present and locating its position. The collection of fluid in the pleural space beneath the inferior surface of the lung (subpulmonic effusion) can mimic an elevated hemidiaphragm. A lateral decubitus X-ray or ultrasound examination confirms the diagnosis of a subpulmonic effusion.

Differential diagnosis

There are many causes of pleural effusion (Table 14.49). The accumulated fluid may be a *transudate*, as a consequence of alteration in the pressure relationships of the pleural space (as in cardiac failure); or it may be an *exudate*, as a result of increased capillary permeability (as in infection).

Transudates have a protein content of less than 3 g/dl, are clear or light yellow, and often bilateral. Exudates have more than 3 g/dl of protein, are dark yellow or orange in colour, often slightly cloudy, may clot on standing and are usually unilateral.

Transudates

Left heart failure, right heart failure, or a combination of both, are common causes of pleural effusion. Initially, the fluid may be unilateral, usually right-sided; when bilateral,

Fig. 14.68 Pleural effusion. A. Small left effusion. The left hemidiaphragm cannot be visualised and the fluid appears to rise laterally and medially: on a lateral chest X-ray it rises anteriorly and posteriorly. (The patient had the yellow nail syndrome.) **B.** Large effusion. Pleural fluid is homogenous and without vascular markings or air bronchogram. The mediastinum is shifted to the right. Note the surgical clips in the axilla and absent breast shadow on the left. (The patient had metastatic pleural disease from breast carcinoma.)

the right effusion is usually larger than the left. In *constrictive pericarditis* the pleural effusions are less significant than the ascites. Any cause of *hypo-albuminaemia* may cause pleural effusion plus oedema and ascites, but most commonly the cause is the nephrotic syndrome. In *Meigs' syndrome* the pleural effusion is associated with ascites due

Table 14.49 Causes of pleural effusion

Transudates (hydrothorax)
Cardiac failure
Constrictive pericarditis
Hypoproteinaemia
Myxoedema
Peritoneal dialysis and ascites (including Meigs' syndrome)
Superior vena cava obstruction

Exudates	
Infections	Asbestos
Malignancy	Sarcoidosis
Pulmonary infarction	Yellow nail syndrome
Rheumatoid arthritis	Familial Mediterranean fever
Systemic lupus erythematosus	Pancreatitis
Acute rheumatic fever	Subphrenic abscess
Polyarteritis nodosa	Hepatic and pulmonary hydatid
Scleroderma	disease
Dermatomyositis	Hepatic amoebiasis
Postmyocardial infarction syndrome	Trauma
	Drugs

to an ovarian tumour (usually a benign fibroma, occasionally malignant disease), and resolution occurs if the tumours are removed. Effusions are more common on the right; they can be large and accumulate quickly. The same syndrome is seen on rare occasions with fibroids and endometriosis. Small bilateral effusions are common with *peritoneal dialysis* but occasionally the fluid collection can be large, usually right-sided and thus similar to Meigs' syndrome and other causes of *ascites* complicated by effusions. The mechanism of the hydrothorax is the direct passage of fluid through the diaphragm into the pleural space. Small communications have been observed at postmortem in patients with hydrothorax and cirrhosis.

Exudates

Post-infective pleural effusions are most common with bacterial infections and, if inadequately treated, may progress to an empyema. Even when not obviously purulent the fluid contains many polymorphonuclear leucocytes and is often associated with persistence of fever and leucocytosis.

Mycoplasma is rarely responsible. Effusions following *viral infections* occasionally occur, particularly as part of the pleuropericardial involvement of coxsackie B infections. Effusions have been described in glandular fever. Rarely, actinomycosis and other fungal infections can cause a pleural effusion. *Tuberculosis*, once a common cause of effusion, is now unusual. An important aspect of diagnosis is pleural biopsy for histological examination and culture of the mycobacterium.

Malignant pleural effusion may be due to *primary pleural tumours*, most commonly mesothelioma (see below) and rarely a benign pleural fibroma. However, the most common cause is *metastatic pleural malignancy* from carcinoma of the bronchus, as well as breast, ovary and other extrathoracic tumours. Effusions, usually bilateral, may complicate *lymphangitis carcinomatosa* (p. 524). Occasionally, *lymphomas* involve the pleura. Involvement of ribs and adjacent parietal pleura by *myeloma* may produce a pleural effusion. It is characteristic of malignant effusions that they develop rapidly and recur quickly after aspiration; they are also commonly, though not invariably, blood-stained.

A pleural effusion is an important clinical feature of *pulmonary infarction* (p. 502). Primary pulmonary thrombosis and infarction with an associated effusion occur occasionally in sickle cell anaemia.

Pleural effusion is relatively common in some of the *collagen vascular disorders* (p. 511). In *systemic lupus erythematosus* and *mixed connective tissue disease* pleurisy and pericarditis are not uncommon, particularly in young and middle-aged females. Aspirated fluid contains lymphocytes, occasionally lupus erythematosus cells and more often antinuclear factor and rheumatoid factor. In active *rheumatoid arthritis* 5% of patients have a pleural effusion (p. 512). Pleural effusions are rather uncommon in *polyarteritis nodosa*, *systemic sclerosis* and *dermatomyositis*. Acute *rheumatic fever* is complicated by pleural effusions, usually small, in 10% of cases, most of which also have pericarditis.

In the *postmyocardial infarction syndrome* pericarditis and fever develop several days or weeks after acute infarction, and occasionally there is also a pleural effusion. Distinct from the pleural effusion associated with *mesothelioma*, benign, sometimes recurrent, pleural effusions develop in occasional patients with *asbestos* exposure. *Sarcoidosis* is a rare cause of pleural effusions. Recurrent, self-limiting effusions can be a feature of *familial Mediterranean fever* (familial paroxysmal polyserositis). In the *yellow nail syndrome* effusions are associated with a yellow discoloration of nails, plus lymphoedema and occasionally bronchiectasis and sinusitis. Lymphatic hypoplasia underlies the disorder and this is thought to explain the effusions. *Drugs* can cause pleurisy with effusions: hydralazine (as part of a lupus syndrome), nitrofurantoin, sulphonamides, PAS, methotrexate, practolol and methysergide have all been incriminated. *Radiotherapy* to the lung can produce a radiation pneumonitis and small bilateral effusions. Following *chest trauma* and *pulmonary contusion* a pleural effusion occasionally collects. However, a haemothorax must first be excluded.

Pathological processes below the diaphragm can cause pleural effusions, a common complication of *acute pancreatitis* when it is usually painless, left-sided and haemorrhagic. The pleural fluid has a high amylase concentration, higher than in the blood. Occasionally similar effusions are seen in patients with chronic pancreatitis or pancreatic pseudocysts.

Subphrenic abscess is frequently accompanied by a pleural effusion, most often on the right, with low lateral chest and shoulder pain as a consequence of diaphragm inflammation. On chest X-ray, in addition to the effusion, there may be elevation of the hemidiaphragm below which there is a fluid level. If treatment is delayed, an empyema develops. Prior antibiotic therapy may produce a chronic clinical picture.

Investigation of pleural fluid

Whenever there is doubt about the cause of an effusion, aspiration should be performed. Loculated or small effusions are best aspirated with ultrasound localisation.

Blood-stained effusions, rather than the frank blood of a haemothorax, are most common with malignancy but also occur in pulmonary infarction and following chest trauma. Rare causes of a bloody effusion include cirrhosis, tuberculosis and leukaemia. *Infected* pleural fluid is turbid and with advanced empyema becomes purulent. With a *chylous* effusion the fluid is a milky white colour.

Analysis of pleural fluid *protein* concentration broadly separates transudates (less than 3 g/dl) from exudates (more than 3 g/dl) but in a large number of cases borderline, unhelpful values are obtained.

Cytology is a key investigation, not simply for malignant cells. The presence of numerous polymorphonuclear leucocytes suggests bacterial infection; lymphocytes predominate in tuberculosis but are also common in any chronic effusion; *eosinophils* are numerous in the effusions of pulmonary eosinophilia, polyarteritis nodosa and Hodgkin's disease. Eosinophils can be the prominent cells following pulmonary infarction and may also accumulate following bleeding into the pleural space from any cause. Pneumonias and rheumatoid arthritis are less usual causes for an eosinophilic effusion. *Malignant* cells are identified in up to half of patients with tumour involving the pleura. *Bacteria* may be demonstrated in postpneumonic effusions, particularly in those progressing to empyema. In tuberculosis acid-fast bacilli are only occasionally identified but culture of pleural fluid for the mycobacteria is often useful.

In rheumatoid arthritis, the pleural fluid contains a characteristically very low concentration of glucose.

When pleural aspiration is not diagnostic, pleural biopsy should be performed. Biopsy is particularly helpful in malignant disease of the pleura and in tuberculosis.

Pleural biopsy

An Abram's biopsy needle is most commonly used and the investigation should not be undertaken when there is no fluid present lest the biopsy needle punctures the visceral pleura. If the pleura is much thickened, biopsy with a cutting needle is safe even in the absence of fluid. Occasionally, diagnosis may require a large biopsy sample; for example, in mesothelioma a surgical biopsy is indicated. Multiple biopsies increase the diagnostic yield and one of the biopsy samples should be sent to the laboratory for culture if a diagnosis of tuberculosis is possible.

Treatment

Whenever pleural fluid is found to be infected, it should be promptly and completely drained, and in most cases this is best done with an intercostal tube. Any pleural effusion causing breathlessness requires drainage. Malignant effusions may be large and recurrent and therefore require pleurodesis. A variety of sclerosing agents can be introduced into the pleural space in an attempt to fuse the visceral and parietal layers, thereby avoiding the re-accumulation of fluid. *Corynebacterium parvum*, tetracycline and bleomycin can all produce satisfactory results.

If a large pleural effusion re-accumulates despite attempts at medical pleurodesis, surgical pleurodesis or pleurectomy should be considered. Medical pleurodesis is successful in approximately 50% of patients whereas surgery is effective in virtually all cases.

CHYLOTHORAX

Chylothorax most frequently follows rupture of the thoracic duct following trauma, particularly during intrathoracic surgery. Damage to the thoracic duct in the lower half of the mediastinum causes a right-sided chylothorax, whereas damage to the duct in the upper mediastium produces a left chylothorax. When not due to trauma, malignancy involving the thoracic duct is the most common cause, particularly metastatic disease from carcinoma of the stomach, and lymphoma. Rarely chylothorax can complicate chylous ascites.

Patients with chylothorax present with symptoms and signs of a large pleural effusion and the diagnosis is only apparent following aspiration. Fluid rapidly re-accumulates and repeated drainage soon leads to severe wasting, hypoproteinaemia and lymphopenia.

In up to 50% of patients with chylothorax there is spontaneous healing of the fistula, but if this does not occur, the prognosis is poor unless the leak of chyle can be stopped. Following diagnosis a lymphangiogram is useful to determine the site of the fistula, and if the leak is demonstrated the patient should be submitted to thoracotomy and ligation of the thoracic duct below the leak. If no leak can be demonstrated at lymphangiography, repeated aspiration is performed, and the patient is supported by parenteral feeding, in the hope that the fistula will heal spontaneously. When healing does not take place, pleural drainage combined with pleurodesis is sometimes successful.

HAEMOTHORAX

Haemothorax is usually the result of a penetrating injury or blunt trauma to the chest. Occasionally, a haemothorax develops without trauma. Such a *spontaneous haemothorax*, almost always left-sided, may occur with acute aortic dissection. Bleeding can occur with a pneumothorax, from the rupture of vessels within pleural adhesions, and in some cases the air may have been absorbed by the time of presentation. Bleeding disorders, heparin therapy, vascular pleural metastases and pleural endometriosis are rare causes of haemothorax. Haemothoraces, unless small and stable, should be drained by a wide-bore intercostal tube introduced in the mid-axilla connected to an underwater seal. If bleeding continues, the patient requires a thoracotomy. If blood is not removed from the pleural space,

14

infection progressing to empyema can be a complication. In the long term an intense fibrous reaction to undrained blood can occasionally lead to a grossly thickened pleura and an encased lung which then requires decortication if there is not to be substantial ventilatory impairment.

EMPYEMA

Empyema refers to infected pleural fluid, whether a turbid effusion or frank pus. In many cases, the diagnosis only becomes apparent upon aspiration of the fluid. Most commonly, an acute empyema complicates a bacterial pneumonia, particularly pneumococcal, but other causes require consideration (Table 14.50).

Staphylococcal pneumonia is an important cause in children. Anaerobic infection is sometimes difficult to diagnose and it is likely that anaerobes are responsible for many 'sterile' empyemas. Tuberculous empyema is now unusual. It is not uncommon for empyema fluid to contain more than one organism. Empyema following thoracic surgery, and also those associated with abdominal sepsis, are frequently due to Gram-negative organisms. Amoebic liver abscess can rarely perforate the diaphragm and enter the pleural space, as can actinomycosis and hydatid disease. The empyema that occasionally complicates the mediastinitis of oesophageal rupture is usually left-sided.

The clinical features of acute empyema include fever, night sweats and chest pain, with signs of a pleural effusion. The most common clinical setting is that of a pneumonia that has failed to respond to therapy. The white cell count is elevated, 15 000–20 000, with a polymorphonuclear leucocytosis. Pleural fluid aspiration is essential and diagnostic; the fluid may be turbid with numerous polymorphs or frank pus. Empyemas are most commonly posterior and lateral above the diaphragm. Initially, the pleural fluid moves freely in the pleural space and the chest X-ray demonstrates the appearances of a simple effusion, but rapidly the infected fluid becomes loculated and the chest X-ray then shows localised collections of fluid (Fig. 14.69).

An acute empyema can breach the lung and enter a bronchus, and thereby produce a bronchopleural fistula. Patients then cough large volumes of purulent sputum and on X-ray the empyema has fluid levels. Untreated, an empyema may discharge through the chest wall (empyema necessitatis). Empyema, particularly when due to staphylococcal infection, can be complicated by a pneumothorax (pyopneumothorax).

Table 14.50 Causes of acute empyema

Pneumonias	Thoracic surgery
Lung abscess	Penetrating chest injuries
Bronchiectasis	Subdiaphragmatic infection
Oesophageal perforation	Haematogenous spread of infection
Pulmonary infarction	

Fig. 14.69 Empyema. A. The PA chest film shows diffuse right lower zone shadowing. **B.** On the lateral chest X-ray the configuration of the posterior loculated pleural fluid is typical of empyema.

Treatment

Antibiotic therapy will depend on the bacteriology of aspirated fluid and regimes will often require metronidazole to cover anaerobic organisms. The pleural fluid must be completely drained as soon as possible. With early infection and freely moving fluid, needle aspiration can be successful. However, in most cases, a large-bore intercostal drain should be inserted. If such treatment fails to produce rapid resolution of symptoms and complete drainage of the empyema, surgery is required. At surgery, the empyema is evacuated and the lung is decorticated so that it may fully expand and thereby obliterate the pleural space.

Chronic empyema

Occasionally, the diagnosis of acute empyema is missed or the condition is inadequately treated and a stable chronic empyema develops. Infection is particularly likely to persist when there is an associated bronchogenic carcinoma or a bronchopleural fistula. Patients are usually not acutely ill. Fever is low-grade and there is likely to be clubbing, weight loss, anaemia and the clinical signs of extensive pleural thickening. The chest X-ray shows dense pleural shadowing, perhaps fluid levels and occasionally periosteal reaction in overlying ribs. A later radiological development is pleural calcification and a late clinical development is secondary amyloidosis. The treatment of chronic empyema is surgical.

DRY PLEURISY

A variety of disorders can cause pleuritic chest pain, often with a pleural rub, but without a pleural effusion. Some of these conditions remain 'dry' but in others fluid may accumulate, and therefore all the causes of a pleural effusion must be considered in the differential diagnosis of dry pleurisy. The most important causes of pleurisy without fluid are listed in Table 14.51.

Pleuritic pain is a common feature of many radiologically obvious pneumonias but can also occur with minor bacterial and viral pulmonary infections, not radiologically apparent. Epidemic myalgia (Bornholm disease), most commonly due to the coxsackie B virus, is primarily an infection of intercostal muscle but occasionally the pleura is involved. The intercostal muscles are tender. There may be associated pericarditis, myocarditis or orchitis. Pain may relapse and remit several times before finally settling. Dry pleurisy is not unusual in rheumatoid arthritis and is a common feature of systemic lupus erythematosus.

Table 14.51 Important causes of dry pleurisy

Pneumonia (particularly pneumococcal pneumonia)	Uraemia
	Coxsackie B virus (Bornholm disease)
Pulmonary infarction	
Bronchogenic carcinoma	Familial Mediterranean fever
Lung abscess	Trauma
Bronchiectasis	Asbestos pleural disease, including mesothelioma
Tuberculosis	
Rheumatoid arthritis	
Systemic lupus erythematosus	

PNEUMOTHORAX

Pneumothorax is air in the pleural space, as a consequence of which there is partial or complete collapse of the lung. Due to the recoil of the chest wall and the lung, the pressure within the pleural space is normally negative. When the pleural membrane (visceral or parietal) is breached, air is therefore sucked into the pleural cavity and the lung collapses. When the defect in the pleura seals, the pneumothorax is *closed* and there is no movement of air in or out of the pleural cavity. When there is a large defect in the pleura the pneumothorax is *open*. When this defect is of the visceral pleura there is then a bronchopleural fistula, and air moves in and out of the pleural space during breathing. Occasionally, the damaged visceral pleura acts as a valve permitting air to enter the pleural space on inspiration but not to leave the space on expiration, leading to a *tension* pneumothorax.

A pneumothorax may be spontaneous, may be secondary to chest trauma, mechanical ventilation or ruptured oesophagus, or may be induced artificially. Causes of traumatic pneumothorax include blunt trauma to the chest, commonly external cardiac massage, and penetrating chest injuries – for example, stab wounds or needle aspiration biopsies that breach the visceral pleura from without – and transbronchial biopsy and positive pressure ventilation that breach the visceral pleura from within. A spontaneous pneumothorax may be primary, in which case the patients are otherwise healthy, or may be secondary to some other disorder (Table 14.52). Of these, airways obstruction, particularly when due to bullous emphysema, is the most common predisposing cause.

Table 14.52 Conditions predisposing to pneumothorax

Chronic bronchitis and emphysema
Asthma
Cystic fibrosis
Tuberculosis
Marfan's syndrome, Ehlers-Danlos syndrome
Congenital cysts
Honeycomb lung

Clinical features

Most commonly, spontaneous pneumothorax develops in an otherwise fit person as a result of the rupture of a small apical pleural bleb, probably congenital in origin. Young adult males are most frequently affected and are often of tall and slim build. Characteristically, there is sudden onset of chest pain, laterally, sometimes radiating to the shoulder. With substantial collapse of the lung there is associated breathlessness, and a dry, irritating cough is common. Sometimes the patient is aware of the partially collapsed lung flopping about within the thorax. On examination, the most striking findings are of reduced breath sounds and hyper-resonant percussion. A small left-sided pneumothorax may be associated with a clicking noise with each heart-beat noted by the patient and on occasions loud enough to be heard by others. A large pneumothorax in a normal person causes breathlessness, and in the presence of pre-existing pulmonary disease a small one may cause severe respiratory distress. Characteristically, breathlessness is greatest immediately the lung collapses and then improves somewhat over a period of several hours, perhaps reflecting the reduction in perfusion of the collapsed lung and an overall improvement in ventilation–perfusion matching.

Tension pneumothorax is a medical emergency. The valve action of the pleural tear results in a progressive increase in the size and pressure of the pneumothorax. The underlying lung is totally collapsed. The mediastinum is shifted to the contralateral side, compromising the function of the opposite lung, and the high intrathoracic pressure elevates the jugular venous pressure, reduces venous return and causes tachycardia, low cardiac output and eventually circulatory collapse and death.

With the exception of a tension pneumothorax, when action may be required immediately, a chest X-ray is necessary in all patients in whom the diagnosis of pneumothorax is a possibility. Small apical pneumothoraces may be difficult to see and an expiratory chest X-ray is helpful. The X-ray allows an assessment of the size and position of the pneumothorax (the air may be loculated if there are pleural adhesions), any abnormality in the underlying lung and the presence of mediastinal or subcutaneous air. A small volume of pleural fluid is commonly seen but when there is a larger collection it should be sampled to exclude bleeding and, occasionally, infection (pyopneumothorax).

Recurrence of pneumothorax is common; a young person with spontaneous pneumothorax has a 20–30% chance of a second one, usually on the same side; with each pneumothorax the probability of further episodes increases. The longer the time that elapses following a pneumothorax, the less chance there is of a recurrence.

Management

Any pneumothorax sufficient to cause or increase breathlessness requires drainage. Many patients, particularly young, otherwise fit males, present with a small or moderate pneumothorax and whatever breathlessness was experienced acutely has settled. Such closed pneumothoraces do not require therapy and the patient can be monitored as an outpatient, provided he is instructed to seek medical advice if breathlessness returns. A 20–30% collapse of a lung normally takes several weeks to expand fully. In a tension pneumothorax, if necessary, prior to the insertion of an intercostal drain, tension can be released by inserting an intravenous cannula into the pleural space in the second interspace in the mid-clavicular line. Unless a pneumothorax is loculated, the best site for a drain is in the mid-axilla at the level of the sixth intercostal space.

When the catheter is connected to the underwater seal drainage bottle, any pleural air under positive pressure bubbles out. Careful and regular inspection of the level and movement of the water meniscus of the draining tube

Fig. 14.70 Pneumothorax. A. In a closed pneumothorax, the meniscus in the drain rises and falls with breathing and at resting end expiration the small negative intrathoracic pressure supports a column of water. **B.** In an open pneumothorax air bubbles into the drainage bottle, with each breath, during active expiration. **C.** If pleural fluid blocks the drainage tube the bubbling of air ceases and there is little movement of the meniscus with breathing. This situation can, therefore, mimic that of a resolved pneumothorax.

provides important information in the management of a pneumothorax (Fig. 14.70). In a closed pneumothorax coughing or other manœuvres that produce a positive intrathoracic pressure drain the air and the pneumothorax rapidly resolves. When there is a large defect in the visceral pleura, producing an open pneumothorax and a bronchopleural fistula, any manœuvre producing positive intrathoracic pressure causes much bubbling, but since the pleural defect remains the pneumothorax does not resolve. The chest drain is kept *in situ* in the hope that the pleural defect will close and the pneumothorax will convert from an open to a closed type and will then resolve. If resolution does not occur within a few days, it is common practice to apply suction to the pneumothorax. In practice, only a minority of open pneumothoraces, usually those in which the pleural leak is small, can be treated in this way. Frequently, the application of suction simply serves to hold the pleural defect open.

When air no longer bubbles from the catheter even when the patient coughs, a chest X-ray should be taken to confirm that the lung has fully expanded. If this is the case, the drain should be clamped for several hours and if the lung remains fully inflated the drain can be removed. Where a drain has been inserted for a recurrent pneumothorax a medical pleurodesis should be undertaken prior to removal of the catheter. If an open pneumothorax persists for a week despite a period of suction the patient should be referred for thoracotomy, closure of the bronchopleural fistula and parietal pleural abrasion or pleurectomy.

Mediastinal emphysema (pneumomediastinum)

Air can enter the mediastinum following penetrating neck injuries, and oesophageal and bronchial rupture, but the most common cause is rupture of alveoli. Air enters the interstitial tissues and tracks to the mediastinum. High intrapulmonary pressures due, for example, to vomiting, are frequently the cause. In asthma, gas trapping, alveolar distension and high intrapulmonary pressures during coughing make mediastinal emphysema a relatively common complication. Positive pressure mechanical ventilation can produce mediastinal emphysema as well as pneumothorax. Mediastinal emphysema is usually asymptomatic but can cause chest pain which may be worse on swallowing or breathing. There may also be a crunching sound coincident with each heart-beat. Radiology may show air in the upper mediastinum, around the heart, within the soft tissues of the neck and, in 30% of cases, an associated pneumothorax. Treatment is of the predisposing cause, following which the mediastinal emphysema rapidly resolves. Resolution can be hastened by breathing a high inspiratory oxygen concentration, during which the more soluble oxygen replaces the insoluble nitrogen.

TUMOURS OF THE PLEURA

The pleura can be the primary site of benign or malignant tumours or, more commonly, the site of metastatic malignant disease.

Fibroma

The pleura, usually the visceral surface, may be the site of a single benign fibrous tumour (localised fibrous mesothelioma). The tumour, which is well encapsulated and often pedunculated, is frequently first noted as a peripheral pleural mass on routine chest X-ray. A pleural effusion is not common. These tumours are not associated with asbestos exposure. Fibromas can become large and thereby cause breathlessness as well as chest pain. Patients are generally middle-aged or elderly and clubbing, as well as hypertrophic pulmonary osteoarthropathy, is a frequent association. A definite diagnosis is seldom possible without thoracotomy and biopsy, and surgical resection is the correct management. If left untreated, these tumours may eventually become locally invasive.

Diffuse mesothelioma

Diffuse mesothelioma, a highly malignant tumour, is related to asbestos exposure in most, perhaps all, cases. The patient's exposure to asbestos is, on average, 30 years prior to the malignancy becoming apparent. Most commonly, exposure to asbestos is in the shipbuilding, construction and demolition industries. Crocidolite (blue asbestos) is most commonly incriminated. In the UK about 300 patients each year are diagnosed as having malignant mesothelioma. The tumour spreads over the pleural surface, causing great thickening of the pleura by malignant tissue, and the lung becomes encased. The tumour spreads into the mediastinum, and through the diaphragm to involve the peritoneum, and invades the chest wall. An effusion is characteristic and is often blood-stained. Distant

metastases occur, although relatively infrequently. The histology is pleomorphic and a definite diagnosis, particularly the distinction from secondary adenocarcinoma, is often difficult on a small biopsy sample.

Patients with malignant mesothelioma present at an average age of 60, most commonly with persistent dull chest pain. There is progressive breathlessness because of pleural thickening and the accumulation of fluid. Finger clubbing is relatively unusual. The chest X-ray commonly shows a large effusion with the pleural tumour often only apparent following aspiration. CT scanning clearly demonstrates the extent of pleural disease, and when pleural calcification is also present, the appearances are highly suggestive of the diagnosis (Fig. 14.71). Although cytology of aspirated fluid may demonstrate malignant cells and Abram's or Trucut pleural biopsy may also show malignancy, a large surgical biopsy is often needed to confirm

Fig. 14.71 Mesothelioma. A. The chest X-ray shows bilateral pleural thickening and fluid. **B.** The CT scan shows extensive pleural thickening, plus fluid, and pleural calcification posteriorly on the right (arrow).

the diagnosis. However, surgical biopsy is not infrequently followed by additional chronic pain and infiltration of the thoracotomy scar by tumour. No therapy, whether surgery, cytotoxic drugs or radiotherapy, has been demonstrated to prolong life. Life expectancy is 1–2 years following presentation. In the UK patients with a definite history of asbestos exposure are eligible for industrial injuries benefit.

Metastatic malignant pleural disease

Pleural metastases with an associated effusion are very common, particularly with bronchial carcinoma. The effusion is usually painless but causes breathlessness and may require pleurodesis (p. 533). Pleural involvement is also common following malignant disease of the breast and ovary. Less commonly, pleural involvement occurs in other carcinomas, lymphangitis carcinomatosa, multiple myeloma, malignant lymphoma (particularly Hodgkin's disease) and Waldenström's macroglobulinaemia.

NEUROMUSCULAR AND SKELETAL DISORDERS

NEUROMUSCULAR DISORDERS

Ventilation depends on adequate central respiratory drive and depression of central nervous system function can therefore cause ventilatory failure. In such patients the diagnosis is usually self-evident and the resulting hypercapnia easily documented. Central nervous system dysfunction may also cause sleep apnoea syndromes (p. 498). In addition to these problems a wide range of neurological and muscular disorders can cause ventilatory impairment on the basis of respiratory muscle weakness (Table 14.53).

Table 14.53 Neuromuscular disorders which cause respiratory muscle weakness

Neurogenic	Myopathic
Motor neurone disease	Muscular dystrophy/atrophy
Surgical trauma of phrenic nerves	Inflammatory myopathies
Polyneuropathy	Myotonic dystrophy
Neuralgic amyotrophy	Acid maltase deficiency
Poliomyelitis	Thyroid myopathy
Multiple sclerosis	Metabolic disturbance (e.g.
Traumatic tetraplegia	hypophosphataemia)
Acute porphyria	
Charcot-Marie-Tooth disease	
Neuromuscular junction	
Myasthenia gravis	
Lambert-Eaton syndrome	

The respiratory muscles

In normal man, at rest, inspiration is active whereas expiration is a passive process; most of the respiratory muscles

are therefore inspiratory in their action.

The *diaphragm* is the principal muscle of inspiration and is responsible for 80% of ventilation at rest. Diaphragm contraction causes descent of the diaphragmatic dome, anterior displacement of the abdominal wall, elevation of the lower ribs and expansion of the lower thorax. At resting lung volume (functional residual capacity) the *external intercostal muscles* are inspiratory and the *internal intercostal muscles* are expiratory. The *abdominal muscles* are the most powerful muscles of expiration. These muscles also return the diaphragm to its optimal resting length prior to inspiration. The *accessory muscles* of respiration are conventionally considered to be the sternomastoid, scalene and pectoral muscles, which act mainly to fix or elevate the upper ribcage. However, many other muscles contract vigorously during maximum respiratory efforts.

The respiratory muscles in neuromuscular disease

Clinical assessment

Isolated involvement of the respiratory muscles by neuromuscular disease is unusual, and most patients will have evidence of more widespread involvement, with, for example, weakness of other muscle groups, bulbar problems and impaired cough, as well as breathlessness. On examination, there may be muscle wasting, weakness and fasciculation. Patients with bilateral severe diaphragm weakness or complete diaphragm paralysis present an unusual and striking clinical picture (Fig. 14.72). Orthopnoea is a prominent symptom of severe diaphragm weakness. When upright, patients frequently manage surprisingly well, but when supine, they become very breathless and exhibit the important physical sign of paradoxical inward movement of the abdomen with inspiration.

Severe weakness of the inspiratory muscles reduces the

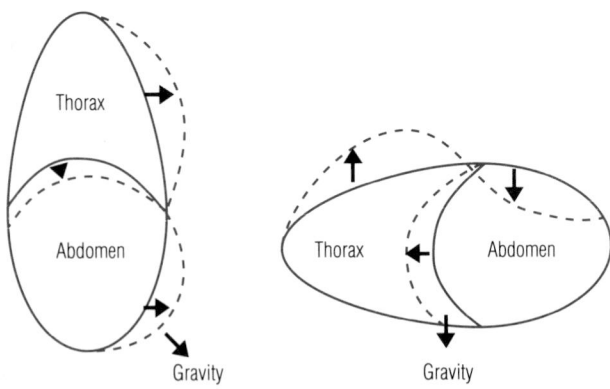

Fig. 14.72 Paralysis or severe weakness of the diaphragm. When upright the thorax is expanded by contraction of the intercostal muscles. The abdominal muscles relax, the diaphragm passively descends, and the anterior abdominal wall moves outwards. When supine the contraction of the intercostal muscles lowers intrathoracic pressure, sucks the diaphragm into the chest and the anterior abdominal wall moves inwards. Patients with diaphragm paralysis therefore have severe orthopnoea.

lung volume on the chest radiograph, but this can be an unreliable sign; furthermore, unless the radiologist is already aware of the diagnosis, it is likely that it will be assumed that the patient has chosen not to take a full inspiration rather than that he is incapable of doing so (Fig. 14.73).

Diaphragm paralysis elevates the hemidiaphragm involved although occasionally there can be similar elevation in normal subjects. Radiological screening, which should be performed with the patient supine, will demonstrate the upward movement of a paralysed hemidiaphragm during a sharp sniff.

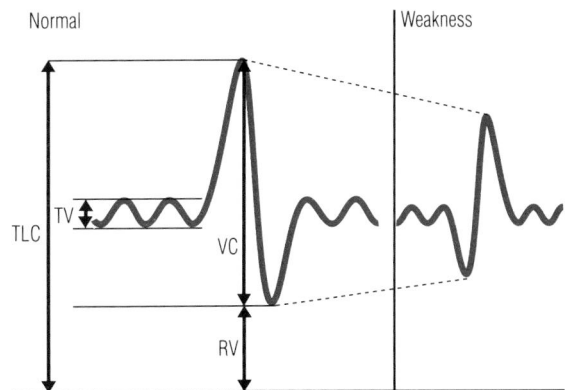

Fig. 14.74 The effect of respiratory muscle weakness on lung volumes. (TLC = total lung capacity; TV = tidal volume; VC = vital capacity; RV = residual volume.)

Fig. 14.73 Severe respiratory muscle weakness in a patient with motor neurone disease. Initially the small-volume lungs on chest X-ray were attributed to poor patient co-operation.

Lung function

Respiratory muscle weakness reduces both inspiratory and expiratory capacity (Fig. 14.74). Total lung capacity (TLC) is reduced, residual volume (RV) is increased and both of these changes decrease vital capacity (VC), and this simple measurement is therefore an excellent one for the detection of respiratory muscle weakness. Vital capacity is an ideal measurement in the follow-up of patients with weakness and in muscular dystrophy; for example, the vital capacity correlates well with both the clinical staging of disease and the assessment of prognosis. In neuromuscular disorders that can cause rapid profound weakness (for example, the Guillain-Barré syndrome) large falls in vital capacity warn that assisted ventilation may be required. The measurement of vital capacity is particularly useful when assessing diaphragm weakness. In the upright posture, vital capacity is reduced, but when the patient lies flat there is a further marked fall in vital capacity, characteristically by 50% with total paralysis of the diaphragm. Lung function in patients with respiratory muscle weakness shows no evidence of airways obstruction and the ratio of FEV_1 to FVC is normal. Although overall gas transfer may be reduced, when corrected for the reduction in lung volume gas transfer is normal or raised. With the progression of neuromuscular disease, patients gradually develop hypoxaemia, but hypercapnia is a late development associated with a poor prognosis. Hypercapnic ventilatory failure is unusual before the vital capacity has fallen to below 50% of normal. With generalised respiratory muscle weakness, particularly when the diaphragm is severely involved, ventilatory failure is more pronounced when supine, and may be particularly severe during sleep.

Respiratory pressure

A normal supine vital capacity excludes severe inspiratory muscle weakness, but a reduced vital capacity is not specific for weakness and must be assessed in the context of possible co-existing respiratory disease. A more specific and sensitive index of global respiratory muscle strength is provided by measurement of maximum static mouth pressures. Pressures are measured by a transducer or gauge; expiratory mouth pressures are taken during a maximum expiratory effort at TLC against an obstructive airway, and inspiratory mouth pressures are measured during a maximum inspiratory effort from residual volume.

In patients with generalised neuromuscular diseases, respiratory pressures are commonly reduced to 50% of normal, even though patients are often not particularly breathless. Hypercapnia is unusual unless inspiratory mouth pressures are reduced to below 30% of normal. A maximum inspiratory pressure of $-80\,cmH_2O$ excludes significant inspiratory muscle weakness but values as low as $-40\,cmH_2O$ are difficult to interpret because of the wide normal range. Experience of measuring oesophageal pressure, a good index of pleural pressure, during a maximum sniff manœuvre (when all inspiratory muscles contract vigorously) suggests that in patients in whom there is difficulty measuring static mouth pressures, sniff oesophageal pressure is a good measurement to quantify inspiratory muscle weakness.

Diaphragm weakness

The phrenic nerves are commonly invaded by tumour, particularly carcinoma of the bronchus. Viral infections, including herpes zoster, can cause a phrenic neuropathy, as can the neurological disorders of motor neurone disease, poliomyelitis, Charcot-Marie-Tooth disease and many peripheral neuropathies. Trauma, particularly surgery, is important, and phrenic nerve dysfunction is quite common following cardiac surgery. In the past, phrenic crush and phrenic avulsion for the treatment of tuberculosis was a common cause of phrenic neuropathy. Unilateral phrenic nerve palsy causes a 20% reduction in ventilatory capacity and a reduction in maximum transdiaphragmatic pressures, but patients have few symptoms: perhaps transient breathlessness, in the absence of additional pathology. Bilateral phrenic nerve paresis, on the other hand, causes shortness of breath on exertion and severe orthopnoea; indeed, patients are quite unable to remain flat for more than a few seconds. Many patients sleep propped up or on their sides to assist ventilation (Fig. 14.71).

Diaphragm strength can be specifically and accurately measured by recording transdiaphragmatic pressure (P_{di}) with oesophageal and gastric balloon catheters. The strength of the diaphragm can be measured for maximum static inspiratory efforts and diaphragm weakness can be quantified for myopathic patients. An alternative manœuvre to assess diaphragm strength and weakness is a maximum sniff.

Management

Respiratory muscle weakness due to neuromuscular disease may spontaneously improve as in the Guillain-Barré syndrome, or may respond to appropriate therapy, as in myasthenia gravis. Prior to improvement, some patients may require a period of mechanical ventilation. In most patients, however, deterioration is relentless, particularly in those with muscular dystrophy or motor neurone disease, and these patients die of respiratory infection and ventilatory failure. In a few patients deterioration may be very slow or a plateau may be reached, with respiratory muscle weakness causing ventilatory failure and disabling breathlessness. For a small number of carefully selected patients, assisted ventilation may be appropriate, particularly at night. Positive pressure ventilation (via tracheostomy or nasal mask) and negative pressure ventilation (with tank ventilators, cuirasses and jackets) can both be used, usually in the patient's home, and long-term survival and quality of life can make this treatment worthwhile.

In patients with quadriplegia from high cervical cord lesions, the diaphragm and other respiratory muscles are paralysed and the patient is dependent on mechanical ventilation. If the phrenic nerves are intact, as shown by adequate diaphragm contraction with percutaneous phrenic nerve stimulation, diaphragm pacing via the phrenic nerves can sustain ventilation and mechanical ventilation is no longer required.

Metabolic disorders causing weakness

Acidosis impairs the contractility of both skeletal and cardiac muscles. Hypercapnia, perhaps mediated through acidosis, adversely affects muscle function and it is probable that the interaction of hypercapnic acidosis and hypoventilation contributes to the rapid deterioration of patients with ventilatory failure and a low pH. Hypophosphataemia is a well-recognised cause of ventilatory failure due to respiratory muscle weakness and is an important factor on the intensive care unit. Reversible weakness of the respiratory muscles also occurs with hypokalaemia and disorders of magnesium and calcium metabolism.

Weight loss and muscle weakness

Patients with a wide variety of medical and surgical illnesses have profound weight loss and muscle atrophy with consequent weakness. This loss of muscle bulk involves the respiratory muscles, which therefore also become weak. Adequate nutrition, particularly in hospitalised patients, can minimise wasting, as will the reversal of catabolic factors such as sepsis, fever, protein-losing states and steroid therapy. Studies of the effectiveness of additional nutritional support designed to improve muscle bulk have yielded conflicting results, but every attempt should be made to optimise the nutrition of all seriously ill patients (p. 554).

Immobilisation leads to rapid atrophy of skeletal muscle, and it is possible that prolonged mechanical ventilation causes disuse atrophy of the respiratory muscles. Recent studies in chronically ventilated animals strongly support the concept of disuse atrophy of the diaphragm. During the 6 months following the initiation of diaphragm pacing, the strength of the paced diaphragm doubles, again suggesting that disuse atrophy can be profound.

Respiratory muscle function in patients with airways obstruction

Chronic bronchitis, emphysema and asthma cause airways obstruction and hyperinflation, both of which require the patient to generate greater than normal pressures during tidal breathing. The capacity of the respiratory muscles to produce the required large negative intrapleural pressure is compromised by muscle shortening, decreased diaphragm curvature, increased velocity of shortening and abnormal ribcage geometry. Respiratory muscle contractility may also be impaired by reduced oxygen delivery to the muscle, as a consequence of hypoxaemia and cardiovascular disease, and also by the respiratory acidosis associated with acute hypercapnia. The increased work of breathing combined with the reduced capacity of the respiratory muscles to generate tensions limits ventilatory reserve, causes breathlessness and may predispose to the development of respiratory muscle fatigue and hypercapnic ventilatory failure as, for example, in severe acute asthma. Patients with airflow limitation require a high respiratory centre output to maintain ventilation, and depression of neural output (for example, by sedatives) can markedly impair breathing. The work of breathing is reduced and the function of the respiratory muscles improved by therapy that reduces airflow limitation and lung volume.

In patients with chronic lung diseases, specific respiratory muscle training has been undertaken with a view to improving both the strength and endurance of the respiratory muscles. Although some studies have reported a modest benefit from training, the overall value of such training programmes remains a matter of debate. Attempts have also been made to improve respiratory muscle contractility with drugs. It has been postulated that theophylline may have a very small inotropic effect but it is doubtful whether under most circumstances this is of any clinical importance.

Respiratory muscle fatigue

All skeletal muscles fatigue when subjected to sufficiently high load, and the respiratory muscles are no exception. Careful studies of the stressed respiratory muscles of normal subjects have demonstrated fatigue in terms of electromyographic changes, slowing of relaxation rate, and reduced contractile response to electrical stimulation. However, these complex techniques have not easily been applied to patients with ventilatory failure and the clinical importance of respiratory muscle fatigue remains to be established. Some authorities, particularly in North America, advocate the 'resting' of the respiratory muscles by assisted ventilation to allow respiratory muscle fatigue to resolve. More clinical studies on the detection of respiratory muscle fatigue and its clinical importance are necessary before widespread use of this approach could be advocated.

THORACIC DEFORMITY

Adequate ventilation requires that the thoracic cage is of adequate volume, rigidity and mobility. Many of the disorders causing thoracic deformity are now rare (for example, rickets) and the most common problems are flail chest (a surgical and anaesthetic emergency), ankylosing spondylitis, scoliosis, thoracoplasty and fibrothorax.

Ankylosing spondylitis

Ankylosis of the ribs is characteristic of ankylosing spondylitis (p. 997) and chest expansion is frequently reduced. Respiratory problems occur relatively late in the course of the disease and most patients are 50–70 years old before developing symptoms. In addition to the classical radiological changes affecting the spine (p. 997), patients can also develop upper zone pulmonary fibrosis with cavitation and occasionally an aspergillus fungal ball (mycetoma). Despite the reduced expansion of the ribcage ventilation

is relatively little impaired because of good diaphragm function and, in the absence of co-existing severe cardiorespiratory disease, ventilatory failure does not occur. As a consequence of the importance of diaphragm function patients tolerate badly upper abdominal surgery or any other factor impairing diaphragm function.

Scoliosis

Scoliosis refers to a lateral curve of the spine and in most cases, perhaps three-quarters, it has no known cause. A wide variety of disorders are responsible for the remaining cases (Table 14.54). Although a congenital vertebral abnormality produces scoliosis in childhood, most scolioses develop in adolescence during the rapid growth spurt. Congenital heart disease is common in scoliotic patients. Scoliosis makes the thoracic cage stiff. The deformity also reduces the volume of the lungs and adversely affects the mechanical advantage of the respiratory muscles. Lung function tests show a restrictive ventilatory defect, the severity of which is related to the angle of scoliosis, with high thoracic curves causing the greatest impairment. Patients with moderate or severe scoliosis are breathless and with more severe deformity they eventually develop hypoxaemia, hypercapnia, pulmonary hypertension and cor pulmonale. Patients with scoliosis secondary to neurological disorders are frequently the most severely affected, particularly if diaphragm function is impaired. Ventilatory failure first becomes apparent during the night, particularly as a consequence of the hypoventilation associated with REM sleep. With the onset of ventilatory failure, the patients require assisted ventilation using negative pressure devices such as a purpose-built cuirass, a Tunnicliffe jacket, pneumosuit or body wrap. Positive pressure ventilation, via a nasal mask, is also very effective. Such domiciliary ventilation is usually only needed at night and can produce remarkable long-term well-being with control of respiratory failure by day, reversal of pulmonary hypertension and resolution of cor pulmonale. During acute episodes of deterioration, more prolonged ventilatory support may be required. From a respiratory point of view, the role of surgery to straighten a scoliosis is controversial. Most surgery is undertaken in adolescence with the aim of avoiding the deterioration of curvature and ventilatory function that otherwise occurs at this time.

Table 14.54 Disorders causing chronic scoliosis

Idiopathic

Disorders of bone (e.g. osteogenesis imperfecta)

Neurological diseases (e.g. cerebral palsy, poliomyelitis)

Muscle disease (e.g. muscular dystrophy)

Connective tissue disorders (e.g. Marfan's syndrome, Ehlers-Danlos syndrome)

Thoracic surgery (e.g. pneumonectomy, thoracoplasty)

Chronic infection (e.g. empyema)

Fig. 14.75 Extensive left thoracoplasty. Also note the apical pleural thickening on the right. The patient had advanced ventilatory failure

Thoracoplasty (Fig. 14.75), a relatively common surgical procedure in the treatment of pulmonary tuberculosis prior to modern drug management, produces a similar ventilatory defect to scoliosis. Many patients with thoraco-plasty develop breathlessness and eventually ventilatory failure in later life. Some of these patients have been treated with nocturnal domiciliary ventilation with excellent long-term results comparable with those for scoliosis. Such is the success of assisted ventilation programmes that all patients with severe or progressive chest wall deformity require careful specialist long-term follow-up.

FURTHER READING

Clark T J H, Godfrey S (eds) 1983 Asthma. 2nd edn. Chapman & Hall, London. *A comprehensive clinical account of all aspects of asthma.*

Fraser R G, Paré J A P 1977 Diagnosis of diseases of the chest. 2nd edn. 4 vols. W B Saunders Company, Philadelphia. *Definitive American text on the diagnosis of chest disease, based on the detailed analysis of the chest X-ray and other imaging techniques.*

Fraser R G, Paré J A P, Paré P D, Fraser R S, Genereux G P 1989 Diagnosis of diseases of the chest. 3rd edn. W B Saunders Company, Philadelphia. *Updated edition of the above; vols 1 and 2 published.*

Murray J F 1986 The normal lung. 2nd edn. W B Saunders Company, Philadelphia. *A comprehensive, well-illustrated account of the structure and function of the respiratory system.*

Murray J F, Nadel J A (eds) 1988 Textbook of respiratory medicine. W B Saunders Company, Philadelphia. *Up-to-date, comprehensive and detailed American text of all aspects of respiratory disease.*

Seaton A, Seaton D, Leitch A G 1988 Crofton and Douglas's respiratory diseases. 4th edn. Blackwell Scientific, Oxford. *The most established and comprehensive British textbook of respiratory medicine.*

Critical Care Medicine

Critical care medicine has its origins in the treatment of failing organ systems; it began with respiratory support, utilising techniques developed in anaesthesia, and was accelerated in the 1950s by the need to ventilate large numbers of patients with paralytic polio. Patients are now admitted to the intensive care unit (ICU), not only to receive mechanical ventilation, but also for the management of a wide variety of severe illnesses, and the role of the 'intensivist' commonly involves the diagnosis of those who are obtunded as well as the management of those in organ failure. The skills required are extensive and the work demands the expertise of a team of medical and nursing staff. This team functions most effectively when led by an enthusiastic and committed critical care specialist.

By necessity, the intensive care unit concentrates facilities in one area, with an array of technology. Facilities are available for immediate resuscitation. Many physiological variables are monitored continuously with the aid of electronic monitors at each bedside (Fig. 15.1). Infusions and fluid balance can be measured over time periods of minutes, as well as hours and days. Routine laboratory investigations are often performed on the ward itself, enabling sequential analysis of arterial blood gases, electrolytes and other biochemical data. Central to this process of monitoring and

Parenteral nutrition

CVP manometer

Drug infusion pump

Haemofiltration (CAVHD)

Cardiovascular monitor (ECG, arterial and PA pressures, PAWP)

Pulse oximeter (oxygen saturation)

CO_2 monitor (end tidal CO_2)

Mechanical ventilator

Cardiac output computer

Fig. 15.1 Patient on the intensive care unit. Physiological monitoring is crucial to the management of failing organ systems. This patient is supported by mechanical ventilation, haemofiltration and parenteral nutrition. Clinical examination is as important as physiological measurement and is easily deterred by the array of equipment. (CVP = central venous pressure; CAVHD = continuous arterio-venous haemodialysis; PA = pulmonary artery; PAWP = pulmonary artery wedge pressure) adjustment of the patient's physiology is the intensive care nurse, usually allocated to the care of a single patient. Specialist skills, formerly undertaken in other units (e.g. angiography, dialysis), are increasingly available on the intensive care unit. Despite advanced technology, basic medical skills still apply, in that all patients require a diagnosis that is based on careful enquiry and examination, supplemented by relevant investigations.

Patients are admitted to the ICU either as a planned extension of their postoperative care, or as a result of a sudden deterioration. The number of postoperative patients has risen as surgical and anaesthetic techniques have advanced, and this has led to competition for intensive care unit facilities. ICUs are provided in most district general hospitals. The number of beds is generally 1 per 100 general beds in the hospital, although in many developed countries the number is substantially greater. The consumption of resources by such units is considerable. The variety of causes for admission to the ICU is wide, but many patients fall within a limited number of clinical categories (Table 15.1).

Table 15.1   Common causes for admission to ICU

- Postoperative care (cardiac, major vascular and abdominal surgery)
- Major trauma, including head injury
- Respiratory failure
- Post-cardiopulmonary resuscitation
- Drug overdose

CARDIOVASCULAR PROBLEMS

Patients admitted to the intensive care unit frequently require assessment, monitoring and therapy directed at the cardiovascular system (CVS). The action of the heart is to deliver oxygenated blood and nutrients to the peripheral organs and tissues. With each contraction, blood is ejected into the aorta (stroke volume) and cardiac output is the product of the stroke volume and heart rate. The effects of disturbances of the CVS are seen in the heart itself and in the peripheral organ systems it supplies.

Some of the mechanical features of the heart can be simply demonstrated by considering a strip of cardiac muscle attached at one end to a transducer that records tension during an electrical stimulation (Fig. 15.2). The other end of the muscle is fixed to a pivoted bar. To the opposite end of the bar, weights can be added, stretching the muscle. The distance the muscle is stretched is limited by a peg.

Ventricular filling pressure (preload)

The muscle is stretched by the weight so that the bar swings upwards, just touching the peg. If the peg is moved, allowing the muscle to lengthen, extra stretch takes place if a slightly greater weight is placed on the end of the bar. The weight stretching the muscle is termed the preload.

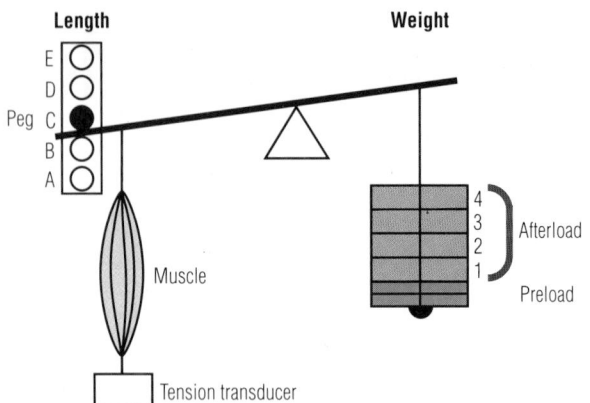

Fig. 15.2   Preload and afterload. The tension generated by the strip of cardiac muscle depends on its length. This is altered by moving the peg up and down (positions A–E). Weights, necessary to lengthen the muscle, are added to the weight hanger (preload). Increasing length initially enhances but eventually impairs contractility. Larger weights added to the hanger are termed the afterload. As these weights are added (1–4), the muscle shortens less during contraction, although it develops greater tension. Eventually the weight (afterload) is so great that no shortening occurs.

The force generated by the muscle can be measured at different muscle lengths. As the muscle is stretched, so the force initially increases, and then declines as the actin–myosin cross-linkages are separated. The length of cardiac muscle cannot be directly measured on the intensive care unit, but during cardiac filling, the ventricular volume and pressure rise as the heart muscle fibres stretch. As the heart fills, the situation is analogous to that depicted in Figure 15.2. Initially the response to raising filling pressure (increased preload) is an increased stroke volume, but excessive pressures result in a fall in output.

In the patient on the ICU the great veins can be cannulated to allow measurement of right heart filling pressures. Central venous pressure (CVP) is related to right ventricular end diastolic pressure (i.e. right ventricular preload). CVP is influenced by the circulating blood volume, and in the hypovolaemic patient, filling pressures may be maintained by increasing the tone of smooth muscle within the walls of the venous circulation. This has the compensatory effect of diverting blood from the venous system, and maintaining cardiac output. Under these circumstances the measurement of a normal CVP may be misleading. In addition, the measurement of CVP does not always closely reflect the filling pressure of the left heart, as, for example, following acute infarction of the left ventricle. An indirect measurement of left ventricular filling pressure is achieved by the insertion of a Swan–Ganz catheter (see below).

Peripheral vascular resistance (afterload)

When the muscle strip depicted in Figure 15.2 is electrically stimulated, little work is performed in lifting a small weight and most of the energy is expended in shortening the muscle quickly. As weights are loaded on to the end of the bar, so the work performed by the muscle increases. The weight lifted by the muscle is termed the afterload, and is the resistance against which the muscle is working. Increasing the weight further eventually results in the muscle's capacity being exceeded, and it is unable to shorten.

Ventricular afterload is the sum of the resistances to blood flow across the circulatory beds of the peripheral organs and tissues. This can be envisaged as if a hosepipe were connected to a pump. As the end of the hosepipe is squeezed, so the resistance to the flow of water increases, decreasing the output of the pump. The work of the pump increases, as witnessed by the strained note of the motor. Without the constriction, flow is enhanced but the pressure in the hosepipe is reduced.

In patients, flow may be enhanced by reducing vaso-constriction, but excessive vasodilation causes a fall in blood pressure. The advantage of reducing afterload has to be judged against the disadvantage of systemic hypo-tension, which if sufficiently severe will itself impair tissue perfusion. Therapeutic intervention in this way therefore requires constant monitoring of circulatory physiology.

Left atrial filling pressure

In most patients, changes in the pressures in the right and left sides of the heart are closely correlated, but in the severely ill this may not be so. In such cases, it is frequently useful to measure separately the filling pressure of the right and the left ventricles. During cardiac surgery there is an opportunity to place a catheter directly into the left atrium, but in the ICU this is not possible and an alternative technique is used. If a catheter is placed peripherally in the pulmonary artery and a small balloon sited near the tip of the catheter is inflated to obstruct the artery, the pressure measured at the end of the catheter will reflect left atrial pressure rather than the pressure within the pulmonary artery. On the ICU, this is achieved by a balloon (Swan–Ganz) catheter, introduced into a central vein and directed into the right atrium. The flow of blood into the right atrium, through the right ventricle, and out into the pul-monary artery carries the catheter into smaller arteries until the balloon, if inflated, can be wedged in a narrow vessel. Running through the catheter is a lumen that emerges at the tip. The pressure at the tip of the catheter is displayed continuously, and as the catheter is advanced, the characteristic pressures of the right atrium, right ven-tricle and pulmonary artery are observed (Fig 15.3). The occluded pressure is termed the pulmonary artery wedge pressure (PAWP) and is related to the filling pressure of the left side of the heart. A pulmonary artery catheter can also be used to measure cardiac output.

Cardiac output

Cardiac output can be measured in patients on the intensive care unit by measuring the rate of disappearance of a dye introduced into the right atrium (*dye dilution technique*).

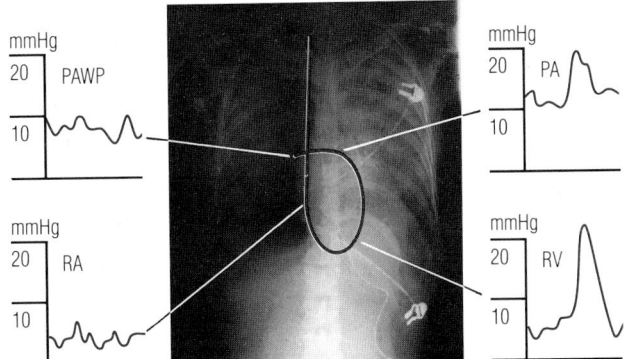

Fig. 15.3 Pulmonary artery (Swan-Ganz) catheter in position in a patient with severe pneumonia. As the catheter is advanced through the great veins into the right atrium (RA), right ventricle (RV) and pulmonary artery (PA), the characteristic pressure waves are displayed. The catheter is sited in the PA, and when measurement of pulmonary artery wedge pressure (PAWP) is required, the balloon at the tip of the catheter is inflated. Note that the chest X-ray confirms the correct positioning of the endotracheal and nasogastric tubes. The patient has a right-sided pneumothorax, with associated surgical emphysema, and an intercostal drain in situ.

The technique can be thought of as if a bath (right heart) were being kept full by a running tap (venous return). The rate of water entering the bath is the same as that being lost from the bath (cardiac output). We wish to know the flow of water through the tap. The dye is added and mixed in the bath (right ventricle), and, if the tap is running fast, the dye will be quickly washed away; the resultant graph of dye concentration against time will show a rapid fall. If the tap is running slowly, the time taken to wash out the dye is prolonged. In practice on the ICU, the indicator 'dye' used is cold saline (*thermodilution technique*), and the change in temperature in the pulmonary artery over time is measured; this technique has the advantage of avoiding the complication of dye recirculation.

CARDIOVASCULAR ASSESSMENT ON ICU

Whether the assessment is by clinical examination or involves complex monitoring, the approach to the cardio-vascular system involves an evaluation of cardiac output and peripheral perfusion in the face of the prevailing filling pressure. The aims are to determine the nature and extent of the cardiovascular disturbance and to monitor the effect of treatment, making adjustments to therapy as appro-priate. The normalisation of cardiac output and peripheral perfusion should be achieved promptly to avoid organ damage. In uncomplicated cases that respond rapidly to treatment, invasive measurements may not be required, but in many patients the need for physiological information to guide treatment requires invasive techniques.

Disorders of the circulation can be considered by con-structing the graph of filling pressure versus cardiac output (Fig. 15.4). In this example we have used the filling pres-sure of the left side of the heart. In order to allow for the

15

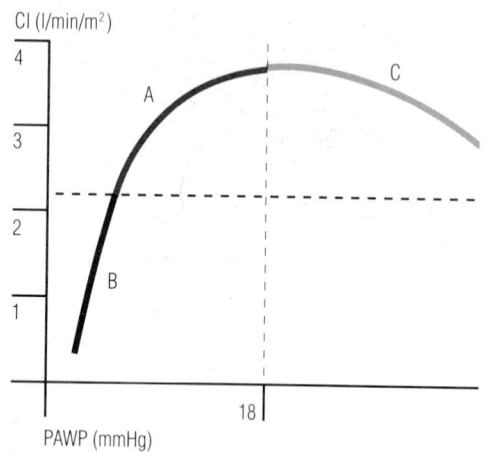

Fig. 15.4   The relationship between cardiac index (CI) and filling pressure (PAWP) for the normal heart. Patients are normally on the curve within square A; with decreased filling pressure, within square B; and with fluid overload, within square C.

differing size of patients, cardiac output is normalised by dividing by body surface area. This number is called the cardiac index (CI), and is expressed as l/min per m². We can see from the graph that, under normal circumstances (within square A), the normal heart responds to a raised filling pressure (increased preload) by a prompt increase in cardiac index. At the upper limits, further stretch or dilation of the heart results in a reduction in cardiac output. The graph can be used to define the cardiovascular problem, monitor the effect of treatment and predict outcome.

Decreased filling pressure

The graph within square B (Fig. 15.4) shows the filling pressure/cardiac index relationship when the filling pressure is reduced. The patient is pushed down the curve and to the left, with the reduction in cardiac index a direct consequence of decreased filling pressure. Filling pressure can be reduced either by a reduction in circulating blood volume due to haemorrhage or severe dehydration, or by loss of venous return if the circulation is suddenly vasodilated. The fall in filling pressure is sensed by barroreceptors, which stimulate the release of catecholamines from the adrenal gland and sympathetic nervous system. Catecholamines act on the myocardium to increase both heart rate and the force of contraction (positive inotropic effect), and on the peripheral vessels to maintain venous return by venoconstriction, and blood pressure by vasoconstriction (increased peripheral vascular resistance). Other neurohormonal reflexes are also stimulated. Fluid loss from the kidney falls, firstly due to a reduction in glomerular filtration rate (GFR). Aldosterone is released, reabsorbing salt and water and further decreasing urinary losses. Metabolism is altered, and glycogenic hormones act to raise blood glucose. Hormones, released locally in the tissues, may also contribute to this 'stress response'.

The vital signs may be surprisingly normal in young, fit patients, who are able to maintain blood pressure despite hypovolaemia. In these patients tachycardia helps to maintain cardiac output. Peripheral blood flow is reduced by the release of catecholamines, and the skin is therefore pale, cold and clammy. The underperfused tissues respire anaerobically, producing lactic acid. With severe volume depletion, the patient may be confused, agitated and hyperventilating.

The important observation is that the filling pressure is low. The urine output is reduced and concentrated, with a high osmolality, and little filtered sodium is excreted. The skin is cold with a marked gradient between skin and central temperature.

Fluid replacement

Restoration of blood volume should be rapid if organ damage is to be avoided. The speed of transfusion is often inadequate, especially in the elderly where there is a fear of precipitating heart failure. As a guide to the adequacy of fluid replacement, a fluid challenge with an aliquot of 200–400 ml is helpful. In the hypovolaemic patient the response to fluid challenge is a transient rise in CVP, falling back to the baseline value in 10–15 minutes. As fluid replacement continues, further volume challenges result in more gradual rises and falls in filling pressure, until the point is reached where an increase in filling pressure is sustained. At this stage fluid replacement is adequate.

Choice of replacement fluid

The choice of replacement fluid depends on the cause of the decreased filling pressure. In haemorrhage, replacement with blood is essential, although blood substitutes may be used until blood is available. Severe dehydration requires predominantly salt and water replacement, and the total body deficit may take some time to correct. Reduction in filling pressure due to vasodilation can be corrected with a plasma substitute. If the circulation is restored quickly, the metabolic effects of an inadequate circulation will reverse spontaneously, but acidosis, hyperkalaemia and hyperglycaemia require careful management in patients in whom hypovolaemia has been prolonged.

Crystalloid solutions are readily available, but once in the circulation, they quickly redistribute away from the circulation and into the interstitial space. Only a small fraction of the volume transfused stays in the circulation. Large volumes are therefore needed to restore circulating volume, and the excess fluid in the interstitial space contributes to tissue oedema (including pulmonary oedema). Oedema is worsened by the dilution of plasma albumin, the major osmotically active component of blood. The subsequent excretion of the excess volume load is often impaired in the critically ill. Crystalloid therapy should usually be avoided and preference given to other solutions that remain in the circulation.

Several solutions are available that contain osmotically

active constituents. Gelatin solutions (e.g. Haemaccel) are maintained within the circulation for 2–3 hours, are stable in solution and have a long shelf life at room temperature; they are therefore immediately available. Starch polymer (hydroxyethyl starch) has a longer half-life (6–9 hours) and is less allergenic than the gelatins. Both these fluids do not carry oxygen, and do not replace clotting factors lost during haemorrhage. Their main value is in the maintenance of filling pressure during resuscitation prior to the availability of blood. The sodium content of these infusions is high, will subsequently need to be cleared by the patient, and can contribute to oedema formation.

Human albumin in solution (plasma protein fraction, PPF) is available and in the isosmotic form (4.5%) is ideal for volume replacement, especially in the critically ill. It is pasturised, avoiding the risk of infection, has a long shelf life and, although more expensive than the other polymer solutions, is better retained in the circulation. It does not contain clotting factors.

Cross-matched blood can be available within 20 minutes in an emergency. Blood is a living tissue, and when stored, metabolites gradually accumulate. It becomes rapidly depleted of clotting factors. The number of damaged cells and debris progressively increases, as well as the acidity and K^+ content. Blood is stored at a low temperature, and rapid transfusion will cool the recipient. The separated constituents of whole blood are available as fresh frozen plasma (FFP), which is frozen to prevent the degradation of clotting factors. FFP is scarce and expensive, and should not be given as routine volume replacement.

Fluid overload

In the muscle strip preparation stretching beyond the relaxed length produces an initial increase in tension, followed by failure as the muscle fibres are pulled apart. In patients, volume overload distends the ventricles, stretching the heart muscle. Volume overload is commonly caused by injudicious intravenous fluid therapy. Critically ill patients often retain fluid due to renal dysfunction, excess ADH secretion or drug therapy (e.g. steroids). Myocardial contractility is normal unless cardiac distension is excessive. Square C of the PAWP/CI graph (Fig. 15.4) shows the position of patients on the curve when the circulation is 'overfilled'. The cardiac index plateaus at high filling pressures, which produce oedema. The clinical signs can be similar to those of the poorly contracting ventricle (see below). Both right- and left-sided filling pressures are raised. Correct assessment commonly requires a pulmonary artery catheter. Treatment is to reduce filling pressures rather than the infusion of inotropes. Diuretic therapy reduces the volume of the circulation and promptly relieves oedema. If filling pressures are critically high, vasodilator therapy can reduce them acutely. Diuretic therapy will only be successful if cardiac output is sufficient to perfuse the kidneys and renal function is not impaired. If renal function is inadequate, volume reduction can be achieved by haemofiltration or veno-venous dialysis (p. 809).

Poor contractility

The relationship between filling pressure and cardiac index when the function of the left ventricle is depressed is shown in Figure 15.5. As filling pressure rises, the response of the ventricle is limited and the cardiac index is low. This commonly occurs after myocardial infarction (cardiogenic shock). The crucial point is that rises in the filling pressure do not improve cardiac index. Pulmonary oedema occurs when the filling pressure is raised (square D). The pressure at which fluid extravasates into the lung is determined by the balance of forces driving the fluid out of the circulation (hydrostatic pressure) and the osmotic pressure of the plasma, acting to retain fluid within the vasculature. As the filling pressures rise, this point is exceeded and oedema fluid develops (p. 520, Fig. 14.56). Oedema develops at low pressure if plasma proteins are reduced or capillary permeability is increased.

Patients with pump failure have a low volume pulse, raised jugular venous pressure, third heart sound and sometimes the signs of pulmonary oedema. As a result of the low cardiac index the urine output may be reduced. In such patients, the monitoring of the circulation is, of necessity, invasive. Continuous monitoring of arterial pressure requires a cannula inserted into a peripheral artery. A pulmonary artery catheter is used to monitor the function of the left and right ventricles, cardiac output, and pulmonary and systemic vascular resistances. A urinary catheter is necessary to measure urine output as an index of renal perfusion.

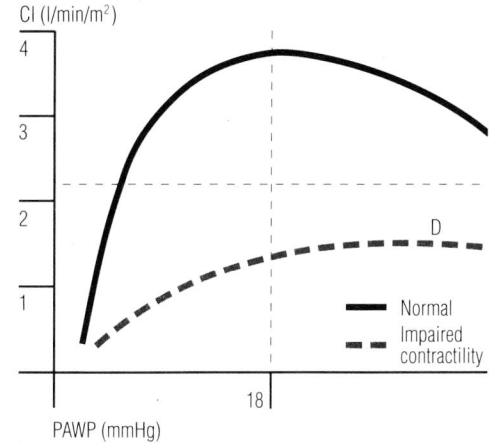

Fig. 15.5 Poor contractility. Compared to normal, the PAWP/CI curve (dashed line) is almost horizontal over a wide range of filling pressures.

Treatment

Whilst both poor contractility and hypovolaemia are characterised by a low cardiac index, the pathophysiology is radically different. In pump failure the aim of treatment is to restore the output of the heart for a given filling pressure, thereby altering the slope of the PAWP/CI curve back towards normal.

15

Positive inotropic agents

The naturally occurring inotropic agents are *adrenaline*, secreted by the adrenal medulla, and *noradrenaline*, produced by the sympathetic nervous system. The action on the heart is mediated via beta receptors and on peripheral blood vessels via alpha receptors. The effect of both of these agents is to increase the force of contraction of the myocardium. In addition, noradrenaline has a greater effect on peripheral blood vessels, causing vasoconstriction. Whilst noradrenaline is more potent in elevating blood pressure, it does so at the expense of decreasing peripheral perfusion.

Synthetic agents

Dopamine, a precursor to adrenaline, has differing effects depending on dose. At low dose the mesenteric circulation is dilated, enhancing flow to the kidney. As the dose increases, dopamine acts as a positive inotrope and chronotrope. At higher doses, peripheral vasoconstriction increases afterload and decreases cardiac index. *Dobutamine* is related to dopamine, but has no dilatory action on the mesenteric vessels. It produces a greater effect on cardiac contractility than dopamine, and may produce less tachycardia. The combination of the two agents permits renal vasodilation and myocardial stimulation.

Diuretic therapy

The potent loop diuretics are frequently used in conjunction with inotropes, when it becomes feasible to lower filling pressure (and reduce pulmonary oedema) without reducing cardiac output. The effect of frusemide is in part due to its minor vasodilating action, reducing filling pressure prior to a reduction in blood volume.

Vasodilators

Both preload and afterload are reduced by vasodilator therapy. Preload reduction is most effective when the filling pressure/cardiac output curve is flat, and reduction in filling pressure produces reversal of pulmonary oedema without large decreases in cardiac index. Careful monitoring of the circulation is essential, as slight alterations in vasodilator dosage may produce catastrophic reductions in cardiac output. All vaso-active drugs should be given by volumetric pumps, and the shorter-acting drugs are an advantage. Alteration in peripheral vascular resistance can be particularly effective if combined with inotropic support, thereby improving forward flow while maintaining myocardial perfusion pressure.

SEPTIC SHOCK

Hypotension as a complication of septicaemia is an important development, indicating the progression of a frequently fatal illness despite antibiotics. Vasodilating fragments and

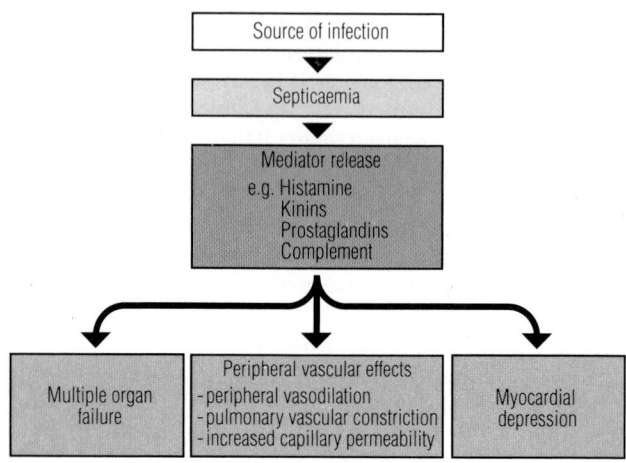

Fig. 15.6 Septic shock.

mediators (Fig. 15.6) cause a fall in peripheral vascular resistance, leading to hypotension despite maintenance of a normal or raised cardiac index. Peripheral blood flow is diverted to the skin and muscle, with poor perfusion of vital organs. In addition, substances released during acute endotoxaemia depress myocardial function. Sudden hypotension may occur, and the peripheral resistance may rapidly fall, possibly due to 'showers' of vaso-active agents released into the circulation.

The patient is vasodilated, with warm peripheries and bounding, high-volume pulses. Pyrexia is usual, but the temperature may, less commonly, be depressed. The cardiac index is high and peripheral resistance is reduced, as are filling pressures. To maintain a high cardiac index, in order to perfuse vital organs, filling pressures are monitored and plasma substitutes (PPF) given, often in large volumes. Despite adequate filling pressures, inotropic support may be required to maintain the cardiac index. Vasoconstricting drugs (alpha agonists) may worsen renal perfusion, but may occasionally be of value in intractable hypotension and increase urine output.

Negative inotropes

The force of contraction of the myocardium is depressed by acidosis, hypokalaemia, hypoxaemia and hypercapnia. These negative inotropes, particularly acidosis, offset the effectiveness of treatment. The dose response of catecholamines is reduced by acidosis. Correction of these disturbances may be dependent on restoring peripheral circulation, although in the short term, reversal of acidosis by hyperventilation (in patients receiving mechanical ventilation) and bicarbonate may be necessary.

The major determinant of oxygen delivery to heart muscle is coronary blood flow, which, if reduced, impairs contractility. Myocardial blood flow, especially to the subendocardial layer, is reduced by an increase in ventricular wall tension. This is the case in the dilated heart and in one contracting against a raised peripheral vascular resistance. Flow to all layers of the myocardium is crucially dependent on diastolic pressure and duration, and both are reduced by tachycardia. Improvement of coronary circulation can be effected by a reduction in afterload (reducing ventricular wall tension), if it is achieved without markedly decreasing diastolic pressure or causing a tachycardia.

Mechanical support

Myocardial function may remain depressed despite conventional therapy. Mechanical devices have been developed to enhance heart action by decreasing left ventricular work, and improving coronary blood flow and oxygenation. One device is the intra-aortic balloon pump (IABP). This pump is connected to a sausage-shaped balloon that is introduced percutaneously into the femoral artery and placed in the descending thoracic aorta. The gas-filled balloon is inflated during diastole, and blood flow in the aorta away from the heart is reversed, increasing coronary blood flow. The collapse of the balloon at the start of systole decreases peripheral vascular resistance. The IABP therefore reduces afterload but maintains coronary perfusion. It has had considerable success in the management of pump failure in the postoperative period following cardiac surgery, but much less success in patients with a low cardiac index after, for example, myocardial infarction. New techniques, including artificial hearts, may in the future allow time to prepare selected patients for cardiac transplantation.

With severe pulmonary oedema, the work of breathing is greatly increased. Overall oxygen consumption (and myocardial work) is reduced by mechanical ventilation. Whilst mechanical ventilation depresses cardiac index, this can be offset by the advantages of controlling pulmonary oedema and reducing oxygen consumption, and may allow for a stable period which will give the opportunity for other therapies to be pursued.

RESPIRATORY PROBLEMS

Respiratory failure has many causes (p. 500, Table 14.31). Severe hypoxaemia with or without hypercapnia is a common indication for the transfer of patients to the ICU, for monitoring and, where necessary, mechanical ventilation.

Assessment of ventilation and tissue oxygen delivery

During steady state conditions, when the amount of CO_2 from the tissues is constant, arterial CO_2 tension is dependent on alveolar ventilation. The adequacy of ventilation can therefore be judged by Pa_{CO_2}. As ventilation becomes inadequate, CO_2 is retained and eventually the patient becomes acidotic. Over many weeks acclimatisation to hypercapnia may occur, and the respiratory acidosis is compensated for by a metabolic alkalosis (p. 854). Despite the undoubted value of CO_2 measurements in the assessment of ventilation, it should be emphasised that in some patients (for example, those with severe asthma) there can be acute respiratory distress with CO_2 levels that are normal or reduced.

Adequacy of oxygenation is more difficult to assess. The arterial oxygen tension should be judged against the added oxygen the patient is breathing. In disease, as gas exchange deteriorates, so the difference between the inspired oxygen tension and that of arterial blood increases (the A–a gradient widens). The size of the A–a difference indicates the failure of the lung to perform gas exchange. The disorder within the lung may be due to impaired diffusion or V/Q mismatch, and added oxygen can correct this defect. However, if the hypoxaemia is due to blood bypassing ventilated alveoli (physiological shunt), then increasing the oxygen fraction will not dramatically improve blood gases. Both the level of added oxygen required, and the rate at which it is necessary to increase this fraction, reflect the severity and progression of disease.

The arterial blood gases provide a single respiratory assessment of the patient, and can be misleading when the patient's circumstances are changing rapidly. Repeated samples are often preferable and require the insertion of an arterial cannula. The clinical context of the arterial sample (e.g. F_{IO_2}, ventilator settings) should always be documented. Oximeters that continuously and non-invasively measure oxygen saturation are very useful.

O_2 must be delivered to the tissues, and therefore the state of oxygen transport and the uptake from the circulation are important. Transport of oxygen depends on the amount of haemoglobin and its ability to take up oxygen (O_2 dissociation curve, p. 453). The cardiac output and the state of the peripheral microcirculation then determine the delivery of oxygen to the respiring cells.

The tissues extract oxygen from the blood and in health the amount of oxygen delivered to the tissues each minute is much greater than is needed. In the critically ill, this may not be the case, and the level of oxygen in the venous blood may be reduced, indicating that not enough oxygen is being supplied. The cause may be failure of the lung to perform gas exchange, or inadequate tissue perfusion. The average O_2 tension in venous blood (mixed venous oxygen) provides useful information and can be measured from samples taken from a pulmonary artery catheter.

Indications for mechanical ventilation

Intubation and ventilation are easier to undertake as a considered manœuvre rather than as an emergency event. The entire clinical situation is relevant, and ventilation is seldom indicated solely on blood gas results. An increasing demand for oxygen over a few hours, or failure adequately to oxygenate the patient with maximum oxygen by mask, or mental deterioration indicates the likely need for mechanical support. Often, patients who are distressed initially have a normal or slightly lowered Pa_{CO_2}, with rapid shallow respirations. Further distress, an increase in the respiratory rate, or increasing sympathetic activity (tachycardia, hypertension) indicates greater difficulty in eliminating

CO_2, and exhaustion, with associated hypercapnia, is a common end point prior to ventilation.

The clearance of secretions by the patient is dependent on the ability to cough vigorously, and sputum retention may worsen or precipitate respiratory failure. Endotracheal intubation allows efficient removal of secretions by suction and also protects the upper airway from aspiration.

Many postoperative patients are ventilated electively to provide a period of stabilisation. Some patients are intubated during resuscitation. Mechanical ventilation is sometimes required to provide a stable setting during the management of another organ failure and is occasionally necessary in the management of the pulmonary oedema of left heart failure.

For artificial ventilation to be initiated, the patient must be anaesthetised and intubated. Patients may already be critically ill; if so, the cardiovascular effects of the anaesthetic agents, lack of reflexes guarding the larynx, mechanical problems in passing the tube, and effects of positive intrathoracic pressure on venous return make intubation and ventilation a potentially dangerous procedure.

Methods of ventilation

The ventilator provides the motive power to drive oxygen-enriched air into the patient's lungs. This may need to be done at high pressure, as, for example, when ventilating an asthmatic with severe bronchoconstriction. With modern ventilators it is possible to determine the respiratory rate, tidal volume, driving pressure and the timing and waveform of the inspiratory cycle. Many patients on ICU are deeply sedated and sometimes paralysed. The ventilatory requirements of such patients are totally provided by the mechanical ventilator: this type of ventilation is termed controlled mandatory ventilation (CMV). Other patients often require partial support from the ventilator, and breathe spontaneously at the same time (intermittent mandatory ventilation, IMV). As the machine and the patient are not synchronised, a machine breath can coincide with the patient's expiratory effort, creating excessive pressures in the airway. By timing the inspiratory cycle of the ventilator to the patient's own inspiratory effort, this can be avoided. The patient's inspiratory effort is sensed at the start of each breath, and the inspiratory cycle of the machine is initiated. The machine rate and tidal volume are set to provide adequate alveolar ventilation; this form of ventilation is termed synchronised intermittent mandatory ventilation (SIMV).

Another feature of ventilators is the addition of positive (greater than atmospheric) pressure throughout the expiratory phase of the respiratory cycle. The purpose of such positive end-expiratory pressure (PEEP) is to prevent collapse of peripheral airways and subsequent atelectasis, thereby improving gas exchange. The addition of PEEP, commonly 5–10 cm H_2O, usually improves arterial oxygen tension, but impedes venous return and can reduce cardiac index. Oxygen delivery to the tissues may therefore be decreased despite an improvement in Pa_{O_2}. PEEP may also increase pressure damage to the lung. The optimum level of PEEP for a particular patient is that which maximises tissue oxygen delivery.

Complications of ventilation

The immediate problems of intubation – for example trauma, aspiration and hypoxaemia – and the initial cardiovascular effects of positive pressure ventilation have already been mentioned. There is significant morbidity and mortality associated with mechanical ventilation.

Pressure damage to the lung is termed barotrauma, and the incidence is increased when high airway pressures are required to ventilate the lungs. Pneumothorax is not uncommon and may present as gas in the pleural space, mediastinum or soft tissues (surgical emphysema). A tension pneumothorax can occur. When drained, the pleural leak may persist (broncho-pleural fistula), and, if severe, the volume of gas escaping from the leak may exceed the capacity of the ventilator, leading to hypoventilation. Selective ventilation of each lung (differential ventilation) can isolate the side with the leak. High levels of oxygen produce lung damage, and cause or exacerbate the adult respiratory distress syndrome (ARDS, p. 518). Patients on ventilators are often deeply sedated and therefore totally dependent on the correct functioning of the equipment. They are also dependent on the supply of humidified, oxygen-enriched air. Constant nursing care is crucial. Secretions in the respiratory tract must be aspirated by the ICU staff, and airway collapse and atelectasis are common complications. The artificial airway is a portal for the entry of pathogens.

With care patients can be ventilated via an endotracheal tube for several weeks, but because the tube is a constant source of irritation to the mouth, a tracheostomy is often performed when it is likely that an artificial airway will be required for a prolonged period (Table 15.2).

Table 15.2 Major indications for tracheostomy

- Provision of prolonged positive pressure ventilation
- Control of secretions
- To prevent aspiration
- To bypass upper airway obstruction

Withdrawal of mechanical ventilation

As patients on the ICU recover, the aim is to withdraw mechanical ventilation. For this to be feasible, the patient's cardiovascular system must be stable, with good peripheral perfusion. Gas exchange must be good, with satisfactory oxygenation and an inspired oxygen concentration of less than 50%. The patient should not be septic. There should be no gross acid–base or electrolyte abnormality.

In those patients where the period of ventilation has been short (hours), the withdrawal of assisted ventilation usually poses few problems. Sedation is withdrawn; the patient wakes up and breathes spontaneously from a source

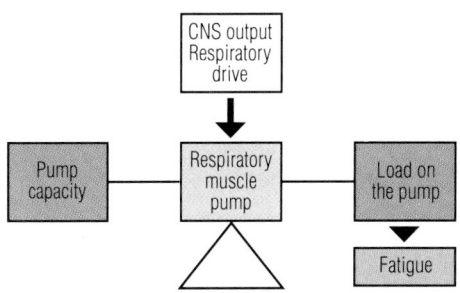

Fig. 15.7 The respiratory muscle pump. When assessing the likelihood of successful weaning from mechanical ventilation the key factors are ventilatory load, drive and capacity. If the demands made of the pump exceed capacity, weaning will fail.

of oxygen, and is then extubated. In those patients who have been ventilated for a number of days, it is frequently not possible to withdraw ventilation suddenly, and a period of gradual withdrawal, or weaning, is necessary. Successful weaning requires careful consideration of the following inter-related questions:

1. Is central drive optimal?
2. Is the respiratory muscle pump as effective as possible?
3. Has the load on the respiratory muscle pump been reduced to the minimum?
4. Given the capacity of the respiratory pump (Fig. 15.7), can the ventilatory load be sustained or is fatigue likely?

Opinions differ as to the best method of weaning. Gradual reduction in the number of machine breaths by using SIMV allows the patient to breathe spontaneously, with a background of support from the ventilator. The alternative is to allow the patient to breathe spontaneously and unaided for successively longer periods of time, alternating with machine ventilation. In some patients the work of breathing can be reduced and weaning facilitated by continuous positive airway pressure (CPAP), which can be continued post-extubation via a face or nasal mask.

During weaning it is important to optimise the function of the respiratory muscle 'pump'. Any metabolic disturbances known to reduce the contractibility of the respiratory muscles should be corrected (Table 15.3). In patients with airways obstruction, bronchodilation is helpful in reducing hyperinflation and improving muscle efficiency, as well as reducing ventilatory load. Treatment of pul-

Table 15.3 Metabolic abnormalities that impair respiratory muscle contractility

● Hypophosphataemia
● Hypomagnesaemia
● Hypokalaemia
● Hyper- and hypothyroidism
● Steroid therapy
● Other drugs. (e.g. drug-induced myasthenic syndromes)
● Hypoxia
● Hypercapnia

monary oedema also reduces the work of breathing. The effort of breathing through the tubing, ventilator and endotracheal tube should be minimised and the airway made as comfortable as possible. The patient should be sitting upright, preferably in a chair. His abdomen should be free to allow the diaphragm to descend. During weaning, nutritional support must be maintained.

A number of factors are known to be useful in predicting weaning outcome (Table 15.4). The patient should not be allowed to become distressed off the ventilator. The sensation of breathlessness is terrifying, especially since the patient has difficulty with communication. Much psychological support is needed. In the early stages of weaning the patient should receive full ventilation during the night, and the benefit of a full night's sleep. Sedative drugs are in general best avoided, but may be required if the patient is sleep-deprived.

Table 15.4 Factors favourable to successful weaning

● Adequate Pa_{O_2} on <40% inspired oxygen ($F_{I_{O_2}}$<0.4)
● Maximum voluntary ventilation >twice resting ventilation
● Respiratory rate <25 breaths/minute
● Minute ventilation <10 l/minute
● Vital capacity >20 ml/kg
● Maximum static inspiratory pressure > 30 cm H_2O

CENTRAL NERVOUS SYSTEM PROBLEMS

Patients are commonly admitted to the ICU after severe trauma, often the result of a road traffic accident. The head may have been injured, and this may be obvious from external wounds or a CSF leak. The brain may be damaged, however, in the absence of external signs. A change in consciousness indicates that the brain is injured, and may be swollen with oedema. In this section the treatment of raised intracranial pressure is outlined. Other neurological problems may require admission to the ICU, and weakness may threaten the function of the respiratory muscles (e.g. myasthenia gravis, Guillain-Barré syndrome).

Pathophysiology

The brain is enclosed in a rigid box. In addition to brain substance, the cranium contains blood and CSF. The ability of the box to accommodate a swollen brain or a space-occupying lesion is, of necessity, dependent on a parallel reduction in the volume of either CSF or blood. This compensation continues until a further increase in the contents of the box produces a sharp and rapid rise in pressure. Initially the change in pressure during the accommodating process is slight, but the response to a small volume of fluid added to the box shows how compliance is falling. At the beginning of the curve illustrated

15

Fig 15.8 Relationship between intracranial volume and pressure (ICP). Initially, increased volume has little effect on pressure but eventually further small increases cause a dramatic rise in ICP. The location of a patient on the curve can be determined by volume challenge (red lines) (see text).

in Figure 15.8 the addition of aliquots of fluid to the box (in this case via a ventricular catheter) produces a slight and transient rise in intracranial pressure. Further along the curve, although the baseline pressure has only risen slightly, the rise in pressure with the added volume is sudden and rapid. Such fluid challenges demonstrate the seriousness of cerebral oedema with greater sensitivity than absolute intracranial pressure measurements.

Sudden rises in pressure reduce brain perfusion. The mean pressure in the cerebral arteries is opposed by the intracranial pressure (ICP), and the balance is the pressure available to perfuse the brain. As ICP rises, so the flow of blood to the brain decreases, and the consequent ischaemia worsens the insult to the already damaged tissue.

Many other factors can raise the pressure within the closed box. Cerebral blood volume can be increased by dilating the cerebral arteries, the calibre of which is greatly affected by CO_2 and O_2 tensions (Fig. 15.9). Increases in CO_2 have a particularly deleterious effect, doubling blood

flow to the brain. Whilst decreasing CO_2 tension reduces flow and therefore lowers pressure in the brain, this is not sustained indefinitely. Severe hypoxaemia increases cerebral blood flow and ICP therefore rises.

Assessment and treatment

Rapid assessment of the patient must, nevertheless, be thorough. The conscious level is determined by grading the response of the patient in terms of best verbal response, best motor response and ability of the patient to speak, according to the Glasgow Coma Scale score (p. 858). The pupillary reflexes, focal neurological signs, blood pressure and pulse are checked and recorded sequentially. The coma score on admission to the ICU and subsequent changes in the score are useful indicators of progress and prognosis (Fig 15.10). Patients admitted after head trauma may also have other injuries that can easily be overlooked.

Therapy of patients with head injury should include the administration of oxygen, as many patients are hypoxaemic. Crystalloid therapy exacerbates oedema, both in the head and the lung. Cardiovascular resuscitation is important, as hypotension may further damage the brain, especially if the ICP is raised. Facilities to reduce or control raised intracranial pressure should be available.

Treatment of patients with severe head injury usually precedes a definitive diagnosis, as diagnostic facilities, particularly CT scanning, are rarely available immediately. Mechanical ventilation may be necessary to reverse hypercapnia as well as to reduce intracranial pressure.

Therapy to reduce ICP

Therapy may be initiated on the assumption that the intracranial pressure is raised, or following ICP measurement. Reduction in pressure may be achieved by reducing the volume of the brain, and reducing cerebral blood volume by controlling cerebral blood flow. Therapy is also aimed at decreasing the requirement of the brain for oxygen by reducing cerebral metabolism and maintaining the perfusion of brain cells.

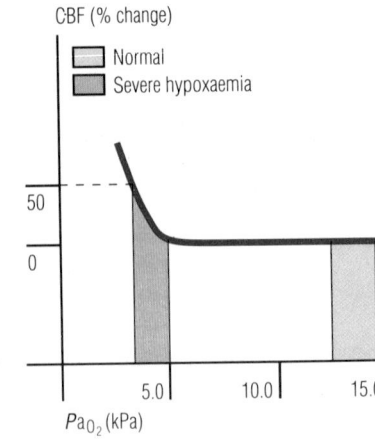

Fig. 15.9 Cerebral blood flow. A. Effect of arterial carbon dioxide tension (Pa_{CO_2}) on cerebral blood flow (CBF). Hypercapnia markedly increases CBF (whereas hypocapnia reduces CBF). **B.** Effect of arterial oxygen tension (Pa_{O_2}) on cerebral blood flow (CBF). Severe hypoxaemia substantially increases CBF.

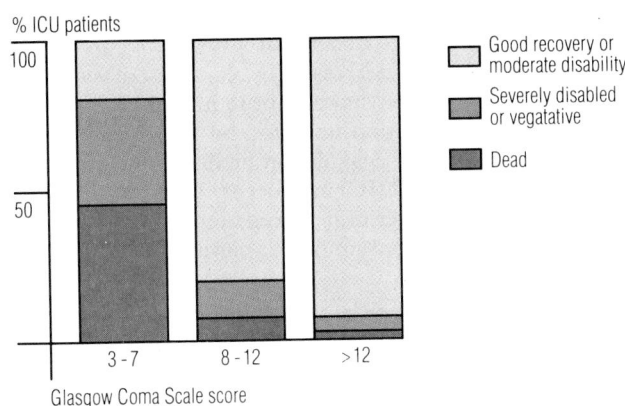

Fig. 15.10 Prognosis following head injury related to Glasgow Coma Scale score.

Reduction in brain size

Decreasing brain water can be achieved by diuretics, most commonly the osmotic diuretic mannitol. Overvigorous treatment can cause severe fluid depletion. If sustained reduction in ICP is not achieved after initial therapy, repeated administration of mannitol should be carefully considered.

Control of cerebral blood volume

Cerebral blood volume is related to the flow of blood to the enclosed box. The lowering of carbon dioxide and the reversal of hypoxaemia reduce cerebral blood volume and intracranial pressure. Mechanical ventilation is necessary for the close control of blood gases.

Reduction in venous drainage transmits pressure retrogradely, raising ICP. A disadvantage of mechanical ventilation is that the positive pressure in the chest raises the venous pressure in the head. Ventilation must be adjusted to ensure that the pressure in the chest is kept as low as practicable.

Cerebral metabolic rate

Damage to surviving neurones occurs due to a reduction in local capillary blood flow. By reducing the requirement for oxygen (by lowering the cerebral metabolic rate), the survival of brain cells is enhanced. Sudden rises in cellular metabolism, during which the consumption of oxygen outstrips supply, must be avoided. Sedative drugs reduce cerebral oxygen consumption. The prevention of convulsions, which dramatically raise cerebral metabolic rate, is essential.

Cerebral perfusion

The blood supply to the brain can be reduced by modest falls in blood pressure when the intracranial pressure is high. Continuous monitoring and maintenance of blood pressure are crucial.

The general care of patients includes:

1. avoiding painful stimuli
2. avoiding overtransfusion of crystalloid solutions
3. moderate fluid restriction
4. maintaining a head-up position to enhance venous drainage.

Monitoring

During appropriate treatment of raised ICP the use of sedation and mechanical ventilation removes many clinical signs that would otherwise indicate changes in the patient's cerebral status. Pupillary and cardiovascular reflexes may be the only signs preserved. Invasive monitoring of ICP is therefore important if changes in the patient's status are to be detected. Intracranial pressure can be measured by several techniques, including a simple manometer system introduced into the cerebral ventricles, or the measurement of pressure at the surface of the brain via intra- or extra-dural probes. Both absolute pressure and response to therapeutic manœuvres are of great help in management.

The detection of grand mal seizures is difficult if the patient is paralysed. However, the electrical activity during fitting is increased, and this can be detected by measuring the electrical activity of the cerebral hemispheres.

RENAL PROBLEMS

The development of renal failure is a common and serious complication in the critically ill, associated with a high mortality. Whilst the major insult to the kidney may have occurred prior to admission, rapid and effective resuscitation may prevent further deterioration of renal function. Incipient or established renal failure requires a diagnosis of the cause and the exclusion of reversible pathology. (The evaluation and diagnosis of renal failure are discussed in Ch. 21.) Sepsis, sometimes occult, is a common cause of renal failure on the ICU.

Commonly, the first indication of renal dysfunction is reduced urinary volume. Assessment and manipulation of the cardiovascular system are often important. Despite hypovolaemia, the blood pressure may be normal due to intense vasoconstriction, and detailed assessment by invasive cardiovascular monitoring is essential in most cases. Renal ultrasound is of value in excluding obstructive lesions.

Once an adequate circulation has been established, urinary output may be enhanced by low-dose dopamine ($<5 \mu g/kg$ per minute). A further reduction in urine output is likely to herald established renal failure, and although output may be enhanced by high-dose frusemide, this may only postpone eventual anuria. Filtration will be depressed by severe acidosis.

Fluid intake should be adjusted to the falling urine

output. The multiplicity of intravenous infusions makes volume overload a common error. Drug dosages should be reviewed in the light of the patient's renal function, and nephrotoxic drugs avoided (e.g. aminoglycoside antibiotics, NSAIDs, frusemide).

The indications for dialysis include the control of extracellular volume, electrolyte imbalance and acidosis, as well as uraemia. Intermittent haemodialysis or peritoneal dialysis can be difficult in the seriously ill. New techniques have greatly improved the management of renal failure. Haemofiltration filters can be perfused with blood and require only a small driving pressure to produce a urine-like filtrate. Whilst this continuous filtration can control extracellular volume, the clearance of urea and electrolytes requires high volumes of filtrate per day and, without skill, imbalance can lead to circulatory collapse. By passing a solution across the membrane against the direction of blood flow, dialysis of urea and other molecules occurs by diffusion and convection gradients. This low-volume continuous arterio-venous haemodialysis (CAVHD) can be enhanced by using a pump to control the flow of dialysis fluid past the filter.

MULTIPLE ORGAN FAILURE

The syndrome of progressive multiple organ failure is not uncommon on the ICU and mortality is very high. The syndrome is characterised by an alteration in tissue blood flow, local release of mediators that are cytotoxic, and an inability of peripheral tissue to utilise oxygen at a mitochondrial level. It is not always associated with sepsis, but failing organs demand a careful and systematic search for infection. Frequent samples of blood and body fluid should be cultured. Repeated pelvic and abdominal ultrasound examinations, echocardiography and CT scanning may be needed. Despite appropriate antibiotic therapy, mortality remains high if any source of infection is not eradicated. In the presence of sepsis, antibiotic therapy should be started immediately. Choice of antibiotics can be made based on the following criteria:

1. the site of infection
2. whether the infection is hospital or community acquired
3. whether the patient has had recent surgery
4. the immunocompetence of the patient
5. the presence of Gram-negative bacilli in infected material.

Treatment with a single agent with a narrow spectrum of activity against a known organism is preferable, but in a severe life-threatening situation multiple antibiotic therapy is difficult to avoid. (Antibiotic therapy is further discussed in Ch. 12.)

As organs fail, progressive hypoxaemia is common. There is a general increase in capillary permeability, and in the lungs the leak of osmotically active fluid at normal or low filling pressures causes pulmonary oedema. This pattern of non-cardiogenic pulmonary oedema is termed the adult respiratory distress syndrome (ARDS, p. 518).

Renal perfusion is decreased by episodes of systemic hypotension. Perfusion may also be reduced by local vaso-constriction and filtration impaired by fibrin deposition. Local disturbances of coagulation or disseminated intravascular coagulation (DIC) may occur. Jaundice develops as hepatic function deteriorates. Hepatic synthetic function declines and serum transaminase is elevated.

NUTRITION

In normal man there is a limited reserve of rapidly available energy substrates (glucose and glycogen), and this is depleted within 24–36 hours of starvation. Prolonged fasting leads to the production of glucose from protein catabolism via gluconeogenesis, and metabolism is shifted towards the utilisation of fats. In starvation the metabolic rate is decreased and nitrogen loss (from protein breakdown) is reduced, with the result that previously well-nourished patients can fast for several weeks. In the severely ill, not only is protein catabolised to glucose at a faster rate, but the calorie requirements are also raised, by as much as 125% in those with extensive burns (Fig. 15.11). Many patients are compromised by a degree of malnutrition prior to admission to the ICU.

Nutritional failure is associated with increased morbidity and mortality. Synthetic capability is reduced, and one of the consequences of this is a decline in immunocompetence and increased susceptibility to infection.

Nutritional status requires careful assessment in the critically ill, and the history and length of illness should be noted. Precise measurement of nutritional status and requirements is difficult. Easily available measurements of synthetic capacity (albumin, total protein) are rather variable and discriminate poorly between nutritional states. (Nutrition is fully discussed in Ch. 8.)

If possible, feeding should be continuous and controlled

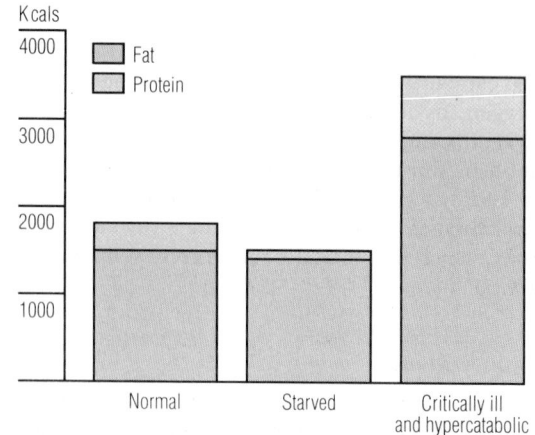

Fig. 15.11 Calorie requirements in normal individuals compared to those starved or critically ill and hypercatabolic.

using a fine-bore nasogastric tube. This route is simple, economical and less likely to lead to infection. The incidence of gastric erosions is reduced in the enterally fed. However, absorption is often decreased by gastric stasis, or the volume that can be given limited by diarrhoea. Parenteral administration is then necessary (p. 134). This involves the placement of a dedicated intravenous line. Peripheral veins can be used, but to provide adequate calorie input the volume of isotonic solution often exceeds 3 litres per day. Hypertonic solutions always require a central line. The constituents of intravenous feeding are ideal culture media and there is always a risk of infection. The volume of fluid, even when made up of highly calorific fats and concentrated glucose solutions, can precipitate volume overload. Careful attention to detail is required to provide appropriate quantities of trace elements and vitamins.

During cellular respiration fats and carbohydrates, when metabolised, produce differing amounts of CO_2 to be excreted mainly by the lungs. High carbohydrate feeds increase CO_2 production and can contribute to carbon dioxide retention and breathlessness in patients with marginal ventilatory function.

GENERAL CARE OF THE CRITICALLY ILL

Care on the ICU must be total as well as intensive. The patient who recovers from serious illness may have decades of life ahead and any residual handicap will be important. Attendant injuries, especially peripheral limb injuries, can be overlooked in the initial effort to resuscitate the patient, but may result in significant disability once the drama of intensive care is over. The maintenance of limb mobility and the prevention of contractures are important in bedbound supine patients. Skin and pressure area care is crucial. Poor peripheral perfusion commonly contributes to skin breakdown. Healing is enhanced when pressure is relieved, and this can be facilitated by air beds. Reflexes are lost during paralysis and sedation. The eyes and mouth are vulnerable. If the patient is ventilated the artificial airway must be kept clear and clean.

There is no ideal sedative drug for patients on the ICU. The administration of sedation does not imply unconsciousness, and the levels of sedation can be difficult to judge if the patient is receiving neuromuscular blocking drugs. For this reason local anaesthesia should always be used during painful procedures. Discussions around the bedside should be conducted as if the patient were aware.

Patients are often mentally obtunded, or may experience hallucinations and paranoia, causing severe agitation. A night-time sleeping regime is of great help in the care of the longer-term patients on the ICU, especially when weaning from mechanical ventilation. It is easy for longer-term ICU patients to become relatively neglected. A general review of all patients on a regular basis will focus attention on organ systems that are assumed to be stable. For example, gastric erosions are a significant cause of sudden bleeding and mortality in the severely ill, and prophylactic protection of the gastrointestinal tract is occasionally overlooked.

The morale of patients and staff is central to the success of an intensive care unit. The sustaining of morale, along with high standards of patient care, is a great challenge for the critical care specialist.

OUTCOME

The outcome of patients admitted to the ICU can be assessed in different ways (Table 15.5). Survival is, in general, related to the severity of the presenting illness and the response to therapy. Patients with multiple organ failure have a particularly poor prognosis. Great care should be taken, however, when judging the prognosis of an individual patient, and the application of scoring systems to assess prognosis for a particular case has limited value. All staff on intensive care units have seen occasional patients survive against massive odds.

Table 15.5 Outcome

Outcome from a single treatment technique for a defined disease

- IPPV for severe asthma: >80% of patients discharged from hospital
- IPPV for poisoning: >80% of patients discharged from hospital
- IPPV for pneumonia or non-traumatic coma: <35% of patients discharged from hospital

Outcome for organ system failure (e.g. cardiac, respiratory or renal failure)

- Failure of one organ system for more than one day: mortality approximately 35%
- Failure of two organ systems for more than one day: mortality approximately 60%
- Failure of three or more organ systems for more than three days: mortality approximately 90%

Assessment of outcome based on past health and present physiological derangement (APACHE score, Knaus et al. 1985)

- APACHE score >35: mortality >80%
- APACHE score <5: mortality 5%

FURTHER READING

Bradley R D 1977 Studies in acute heart failure. Edward Arnold, London. *Essential monograph of disorders of the circulation*

Knaus W A, Draper E A, Wagner D P, Zimmermen J E 1985 APACHE II: A severity of disease classification system. Crit Care Med. 13: 818–829. *A description of the APACHE II score which can be used to predict outcome*

Ledingham I McA, Hanning C D 1983 Recent advances in critical care medicine. Churchill Livingstone, Edinburgh. *Contains good accounts of many of the important topics in critical care medicine*

Tinker J, Rapin M 1983 Care of the critically ill patient. Springer Verlag, Berlin. *Comprehensive textbook of critical care medicine*

Gastrointestinal Disease

INTRODUCTION

The purpose of this chapter is to give an outline of the diseases that affect the gastrointestinal tract from mouth to anus. In the last decade, there have been great advances in clinical gastroenterology, particularly with regard to endoscopic examination. Initially, this technique resulted in improved diagnosis but now, increasingly, treatment too can be done via an endoscope. There have also been major advances in drug treatment, for example of peptic ulcers.

CLINICAL FEATURES OF GASTROINTESTINAL DISEASE

The initial approach to a patient with gastrointestinal disease is to take a careful history and then to perform a full examination. Many patients can be treated on the basis of this alone and do not need further tests.

Typical symptoms are shown in Table 16.1. General symptoms are useful in assessing the state of health of many patients with gastrointestinal symptoms. Patients commonly complain of non-specific symptoms, but these are rarely associated with serious disease. Proctalgia fugax is a transient shooting pain in the rectum. Tenesmus, an uncomfortable desire to defaecate often when there is no stool in the rectum, may be associated with rectal inflammation.

Abnormal signs in patients with gastrointestinal disease are summarised in Table 16.2. Diseases of the gut can

Table 16.1   Symptoms of gut disease

General symptoms	Small intestinal symptoms
Anorexia	Steatorrhoea
Weight loss	Diarrhoea
Nausea and vomiting	Malaise and dyspnoea due to anaemia
Non-specific symptoms	Abdominal colic
Flatulence	Abdominal distension
Abdominal bloating	**Large intestinal symptoms**
Poorly or variably localised pain	Malaise and dyspnoea due to anaemia
Oesophageal symptoms	Diarrhoea
Dysphagia	Constipation
Heartburn	Abdominal colic
Regurgitation and waterbrash	Blood per rectum
Gastroduodenal symptoms	Tenesmus
Upper abdominal pain	
Haematemesis and melaena	

Table 16.2   Signs of gut disease

General	Gastroduodenal
Nutrition	Epigastric tenderness
Hydration	Epigastric mass
Oedema	Succussion splash
Glossitis	
Bone tenderness ⎫	**Small intestinal**
Chvostek's sign ⎬ Hypocalcaemia	Steatorrhoea
Trousseau's sign ⎭	Diarrhoea
Nails	Mass (often in right iliac fossa)
Clubbing	Intestinal obstruction
Leuconychia	
Koilonychia	**Colonic**
	Colonic mass
Orofacial	Colonic obstruction
Anaemia	
Aphthous ulcers	**Anorectal**
Other oral ulcers	Anal lesions: fissures, tags
Angular cheilitis	Rectal examination: mass
Stomatitis	Sigmoidoscopy: proctitis, ulcers,
Telangiectasia	tumours and melanosis

result in malnutrition, while a failure of fluid intake or increased loss due to vomiting or diarrhoea results in dehydration. Peripheral oedema and ascites occur because of hypoproteinaemia due to protein loss or malnutrition. Vitamin D and calcium malabsorption result in hypocalcaemia and osteomalacia (Ch. 19). Nail clubbing is associated with inflammatory bowel disease and intra-abdominal sepsis, leuconychia (white nails) with hypoalbuminaemia, and koilonychia (spoon-shaped nails) with chronic iron deficiency anaemia. Aphthous ulcers can occur in increased numbers in patients with coeliac disease, and more indolent mouth ulcers in Crohn's disease. Angular cheilitis, stomatitis and glossitis may occur in patients with iron and water-soluble vitamin deficiencies. Facial and oral telangiectasia are associated with telangiectasia lower in the gut and these may bleed. Rectal examination and sigmoidoscopy are an essential part of the initial examination in patients with a change in bowel habit.

INVESTIGATION OF GASTROINTESTINAL DISEASE

Haematological and biochemical abnormalities

Diseases of the gastrointestinal tract are often accompanied by changes in the blood.

Iron and folic acid are absorbed from the upper small intestine, and malabsorption of either results in characteristic haematological changes (Table 16.3). In some patients with upper intestinal malabsorption (especially coeliac disease), a mixed folate and iron malabsorption may be seen. Dietary iron deficiency can occur in patients with diets low in meat, and is particularly common in the elderly and in Asian vegans. Blood loss can occur throughout the gut with consequent iron deficiency and anaemia. Gastric surgery can cause iron deficiency by reduced acid secretion impairing absorption, by bypassing the upper small intestinal mucosa, and by intestinal hurry. Folic acid is present in large amounts in green vegetables and liver but dietary deficiency may occur if the diet is inadequate.

Vitamin B$_{12}$ is bound to intrinsic factor in the stomach and is absorbed specifically in the terminal ileum (along with bile acids). Intrinsic factor deficiency can be congenital or secondary to pernicious anaemia or gastrectomy. Malabsorption of the B$_{12}$-intrinsic factor complex is generally due to terminal ileal resection (usually secondary to Crohn's disease). However, it can also occur (rarely) secondary to infestation with the fish tapeworm (*Diphyllobothrium latum*), to intestinal fistulas and blind loops, or (again rarely) with chronic pancreatitis (p. 617). The double isotope Schilling test (p. 1046) is used to determine whether B$_{12}$ deficiency is due to lack of intrinsic factor or to malabsorption of the intrinsic factor-B$_{12}$ complex.

Hyposplenism is a feature of some bowel disorders, particularly coeliac disease. The typical finding on a blood film is of Howell-Jolly bodies (red cells containing small nuclear fragments). It also occurs in some patients with inflammatory bowel disease.

Neutrophil leucocytosis, a *high ESR* and a high C-reactive protein are useful non-specific markers of intra-abdominal

Table 16.3 Haematological abnormalities in gut disease

Abnormality	Laboratory changes	Causes
Anaemia		

Iron deficiency	Blood film: hypochromic microcytic red cells
	 Low MCV, MCH and MCHC
	 Low serum iron and high total iron binding capacity
		Dietary
		 Blood loss
		 Malabsorption
		   Postgastrectomy
		   Upper small bowel disease

Folate deficiency	Blood film: macrocytic red cells High MCV, MCH and MCHC Low red cell folate	Dietary Upper small bowel disease
B$_{12}$ deficiency	Blood film: macrocytic red cells High MCV, MCH and MCHC Low serum B$_{12}$	Pernicious anaemia Terminal ileal disease Pancreatic disease Fish tapeworm (*Diphyllobothrium latum*)
Hyposplenism	Howell-Jolly bodies Giant platelets	Coeliac disease Tropical sprue Crohn's disease
Neutrophil leucocytosis and high ESR		Chronic inflammation (e.g. inflammatory bowel disease, abscess etc.)

inflammation, particularly inflammatory bowel disease.

A *low serum albumin* is commonly seen in patients with bowel disease (Table 16.4) and usually reflects protein

Table 16.4 Gastrointestinal causes of a low serum albumin

Increased loss (protein-losing enteropathy)
Stomach
  Ménétrièr's disease (giant rugae)
  Multiple gastric ulcers
  Gastric tumours

Small intestine
  Coeliac disease
  Crohn's disease
  Tropical sprue
  Lymphoma
  Lymphangiectasia

Large intestine
  Crohn's disease
  Ulcerative colitis
  Colonic tumours

Decreased intake
Anorexia
Protein deficient diet

Decreased synthesis
Associated liver disease (as can occur in inflammatory bowel disease)

leakage into the gut. Decreased intake and, rarely, decreased synthesis, may contribute. Albumin has a plasma half-life of about 23 days. Proteins such as transferrin and pre-albumin have a shorter half-life and plasma levels consequently fall earlier.

Electrolytes may be deranged. In patients with gastric outflow obstruction (pyloric stenosis), a hypochloraemic hypokalaemic alkalosis may occur. Diarrhoea may result in dehydration and electrolyte loss, particularly potassium.

Post-gastrectomy patients and patients with severe bowel disease (usually coeliac or Crohn's disease) may have a *low serum calcium*, even after correction for a low serum albumin. This is caused by malabsorption. Osteomalacia may develop and be associated with raised bone alkaline phosphatase levels in plasma. As a result of efforts to maintain serum calcium concentration, these patients develop secondary hyperparathyroidism, hyperphosphaturia and thus hypophosphataemia.

Endoscopy

Rigid endoscopes for examination of the oesophagus, stomach and sigmoid colon have been available for many years. However, the development of flexible fibre-optic endoscopes, in the 1970's, revolutionised the gastroenterologist's view of the gut. Endoscopy is generally superior to radiology as an investigative technique, as it provides a direct mucosal view; it also enables biopsies to be taken for histological and biochemical analysis, and therapeutic manoeuvres.

Endoscopes are used in the upper gut to examine the oesophagus, stomach and duodenum. Oesophageal strictures can be dilated using bougies, and prosthetic tubes can be put through strictures (usually malignant) in the oesophagus and stomach. Bleeding lesions can be cauterised by electric current or lasers. With a side-viewing endoscope, the ampulla of Vater can be cannulated and contrast medium injected to reveal the anatomy of the pancreatic ducts and biliary tree; this is endoscopic retrograde cholangiopancreatography (ERCP). If there are stones in the biliary tree, a sphincterotomy can be performed to allow them to fall out or be extracted by baskets or balloons. Malignant strictures in the common bile duct can be bypassed by teflon stents passed endoscopically, or percutaneously, through the liver.

The lower rectum can be examined by a rigid proctoscope (this is particularly useful for demonstrating haemorrhoids), and the rectum and lower sigmoid colon by a 25 cm rigid sigmoidoscope. A flexible fibre-optic sigmoidoscope can be used for the distal colon and rectum, and can usually be advanced further than the rigid instrument (Fig. 16.1). Colonoscopes can be passed round the colon to the caecum and thence, via the ileocaecal valve, into the terminal ileum. Biopsies of suspicious lesions can be taken and polypoid lesions can be snared, or excised and removed by excision diathermy. Abnormal colonic blood vessels (angiodysplasia) can be cauterised. The small bowel mucosa from the end of the second part of the duodenum to the terminal ileum cannot normally be

A

B

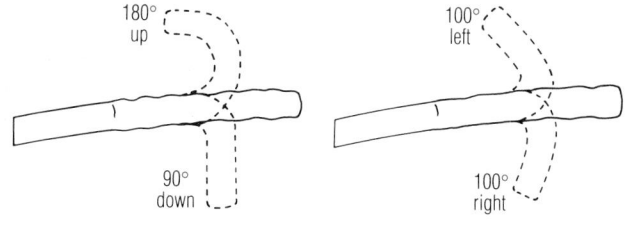

C

Fig. 16.1 Endoscopic instruments. A. A rigid proctoscope and sigmoidoscope with their respective trocars removed are seen centrally. They are surrounded by a diagram of a typical fibre-optic gastroscope. **B.** Diagram of the distal end of a typical fibre-optic gastroscope. Light is provided by the guides and the image is transmitted via the objective lens to the operator. The air and water outlets allow insufflation of the gut with air and cleansing of the lens with water. Gastric contents and secretions can be removed via the suction channel and biopsy forceps and cytology brushes can also be passed by this route. **C.** Diagram of the movements which the tip of a typical fibre-optic endoscope can achieve.

viewed endoscopically; at laparotomy, however, it is possible to make an enterotomy and inspect the whole small bowel.

Barium studies

If a patient has difficulty with swallowing (dysphagia), a barium swallow is needed before endoscopy to outline the anatomy and to avoid possible endoscopic perforation. A barium swallow on video is very helpful in elucidating motor problems of the oesophagus, such as bulbar palsy, spasm and achalasia. In the investigation of dyspepsia, upper gastrointestinal endoscopy is preferred as it is more accurate and allows biopsy and cytology specimens to be obtained.

The small intestine can be examined by a barium follow-through, in which barium is swallowed and its progress followed to the terminal ileum. Better views, particularly of ileal disease, can be obtained by a small bowel enema in which contrast is placed directly into the upper jejunum via a nasal tube (Fig. 16.2).

Double-contrast air and barium enemas after careful laxative preparation are useful in demonstrating colonic lesions such as carcinomas, polyps and inflammatory bowel disease. Barium enema should be delayed for at least one week after rectal biopsy to avoid the risk of perforation. If there is doubt about the barium appearances, or if angiodysplasia is suspected, colonoscopy should be performed.

Fig. 16.2   A normal small bowel enema, showing jejunum and ileum in the upper and lower parts of the picture respectively. Pressure with a leaded glove can be used to separate overlapping loops of ileum.

Imaging techniques

Ultrasound, computerised tomography (CT scanning) and nuclear magnetic resonance (NMR) are all useful in imaging the liver, biliary tree, spleen, pancreas, pelvis and retroperitoneal structures. They are helpful in demonstrating tumours, abscesses and stones, but are of little help in outlining the bowel.

Isotopic techniques can be used to investigate gut disease. ^{99m}Technetium sulphur colloid can be used to monitor the liquid and solid phase of gastric emptying (in general, liquids empty faster) and to measure the time taken by nutrients to pass through the small bowel (small bowel transit). Red cells can be radiolabelled with ^{51}chromium to demonstrate gastrointestinal blood loss, especially when this cannot be demonstrated by conventional endoscopic and radiological means. White cells can be radiolabelled with ^{111}indium to demonstrate abscesses and areas of active inflammatory bowel disease. Meckel's diverticula often contain gastric epithelium and can be localised by radiolabelled pertechnate, which is secreted by the parietal cells.

Arteriography is useful in outlining the coeliac and superior and inferior mesenteric arteries. Using this technique, stenosis or occlusion of these arteries can be defined in patients with pain after eating (mesenteric angina); bleeding lesions (e.g. tumours and angiodysplasia) can also be defined. If the patient is losing blood at the rate of more than 2 ml/min, a blush of contrast should also be seen in the bowel lumen.

Gut regulatory peptides

Three classes of regulatory peptides have been defined.

1. *Hormones.* It has long been recognised that there are hormones, such as secretin and gastrin, which are released as a result of food in the gut and which have effects at distant sites.
2. *Paracrine regulatory peptides.* Subsequently, paracrine regulatory peptides have been discovered in the gut mucosa; these are released locally and have profound effects on neighbouring cells.
3. *Neurotransmitters.* Finally, immunocytochemistry has demonstrated some peptides in the nerves of the gut, e.g. somatostatin, vasoactive intestinal polypeptide (VIP) and substance P, which are thought to act as non-adrenergic non-cholinergic neurotransmitters.

The site of origin, mechanism of action and main physiological effects of the best documented regulatory peptides are summarised in Table 16.5. Clinically, the most important aspects of these hormones are their use in diagnostic tests (e.g. the pentagastrin test for gastric acid secretion and the secretin-cholecystokinin test for pancreatic function) and their role in tumour syndromes (p. 620). Measurement of the peptides in plasma or tissue can be performed by radioimmunoassay. The following abnormal results may have a role in diagnosis:

1. In untreated coeliac disease (which results in upper small intestinal atrophy), meal-stimulated plasma levels of the upper small intestinal hormones, secretin, cholecystokinin and gastric inhibitory polypeptide, are

Table 16.5 Origin and action of some gastrointestinal regulatory peptides

Regulatory peptide	Site of origin	Mechanism of action	Main physiological effect
Gastrin	Gastric antrum	Hormone	Stimulates gastric acid secretion
Secretin	Duodenum	Hormone	Stimulates pancreatic bicarbonate secretion
Cholecystokinin	Duodenum	Hormone	Stimulates pancreatic enzyme secretion and gallbladder contraction
Motilin	Upper small bowel	Hormone	Increases gastric emptying and gut motility
Gastric inhibitory polypeptide (GIP)	Upper small bowel	Hormone	Stimulates insulin secretion
Enteroglucagon	Terminal ileum and colon	Hormone	Delays gastric emptying; trophic effects on gut mucosa
Neurotensin	Terminal ileum	Hormone	Delays gastric emptying
Pancreatic polypeptide	Pancreas	Hormone	Decreases pancreatic and biliary secretion
Somatostatin	Pancreas and all the gut	Hormone Paracrine ? Neurotransmitter	Reduces hormonal and intestinal secretions
Vasoactive intestinal polypeptide (VIP)	Pancreas and all the gut	Neurotransmitter	Increases intestinal secretion

low. The terminal ileal hormones, neurotensin and enteroglucagon, are increased.

2. In chronic pancreatitis with steatorrhoea, levels of meal-stimulated plasma pancreatic polypeptide are reduced.

3. In idiopathic neonatal hypoglycaemia, plasma and pancreatic somatostatin levels are low, resulting in hyperinsulinism.

4. In neuropathic diseases, such as Hirschsprung's disease and Chagas' disease, tissue vasoactive intestinal polypeptide levels are reduced.

Specific function tests

Gastric acid secretion can be assessed via a nasogastric tube first in the fasting state (basal acid output) and then after stimulation with a gastrin analogue, pentagastrin, to assess maximal acid output. Very high levels of basal acid secretion are seen in patients with gastrin-secreting tumours (gastrinomas), and high stimulated levels also often occur in patients with duodenal ulcers. Twenty-four-hour acid secretion can also be monitored, to assess the effects of drugs which reduce acid secretion. Insulin hypoglycaemia stimulates gastric acid secretion via the vagus and can therefore be used postoperatively to assess the efficacy of surgical vagotomy. pH probes can also be placed in the oesophagus to monitor acid reflux, and in the stomach to monitor the effects of treatment.

Small bowel function has traditionally been assessed by xylose and glucose absorption tests; plasma levels of the sugars are reduced in some patients with small bowel malabsorption. However, these tests are unreliable, and can be replaced by assessing both reduced absorption of small hydrophilic molecules (e.g. L-rhamnose and mannitol) and increased permeability to and thus absorption of larger molecules such as lactulose, cellobiose and ^{51}Cr-EDTA. It is also possible to place a triple lumen tube in the intestine and, by infusing at the top and extracting at the distal end, to assess the absorption and secretion of different solutes over a given length of small intestinal mucosa. These tests are complicated and time-consuming, however. Thus, in clinical practice, assessment of the small bowel by endoscopic biopsy and small bowel barium enema X-rays is most rewarding.

Motility

The purpose of normal gut motility is to pass food and excreta along the lumen at a rate that allows the appropriate physiological processes to take place. Well-regulated 'brakes' occur at the gastro-oesophageal junction, the pylorus, the ileocaecal valve and the rectum. Control of gut motility is thought to be mainly neural but hormones, in particular motilin, may also play a role. The stomach plays a major role in grinding food to small particles and in controlling the exit of contents into the duodenum (this may take up to five hours after a large meal). In the fasting state, the stomach and small intestine are kept empty by the 'migrating myoelectric complex', which passes a peristaltic wave down the small bowel at approximately 90 minute intervals.

Oesophageal motility can be investigated by a barium study on video, by manometric pressure studies, and by a pH probe in the lower oesophagus to assess gastro-oesophageal acid reflux. Gastric emptying can be investigated by labelling the solid or the liquid phase with an isotope. Small intestinal motility can be assessed through the time taken for isotopes to reach the caecum, or by demonstrating a peak of breath hydrogen excretion liberated from bacterial breakdown of a carbohydrate load when a test meal

Table 16.6 Disorders of gut motility

Oesophagus	Stomach	Small bowel	Colon
Anatomical			
Tumours ↓	Tumours ↓	Tumours ↓	Tumours ↓
Inflammatory stricture (e.g. acid reflux and acid/alkali burns) ↓	Pyloric stenosis ↓	Inflammatory stricture (e.g. Crohn's disease and tuberculosis) ↓	Inflammatory strictures (e.g. Crohn's disease) and ischaemic colon ↓
	Post-gastrectomy ↑↓	Post-surgical resection ↑	Post-surgical resection ↑
Neuropathic			
Achalasia ↓	Postvagotomy ↓		Hirschsprung's and Chagas' disease ↓
	Diabetes mellitus ↓		
Psychosomatic			
Globus hystericus	Vomiting	Irritable bowel syndrome ↑	Irritable colon syndrome ↑↓
	Aerophagy		Simple constipation ↓

↑ increased motility   ↓ decreased motility

reaches the distal ileum and caecum. Mouth to anus motility can be assessed by marker beads or by non-absorbable dyes.

A variety of clinical syndromes give rise to abnormal motility (Table 16.6). This most commonly causes a delay in transit, but gastric and other surgery can result in excessively rapid transit.

Gastrointestinal secretion

The salivary glands, stomach, pancreas, biliary tree and intestine all produce a large volume of secretions; these change the pH and produce enzymes which allow digestion of food and thus absorption of nutrients (Fig. 16.3). The secretions are controlled by vagal nerves including non-cholinergic non-adrenergic fibres, by local paracrine substances and by classical hormones.

Modes of investigations and abnormalities of secretion are shown in Table 16.7. In general, meal tests are more physiological than hormonal tests, e.g. the pentagastrin and secretin-cholecystokinin tests, where pharmacological doses of hormones are given intravenously. The triple lumen tube can be passed perorally into the intestine and

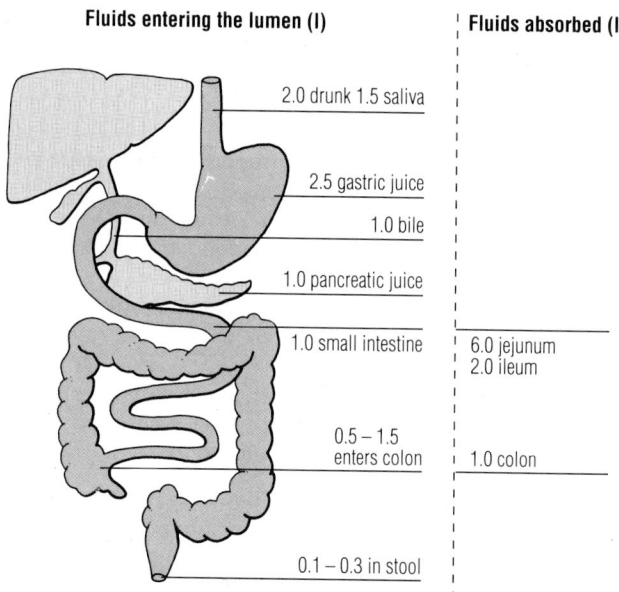

Fluids entering the lumen (l) | **Fluids absorbed (l)**

2.0 drunk 1.5 saliva

2.5 gastric juice

1.0 bile

1.0 pancreatic juice

1.0 small intestine | 6.0 jejunum 2.0 ileum

0.5 – 1.5 enters colon | 1.0 colon

0.1 – 0.3 in stool

Fig. 16.3 The typical daily fluid intake, secretions and absorption in a healthy person.

Table 16.7 Investigation and examples of important hyper- and hyposecretion syndromes

Type of secretion	Modes of investigation	Examples of increased secretion	Examples of reduced secretion
Salivary glands	Volume, pH and amylase levels, with or without local oral stimulant	Sialorrhoea	Sjögren's disease
Stomach	Pentagastrin and meal-stimulated acid output	Duodenal ulcer Gastrinoma	Carcinoma of stomach Atrophic gastritis
Pancreas	Lundh test meal and secretin-cholecystokinin stimulation		Chronic pancreatitis with exocrine insufficiency
Small intestine	Triple lumen tube and assessment of secretion/absorption over given length of intestine	VIP-secreting tumours Cholera Phenolphthalein	
Large intestine	Triple lumen tube	VIP-secreting tumours Dihydroxy bile acids	

various solutions containing a non-absorbable marker may then be perfused. By sampling at the end of the tube, the amount of secretion or absorption can be assessed.

Intestinal digestion and absorption

Small molecules may be absorbed from the mouth and nose. The stomach secretes acid and pepsin and, by physical churning and mixing, breaks down food into proportions which allow pancreatic and brush border enzymes to digest it ready for absorption. Fat and fat-soluble vitamins require bile acids, lipase and micellar formation to permit absorption. Proteins require gastric pepsin, pancreatic trypsin and brush border peptidases to break down proteins to absorbable single amino acids or 2–4 amino acid peptides. Carbohydrates require amylase, and then brush border disaccharidases, to form monosaccharides which can be absorbed (Fig. 16.4). Calcium, iron and folic acid are absorbed in the duodenum and upper jejunum, while vitamin B_{12} and bile acids are absorbed in the terminal ileum; all other nutrients are absorbed throughout the small intestine. Small intestinal absorption requires active or passive transport across the brush border membrane, transport through the cell (often in Golgi or mitochondria) and then extrusion through the cell's basolateral membrane.

The colon is primarily involved in the absorption of water and electrolytes. Normally, up to 1500 ml of fluid passes through the ileocaecal valve daily, and this is concentrated to a 100 g formed stool. Small amounts of other nutrients, often partially metabolised by intracolonic bacteria, may also be absorbed.

THE MOUTH

The subspeciality of stomatology sits uneasily between dentistry and gastroenterology. This may, and sometimes should, result in cross-referral of patients.

Normal and abnormal function

The importance of the mouth, tongue, teeth and secretions of the salivary glands (parotid and submandibular) in starting the digestive process is often overlooked. Mastication and lubrication of the food bolus is desirable, if not essential, to facilitate its painless progression. Once swallowing has been voluntarily initiated, the rest of the act is reflex and automatic. Coordination of the soft palate rising to occlude the nasopharynx, the epiglottis tilting backwards to occlude the larynx, and the temporary cessation of respiration, is under complex neurological control, principally by the brainstem.

Afferent pathways from taste and olfactory receptors initiate the cephalic phase of vagally-mediated gastric secretion. Inadequate salivary secretion will prevent sapid substances dissolving to provide this stimulus. Saliva also contains two digestive enzymes – an α-amylase (ptyalin) which digests starch, and a lipase. Ptyalin is relatively inactive at gastric pH. Lingual lipase becomes important in patients with chronic pancreatic insufficiency, such as occurs, for example, in cystic fibrosis. Here, its normally very small contribution to total lipase output increases; lingual lipase is also able to function in the more acid milieu often present because of the impairment of pancreatic bicarbonate secretion, which often renders exogenous lipase extracts relatively ineffectual.

Xerostoma (dry mouth) can occasionally be severe enough to cause problems in initiating swallowing. Normally, it is an important stimulus in creating the sensation of thirst, and thus in correcting dehydration. Lack of saliva may predispose to ascending bacterial infections of the salivary glands (sialadenitis), especially the parotid glands (parotitis).

Saliva also contributes to the prevention of dental caries, the pathogenesis of which involves the facultative anaerobe, *Streptococcus mutans*, together with carbohydrate (mainly sucrose) and the formation of dental plaque. Bacterial metabolism converts plaque to lactic and other organic acids, which demineralise the enamel, decalcify the dentine and then give rise to necrosis and infection of the pulp. Fluoridation of drinking water to the harmless

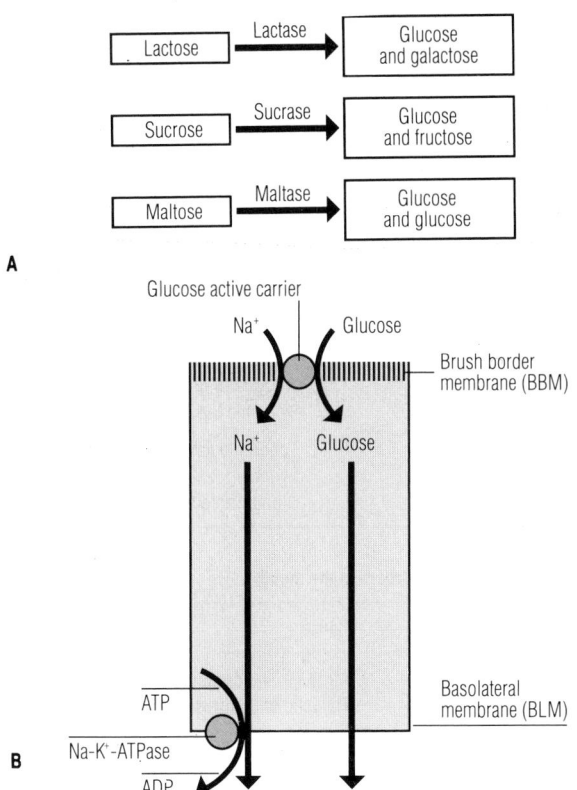

Fig. 16.4 Intestinal digestion and absorption. A. Enzyme activity allowing the conversion of major unabsorbable disaccharides to monosaccharides, which the enterocyte then can absorb. **B.** Glucose is transported by an active carrier with sodium at the brush border membrane. The gradient of sodium across the enterocyte is maintained by the Na^+-K^+-ATPase at the basolateral membrane, which allows sodium to pass out of the cell in exchange for potassium. Glucose leaves the cell at the basolateral membrane by a Na^+-independent carrier

Gastrointestinal Disease

level of one part per million can reduce the incidence of
caries in children by 60%, but has not yet achieved universal approval.

Both the edentulous and patients with ill-fitting or
painful dentures may limit their food intake, often unconsciously, and thus lose weight. Other painful lesions of the
mouth or tongue may have a similar effect but, being more
obvious, come more readily to medical attention.

Diseases of the mouth

Disease of the mouth may be of importance for the following reasons:

1. The disease, although confined to the mouth, may give
rise to unpleasant symptoms and disordered function
(Table 16.8).
2. It may represent mucous membrane involvement of a
generalised dermatological condition. Sometimes the
mouth may be the first or only site (Table 16.9).
3. Involvement of the mouth may be part of a systemic
disease and a valuable diagnostic indicator even if not
troublesome in its own right (Table 16.10).
4. The condition may be iatrogenic (Table 16.11).

ORAL ULCERATION

Recurrent aphthous ulcers

There are many possible causes of oral ulceration (Tables
16.8–16.11) but the commonest is *idiopathic aphthous ulceration*. This occurs in up to 20% of patients seen in hospital
and 10% in general practice. It often begins in late childhood or the early teens and frequently recurs. In about
80% of cases the condition (though still unpleasant) is
regarded as minor with up to five ulcers, less than 1 cm
diameter, affecting lips, cheeks and tongue and healing
within a week. Major ulcers are larger, often more numer-

Table 16.8 Diseases confined to the mouth

Ulceration
Herpes simplex (HSV1)
   Recurrent herpes labialis
   Primary gingivostomatitis
Acute ulcerative gingivitis (Vincent's angina, caused by *Fusobacterium fusiformis* and *Borrelia vincenti*)
   Cancrum oris
Coxsackie A
   Herpangina
   Hand, foot and mouth disease
Recurrent aphthous ulcers
   Minor
   Major
Denture gingivitis

Plaques
Candida
Leucoplakia
Carcinoma

Table 16.9 Dermatological conditions involving the mouth

Ulceration (burst bullae)	Plaques
Pemphigus vulgaris	Lichen planus
Pemphigoid	Psoriasis
Erythema multiforme	
Lichen planus	

Table 16.10 Mouth involvement in systemic disorders

Mouth involvement	Systemic disorder
Mucocutaneous pigmentation of lips	Peutz-Jegher's syndrome
Telangiectasia (lips)	Scleroderma (CRST syndrome) Hereditary haemorrhagic telangiectasia (Osler Weber Rendu syndrome)
Buccal pigmentation	Addison's disease ACTH-producing tumour
Macroglossia	Hypothyroidism Acromegaly Amyloid
Glossitis	Iron deficiency (also angular cheilitis) Folate and vitamin B_{12} deficiency
Gingival hypertrophy	Acute leukaemia Amyloid
Gingivitis (with or without bleeding)	Acute leukaemia Scurvy Thrombocytopenia Agranulocytosis
Oral ulceration	Behçet's disease Reiter's syndrome Erythema multiforme Crohn's disease Coeliac disease Wegener's granulomatosis Systemic lupus erythematosus Tuberculosis Syphilis Glandular fever

Table 16.11 Iatrogenic disorders of the mouth

Iatrogenic disorder	Cause
Xerostomia	Atropine-like drugs Tricyclic antidepressants
Gingival hyperplasia	Phenytoin, primidone, phenobarbitone, cyclosporin
Gingival pigmentation	Bismuth, mercury, lead, arsenic, silver
Ulceration	Sulphonamides, barbiturates, penicillin (cause erythema multiforme) Gold Penicillamine Cytotoxics Drugs causing agranulocytosis, e.g. carbimazole, sulphasalazine

ous, and may involve the pharynx and palate. Cervical lymph node enlargement may occur, and healing may be delayed for several weeks, leaving scarring. A variant of this condition is herpetiform ulcers, where crops of small ulcers may coalesce; despite the descriptive title, the herpes virus has not been implicated. The aetiology of aphthous ulcers is unknown. The preponderance of the disease in females, its onset at the menarche, relationship to menstruation and improvement in pregnancy have led to the obvious postulation of hormonal factors (in women at least!). There is often a positive family history. When all obvious associated conditions have been excluded, the possibility of occult disease remains. A proportion of asymptomatic patients with coeliac disease present in this way, and a haematological screen, looking for a macrocytosis, is therefore justified. Red cell folate is a sensitive test before considering jejunal biopsy. Recurrent aphthous ulcers are best treated by local steroids, such as hydrocortisone pellets, or tetracycline solution.

Herpes simplex

The commonest manifestation of *Herpes simplex* (HSV1) is of recurrent herpes labialis or cold sore. The virus lies dormant in the trigeminal ganglion. Antiviral therapy with local idoxuridine or acycloguanosine (acyclovir) is probably only necessary in the severely immunocompromised patient.

A rarer, more severe and usually non-recurrent infection is primary herpetic gingivostomatitis. It occurs primarily in childhood and the sore mouth and gums, with vesicles preceding ulceration, is accompanied by fever and regional lymphadenitis.

Acute ulcerative gingivitis

Primary herpetic gingivostomatitis must be distinguished from acute ulcerative gingivitis (Vincent's angina) which is thought to be due to bacterial infection; *Fusobacterium fusiformis* and *Borrelia vincenti* are the currently incriminated organisms. This disease affects young adults and the immunosuppressed, and is again accompanied by fever and lymphadenitis. The painful gums may bleed. Vincent's angina may be distinguished from herpes by the foul fetor and absence of vesicles. Penicillin or metronidazole are usually effective treatments but, in the severely ill, immunosuppressed patient, gangrene spreading to lips and cheeks (cancrum oris) may occur.

Coxsackie A

Both herpangina and hand, foot and mouth disease are due to Coxsackie group A viruses. They affect children and may be difficult to distinguish from HSV infection, unless the virus is isolated or rising antibody titres found.

Other causes of ulceration

Oral ulceration may predominate in Behçet's disease, Reiter's syndrome and erythema multiforme. In all three conditions, ocular and genital lesions may be present. Although many cases of erythema multiforme have no apparent cause, some are induced by Herpes simplex and drugs, such as sulphonamides, barbiturates and penicillin.

Bullous disorders of mucous membranes result in their rupture to form ulcers in the mouth. As at other sites, differentiating the intraepithelial bullae of pemphigus from the subepithelial bullae of pemphigoid may be difficult (p. 1133). Lichen planus may also present with erosion of vesicles causing ulceration and, in a significant number of patients, the mouth may be the only site of the disease (p. 1134).

PLAQUE LESIONS

The commonest form of lichen planus is the hyperkeratotic lesion, rather than the bullous and erosive. This form is often asymptomatic and longstanding; the furry thickening or white criss-cross striae on the buccal mucosa, lips, gums and tongue may first be noted by the dentist.

Candida

Candidiasis, giving rise to thrush, usually arises as a result of a defect in immunity, since the causative fungus is a common commensal. Candidiasis may complicate HIV infection and is common in poorly controlled diabetics. Beneath the creamy exudate the mucosa may be inflamed and painful. In denture wearers, a more chronic form is seen usually limited to the area covered by the upper plate. Antifungal agents, such as nystatin and amphotericin B, applied locally are usually effective in acute cases. However, in more chronic cases or in severely immunocompromised patients, the disease may spread to the oesophagus or penetrate the basement membrane to enter the bloodstream, causing infective endocarditis, and renal and brain involvement. Treatment with more toxic agents such as ketoconazole, clotrimazole, miconazole or intravenous amphotericin may be needed.

Leucoplakia

Leucoplakia is a serious condition because of its propensity for malignant transformation in about 5% of cases. The white patches can occur anywhere within the oral cavity. Biopsy, which must be regularly repeated to detect atypia or early cancer, confirms the diagnosis by showing epithelial keratosis and hyperplasia. The aetiology is multifactorial, but idiopathic cases do occur. There is no specific treatment other than excision and avoiding the presumed causative factors. These include smoking, local friction and chronic infection – chronic candidiasis or tertiary syphilis; the latter has a worse prognosis regarding malignant change. Leucoplakia is an important manifestation of HIV infection (p. 252).

Carcinoma

Squamous carcinoma of the oral cavity may affect the lips, tongue or any other part of the mouth, and may present as a nodular or ulcerating lesion. As with leucoplakia, its incidence appears to be declining, emphasising the important association between the two conditions. Pipe and cigar smoking are strongly associated with oral cavity carcinoma, and other causative factors are also similar to those of leucoplakia. A particular local irritant in the Indian subcontinent is the eating and chewing of chillis; this gives rise to submucosal fibrosis which may predispose to cancer, as does the chewing of tobacco.

OTHER LESIONS

Other disorders of the mouth are listed in Tables 16.8 to 16.11. Minor abnormalities of the tongue may, because easily seen by the patient, give rise to considerable anxiety.

Geographic tongue (benign migratory glossitis) is caused by shifting areas of desquamation of short duration in any one location. It is invariably symptomless and the patient should be reassured of this.

Fissure tongue may be associated with symptomatic glossitis but, if symptomless, the patient can be reassured.

Black hairy tongue can be as spectacular as it is asymptomatic. The filliform papillae hypertrophy and normal desquamation does not occur but can be encouraged by brushing the tongue with a toothbrush. Tripotassium dicitrate bismuthate (De-nol) in the liquid form is an obvious cause and the disorder may also follow antibiotics, but the aetiology is usually unknown. Reassurance is required.

THE OESOPHAGUS

Normal swallowing involves coordinated action of the oropharynx, relaxation of the cricopharyngeus, passage down the oesophagus (upper one-third striated muscle, lower two-thirds non-striated muscle) and relaxation of the lower oesophageal sphincter. Fluids or solids then come to rest in the stomach.

Clinical features of oesophageal pathology

Typical symptoms of patients with oesophageal pathology are listed in Summary 1.

Dysphagia

Difficulty with swallowing (dysphagia or 'food sticking') is the most important symptom, and must always be investigated early, initially by a barium swallow, to prevent progression of treatable disease. Some of the causes (in approximate order of frequency) are shown in Table 16.12 (see also p. 20, Fig. 2.1). When there are obstructive lesions such as carcinoma, dysphagia is initially for large boluses of food, but then progresses to less solid food and finally to liquids ('total dysphagia'). Most of the causes can be elucidated by a good history (p. 18), examination, barium swallow and endoscopy. Patients with central and peripheral nervous system, and primary muscle disorders,

> **Summary 1   The main symptoms, signs and investigations of oesophageal disease**
>
> *Symptoms*
> Difficulty with swallowing (dysphagia)
> Painful swallowing
> Heartburn
> Regurgitation (including waterbrash)
> Vomiting
> Weight loss
> Gastrointestinal bleeding
>
> *Signs*
> Epigastric tenderness
> Abnormal palatal movement
> Presence of a mass (epigastric or supraclavicular fossa)
> Chest signs due to aspiration
>
> *Investigations*
> Full blood count
> Barium swallow
> Chest X-ray
> Endoscopy
> Manometry
> Acid monitoring

Table 16.12   Causes of dysphagia

- Local oropharyngeal problems, e.g. infections, tumours
- Central nervous system disorders affecting oropharyngeal function, e.g. brainstem lesions associated with multiple sclerosis, cerebrovascular disease, Parkinson's disease, Huntington's chorea and motor neurone disease
- Malignant and benign oesophageal strictures
- Other local oesophageal problems, e.g. infections, web, diverticulum
- Peripheral nervous system disorders affecting oesophageal striated muscle, e.g. chronic alcoholism, diabetes mellitus
- Peripheral nervous system disorders affecting oesophageal unstriated muscle, e.g. achalasia
- Striated muscle diseases e.g. myasthenia gravis, dystrophia myotonica
- Psychiatric, i.e. globus hystericus

usually have other neuromuscular symptoms and signs. Hysterical dysphagia is a diagnosis of exclusion and usually occurs in psychiatrically disturbed patients.

Other symptoms

Painful swallowing and retrosternal pain associated with swallowing, or gastro-oesophageal reflux (heartburn) are also serious symptoms. On occasions, it may be difficult to differentiate oesophageal and cardiac pain and there is evidence that reflux may lower the threshold for angina. Regurgitation of gastric juice into the lower oesophagus and the back of the mouth (waterbrash) are due to an incompetent lower oesophageal sphincter; this is commonly precipitated by raising the intra-abdominal pressure (lifting, pregnancy). If food accumulates in the oesophagus, nausea, vomiting and weight loss may occur. The oesophagus is also a site of bleeding from varices, ulcers and inflammmatory lesions (oesophagitis).

Signs

Abnormal physical signs are often absent in patients with oesophageal disease, but epigastric tenderness may indicate oesophagitis, peptic ulceration or a carcinoma. Neurological examination of palatal movement and the gag reflex are important when dysphagia could be due to a neurological cause. An epigastric mass or palpable supraclavicular lymph nodes suggests a neoplasm. Decreased oesophageal clearance of solids and fluids (especially in patients with achalasia and carcinomas) may cause pulmonary aspiration.

Investigation of oesophageal pathology

A barium swallow outlines the oropharyngeal and oesophageal anatomy, and a video can be taken to look for disordered motility. A chest X-ray helps to assess oesophageal dilatation. If a patient has dysphagia, a barium swallow is done before an endoscopy; this is because patients' symptoms alone cannot localise the site of the lesion and, if the endoscopist is unprepared for the abnormal anatomy, perforation of an oesophageal carcinoma or diverticulum may occur. If there is a risk of pulmonary aspiration, a less hyperosmolar contrast medium is used. The endoscope can be used for inspection, biopsy and treatment (e.g. variceal sclerosis, tumour lasering and the diathermy of bleeding points respectively). Manometry is useful in reflux and achalasia to assess the lower oesophageal sphincter pressure. Acid reflux can be monitored by a pH-sensitive probe in the distal oesophagus.

OESOPHAGEAL REFLUX

In normal people, oesophageal reflux is prevented by the gastro-oesophageal sphincter, aided by the diaphragm. In patients with reflux, there are repeated episodes of significant quantities of acid, bile and food regurgitating into the lower oesophagus. This leads to inflammatory change (oesophagitis). Oesophagitis is associated with decreased oesophageal clearance of liquids and solids.

Aetiology

The most common cause of oesophageal reflux (Table 16.13) is a hiatus hernia. Pregnancy is commonly associated with reflux, due partly to sex hormones lowering the gastro-oesophageal sphincter pressure, and partly to pressure from the intra-abdominal mass. Smoking, eating fat and chocolate, drinking coffee, tea and alcohol, and certain drugs (e.g. calcium antagonists) act by reducing the lower oesophageal sphincter pressure.

Clinical features

Reflux can give rise to the symptoms of regurgitation, oesophageal pain and heartburn. The symptoms are often

Table 16.13 Causes of oesophageal reflux

Cause	Example
Disordered anatomy	Hiatus hernia Obesity Post-surgical treatment of achalasia Presence of tube for treating carcinoma
Myogenic	Systemic sclerosis Oesophagitis
Hormonal	Pregnancy Menstruation
External influences	Smoking Eating fat/chocolate Coffee/tea Large meals Alcohol Drugs

aggravated by bending down or raising intra-abdominal pressure (e.g. by lifting). If it is complicated by oesophagitis or stricture formation, vomiting, haemorrhage, dysphagia and pulmonary aspiration may occur.

Investigation

Oesophageal reflux, if the symptoms are typical, requires little investigation. However, if the symptoms are less typical, severe, or include gastrointestinal bleeding or dysphagia, further investigation is indicated. Endoscopy is preferred, as this allows more accurate visualisation of associated lesions (oesophagitis, ulcers, stricture formation etc.) and permits biopsies of inflamed, ulcerated or questionably malignant areas. However, endoscopy does not permit satisfactory demonstration of reflux itself; this can be done by a barium swallow or ingestion of a radioisotope. A very good objective assessment of reflux can be obtained by placing a pH probe in the lower oesophagus and measuring falls in pH due to acid regurgitation over a 24-hour period. If the patient's symptoms correlate with a fall in pH, the diagnosis is confirmed. Oesophageal manometry is of little use in the diagnosis of reflux. The pressure in the lower oesophagus in patients who reflux tends to be reduced, but is often still in the same range as that of normal individuals. Manometry is, however, useful in distinguishing reflux from other conditions where symptoms can be similar, such as achalasia, systemic sclerosis and diffuse oesophageal spasm.

REFLUX OESOPHAGITIS

Oesophagitis is an inflammatory response secondary to reflux.

Clinical features

Typical symptoms are heartburn, retrosternal pain and vomiting, which may be blood-stained. Endoscopically, it can be graded into four stages.

1. *Mild.* Single or nonconfluent areas of superficial mucosal erosions and erythema.
2. *Moderate.* Confluent erosions not including the whole circumference of the oesophagus.
3. *Severe.* Confluent erosions including the whole oesophageal circumference.
4. *Complicated.* Oesophagitis with additional complications, e.g. peptic ulcers, strictures, gastric mucosa in oesophagus (Barrett's syndrome).

Treatment

Medical

The treatment of oesophageal reflux and oesophagitis is outlined in Summary 2. Obesity is frequently a major causal factor, and weight loss is then a priority. Raising the head of the bed on blocks of wood or bricks by 20 cm or more discourages nocturnal acid regurgitation, and is more satisfactory than increasing the number of pillows. The avoidance of precipitating foods and drinks also often helps. In mild cases, a mixture of alginic acid, which coats and forms a barrier over the oesophageal mucosa, and a simple antacid is effective. In patients with troublesome symptoms (especially if there is coexistant oesophagitis), a six-week course of metoclopramide before meals, full dose H_2-receptor antagonists (taken twice daily or all at night), and an alginic acid and antacid mixture is usually effective. The metoclopramide increases gastric emptying, the H_2-receptor antagonist reduces gastric acid secretion, and the alginic acid forms a protective coat over the oesophageal mucosa. An effective alternative is to use low dose car-benoxolone (a mucosal protection agent) combined with an alginic acid/antacid mixture. However, this has the disadvantage that, especially in the elderly, carbenoxolone can cause sodium retention and lead to hypertension and heart failure. In refractory cases, the parietal cell proton pump inhibitor, omeprazole, should be considered.

Surgical

Surgery is indicated in patients with large hiatus hernias and severe symptoms of reflux or dysphagia unresponsive to medical treatment. Selected patients should preferably be non-obese, free of other serious medical problems and be under 70 years of age. Surgery usually involves an anti-reflux procedure (e.g. fundoplication) and vagotomy to reduce gastric acid secretion. Recently, attempts have been made, in frail elderly patients, to prevent gastric herniation and reflux by fastening a silicone ring around the gastro-oesophageal junction below the diaphragm, through a small incision (Angelchik prosthesis). If bile reflux is a problem (e.g. after a previous partial gastrectomy), a procedure to divert bile lower down the intestine using a Roux-en-Y anastomosis should be considered.

HIATUS HERNIA

Hiatus hernias can be congenital, in which case they usually present, and are treated, during childhood. Acquired hiatus hernias are often of the sliding type and result in varying lengths of the stomach being in the chest (Fig. 16.5). The rolling type is less common, and occurs when a portion of the fundus of the stomach lies anterior to the oesophagus.

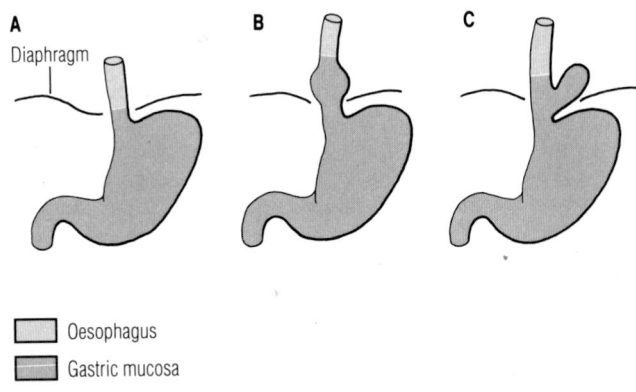

Oesophagus

Gastric mucosa

Fig. 16.5 Diagram of (A) normal anatomy, (B) sliding hiatus hernia and (C) rolling hiatus hernia.

Clinical features

Sliding hiatus hernias present with symptoms of reflux. Difficulty with swallowing suggests the presence of a complicating stricture.

The symptoms of rolling hiatus hernias do not include reflux and are commonly very non-specific, such as vague upper abdominal discomfort, nausea and fullness after

---

Summary 2 Treatment of oesophageal reflux and oesophagitis

- Simple measures
  - Lose weight
  - Raise head of bed on blocks
  - Avoid bending

- Avoid possible aetiological factors which reduce lower oesophageal sphincter pressure
  - Smoking
  - Eating fat/chocolate
  - Coffee/tea
  - Alcohol

- Drugs to reduce gastric acid secretion
  - H_2-receptor antagonists

- Drugs to increase gastric emptying
  - Metoclopramide
  - Domperidone

- Drugs to protect mucosal lining
  - Alginic acid containing antacid
  - Carbenoxolone

- Drugs to neutralise gastric acid
  - Simple antacids

- Surgery

eating. Complications include bleeding from gastritis or a gastric ulcer (sometimes presenting as an iron deficiency anaemia), gastric volvulus and hernial strangulation.

Investigation

Investigations should include a haemoglobin to look for an anaemia secondary to blood loss. If a sliding hiatus hernia is large, it may be seen on chest X-ray as a retrocardiac shadow with a fluid level. Endoscopy is the diagnostic procedure of choice, as this allows direct assessment of hernial size, oesophagitis and stricture formation, the taking of diagnostic biopsies and the passage of dilating bougies to treat a stricture. Alternatively, a barium swallow can be used to assess hernia size and the development of complications.

Treatment

Treatment of a sliding hiatus hernia is generally the treatment of its complications, such as reflux, oesophagitis and stricture formation. Surgery is sometimes indicated to reduce a large hernia and also, in view of the risk of strangulation, where a rolling hernia occurs. However, as rolling hernias are often found in the very elderly, surgery may be postponed until a major complication occurs.

BARRETT'S OESOPHAGUS

Barrett's oesophagus is a complication of oesophagitis where a portion of the lower oesophagus is lined by gastric columnar epithelium instead of normal squamous epithelium. It presents as oesophagitis and is thought to be premalignant, giving rise to an adenocarcinoma of the lower one-third. The disorder therefore requires regular annual endoscopic inspection and biopsy in patients under 70 years of age.

PEPTIC OESOPHAGEAL STRICTURE

Peptic oesophageal strictures are fibrous strictures which occur at the lower end of the oesophagus as a result of persistent oesophageal reflux usually due to a sliding hiatus hernia. The main symptom is progressive dysphagia, first for solids and then for liquids. The patients become frightened to eat, develop increasing pain and sometimes aspiration and, as a result, become anorexic and lose weight.

Treatment is by passage of an endoscope or, if the stricture is tight, by metal dilators (Fig. 16.6). Treatment can be repeated if symptoms recur, but many patients only require it once or every few years. Patients should be encouraged to return to eating solids after the procedure. Oesophageal perforation is rare. Surgery is seldom indicated and, in particular, is best avoided in the elderly.

CORROSIVE AND FOREIGN BODY INGESTION

In certain parts of the world (e.g. India and South America), strong acid or alkali solutions are commonly

Fig. 16.6 Instruments used in treatment of oesophageal strictures. A. Prosthetic tubes used for carcinomas: the Celestin tube (above) and the Atkinson (Nottingham) tube (below). **B.** An Eder-Prestow metal dilator (above) used for benign and malignant strictures; and (below) a Rider-Moeller bag dilator used in achalasia.

taken with suicidal intent. This most commonly affects the oesophagus, though the stomach and duodenum can also be damaged. In some patients, oesophageal perforation requires urgent surgery. In patients without perforation, conservative treatment with neutralising lavage can be successful without long-term complications, but in others a stricture develops. Gastric or duodenal strictures usually require surgical intervention.

Foreign bodies (e.g. fish bones, coins) may stick in the gut, usually the oesophagus, and cause dysphagia. Small articles can be extracted endoscopically. A bolus of food often obstructs the oesophagus of patients with benign or malignant strictures, and this can usually be treated by using the endoscope to push the bolus distal to the obstruction. When larger solid articles are swallowed and are thought likely to obstruct the bowel or cause perforation, a laparotomy should be considered.

OESOPHAGEAL TUMOURS

A basic classification of oesophageal tumours is shown in Table 16.14. Benign tumours are rare. Malignant tumours occur in the upper third of the oesophagus (about 15%) but are more common in the middle (about 40%) and lower third (about 45%). The majority of oesophageal tumours are squamous cell in origin (if adenocarcinomas which arise in the stomach and invade upwards are excluded). The

Table 16.14 Basic classification of oesophageal tumours

Class	Example
Malignant	Squamous cell carcinoma
	Adenocarcinoma
	Melanoma
	Sarcoma (usually leiomyosarcoma)
Benign	Leiomyoma
	Adenoma
	Cysts

tumours spread early by local invasion and lymphatic metastases.

The incidence of oesophageal cancer varies greatly in different regions of the world, with a high incidence in Central Asia, the Far East and Transkei (Fig. 16.7). The age-specific incidence is shown in Figure 16.8.

Fig. 16.7   Areas of high incidence of oesophageal carcinoma worldwide.

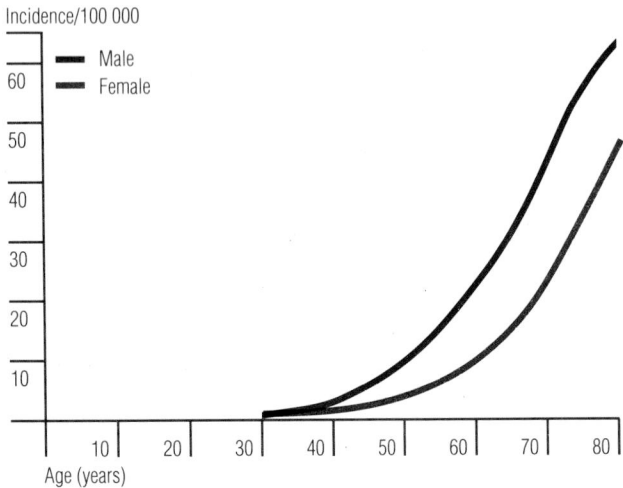

Fig. 16.8   Age-specific incidence of carcinoma of the oesophagus in the UK.

Aetiology

In the UK, aetiological factors in squamous cell carcinomas of the oesophagus are cigarette smoking, high alcohol intake, coeliac disease, achalasia, ingestion of strong acids and alkalis and, possibly, oesophagitis. Such carcinomas are often preceded by histological dysplasia which can be detected by endoscopic biopsies. Islands of gastric-type mucosa in the oesophagus (Barrett's oesophagus) predispose to the development of adenocarcinomas. The Plummer-Vinson syndrome, which occurs in long-stand-

ing iron deficiency anaemia is, rarely, associated with post-cricoid carcinoma. A rare inherited syndrome of palmar hyperkeratosis (tylosis palmaris) is associated with oesophageal cancer.

Clinical features

The symptoms and signs of oesophageal carcinomas are listed in Summary 3. Dysphagia is the main symptom of oesophageal carcinomas, whether the pathology is an ulcer, a polypoid mass or a scirrhous lesion encircling the whole lumen. The dysphagia is rapidly progressive. Pain is usually retrosternal and is due to invasion through the oesophagus into the mediastinum. A cough productive of sputum may reflect aspiration, or erosion into a bronchus (broncho-oesophageal fistula). On examination, weight loss is often obvious. Anaemia usually reflects bleeding. Lymph node enlargement and hepatomegaly due to distant spread are late signs.

Summary 3 Symptoms and signs of oesophageal carcinoma	
Symptoms	*Signs*
Dysphagia (Initially solids, then liquids, then complete)	Weight loss
	Anaemia
Pain	Enlarged cervical lymph nodes
Weight loss	Hepatomegaly
Cough	

Investigation

Patients who present with dysphagia often localise the point where food sticks, but this does not correlate with the anatomical site of obstruction. It is dangerous for patients to be endoscoped without knowing the level of the lesion as perforation may result. The first investigation for dysphagia is therefore a barium swallow (Fig. 16.9). Endoscopy and biopsy to ascertain cell type follows. A chest X-ray is done to assess mediastinal spread, and liver function tests and ultrasound are performed to detect metastases. If curative surgery is contemplated, a CT scan of the chest is necessary to define the degree of local infiltration.

Treatment

The treatment of oesophageal carcinoma (Table 16.15) is controversial and results are poor. Surgery is effective in patients who are fit, with no involved nodes or metastases, but these patients make up only about 10% of those presenting with the disease.

In the upper third, radiotherapy is usually the preferred treatment but radical treatments are technically very difficult to give. Surgery involves total oesophagectomy and colonic interposition. In the middle and lower thirds, surgery is preferred to radiotherapy if the patient is fit enough. The stomach is mobilised and anastomosed to the oesophagus in the chest. Radiation may be complicated

Fig. 16.9 Barium swallow examinations.
A. A smooth benign oesophageal stricture above a hiatus hernia. **B.** A typical carcinoma with destruction of the oesophageal lumen.

Table 16.15 Treatment of oesophageal carcinoma

Aim	Treatment modality	Criteria	Result
'Curative'	Radical surgery (with or without pre- or postoperative radiotherapy)	Tumour localised to oesophagus	Overall 5% five-year survival
	Radical radiotherapy	Tumour localised to oesophagus	Similar results to surgery
Palliative	Radiotherapy Dilatation Intubation Laser therapy Pain relief and general nutritional support	Widespread local tumour; distant metastases; other medical conditions preclude surgery or radical radiotherapy	Good palliation

by oesophagitis and stricture, and surgery by stricture, mediastinitis, and anastomotic leaks. Overall survival for either treatment is less than 5% at five years.

Malignant stricture formation can be palliated by repeated endoscopic dilatations; when these are needed more than once every six weeks, it is useful to insert a tube to keep the lumen open and to allow liquidised food to pass. The tube can be placed using a fibre-optic endoscope under local or general anaesthesia, and is also useful for sealing off fistulas with bronchi or the trachea. Tubes can be replaced as necessary; if they become blocked by food, fizzy drinks can be tried first, and then endoscopic procedures. With intubation, good pain relief and general supportive care, patients with advanced carcinoma of the oesophagus should be able to swallow and be comfortable up to the time of death. Repeated endoscopic laser treatments are an alternative approach.

ACHALASIA

Achalasia is obstruction at the level of the lower oesophageal sphincter due to a failure of relaxation. It results in progressive dilatation of the oesophagus proximal to the obstruction. Achalasia is caused by degeneration of ganglion cells in the muscle of the mid and lower oesophagus. In the West, the aetiology is obscure although the disease is sometimes familial. In South America, a similar problem occurs as a late result of destruction of the ganglion cells by the protozoon *Trypanosoma cruzi* (Chagas' disease; see p. 304).

Clinical features and investigation

Initial presentation is usually with slowly progressive dysphagia for both solids and liquids; there may be associated

Fig. 16.10 Barium swallow examination showing oesophageal achalasia. There is hold-up of barium at the level of the gastro-oesophageal junction, and oesophageal dilation and lack of contractions above. Advanced cases also have a fluid level which may be seen on a chest X-ray.

pain. Regurgitation of food swallowed some hours before may occur, but heartburn is unusual. Anorexia and weight loss may also occur and some patients develop pulmonary aspiration.

The diagnosis is best made radiologically. If gross oesophageal dilatation has occurred, a dilated oesophagus with a fluid level is seen on chest X-ray. A barium swallow reveals a failure of the lower oesophageal sphincter to relax, and sometimes proximal dilatation with food and fluid in the lumen (Fig. 16.10). The gastric air bubble is usually absent on initial erect films. Manometry confirms the diagnosis, with an elevated lower oesophageal sphincter pressure and weak contractions of the oesophagus above.

Treatment

Treatment of achalasia can be with either pneumatic balloon dilatation under endoscopic control or oesophageal myotomy (Heller's operation). Both these treatments are effective, but balloon dilatation has the advantage of being

Fig. 16.11 Barium swallow examination showing oesophageal spasm ('the nutcracker oesophagus').

less invasive. Carcinoma of the oesophagus is a rare complication of achalasia.

OESOPHAGEAL SPASM

Oesophageal spasm presents with chest pain and/or dysphagia. A barium swallow shows a normal oesophagus, but the oesophagus may undergo diffuse spasm during the investigation to produce a corkscrew configuration (Fig. 16.11). Manometry shows intermediate bursts of high amplitude contractions often unrelated to swallowing. Angina is a major differential diagnosis, but oesophageal spasm is not precipitated by exertion and stress.

Treatment is also similar to angina since glyceryl trinitrate sublingually (as necessary), and regular isosorbide dinitrate or nifedipine often help. In resistant cases, balloon dilatation or myotomy can be considered, but the results are not as good as for achalasia.

SYSTEMIC SCLEROSIS

Systemic sclerosis causes loss of oesophageal contractions (which may also occur in patients with Raynaud's phenomenon, systemic lupus erythematosus and polymyositis). Dysphagia and heartburn may occur. A barium swallow shows lack of peristalsis, and thus failure of the barium to move if the patient lies flat. The gastro-oesophageal junction may become incompetent, with consequent reflux, oesophagitis and peptic stricture.

ANATOMICAL ABNORMALITIES

Oesophageal diverticula are outpouchings of the oesophageal wall that can occur at any position in the oesophagus. Dysphagia and regurgitation are both typical symptoms. If symptoms become severe, corrective surgery may be necessary.

Oesophageal webs are thin structures impinging a few millimetres into the lumen and consisting of mucosa and submucosa. They occur throughout the oesophagus and can be multiple. An association with chronic iron deficiency is now rare; treatment of the latter may prevent an associated postcricoid carcinoma. Dilatation helps if dysphagia occurs.

Oesophageal rings occur at the lower end of the oesophagus and contain muscle as well as mucosa and submucosa. They present with intermittent dysphagia, which may become more common as the years pass. If symptoms are serious, endoscopic dilatation usually relieves them.

OESOPHAGEAL INFECTIONS

The most important oesophageal infections are candidiasis and *Herpes simplex*. Both occur in patients who are immunosuppressed, e.g. in patients who are receiving corticosteroids or cytotoxic drugs, or who have AIDS. Antibiotic treatment predisposes to monilial infections.

Patients with oesophageal infections usually present with dysphagia which may be painful. Diagnosis of candidiasis is by endoscopic demonstration of the creamy exudates on the oesophageal wall (the mouth and pharynx are often also involved) and by demonstration of the typical yeast hyphae on microscopy. *Herpes simplex* appears similar on endoscopy, but can be confirmed by histological demonstration of inclusion bodies in epithelial cells and by viral culture.

The treatment of oesophageal candida infection is initially with nystatin or amphotericin in the form of lozenges. Herpes simplex is treated symptomatically with local anaesthetic drinks, although acyclovir is necessary in patients who are severely immunosuppressed. Candidiasis responds quickly to adequate treatment unless there is severe immune suppression, in which case ketoconazole is helpful; herpes usually settles over 1–2 weeks.

GASTROINTESTINAL BLEEDING

ACUTE GASTROINTESTINAL BLEEDING

Upper gastrointestinal bleeding presenting with haematemesis (vomiting blood or altered 'coffee ground'

material) and/or melaena (the passage of black tarry faeces) is a common medical emergency. In the United Kingdom, it has an annual prevalence of about 50 cases per 100 000 population. The different sites of gastrointestinal bleeding and approximate mortality rates in the UK are shown in Figure 16.12.

Fig. 16.12 Gastrointestinal bleeding: sites of origin and mortality rates in the UK. A. Typical values for the site of origin of gastrointestinal bleeding. **B.** Approximate mortality rates for different causes of gastrointestinal bleeding. **C.** Mortality rates related to age showing a rise from 60 years of age onwards.

Aetiology

The causes of gastrointestinal bleeding are shown in Table 16.16. Peptic ulcers, gastritis, Mallory-Weiss tears, varices and tumours account for the majority of patients. Bleeding may be provoked by ingestion of alcohol, aspirin, corticosteroids and non-steroidal anti-inflammatory drugs (NSAIDs). A Mallory-Weiss tear is a small lesion at the gastro-oesophageal junction, which usually follows vomiting and causes an episode of self-limiting bleeding. Systemic and vascular causes are rare. Occasionally, patients are seen who invent the symptoms, ingest blood from

Gastrointestinal Disease

Table 16.16 Causes of gastrointestinal bleeding (brackets indicate rare cause)

Causes of haematemesis

Oesophagus
  Carcinoma
  Oesophagitis ⎱ usually associated
  Peptic ulcer ⎰ with hiatus hernia
  Varices

Stomach
  Peptic ulcer
  Carcinoma
  Acute gastritis
  Mallory-Weiss tear
  (Other tumours)
  (Angiodysplasia)

Duodenum
  Peptic ulcer
  (Tumours)

Systemic causes
  Chronic renal failure
  Thrombocytopenia
  (Clotting factor deficiency)

Vascular causes
  (Mesenteric ischaemia)
  (Hereditary telangiectasia)

Swallowed blood
  from oropharynx and nose

(Munchausen's syndrome)
  – symptom invented
  – ingested blood
  – self-induced

Causes of melaena

Causes of haematemesis (see above)

Jejunum and ileum
  (Meckel's diverticulum)
  (angiodysplasia)
  (tumours)
  (Crohn's disease)
  (infarction of bowel)

Colon
  Higher tumours
  Angiodysplasia
  Inflammatory bowel disease

Causes of blood intermixed with stool

Colon
  Left-sided colonic tumours
  Inflammatory bowel disease
  Diverticular disease
  Infective colitis
  Angiodysplasia
  Ischaemic colitis

Causes of fresh blood per rectum

Anus and rectum
  Haemorrhoids
  Proctitis of any cause
  Carcinoma of anus or rectum
  Crohn's disease of anus

outside (for example, from animals) or deliberately break their mucosa to cause bleeding.

Haematemesis is usually from a bleeding site proximal to the distal duodenum. If there is rapid intestinal transit, fresh blood per rectum may be passed from upper gastrointestinal lesions. Melaena is altered, partially digested blood passed per rectum. It can result from any cause of haematemesis. Meckel's diverticula are uncommon developmental abnormalities in the distal ileum; these frequently contain gastric acid-secreting cells, and usually present with recurrent melaena before adolescence. Angio-

dysplasia is increasingly recognised as a cause of melaena. In this condition, there are leashes of dilated submucosal vessels which usually occur in the ileum and right side of colon, although the stomach and upper small bowel may be involved.

Clinical features

The history is important in diagnosis, particularly with regard to previous symptoms (e.g. pain, vomiting, weight loss), past medical history (e.g. previous episodes, ulcers, liver disease) and ingestion of alcohol, aspirin, steroids and NSAIDs.

Frank gastrointestinal bleeding may present with haematemesis and melaena. With severe bleeding there will be signs of shock, with a tachycardia and hypotension (particularly a postural drop in blood pressure). Anaemia suggests either acute bleeding over several days with time for haemodilution, or an underlying chronic disease which has been causing blood loss over weeks or months. Spooning of the nails (koilonychia) infers years of iron deficiency. Signs of chronic liver disease suggest varices as the aetiology. Vascular malformations on the face and mucous membranes of the lips or mouth suggest hereditary telangiectasia.

Investigation

The most precise investigation for making a diagnosis is an upper gastrointestinal endoscopy within 24 hours of the bleeding starting. The patient should be resuscitated and endoscoped as soon as practicable. At this stage, most Mallory-Weiss tears, acute ulcers and areas of acute inflammation are obvious and the bleeding point may be identified. Perendoscopic thermal coagulation or laser therapy may be used on any bleeding vessels seen.

The small intestine, beyond the distal duodenum and proximal to the distal terminal ileum, can only be reached by an endoscope during a laparotomy. Small intestinal bleeding may, however, be identified preoperatively by arteriography. Colonic bleeding may be identified by sigmoidoscopy or colonoscopy, or by arteriography if the bleeding is sufficiently profuse.

Treatment

A joint medical and surgical approach to acute gastrointestinal bleeding is important. Before investigation takes place, if there are signs of shock, a central venous pressure line is essential. Blood should be given if the haemoglobin is less than 10 g/dl or, if there is a tachycardia or hypotension, to restore the blood volume. H_2-receptor antagonist drugs are widely used, but there is little evidence that they reduce operation rates or mortality. Tranexamic acid (which enhances coagulation) and somatostatin (which reduces acid secretion and splanchnic blood flow) may have a role in controlling bleeding. Vasopressin, which also reduces splanchnic blood flow, is usually reserved for variceal bleeding (Ch. 17, p. 654).

Surgery is indicated if the bleeding is life-threatening or when it is persistent despite receiving three or more litres of blood, especially if the patient is over 60 years of age. Early surgery is indicated if there is a visible vessel at the base of an ulcer or if an operable carcinoma is present. Surgery is best avoided in self-limiting conditions, such as gastritis and a Mallory-Weiss tear, if there is a clotting disorder or if varices are present (Ch. 17, p. 654).

The mortality of acute gastrointestinal bleeding is up to 10% with each episode. However, this relatively high mortality is mostly due to deaths in patients aged over 65 (Fig. 16.12) from associated causes (such as vascular, pulmonary or renal diseases), rather than from exsanguination.

CHRONIC GASTROINTESTINAL BLEEDING

Aetiology and clinical features

A microcytic hypochromic anaemia is a common presentation of chronic gut blood loss. The commonest causes are shown in Table 16.17. Patients often present with symptoms of anaemia – malaise, dyspnoea and angina. Clinical examination usually shows signs of anaemia, but the classical signs of iron deficiency, glossitis, cheilitis and koilonychia, are often not present.

Table 16.17 Causes of chronic occult gastrointestinal bleeding (in approximate order of frequency)

- Colonic neoplasm
- Duodenal ulcer
- Complicated hiatus hernia
- Gastric ulcer
- NSAIDs
- Meckel's diverticulum
- Angiodysplasia

Investigation

The purpose of investigations is to identify the cause of the iron deficiency anaemia. Positive faecal occult blood testing suggests gastrointestinal blood loss, but bleeding may be spasmodic so false negatives can occur. False positives may occur with meat ingestion, and bleeding gums.

In the presence of upper gastrointestinal symptoms, or if there are no specific symptoms and signs, upper gut endoscopy is usually performed first. This may be combined with duodenal biopsy if there is a possibility of an underlying malabsorption syndrome. If no abnormality is found in the upper gut, double contrast air and barium enema is the next investigation. If still no cause is evident, colonoscopy and investigation of the small bowel, e.g. small bowel enema, Meckel scan (p. 560) or arteriography, must be considered.

Treatment

Wherever possible, the primary cause of the bleeding is treated. The iron stores are replenished by giving oral iron in the form of ferrous sulphate, fumarate or gluconate. Oral iron can cause nausea, dyspepsia and altered bowel habit. If these side-effects develop, a lower dose or a different preparation should be tried. If the patient is unable to tolerate oral iron, a total dose infusion of intravenous iron dextran, or intra-muscular doses of smaller amounts of iron sorbitol, can be used (p. 1045). Severe symptomatic anaemia may require blood transfusion; this is especially likely to occur if the primary cause cannot be found or treated successfully. If no cause is found, the patient is followed carefully and reinvestigated if the problem recurs.

THE STOMACH AND DUODENUM

Anatomy and physiology

The lower end of the oesophagus and the fundus of the stomach are separated by the gastro-oesophageal sphincter, which normally prevents reflux and allows the downward passage of food. The stomach is arbitrarily divided into three parts: fundus, body and antrum. The incisura is an angle on the lesser curve which is an important endoscopic landmark, as the endoscope has to be pointed upwards to negotiate it. The pylorus is a sphincter that controls passage of gastric contents into the first part of the duodenum. Parietal cells synthesising hydrochloric acid are in the fundus and body of the stomach; gastrin is synthesised in the antral G-cells. Pepsinogens are produced by the chief cells in the crypts.

The stomach has three main functions.

1. *The secretion of HCl*, to hydrolyse food and convert pepsinogen to pepsin to initiate protein digestion into polypeptides. The pH is kept around 2 and this is bacteriostatic. In man, HCl secretion is mainly stimulated by the antral hormone gastrin, which is released in response to dietary protein, gastric distension, and vagal stimulation. At the level of the parietal cell, there is an H_2-receptor which is a final common pathway for HCl synthesis and a K^+-H^+-ATPase which pumps H^+ ions into the lumen of the stomach. The inter-relationships of these stimuli are shown in Figure 16.13.

2. *As a reservoir.* The stomach acts as a reservoir, and constant churning allows breakdown of food into small particles. Gastric emptying proceeds slowly so that the small bowel can digest and absorb maximally. Gastric emptying is a complex process, dependent on duodenal receptors; it is, for example, slower for fats than protein. Control is partly vagal and partly hormonal (motilin accelerates the process, while enteroglucagon and neurotensin slow it down).

3. *Secretion of intrinsic factor*, by the parietal cells.

575

Gastrointestinal Disease

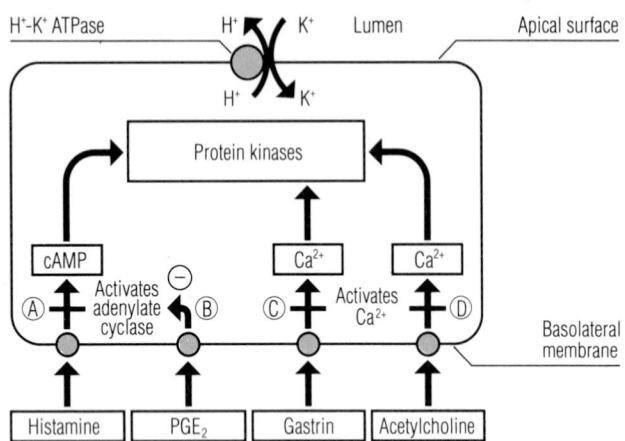

Fig. 16.13 Diagram showing secretion of H$^+$ by a gastric parietal cell. There are receptors on the basolateral membrane for histamine (H$_2$), gastrin and acetylcholine, all of which can mediate the activation of second messengers. A complex series of metabolic events then occurs with the result that H$^+$-K$^+$-ATPase at the apical surface pumps H$^+$ into the gastric lumen in exchange for K$^+$. Antagonists exist for each of the three basolateral receptors (e.g. cimetidine (A), proglumide (C) and pirenzipine (D) and for H$^+$,K$^+$,ATPase (omeprazole). The prostaglandin E$_2$ receptor inhibits the stimulatory effect of histamine on cAMP; misoprostol (B) is a PGE$_2$ analogue.

The duodenum is largely retroperitoneal and is divided into first, second, third and fourth parts. The pH is lowest in the first part and nearly all duodenal ulcers are sited here. The medial border of the second part of the duodenum receives alkaline biliary and pancreatic secretions. The first and second parts contain Brunner glands, which secrete bicarbonate and help bring the pH up to around neutral. Villi are present throughout the duodenum and increase in size down its length. Enzyme digestion and absorption of small molecules not needing digestion (e.g. calcium, iron, folic acid) occur in the duodenum.

Clinical features of gastroduodenal pathology

The main symptoms, signs and investigations of gastroduodenal disease are listed in Summary 4. The site of gastroduodenal pain is usually epigastric, but may radiate through to the back and to the right and left hypochondria. Duodenal ulcer pain is typically relieved by food and simple antacids. Functional dyspepsia usually occurs at the time of maximal stress. Nausea, vomiting, anorexia and weight loss raise the possibility of luminal obstruction or a carcinoma. Bleeding can cause haematemesis and melaena.

Epigastric tenderness may be present on superficial or deep palpation. An epigastric mass may be palpable, and can be difficult to distinguish from the liver. With gastric carcinoma, metastatic supraclavicular nodes may be palpable. A succussion splash, present three or more hours after the last drink or meal, suggests delayed gastric emptying commonly due to pyloric obstruction. It is elicited by shaking the patient's upper abdomen while listening over the epigastrium.

Summary 4   The main symptoms, signs and investigations in the diagnosis of gastroduodenal disease

Symptoms	Signs
Pain	Tenderness
Site	Presence of a mass (epigastric
Relationship with food, drugs,	or supraclavicular fossa)
stress	Succussion splash
Nausea and vomiting	
Haematemesis and melaena	
Anorexia	
Weight loss	
Oesophageal reflux	

Investigations

Endoscopy
Barium meal
Gastric acid secretion
Full blood count
Liver function tests

Investigation of gastroduodenal pathology

An endoscopy is the preferred procedure for the investigation of possible gastroduodenal disease. A barium meal is reserved for the patients who are frail, have poor lung function, refuse endoscopy or cannot swallow the endoscope. The clinical indications for measuring gastric acid secretion are to exclude a gastrinoma (when the basal acid secretion is very high) and to confirm that parietal cell innervation has been lost after a surgical vagotomy. After successful vagotomy, insulin-induced hypoglycaemia no longer causes acid secretion. A haemoglobin is performed to detect anaemia, and plasma liver enzyme tests for coexisting liver disease.

PEPTIC ULCERS

Peptic ulcers can occur in the oesophagus (usually in association with a hiatus hernia), in the stomach (gastric ulcer, GU) and in the duodenum (duodenal ulcer, DU). An erosion is present when the mucosal surface is broken. Ulcers are present when the muscularis mucosae is penetrated. In practice, it is difficult to tell the difference at endoscopy. Lesions may vary in size from 1 mm to several centimetres in diameter.

Aetiology

The aetiological factors in peptic ulceration are shown in Table 16.18. The aphorism 'no acid: no ulcer' is true for benign peptic ulcers. Gastric ulcers, however, are usually associated with normal or low acid outputs, although this may partly reflect duodenogastric reflux of alkaline juice. The combination of high gastric acid outputs, rapid gastric emptying, and possibly reduced duodenal bicarbonate production are important in the pathogenesis of duodenal ulcers. Duodenogastric reflux of alkaline juice, bile and

Table 16.18 Aetiological factors in peptic ulceration

Causal factor	Gastric ulcer	Duodenal ulcer
Acid	Normal or low acid output	High acid output
Duodenogastric reflux	Important	Unimportant
Gastric emptying	Delayed	Increased
Steroids and NSAIDs	Small role	Small role
Smoking	Important	Important
Stress	Evidence for head injuries and burns only	
Family history	Uncommon	Common

pancreatic enzymes is thought to be important for gastric ulcers. Corticosteroids, aspirin and NSAIDs are associated with an increased incidence of peptic ulcers and of the complications of bleeding and perforation. Smoking plays a role in pathogenesis and delays healing of duodenal ulcers. The objective evidence that ordinary stress causes ulcers is poor, but severe head injuries (Cushing's ulcer) and burns (Curling's ulcer) are associated with the development of acute ulcers. Duodenal ulcers are often familial and are associated with blood group O. The factors involved in mucosal cell resistance or liability to ulceration are not understood. Possibly important factors are gastric mucus, gastric bicarbonate secretion and the organism, *Campylobacter pylori*, which is present in many patients with gastritis and peptic ulcer disease. An additional, and rare, cause of peptic ulceration is gastrinoma (p. 579).

Duodenal ulcers are approximately four times as common as gastric ulcer. Whereas there appears to be a tendency for spontaneous remission with duodenal ulcers the prevalence of gastric ulcer progressively increases with age (Fig. 16.14).

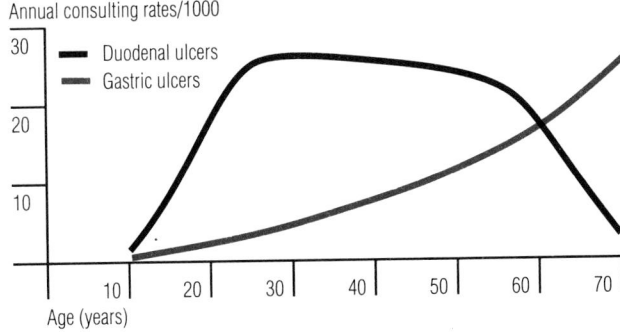

Fig. 16.14 Incidence of peptic ulcer related to age, UK.

Clinical features

The symptoms and signs of ulcer disease are non-specific for each type of ulcer and commonly overlap those found in patients with cholelithiasis, oesophagitis, pancreatitis

and no demonstrable organic disease. Duodenal ulcer patients tend to have epigastric pain which is worse with fasting, better with antacids and food, and wakes them at 2–4 am. Gastric ulcer patients' epigastric pain is sometimes worse with food. Nausea and vomiting are relatively unusual and imply outlet obstruction. Anorexia and weight loss can occur with both gastric and duodenal ulcers. Many ulcers are asymptomatic.

In an uncomplicated peptic ulcer patient, epigastric tenderness is usually the only abnormal sign, and even this is often absent. If there is gastric outflow obstruction, a succussion splash is present.

Investigation

Endoscopy is more accurate than barium studies in the diagnosis of peptic ulcers (Table 16.19 and Fig. 16.15). It also enables accurate histological diagnosis of malignancy, and treatment with electrocautery and lasers as necessary. Barium meals are, however, useful in patients who will not swallow the endoscope, or who have poor respiratory function. Endoscopic complications are rare, but sedation can cause respiratory depression, biopsy can cause bleeding and air insufflation can cause perforation.

Table 16.19 Relative merits of endoscopy and barium studies in diagnosis of peptic ulcer

Merit	Endoscopy	Barium study
Accuracy	Almost 100%	Lower, especially for superficial lesions
Ability to obtain biopsies and brush cytology	Yes	No
Enables other treatments (e.g. diathermy, lasers)	Yes	No
Detection of bleeding	Yes	No
Complications	Small	Small

Complications

There are three main complications of peptic ulcers:

1. *Gastrointestinal bleeding* (p. 573). In a small proportion of patients gastrointestinal bleeding is the first symptom of a peptic ulcer, but usually there is a variable period of preceding dyspepsia.
2. *Perforation* of an ulcer usually presents with acute severe upper abdominal pain, and circulatory collapse may rapidly develop. Specific symptoms may be minimal or absent in the elderly and in patients on corticosteroid therapy. After resuscitation, surgery should be performed to clean the peritoneum and oversew the ulcer; a procedure may also be performed to prevent further ulcers, e.g. a vagotomy with or

16

Fig. 16.15 Barium studies and endoscopy in diagnosis of peptic ulcer. A. Barium meal demonstrating a large gastric ulcer filled with barium. **B.** Typical duodenal ulcer with pyloric stenosis. **C.** Endoscopic appearance of a chronic prepyloric ulcer.

without a drainage procedure. Rarely, surgery may be contraindicated by high anaesthetic risks, such as respiratory failure or a recent myocardial infarct. Under these circumstances, the perforation can sometimes be healed using conservative methods such as nasogastric suction, intravenous nutrition, antibiotics and nursing in the upright position (so that any abscess forms in the pelvis where it can be more easily drained).

3. *Pyloric stenosis* usually follows longstanding duodenal ulcer disease and is due to narrowing of the pyloric canal by fibrosis. The patients complain of vomiting food eaten many hours before. The failure of gastric emptying results in postprandial fullness, anorexia and weight loss. A succussion splash may be heard many hours after the last meal. If the patient is slow to seek medical help, dehydration, alkalosis and electrolyte deficiency may develop.

If there is an active ulcer, pyloric stenosis may respond to medical treatment. Otherwise, surgical treatment via a laparotomy is necessary although, in a medically very sick patient, endoscopic dilation with a balloon can be considered.

Treatment

Medical

Before a definite diagnosis is made, patients can be treated by simple antacids. In standard doses these are effective symptomatically, but rarely heal significant ulcers. When a diagnosis is made, patients should be encouraged to give up smoking as this will improve their chance of healing and reduce relapse rate. Minimisation of alcohol intake should also be encouraged.

Many effective medical treatments are now available (Table 16.20). The H_2-receptor antagonists are now the treatment of choice, and heal about 80% of ulcers within six weeks. Acid secretion at night is particularly damaging and so taking all the tablets at bedtime is as effective as splitting them during the day. Other drugs, except omeprazole, are marginally less effective and tend to have more side-effects. Gastric ulcers should be followed up by endoscopy at six weeks to check healing, and by rebiopsy to exclude a tumour if unhealed; repeat endoscopy is less important in duodenal ulcers but is helpful in some patients.

If gastric ulcers are healed, half the standard dose of an H_2-receptor antagonist is taken at night for six weeks; the treatment is then usually stopped. The relapse rate for duodenal ulcers is so high that a maintenance dose of half the standard dose can be justified for some months if it is the first attack, and for years if it is a recurrence. If ulcers have not healed, it is best to change to a second agent with a different mode of action (usually bismuth chelate or sucralfate, see Table 16.20), and recheck endoscopically in a further six weeks (when healing is usually found).

Surgical

The indications for surgery for peptic ulcers are shown in

Table 16.20 Main drugs used in treatment of peptic ulcers

Drug	Mode of action	Efficacy	Main side-effects
Cimetidine	H_2-receptor antagonist	Good (80% healing)	Anti-androgenic effects (e.g. impotence, gynaecomastia) Enzyme induction
Ranitidine	H_2-receptor antagonist	Good (80% healing)	Mild rashes
Omeprazole	Proton pump inhibitor	Good	Gastric carcinoid tumours in animals
Aluminium hydroxide	Simple antacid	Good for symptoms; poor for healing	Constipation
Magnesium trisilicate	Simple antacid	Good for symptoms; poor for healing	Diarrhoea
Pirenzipine	Anticholinergic	Good	Dry mouth
Bismuth	Mucosal protection	Good	Unpleasant taste Constipation
Carbenoxolone	Mucosal protection	Good	Sodium retention leading to heart failure, hypertension and potassium loss
Sucralfate	Mucosal protection	Good	Constipation
Misoprostal	Prostaglandin E_2 analogues; mucosal protection; acid and gastrin reduction	Good	Diarrhoea Abortion

---

Summary 5   Indications for surgery for peptic ulcers

- Failure of medical treatment
- Repeated relapses
- Severe haemorrhage
- Perforation
- Pyloric stenosis

Summary 5. The number of patients coming to surgery has reduced since the introduction of H_2-receptor antagonists in the 1970s. Failure of medical treatment or repeated recurrences are relative indications, but such patients should preferably be compliant, non-smokers, not heavy drinkers and thin. Severe haemorrhage and perforation are indications for surgery unless the patient is thought unfit for a general anaesthetic. Pyloric stenosis also usually requires surgery, although occasionally medical treatment of an active ulcer may improve symptoms.

Complications of gastric surgery

Surgery for gastric and duodenal ulcers is usually successful, but the ulcer may recur in that 15% of patients who have a highly selective vagotomy for a duodenal ulcer. Postoperative weight loss is a common symptom but usually stabilises. If a partial gastrectomy is performed, bile reflux may result and cause gastritis in the remnant.

Following gastric surgery, gastric emptying into the small intestine may become very rapid. Hyperosmolar contents cause fluid to be secreted into the jejunum, the plasma compartment contracts and the haematocrit rises. This results in 'early dumping', and the patient complains about 30 minutes after a meal of sweating, palpitations, faintness and abdominal distension. These symptoms may be mediated in part by the vasomotor peptides, neurotensin and vasoactive intestinal polypeptide (VIP, p. 560). The rapid emptying also results in increased early insulin secretion, so that reactive hypoglycaemia may occur 3–4 hours after a meal ('late dumping'). As a result of the rapid gastric emptying, there may be small bowel malabsorption, causing diarrhoea associated with raised faecal fat excretion (steatorrhoea). All these problems can be improved by small, regular and relatively iso-osmolar meals.

After partial and total gastrectomy, some patients become iron, vitamin B_{12}, calcium and vitamin D deficient. A full blood count and plasma calcium, phosphate and alkaline phosphatase should be checked regularly, and life-long supplementary treatment initiated as necessary.

Carcinoma of the stomach is more common after partial gastrectomy, particularly after 20 years. There is no evidence that early diagnosis by regular check endoscopies reduces the very high mortality associated with this problem.

Prognosis of peptic ulcers

The morbidity from peptic ulcer disease is substantial. Despite the fact that nearly 10% of patients with peptic ulcer bleeding die, the overall mortality is low; the majority of patients die of other, unrelated, disease.

GASTRINOMA

Rarely, tumours secreting gastrin stimulate gastric acid secretion, resulting in severe duodenal and upper small

16

bowel ulceration. The primary tumours are usually in the pancreas or duodenum. The tumours may be malignant, and 50% have metastasised at the time of diagnosis. The gastrinoma syndrome (originally described by Zollinger and Ellison in 1955) is characterised by severe peptic ulceration and, in 40% of patients, by diarrhoea, occasionally with malabsorption. The duodenal ulcers are often multiple and may be associated with perforation, bleeding and pyloric stenosis. The acid may also reflux into the oesophagus and cause oesophagitis and oesophageal strictures. About a third of the patients have a functioning parathyroid tumour causing hypercalcaemia, and adenomas also occur in the pituitary, adrenal and thyroid (Multiple Endocrine Neoplasia Type 1, see p. 712). Diagnosis is by demonstrating gastric hyperacidity and a high fasting plasma gastrin. Localisation of the tumour(s) is by CT scanning, arteriography and, if there is still doubt, portal venous sampling.

The tumours are usually slowly progressive, and should only be resected if they are thought to be single and non-metastatic. At one time, total gastrectomy was used as a way of ablating the target organ of the gastrin; now, the acid hypersecretion may be controlled by high dose H_2-receptor antagonists or omeprazole (Table 16.20).

GASTRITIS

In acute gastritis, there are areas of inflamed red oedematous mucosa. The diagnosis can be confirmed by biopsy showing an acute inflammatory infiltrate.

Acute

Acute gastritis is commonly associated with non-steroidal anti-inflammatory drugs (NSAIDs), excessive alcohol and iron intake, and renal failure. It may cause dyspepsia and often presents with gastrointestinal bleeding. It can be diagnosed by direct vision with an endoscope, but not by a barium meal. Treatment is by removing the cause, together with simple antacids. Patients with renal disease have a poor prognosis if they bleed; prophylactic H_2-receptor antagonists are therefore used in patients with dyspeptic symptoms or inflammatory changes on endoscopy.

Chronic

Chronic gastritis is a pathological, rather than endoscopic, diagnosis. It does not usually give rise to symptoms although occasionally it may be associated with dyspepsia. Chronic gastritis may lead to pernicious anaemia and there is an increased incidence of gastric adenocarcinoma.

MÉNÉTRIÈR'S DISEASE

Ménétrièr's disease is a very rare condition, where the normal gastric rugae are increased in height to 1–2 cm. The aetiology is unknown. The main problem is gastric protein loss leading to peripheral oedema (Table 16.4). Reduced

acid secretion, iron and vitamin B_{12} deficiency occur; occasionally, a gastric ulcer develops.

In some patients, the condition may improve with a high protein diet and antacids. Anticholinergics may reduce protein loss, and cimetidine is useful if there is a gastric ulcer. There is a tendency to spontaneous remission. In some patients, however, only total gastrectomy relieves the problem.

DUODENITIS

Duodenitis is an endoscopic or surgical appearance where the mucosa appears inflamed, reddened and sometimes haemorrhagic. It may be seen in isolation or around ulcer craters and may follow or precede the development of duodenal ulcers. When no break in the mucosa (i.e. ulcer) is present, histology shows acute and chronic inflammation. The relationship of duodenitis to symptoms is variable; sometimes patients are asymptomatic and sometimes they have severe pain.

Treatment is by avoiding potential aetiological factors such as smoking, alcohol and NSAIDs, and with simple antacids. Many patients do not need more potent drugs but, if symptoms are severe, H_2-receptor antagonists may help.

MALIGNANT TUMOURS OF THE STOMACH: ADENOCARCINOMA

The commonest gastric cancer is adenocarcinoma. (Lymphomas of the stomach account for less than 3% of all malignant gastric neoplasms.)

There are marked geographic variations in the incidence of adenocarcinoma (Fig. 16.16). In the UK, the incidence is 30 per 100 000 for men and 20 per 100 000 for women. As in other Western countries, there has been a gradual decline in death rate in the last 20 years.

Aetiology and pathology

Gastric carcinoma is five times more common in patients with pernicious anaemia. Other risk factors include achlorhydria, previous partial gastrectomy and blood group A. It has been postulated that gastric atrophy leads to a fall in acid production which allows colonisation of the stomach with bacteria. The result of bacterial growth may be to convert dietary nitrates to nitrites which then react with amino acids in food to form N-nitroso compounds. These have been shown to be carcinogens in animals.

The typical tumour is a diffuse infiltrating carcinoma of variable size with a rolled edge and a central ulcer. It spreads through the gastric wall, invades lymph nodes, and metastasises to the liver via the bloodstream. It may also seed into the peritoneal cavity giving rise to abdominal and pelvic tumours and ascites. Less commonly, the tumour infiltrates diffusely through the stomach wall (linitis plastica or 'leather bottle stomach'). Microscopically, the carcinomas may resemble intestinal cells or may be diffusely infiltrating tumours. The 'intestinal' type of tumour has a

A
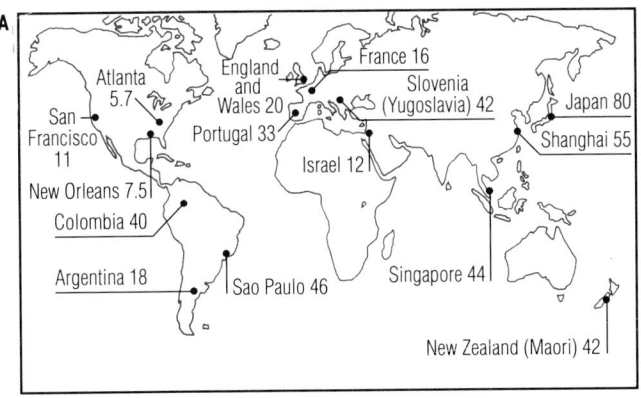

Fig. 16.16 Gastric adenocarcinoma: incidence and mortality. A. Worldwide incidence per 100 000. **B.** Gastric adenocarcinoma mortality related to social class. Figures are for men aged 15–64 in England and Wales in 1970–72 (OPCS data, 1978). Values for each social class are in proportion to 100 which represents all social classes combined. **C.** Age adjusted incidence of gastric carcinoma in England.

B

C
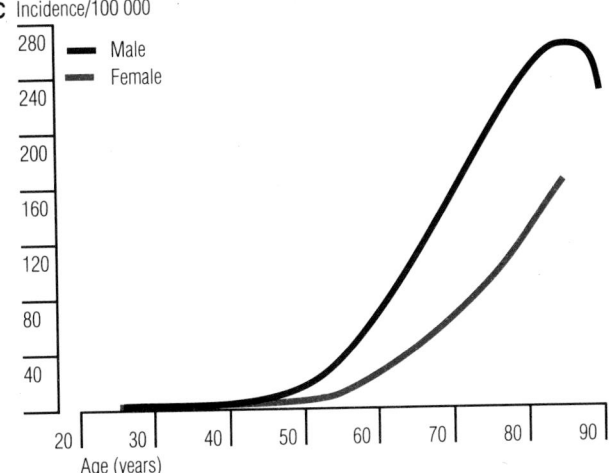

better prognosis and is more frequent in areas of high incidence such as Japan. In Japan, screening for gastric carcinoma has led to the detection of early stage tumours limited to the mucosa or submucosa; such tumours have a good prognosis.

Clinical features

Typically, the patient presents with anorexia, nausea and vague abdominal discomfort. Bleeding is common, leading to iron deficiency and, occasionally, frank haematemesis or melaena. There may be dysphagia if the tumour involves the gastro-oesophageal junction, and vomiting if there is outflow obstruction. Non-metastatic, paraneoplastic manifestations (p. 146) are unusual and include acanthosis nigricans (of which it is the commonest cause), venous thrombosis and dermatomyositis. Physical examination may reveal evidence of weight loss, anaemia and an epigastric mass. Enlarged lymph nodes may be palpable in the supraclavicular region.

Investigation

Diagnosis is usually made at endoscopy when an ulcer is found. It is safest to assume that every gastric ulcer is malignant until proved otherwise. Diffusely infiltrating tumours of the *linitis plastica* type may be more easily diagnosed on a barium meal, when the stomach appears contracted and non-distensible. On barium meal, the ulcerative neoplasms appear as an ulcer with irregular borders and disruption of the normal mucosal folds (Fig. 16.17). If there are no clinically evident metastases, and surgery is a possible treatment, it is essential to stage the tumour further. This will include chest X-ray, liver enzyme measurement and liver ultrasound. Tumour markers are not helpful in diagnosis or management.

Treatment

Surgical resection is the only curative treatment for adenocarcinoma and a total or partial gastrectomy is performed.

581

Fig. 16.17 Barium meal examination showing typical gastric carcinoma.

The prognosis is directly related to stage, being good (five year survival, 55%) when the tumour is confined to the mucosa or submucosa. Only 2.5% of tumours are in this category. If the tumour has spread through the stomach wall (but no further), the survival falls to 25%; and if the lymph nodes are involved few patients will survive five years. Overall, only 60% of patients undergoing surgery have resectable tumours and of these, only 20% will live five years.

In recent years, gastric carcinoma has been shown to respond occasionally to chemotherapy which may sometimes be helpful in palliating symptoms of metastatic disease. However, adjuvant chemotherapy has not yet improved the outlook after gastric resection. Radiotherapy may be helpful in palliation of symptoms resulting from local recurrence.

MALIGNANT TUMOURS OF THE STOMACH: GASTRIC LYMPHOMA

Although uncommon, gastric lymphoma is of interest because it remains localised for a considerable period. It typically presents with upper abdominal discomfort, nausea or gastrointestinal bleeding, and an ulcer is found endoscopically. The histological appearances may be misinterpreted as inflammatory infiltrate, and the diagnosis established only later when the disease is more florid. Gastric lymphoma is a tumour of B lymphocytes (centrocytes and centroblasts, see Ch. 25) and remains localised to the gastric mucosa for months or years before involving the lymph nodes.

Surgical resection may be curative in the early stages, but the prognosis with surgery alone is worse if local nodes are involved. These patients should receive combination chemotherapy following surgery.

BENIGN TUMOURS OF THE STOMACH

Gastric leiomyomas

Gastric leiomyomas are benign submucosal tumours which rarely become sarcomatous. They arise from the muscularis mucosae. The aetiology is unknown. In many patients they are asymptomatic but, in others, may present with non-specific features such as epigastric pain. The centre of the tumour often ulcerates and patients can present with haematemesis and melaena. In this situation, surgical resection is indicated.

Gastric polyps

Gastric polyps may also occur and should be biopsied endoscopically. Hyperplastic polyps are not known to be associated with specific symptoms, have no malignant potential and can therefore be ignored. Adenomatous polyps may be premalignant (although the malignant association is not as strong as with the adenomatous polyp-carcinoma sequence in the colon) and should be removed endoscopically or surgically. Adenomatous polyps are usually asymptomatic but can be associated with dyspepsia, gastrointestinal bleeding or pyloric obstruction.

THE SMALL INTESTINE

The small intestine is the prime site of nutrient digestion and absorption. It is also a site of water and electrolyte secretion and consequent marked fluid fluxes.

Clinical features of small bowel disease

The most common symptom of small intestinal disease is loose stools, which may be steatorrhoeic due to malabsorption of fat, or watery due to increased secretion or osmosis of water. Pain is usually colicky and a feature of obstruction. Malabsorption of folic acid, iron and vitamin B_{12} results in anaemia. Fat-soluble vitamin deficiency and hypokalaemia also occur. The faeces must be examined for colour, consistency and amount, and a sigmoidoscopy performed to exclude rectal disease.

Investigation of small bowel disease

The investigations of small bowel disease are listed in Summary 6.

Summary 6   Investigation of small bowel disease

Investigation of systemic effects

Haemoglobin and blood film
White cell count and ESR
Plasma proteins
Plasma urea and electrolytes
Plasma calcium, phosphate and alkaline phosphatase
Plasma liver function tests
Fat-soluble vitamin deficiency (vitamin A, K)
Faecal weight and fat content

Tests of small bowel function

Small bowel histology and biochemistry
Absorption tests
Triple lumen tube tests
Breath tests

Radiology

Small bowel enema
Barium follow-through
Arteriography

Radio-isotopes

Radiolabelled albumin for protein loss
Radiolabelled white cells for sites of inflammation
Radiolabelled red cells for sites of bleeding

Investigation of systemic effects

The haemoglobin and blood film assess haematinic deficiency and hyposplenism. A raised white cell count, C-reactive protein or ESR is a non-specific indicator of underlying inflammation. The albumin is measured to look for protein-losing enteropathy and nitrogen deficiency. The plasma urea and electrolytes are measured to assess renal function and hypokalaemia. A low plasma calcium usually indicates calcium deficiency which is due in part to malabsorption of vitamin D which is fat-soluble. This may be associated with low plasma 25-hydroxy and 1,25-dihydroxy vitamin D levels. As a consequence, there may be increased parathyroid hormone secretion (secondary hyperparathyroidism) resulting in hypophosphataemia and a rise in the plasma bone alkaline phosphatase. Abnormal liver function tests are associated with the hepatic complications of Crohn's disease. With steatorrhoea, malabsorption of the fat-soluble vitamins (A, D, E and K) may lead to a low plasma vitamin A and vitamin E, and the prothrombin time may be prolonged due to vitamin K deficiency. Water-soluble vitamin deficiencies are rare; thiamine can be assessed by the red cell transketolase level. The 24-hour faecal weight can be calculated on the mean of a three-day collection.

Tests of function

Many causes of malabsorption can be diagnosed by small bowel histology (p. 538). Until recently, this test was performed by passing a Crosby capsule to the duodenojejunal junction, but direct endoscopic biopsies from the second part of the duodenum are easier to perform. The biopsy material can be analysed for enzymes, such as lactase. Sugar (e.g. D-xylose) and fat absorption (e.g. radiolabelled palmitic or oleic acid) tests have been used but are of little help in making a precise diagnosis. The triple lumen tube tests involve passing a tube into the small bowel and infusing physiological solutions through the upper opening; the fluid is then aspirated from the distal orifice and the amount of water and electrolytes absorbed or secreted over a given length of bowel can be calculated. The hydrogen breath test is used to estimate oro-caecal transit time, as breath hydrogen rises when non-absorbable carbohydrates reach bacteria in the caecum. The ^{14}C-glycocholate breath test is used to assess bacterial deconjugation of bile acids.

Radiology

The small bowel is best outlined by placing a tube at the duodenojejunal junction and infusing dilute barium (a small bowel enema). If the patient cannot swallow the tube, barium may be taken orally and X-rays taken as it passes through the gut. Arteriography is used to assess ischaemia and demonstrate bleeding sites. The small bowel cannot be satisfactorily imaged by ultrasound or CAT scan techniques.

Radio-isotopes

Radiolabelled albumin is used to assess protein-losing enteropathy and radiolabelled (e.g. indium) white cells are used to indicate the site of active inflammation in patients with Crohn's disease. ^{51}Chromium labelled red cells can be used to indicate the site of small intestinal bleeding, if this is more than 1 ml blood per minute.

MALABSORPTION

A simple classification of small intestinal malabsorption is shown in Table 16.21. Osmotic diarrhoea occurs when the luminal contents are osmotically active and draw pathologically large amounts of water into the small bowel. Secretory diarrhoea occurs when small intestinal water and electrolyte secretion is increased and overcomes absorptive capacity. A number of drugs can cause malabsorption.

The most severe steatorrhoea (more than 100 g fat/24 h) is seen in patients with very short small intestines or in pancreatic exocrine failure. The amount of fat malabsorption in most patients with small intestinal malabsorption is less than 40 g/24 h. Steatorrhoea is minimal or absent in patients with both osmotic and secretory diarrhoea.

Large volumes of stool (more than 1 kg/24 h) are usually seen in patients with secretory diarrhoea, and occasionally in patients with osmotic diarrhoea and in those with substantially reduced lengths of functional small intestine.

Table 16.21   Classification of small intestinal malabsorption

Abnormality	Causes	Steatorrhoea	Watery stool	Other results
Upper small bowel disease	Coeliac disease Giardia etc.	+	+	Iron ↓ Folate ↓ Calcium ↓
Osmotic diarrhoea	Enzyme deficiencies Magnesium sulphate	−	+ +	
Secretory diarrhoea	Cholera VIP Phenolphthalein	−	+ + +	Dehydration Hypokalaemia
Rapid transit	Postgastrectomy Thyrotoxicosis	+	+	
Short gut	Surgery Fistula	+ +	+ +	
Lower small bowel disease	Crohn's disease Tuberculosis etc.	+	+	Vitamin B$_{12}$ ↓ Bile acids ↓
Drug-induced	Neomycin Cholestyramine Alcohol	+	±	

COELIAC DISEASE

Coeliac disease is also known as gluten-sensitive enteropathy and non-tropical sprue. The disorder results in abnormal small bowel mucosa, with loss of villi, crypt hyperplasia and infiltration with chronic inflammatory cells. The clinical syndrome and small bowel histology improve with removal of dietary gluten and return if gluten is eaten again.

Aetiology

The aetiology of coeliac disease became clear at the end of World War II when it was realised that Dutch coeliac children improved when wheat was unavailable (they subsisted on tulips and sugar-beet) but deteriorated when wheat was reintroduced into their diets. Wheat, rye and barley (but probably not oats) contain gluten. During milling, bran is separated from flour (Fig. 16.18). Gluten is contained in the water-insoluble portion of flour; the toxic moiety is present in an alcohol-soluble portion of gluten, known as gliadin. Digestion of gliadin with pepsin and trypsin results in smaller toxic subunits. The mode of gluten's toxicity is uncertain but there are three main hypotheses:

1. *Immunological.* The strong association of coeliac disease with the HLA B8-DRW3 haplotype links it with many of the autoimmune diseases (see p. 113) and suggests a possible immunological origin. This is consistent with the finding of a predominantly T lymphocyte infiltration of the mucosal lesions, and the local production of anti-gluten antibody. However, neither humoral nor cellular tests show any consistent changes to distinguish coeliac disease from other inflammatory bowel conditions or to suggest a mechanism for the damage. It has recently been shown that the α-gliadin molecule shares an amino acid sequence with type 12 adenovirus, suggesting that coeliac disease may represent an abnormal response to a common infectious agent.

2. *Peptidase deficiency.* It has been suggested that coeliac disease is due to a lack of an intestinal peptidase, leading to accumulation of gliadin and gluten which are directly toxic to small intestinal mucosal cells. However, the discordance of 30% among identical twins does not support such a simple enzymatic deficiency theory; if coeliac disease were solely a hereditary defect, both or neither identical twins would be expected to be affected in each case.

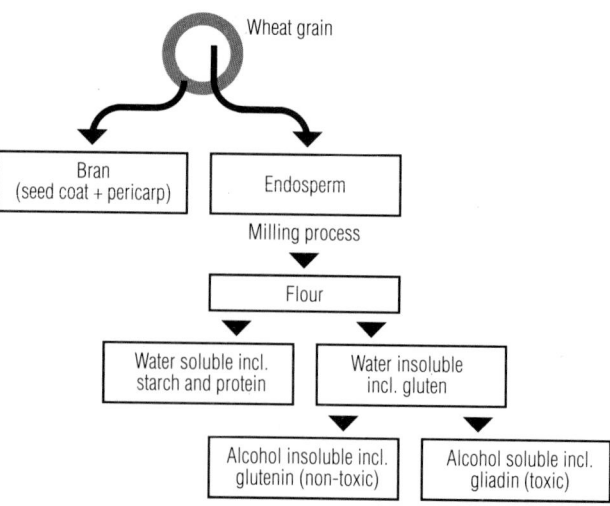

Fig. 16.18   The wheat grain as a source of gluten. The wheat germ has an inner endosperm which is the source of gluten and gliadin.

3. *Enterocyte membrane defect.* This hypothesis suggests that there is a defect in the glycoprotein structure of the brush border membrane which allows gluten to bind to it and cause cell damage and death.

The true prevalence of coeliac disease is unknown as this would involve performing small bowel biopsies on asymptomatic individuals who do not have haematological or biochemical abnormalities. The highest recorded incidence of coeliac disease is in the west of Ireland where it is one in 300. In the UK, the incidence is about one in 2000. The disease is unusual in Negroes and the Japanese. There is evidence that the incidence in children is falling in the UK and this may reflect the fact that most infant feeds are now gluten-free. There is a modest female preponderance. About 10% of asymptomatic first degree relatives have the disorder, but the mode of inheritance is unknown.

Clinical features

Coeliac disease can present at any age, but there are peaks between 1–5 years of age and in the third and fourth decades. Typically, the disease is now diagnosed in patients who are found to be iron or folate deficient when being investigated for rather non-specific symptoms. The extreme case of a cachectic, oedematous, clubbed, pigmented, dying patient with multiple vitamin deficiencies is now rare.

The main symptoms and signs are shown in Table 16.22. In children, the symptoms are often non-specific, with failure to thrive in infancy or growth retardation. Presentation in adolescence is unusual. Diarrhoea is more common in adults than children, where an accurate history of bowel habit may be difficult to obtain. Diarrhoea is not universal and coeliacs may, rarely, present with constipation. Abdominal pain is usually mild. About 30% of patients have aphthous ulcers which are usually severe and recurrent but respond to a gluten-free diet. Dermatitis herpetiformis is an itchy vesicular rash which is usually predominant on extensor surfaces such as the elbows and knees (p. 587).

Examination is often non-contributory, with mild anaemia, weight loss, and diarrhoea or steatorrhoea on rectal examination being the most common physical signs. Hypocalcaemia may develop relatively quickly, but bone tenderness and proximal myopathy imply longstanding hypocalcaemia with osteomalacia.

Investigations

Small bowel histology

The diagnosis is made by a characteristic small bowel biopsy which improves on gluten withdrawal. It is not reasonable to advocate a gluten-free diet without it. The villi may be totally or partially lost (total or partial villous atrophy, see Fig. 16.19). The duodenum and jejunum are predominantly affected but, in severe cases, villous abnor-

Table 16.22 Clinical manifestations of coeliac disease

Symptom/sign	Mechanism
History	
Non-specific, e.g. malaise, anorexia	Iron, folate or calcium deficiency
Diarrhoea and steatorrhoea	Water, electrolyte and fat malabsorption
Weight loss	Fat and carbohydrate malabsorption
Abdominal pain and bloating	Distended bowel loops
Aphthous ulcers	
Nausea and vomiting	
Itchy spots on extensor surfaces (dermatitis herpetiformis)	
Positive family history; Irish background	
Oedema	Hypoproteinaemia
Pigmentation	
Tetany	Vitamin D and calcium deficiency
Bone pains; muscle weakness	
Bleeding tendency	Vitamin K deficiency
Night blindness	Vitamin A deficiency
In children	
Failure to thrive	Malabsorption
Irritability	
Growth failure	
Delayed puberty	
Examination	
Anaemia	Iron and folate (and, rarely, vitamin B_{12}) deficiency
Weight loss	Malabsorption
Pigmentation	Unknown
Glossitis	Iron and folate deficiency
Angular cheilitis	
Aphthous ulcers	Unknown
Koilonychia	Iron deficiency
Clubbing	Unknown
Oedema	Hypoproteinaemia
Bruising	Vitamin K deficiency
Abdominal distension	Distended bowel loops
Positive Chvostek's and Trousseau's signs	Hypocalcaemia
Bone tenderness; proximal myopathy	Osteomalacia
Reduced light adaptation	Vitamin A deficiency

malities may also be seen in the ileum. Villous atrophy commonly results in nutrient malabsorption and the characteristic syndrome, but total villous atrophy can occur in an asymptomatic patient with normal blood tests.

Villous atrophy usually indicates coeliac disease. However, in the absence of a response to a gluten-free diet, conditions such as giardiasis, tropical sprue, malnutrition, small bowel ischaemia, severe skin disease, gastrinomas and malignancy elsewhere in the body must also be considered.

Gastrointestinal Disease

Fig. 16.19 Comparison of normal small bowel histology with that of a patient with coeliac disease. A. Photomicrograph of normal small intestinal finger-like villi with columnar surface cells. **B.** Photomicrograph of small bowel biopsy in a patient with coeliac disease. There is total villous atrophy with complete loss of the villi, cuboidal surface cells, crypt hyperplasia and an increased number of lymphocytes.

Haematology

The most common haematological abnormality is anaemia due to iron and/or folate deficiency as a consequence of malabsorption. Folate deficiency is most reliably characterised by a low red blood cell folate which reflects long-standing folate deficiency. Serum B_{12} levels are quite often low, often secondary to a defect in mucosal absorption as a result of folate deficiency. Hyposplenism is present in most patients, and Howell-Jolly bodies may be seen on the blood film. The ESR is raised in a minority of patients. Sideroblastic anaemia may occur due to vitamin B_6 deficiency. If there is severe malabsorption of vitamin K, the prothrombin time may be prolonged.

Biochemistry

Hypoalbuminaemia is relatively common and is due to protein loss from the small intestine and amino acid malabsorption. Faecal fat levels are usually raised. Hypocalcaemia due to malabsorption of calcium is common, with consequent secondary hyperparathyroidism. In chronic hypocalcaemia, the serum bone alkaline phosphatase rises. Some patients are vitamin D deficient and this is best demonstrated by a low serum 25-hydroxy vitamin D. Serum vitamin A and magnesium levels may also be low. Zinc deficiency is rare.

Absorption tests

The absorption tests are non-specific, reflecting a variety of upper small bowel diseases. Tritium-labelled fat can be used to assess fat absorption and these tests are less unpleasant for laboratory personnel than faecal fat estimation. Low molecular weight sugars such as glucose, xylose and rhamnose are malabsorbed as a consequence of mucosal damage; whereas the bowel is pathologically permeable to larger molecules, such as lactulose and ^{51}Cr-labelled EDTA.

Radiology

Small bowel radiology may show non-specific jejunal dilatation and flocculation of barium; its main value is in excluding anatomical abnormalities. Bone radiology may show signs of osteomalacia (bone thinning and pseudo-fractures) and secondary hyperparathyroidism (subperiosteal erosions; see Ch. 19).

Treatment

Treatment is with a strict gluten-free diet, avoiding flour from wheat, rye, barley and, occasionally, oats. This means the avoidance of most bread, cakes and biscuits as well as foods where flour has been used as a thickening agent (e.g. gravy). Rice and maize can be used as substitutes. In the UK, gluten-free foods can be obtained on prescription. Such a diet allows the small bowel mucosa to return almost to normal.

A strict diet is essential in children (to promote normal development), in patients with severe symptoms, and in women who have problems with fertility. It should also be encouraged in other young people as it improves general wellbeing and avoids deficiency states. It may also reduce the chance of malignancy developing in the small bowel. In the newly diagnosed elderly patient with minor symptoms, strict adherence to diet is less essential. In the UK, membership of the Coeliac Society should be encouraged.

Supplements of folic acid, iron, vitamin B_{12}, calcium, vitamin D etc. should be given to correct deficiency states. Most patients make a good response to the diet and nutritional supplements. Rarely, corticosteroids are indicated in patients who have a poor initial response to a gluten-free diet.

Children require frequent follow-up. Small bowel biopsies are repeated after 3–6 months of a gluten-free diet in children, and are also helpful in adults. Biopsy after a gluten challenge may be used to confirm the diagnosis. For adults stable on a gluten-free diet, an annual review is useful to check the patient's weight and exclude deficiency states.

Development of malignancy

There is an increased risk in coeliac disease of small intestinal lymphoma and adenocarcinoma. The former was originally termed 'malignant histiocytosis of the intestine' but is now thought to be a tumour of T lymphocytes. It is usually widespread throughout the small bowel and responds poorly to chemotherapy. There is also a higher incidence of some other malignancies, in particular squamous cell carcinomas of the oesophagus and pharynx.

DERMATITIS HERPETIFORMIS

Dermatitis herpetiformis is a blistering and pruritic skin eruption which particularly affects the extensor surface of the knees and elbows (p. 1134). The majority of patients have associated small intestinal villous atrophy and may also develop the other complications of coeliac disease. Histology of the skin lesions shows blister cavities, while immunofluorescence shows IgA deposits at and just below the dermo-epidermal junction (p. 1133, Fig. 26.13). Both the rash and intestinal lesion improve with gluten withdrawal. The rash is also helped by treatment with oral dapsone.

BACTERIAL OVERGROWTH

Aetiology

Under normal circumstances, the stomach and upper intestine have a low concentration of bacteria, due to gastric acid secretion and normal small bowel motility. Greater numbers of bacteria, intermediate in amount between the jejunum and the colon, are found in the ileum. Bacterial overgrowth of the upper small bowel is most commonly associated with jejunal diverticular disease (Fig. 16.20A), but other causes include reduced or absent gastric acid secretion, Polya gastrectomy, small bowel stasis (due to strictures, systemic sclerosis, diabetic neuropathy or adhesions) and fistulas from the small to the large bowel. Bacterial deconjugation and dehydroxylation of bile acids is thought to be the main mechanism of the steatorrhoea, but there is also some damage to the small intestinal mucosa.

Clinical features and investigation

Patients present with weight loss, anorexia, nausea, diarrhoea (but sometimes constipation) and increased flatulence. Steatorrhoea and B_{12} malabsorption (resulting in red cell macrocytosis) are the commonest laboratory abnormalities. Deficiencies of iron, protein and calcium may occur. The red cell folate levels can be high because of bacterial synthesis of folic acid.

The diagnosis can be confirmed by demonstrating increased numbers of bacteria in upper small bowel aspi-

rates. This is technically difficult, however, and instead the ^{14}C-glycocholate breath test is often used to demonstrate early deconjugation of bile acids by bacteria (Fig. 16.20B). The diagnosis is supported by finding a high fasting breath hydrogen. The many other tests devised include demonstrating increased deconjugated bile acids in small bowel aspirates, and increased urinary excretion of indoles and phenols synthesised by the bacteria. It is also important to

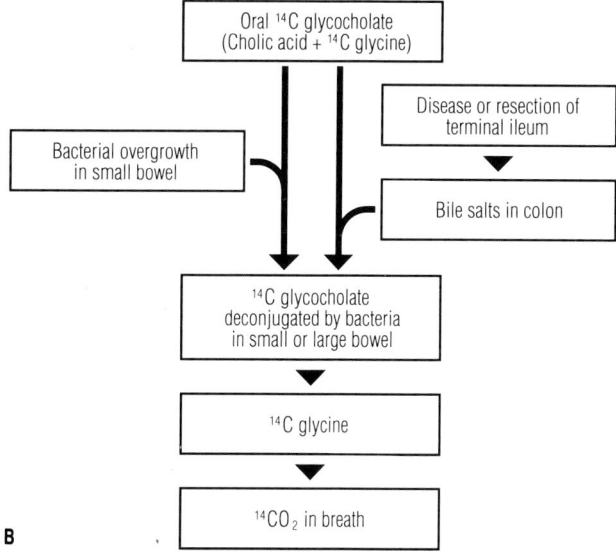

Fig. 16.20 Diagnostic findings in bacterial overgrowth. A. Small bowel enema showing multiple small bowel diverticula. **B.** In the normal ^{14}C glycocholate breath test, little $^{14}CO_2$ appears in the breath until 4–5 hours after ingestion. In the presence of small bowel bacterial overgrowth, there is early cleavage of glycine and thus an early peak of $^{14}CO_2$ at 1–2 hours.

demonstrate the cause of the overgrowth. This may be obvious from the history (such as a Polya gastrectomy) or may require a small bowel enema, e.g. to show diverticular disease, systemic sclerosis or fistula formation.

Treatment

The treatment of bacterial overgrowth is, if feasible, of the underlying cause, e.g. surgical correction of adhesions, fistulae and blind loops. Non-correctable upper small bowel abnormalities, such as multiple diverticula and scleroderma, have to be treated medically with broad-spectrum or anaerobe-directed antibiotics. Tetracycline, ampicillin, metronidazole and lincomycin may all be effective. There is a tendency for the problem to recur and, if one antibiotic is ineffective, another should be tried (there is little evidence that bacterial aspirate sensitivities help in the choice of antibiotics). Deficiencies, in particular that of vitamin B_{12}, should be corrected. In severe cases, there must be careful attention to nutrition with the avoidance of dietary fats and their substitution with mid-chain triglycerides.

GIARDIASIS

Giardia lamblia is a protozoon which colonises the bowel, especially the upper small intestine (p. 289).

Aetiology and pathology

Trophozoites are active in the bowel, and produce oval cysts which are passed in the faeces and are potentially infective. The organism is thought to produce its effects by adhering to the villi and blocking absorption, both by competing for nutrients and by direct mucosal damage (including partial villous atrophy). The parasites adhere to enterocyte surface glycoproteins and, when they move to another site, the glycoproteins are avulsed and membrane function reduced. Infection is transmitted by the faeco-oral route from contaminated water as well as by person-to-person transmission in male homosexuals and the mentally handicapped. Hypogammaglobulinaemia and reduced gastric acid secretion both increase host susceptibility.

The incidence is particularly high in Eastern Europe, the USSR, and parts of Africa and Asia, where up to 20% of stools may be positive. As duodenal aspirates give a higher yield of positive results, the true incidence may be yet higher. The organism can be removed by sand-filtering water supplies.

Clinical features and investigation

The majority of patients with giardia are asymptomatic. Most symptomatic patients present acutely with diarrhoea, abdominal pain and distension and malaise; in many cases, the symptoms settle spontaneously in a few weeks without treatment. Patients may also present with chronic malabsorption, with steatorrhoea, weight loss, abdominal pain, anaemia and (in children) failure to thrive and grow. Investigations may show steatorrhoea, anaemia due to vitamin

B_{12} and folic acid deficiency, and xylose malabsorption.

Diagnosis is by identifying cysts in the stool, or trophozoites in duodenal aspirates or on small bowel biopsies.

Treatment

Effective treatment is metronidazole (400 mg tds) for 3–7 days to eradicate the organism. As this drug has a disulfiram effect, alcohol must be avoided. It should also be avoided in the first trimester of pregnancy because of its potential mutagenic effect. If patients develop side-effects such as anorexia or vomiting, the dose should be reduced and the duration of treatment prolonged. Alternative drugs are tinidazole, which can be given as a single dose, and mepacrine.

TROPICAL SPRUE

Tropical sprue is a chronic malabsorption syndrome which occurs only in patients who live, or have lived, in the tropics (in particular, the Middle and Far East, and the Caribbean). The aetiology is unknown, although toxin-forming coliform bacteria have been implicated in some patients. Tropical sprue results in upper intestinal villous atrophy similar to that seen in coeliac disease.

Clinical features, investigation and treatment

Symptoms include diarrhoea, steatorrhoea, weight loss and abdominal distension, and also those of nutritional deficiency and of hypoproteinaemia.

The diagnosis is made on the basis of the history, particularly foreign travel; the presence of vitamin deficiencies; evidence of malabsorption of fat, vitamin B_{12} and xylose; and a small bowel biopsy showing villous atrophy.

Many patients are cured by a one-month course of oxytetracyline with folic acid and vitamin B_{12} supplements; any other deficiencies should be treated as necessary. The diarrhoea may be treated symptomatically with codeine phosphate or loperamide. There is a tendency to spontaneous remissions and relapses. Untreated patients may die of chronic malnutrition, or secondary infections such as tuberculosis.

WHIPPLE'S DISEASE

Whipple's disease is a rare disease characterised by large, foamy periodic acid Schiff (PAS)-positive macrophages, containing glycoprotein within the lamina propria. The overlying villi are distorted and upper small bowel radiology shows thickened and oedematous mucosa. The patients are often iron or folate deficient. Whipple's disease is thought to be due to a bacterial infection, as rods are often seen in affected tissue; the precise organism is, however, unknown.

Clinical features, investigation and treatment

The disease usually affects middle-aged men. Early symptoms are arthritis, fever, malaise, recurrent cough, pleuritic chest pain and lymphadenopathy. Intestinal symptoms such as diarrhoea, steatorrhoea, weight loss and abdominal pain occur 1–10 years later. Small bowel biopsy is diagnostic even before intestinal symptoms develop. Associated features are nail-clubbing, cutaneous pigmentation, cardiac complications (such as pericarditis, myocarditis and left-sided valvular lesions) and central nervous system complications, such as depression, dementia and fits.

Broad-spectrum antibiotics are rapidly effective in abolishing all the problems and are life-saving. It is generally suggested that intramuscular penicillin and streptomycin are used for two weeks and then replaced by tetracycline continued for one year. About 30% of patients subsequently relapse, and so long-term follow-up is recommended.

LYMPHANGIECTASIA

Lymphangiectasia is a rare idiopathic condition of children and young adults, associated with dilated lacteals in the villi due to hypoplasia of the lymphatics. It may also be acquired as a result of intra-abdominal malignancy or constrictive pericarditis.

Clinical features, investigation and treatment

The most common symptom is peripheral oedema secondary to hypoproteinaemia; this is due to a protein-losing enteropathy. Diarrhoea, steatorrhoea, abdominal pain, hypocalcaemia and growth retardation occur. Protein loss leads to an immune-deficiency state which predisposes to infection.

Diagnosis is by small bowel biopsy which shows dilated lymphatics throughout the villi. A small bowel enema shows large intestinal folds, mucosal nodularity and contrast flocculation.

The idiopathic variant should be treated with a low fat diet and possibly substitution of dietary fat by mid-chain triglycerides. Occasionally, only a small segment of bowel is involved and this can be excised. Pericardectomy may result in complete resolution of the syndrome if constrictive pericarditis is the problem.

ABETALIPOPROTEINAEMIA

Abetalipoproteinaemia is a rare disorder, inherited as an autosomal recessive and usually presenting in childhood. Plasma betalipoproteins are absent and plasma cholesterol, triglycerides and phospholipid are low. The defect appears to be a failure of synthesis of apoprotein B, with defective transport of triglyceride from the liver and gut (p. 778). The red cells show spiked acanthocytes. The patients initially have mild diarrhoea and steatorrhoea but, by 20 years of age, most have developed progressive neurological deficits with peripheral neuropathy and cerebellar ataxia. A small bowel biopsy shows cytoplasmic fatty vacuolation of the enterocytes at the apex of the villi.

No treatment is known to affect the underlying problem but a low fat diet is usually given and deficiencies of fat-soluble vitamin deficiencies are corrected.

SYSTEMIC SCLEROSIS

Systemic sclerosis (p. 1020) may affect the small bowel as well as the oesophagus. It is associated with poor motility, duodenal dilatation, and a distended jejunum with prominent folds. Full thickness histology shows submucosal collagen and muscle atrophy. Bacterial overgrowth often occurs. Symptoms include weight loss, nausea, abdominal distension, diarrhoea and constipation (if there is colonic involvement).

Treatment is of the nutritional deficiencies and bacterial overgrowth with antibiotics. No treatment has been found to influence the underlying gastrointestinal process.

RADIATION ENTERITIS

Radiation enteritis usually occurs in the small intestine in patients who have undergone radiation treatment for gynaecological, bladder and rectal carcinomas, and for retroperitoneal tumours. In the early phases of treatment, there is cell necrosis and shortening of the villi; with increasing dose, polymorphs become prominent. Oedema, collagen formation and telangiectatic blood vessels develop as long-term sequelae.

During treatment, patients develop anorexia, nausea and diarrhoea; this usually settles when treatment stops. Chronic complications are unusual, but include diarrhoea, steatorrhoea, intestinal obstruction from stricture formation, intestinal ulceration with haemorrhage or perforation, bleeding from telangiectatic vessels, fistula formation or infarction.

Medical treatment of the chronic diarrhoea is unsatisfactory, but attention to diet, cholestyramine, corticosteroids and broad-spectrum antibiotics may help. Some patients require surgery for strictures and, in severe acute cases, parenteral nutrition may be necessary.

OSMOTIC DIARRHOEA

The two major causes of osmotic diarrhoea are enzyme deficiencies and purgative abuse.

Enzyme deficiencies

The commonest cause of osmotic diarrhoea is an acquired deficiency of the brush border membrane enzyme, lactase. This means that lactose is not split into its constituent monosaccharides, galactose and glucose, and so becomes osmotically active.

Clinical features

An oral load of dairy products (which are rich in lactose) results in loose stools, abdominal distension, borborygmi, colic and increased rectal flatus. The distension and flatus are due to colonic bacterial digestion of lactose.

Most Negroes and Asians have primary hypolactasia and may suffer diarrhoea, bloating and flatulence if they eat lactose. The incidence of primary alactasia in the Caucasian population in Europe and North America is up to 20% (about 6% in the UK). Secondary hypolactasia may also occur as a result of small bowel diseases (such as coeliac disease and Crohn's disease), in patients with ulcerative colitis, and during and after bowel infections. Patients with secondary hypolactasia also have reduced levels of other disaccharidases, such as maltase and sucrase, but these deficiencies rarely produce symptoms.

Investigation

In many patients, where the symptoms occur following an acute infection, it is unnecessary to make a definitive diagnosis. If definitive diagnosis is necessary, the best test is to measure lactase activity in a small bowel biopsy specimen. Measurement of the rise of blood glucose after oral lactose correlates poorly with mucosal lactase levels. However, bacterial breakdown of unabsorbed lactose in the colon results in abnormally high hydrogen excretion in the breath, so that measurement of exhaled hydrogen is a more reliable index of lactase deficiency.

Treatment

Treatment is by elimination of lactose from the diet. An underlying cause should be sought if symptoms persist. The majority of patients with secondary hypolactasia can resume lactose some weeks after treatment.

Sucrase-isomaltase deficiency is a rare enzyme deficiency which results in diarrhoea as soon as sucrose is introduced into the diet in infancy. It responds to elimination of sucrose, and tolerance may improve later in life. Very rarely, the small intestinal glucose and galactose transport system itself is ineffective; this results in an infant with watery motions and glucose in the faeces. Treatment is by avoidance of glucose- and galactose-containing foods.

Purgative abuse

The laxatives magnesium sulphate, magnesium hydroxide, magnesium carbonate and lactulose act by osmosis. Magnesium salts may be used for bowel preparation for surgery and colonoscopy, while lactulose (a synthetic disaccharide) is used for mild constipation and portosystemic encephalopathy. Patients may secretly take these drugs in excess (see also p. 613) to produce watery diarroea of unknown cause, but a diagnosis can be made by finding high faecal magnesium levels for the magnesium salts, and a low faecal pH for lactulose.

SECRETORY DIARRHOEA

Under normal circumstances, there is a daily flux of about eight litres of water and electrolytes across the small intestinal mucosa, but only about 1000 ml of this passes through the ileocaecal valve.

Secretory diarrhoea is due to absorption being exceeded by active secretion, leading to profuse watery diarrhoea, often more than 1 kg per 24 hours. In the Western World,

---

> **Summary 7   Causes of secretory diarrhoea**
> - Infection – e.g. cholera
> - Purgative abuse
> - Hormonal – VIPoma
>   – Carcinoid syndrome
>   – Medullary carcinoma of the thyroid
>   – Gastrinoma

secretory diarrhoea is usually due to a vasoactive intestinal polypeptide (VIP)-secreting tumour (p. 620) or laxative abuse, especially phenolphthalein (p. 613). The enterotoxin of *Vibrio cholerae* (cholera) is also an important cause. Secretory diarrhoea may also occur with the carcinoid syndrome associated with small intestinal primary tumours, medullary carcinoma of the thyroid, and gastrinomas (Summary 7). The clinical features and management of cholera are discussed in Chapter 12, page 275.

Investigation

Confirmation of excess secretion can best be obtained by placing a triple lumen tube in the small intestine, and measuring the absorptive and secretory response to various physiological solutions over a defined segment. Normally, there is water and electrolyte absorption but, under these circumstances, the solutions are further diluted by active intestinal secretion of water and electrolytes.

DIARRHOEA DUE TO RAPID TRANSIT

Diarrhoea due to rapid transit may be caused by rapid gastric emptying due to previous gastric surgery, which results in intestinal hurry, mild steatorrhoea and reactive hypoglycaemia (p. 579). Thyrotoxicosis also causes rapid small intestinal transit, and may be associated with mild diarrhoea and steatorrhoea.

In addition, rapid transit may occur as a result of fistulas which are due to Crohn's disease, peptic ulcers or carcinomas. These may be gastro-colic, entero-enteric or entero-colic. The diagnosis of such fistulas is by barium meal, small bowel enema or barium enema.

Corrective surgery is usually needed, but gastro-colic fistulas due to peptic ulceration may respond to H_2-receptor antagonists, and Crohn's fistulas to parenteral nutrition.

SHORT GUT

Diarrhoea and malabsorption may follow small intestinal resection. This is most commonly due to Crohn's disease, ischaemia due to superior mesenteric artery infarction or radiation damage. The greatest problems with water and electrolyte handling occur with loss of the duodenum or upper small intestine.

Some patients can be managed by regular small meals, and isotonic glucose and electrolyte solutions. If the patient continues to produce several litres of stool daily and to lose weight, long-term total parenteral nutrition must be considered.

LOWER SMALL BOWEL DISEASE

The terminal ileum is the primary site of absorption of vitamin B_{12} and bile acids and is part of the enterohepatic circulation (Ch. 17).

The commonest cause of terminal ileal disease in the Western World is Crohn's disease, while in parts of Asia it is tuberculosis. Rare causes include tumours and radiation damage. All of these lesions may require surgical resection which unfortunately perpetuates the problems of malabsorption.

Clinical features

B_{12} deficiency due to ileal disease is unresponsive to intrinsic factor in the Schilling test (Ch. 25, p. 1046). If there is malabsorption of bile acids, the following complications may arise:

1. *Diarrhoea.* Excess bile acids in the intestinal lumen reduce the colonic absorption of water and electrolytes, and may induce net secretion.
2. *Depletion of the bile acid pool.* This can result in small intestinal fat malaborption and an increase in the cholesterol:bile acid ratio in the bile. Bile supersaturated with cholesterol increases the incidence of gallstones.
3. *Oxalate renal stones.* The increased intracolonic bile acid concentration results in increased absorption of oxalic acid; this is excreted by the kidneys and may result in oxalate renal stones.

Treatment

Treatment is firstly of the causative disease process. Vitamin B_{12} deficiency is treated with an intramuscular loading dose of 1 mg daily for five days; thereafter, 1 mg at three-monthly intervals is adequate. Cholestyramine is an anion exchange resin which can alleviate bile acid-induced diarrhoea by binding bile acids and reducing intracolonic free bile acid concentrations. Unfortunately, this often fails to cure the diarrhoea and results in further depletion of the bile acid pool, and hence a greater tendency to cholelithiasis. Gallstones should be treated surgically. Hyperoxaluria should be treated with a low oxalate diet which includes avoiding fruits such as strawberries; surgical treatment may be necessary for renal stones.

DRUG-INDUCED MALABSORPTION

Numerous drugs have been implicated (Table 16.23); the effects are all dose-related and reversible.

Cholestyramine has few side effects when used in hyperlipidaemic patients but, in patients with biliary disease (when there are reduced bile acids) and in patients with terminal ileal disease with a reduced bile acid pool size, fat malabsorption and cholesterol gallstones may result. These

Table 16.23 Examples of drugs causing malabsorption

Drug	Mechanism of action	Results
Cholestyramine	Binds bile acids	Steatorrhoea Gallstones Malabsorption of fat-soluble vitamins
Colchicine and cytotoxic drugs	Arrest enterocyte mitosis	Steatorrhoea
Neomycin	Causes partial villous atrophy and enzyme inhibition	Steatorrhoea Iron, vitamin B_{12} and glucose malabsorption
Methyldopa	Causes partial villous atrophy	Steatorrhoea
Ferrous sulphate	Binds with tetracycline	Malabsorption of both drugs
Ethanol	Damage to enterocyte subcellular organelles	Folate deficiency and steatorrhoea

patients are already at risk of fat-soluble vitamin malabsorption, and this may be aggravated by the drug binding more of these vitamins.

High doses of colchicine, taken for acute gout, may cause steatorrhoea. It is also common for patients on combination cytotoxic chemotherapy regimes to develop diarrhoea and mild steatorrhoea; this may be further aggravated by the use of broad-spectrum antibiotics during periods of neutropenia.

Neomycin, para-aminosalicylic acid and methyldopa cause partial villous atrophy and their longstanding use can result in nutrient malabsorption, particularly of fats.

Drugs may interact within the gut. Ferrous sulphate binds to tetracycline and both are then malabsorbed. Cholestyramine binds acidic drugs such as digoxin, warfarin and penicillin. Broad-spectrum antibiotics are sometimes associated with increased plasma digoxin levels; this is thought to be due to the loss of bacteria which were previously metabolising some of the digoxin.

Ethanol probably affects the small intestine directly both by damaging subcellular organelles, and by causing leaky enterocyte membranes. Malabsorption of fat, folic acid, vitamin B_{12}, fat-soluble vitamins and carbohydrates may all occur.

SMALL BOWEL ISCHAEMIA

Aetiology

Aetiological factors in small intestinal ischaemia are shown in Table 16.24; experimentally, venous occlusion can cause infarction but it is not known whether this is the case in man.

Clinical features and treatment

Small bowel ischaemia may present acutely, with gut infarction following occlusion of the coeliac and superior

16

Table 16.24 Aetiology of small bowel ischaemia

- Arterial atheroma
- Arterial thrombosis
- Arterial emboli (usually from the heart)
- Vasculitis due to collagen disorders
- External compression of arteries (e.g. tumours, aneurysms)
- ? Venous thrombosis

mesenteric arteries, or chronically, with postprandial pain and weight loss.

Acute ischaemia

Acute ischaemia presents with pain, diarrhoea, vomiting and an acute abdomen. The patient should be resuscitated with fluids and treated with antibiotics and urgent laparotomy performed. At operation, an attempt is made to restore patency to embolised or thrombosed major arteries and all non-viable bowel is resected. The mortality is high and, if a large proportion of the upper jejunum and/or duodenum is removed, the patient has severe malabsorption, often with profuse diarrhoea. Such patients may require long-term total parenteral nutrition.

Chronic ischaemia

Chronic ischaemia is usually due to atheroma and, if undiagnosed, may progress to acute ischaemia. The patient is usually middle-aged or elderly and complains of colicky abdominal pain after eating ('intestinal angina'). This may be relieved by analgesics or vasodilating drugs (e.g. trinitrin). Weight loss follows, mainly due to a fear of eating, but malabsorption may also occur. Examination is relatively unhelpful; an abdominal arterial bruit may be heard in normal people and is thus a non-specific finding. There may be other evidence of arteriopathy. Investigation is by arteriography which may show a localised narrowing at the origin of a major artery off the aorta. Reconstruction of stenoses can help some patients.

SMALL BOWEL TUMOURS

Despite its long length, the small intestine is the site of less than 1% of all malignant tumours and less than 5% of

gastrointestinal neoplasms. Malignant tumours occur more frequently in the duodenum and jejunum, and benign lesions, such as leiomyomas and adenomas, in the jejunum. Small bowel malignancy is more common in patients with Crohn's disease and Gardner's syndrome (p. 596). The commonest tumours are adenocarcinomas (50%), carcinoid tumours (30%), lymphomas (15%) and sarcomas (5%).

Adenocarcinomas

Aetiology and pathology

The tumours usually occur in the upper small bowel and are more common in patients with coeliac disease, Crohn's disease and dermatitis herpetiformis. Histologically, these are mucus-secreting adenocarcinomas which present as ulcerating obstructing neoplasms. They metastasise to regional lymph nodes and the liver.

Clinical features and investigation

Patients usually present with abdominal pain, and intussusception may occur causing acute obstruction. Chronic blood loss is frequent and there may be melaena. The diagnosis can sometimes be made by small bowel enema and, occasionally, endoscopically (if in the duodenum) or by colonoscopy (if in the terminal ileum).

Treatment

Surgical excision is the treatment of choice but only 70% are resectable. In the duodenum, pancreatico-duodenectomy may be necessary, with hemicolectomy for terminal ileal lesions. The regional lymph nodes are resected where possible. Metastatic lesions respond poorly to cytotoxic chemotherapy.

Carcinoid tumours

Gut carcinoid tumours are rare; their behaviour is to some extent dependent on the part of the gut from which they are embryologically derived (Table 16.25). Histology shows sheets of neuroendocrine cells which are usually of low-grade malignancy. Immunocytochemistry shows positive silver staining for amines, and mid-gut tumours are often also positive for gut regulatory peptides such as neuro-

Table 16.25 Clinical features of gut carcinoids according to embryological origin

Embryological origin	Usual primary site	Principal active substance	Diagnosis	Specific treatment
Foregut	Stomach	Histamine	Raised urinary 5-HIAA	Surgery H_1- and H_2-receptor antagonists
Mid-gut	Terminal ileum	5-hydroxytryptamine	Raised urinary 5-HIAA	Surgery Cyproheptadine, methysergide and somatostatin
Hind-gut	Colon and rectum	None	Histology	Surgery only

tensin. Foregut tumours usually originate in the stomach and predominantly secrete histamine. Appendiceal carcinoid tumours are commonly found in appendicectomy specimens but do not metastasise or cause clinical problems. Terminal ileal carcinoids are those most likely to metastasise. They cause the *carcinoid syndrome* and predominantly secrete 5-hydroxytryptamine. Hind-gut tumours do not produce the syndrome and behave similarly to colonic adenocarcinomas.

Carcinoid syndrome

Aetiology

The carcinoid syndrome only occurs when the liver is bypassed and cannot metabolise tumour products. Symptoms thus arise when there are hepatic metastases which drain direct into the hepatic vein. Symptoms can also be seen in the absence of hepatic metastases with primary pulmonary, testicular and ovarian tumours whose venous drainage is directly into the systemic circulation.

Clinical features

The most characteristic symptom of the carcinoid syndrome is a flush, usually of the face and upper trunk. Provoking agents include stress (via noradrenaline), alcohol and food (possibly via gastrin). Other symptoms include secretory diarrhoea, weight loss, wheezing dyspnoea, pellagra and right hypochondrial pain. This is due to the marked hepatomegaly which is usually the main clinical sign. Other signs include a flushed (often cyanosed) face and signs of fibrotic right heart valves (giving both stenosis and regurgitation).

Mid-gut carcinoid tumours produce large amounts of 5-hydroxytryptamine (5-HT, serotonin; see Table 16.26). This substance is thought to play a part in the pathogenesis of carcinoid syndrome symptoms such as flushing and diarrhoea. Foregut tumours may secrete histamine and this produces a pink, weal-like flush which may itch and migrate. Metabolically active tumours may also produce other substances, e.g. enteroglucagon and neurotensin, but their role is uncertain. Pellagra due to nicotinic acid

deficiency (resulting from tryptophan consumption by the tumour) may occur. The cause of the right-sided cardiac fibrosis is unknown, but serotonin has been suggested as a possibility.

Investigation

Functioning carcinoid tumours can be diagnosed by demonstrating raised 24-hour urinary 5-HIAA levels or by whole blood 5-HT. The majority of 5-HT is bound to platelets and plasma levels are thus unhelpful. False positive results may be obtained by eating bananas, pineapples and walnuts, and false negative results by phenothiazines. If the diagnosis is confirmed by urine 5-HIAA, but no liver metastases are demonstrable, a bronchial carcinoid should be suspected.

Treatment

Surgical removal of primary tumours may be helpful, but is rarely so in patients with terminal ileal tumours, where the primaries are usually small and multiple. Symptoms of the carcinoid syndrome may be controlled by 5-HT antagonists such as cyproheptadine. Methysergide is also a 5-HT antagonist, but has the disadvantage of causing retroperitoneal fibrosis. The symptoms of histamine-producing gastric carcinoids can be blocked by a combination of H_1- and H_2-receptor antagonists. Somatostatin or its analogues prevents flushing and diarrhoea, presumably by inhibiting the release of provoking agents from carcinoid cells. Diarrhoea may be helped by simple agents such as loperamide and codeine phosphate. Pellagra responds to large doses of nicotinamide. There is no definite role for cytotoxic drugs or radiotherapy, but hepatic arterial catheterisation and embolisation or surgical tumour debulking may help. In a carcinoid crisis, when the flushing is so severe that arterial hypotension develops, corticosteroids and plasma volume expansion may be necessary.

Lymphomas

Lymphomas are the commonest gut tumours in children and a common small bowel tumour in adults.

Aetiology

In the West, most cases arise without any predisposing cause, but coeliac disease may be complicated by a diffuse ulcerating lymphoma. In the Middle East, an immune proliferative disease of the small intestine, of unknown aetiology, frequently develops into a non-Hodgkin's lymphoma of B lymphocytes, which secretes free α heavy chains (α-chain disease).

Most cases in the West are of non-Hodgkin's lymphoma and are B cell in origin. The histology usually shows diffuse infiltration of the bowel wall; nodular forms are rare. The lower small bowel is involved most frequently. The disease spreads early to involve local nodes but distant dissemination is late.

Table 16.26 Biochemical pathway for the synthesis and degradation of 5-hydroxytryptamine

Tryptophan
↓
5-hydroxytryptophan
↓
5-hydroxytryptamine (5-HT, serotonin)
↓
5-hydroxyindole acetaldehyde
↓
5-hydroxyindole acetic acid* (5-HIAA)

*24-hour urinary 5-HIAA levels are raised in mid-gut and foregut carcinoids.

16

Clinical features

The presentation is with subacute intestinal obstruction with pain and vomiting. Bleeding may occur and is usually chronic. Perforation is not unusual and is often above the site of the tumour. When extensive, the disease may present as a fever of unknown origin.

Treatment

The most important aspect of treatment is surgical resection of the tumour. Further treatment is not required if there is no evidence of spread, but involvement of nodes or distant spread are indications for intensive combination chemotherapy. In childhood, the risk of CNS involvement is small (this is in contrast to other childhood lymphomas).

The prognosis of localised resected gut lymphoma is good, with over 60% of patients alive at five years. It is not yet clear what impact modern chemotherapy will have on survival in more advanced cases. Malignant lymphoma complicating coeliac disease has a poor prognosis.

COLORECTAL DISEASE

The colon and rectum act to reduce up to 1500 ml of fluid material per day passing through the ileocaecal valve to a formed stool of 50–200 g. Important symptoms of colorectal disease are constipation, diarrhoea, blood per rectum, tenesmus, colicky abdominal pain and the symptoms of iron deficiency anaemia. Important signs are abdominal masses and abnormalities on rectal examination. Radiologically, the rectum and colon can be visualised by the plain abdominal X-ray and double contrast barium enema. Endoscopically, the rigid sigmoidoscope, flexible fibre-optic sigmoidoscope and flexible fibre-optic colonoscope are used to view the mucosa directly and to take biopsies.

CONSTIPATION

The normal person opens his bowels with a frequency of from two to three times a day to once every two to three days. The normal daily stool weight in the West is 50–200 g, but 500 g is more usual in countries where a much higher fibre intake is consumed. Constipation can be considered to be present when a patient defaecates twice a week or less. Faecal consistency is also a component in the patient's awareness of constipation. Many patients complain of constipation but, when a careful history is taken, do not fulfil these criteria. Nevertheless, the complaint of constipation is extremely common in the Western World, and vast quantities of laxatives are purchased annually to treat the symptoms.

Aetiology and diagnosis

Some of the many causes of constipation are listed in Table 16.27. Simple constipation is a diagnosis of exclusion where

594

Table 16.27 Causes of constipation

Simple constipation	**Drugs**
	Anticholinergics
Colonic obstruction	Antidepressants
Tumours	Anticonvulsants
Encarceration in hernias	Antacids (aluminium and calcium
Volvulus	salts)
Diverticular disease	Diuretics
	Analgesics
Abnormal muscle function	Iron
Old age	
Irritable bowel syndrome	**Metabolic and endocrine problems**
Crohn's and ulcerative colitis	Diabetes
Ischaemic colitis	Hypothyroidism
Systemic sclerosis	Hypercalcaemia
	Pregnancy
Anorectal problems	Chronic renal failure
Ulcerative proctitis	Hypokalaemia
Anal fissure	Porphyria
Thrombosed haemorrhoid	Lead poisoning
Neuro-psychiatric disorders	
Depression	
Spinal cord injury	
Cauda equina lesions	
Hirschsprung's disease	
Multiple sclerosis	
Parkinson's disease	
Some cerebral tumours and cerebrovascular accidents	

no other cause than a low fibre diet is present. It is common in women and, in young women in good health on a low fibre diet, it is usually not necessary to search further. Constipation is common in old age, when impaired colonic muscle function may contribute to the problem. Anorectal problems are associated with constipation because the patients delay defaecating to avoid pain. Inflammatory proctitis may result in faecal loading proximal to the inflamed mucosa (this is best seen on plain abdominal X-ray); the patient usually complains of passing small amounts of faeces frequently. Hypothyroidism, hypopituitarism and hypercalcaemia may have constipation as one of their earliest features. A careful drug history should be taken. Peripheral and central nervous system diseases (apart from Hirschsprung's, which usually presents in early childhood), commonly have obvious manifestations before constipation develops. Constipation may be the presenting symptom of depression.

Treatment

Wherever possible, the treatment of constipation is of the underlying cause. In simple constipation and in other situations where a low residue diet is being consumed, a high fibre diet should be recommended. Diet sheets can be useful, as can the help of a dietician (Table 16.28). Bran is the best source of fibre as it absorbs a large amount of water and allows the passage of larger amounts of soft stool. Beans, dried fruits, some nuts and pasta also contain large

Table 16.28 Dietary fibre content of foods

Fibre content	g fibre/100 g food
High (more than 10g/100 g food)	
Bran	44.0
Partially purified bran	26.7
Haricot and kidney beans	25.0
Dried apricots	24.0
Desiccated coconut	23.5
Almonds	14.3
Potato crisps	11.9
Lentils	11.7
Spaghetti, macaroni, lasagne	10.0
Medium (5–10 g/100 g food)	
Wholemeal bread	8.5
Peas	7.8
Peanuts	7.6
Raspberries	7.4
Muesli	7.4
Sultanas	7.0
Chestnuts	6.8
Spinach	6.0
Low (below 5 g/100 g food)	
Cornflakes	3.0
White bread	2.7
Boiled potato	2.4
White rice	2.4
Cauliflower	1.8
Lettuce	1.5
Jam	1.1
Grapes	0.9

amounts of fibre, and fruit and vegetables contain non-absorbable polysaccharides, such as cellulose and pectins, which are also useful. Pharmacological preparations of agents such as methylcellulose, isphaghula husk, sterculia and, possibly, guar are helpful if patients cannot remedy the situation by diet alone. The osmotically active disaccharide lactulose can be used as a mild laxative. If possible, the stimulant laxatives which increase intestinal motility (e.g. senna, cascara, castor oil, bisacodyl and danthron) should be avoided, as it is thought they can cause ganglion degeneration and an acquired megacolon, thus perpetuating constipation. Stimulant laxatives also tend to cause abdominal colic and hypokalaemia. Faecal softeners (e.g. liquid paraffin and dioctyl sodium sulphosuccinate) have a short-term role in softening stool in the presence of anal disease. Regular use should be avoided, however, as this tends to cause incontinence and lead to pruritus ani; on rare occasions, they cause lipoid pneumonia and malabsorption of fat-soluble vitamins.

NEUROPATHIC COLON

Neuropathic colon occurs as a result of a loss of Auerbach's and Meissner's plexuses along with the associated intrinsic neurones. This results in failure of colonic motility and constipation.

Hirschsprung's disease

The most common cause is Hirschsprung's disease, which usually presents in early childhood but has been reported in patients up to the age of 70. Constipation and abdominal distension are the most usual symptoms. Barium enema shows a narrow aganglionic segment with grossly dilated proximal colon. The diagnosis can be confirmed by demonstrating lack of ganglia and neurones and high acetylcholinesterase activities in rectal biopsies. Treatment is by surgical resection.

Chagas' disease

Chagas' disease is endemic in South America and is due to infection with the protozoon, *Trypanosoma cruzi* (p. 304). Chronic myocarditis, megaoesophagus and megacolon are late symptoms of the disease. Destruction of the ganglia produces a dilated and atonic colon. Treatment is with bulking agents and laxatives but, occasionally, panproctocolectomy and ileostomy may be necessary.

Other causes

Other cases of ganglionic destruction sometimes occur where the aetiology is uncertain. The possible role of irritant laxatives, senna in particular, is controversial. Treatment is usually medical as for Chagas' disease but, on rare occasions, surgical resection may become necessary.

BENIGN TUMOURS OF THE LARGE BOWEL

Large bowel polyps

Medical interest in rectal and colonic polyps has increased since the 1970's for two reasons. Firstly, it is now better appreciated that some polyps may progress to carcinomas, and that early diagnosis and removal therefore have the potential to prevent the many premature deaths associated with advanced colonic carcinoma. Secondly, fibre-optic instruments (colonoscopes) have been developed to inspect the rectum, colon and terminal ileum. These instruments allow the passage of wire snares which can be pulled tight around the stalk of polyps. A diathermy current can then be passed through the polyp enabling its removal for histological analysis. Many laparotomies have been avoided by the use of this technique.

Classification

A classification of colonic polyps is shown in Table 16.29. The adenomas are all potentially malignant. Colonic carcinoid tumours are relatively rare and do not produce biologically active amines or peptides. Metaplastic polyps are usually small (less than 1 cm), whereas adenomas may grow to several cms in diameter. Small adenomatous and metaplastic polyps cannot be differentiated however and, as subsequent management is different, all polyps must therefore be submitted to histological

Table 16.29 Histological classification of colonic polyps

Potentially malignant
Adenomas
  Tubular
  Villous
  Tubulovillous
  May be simple or multiple (e.g. Gardner's syndrome)

Carcinoid

No malignant potential
Metaplastic (hyperplastic polyps)

Connective tissue polyps
  Lipomas
  Fibromas
  Leiomyomas

Inflammatory
  Ulcerative colitis
  Crohn's disease

Hamartomas
  Peutz-Jegher's
  Juvenile

A

B

Fig. 16.21 Demonstration of colonic polyps. A. Double-contrast barium enema showing colonic polyps. **B.** Colonoscopic appearance of a polyp being snared prior to excision diathermy.

assessment. Inflammatory polyps are islands of regenerating mucosa which occur with severe ulcerative or Crohn's colitis. Hamartomas are heaped-up areas of normal tissues arranged in a disorganised way; they are commonest in children but may be seen in patients of any age. *Peutz-Jegher's syndrome* is a dominantly inherited disease associated with pigmentation of the skin and mucous membranes, and hamartomatous polyps in the stomach and small and large intestines. The polyps only rarely undergo malignant change, but cause symptoms through slow blood loss.

Clinical features and investigation

Many polyps are asymptomatic. When symptoms do occur, the most common is the passage of blood per rectum; altered bowel habit, colicky abdominal pain and, rarely, anorexia and weight loss may also be seen. For non-malignant polyps, the only physical signs are anaemia due to blood loss, mucocutaneous pigmentation (in Peutz-Jegher's syndrome) or polyps discovered by chance at sigmoidoscopy.

A double-contrast barium enema shows most polyps (Fig. 16.21). Colonoscopy is performed when the barium enema is equivocal, or when it is normal but doubt remains because of continued rectal bleeding or other problems. Colonoscopy is also essential for biopsy and treatment. If potentially, or frankly, malignant polyps are removed, long-term colonoscopic follow-up is required, initially annually and then perhaps trienially, to detect recurrent or new lesions.

Multiple polyposis coli

Familial adenomatous polyposis is a dominantly inherited condition where affected individuals develop multiple (usually more than 100) adenomatous colonic polyps. A variant of this condition, associated with epidermoid cysts and osteomas, is known as *Gardner's syndrome*. Most patients develop carcinomatous change in their polyps before the age of 40 and, if not treated early, have a poor prognosis. Panproctocolectomy with ileostomy formation, or ileoanal anastomosis with a pelvic ileal pouch, is therefore recommended in affected individuals in their late teens. Family screening for affected siblings is essential.

Some of the patients also develop adenomas of their small intestine and stomach and these may rarely become malignant.

CARCINOMA OF THE LARGE BOWEL

Colorectal carcinoma is primarily a disease of Western Europe and North America (Fig. 16.22). In England and Wales, it accounts for approximately 17 000 deaths annually, and is thus second only to carcinoma of the bronchus as a cause of death from malignant disease. Carcinoma of the colon affects the sexes equally, but carcinoma of the rectum has a higher incidence in men.

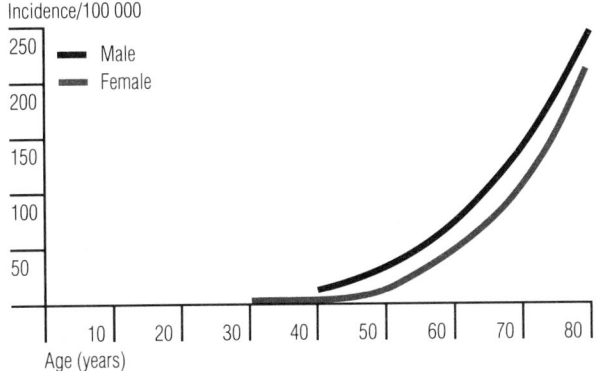

Fig. 16.22 Age-specific incidence of carcinoma of the large bowel in the Western World.

Aetiology

The aetiology is unknown although clearly there are factors associated with a Western life style. For example, the incidence is low in Japan but Japanese who move to the USA then have a much higher incidence. Diet has been implicated in the aetiology with the suggestions that high animal fat and low fibre intake is important. Altered colonic bacterial flora and changes in bile acid secretion may be important in pathogenesis. Genetic factors are important in familial polyposis and Gardner's syndrome, both of which are inherited as autosomal dominant traits. Adenomatous polyps and ulcerative and Crohn's colitis are well established precursors.

Pathology

The pathology is a malignant epithelial tumour of the rectum or colon. Macroscopically, there are three main appearances: cauliflower, ulcerative and annular lesions. The primary site is most commonly the rectum, followed by the sigmoid colon and the right side of the colon. These tumours then spread outwards through the wall of the bowel and invade local tissues, lymphatics and the blood

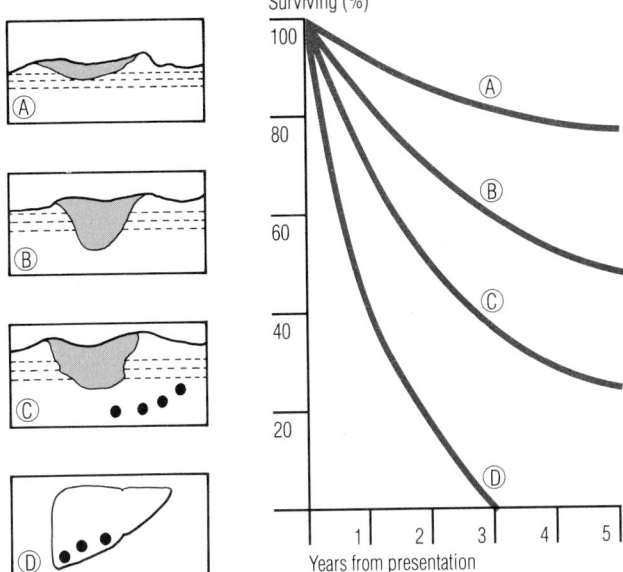

Fig. 16.23 Dukes' staging of carcinoma of the colon. (A) Tumour involves mucosa and submucosa only, good prognosis. (B) Tumour has penetrated muscle, moderate prognosis. (C) Tumour has spread to lymph nodes, poor prognosis. (D) Distant metastases are present. The corresponding five-year survival rates are also shown.

vessels. The staging of the tumour is important in predicting prognosis and is done by Dukes' classification (Fig. 16.23).

Clinical features

Many tumours are initially asymptomatic or their symptoms (rectal blood loss, constipation) are misinterpreted by the patient, resulting in a delay in diagnosis. The change in bowel habit may be constipation, diarrhoea or one alternating with the other. If the lesion is in the rectum, the blood is usually fresh and similar to that seen with haemorrhoids; if higher in the left side of the colon, it is fairly fresh and intermixed with stool; if in the right side of the colon, it may be stale blood or even melaena. Colicky abdominal pain is usually associated with colonic obstruction, whilst a constant pain implies local invasion. Tenesmus suggests a rectal carcinoma, whilst anal pain suggests local invasion down towards the anus. Air and faeces being passed via the urethra or the vagina imply local invasion anteriorly from the rectum with fistula formation; posterior invasion may result in sacral pain.

Signs are unusual in early disease unless the lesion is palpable per rectum or can be seen by a sigmoidoscope. Tumour bleeding may cause anaemia. Liver metastases may give rise to hepatomegaly, with jaundice as a late sign. Lymphatic spread is usually to para-aortic nodes and may cause extra-hepatic biliary obstruction. Ascites may occur due to peritoneal carcinomatosis. The tumour may be palpable and, if it is obstructing the bowel lumen, there will be proximal faecal loading. Rectal examination and sig-

16

moidoscopy are essential as part of the initial assessment. The fibre-optic sigmoidoscope can visualise the whole of the left side of the colon. Patients may present with large bowel obstruction or perforation in which case urgent surgery is required.

Investigation

If colorectal carcinoma is suspected, a double contrast barium enema is carried out. However, non-malignant lesions, particularly those due to inflammatory disease, can mimic tumour. In doubtful cases, colonoscopy can be of great value. Investigations are necessary to determine the extent of spread of the tumour.

Treatment

A laparotomy is indicated unless a carcinoma is localised within a resectable polyp. For right-sided tumours, a right hemicolectomy is performed, and a left hemicolectomy for left-sided tumours. Rectal tumours are usually treated with abdominoperineal resection of the tumour and rectum. There is some interest in treating very small rectal tumours by local diathermy or laser techniques. These techniques may also be used palliatively in advanced inoperable lesions causing obstruction or bleeding. For operable lesions, the role of pre- or postoperative radiotherapy is still being assessed. There is no evidence that adjuvant chemotherapy postoperatively improves the prognosis. Treatment of metastatic disease is unsatisfactory and response rates to cytotoxic drugs are low. Embolisation of hepatic metastases can be helpful for pain, as can external beam irradiation.

The prognosis depends on the extent of spread at the time of surgery. The overall five-year survival rate in the UK is approximately 25% (80% for Dukes' stage A, 60% for stage B and 20% for stage C). Most patients with Dukes' stage D die within a year. Early diagnosis is therefore critical, and this has led to a search for effective screening procedures.

OTHER MALIGNANT COLORECTAL TUMOURS

Malignant colorectal tumours other than adenocarcinomas form less than 5% of primary malignant colorectal neoplasms. They behave in a similar way to adenocarcinomas, and include carcinoids, lymphomas, leiomyosarcomas, fibrosarcomas and melanomas. Squamous carcinoma of the anus may also invade the rectum and be clinically indistinguishable from a rectal adenocarcinoma.

Screening for colorectal tumours

In view of the late presentation and consequent poor prognosis of patients with colorectal tumours, screening programmes for asymptomatic patients have been developed. These aim at diagnosing the tumour at the premalignant adenomatous polyp stage or whilst the carcinoma is still at

Dukes' stage A. The screening has been based on the faecal occult blood test. False positive results may be obtained with raw meat, iron therapy, blood loss from other sites, and vegetables containing peroxidase (e.g. cauliflower and radishes). False negative results are obtained because the tumours sometimes do not bleed, or bleed only irregularly. Follow-up of positive tests is usually by colonoscopy. The precise role of screening programmes has yet to be determined.

DIVERTICULAR DISEASE

Incidence and aetiology

Colonic diverticula are herniations of mucosa and submucosa through the wall of the large bowel, usually at the point where arteries pass through the submucosa. The most common site is the sigmoid colon, but colonic diverticula may occur throughout the large bowel and can be very numerous. They are rare before the age of 30 but occur in about 50% of people by the age of 70. They are uncommon in the Middle and Far East and in Africa.

Diverticula occur because of a weakness in the bowel wall and increased intracolonic pressure. The former is associated with an age-related reduction in strength of colonic connective tissue. The latter is thought to be due to reduced colonic contents due to a low dietary fibre intake.

Clinical features

Uncomplicated diverticulosis is asymptomatic. Symptoms may arise due to the complications of diverticular disease, the most important of which is an inflammatory mass (diverticulitis). This may result in an abscess which presents with abdominal pain and fever and, sometimes, as an emergency with ileus and septicaemic shock. Perforation may take place with leakage of faeces into the peritoneum. This may occur through a solitary diverticulum or through an inflammatory mass. In diverticular disease, there may be profuse colonic bleeding or a chronic iron deficiency anaemia. The differential diagnosis will then include other causes of chronic blood loss, such as a carcinoma.

Investigation

Anaemia suggests blood loss, and a raised white cell count and ESR suggest infection. If patients are acutely unwell, plain abdominal and chest X-rays may be helpful in detecting subdiaphragmatic gas due to a perforation. When the problem is not acute, a double contrast barium enema is useful to show the extent of the diverticula (Fig. 16.24). If the patient is persistently unwell, with a pyrexia, an ultrasound should be performed to detect an abscess following a localised perforation. A difficult diagnostic problem is the presence of a carcinoma in a segment of colon badly affected by diverticular disease. If the barium enema is difficult to interpret, a careful colonoscopy is indicated.

there may be no evidence of a mucosal break, and the majority of these have chronic obstructive airways disease.

Most patients are asymptomatic, but symptoms can include bloody diarrhoea, lower abdominal pain and increased rectal flatus. The cysts may be palpable rectally and sigmoidoscopy usually shows them as multiple blue swellings. Biopsy causes deflation, and the biopsy specimen often floats on the surface of the formol saline fixative. Plain abdominal X-ray shows multiple translucent cysts along the course of the colon and may be used to follow progress.

Treatment

Treatment is symptomatic, but breathing high concentrations of oxygen accelerates resorption of the cysts. This treatment is usually effective within five days but there is a tendency to relapse.

PRURITUS ANI

Itching around the anus is a common symptom and can have a number of causes (Table 16.30). A careful history should therefore be taken to identify an aetiological factor. This is followed by anal inspection, rectal examination and, if necessary, proctoscopy or sigmoidoscopy. In the UK, many patients use proprietary ointments and creams for their 'piles'. Various constituents of these treatments commonly produce contact dermatitis and pruritus. Unless there is a thrombosed pile or hygiene is poor, pruritus rarely complicates haemorrhoids.

Investigation of infections requires the laboratory examination of anal smears and, sometimes, faeces for threadworms and infections such as candida. Tight-fitting clothing and obesity cause local warmth and moisture, and predispose to skin infection and inflammation. In some patients, no cause can be identified; some of these have an obsessive and neurotic attitude which may be the primary problem.

Treatment

Treatment is directed at the underlying cause. The patient is reassured and encouraged to take a high fibre diet to

Fig. 16.24 Double contrast barium enema showing widespread diverticula, worst in the visible descending and sigmoid colon.

Treatment

There is no specific treatment for uncomplicated diverticular disease, although a high fibre diet may be recommended on the basis that it may prevent further diverticula developing. In general, the patient with uncomplicated diverticular disease should be strongly reassured there is nothing serious amiss and told that the probability is that he will not develop significant complications. Antispasmodic drugs such as mebeverine may help some patients with colicky pains.

Surgery is indicated for severe haemorrhage, treatment of a local abscess and treatment of perforation. In addition to resection of the diseased bowel and peritoneal lavage after perforation, antibiotics to eradicate coliforms and anaerobic bacteria should be used (e.g. a combination of intravenous gentamicin, ampicillin and metronidazole). Rarely, surgery may be indicated for pain due to a diverticular stricture.

PNEUMATOSIS COLI

Pneumatosis coli is a rare syndrome where cysts of gas up to 2 cm in diameter form in the submucous and subserous areas of the colon (and occasionally the small intestine). It can occur as a result of a peptic ulcer. In some patients

Table 16.30 Causes of pruritus ani

- Anorectal disease (fistulas, fissures, skin tags, haemorrhoids)
- Vaginal discharge
- Primary skin disease (psoriasis, eczema, lichen planus)
- Contact dermatitis (secondary to soaps, ointments, powders)
- Infections (candida, scabies, pediculosis pubis, worms)
- Poor hygiene
- Warmth and moisture
- Psychological

16

avoid constipation. The anus is kept clean by washing twice daily without use of strong soaps, ointments etc. If the problem is persistent and there is no obvious treatable cause, local 1% hydrocortisone and oral antihistamines may help.

INFLAMMATORY BOWEL DISEASE

Inflammatory bowel disease can be defined as chronic inflammatory disease of the gut of uncertain aetiology. It is divided into two types:

1. *Crohn's disease*, which affects the gut from mouth to anus and is pathologically characterised by non-caseating giant cell granulomata
2. *ulcerative colitis*, which affects only the large bowel.

Macroscopically, in Crohn's disease, small aphthoid ulcers, larger ulcers and strictures are seen. Histology shows the whole bowel wall to be infiltrated by lymphocytes and plasma cells. In contrast, ulcerative colitis is primarily a superficial mucosal inflammation. In both diseases, the large bowel may initially be the only site of involvement, and differentiation of the two is then of less importance, as the presentation, complications and treatment of the colitis are very similar. It is possible that the two diseases are different responses to the same aetiological agent.

CROHN'S DISEASE

Crohn's disease is a granulomatous disease most commonly affecting the terminal ileum and right side of the colon. It is named after Dr Burrill Crohn of New York, who described 52 cases in 1932. He spoke of a 'terminal ileitis' but it has subsequently become clear that the gut may be involved from mouth to anus; this has led to the term 'regional enteritis' as a synonym for the disease.

Crohn's disease is common in the Western World but rare in underdeveloped countries. This is in contradistinction to tuberculosis, the bovine form of which also affects the terminal ileum and is relatively common in the developing world. The annual incidence of new cases appears to be rising in all countries studied (England, Wales, Scotland, Scandinavia and North America) and is currently 3–6 per 100 000 population (Fig. 16.25). It occurs equally in the sexes. The initial presentation can be at any age but is most common in early adult life.

Aetiology

The aetiology is unknown but the evidence suggests that the cause is largely environmental. For example, when a population migrates from areas of low to high incidence, the incidence in that population subsequently rises. The following theories have been put forward:

1. *Infection.* No infectious agent has yet been shown to transmit the disease or produce similar granulomatous reaction in animals. In the past, viruses, bacterial L forms and cell wall deficient pseudomonads have been suggested as causes, but their role has not been substantiated. At present there is interest in the possible role of mycobacteria and campylobacter.
2. *Immunological.* The characteristic granuloma of Crohn's disease suggests a possible immunological origin. Both food and bacterial antigens have been implicated, but there is no clear evidence for either. As with other inflammatory bowel diseases, minor, non-specific, immunological changes have been reported – T cells cytotoxic to colon epithelium, circulating immune complexes, and anti-colon antibodies.
3. *Dietary.* A high intake of refined sugars and a low intake of fibre have been suggested as aetiological factors, but the evidence that they are primary factors is not strong.
4. *Genetic.* There is a higher incidence of both Crohn's disease and ulcerative colitis in relatives of patients with Crohn's disease.
5. *Smoking.* In direct contrast to ulcerative colitis, patients with Crohn's disease are more likely to be cigarette smokers than appropriate controls.
6. *Others.* Oral contraceptives, detergents, mercury and psychological trauma have all been proposed as aetiological agents, but with little firm foundation.

Pathology

At laparotomy, Crohn's disease is seen as thickened bowel with associated enlarged lymph nodes. Microscopically, the inflammation is transmural, in contrast to ulcerative colitis where the mucosa only is usually involved. The other hallmark of Crohn's is the microscopic finding of non-caseating granulomas. As a result of the transmural inflammation, there may be local abscesses or fistulae between two pieces of bowel (entero-entero or entero-colonic) or between the bowel and the skin (entero-

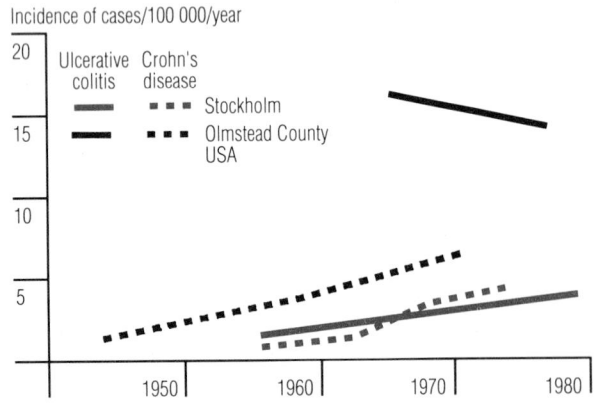

Fig. 16.25 Incidence of ulcerative colitis and Crohn's disease in two centres in Sweden and the USA.

cutaneous), usually in the anterior abdominal wall or around the anus. Fistulae may also form between the bowel and bladder or vagina.

Clinical features

The symptoms and signs of Crohn's disease are shown in Summary 8. The commonest initial presentation is terminal ileal disease, often with coexistent oral and anal involvement. Less common initial presentations are acute right iliac fossa pain, simulating acute appendicitis, and acute colitis identical to ulcerative colitis.

General symptoms

When the disease is active the majority of patients have a mild fever and general malaise. Loss of appetite and malabsorption contribute to weight loss. Amenorrhoea may occur when there is weight loss and constitutional symptoms.

In prepubertal and pubertal children, there may be no history of diarrhoea or abdominal pain. Commonly, the patients present with non-specific symptoms – failure to thrive, decreased growth velocity and possibly delayed puberty.

Gastrointestinal symptoms

The gastrointestinal symptoms depend primarily on the site of disease. As a result of stricture formation, many patients with ileal disease complain of colicky abdominal pain, usually in the right iliac fossa. Diarrhoea, usually modest and containing excess fat, is usual. Disease in the right side of the colon produces similar symptoms, although colonic disease alone does not cause steatorrhoea. It is often combined with ileal disease. Left-sided colonic disease results in diarrhoea without steatorrhoea but with blood per rectum.

Urinary frequency and dysuria may result from inflamed bowel adjacent to the urinary tract (especially the right ureter and bladder). Pneumaturia (air in the urine), and faeces via the urethra or vagina indicate a fistula from bowel to the genito-urinary tract.

Complications due to nutritional deficiency

General complications due to nutritional deficiency may cause symptoms (Summary 8). Anaemia may be due to blood loss or reduced absorption of iron, folate and vitamin B_{12}. Oedema secondary to hypoproteinaemia is a consequence of both protein loss into the lumen of the gut (protein-losing enteropathy) and reduced dietary intake. Gallstones are due to terminal ileal bile acid malabsorption which results in cholesterol-supersaturated bile and causes cholesterol gallstones. Vitamin D and calcium malabsorption can result in hypocalcaemia (manifest as tetany) or, when long-standing, pseudofractures (Looser's zones) or fractures due to osteomalacia (p. 735). Night blindness and spontaneous bleeding may rarely occur due to vitamin

Summary 8	Clinical presentation of Crohn's disease
General	*Mouth*
Fever	Cobblestone ulcers
Malaise	Aphthous ulcers
Weight loss	Glossitis
Amenorrhoea	Stomatitis
In children: failure to thrive, growth retardation, delayed puberty	
	Fistula formation
	Entero-enteric or entero-cutaneous
Terminal ileal disease	
Abdominal pain	Urinary frequency, dysuria, haematuria and pneumaturia
Diarrhoea (with or without steatorrhoea)	Faeces per vaginam and per urethram
Right iliac fossa tenderness, mass, possibly signs of small intestinal obstruction	
	Complications due to nutritional deficiencies
Colonic disease	Anaemia
Abdominal pain	Oedema due to hypoproteinaemia
Diarrhoea	Gallstones
Blood and mucus per rectum	Tetany
Tenesmus	Osteomalacia
Abdominal tenderness, possibly abnormal sigmoidoscopy	Vitamins A and K deficiency
	Water-soluble vitamin deficiency
Anal disease	Ion deficiencies (potassium, magnesium and zinc)
Skin tags, fissures and abscesses	
Incontinence	
Fistulae between anal canal and skin	

A and K malabsorption. Angular cheilitis, glossitis and even scurvy can result from vitamin B and C deficiency. Hypokalaemia results in malaise and muscle weakness and hypomagnesaemia can cause tetany. Zinc deficiency can cause a rash similar to that seen in zinc-deficient children with acrodermatitis enteropathica.

Non-intestinal manifestations

Both Crohn's disease and ulcerative colitis may be associated with non-intestinal manifestations (Table 16.31), which usually indicate colonic disease. The acute large joint arthritis seen commonly affects the knees and ankles. Erythema nodosum and pyoderma gangrenosum usually affect the limbs, particularly the legs (p. 1129). If urticaria and erythema multiforme are seen, they should be assumed initially to be due to sulphasalazine. If there are ophthalmic symptoms, an assessment with a slit lamp is needed to exclude uveitis. Sacro-iliitis occurs in up to 10% of patients, and may produce severe low back pain. The association with ankylosing spondylitis is rare. Abnormal liver function tests occur in about 10% of patients with colitis and are usually asymptomatic. The mildest lesion is fatty infiltration, and this and intrahepatic pericholangitis are the two commonest abnormalities (Ch. 17, p. 642). Primary sclerosing cholangitis is a rare disease charac-

Table 16.31 Non-intestinal manifestations of inflammatory bowel disease

Affected part	Manifestation
Reflecting acute illness	
Joints	Acute large joint arthritis
Skin	Pyoderma gangrenosum
	Erythema nodosum
	Urticaria ⎱ often secondary to
	Erythema multiforme ⎰ sulphasalazine therapy
Eyes	Conjunctivitis
	Episcleritis
	Uveitis
Not reflecting acute illness	
Joints	Sacro-iliitis
	Ankylosing spondylitis
Liver	Fatty change
	Pericholangitis
	Primary sclerosing cholangitis
	Carcinoma of bile duct (cholangiocarcinoma)
	Autoimmune chronic active hepatitis

Summary 9   Investigation of Crohn's disease

- Sigmoidoscopy and rectal biopsy
- Stool culture and microscopy
- Abdominal and chest X-ray
  Small bowel enema
  Barium enema
- Colonoscopy (when indicated)
  Upper gastrointestinal endoscopy (when indicated)
- Full blood count, ESR
  Serum iron, iron binding capacity, folate and B_{12}
  Liver function tests including serum albumin
- Indium-labelled white blood cells (when indicated)

terised by alternating strictures and dilatations of major bile ducts. It may be asymptomatic or present with pruritus or jaundice. Cholangio-carcinoma and autoimmune chronic active hepatitis are rare.

Signs

Physical examination of a patient with Crohn's disease should start with a search for nail changes (including clubbing, leuconychia and koilonychia), anaemia, pyrexia, a tachycardia and mouth ulcers. Non-intestinal manifestations should be looked for. In the abdomen, there may be operation scars, evidence of fistulae and signs of intestinal obstruction with visible peristalsis. Palpation may reveal a mass, most commonly in the right iliac fossa, due to disease in the terminal ileum and the right side of the colon. Auscultation may suggest intestinal obstruction. Sigmoidoscopy and rectal biopsy are essential. Sigmoidoscopy may show granular inflamed mucosa, sometimes with spontaneous bleeding and increased mucus formation. Even in the absence of obvious inflammatory changes, the rectal biopsy may demonstrate diagnostic granulomas.

Investigation

The purpose of investigations is to make a definite diagnosis and to assess the severity and extent of disease (Summary 9). The diagnosis is confirmed by demonstrating the characteristic granulomatous histology, often by rectal biopsy. In the presence of active disease, the haemoglobin is usually low and the neutrophil count and ESR are raised. The plasma albumin is low if there is widespread disease. Stool culture and microscopy should be performed; infections, particularly *Yersinia* (p. 272) and *Campylobacter* (p. 276) may mimic Crohn's ileitis.

A plain abdominal X-ray should be done initially to determine if there is any colonic dilatation. A chest X-ray may reveal tuberculosis, which may present with ileal disease similar to Crohn's disease. A small bowel enema involves passing a nasogastric tube into the upper jejunum and passing barium and air through it to outline the jejunum and ileum. Involvement of the small bowel is characterised by stricture formation, rose-thorn ulcers, proximal dilatation and fistula formation (Fig. 16.26A). The colon and caecum (and often also the terminal ileum) are visualised by a double-contrast barium enema (Fig. 16.26B). Colonic changes include thickening of the wall, deep ulcers (rose-thorn and collar-stud ulcers) and skip lesions, with areas of normal bowel interspersed between diseased segments. Colonoscopy allows direct inspection and biopsy of the colon and terminal ileum, thereby confirming the diagnosis of Crohn's disease and excluding dysplastic and carcinomatous change. A new and potentially useful technique is to label the patient's white cells *in vitro* with an isotope such as [111]indium. After reinjecting them into the patient, the localisation and activity of the disease can be assessed by following the site of migration using a gamma camera.

Differential diagnosis

The differential diagnosis of Crohn's disease is shown in Table 16.32. In many parts of the Middle and Far East, bovine tuberculosis of the terminal ileum is quite common and Crohn's disease is rare. In the UK, bovine tuberculosis has been eradicated in milk herds and tuberculous ileitis is seen only in immigrants or in foreign travellers. The barium radiological appearance is similar to that of Crohn's disease; however, in the case of tuberculosis, caseating granulomas are found on histology, acid-fast bacilli may be seen on microscopy, and mycobacteria are isolated on culture of the biopsy.

Yersinia can present with an acute ileitis in young people, but signs disappear within three months.

Some patients with Crohn's are inappropriately diagnosed and treated for anorexia nervosa. Addison's disease and hypopituitarism can also present as weight loss and diarrhoea.

Fig. 16.26 Barium enemas demonstrating Crohn's ileitis and colitis. A. Small bowel enema showing stricture formation and ulceration of the terminal ileum, typical of Crohn's ileitis. **B.** Barium enema showing deep ulceration of the distal colon suggesting Crohn's colitis.

Table 16.32 Differential diagnosis of Crohn's disease

Symptoms	Differential diagnosis
Terminal ileal disease	Tuberculosis
	Yersinia
	Tumours, especially lymphoma and primary carcinoid
Colitis	Ulcerative colitis
	Infective colitis
	Ischaemic colitis
Weight loss and diarrhoea	Carcinoma especially of the large bowel in older people
	Other causes of malabsorption e.g. coeliac disease
	Hyperthyroidism
	Anorexia nervosa (with or without surreptitious purgative abuse)
	Addison's disease
	Hypopituitarism

Complications

There are a number of complications of Crohn's disease.

1. *Acute colonic dilatation*, indistinguishable from that seen with ulcerative colitis and sometimes complicated by perforation and haemorrhage.

2. *Subacute small bowel obstruction*, due to stricture formation and obstruction by solid foods.
3. *Fistula formation*.
4. *Renal stones*. Oxalate stones due to increased urinary oxalate excretion is a complication of terminal ileal disease because of increased colonic bile acids enhancing oxalate absorption.
5. *Carcinoma of the colon* may complicate long-standing (usually more than 20 years) Crohn's colitis. Small intestinal carcinomas may complicate ileal Crohn's.
6. *Amyloid* may occur in the bowel and other organs and may regress with resection of diseased bowel.

Treatment

Crohn's disease can cause considerable morbidity but, with joint medical and surgical specialist care, the overall quality of life should be good. The mortality rate is about twice that of normal controls.

Medical

The treatment of patients with Crohn's disease depends on the site, severity and extent of disease (Table 16.33). In general, patients should be encouraged to take a balanced diet with an adequate amount of fibre. Dietary fibre should only be restricted when there is stricture formation, as it

Table 16.33 Medical treatment of Crohn's disease

Symptoms	Treatment
Nutritional deficiencies	Good balanced diet Folic acid Vitamin B_{12} Iron Vitamins A, D, E and K Potassium, zinc and calcium
Ileal disease	Prednisolone Elemental diet Azathioprine
Colonic disease	Prednisolone Sulphasalazine Azathioprine
Severe active ileitis and/or colitis	Intravenous hydrocortisone Intravenous fluids or total parenteral nutrition Antibiotics
Anal disease and fistulae	Metronidazole Azathioprine Elemental diet/total parenteral nutrition and nil by mouth
Non-intestinal manifestations	Local measures Prednisolone (if acute illness)

Table 16.34 Role and side-effects of salicylate drugs used in Crohn's disease and ulcerative colitis

Drug	Side-effects	Role
Sulphasalazine	Skin rashes Marrow suppression Haemolysis Male subfertility Gastrointestinal symptoms Orange urine	Prevention of relapse in UC Some use in colonic Crohn's disease
5-aminosalicylic acid (mesalazine)	Headache	Alternative to sulphasalazine
Azodisalicylate (olsalazine)	Headache	Alternative to sulphasalazine
5-aminosalicylic acid enemas	Headache	Alternative to sulphasalazine

may then contribute to intestinal obstruction. Replacements are given if there is evidence of haematinic, fat-soluble vitamin or mineral deficiency.

Active ileitis and colitis

Active ileal disease causing diarrhoea, abdominal pain and a right iliac fossa mass is usually treated with a three-month course of oral prednisolone (starting at 30–40 mg/day). If the disease is resistant, azathioprine (2 mg/kg) may be used, with regular blood counts to detect marrow suppression. Clinical trials have shown that sulphasalazine is of little value when the disease is restricted to the ileum, but it should be tried in difficult cases. An elemental diet (a solution of essential amino acids, carbohydrate, fat, vitamins and trace elements) may also be of value in the treatment of active ileal disease.

Active colonic disease is also treated with prednisolone. Sulphasalazine, which is 5-aminosalicylic acid bound to a sulphonamide (sulphapyridine), may be of some use in Crohn's colitis although its main role is in the prevention of relapse in ulcerative colitis. The sulphonamide is cleaved from the 5-aminosalicylic acid in the terminal ileum and colon by bacteria and it is the latter which is the active moiety. However, because of the numerous and potentially serious side-effects (Table 16.34), mostly due to the sulphonamide, alternatives to sulphasalazine have been developed. One of the enteric coated preparations uses an acrylic-based resin outer coat (mesalazine) which, like the semi-permeable membrane of the slow-release preparation of sulphalazine, is pH-dependent and allows release

of 5-aminosalicylic acid into the ileum and colon. Azo-disalicylate consists of two molecules of 5-aminosalicylic acid bound by an azo bond which is split by lower intestinal bacteria. Another option is the use of 5-aminosalicylic acid enemas. It seems probable that sulphasalazine will be replaced by aminosalicylic acid or azodisalicylate in the near future; both are currently in clinical trials.

Patients with severe active ileitis and/or colitis have constitutional symptoms and require hospital admission. Intravenous hydrocortisone sodium succinate (usually 100 mg 8-hourly) is usually given for about 5 days and then oral prednisolone is substituted. Intravenous fluids are needed and, if the patient is malnourished, total parenteral nutrition should be undertaken. If there is a possibility of infection, the patient is treated with intravenous broad-spectrum antibiotics (e.g. ampicillin, gentamicin and metronidazole).

Anal disease

Anal disease should be treated with metronidazole for several weeks, but the patient should be warned to report any symptoms suggestive of peripheral neuropathy.

Resistant anal disease may respond to dietary measures or require surgical resection with formation of a stoma. In severe cases, an elemental diet will greatly reduce stool frequency and help healing. Entero-cutaneous and entero-entero fistulae usually require surgery, but an elemental diet or total parenteral nutrition with nil by mouth ('bowel rest') for a few weeks may promote temporary or permanent closure.

Non-intestinal manifestations

Non-intestinal manifestations may require specific treatment. Severe joint, skin or eye disease requires prednisolone. The diseases reflecting acute illness settle with removal of the affected bowel (usually colon) but those due to the chronic illness do not. The treatment of sacro-iliitis and ankylosing spondylitis is described in Chapter 24, page

997. The liver changes are little affected by medication apart from chronic active hepatitis, which requires prednisolone with or without azathioprine.

Surgical

Surgery is reserved for attacks resistant to corticosteroids and other forms of treatment. Most Crohn's patients will at some time require intestinal surgery. Limited resections and end-to-end anastomoses are performed as necessary, usually to relieve obstruction or fistula formation. Occasionally, panproctocolectomy with formation of an ileostomy is indicated for severe colitis. The complications of ileostomy are discussed on page 607.

ULCERATIVE COLITIS

Ulcerative colitis (UC) is a chronic inflammatory condition of unknown aetiology affecting the colon and rectum. Like Crohn's disease, it is most common in the Western World. In 1971–77 the annual incidence of UC in the North Tees region of the UK was 15.1 per 100 000 and the prevalence rate for the same area was 99.0 per 100 000 population. These are slightly higher levels than those of other studies (Fig. 16.25). The incidence of UC appears to be stable. It is slightly more common in women than men. Most patients present in early adult life, but all ages can be affected.

Aetiology and pathology

Aetiological factors are similar to those for Crohn's disease (p. 600). There is recent evidence that relapses can be associated with stopping smoking cigarettes; the explanation for this is not known.

Ulcerative colitis primarily involves the mucosa; only in very severe disease is the muscularis mucosae penetrated. Microscopy shows plasma cells and neutrophils, particularly in the crypts of Lieberkühn, which can break down to form 'crypt abscesses' communicating with the luminal surface. If the disease is confined to the rectum (proctitis), it is clinically less severe and there is no increased long-term risk of carcinomatous change.

Clinical features

Acute attack

The usual presenting symptom of acute attacks is the passage of frequent loose, small-volume, brown motions with fresh blood and mucus either on the surface of the stools or intermixed with them. There is usually no history to suggest infection (e.g. foreign travel). Blood per rectum alone or diarrhoea alone are common first symptoms. Attacks can be usefully divided into mild, moderate and severe (Table 16.35). Patients with mild attacks open their bowels up to five times a day, with moderate attacks up to ten times a day, and with severe attacks over ten times a day. The faeces become increasingly soft with more severe relapses. Cramping abdominal pains are common in attacks of moderate severity, while rectal pain and a painful feeling of incomplete evacuation (tenesmus) are common in the more severe cases.

Fever and tachycardia indicate severe disease – usually widespread and active – rather than infection. Anaemia, if present, is usually hypochromic and microcytic and due to blood loss.

Colonic blood loss causes anaemia, while protein loss leads to hypoproteinaemia and peripheral oedema. With

Table 16.35 Ulcerative colitis: clinical features of mild, moderate and severe attacks

Clinical feature	Mild	Moderate	Severe
Diarrhoea	+	++	+++
Blood per rectum	+	++	+++
Mucus	+	++	+++
Abdominal pain	−	+	++
Tenesmus	±	+	++
Anorexia	−	+	++
Weight loss	±	+	++
Acute extracolonic manifestations	+	+	++
Fever	−	±	+
Tachycardia	−	±	++
Anaemia	±	+	+
Distended abdomen	−	±	+
Abdominal tenderness	−	±	+
Sigmoidoscopy	Fine granularity	Coarse granularity Spontaneous bleeding	Friable Pseudopolyps Mucopus
Abnormal plain abdominal X-ray	−	−	+
High ESR	±	+	++
High neutrophil count	±	+	++
Hypoproteinaemia	−	+	++

acute colonic dilatation, the patient becomes very unwell, febrile with abdominal tenderness and reduced bowel sounds. Signs of peritonitis (abdominal rigidity, extreme tenderness and absent bowel sounds) suggests colonic perforation, a complication with a mortality rate approaching 50%. Colectomy may therefore be necessary in acute colonic dilatation to avoid this complication.

Chronic ulcerative colitis

Following recovery from an acute attack, patients may return to a normal bowel habit. Acute exacerbations of varying severity usually occur intermittently. In some patients, these periods of remission may be very short so that treatment becomes almost continuous. Other patients have persistent symptoms which typically become worse when their prednisolone dose is reduced.

Development of malignant change

Patients with pancolitis for more than 10 years are at an increased risk of developing carcinoma of the colon – hence the need for regular colonoscopic screening.

Non-intestinal manifestations

The non-intestinal manifestations of ulcerative colitis are similar to those of Crohn's disease (p. 604 and listed in Table 16.31).

Sigmoidoscopy and rectal biopsy are essential for the assessment of proctocolitis and should be performed as part of the initial examination of the patient. Normal sigmoidoscopy shows smooth, pink, 'wet' mucosa with visible submucosal vessels and rectal folds. In proctitis, the mucosa becomes oedematous, diffusely reddened, and granular when it loses its 'wet' appearance. The blood vessels and mucosal folds are lost, and contact bleeding and spontaneous haemorrhages may be present. 'Pseudo-polyps' are islands of residual mucosa around which mucosa has been lost. Sigmoidoscopy in active proctitis should be brief; no attempt should be made to insert the instrument far into the rectum and only a little air insufflated.

Investigation

The relevant investigations in ulcerative colitis are shown in Table 16.36. Stool microscopy and culture are necessary

Table 16.36 Investigation of acute attack of presumed ulcerative colitis

- Rectal biopsy
- Haemoglobin, white cell count, ESR, C-reactive protein
- Liver function tests, plasma proteins
- Stool microscopy and culture
- Plain abdominal X-ray
- Barium enema (delay)
- Radiolabelled white cell scan (selected cases)

Fig. 16.27 Plain abdominal X-ray showing a dilated transverse colon outlined by air – the toxic megacolon of colitis.

to exclude infection. A plain abdominal X-ray may demonstrate the degree of colonic dilatation; this is usually best seen in the transverse colon (Fig. 16.27). Barium enemas can precipitate toxic dilatation. They should therefore be avoided in acute disease but, when used, show loss of haustra, dilatation of the lumen and superficial ulceration.

Treatment

Acute attack

The most important treatment for acute episodes of colitis is corticosteroids. In mild attacks, rectal hydrocortisone or prednisolone is usually effective. In moderately severe attacks, oral prednisolone (30–40 mg daily) is the usual therapy, with the dose then being tapered off over three months. In severe attacks, intravenous hydrocortisone (100 mg tds) is given. When the patient improves, prednisolone can be given orally and the dose slowly reduced.

Sulphasalazine (1 g bd) or other 5-amino salicylic acid compounds, such as mesalazine (400 mg tds) reduce symptoms in patients with mild attacks. Some patients benefit from the exclusion of dietary milk products. Total parenteral nutrition with only sips of water by mouth (bowel rest) and antibiotics have been advocated in severe cases, but there is little evidence that these measures improve results.

Maintenance treatment

Numerous studies have shown that long-term sulphasalazine (1 g bd) reduces the relapse rates of patients in remission. (For the side-effects and possible alternatives to this drug, see p. 604.) There is no indication for steroids in patients in remission.

Treatment in pregnancy

Most patients with inflammatory bowel disease improve during pregnancy, although a minority (about 20%) have relapses. There is no contraindication to the use of sulphasalazine and prednisolone in any trimester, and they should therefore be used in the normal way. Azathioprine and metronidazole, however, may adversely affect the fetus and should be avoided. Patients tend to relapse postpartum because of a fall in plasma steroid levels. Patients should be warned of this possibility and the disease treated vigorously if it occurs.

Treatment in childhood

Children should be treated actively in the same way as adults to maximise growth. Prednisolone should be used sparingly because, although it reduces disease activity, it tends to inhibit growth. Particular attention should be paid to diet. In medically resistant disease, a colectomy should be performed.

Ileostomy

There are three major complications of UC which are indications for panproctocolectomy and formation of an ileostomy:

1. Patients with severe acute disease where the colon is dilated more than six cm on plain abdominal X-ray and the patient is toxic with a pyrexia and tachycardia. The operative mortality becomes much higher (50%) if patients perforate their colon and develop a faecal peritonitis (compared to 3% for elective and 10% for urgent operations). Acute severe colonic bleeding is also an indication for surgery.
2. Patients with chronic severe disease which persistently requires high dose corticosteroid treatment. Diarrhoea and blood and protein loss lead to chronic ill-health. A barium enema (Fig. 16.28) usually shows a pancolitis. Patients usually feel dramatically better after colectomy, which also avoids the development of further complications (apart from chronic liver disease).
3. In patients with pancolitis for more than 10 years, there is a significant risk of carcinomatous change; this has a poor prognosis if not recognised early. Carcinomas may be multifocal and are often preceded by the development of mucosal cellular dysplasia in rectal and colonic biopsies. After 10 years' pancolitis, regular colonoscopies are therefore indicated. Severe dysplasia or carcinoma are indications for total colectomy.

Complications of an ileostomy

Complications of ileostomy are usually minimal apart from minor problems with the abdominal wall around the stoma. There may be high effluent outputs (more than one l/day), especially if there has been small bowel surgery or there is active Crohn's disease. This can be helped by avoiding hyperosmolar food and by the use of drugs which slow intestinal motility (e.g. loperamide, codeine phosphate). Impotence due to damage to the sacral nerves is unusual.

Fig. 16.28 Barium enema findings with pancolitis. Long-standing ulcerative colitis, with disease throughout the colon, mucosal ulceration and loss of haustrations. There is an 'apple-core' lesion of the ascending colon typical of carcinoma.

The great majority of patients with an ileostomy have excellent health.

Psychological problems can be severe and patients require sensitive handling and counselling by medical and nursing staff. Many hospitals have full time 'stoma nurses', who care for patients' equipment and basic medical and psychological needs both in and out of hospital. Many patients also find it helpful to meet other stoma patients. Colitis and stoma societies and self-help groups are of great value in helping patients to lead a normal life.

Alternative surgical procedures to ileostomy have been developed. Direct ileorectal anastomosis is often unsatisfactory, as inflammatory and neoplastic complications may occur in the rectum and the fluid stool often makes the anus sore. A Koch's continent ileostomy allows the ileal effluent to collect in an ileal sump, and thus be released intermittently rather than to ooze continuously. Recently, an operation has been devised in which a pouch of the terminal ileum is formed in the pelvis and anastomosed to the anus. This can be emptied by the patient spontaneously or by using a catheter. This operation is technically difficult and is being developed in a few specialist centres.

Prognosis

Less than 5% of patients suffering from ulcerative colitis die within a year of presentation. In contrast, after their first attack settles, 10% of patients will have at least 15 subsequent asymptomatic years. Up to 25% of patients require colectomy within 5–10 years of developing the disease. Deaths can be avoided by performing colectomies before advanced carcinomas develop. Overall, the mortality rate is about twice that of the normal population.

INFECTIVE, ISCHAEMIC AND RADIATION COLITIDES

PSEUDOMEMBRANOUS COLITIS

Pseudomembranous colitis is due to a toxin produced by *Clostridium difficile* and nearly always follows the use of broad-spectrum antibiotics. The symptoms develop from four days to six weeks after starting the drugs.

Clinical features and investigation

The patients develop cramping abdominal pains and diarrhoea with mucus and, sometimes, blood. Sigmoidoscopy reveals diarrhoea, a proctitis and, sometimes, multiple yellow elevated plaques up to 20 mm in diameter. Investigations may demonstrate *C. difficile* toxin in the faeces. In severe cases, there is a dilated oedematous colon on plain abdominal X-ray. A rectal biopsy is usually diagnostic and shows necrotic foci with inflammatory cells migrating through to the lesion ('the summit lesion') and pseudomembranes.

Treatment

Treatment is with vancomycin or metronidazole. Cholestyramine, an anion-exchange resin, can be used to bind the toxin and reduce diarrhoea. Supportive measures, which often include intravenous fluids, are important. The prognosis is usually good, except in the elderly or if there is a delay in making the diagnosis.

YERSINIA

Yersinia enterocolitica and *pseudotuberculosis* are organisms which may cause an acute ulcerative inflammation of the ileum, appendix and caecum. They may be associated with erythema nodosum and an acute arthritis. Barium studies show a swollen terminal ileum with tortuous folds and filling defects giving a cobblestone appearance. Some of the patients have a laparotomy because a mistaken diagnosis of acute appendicitis is made. The condition is self-limiting and resolves completely within three months.

INTESTINAL TUBERCULOSIS

Mycobacterium tuberculosis can cause: ileocaecal disease similar to Crohn's disease; colonic strictures; or peritoneal disease, which may be 'wet' and associated with exudative ascites, or 'dry' with fibrous omental adhesions and thickening. In the UK, the majority of patients are Asian immigrants; it is a common problem in developing countries where inflammatory bowel disease is rare. About one-third of the patients have evidence of active tuberculosis on the chest X-ray. The diagnosis is made by histological examination and culture, and may require a laparotomy to obtain tissue.

Treatment is with antituberculous chemotherapy (p. 480); the patient usually responds well.

GAY BOWEL SYNDROME

Homosexuals have an increased incidence of diarrhoea from infections such as shigella, campylobacter, giardia, amoeba, and cryptosporidium. They also commonly develop perianal warts (condylomata acuminata). These patients may have a proctitis due to gonococcal and *Herpes simplex* type 2 infection and, occasionally, anal syphilis. Warts can be treated with local podophyllin or silver nitrate. Syphilis, gonorrhoea and most of the other infections are treated in the standard manner (Ch. 12). Identification of contacts is important to avoid early reinfection. Acyclovir is used for herpetic infections, together with analgesia and stool softeners.

The acquired immune deficiency syndrome (AIDS) can be associated with fulminant bowel infections as well as the development of plaques of Kaposi sarcoma throughout the bowel (p. 251). Eating and swallowing may be painful due to oral and oesophageal candida infection.

ISCHAEMIC COLITIS

Aetiology and pathology

Ischaemic colitis usually affects the area of the splenic flexure and descending colon. Rarely, ischaemia of the superior mesenteric artery may affect the ascending and proximal transverse colon. Atheroma is a more common cause than embolus; but aetiological factors are otherwise similar to those seen in small bowel ischaemia (p. 591).

Clinical features and investigation

The patients are usually elderly and present with bloody diarrhoea and abdominal pain. Examination shows mild peritonism and normal rectal mucosa at sigmoidoscopy. Investigations may show a low haemoglobin because of blood loss, a high ESR and neutrophil leucocytosis. Sometimes, a plain abdominal X-ray shows a dilated colon with 'thumb printing'. A barium enema confirms this.

Treatment

In most patients, the symptoms resolve with analgesia and intravenous fluids. Perforation is rare. A late complication is benign stricture formation and this may occasionally require resection because of intestinal obstruction.

RADIATION COLITIS

Damage to the transverse colon may occur during upper abdominal radiotherapy and damage to the sigmoid colon and rectum during gynaecological treatment. In the acute phase (during or immediately after treatment) the symptoms are bloody diarrhoea, tenesmus and abdominal pain. These are treated with a low residue diet and rectal steroids if there is a proctitis. Later complications include the development of a chronic proctitis with telangiectatic lesions which may bleed, benign ulcers and stricture formation. The proctitis and ulcers may sometimes improve with rectal steroids.

FUNCTIONAL BOWEL DISORDERS

Incidence

In the UK, it is estimated that some 15% of the population have symptoms of a functional disorder of the bowel. These patients have abdominal symptoms without any evidence of underlying organic pathology. Many individuals do not seek medical advice, presumably because they understand the nature of their symptoms and may be able to attribute them to a particular cause; they thereby learn to avoid or live with them. Others will consult their general practitioner, sometimes because of the discomfort experienced but often out of fear that the symptoms might indicate more serious disease. Some will then be referred to a specialist. This may be because of the severity or intractability of the symptoms or because the presence of atypical features causes concern. More often, however, the referral will be made in order to reinforce the reassurance already given and, hopefully, to make treatment more effective. Specialists thus tend to see a selected sample of patients who will often form the basis of clinical studies.

Because the cause or causes are not known, and because the range of symptoms is wide and relates to the whole of the gastrointestinal tract, it is sensible to consider all the manifestations of functional bowel disorder as a single entity due to multiple factors. At different times, the same patient may experience either predominantly lower gastrointestinal symptoms (irritable bowel syndrome, IBS), or upper gastrointestinal symptoms (functional dyspepsia).

Functional bowel disorders commonly present in the third and fourth decades with a slight predominance in women. In retrospect, many patients can recall intermittent symptoms in childhood, often at times of stress, to which various labels may have been applied, e.g. bilious vomiting, grumbling appendix, abdominal migraine. This gives rise to the aphorism that 'little bellyachers grow into big ones'. Suggestive symptoms first presenting in the mid-forties onwards should be regarded more seriously, as possibly indicating organic disease. Many of these older patients will, nonetheless, be found to have sigmoid diverticular disease which has pathophysiological features in common with IBS. However, there is no convincing evidence that IBS of young adults progresses to diverticular disease in the middle-aged.

Surveys of the population which does not complain to doctors of the symptoms comprising IBS show that these are, nonetheless, commonly experienced; 30% of such a sample of 301 apparently healthy people had either abdominal pain, constipation or diarrhoea. When 2000 new attenders at a gastroenterology outpatient clinic in Bristol were prospectively studied over a five-year period, about half turned out to have functional disorders. It is interesting to contrast these patients with the remainder found to have organic disease, as many of the organic conditions have to be considered in the differential diagnosis of functional bowel disorders (Table 16.37).

Table 16.37 Organic vs functional disorders in a sample of 2000 gastroenterology outpatients*

Diagnosis	Number of patients
Definite non-organic	888
Spastic colon	449
Painless diarrhoea	107
Painless constipation	39
Depression and pain	50
Anxiety and GI symptoms	24
Functional dyspepsia	77
Others	59
Definite organic	980
Peptic ulcer	197
(Duodenal ulcer)	(135)
(Gastric ulcer)	(62)
Oesophagitis	188
Carcinoma of stomach	13
Postgastrectomy	14
Inflammatory bowel disease	168
(Crohn's disease)	(57)
(Ulcerative colitis)	(111)
Coeliac disease	26
Infective diarrhoea	21
Carcinoma of colon	28
Gallstones	48
Hepatitis	11
Cirrhosis	21
Alcoholism	16
Other	229

* After Harvey, Salih and Read 1983. Lancet 1: 632–634. The study was based on 2000 new attenders at a gastroenterology outpatient clinic over a period of five years. Of these, 57 had a non-gastroenterological diagnosis and 75 remained undiagnosed.

Aetiology

Many aetiological factors have been postulated for functional bowel disorders (Summary 10). Whether the bowel is inherently irritable or normal until irritated cannot be determined. Analogies might be drawn with duodenal ulcer where, though an individual may be born with a greater parietal cell mass of acid secretory cells than normal, he will only develop an ulcer if certain environmental factors supervene. No clear pattern of inheritance of functional bowel disorders has been demonstrated; while it may sometimes appear to be familial, this can probably be explained by the similar environmental factors.

> **Summary 10 Contributory factors in functional bowel disorders**
>
> - Motility disturbance
> - Altered sensory threshold
> - Previous gut infections
> - Altered gut flora
> - Dietary
>   Fibre
>   Food intolerance – Immunological ('allergy')
>   – Non-immunological
>   Food additives
> - Psychological
>   Anxiety
>   Depression

Motility disturbance

Hyper-reactivity of the gut, both in the sense of provoking reflex contraction and of a lowering of the threshold to stimuli causing pain, has been demonstrated in many ways, including balloon distension studies. Pressure transducer studies have shown that some patients have increased frequency and strength of small intestine motility. Apart from there being an inherent hyper-reactivity, various possible acquired causes may also be responsible for the condition.

Previous gut infection

The post-infective diarrhoeal variant of IBS may comprise up to a third of all patients. Damage to the epithelium by microorganisms, their toxins or bile acids may allow stimulation of mast cells or paracrine cells initiating the syndrome.

Dietary factors

Food intolerance is often suspected by patients. In different studies, its estimated frequency varies between 6% and 60%. Although exclusion diets, with recurrence of symptoms when the suspected food is reintroduced, would seem to support this possibility relatively few studies of double blind challenge have been undertaken. True allergy, in an immunological sense (using such criteria as a rapid reaction to small doses of antigen accompanied by raised IgE levels and positive skin prick tests), is exceedingly rare. The usually transient cows' milk intolerance of infants is the best-known example. Alternative non-immunological mechanisms have been postulated to account for some apparent reactions which require large amounts of the suspect food and come on so slowly that the offending food may not be recognised. Prostaglandin release or alterations in gut hormone profiles seem unlikely. It has recently been suggested that changes in gut flora to give high counts of facultative anaerobes (analogous to changes produced by antibiotic therapy) may enhance the production of toxic metabolites from undigested food residues.

Psychological

The psychosomatic mechanisms postulated seem to be borne out by the frequently found evidence of stress and anxiety. Nonetheless, attempts to modify autonomic nervous activity pharmacologically have met with limited success, perhaps in part because the less accessible enteric nervous reflexes may be at fault.

Much remains unexplained. It is not known what determines which of the various symptom patterns will develop in an individual patient, nor what makes some individuals accept the situation without recourse to orthodox, or even complementary, medical advice. A study screening consecutive non-complaining blood donors showed that the psychoneurotic symptomatology in the non-complaining IBS subjects more closely matched that of IBS patients than that of the remaining blood donors. It is not clear whether the differences between patients and the normal population are quantitative or qualitative.

Clinical features

The descriptive names given to functional bowel disorders indicate many of the symptoms – spastic colon, mucous colitis (in fact, a misnomer as the colon is not inflamed), and functional dyspepsia. Globus hystericus is difficulty with swallowing on a non-organic basis. Most patients will experience alteration of bowel habit, many will have pain and bloating, and distension and excess flatus are common in the predominant lower gastrointestinal IBS.

Pain after food, with nausea, distension, belching and regurgitation, in patients who have had negative gastroscopy and barium meal studies, are the hallmarks of functional dyspepsia, though the symptoms may overlap those of IBS. Unlike IBS, which does not progress to any other condition, up to 20% of patients with functional dyspepsia may subsequently develop demonstrable peptic ulceration or oesophagitis.

Pain

It has long been recognised that pain arising from the gut is not always localised to the midline. In addition to 'classical' subumbilical griping, pain in many other sites and radiations, sometimes extra-abdominal, can occur. This can lead to a wide differential diagnosis (Table 16.38). Although not feasible as a routine diagnostic procedure, it is useful to perform studies in which a balloon attached to a colonoscope is inflated at different sites as it is withdrawn from the caecum. This not only confirms that colonic distension can produce pain at both conventional and unconventional sites, but may also exactly reproduce a patient's pain. Severity and quality of pain may vary considerably, even mimicking biliary colic and other acute abdominal emergencies. Palpable and tender bowel in the left iliac fossa is a relatively non-specific finding, but evidence of spasm (by feeling transmitted pressure waves in the reservoir bulb on sigmoidoscopy) or reproduction of pain by the above procedure are particularly helpful in making a

Table 16.38 Differential diagnosis of typical and atypical IBS and functional dyspepsia

Functional bowel disorder	Differential diagnosis
Typical IBS	Inflammatory bowel disease (Crohn's > ulcerative colitis)
	Colorectal cancer
	Diverticular disease
	Infective diarrhoea
	Malabsorption (coeliac disease)
	Endocrinopathies
	Thyrotoxicosis
	Hypothyroidism
	Carcinoid syndrome
Atypical IBS	
Right iliac fossa pain	Appendicitis
Right hypochondrial pain	Gallstones
Left hypochondrial pain	Ischaemic heart disease
Back pain	Pancreatic disease
	Spinal osteoarthritis
Loin pain	Renal disease
Menstrual exacerbation	Endometriosis
Dyspareunia	Pelvic inflammatory disease
Functional dyspepsia	Peptic ulcer
	Oesophagitis
	Gastric cancer
	Ischaemic heart disease

positive diagnosis. Proctalgia fugax is a transient shooting pain in the rectum; the cause is unknown.

Constipation

Constipation may be the predominant presenting symptom in functional bowel disorders, but often alternates with diarrhoea and may be associated with pain. The stools may be pellet- or ribbon-like and be commonly associated with the passage of mucus. Rectal bleeding must always be fully investigated, even if only to confirm that it is due to haemorrhoids. Although some patients may have large amounts of dry stool in the rectum with little awareness of its presence there, others, despite not having a bowel action for several days, may have an empty rectum with greatly delayed colonic transit. Constipation dating back to childhood commonly emerges in the history, when 'potty training' may have been at fault, the urge to defaecate repeatedly ignored, and purgatives regularly administered. Melanosis coli (the deposition of dark pigment in the submucosa due to prolonged use of anthracene derivatives) may rarely be seen on sigmoidoscopy.

Diarrhoea

Diarrhoea is often a distressing symptom because of the uncertainty and anxiety which it may generate in an already anxious patient. The fear of faecal incontinence is a real one and, as the diarrhoea frequently occurs mainly during the morning, the journey to work may be dreaded. The stool may vary between liquid and semi-formed. There is often much flatus and another uncertainty is thus whether the urge to pass wind may result in passage of diarrhoea and consequent soiling. The patient may be greatly relieved to be asked about this as he may be too embarrassed to volunteer the symptom. A sense of wanting to evacuate when there is nothing there (tenesmus) or of incomplete defaecation is also particularly common. Although the patient may think large amounts are being passed, stool weights are in fact within the normal range. Diarrhoea occurs less commonly at other times of the day and, unlike inflammatory bowel disease or other organic diarrhoeas, does not usually disturb sleep. Rumbling and gurgling (borborygmi) accompany diarrhoea and flatus.

Dyspepsia

Functional dyspepsia may predominantly cause pain (mimicking an ulcer or oesophagitis), distension, flatulence with belching, and nausea. The symptoms are more clearly related to eating than in IBS. An important differential diagnosis is oesophageal reflux, which may occur without a hiatus hernia or endoscopic evidence of oesophagitis. If oesophageal reflux is suspected, 24-hour oesophageal pH monitoring can be performed. If there is a good correlation between episodes of reflux and the patients having symptoms, the problem is not functional and the reflux should be treated (p. 567).

Other symptoms

Other associated, non-specific symptoms may confuse the diagnosis. Sweating, tremor, hyper-reflexia and tachycardia in association with diarrhoea are usually due to anxiety rather than thyrotoxicosis; a marked sinus arrhythmia, indicating autonomic overactivity, is frequently present.

Psychological symptoms are common, and underlying stress and disorders of mood and personality are frequently invoked as major factors in pathogenesis. Nonetheless, the results of formal studies have often been conflicting. The perennial problem of whether anxiety provokes symptoms or vice-versa cannot be clearly resolved, although the vicious circle of symptoms – anxiety – more symptoms – more anxiety, is real enough. Although depression may present with predominantly functional bowel symptoms (which regress with antidepressants), this is not as common as was once thought. Even if there were initially other reasons for a patient's anxiety, the symptoms frequently reinforce it. An important part in history-taking is to ask the patient what she considers the cause to be. Frequently, a fear of cancer, which the patient was reluctant to voice, will be revealed. Many will also be worried about inflammatory bowel disease, a worry perhaps reinforced by a previous vague diagnosis of mucous colitis, or peptic ulcer.

Prognosis

Morbidity from functional bowel disorders can be considerable. There have been few long-term studies, but in one such study, of 77 of 91 patients recalled after six years, 29 had no bowel problems and many of the 44 who still had IBS symptoms found the condition easier to cope with. In view of the difficulties in making a positive diagnosis, it is of note that only four patients had had a new diagnosis made, invariably prompted by a change in the clinical picture.

Investigation and treatment

The first problem that arises in the management of functional bowel disorder is the confidence with which one can make the diagnosis and the extent to which further investigation should be undertaken. The need for a full history and examination (including sigmoidoscopy) is self-evident; the history may be further supplemented at the follow-up appointment, which should be given to every patient. Many important psychological and social factors may then be disclosed to a doctor who has earned the patient's confidence. All investigations should be ordered at the first visit and the patient told that they are expected to be normal. To go on asking for 'just another test' counters the essential reassurance given by the doctor. In hospital practice, the stool should be examined for pathogens and parasites if the history is of recent diarrhoea, especially after foreign travel. A barium enema or colonoscopy, to exclude other colonic disease, is not necessary in all patients, particularly if they are young with typical symptoms. Sometimes, however, the patient will require this investigation for complete reassurance.

The less typical the clinical presentation the more the exclusion of other diseases may be necessary, but a positive diagnosis should be made rather than one arrived at purely by exclusion.

Such a minimalist approach is therapeutically effective and safe with the proviso that fuller investigation or even re-investigation is undertaken under the following circumstances:

1. patients over 40 years of age presenting with symptoms for the first time
2. any change in the pattern of symptoms or development of new symptoms which sound organic
3. presence of additional symptoms which are not part of IBS, such as weight loss, rectal bleeding or fever.

At the end of the first consultation, the physician should be able to make a positive diagnosis and suggest an explanation for the cause of the symptoms. Even if the symptoms are bizarre, their existence should not be questioned. He should ask the patient what he feared might be the cause and be able to reassure him, pointing out how common the problem is and the generally good prognosis.

After identifying any provocative factors, the doctor should suggest modifications in the patient's life style that might be beneficial. The constipated may need to increase dietary fibre and also ensure an adequate daily fluid intake. Smoking and excess alcohol consumption should be stopped and the effects of other medications reviewed. At a subsequent interview, the results of normal tests can be used to reinforce the fact that there is no serious underlying cause for the symptoms.

Medication

Drugs play only a minor role in management. They should be props for intermittent rather than continual usage, except when stool bulking agents are necessary to supplement dietary fibre because the patient cannot cope with a change in diet.

When properly conducted, all drug trials in IBS and functional dyspepsia have shown very high rates of response to placebo (often over 50%).

Antispasmodics. Anticholinergic drugs may relieve pain but are limited in dosage by their side-effects. Buscopan, though effective intravenously, is too unreliable in its absorption to be used orally. The directly acting smooth muscle relaxant mebeverine is widely used and, in some studies, has been shown to be superior to placebo. An old remedy, peppermint oil, in a new colonic release capsule is probably as effective.

Antidiarrhoeals. Disabling morning diarrhoea can be treated with codeine phosphate on rising and repeated if necessary. If not effective, loperamide can be substituted. Constipation should be avoided.

Laxatives and purgatives. Only bulking agents should be encouraged. Many constipated patients may have been using purgatives for many years and these should be stopped, despite the fears and reluctance of patients to abandon them. Simple suppositories, or even periodic enemas, may have to be given temporarily while attempts are made to re-educate the bowel.

Psychotropics. Long-term use of benzodiazepine or other tranquillisers must be avoided, but they may be necessary as a short-term measure to combat periods of stress. Antidepressants, usually given at night, should also only be considered if there are clear depressive symptoms.

Antinauseants. The post-prandial distension and nausea of functional dyspepsia is often greatly helped by metoclopramide syrup or tablets before meals. If ineffective, or if the drug is not tolerated because of somnolence or dyskinetic movements, domperidone or cisapride should be substituted.

SELF-INDUCED BOWEL DISEASE

Self-induced bowel disease may be a variant of the Munchausen syndrome, where patients deliberately invent symptoms (p. 201), or be a result of drug abuse. Both problems are rare. They tend to occur in young female patients. The diagnosis is often well disguised.

Invention of symptoms

The patient who is inventing symptoms most commonly presents with severe abdominal pain or with gastrointestinal bleeding (sometimes fictitious and sometimes simulated by the ingestion of animal blood). The history may be convincing but background information is vague. Examination often reveals an abdomen with multiple scars from when previous surgeons have been misled in the past. If this diagnosis is suspected, investigations should be minimal and the treatment is observation and reassurance. Psychiatric support rarely helps.

Drug abuse

The patient abusing drugs usually presents with profuse watery diarrhoea secondary to purgative abuse. There may be several litres of watery diarrhoea a day with consequent weight loss, dehydration and hypokalaemia. The diagnosis may be suggested by the appearance of pigment deposition in the rectal mucosa at sigmoidoscopy (melanosis coli). It may be confirmed by demonstrating by chemical analysis that purgatives are present in the faeces or urine, or by finding the patient surreptitiously taking them. Confrontation should be avoided, and treatment offered in conjunction with a psychiatrist.

THE PANCREAS

The pancreas is a retroperitoneal organ which, along with the common bile duct, drains through the medial wall of the second part of the duodenum.

The pancreas has exocrine and endocrine functions. Duodenal release of the hormone secretin results in acinar bicarbonate secretion. The pancreatic enzymes trypsin and chymotrypsin break down proteins, lipase digests fats, and amylase acts on starch. These enzymes are released in response to cholecystokinin and activity of the parasympathetic nervous system. The endocrine cells of the pancreas are localised to the islets of Langerhans and make up about 1% by volume of the pancreas. The most numerous endocrine cells are the beta cells secreting insulin but also present are alpha cells secreting pancreatic glucagon, D cells secreting somatostatin and PP cells secreting pancreatic polypeptide. When there is damage to the pancreas (for example chronic pancreatitis), exocrine function is usually lost before endocrine function.

Clinical features of pancreatic disease

The symptoms of pancreatic disease include pain (severe, epigastric or central abdominal, and often radiating to the back), steatorrhoea (indicating lipase deficiency), weight loss, nausea, vomiting and those of hyperglycaemia. Patients with acute pancreatitis may present with an acute abdomen with peritonism and absent bowel sounds. Other features of pancreatic disease include anaemia, jaundice due to common bile duct obstruction or associated liver disease, an abdominal mass, ascites and a pleural effusion (usually left-sided).

Investigation of pancreatic disease

The investigations of pancreatic disease are listed in Summary 11.

Summary 11 Investigations of pancreatic disease

General

Full blood count
Liver function tests and proteins
Serum amylase
Blood glucose
Serum B$_{12}$
Three-day faecal fats

Tube pancreatic function tests

Cholecystokinin-secretin test
Lundh meal

Tubeless pancreatic function tests

PABA test
Fluorescein dilaurate test

Imaging techniques

Plain abdominal X-ray
Ultrasound
CT scan
ERCP

General

A full blood count is done primarily to look for an anaemia and for the white cell count (high in acute pancreatitis and abscesses etc., low in the Shwachman syndrome; see p. 615). A serum amylase is only indicated if the diagnosis of acute pancreatitis or continuing pancreatic obstruction due to an abscess or pseudocyst is being considered. If there is doubt about the significance of a serum amylase result, plasma chromatography can detect macroamylasaemia; alternatively, the urinary creatinine:amylase ratio can be used, to assess how much normal molecular weight amylase is being excreted. Blood glucose estimations are performed to assess the presence and severity of diabetes due to beta cell loss. The pancreas produces a protease essential for the binding of vitamin B$_{12}$ to intrinsic factor, and a deficiency of this enzyme may result in megaloblastic anaemia. Three-day faecal fats are useful to assess the degree of steatorrhoea, and very high levels (more than 100 g fat per day) may be seen with pancreatic insufficiency.

Tube pancreatic function tests

Tube pancreatic function tests involve the passage of a thin catheter into the second part of the duodenum. The duodenal contents are then aspirated for measurement of bicarbonate and pancreatic enzymes, after a pharmacological dose of intravenous cholecystokinin and secretin, or a Lundh test meal which consists of a 500 ml mixture of fat, protein and carbohydrate.

Tubeless pancreatic function tests

Tube tests are uncomfortable for patients and oral tests (Fig. 16.29) are fortunately now available. In the PABA test, pancreatic chymotrypsin cleaves N-benzoyl-L tyrosyl-p-amino-benzoic acid; the resulting para-amino-benzoic acid (PABA) is absorbed and the urinary PABA is measured in a six-hour collection. To assess possible intestinal malabsorption, a trace dose of ^{14}C-PABA is given at the same time and urinary radioactivity measured. The test is invalidated by paracetamol and cotrimoxazole and is dependent on normal gastric emptying and renal function. A similar test involves the cleavage of fluorescein dilaurate by pancreatic esterase, and subsequent measurement of urinary fluorescein.

Fig. 16.29 Tubeless pancreatic function tests. A. The PABA test involves chymotrypsin cleavage of N-benzoyl-L-tyrosyl and the subsequent measurement of PABA in urine or plasma. **B.** The fluorescein test involves esterase cleavage and the subsequent measurement of fluorescein in urine. If either test is abnormal, the basic chemical (i.e. PABA and fluorescein) should be given on a separate day to exclude a problem with intestinal malabsorption.

Imaging techniques

The pancreas is relatively difficult to image because of its retroperitoneal location. The plain abdominal X-ray is usually unhelpful, but pancreatic calcification may be seen with chronic pancreatitis and a 'sentinel loop' of dilated small intestine may be seen over the pancreas in acute pancreatitis. An ultrasound or CT scan is potentially very useful in delineating abnormal anatomy and can be used to direct needle biopsies. Endoscopic retrograde pancreatography (ERP) is usually combined with cholangiography (ERCP). These techniques involve cannulating the ampulla of Vater and injecting X-ray contrast under screening into the pancreatic and bile ducts. ERP is particularly useful in demonstrating abnormalities due to chronic pancreatitis or carcinoma.

CONGENITAL PANCREATIC ANATOMICAL ABNORMALITIES

The pancreas is subject to several congenital disorders. Embryologically, it is derived from an anterior and a posterior bud which normally fuse and drain into the medial wall of the duodenum. The developmental abnormalities include:

1. *Accessory pancreatic tissue*, which is separate from the body of the pancreas. This is found in about 10% of autopsies, with ectopic tissue most commonly located in the wall of the stomach and intestine. Rarely, it may ulcerate and cause gastrointestinal bleeding or be the site of carcinomatous change.
2. *Annular pancreas*, where the second part of the duodenum is encircled by pancreatic tissue. This is a rare abnormality which usually presents in the first months of life with duodenal obstruction; it requires a bypass gastrojejunostomy. Mild cases are asymptomatic, but the condition may present for the first time in adults with abdominal pain and vomiting, sometimes associated with peptic ulcer or obstructive jaundice.
3. *Pancreas divisum*, due to failure of the two pancreatic ducts to fuse. The majority of the gland is drained through the accessory ampulla. It is associated with an increased incidence of acute pancreatitis. Sphincterotomy of the accessory ampulla may reduce the number of attacks.

CONGENITAL PANCREATIC FUNCTIONAL ABNORMALITIES

Cystic fibrosis

Cystic fibrosis is the most important congenital disease of the pancreas. It also affects the lungs and is inherited as an autosomal recessive; the abnormal gene is in the middle of the long arm of chromosome 7. Cystic fibrosis is most common in Caucasians, where it has an asymptomatic heterozygote gene frequency of one in 20; one in 2000 live births are homozygotes. In the past, most homozygote children died before the age of 10 but, with improving care, many children are now surviving to adulthood. The pancreatic and intestinal effects of the disease are summarised in Table 16.39. Other complications include cirrhosis of the liver (Ch. 17), pulmonary disease (Ch. 14) and male infertility due to atrophy or absence of the vas deferens, seminal vesicles and epididymis.

Cystic fibrosis is characterised by high sweat sodium and chloride concentrations and hyperviscous secretions, containing mucus and protein, from exocrine glands. The high sweat sodium and chloride is used as a diagnostic test. The hyperviscous secretions result in plugging of ducts and bronchi, leading to destruction of glandular tissue and bronchiectasis (Table 16.39).

Table 16.39 Pancreatic and intestinal complications of cystic fibrosis

Effect	Complication
Pancreatic insufficiency	Enzyme deficiency Diabetes mellitus
Meconium ileus	Intestinal obstruction Volvulus Peritonitis following perforation Polyhydramnios in utero
Meconium ileus equivalent	Intussusception Intestinal obstruction

Pancreatic insufficiency

The destruction of pancreatic exocrine acini is often rapid. The patient develops steatorrhoea and oedema secondary to hypoproteinaemia. A good response is seen with the introduction of pancreatic enzyme supplements taken with each meal, and H_2-receptor antagonists can help by raising duodenal pH to increase pancreatic enzyme activity. Supplements of vitamins A, D, E and K also have a role in the presence of steatorrhoea. With severe malnutrition, dietary supplements of easily absorbed mid-chain triglycerides and protein hydrolysates in the form of milk-shakes or cooking additives may be helpful.

Diabetes mellitus due to destruction of pancreatic endocrine tissue is a late event.

Meconium ileus

In cystic fibrosis, the meconium protein content at birth is about eight times the normal level. As a result, neonates with cystic fibrosis often present with intestinal obstruction and this may be complicated by a volvulus or peritonitis due to a perforation. Treatment is with instillation of high osmolarity diatrizoate (e.g. Gastrografin) which causes shrinkage of the plug and allows its passage down the gut. If a perforation or volvulus has occurred, surgery is usually needed. Maternal polyhydramnios is due to fetal meconium ileus *in utero*.

Meconium ileus equivalent

'Meconium ileus equivalent' is, as the name suggests, a problem similar to meconium ileus, but it occurs later in life and is complicated by the presence of faeces. A high fibre diet to soften the stool, and laxatives are effective in mild cases. N-acetylcysteine can be used as a mucus-clearing agent. In severe cases, diatrizoate is usually effective in shrinking the faecal mass; surgery should be avoided if possible, because of the high mortality from intestinal and pulmonary complications.

Prognosis

The prognosis is variable, but many affected children are now surviving into their twenties and thirties. Patients may rarely present as young adults. Infertility is not always present. Males tend to survive longer than females.

Macroamylasaemia

Macroamylasaemia is a condition of unknown aetiology characterised by large molecular weight amylase in the serum. It accounts for 2.6% of elevated serum amylase levels. The amylase may be bound to immunoglobulins or glycoproteins and is too large to be excreted by the glomerulus like normal amylase. Consequently, very high serum amylase levels occur. The diagnosis can be confirmed by chromatography and by showing low urinary amylase and normal plasma trypsin and lipase levels. It is important to make the diagnosis to avoid mistaking the condition for acute pancreatitis.

No treatment is needed for macroamylasaemia. The patient should be reassured and the problem explained so that he can inform future medical attendants.

Shwachman syndrome

Shwachman syndrome is the association of pancreatic enzyme deficiency, neutropenia, short stature, and metaphyseal dysostosis. Sometimes there is also an anaemia, thrombocytopenia and low intelligence. It is inherited as an autosomal recessive. The usual presentation is steatorrhoea and failure to thrive; a normal sweat sodium and chloride excludes cystic fibrosis.

Treatment is of the pancreatic insufficiency with pancreatic enzyme supplements and possibly H_2-receptor antagonists. Infections should be treated aggressively in the presence of the neutropenia, which is associated with a deficiency of white cell precursors. The prognosis is usually good.

ACUTE PANCREATITIS

Acute pancreatitis is an acute inflammatory condition of the pancreas which results in necrosis of exocrine tissue. It causes abdominal pain and is associated with high plasma and urinary pancreatic enzyme levels.

The incidence is 10 per 100 000 per annum in the UK and North America and 28.1 per 100 000 in people over the age of 20 in Copenhagen in 1979–80. The median age is 53 years, with an equal incidence in males and females.

Aetiology

Summary 12 shows the aetiological factors. Pancreatitis occurs as a result of pancreatic duct obstruction, bile and duodenal content reflux and direct action of toxins. In the UK, about 80% of cases are due to gallstones or alcohol abuse. In some parts of the world (e.g. South America), alcohol abuse is the most important factor. Gallstones are thought to block pancreatic enzyme outflow, but may be passed via the ampulla of Vater before investigations are undertaken. In this situation, further gallstones are usually found in the gallbladder or in the common bile duct. The

16

Summary 12 Aetiology of acute pancreatitis

- Gallstones in common bile duct
- Alcoholism
- Iatrogenic – usually post-ERCP
- Trauma
- Viral – mumps and coxsackie B
- Pancreatic tumours
- Drugs, e.g. corticosteroids, oral contraceptives, thiazide diuretics
- Possibly hyperlipoproteinaemia and primary hyperparathyroidism
- Idiopathic

Table 16.40   Complications of acute pancreatitis

Early complications

Clinical	Biochemical
Cardiac failure	Uraemia
Renal failure	Hypocalcaemia
Respiratory failure (ARDS)	Hypoalbuminaemia
Hyperglycaemia	Abnormal liver function
Anaemia	Hyperglycaemia
Jaundice	Metabolic acidosis
Disseminated intravascular coagulation	Hypoxaemia

Late complications
Pseudocyst
Abscess
Pancreatic duct stricture
Ascites/pleural effusion
Diabetes mellitus

---

mechanism by which alcohol causes acute pancreatitis is controversial. It may be due to a rise in pancreatic duct pressure or to a direct action of alcohol on the acinar cell membranes.

Endoscopic retrograde pancreatography may cause acute pancreatitis, possibly as a result of increased pressure in the pancreatic duct. Exploratory laparotomy, other intra-abdominal operations and translumbar aortography may also be complicated by acute pancreatitis. Patients with a Polya gastrectomy with a 'blind' duodenal loop are at increased long-term risk. Acute pancreatitis due to viral infection is rare, and is caused by viral destruction of acinar cells. Pancreatic tumours may cause pancreatitis by ductular obstruction. Many drugs have been reported as possible causes. It is often stated that types I, IV and V hyperlipoproteinaemia and hypercalcaemia (usually due to primary hyperparathyroidism) are causes of acute pancreatitis; however, recent studies have suggested that the association is doubtful.

Clinical features

The main symptom of acute pancreatitis is severe abdominal pain. Its usual site is epigastric or hypochondrial, but it may occur around the umbilicus. In about half the patients, it radiates to the lower thoracic and upper lumbar area of the back. The onset is usually sudden, such that the main differential diagnosis is intestinal perforation. The pain settles within 48 hours in most patients. The other common initial symptom is vomiting.

Examination reveals a patient in great pain with severe abdominal tenderness and often guarding and rigidity. Bowel sounds are usually reduced. Extra-abdominal signs may include a tachycardia and hypotension. In severe cases, signs of the complications of acute pancreatitis may be present (Table 16.40).

Investigation

The diagnosis is made by finding a serum amylase at least four times the upper limit of normal. A smaller rise in serum amylase may be seen in patients with perforated ulcers, intestinal obstruction, other intra-abdominal

emergencies, diabetic ketoacidosis, after opiate analgesia, and in macroamylasaemia and renal and hepatic failure. If the serum amylase is less than four times the upper limit of normal, or if it is thought that the high amylase may be due to macroamylasaemia, a high amylase:creatinine urinary excretion, serum lipase and serum trypsin may be used as confirmatory evidence of acute pancreatitis. A plain abdominal X-ray may show a 'sentinel loop' of air-filled small intestine lying over the pancreas. It may also show evidence of ascites or intestinal ileus, which may complicate acute pancreatitis. Ultrasound and CT scanning may demonstrate an oedematous enlarged gland, gallstones and complications such as pseudocysts.

The differential diagnosis of acute pancreatitis includes gastric or intestinal perforation, peptic ulcer disease, acute cholecystitis, intestinal obstruction, acute mesenteric ischaemia, ruptured aortic aneurysm and myocardial infarction.

Treatment

Acute pancreatitis may have a self-limiting short course, be associated with the development of late complications or be very severe and result in early death from circulatory collapse. In order to predict severity and prognosis, a number of parameters are helpful (Table 16.41); if more than three of these indicators are present, the acute pancreatitis is severe and there is a significant risk of early death or complications.

Initial treatment is to restore fluid and electrolytes by intravenous infusion. A central venous pressure line is helpful to monitor fluid replacement. Analgesia should be maintained with pethidine or buprenorphine; morphine is contraindicated because it causes spasm of the sphincter of Oddi. A sedative such as diazepam may be helpful. Nasogastric suction is indicated initially, and should be continued until there is evidence that gastric emptying is normal and there is no intestinal ileus. Neither drugs such as cimetidine, anticholinergics, aprotinin (a trypsin and

Table 16.41   Indicators of severe acute pancreatitis

- White blood cell count over $15 \times 10^9/l$
- Glucose over 10 mmol/l
- Urea over 16 mmol/l
- Pa_{O_2} below 8.0 kPa
- Calcium below 2.0 mmol/l
- Albumin below 32 g/l
- LDH over 600 units/l
- SGOT over 100 units/l
- Over 55 years of age

kinin inhibitor), antibiotics and calcitonin, nor parenteral nutrition have been shown to have overall benefit when subjected to clinical trial.

Complications of acute pancreatitis

More than one complication (Table 16.40) may be present in an individual patient. The treatment of these severe problems is supportive (usually in an intensive care unit) with fluids, cardiac inotropes, oxygen, ventilation, dialysis, calcium and insulin as necessary. Pseudocysts are collections of pancreatic juice in the lesser sac, and may need surgical drainage into the stomach. Pancreatic abscesses are usually due to *E. coli* infection and require surgical drainage and antibiotics. Ascites and pleural effusions due to a fistula from the pancreatic duct system into the peritoneal or pleural spaces are characterised by very high amylase concentrations in the fluid aspirate. The effusions can often be treated with drainage via a cannula, but sometimes surgical closure is required. Diabetes mellitus varies in severity and may be controlled by diet alone, oral hypoglycaemic drugs or insulin.

The overall mortality rate is about 10% per attack; this rises with age and other parameters of severity. The mortality of initial attacks is more than ten times higher than that of recurrent attacks, and is twice as high with gallstones compared to that with alcoholism. The recurrence rate is greatly reduced by successful treatment of gallstones or alcoholism.

CHRONIC PANCREATITIS

Chronic pancreatitis is associated with destruction of pancreatic exocrine tissue which persists even when the underlying cause has been removed. Inflammation is followed by fibrosis and atrophy. Chronic relapsing pancreatitis is a variant in which symptoms such as pain, nausea and vomiting are intermittent. The disease may be further classified according to its aetiology and whether steatorrhoea or diabetes mellitus is present. Steatorrhoea implies loss of lipase due to advanced acinar damage; diabetes mellitus indicates severe loss of islet tissue and advanced disease.

In 1978–79 the prevalence of chronic pancreatitis in Copenhagen was 27.4 per 100 000 adult population per year. There was a 3:1 male preponderance. The median age at onset was 39. The annual incidence in Minnesota in 1960–69 was 3.5 per 100 000 population. The incidence rises in areas with high alcohol intakes.

Aetiology

The aetiology of chronic pancreatitis is shown in Summary 13. Alcohol is by far the most important factor in those cases where a cause can be identified. Protein precipitates have been found in the pancreatic juice of alcoholics with chronic pancreatitis, and it is suggested that these form plugs which block the small pancreatic ducts and cause acinar damage. Gallstones are a common cause of acute pancreatitis but a rare cause of the chronic form.

In the hereditary form of chronic pancreatitis, the children in affected families usually present in adolescence. It is inherited as an autosomal dominant but penetrance is variable. Pancreas divisum, which occurs when the ventral and dorsal embryological buds do not join, is a rare cause of chronic pancreatitis, as are hyperlipidaemia and hypercalcaemia. The disease may also occur in primary biliary cirrhosis, sclerosing cholangitis and with choledochal cysts. In a significant number of patients no cause can be found.

Summary 13   Aetiology of chronic pancreatitis

- Alcohol
- Gallstones
- Hereditary
- Pancreas divisum
- Hyperlipidaemia
- Hypercalcaemia
- Idiopathic

Clinical features

The main symptom of chronic pancreatitis is upper abdominal pain. This is usually severe, chronic and often debilitating although, in about 10% of patients, pain is not a feature. Radiation to the lower thoracic and upper lumbar spine is common and sometimes the pain can be relieved by leaning forward. It may be exacerbated by eating. Anorexia, nausea and vomiting may be prominent. Steatorrhoea occurs with very high faecal fat output, and is associated with weight loss despite a good appetite. After eight years of symptoms, about 70% of patients have steatorrhoea. If there is gross steatorrhoea, deficiencies of vitamins A, D, E and K may occur. The pancreas secretes a protease which is important for absorption of vitamin B_{12}, and a B_{12} deficiency anaemia may therefore rarely occur. Oesophageal and gastric varices may be present as a result of coexistent alcoholic cirrhosis, or of thrombosis of the portal or splenic vein as a direct complication of pancreatitis. Gastric outflow obstruction due to swelling of the pancreatic head or a pseudocyst, and pancreatic ascites due to a fistula from the pancreatic duct to the peritoneum, occasionally occur. About a third of patients develop the symptoms of diabetes mellitus.

Investigation

The investigations for chronic pancreatitis are shown in Summary 14.

Summary 14   Investigations for chronic pancreatitis

Biochemical

Faecal fat estimation and other tests for malabsorption
Secretin-cholecystokinin test
Lundh test
PABA test
Liver function tests
Blood glucose
Serum amylase (only useful in acute attacks)

Radiological

Plain abdominal X-ray
Ultrasound, possibly CT scanning
Endoscopic retrograde pancreatography (ERCP)

Biochemical

Serum amylase levels are high in acute or recurrent acute pancreatitis but not in chronic pancreatitis. Although faecal fat excretion may be very high (more than 100 g/24 hours), this is not diagnostic of pancreatic disease, as amounts approaching this level may be seen in patients with small bowel disease.

Low pancreatic enzyme and bicarbonate outputs can be measured by aspirating a nasoduodenal tube in the second part of duodenum after secretin and cholecystokinin, or after a standardised test (Lundh) meal. The PABA test has been used to circumvent the use of nasoduodenal tubes; in this test patients are given para-amino-benzoic acid (PABA) bound to N-benzoyl-L-tyrosyl which requires chymotrypsin for cleavage of the bond. If chymotrypsin is present, the PABA is liberated, absorbed by the small intestine and excreted in the urine. Low levels indicate chymotrypsin (and usually other pancreatic enzyme) deficiency (p. 614).

Mild abnormalities of liver function tests are common. Rarely, the head of the pancreas may swell and cause an obstruction to the lower end of the common bile duct; this results in jaundice and cholestatic liver function tests.

Radiological

A plain abdominal X-ray may show pancreatic calcification (Fig. 16.30A). Ultrasound and CT scanning may show swelling and dilatation of the main pancreatic duct. The diagnostic investigation of choice in chronic pancreatitis is endoscopic retrograde pancreatography (Fig. 16.30B).

A

B

Fig. 16.30   Chronic pancreatitis. A. Plain X-ray showing pancreatic calcification. **B.** ERCP in chronic pancreatitis showing a dilated main pancreatic duct with associated dilated side branches.

Treatment

The treatment of chronic pancreatitis is summarised in Summary 15. It is important to treat the underlying cause, although this may not prevent progression and pain and is

Summary 15   Treatment of chronic pancreatitis

- Treatment of aetiological problem. No alcohol.

- *Pain* – Aspirin/NSAIDs/paracetamol
  - Codeine/pethidine/buprenorphine
  - Splanchnic nerve block
  - Methadone

- *Steatorrhoea* – Low fat/high carbohydrate diet
  - Enzyme supplements
  - H$_2$-receptor antagonists
  - MCTs/fat-soluble vitamins

- *Diabetes mellitus* – Diet
  - Oral hypoglycaemics
  - Insulin

- *Metabolic complications* – Protein supplements
  - Vitamin B$_{12}$

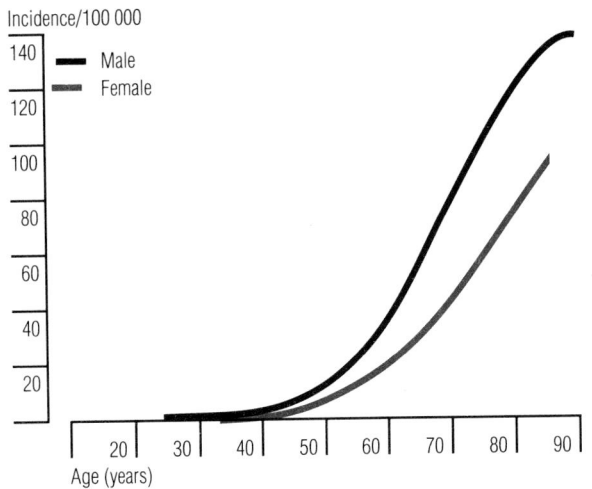

Fig. 16.31   Age-specific incidence of pancreatic carcinoma per 100 000 population in the UK. It is commoner in males and the incidence increases with age.

not always possible (e.g. alcoholics often continue drinking). Mild analgesia is rarely effective. Codeine, pethidine or buprenorphine may control pain, and destruction of the splanchnic nerve with injection of 100% alcohol may give relief. A minority of patients require regular methadone.

Steatorrhoea and the resulting malnutrition may be helped by a low fat and high carbohydrate diet. Pancreatic enzyme supplements should be taken with food. H$_2$-receptor antagonists raise the intraduodenal pH which is otherwise pathologically low due to lack of bicarbonate. Food may be cooked in, or be supplemented by, mid-chain triglycerides (MCTs) as these can be absorbed directly without lipolysis. Supplements of vitamins A, D, E and K should be prescribed as necessary.

Diabetes mellitus requires standard treatment. A particular problem is variable absorption of carbohydrate due to exocrine deficiency or after surgical procedures, as this may result in poor control of blood glucose ('brittle diabetes'). Protein supplements may help raise plasma proteins, and parenteral vitamin B$_{12}$ is occasionally required.

Prognosis

The prognosis, if not the quality of life, of patients with chronic pancreatitis is generally good. Patients rarely die directly of the complications and most survive 20 years from the onset. In some cases, the pain settles spontaneously; this may reflect 'burning out' of the pancreas and be complicated by steatorrhoea and diabetes. Sometimes, patients whose pain is poorly controlled become dependent on narcotics or, occasionally, commit suicide.

TUMOURS OF THE EXOCRINE PANCREAS

The commonest pancreatic tumour is carcinoma of the exocrine pancreas; this is a major cause of mortality in the Western World. (Tumours of the endocrine pancreas (p. 620) are rare, but of considerable interest because of the range of hormones they secrete.) The overall incidence

of carcinoma of the pancreas is about 10 per 100 000 per year, but this rises to 100 per 100 000 in those over 65 years of age (Fig. 16.31). It accounts for 5.5% of cancer deaths and is the fourth most common cause of such deaths in men. The incidence is rising throughout the world, with particularly high rates seen in American Negroes and New Zealand Maoris.

Aetiology and pathology

The aetiology is unknown. The disease is twice as common in cigarette smokers and in patients with diabetes mellitus; chemists and non-oven coke workers also have an increased incidence. There is no definite association with alcoholism, coffee drinking or acute or chronic pancreatitis (except of the rare familial chronic type). However, there may be an increased incidence in chronic calcific pancreatitis.

In those cases where a histological diagnosis is established, the tumour is almost always an adenocarcinoma. The carcinoma arises from the ductular epithelium and may be mucin-producing. About 5% of tumours arise from the acinar cells and, rarely, sarcomas may occur. The tumour metastasises to local lymph nodes adjacent to the vascular supply and, by invasion of blood vessels, to the liver and distant sites. Sixty-five per cent of tumours occur in the head of the pancreas, 30% in the body and 5% in the tail. The tumour infiltrates locally into the duodenum and the retroperitoneal space. It may involve the portal vein, causing thrombosis and splenomegaly, and may also seed into the peritoneal cavity causing ascites.

Clinical features

Symptoms tend to occur late, and are often non-specific (Summary 16). Consequently, there may be a delay in diagnosis, and the majority of patients already have inoperable

16

large tumours and/or metastases by the time the diagnosis is made. Jaundice and pruritus indicate obstruction to the common bile duct or multiple hepatic metastases. Vomiting may be due to gastric or duodenal invasion or peritoneal metastases. Haematemesis and melaena may also occur as a result of invasion of the stomach or intestine. Steatorrhoea may occur as a result of bile duct obstruction. Hepatomegaly and/or jaundice are found in the majority of patients at presentation, and the coexistence of a palpable distended gallbladder suggests the presence of a carcinoma obstructing the lower end of the common bile duct (Courvoisier's sign). This is, however, an unreliable sign as it can also occur with cholelithiasis and is often absent with pancreatic cancer. Thrombophlebitis at remote sites, or deep venous thrombosis, occur in about 10% of patients as a paraneoplastic syndrome (Ch. 9, p. 146).

Investigation

A full blood count and liver enzyme tests may show anaemia and an obstructive jaundice, but these are non-specific and do not help make the diagnosis. In experienced hands, ultrasonography can be diagnostic; it also allows the passage of an ultrasound-directed thin needle to aspirate cells from the tumour for cytology. CT scanning (Fig. 16.32) has an equal or greater accuracy and is of great

Fig. 16.32 CT scan of abdomen demonstrating a dilated gallbladder (filled with contrast following an ERCP) and a large tumour mass in the head of the pancreas (arrowed).

help if ultrasound is negative or equivocal. Endoscopy may allow a direct view and biopsy of ampullary lesions, while ERCP often demonstrates main duct lesions and gives information about the biliary tree. In the case of ductular lesions, pancreatic juice may be aspirated for cytology. Laparoscopy and biopsy under direct vision are helpful in some difficult cases. Hepatic metastases and portal vein thrombosis are contraindications for surgery. Plasma tumour markers, such as carcinoembryonic antigen, are of little value in diagnosis or for the detection of recurrence.

Treatment

The surgical treatment of carcinoma of the pancreas is very unsatisfactory due to the organ's inaccessibility, the frequency of local spread and metastases. Radical surgery may be performed for localised tumours, especially of the ampulla, and a small number of patients are cured. However, even in operable cases, the five-year survival is less than 15%. If there is obstruction to the common bile duct, a palliative bypass procedure relieves jaundice and pruritus.

For most patients with carcinoma of the pancreas, treatment is directed to symptomatic relief. Palliation of pain can be achieved by radiotherapy. The dose required with external beam irradiation is high (55 Gy) and interstitial implants of ^{125}I can also produce satisfactory palliation. Analgesics and coeliac plexus block may be needed. There are few cytotoxic drugs which are effective in pancreatic carcinoma, although responses are sometimes seen with the alkylating agents, nitrosoureas and 5-fluorouracil. If a blocked bile duct is causing jaundice and itching, a stent should be used to bypass the obstruction; this may be done from below via an endoscope, or from above by the percutaneous trans-hepatic route. Use of these techniques reduces the need for laparotomy and surgical bypass (e.g. cholecystojejunostomy).

PANCREATIC ENDOCRINE TUMOURS

The pancreas is the primary site for a number of rare functioning endocrine tumours (Table 16.42) which produce characteristic syndromes. These tumours are important, because surgical cure by resection may be possible. The symptoms caused can be predicted by the known physiological action of the hormone produced, the exception to this being pancreatic polypeptide which is secreted by many of these tumours and can be used as a tumour marker. Multiple Endocrine Adenomatosis Type I (MEA Type I, or Wermer's syndrome) is inherited on an autosomal dominant basis, and is the association of hormone-synthesising parathyroid adenomas (parathyroid hormone), pituitary adenomas (such as prolactin, growth hormone) and pancreatic endocrine tumours. Multiple Endocrine Adenomatosis Type II (MEA Type II, or Sipple's syndrome) is similarly inherited, and is the association of hormone-synthesising parathyroid adenomas (parathyroid hormone), phaeochromocytomas (catecholamines) and medullary carcinoma of the thyroid (calcitonin).

Table 16.42 Pancreatic endocrine tumours

Peptide	Cellular source	Title	Clinical syndrome
Pancreatic glucagon	Alpha cell	Glucagonoma	Necrolytic migratory erythema Diabetes mellitus
Insulin	Beta cell	Insulinoma	Hypoglycaemia
Somatostatin	D cell	Somatostatinoma	Diabetes mellitus Steatorrhoea Cholelithiasis
Gastrin	G cell	Gastrinoma (Zollinger-Ellison syndrome)	Duodenal ulcers and malabsorption secondary to gastric hyperacidity
Pancreatic polypeptide	Pancreatic polypeptide cell	PP-oma	None
Vasoactive intestinal polypeptide	Nerves	VIP-oma (Verner-Morrison syndrome)	Watery diarrhoea, hypokalaemia and acidosis (WDHA syndrome)
Adrenocorticotrophic hormone	Unknown	Cushing's syndrome	Cushing's syndrome (p. 708)
Parathyroid hormone	Unknown	Ectopic hyperparathyroidism	Hypercalcaemia
Growth hormone releasing hormone	Unknown	Pituitary acidophil hyperplasia	Acromegaly

Investigation

Diagnosis of these tumours is by demonstrating a high plasma level of the appropriate peptide by radio-immunoassay. The tumours can often be demonstrated by ultrasound or CT scanning. On occasions, it is necessary to sample blood along the portal vein and to demonstrate a peak of hormone secretion corresponding to the site of tumour venous drainage. Arteriography can also be used, and is helpful in demonstrating multiple primary tumours (common with gastrinomas) and hepatic metastases.

Treatment

Treatment is by surgical resection if possible, and this often results in cure. In the presence of metastatic disease, the cytotoxic drugs streptozotocin and 5-fluorouracil can produce worthwhile remissions. The symptoms of most of the tumours may be helped by somatostatin therapy. The rash of the glucagonoma syndrome can be improved by zinc, and the hypoglycaemia of insulinomas by diazoxide. The symptoms of gastrinomas are helped by high dose H_2-receptor blocking agents or omeprazole, and the diarrhoea of VIP-omas by a variety of agents including corticosteroids, metoclopramide and trifluoperazine.

FURTHER READING

Collins R, Langman M 1985 Treatment with histamine H_2 antagonists in acute upper gastrointestinal haemorrhage: implications of randomized trials. New England Journal of Medicine 313: 660–666. *Overview of the use of drugs for gastrointestinal bleeding.*

Corfield A P, Cooper M J, Williamson R C N et al 1985 Prediction of severity in acute pancreatitis: prospective comparison of three prognostic indices. Lancet 2: 403–407. *Assessment of the severity of acute pancreatitis.*

De Caesteker J S, Blackwell J N, Brown J, Heading R C 1985 The oesophagus as a cause of recurrent chest pain: which patients should be investigated and which tests should be used? Lancet 2: 1143–1146. *Discussion of cardiac and oesophageal causes of chest pain, with special reference to the oesophagus.*

Field M, Rao M C, Chang E B 1989 Intestinal electrolyte transport and diarrheal disease. New England Journal of Medicine 321: 800–806 and 879–883. *Scientific background to abnormal intestinal secretion.*

Forman D, Adabbag S, Doll R 1985 Nitrates, nitrites and gastric cancer in Great Britain. Nature 313: 620–625. *Review of the possible role of nitrates in the pathogenesis of gastric cancer.*

Foster P N, Mitchell C J, Robertson D R C et al 1984 Prospective comparison of three non-invasive tests for pancreatic disease. British Medical Journal 289: 13–16. *A study of non-invasive techniques which avoid intubation and X-rays.*

Kumar D, Wingate D L 1985 The irritable bowel syndrome: a paroxysmal motor disorder. Lancet 2: 973–977. *An attempt to give an organic basis to the irritable bowel syndrome.*

Liver and Biliary Tract Disease

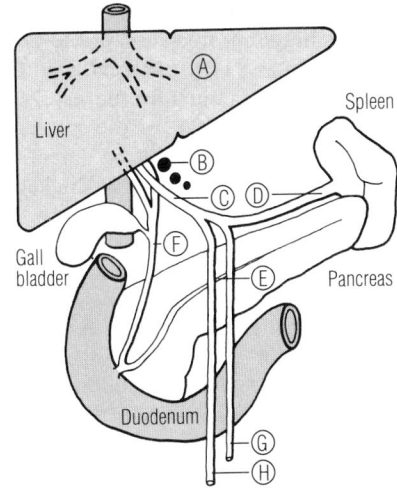

Fig. 17.1   A simplified view of the gross anatomy of the liver and its major relationships. Hepatic veins (A); hilar lymph nodes (B); portal vein (C); splenic vein (D); pancreatic duct (E); bile duct (F); inferior mesenteric vein (G); superior mesenteric vein (H).

STRUCTURE AND FUNCTION

Anatomy

The liver, weighing from 1200–1500 g, is the largest solid organ in the body (Fig. 17.1). It lies in the right hypochondrium and is roughly wedge-shaped, with the apex to the left and the base to the right. Although there is a classical division into a large right lobe and smaller left lobe, this bears no relationship to the true functional division, on the basis of blood supply, into almost equal right and left lobes. The inferior surface is concave and slopes obliquely upwards from front to back, forming the characteristic sharp anterior margin of the organ. The anterior and superior surfaces are convex and closely applied to the posterior aspect of the anterior abdominal wall and the lower surface of the right hemidiaphragm respectively. It is attached to and suspended from these structures by a reflection of the peritoneum, the falciform ligament. Elsewhere, the peritoneum almost completely covers the liver surface, apart from further reflections post-

eriorly and inferiorly, which form the lesser omentum, joining the liver to the stomach.

The liver has a dual blood supply, from the hepatic artery, which is usually a branch of the coeliac axis, and from the portal vein, formed from the mesenteric vein and splenic vein. The total liver blood flow is about 1300 ml/min, one-quarter of the resting cardiac output. The hepatic artery supplies about 25% of the total liver blood flow but 50% of the oxygen, while the remaining 75% of the volume and the other half of the oxygen comes from the relatively deoxygenated, low-pressure portal vein supply. Both vessels run in the free edge of the lesser omentum to the liver hilum before dividing into major right and left branches. The hepatic veins drain directly into the inferior vena cava, which runs in a groove along the back of the liver between the functional right and left lobes. Three large veins enter just below the diaphragm, but there are a number of smaller veins draining the posterior aspect of the right lobe which enter the vena cava directly.

These assume importance in two clinical situations: they may be the only remaining draining vessels if there is thrombosis of the main hepatic veins (the Budd-Chiari syndrome), and they are particularly difficult to dissect during a right hemihepatectomy.

The biliary system collects bile, stores and concentrates it in the gall bladder, and delivers it to the duodenum when required. The main right and left hepatic ducts join in the hilum of the liver to form the common hepatic duct. The gall bladder lies on the under-surface of the right lobe of the liver with its fundus usually projecting slightly below the lower edge. The cystic duct runs upwards and backwards to join the common hepatic duct, and the resulting common bile duct then runs with the hepatic artery and portal vein in the free edge of the lesser omentum to pass behind the first part of the duodenum and the head of the pancreas before turning to the right to enter the duodenum. This part of the duct is often completely buried in the pancreas and it is here that it is susceptible to obstruction by pancreatic tumours. The pancreatic and bile ducts usually share a common channel for the last 2–7 mm which opens through a small papilla on the inner wall of the duodenum (the ampulla and papilla of Vater). In this part of the duct the choledochal muscle is thickened to form the sphincter of Oddi.

Micro-anatomy

At a micro-anatomical level, the liver essentially consists of a series of channels, or sinusoids, running between plates of hepatocytes. These are lined by endothelial cells which have unusually large fenestrations in them, allowing the sinusoidal part of each hepatocyte surface to have free access to almost all the constituents in plasma (Fig. 17.2). Specialised phagocytic cells (Kupffer cells) are also present in the sinusoids. Biliary canaliculi form between the contiguous surfaces of hepatocytes, and here, and on the sinusoidal surface, there are extensive microvilli in the cell membrane to increase the capacity for transmembrane transfer.

Branches of the hepatic artery, portal vein and bile duct within the liver are carried in portal tracts. The smallest of these, carrying terminal branches, supply groups of sinusoids which together form a functional unit, the acinus. Blood from each acinus then passes into a number of efferent veins. While the concept of the acinus as a functional unit has proved useful in understanding patterns of liver injury, it is still useful for descriptive purposes to refer to the lobule as the classical structural unit of the liver. Each lobule is centred on an efferent (or central) vein surrounded by radially orientated sinusoids and with five or six portal tracts at the periphery.

Physiology

Essentially the liver has four quite distinct functions:

1. It supplies bile salts and bicarbonate to assist in digestion.
2. It acts as a buffer between the gut and the systemic

Fig. 17.2 **The micro-anatomy of the liver. A.** The classical liver lobule is centred on the central vein with the portal tracts at its periphery. The concept of the functional lobule emphasises the portal tract as the point of entry of the arterial and portal venous blood, with the sinusoids then extending from there to the 'central veins'. **B.** A liver sinusoid with liver cell plates separated from the lining endothelial cells by the space of Disse. The Kupffer cells straddle the blood-filled centre of the sinusoid. **C.** The endothelial cells riddled with fenestrations allow macromolecules to pass between the blood and the hepatocytes. The biliary canaliculi run between the hepatocytes in the liver cell plates.

circulation, maintaining stable levels of amino acids and glucose.
3. It synthesises a large number of specialised proteins, carbohydrates and lipids.
4. It is a major excretory pathway for larger and more hydrophobic metabolites, foreign substances and drugs.

Bile acid metabolism and secretion

The primary bile acids, *cholic and chenodeoxycholic acid,* are synthesised from cholesterol in the liver, conjugated with taurine or glycine to form bile salts and then excreted by an active transport mechanism into the bile canaliculi, and eventually into the duodenum. In the distal ileum,

Summary 1	Liver physiology
Normal function	*Consequence in disease*
Bile acid metabolism	Fat malabsorption
Glucose and amino acid homeostasis	Encephalopathy
Synthesis of plasma proteins, clotting factors, lipids	Ascites, bleeding, xanthalasmata
Metabolism/excretion of bilirubin, ammonia/urea, drugs	Jaundice, encephalopathy, drug toxicity

may then occur, particularly if a nidus for crystal formation is present. This is the pathophysiological basis for gallstone formation which is discussed further on page 641.

The active transport of bile salts is the main driving force for bile secretion, and its failure may be an important cause of intrahepatic cholestasis. Bile salts accumulate in cholestasis, whether due to mechanical obstruction or a defect in excretion, and deposition in the skin may account for the pruritus which is often a troublesome symptom. There is also a bile salt independent contribution to bile secretion which is probably driven by active sodium transport in the distal canaliculus. Bicarbonate is added in the small bile ductules and this process is stimulated by the hormone secretin. Cholecystokinin principally stimulates gall bladder contraction.

Protein metabolism

The liver receives amino acids from the gut and the muscles and regulates their levels in plasma by controlling the rate of gluconeogenesis and transamination. It also converts ammonia into urea by the urea cycle. Ammonia is produced intrahepatically by de-amination, in other tissues by nucleotide metabolism, and by bacterial action on proteins or urea in the colon. The liver is the major site of synthesis of almost all the plasma proteins, and, for many, is also the principal site of degradation.

In an average 70 kg adult, total body protein is about 12 kg, and turns over at a rate of about 250 g/day. There is a close relationship between the muscles, liver and gut with respect to amino acid fluxes (Fig. 17.4). Muscle contributes

there is another active transport system which ensures conservation of bile salts when they have fulfilled their digestive function (Fig. 17.3). This system of enterohepatic circulation is extremely efficient. The entire body pool of bile salts is circulated through the gut about twice in each main meal and only about 5% is newly synthesised in the liver. The small fraction reaching the colon is modified by bacteria, which perform 7-alpha-dehydroxylation, producing the secondary bile acids, *deoxycholic and lithocholic acid*. All bile salts are powerful detergents, solubilising lipids by enclosing them in bile salt aggregates called micelles. These are organised so that hydrophobic groups are orientated into the lipid-rich interior while the hydrophilic hydroxyl and carboxyl groups are on the outside. Cholesterol and lecithin in bile itself are carried in such micelles, and, if the concentration of these molecules rises too high relative to the concentration of bile salts, then the bile becomes supersaturated. Precipitation of cholesterol

Fig. 17.3 Enterohepatic circulation of bile acids. Bile salts entering the duodenum via the bile duct (A); absorption of bile salts in the terminal ileum (B); secondary bile acids formed by bacterial degradation (C); uptake and re-excretion of bile salts by liver (D).

Fig. 17.4 Amino acid and protein metabolism in health. Branched chain amino acids (BCAA), marked in red, constitute only 20% of the dietary intake, while aromatic amino acids (AAA), marked in black, make up 80%. The liver preferentially metabolises AAA rather than BCAA which are passed to the tissues (particularly muscles). The thickness of the red and black lines represents the relative amounts of the amino acids in the different body compartments.

the biggest source of protein turnover, about 130 g/day, while dietary intake is about 90 g/day. Only 23% of amino acid nitrogen absorbed into the portal bloodstream after a meal is passed on to the peripheral tissues, and in exercising this gate function, the liver is responsible for extensively modifying the blood amino acid composition. The aromatic amino acids – phenylalanine, tyrosine and methionine – are preferentially processed to urea, while the branched chain amino acids – valine, leucine and isoleucine – are selectively passed to the periphery where they are predominantly metabolised by muscle. This selectivity is lost in severe liver disease and it is possible that the resulting change in the ratio of the plasma concentrations of these two groups of amino acids may alter cerebral neurotransmitter metabolism and contribute to the pathophysiology of portosystemic encephalopathy (p. 655).

Of the many proteins synthesised in the liver, *albumin* and *prothrombin* are of particular interest in relation to liver disease and are discussed as liver function tests on page 628. Since albumin is also the most important mediator of the plasma colloid osmotic pressure, the fall in albumin concentration which accompanies chronic liver disease is of relevance to the pathophysiology of ascites, one of the frequent complications of cirrhosis (p. 652).

Carbohydrate metabolism

The liver acts as a gate for the large amounts of glucose delivered from the gut during digestion, by storing it as glycogen, and is also the main source of glucose during starvation. Initially, glycogenolysis is the principal metabolic pathway used, but, as the glycogen stores become depleted, gluconeogenesis assumes greater importance. The main substrates for this pathway are lactate, pyruvate, glucogenic amino acids (mainly alanine from muscle) and glycerol (from lipolysis in fat stores). In the fed state, about 160 g/day of glucose are needed for those tissues with an obligatory requirement for this substrate, principally the brain and haemopoietic tissues. During prolonged starvation, the brain adapts to ketone bodies as an alternative energy source, and the total body requirement for glucose drops to about 40 g/day. Although blood glucose levels may directly influence carbohydrate metabolism in the liver, the principal instruments for metabolic control are the hormones, insulin, glucagon, catecholamines and glucocorticoids (Fig. 17.5). The fall in insulin levels during starvation releases glycogenolysis and gluconeogenesis from the inhibitory effects of this hormone, with glycogenolysis being particularly sensitive. The increasing glucagon and catecholamine levels act directly to stimulate glycogenolysis. In the periphery, the relative excess of glucocorticoids compared to insulin leads to increased release of amino acids into the circulation, and high glucagon levels stimulate alanine uptake by the liver.

In liver disease, the supply of glucose by gluconeogenesis is generally well preserved, and hypoglycaemia is only usually a problem in severe (fulminant) liver failure. Glucose intolerance is more common but rarely a clinical problem.

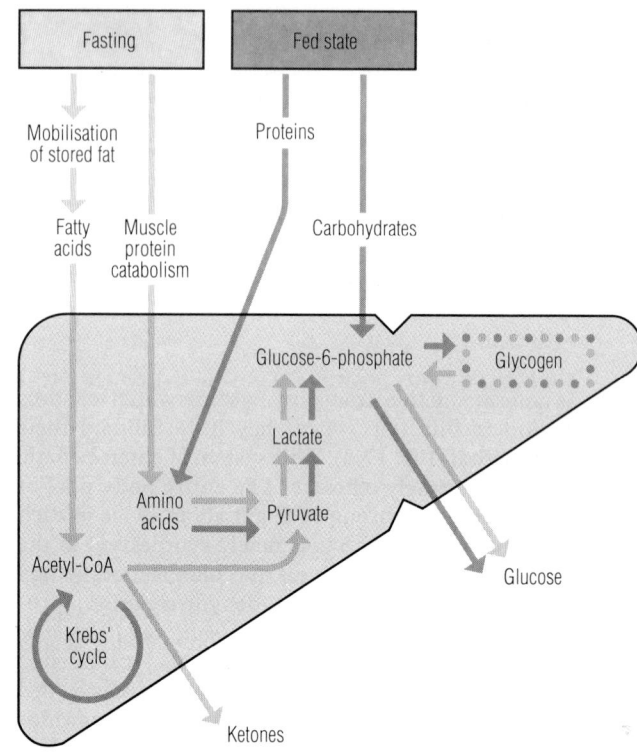

Fig. 17.5   The main routes of carbohydrate metabolism in the fed state and fasting.

Lipid metabolism

The major plasma lipids, *cholesterol, cholesterol esters, phospholipids* and *triglycerides*, are highly insoluble in water and are carried in macromolecular complexes, of lipid and a protein carrier (apoprotein) called plasma lipoproteins. Only the intestine and liver synthesise and secrete plasma lipoproteins. There are four main classes, differing in size and density, and having different proportions of the main lipids:

1. *Chylomicrons* are made in the mucosal cells of the small intestine during dietary fat absorption, and are the main carriers of triglyceride.
2. *Very low density lipoproteins (VLDL)* are produced in the liver and intestine and have a core which contains 50–60% triglyceride. Their apoprotein content is low (about 10%).
3. *Low density lipoproteins (LDL)* are formed in the plasma by catabolism of VLDL. They have a higher protein content (22%) and lower triglyceride proportion (10%) than VLDL.
4. *High density lipoproteins (HDL)* are made to some extent within the plasma, but are also synthesised in the liver and intestine. They have the highest protein content (50%) and lowest triglyceride proportion (5%).

Hypercholesterolaemia is a feature of any liver disease

in which there is obstruction to bile flow, whether this is intra- or extrahepatic. The increase is due to a rise in free cholesterol levels. Although total plasma phospholipids are often normal, lecithin levels are increased, due to regurgitation back into the blood from the obstructed biliary tree. Although the elevated free cholesterol levels may also be due to regurgitation, there is some evidence to suggest that the increased plasma lecithin stimulates hepatic cholesterol synthesis. A marked increase in LDL levels, and the appearance of an abnormal lipoprotein, lipoprotein X, are due to the lipids providing increased substrate drive. Among the clinical effects of these lipid changes are the yellowish plaques of cholesterol deposited in the skin (xanthomata) in longstanding biliary obstruction, and the appearance of 'target' red cells in the peripheral blood film, probably a reflection of altered membrane fluidity.

Drug metabolism

The liver is an important site for the clearance of many drugs. In general the more lipophilic and the higher the molecular weight, the more likely the drug is to be cleared by the liver rather than the kidney. Such hepatic clearance usually involves metabolic biotransformation with or without conjugation. In liver disease alteration of drug handling can have clinically important consequences (Ch. 3).

INVESTIGATIONS IN LIVER DISEASE

LIVER FUNCTION TESTS

The conventional profile of blood tests often described as 'standard' liver function tests are not true tests of the function of the liver, but reflect present or previous liver cell damage and biliary obstruction. Although they are useful in differential diagnosis, and may be the first indication of liver disease, they are rarely of diagnostic value

alone. It is also important to realise that most of these tests are not specific indicators of liver damage. The influence of disease in other organs needs to be carefully considered when evaluating their significance (Table 17.1).

Serum bilirubin

The main source of bilirubin is the reticulo-endothelial system, where haemoglobin from effete red blood cells is split to haem, then bilirubin. This is lipophilic, and is carried in the plasma, tightly bound to albumin. Uptake into the hepatocytes is mediated by a carrier system in the liver cell membrane, and ligands in the cytosol (Fig. 17.6). Bilirubin is then converted to a water-soluble compound by conjugation with glucuronic acid, and excreted, as the diglucuronide, into bile. Conjugated bilirubin refluxing back into the blood can be excreted by the kidney, but the water-insoluble unconjugated bilirubin cannot. Hence jaundice without bilirubinuria indicating high serum levels of *unconjugated* bilirubin is a feature of haemolysis (increased formation), or failure of bilirubin uptake or conjugation in the liver. Excess *conjugated* bilirubin in serum occurs with cholestasis. In hepatitis there is intrahepatic cholestasis in addition to liver cell injury but conjugated bilirubin is found in the plasma since conjugation is preserved even with severe liver damage.

Table 17.1 Non-hepatic causes of impaired liver function tests

Cause	Nature of abnormality
Haemolysis	Isolated hyperbilirubinaemia
Adolescence, Paget's disease, osteomalacia, bone tumours	Isolated elevation in (bone) alkaline phosphatase
Enzyme-inducing drugs (and alcohol)	Increased gamma glutamyl transpeptidase (GT) levels
Malnutrition, malabsorption, protein loss and chronic illness	Decreased serum albumin
Fat malabsorption	Prolonged prothrombin time
Myocardial infarction, myositis	High serum aspartate aminotransferase (AST) levels

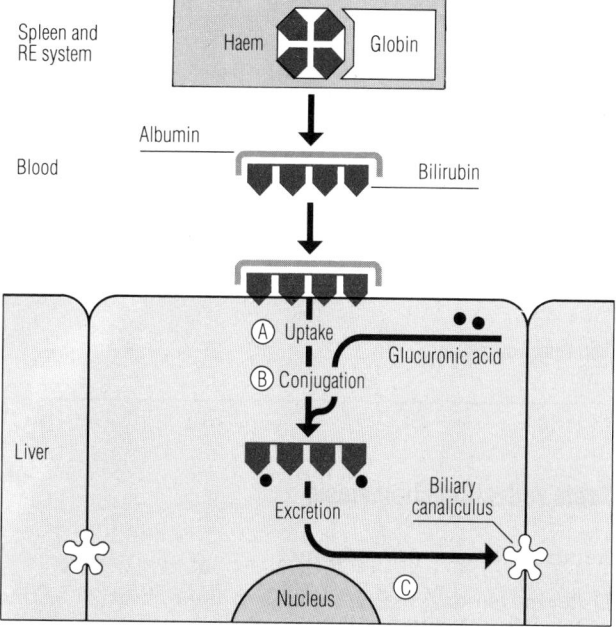

Fig. 17.6 The formation and metabolism of bilirubin. The main sites of congenital defects leading to jaundice are indicated. Failure of uptake into hepatocytes; probably the main abnormality in Gilbert's syndrome (A). Failure of conjugation; the main abnormality in more serious cases of unconjugated hyperbilirubinaemia in childhood (e.g. Crigler-Najjar syndrome) (B). Failure of excretion can occur in some rare congenital causes of conjugated hyperbilirubinaemia such as Dubin-Johnson syndrome (C).

Liver and Biliary Tract Disease

Tests reflecting synthetic function

Serum albumin

Although low albumin levels may be due to malnutrition, malabsorption, increased loss and hypercatabolism, as well as decreased liver synthesis, serum levels can be useful as a guide to functioning liver cell mass. Its relatively long half-life (about 21 days), means that serum albumin is often normal in acute hepatitis, and is of most value in assessing the severity of chronic liver disease.

Prothrombin time

The one-stage prothrombin time test is dependent on the function of several clotting factors, many of which are synthesised in the liver (Table 17.2). It is a relatively insensitive test of liver function, but because of the short half-life of many of the clotting factors, it is an early indicator of severe acute liver damage. In chronic liver disease, it tends to parallel changes in serum albumin levels. In cholestasis, the prothrombin time is often prolonged, even though synthetic liver function is intact. This is because several of the factors evaluated in the test are dependent for their activity on vitamin K, one of the fat-soluble vitamins which is poorly absorbed when bile salts are not reaching the intestine. Giving vitamin K parenterally (10 mg daily for 3 days) is, therefore, a clinically useful test of liver synthetic function. The prothrombin time corrects completely in cholestasis but remains abnormal in severe hepatitis or chronic liver disease.

Table 17.2 Clotting factors synthesised in the liver

Fibrinogen

Vitamin K-dependent factors
  II, VII, IX and X

Labile factors
  V and VIII

Contact factors
  XI and XII

Fibrin stabilising factor
  XIII

Tests reflecting cholestasis

Serum alkaline phosphatase

Different iso-enzymes are found in bone, liver, intestine and placenta, and serum electrophoresis can be useful to identify the source of elevated levels. The liver iso-enzyme is located mainly in the bile canalicular region of the hepatocyte surface membrane, and high serum levels are a sensitive indicator of segmental or global biliary obstruction whether within or outside the liver. Much of the rise is due to increased production of the enzyme in areas of the liver proximal to an obstruction, together with reflux

Summary 2 Liver function tests

All non-specific – so think of disease in other organs

Synthesis
Albumin – long half-life, so slow response = chronic liver disease
Prothrombin time – short half-life, so fast response = acute and chronic liver disease

Excretion
Bilirubin – conjugated bilirubin elevated in liver disease, whatever the cause
Alkaline phosphatase – sensitive indicator of cholestasis
Gamma GT – not so sensitive, but elevated with enzyme induction including alcohol

Cell damage
AST/ALT – released from damaged liver cells = active liver inflammation

of a high molecular weight form of the liver type of iso-enzyme, the 'biliary iso-enzyme'. This is associated with vesicular structures which may be actual fragments of the canalicular membrane. Although high plasma bilirubin levels often accompany high alkaline phosphatase levels, there can be a marked discrepancy, with normal bilirubin values in spite of markedly raised serum alkaline phosphatase levels. This usually indicates a patchy or incomplete obstructive lesion, with bilirubin being excreted by the non-obstructed areas. This pattern is a feature of space-occupying lesions in the liver, including granulomata, cysts and abscesses, as well as secondary deposits.

Serum gamma-glutamyl transpeptidase

Serum gamma-glutamyl transpeptidase (gamma GT) is a more liver-specific enzyme than alkaline phosphatase and one which also reflects cholestasis. However, it is less sensitive to biliary obstruction, and an important clinical point is its sensitivity to enzyme-inducing drugs and alcohol, both of which can cause quite marked elevations in serum levels in the absence of significant liver damage. A useful practical guide to interpretation is to compare the levels of gamma GT and alkaline phosphatase in serum. In cholestasis, the alkaline phosphatase is usually higher than the gamma GT, while the reverse is usually true in alcoholic liver disease or in patients taking enzyme-inducing agents.

Tests reflecting liver cell injury

Serum aspartate aminotransferase

Serum aspartate aminotransferase (AST) is found in particularly high levels in liver and in skeletal and cardiac muscle, and serum levels can rise after injury to any of these tissues. High levels in liver disease are classically associated with liver cell necrosis in acute or chronic hepatitis, but membrane damage without cell death may also allow enzyme to leak out into the circulation. Thus, high levels of serum AST can occur in conditions like acute left ventricular failure and septicaemia, in which hypo-

628

perfusion and anoxia lead to transient liver cell injury. Correction of the circulatory disturbance often results in a very rapid fall in AST levels.

Serum alanine aminotransferase

Although more liver-specific, changes in serum levels of serum alanine aminotransferase (ALT) tend to parallel those of serum AST.

SPECIAL INVESTIGATIONS

Imaging techniques

Plain X-ray of the abdomen

Taking a plain X-ray of the abdomen is a simple technique which may allow an assessment of liver and spleen size, and show calcified gallstones and cysts, or gas in the biliary tree.

Ultrasound scanning

Ultrasound scanning enables a rapid assessment of liver and spleen size, vessel size and patency, the calibre of bile ducts (Fig. 17.7) and cysts. It is particularly good at detecting gallstones, as they are so echogenic (p. 25, Fig. 2.5), it may, however, be less successful at detecting some tumours in the liver, and can be technically difficult in the presence of extensive bowel gas, ascites or obesity. Considerable skill is needed for accurate interpretation of the findings.

Fig. 17.7 Ultrasound of the liver demonstrating dilated intrahepatic and common duct.

Liver scintiscanning

Liver scintiscanning can be obtained by gamma camera imaging of the upper abdomen after the intravenous injec-tion of 99m technetium-labelled sulphur colloid which is taken up by Kupffer cells in liver sinusoids. Liver and spleen size can be accurately assessed and most space-occupying lesions larger than 2 cm in diameter located. In cirrhosis, effective hepatic (sinusoidal) blood flow is reduced, and other parts of the reticulo-endothelial system, notably the spleen and bone marrow, show markedly increased isotope uptake.

Computed axial tomography

Computed axial tomography (CT scanning) is capable of providing high-resolution sectional views of the liver and surrounding structures in the upper abdomen (Fig. 17.23B, p. 660). Contrast enhancement is of value in further defin-ing the nature of abnormal areas. Because of its high cost and limited availability, the technique is best used for difficult cases where ultrasound has failed to provide the expected morphological information.

Contrast radiology

Although ultrasound scanning is the best technique for detecting gallstones and dilated bile ducts, radiological contrast studies are of great value in further defining the morphology of the biliary tree. In some cases therapeutic procedures for long-term biliary drainage and treatment of bile duct tumours have been developed from these inves-tigative techniques.

Oral cholecystography

Oral cholecystography may be used as a screening pro-cedure in patients with suspected gall bladder disease. Like all procedures which rely on excretion of contrast material by the liver, poor results are obtained in the presence of liver disease, particularly cholestasis.

Intravenous cholangiography

Intravenous cholangiography is the demonstration of the biliary tree following the intravenous injection of contrast material. It is rarely used now that ultrasound and direct cholangiography have become more widely available.

Percutaneous transhepatic cholangiography

In percutaneous transhepatic cholangiography (PTC), a very fine flexible needle is introduced into the liver sub-stance until a bile duct is punctured. Contrast is then injected to fill the biliary system. It is successful in almost all cases with dilated intrahepatic bile ducts, and in about two-thirds of those with ducts of normal size. Bleeding and biliary peritonitis are rare complications. Antibiotics are often given just before the procedure to reduce the risk of cholangitis.

Fig. 17.8 Endoscopic retrograde cholangiopancreatography. A. ERCP demonstrating a normal duct system in a patient who has had a previous cholecystectomy. **B.** ERCP in a patient immediately following cholecystectomy (note T-tube). There is a stone (arrowed) at the lower end of the common bile duct which is dilated.

Endoscopic retrograde cholangiopancreatography

Endoscopic retrograde cholangiopancreatography (ERCP) involves cannulation of the ampulla of Vater via an endoscope, followed by the injection of contrast medium into the bile ducts; it allows excellent pictures of the biliary tree to be obtained (Fig. 17.8) and is the procedure of choice in patients with non-dilated bile ducts.

Liver biopsy

Percutaneous needle biopsy of the liver has been increasingly accepted as part of the routine investigation of patients with liver disease since the 1940s, when it became firmly established in clinical practice. In experienced centres it is an extremely safe procedure, the overall mortality in one of the largest published series (79 381 liver biopsies) being 0.015%. Nevertheless it is an invasive procedure which needs to be approached with care.

Indications

Although on many occasions the biopsy will be used to obtain information for diagnostic or follow-up purposes in a patient with suspected primary liver disease, liver biopsy is often of great value in the investigation of multisystem disease (Table 17.3).

Contra-indications and precautions

These are equally important in a potentially hazardous procedure. The patient must be able to understand the instructions, particularly to hold his breath at the appro-

---

Table 17.3 Indications and contra-indications for liver biopsy

Indications

For diagnosis of
  Primary liver disease
  Multisystem disease commonly affecting the liver, e.g. sarcoidosis, lymphoma
  Pyrexia of unknown origin and disseminated infection, e.g. tuberculosis
  Malignant disease
  Metabolic disease, e.g. glycogen storage disease

For assessment of
  Progression of disease and response to treatment

Contra-indications

Clotting defect
  Prothrombin ratio greater than 1.3 (not more than 4 secs prolonged)
  Platelet count less than 50 ×10⁹/l

Hydatid cyst
  Risk of dissemination

Haemangioma or amyloid
  Increased risk of bleeding

Biliary obstruction
  Risk of biliary leak, cholangitis and peritonitis

---

priate moment. The clotting system must be able to seal the puncture site effectively, and a prothrombin time and platelet count are essential preliminary investigations. The prothrombin time should not be prolonged by more than 4 seconds and the platelet count should be greater than $50 \times 10^9/l$. Determination of the patient's blood group is a sensible precaution, with some serum being saved for cross-matching should transfusion be required. The contra-indications (Table 17.3) are not absolute, but in the presence of any of these risk factors the chance of complications is considerably increased.

Technique

A skilled operator and a co-operative patient are required. Sedation is rarely necessary, except in young children where general anaesthesia is often used. The lateral intercostal route is usually preferred, although an anterior approach can be useful in specific lesions in the left lobe, particularly when combined with ultrasound guidance. Two different types of needle are used: one in which the biopsy is aspirated into the lumen of a large-bore needle (the *Menghini needle*), and one where a core of liver tissue is cut out by a needle sheath sliding over a notched introducer (the *Tru Cut needle*). The latter is often preferred because of the good preservation of the integrity of the specimen in hard fibrotic or cirrhotic livers, although technically the Menghini is easier to use.

After the biopsy, the patient is advised to lie on the right side for 2 hours, and during this time quarter-hourly pulse and blood pressure measurements are recorded. It is customary in the United Kingdom to keep the patient in hospital overnight, although there have been some reports elsewhere of the use of this procedure in outpatients.

Complications

Some *bleeding* at the site of liver puncture is inevitable and this usually causes some mild pain, either locally, or at the right shoulder tip because of diaphragmatic irritation. Persistent bleeding into the peritoneum or biliary tree (*haemobilia*) is much rarer and more serious, and laparotomy is needed to secure haemostasis. *Sudden transient hypotension* immediately after the biopsy, probably due to vagal stimulation, is not uncommon. Occasionally it may be dramatic and lead to loss of consciousness but rapid recovery can be confidently anticipated. *Perforation* of the colon, or *puncture* of the kidney or pancreas, is rare, but can usually be managed conservatively. *Pneumothorax* may occur in patients with obstructive airways disease and hyperinflated lungs, and in those who have been unable to co-operate at the time of the biopsy. *Biliary peritonitis* can usually be avoided if biopsies are not performed in patients with biliary obstruction. It is a potentially very serious complication with a high mortality. Early laparotomy is indicated. Introduction of a needle into an obstructed biliary tree also carries a high risk of *cholangitis* and *septicaemia*, another reason for avoiding biopsy in these patients.

THE JAUNDICED PATIENT

17

Differential diagnosis

There are four broad categories of disease which can lead to a patient presenting with jaundice:

1. pre-hepatic (unconjugated hyperbilirubinaemia)
2. hepatitis
3. intra- or extrahepatic obstructive jaundice
4. chronic liver disease.

The initial aim should be to use the clinical history, physical examination, liver function tests and special investigations to establish a working diagnosis in terms of one of these broad groupings. This will then determine the next steps to be taken in establishing the final diagnosis and treatment. The organisation of this chapter reflects this clinical approach. After discussing the presentation and special investigations, each of the four broad categories of disease presenting with jaundice will be discussed in detail.

Clinical features

While the jaundice itself is often the dominant feature of the illness for the patient, it is important to explore the first symptoms in detail as these often contain the most reliable clues to the diagnosis. A prodromal ''flu-like' illness with anorexia and myalgia is characteristic of acute viral hepatitis and usually starts from a few days to 2 weeks before the onset of jaundice. A longer history of mild malaise and anorexia (often 3–6 months in duration), associated with weight loss of more than 3 kg, is common with carcinoma of the pancreas. Biliary colic with pain referred to the right scapula and shoulder a day or two before the jaundice suggests passage of a stone down the common bile duct.

Generalised itching is another symptom of considerable importance. It often precedes or parallels the jaundice in patients with biliary obstruction, but is usually absent or delayed in acute hepatitis, only becoming of major clinical importance in those with an unusually prolonged cholestatic phase during recovery. Important exceptions to this general rule are acute alcoholic hepatitis, where cholestasis is sometimes a dominant early feature, and hepatitis associated with some drugs and chemicals, in which the dominant feature is a disturbance of biliary secretion rather than hepatocellular damage.

Pale stools and dark urine are to be expected in jaundice due to obstruction, and in acute and chronic hepatitis. This finding is therefore of no help in differential diagnosis. In contrast, normal-coloured urine and stools in the presence of obvious jaundice strongly suggests a prehepatic cause.

In addition to these general features, specific risk factors should be identified, including homosexuality, drug addiction, foreign travel and contact with jaundiced patients, as well as alcohol intake. It is essential to take a complete drug history. Drug-induced hepatitis can mimic a viral hepatitis,

Liver and Biliary Tract Disease

including a prodromal illness, or can present with all the features of a pure obstructive jaundice.

Physical examination

In contrast to the history, which may point strongly to the diagnosis, the physical examination usually gives less specific information. Tender hepatomegaly is often present in both acute hepatitis and obstructive jaundice, while minor splenomegaly is present in a small proportion of patients with viral hepatitis. The finding of a palpable gall bladder is well recognised as a classical sign of carcinoma of the head of the pancreas, but is not often present. If jaundice is due to hepatic metastases, hard, irregular and sometimes tender hepatomegaly is usually a prominent feature. Cutaneous stigmata of chronic liver disease, such as spider naevi, liver palms, leuchonychia and Dupuytren's contracture, should be looked for carefully, since these are important clues that an apparently acute episode may instead be a manifestation of chronic liver disease. Conversely, in acute alcoholic hepatitis there may be signs suggestive of chronic liver disease, including splenomegaly, ascites and florid cutaneous stigmata, but no histopathological features of cirrhosis. If the patient survives the acute episode and remains abstinent, he can be expected to make a complete clinical and biochemical recovery.

Liver function tests

While it is generally true that the ratio between the serum AST (or ALT) and alkaline phosphatase helps to distinguish between hepatitic (ratio high) and cholestatic (ratio low) types of jaundice, there is a large 'grey area', and the results of these tests are best thought of as an extension to the evidence from the history and examination, rather than being diagnostic in their own right. The finding of a prolonged prothrombin time is an exception, for the response to parenteral vitamin K clearly distinguishes between a hepatitic and cholestatic cause. In isolated hyperbilirubinaemia, the determination of conjugated and unconjugated serum bilirubin levels is of considerable value in confirming a diagnosis of prehepatic jaundice.

Special investigations

The most useful of the special tests in the jaundiced patient is an ultrasound scan. The aim should be to concentrate on determining whether or not the intrahepatic biliary system is dilated, for this is one of the most reliable guides to the presence of extrahepatic obstruction. However, the ducts take a few days to become dilated, and if the history strongly suggests the recent onset of large duct obstruction, then the test should be repeated 3 or 4 days later. If duct dilatation is detected, then it is usual to proceed to ERCP or PTC (pp. 629, 630) to define the morphology of the bile ducts and identify the site of the obstruction prior to surgery or interventional radiology. If the ducts are of

normal calibre and the history is consistent with an acute hepatitis, then the specific diagnosis should be established with the appropriate virological tests. Liver biopsy is only indicated if there is real doubt as to the diagnosis, or if chronic liver disease is suspected.

UNCONJUGATED HYPERBILIRUBINAEMIA

The two principal diagnostic categories are haemolysis and congenital defects in bilirubin uptake or conjugation.

Haemolytic jaundice

The diagnostic features of haemolytic jaundice are acholuric jaundice (jaundice without bilirubinuria), unconjugated hyperbilirubinaemia and a raised reticulocyte count. The differential diagnosis, further investigation and treatment are discussed on page 1050.

Defects in bilirubin uptake or conjugation

The commonest defect in bilirubin uptake or conjugation (Fig. 17.6) is *Gilbert's syndrome*, probably due to defective uptake of bilirubin into hepatocytes and secondary deficiency of hepatic glucuronyl transferase, although many cases have a minor decrease in red cell survival which could contribute to the bilirubin load. The condition is of no functional significance, and is thought by some to represent the upper end of the normal curve for the distribution of bilirubin values in the population. It is, however, frequently the cause of much diagnostic confusion, with 'recurrent hepatitis' being the commonest misleading label. The finding of unconjugated hyperbilirubinaemia, rising further after a 48-hour fast, and a normal reticulocyte count, with no other abnormalities on the standard tests of liver function, is sufficient to make the diagnosis with confidence. A full explanation to the patient is all that is required for successful management. More serious congenital defects in bilirubin conjugation, such as the *Crigler-Najjar syndrome* (Fig. 17.6) can produce higher unconjugated bilirubin levels in the blood and kernicterus in infants, but are rare.

ACUTE HEPATITIS

The term 'viral hepatitis' is often used rather loosely to mean infection with one of the hepatotropic viruses, although jaundice can occur as part of a systemic infection with several other viruses (Table 17.4), or as a reaction to drugs or alcohol. The general features of hepatitis described earlier are rather similar whichever virus is responsible, but there are major differences in epidemiology and prognosis between the various hepatotropic viruses. Identification of the responsible agent by sero-

Table 17.4 Viral causes of hepatitis

Virus	Features
Hepatotropic viruses	
Hepatitis A virus (HAV)	RNA virus; faecal/oral transmission; 1-month incubation
Hepatitis B virus (HBV)	DNA virus; blood and sexual transmission; 3-month incubation
Hepatitis Delta virus (HDV)	RNA virus; blood (and sexual?) transmission; needs HBV
Non-A, non-B virus (NANB)	Unknown structure; several types; faecal/oral and blood transmission; 2-month incubation
Other viruses which can cause hepatitis	
Epstein-Barr virus (EBV) (infectious mononucleosis)	DNA herpes-type virus; close contact and aerosol transmission; liver function tests abnormal in most cases, but jaundice in only 15%
Cytomegalovirus (CMV)	DNA herpes-type virus; blood and close contact transmission; behaves like EBV infection
Herpes simplex and H. zoster	Rarely involves the liver, but may cause severe liver damage in immunosuppressed patients
Lassa fever, Marburg virus and Ebola virus	Rare diseases; imported from Africa; severe organ damage, including liver

logical tests is therefore of considerable help in management.

Treatment is in general supportive, and in controlled clinical trials neither bed rest nor low fat diets, which are often advised, have been shown to be of any value in speeding recovery. Similarly, although abstinence from alcohol is usually advised for about 6 months after recovery from the acute illness, there is no hard evidence that this makes any difference to the outcome. There is anecdotal evidence that vigorous exercise in the prodromal phase may increase the severity of the illness.

HEPATITIS A VIRUS

Virology

Hepatitis A virus (HAV) is an RNA virus whose major polypeptides are similar to the enterovirus group (Fig. 17.9). Serologically the diagnosis of acute HAV infection is usually made by testing for the presence of specific IgM anti-HAV antibodies which are present in serum for about 80 days after the acute illness.

Little is known of the mechanisms leading to cell necrosis. The virus is not cytopathic in tissue culture.

Epidemiology

HAV is transmitted by the faecal/oral route and rarely, if ever, parenterally. It may be endemic or sporadic and epidemics sometimes occur. Although direct contact, often during travel abroad, is the usual source of infection,

Fig. 17.9 The structure of the hepatitis viruses. A. Hepatitis A. **B.** Hepatitis B.

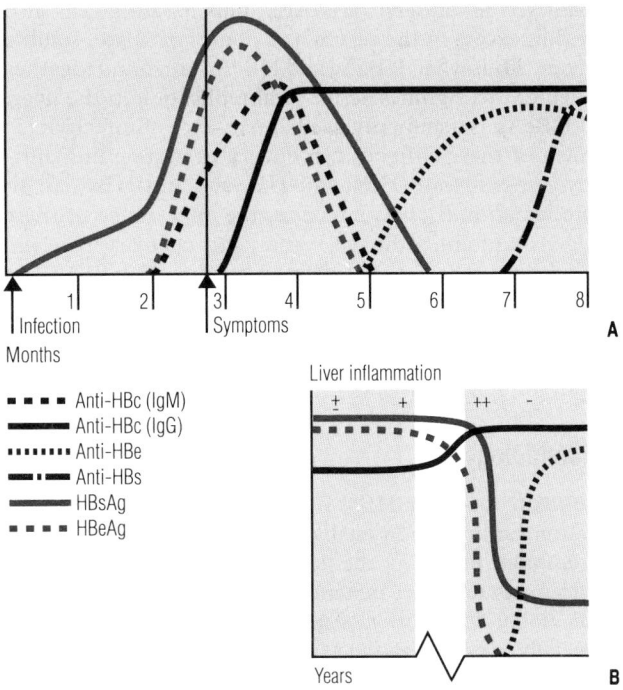

- ▪ ▪ ▪ ▪ Anti-HBc (IgM)
- ─── Anti-HBc (IgG)
- ▪▪▪▪▪▪ Anti-HBe
- ─ ▪ ─ ▪ Anti-HBs
- ─── HBsAg
- ▪ ▪ ▪ ▪ HBeAg

Fig. 17.10 The main serological changes in acute HBV (A) and chronic HBV (B) infection. The break in the x-axis of B has been used to indicate the very variable length of time which can elapse between the establishment of the chronic carrier state and the spontaneous cessation of viral replication.

17

asymptomatic cases are very common and a history of contact is often not obtained. Contaminated food, particularly fresh seafood, is a well-recognised source of infection. The incubation period is about 1 month (2–7 weeks). Carriers have not been detected.

Clinical features

Acute hepatitis A is usually a mild illness preceded by a typical prodrome. This may be so similar to 'flu', with prominent myalgia, that the patient does not connect the prodrome with the jaundice and the patient should be asked about a preceding febrile illness. Fulminant hepatic failure is a rare complication and progression to chronic liver disease does not occur. Aplastic anaemia, particularly in children, is a rare complication with a high mortality.

HEPATITIS B

Virology

The hepatitis B virus is a member of an unusual group, called the HepaDNA viruses. It has an outer and inner protein coat, with double-stranded DNA and a DNA polymerase in the nucleocapsid (Fig. 17.9). The main antigenic protein of the outer coat, the hepatitis B surface antigen (HBsAg), is produced in excess during viral replication, and forms large numbers of smaller empty particles in the serum. The complete core protein coat reacts antigenically as hepatitis B core antigen (HBcAg), but its constituent polypeptides alone have a different antigenic reactivity, the hepatitis B 'e' antigen (HBeAg). This 'e' antigen is also found in excess in the serum as a non-particulate, soluble antigen. Thus when HBsAg and HBeAg are found together in serum, this signifies active viral replication in the liver, and HBeAg is commonly used as a marker of infectivity.

Each of these antigens can elicit a corresponding antibody response (anti-HBs, anti-HBe and anti-HBc). In an acute hepatitis B virus infection, the appearance of these antigens and antibodies in serum, and changes in serum AST levels, follow a well-defined pattern (Fig. 17.10). In the majority of cases, hepatitis B infection is detected by finding HBsAg in serum. The diagnosis of acute, as opposed to chronic, HBV infection is best made by testing serum for IgM-class anti-HBc antibodies.

Epidemiology

The main route for HBV infection is by parenteral inoculation, although direct blood transfusion is now very uncommon, following the development of sensitive serological tests to detect infectious material. The virus has a wide global distribution (Fig. 17.11). Chronic carriers are especially prevalent in the Middle and Far East and in sub-Saharan Africa, where they may constitute up to 30% of the population. In these areas vertical transmission from mothers to their children and horizontal spread in early childhood seem to be the principal modes of infection. In northern Europe and the USA, where chronic carriers are

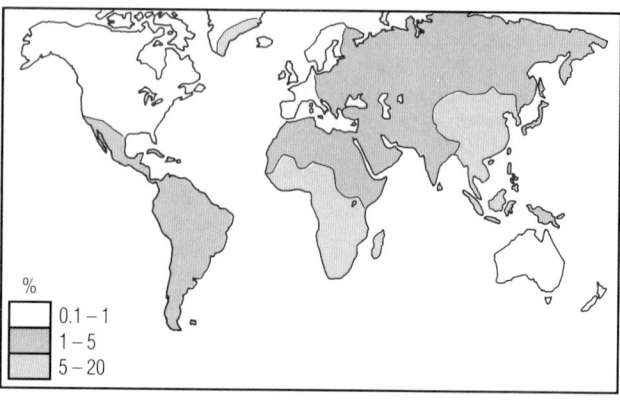

%
☐ 0.1 – 1
▨ 1 – 5
▥ 5 – 20

Fig. 17.11 The distribution of hepatitis B virus infection in the world as judged by the prevalence of hepatitis B surface antigen (HBsAg) in different populations.

less common and where the screening of blood donations is accepted practice, the main reservoirs for the virus are urban homosexual communities and intravenous drug abusers. The virus seems to be readily transmitted by rectal intercourse.

Immunopathology

Recent evidence suggests that the complete hepatitis B virion has binding sites on its surface for polymerised human serum albumin, and that similar receptors are present on the surface of hepatocytes. Polyalbumin-coated virions may thus gain access to hepatocytes by using the albumin as a bridge. This probably explains the hepatotropism of HBV. During replication of the virus, viral antigens, principally HBsAg and HBcAg, appear on the surface membrane of infected hepatocytes and trigger a cytotoxic T lymphocyte response (Fig. 17.12). This is largely directed at HBcAg, and leads to cytolysis, seen clinically as acute liver damage (jaundice and AST elevation), and histologically as spotty necrosis of hepatocytes scattered throughout the liver lobules. Released virions are then neutralised by antibodies directed at the polyalbumin receptor sites. Complete recovery involves a co-ordinated T cell and antibody response to different viral antigens. Failure of these complex mechanisms results in about 5% of apparently normal individuals not clearing the virus, and becoming chronic carriers (Fig. 17.10).

The carrier state is commoner in infancy and childhood, and in those with an associated immunodeficiency, whether this is congenital; due to drugs, as in immunosuppressed transplant recipients; or secondary to other diseases, such as immunosuppressive viral infections in promiscuous homosexuals. The human immunodeficiency virus (HIV) is the most dramatic of these associated virus infections, and AIDS and hepatitis B infection often co-exist in homosexuals. In both these conditions, a reduction in promiscuity is an important preventive measure. In the case of hepatitis B, an effective vaccine made by purifying HBsAg

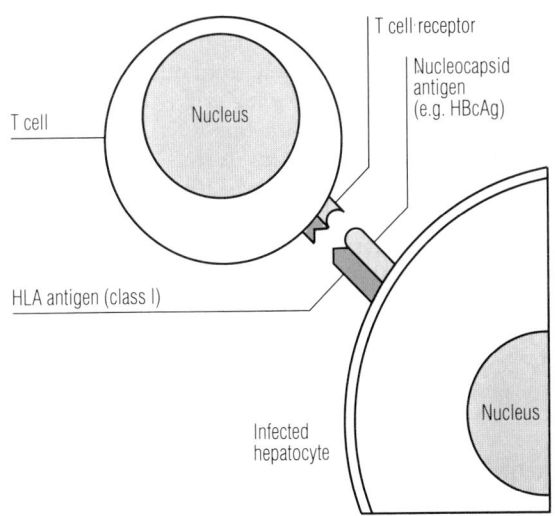

Fig. 17.12 The immunopathology of hepatitis B. Liver cell damage in HBV infection is due to an immune attack by T cells against viral antigens expressed on the surface of infected hepatocytes. The T cells recognise the foreign viral antigens as small peptides bound to class I histocompatibility antigens (HLA class I).

from the plasma of carriers is available for those at increased risk. These include sexual and family contacts of carriers, as well as health-care workers and children born to carrier mothers.

Clinical features

The prodromal illness may be particularly severe, with arthralgia, urticaria and occasionally a full 'serum sickness' syndrome with associated glomerulonephritis. Fulminant hepatic failure is a rare complication, and the main clinical concern is the relatively high rate of progression to a chronic carrier state. The resulting liver lesions are described on page 647. Careful follow-up with repeated serological tests is an essential part of the management. While persistence of HBsAg for more than 6 months is the usual criterion for chronicity, persistence of HBeAg in serum for more than 8 weeks may give an earlier indication of failure to clear the virus normally.

DELTA VIRUS

Virology

This is a small RNA virus with a genome which does not code for its own protein coat; instead it borrows HBsAg provided by a concurrent HBV infection (Fig. 17.13). Serologically, Delta infection can be detected by testing for anti-Delta antibodies in serum. These appear early in the course of the infection but may not persist. Tests for Delta antigen in serum are also being developed, and look promising as diagnostic aids.

Fig. 17.13 The Delta virus. The Delta virus is a strange structure. It borrows its coat from the hepatitis B virus (HBsAG), so HBV must also be present in hepatocytes. The infective material of Delta is a small circular strand of RNA.

Epidemiology

Delta infection is absolutely dependent on a helper function of HBV, and so is only found in two settings: either

Summary 3 Clinical aspects of viral hepatitis				
Type	Incubation period	Clinical features	Outcome	Vaccines
A	4 weeks	Mild often subclinical	No chronic disease	First clinical trials successful
Enteric non-A, non-B	6 weeks	High mortality in pregnancy	No chronic disease	None
Parenteral non-A, non-B	8 weeks	Mild often subclinical	20–40% progress to chronic disease	None
B	12 weeks	Variable severity	Neonatal 90% carriers Childhood 10–40% carriers Adult 1–10% carriers	Widely available and in national programmes
Delta	4–12 weeks	Severe in HBV carriers	Carrier on chronic HBV; recovery in most co-infections	None

Liver and Biliary Tract Disease

17

there is a dual acute infection of HBV and Delta virus, or Delta virus infects an existing HBsAg carrier. Like HBV it is spread by the parenteral route or intimate contact. It is endemic in countries around the Mediterranean basin, and in northern Europe and the USA is mainly found in drug abusers.

Immunopathology

Clinical evidence and studies in primates suggest that the Delta virus is directly cytopathic to the cells it infects. The contribution of immune responses to cell damage and recovery is not known.

Clinical features

Co-infection produces an acute hepatitis, clinically indistinguishable from HBV infection alone, although there is some suggestion that the illness may be more severe. Recovery from the HBV infection is always associated with the disappearance of Delta. Infection in an HBsAg carrier can produce a severe acute hepatitis, and in some cases fulminant hepatic failure. Chronic Delta infection is also more likely to occur and this carries a bad prognosis (p. 648).

NON-A, NON-B VIRUSES

Virology

When all known virus infections of the liver and possible hepatotoxins have been excluded, there remain a number of cases with clinical features typical of viral hepatitis. The presumed viral agents responsible have been called 'non-A, non-B'. On the basis of experimental transmission studies in primates, it seems likely that several different viruses are present in this group. One enterically transmitted virus has been visualised in faeces from acute cases, but no generally available serological test has yet been developed. Very recently, one of the parenterally transmitted agents has been cloned, sequenced and its major surface proteins expressed in yeast. It seems to be a single-stranded RNA virus belonging to the flavivirus group. Based on this work, a serological assay has been developed which is expected to be commercially available soon.

Epidemiology

Apart from the enterically transmitted virus discussed above, the other non-A, non-B viruses appear to be transmitted by parenteral inoculation. Apparently healthy carriers must exist in the population since blood transfusions and blood products, such as factor VIII, are important sources of infection. Sporadic cases may follow travel abroad, and drug abusers are another group at high risk of infection. Promiscuous homosexuality does not seem to be a risk factor, possibly because of the relatively high doses of infectious material required to transmit the infection.

Clinical features

The illness is indistinguishable from other forms of acute viral hepatitis (p. 634). Histologically, there is often an emphasis on cholestasis, with bile duct damage in some cases, but this is not a striking feature clinically. In the absence of reliable serological tests, little progress has been made in understanding the pathological process, although there is evidence that cellular immune responses may be involved in the pathogenesis of liver cell damage. The major clinical concern is the relatively high rate of progression to chronic liver disease (10–40% of cases), particularly in those who have acquired the infection from blood transfusion or blood products.

NON-HEPATOTROPIC VIRUSES

Epstein–Barr virus

Liver function tests are often abnormal in glandular fever, but jaundice occurs in less than 10% of cases. The Epstein–Barr virus (p. 240) does not seem to infect hepatocytes and pathologically, portal, sinusoidal and focal infiltrates of lymphoid cells are prominent features, while liver cell necrosis is minimal. Recovery is almost always uneventful, although fatigue, as part of a postviral syndrome, can be troublesome for a few months.

Cytomegalovirus

In adults cytomegalovirus (p. 241) can produce an illness like glandular fever, with accompanying jaundice in some cases, but recovery is usually rapid. Liver biopsy, although not required to make the diagnosis (which is made serologically), may show the characteristic eosinophilic nuclear inclusions in infected hepatocytes.

Herpes simplex

Herpes simplex (p. 239) is a rare cause of severe acute hepatitis, usually affecting immunosuppressed patients. There is usually a local oral lesion, but the striking feature is disseminated infection with encephalitis or myocarditis, in addition to hepatitis.

DRUG-INDUCED JAUNDICE

The continued production of new drugs has been accompanied by an increasing problem with drug-induced liver damage (Table 17.5). It is generally stated that about 10% of cases of jaundice in hospital practice are due to medication. There are two main types of adverse reaction: *predictable or dose-dependent* (type A), and *idiosyncratic or dose-independent* (type B). In the former, liver damage is dose-dependent and relatively common, and can usually be reproduced in laboratory animals. Idiosyncratic cases are infrequent, not related to dose and not usually repro-

636

Table 17.5 Drugs causing liver damage

Drug	Comments
Antituberculous	
Para-aminosalicylic acid (PAS)	Idiosyncratic type; 1% get drug hepatitis in first 2 months
Isoniazid (INAH)	Raised transaminases in 10%; 1% jaundice in first 2 months
Rifampicin	Up to 4% develop hepatitis; ?increases isoniazid toxicity
Pyrazinamide and ethionamide	Late-onset hepatitis in 1%
Other antibiotics	
Tetracycline	Microvesicular fatty liver
Sulphonamides including co-trimoxazole	Idiosyncratic; mimics viral hepatitis
Erythromycin	Cholestasis; especially estolate
Ketoconazole	Hepatitis in 0.1%
Nitrofurantoin	Cholestasis and chronic hepatitis
Psychotropic drugs	
Monoamine oxidase inhibitors	Viral hepatitis look-alike in 1–2% after about 4 months
Phenothiazines	Mixed cholestatic and hepatitic picture in 1–2% after 2–4 months; can persist
Tricyclic antidepressants	Rare cholestatic hepatitis
Analgesics	
Paracetamol	Predictable liver necrosis in overdose (more than 10 g); methionine/cysteamine antidote
Aspirin	Acute anicteric hepatitis, especially in children; may cause Reye's syndrome
Non-steroidal analgesics	Three withdrawn because of hepatotoxicity (benoxaprofen, ibufenac and aclofenac)
Steroid drugs and hormones	
17-alkyl/ethynyl substituted steroids (including contraceptive pill)	Predictable (dose/duration-dependent) cholestasis, especially the 19-nortestosterones; increased risk of adenoma
Anaesthetic agents	
Halothane	Commonly produces minor increase in transaminases; very rarely fatal hepatitis
Immunosuppressive drugs	
Azathioprine	Rare cholestasis
Methotrexate	Long continued treatment, as in psoriasis, may cause fibrosis and cirrhosis
Corticosteroids	Fatty infiltration
Cardiovascular drugs	
Methyldopa	Acute and chronic hepatitis starting after 2–5 months
Perhexilene	Rare hepatitic illness, looks like alcoholic liver damage
Thiazide diuretics	Cholestatic hepatitis; may be prolonged
Oral hypoglycaemic drugs	
Chlorpropamide	Cholestatic hepatitis in 5%, with granulomatous reaction

ducible experimentally. Recognition of these cases is important for two main reasons: withdrawal of the drug usually leads to rapid recovery, and repeat prescription, which may be associated with a more severe reaction, can be avoided. Proof of an association between a particular drug and idiosyncratic hepatotoxicity can be difficult, since it is almost impossible to exclude a coincidental non-A, non-B hepatitis. Systematic reporting of suspected reactions is the only way in which sufficient evidence can be accumulated to suggest a true association. In the UK this is done by a system of postal reporting of adverse reactions (the yellow card) to the Committee on Safety of Medicines (CSM) (p. 30). Over the last 20 years reports to the CSM have indicated that between 10 and 24 adult patients have died each year from drug-induced liver disease.

The liver damage produced by drugs can mimic almost any acute or chronic hepatic or biliary disorder, and thinking of drugs as a possible cause of a liver illness is the first vital step to the correct diagnosis. In most cases, liver damage is predominantly hepatitic or cholestatic.

Drug-induced hepatitis

Paracetamol- and halothane-induced liver damage are two examples of drug-induced hepatitis; both are potentially fatal. Paracetamol is a predictable hepatotoxin, while the liver damage induced by halothane occurs idiosyncratically.

Paracetamol

Paracetamol is safe in normal therapeutic doses but produces a severe hepatitis if taken in overdose (more than 10 g or 20 tablets), usually with suicidal intent. Liver damage is due to the formation of highly reactive metabolites (Fig. 17.14). At normal dose levels these are inactivated by conjugation with glutathione. Insufficient glutathione is available for detoxification when a large amount of drug is taken, and the metabolites damage the cell by binding to cellular macromolecules. Compounds acting as -SH donors can prevent this process. The most effective and non-toxic of these is N-acetyl cysteine given intravenously (p. 56).

Halothane

Halothane is an example of an unpredictable (idiosyncratic) hepatotoxin. Significant liver damage is very rare (1 in 30 000 halothane anaesthetics), but when it occurs it is often fatal. It is more common after repeated halothane anaesthesia, often for minor surgical procedures such as repeated cystoscopies. The clinical picture is very similar to viral hepatitis, with a prodromal illness starting a few days after the surgical procedure. In about one-third of cases unexplained pyrexia has been noted following a previous halothane anaesthetic. Progression to fulminant hepatic failure is common, although the exact frequency of this complication is difficult to assess because of uncer-

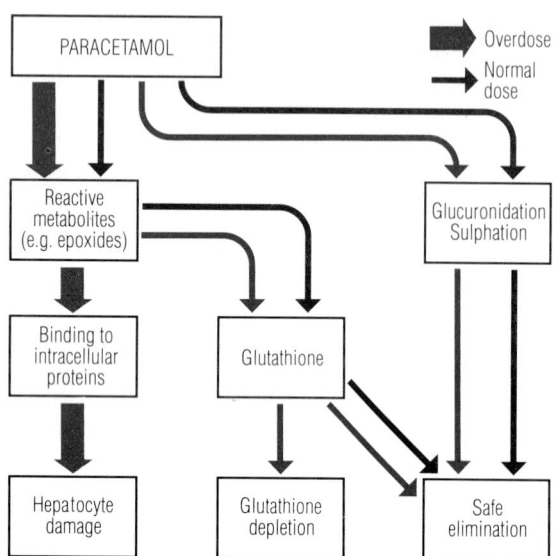

Fig. 17.14 Paracetamol overdose. Paracetamol is normally safe to take because the metabolites are inactivated by conjugation. After an overdose the conjugating material, particularly glutathione, is used up and reactive metabolites damage the liver cell proteins.

tainty about the diagnosis in mild cases. The mechanism of liver damage is thought to be immunological. A reactive metabolite, produced during oxidative metabolism of halothane, alters the normal antigens on the liver cell membrane. In patients with halothane hepatitis these new antigens have been shown to stimulate an immune response, which may produce the liver damage. The idiosyncrasy seems to be related to the ability to recognise these subtle antigenic alterations.

Drug-induced cholestasis

The cholestatic jaundice induced by C17 substituted testosterone derivatives and chlorpromazine are examples of predictable and idiosyncratic hepatotoxicity.

C17 substituted testosterone derivatives

C17 substituted testosterone derivatives produce liver damage by direct hepatotoxicity. The agents include androgenic and anabolic steroids, progestogens and oestrogens. The cholestatic effect is dose-related. The obstructive jaundice resolves following cessation of treatment. Histologically, there is evidence of centrilobular cholestasis, without obvious hepatocellular damage. The exact mechanism is unknown.

Chlorpromazine

Chlorpromazine is a rather dramatic example of an idiosyncratic reaction. About 1–2% of those taking this drug develop a severe cholestasis, which may persist for weeks after the drug has been withdrawn. The reaction has been

described following only one dose. The mechanism responsible for the cholestasis is unknown. The finding of eosinophilia has led to the suggestion that this may be an example of a hypersensitivity reaction, but there is no immunological evidence to support this.

FULMINANT HEPATIC FAILURE

Pathophysiology

Rarely, liver damage in the course of acute hepatitis is very severe, and leads to secondary disturbance of function in other organ systems. This complex and potentially serious development is recognised clinically as fulminant hepatic failure. *Encephalopathy* is the commonest and most obvious complication. Although the exact cause is unknown, some of the potential factors include release of toxins from the damaged liver, failure to detoxify metabolites, and alterations in cerebral neurotransmitters due to amino acid imbalances (p. 655). *Renal failure* is also common and carries a particularly bad prognosis. It may be due to endotoxaemia or septicaemia.

Epidemiology

Fulminant hepatic failure is a rare complication of almost any of the causes of acute hepatitis. About half the cases in the UK are due to paracetamol poisoning, with most of the remainder being associated with a hepatitis virus infection (about one-third each of A, B and non-A, non-B). A small proportion are due to other drugs such as halothane, isoniazid and rifampicin. In France ingestion of the poisonous mushroom *Amanita phalloides* is an important cause.

Clinical features

Patients will develop the signs of fulminant hepatic failure within 8 weeks of the onset of the illness and have no previous history of liver disease. This distinguishes fulminant hepatic failure from rapidly progressive chronic liver disease. The first signs of the disease often relate to the encephalopathy with the appearance of mild confusion, irrational behaviour or even euphoria. A confusing early feature can be an agitated noisy phase, when the use of sedatives may seem necessary but must be avoided. A widely fluctuating but progressive deterioration in mental condition then follows, leading to coma. The usual grading of the level of coma is according to a four-stage model (Table 17.6). In some rapidly progressive cases, jaundice may never be apparent and the whole illness, from first symptoms to death, may last less than a week. Important signs on examination include fetor hepaticus (a rather sweet and sickly odour on the breath), a flapping tremor (asterixis), slurred speech, and difficulty in writing and copying simple diagrams (constructional apraxia). At this stage, serum aminotransferase (AST or ALT) is often

Table 17.6 Grades of coma in liver failure

Grade	Clinical features
I	Slowness of mentation and affect; fluctuant mild confusion; reversed sleep rhythm; slurred speech; alternating euphoria and depression; untidiness
II	Accentuation of grade I; inappropriate behaviour; drowsy
III	Marked confusion; sleeps most of the time but rousable; incoherent speech
IV	Unrousable; may or may not respond to noxious stimuli

elevated by 40-fold or more, and the prothrombin time is usually more than 20 seconds prolonged. In the early stages of grade IV coma, hyperventilation is common, and the pupils are dilated and react sluggishly to light. Hypertonia and grasp reflex are readily elicited, and in deep coma, decerebrate postures are seen. Terminally, the oculo-vestibular reflex is lost and hypotension, cardiac arrhythmias and respiratory arrest occur.

Complications and management

Complications and management of acute liver failure are listed in Table 17.7. Treatment consists of skilled supportive therapy based on a sound knowledge of the expected course of the disease and its complications. Admission to an intensive care area is essential. The encephalopathy is treated by withdrawal of dietary protein, emptying of the large bowel using a magnesium sulphate enema, and administration of lactulose orally. Intravenous nutritional support is with 10% dextrose. Serum sodium and potassium levels are measured daily and any abnormalities corrected. Hypoglycaemia and hypokalaemia are early life-threatening abnormalities which must be detected and corrected quickly. Erosive oesophagitis and gastritis leading to severe gastrointestinal haemorrhage

Table 17.7 Complications and management of acute liver failure

Problem	Treatment
Coma	Lactulose, neomycin and magnesium sulphate enemas to reduce gut ammonia load
Cerebral oedema	Mannitol infusions given promptly reverse pressure rises
Nutrition, fluid and electrolytes	10% dextrose into a central vein; extra potassium needed; low sodium is usually dilutional
Renal failure	Common problem; half have 'function renal failure', others acute tubular necrosis. Attention to fluid balance may help, but dialysis may be needed
Gastrointestinal haemorrhage	H_2-receptor antagonists significantly reduce risk, and are given routinely
Respiratory failure	Common late complication. Intubate early to protect airway

used to be a major problem, but the prophylactic use of H_2-receptor antagonists has proved very effective. Renal failure is common, and haemodialysis may be needed. Coagulation disorders are also common, due to failure of synthesis of clotting factors and, in some cases, the occurrence of disseminated intravascular coagulation (p. 1103). Fresh frozen plasma is the usual treatment for the clotting disturbance. Cerebral oedema is an important cause of death, and mannitol infusions are useful in reducing increased intracranial pressure. Liver support systems based on charcoal haemoperfusion, with prostacyclin infusion to reduce platelet consumption and improve biocompatibility, are being developed but have not yet been evaluated in controlled clinical trials. Rarely a suitable donor may become available and liver transplantation then becomes another treatment option.

Even with the most skilful intensive care support the mortality of fulminant hepatic failure is high, with most centres reporting mortality rates of more than 80% in those who develop grade IV encephalopathy. However, survivors rarely develop cirrhosis or chronic liver disease, probably because of the remarkable regenerative capacity of the liver, and this continues to encourage efforts to improve supportive care, to allow more time for regeneration to overtake cell destruction.

JAUNDICE IN PREGNANCY

There are two causes of jaundice which are peculiar to pregnancy.

Cholestasis of pregnancy

Cholestasis of pregnancy is a rare condition, in which pruritus, with or without painless jaundice, occurs in the last trimester of pregnancy. Some women taking the oral contraceptive pill seem to develop a similar condition, suggesting that it represents an unusual response to high oestrogen levels. The alkaline phosphatase is always elevated. It is useful to exclude extrahepatic obstruction by showing that the bile ducts are not dilated on ultrasound, but liver biopsy is rarely justified. The itching can be very troublesome, but usually responds to cholestyramine. The symptoms disappear following the birth, and the liver function tests return to normal. The cholestasis tends to recur with each pregnancy.

Acute fatty liver of pregnancy

Acute fatty liver of pregnancy is a serious but rare condition. It presents in the last trimester with a prodromal illness which is similar to acute viral hepatitis, and which starts about a week before the jaundice appears. The histological changes are quite distinct from viral hepatitis. There is a widespread, centrilobular, microvesicular fatty change in hepatocytes. The aetiology is unknown, although identical changes are rarely seen following tetracycline treatment. Serum transaminases are usually very high, and the prothrombin time is markedly prolonged. Maternal and fetal mortality is high, even with full intensive care support. Urgent delivery is recommended, as dramatic recovery can occur in some cases following the birth.

Neonatal hepatitis

Jaundice due to increased plasma levels of unconjugated bilirubin occurs in up to 90% of healthy newborn infants, and in the majority is due to a temporary inefficiency of hepatic excretion of bilirubin. Conjugated hyper-bilirubinaemia in infancy is always pathological. Neonatal hepatitis, better called the hepatitis syndrome in infancy, is the commonest cause of elevated plasma levels of conjugated bilirubin. The standard liver function tests often show a rather mixed picture of obstruction and liver cell damage. There are many causes, including viral infections, metabolic disorders, bile duct abnormalities and vascular lesions.

ACUTE ALCOHOLIC HEPATITIS

Clinical features

The term 'alcoholic hepatitis' has two quite different meanings. To the histopathologist, it indicates certain specific features found in some patients with alcoholic liver disease, particularly perinuclear eosinophilic hyaline inclusion bodies (Mallory's hyaline) in hepatocytes in, or near to, areas of spotty parenchymal necrosis. An associated inflammatory infiltrate consists largely of polymorpho-nuclear leucocytes. There may or may not be associated fibrosis or cirrhosis. Although some patients with these changes on liver biopsy are entirely asymptomatic, the pathological features are important as they indicate a greatly increased chance of the development of cirrhosis. This progression occurs in 90% of patients with features of alcoholic hepatitis on liver biopsy if they continue to drink, while complete regression is the rule in 90% of those who subsequently remain abstinent.

To the clinician, the term 'alcoholic hepatitis' is also used to describe an acute illness associated with alcohol abuse, in which deep jaundice, abdominal pain, fever, marked polymorphonuclear leucocytosis, and elevated prothrombin time are the principal features. Cutaneous stigmata of chronic liver disease are common, even in the absence of cirrhosis. Cholestasis is often prominent and may lead to a mistaken diagnosis of extrahepatic obstructive jaundice, and possibly a laparotomy, which can be fatal. The mortality of the condition is high (30–60%).

Both the clinical illness and the pathological changes are commoner and more severe in women, and in people of northern European origin (including America). Although the histological changes can be found in southern European

patients, the severe acute clinical illness is uncommon. There is no definite relation to the pattern of drinking or the type of alcoholic drink.

Treatment

Trials of specific drug treatments have proved disappointing, and abstinence remains the most effective therapy. For a discussion of methods which can help to achieve this goal, see page 74.

OBSTRUCTIVE JAUNDICE

As with the diagnosis of acute hepatitis, a good history is the key to identification of obstructive jaundice. While pale stools and dark urine are common to both, the early appearance of itching and, more rarely, high fevers with rigor (ascending cholangitis) are general pointers to extrahepatic bile duct obstruction. The commonest causes are outlined in Table 17.8 and the specialised investigations which may be required to identify the site and cause of the obstruction are described on page 629. An essential early investigation is an ultrasound scan of the upper abdomen. The presence of dilated bile ducts (which can be identified with great confidence by this procedure) is an almost certain indication of major duct obstruction. Gallstones, which are echo-dense, are also detected easily, but it can be more difficult to comment with certainty on the pancreas and other retroperitoneal structures. In some cases, a CT scan may be helpful. The final determination of the site of obstruction is best made by ERCP or percutaneous cholangiography.

Table 17.8 Causes of obstructive jaundice

Intrahepatic

Metabolic/unknown cause	Liver damage
Pregnancy	Primary biliary cirrhosis
Contraceptive pill;	Late viral hepatitis
Methyltestosterone	Alcoholic hepatitis
Parenteral nutrition	Biliary hypoplasia
Lymphoma	Secondary deposits
Benign recurrent intrahepatic, and postoperative cholestasis	

Extrahepatic

Benign	Malignant
Gallstones in bile duct	Carcinoma of the gall bladder
Post-traumatic stricture	Carcinoma of the bile duct
Sclerosing cholangitis	Hilar lymphadenopathy
Biliary atresia	Carcinoma of the ampulla of Vater
Choledochal cyst	Carcinoma of the pancreas
Acute and chronic pancreatitis	
Retroperitoneal fibrosis	
Ascending cholangitis	
Haemobilia	

GALLSTONES

Pathophysiology

Mixed cholesterol stones

Mixed cholesterol stones are the commonest variety in the Western world, and consist largely of cholesterol crystals with a variable proportion of calcium salts. The main constituents of bile are cholesterol, phospholipids and bile salts. The ratio between cholesterol and the other constituents is crucial in maintaining cholesterol in solution. Bile supersaturated with cholesterol can develop because of an increased cholesterol concentration, or decreased bile salt content. These changes in the constituents can be due to altered rates of secretion, either congenital or acquired, or changes in the relative proportions during concentration and storage of bile in the gall bladder.

Pigment stones

Pigment stones consist of bilirubin and salts such as phosphates and carbonates. They are common in the Far East. Increased delivery of bilirubin in chronic haemolytic anaemias is a frequent cause in the United Kingdom, while in the Far East parasitic and bacterial infection of the bile is the usual causative factor. These organisms promote the formation of insoluble deconjugated bilirubin by the release of enzymes such as glucuronidase.

Epidemiology

The epidemiology of gallstone disease is changing. Cholesterol gallstones occur more often in women than in men (Fig. 17.15), and the prevalence increases with age, obesity and parity. Other suggested risk factors are diet (a vegetarian diet appears protective), a positive family history, social class (low social class being linked to an increase in risk) and use of oral contraceptives. There are marked racial differences in prevalence, with American Indians being particularly susceptible. There is a predisposition to cholesterol stone formation in patients with chronic liver disease where there is reduced excretion of bile salts, and also in patients with a resection or disease of the terminal ileum. In these cases there is reduced bile salt re-absorption from the gut and a consequent fall in bile salt excretion into the bile.

Detection

Only 10% of cholesterol gallstones contain enough calcium salts to be visualised on plain X-ray of the abdomen, and in most cases it is necessary to employ further investigative techniques to confirm the diagnosis. Oral cholecystography uses a radio-opaque contrast which is concentrated in the gall bladder to show the stones as lucent areas. One of the major problems with this technique is that it is dependent on intact gall bladder function to concentrate the contrast and in the presence of gallstones this function is sometimes disturbed. Ultrasound is gradually replacing oral cholecystography as the investigation of choice to detect stones in the gall bladder. Gallstones are so echo-dense that they are associated with a characteristic acoustic shadow (p. 25, Fig. 2.5). Several studies have shown that using ultrasound, stones can be detected with an accuracy of more than 95%.

Clinical features

Stones in the gall bladder are a common incidental finding and, if they remain there, may never give rise to symptoms. Stones in the biliary tree may cause biliary colic. Impaction in the cystic duct followed by infection produces acute cholecystitis, while passage down the common bile duct produces biliary colic, obstructive jaundice and cholangitis.

Acute cholecystitis

The presenting symptoms of acute cholecystitis are malaise, anorexia and pyrexia, with pain in the right hypochondrium sometimes radiating to the right shoulder. There is guarding and rigidity in the right upper quadrant. Tenderness on inspiration over the gall bladder area (Murphy's sign) is usually present. Jaundice suggests stones in the common bile duct.

A polymorphonuclear leucocytosis is usually present, but does not help in the differential diagnosis, which includes acute appendicitis and pancreatitis. Ultrasound is the best investigation to confirm the presence of gallstones.

There are two different approaches to treatment: either *early cholecystectomy* in all cases, or initial *broad-spectrum antibiotic therapy* (such as a cephalosporin with metronidazole), *fluid replacement* and *analgesia*, followed by elective cholecystectomy several weeks later. Exploration of the common bile duct, with operative cholangiography, should be undertaken if there is jaundice, dilatation of the duct or evidence on previous investigations of stones in the common bile duct.

Complications include empyema and perforation of the gall bladder, and liver abscesses following portal pyaemia. Perforation is particularly frequent in the elderly. The signs are those of generalised peritonitis, unless previous

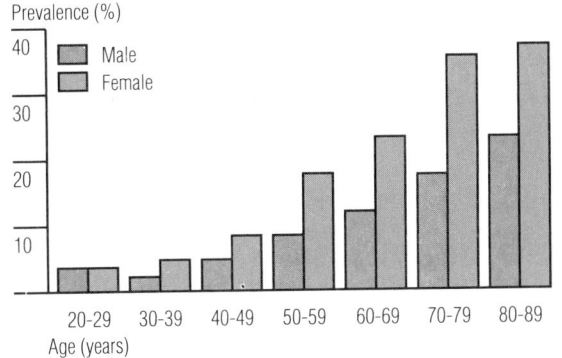

Fig. 17.15 **The increasing prevalence of gallstones with age in both men and women.**

episodes of cholecystitis have led to dense adhesions, when a localised abscess may be produced. Empyema results from infection of obstructed bile in the gall bladder, which fills with pus. There is a very tender mass in the right hypochondrium, with fever and sometimes Gram-negative septicaemia. Treatment is by emergency drainage of the biliary system under broad-spectrum antibiotic cover.

Stones in the common bile duct

Although the classical symptoms of biliary colic, followed by jaundice, might be expected to accompany the passage of a stone down the common bile duct, it is important to realise that a substantial proportion of patients with biliary obstruction due to gallstones may present with painless jaundice. Cholangitis and Gram-negative septicaemia are frequent and dangerous complications, and the diagnosis must be established quickly.

Ultrasound is again of great value in demonstrating a dilated biliary system, and may also show the stone in the common bile duct. It is usually necessary to proceed to cholangiography (PTC or ERCP, pp. 629, 630) to confirm the diagnosis, but antibiotics should be given first to minimise the risk of cholangitis.

Treatment is usually surgical, involving exploration of the duct, removal of stones and temporary T-tube drainage. It is best to start antibiotics, give intramuscular vitamin K, and correct fluid balance or electrolyte abnormalities before surgery. Many broad-spectrum antibiotics have been shown to be effective in this prophylactic setting, and cephalosporins with their low incidence of toxic reactions are usually favoured. Mannitol infusion has been shown to reduce the incidence of postoperative renal failure. In the elderly or bad-risk patients, endoscopic sphincterotomy followed by removal of any remaining stones with a basket or balloon via the endoscope, is an alternative procedure.

Acute cholangitis

In any patient with obstructive jaundice the biliary system can become infected, often with dramatic clinical consequences. Rigors usually accompany a high fever, and this in the presence of jaundice is sometimes known as *Charcot's intermittent biliary* fever, or more simply *ascending cholangitis*. Vascular collapse and renal failure are common complications, reflecting the high incidence of Gram-negative septicaemia. Urgent broad-spectrum antibiotic therapy, after taking blood cultures, is essential, and must be coupled with early relief of the biliary obstruction. A combination of antibiotics active against aerobic and anaerobic organisms is usually chosen. A suitable combination is gentamicin, ampicillin and metronidazole, although it is usually necessary to monitor the serum gentamicin levels carefully as renal impairment is common.

Chronic cholecystitis

Chronic inflammation of the gall bladder is usually found in association with gallstones, but whether or not this produces symptoms, and what these are, is a subject of continuing debate. The diagnosis of chronic cholecystitis is almost certainly made too frequently. The symptoms are often vague, with 'flatulent dyspepsia', fullness in the upper abdomen and excessive eructations (belching). In a sizeable minority of cases, treatment, by cholecystectomy, does not alter these complaints. Other conditions, like the irritable bowel syndrome (p. 609), can produce identical symptoms. Nausea is the commonest single symptom and is often triggered by fatty food. Gallstones are best detected by ultrasound or oral cholangiography, but are common in older women and should not be used as the sole criterion for making a diagnosis of chronic cholecystitis. Careful investigation of the upper abdomen by endoscopy is often helpful. In the elderly medical dissolution of gallstones with bile salts is an alternative to cholecystectomy, but the rate of dissolution is slow and the stones usually return after withdrawal of treatment.

BENIGN BILE DUCT STRICTURE

Benign bile duct stricture is almost always a consequence of prior surgical intervention. The bile duct may have been cut and repaired, or stenosis may develop after interference with its blood supply, or be secondary to local sepsis.

Clinical features

The usual history is of recurrent episodes of obstructive jaundice, fever and rigors, due to ascending cholangitis. After many months of recurrent symptoms progressive fibrosis and secondary biliary cirrhosis may develop.

Diagnosis and treatment

Good-quality cholangiography, often using a combination of PTC and ERCP, is essential in making the diagnosis and in planning treatment. Antibiotic cover for these procedures is a sensible precaution. Surgical relief of the obstruction offers the best chance of long-term relief of symptoms, but it is often difficult to find suitable sites in the biliary tree for an adequate by-pass anastamosis. Fat malabsorption is common, and should be treated with replacement of the fat-soluble vitamins A, D and K. Sequential use of antibiotics can reduce the number of disabling and potentially dangerous attacks of ascending cholangitis.

SCLEROSING CHOLANGITIS

In sclerosing cholangitis, short strictures form in the intrahepatic and extrahepatic biliary system. It is of unknown cause, although about 70% of cases have mild ulcerative colitis. Episodes of ascending cholangitis and jaundice are common. ERCP shows a characteristic beaded appearance of the bile ducts, and liver biopsy typically shows concentric, onion-skin fibrosis around the bile ducts. Drainage procedures are rarely possible. Corticosteroids and penicillamine have been tried, but are of no proven benefit. The disease is slowly progressive and secondary biliary cirrhosis usually develops.

Carcinoma of the pancreas

A full discussion of carcinoma of the pancreas is included on p. 619.

CANCER OF THE BILE DUCTS AND GALL BLADDER

Incidence and aetiology

Tumours of the bile duct and gall bladder have an equal sex incidence and occur most frequently over the age of 60 (Fig. 17.16), when they are commoner than hepatoma. Known aetiological factors include liver flukes (*Opisthorchis felineus* and *Clonorchia sinensis*) and gallstones. The risk of these tumours in patients with longstanding gallstones is about 2%. Bile duct cancer is more common in longstanding ulcerative colitis, occurring in about 1 in 200 of all cases.

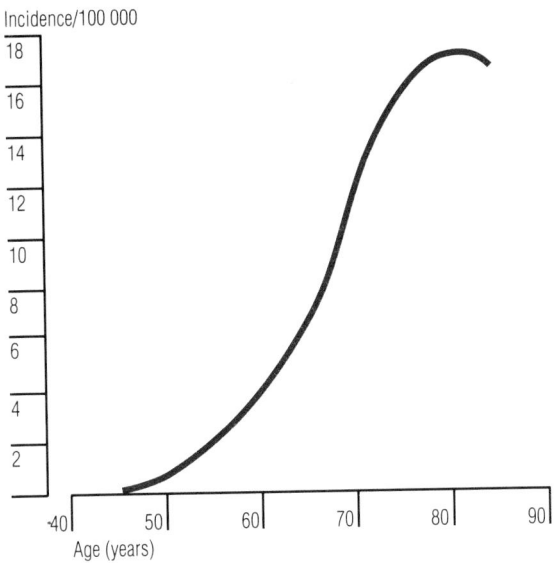

Fig. 17.16 The steep rise in the incidence of gall bladder cancer with age.

Pathology

In the biliary tree the distal common bile duct is the commonest site (50% of cases) and the ampulla of Vater is the most usual location. Of the remainder, 20% of cases arise from the small intrahepatic biliary ducts, and 30% from the proximal extrahepatic duct. Gall bladder cancers usually arise in the body (95% of cases).

Bile duct cancers are adenocarcinomas which usually provoke a fibrous reaction. In the liver they may sometimes be difficult to distinguish from hepatoma. Gall bladder cancers are usually adenocarcinomas (85%), with occasional squamous and anaplastic forms. The tumours infiltrate locally and metastasise to regional lymph nodes. They spread to involve the liver both by local infiltration and by metastases.

Clinical features

Bile duct tumours grow slowly and cause obstructive jaundice with pruritus. The jaundice may fluctuate if the tumour sloughs and obstruction is temporarily diminished. The gall bladder may be distended if the tumour is distal to the junction of hepatic and cystic ducts. Intrahepatic tumours may not cause jaundice until they are very large. Right upper quadrant pain is common. Carcinoma of the gall bladder causes similar pain, with obstructive jaundice occurring later.

Diagnosis and investigation

The presentation with pain may lead to a diagnosis of gallstones. A palpable mass usually means the tumours are inoperable. With gall bladder cancer, ultrasound and CT scanning may show a mass, but the diagnosis is frequently made at laparotomy. With bile duct cancer, percutaneous transhepatic cholangiography (PTC) is usually carried out before surgery and will show the dilated proximal ducts and the upper limit of the block. ERCP may be used to demonstrate the distal extent.

Management

Gall bladder cancer is often unresectable, and a biliary decompression operation is undertaken when technically possible. Resection may involve removal of part of the liver as well as the gall bladder. Only 20% of carcinomas of the biliary tree are operable, and major resections carry a high operative mortality (10–15%). Biliary bypass procedures are effective in palliation and this may be accomplished during PTC, with the passage of a cannula (stent) through the site of the obstruction. Radiotherapy can be used to reduce tumour size, and may relieve obstruction and pain for a considerable time.

CIRRHOSIS

Definition

Cirrhosis (Table 17.9) is an irreversible change in liver structure, the essential features being disorganisation of the lobular architecture, the presence of regeneration nodules and increased fibrosis. The size of the regeneration nodules can be smaller than the size of a normal liver lobule (micronodular cirrhosis) or embracing several portal tracts and central veins (macronodular cirrhosis). These are not separate varieties. The nodules tend to be small when there is active, continuing liver cell destruction, and larger when there is low-grade inflammation and necrosis. The most important pathological distinction is from portal fibrosis, which is a reversible increase in collagen deposition in and between portal tracts.

Classification

Table 17.9 gives a classification of cirrhosis based on aetiology. Although pathogenetic mechanisms are often poorly understood, this is a useful way of grouping cases with similar aetiology. The relative importance of the various types depends very much on geography and social factors. For example, in the developed countries of the West, alcohol is the commonest cause of cirrhosis (about 80% of cases in the UK), but is relatively less frequent in Africa and Asia. Cirrhosis due to chronic hepatitis B virus infection dominates the picture in the Middle and Far East and in many places in Africa, while both these main causes are common in southern Europe.

Whatever the cause, cirrhosis produces common complications (p. 652).

Table 17.9 Classification and distribution of cirrhosis

Common causes

Alcoholism	Primary biliary cirrhosis
The commonest cause in the Western world	Broad geographical spread, 90% female
Chronic active hepatitis	Schistosomiasis
Chronic virus infection (HBV, Delta, NANB)	Equatorial and in the Middle and Far East; fibrosis is usual, but cirrhosis is found in *S. japanicum*
The commonest cause in the Middle and Far East	
Autoimmune	
Almost restricted to north European caucasians	

Rare but potentially reversible causes

Wilson's disease (hepatolenticular degeneration)	Drug-induced
Early copper chelation can reverse liver damage	Methotrexate, methyldopa, isoniazid, perhexiline
Haemochromatosis	Galactosaemia and fructosaemia
Venesection removes iron, improves liver function	Genetically determined metabolic disorders; diet can prevent cirrhosis
Constrictive pericarditis, congenital venous web	Biliary atresia
Two examples of chronic venous congestion, often completely reversible	Early porto-enterostomy can prevent cirrhosis

Rarities

Secondary biliary cirrhosis	Sclerosing cholangitis
Cystic fibrosis	Neonatal hepatitis syndrome
Glycogen storage disease	Alpha-1-antitrypsin deficiency
Indian childhood cirrhosis	Veno-occlusive disease

Presentation and general clinical features

If the process causing the cirrhotic transformation is inactive, presentation is usually delayed until portal hypertension and liver cell failure produce symptoms of ascites, haematemesis from bleeding varices, or encephalopathy. In older males, primary hepatocellular carcinoma (primary hepatoma) is a frequent complication, usually associated with an underlying inactive, macronodular cirrhosis. In some cases the disease is detected at an asymptomatic stage during routine physical examination or biochemical screening. Some of the causes of cirrhosis produce more florid liver damage, and may present with jaundice, pruritus or symptoms of other organ involvement before cirrhosis has become established.

On examination, cutaneous stigmata of chronic liver disease are usually prominent. Spider naevi are restricted to the upper half of the body. Possible causal mechanisms are inappropriate vasodilatation or high oestrogenic activity. They are normal features of pregnancy and are sometimes found in females taking oral contraceptives. Leuconychia is a manifestation of low serum albumin levels and is not specific for liver disease. The term 'liver palms' refers to a blotchy erythema of the thenar and hypothenar eminences, and may be a visible manifestation of a widespread disturbance in vasomotor tone. Dupuytren's contracture is due to a thickening of the palmar fascia and is particularly common in alcoholic liver disease. It can, however, be idiopathic, or secondary to chronic occupational trauma to the palms of the hands. A flapping tremor of the outstretched hands (asterixis), best seen when the wrists are extended, is a feature of hepatic encephalopathy, but is also found in CO_2 retention and in renal failure. It may be due to sudden, intermittent inhibition of motor tone, rather than active muscle contractions. Feminisation in males, with gynaecomastia, testicular atrophy and loss of body hair, is particularly common in alcoholic liver disease and haemochromatosis. It is not due to high oestrogen levels alone but also to more complex gonadal and hypothalamic dysfunction. Female patients with cirrhosis may develop amenorrhoea. Examination of the abdomen usually reveals hepatosplenomegaly, although the liver may become very small in advanced cirrhosis. Ascites may be present, and striae may be a sign of previous abdominal distension. Patients with portal hypertension may have dilated veins on the abdominal wall.

CHRONIC ALCOHOLIC LIVER DISEASE

Epidemiology

Chronic alcoholic liver disease is the commonest cause of cirrhosis in Europe, and is increasing in prevalence in most countries (Fig. 17.17). In district general hospitals in Britain, 80% of all cases of cirrhosis are associated with alcohol abuse. In the USA, deaths from cirrhosis, mostly alcohol-related, increased by 72% between 1950 and 1974,

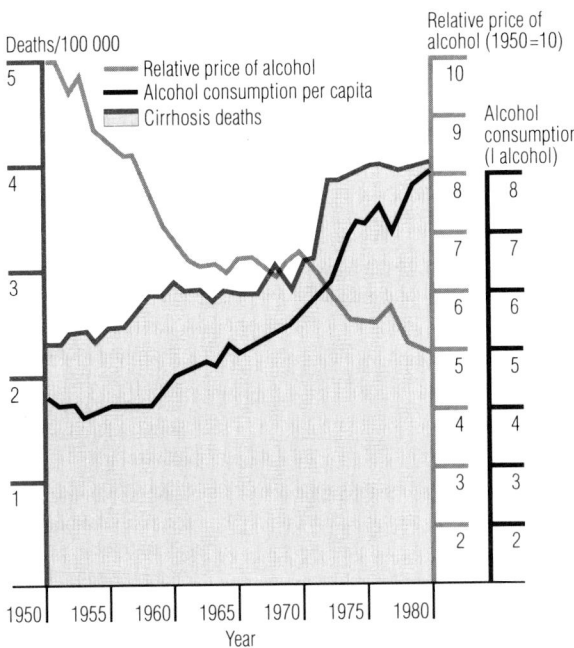

Deaths/100 000

Relative price of alcohol (1950=10)

— Relative price of alcohol
— Alcohol consumption per capita
▨ Cirrhosis deaths

Alcohol consumption (l alcohol)

Year

Fig. 17.17 Chronic alcoholic liver disease. The steady increase in alcohol consumption in the UK from 1950 to 1980 was accompanied by an increase in deaths from cirrhosis of the liver, and a fall in the relative price of alcohol as a fraction of average income.

making it the fourth commonest cause of death in white male adults.

Pathology

There is a striking range of histopathological changes produced by alcohol. The most consistent is increased fat deposition (steatosis), which is almost invariably present in those drinking more than 80 g (1 bottle of wine or 3 pints of beer – 6 units, p. 72) of alcohol per day. Although a large proportion of the cytoplasm of affected hepatocytes is occupied by a single large triglyceride inclusion, liver function is surprisingly normal. The fatty change is rapidly reversible during abstinence. In the majority of cases, isolated steatosis does not progress to cirrhosis, although in some there may be slowly increasing fibrosis around central veins, leading to stellate scarring and incomplete septum formation. It is possible that this could eventually lead to cirrhosis. The particular histological changes seen in alcoholic hepatitis (p. 640) are thought to be of fundamental importance in determining progression to cirrhosis. The perinuclear eosinophilic inclusion bodies (Mallory's hyaline), one of the most obvious features, are probably condensed and disorganised fragments of the cytoskeletal framework of the hepatocyte. They are not specific to alcoholic liver disease, but may also be seen in Wilson's disease, primary biliary cirrhosis, Indian childhood cirrhosis and perhexiline-induced liver injury. Collagen deposition is another striking feature of alcoholic hepatitis. It can be pericellular, in the space of Disse, and around

central veins (central hyaline sclerosis). This latter lesion is particularly associated with rapid progression to cirrhosis, and is commoner and more severe in women than in men. Collagen bridges eventually develop between central veins and portal tracts, isolating groups of hepatocytes which form the regeneration nodules characteristic of cirrhosis.

Pathogenesis

The metabolism of ethanol to acetaldehyde and acetate is normally dependent on the enzymes alcohol dehydrogenase and acetaldehyde dehydrogenase (Fig. 17.18). These oxidation reactions are associated with the formation of NADH from NAD and alter the redox state of the cell. This in turn has profound effects on lipid and carbohydrate metabolism, one of which results in steatosis. In habitual drinkers, a microsomal mixed function oxidase, the microsomal ethanol oxidising system (MEOS), is increased by enzyme induction, and is also responsible for the production of acetaldehyde. Breakdown of acetaldehyde may then become the rate-limiting step in ethanol metabolism, and it is now thought that this toxic metabolite may be responsible for the liver cell injury.

The direct correlation, in populations, between alcohol intake and risk of cirrhosis obscures the wide individual variation in susceptibility, for which there is at present no satisfactory explanation. An attractive hypothesis is that the rate of removal of acetaldehyde is one factor determining individual susceptibility to ethanol-induced liver damage and cirrhosis, but this is not yet proven. Concomitant malnutrition may exacerbate existing liver injury, but is not now thought to be primarily responsible for changes in susceptibility to alcoholic liver disease. Retrospective analyses of lifetime alcohol consumption in patients with cirrhosis have shown that women develop

Fig. 17.18 The metabolism of ethanol. Ethanol metabolism largely takes place in the mitochondria. The main product is acetaldehyde (A) which may itself be damaging. Hydrogen ions (B) are an important by-product which can drive many metabolic reactions in the liver cell cytosol to create harmful effects (C, D).

cirrhosis about twice as fast as men, and that those individuals who have inherited the histocompatibility antigen HLA B8 have a much shorter history of heavy drinking. This particular HLA antigen is strongly associated with organ-specific autoimmunity, and there is other evidence suggesting that immune reactions against Mallory's hyaline, or against new antigens on the surface of hepatocytes, induced by acetaldehyde, could be responsible for liver cell damage. However, it is always difficult in patients with liver necrosis to distinguish between immune reactions which might be the cause of the damage, and those which are secondary to it.

Diagnosis

The presenting features of cirrhosis and alcoholic hepatitis have already been discussed. However, some cases with significant liver damage are asymptomatic, and liver biopsy is the only way reliably to assess the degree of liver injury. Recognition of alcohol abuse is crucial so that disease can be detected at a stage where abstinence can still lead to complete resolution of tissue damage. Important points in the history and examination are discussed on page 72. A high mean corpuscular volume and serum gamma glutamyl transpeptidase are important clues from laboratory tests.

Treatment

Malnutrition is common in those with alcohol addiction, and should be treated with vitamin supplements and a high protein diet. Withdrawal from alcohol is best initiated in hospital, where appropriate physical support is available. Fits are best controlled with diazepam, and delirium tremens prevented and treated with chlormethiazole, either orally or by slow intravenous infusion. The drug should be gradually withdrawn over 2 or 3 weeks. Other causes of confusion and coma, such as Wernicke's syndrome, subdural haematoma, hypoglycaemia and hepatic encephalopathy, must be excluded.

Abstinence is the key to successful long-term management. Ninety per cent of patients with alcoholic hepatitis alone will show complete regression of the liver damage, while those with cirrhosis who remain abstinent have a much better prognosis than those who continue to drink. In the UK many patients presenting with alcoholic liver disease are not physically addicted, and achieving sustained abstinence is possible with careful and caring support. For further details see page 74.

CHRONIC ACTIVE HEPATITIS

Chronic active hepatitis is a syndrome consisting of several different diseases with similar histological appearances on liver biopsy (Table 17.10). Portal tracts are enlarged, and contain a chronic inflammatory cell infiltrate of lympho-

Table 17.10 Classification of chronic active hepatitis

Type	Distribution	Features
Autoimmune	Northern Europe, USA, Australia, South Africa	Female/male ratio 7:3; high titre antinuclear antibodies
Chronic virus infection		
Hepatitis B	Mediterranean, Middle and Far East	Female/male ratio 1:9; low titre antinuclear antibodies
Delta hepatitis	Mediterranean and Middle East	Endemic in HBV carriers in Mediterranean; intravenous drug abusers in northern Europe
Non-A, non-B	Wide distribution	Commonest post-transfusion hepatitis; also transmitted by blood products
Drug-induced	A phenomenon of the developed world	Examples are methyldopa, isoniazid, nitrofurantoin and dantrolene; usually like autoimmune chronic active hepatitis
Metabolic		
Wilson's disease	Wide distribution	Can mimic any liver disease, so easily missed
Haemochromatosis	Wide distribution, but note Brittany and Utah Mormons	Usually inactive fibrosis, but rarely resembles chronic active hepatitis, almost exclusively males affected
Alcohol	Wide distribution, but particularly the developed world	Controversial as a cause of chronic active hepatitis; may be in recovery phase of alcoholic hepatitis

cytes, plasma cells and macrophages. The cells extend beyond the edges of the portal tracts, through the limiting plate of periportal hepatocytes, and there is 'piecemeal necrosis' of liver cells in this part of the lobule. Collagen deposition is prominent in the areas of liver cell damage, and this leads to the formation of fibrous septa linking portal tracts to each other and to central veins. If the disease process continues unchecked, cirrhosis is an inevitable consequence.

AUTOIMMUNE

Aetiology and pathogenesis

Autoimmune chronic active hepatitis is the commonest cause of the syndrome in northern Europe and Australia, and was the first to be described. It is best considered as one of the organ-specific autoimmune diseases. Women are affected more commonly than men, antinuclear and smooth muscle antibodies are commonly found in serum, serum total globulin and IgG levels are high, and there is evidence of both cellular and humoral liver-specific autoimmune reactions directed at normal antigens on the surface of hepatocytes. The histocompatibility antigens (HLA) B8 and DR3 are found in a high proportion of cases.

Antibodies reacting with liver cell membrane components are almost always present, and probably damage hepatocytes in co-operation with cytotoxic lymphocytes bearing receptors for the Fc end of the antibody molecules. There is a profound disturbance in immunoregulation associated with functionally abnormal suppressor T cells.

Clinical features

Two-thirds of patients present with an illness indistinguishable from acute viral hepatitis, although the causative agent is not usually identified. The remainder have symptoms due to an already established cirrhosis, such as ascites, haematemesis from bleeding varices, or encephalopathy. Half of those with an initial acute hepatitis remain jaundiced and have biochemical evidence of continued liver necrosis. The others appear to recover normally, but develop a second episode of jaundice some months later. Multisystem involvement is common, and includes arthralgia, ulcerative colitis, autoimmune thyroid disease and haemolytic anaemia. Cutaneous stigmata of chronic liver disease are often present, and more than 70% of patients already have cirrhosis when the diagnosis is first made.

Investigations

Liver function tests usually show a hepatitic picture with high serum transaminases. A marked elevation in the total globulin (more than 40 g/l), with a high IgG, is a useful pointer to this subgroup. The diagnosis is made on liver biopsy, while the presence of the appropriate non-organ-specific autoantibodies indicates the correct classification.

Treatment

The response to corticosteroids is excellent. The survival rate is greatly increased, with more than 60% alive at 10 years, although cirrhosis, if absent initially, may still develop. Azathioprine in a dose of 1–2 mg/kg is a useful adjunct to steroid therapy and may allow a lower dose of steroid to be used. This can be particularly important in older women who are prone to osteoporosis. Although serum transaminase levels are often used to monitor progress, liver biopsy is useful in establishing the activity of the disease during follow-up. If the disease has remained inactive for more than 2 years, steroid treatment can be cautiously withdrawn. However, relapse is very common (60–80%) and can be severe, necessitating prompt re-introduction of corticosteroids.

CHRONIC HEPATITIS B VIRUS INFECTION

Worldwide, hepatitis B virus is the commonest type of chronic active hepatitis, being particularly prevalent in the Mediterranean, the Middle and Far East, and tropical Africa. The serology and structure of the hepatitis B virus have been described earlier (p. 634).

Clinical features

Many patients are asymptomatic, the chronic virus infection being detected on screening for blood donations or investigation of other diseases. When symptoms do occur, they are often mild and non-specific, malaise being the commonest. Some progress from an acute HBV infection. There is a striking male preponderance. The incidence of multisystem disease is lower than that found in the autoimmune variety. The liver function tests usually show a relatively mild hepatitic picture, with only moderately raised levels of serum transaminase. Antinuclear antibodies are not usually present in serum, although smooth muscle antibodies may be detected in low titre.

Serological markers

There are two phases to the infection. Initially, there is active viral replication, with HBsAg, HBeAg, HBV DNA, and the DNA polymerase of the virus detectable in the serum. In this phase the histological features of chronic active hepatitis are most often present. After several years, there may be a rather abrupt cessation of viral replication, with loss of serum HBeAg, HBV DNA and DNA polymerase. This change is often preceded by a rise in the levels of serum aminotransferase, but is frequently followed by a striking decrease in the activity of the disease, with reduction in the extent of the inflammatory infiltrate in the liver. HBsAg levels in serum decrease because free viral DNA has been lost, but this surface protein of the virus usually remains detectable in serum, probably because there has been integration of the viral genome into the hepatocyte DNA.

The defect responsible for the failure to clear the virus after the initial infection has not been identified. However, most patients do not have detectable antibodies to the receptor for polymerised albumin on the surface of the virions, and it is possible that the absence of this neutralising antibody allows continued viral penetration of uninfected hepatocytes. Cellular immunity to HBcAg on the surface of infected liver cells, which is probably responsible for liver cell necrosis in acute HBV infection, is present, and may be a component of the inflammatory liver lesion. On the other hand, some factors must be present which interfere with effective clearance of infected cells. Autoimmune reactions to normal liver cell membrane antigens, similar to those found in 'autoimmune' chronic active hepatitis, can be demonstrated, and these could be the explanation for the similarity of the periportal histological changes in two diseases with quite distinct aetiological backgrounds.

Treatment

Corticosteroids are of no benefit in the phase of active viral replication, and may be harmful. There is current interest in antiviral agents, such as adenine arabinoside, acyclovir and interferons. Although immediate effects on viral replication can be convincingly demonstrated, only 20–40% of cases show long-lasting benefit.

CHRONIC DELTA VIRUS INFECTION

The histological changes of chronic active hepatitis are often present in chronic Delta virus infection (p. 635). The diagnosis is made by finding anti-Delta antibodies in serum or demonstrating Delta antigen in the nuclei of liver cells by immunofluorescence. Progression to cirrhosis seems to occur quite rapidly, and the prognosis is poor. Little is known about the mechanisms of tissue damage, and no specific treatment has been shown to be effective.

CHRONIC NON-A, NON-B VIRUS INFECTION

Since a specific serological test for one of these non-A, non-B viruses has only recently become available (p. 636), most of the information on the existence and natural history of this type of chronic active liver disease has come from follow-up of cases with acute non-A, non-B hepatitis acquired from blood transfusion or blood products. The clinical and immunological features are more like those of chronic HBV infection rather than the 'autoimmune' cases. Thus, smooth muscle antibodies may be present in low titre, but antinuclear antibodies are usually absent. The disease activity is usually mild, and seems to become less severe with time. In some cases, cirrhosis may not develop. Corticosteroids are of no benefit but low-dose α-interferons suppress virus replication; and if continued for a year, may be of lasting benefit in some cases.

DRUG-INDUCED CHRONIC ACTIVE HEPATITIS

Although rare, these cases are important, as the disease almost always responds to drug withdrawal. All reported cases are examples of idiosyncratic reactions, which have not been reproduced experimentally. The drugs most frequently implicated are isoniazid, alpha methyldopa, nitrofurantoin and the laxative oxyphenisatin. In many cases, the disease is very similar to the 'autoimmune' type, with antinuclear and smooth muscle antibodies present in serum.

OTHER CAUSES

The most important of the other causes of chronic active hepatitis is Wilson's disease (p. 650), which can mimic the changes seen in viral or autoimmune cases. Since long-term survival on D-penicillamine is possible, it is clearly of great importance to exclude this condition in all cases of chronic active hepatitis in children and young adults. The histological features of chronic active hepatitis can also be found in some cases of alpha-1 antitrypsin deficiency, and in alcoholic liver disease.

PRIMARY BILIARY CIRRHOSIS

Like chronic active hepatitis, primary biliary cirrhosis is a condition which is not necessarily associated with cirrhosis at presentation, although this frequently develops later in the course of the disease. The essence of the disease is a slowly progressive destruction of intrahepatic bile ducts, possibly due to immune-mediated injury.

Incidence and aetiology

In most series more than 90% of patients are women, with most being in middle age. In the UK the incidence is between 6 and 12 per million, with a prevalence of 40–80 per million. There is no definite HLA association but familial cases are well described. The antibodies in serum reacting with mitochondria, which are such a strong feature of the disease, are also found in family members, but in most cases there is no apparent liver or bile duct injury associated with this finding. There is one report of the disease developing in a daughter, her mother and a close friend who nursed the daughter, suggesting that environmental factors may play a role, and this was supported by the finding that in Sheffield, 90% of the patients came from an area of the city with only 4% of the population, and were supplied with water from one reservoir.

Pathology

Four stages in the histopathology of the disease have been described. They are not necessarily sequential, and there is considerable overlap between them.

1. *First stage*. There is focal damage to the larger intrahepatic bile ducts, with a surrounding chronic inflammatory infiltrate of lymphocytes, plasma cells, eosinophils and macrophages. In some areas the infiltrate may be organised into an epithelioid cell granuloma, lying close to a damaged duct.
2. *Second stage*. Some of the larger ducts are replaced by lymphoid aggregates, and there is proliferation of smaller ductules. Fibrosis is present.
3. *Third stage*. Fibrosis extends beyond the edges of the portal tracts. There is often periportal cholestasis, and accumulation of copper-binding proteins.
4. *Final stage*. The features are those of an established cirrhosis. Ill-defined collections of lymphocytes and a paucity of bile ducts may be the only clues to the aetiology.

Immunopathogenesis

Antimitochondrial antibodies are directed at an antigen on the inner membrane of the mitochondrium, and are unlikely to be of pathogenetic importance. However, they are clearly an important feature of the disease. An attractive but unproven hypothesis is that they are cross-reactive antibodies generated by an immune response to an as yet unidentified bacterium which is in some way responsible for the bile duct destruction. This hypothesis has been reinforced by the finding that the antimitochondrial antibodies are directed at the pyruvate dehydrogenase complex and cross-react extensively with the corresponding bacterial enzyme complex in *E. coli*. Granulomas are usually indicative of a cellular immune reaction, but it is not clear what the antigenic stimulus could be. T cells sensitised to antigenic components in bile ducts are often present, but could be secondary to the bile duct destruction. The disease in other organs may be an indication of a generalised disturbance in immunoregulation, but could also be due to an observed antigenic cross-reactivity between bile duct antigens and secretory duct epithelium in other organs.

Clinical features

The disease is much commoner in females than males (9 to 1), and usually presents in the fifth and sixth decades. Pruritus is often the first symptom, and may lead to a dermatological consultation. Weight is usually well maintained and abdominal pain is unusual. Jaundice is a late feature. On examination there is often quite marked hepatosplenomegaly and skin pigmentation. Skin xanthomas are common.

With the increasing availability of automated biochemical profiles, and screening tests for non-organ-specific auto-antibodies in serum, asymptomatic cases are being seen more frequently. In these patients, minor hepatomegaly may be the only abnormality.

The most striking serological feature is the presence of antimitochondrial antibodies in serum. These are of considerable help in the differential diagnosis, as they are found in 95% of patients with primary biliary cirrhosis, but are usually absent in prolonged extrahepatic obstruction.

Associated diseases

Disease in other organs is very common, and includes one or more of the components of the CRST syndrome (calcinosis, Raynaud's phenomenon, sclerodactyly, telangiectasia), autoimmune thyroiditis, renal tubular acidosis, rheumatoid arthritis and the 'sicca complex' (dry eyes and dry mouth).

Course and treatment

In symptomatic cases, average survival is 6 years, but it is difficult to give an accurate prognosis in individual cases. The bile duct destruction is slowly progressive, but bilirubin levels usually remain stable for several years, before rising steadily in the last year or two of the illness. Steatorrhoea with malabsorption of fat-soluble vitamins can be a problem, and it is important to give supplements of calcium and vitamins D and K. Cholestyramine usually controls pruritus. Corticosteroids are not usually given because of the likely exacerbation of osteoporosis in postmenopausal women. D-penicillamine has several potentially useful effects, including chelation of copper, which slowly accumulates in chronic cholestasis, interference with collagen synthesis, and immunosuppression. However, controlled clinical trials have provided conflicting evidence of benefit, and side-effects such as skin rashes, nausea and vomiting, proteinuria and bone marrow

suppression are common. Cyclosporin A is now being evaluated as a possible therapeutic agent. This is an immunosuppressive drug which acts by interfering with the production of interleukin 2, an important stimulator of lymphocyte proliferation. Colchicine and ursodeoxycholic acid also seem to be beneficial in controlled trials, and in very advanced cases liver transplantation is a useful and successful treatment option.

An important finding is that asymptomatic cases often have an excellent prognosis. In some of these patients, serial observations over several years have shown no evidence of any deterioration in liver function tests or liver histology.

HAEMOCHROMATOSIS

Increased iron deposition in hepatocytes is the hallmark of haemochromatosis. In idiopathic haemochromatosis this is due to a genetically determined increase in iron absorption. The inheritance is now known to be autosomal recessive and is associated with an increased frequency of HLA A3 (75% of patients, compared with 25% of controls). The exact mechanism of the defect in control of iron absorption is not understood.

Haemosiderosis, secondary iron overload, is usually due to a chronic haemolytic anaemia such as thalassaemia. The increased liver iron content is due to both increased iron release and repeated blood transfusions (p. 1066).

Clinical features

There is a striking male preponderance, almost certainly because menstruation in women prevents a significant rise in iron stores. The disease usually presents in middle age. 'Bronzed diabetes' is a useful reminder of two of the important clinical features. The pigmentation is due to *increased melanin* in the skin, and is often seen best over the shins where it gives a slate-grey appearance. Patients may present with *diabetes*, sometimes well before the liver disease becomes symptomatic. It is associated with iron deposition in the pancreas. An *arthritis*, particularly affecting the knees and metacarpophalangeal joints, can also be a presenting feature, and is associated with the deposition of calcium pyrophosphate crystals in the affected joints.

On examination, *gynaecomastia, testicular atrophy* and *loss of body hair* are often present, and seem to be due to a combination of partial testicular and pituitary failure, associated with iron deposition in these areas. *Hepatomegaly* is invariably present, but splenomegaly is uncommon. In younger patients, *congestive cardiomyopathy* can be an unusual but troublesome complication.

Diagnosis

Liver function tests can be entirely normal and haemochromatosis is a good example of a disease which must be considered before it can be diagnosed. Liver biopsy allows demonstration of the iron deposition in liver cells, usually in a periportal distribution. Extensive portal fibrosis develops before there is progression to a true cirrhosis, with regeneration nodules. Serum iron levels are high, with greater than 90% saturation of the total iron binding capacity. Serum ferritin levels are a good reflection of total body iron content, but do not correlate precisely with the concentration of liver iron.

Treatment and prognosis

Gradual depletion of the body iron stores is best achieved by regular venesection, initially 1 unit weekly. Serum ferritin and a repeat liver biopsy are the most useful markers of complete removal of the excessive iron deposits. The severity of the associated diabetes tends to decrease, and there is a general improvement in malaise and decrease in liver size. The changes of cirrhosis in the liver are, of course, not reversible, and one of the long-term risks is the development of primary hepatocellular carcinoma. Venesection is most effective when started early in the course of the disease, before the development of diabetes or cirrhosis, and investigation of the patient's relatives is an essential part of management. Undiagnosed cases may be detected by the combination of HLA A3 and a high serum ferritin. In 1935 the mean survival after diagnosis was 4.4 years, in 1969 the 5-year survival rate was 89%, and as more asymptomatic family members are picked up and treated, it is becoming clear that the disease can be prevented if excess iron is removed at an early stage and future accumulation of iron prevented.

WILSON'S DISEASE

In this disease, genetically determined accumulation of copper in the liver, basal ganglia, kidney and cornea can produce a wide variety of liver lesions with or without associated extrapyramidal dysfunction. It is an autosomal recessive condition with an incidence of about 1 in 50 000. Heterozygous individuals remain in virtually zero copper balance throughout their life and show no clinical features of the disease. Radiocopper studies indicate that the inherited defect in copper metabolism principally affects copper excretion from hepatic lysosomes to bile (Fig. 17.19). Pathologically and clinically the liver is the first organ to be affected. The appearance of lipid droplets in the liver cell cytoplasm is the first abnormality, followed by increasing fibrosis and cirrhosis.

Clinical features

Wilson's disease is a great mimic of many other liver diseases, and because of the excellent response to D-pen-

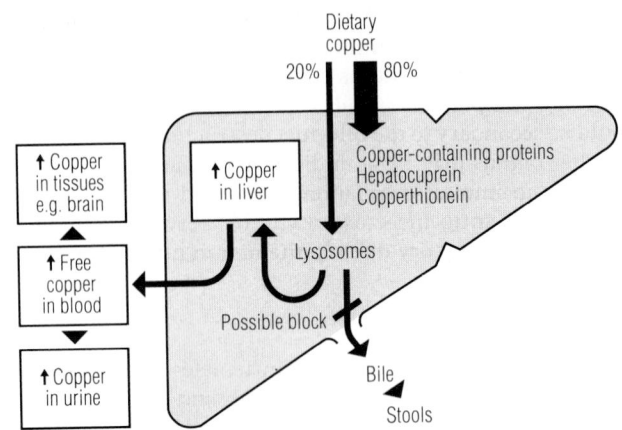

Fig. 17.19 Wilson's disease. The postulated block in copper metabolism in Wilson's disease is a failure to excrete copper from lysosomes into bile. This leads to a build-up of the toxic metal in the liver and other tissues, particularly the basal ganglia in the brain.

icillamine in the early stages of the disease, must always be thought of and excluded in any child or young adult with chronic liver disease. In some cases there is a combination of fatty change, Mallory's hyaline, and fibrosis, and this may be wrongly attributed to the effects of social drinking. In others, there is a mononuclear infiltrate in the portal tracts with piecemeal necrosis of periportal hepatocytes, and this can lead to a diagnosis of non-A, non-B, or autoimmune chronic active hepatitis. In children, an 'acute hepatitis', sometimes progressing to fulminant hepatic failure, may be a presenting feature. This may be accompanied by acute haemolysis. At the other extreme, the disease may remain silent until a slowly progressive, inactive cirrhosis presents with haematemesis, ascites or encephalopathy. Neurological abnormalities may be absent in younger patients; when present, they are often subtle. They include deteriorating school performance, changes in personality, slurring of speech, clumsiness and difficulties with fine movements. In adults, dysarthria and bulbar palsy may accompany more classical extrapyramidal signs and symptoms.

Diagnosis

Brown deposits of copper in the margins of the cornea, called *Kayser-Fleischer rings*, are diagnostic. They are always present in patients with neurological symptoms, but can be absent in young patients presenting with liver disease. They are best seen on slit-lamp examination. Serum caeruloplasmin levels are typically low, but may also be decreased in chronic active hepatitis and fulminant liver failure as well as in about 10% of healthy heterozygotes. Urinary copper excretion is high, and rises dramatically after a test dose of D-penicillamine. Liver copper levels are between one-and-a-half and 25 times the upper limit of normal, but are also increased in some conditions with chronic cholestasis, such as primary biliary cirrhosis.

Treatment

The chelating agent, D-penicillamine, gradually depletes the copper stores, and is the mainstay of treatment. In cases picked up early, and in those with a relatively inactive well-compensated liver lesion, there is usually some improvement in liver function and no further progression of the liver disease. Patients who present with fulminant hepatic failure of decompensated cirrhosis show little response to chelation therapy, and have a poor prognosis.

OTHER CAUSES OF CIRRHOSIS

Alpha-1 antitrypsin deficiency

Alpha-1 antitrypsin, a protease inhibitor, is remarkably polymorphic, with more than 30 different variants now recognised. The inheritance of these alleles is autosomal and codominant, with the normal phenotype being designated MM. The clinically important variant is called Z. This codes for a defective protein core which has altered carbohydrate side chains, and cannot be excreted from hepatocytes. It can be seen in liver biopsies as diastase-resistant, PAS-positive granules in periportal hepatocytes. Heterozygotes, with an MZ phenotype, have about half the normal circulating levels of alpha-1 antitrypsin, while none can be detected in ZZ homozygotes. It is these ZZ individuals who are susceptible to the development of emphysema (p. 493) and cirrhosis, but the mechanisms responsible are not understood.

The liver disease usually presents in infancy, with symptoms of the neonatal hepatitis syndrome (conjugated hyperbilirubinaemia with pale stools, dark urine and hepatomegaly). At this stage, cirrhosis may already be present on liver biopsy, although varying degrees of hepatocellular damage and fibrosis are more usual. In those who survive, cirrhosis usually develops, and about a quarter will die in early childhood. The clinical course in the remainder may be relatively long, although decompensation can occur in adolescence or early adult life. There is no specific treatment. Some adults with alpha-1 antitrypsin deficiency can present with cirrhosis without a history of jaundice in infancy. In these patients, primary hepatoma is a recognised complication.

Cystic fibrosis

Cystic fibrosis is considered in detail in Chapter 14. There is a generalised disorder of exocrine secretory glands, whose ducts become blocked with viscid, tenacious secretions. The liver can be involved in this process, with mild focal biliary obstruction due to inspissated bile being found in almost all cases. In some, for unknown reasons,

this process slowly progresses to a relatively inactive cirrhosis. This is present in about 10–15% of adolescents with cystic fibrosis, and can present with the complications of portal hypertension.

Secondary biliary cirrhosis

Secondary biliary cirrhosis can be a complication of any disease in which there is prolonged biliary obstruction. For example, it may arise as a long-term complication of biliary stricture due to operative damage to the bile duct, or in sclerosing cholangitis (p. 642). There is slowly progressive portal fibrosis, often for several years before the development of true cirrhosis. If adequate biliary drainage can be restored during the earlier stages there may be substantial regression of the portal fibrosis and a fall in portal pressure.

Hepatic venous congestion

'Cardiac cirrhosis' occurs in patients with chronic right heart failure. It is a progressive liver fibrosis due to chronic centrilobular congestion. It has become uncommon since the development of powerful diuretics. An important exception is constrictive pericarditis, where the absence of attacks of acute left ventricular failure, and the delayed onset of peripheral oedema may postpone presentation until extensive liver fibrosis has developed. At this stage, ascites is often a presenting symptom, and the underlying cardiac condition can easily be overlooked. Treatment, by surgical removal of the pericardium, usually leads to resolution of the ascites and regression of the liver fibrosis.

A congenital web in the inferior vena cava at, or above, the level of the diaphragm, is another rare but correctable cause.

A more dramatic cause of hepatic venous congestion is sudden occlusion of the main hepatic veins: the *Budd-Chiari syndrome*. The presenting features, of pain and tenderness over a large liver and tense ascites, are due to the marked elevation in portal pressure, the severe hepatic congestion and liver cell necrosis. In some cases the onset is more gradual, with refractory ascites being the dominant clinical feature. The occlusion of the hepatic veins is occasionally due to obstruction by tumour tissue extending up the vena cava from a hypernephroma, but is usually thrombotic. This may be initiated by trauma, or due to a thrombotic tendency in diseases such as polycythaemia rubra vera, primary thrombocythaemia, paroxysmal nocturnal haemoglobinuria and chronic myeloid leukaemia. A number of cases have been reported in young women taking the oral contraceptive pill, but since its oestrogen content has been reduced, this association seems to have become less frequent. A liver scintiscan can be helpful in establishing the diagnosis. The characteristic finding is reduced liver activity, except for a central area where uptake is well preserved. This is probably the caudate lobe, which often has a separate venous drainage. The patency of the main hepatic veins may be investigated by ultrasound, but radiological contrast studies are more definitive. Direct injection into hepatic venous radicles can show a network of collateral veins, or it may be possible to insert a catheter from the vena cava into the end of one of the hepatic veins. Treatment is difficult, with control of the ascites being a particular problem. Cases with an acute onset have a high mortality. If the vena cava is patent, liver transplantation should be considered.

Childhood metabolic diseases

Type IV glycogen storage disease, galactosaemia, fructosaemia and tyrosinaemia are all rare causes of cirrhosis in infancy and childhood. The clinical presentation and underlying metabolic defects are described in Chapter 20.

CONGENITAL HEPATIC FIBROSIS

Although this inherited condition is not a cause of cirrhosis, the presentation, with the symptoms and signs of portal hypertension, place it firmly in this context with respect to differential diagnosis. The basic hepatic architecture is preserved, but portal tracts are linked by broad bands of fibrous tissue. Increased numbers of bile ductules are seen in the portal areas, and some may appear cystic. The presentation is usually in childhood with hepatosplenomegaly, and haematemesis from bleeding oesophageal varices. Liver function tends to be well preserved, and a portosystemic shunt operation is usually performed to reduce portal vein pressure. The prognosis is good.

COMPLICATIONS OF CIRRHOSIS

Although there is no specific therapy for many types of cirrhosis, skilled management of the complications can often provide prolonged relief from disabling symptoms.

ASCITES

Pathophysiology

There are two main hypotheses which seek to explain the formation of ascitic fluid in cirrhosis (Fig. 17.20). The first, sometimes referred to as the *'underfill theory'*, suggests that the reduction in plasma colloid osmotic pressure, due to a fall in serum albumin concentration, together with raised portal pressure, leads to a net extravasation of capillary filtrate from the splanchnic circulation. This in turn reduces the circulating plasma volume, and promotes secondary hyperaldosteronism with retention of sodium and water in the kidneys. This theory predicts a normal or reduced cardiac output, decreased plasma volume and peripheral vasoconstriction. The observations that cardiac output is usually increased, that plasma volume is high and that there is peripheral vasodilatation in most patients with cirrhosis and ascites prompted the development of an alternative view, sometimes known as the *'overflow theory'*. This suggests that the primary abnormality is increased

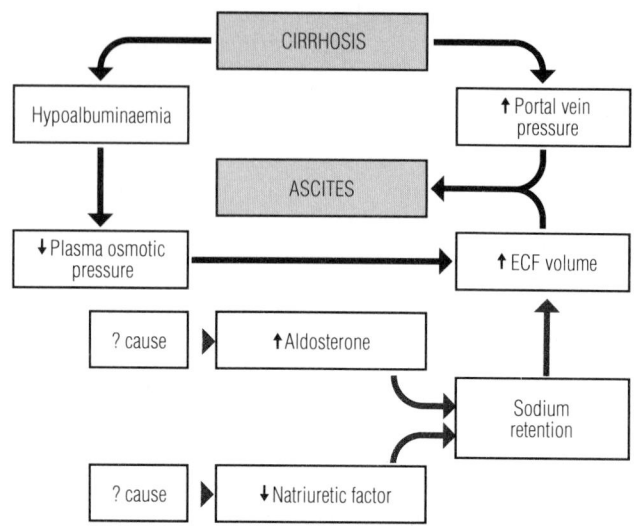

Fig. 17.20 The pathophysiology of ascites formation in cirrhosis. In addition to direct effects of the cirrhotic process leading to ascites, such as increased pressure in the portal vein and decreased albumin lowering the plasma osmotic pressure, there is also an aldosterone-driven increase in sodium retention.

renin and aldosterone levels producing inappropriate sodium and water retention. The plasma volume and cardiac output are increased. Formation of oedema is a secondary event which is encouraged by the low colloid osmotic pressure in plasma, and tends to be localised to the ascitic compartment because of the portal hypertension. Although this theory fits better with the clinical measurements, it does not explain why there should be a primary increase in renin and aldosterone levels in some patients with cirrhosis. Renal haemodynamics are certainly altered, with a tendency for redistribution of blood flow from cortical to juxtamedullary nephrons, a tendency which is opposed in many patients by an increase in renal prostaglandin synthesis. However, the relationship between these changes and the liver disease is not clear.

Clinical features

Fullness in the flanks, with dullness on percussion which shifts with a change of position, is the earliest sign of ascites and is often asymptomatic. Ultrasound can reveal small amounts of fluid. Later the abdomen becomes tense and uncomfortable. At this stage, a fluid thrill is more useful than shifting dullness in confirming the presence of fluid. It can be difficult to palpate the liver and spleen, although ballotting through the fluid may reveal them. A pleural effusion, particularly on the right side, may be present, and peripheral oedema often develops.

Spontaneous bacterial peritonitis is a serious complication, with a high mortality. It can be asymptomatic, although fever, abdominal pain and a general deterioration in well-being, with encephalopathy and renal failure, may be accompanying features.

Treatment

A diagnostic paracentesis is first performed to exclude bacterial peritonitis. The fluid should be clear or straw-coloured and any cloudiness should lead to suspicions of infection. Bacterial culture may be negative, and the most frequent abnormal finding is a polymorph count of more than 500 per mm³. The causative organisms are usually coliforms or streptococci, including anaerobes, and broad-spectrum antibiotics should be started as early as possible. Tuberculous peritonitis is rare, but should be considered, particularly in a malnourished alcoholic, and when the ascitic leucocytes are predominately mononuclear.

Diuretics

Treatment of the ascites is only necessary if it is producing symptoms. *Diuretics* are the mainstay of treatment, but care is necessary since overdiuresis precipitates renal failure and encephalopathy and must be avoided. Therapeutic paracentesis is possible but usually unnecessary. The diuretic of choice is the aldosterone antagonist spironolactone in a starting dose of 100 mg per day. In addition to being a logical choice to combat the high aldosterone levels, it is also potassium-sparing. Total body potassium levels are usually low, and hypokalaemia not only increases the risk of a cardiac arrhythmia, but also exacerbates encephalopathy. The rate of fluid loss is best assessed by changes in daily weight. A figure of half a kilogram per day is ideal, as the maximum rate of transfer of fluid from the ascitic to the vascular compartment is only about 700 ml per day. If a satisfactory response is not forthcoming in a few days, the daily dose of spironolactone should be increased in 100 mg increments to a maximum of 600 mg per day. It is not usually necessary to add loop diuretics. If they are used, the rate of weight loss, renal function and plasma potassium levels must be carefully monitored. Measurement of urinary sodium concentration can be helpful in assessing the effectiveness of diuretic therapy. Strict control of sodium intake is not always necessary, but does allow lower doses of spironolactone to be effective.

Additional medications should be reviewed with care. Several antacid preparations contain enough sodium to counteract the effect of the diuretic, while non-steroidal anti-inflammatory drugs can precipitate renal failure (hepatorenal syndrome) by reducing the intrarenal levels of vasodilating prostaglandins. The aim of the treatment is to relieve symptoms, not to remove all the ascitic fluid. Complications are more common if high doses of diuretic are continued. Reduction to maintenance doses should be started before the ascites has disappeared.

Further measures

Failure of response to these treatment measures is unusual. It often indicates severe liver disease and carries a bad prognosis. Hyponatraemia can be a problem, and is usually due to impaired renal free water clearance. Restriction of fluid intake is an appropriate therapeutic measure; sodium infusion simply increases fluid retention.

Direct removal of ascitic fluid is safe if decompression is gradual and electrolyte levels are monitored and corrected. Maintenance diuretic therapy can then be used to prevent re-accumulation of fluid. Alternatives include ascites re-infusion, either via external ultrafiltration apparatus, which concentrates the ascitic fluid before it is returned to the patient intravenously, or by a Le Veen peritoneal venous shunt, which transfers the ascitic fluid directly from the peritoneal cavity to the superior vena cava. Both techniques have a high incidence of complications, including Gram-negative septicaemia, disseminated intravascular coagulation, and fibrinolysis. They should only be used if conventional therapy has been ineffective.

VARICEAL HAEMORRHAGE

Distortion of the lobular architecture in cirrhosis almost always produces raised portal venous pressure. Collateral veins develop between the portal and systemic systems. The most important clinically are those which run beneath the oesophageal mucosa, as these frequently rupture, producing life-threatening haematemesis (variceal haemorrhage).

Clinical features

Evidence of portal hypertension may be detected on examination. Splenomegaly is almost invariable. Dilated collateral veins may be seen in the abdominal wall, and may radiate outwards from the umbilicus. In rare cases these may be especially prominent, forming a caput medusa. The obliterated umbilical vein may recanalise, and flow through it sometimes produces a venous hum heard best in the epigastrium or around the umbilicus.

Treatment

This consists of:

1. immediate measures to deal with the variceal haemorrhage

Summary 4	Management of ascites	
Treatment	Indication	Problems
Spironolactone	Main treatment	Gynaecomastia
Other diuretics	Not alone; give with spironolactone if necessary	K⁺ depletion; renal failure; encephalopathy
Salt restriction	If unable to get control with diuretics	Unpalatable diet leads to weight loss; hyponatraemia more likely
Fluid restriction	Only if hyponatraemic	Compliance
Paracentesis	Only in 3–5 l amounts with iv albumin	Renal failure

2. consideration of appropriate longer-term treatment to prevent rebleeding.

Immediate measures

The first priority is resuscitation. Blood transfusion is usually necessary, often with large quantities. The next step is to establish the source of the bleeding. Peptic ulceration is common in cirrhosis, and acute erosive gastritis and oesophagitis are often present, particularly in alcoholics. These lesions are often found to be the site of the blood loss, even in cirrhotics with known oesophageal varices. Early endoscopy is therefore helpful in demonstrating the likely bleeding site. Most patients stop bleeding spontaneously after resuscitation. In those who do not, two immediate treatment options are available:

1. *Vasopressin* (initially 0.4 units per minute intravenously for 1–2 hours) is a powerful vasoconstrictor of the splanchnic bed, which reduces portal vein pressure and flow through the portosystemic collateral veins. It also produces coronary vasoconstriction, and can trigger cardiac arrhythmias or precipitate myocardial infarction. Recently a glyceryl trinitrate infusion has been added to counteract the systemic vasoconstriction and appears to offer some benefit.
2. *A Sengstaken-Blakemore tube* is an alternative. This has a long oesophageal balloon which can be inflated to compress the varices, and a gastric balloon which anchors the lower end in the fundus of the stomach, and which may assist in reducing variceal flow by compressing gastric varices. It is very effective, but skill is needed in its introduction and in maintaining it in position with safety. The airway is in danger both from saliva, which must be aspirated from the upper oesophagus at frequent intervals, and from the balloons themselves. The tube can sometimes work its way up the oesophagus until the oesophageal balloon obstructs the upper pharynx. Its position needs to be carefully checked. Oesophageal ulceration can occur, but the risk is minimised if the oesophageal balloon is decompressed for 5 minutes every hour, and the tube itself is not kept in place for longer than 48 hours.

The decision whether or not to give longer-term treatment is dependent on an assessment of the risk of early rebleeding. The Child's classification is useful. This is a scoring system where points are given for adverse factors (Table 17.11). These include the serum bilirubin and albumin levels, the prothrombin time and the presence of ascites or encephalopathy. On the basis of the total score the patient is classified in one of three grades: A, B or C. Those with Child's grade A almost all stop bleeding soon after admission and may not rebleed for many months, while the grade C patient is likely to have a serious rebleed during the same hospital admission. In these cases, the mortality in the first admission due to variceal haemorrhage may be as high as 80%. Another important factor to be considered is the pattern of admissions in individual patients. Those with infrequent episodes usually retain

Table 17.11 Child's classification of severity of cirrhosis

Feature	Points scored for increasing abnormalities		
	1	2	3
Encephalopathy (grade)	None	1 and 2	3 and 4
Ascites	None	Mild	Moderate/ severe
Plasma bilirubin (mol/l)	less than 25	25–40	more than 40
Plasma albumin (g/l)	more than 35	28–35	less than 28
Prothrombin time (secs prolonged)	1–4	4–6	more than 6

Total score: 5–6 = grade A; 7–9 = grade B; 10–15 = grade C

this pattern and it may be worth adopting a conservative approach.

Longer-term treatment

If, after full assessment, further treatment is considered desirable, then there are again two main options:

1. The varices can be obliterated by a direct approach
2. The portal pressure can be reduced by some form of surgical portosystemic shunt.

The shunt approach is becoming less popular, as several controlled trials have shown no benefit for porto-caval shunting in terms of mortality at any stage. Reduced deaths from rebleeding were offset by an increased incidence of liver failure and encephalopathy, presumably due to the reduction in liver blood flow and increased amount of blood bypassing the liver after the shunt procedure. The distal spleno-renal shunt (or Warren shunt) aims to preserve the portal blood flow to the liver: while decompressing the varices, the distal splenic vein is isolated from the main portal system, before making a spleno-renal anastamosis. The operation is technically difficult, and while the immediate results seemed promising, further studies have shown a rising incidence of encephalopathy, probably due to the formation of new collaterals between the distal splenic vein and the portal vein systems.

Summary 5 Management of haematemesis in cirrhosis

1. Resuscitate – blood, blood substitutes
2. Stop bleeding – endoscopy (haemorrhagic gastritis and ulcers common)
3. If varices bleeding, either:
   Sengstaken-Blakemore tube (difficult to pass; can be dangerous)
   Vasopressin infusion (effective, but intestinal colic and coronary vasoconstriction)
4. Long-term:
   Sclerotherapy (effective but manpower-intensive)
   Shunts not usually used because of increased liver failure

---

The most successful form of direct variceal attack is by *endoscopic sclerotherapy*. Sclerosant solution is injected under direct vision into or around the varices at repeated endoscopy sessions until the varices have been obliterated. Recanalisation and formation of new collaterals does occur, and regular follow-up treatments are necessary. Complications include oesophageal ulceration, perforation and stricture formation, but are infrequent. This is the only procedure to have been shown in controlled clinical trials to prolong survival significantly.

Extrahepatic portal vein obstruction

Although relatively uncommon, this is a condition with a good prognosis which often presents with variceal haemorrhage, and must be distinguished from cirrhosis. The cause of the portal vein obstruction is often not apparent and in many cases is thought to be due to portal vein thrombosis in infancy, possibly secondary to umbilical sepsis. Patients first present with haematemesis from bleeding oesophageal varices in childhood, adolescence or early adult life. Clinically, there are no cutaneous stigmata of chronic liver disease, and although splenomegaly is often marked, the liver is usually impalpable. Liver function tests are normal, and ascites does not occur. Liver biopsy is helpful in excluding cirrhosis, and ultrasound can often determine the patency of the portal vein. Direct confirmation of the diagnosis is best obtained from the venous phase of selective coeliac axis and superior mesenteric angiograms. These usually show a leash of collateral vessels in the porta hepatis where the portal vein would normally be seen. In adults portal vein thrombosis can be a complication of intra-abdominal sepsis or carcinoma of the pancreas.

Treatment is made easier by the excellent liver function. Most patients stop bleeding after resuscitation. Portosystemic shunts can be technically difficult, although if successful the risk of encephalopathy is much less than in patients with cirrhosis because liver cell function is not impaired. Endoscopic sclerotherapy is a suitable alternative.

ENCEPHALOPATHY

Development of this complication of cirrhosis is a sign of severe liver cell failure, and is usually associated with a bad prognosis. However, a treatable precipitating factor is often present, and its identification and correction is one of the important clinical objectives.

Pathophysiology

A reduction in functioning liver cell mass, and diversion of portal blood past the liver via portosystemic collaterals, are the two important ingredients which predispose to the disturbance in cerebral function, but the precise mechanisms involved are not known. There are two main theories:

1. Toxic substances normally detoxified by the liver are thought to gain access to the systemic circulation and thus the brain where they alter cerebral metabolism.
2. An alteration in the balance between cerebral neurotransmitters is postulated with formation of false neurotransmitters, possibly because of altered amino acid levels in the circulation, which in turn alter the levels of these neurotransmitter substrates in the brain.

Possible candidates as toxins in the first theory include ammonia, mercaptans, amines and indoles. All can be shown to induce encephalopathy in experimental animals, but in concentrations higher than those found in hepatic encephalopathy. Increased serum levels of the aromatic amino acids, and decreased levels of branched chain amino acids, have promoted the concepts outlined in the second theory. There have been attempts to treat the encephalopathy by correcting the balance between the aromatic and branched chain amino acids, but the place of this therapy in clinical practice is not established.

Recently changes in the relative proportions of high and low affinity receptors for some of the cerebral neurotransmitters have been demonstrated in animal models of hepatic encephalopathy, and this seems to be a fruitful area for further research.

Clinical features

The main difference between the encephalopathy seen in chronic liver disease from that already described in fulminant hepatic failure is the relapsing acute on chronic course and the consequent emphasis on the search for, and correction of, precipitating factors. The prodromal phase of an acute on chronic episode may be very gradual. Impairment of judgment can be an early sign. Anorexia is common and the reversal of sleep pattern may be troublesome. Fatigue, withdrawal, apathy and slowness of response often precede a more profound disturbance in consciousness (Table 17.6). There may be spatial disorientation with confusion as to place, time and person. The flapping tremor of the outstretched, extended hands, due to periodic loss of muscle tone, is also seen in uraemia, ventilatory failure, hypokalaemia and congestive heart failure.

Although not specific to liver disease, changes in the EEG can be helpful in identification and management. There is generalised slowing of the main components, with a resulting fall in the mean dominant frequency. Serial recordings are one objective way of following progress during treatment, although simple bedside tests for constructional apraxia, such as the copying of a five-pointed star, are sufficiently reliable and sensitive in practice.

Treatment

An important objective, as mentioned earlier, is to search carefully for a possible precipitating cause (Table 17.12). Intercurrent infection may be identified by culturing blood, ascitic fluid and urine. Occult gastrointestinal bleeding may be detected on rectal examination or on testing

Liver and Biliary Tract Disease

17

Table 17.12 Factors precipitating encephalopathy in cirrhosis

Intercurrent infections
Urinary tract
Chest
Upper respiratory tract
Genito-urinary tract
Spontaneous bacterial peritonitis
Septicaemia

Dietary indiscretion
High-protein meal
Alcohol binge

Gastro-intestinal haemorrhage
Blood acts as protein load, and hypotension impairs liver function (may be occult; melaena on rectal examination)

Electrolyte imbalance
Hyponatraemia or hypokalaemia (possibly due to vomiting, reduced free water clearance or effect of diuretics)

Drugs
Usual candidates are sedatives (increased end-organ sensitivity and reduced clearance) and diuretics (electrolyte imbalance)

Primary hepatocellular carcinoma
Worsening of encephalopathy may be the first indication

stools for blood. Alcohol abuse, and changes in medication and diet, should be identified from the clinical history, particularly if a close relative is available, or by contacting the family doctor. Mild anxiolytics, such as diazepam and night-time sedatives, are common causes, as is a change in diuretic treatment.

Treatment of the encephalopathy is mainly directed at minimising the absorption of nitrogenous material, particularly ammonia, from the bowel. Protein is removed from the diet, the colon is emptied using a magnesium sulphate enema, and ammonia-producing colonic bacteria are reduced in number by giving oral neomycin and lactulose. Lactulose is a synthetic disaccharide which is broken down into its constituent monosaccharides by bacteria in the colon, and then into lactic acid. This not only acts as a purgative, but also discourages the growth of ammonia-producing bacteria. Because of the change in pH, ammonia may also be fixed in the colon as ammonium ions.

HEPATOCELLULAR CARCINOMA

Often referred to as hepatoma, hepatocellular carcinoma arises from the hepatic parenchymal cells.

Incidence, epidemiology and aetiology

In Africa and the Far East, hepatocellular carcinoma is one of the commonest tumours, while it is unusual in Europe and the USA (Fig. 17.21).

Hepatocellular carcinoma usually arises in a cirrhotic liver, and in this setting is commoner in males than females. In Europe and North America, the peak incidence is from 50–70 years of age (Fig. 17.22), but in high-incidence areas patients are often in their twenties or thirties. When there

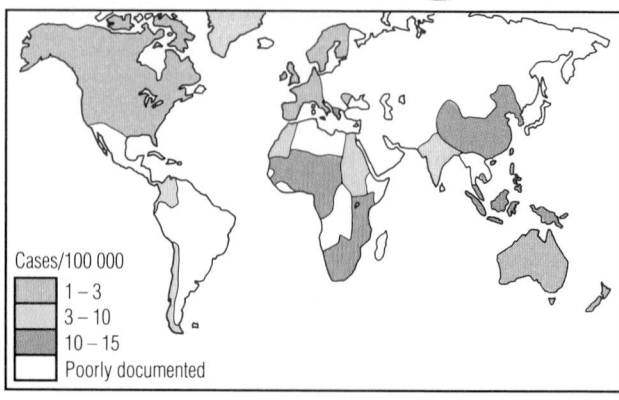

Fig. 17.21 The distribution of hepatocellular carcinoma in the world. It almost parallels the distribution of hepatitis B virus infection (Fig. 17.11).

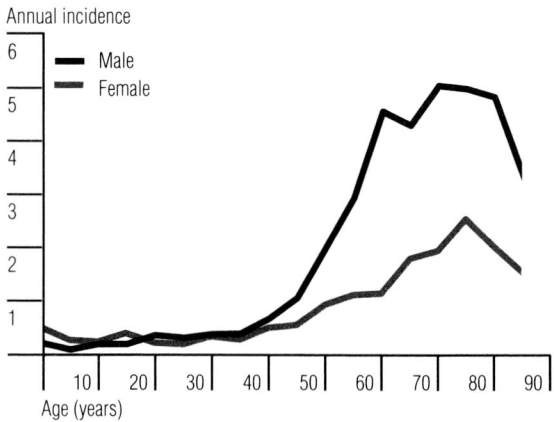

Fig. 17.22 Primary hepatocellular carcinoma. The average number of cases of primary hepatocellular carcinoma seen each year in the south-east of England between the years 1965 and 1984 in men and women by age group (per 100,000).

is no underlying cirrhosis, the sex ratio is equal, and the tumour usually presents in teenagers and young adults.

Chronic hepatitis B virus infection is strongly associated with the development of the tumour, particularly in areas with a high HBsAg carrier rate. The finding of subgenomic fragments of HBV DNA in liver cell and tumour DNA, even in some patients without serological markers of previous HBV infection, has led to the suggestion that the virus may be directly oncogenic. However, the pattern of integration of viral DNA appears to be random and molecular mechanisms which could be responsible for oncogenesis have not yet been identified. Careful prospective studies of hepatoma development in patients with cirrhosis in the UK have shown that previous HBV infection, as detected serologically, is not a significant independent risk factor.

Aflatoxin, a product of the fungal mould *Aspergillus flavus*, can induce liver damage and hepatocellular carcinoma in animals, and is a food contaminant in many tropical countries. Very rarely, hepatocellular carcinoma has been described following prolonged use of the oral

656

contraceptive pill, and in individuals exposed to Thorotrast, an early radioactive X-ray contrast material. It is likely that several factors combine to increase the risk of tumour development, but longstanding cirrhosis and male sex are the most important.

Pathology

The commonest microscopic pattern of hepatocellular carcinoma is the characteristic trabecular or sinusoidal pattern, which reproduces the normal relationship between clusters of liver cells and a flat endothelial cell covering (Fig. 17.2).

Fibrolamellar carcinoma is a distinct variant with a better prognosis, found in mainly young female non-cirrhotic patients. The tumour cells are large and polygonal and are arranged in trabeculae separated by parallel bundles of collagen which merge in places to form broader bands of fibrous tissue.

Clinical features

In the UK, there is usually a slow deterioration in well-being, with anorexia, weight loss and abdominal pain in a patient known to have cirrhosis. Rare, non-metastatic systemic manifestations can occur, and include hypercalcaemia, hypoglycaemia and porphyria cutanea tarda. There may be no specific signs on examination. Hepatomegaly is usually present and there may be an arterial bruit and a friction rub over the tumour. In high-incidence areas, the presentation is often more dramatic, with pain over the tumour, fever and weight loss. The deterioration in liver function is more profound in the patient with pre-existing cirrhosis.

Diagnosis

The routine liver function tests are unhelpful, reflecting the underlying cirrhosis and some cholestasis due to the space-occupying lesion. The most important biochemical marker of the tumour is alpha-fetoprotein (AFP). This is a glycoprotein, which can be thought of as a fetal albumin. It is synthesised by the fetal liver, but levels fall rapidly after birth. In adults it is present in serum in a concentration of less than 10 ng/ml. About 80% of patients with hepatocellular carcinoma arising in a cirrhotic liver, and 50% of those without an underlying cirrhosis, will show elevated AFP levels in serum. In a cirrhotic, levels above 1000 ng/ml are almost diagnostic of hepatocellular carcinoma. AFP is also greatly elevated in patients with germ cell tumours of the testis and ovary but this will not be a diagnostic problem. Some patients with hepatic metastases can also have elevated AFP levels, but not as high as those found in hepatoma. In active cirrhosis, levels of AFP can, on occasions, rise above the normal adult range, probably reflecting increased liver cell regeneration, but a rapid, sustained rise in the serum levels on serial estimations is typical of hepatoma.

Ultrasound, computerised tomography and scinti-scanning are all capable of visualising hepatocellular carcinoma. In practice, CT scans are rarely necessary, but the other two techniques often give complementary information about the tumour and the underlying cirrhosis. Selective hepatic arteriography is a very useful diagnostic technique, and also provides information on the distribution of the tumour within the liver. There is usually a well-defined tumour circulation, with new vessel formation. Although the definitive diagnosis can only be made by histological examination of tumour tissue, in practice liver biopsy may not always be possible because of a prolonged prothrombin time. In these cases a working diagnosis is established from a combination of elevated alpha-fetoprotein levels in serum and the demonstration of a tumour circulation on arteriography.

Treatment

Hepatocellular carcinoma is usually a rapidly growing tumour which presents late. The prognosis is poor, with a mean survival of about 4 months. Resection is potentially curative but is only possible in those cases where tumour is limited to one lobe of the liver and where there is no underlying cirrhosis. The long-term outlook following successful resection is good, with local recurrence being much commoner than distant metastases. On the basis of this experience, it might be expected that liver transplantation would be another effective treatment, also applicable to those with cirrhosis. However, both tumour recurrence in the liver graft and distant metastases are commonly observed within a year or two of the procedure. It is not clear whether this is due to immunosuppressive therapy, or that the tumours are often more advanced than initially suspected.

The only cytotoxic drug to show any benefit so far is adriamycin (doxorubicin). About one-third of those treated show a response, with shrinkage of the tumour and a fall in AFP level, but in most of these survival is only prolonged by a few months. Cardiotoxicity and bone marrow depression are the most serious drug-induced complications, although the former can usually be avoided by limiting the total dose given. Hair loss is a common side-effect. Embolisation of the hepatic artery or the branches supplying the tumour with gelatin foam can give useful pain relief, and is often used before cytotoxic drug therapy to reduce tumour mass.

LIVER METASTASES

Many tumours metastasise to the liver, particularly those arising in the abdomen; in Western societies, this is the commonest cause of malignancy within the liver.

Clinical features

Although the primary tumour may have already been identified, in some cases the metastatic tumour may be the cause of the presentation. In these cases, malaise, weight loss, pain over the liver and abdominal distension are the likely symptoms. Examination often confirms substantial weight loss and usually demonstrates a hard enlarged liver with an irregular surface and edge.

Investigations

The serum alkaline phosphatase is often elevated in patients with liver metastases, and is the most sensitive of the standard liver function tests. Jaundice is usually a late occurrence, and carries a particularly bad prognosis. Ultrasound and scintiscans frequently confirm the presence of filling defects in the liver, and the definitive diagnosis can then be made on liver biopsy. Tumour tissue can be expected on liver biopsy in more than 70% of cases, and the success rate can be further enhanced by using ultrasound to indicate where the biopsy should be taken.

Differential diagnosis

Because of the importance of the diagnosis of metastatic liver cancer, it is usually necessary to obtain histological proof of malignancy. The conditions most likely to be misdiagnosed are cysts, abscesses and granulomas. In areas where hepatoma is common, the pain, fever and rapidly enlarging liver make amoebic abscess and hydatid disease important treatable conditions to be considered in the differential diagnosis.

Treatment

Treatment depends on the nature of the primary tumour. For certain tumours, such as small cell carcinoma of the lung, breast cancer and lymphoma, chemotherapy may be highly effective in producing regression of metastases and symptomatic improvement. With other tumours, such as metastatic gastrointestinal and pancreatic cancer, chemotherapy is usually ineffective, although infusion of cytotoxic drugs such as 5 fluorouracil into the hepatic artery occasionally relieves pain and produces regression. It is questionable whether this complex procedure is more effective than intravenous administration. Pain in the liver is usually controlled by analgesics, but occasionally severe pain can be helped by external irradiation and even hepatic artery ligation or tumour embolisation. Rarely resection of an isolated metastasis may be feasible; carcinoid tumour (p. 592) is a slow-growing tumour where this approach may be valuable.

Symptoms of pain, nausea and anorexia are best treated by palliative measures including analgesics, anti-emetics such as metaclopramide, and corticosteroids.

LYMPHOMA

The liver is often directly involved with infiltration of lymphoma cells. Liver biopsy can therefore be helpful in diagnosis. Documenting liver involvement is also important in staging the disease before deciding on appropriate therapy. Serum alkaline phosphatase levels may be increased and jaundice can occur. In Hodgkin's disease a cholestatic jaundice may appear before there is obvious lymph node involvement, and occasionally in the absence of any evidence of direct hepatic involvement.

THE LIVER IN SYSTEMIC DISEASE

Rheumatoid arthritis

Increased serum alkaline phosphatase levels are frequently seen in rheumatoid arthritis, and are often due to an increase in the liver iso-enzyme. Histological changes on liver biopsy are often non-specific and unremarkable. The condition has sometimes been called 'rheumatoid liver', but the aetiology of the condition, if it really exists, is not understood. It is possible that the mild cholestasis is really due to anti-inflammatory drugs. Amyloidosis and primary biliary cirrhosis are well defined but infrequent associations. Nodular regenerative hyperplasia is sometimes found in Felty's syndrome (p. 980).

Systemic lupus erythematosus

The early finding of lupus erythematosus (LE) cells in about 10% of cases of autoimmune chronic active hepatitis, and the use of the term 'lupoid hepatitis' to describe these patients, created considerable confusion concerning the relationship between chronic active hepatitis and systemic lupus erythematosus (SLE). Although anti-DNA antibodies are frequently present in autoimmune chronic active hepatitis, it is now clear that the two conditions are quite distinct. In particular, clinically significant renal involvement, an important feature in SLE, is very rare in chronic active hepatitis. Furthermore, careful studies of liver involvement in SLE have in most cases shown only minor portal tract inflammation.

Polyarteritis nodosa

Chronic hepatitis B virus infection has been reported in up to 40% of cases of polyarteritis nodosa, but this is not a consistent finding. The associated liver disease in these cases is usually very mild, with minor histological changes on liver biopsy. The appearance of the characteristic arterial lesions in biopsy material is sometimes of help in making the diagnosis.

Scleroderma

As already mentioned, there is a well-recognised association between scleroderma (sometimes called systemic sclerosis) and primary biliary cirrhosis (PBC). In some cases of PBC the associated sclerosis is truly systemic but in most it is limited to the skin of the terminal phalanges (sclerodactyly), and may be part of the CRST syndrome (calcinosis, Raynaud's phenomenon, sclerodactyly, telangiectasia).

Amyloidosis

The liver is often involved in systemic amyloidosis (p. 1092) but this does not produce clinically significant liver disease. Rectal biopsy is safer than liver biopsy in establishing the diagnosis, as haemorrhage is a well-recognised complication.

Porphyria

The metabolic abnormalities responsible for the various types of porphyria and their clinical features are described in Chapter 20. Porphyria cutanea tarda may be associated with alcoholic liver disease, and sometimes hepatoma, and the accumulation of protoporphyrin in the liver in erythropoietic protoporphyria may eventually lead to cirrhosis and liver failure.

Granulomatous conditions

The finding of granulomata in liver biopsy specimens is relatively common. Although they are a feature of some primary liver diseases, particularly primary biliary cirrhosis, they are more often a reflection of a systemic condition (Table 17.13). In the UK the commonest causes are sarcoidosis, tuberculosis, and drug reactions. There is usually hepatomegaly, with a raised serum alkaline phosphatase but a normal serum bilirubin level. In up to 30% of cases the cause of the hepatic granulomata cannot be determined in spite of rigorous investigation. Occasionally portal hypertension may develop either because of a direct effect of the granulomata on liver blood flow or in association with increasing liver fibrosis. In these cases a trial of steroids is justified to try to halt the progress of the disease.

Granulomatous hepatitis is a term used to denote the presence of focal parenchymal liver damage in association with multiple granulomata. In some cases of unknown aetiology there may be quite striking symptoms of a systemic illness, including fever, malaise and weight loss. There is often a dramatic improvement on corticosteroid therapy.

Table 17.13   Causes of granulomatous liver disease

Infections	**Neoplasms**
Bacterial	Hodgkin's lymphoma*
Usually chronic intracellular	Adenocarcinoma
infections	Hepatocellular carcinoma
Mycobacterial including	
tuberculosis*	**Multisystem diseases**
Brucellosis*	Collagen-vascular disease
Leprosy	Polymyalgia rheumatica*
Listerosis	Systemic lupus erythematosus
Fungal	Others
Histoplasmosis*	Sarcoidosis*
Nocardia	Whipple's disease
Candidiasis	Wegener's granulomatosis
Actinomycosis	Granulomatous disease of
Parasitic	childhood
Schistosomiasis*	
Ascariasis	**Miscellaneous**
Toxacara	Primary biliary cirrhosis*
Amoebiasis	Crohn's disease*
Strongyloides	IV drug abusers
Giardiasis	Patients on haemodialysis
Viral	Haemophilia
Cytomegalovirus	After ileal bypass surgery
Lymphogranuloma venereum	Erythema nodosum
Infectious mononucleosis	
Other	
Syphilis	
Q fever	
Drug-induced	
Sulphonamides and derivatives	
Sulphonamide-containing	
antibiotics* and anti-diabetics like	
chlorpropamide*	
Others	
e.g. Phenylbutazone*	
Allopurinol	
Hydralazine	
Carbamazepine	
Quinidine	

* Common causes of liver granulomata

NON-VIRAL INFECTIONS INVOLVING THE LIVER

Schistosomiasis

Worldwide schistosomiasis (p. 318) is a common cause of chronic liver disease. Adult worms live in small veins of the colon (*Schistosoma mansoni*) and the small intestine and colon (*S. japonicum*). The liver damage is due to granulomatous reactions to eggs which have embolised in the liver, and impacted in pre-sinusoidal branches of the portal vein. Resolution of granulomata leads to severe periportal fibrosis in patients with heavy infections. Portal hypertension usually accompanies the developing fibrosis, but liver cell function is well preserved unless there is coexisting cirrhosis from another cause. Patients often present with haematemesis from ruptured oesophageal varices. Gross splenomegaly is common and ascites occurs. The prognosis is fairly good. Diagnosis and management are discussed in Chapter 12.

Liver flukes

Fasciola hepatica is a flatworm which is common in sheep, and to a lesser extent, cattle worldwide. It lives in the biliary tree and sheds its ova into the stools. Infection is acquired by eating watercress on which metacercariae are encysted. These excyst, penetrate the wall of the intestine and migrate across the peritoneal cavity to the liver. (See also p. 322.)

The liver damage is caused by the worms in the biliary system. In severe infections there is intermittent obstructive jaundice with high fever, painful hepatomegaly, and jaundice. Eosinophilia is common, and a complement fixation test is usually positive in high titre. The definitive diagnosis is made by finding ova in stool concentrates. The infection responds to treatment with praziquantel.

Clonorchis sinensis is found in the Far East. Its life cycle is similar to fasciola except that the cercariae released from snails form cysts in freshwater fish. If this is eaten raw, the worms eventually reach the biliary system. Symptoms are usually mild, except in heavy infections when there may be upper abdominal pain, tender hepatomegaly and diarrhoea. Praziquantel is an effective treatment. Late complications include obstructive jaundice, cholangitis, stones in the common bile duct and cholangiocarcinoma (p. 643).

Hydatid cysts

Hydatid cysts (p. 325) are cysts in the liver formed by the larval stages of two tapeworms, *Echinococcus granulosus* and *Echinococcus multilocularis*, which normally live in dogs and wild carnivores respectively. Although man is not the usual intermediate host, the larval stages can infect the liver, and sometimes the lungs, brain, bones and spleen. *Echinococcus granulosus*, which has a wide geographical distribution, forms well-defined single or multiple cysts, with a thick fibrous capsule and an inner germinal layer from which daughter cysts bud off internally. The daughter cysts from *Echinococcus multilocularis* proliferate external to the main cyst, and this is an invasive lesion. It is mainly found in central and eastern Europe.

Cysts may be asymptomatic or may present with pain in the right hypochondrium. If they are very large, they can cause abdominal distension and discomfort. Secondary infection in a cyst is a serious complication, presenting with fever and pain like other pyogenic liver abscesses.

Ultrasound and CT scanning are the most useful investigations and can be diagnostic if the 'daughter' cysts can be identified (Fig. 17.23). Complement fixation and haemagglutination tests for antibodies to hydatid material can also be helpful in making a specific diagnosis, although negative results can occur, particularly in asymptomatic cases.

Mebendazole and more recently albendazole have been used for treatment and information is now available regarding the relationship between serum and cyst concentrations. Drug treatment may become the first line of therapy. Surgical removal of the cysts still offers the best chance of cure but great care must be taken to prevent rupturing of the cysts, which leads to dissemination of daughter cysts into the peritoneal cavity. This risk is minimised by injecting formalin, alcohol or hypertonic saline into the cyst before attempting removal. It is wise to leave asymptomatic cysts alone.

Amoebiasis

In some cases of amoebic colitis, and in others without bowel symptoms, the organisms reach the liver through the portal venous system and form intrahepatic amoebic

Fig. 17.23 Hydatid disease of the liver. A. Ultrasound demonstrating multiple cysts. **B.** CT scan demonstrating 'daughter' cysts in the liver. There is calcification within the cyst wall.

abscesses. Pain in the right hypochondrium, with tender hepatomegaly and fever, are the usual manifestations. A right-sided pleural effusion can also occur if an abscess has ruptured through the diaphragm. Ultrasound and CT scans are very useful investigations, and antibody tests are almost always positive. A week's course of metronidazole is a very effective treatment and can be used as a therapeutic test of the diagnosis; however, anaerobic pyogenic liver abscess will also respond. (See also p. 661.)

Weil's disease

The spirochaete *Leptospira icterohaemorrhagica* can be transmitted to man from infested rats' urine. Those in contact with sewage and rat-infected water are at highest risk. The incubation period is 1–2 weeks. At first the illness may resemble a prodromal stage of viral hepatitis, with mild fever and malaise, but it is often more severe, with myalgia and high fever. This may progress to prostration, jaundice and renal failure. Headache, confusion and meningism are often present. Epistaxis, haematuria and petechiae occur. There is often a prominent leucocytosis, and the urine contains red cells and albumin. Identification of the causative organism in blood or urine is the definitive diagnostic test although there is a rise in serum IgM antibody at the end of the acute phase of the disease. Although the jaundice may be deep, liver failure does not occur, and general toxaemia and renal failure are the usual problems in management. The organism is sensitive to benzyl penicillin and large doses are usually given. However, there is no convincing evidence that this contributes to the resolution of the disease, and skilled intensive care is essential. The reported mortality varies from 4–40%.

Septicaemia

Cholestasis is not uncommon in severe sepsis. A rise in serum bilirubin occurs in 25–50% of cases, but serum aminotransferase and alkaline phosphatase are often normal. The pathogenesis is not understood but there is no evidence of gross liver damage and there is usually rapid resolution with appropriate antibiotic therapy. In jaundice due to staphylococcal sepsis, treatment with fucidic acid should be avoided as this interferes with bilirubin excretion.

PYOGENIC LIVER ABSCESS

The commonest cause of liver abscess worldwide is amoebiasis, but in the developed world pyogenic causes are becoming of increasing importance. In the past pyogenic liver abscess was most commonly seen in children or young adults in association with appendicitis. However, as antibiotics have become more widely prescribed, the condition is now most often seen in the elderly, due to incomplete treatment of biliary tract disease or diverticulitis. In these patients, the presenting symptoms are often non-specific and the diagnosis is often delayed.

Aetiology

There are many possible causes of pyogenic liver abscess (Table 17.14). Infection in any site drained by the portal vein can cause portal pyaemia and this can then seed the liver with abscesses. These are usually multiple and often concentrated in the right lobe. The primary site, particularly in diverticular disease, may be relatively silent. Direct spread of infection from the biliary tree is the presumed route of entry of the bacteria in those cases where abscess complicates biliary tract disease. Trauma and hepatic malignancy are uncommon causes.

Bacteriology

The dominant organism isolated from hepatic abscess has changed over the last few years. While aerobic Gram-

Table 17.14 Causes of pyogenic liver abscess

Biliary tract disease
Ascending cholangitis is the commonest cause and may be a complication of any obstruction in the biliary tract; it can also follow cholecystitis

Portal phlebitis
Any primary septic focus within the abdomen (diverticulitis, appendicitis, infected haemorrhoids, etc.) can cause thrombophlebitis in the local branches of the portal vein, and infect the liver

Septicaemia
Severe generalised sepsis can infect the liver via the hepatic artery

Trauma
Secondary infection of a damaged area of liver or a haematoma can lead to abscess formation

Malignancy
Some tumours develop areas of central necrosis, and pyogenic infection can then follow

Extension of local infection
e.g. Subphrenic abscess and empyema of the gall bladder

negative organisms, especially *Escherichia coli*, used to predominate, anaerobes, particularly *Streptococcus milleri*, are now found in up to 50% of abscesses. Mixed infections are identified in about one-third of cases.

Presentation

Classically there is upper abdominal pain, swinging pyrexia, anorexia, malaise and weight loss. However, in many older patients the symptoms and signs may be much less dramatic, and pain and hepatomegaly may not be present. This is one of the causes of pyrexia of unknown origin which must not be overlooked.

Investigations

A polymorphonuclear leucocytosis is usually present and the routine liver function tests often show a high serum alkaline phosphatase. The most useful investigation, which is often diagnostic, is an ultrasound scan. If there has been no previous antibiotic treatment, aerobic and anaerobic cultures of blood or direct aspirates of pus under ultrasound control will usually reveal the causative organism.

Treatment

Antibiotics are always needed and are best chosen according to the bacteriological findings. In cases where these are unhelpful or where sepsis is life-threatening and treatment has to be given before the results are available, then a combination of gentamicin (or a broad-spectrum cephalosporin), metronidazole and flucloxacillin will cover most of the likely organisms. In cases with very small multiple abscesses, appropriate antibiotic treatment alone may be adequate therapy but in most cases drainage is also required. In a solitary abscess or where the number is small it may be possible to achieve satisfactory percutaneous drainage by repeated needle aspiration. In elderly patients the first line of treatment is usually closed aspiration combined with antibiotics instilled into the abscess cavity and given intravenously. When the abscesses are difficult to approach, open surgical drainage is used. Soft pliable drains are placed in the largest cavities and intensive broad-spectrum antibiotic treatment started. Whichever approach to drainage is used, the antibiotics need to be continued for 6 weeks to ensure resolution of infection.

Prognosis

Unfortunately the diagnosis of pyogenic liver abscess is often delayed, and under these circumstances the mortality may be as high as 80%. With a high index of suspicion and early diagnosis the mortality has been as low as 10% in some series. Co-existent biliary tract disease, old age and multiple abscesses are associated with a poor prognosis.

CONGENITAL BILIARY AND HEPATIC DISORDERS

Caroli's disease

Caroli's disease is a rare condition in which saccular dilatations of the intrahepatic biliary tree predispose to ascending cholangitis. Symptoms usually begin in childhood or early adult life. Long-term antibiotic treatment reduces the frequency of attacks.

Choledochal cyst

Choledochal cyst is a gross dilatation or diverticulum of the common bile duct, which obstructs normal bile flow and presents as cholestatic jaundice in childhood. The diagnosis is made on ultrasound and cholangiography. Treatment is by surgical resection and drainage, usually via a Roux-en-Y anastomosis.

Biliary atresia

Originally thought to be a congenital anomaly, with failure of development of the extrahepatic biliary system, biliary atresia is now recognised as an acquired condition in many cases. There is gradual destruction of the common bile duct soon after birth, leading to deepening jaundice and secondary biliary cirrhosis. Early surgical intervention, with a bypass anastamosis high in the porta hepatis, has proved remarkably successful in some cases. More recently, liver transplantation has also produced promising results.

Polycystic disease of the liver

Polycystic disease of the liver may be a congenital anomaly related to biliary atresia, but rarely presents with jaundice. Large cysts, similar to those seen in polycystic kidney disease and often associated with them, may be found throughout the liver. Gross nodular hepatomegaly, often asymptomatic, is the usual finding on examination. Although pain, due to haemorrhage or infection in a cyst, can occur, the prognosis with respect to the liver lesions is excellent.

LIVER TRANSPLANTATION

Replacement of the liver by an orthotopic graft is a technically difficult procedure but one that is now accepted as a feasible and appropriate treatment for advanced liver disease.

Selection of suitable patients is difficult (Table 17.15). If the disease process is too advanced then the operative mortality will be unacceptably high. Survival figures (Fig. 17.24), although improving, are not as good as after renal transplantation, and a skilled assessment of the patient's prognosis is essential to balance the likely benefit of the operation with its considerable risks. Hepatocellular carcinoma, with its very poor prognosis, would seem to be an obvious choice. However, even with careful patient selection to exclude those with extrahepatic spread, recurrence of tumour in the graft and distant metastases have occurred in about 60% of cases, and transplantation is no longer considered to be a useful treatment option. Currently the best results are obtained in patients with advanced cirrhosis, either cryptogenic or due to chronic active hepatitis or primary biliary cirrhosis. Many of these patients have severe portal hypertension, with encephalopathy and bleeding varices, but these are not contraindications to the procedure. The reversal of encepha-

Table 17.15 Common indications for liver transplantation

Disease	Comments
Cirrhosis	
Primary biliary cirrhosis	Increasing bilirubin a good indication of advanced disease; results excellent
Chronic active hepatitis	
Autoimmune	Good results; not so easy timing transplant
HBV	Frequent recurrence of HBV infection in transplant but resulting disease mild
Cryptogenic	Timing difficult; results good if not too advanced
Fulminant hepatic failure	Simple tests can indicate prognosis and need for transplant; urgent need for donor organ makes organisation difficult but results good
Biliary atresia	Transplantation of half a liver makes a wider range of donor organs available; early Kasai operation (porto-enterostomy) may make later transplant unnecessary

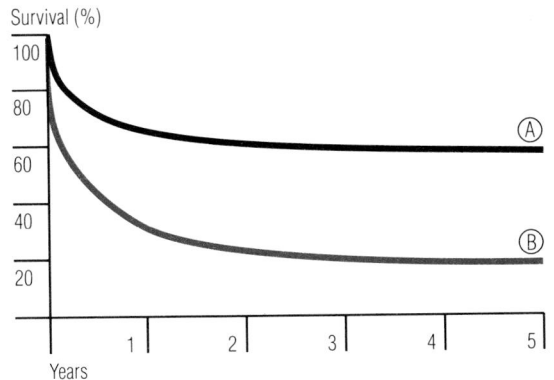

Survival (%)

Ⓐ

Ⓑ

Years

Fig. 17.24 Liver transplant survival rates. The dramatic improvement in the survival of liver transplants after 1978 (A) compared to before 1978 (B) is partly due to improved surgical techniques, but also better patient selection and better immunosuppression following the introduction of cyclosporin A. Many centres are now reporting results as good as those shown in curve A.

lopathy is often dramatic, even in those in whom it has been present for many months. In acute liver failure there are difficulties in obtaining donor organs at an appropriate time, but patients with subacute hepatic necrosis and the Budd-Chiari syndrome have been successfully treated. In America, children with biliary atresia have been successfully treated by liver transplantation for many years. In the UK donors of a suitable age have only recently become more readily available, and the operation is proving useful in those cases presenting too late for a successful biliary drainage procedure.

The postoperative period

The immediate postoperative period is often remarkably uneventful in those patients who have received a well-preserved donor liver. In experimental animals the liver is rejected less vigorously than other organs and this also seems to be true in man. Cyclosporin A, a potent inhibitor of antigen-induced lymphocyte proliferation, has reduced the severity of rejection even further, although nephrotoxicity, its most important side-effect in man, is a continuing problem. Biliary obstruction and fistulae were important early problems, but changes in technique have led to some improvements in this area.

Overall, 1-year survival rates are now between 40% and 70% in most series. The quality of life is usually excellent and many patients have survived for more than 5 years.

FURTHER READING

Schiff L, Schiff E R 1982 Diseases of the liver. 5th edn. J P Lippincott Co., Philadelphia. *A major US text. Heavy but complete.*

Sherlock S 1985 Diseases of the liver and biliary system. 7th edn. Blackwell Scientific Publications, Oxford. *The latest edition of the 'standard' liver text.*

Wright R, Millward-Sadler G H, Alberti K G M M, Kattin S J (1985) Liver and biliary disease. 2nd edn. Baillière-Tindall, London. *The modern British composite liver textbook. Readable, accurate and combining basic science with clinical medicine.*

Endocrine Diseases

18

HISTORICAL INTRODUCTION

The history of endocrinology, although interesting, can seldom be said to have followed a logical and coherent progression. Certain landmarks only will be mentioned here – historical notes where appropriate are given for individual hormones.

Aristotle had suggested that certain organs (such as the testes) produced substances which travelled through the bloodstream and acted at distant sites. However, it was not until the 19th century that endocrinology began to emerge as a medical discipline. Berthold of Göttingen, in 1849, was the first to provide 'experimental proof' for the existence of an internal secretion, by demonstrating that transplantation of the testis to another part of the bird's body prevented atrophy of the cock's comb, known to be caused by castration. In 1855, Thomas Addison described the clinical picture which resulted from destruction of the adrenal glands in man. The first clear demonstration that an extract of a gland could correct a deficiency disease was provided by Murray and others, who showed that the administration of sheep thyroid extract would cure myxoedema and its childhood equivalent, cretinism, and the effects of thyroidectomy. In 1915 Kendall isolated the active principle and named it thyroxine. By then, the first demonstration of a hormone had been made in 1902, by Baylis and Starling, who extracted the hormone they termed secretin from the duodenum, and found that it promoted pancreatic enzyme secretion. Adrenaline was extracted from the adrenal glands at about the same time, causing considerable confusion regarding the endocrine role of the adrenal glands until the discovery of the corticosteroid hormones in the 1930s and 1940s. By the mid-1930s, German chemists had isolated and later synthesised testosterone and the main oestrogen, oestradiol, followed shortly after in the 1940s by the adrenal glucocorticoids, cortisone and cortisol. Because of its unusual chemical structure and high potency, the main mineralocorticoid, aldosterone, was not discovered until the mid 1950s. The major pathways of steroid synthesis were not completely identified, nor the inborn errors of steroid production recognised, until this time.

From an early stage, clinical observation has had a major impact on the development of the science of endocrinology and the recognition of different hormones. This is particularly true of the pituitary gland and its subservient endocrine glands. Early this century, Harvey Cushing, the father of pituitary surgery, recognised that some features of pituitary disease were due to deficiencies, and others (for example in acromegaly) to hormone excess (in this case, growth hormone).

Geoffrey Harris, working in Cambridge, was responsible for the concept that the anterior pituitary gland was controlled by secretions coming to it through a portal blood supply from the hypothalamus. Since the late 1960s, we have seen the isolation and synthesis of several of these releasing factors and their entry into clinical practice.

Recently, the pace of development of our understanding of basic and clinical endocrinology has been truly staggering. Much has come from advances in methods for measuring the minute concentrations of hormones in body fluids. In many instances, the concentration of active hormones in the circulation is in the range of picogrammes (10^{-12}g) per ml. In the 1960s, initial bioassay and chemical methods gave way to protein-binding assays of which the most widely used have been radioimmunoassays. These depend upon developing highly specific antibodies to hormones, coupled if necessary (e.g. for steroids) to a protein.

Endocrine Diseases

A further essential development was the capacity to make radiolabelled hormones. Such methods have demonstrated, amongst other phenomena, the episodic nature of release of certain hormones. Thus, administration of gonadotrophin-releasing hormone GnRH (initially to monkeys) showed the importance of pulsatile secretion of GnRH in transmitting the correct message. Continuous administration was found to switch off secretion of the hormones that it stimulates when given episodically.

Recently, very sensitive bioassay methods have been developed, such as those using isolated cells; these are especially important for polypeptide hormones. Furthermore, immunoradiometric assays for many polypeptide hormones have now become available, with even greater sensitivity and specificity than radioimmunoassays.

THE PHYSIOLOGY OF HORMONE ACTION

THE TARGET ORGAN ACTION OF HORMONES

The growing edge of research into endocrinology and endocrine disease is now undoubtedly at the site of action of hormones, rather than at their sites of biosynthesis.

Hormone action through cell surface receptors

Target cell responses to hormones can be divided into two broad groups depending upon where the receptors are located. Some hormones bind to receptors in the cell membrane, and others to receptors in the cell cytoplasm or nucleus. All receptors contain a binding site of high affinity and specificity for the relevant hormone, whose binding changes the conformation of the receptor. With cell surface receptors, this change is coupled to one or more effector systems inside the membrane.

Actions mediated by adenylate cyclase

The first such effector mechanism to be recognised was the adenylate cyclase system which, when activated, generates cyclic-AMP (from ATP) as second messenger (Fig. 18.1).

It is now recognised that hormones can either activate or inhibit this enzyme, depending upon whether they are linked to it via a stimulatory (Ns) or inhibitory (Ni) guanosine triphosphate (GTP)-containing coupling protein. The N (or G) protein consists of three subunits, α, β and γ. When the receptor is activated by the hormone, it associates with an Ns coupling protein; the α-subunit dissociates and activates adenylate cyclase. The α-subunit is also a guanosine triphosphatase (GTPase), and its activation leads to a simultaneous breakdown of GTP to GDP, switching-off adenylate cyclase. Cholera toxin permanently activates Ns by causing its linkage to ADP-ribose via the α-subunit, while pertussis toxin permanently activates Ni by a similar mechanism. These ADP-ribosylated forms lose their GTPase function.

Cyclic-AMP, in turn, binds to and activates certain intracellular kinases which then activate other enzymes and proteins by phosphorylation. The concentration of cyclic AMP is determined by the combined activity of adenylate cyclase and the enzyme that destroys cyclic-AMP, phosphodiesterase.

Many hormones are now known to act wholly or in part via the second messenger cyclic-AMP. These include many *polypeptide hormones* such as adrenocorticotrophic hormone (ACTH), luteinising hormone (LH), follicle stimulating hormone (FSH), thyroid stimulating hormone (TSH), parathyroid hormone, calcitonin and antidiuretic hormone (vasopressin). The effects of the catecholamine hormone adrenaline (also called epinephrine), mediated by the β-receptor, are also produced by activation of adenylate cyclase. On the other hand, its alpha-adrenergic effects are mediated, in part at least, by *inhibiting* adenylate cyclase (via the Ni coupling protein discussed above). This accounts in part for the mutually antagonistic α and β effects of adrenaline, at least in tissues that possess both types of receptors. Many of the effects of *prostaglandins*, which are not systemic hormones but do act via cell surface receptors, are also mediated by adenylate cyclase.

Actions mediated by calcium transport

Since the early eighties it has become increasingly apparent

Fig. 18.1 Mechanism of action of hormones that activate adenylate cyclase. A. State of cell membrane when hormone is not bound. **B.** Hormone (H) binds to receptor (R); GTP binds to α subunit of coupling protein. **C.** Alpha subunit dissociates and binds to adenylate cyclase (C) which is activated. GTP breaks down to GDP by α subunit enzyme activity. H dissociates from R. **D.** Dissociation of α subunit from C. Activation ceases. State returns to **A.**

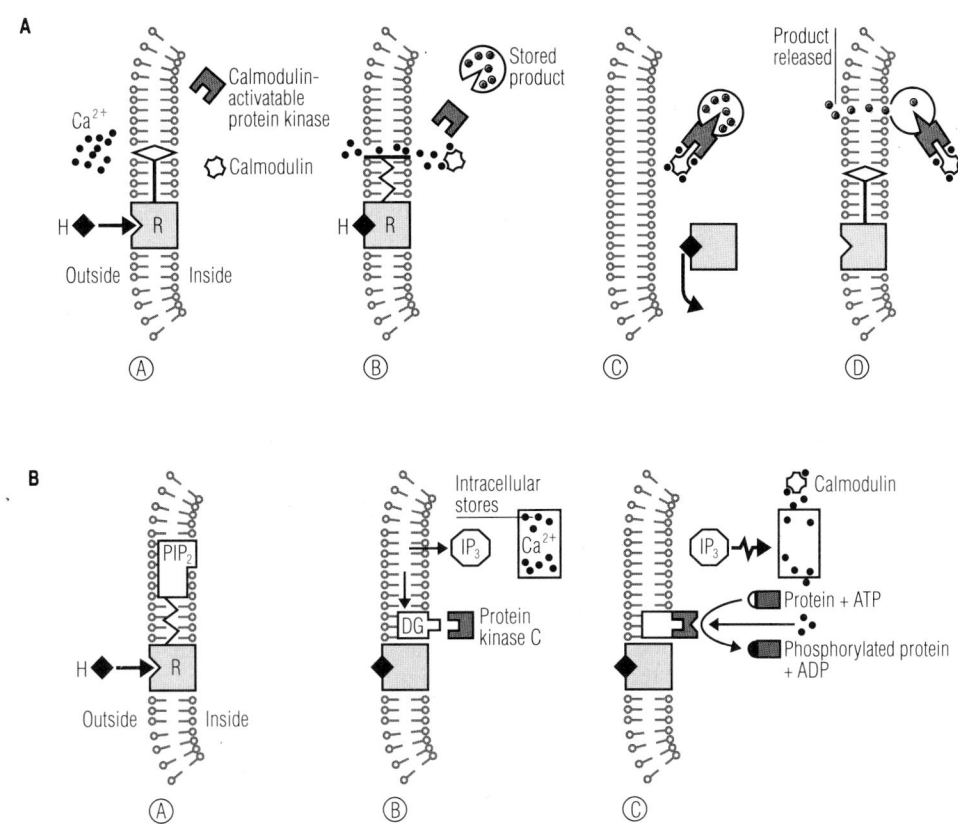

Fig. 18.2 Mechanisms of hormone actions mediated by calcium transport or release. A. Hormones that promote calcium transport into the cell. (A) Absence of hormone. (B) Hormone (H) binds to receptor and (R) opens up Ca^{2+} channel. (C) Ca^{2+} binds to calmodulin, which binds to secretory granule. (D) Secretory granule fuses with cell surface and releases product. **B.** Hormones that act via cleavage of phosphatidyl inositol bisphosphate (PIP_2). (A) Hormone binds to receptor. (B) Receptor (activated) cleaves PIP_2 to diacylglycerol (DG) and inositol trisphosphate (IP_3). (C) IP_3 causes Ca^{2+} release from microsomes; Ca^{2+} binds to calmodulin. DG binds and activates protein kinase C (PKC). PKC action, potentiated by Ca^{2+}, phosphorylates protein.

that many hormones act through cell surface receptors independently of adenylate cyclase. These include insulin and related growth factors, and some or all of the hypothalamic releasing hormones. It is now clear that many such effects are due to activation of calcium transport into the cell or its release from intracellular stores, and/or to cleavage of cell membrane phospholipids to generate two further second messengers, inositol 1,3,4 triphosphate (IP_3) and diacylglycerol (DG) (Fig. 18.2).

IP_3 is believed to act principally by stimulating calcium release from the microsomal pool of calcium. In the inactive state, calcium levels inside the cell are kept extremely low. A transient rise in intracellular calcium is capable of activating intracellular proteins, notably calmodulin, which has four binding sites for calcium. In its activated state, calmodulin will activate certain protein kinases which, using ATP as substrate, will then phosphorylate other proteins, thus activating them. Analogues of DG (the phorbol esters) will stimulate prolonged cell growth and proliferation and promote tumour growth.

Many hormones act through more than one of these mechanisms. There is a wide variety of possible combinations of different effects involving these simple organic compounds and calcium. An appreciation of the general

structure of the system is of increasing importance not only in endocrinology, but also in our understanding of tumour growth and development.

The insulin receptor is now well characterised; it consists of four subunits, two α and two β. The β-subunit acts as a tyrosine kinase, which is capable of phosphorylating and thereby activating a number of intracellular enzymes (Fig. 18.3). These include serine kinases and ser-

Fig. 18.3 Mechanism of action of insulin. Binding to subunit(s) alters conformation of β subunit and switches on its protein kinase activity.

18

ine/threonine phosphatases, which in turn activate their substrates. One of these substrates is the insulin-related growth factor II (IGF II) receptor, which cycles from the cell surface to microsomes and back again, carrying IGF II into the cell in the process. Insulin greatly reduces the amount of this receptor on the cell surface. It is probable that phosphorylation and dephosphorylation of the IGF II receptor provides the driving force for this cycle of endocytosis and exocytosis. It seems likely that the action of insulin in promoting glucose uptake depends upon a similar effect of altering the phosphorylation state of the glucose transporter molecule.

Hormone action through intracellular receptors

Receptors for steroid hormones (including vitamin D) and thyroid hormones are located in the cell cytoplasm and (principally) nucleus. In the presence of its ligand, the receptor binds with high affinity to specific promotor sites on DNA. Specific regions of DNA are then 'read' by the enzyme RNA polymerase, with consequent synthesis of messenger RNA and specific proteins important for cell function (Fig. 18.4). Most of the actions of steroid hormones are believed to be mediated by such receptors, although at high concentrations (such as are seen within steroid-producing tissues), non-receptor-mediated effects may also operate.

Some hormones are made from conversion of less active precursors in target tissues. The clearest example of this is dihydrotestosterone, which is synthesised from testosterone (the circulating form) by the enzyme 5-α-reductase. This transformation is essential for many of the actions of testosterone.

CIRCULATION AND METABOLISM OF HORMONES

The fate of hormones in the circulation varies widely. Most polypeptide hormones have a relatively short half-life (minutes) in the circulation, before they are degraded by proteases in the liver, kidneys, lungs and elsewhere. As implied above, some of the hormone is also internalised in target tissues. Exceptions to the short half-life are the glycosylated peptides – TSH, LH, FSH and human chorionic gonadotrophin (HCG) – where a coating of sugar

residues partially protects the protein from degradation, without apparently affecting its binding to the receptor. In some instances, such as FSH, the hormone is secreted episodically, but this is difficult to demonstrate because of its long half-life (several hours). LH, on the other hand, has a much shorter half-life, so episodic secretion is easily detected, with 'pulses' occurring up to once every 60 minutes.

The steroid and thyroid hormones are partially protected from degradation by the liver and from renal excretion, by circulating binding proteins, the most important of which are corticosteroid binding globulin (CBG), sex-hormone globulin (SHBG), vitamin D-binding protein (DBP), and thyroxine binding globulin (TBG). These proteins are less specific than the receptors; indeed, no general rules can be made for the relation between the affinity of a compound for its binding protein and its biological activity except to say that these proteins generally bind biologically active compounds. In addition, a substantial fraction of many of these hormones bind to albumin and, in some cases, to other proteins with low affinity. Since the concentration of albumin is high, albumin binding is, in some cases, quantitatively important.

Most of the evidence suggests that hormone-binding proteins serve a damping role, reducing the fluctuations produced by episodic secretion of hormones, and reducing their rate of degradation. The small fraction (0.1–5%) of total hormone in free solution (unbound) is believed to be the 'biologically active' fraction – that is, to determine the free concentration inside the cells and so the amount available to activate cellular receptors. In the case of steroid hormones, it is probably also the unbound plasma steroid that is monitored as part of the feedback control mechanism.

INTERACTIONS BETWEEN DIFFERENT HORMONES

Nature is economical, and two hormones acting together may transmit information differing both qualitatively and quantitatively from that conveyed by either separately. For example, glucocorticoids and adrenaline interact strikingly at the levels of both production and action. Glucocorticoids induce the last enzyme necessary for adrenaline synthesis; they also promote production of the β-adrenergic receptor

Fig. 18.4 Mechanism of action of steroid and thyroid hormones. A. Hormone (H) binds to nuclear receptor (R). **B.** Activated receptor now binds to specific promoter on DNA, allowing access of RNA polymerase. **C. and D.** RNA transcript is processed by removal of introns and splicing. **E.** Messenger RNA (mRNA) is translated in cytoplasm by ribosomes which synthesise proteins.

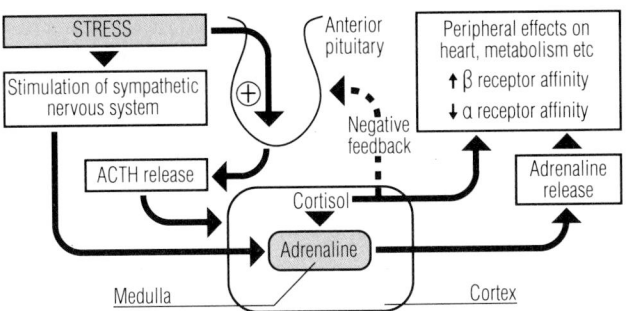

Fig. 18.5 Interactions between glucocorticoids and adrenaline at levels of production and action.

and so enhance some target hormone responses to β-adrenergic agonists (Fig. 18.5). The two hormones act together, for example, to enhance fetal lung maturation at birth. This may have therapeutic importance in treating respiratory distress syndrome and, in later life, in treating bronchial asthma, when analogues of glucocorticoids and adrenaline act synergistically.

Many of the symptoms and signs of thyroid hormone excess result from an augmented sensitivity to adrenaline, thought to result from enhanced responsiveness to β-adrenergic effects. The mechanism which enhances β (and probably diminishes α) agonist activity is not yet clear. Many of these effects (excess sweating, lid lag, tachycardia, and tremor) can be blocked acutely by administering a β-adrenergic blocking agent while the thyroid hormone excess persists.

A third example of hormone-hormone interaction is that between oestrogens and progestogens. One of the effects of the natural oestrogen oestradiol (and its synthetic counterparts) is to induce production of the progesterone receptor. Indeed, in the absence of previous oestrogen, exposure to progesterone has little if any effect on the uterine endometrium or the breast. The presence of progesterone receptors in breast cancer is among the best available evidence that the tumour is oestrogen-dependent, and should therefore respond to treatment with an anti-oestrogen, such as tamoxifen.

CLASSIFICATION OF ENDOCRINE DISEASES

Hyper-, hypo- and dysfunction

As our knowledge of the anatomy, physiology and biochemistry of the endocrine system has increased over the last century, so our appreciation of the mechanisms and treatment of its disorders has changed. With most of the endocrine glands, both excess and deficiency of hormone production occur and are associated with particular constellations of symptoms and physical signs.

Although excess and deficiency diseases still form the basis of endocrine practice, it is an oversimplification to think merely in terms of 'too much or too little hormone'.

It is true that with some systems, e.g. the thyroid gland, normal production of the hormone(s) is relatively steady and the concept of pure excess or deficiency approximates to the truth. However, in other systems, e.g. the adult female reproductive system, there is an inbuilt and complex rhythm. Each of the major components of this system (hypothalamus, pituitary and ovary) secretes hormones and responds to those produced by other components. The interactions depend on both the levels of hormone (often more than one), and the very important dimension of time. Here, the capacity for responses to become out of phase with one another is considerable, and many of the syndromes that we see with this system have features which suggest dysfunction rather than simple hyper- or hypofunction. Since one abnormality may lead to another, with endocrine dysfunction we are in many instances still unable to dissect out the primary abnormality. Our only hope of doing so is to use the model of the normal system as a starting point.

Primary vs secondary abnormalities

When considering malfunction of endocrine glands it is obviously useful to identify whether the abnormality of production is primary or secondary. Adrenal or thyroid insufficiency, for example, may be due either to intrinsic disease of these glands, or to a failure of secretion of the trophic hormone (ACTH and TSH respectively) by the pituitary. Pituitary deficiency in turn may also be intrinsic, or due to damage to the hypothalamus. The distinction may be important from the point of view of treatment (although in both of these instances the products of the subservient endocrine glands would be replaced even when the primary defect lies in the controlling pituitary). It is certainly important to make the distinction when predicting and treating accompanying features, including other hormone deficiencies.

Target organ disease

With respect to events after the secretion of a hormone, we are increasingly coming to recognise conditions in which the basic abnormality lies in the target organ detection system. This process generally involves receptor proteins with a binding site for the hormone, linked to an effector system. There are many instances of 'target organ' endocrine diseases, and although major disorders due to problems at this level are rare they are well documented and minor problems are quite common. Only recently have the methods become available for examining such defects.

THE AETIOLOGY OF ENDOCRINE DISEASES

Tumours

Neoplasms of endocrine tissue are extremely common; they are usually benign and may secrete one or more hormones or be apparently functionless. Such tumours cause problems for one of three reasons:

1. They may present as a local space-occupying lesion. This is particularly true of tumours of the pituitary gland because there is very little room for expansion without producing pressure effects on important surrounding structures.
2. By secreting a hormone, or hormones, they may produce the syndrome associated with excess of that hormone or of the gland that it controls.
3. They may destroy or compress the normal gland and lead to underproduction of other hormones (again this applies almost exclusively to the pituitary gland).

Malignant tumours of endocrine tissue share many of the properties common to other cancers. With some (such as the pituitary) distant metastases are infrequent.

With endocrine tumours, hormone production may continue, or be abnormal; for example carcinomas of the adrenal cortex may secrete the normal product cortisol, or precursor steroids, or no steroids at all. The control mechanisms of hormone secretion for malignant tumours are generally more disturbed than are those of benign tumours. Occasionally, the properties of the normal gland can be used to treat the tumour; thus, for example, the uptake of radioactive iodine by the tumour can be used very effectively to treat metastases in papillary and follicular carcinomas of the thyroid gland.

In some familial syndromes, in which tumours occur in more than one endocrine gland (so-called multiple endocrine neoplasia syndrome, MEN), an underlying fundamental defect in cell regulation is suspected (p. 713).

Primary, secondary and tertiary hyperfunction

The concepts of primary, secondary and tertiary hyperfunction can be readily appreciated in the case of the parathyroid glands.

Primary hyperparathyroidism exists when excess secretion of parathyroid hormone, not apparently secondary to any other process, leads to hypercalcaemia and other metabolic changes. It may be due to parathyroid adenoma, or to 'primary hyperplasia'.

Secondary hyperparathyroidism is a physiological adaptation to hypocalcaemia. For example, in vitamin D deficiency, calcium malabsorption leads to hypocalcaemia and secondary increased parathyroid hormone (PTH) secretion. This exerts effects on kidneys and bone which restore the plasma calcium level to normal, while increasing phosphate excretion. In chronic renal failure, other factors make this a less efficient process (p. 805), and so the parathyroid hyperplasia and PTH excess tends to be more prolonged and more extreme.

If this secondary hypoparathyroidism leads to the development of an autonomous parathyroid tumour or tumours, *tertiary hyperparathyroidism* is said to have developed. After renal transplantation temporary hypercalcaemia is quite common; although often referred to as tertiary hyperparathyroidism, it is usually due to the increased bulk of hyperplastic parathyroid tissue which has developed during prolonged renal failure and which cannot be completely switched off or does not atrophy immediately, rather than to true autonomous tumour development.

Abnormalities of hormone biosynthesis and function

One of the great intellectual satisfactions of endocrinology is that, as the pathways of production and action of the major hormones have been defined, so defects in these pathways leading to specific clinical syndromes have been discovered. Often, logical and effective treatment of the condition has resulted. The defects may be inborn, due to single point mutations, or they may be produced by pharmacologists developing new drugs.

Most of the inborn errors described below occur in the peripheral rather than the central (hypothalamus and pituitary) endocrine glands. A single example will illustrate some general principles. The commonest inborn error of adrenal cortex function is 21-hydroxylase deficiency (Fig. 18.31, p. 708) which is inherited as an autosomal recessive condition (p. 88). In its extreme (salt-losing) form, it is associated with blocks in the conversion of progesterone to aldosterone, as well as in the conversion of 17-hydroxyprogesterone to cortisol. This leads to both mineralocorticoid and glucocorticoid deficiency. Clinical disease results in part from deficiencies of these two hormones, and in part from the build-up of precursors and their androgenic by-products. Finally, excess ACTH secretion (in response to cortisol deficiency) and excess renin and angiotensin secretion (in response to aldosterone deficiency) also result. These tend to restore a new steady state, but at the expense of marked adrenal hyperplasia and even greater secretion of androgenic by-products.

The less common inborn error of 11-hydroxylase deficiency (p. 708) brings its own particular distinctive cluster of (largely predictable) symptoms and physical signs. The drug metyrapone, which competes with cytochrome P-450 11-α-hydroxylase, is used clinically and in testing pituitary-adrenal function to produce an enzyme block at the same site (Fig. 18.29, p. 705).

Similarly, with recent advances in our knowledge of the target organ mechanisms of action of hormones, so increasing numbers of 'target organ' endocrine diseases have been characterised, e.g. the androgen receptor defect (which causes testicular feminisation) and 5-α-reductase deficiency (which causes a particular form of male pseudo-hermaphroditism, see p. 723).

Autoimmune endocrine disease

In recent years, the role of the immune system in causing destruction and malfunction of parts of the endocrine system has become increasingly apparent. It is evident that both antibody-mediated and cell-mediated immunity may be involved, but much more is understood about the former. A wide range of antibodies may be involved which may be directed at components of the cell surface, or at microsomes, mitochondria and other intracellular organelles. In many cases, it is not clear which, if any, of the antibodies are causes of tissue damage and which are produced in response to cell destruction.

The immune disturbance may lead to:

1. *Destruction of the gland*, e.g. in autoimmune Addison's disease (where anti-adrenal antibodies are generally present in plasma) or in primary autoimmune hypothyroidism.
2. *Lymphocytic infiltration of the gland*, as in Hashimoto's thyroiditis (where a high titre of anti-microsomal and anti-thyroglobulin antibodies is invariably present).
3. *Uncontrolled stimulation of the gland*. This occurs particularly in the case of the thyroid gland. In thyrotoxic Graves' disease, this is due to production of antibodies which mimic TSH sufficiently closely to bind to, and activate, the TSH receptor.

There is no doubt that different individuals vary greatly in their inherited tendency to develop autoimmune endocrine disease. The full basis for individual susceptibility is not known, but an undoubted factor is the histocompatibility (HLA) antigen status of the individual. Certain HLA types, particularly those expressed normally only on lymphocytes (the so-called DR antigens) confer particular susceptibility. Acquired factors, such as virus infections, may initiate the process. One hypothesis is that, in autoimmune thyroid disease, certain DR antigens necessary for immune recognition are exposed on the external surface of the thyroid follicle cells and activate an immune response against the cells (p. 104).

The term *organ-specific autoimmune disease* encompasses both endocrine and non-endocrine diseases, and includes autoimmune Addison's disease, Graves' disease, Hashimoto's disease, autoimmune hypothyroidism, myasthenia gravis, hypoparathyroidism, true autoimmune diabetes mellitus, pernicious anaemia, autoimmune ovarian failure and vitiligo (autoimmune skin depigmentation). As a general rule, individuals with one such disease are more likely than normal individuals to develop another.

SYSTEMIC EFFECTS OF ENDOCRINE DISORDERS

Central nervous system

Local expansion of pituitary tumours commonly causes headache (due probably to tension on the diaphragma sellae) and damage to adjacent structures. The optic nerves are particularly vulnerable to pressure, especially at the optic chiasm, and bitemporal hemianopia may result. Less frequently, pituitary or suprapituitary tumours may cause damage in the region of the fourth ventricle, resulting in a syndrome of recent memory loss similar to Korsakoff's psychosis (p. 972); this may be reversible with treatment of the tumour.

Both *hyper-* and *hypocalcaemia* may present with neuro-

logical or psychiatric disorders; either may precipitate any psychosis to which that individual is predisposed or cause neuro-psychiatric symptoms de novo. Hypocalcaemia may be associated with raised intracranial pressure, epileptic fits and, of course, tetany. The latter is extremely disturbing psychologically if undiagnosed and untreated.

Hyperfunction of both the adrenal cortex and the adrenal medulla may present with *psychiatric manifestations*. In Cushing's syndrome, the individual may present with depression or with a schizophrenia-like syndrome. Excess cortisol secretion may occur in severe depression per se, so it can be very difficult to establish whether the patient has Cushing's syndrome or not. Many of the symptoms and signs of emotional or physical stress result from release of hormones, notably adrenaline, from the adrenal medulla. Tumours of the adrenal medulla (phaeochromocytomas) usually secrete predominantly noradrenaline, thus causing hypertension, but sweating and anxiety attacks are often an accompanying feature.

Thyroid disease may also be accompanied by a variety of neuropsychiatric features. Thyrotoxicosis may present to the psychiatrist as anxiety, depression or behavioural disturbance, although the warm sweaty hands and rapid pulse usually distinguish the condition from a simple anxiety state. Occasionally, the patient appears unduly apathetic. Proximal muscle weakness is another common feature of thyrotoxicosis. Accompanying exophthalmos due to ocular muscle infiltration may cause diplopia. Hypothyroidism may also present with depression. Its other neurological manifestations include carpal tunnel syndrome, myotonia, and cerebellar dysfunction.

Coma may be the presenting sign of a number of endocrine disorders. These (and other) manifestations of hyper- and hypoglycaemia are considered in Chapter 20. In profound hypothyroidism, coma is likely to be due to hypothermia. In severe hypopituitarism, stupor leading to coma commonly follows a relatively minor disturbance (such as a trivial accident or infection). It is due in part to profound cortisol deficiency, in part to hypothyroidism, and is usually associated with hyponatraemia due to excess secretion of antidiuretic hormone. The patient is usually hypotensive and responds rapidly to hydrocortisone therapy. In diabetes insipidus (DI), hypernatraemia may occur rapidly and produce convulsions or irreversible brain damage if access to water is restricted (for example postoperatively). Conversely, in the treated patient with DI, unlimited drinking may lead to cerebral dysfunction and fits from hyponatraemia (water intoxication).

Cardiovascular system

Hypotension, especially in the upright posture, commonly results from either glucocorticoid or mineralocorticoid deficiency, while hypertension, usually of mild degree, may result from mineralocorticoid excess. Endocrine diseases leading to electrolyte disturbances such as hyper- or hypocalcaemia or -kalaemia may present with dysrhythmias and/or characteristic ECG abnormalities. Prolonged hypercalcaemia and prolonged glucocorticoid excess are associated with an increased incidence of arterial calcification. Patients with primary hypothyroidism have a high incidence of ischaemic heart disease, which is in part due to hypercholesterolaemia. Those with angina are particularly vulnerable to myocardial infarction when treated with thyroxine. Acromegaly is associated with cardiac enlargement, hypertension and a form of cardiomyopathy.

Skeletal system

Skeletal manifestations of endocrine disease are commonly caused by osteoporosis, as in Cushing's syndrome, sex hormone deficiency, or prolonged hyperthyroidism. Primary hyperparathyroidism may also produce the clinical picture of osteoporosis with pathological fractures; it may also lead to calcification of articular cartilage, and present with calcium pyrophosphate crystal arthropathy (pseudogout, see p. 1014). The classical bone disease of Von Recklinghausen, with giant cell tumours of bone due to primary hyperparathyroidism, is now exceptionally rare. Occasionally, autoimmune thyrotoxicosis is associated with finger clubbing and periosteal new bone growth (so called thyroid acropachy). In mild acromegaly, peri-articular overgrowth of new bone and increased cartilage quite commonly lead to osteoarthritis. In severe acromegaly and gigantism, skeletal abnormalities may be gross.

Genito-urinary and reproductive systems

Conditions which affect sex hormone secretion in utero produce malformation of the external and internal genitalia (p. 722). Renal function may be disturbed by a number of metabolic disorders, some of which are of endocrine origin. For example, both hypercalcaemia and hypokalaemia may present with a form of (nephrogenic) diabetes insipidus and polyuria due to a water diuresis.

Integumentary system

Hirsutism and acne are common manifestations of androgen excess in the female. Of other endocrine disorders presenting with skin manifestations, the glucagonoma syndrome, which causes migratory necrolytic erythema, is probably the most striking (p. 620).

Alimentary system

Thyrotoxicosis commonly causes diarrhoea and sometimes malabsorption. Hypothyroidism causes constipation. Conditions such as Addison's disease, hypopituitarism and diabetic ketoacidosis may present as apparent upper abdominal emergencies with epigastric pain and rigidity. Hypercalcaemia commonly causes vomiting, constipation and abdominal pain.

ENDOCRINE FUNCTION TESTING

In carrying out tests of endocrine function, it is important to have a clear idea why they are being performed; it may be to establish or refine the diagnosis, to monitor the response to treatment, to assess the prognosis, or to establish the pathogenesis of the condition. Clearly, it is important to understand both the underlying physiology on which the test is based, and the limitations of the assay method. As a general rule, the minimum number of tests should be made to answer a particular question. The student is readily confused by the fact that different centres will often adopt equally valid but different approaches, depending upon the local laboratory expertise as well as local prejudices. In a field developing as rapidly as endocrinology, old tests are rapidly being superseded by new and better methods.

Basal measurements

Much can be learnt by *basal measurements* of so-called routine biochemistry (Table 18.1). Where endocrine disease involves hormones that control the electrolytes, these measurements remain the mainstay. Thus, a parathyroid tumour is most unlikely unless the serum calcium level is raised, and a low serum phosphate further suggests the diagnosis. Aldosterone deficiency in Addison's disease is suggested by the finding of a high serum potassium level, usually associated with a low sodium and elevated urea, due to extracellular fluid depletion.

In assessing posterior pituitary function, the tests (fluid deprivation) depend upon assessing the renal response, mediated by vasopressin, to deliberate but controlled withholding of fluids. In most cases, and certainly to exclude diabetes insipidus, simple study of the relationships of fluid loss to serum and urine osmolality suffice, without the need for difficult assays of vasopressin.

Basal measurements of hormone levels or metabolites are most practical when they can be conducted on serum or urine samples collected at random. Nowadays, the wide-

Table 18.1 'Routine' biochemical pointers in blood plasma to endocrine disorders

Pointers	Condition
Hyperkalaemia, hyponatraemia	Addison's disease
Hypokalaemia, metabolic alkalosis (high serum bicarbonate)	Conn's syndrome Cushing's syndrome (severe)
Hyponatraemia, hypochloraemia	Inappropriate ADH secretion Hypopituitarism Severe hypothyroidism
Hypernatraemia, hypochloraemia	Diabetes insipidus
Hyperglycaemia, hyperchloraemia, metabolic acidosis (low serum bicarbonate)	Diabetic ketoacidosis
Hyperglycaemia, uraemia hypernatraemia, hyperchloraemia	Diabetic-hyperosmolar
Hypercalcaemia, hypophosphataemia, hyperchloraemia	Primary hyperparathyroidism
Hypocalcaemia, hyperphosphataemia	Hypoparathyroidism

spread development and application of radioimmunoassay has helped enormously, especially for those hormones that are relatively stable in body fluids. This applies to the steroid hormones, thyroid hormones, and to most of the pituitary hormones (with the exception of ACTH). In most cases, serum is preferred to plasma; clotted blood can be left for 1–2 hours before centrifugation, and serum stored indefinitely at −20°C. Economic and methodological considerations dictate that samples are assayed batch-wise, so that the result is often not available at once. It may therefore be necessary to start treatment while the result is awaited. Urine sometimes has the advantage of reflecting integrated secretion and the 'free' (unbound) level (e.g. with cortisol). However, the major steroids in urine are metabolites several steps away from the biologically active compound.

Dynamic function tests

The static nature of information obtained by basal measurements has led to the development of a whole range of *dynamic function tests*, where the system under study is deliberately driven, usually by interrupting negative feedback or by stimulation at one or more levels. In testing anterior pituitary function, there is a bewildering array of possible tests, not all of which are useful. For example stimulation tests for ACTH (and so cortisol) with insulin-hypoglycaemia, glucagon, vasopressin, and CRH have all been devised, in addition to direct adrenal stimulation with synthetic ACTH (synacthen). With TSH and the thyroid hormones, marked episodic and diurnal variation – a problem inherent in assessing the ACTH-cortisol axis – is missing and, especially with new sensitive TSH assays, dynamic testing with TRH is thus seldom needed. Sometimes, two or more tests can be carried out simultaneously, e.g. insulin, TRH and GnRH can all be given together to assess the extent of hypopituitarism. An example of a test

used to monitor or predict response to treatment is the measurement of serum prolactin or growth hormone levels after a single dose of bromocriptine, in patients with prolactinoma or acromegaly respectively. In complex endocrine systems such as the menstrual cycle, repeated samples over the cycle of more than one hormone may be necessary to understand what is wrong; this may be much more useful than contrived 'dynamic function tests' (see Fig. 18.6).

THE PITUITARY GLAND

The pituitary gland is composed of two principal lobes, the anterior and the posterior (pars nervosa) with an intermediate lobe which is vestigial in man. The gland is derived from a down-growth from the floor of the third ventricle and from Rathke's pouch, which is formed by invagination of part of the roof of the primitive nasopharynx. Although there are important interactions between the products of the anterior and posterior lobes, for practical purposes they are usually considered as functionally separate. There is little if any blood flow between the two.

The pituitary gland is almost entirely enclosed in a bony box, the sella turcica; this has a floor and an anterior and posterior wall, the lateral extremities of which become the anterior and posterior clinoid processes. Immediately lateral to the pituitary gland are the two cavernous sinuses, with the IIIrd, IVth and Vth cranial nerves sandwiched

A

Optic nerve

Anterior clinoid processes

Pituitary gland

Optic chiasm

Posterior clinoid processes

Pituitary stalk

Optic tract

Dorsum sellae

B

Pituitary gland

II

Carotid artery

III

IV

Sphenoidal sinus

V¹

VI

Bone

V²

Cavernous sinus

V³

Fig. 18.6 Principles of dynamic endocrine function testing. Hypothalamic hormone A stimulates pituitary to produce pituitary hormone B which then stimulates peripheral gland to produce C. Hormone C (or a synthetic analogue) inhibits production of A and/or B by negative feedback.

Hypothalamus

Hormone A

Pituitary

Hormone B

Negative feedback

Peripheral gland

Hormone C

Metabolites of C (urine)

Peripheral effects

Fig. 18.7 Gross anatomy and relations of the pituitary gland. A. View of pituitary glands, anterior clinoids, dorsum sellae and optic chiasm from above. **B.** Coronal cross-section through pituitary gland to show relation to important structures nearby.

between; the carotid syphon courses through the cavernous sinus (Fig. 18.7). Overlying the pituitary is a fibrous sheet, the diaphragma sellae, which is pierced by the pituitary stalk; this slender structure carries the nerve fibres to the posterior pituitary gland and the blood supply, including the portal blood vessels draining from the median eminence of the hypothalamus.

Terminology of hypothalamic and pituitary hormones

The terminology of hypothalamic and pituitary hormones is a complex subject, made more so by the wide range of acronyms and synonyms for the various hormones. In the case of those peptides produced in the hypothalamus which act locally on the pituitary gland, there is little consistency in the use of the term 'factor' or 'hormone'. In this chapter, most are referred to as hormones, as this is what they are, albeit in a local context. Although still commonly referred to as prolactin inhibitory factor (PIF) this substance has now been identified as dopamine and should probably be referred to as such. Some of the more important interchangeable terms are given in Table 18.2.

Table 18.2 Terminology of hypothalamic and anterior pituitary hormones

Hypothalamic hormone	Effect (stimulation or inhibition)	Pituitary hormone
Gonadotrophin-releasing hormone (GnRH, LH-releasing hormone/factor, LH-FSH releasing hormone)	+	Luteinising hormone (LH) Follicle stimulating hormone (FSH)
Corticotrophin-releasing hormone/factor (CRF)	+	Adrenocorticotrophic hormone (ACTH corticotrophin)
Vasopressin (ADH)	+	
Somatostatin (growth hormone/ somatotrophin release inhibiting hormone)	−	Growth hormone (GH somatotrophin)
Growth hormone releasing hormone (GHRH)	+	
Thyrotrophin releasing hormone (TRH)	+	Thyroid stimulating hormone (TSH, thyrotrophin)
Dopamine (prolactin inhibiting factor, PIF)	−	Prolactin

THE ANTERIOR PITUITARY GLAND

SYNTHESIS AND SECRETION OF THE MAIN HORMONES

Much is now known about how the synthesis and secretion of anterior pituitary hormones is controlled, and this is summarised in Table 18.3.

Table 18.3 Factors directly affecting anterior pituitary hormone synthesis and release

Pituitary hormone	Stimuli	Inhibitors
ACTH	CRF Vasopressin (ADH) Interleukin I IL-1*	Cortisol
GH	GHRH	Somatostatin Insulin-like growth factor I (IGF1) Cortisol
TSH	TRH	T3, T4
LH	GnRH Oestradiol (+ve feedback)	Oestradiol Progesterone
FSH	GnRH	Inhibin Oestradiol Progesterone
Prolactin	TRH Oestradiol**	Dopamine

* Effect probably via CRF
** Increases prolactin synthesis, produces lactotroph hyperplasia but inhibits milk secretion

Adrenocorticotrophic hormone

Adrenocorticotrophic hormone (ACTH) is synthesised in specific cells (the corticotrophs) from a large precursor molecule called pro-opiomelanocortin (POMC, Fig.18.8). It is produced in both the anterior and intermediate lobe of the pituitary, but the final processing is different in the two. Of the other ACTH-related peptides, important ones are β lipotrophin (LPH), β endorphin, and α MSH. LPH and β endorphin are synthesised and secreted with ACTH. Beta endorphin may have a role as an opiate in modifying the response to pain at times of stress.

The synthesis and release of ACTH is controlled by corticotrophin-releasing factor (CRF), which acts synergistically with antidiuretic hormone (ADH) and probably also another hypothalamic factor. There are at least two basic rhythms of ACTH secretion; episodes of secretion every 1–3 hours and at meal times are superimposed on a

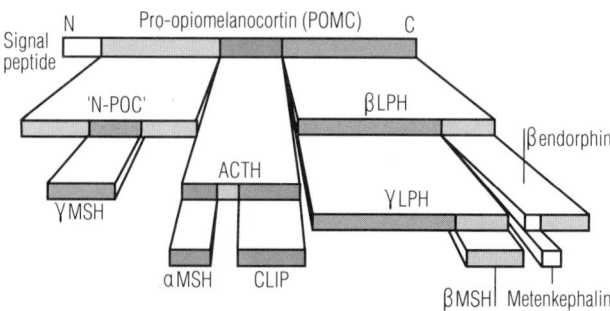

Fig. 18.8 Relationship between pro-opiomelanocortin (POMC) and the various intermediates and end-products of its processing in the pituitary gland. LPH = lipotrophin; N-POC = N-propiomelanocortin; MSH = melanocyte stimulating hormone; CLIP = corticotrophin-like intermediate lobe peptide.

Fig. 18.9 Plasma cortisol levels through the 24-hour cycle to show circadian variation, pulsatile secretion and influence of meals and stress.

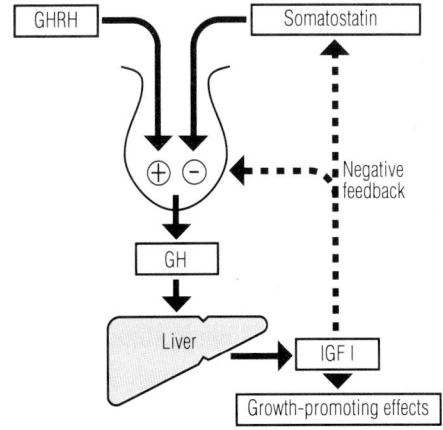

Fig. 18.10 Control of growth hormone and IGFI secretion.

24-hour rhythm, with lowest levels during the earliest hours of sleep, and peak secretion just before wakening (Fig. 18.9). At any time, exposure to sudden physical or mental stress will overcome this rhythm and lead to a pulse of ACTH secretion. The adrenal cortex responds in turn with a pulse of cortisol secretion within minutes, so that the 24-hour plasma profile of cortisol is a somewhat dampened version of the 24-hour ACTH profile.

The most important role of ACTH is to control the synthesis and secretion of the glucocorticoid cortisol. As would be expected from its relationship to melanocyte stimulating hormone (MSH, see Fig. 18.8), ACTH possesses MSH activity, and will directly stimulate the melanocytes of the skin and buccal mucosa when secreted in excessive amounts. This accounts for the increase in pigmentation to above normal (for that individual) seen in Addison's disease (p. 706) and Nelson's syndrome (pp. 685 and 710).

Growth hormone

Growth hormone (GH), human placental lactogen (HPL) and prolactin (PRL) belong to a family of polypeptide hormones. GH and HPL both contain 191 amino acids, and PRL 199. GH and HPL are closely homologous (with 85% identical residues) and probably arose by gene duplication relatively recently in evolution; their genes are located on chromosome 17. PRL is much less closely related.

Growth hormone is synthesised in specific cells (known as somatotrophs), where it is stored in granules and released episodically in response to peaks of hypothalamic secretion of GHRH (Fig. 18.10). The precise physiological interactions of GHRH with somatostatin, which inhibits its release, are complex. Much of the GH is secreted at night and episodically. Its secretion is inhibited by a rise in blood glucose (the basis of a useful suppression test) and

stimulated by hypoglycaemic stress and by amino acids such as arginine (which are the basis of stimulation tests). GH is believed to act principally on the liver, where it controls the secretion of an insulin-like growth factor, somatomedin C (otherwise known as IGF I). This compound appears to function as a hormone controlling the growth of cartilage and soft tissues. During puberty, secretion of sex hormones appears to increase the pituitary secretion of GH, which is probably important in promoting growth before the sex hormones lead to closure of the epiphyses.

Prolactin

Prolactin (PRL) is produced in specific cells, the lactotrophs, under stimulation by TRH, and under tonic inhibition by dopamine. PRL has a basically nocturnal pattern of secretion and is also released in response to stress.

Table 18.4 Action of hormones on the human breast

Hormone	Action
Polypeptide hormones	
Prolactin	Milk protein synthesis and excretion in ducts and lobules
Oxytocin	Milk ejection. Contraction of myoepithelial cells
Human placental lactogen	Similar to prolactin
Growth hormone	'Permissive' effects
Insulin	'Permissive' effects
Steroid hormones	
Oestrogens	Increase duct and breast fat growth. Inhibit prolactin–induced milk secretion.
Progestogens	Inhibit lactation. (Effect requires oestrogen.)
Cortisol	'Permissive' effects.
Androgens	Inhibitory effects on ? stroma.

Oestrogens probably act directly on the lactotrophs, increasing their number and activity. In pregnancy, PRL levels are high and so lead to hypertrophy of the breast epithelium (Table 18.4). However, high oestrogen and progesterone levels partially block this effect so that milk production only starts in quantity after delivery of the baby. During lactation, suckling stimulates secretion of prolactin via a reflex arc. High prolactin levels have a contraceptive effect, probably by inhibiting cyclical gonadotrophin release.

Luteinising hormone and follicle stimulating hormone

Luteinising hormone (LH) and follicle stimulating hormone (FSH) appear to be controlled by the same releasing hormone and produced in the same cell type (the gonadotroph). The two hormones resemble TSH and HCG in being two-subunit polypeptides, and in possessing a sugar 'coat'. The α-subunits of these peptides differ very little, but the β-subunits differ greatly and confer the specificity. The sugar 'coat' of these glycoproteins is important in protecting them from enzymic degradation in the circulation. The ratio and absolute amount of LH and FSH secreted in response to a single pulse of GnRH varies greatly under different circumstances. In both sexes, it appears to be modified by age, by sex hormone secretion by the gonads, and by the preceding pattern of discharge of GnRH. Low frequency discharge seems to favour FSH synthesis and release. In females, a rise in oestrogen level differentially reduces FSH and eventually promotes LH release ('positive feedback', see Fig. 18.35A). These interactions and their significance are discussed on page 718. The gonads also appear to produce a polypeptide hormone (inhibin) which feeds back to the pituitary to switch off FSH synthesis and secretion selectively.

Thyroid stimulating hormone

Thyroid stimulating hormone (TSH) promotes the synthesis and secretion of thyroid hormones, and the growth of the thyroid gland. Only recently have methods been developed that allow measurement of normal circulating levels of TSH, so its physiology is not yet fully understood. The principal hypothalamic control is from thyrotrophin releasing hormone (TRH), whose secretion, as with GnRH, is apparently pulsatile. The thyroid hormones are thought to feed back principally on the pituitary gland, inhibiting the response of TSH to TRH.

ANTERIOR PITUITARY HYPOFUNCTION

Anterior pituitary hypofunction may develop rapidly or insidiously, and may affect all the pituitary hormones, a few, or only one. We consider here those causes associated with partial or complete loss of all the anterior pituitary hormones, causing a state of so-called (anterior) panhypopituitarism. This will, in some cases, be associated with diabetes insipidus, where vasopressin secretion from the posterior pituitary is also impaired.

Aetiology

The causes of panhypopituitarism are listed in Table 18.5. The commonest *vascular* cause is Sheehan's syndrome, in which hypopituitarism occurs following a pregnancy which has been complicated by a period of shock and hypotension, commonly due to post-partum haemorrhage. The pituitary normally enlarges during pregnancy under the action of oestrogens on the lactotrophs, but the blood supply does not; it is therefore particularly vulnerable to a fall in blood pressure. There are usually no symptoms (such as headache) directly related to the infarction, but lactation does not occur, and the symptoms of hypopituitarism soon follow. Menstrual periods do not return. Rarely, prolonged shock in other situations may precede the development of panhypopituitarism. Similarly, *meningitis* in pregnancy (tuberculous or otherwise) is more likely to be followed by pituitary deficiency.

Tumours, both within the pituitary and suprasellar in location (such as the craniopharyngioma, which develops from Rathke's pouch) are common causes of panhypopituitarism. In these cases, the clinical features include pressure effects on surrounding structures, including the optic chiasm and the hypothalamus. In the case of *intrasellar* tumours, panhypopituitarism is usually a late development, since some normal pituitary tissue remains. If the tumour is functional, there may be additional features, other than those from pressure on the remaining normal pituitary. A prolactinoma, for example, may cause hypopituitarism and hyperprolactinaemia. Suprasellar tumours are more likely to affect the pituitary stalk, and thereby the posterior pituitary gland. If a large pituitary tumour becomes infarcted, it will cause the syndrome of 'pituitary apoplexy' (severe headache, neck stiffness, vomiting), which may be followed by hypopituitarism if the normal tissue is compromised.

Granulomatous conditions that may occasionally be responsible include eosinophilic granuloma and sarcoidosis. Carotid aneurysms may occasionally damage the pituitary. A common situation is for panhypopituitarism to develop long after pituitary irradiation (for example for a growth-hormone secreting tumour). The hypopituitarism is in part a consequence of hypothalamic rather than pituitary damage, and commonly affects growth hormone and gonadotrophin secretion before other hormones.

In many cases of panhypopituitarism, the aetiology is obscure; some may be autoimmune. In some cases, there is an empty sella turcica and a defective diaphragma. It is still undecided whether the so-called 'empty sella syndrome' can be a primary cause of hypopituitarism.

Local pressure effects of pituitary and suprasellar tumours

The principal symptoms arising from local pressure effects of pituitary and suprasellar tumours are headache and visual field disturbances. The headaches may be severe and persistent. The characteristic visual field disturbance is a bitemporal hemianopia which starts with loss of the upper

Table 18.5 Causes of panhypopituitarism

Cause	Mechanism	Associated features
Developmental abnormalities	Failure of hypothalamic or pituitary development Perinatal asphyxia	Severe cranial abnormalities (e.g. anencephaly, hydrocephalus) Midline facial abnormalities GH deficiency predominant
Infection Encephalitis Bacterial meningitis	Hypothalamus or stalk damage, or pituitary destruction	History of encephalitis or bacterial meningitis
Granulomata Eosinophilic granuloma Sarcoidosis	Infiltration of pituitary/hypothalamus	Eosinophilic granuloma Sarcoidosis (p. 506)
Vascular Infarction	Hypotension, especially when the pituitary is enlarged, e.g. by pregnancy or tumour	Sheehan's syndrome from antepartum or postpartum haemorrhage Hypotension (surgical or traumatic)
Haemorrhage	Pituitary apoplexy Subarachnoid haemorrhage	Pituitary enlargement/tumour Cranial nerve lesions Apoplexy simulates subarachnoid
Aneurysms	Pressure	Ballooning of pituitary fossa
Tumour Suprapituitary (craniopharyngioma)	Pressure on stalk	Pressure on optic chiasm or brain stem Suprasellar calcification (craniopharyngioma)
Pituitary	Pressure or invasion of normal gland	Large pituitary fossa Hormone excess if tumour functional
Empty sella	Mechanism uncertain	Ballooning of pituitary fossa
Autoimmune	Antibodies to pituicytes	Other organ-specific autoimmune disease Anti-pituitary antibodies
Trauma	Severe head injury causing stalk damage	Brain and cranial nerve damage

---

Summary 1   Clinical features of hormone-producing pituitary tumours

- Local symptoms are headache and visual disturbance

- In acromegaly the tumour is usually large, but small in Cushing's disease.

- Incipient visual loss may merit an immediate trial of bromocriptine.

- Macroprolactinomas occur equally in men and women. Microprolactinomas in women only.

---

quadrant (if the tumour is below the chiasm). The patient may notice loss of the lateral part of the visual fields; the defect will not at first be detectable by confrontation, but can be shown by formal perimetry with a Bjerrum's screen, and may be most obvious if a red object is used. Fundoscopy may reveal bi- or unilateral optic atrophy. Other field defects are also quite common. More rarely, other cranial nerves (the IIIrd, IVth, Vth and VIth) are involved.

A syndrome reminiscent of Korsakoff's syndrome with recent memory loss may occur if there is pressure on the floor of the third ventricle. Disturbances of appetite (causing hyperphagia), and of thirst, may be seen. The latter causes particular problems if diabetes insipidus is also present, since the patient does not drink enough to prevent hyperosmolarity. The occurrence of pressure effects depends mainly on the size of the tumour, for example GH-secreting pituitary tumours (in acromegaly) are generally much larger than ACTH-secreting tumours (in Cushing's disease). Non-functioning tumours and prolactinomas are the two other intrasellar lesions which commonly cause pressure symptoms.

Clinical features of anterior pituitary hypofunction

The clinical features of anterior pituitary hypofunction depend in part upon the age of onset.

Childhood

If the onset of panhypopituitarism is before growth is completed, the patient will have the features of hypopituitary dwarfism, i.e. normal body proportions but failure to grow. The latter is detected and documented by careful measurements of height using a stadiometer recorded on standard growth charts (Fig. 18.11). From serial measurements, growth velocity (cm/year) can be calculated and related to standard rates of growth. Panhypopituitarism in childhood is also associated with failure of pubertal development.

Other common features of hypopituitarism in childhood include a tendency to hypoglycaemia and other general features discussed below.

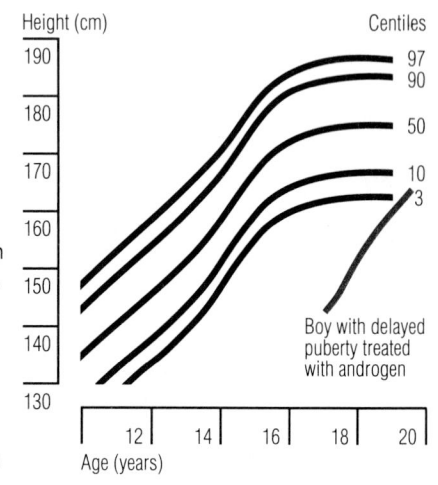

Fig. 18.11 Hypopituitarism in childhood. A. Child aged $5\frac{1}{2}$ years (before GH therapy) and **B.** aged $6\frac{1}{2}$ years, after 9 months GH therapy, when he had grown 11 cm. **C.** Height measurements of the boy illustrated in **A** and **B** before (black line) and during (red line) GH treatment. Normal values for each centile are also shown (courtesy of Dr S M Shalet). **D.** Height measurements in a boy with delayed puberty treated with androgens. Normal values for each centile are also shown (courtesy of Dr S M Shalet).

Adult life

In panhypopituitarism developing in adult life, the patient usually feels unwell in a non-specific way. They appear pale without being anaemic and the skin has a 'waxen doll' appearance. They notice the cold, although features of hypothyroidism are often not as gross or obvious as in myxoedema. Women have amenorrhoea and men lose their sex drive and potency. Loss of secondary sexual hair and decline of other secondary sexual characteristics is a feature in both sexes. The patients may present with a 'hypopituitary crisis' when challenged by trivial stress, which would normally be met by increased secretion of ACTH and cortisol. In a hypopituitary crisis there may be acute abdominal pain mimicking an acute abdominal emergency. This syndrome responds rapidly to cortisol administration. Patients commonly develop hypoglycaemia but, because of an associated lack of adrenaline secretion (see Figure 18.5, p. 669), they do not develop symptoms of 'classical' hypoglycaemia, i.e. a sympathetic response to the low blood sugar. They may therefore present with coma due to hypoglycaemia. Coma may also be due to hyponatraemia, since there is commonly an excess of vasopressin secretion (cortisol inhibits vasopressin secretion and the renal response to it).

Manifestations of *growth hormone deficiency* include pallor, thin skin, and hypoglycaemia. Those of *ACTH* (and thus cortisol) *deficiency* include malaise, somnolence, hyponatraemia, poor response to stress, hypoglycaemia, confusion, coma, hypotension and fever.

Effects of *sex hormone deficiency* include delayed puberty, sexual infantilism, amenorrhoea and lack of breast development. Men show abnormal 'puppy fat' distribution of body fat, and lack of muscular development. Loss of secondary sexual hair is much more marked in panhypopituitarism than in conditions where there is only lack of gonadal sex hormones. As with other causes of androgen deficiency in men, the patient's partner may complain more than him. Loss of sex drive is also common in hypopituitary women. Features due to *TSH deficiency* include cold intolerance and dry skin, although hypothyroidism may be masked by other deficiencies. It is most important not to replace thyroid hormones first, since the increased metabolic rate will cause increased metabolism of cortisol and so precipitate an adrenal crisis. *Diabetes insipidus* is discussed on page 689; its effects are often less marked when cortisol is also deficient, since the latter is necessary for a water diuresis in vasopressin deficiency. *Prolactin deficiency* leads to failure of milk production, which is of importance only to the lactating woman.

Investigation of suspected pituitary hypofunction

If hypopituitarism is suspected, a clotted blood sample is taken for later hormone analysis and glucocorticoid treatment commenced at once, most conveniently by giving 100 mg hydrocortisone intravenously, followed by 50 mg six hours later and then a normal regular replacement dose. If the patient does not have pituitary or adrenal insufficiency, such treatment is unlikely to be harmful, and if they do it may be life-saving. There is a risk of precipitating adrenal insufficiency or coma with stress tests, or by starting thyroid hormone without hydrocortisone (p. 671 above).

Much of value can be learnt from *basal measurements* of serum urea and electrolytes, LH and FSH, testosterone (in men), progesterone and oestradiol (in women), cortisol, thyroxine (T4) and triodothyronine (T3), GH and prolactin. These measurements will go a considerable way to establish the diagnosis, and possibly its cause.

Dynamic hormone tests are conventionally used as the 'gold standard' for assessing pituitary function (Fig. 18.12). Insulin should be given in a low dose (0.1 unit per kg) with close observation by a doctor throughout. An ECG should be done first, and the test not undertaken in the elderly or those with heart disease. In this situation, glucagon (1 mg) can be used as an alternative stimulus to ACTH and cortisol secretion. Glucose for intravenous injection, or glucagon, should be available, and given early rather than late. GH and cortisol measurements are made serially over two hours. For convenience, GnRH, TRH and insulin can be given simultaneously (Fig. 18.12).

Investigations to establish the underlying cause of hypopituitarism

The history and physical examination may point to a particular cause of hypopituitarism, such as previous infarction, meningitis or radiotherapy.

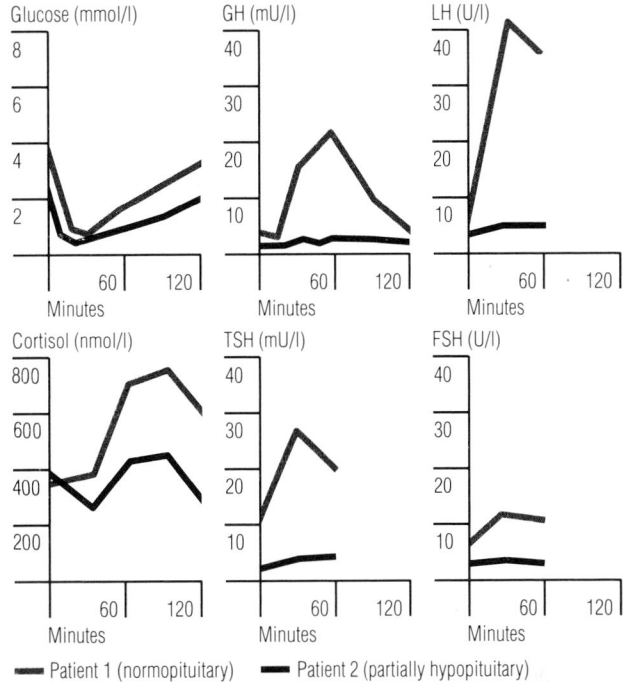

— Patient 1 (normopituitary)   — Patient 2 (partially hypopituitary)

Fig. 18.12   Responses in two patients to combined pituitary stimulation with insulin (0.15 U/kg), GnRH (100 μg) and TRH (200 μg) given iv as a bolus at time 0. Patient 1 is a woman with amenorrhoea. She has normal responses despite previous operation for a functionless pituitary adenoma. Patient 2 is a man, also with a functionless pituitary tumour. He has absent responses for all except cortisol, which is blunted. The diagnosis is panhypopituitarism, requiring replacement therapy.

Imaging

Carefully taken lateral and antero-posterior X-ray views of the skull may reveal expansion of the pituitary fossa and erosion of the dorsum sellae and anterior or posterior clinoids (Fig. 18.13) although such changes do not indicate that the tumour responsible still exists – the fossa may be empty. For this reason, a CT scan is essential (Fig. 18.14),

Fig. 18.13   Lateral X-rays of skulls of patients with pituitary tumours. A. Expansion of pituitary fossa and a 'double floor' due to asymmetrical enlargement. **B.** 'Copper-beaten' skull with expanded sutures due to obstructive hydrocephalus in a girl of 15. (Courtesy of Dr St Clair Forbes). **C.** Complete destruction of pituitary fossa and dorsum sellae.

Fig. 18.14 CT scan of pituitary tumour eroding floor of fossa (black arrow), and expanding upwards (white arrows).

and this has now largely superseded more invasive studies with injection of contrast media such as metrizamide or air into the subarachnoid space. Conventional tomography is also now largely redundant, although angiography still has a role in defining the relationship of major blood vessels before surgery.

Plain X-ray may sometimes give specific diagnostic clues, e.g. suprasellar calcification suggests a craniopharyngioma. Rarer causes include eosinophilic granuloma, in which case 'punched out' bone lesions may be present in the skull or elsewhere and there may be a reticular lung pattern on the chest radiograph. The pituitary gland may be the site of a metastasis from a carcinoma, in which case the skull X-ray may show bone destruction; the history and general examination may point to the site of the primary. Where there is no evident cause, and no history to suggest Sheehan's syndrome or an infarcted pituitary tumour, the condition may be due to organ-specific autoimmune disease, with antibodies directed against the pituitary cells. The 'empty sella' syndrome, in which CT scan shows an absent pituitary gland, is usually a diagnosis of exclusion after the relevant radiological studies. In some cases the syndrome follows infarction of a tumour, while others are possibly due to the transmission of cerebro-spinal fluid (CSF) pressure to the pituitary fossa as a result of a defective diaphragma sellae.

Hormone measurements

Hormone measurements (prolactin, GH, gonadotrophins,

TSH) will indicate the nature of a functioning pituitary tumour, but there may still be major difficulties in diagnosis. For example, modest elevation of prolactin may be due simply to stalk damage, and not to prolactinoma. Levels more than about 10 times the upper limit of normal are, however, always due to a prolactinoma. Similarly, the levels of the gonadotrophins are normally elevated after the menopause. If TSH is raised this is most likely to be due to primary myxoedema rather than a TSH-producing pituitary tumour. In the former case, serum T3 and T4 levels will be very low. ('Feedback tumours' secreting TSH are, however, a well recognised complication of long-standing untreated myxoedema; they will usually shrink with thyroid hormone replacement.)

Treatment of anterior hypopituitarism

It is important to realise that although patients with hypopituitarism may have been ACTH- (and therefore cortisol) deficient for many months or years without severe illness, they are, nevertheless, extremely vulnerable to even minor stress. A minor infection, illness or trauma may precipitate acute glucocorticoid deficiency, as may ill-advised prior treatment of hypothyroidism.

Immediate

The patient with pituitary collapse or coma should be given intravenous hydrocortisone (100–200 mg repeated in 2–4 hours), which will generally lead to rapid improvement in the clinical condition, a rise in blood pressure and a fall in temperature. In some cases, volume expansion may be necessary and, if the serum sodium level is very low (below 115 mmol/l) because of inappropriate ADH secretion (p. 690), judicious correction to above 120 mmol/l may be indicated by means of small amounts of hypertonic saline. Steroids should always be replaced before thyroid hormones, which can generally be given orally from the outset. Sex hormone replacement therapy, particularly (in men) testosterone therapy, should be considered and generally instituted without delay, since this will greatly hasten the return of strength and well-being.

Where occult posterior pituitary hormone deficiency co-exists, it may be uncovered by glucocorticoid therapy. This should be suspected when there is marked and continuing water diuresis in the recovery phase, with low urine and rising serum osmolality. It is best corrected with the synthetic ADH analogue, desmopressin (DDAVP, p. 689).

Long-term

Steroid therapy

There is no convenient way of mimicking the episodic secretion of glucocorticoids. Fortunately, however, this does not seem to matter, and oral treatment with hydrocortisone (cortisol) in a total daily dose of 20–40 mg given in two or three divided doses (to approximate the normal diurnal variation) is usually quite satisfactory. At least half the dose is given on waking in the morning (with reversal for anyone working on a night shift). Cortisone acetate is generally equally effective, since the acetate is hydrolysed and cortisone converted to cortisol by the liver. However, a possible disadvantage of cortisone over cortisol is that the plasma cortisol level rises to a peak more gradually on treatment with the former. In addition, some individuals, especially those with liver disease, have impaired conversion of cortisone to cortisol. Prednisolone is a suitable alternative (5 mg being roughly equivalent to 20 mg hydrocortisone); but dexamethasone – an even more potent halogenated glucocorticoid – should probably be avoided for long-term treatment because its much longer half-life means that glucocorticoid levels do not fall at night. Low levels then probably permit normal processes of collagen repair, which are inhibited by glucocorticoids.

Thyroid hormones

Thyroid hormones are best replaced as oral thyroxine (100–200 μg once daily). This is converted to the more active triiodothyronine in the liver.

Sex hormone replacement

In *men* testosterone is given in one of three ways, none of which is ideal. It may be implanted subcutaneously in the abdominal wall as fused pellets of testosterone (600–800 mg every 4–6 months). More commonly, but with wider fluctuation in plasma testosterone levels, it may be given as testosterone esters – Sustanon (mixed testosterone esters) or Primoteston depot (testosterone enanthate, 250 mg im every 2–4 weeks). Finally, it may be given as the orally absorbed ester testosterone undecanoate (40–80 mg twice daily), but this has the disadvantage of high price, and the capsules may cause gastrointestinal symptoms, perhaps due to the oleic acid vehicle.

In *women*, where the uterus is present, cyclical oestrogen replacement therapy is required. This is because continuous oestrogen administration leads to hyperplasia of endometrium, and eventually 'break-through' bleeding. There is also a strong suspicion that oestrogen unopposed by progesterone may predispose to endometrial cancer. It is therefore necessary to give a progestogen (such as norethisterone 1–5 mg daily) for 10–14 days, regularly every 1–2 months. Conventionally, the oestrogen is stopped for a week once the progestogen is discontinued. However, cyclical menstruation can be produced quite satisfactorily by giving a progestogen in this way to women receiving oestrogen continuosly (for instance by implantation of oestradiol pellets).

Restoration of fertility

In hypopituitary patients of either sex, restoration of fertility can usually be achieved by administering gonadotrophins. In men HCG (1500–2000 IU im weekly) is given to simulate Leydig cell testosterone production, and after some three months or more this is combined with three times weekly injections of 225 units of FSH (Per-gonal). Spermatogenesis should be evident after three months, as indicated by increased testicular volume and the appearance of motile spermatozoa in the ejaculate. Gonadotrophin therapy in women is much more complex, since FSH must be given early in the cycle and the follicular response followed by ultrasound scanning and serum or urinary oestrogen measurements (p. 673). When one or two follicles have achieved a diameter of 2 cm, ovulation is produced by giving intramuscular HCG (5000 units). This treatment should only be undertaken in units with facilities for ultrasound and rapid oestrogen assays, and with expertise in this area. An alternative treatment, effective in some cases, is to administer GnRH in a pulsatile fashion through a pump connected to a subcutaneous needle.

Posterior pituitary hormone replacement

Posterior pituitary hormone replacement is discussed on page 689.

ISOLATED GROWTH HORMONE DEFICIENCY AND RELATED SYNDROMES

Growth hormone deficiency only produces clinically obvious manifestations when it occurs in childhood. Although GH is secreted from early fetal life, it is not until infancy that its deficiency leads to impaired growth.

Aetiology

In most cases of isolated GH deficiency, the cause is unknown. There are, however, several familial syndromes inherited as autosomal recessive conditions with defective GH secretion. Recent evidence indicates that in one of these, pituitary somatotrophs synthesise GH but there is failure to respond to the releasing hormone, GHRH. In others, the abnormality appears to be a deletion of the GH gene. Patients in the latter group in particular may respond to injected GH as if it were a foreign protein and develop antibodies to it. In some cases of GH deficiency, it may become apparent after GH therapy is initiated that TSH synthesis is also impaired; it appears that GH therapy accelerates the metabolism of TSH.

Laron dwarfism is the term given to a syndrome which mimics GH deficiency, but in which GH levels are high and IGF I levels low (p. 675). It is apparently due to failure of a target organ to respond to GH. Some cases of short stature may also be due to failure to respond to IGF I. In Pygmies, the short stature and other somatic features appear to be due in part to low levels of IGF I.

Clinical features

Abnormally low rates of overall growth, leading to short stature, are associated with typical somatic abnormalities. In particular, the face appears baby-like, with persistence of a small nose, poorly developed nasal bridge and small chin. The dentition may be delayed with later crowding of teeth. Muscle development is poor, with excess subcutaneous fat, thin hair and skin, small larynx and high-pitched voice. Puberty is typically delayed until 18–20 years. Even in patients with complete GH deficiency, longitudinal growth occurs, but at only about one-third of the normal rate. With the onset of puberty, there is a very small growth spurt. There is an increased tendency to hypoglycaemia, and this may be the most obvious feature in the neonate. GH deficiency developing in adult life does not present a clinical problem or require replacement.

Treatment

The diagnosis of GH deficiency is established by a combination of clinical observation (including serial measurements of growth and assessment of growth velocity) and provocative testing with insulin injection or arginine infusion. GH therapy is then initiated. In the past, this was with purified pituitary GH obtained from pituitaries removed at autopsy; this was possible because GH is resistant to post-mortem autolysis. Recently, however, cases of Jacob-Creutzfeldt disease (p. 964), caused by slow-virus infection, have been linked to previous GH therapy; this led to a complete halt in treatment until supplies of biosynthetic human GH became available. Treatment is with 30–100 mu/kg body weight given three times per week by sc injection. There seems to be little additional benefit in giving GH by sc infusion. Recent work indicates that the response can be improved in boys by addition of small doses of synthetic androgens. There is currently no treatment for Laron dwarfism, although IGF I may soon become available.

The response is monitored by frequent measurements of height, and calculation of growth velocity (Fig. 18.11, p. 678). There is an initial 'catch-up' period, followed by more steady growth.

Growth retardation in other conditions

It is often difficult to distinguish partial idiopathic GH deficiency from other states in which GH or IGF I secretion is secondarily impaired. These states include psychological deprivation, growth failure due to inadequate nutrition, e.g. in malabsorption due to coeliac disease, and chronic liver and kidney disease. Not infrequently, simple delayed puberty may present with growth failure. In these cases, if GH secretion in response to insulin is low, the test will usually become normal when repeated after a short course of androgen (or oestrogen) replacement therapy. In prepubertal teenage boys with delayed stature, it is often justified to give a 3–6 month course of treatment with HCG or androgens. The resulting growth spurt results in part from the androgens and in part from the augmentation of (nocturnal) GH secretion that they cause.

GROWTH HORMONE EXCESS

The term *acromegaly* refers to the syndrome of GH excess when it develops in adult life. *Gigantism* is when its onset

in childhood also leads to excessive height. At the turn of this century, Harvey Cushing recognised that acromegaly and gigantism were due to acidophil tumours of the pituitary gland that produce growth hormone. He was the first clinician to recognise and distinguish features of pituitary disease that were due to hyperpituitarism (hormone excess) from those due to hypopituitarism.

Clinical GH excess is almost always due to a pituitary tumour, but there are two exceptions to this. Firstly, tall stature in boys may be linked to episodic high GH secretion without a tumour. Secondly, it has recently been recognised that pancreatic tumours secreting GHRH may lead to the syndrome of acromegaly by stimulating the pituitary gland to produce GH. Indeed, it was recognition of this syndrome that led recently to the extraction and purification of pancreatic GHRH which was rapidly shown to be present in identical form in the hypothalamus.

Aetiology

Little is known of the factors leading to the development of a GH-secreting adenoma. Most such tumours are benign and secrete GH alone, although occasional mixed tumours also synthesise and secrete prolactin.

Normally GH release is stimulated by dopamine, probably acting via the hypothalamus. Dopamine administration will therefore cause a rise in serum GH in normal individuals, presumably due to suppression of somatostatin, and/or to stimulation of hypothalamic GHRH release. GH secretion in acromegaly can be rapidly but transiently inhibited by somatostatin or its synthetic analogues. Of more practical benefit is the paradoxical observation that the dopaminergic agent bromocriptine usually has a modest, but significant, inhibitory effect on GH secretion. In some cases, especially in individuals with mixed GH and PRL-secreting tumours, this effect may be very marked and lead to complete inhibition of secretion. It is probable that the inhibitory effect of bromocriptine requires both the presence of dopamine receptors on the surface of the tumour cells, and their coupling to hormone release by an inhibitory mechanism.

Clinical features

The clinical features of acromegaly and gigantism may be considered under three headings:

1. features due to GH excess
2. those due to a local space-occupying lesion arising from the pituitary fossa
3. those due to other hormone deficiencies.

Except where the tumour is large and growing rapidly, the latter usually occur late in the disease as a result of attempted treatment (radiotherapy or surgery), especially transfrontal surgery.

Gigantism

Gigantism is the most obvious and serious consequence of GH excess in childhood and adolescence. Normally, GH secretion occurs at a low level throughout childhood, and increases with the rise in sex hormones at the time of puberty. With a GH-secreting tumour in childhood, however, inappropriate GH secretion occurs out of phase with the stage of puberty. The growth of cartilage at the epiphyseal plates is greatly stimulated due to the action of IGF I (p. 675). Normally, this effect is held in check by an inhibitory action of sex hormones on the epiphyseal cartilage stem cell.

The first feature of gigantism is therefore the onset of an inappropriate, continuing and excessive growth spurt, coupled with increased hand and foot size and general skeletal enlargement. Later, other features (increased skin and soft tissue growth) become evident. The most devastating skeletal deformities affect the chest wall, and are probably due to the combination of GH excess and sex hormone deficiency which together predispose to osteoporosis. Severe kyphosis may result.

In childhood, as in adult life, the pituitary tumour is commonly quite large at the time of presentation, and may lead to local pressure effects. These include headache (thought to be due to pressure on the diaphragma sellae) and visual field defects due to pressure on the optic chiasm (p. 676).

If pubertal failure results, either as a direct effect of a large tumour or as a result of treatment, epiphyseal closure will be delayed and the ultimate height attained even more extreme.

Acromegaly

There is a highly variable time between the onset of symptoms and signs and the diagnosis of growth hormone excess in adults. This is dependent, among other things, upon chance and the index of suspicion of any doctor who encounters the patient, often for an unrelated problem. In general, the greater the experience of the doctor, the more likely he is to make a confident and correct diagnosis early. Clinical features due to the *local tumour* include headache and visual field defects (most commonly bitemporal hemianopia).

Features due to GH excess may occur in many organs, but the most obviously apparent on casual observation involve the soft tissues and skin, and the skeleton. Together, these give the classical *acromegalic facies* (Fig. 18.15), with prominent orbital margins, large nose, prominence of the lower jaw (prognathism) and thickening of the skin and soft tissues, including the lips and tongue. In men especially, there is often a typical rather rough vibrant voice, presumably due to thickening of the vocal cords, enlargement of the sinuses and changes in other tissues in the nasopharynx and larynx. As a consequence of prognathism there is often dental malocclusion, with protrusion of the teeth of the lower jaw on the upper. The teeth may become more widely spaced or dentures may need to be changed.

There is obvious enlargement of the hands and feet. The wide 'spade-like' hands are due to increased thickness and volume of skin and soft tissues and growth of periarticular

Fig. 18.15 Typical appearance of acromegaly.

cartilage. Ring, glove, shoe and hat sizes increase. In longstanding and severe acromegaly, there are commonly major skeletal deformities. Severe thoracic kyphosis and accompanying respiratory disease are common in acromegalic giants. In acromegalics with onset of the disease in adult life, growth of articular cartilage and soft tissues in and around a joint commonly leads to secondary osteoarthritis, which may be compounded by necrosis of articular cartilage.

Neurological problems include carpal tunnel syndrome and, in advanced gigantism, peripheral neuropathy. The age-related mortality rate of patients with untreated acromegaly is probably twice normal, largely attributable to cardiovascular disease – hypertension, cardiac muscle hypertrophy, cardiomyopathy and ischaemic heart disease. The latter is particularly likely in acromegalics with diabetes mellitus. Overt diabetes probably occurs in about 10% of acromegalics, although insulin secretion is increased in most because growth hormone antagonises the effects of insulin.

A common early complaint in acromegaly is increased sweating, due to an increase in both number and activity of sweat glands. About one-quarter of patients have a goitre, which is commonly multinodular and which may, together with increased sweating, lead to an erroneous

18

> **Summary 2   Clinical features of acromegaly**
>
> - Symptoms and signs are due to local tumour, growth hormone excess and deficiency of other hormones.
>
> - Prognathism, enlarged soft tissues, skeletal deformity, nerve entrapment occur.
>
> - Hypertension and diabetes mellitus contribute to mortality.

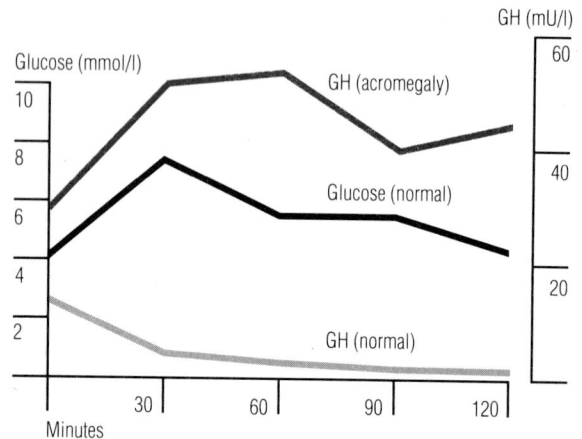

Fig. 18.16   GH response to oral glucose load in a normal subject (suppression) and a man with acromegaly (no suppression or paradoxical rise).

diagnosis of thyrotoxicosis (although the two conditions may coexist). Macroglossia may lead to sleep apnoea, due to obstruction of the airway at night; this commonly presents with daytime somnolence. Enlargement of the liver, spleen, pancreas and kidneys seldom causes problems, although the glomerular filtration rate may be increased due to the latter.

Patients with acromegaly are quite often labelled as neurotic before the diagnosis is made, because many of the symptoms, such as headache, sweating and somnolence, are rather vague. Impotence is a common complaint, which only rarely appears to be due to hypogonadism. Women commonly have menstrual irregularities, and some are hirsute. Galactorrhoea due to accompanying hyperprolactinaemia occurs in about one acromegalic woman in five. In some, this is due to a mixed prolactin and GH-secreting tumour; in others, to damage to the pituitary stalk.

Investigation

Clearly, the association of classical clinical features with evidence of local pressure effects will lead to a confident and accurate diagnosis at the time of presentation. However, it is clearly preferable to make the diagnosis before it is grossly obvious clinically. Furthermore, there are cases where 'acromegaloid' features may occur without GH excess. In some of these, the primary abnormality may be excess production of IGF I (somatomedin C), which mediates many of the effects of GH.

GH suppression test. Baseline GH levels are of limited value in diagnosis because GH is normally secreted episodically. The best screening test in suspected cases remains the oral glucose load (50–75 g) with accompanying measurements of GH (Fig. 18.16). Normally, GH suppresses to below 2 mu/l after 50 g oral glucose load, probably as an effect of central inhibition of GHRH secretion. In acromegaly, levels either fail to suppress, or show a paradoxical rise. About 30–40% of cases also show a paradoxical rise of GH in response to TRH or GnRH given intravenously, presumably because the tumour possesses receptors for these hormones. Dopamine infusion in acromegaly often inhibits GH secretion, again in contrast to the normal response which is of stimulation. Bromocriptine suppresses GH in the majority of acromegalics, though it is only clinically useful in a minority. An indication of its potential usefulness in an individual case is obtained from measurement of GH hourly for 4–6 hours after 5 mg bromocriptine orally.

IGF I assay. The normal response of GH to hypo-

glycaemia is for the level to rise acutely; this response is commonly absent in acromegaly. An important new development is the availability of reliable assays for circulating levels of IGF I. Levels in gigantism and acromegaly are almost always elevated, and the measurement may be particularly informative in cases with equivocal results to conventional tests, for example relatively low GH levels which fail to suppress with oral glucose.

GHRH assay. In occasional cases with normal pituitary radiology or other atypical features, it is possible to measure circulating levels of GHRH which, if elevated, point to a rare extra-hypothalamic GHRH-secreting tumour (e.g. in the pancreas). Injection of GHRH or somatostatin and measurement of the subsequent GH response appears to be of little practical value.

The rapidly growing tall child presents a particular problem, for whom a number of the above tests, perhaps combined with measurements of normal GH secretion, may be indicated. Recent evidence indicates that very tall children may secrete excess GH in a physiological but exaggerated way at night, and after initial suppression following food or glucose.

Radiological investigations are as outlined on pages 679–80.

Treatment

The aim of treatment of GH excess is to arrest and, where possible, to reverse the local and systemic effects of the tumour. Except in the growing child, correction of GH excess is seldom urgent. Visual field defects, however, present an immediate and compelling indication for surgery.

Surgery

Surgery is now usually carried out through a midline, trans-sphenoidal route, approaching the pituitary gland through an incision in the mouth, and removing part of the nasal septum or deflecting it. Some surgeons approach the pituitary through the medial wall of the orbit and ethmoid sinuses. Even when there is a large suprasellar tumour, trans-sphenoidal surgery may relieve pressure on the optic chiasm and allow the suprasellar part of the tumour to fall into the fossa. The transfrontal approach, which almost inevitably causes hypopituitarism, is therefore seldom needed.

With small tumours, the best centres now achieve 70% cure rates by trans-sphenoidal resection, without causing hypopituitarism, although the balance between endocrine benefit and penalty shifts unfavourably with increasing tumour size.

Drug therapy

Bromocriptine does not cause tumour shrinkage in acromegaly, but is indicated when surgery is not thought desirable (for example in mild disease or the elderly) or when GH is effectively suppressed by the drug. Usual doses needed are 10–30 mg daily, divided into four doses, although additional benefit with higher doses has been reported. The clinical effect often exceeds the biochemical response, possibly because of a direct suppressive effect on IGF I secretion. Somatostatin, given by frequent sc injection, effectively lowers GH in many acromegalic subjects. Cost, however, may limit the therapeutic value of both somatostatin and its analogue octreotide.

Radiotherapy

External radiotherapy can be used to produce tumour regression. It requires careful planning and megavoltage machinery. The treatment is remarkably safe but its effect is delayed, with a gradual and progressive benefit over 2–5 years. Interstitial radiotherapy by pituitary implantation of ^{90}yttrium has proved effective, and is more akin to surgery than radiotherapy in the rapidity of its effect. However, it is now practised by few centres having been largely superseded by improved neurosurgery.

Complications of treatment

The complications following surgery and radiotherapy vary greatly with the skill and technique of the operator. After surgery by the trans-sphenoidal route, panhypopituitarism is quite rare, except where radical removal of a large tumour has been attempted. Postoperative diabetes insipidus is usually transient. If anterior hypopituitarism is suspected in the recovery period, full replacement therapy should be initiated and combined pituitary function tests conducted about six weeks postoperatively. After external radiotherapy, the onset of hypopituitarism should be suspected if the patient complains of lassitude, lethargy and/or impotence. If in doubt, pituitary function tests should be performed and replacement therapy initiated without waiting for the results. One should not wait for gross hormone deficiencies to develop.

ACTH DISORDERS

Physiology

Adrenocorticotrophic hormone (ACTH) is the most important hormone synthesised and secreted by the corticotrophic cells; these may appear basophilic on staining due to the glycoprotein nature of pro-opiomelanocortin (POMC), the ACTH precursor. Processing of POMC to produce the hormone ACTH (39 amino acid residues) occurs as a result of selective enzymatic cleavage within the cells' hormone-containing granules; the relationship of the principal cleavage products is shown in Fig. 18.8 (p. 674). It will be apparent that ACTH, β LPH, and their cleavage product β endorphin, are secreted simultaneously in response to CRF and other 'physiological' stimulants, such as insulin-induced hypoglycaemia.

The principal hormonal action of ACTH is to stimulate cortisol secretion from the cells of the adrenal cortex, particularly those of the zona fasciculata. Its action is via cell surface receptors which act in part by activation of adenylate cyclase, but also by inducing changes in cell membrane phospholipids and consequent calcium fluxes into the cell (p. 666). ACTH secretion is under complex control from several hypothalamic factors which act synergistically, including corticotrophin-releasing hormone (CRF, a 41 amino acid neuropeptide), vasopressin and, probably, bombesin. The factors that influence ACTH and hence cortisol secretion are shown in Fig. 18.9 (p. 675); they include circadian rhythm (which affects both pulse amplitude and frequency), stress and food.

Isolated ACTH deficiency

Isolated ACTH deficiency is uncommon and may be difficult to diagnose. Patients are usually middle-aged at time of presentation with weakness, lethargy, hypoglycaemia, and sometimes hyponatraemia. The diagnosis is confirmed by a low urinary free cortisol excretion, and a low plasma ACTH and cortisol level which do not rise normally in response to insulin hypoglycaemia. The defect may result either from CRF deficiency or from isolated failure of corticotroph function. Treatment is with glucocorticoid replacement.

ACTH excess

ACTH excess due to hypothalamic defect or to an ACTH-secreting microadenoma leads to pituitary-dependent Cushing's syndrome (p. 708). 'Physiological' ACTH excess occurs when the adrenal glands fail due either to an inborn error of secretion, or to destruction by disease. Under these circumstances, the normal episodic and circadian fluctuations in ACTH secretion occur at much higher than normal levels. Rarely, sustained stimulation of ACTH secretion may lead to development of a 'feedback tumour'.

Nelson's syndrome is the name given to hyperpigmentation, ACTH excess and pituitary expansion that may follow bilateral adrenalectomy for Cushing's syndrome due to a pituitary adenoma. It is presumed to result from removal of negative feedback inhibition of a semi-autonomous pituitary adenoma that was previously subject to some restraint by the high circulating levels of cortisol.

PROLACTIN DISORDERS

Physiology

Prolactin (PRL) is a polypeptide hormone of 199 amino acid residues.

Secretion of prolactin

PRL is synthesised and secreted by cells of the pituitary (lactotrophs), which are mainly located laterally in the gland and are chromophobe in staining. There is little prolactin stored in the pituitary. The lactotrophs secrete prolactin in the absence of stimuli, and the predominant influence of the hypothalamus is to restrain this by secretion of dopamine. Besides causing TSH release, TRH also stimulates prolactin secretion. Prolactin secretion is episodic and increases at night; in females, the level increases at the time of puberty. Androgens probably have a modest inhibitory effect, both on its secretion and on the response of the breast.

Physiologically, the most important change in PRL secretion occurs during pregnancy, when levels rise about five-fold. During pregnancy, oestrogens, probably together with progesterone, cause hyperplasia of the lactotrophs and enhance prolactin secretion, while inhibiting its effect on the breast epithelium. The decline in sex hormones after delivery, coupled with the stimulus of suckling, is responsible for post-partum lactation. (Breast manipulation also enhances PRL levels in a minority of non-pregnant women.) Post-partum breast-feeding causes a marked increase in PRL secretion, as a result of a reflex involving sensory fibres from the breast, the dorsal nerve roots and the hypothalamus. This is probably important in maintaining milk production for weeks and months after delivery, when baseline PRL levels have declined to normal. Another reflex arc is responsible for suckling-induced oxytocin secretion, which is important in stimulating myo-epithelial cells of the breast and so causing milk-ejection from the ducts.

Action of prolactin and other hormones on the breast

Prolactin has an action on the breast that is essential for lactation (Table 18.4). Oestrogens promote ductal growth, while prolactin and progesterone promote growth of the lobules and alveoli. Progesterone enhances the synthesis of β-lactalbumin, a non-catalytic subunit that converts the function of the enzyme galactose synthetase to lactose synthesis. Other hormones with important effects on the breast include insulin and cortisol (which are permissive or facilitatory), growth hormone and placental lactogen. The decline in oestrogen and progesterone levels after delivery releases the brake on prolactin-stimulated lobulo-alveolar milk production.

Pathology

Prolactin deficiency occurs in Sheehan's syndrome when pituitary infarction results from post-partum haemorrhage and consequent hypotension. It results in failure of lactation.

Prolactin excess. Hyperprolactinaemia and associated disorders are common, particularly in women. The low incidence in men is a reflection of the inhibitory effects of androgens both on the lactotrophs and on the breast. Unlike the situation in women, the occurrence of hyperprolactinaemia and/or galactorrhoea in men is almost always of pathological significance.

HYPERPROLACTINAEMIA

Aetiology

The causes of hyperprolactinaemia are best considered in relation to the physiology of prolactin. Table 18.6 lists the principal causes, most of which lead to only mild to moderate hyperprolactinaemia (levels up to 5–10 times normal).

Drugs that inhibit the secretion or action of dopamine are commonly implicated in hyperprolactinaemia. Oestrogens may stimulate lactotroph growth, and (in subjects on the

Table 18.6 Classification of causes of hyperprolactinaemia

Cause	Example
Pituitary lactotroph excess	
Physiological	Pregnancy
Drug-induced	Oestrogens
Pathological	Tumour – microprolactinoma
	– macroprolactinoma
	– mixed GH and prolactin tumour
Inhibition of dopamine secretion	
Neurogenic	Thoracic sensory nerve stimulation
	Chest wall burns/incisions
	Suckling/nipple stimulation
Pituitary stalk damage	Stalk section
	Stalk/hypothalamic tumour
Drug-induced	Methyldopa, reserpine, opiates, H_2-receptor blockers
Inhibition of dopamine action	
Neuroleptic drugs	Phenothiazines, e.g. chlorpromazine
	Butyrophenones, e.g. haloperidol
Anti-emetics	Metoclopramide
Endocrine disorders	TRH-mediated, e.g. primary hypothyroidism.
	Miscellaneous, e.g. adrenal insufficiency
	Cushing's syndrome

contraceptive pill, or during pregnancy) a modest elevation of prolactin secretion. Primary *hypothyroidism* may cause modest hyperprolactinaemia, probably as a consequence of increased TRH secretion. *Cushing's syndrome* and adrenal insufficiency may both be associated with mild hyperprolactinaemia.

Pituitary tumours may lead to hyperprolactinaemia for one of two reasons – they may interfere with the pituitary stalk and so produce local dopamine deficiency, or they may secrete prolactin. Pure *prolactinomas* are classified into two broad categories: the *microprolactinoma*, which is less than one cm in diameter, and is associated with mild to modest hyperprolactinaemia and no pressure symptoms, and the *macroprolactinoma*. In many instances, the diagnosis of microprolactinoma is presumptive, and based on exclusion of other causes; some such cases may simply have hyperplasia or malfunction of lactotrophs. Some patients with *acromegaly* have coincident hyperprolactinaemia, in which case a mixed tumour containing GH- and PRL-secreting cells is suspected. Such cases usually respond well to bromocriptine, in terms of both GH and PRL suppression.

Clinical features and treatment

The unwanted *secretion of milk* (galactorrhoea) is a common disorder in women, but in only about one-third of cases is it due to prolactin excess. If treatment is required, bromocriptine may be effective, even when PRL levels are normal. Increased secretion of prolactin has an inhibitory effect on cyclic ovarian function, probably due to a direct effect of PRL in inhibiting secretion of GnRH in hypothalamic neurones. Erratic and anovulatory cycles or amenorrhoea result. Treatment with a dopaminergic drug such as bromocriptine results in a drop in PRL and resumption of normal ovulatory cycles. It should be remembered that the commonest cause of hyperprolactinaemic amenorrhoea is, of course, pregnancy!

Microprolactinoma

Clinical features

Classical presentations of microprolactinoma are with erratic menstrual cycles or amenorrhoea, with or without galactorrhoea. In some patients, presentation is because of infertility, usually associated with amenorrhoea (primary or secondary). Frequently, presentation follows cessation of the pill (post-pill amenorrhoea) or pregnancy. Patients with microprolactinoma never present with visual field defects or other pressure effects. Indeed, the presence of these effects associated with modest prolactin excess indicates dopamine deficiency due to a non-prolactin secreting tumour in the pituitary stalk or above (e.g. a craniopharyngioma).

Investigation

Diagnosis depends upon demonstration, in several serum samples, of hyperprolactinaemia, in the absence of other causes of prolactin excess. Pituitary radiology is (by definition) normal or borderline abnormal. It is doubtful if the resolution power of CT scans is yet adequate to allow a confident demonstration of microadenomas of any kind, and the issue is further confused by the high incidence of small pituitary adenomas (some of which stain for prolactin) at autopsy in normal individuals.

Treatment

Treatment should generally be conservative, using bromocriptine or other dopaminergic agents such as pergolide or lisuride. Since bromocriptine may cause nausea and postural hypotension at first, the drug should be started in a low dose (1.25 mg bd) with food, and increased gradually over one to two weeks to 2.5 mg three times daily. In most cases, this is highly effective both in suppressing PRL, and in resolving the amenorrhoea and galactorrhoea. If pregnancy is desired, it may be sensible to advise contraception for six months, in order to allow reduction in adenoma size. In contrast to the situation with acromegaly, prolactin-secreting tumours commonly shrink in size with bromocriptine. Bromocriptine may be safely taken during pregnancy but is conventionally stopped once the pregnancy test is positive. With a microprolactinoma, the risk of tumour expansion sufficient to cause visual field defects is probably negligible.

In many cases, mild hyperprolactinaemia continues without progression for years and may remit spontaneously. Surgery (trans-sphenoidal) or radiotherapy are probably seldom indicated, except if there is clear biochemical or radiological evidence of progression. It is as yet uncertain for how long dopaminergic therapy should be given in such cases. A reasonable policy, if pregnancy is not desired, is to treat for one to two years, and then to repeat prolactin levels one week after stopping the drug. Sustained normal levels would suggest that the tumour has regressed and that treatment can be safely stopped and the patient observed. Not infrequently, patients with hyperprolactinaemia are happy to be amenorrhoeic. However, this state is associated with oestrogen deficiency and so a long-term risk of osteoporosis.

If contraception is desired by a patient with microprolactinoma, bromocriptine may be combined safely with the contraceptive pill, the combination protecting against the short- and long-term ill-effects of oestrogen deficiency.

Macroprolactinoma

The definition of macroprolactinoma is arbitrary, but any non-pregnant patient with circulating PRL levels in excess of ten times the upper limit of normal (over 5000 mU/l, 200 ng/ml) probably has a more aggressive prolactinoma which is potentially or actually large and expanding. Virtually all detected prolactinomas in men and about one-fifth of those in women fall into this category.

Clinical features

All features are likely to be more extreme than with a microprolactinoma. These include the endocrine consequences of prolactin excess (galactorrhoea, amenorrhoea, and, in the case of men, impotence). The latter is principally due to gonadotrophin (and so testosterone) deficiency, suggested also by lethargy, depression and loss of secondary sexual hair. Rarely, presentation may be with infertility and oligo- or azoospermia. Local pressure effects – headache, visual field defects and other cranial nerve lesions – are often present at the time of diagnosis. As with other pituitary tumours, the occurrence of panhypopituitarism in the untreated patient indicates the presence of a large and destructive tumour. In the male, galactorrhoea may be present even in the absence of gynaecomastia.

Investigation

Radioimmunoassay measurement of serum prolactin shows levels often 10–200 times normal. Plain X-ray of the pituitary gland will usually show enlargement, an apparent 'double floor', and erosion of the dorsum sellae (Fig. 18.13, p. 679). CT scanning will show the full extent of the tumour, superseding more invasive methods of soft tissue imaging.

Treatment

The urgency of treatment depends upon the severity of local pressure effects. Significant changes have taken place in recent years. Transfrontal surgery (which almost invariably causes hypopituitarism) is now seldom conducted, even when the tumour is expanding upwards; instead, decompression can often be achieved rapidly either with bromocriptine or with trans-sphenoidal surgery. Most would agree that a therapeutic trial of bromocriptine (2.5–5 mg three times daily), with daily measurement of visual fields and acuity, is the initial treatment of choice, followed if necessary by trans-sphenoidal decompression. In macroprolactinomas, it is impossible to eradicate the tumour surgically, and external radiotherapy in a specialist unit is ultimately indicated in every case, regardless of whether or not an operation has been performed.

GONADOTROPHIN DISORDERS

Gonadotrophin disorders are considered in more detail under the section on gonads (p. 713–26). *Gonadotrophin secreting tumours* are rarely diagnosed. Most published cases have been FSH-secreting tumours, although this may simply be because these tend to be larger than LH-secreting tumours and so more obvious. Some 'functionless' pituitary tumours stain for LH and FSH or their subunits, and so may be non-secreting gonadotrophinomas.

Ectopic secretion of gonadotrophins appears to be confined to HCG, which is a normal product of the placenta and a tumour marker for hydatiform mole and its malignant counterpart the choriocarcinoma (a tumour which can now be cured by intensive chemotherapy). Germ cell tumours of the testis and ovary often secrete HCG, as may some carcinomas (e.g. adenocarcinoma of the lung). This leads to excess testicular oestrogen secretion and gynaecomastia. In children, hepatoblastomas may produce pseudo-precocious puberty by HCG secretion.

TSH DISORDERS

Thyroid stimulating hormone (TSH) disorders are principally discussed under panhypopituitarism (p. 676) and thyroid disorders (pp. 690–701). Isolated TSH deficiency is a rare cause of secondary hypothyroidism. Curiously, pituitary tumours leading to secondary hypothyroidism may be associated with detectable immunoreactive TSH (which is presumably not bioactive).

Primary TSH excess due to a *thyrotrophinoma* is a rare cause of hyperthyroidism. Patients with long-standing severe primary hypothyroidism (myxoedema) often develop pituitary enlargement due to thyrotroph hyperplasia and, occasionally, TSH-secreting pituitary ('feedback') tumours. However, the latter usually shrink with thyroxine replacement therapy and probably do not become autonomous.

THE POSTERIOR PITUITARY GLAND

The posterior lobe of the pituitary gland is embryologically and anatomically quite distinct from the anterior; it consists principally of the secretory terminal extensions of neurones that arise in the pre-optic nucleus of the hypothalamus. Its blood supply is derived principally from the hypophyseal arteries, rather than from the hypothalamus-pituitary portal circulation.

SYNTHESIS AND SECRETION OF THE MAIN HORMONES

The posterior pituitary gland secretes two principal octapeptide hormones, vasopressin and oxytocin. In man, the vasopressin produced is arginine vasopressin (AVP; also known as ADH). Both hormones are synthesised in specialised neurones in the pre-optic and ventromedial nuclei as part of a larger precursor which, in each case, also includes the sequence of another protein (a neurophysin). Axonal flow carries the normal precursors to the specialised nerve terminals in the posterior pituitary gland, where they are stored in cytoplasmic granules. Neuronal activation leads to the release of the hormone and its neurophysin into the hypophyseal capillaries and hence into the general circulation. Despite these overall similarities, separate neurones are believed to synthesise oxytocin and vasopressin and the circumstances and purposes of their release are different.

Control mechanisms

ADH secretion is stimulated by an increase in osmolality, and by 'stress' stimuli such as hypoglycaemia (Fig. 18.17). Glucocorticoids exert an inhibitory effect on its release and also interact with ADH at the renal tubule so that, in the presence of glucocorticoid insufficiency, diabetes insipidus may be masked. ADH acts on two different kinds of receptors, those on the renal tubules (type I) and those on blood vessels (type II). The action of ADH on the former is mediated by cyclic-AMP; ADH opens up pores in the basolateral membrane for water and urea.

Oxytocin acts on the smooth muscle of the uterus and mammary ducts (to cause milk ejection). It also causes contraction of myo-epithelial cells of the seminiferous tubules.

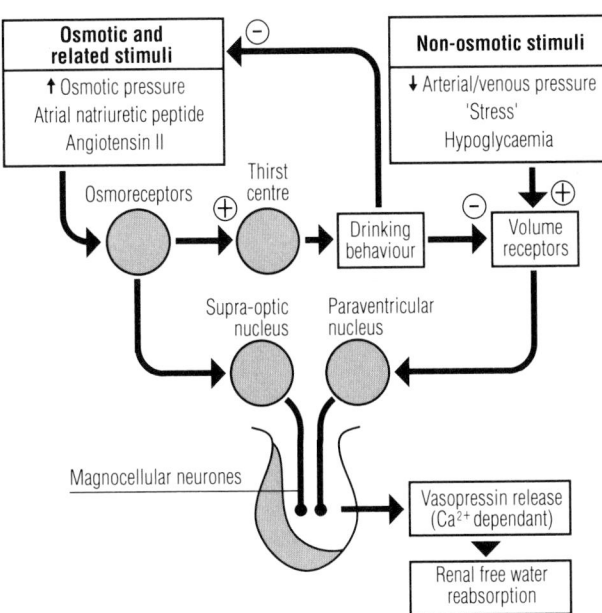

Fig. 18.17   Factors stimulating vasopressin secretion by osmotic and non-osmotic mechanisms. Osmoreceptors also activate the thirst centre to stimulate drinking.

ADH DEFICIENCY

Deficiency of ADH causes the syndrome of diabetes insipidus (Ch. 22, pp. 343–45).

Aetiology

ADH deficiency may be caused by trauma (head injury or neurosurgery); primary or secondary neoplasms of the pituitary, pituitary stalk or hypothalamus; inflammatory disorders such as sarcoidosis; and eosinophilic granuloma. It may be part of a familial syndrome of diabetes mellitus, diabetes insipidus, optic atrophy and nerve deafness. In addition, the condition may be simulated by disorders which lead to renal resistance to vasopressin. These include

X-linked nephrogenic diabetes insipidus (confined to males), and hypercalcaemia and hypokalaemia, both of which lead to a water diuresis from resistance to ADH.

Clinical features

The principal symptom of ADH deficiency is thirst and incidental polyuria, since the patient is forced by the osmotic stimulus to drink large volumes of water or other fluids. It is not uncommon for patients to pass in excess of 10 litres of urine a day, of very low specific gravity (1.003 or less, osmolality less than 100 mosmol/kg). The serum sodium concentration is generally moderately raised, but seldom over 150 mmol/l provided the patient has free access to water. The major danger is when such access is denied, or when the patient is unconscious, e.g. due to an anaesthetic or head injury. Under these circumstances, the osmolality and sodium concentration climbs rapidly. A serum sodium concentration over 160–170 mmol/l may lead to severe and irreversible brain damage.

Investigation

The major differential diagnosis is from psychogenic polydipsia and from other causes of thirst and polyuria (Ch. 21, Table. 21.10). The mainstay of diagnosis is measurement of serum and urine osmolality, serum sodium concentration (more reliable than the osmolality), and urine specific gravity (approximately 0.010 above that of water (1.00) for every 300 mosmol/l of urine solutes). Vasopressin assays are not widely available and seldom needed.

The formal water deprivation test is conducted once the serum sodium concentration and osmolality are known (and shown to be normal). Free access to water is allowed up to the start of the test at 8 am, when the patient is weighed and blood and urine samples taken for osmolality. Timed hourly urine collections, serum osmolality measurements and body weight recordings are made. For safety, the test is discontinued if 3% of body weight is lost or 3 litres of urine are passed. At the end of 8 hours, if urine concentration has not occurred, 1 μg of the analogue DDAVP is given iv, and further samples taken; in true diabetes insipidus this leads to prompt urine concentration. Further details are given in Chapter 22, p. 344.

Treatment of diabetes insipidus

A major advance in the treatment of diabetes insipidus came in the early 1970s, with the development of the long-acting vasopressin analogue, desamino-D-arginine vasopressin (DDAVP, desmopressin). This acts almost exclusively on the (type I) receptors of the renal tubule, and so does not cause hypertension and constriction of the splanchnic circulation. It is also resistant to enzyme degradation in the circulation or peripheral tissues and has a greatly prolonged half-life. DDAVP is given once or twice a day intranasally (10–20 ug) or, for the post-operative patient, intravenously (1–2 mg). With the introduction of desmopressin, diabetes insipidus is no longer a problem of

18

management, provided the patient has an intact thirst centre and does not drink excessive volumes. Chlorpropamide enhances the renal response to ADH, but is now seldom used in its treatment.

'INAPPROPRIATE' SECRETION OF ADH

Aetiology

The syndrome of inappropriate secretion of ADH is frequently encountered in a variety of different conditions (Ch. 22, p. 846). These include acute and chronic pulmonary disease, congestive cardiac failure, small-cell carcinoma of bronchus, cerebral disease, hypoglycaemia, hypopituitarism, and hypothyroidism. ADH secretion is a transient accompaniment of surgery for 24–48 hours. Of the above conditions, only small-cell carcinoma of bronchus is ever associated with true ectopic tumour synthesis and secretion of vasopressin. Even in this condition, however, hyponatraemia is often caused by excess hypothalamo-pituitary ADH secretion, rather than an ectopic source.

Clinical features, investigation and treatment

The hallmark of excessive ADH secretion is a low serum sodium concentration (below 135 mmol/l), and serum osmolality (below 270 mosmol/kg), associated with an inappropriately high urine osmolality (well in excess of 295 mosmol/kg), in a patient who is not clinically volume depleted. It should be recalled that volume depletion from any cause is a stimulus to ADH secretion, so that these biochemical abnormalities would be appropriate in, for example, a patient overtreated with diuretics, a common cause of hyponatraemia in the elderly.

The major clinical features are confusion, coma and fits (water intoxication) if the serum sodium falls much below 120 mmol/l (osmolality below 250 mosmol/kg). Treatment is with fluid restriction and by correction of the underlying cause. If this is not possible, the patient can be treated with small volumes of hypertonic (1.8%) sodium chloride (in severe cases), or with the tetracyclic antibiotic demethylchlortetracycline which diminishes the renal response to ADH. For further details, see Chapter 22, p. 847.

THE THYROID GLAND

EMBRYOLOGY, ANATOMY AND PHYSIOLOGY

The thyroid gland is derived in early embryonic life from an outpouching of the floor of the pharynx which becomes displaced caudally and fuses with the fourth pharyngeal pouch. During its caudal displacement, it leaves the thyroglossal duct, which usually becomes fragmented and resorbed, but may persist to form thyroglossal cysts. If migration is incomplete, ectopic thyroid tissue may lie at the base of the tongue. In adults, the thyroid gland weighs about 20 g and lies in front of the thyroid cartilage, its two lobes connected by a narrow isthmus. It moves upwards with the thyroid cartilage on swallowing.

Histologically, the thyroid gland is composed of follicles of varying diameter lined by a single-layered epithelium; these are arranged into lobules of 10–12 follicles, each served by a common blood supply. The gland is highly vascular, being supplied by two pairs of thyroid arteries which arise from external carotid (superior) and subclavian (inferior) arteries. There is a rich lymphatic drainage and adrenergic and cholinergic innervation. In addition to follicle cells, the thyroid gland also contains *parafollicular* or *C-cells*, which lie next to the follicle but do not abut the colloid. These cells, which arise from the last pair of pharyngeal pouches, secrete the calcium-lowering hormone calcitonin.

The follicles themselves contain a protein-rich colloid, of which the major constituent is the glycoprotein thyroglobulin, which is rich in thyroxine residues. The thyroid epithelial cells synthesise and secrete thyroglobulin into the colloid. Later, they resorb it, cleave the thyroid hormones from the glycoprotein backbone and secrete them into the circulation. Thyroglobulin is both an integral part of the process of thyroid hormone synthesis, and a major storage form of iodine and thyroid hormones within the thyroid.

Synthesis and secretion of thyroid hormones

The unique feature of the thyroid hormones is their content of iodine. The thyroid gland contains about 90% of the body's total iodine, mainly in organic form. The thyroid cells actively transport the iodide into the cells by a process which is competitively inhibited by other anions of similar size, such as perchlorate. Iodide is then oxidised to iodine and incorporated into mono- and di-iodotyrosine (MIT and DIT) residues on thyroglobulin. Favoured residues at particular sites on the thyroglobulin molecule are then converted to thyroxine (T4) and tri-iodothyronine (T3) residues (principally the former) either by interaction with other DIT and MIT residues, or by interaction with an oxidation product of DIT and MIT themselves. This process of 'organification' of iodine (which requires the action of a peroxidase) is believed to take place principally at the basal membrane of the thyroid cell, as thyroglobulin is being formed and secreted into the colloid (Fig. 18.18).

The availability of iodide exerts a direct regulatory effect independent of TSH levels; thus, iodination is most active when iodide levels are low. TSH is the principal active regulator, and exerts its action via a cell-surface receptor; at least part of its effect is mediated via adenylate cyclase. TSH causes acceleration of the process of iodoprotein synthesis, and resorption of colloid by a phagocytic process, followed by fusion with lysosomes. Thyroglobulin is then hydrolysed, facilitated by reduction of disulphide bonds in the molecule. De-iodinases remove iodine from the iodotyrosine residues, and this iodine returns to the iodide pool for iodination of more thyronine residues. The principal thyroid hormone secreted is T4, most circulating T3 arising from its peripheral de-iodination.

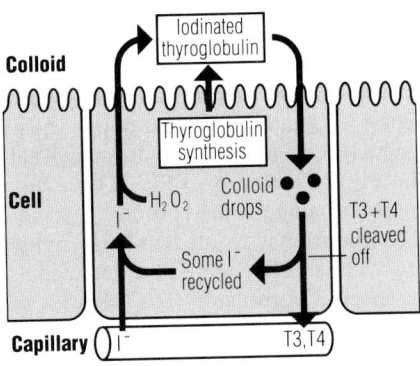

Fig. 18.18 Thyroid hormone synthesis and release (see text for details).

Circulation, action and metabolism of thyroid hormones

Thyroxine (T4) is the major form of thyroid hormone secreted by the thyroid; it is converted enzymatically to either T3 or reverse T3 (rT3) (Fig. 18.19), of which only the former is biologically active. Regulation of the activity of the relevant de-iodinases, in the liver and in other tissues, appears to be important both in health and disease. Generally, the production of T3 and/or rT3 appears to be reciprocally controlled. Although T4 itself has some biological activity in target tissues, it is probably largely active by virtue of its conversion to T3. It is, however, the principal circulating form of thyroid hormone and is more than 99% bound to three plasma proteins – thyroxine binding globulin (TBG), thyroxine binding prealbumin (TBPA) and albumin. TBG has the highest affinity but the lowest capacity, followed by TBPA. T3 binds with lower affinity to TBG, also binds to albumin, but not at all to TBPA. In their bound state(s), T3 and T4 are not biologically active. It is the concentration of unbound hormone which determines the level to which the target cells are exposed (the biologically active fraction).

The liver is the major site of degradation of thyroid hormones. Although much of the iodine is recycled, some is inevitably wasted, being excreted principally in the urine as iodinated degradation products and as inorganic iodide. Under normal circumstances, this is matched by a daily intake of iodide of about 500 μg.

The normal circulating level of T4 (50–150 nmol/l) exceeds that of T3 (1–3 nmol/l) by 50-fold; the difference in their unbound concentrations is about 10 times less than this, because of both the lower binding of T3 to TBG, and its failure to bind to TBPA.

Physiological changes in thyroid hormones

The physiological changes in thyroid hormones of different ages and in various physiological states are shown in Fig. 18.20. The fetus derives little of its thyroid hormones and no TSH from the mother. During the second trimester, the fetal pituitary-thyroid axis becomes active, although it appears that hypothyroidism up to the time of birth does not greatly impair fetal development; the exception to this is retardation in the appearance of some of the ossification centres. Although T4 is secreted in the fetus, very little T3 is produced before birth, rT3 being the major product. At birth, however, there is an immediate switch of hepatic metabolism of T4 from rT3 to T3, so that levels of T3 rise briskly during the first week of life. This change may well be important in adaptation in post-fetal life (in the same way that thyroid hormones are critical for the metamorphosis of amphibians). TBG levels in the fetus are low, and rise after birth. T3 levels throughout infancy and childhood tend to be higher than those of the adult.

In adults, a change occurs during pregnancy when total T4 and T3 levels rise passively in response to an oestrogen-induced rise in TBG. A similar change is produced by the oestrogen-containing oral contraceptive pill. In a wide variety of conditions of stress and ill-health, hepatic pro-

Thyroxine T4

HO—⬡—O—⬡—R

3',3,5-tri-iodothyronine
T3 (active)

HO—⬡—O—⬡—R

3',5',3-tri-iodothyronine
reverse T3 (inactive)

HO—⬡—O—⬡—R

Fig. 18.19 Structures of T4, T3 and reverse T3. R is the alanine residue (—CH₂-CHNH₂-COOH).

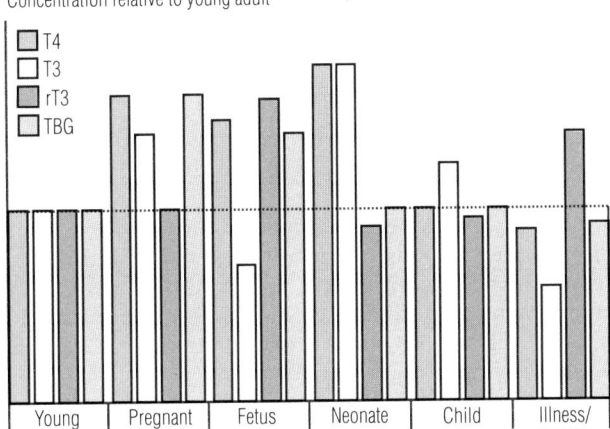

Fig. 18.20 Relative changes of serum T4, T3, reverse T3 and thyroxine binding globulin (TBG) in different physiological states and in illness.

Endocrine Diseases

duction of T3 declines and of rT3 increases. This decline in T3 production also occurs in old age. It is of uncertain biological significance, since T4 itself has some direct biological effect and conversion of T4 to T3 still occurs in some target tissues. Exposure to extreme cold is associated with reduced production of rT3 and increased production of T3.

PATHOLOGY OF THYROID DISEASE

The thyroid gland is among the endocrine glands most likely to be affected by disease. It may be the subject of defective development, of inborn biosynthetic errors, of toxic or nutritional damage, of autoimmune disease, and of benign and malignant tumours. Many of these abnormalities give rise to enlargement of the gland and to the appearance of a goitre (thyroid enlargement).

Goitre. Thyroid enlargement may be focal (as in adenoma, cyst, or carcinoma) or generalised, in which case it may be either multinodular or diffuse and smooth. Clinical assessment alone will often allow an accurate assessment of the cause of the goitre.

Autoimmune disease and the thyroid

The thyroid is the endocrine gland most commonly affected by autoimmune disease. Immune mechanisms are involved in the pathogenesis of Graves' disease, Hashimoto's thyroiditis, and primary myxoedema. For reasons yet unclear, these disorders are about five times commoner in women than in men. It is probable that viral or other damage may result in the thyroid cell presenting HLA antigens on the external surface of the follicle; these may then set in motion an autoimmune response, which is partly humoral and partly cellular. In Graves' disease, the TSH receptor is an important antigen to which antibodies may be produced. These antibodies may bind to the receptor, causing stimulation. Growth-promoting antibodies may also be produced, as are antibodies to thyroid microsomes and to thyroglobulin. The factors which determine what antibodies are produced in an individual case are uncertain.

Measurement of circulating levels of relevant antibodies may be of diagnostic value. In general, however, both the presence of antibody and its titre are disappointingly non-specific. The most commonly measured antibodies (which are of the IgG subclass) are those against thyroid cell microsomes, thyroglobulin (Tg) and the TSH receptor. Antibodies to microsomes, Tg or both are present in about 10% of apparently healthy individuals, usually women. In disease, they are most commonly detected against microsomes, being present in 85% or more of patients with autoimmune thyroid disease. Very high titres indicate the presence of foci of lymphocytic infiltration and Hashimoto's thyroiditis.

There is a significant association of autoimmune thyroid disease with certain HLA types, most strikingly DW3 and DR3. It has been suggested that the presence of this tissue type predicts a high chance of recurrence in a patient with Graves' disease (p. 671).

Antibodies to the TSH receptor

Antibodies to the TSH receptor are of importance in the pathogenesis of Graves' disease and of hypothyroidism. Thyrotoxicosis in Graves' disease is due to the presence of antibodies which bind to, and activate, the TSH receptor, thus simulating the action of TSH. These are now best detected in assays using purified porcine thyroid cell membranes and competition with labelled TSH, or by activation of adenylate cyclase. They were first detected as so-called long-acting thyroid stimulator (LATS) in a mouse bioassay. Other antibodies bind to the TSH receptor but do not activate it, and so cause hypothyroidism, often in the presence of a goitre. (In most cases of myxoedema, however, the thyroid dysfunction is due to the destructive effect of cell-mediated immunity and cytotoxic antibodies.)

Antibodies can cross the placenta and cause thyrotoxicosis in the newborn infant. Measurement of anti-receptor antibody in the mother allows detection of babies at risk. Otherwise, there is a generally poor correlation between the circulating titre of thyroid-stimulating antibodies and the activity of Graves' thyrotoxicosis; this is probably because the antibodies are produced largely within the thyroid gland itself and spill over into the circulation.

Nutrition and thyroid disease

There is a wide geographical variation in the incidence of endemic goitre which is only partly understood. The major factors responsible for goitre appear to be dietary iodine deficiency and ingestion of goitrogenic substances which interfere with either uptake or organification of iodine. For example, cassava, a root crop eaten extensively in Africa, is rich in goitrogens. Women are particularly susceptible to goitre because of the demands of the fetus for iodine. Endemic cretinism is a neurological disease which afflicts the offspring of goitrous mothers in parts of the world where iodine is deficient, especially in the mountainous regions of New Guinea. It appears to be due to fetal iodide deficiency at the stage of early brain development, rather than to thyroid hormone deficiency. It is completely prevented by providing the mother with iodised salt.

INVESTIGATION OF THYROID DISEASE

Examination of the thyroid gland

The thyroid should be carefully examined by observation from the front, and by palpation from behind while swallowing. The consistency of the gland should be assessed. In Graves' disease, the gland is typically either diffusely enlarged or slightly asymmetrical. The swelling is firmer with a carcinoma and associated with enlargement of local lymph nodes. A midline swelling that moves up with protrusion of the tongue is likely to be a thyroglossal cyst or ectopic thyroid. The gland, if enlarged, should be auscultated; a bruit, which may be diastolic as well as systolic, indicates a vascular gland and usually points to Graves' disease.

Laboratory assessment of hypo- and hyperthyroidism

Radioimmunoassay

In most cases, the laboratory assessment of hypo- and hyperthyroidism is now extremely simple, thanks to specific radioimmunoassays for T3, T4 and TSH, and (where relevant) methods of assessing thyroid hormone binding. In most cases, clinical assessment combined with a single measurement of serum T3, T4 and TSH levels is sufficient.

In *primary hypothyroidism*, T4 and T3 levels are low and TSH rises markedly. In the early stages, or in patients who have had a subtotal thyroidectomy, T4 and T3 levels are normal, and TSH modestly raised. In most cases of symptomatic hypothyroidism, TSH will be more than five times the upper limit of normal. Serum T4 is more reliable for the assessment of early cases than T3 which may be low as a non-specific consequence of illness.

In *secondary (pituitary) hypothyroidism* one would expect the TSH to be undetectable, but this is frequently not the case. In some cases an abnormal TSH that is detectable on immunoassay but not biologically active may be produced.

In *hyperthyroidism* serum T3 and T4 levels are elevated. In mild cases, serum T3 may be raised before T4 and so is a more reliable test for early detection of thyrotoxicosis. TSH levels are low but, until recently, assays were not sufficiently reliable to detect this. It was therefore necessary to inject thyrotrophic releasing hormone (TRH 200 μg iv), and to demonstrate an absent TSH response over the next 60 minutes. Recently, highly sensitive and specific two-site immunoradiometric assays have been introduced which allow subnormal TSH levels to be detected and so have largely eliminated the need for the TRH test.

Protein-binding tests

Tests of protein binding are widely used. TBG levels are generally reduced in hyperthyroidism, and increased in hypothyroidism. Oestrogens promote the hepatic synthesis of TBG along with other binding proteins; thus, the situation most commonly encountered where the T4 is raised and protein binding has to be taken into account is in a woman during pregnancy or while on the contraceptive pill. The most widely used test to elucidate this problem is an *in vitro* thyroid hormone-uptake test, in which TBG in dilute serum and sephadex compete to bind radiolabelled T3 (Fig. 18.21).

Recently, a *direct free T4 assay* has become commercially available. This assay uses a synthetic ligand which binds to the T4 antibody but not to TBG, and thus allows assessment of the actual unbound T4. All tests, including this one, have pitfalls for the unwary and require expert assessment whenever the clinical features and biochemical results are out of line with one another.

Radioactive uptake tests

Historically, ^{131}I uptake was routinely carried out to confirm the diagnosis of hyper- and hypothyroidism. This

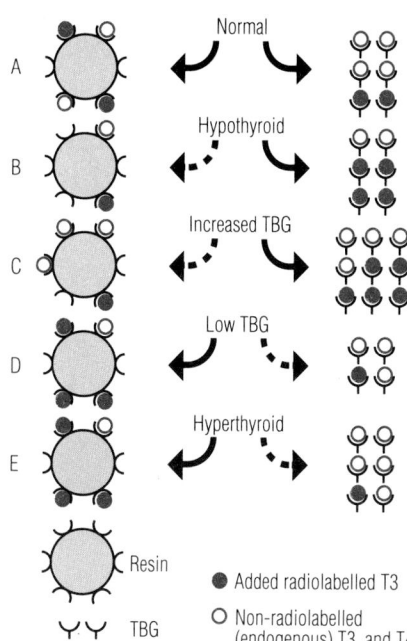

Fig. 18.21 Distribution of radiolabelled triiodothyrone between resin (left) and binding proteins (right), in different clinical states. Arrows indicate direction of distribution.

test was tedious however as, to be reliable, it required serial measurements of uptake over 1–2 days, to allow a curve to be plotted. In thyrotoxicosis, both uptake and discharge are more rapid than normal so that the protein bound ^{131}I level at 48 hours was perhaps the most reliable measurement. A major problem with all quantitative uptake tests is that they are conducted against a variable background concentration of circulating inorganic iodide, which competes with the isotope and is generally an unknown quantity in the calculation.

Nowadays, virtually the only isotope to be used diagnostically is [99]Tc (as radiolabelled pertechnate), a short-lived gamma-emitter with a half-life of six hours. Scans are of great value in assessing the distribution of uptake within the gland. Uptake may be confined to one area in a functioning autonomous adenoma, since uptake by the rest of the gland is suppressed; conversely, uptake is absent in an area occupied by a cyst or carcinoma. Even a well-differentiated carcinoma will seldom take up isotope in the presence of a normally functioning gland.

Ultrasound

Ultrasound is a useful technique, particularly for demonstrating the cystic nature of a lesion. Unfortunately, some tumours may also be cystic, so the test is not completely reliable.

Needle aspiration

Needle aspiration of the thyroid is also a simple and useful technique for non-invasive diagnosis of thyroid masses.

Fig. 18.22 ^{99}Tc-labelled pertechnetate isotope scan showing asymmetrical uptake in the thyroid (dashed outline) with one particularly large 'hot' nodule. The dark spot below the thyroid is the suprasternal notch, marked with the isotope. The two areas of uptake visible above the thyroid are the submandibular glands.

Interpretation requires a degree of expertise on the part of the histopathologist, particularly if there is a suspected carcinoma. However, once the technique is mastered, it greatly reduces the need for thyroid scans, and for surgery on benign nodules.

PRIMARY HYPOTHYROIDISM: CONGENITAL AND JUVENILE

Hypothyroidism may be present before birth (although it is probably not of great importance until immediately after birth) or may develop at any time thereafter.

Congenital hypothyroidism

The causes of congenital hypothyroidism are listed in Table 18.7. Endemic cretinism is a severe developmental disorder which occurs in areas of endemic goitre in children born to goitrous and iodine-deficient mothers. Severe neurological defects (deaf mutism, spasticity and motor impairment) are associated with variable hypothyroidism

Table 18.7 Causes of congenital hypothyroidism
Non-goitrous
Complete failure of thyroid development
Ectopic thyroid
Endemic cretinism
Pituitary or hypothalamic insufficiency
Goitrous
Maternal antithyroid drugs
Endemic cretinism
Iodine treatment of mother
Defects in thyroid hormone biosynthesis
Iodide transport, organic binding defects
Iodotyronine coupling defect
Iodotyronine dehydrogenase (iodine recycling) defect
Abnormal iodoprotein secretion
Thyroid hormone resistance

and goitre. In non-goitrous areas, congenital hypothyroidism occurs with a frequency of around 1 in 5000 births, and is most frequently due to failure of normal development or to atrophy of the thyroid. It is usually not clinically apparent at birth, but may be diagnosed reliably within 1–2 weeks by TSH assay on a blood spot dried on filter paper.

Diagnosis is difficult at birth. Suggestive features include postmaturity, hypothermia, enlargement of the posterior fontanelle, neonatal jaundice, and delayed passage of meconium. Failure to diagnose and treat leads to retardation of physical growth and mental development, which becomes gross by late infancy. Early signs are feeding difficulty, failure to thrive, protuberant abdomen, dry skin and hair, and delayed eruption of teeth. The infant is slow to reach the usual milestones. Radiological abnormalities include delayed development and 'stippling' of the epiphyses. The longer treatment is delayed, the greater is the likelihood of permanent mental retardation; any delay is likely to result in a lower than maximum potential IQ.

Juvenile hypothyroidism

Hypothyroidism starting in childhood results in mental slowness but no permanent mental retardation. Features seen are less obvious than in the myxoedematous adult, but growth and sexual development are retarded, often markedly. Delay in body development principally affects the long bones and the bones of the face which therefore appears immature. Epiphyseal dysgenesis with 'stippling' of the epiphyses on X-ray is common, and epiphyseal closure is delayed. Puberty is usually delayed, although, paradoxically, precocious puberty may also occur. Replacement therapy results in some catch-up growth and in spontaneous puberty (if this was delayed).

PRIMARY HYPOTHYROIDISM DEVELOPING IN ADULT LIFE

Hypothyroidism with onset in adult life is almost always

due to autoimmunity, unless it results from previous treatment of thyrotoxicosis.

Clinical features

The onset of hypothyroidism is usually gradual, and the symptoms are often attributed incorrectly by the patient and relatives to increasing age. Symptoms, especially in the early stages, are frequently vague. Increasing lethargy, slowness, memory loss, and depression are often coupled with increasing weight (without eating more) and cold intolerance. The skin becomes dry and the hair 'lifeless'. Puffiness below the eyes, especially in the morning, is frequently noted. Symptoms are referred to many systems; constipation is common, and may be associated with abdominal distension; in the nervous system, symptoms of carpal tunnel syndrome are common, as is a complaint of dizziness. Deafness is a frequent symptom due to fluid in the middle ear. The patient may have noticed a change in the voice with deepening or 'gruffness'. Rarely, the patient develops cerebellar ataxia. Myotonia is a rare complication.

Hypercholesterolaemia predisposes to vascular atheroma, and angina in the untreated patient is particularly important, as treatment in such a patient may precipitate myocardial infarction. Effusions may occur into any serous cavity – pericardial, pleural, peritoneal or joint spaces. Mild anaemia of macrocytic type is quite common; megaloblastic anaemia suggests coincidental pernicious anaemia. Other organ-specific autoimmune diseases, such as vitiligo and Addison's disease, may be associated. Rheumatoid arthritis and polymyalgia rheumatica are also significantly associated with autoimmune thyroid disease. In severe myxoedema, the patient is grossly retarded and may become psychotic when treated; rarely, however, they paradoxically appear mentally hyperactive (myxoedema madness). Hypothyroidism predisposes to hypothermia. It may cause hyponatraemia, since hypothyroidism predisposes to inappropriate secretion of ADH. If hypothyroidism is suspected, a past history of thyrotoxicosis (with surgery or ^{131}I therapy) and a family history of thyroid disease should be sought.

With experience, a confident clinical diagnosis of hypothyroidism can often be made from the history and physical examination. However, the aim should be to make the diagnosis before it is clinically obvious, and serum T3, T4 and TSH estimation allows this to be done. Early signs are lethargy, depression, slowness in answering questions, a malar flush, puffy eyes, dry skin, and delayed relaxation of the tendon reflexes (e.g. ankle jerks, if present, or biceps jerks). The voice may be husky or 'gruff'. There is usually a relative or absolute bradycardia. The patient may have gained weight.

The commonest conditions with which hypothyroidism is confused are obesity and depression. With good clinical practice, gross myxoedema should be a thing of the past. In any case where there is doubt, thyroid function tests should be measured on a blood (serum) sample. The thyroid is usually impalpable, except where hypothyroidism is due to an enzyme deficiency or to TSH receptor-blocking antibodies, rather than destruction of the gland.

Investigation

T4 and T3 are low (the former being more reliable) and TSH greatly raised. Free T4 is reduced. Investigations to establish the aetiology depend upon the clinical setting. In a child, a thyroid scan may demonstrate ectopic tissue and, if a goitre is present, a perchlorate discharge test may uncover an organification deficit. This test depends on the failure of iodide to be used in thyroxine synthesis; free (labelled) iodide can therefore be discharged from the gland when perchlorate is administered. Antithyroid antibodies, if present, point to an autoimmune aetiology.

It is important to carry out investigations to determine the extent of damage that has resulted from the hypothyroidism, such as X-rays of bones in a child, and endocrine tests to assess pubertal stage. Juvenile hypothyroidism is commonly confused with panhypopituitarism, but TSH will be low in the latter and high in the former. Chest X-ray may reveal a pleural or pericardial effusion. An ECG is important, especially in the elderly patient with angina or ischaemic heart disease, in which case thyroxine replacement should be started cautiously and under β-adrenergic blockade. Measurement of serum electrolyte levels may reveal hyponatraemia due to inappropriate ADH secretion.

Treatment

In treating hypothyroidism, it is important to be certain before commencing thyroid hormones that the patient is not hypopituitary. If in doubt, hydrocortisone replacement should be given as well, until ACTH and cortisol deficiency have been excluded. In mild cases, the patient can be commenced forthwith on a full replacement dose of thyroxine (100–200 μg/daily). In an adult, the median dose required to suppress TSH to normal is about 125 μg/day. In severe cases, especially if there is ischaemic heart disease, replacement should be more cautious, with 5 mcg bd of tri-iodothyronine or 25–50 μg of thyroxine. Myxoedema coma and hypothermia carries a poor prognosis and requires rewarming, cardiovascular support, hydrocortisone, parenteral tri-iodothyronine (15–30 μg daily) and antibiotics if there is infection. In hypothyroidism there is no advantage to be gained long-term from giving tri-iodothyronine or T3-T4 mixtures.

Summary 3 Clinical features of myxoedema

- Symptoms include lethargy, increased weight, cold intolerance, mental slowing.

- Signs include dry skin, puffy face, gruff voice.

- Complications include serous effusions, vascular disease, psychosis.

Prevention

At present, nothing can be done to prevent thyroid failure from developing; however, much can be done to ensure its early detection and treatment. Thyroid hormone replacement is the simplest form of endocrine therapy so, for practical purposes, prevention is by early detection. Patients with any form of autoimmune thyroid disease, such as Graves' disease, should be told that there is an increased chance of developing thyroid failure later, and that if there is clinical suspicion they should therefore ask for thyroid function tests to be performed. Patients who have had radioactive iodine therapy are at particular risk and should be told of this, as should thyrotoxic patients who have had subtotal thyroidectomy. The earliest biochemical change is a rise in serum TSH although, particularly after thyroid surgery, this may simply indicate a new steady state, with normal T3 and T4 being produced under modestly increased TSH drive. Borderline thyroid function tests may present a problem; in such cases, the tests can be repeated after an interval and, if thyroid failure is developing, TSH will rise progressively.

Once on thyroxine, patients must be told to stay on it for life, advice that may easily be ignored, especially by the elderly and the confused. Sadly, many early cases of hypothyroidism are still missed by doctors each year, perhaps because they expect the patient to have 'textbook' myxoedema. Every such case is to be regarded as a major failure of preventative medicine, and the aim should be to diagnose hypothyroidism *before there are any physical signs*. As always, taking a careful history and having a high index of suspicion is the key. The time to check the thyroid function tests is when you first think of the possibility of hypothyroidism. Thyrotoxic patients on antithyroid drugs should be monitored carefully both clinically and biochemically, since the dose needed varies considerably and a patient may develop a lower requirement with time.

Prevention of cretinism now depends upon TSH assays done on blood spots in the neonatal period as a screening test. High or borderline levels lead to more detailed clinical and biochemical screening.

HYPERTHYROIDISM

In areas where iodine is abundant, most patients with thyrotoxicosis have autoimmune thyroid disease (Graves' disease). Thyrotoxicosis due to multinodular goitre, or to a toxic adenoma, is less common.

There is a wide clinical spectrum of severity of thyroid hormone excess, of the systemic manifestations of the disease, the size and vascularity of the thyroid gland, and the extent to which other systems, notably the extraocular muscles and the skin, are involved in associated autoimmune disorders. The clinician should therefore consider separately those features which are directly or indirectly due to thyroid hormone excess, from associated abnormalities (such as some of the eye signs).

Toxic multinodular goitre usually develops after the age of 50 against a background of many years of non-toxic goitre. It is therefore much more common in areas of endemic goitre. For reasons that are not clear, diffuse or focal autonomous nodule formation develops in the enlarged thyroid (detected as areas of increased radioiodine uptake), with associated thyrotoxicosis which is generally of a relatively mild degree and associated with suppressed TSH. This disorder is not associated with infiltrative ophthalmopathy.

In *toxic adenoma*, an autonomous nodule (follicular adenoma) develops and progressively enlarges. It secretes an increasing amount of the total thyroid hormone until TSH is switched off completely and (generally mild) thyrotoxicosis develops. This usually happens only when the nodule reaches 2.5 cm diameter or more.

In *Graves' disease*, antibodies to the TSH receptor stimulate the thyroid gland in ways analogous to the normal action of TSH. The disease presents most commonly in the third and fourth decades of life. As with many organ-specific autoimmune diseases, Graves' disease is much commoner in women than in men; this also applies to toxic multinodular goitre. Especially in the latter disorder, hyperthyroidism may be induced by high doses of iodine or iodine-containing drugs (the Jod-Basedow phenomenon). Hashimoto's disease, which is also of autoimmune aetiology, may also be associated with mild thyrotoxicosis in the early stages. Occasionally, the thyrotoxicosis is due to exogenous hormone consumption; this is known as *thyrotoxicosis factitia*.

Clinical features due to thyroid hormone excess

History

The history of the patient with thyroid hormone excess is variable. Typically, the patient develops weight loss, increased appetite, heat intolerance and sweating. She becomes anxious, nervous, restless, depressed, irritable and difficult to live with. A fine tremor is common, and proximal myopathy may cause muscle weakness, especially in the elderly. In women, menstrual disturbances such as oligomenorrhoea and menorrhagia are common. Increased gut motility may lead to diarrhoea. Palpitations are common and symptoms of heart failure are especially likely in the elderly, often precipitated by atrial fibrillation. A goitre may be noted, and complained of, especially if the gland is large and vascular. It rarely obstructs swallowing or breathing unless it is retrosternal. To assess the patient quickly when thyrotoxicosis is suspected, a clinical checklist is useful, such as that given in Table 18.8.

Examination

Most of the features of thyroid hormone excess are due to increased sensitivity to circulating catecholamines. Part of the levator palpebrae superioris (called Müller's muscle) is sympathetically innervated, and catecholamine excess causes a staring appearance, lid lag, lid retraction, and infrequent blinking. This may be associated with feelings of anxiety, nervousness, tremor, sweating, tachycardia, and

Table 18.8 Symptoms and signs of thyrotoxicosis (Graves' disease)

Mechanisms	Symptoms	Signs
Primary autoimmune process	Swelling, dysphagia, pain	Goitre, bruit
	Exophthalmos, discomfort	Exophthalmos, ocular palsies
	Diplopia etc.	Congestion, papilloedema, etc.
	Itchy/painful rash on legs	Pretibial myxoedema (rare)
Thyroid hormone excess		
Combination of catecholamine sensitivity, thyroid hormone excess and metabolism	Palpitations* Breathlessness	Resting tachycardia*, atrial fibrillation, other arrhythmias* Heart failure
	Heat intolerance* Sweating*	Warm and sweaty*
	Increased appetite Weight loss Diarrhoea*	Bowel sounds Malabsorption
	Weakness	Proximal myopathy
	Nervousness and irritability*	Inability to sit still Emotional lability* Tremor*
	'Staring' eyes*	Infrequent blinking* Lid lag* Lid retraction*

*Signs and associated symptoms (partially) blocked by beta-blockers

supraventricular arrhythmias (notably atrial fibrillation).

Thyroid hormones also stimulate the metabolic rate, probably both directly by inducing a number of metabolic enzymes, and also indirectly, through catecholamine sensitivity. Heat intolerance and weight loss (in spite of increased appetite) result.

Features that may occur and are of uncertain pathogenesis include myopathy, cardiac failure, hypercalcaemia, gynaecomastia and female infertility. The hypercalcaemia is usually mild and does not always respond to rendering the patient euthyroid. Gynaecomastia probably results from metabolic alterations of androgen and oestrogen metabolism, and increased sex hormone binding globulin (SHBG) levels, which lead to an increased ratio of free oestradiol to testosterone.

Natural history of thyrotoxicosis

Graves' disease. While it is difficult to be certain, it seems likely that, before treatment became available, one-third to one-half of patients with Graves' disease had a spontaneous remission of their thyrotoxicosis. This applied particularly to thyrotoxic patients during pregnancy, possibly because of the weak glucocorticoid-like effect of progesterone. An uncertain proportion (perhaps 20%) of patients will spontaneously become hypothyroid if followed long enough.

The reverse pattern – hypothyroidism progressing to hyperthyroidism – is a rare but recognised presentation of Graves' disease. The prognosis for relapse after medical treatment is probably worst if there is a large vascular goitre.

Hashimoto's disease. In Hashimoto's disease, a similar percentage of patients to that seen in Graves' will go into remission spontaneously. In others, an early thyrotoxic phase is followed by progressive hypothyroidism.

Toxic adenoma. Occasionally, patients with toxic adenoma treat themselves by infarcting the tumour, a condition associated with sudden development of pain and swelling of a thyroid nodule. Usually, the condition gradually progresses until the patient becomes overtly toxic.

Dysthyroid eye disease

Dysthyroid eye disease (infiltrative ophthalmopathy) remains one of the more puzzling clinical features of endocrinology.

Aetiology

Dysthyroid eye disease occurs in Graves' disease but not in other causes of thyrotoxicosis, such as toxic adenoma. There is little doubt that the condition – fortunately only rarely sufficiently severe to threaten eyesight – is due to an autoimmune process which involves the extra-ocular muscles and appears to be indirectly linked with that causing the thyroid disease. Recent evidence indicates that antibodies are directed against specific antigens on the eye muscles. These become infiltrated with lymphocytes and swollen; in the later stages of the disease, they may be destroyed and become fibrosed. Later, there is involvement of the retro-orbital fat in the inflammatory process.

Clinical features

The clinical features of dysthyroid eye disease are to be distinguished from those due to thyrotoxicosis. The latter – lid lag, lid retraction, infrequent blinking – are principally due to increased sympathetic activity and become less marked on treatment with beta-adrenergic blockers (Table 18.8). Protrusion of the eyeball (Fig. 18.23) is most obvious if the orbits are shallow. It is usually, but not invariably, symmetrical. If marked, it leads to inability to close the eye fully, corneal damage (exposure keratitis) and a risk of secondary infection. Increased orbital pressure leads to suffusion of the ocular and orbital circulation with conjunctival oedema, retinal venous congestion, raised intraocular pressure (glaucoma), and papilloedema. Ocular muscle paresis is common and leads to troublesome diplopia. Ocular muscles frequently become tethered to surrounding soft tissues; this is particularly so for the inferior rectus muscles, so that diplopia is often most marked upon looking upwards. Conjugate deviation may be impossible.

The symptoms of dysthyroid eye disease include discomfort, grittiness, swelling, redness and pain in the eyes

Fig. 18.23 Eye signs in thyrotoxicosis and dysthyroid eye disease. A. Eye signs in thyrotoxicosis – (A) Lid retraction. (B) Lid lag. (C) Exophthalmos with conjunctival oedema. (D) Strabismus with diplopia due to paralysis/tethering. Arrows indicate direction of gaze. **B.** CT scan through orbits in a case of exophthalmos. Note oedematous and enlarged extraocular muscles. **C.** Patient with typical features of dysthyroid eye disease with exophthalmos.

which is often most marked on wakening (because of orbital congestion on recumbency and exposure of the cornea during sleep). The patient or relatives may have noticed the development of 'bulging eyes'. Occasionally, presentation may be with visual failure due to glaucoma or optic nerve damage (e.g. retinal vein thrombosis). The signs of a dangerous rise in ocular and orbital pressure are obvious conjunctival or periorbital oedema, painful eyes, exposure keratitis, retinal venous congestion and papilloedema. These should lead to urgent specialist referral to an endocrinologist working closely with an ophthalmologist experienced with the condition.

Treatment

In most cases no specific treatment is indicated and, in 90% of individuals, the eye condition will settle spontaneously. Local use of artificial tears at night is helpful if there is corneal exposure with the eyelids closed. Ocular congestion is an indication for use of diuretics to cause minimal sodium depletion and, in more severe cases, admission to hospital and treatment with systemic steroids in high dosage (e.g. prednisolone, 60–80 mg daily). In severe cases, if improvement does not occur, or if deterioration follows gradual reduction in dosage, orbital decompression may save vision. This is carried out by a neurosurgeon or ophthalmic surgeon and involves removal of part of the wall or roof of the orbit. Later (but only after the condition has been stable for six months or more), ocular surgery may be indicated for diplopia that cannot be managed by refractive means (e.g. use of prismatic spectacles). It is important, in patients with dysthyroid eye disease, to avoid overtreatment of thyrotoxicosis, since treatment-induced hypothyroidism can lead to rapid deterioration in the eyes; this is probably because myxoedematous congestion is added to an already critical situation. Orbital radiotherapy also has a part to play in the management of severe dysthyroid eye disease.

Pretibial myxoedema and thyroid acropachy

Pretibial myxoedema is a rare feature of Graves' disease. It is the name given to purplish infiltration of the dermis of the skin over the anterolateral aspect of the lower legs.

It is of unknown aetiology. In texture, the surface resembles the skin of an orange. Pathology shows deposition of mucin between collagen bundles. Pretibial myxoedema may present incidentally, for cosmetic reasons or because the lesion is itchy.

Thyroid acropachy is usually associated with pretibial myxoedema, and is the association of Graves' disease with extreme finger clubbing and periosteal reaction in the bones of the forearm.

Treatment of thyrotoxicosis

Traditionally, young patients have been treated with antithyroid drugs (carbimazole or propylthiouracil). If the condition relapses, they have been subjected to subtotal thyroidectomy, while patients over about 40 years of age have been given radioactive iodine therapy. Nowadays, however, a range of different guidelines are used in different centres, with some physicians prescribing ^{131}I as definitive treatment even for young patients, and others giving carbimazole long-term. Much depends on the local expertise available. As a good general principle, surgery should not be undertaken, nor ^{131}I given, while the patient is grossly thyrotoxic. The patient should first be made euthyroid with antithyroid drugs because there is a risk of precipitating a thyrotoxic 'storm' with ^{131}I or surgery when the patient is still thyrotoxic.

Drug therapy

The major antithyroid drugs used are *thiourea compounds* of which carbimazole is usually used in the United Kingdom and methimazole and propylthiouracil in the USA. These drugs were introduced in the early 1950s and represented a major advance in the treatment of thyrotoxicosis. They are generally well tolerated, with reversible leucopenia or skin rashes developing in only about one per cent of cases, usually during the first six weeks of therapy. During this time, the white blood count should be checked every two weeks or if a sore throat develops. The drugs are usually given initially at high dosage. Thus, carbimazole is given at first in a dose of 40–60 mg daily, in 3 or 4 divided doses because of its short half-life. This is tapered off after 3–4 weeks to a maintenance dose of 5–30 mg daily. This tapering regimen is probably not necessary. An alternative policy is to start straightaway with the likely maintenance dose (higher for gross thyrotoxicosis, with a large vascular gland) and to titrate this against the circulating T3 and T4 level. On treatment, the ratio of T3 to T4 is higher than normal, because of preferential suppression of T4 formation, but this does not seem to matter clinically. It is important to realise that there is a lag of 1–2 weeks between the achievement of biochemical and that of clinical euthyroidism. It is easy to overtreat if this is not appreciated, and to have a patient who is biochemically hypothyroid while still clinically thyrotoxic; such a patient will eventually and rapidly become clinically hypothyroid. It appears satisfactory to maintain patients on a daily dose of carbimazole. In some centres, a high dose of carbimazole is

routinely combined with replacement doses of thyroxine. Since most of the adverse effects of the thiourea drugs occur during the first few weeks of treatment, patients stabilised on a small dose but who relapse when taken off it can safely be maintained on the drug long-term.

Beta-adrenergic blocking drugs are useful for symptomatic treatment during the first 4–8 weeks until several weeks after biochemical euthyroidism is achieved. Usually, small doses (e.g. 20–40 mg of propranolol twice daily) are sufficient. In mild cases, beta-blockers alone may be used while the effect of ^{131}I therapy is awaited.

Potassium perchlorate is now no longer used because of a high incidence of toxic reactions.

The optimal duration of antithyroid drug therapy is open to question, but is probably 12–18 months. There is some evidence that the drugs act in part by exerting an immunosuppressive effect within the thyroid, thereby preventing relapse, and this may be an argument for prolonging treatment. It has also been used as an argument for giving all patients high doses of carbimazole therapy, 'covered' with thyroxine (100–150 µg daily) to prevent the otherwise inevitable development of hypothyroidism. Alternatively, the apparent immunosuppressive effects of these drugs may be due to resolution of the thyroid hormone excess, which itself activates the immune system.

Thyroid surgery

The indications for thyroid surgery are not clear-cut. Where patients are referred first to a surgeon, the operation rate tends to be high. In centres where radio-iodine therapy is given the frequency of surgery is lower. Patients should be rendered euthyroid medically for three months before surgery is undertaken (see above). Surgery should probably not be considered in Graves' disease before a proper trial of medical therapy (except in cases where thyrotoxicosis is excessively difficult to control). Other exceptions are where the goitre is unusually large or painful, or is causing tracheal obstruction.

Pre- and postoperative management

Potassium iodide is generally administered by mouth in a dose of at least 5 mg daily (many surgeons use much more) for 7–10 days before operation. This blocks the release of thyroid hormones but also, more importantly, leads to a marked accumulation of colloid in the thyroid follicles and, partly as a consequence of this, reduces the vascularity of the gland. Laryngoscopic examination of the cords is undertaken routinely before surgery. Most surgeons

---

Summary 4 Management of hyperthyroidism

- Carbimazole is usually the first treatment for patients of all ages.
- Beta-blockers are useful symptomatically for the first 1–2 months.
- Surgery is considered for failed medical treatment and large goitres.
- [131]I is considered for older patients and for toxic adenomas.

remove about seven-eighths of the gland, taking care to identify and preserve the parathyroid glands and, of course, the left recurrent laryngeal nerve. Nevertheless, there is a significant incidence (5–10%) of postoperative hypocalcaemia from hypoparathyroidism, as some vascular damage to these glands is probably inevitable. It is usually transient, however. Serum calcium levels should be checked 12 and 24 hours after surgery.

Radio-iodine treatment

It is impossible to judge accurately the optimum dose of ^{131}I to be given in radio-iodine treatment although, in general, large vascular glands are more resistant than small avascular glands. The usual dose for an adult is 15 mCi given by mouth. Antithyroid drugs should be stopped for a few days beforehand and can then be restarted 7–10 days afterwards. There is an acute effect in the first few weeks or months and a more prolonged effect thereafter. The latter means that any patient rendered euthyroid by ^{131}I is at long-term risk of developing hypothyroidism (sometimes as much as 20 years later). Patients should be told of this possibility and reassured that it is easily treated if it occurs. There does not appear to be any increased risk of thyroid or other cancer after ^{131}I therapy. The treatment is obviously contra-indicated in pregnancy, or where there is a significant likelihood of pregnancy.

Follow-up of patients who have been thyrotoxic is important, regardless of the treatment used, as both recurrence and hypothyroidism are difficult to predict and best spotted early. After ^{131}I therapy, patients should have T3, T4 and TSH estimations at lengthening intervals; a rising TSH should warn of the likelihood of impending overt hypothyroidism. Once thyroxine therapy has been started, no special follow-up is needed.

Management of thyrotoxicosis in the elderly

In the elderly, the same principles of management of thyrotoxicosis apply, except that surgery is rarely indicated. Where atrial fibrillation is present, it is advisable to anticoagulate the patient (if there is no contra-indication such as hypertension). Atrial defibrillation may be undertaken, if the patient is off digoxin and does not revert to sinus rhythm spontaneously.

Treatment of toxic adenoma is usually by surgical excision, although in the elderly or frail ^{131}I or long-term drug therapy may be used.

Thyrotoxicosis and pregnancy

A number of autoimmune conditions commonly improve during pregnancy, probably due in part to the high levels of progesterone (which has a mild glucocorticoid action) and in part to increased cortisol production. Thyrotoxicosis often enters remission during pregnancy, and relapses in the puerperium. It is important to avoid overtreatment with antithyroid drugs during pregnancy. In the fetus, these can cause hypothyroidism, increased TSH secretion and thyroid enlargement (which may cause respiratory obstruction in the newborn). It is therefore the rule to keep the mother on the minimum dose needed to maintain euthyroidism, and usually to discontinue the drug in the last four weeks or so of pregnancy.

If the titre of thyroid stimulating antibodies (which can cross the placenta) is high, this may lead to significant thyroid stimulation in the baby, and neonatal thyrotoxicosis. As the titre of antibodies (principally of the IgG subclass) declines, so does the thyrotoxicosis. The infant is treated with beta-blockers and carbimazole until the condition subsides spontaneously. Neonatal thyrotoxicosis can be predicted by measuring maternal TSI. The clinical manifestations do not occur until 1–2 weeks after birth, so prolonged hospital observation of the at-risk neonate is essential.

OTHER THYROID DISORDERS

Simple diffuse goitre

Simple diffuse goitre with euthyroidism is extremely common, especially in women, and seldom requires treatment. The aetiology is poorly understood but, since it usually develops at puberty, oestrogens may be partly responsible. It is TSH-dependent and generally diminishes on treatment with thyroxine in replacement doses. Pseudo-goitre is also common. Here, a normal-sized gland is readily visible because it is high-lying, usually in a girl with a long neck.

Diffuse multinodular goitre

Diffuse multinodular goitre is common, but poorly understood. In Western countries, where salt is iodised, it is now seldom due to iodine deficiency. The high incidence in many underdeveloped parts of the world is almost certainly due to the ingestion of goitrogens, e.g. from the cassava root, which apparently interfere with the organification of iodine. In a goitrous area, there are also other factors (such as mild enzyme deficiencies, and the iodine-drain of recurrent pregnancies) which predispose certain individuals (usually women) to gross degrees of goitre. Eventually, the nodules (which are initially TSH-dependent) may become autonomous. Sudden introduction of high levels of iodine in the diet in such communities has led to epidemics of thyrotoxicosis (the so-called Jod-Basedow phenomenon). This is due in part to unmasking cases of Graves' disease, and in part to cases of multinodular goitre.

Management of multinodular goitre

In the early stages, non-toxic goitre will respond either to suppressing TSH by giving exogenous thyroid hormones, or to removing the cause (goitrogens or iodine deficiency). Once autonomous nodules have developed, TSH suppression with thyroxine is much less effective, and iodine administration carries the risk of precipitating hyperthyroidism. The chances of successful response are highest

Fig. 18.24 Large multinodular goitre.

if TSH levels are not completely suppressed.

Toxic multinodular goitre is usually treated with ^{131}I therapy, though it is often relatively resistant and repeated doses may be needed. Patients should generally be rendered euthyroid with carbimazole first. Where the goitre is large (Fig. 18.24) or causing severe obstructive symptoms (especially pressure on the trachea), surgery is the treatment of choice, especially since ^{131}I therapy may temporarily cause further thyroid enlargement. Tracheal compression is confirmed by soft tissue X-rays of the neck.

Riedel's thyroiditis

Riedel's thyroiditis is a peculiar condition of unknown aetiology associated with woody fibrous infiltration of the thyroid gland and surrounding tissues.

Viral thyroiditis

The condition of viral thyroiditis commonly presents with acute painful generalised swelling of the thyroid gland, fever, elevated protein-bound iodine (due to release of thyroglobulin) and mild transient hypothyroidism. Some cases appear to be due to Coxsackie B viruses.

Localised thyroid swellings

The most important of the localised thyroid swellings is thyroid carcinoma which, however, only accounts for 1–2% of such lesions. Well-differentiated carcinomas may be papillary, follicular or mixed. Anaplastic carcinomas

account for 15% of tumours and are commonest in the elderly. All these tumours are derived from the thyroid epithelial cell and, since they are less efficient than the surrounding normal gland at concentrating iodine, show on thyroid scans as 'cold' nodules. About 5% of thyroid carcinomas are of different origin, being derived from the calcitonin-secreting parafollicular C-cells. These are the medullary carcinomas, associated with high circulating levels of calcitonin. They are sometimes familial and associated with phaeochromocytomas, with or without neurofibromas in the mouth (multiple endocrine adenomatosis type II, see p. 712). Many thyroid adenomas are also cold on scan, but a 'hot' nodule (Fig. 18.22, p. 694) is virtually always benign. Here, the (autonomous) adenoma synthesises and secretes thyroid hormones without the need for TSH stimulation. TSH secretion is switched off, and so the rest of the gland becomes atrophic and inactive. Simple thyroid cysts are common, and also show up on scan as a 'cold' nodule that is cystic on ultrasound. A cystic nodule is not, however, necessarily benign.

Thyroid scans, ultrasound, and fine-needle aspiration with expert cytology are all useful techniques in the differential diagnosis of isolated thyroid swellings. If doubt remains, the nodule is removed surgically. 'Hot' nodules respond well to ^{131}I therapy (p. 700).

Treatment of thyroid cancer

Where possible, thyroid carcinomas are treated surgically. ^{131}I therapy is of value if the carcinoma takes up the isotope, and is required for patients with residual and metastatic disease. Uptake usually only occurs in papillary and follicular tumours. If the patient has had a subtotal thyroidectomy, the remaining normal thyroid is ablated with a high dose of ^{131}I. Replacement therapy is then started and continued for six weeks. It is then withdrawn to allow TSH levels to rise, following which an ablative dose of ^{131}I is given to treat metastatic or persistent local disease. This treatment can be repeated 3–4 monthly as long as isotope scans show persistent metastatic or local disease. Poorly differentiated cancers, and those which do not take up ^{131}I, are treated with radiotherapy to the local tumour. Results of treatment of metastatic disease with chemotherapy are disappointing.

THE ADRENAL GLANDS

ANATOMY AND PHYSIOLOGY

The gross anatomy of the adrenal glands is shown in Fig. 18.25. The adult adrenal glands weigh 4–5 g each, and are situated at the upper poles of the kidneys.

The adrenal cortex

The cortex, whose role is to secrete steroid hormones, consists of a capsule, a subcapsular layer (the zona glo-

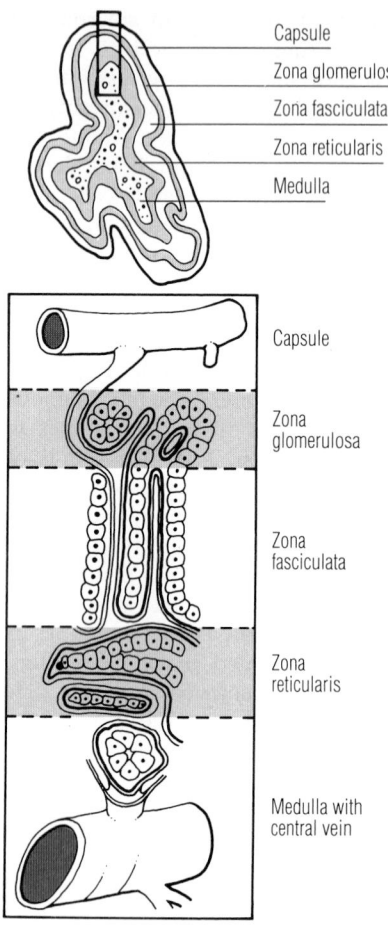

Fig. 18.25 Coronal section through the adrenal gland.

merulosa), the middle zone (zona fasciculata) and a zona reticularis. The latter envelops the adrenal medulla. The blood supply is centripetal, running from the cortex to the medulla; this is probably of great importance in maintaining the structure of the gland, since all the steroid-secreting cells appear to be of common origin. The terminal differentiation of these cells is determined by their location, and by other factors such as local oxygen tension and gradients of steroids. In utero, the glands are much larger, and the cortex is dominated by a large innermost (fetal) zone, which degenerates shortly after birth.

The zona glomerulosa synthesises and secretes mineralocorticoids, of which the most important is aldosterone. The zona fasciculata synthesises cortisol, and the reticularis and fetal zone the weak adrenal androgens, notably dehydroepiandrosterone (DHEA) and its sulphate. The fetal zone appears to develop as a consequence of the high levels of ACTH and oestrogen in utero. Oestrogens impair cortisol synthesis by inhibiting the action of the enzyme 3-β-hydroxysteroid dehydrogenase. On present evidence the existence of a separate adrenal androgen-stimulating hormone seems unlikely. The two-dimensional structures of aldosterone, cortisol and dehydroepiandrosterone sul-

phate are shown in Figure 18.26.

The basic pathways of steroidogenesis in the adrenal cortex are set out in Figure 18.27 (opposite). The differences between the three zones and their function can be narrowed down to the presence or absence of a few critical enzymes.

Fig. 18.26 Two-dimensional structures of three adrenal steroids – aldosterone, cortisol and dehydroepiandrosterone sulphate.

Physiological control of the adrenal cortex

Mineralocorticoids

Aldosterone is much the most potent adrenal steroid on a molar basis; about $100\,\mu g$ is secreted per day as compared to $10\,mg$ for cortisol. Aldosterone acts on intranuclear mineralocorticoid receptors in the distal renal tubule to promote sodium uptake and potassium secretion. Interactions between this sodium retaining system and the secretion and action of the newly discovered atrial natriuretic peptide (ANP) are still being elucidated.

The synthesis and secretion of aldosterone are relatively independent of ACTH secretion. The major control factors are angiotensin II and the extracellular sodium and potassium concentration (Ch. 21, Fig. 21.19). Angiotensin II acts through cell surface receptors, but not by activation of adenylate cyclase (p. 666), and principally stimulates enzymes late in the biosynthetic pathway. The hormonal control of this system is most unusual, since renin is an enzyme secreted by the juxtaglomerular apparatus, which acts on a circulating substrate of hepatic origin to release the decapeptide angiotensin I. This is then converted to the active octapeptide angiotensin II in peripheral tissues, including lung, by angiotensin converting enzyme (ACE).

Glucocorticoids

Glucocorticoids, of which the main one in man is cortisol (hydrocortisone), have a wide range of actions on many

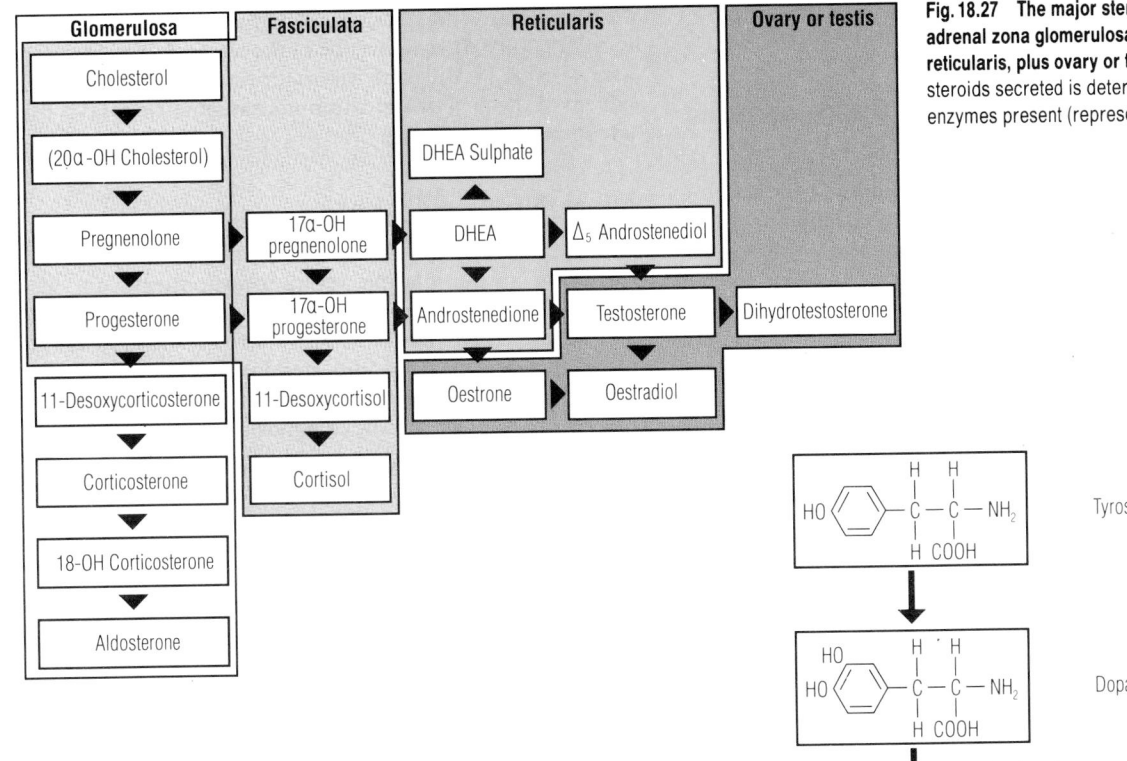

Fig. 18.27 The major steroid pathways in adrenal zona glomerulosa, fasciculata and reticularis, plus ovary or testis. The balance of steroids secreted is determined by the enzymes present (represented by arrows).

Fig. 18.28 Pathway for the biosynthesis of adrenal catecholamines.

different cells and tissues. As their name suggests, they have a major influence on glucose homeostasis, with catabolic actions on tissues such as muscle, and an action on the liver to enhance gluconeogenesis. In their absence, the response to stress of any kind is greatly impaired. Glucocorticoids inhibit the immune system, repair processes and collagen synthesis in bone and soft tissues. They also modify the effect of many other hormones on a range of cell types. Whereas it is relatively easy to define the endocrine role of the gonadal sex steroids (since they clearly integrate a pattern of responses directed at a single common aim), this is more difficult with glucocorticoids, since their actions are very diverse. Glucocorticoids are secreted episodically with a very pronounced diurnal variation. It is probable that glucocorticoids facilitate the immediate requirements of daytime activity while inhibiting other processes, such as tissue repair, which then occur at night.

Adrenal androgens

Apart from their role as oestrogen precursors *in utero*, adrenal androgens appear to be of relatively trivial importance. Increased synthesis before puberty (the adrenarche) contributes to the development of secondary sexual hair. Their control is a matter of continuing controversy.

The adrenal medulla

The adrenal medulla receives a sympathetic nerve supply, which is responsible for initiating adrenaline (epinephrine) secretion in response to stress. Its blood supply comes largely from the adrenal cortex and is therefore very rich

in cortisol. The pathway of adrenaline synthesis from phenylalanine is indicated in Figure 18.28. The last stage of adrenaline synthesis (the methylation of noradrenaline) is cortisol-dependent – cortisol appears to control the synthesis of the enzyme phenylalanine N-methyl transferase. As a consequence of this dependence, pituitary ACTH and adrenal cortisol deficiency also leads to adrenaline deficiency. Glucocorticoids and adrenaline (particularly its α-receptor-mediated effects) also interact in other ways, including at target tissues; indeed in many conditions (e.g.

bronchial asthma) synthetic analogues of these hormones are used together therapeutically.

Adrenal glands and the response to changes in trophic hormones

Chronic ACTH excess leads to hypertrophy of the adrenal cortex, particularly the zona fasciculata-reticularis, and to alterations in the blood vessels. In some individuals, the chronic consequence appears to be multinodular hyperplasia, in which the nodules of hyperplastic tissue tend to become semi-autonomous; rarely, malignant tumours may develop in these nodules.

Chronic ACTH insufficiency leads to adrenal atrophy – particularly of the androgen-secreting zona reticularis. The zona glomerulosa continues to function under the trophic stimulation of angiotensin II, so that the picture is predominantly one of glucocorticoid (and adrenal androgen) deficiency, rather than of mineralocorticoid lack.

INVESTIGATION OF ADRENAL DISORDERS

Recent years have seen dramatic advances in the techniques available for investigating adrenal disorders. Methods once considered essential have been supplanted by more direct, simple, cheap and reliable techniques. For example, chemical methods for the analysis of steroid metabolites have now been largely replaced by radioimmunoassay of the levels of the steroids themselves. The clinical investigator should start with a particular question, (for example, is there primary adrenal insufficiency?) and only use such tests as are necessary to answer the question beyond reasonable doubt.

Cortisol assay

Cortisol assay is useful in many situations and can be conducted directly or indirectly, in plasma, serum or urine. Since direct radioimmunoassays are readily available, the older indirect methods of assessing metabolites (e.g. the urinary 17-hydroxycorticosteroids, and 17-oxogenic steroids) are not often used now. The urinary free cortisol excretion in 24 hours correlates very well with both the cortisol secretion rate (a tedious radio-isotopic measurement) and the mean 24-hour free plasma cortisol level. It is more widely used to diagnose hyper- than hypocortisolism. Serum cortisol assays have the disadvantage that the hormone is normally secreted episodically, so that repeated measurements are usually needed for reliable interpretation. The 11 pm or midnight cortisol assay (often used in the investigation of Cushing's syndrome) has the disadvantage that stress can cause its elevation, even in normal individuals. Also, the patient has to be admitted to hospital first, which makes this an extremely expensive assay to perform.

Assays for precursors of cortisol are of use in diagnosing enzyme deficiencies or assessing drug-induced enzyme blocks; they include 17-hydroxyprogesterone (or its urinary metabolite pregnanetriol) and 11-desoxycortisol.

Unfortunately, the plasma ACTH assay is still fraught with difficulty. It remains one of the least reliable hormone assays even in the best laboratories although, with the advent of the new two-site immunoradiometric assays, this situation should change.

Mineralocorticoid assays

Aldosterone can be measured by radioimmunoassay in serum or urine; plasma renin measurements are also reasonably reliable. Provided the patient is not on diuretics, and the electrolyte levels are known, renin and aldosterone measurements in lying and standing positions are very helpful in the investigation of suspected mineralocorticoid disorders, notably in the diagnosis of primary hyperaldosteronism.

Adrenal androgen assays

Urinary 17-oxosteroid levels are still of use in investigating virilisation. High levels point to excess secretion of (weak) adrenal androgens and a possible adrenal tumour or enzyme defect. Plasma androstenedione and testosterone levels should also be assayed. The serum level of DHEA sulphate is also of value, high levels pointing to an adrenal source of androgen excess.

Use of dynamic function tests

Adrenal function is intrinsically dynamic, and much can be learnt from examining spontaneous changes in activity, e.g. by the serial measurement of serum cortisol levels and its diurnal changes. Several morning and evening samples will be helpful in diagnosing Cushing's syndrome, where there is loss of the diurnal rhythm and levels remain high in the evening. In contrast, there is little point in taking late evening samples in a patient with suspected cortisol deficiency, since cortisol levels are normally low at that time.

Suppression tests

The most useful suppression test involves the administration of dexamethasone (chosen because it does not cross-react with the cortisol assay), with subsequent measurement of serum and urinary cortisol. The *overnight dexamethasone suppression test* involves the patient taking 1–2 mg of dexamethasone orally at 11 pm, with a serum sample taken for cortisol assay the following morning. In a normal individual, dexamethasone suppresses the morning secretion of ACTH so that the morning serum cortisol value is low. This simple overnight test is a useful screening test for Cushing's syndrome. Failure to suppress indicates Cushing's syndrome or excess metabolism of dexamethasone due to enzyme induction by alcohol, or drugs such as phenytoin and carbamazepine. Traditionally, investigation of Cushing's syndrome involves the use of low dose (0.5 mg 6-hourly for 48 hours) and high dose (2 mg, 6-hourly for 48 hours) suppression with dexamethasone;

urine and serum cortisol levels are assayed. In theory (but sometimes not in practice), there is partial suppression on the high dose in pituitary-dependent, but not in other forms of, Cushing's syndrome.

Stimulation tests

Insulin-induced hypoglycaemia is a potent stimulus to ACTH (and hence cortisol) release in normal individuals. Provided its use is not contraindicated, it is the final arbiter in diagnosing ACTH deficiency. A convincing rise in serum cortisol levels to above about 500 nmol/l in the presence of hypoglycaemia indicates that the hypothalamic-pituitary-adrenal axis is intact. Since the stimulus is also effective for testing GH secretion, this test is very useful.

Corticotrophin-releasing factor (CRF) has not so far proved a useful addition to tests of pituitary-adrenal function except, possibly, to distinguish pituitary-dependent ACTH secretion (where ACTH responds to CRF) from ectopic ACTH secretion.

The adrenal can be stimulated directly with ACTH – usually *synthetic 1–24 ACTH* (synacthen) – and the response measured 30–60 minutes after an im dose of 250 μg. Occasional fatal anaphylactic reactions have followed depot-synacthen so, for prolonged stimulation (which is rarely needed), ACTH gel should be used instead.

Metyrapone blocks the last stage in cortisol biosynthesis (Fig. 18.29); ACTH levels rise and the adrenal gland normally responds with increased production of the cortisol precursor 11-desoxycortisol. This in turn is metabolised and excreted as urinary 17-hydroxycorticosteroids. The response is exaggerated in pituitary-dependent Cushing's syndrome. The test can be refined by measurement of ACTH, serum or urine 11-desoxycortisol and cortisol.

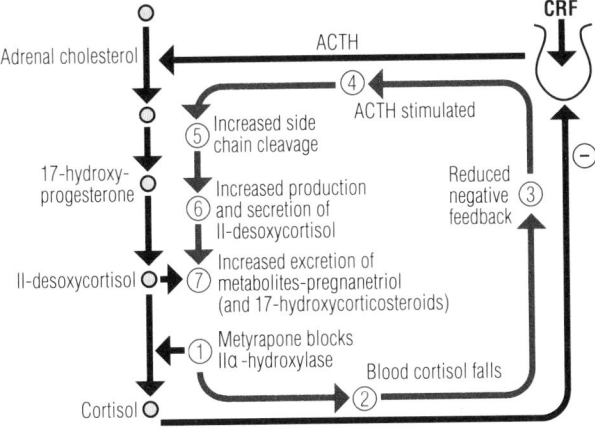

Fig. 18.29 Principles behind the metyrapone test. Metyrapone competitively blocks adrenal 11α-hydroxylase (1). In a normal individual, cortisol falls (2), ACTH rises (3–4) and increased production of precursors (5–7) leads to a rise in 11-desoxycortisol, and increased excretion of metabolites (17-hydroxycorticoids). In Cushing's due to adrenal tumour, no such increase occurs as ACTH is suppressed. In Cushing's disease, there is classically an exaggerated response to metyrapone as tumour-derived ACTH 'drives' the hyperplastic adrenal glands.

However, its diagnostic usefulness is limited and there is a serious risk of producing adrenal insufficiency in cases of primary adrenal tumour where ACTH levels do not rise and partly overcome the effect of the block.

Investigation of the adrenal medulla

The diagnosis of phaeochromocytoma is confirmed by one or more of a number of methods for measuring catecholamines or their metabolites. The simplest is the urinary excretion of vanyl mandelic acid, followed by urinary normetadrenaline. Serum assays for noradrenaline (by a radioenzymatic method) and adrenaline taken lying and standing are also of considerable diagnostic value.

Radiological methods

The advent of *CT scanning* in recent years has constituted a considerable advance in radiological method. It is particularly useful for localising adrenal tumours of the cortex and medulla (Fig. 18.30). Angiographic methods are now seldom required. *Radio-isotope scans* are sometimes of use; those for cortical tumours involve use of a selenium-labelled cholesterol derivative, while those for the medulla use labelled catecholamine precursors.

DISEASES OF THE ADRENAL CORTEX

ADRENO-CORTICAL INSUFFICIENCY

Aetiology

The major causes of adrenal insufficiency are shown in Table 18.9. It may be due to ACTH deficiency, or congenital disorders (notably enzyme defects) or destruction of the adrenal glands. The adrenal glands can be destroyed rapidly or slowly. Acute destruction occurs in septicaemia, particularly due to the meningococcus, and this is responsible for the so-called Waterhouse-Friderichsen syndrome. Meningococcal septicaemia is associated with purpura and haemorrhage, including massive haemorrhagic destruction of the adrenals. (The adrenal glands are particularly susceptible to haemorrhage within them; indeed, ACTH treatment alone causes marked vascular engorgement, and enlargement of perivascular spaces.) Untreated, it leads rapidly to circulatory collapse and death. Recently, introduction of the anaesthetic agent etomidate, which was not previously recognised as an enzyme inhibitor, led to deaths from adrenal insufficiency. Chronic destruction of the adrenal glands is most commonly due to tuberculosis or autoimmune disease, leading to the clinical features of Addison's disease (see below).

The possibility of adrenal insufficiency should always be considered in any patient with circulatory collapse; the picture will vary somewhat depending on whether it is primary or secondary (p. 669). Other causes of adrenal insufficiency tend to be much more insidious. Tuberculosis

705

Table 18.9 Causes of adrenocortical insufficiency

Primary (High ACTH)

Congenital/familial
   Adrenal enzyme defects (usually 21-hydroxylase deficiency)
   Congenital adrenal hypoplasia
   Adrenal leukodystrophy

Acquired
   Infections – tuberculosis†
           – histoplasmosis
   Autoimmune†
   Vascular – meningococcal septicaemia
           and haemorrhagic destruction
         – thrombosis (adrenal vein catheterisation)
   Neoplastic – secondary carcinoma
   Degenerative – amyloid

Secondary (low ACTH)

Hypopituitarism
Isolated ACTH deficiency
Glucocorticoid therapy

Enhanced glucocorticoid metabolism

Drug-induced, e.g. rifampicin*, carbamazepine

* Important – may precipitate adrenal failure if already compromised, e.g. in tuberculosis, accelerated hepatic steroid metabolism. Enhances steroid requirements.
†These commonly present as Addison's disease (chronic adrenal insufficiency with pigmentation).

---

leads to enlargement of the adrenals and, eventually, total destruction of the normal tissue and caseation. Possibly, the high cortisol levels within the adrenal make it difficult to mount the necessary cellular immune response to eradicate the bacteria. In Western countries, the decline in tuberculosis makes autoimmune destruction of the adrenals the commonest cause of chronic adrenal insufficiency.

Adrenal insufficiency is often familial, and associated with a high incidence of other organ-specific autoimmune disease, especially thyroid failure (Schmidt syndrome). There is an association with HLA-B8, which increases the relative risk of developing the disease about twelve-fold.

In the presence of chronic primary adrenocortical insufficiency, there is usually an increase in the individual's normal level of pigmentation, sodium and water depletion, postural hypotension and hyperkalaemia.

Secondary adrenal insufficiency due to hypopituitarism and isolated ACTH deficiency is discussed on page 685.

ADDISON'S DISEASE

Clinical features

The original description of *Addison's disease* was given by Thomas Addison in 1857, and this remains an admirable account of the main features of chronic primary adrenal insufficiency. The speed of onset varies from insidious to sudden. When the onset is insidious, the early symptoms are often extreme and unaccustomed lassitude, somnolence

---

Summary 5 Clinical features of Addison's disease

- Increased pigmentation in mouth, skin creases, pressure areas.
- Crises of hypotension, salt and water loss, hyperkalaemia, hypercalcaemia, hypoglycaemia.
- Associated vitiligo, myxoedema or pernicious anaemia.

---

and depression. Dizziness due to postural hypotension or fasting hypoglycaemia, and nocturia may occur, due to failure to excrete a waterload in the daytime. Frequently, the patient notices an increased pigmentation or simply retention of the summer suntan; as a result the patient may appear 'healthy' to relatives.

In its most dramatic form, the disease presents with Addisonian crisis which, in the absence of effective treatment, is also the terminal picture. The patient is ill and anorexic, with vomiting and abdominal pain, often with rigidity simulating an abdominal emergency. There is usually a fever, tachycardia, hypotension (with a marked postural drop in blood pressure), cramps and postural dizziness, and signs of sodium and water depletion. There is marked loss of skin turgor with loose skin like damp leather and sunken eyes. The blood urea rises because of poor renal perfusion, and the serum potassium concentration is raised. There may be hypercalcaemia, and there is commonly hypoglycaemia.

The features of the associated ACTH excess are variable, and consist of increased pigmentation of skin (especially exposed areas, pressure points, skin creases and recent scars), buccal mucous membrane and sometimes sclerae, and streaked pigmentation of the nail beds. These changes are due to stimulation of melanocytes by ACTH and related peptides with melanocyte-stimulating activity.

Of the other clinical features, those due to mineralocorticoid deficiency – principally the sodium and water depletion, hyperkalaemia and hypercalcaemia – are unique to primary adrenal failure, and are absent or much less marked in secondary adrenal failure. The serum sodium concentration is usually low in both conditions, in part due to excessive secretion of ADH. Features due to glucocorticoid deficiency include hypoglycaemia (more marked in pituitary insufficiency since growth hormone is also usually lacking), inability to respond to stress and infection, and also, in part at least, hypotension and pyrexia. The white cell count is usually elevated, with a neutrophil leukocytosis and an elevated eosinophil count.

Other clinical features which should immediately suggest a diagnosis of adrenal insufficiency are the presence of other forms of organ-specific autoimmune disease (e.g. hypothyroidism, pernicious anaemia, or vitiligo) or a history, or signs of, tuberculosis.

Investigation

A high index of suspicion is important in the diagnosis of Addison's disease. Once suspected, the appropriate blood samples should be taken for electrolyte and cortisol assay, and treatment instituted forthwith. Hyperkalaemia (with or without a low serum sodium concentration) in a patient with Addisonian-type pigmentation, hypotension and fluid depletion, is suggestive of primary adrenal insufficiency. In pituitary insufficiency, aldosterone secretion generally persists, and so hyperkalaemia is not usually seen. Inappropriate ADH secretion is common in pituitary insufficiency, however, and leads to a low serum sodium concentration. In Addison's disease, circulatory collapse and unexplained pyrexia are common, as are non-specific T wave abnormalities on ECG.

Clotted blood should be taken for a serum cortisol assay. If time permits, synacthen (250mg im) may be given and the sampling for cortisol assay repeated after 30–60 minutes. There will be a poor or absent response to this short synacthen test in both primary and secondary insufficiency since, in the latter, long-standing ACTH deficiency makes the gland slow to respond. Immediate treatment should be instituted forthwith (see below). The diagnosis can always be confirmed or refuted the next day.

Further investigations include tests for adrenal (and other) auto-antibodies, plain X-ray of abdomen (to show adrenal calcification due to tuberculosis) and CT scanning of the adrenals (Fig. 18.30).

Fig. 18.30 CT scan of the adrenal glands. The scan shows a tumour (arrowed) in a patient with Cushing's syndrome.

Treatment

Immediate treatment is with fluids, electrolytes and hydrocortisone (100–200 mg iv, then 100 mg in 6 hours, with subsequent doses tapered down to replacement doses). Mineralocorticoid therapy is only required when the dose of hydrocortisone is being reduced to 2–3 times normal replacement doses (i.e. about 60 mg/day), and then only in primary adrenal insufficiency.

Long-term management of adrenal failure is generally simple if the patient is co-operative. Glucocorticoid and mineralocorticoid replacement are required. It is not possible to simulate precisely the normal pattern of hormone secretion, since cortisol is normally secreted episodically. Cortisol itself can be conveniently given as hydrocortisone in a split dose which, for an adult, is normally 20 mg on rising, and 10 mg at about 5 pm. Alternatively, cortisone acetate can be used (equivalent doses being 25 and 12.5 mg). The only disadvantage is that, with this form of replacement, peak cortisol levels occur a little later, since the drug has to be converted to cortisol by the liver. The process may thus be disturbed in liver disease. There is generally little advantage in using synthetic glucocorticoids, such as prednisolone or dexamethasone.

Aldosterone is inactive when given by mouth, so mineralocorticoid replacement is normally given with the synthetic mineralocorticoid fludrocortisone (0.05–0.2 mg daily). The dose is normally adjusted empirically according to blood pressure and serum potassium levels. About half of Addisonian patients do not need mineralocorticoid therapy, because zona glomerulosa function may be spared and replacement glucocorticoids have a weak mineralocorticoid effect.

Patients on long-term steroid replacement should be given a special card clearly stating the steroids that they are on, and asked to ensure that they keep it with them at all times. It is important that additional glucocorticoid is given in emergencies. If the patient has a gastrointestinal upset he should be given an increased dose parenterally.

Some drugs increase steroid requirements because they accelerate steroid metabolism; this occurs particularly with anticonvulsants and the antituberculous drug rifampicin, which is given as part of triple chemotherapy if tuberculosis is the cause of Addison's disease.

ADRENAL ENZYME DEFECTS

Adrenal enzyme defects are rare disorders which should be managed by the endocrine specialist. The pathways of steroidogenesis and the defects associated with them are discussed on pages 702–704. The principle defects affecting the adrenal glands exclusively are 21-hydroxylase and 11-hydroxylase deficiency (Fig. 18.31).

21-hydroxylase deficiency

21-hydroxylase deficiency is inherited as a recessive condition. It is due to a mutation in the gene for 21-hydroxylase, which gene is located on chromosome 6, close to the HLA tissue-type locus. The frequency of the defective gene is about one in 40, which gives a frequency of the disorder of $1/4 \times (1/40)^2$, or about one in 7400 births. Almost one-third of cases have a severe form and, if untreated, develop severe mineralocorticoid deficiency and salt loss. The remaining two-thirds are able to maintain adequate aldosterone secretion and generally present with the side-effects of androgen excess, or with glucocorticoid insufficiency in the face of stress.

Female infants with the condition are usually recognised

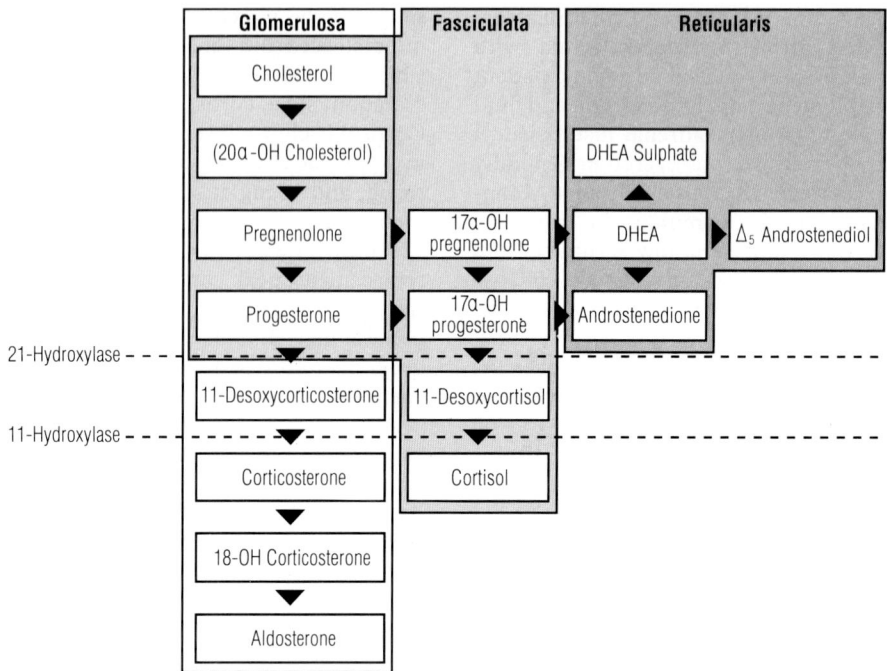

Fig. 18.31 Normal adrenal steroid pathways with sites of action of 21-hydroxylase and 11-hydroxylase, the two enzymes most commonly defective in congenital adrenal hyperplasia.

at birth, because of their ambiguous (virilised) external genitalia, before salt deficiency can develop. Some mildly affected females do not have any genital virilisation at birth, but develop it instead at puberty, when they present with hirsutism, amenorrhoea and clitoral enlargement. This situation is, however, extremely uncommon.

Male infants appear normally virilised. Salt-losing males present with acute adrenal insufficiency and sodium and water depletion, usually within the first few weeks of life. The mortality is therefore much higher with male infants and the cause of death may not be recognised unless previous affected siblings have drawn attention to its likelihood. Non-salt-losing males will present with accelerated growth and sexual development but small testes (sexual precocity and pseudo-puberty). Ultimate height is reduced and, if treatment with replacement glucocorticoids is delayed until the epiphyseal bone age has advanced to 11 years or more, affected males often undergo true precocious puberty.

Once suspected, the diagnosis is easily made by measurement of plasma, salivary or urinary levels of 17-hydroxy-progesterone or its urinary metabolite pregnanetriol, with or without ACTH stimulation.

The importance of early diagnosis in female infants, and the use of corrective genital surgery are discussed on page 723 under disorders of sex differentiation. Replacement therapy is with glucocorticoids and mineralocorticoids as for Addison's disease. A middle way must be found between over-treatment (with the associated side-effects, especially for glucocorticoids) and under-treatment (with consequent androgen excess).

11-hydroxylase deficiency

Deficiency of 11-hydroxylase (Fig. 18.31) is only about a fifth as common as 21-hydroxylase deficiency. It also causes the 'adreno-genital syndrome', but the androgen excess is generally less marked and the picture is dominated instead by the presence of hypertension. This is due to ACTH-induced excessive secretion of 11-desoxy-corticosterone (DOC). When glucocorticoid therapy is introduced, ACTH and DOC levels fall, and insufficiency of the zona glomerulosa is uncovered. The blood pressure falls and sodium depletion and potassium excess may result unless the condition is also treated with fludrocortisone.

ADRENO-CORTICAL EXCESS (CUSHING'S SYNDROME)

The diagnosis and treatment of the disorders which lead to adrenal glucocorticoid excess (Cushing's syndrome) remain problematic, and are therefore best conducted in specialist endocrinology units. The conditions are relatively rare, but very troublesome.

Aetiology

Cushing's syndrome is either ACTH-dependent, or independent (Table 18.10). In the latter event, it is either caused by a steroid-secreting tumour (carcinoma or adenoma) of the adrenal cortex or else is iatrogenic (due to excessive glucocorticoid therapy). Adrenal tumours generally predominate in children and young adults; adenoma

Table 18.10 Causes of Cushing's syndrome

Cause	Example
ACTH-driven	
Pituitary-dependent	Pituitary hyperplasia
	Pituitary adenoma*
	Pituitary carcinoma
	CRF-secreting tumour**
	Hypothalamic
	Ectopic
Ectopic ACTH secretion	Tumours
	Oat cell carcinoma
	Bronchial carcinoid
	Medullary thyroid carcinoma
	Pancreatic carcinoma
	Phaeochromocytoma
ACTH therapy	
Non-ACTH-driven	Adrenal adenoma
	Adrenal carcinoma
	Glucocorticoid therapy
Doubtful or mixed aetiology	Multinodular hyperplasia
	Alcohol-induced 'pseudo'-Cushing's

* 'Cushing's disease'
** Very rare

is the easiest form of the syndrome to treat.

ACTH-dependent causes are of pituitary or non-pituitary origin. Pituitary Cushing's syndrome is due to a pituitary basophil adenoma (*Cushing's disease*), or to hyperplasia. The latter may be due to intrinsic hypothalamic disease, chronic alcoholism or endogenous depression. Since depression is, in turn, a common result of ACTH excess, it can cause obvious diagnostic difficulties. Some rare cases are due to secretion of a corticotrophin-releasing factor by a hypothalamic or extra-hypothalamic tumour.

Ectopic ACTH syndrome is the term given to Cushing's syndrome caused by ACTH secretion from a tumour outside the pituitary gland. The commonest types are carcinoid tumours in the bronchus, thymus and pancreas, small cell lung cancer and thymoma. Pancreatic carcinoma, medullary thyroid carcinoma and phaeochromocytoma are other rare causes. It is now recognised that non-endocrine tissues can synthesise a variety of peptide and non-peptide hormones and growth factors. Indeed, tumours that occasionally secrete ACTH, such as small cell lung cancer, sometimes also secrete other ACTH-related peptides, as well as calcitonin and bombesin. Bombesin may act as an autocrine growth factor, and stimulate cell growth by binding to receptors on the same cell.

Multinodular adrenal hyperplasia is a rare variant of pituitary-dependent Cushing's syndrome in which, probably as a long-term consequence of high ACTH levels, the adrenal glands become hyperplastic with semi-autonomous or autonomous nodules. Occasionally, frank carcinoma may develop in one of the nodules.

Clinical features

Common features

Features common to all forms of Cushing's syndrome are those due to glucocorticoid excess. These include centripetal obesity, proximal muscle weakness and wasting, thin skin, increased sebaceous gland activity and acne (p. 1147), striae, poor wound healing, thin bones due to osteoporosis, hypertension, vascular calcification, diabetes mellitus, peptic ulceration, depression and psychosis (Fig. 18.32). Because they lack the protective effect of androgens, women (and especially post-menopausal women), are particularly susceptible to the catabolic effect of glucocorticoid excess. Mild hirsutism is common and is due to adrenal androgen as well as glucocorticoid excess. In men, LH and testosterone secretion may be inhibited, and libido consequently reduced.

Features unique to specific forms

Cushing's syndrome that disappears or diminishes under hospital scrutiny is commonly alcohol-induced. Some

Fig. 18.32 Classical features of severe Cushing's syndrome.

Summary 6 Clinical features of Cushing's syndrome

- Central obesity, moon face, buffalo hump
- Proximal myopathy
- Osteoporosis
- Striae and poor wound healing
- Depression and psychosis
- Hypertension
- Diabetes mellitus

Table 18.11 Investigation of suspected Cushing's syndrome

1. **Clinical assessment**	
2. **If suspicion:**	24-hour urine free cortisol Overnight dexamethasone suppression
If no suspicion:	No tests necessary
3. **If one or both abnormal:**	Admit Plasma electrolytes Further 24-hour cortisol Circadian blood cortisol ACTH levels Formal dexamethadone suppression (2 mg/day)
If both normal:	Reassure

4. **If abnormal, find cause:**	Alcohol? – Withdraw and reassess
	Ectopic ACTH? – CXR and mediastinal CT
	Adrenal tumour? – Adrenal CT
	  Steroid metabolites
	  ACTH levels
	Pituitary dependent? – High dose dexamethasone
	  Pituitary CT
	  Metyrapone test

If normal:	Reassure/observe
5. **Treat**	

other forms of pituitary-dependent Cushing's syndrome may be cyclical. Addisonian-type pigmentation suggests marked ACTH excess, which is found most often with the ectopic ACTH syndrome (unless the adrenals have been removed, when it suggests Nelson's syndrome; see below and p. 685). The presence of profound hypokalaemia suggests the ectopic ACTH syndrome. Abnormalities on pituitary X-ray are extremely uncommon, even with a pituitary adenoma, except after bilateral adrenalectomy. The ectopic ACTH syndrome due to a small cell carcinoma of lung may not be attended by centripetal obesity, because of cachexia and rapid dissemination of the tumour.

Investigation

The investigation of suspected Cushing's syndrome is summarised in Table 18.11. The difficulties have been discussed under dynamic testing. The low 24-hour urinary free cortisol excretion and overnight low dose dexamethasone test (p. 704) are the mainstays of initial diagnosis. Adrenal radiology with a CT scan (Fig. 18.30, p. 707) is of great importance in diagnosis and localisation of adrenal tumours, as is the (suppressed) plasma ACTH level. Pituitary radiology – including high resolution CT scanning with iv injection of contrast medium – is often surprisingly unhelpful (and occasionally misleading) in the investigation of Cushing's syndrome. Pituitary tumours are usually small, and rarely cause any distortion of the pituitary fossa. CT scan of the thorax may reveal a small bronchial or thymic carcinoid which is the source of ectopic ACTH.

Treatment

Drug therapy

Drugs, such as metyrapone and aminoglutethimide, that inhibit adrenal steroidogenesis, have a place in the preoperative, and occasionally also the long-term, management of Cushing's syndrome. Steroid production can readily be inhibited in patients with adrenal tumours by the 11-hydroxylase inhibitor metyrapone. Indeed, there is real risk of inducing adrenal insufficiency. The dose (250–750 mg every 4 hours, omitting 4 am dosage) should be titrated against the serum and urinary cortisol response. Before surgery, it is wise for the patient to be treated with metyrapone for several weeks to improve wound healing.

Palliative drug therapy in ectopic ACTH syndrome generally requires the simultaneous use of metyrapone and aminoglutethimide to block biosynthesis of cortisol; the dose is titrated against cortisol secretion. The DDT analogue ortho, para, dichloro-diphenyl-dichlorophenazone (O'p'DDD) also has an established place in the management of adrenal carcinoma; it induces adrenal cell necrosis and may produce prolonged remissions. Cytotoxic chemotherapy is the treatment of choice for small cell lung cancer, but the prognosis of the disease is especially poor when accompanied by ectopic ACTH secretion.

Adrenal surgery

Surgery is clearly indicated for an adrenal adenoma or carcinoma, where this is thought to be operable. In a young person, and even when not totally resectable, removal of the bulk of a carcinoma may be indicated in order to maximise the efficacy of chemotherapy. Surgery is also the treatment of choice for carcinoid tumours causing ectopic ACTH secretion.

Bilateral adrenalectomy was formerly the preferred treatment for Cushing's disease. This has the advantage of eliminating the possibility of cortisol excess (provided no remnant is left behind). The disadvantages are that it involves major surgery, with a significant mortality, and also a significant (10–20%) risk of developing *Nelson's syndrome* – the condition of hyperpigmentation, increasing ACTH excess, and an expanding pituitary tumour. The syndrome probably only develops where there is already a semi-autonomous ACTH-secreting pituitary tumour, which has previously been kept under partial restraint by the high circulating cortisol levels. Many centres now combine bilateral adrenalectomy for Cushing's disease with external pituitary radiation, to minimise the risk of this unpleasant complication. Bilateral adrenalectomy is probably the treatment of choice in multinodular adrenal hyperplasia.

Pituitary surgery

Having excluded, as far as is possible, the ectopic ACTH syndrome and an adrenal tumour, most endocrinologists would now refer the patient with pituitary-dependent Cushing's syndrome (Cushing's disease) to an expert centre for surgery by the trans-sphenoidal route. If a tumour is present it is removed; if not, then as much as possible of the pituitary gland is resected. Hypopituitarism (with replacement therapy) is generally preferable to continuing active Cushing's syndrome.

Pituitary radiotherapy

Pituitary radiotherapy can be an effective treatment for Cushing's disease and may be given either by external irradiation or by pituitary implantation of radioactive seeds of ^{90}yttrium. The latter is now rarely used. The major problems of external radiotherapy are slow onset of action for a disease where treatment is relatively urgent. Radiotherapy may be particularly useful in the elderly or frail patient with moderately active disease, who has shown some hormonal response to drug therapy.

In summary, there is no single universally effective treatment, probably because Cushing's syndrome is not a single condition but a group of conditions. Practices vary in different places, often depending upon the relevant therapeutic expertise available locally.

TUMOURS OF THE ADRENAL CORTEX

Tumours of the adrenal cortex may be functioning or non-functioning; the latter secrete either no steroids, or weak steroids (for example pregnenolone) with little or no biological activity. The mode of presentation of the tumour generally depends upon the nature and amount of steroid being produced. Recognised consequences are Cushing's syndrome (cortisol secretion), Conn's syndrome (mineralocorticoid), virilisation (usually weak adrenal androgens, but sometimes testosterone) and feminisation (oestrogens). With the exception of aldosterone-secreting tumours, the tumour is likely to be quite large by the time of presentation and readily detectable on an adrenal CT scan. Sometimes, other techniques are indicated to establish the diagnosis, such as scanning with radio-labelled cholesterol, or adrenal vein catheterisation and blood sampling for hormone assay. Treatment is by surgery, after appropriate medical treatment.

DISORDERS OF ALDOSTERONE SECRETION

The basic components (renin, angiotensin and aldosterone) of the mineralocorticoid system are discussed on page 702. In addition, the heart is also now known to be involved in salt and water homeostasis, through the recently discovered atrial natriuretic peptide (ANP). This peptide is produced by endocrine cells in the right atrium, and acts on the renal tubule to cause a sodium diuresis (Ch. 21, p. 789). The principal recognised disorders of aldosterone secretion are hypo- and hyperaldosteronism.

Hypoaldosteronism

Hypoaldosteronism may be a result of general adrenal insufficiency due to destruction of the adrenal glands (p. 705), or it may occur in the presence of normal secretion of other adrenal steroids. The disorder may be primary, due to a selective adrenal enzyme deficiency late in the aldosterone pathway, or secondary to isolated renin deficiency. This occurs quite commonly in long-standing diabetes mellitus, and may be a consequence of autonomic neuropathy, since beta-adrenergic stimulation is normally a stimulus to renin secretion from the juxta-glomerular apparatus. Aldosterone deficiency is manifested by a tendency to sodium depletion, hypotension and hyperkalaemia. Treatment is with fludrocortisone.

Hyperaldosteronism

Primary hyperaldosteronism (Conn's syndrome) is a rare cause of a generally mild hypertension and hypokalaemia. It is caused either by an adrenal adenoma, or by zona glomerulosa hyperplasia. The diagnosis is confirmed by the finding of elevated serum aldosterone, and low renin levels, and by the clinical response to a therapeutic trial of spironolactone. Treatment is with spironolactone or (in the case of definite adenoma) adrenal surgery. Some cases respond to low doses of dexamethasone.

Secondary hyperaldosteronism is a common physiological adaptation seen in such disorders as congestive cardiac failure, accelerated hypertension, cirrhosis of the liver and nephrotic syndrome. Reduced renal perfusion is the major stimulus to increased renin secretion, angiotensin II production and aldosterone secretion, and thus to sodium retention and potassium excretion. Aldosterone antagonists, such as spironolactone, or drugs which act on the distal tubule sodium pump (such as amiloride) are commonly used in its treatment. Rarely, hyperaldosteronism is caused by a renin-secreting tumour of the kidney.

THE ADRENAL MEDULLA

Adrenaline (epinephrine) is the major product of the normal adrenal medulla; 90% of the adrenaline in the circulation arises from this gland; the remainder is produced in the central nervous system. The main path-

Endocrine Diseases

ways of adrenal catecholamine synthesis are shown in Fig. 18.28. It is of particular importance in the acute response to stress, causing increased alertness, tachycardia, nervousness, glucose and fat mobilisation and inhibition of insulin secretion.

Adrenal medullary insufficiency is of importance in the impairment of the response to hypoglycaemia in hypopituitarism and in generalised autonomic neuropathy (the Shy-Drager syndrome). It may play a part in so-called idiopathic hypoglycaemia of infancy.

ADRENAL MEDULLARY EXCESS

There is no doubt that the adrenal cortex and medulla are integrated in their response to stress. The stimulus is ACTH secretion for the cortex and neural activation for the adrenal medulla. Cortisol is necessary for adrenaline biosynthesis, and glucocorticoids and catecholamines interact at the target tissues, the former potentiating beta-adrenergic effects, for example. In thyrotoxicosis, many of the effects (symptoms and signs) are those of catecholamine excess. This is not because adrenaline secretion is increased (it is normal), but because thyroid hormones augment the target organ sensitivity to catecholamines, particularly their beta-adrenergic effects. Many of the symptoms and signs of thyrotoxicosis – nervousness, tremor, palpitations, sweating, lid retraction and lid lag – can be blocked by administration of a small dose of a beta-blocking drug.

Phaeochromocytoma

Phaeochromocytomas are tumours of the adrenal medulla and are, fortunately, rare. The usual figure quoted is 1 per 1000 cases of hypertension; however, in a large autopsy series from the Mayo Clinic, three-quarters of the patients found to have had phaeochromocytoma were undiagnosed during life, so the true incidence may be considerably higher. Death in cases previously undiagnosed is commonly from cardiovascular disease or cerebral haemorrhage. The tumours are usually located in the adrenal medulla, with 10% being in extra adrenal chromaffin tissue, usually in the sympathetic chain in the abdomen. Most predominantly secrete noradrenaline. Ten per cent of all phaeochromocytomas are malignant. They can occur at any age but present most commonly between 40 and 60 years of age. They may be associated with neuro-fibromatosis, tuberous sclerosis, and with the Sturge-Weber (p. 900) and von Hippel-Lindau syndromes (p. 900). They may be multiple, and are a component of one form (type II) of the syndrome of multiple endocrine neoplasia (MEN, see below). Other components of this syndrome are medullary thyroid carcinoma, hyperparathyroidism, and neurofibromas of the tongue.

Clinical features

The history is of 'attacks' of headache, sweating, palpitations, flushing and nervousness. The blood pressure is generally moderately raised and becomes grossly so during 'attacks', which may be precipitated by exercise or abdominal palpation. Because the hypertension is accompanied by secondary volume depletion, there is commonly a significant drop in blood pressure on standing; this is unusual in untreated hypertension from other causes.

Investigation

Diagnosis of phaeochromocytoma is made by measurement of plasma levels of noradrenaline, or its urinary precursors or metabolites – vanylmandelic acid (VMA), and normetadrenaline. When carried out in specialised laboratories these tests, particularly plasma noradrenaline, are very reliable. The paroxysmal nature of the secretion may lead to normal plasma levels being obtained at times and repeated blood and urine measurements may therefore be necessary. The tumour can be localised by adrenal CT scan. Occasionally, radio-isotope scanning with a radio-labelled catecholamine precursor is helpful to demonstrate an ectopic site. Pharmacological tests using the α-adrenergic blocker phentolamine with blood pressure monitoring are seldom used, because the response to them is erratic and sometimes excessive.

Treatment

The principles of treatment of phaeochromocytoma are to start with pharmacological measures, namely adrenergic blockade (initially with the α-adrenoreceptor blocking agent phenoxybenzamine), followed a few days later by beta-blockade (e.g. with propranolol). Seven to ten days should be allowed before surgery for volume repletion. During surgery, blood pressure is closely monitored and any elevation treated with an intravenous infusion of phentolamine (an α-adrenoreceptor antagonist).

Multiple endocrine neoplasia (MEN)

There are at least three different syndromes associated with multiple neoplasia of endocrine glands (Table 18.12); in each case, inheritance is autosomal dominant. The involved glands may be the subject of hyperplasia, adenoma, or carcinoma development, and different glands may be involved in different individuals in the same family.

In MEN type I (Wermer's syndrome), hyperparathyroidism due to parathyroid hyperplasia is present in 95% of cases at the time of diagnosis. Major morbidity and mortality results from the development of pancreatic tumour, notably insulin-secreting islet cell tumours causing hypoglycaemia, and gastrinomas causing intractable peptic ulceration (Zollinger-Ellison syndrome). Pituitary tumours (prolactinomas, growth hormone or ACTH-secreting) are also common, and carcinoid tumours too are recognised as part of the syndrome.

MEN types II and III share, in common with type I, the occurrence of hypercalcaemia due to parathyroid hyperplasia. In both, the components include medullary cell thyroid carcinoma (calcitonin-secreting) and phaeochromocytoma. The former occurs in virtually all cases,

Table 18.12 Multiple endocrine neoplasia (MEN)

Type	Inheritance	Major glands/areas involved	Clinical features
I (Wermer)	Autosomal dominant	Parathyroid Pancreas Anterior pituitary Bronchus, bowel	Hypercalcaemia Insulinoma Gastrinoma Glucagonoma Prolactinoma Acromegaly Cushing's syndrome Carcinoid tumours
II (Sipple)*	Autosomal dominant	Thyroid (C cell) Adrenal medulla Parathyroid	Medullary carcinoma (High calcitonin) Phaeochromocytoma Hypercalcaemia
III (mucosal neurinoma)**	Autosomal dominant	Thyroid (C cell) Adrenal medulla Tongue etc.	Medullary carcinoma (high calcitonin) Phaeochromocytoma Mucosal neurinoma Marfanoid habitus

* Sometimes referred to as IIa
** Sometimes referred to as IIb

and the latter in about half. MEN type III is similar to type II but does not include hyperparathyroidism and is associated with mucosal neurinomas and with a body habitus similar to Marfan's syndrome (p. 93), but without the lens subluxation and cardiovascular problems.

Families with hypercalcaemic MEN type I or II should be distinguished from familial hypocalciuric hypercalcaemia (p. 741); this condition is also inherited as an autosomal dominant but lacks the association with endocrine tumours.

The MEN syndromes appear to be related to deletions of a regulating gene or genes, such that a further mutation of its pair in an endocrine cell can lead to the cell's uncontrolled proliferation.

THE TESTES

ANATOMY AND PHYSIOLOGY

The testes have a crucial early role in the male fetus in determining that primary sex differentiation is male. After puberty, they serve the dual function of spermatogenesis and androgen (testosterone) production. The initial gonadotrophin stimulation in utero comes principally from the placental hormone human chorionic gonadotrophin (HCG). However, during and after puberty, the stimulation comes from the pituitary via its two gonadotrophins, follicle stimulating hormone (FSH) and luteinising hormone (LH).

The testes in utero: sex differentiation

After the primitive germ cells have been joined by steroid-producing cells, the primitive 'indifferent' gonads develop in fetuses of both sexes. Much of the current knowledge on the role of the testes was obtained more than 40 years ago, in pioneering experiments by the French biologist Alfred Jost on rabbit fetuses. The presence of the Y chromosome is believed to determine the production of the so-called HY antigen which dictates early in utero (at around 6–7 weeks in man) that the 'indifferent' gonad becomes a testis. Shortly thereafter, two pairs of duct systems, the Müllerian and the Wolffian, extend from the region of the gonads to the genital groove. The basic pattern of sex differentiation, which requires no hormonal function for its persistence, is female. In the absence of testes, the Müllerian ducts persist and become the uterus and Fallopian tubes, and the Wolffian ducts disappear. The Sertoli cells of the developing testes produce a peptide hormone, the anti-Müllerian hormone, which causes the Müllerian ducts to disappear permanently.

The major pathway of steroidogenesis that leads to testosterone production occurs in the Leydig cells and is shown in Figure 18.27 (p. 703). At around 12 weeks, testosterone is secreted, under stimulation from HCG, and acts on the Wolffian ducts which contain androgen receptors. This permanently 'imprints' a message on the cells of the Wolffian ducts that ensures they persist to form the male internal genital ducts. If testosterone is absent at this time, the Wolffian duct cells die and are resorbed. Persistence of the Wolffian ducts does not require conversion of testosterone to dihydrotestosterone.

The development of the external genitalia is also dictated by androgen secretion from the Leydig cells at around 12–14 weeks. Full virilisation involves fusion of the labioscrotal folds to form a scrotum, enlargement of the genital tubercle (to become a penis) and the incorporation into the latter of a penile urethra. Both these effects and development of the prostate require conversion of testosterone to 5-α-dihydrotestosterone; this occurs by local action of the enzyme 5-α-reductase in target tissues.

713

18

Later in utero, at around 20 weeks, pituitary secretion of LH and FSH commences. HCG secretion reaches a peak at around 12 weeks and subsequently declines.

The testes in infancy and childhood

Late in utero or shortly after birth the testes, guided by the gubernaculum to the inguinal canal, descend to their final site in the scrotum. During the first six months of extra-uterine life, there is a transient rise in plasma levels of LH and secretion of testosterone. Since levels of the plasma binding protein, sex hormone binding globulin (SHBG) also rise during the first week of life (for reasons as yet uncertain), plasma testosterone levels in early infancy are in the low adult male range (although free testosterone levels are lower). Gradually, however, and probably under the influence of the pineal gland, activity of the hypo-thalamo-pituitary-testis axis subsides, and remains low throughout childhood.

The testes in puberty

The first endocrine event of puberty is the onset of pulsatile secretion of LH during sleep; this initiates pulsatile noc-turnal secretion of testosterone (Table 18.13). Levels of FSH also rise and this, together with testosterone from the Leydig cells, stimulates spermatogenesis. During the course of puberty, the volume of the testes increases some 20-fold from about 1 ml to 15–25 ml each; 95% of the volume of the testes consists of the tubules and their con-tents. The interstitial (Leydig) cells are the sole source of de novo steroidogenesis, which occurs under stimulation of LH. The action of LH is via specific cell surface receptors, mediated principally by cyclic-AMP. FSH also acts via surface receptors and cyclic-AMP, but on the Sertoli cells. The Sertoli cells are now known to be crucial in the control of spermatogenesis. Beyond the stage of Type A spermatogonia, the germ cells are enclosed in the cytoplasm of Sertoli cells (Fig. 18.33). Adjacent Sertoli cells form tight junctions which ensure that the germ cells and con-tents of the tubule are kept secluded by a very effective 'blood-testis barrier'.

During puberty, systemic secretion of testosterone initially occurs only at night-time, but later, as LH levels rise during the day, throughout the 24 hours. Testosterone and, in some tissues, dihydrotestosterone, leads to pro-

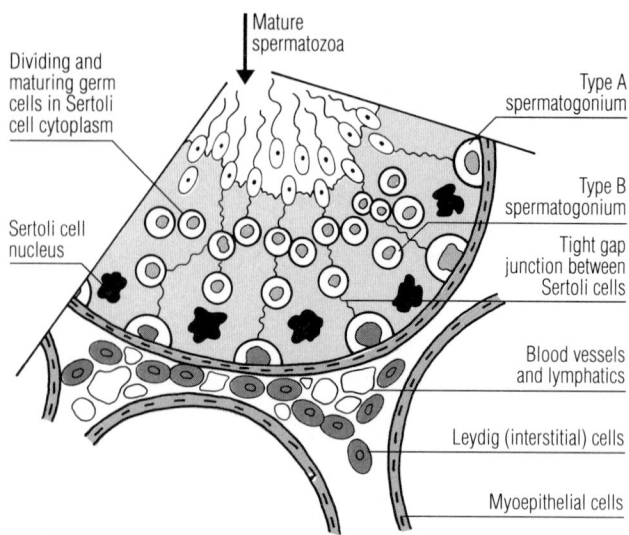

Fig. 18.33 Relationship between testicular tubules (cut in cross-section) and interstitial (Leydig) cells. Only type A spermatogonia lie outside the Sertoli cells (pink) and so outside the blood-testis barrier.

gressive development of secondary sexual characteristics. In man, these include: enlargement and development of external and internal genitalia; muscular development; growth of long bones followed by closure of the epiphyses; and male sex drive and sexual behaviour including noc-turnal emissions and masturbation. There is no evidence that homosexuality is in any way related to abnormal sex hormone levels. Since oestradiol is also produced by con-version from testosterone, in amounts otherwise sufficient to cause breast development, there is strong evidence to suggest that testosterone is responsible for inhibiting breast development in males. Plasma SHBG levels decline by about 50% during male puberty.

The testes in adult life

In men, there is no evidence of an abrupt decline in gonadal function in old age equivalent to that of the female meno-pause. This is because there is a constant supply of new germ cells from mitotic division of Type A spermatogonia; in women, the supply of oöcytes declines progressively even from before birth, and eventually none remain.

Table 18.13 Actions of luteinising hormone (LH) and follicle stimulating hormone (FSH)

Hormone	Effect on testis	Effect on ovary		
		Follicular phase	Midcycle	Luteal
LH	Stimulates Leydig cells to produce testosterone, which has local and general effects	Theca cell androgen secretion	Midcycle surge induces ovulation and luteinisation	Sustains corpus luteum until HCG from blastocyst takes over
FSH	Stimulates Sertoli cells. With local testosterone, regulates spermatogenesis	Stimulates next cohort of follicles, and growth of dominant follicle	Small midcycle surge possibly helps ovum maturation	FSH prepares next crop of follicles if no pregnancy

CLINICAL ASSESSMENT OF TESTICULAR FUNCTION

The clinical assessment of testicular function depends upon the age of the subject. A detailed history of sexual activity is important. For example, if a patient has normal nocturnal erections and ejaculation (wet dreams or masturbation), a complaint of lack of potency (erection or ejaculation) during intercourse is unlikely to be due to androgen deficiency. Assessment of testicular size can best be made by reference to an orchidometer – a series of ovoids of known volume. Small testes are usually a sign of damage to the seminiferous tubules. Examination of external genitalia will also determine if there has been any failure of intra-uterine virilisation. Failure of normal pubertal development may be associated with a degree of growth failure or, conversely, with excessive growth of the long bones before epiphyses close so that span exceeds height. Female fat distribution, gynaecomastia and failure of development of secondary sexual hair are also features of failure of pubertal development, but the latter is most difficult to interpret in view of great inherited variability in potential for body hair.

Where the patient is normally virilised and the clinical problem is subfertility, examination for proper scrotal descent or previous damage (leading to a small testis or testes) and varicocele (which may depress the sperm count) is important. Phimosis should be specifically excluded.

DEFECTIVE TESTICULAR FUNCTION IN UTERO

Defective testicular function in utero leads to male pseudo-hermaphroditism. The major causes are listed in Table 18.14. The defects in testosterone and dihydrotestosterone biosynthesis are inherited as autosomal recessive disorders and are extremely rare. They are discussed below, under disorders of sex differentiation (p. 723).

DEFECTIVE TESTICULAR FUNCTION IN ADULT LIFE

Male infertility without androgen deficiency

In at least one-third of couples presenting with infertility, the condition is attributable largely or entirely to abnormalities in the male, leading either to azoospermia, oligospermia or abnormal sperm. A general classification of causes is given in Table 18.15. Management is in most cases unsatisfactory and is beyond the scope of this book.

In general, if the serum level of FSH is elevated in a patient with azoospermia or severe oligospermia, severe irreversible testicular damage will be present on biopsy and no treatment will be effective. Recently, it has been recognised that, in many men with normal sperm counts but poor virility, there are antibodies in semen which are impairing fertility. Antibodies can also be detected in serum. There is at present no effective treatment.

Androgen deficiency (male hypogonadism)

The presentation of testicular dysfunction with androgen

Table 18.14   Causes of male pseudohermaphroditism

Pure XY gonadal dysgenesis

Testicular enzyme deficiencies

With adrenal enzyme deficiency
  Cholesterol desmolase
  $\Delta_5,3\beta$-hydroxysteroid dehydrogenase
  17-hydroxylase
Without adrenal deficiency
  17,20-desmolase
  17-ketosteroid oxidoreductase

Target organ abnormalities

5-α-reductase deficiency
Androgen receptor defect – testicular feminisation, complete or partial

Table 18.15   Causes of male infertility

Level of dysfunction	Cause

Pituitary	Gonadotrophin deficiency
	  Primary*†
	  Secondary, e.g. tumour*†, radiation etc.
	Gonadotrophin suppression
	  Exogenous androgens (e.g. body builders)*
	  Endogenous, e.g. 21-hydroxylase deficiency*

Testicular	Chromosomal defect, e.g. Klinefelter's syndrome†
	Germ cell damage, e.g. Sertoli cell only syndrome
	Undescended testes
	Radiotherapy†
	Drugs
	  Cytotoxic†
	  Sulphasalazine*
	Temperature-induced damage
	  Varicocoele*
	  Exogenous*
	  Pyrexia*
	Castration†
	Anorchia†

Post-testicular	Absent or obstructed vasa Vasectomy* Epididymal damage Prostatitis, orchitis*

Ejaculatory failure	Erectile failure
	  Psychogenic
	  Vascular
	  Neurogenic
	Retrograde ejaculation
	Spinal cord or cauda equina damage

Spermatozoal dysfunction	Infection* Antisperm antibodies Failure to penetrate mucus/poor viability Miscellaneous, e.g. defects in sperm structure

*Partially or totally treatable or reversible
†Associated with androgen deficiency and therefore also with infrequent or absent intercourse

deficiency may be at the time of puberty, or much later. A small minority of men presenting with infertility have a mild degree of androgen deficiency and associated oligo- or azoospermia; most such men, and all who are severely androgen-deficient are sexually inactive. The causes of androgen deficiency, classified according to whether the gonadotrophin levels are low (hypogonadotrophic) or high (hypergonadotrophic), are given in Table 18.16. In both groups, the severity of the androgen deficiency can vary considerably; it is usually least severe in Klinefelter's syndrome (which in most cases is associated with an XXY chromosomal constitution) and where the Leydig cells continue to function (although subnormally) despite severely damaged tubules. In this condition, the testes are usually firm and pea-sized. Gynaecomastia may occur in any form of hypogonadism, due in part to increased oestrogen but mainly to reduced testosterone action on the breasts. If the condition dates from before puberty, the limbs continue to grow, so that the final height is increased, with long extremities ('eunuchoidal proportions', Fig. 18.34). Isolated gonadotrophin deficiency (due usually to GnRH

Table 18.16 Causes of androgen deficiency in phenotypically normal adult men

Gonadotrophin levels	Cause of androgen deficiency
Low LH and FSH	Simple delayed puberty
	Illness and malnutrition
	Anorexia nervosa
	Isolated gonadotrophin/GnRH deficiency
	Normal sense of smell
	Anosmia (Kallman's syndrome)
	Panhypopituitarism
	Tumour – suprapituitary
	(craniopharyngioma)
	– pituitary
	Infarction
	Haemochromatosis
	Drugs – cyproterone acetate*
High LH and FSH	**Developmental**
	Klinefelter's syndrome (XXY and its variants)
	Acquired
	Trauma
	Castration
	Injury
	Torsion
	Anorchia (testicular degeneration)
	Viral orchitis (mumps)
	Radiation
	Drugs, e.g. cyclophosphamide
	Dystrophia myotonica
Variable LH and FSH	Prader-Willi syndrome
	Hyperprolactinaemia
	Noonan's syndrome
	Cirrhosis of liver
	Drugs, e.g. spironolactone, alcohol
	Cushing's syndrome

*Gonadotrophin suppression combined with androgen resistance

deficiency) may be sporadic or familial (X-linked or X-limited). When associated with anosmia, it is termed Kallman's syndrome. The anosmia is due to failure of development of the amygdala. When hypogonadism develops after puberty, it is highly likely that a pituitary tumour or craniopharyngioma is responsible, a suspicion that can be confirmed by appropriate radiology and hormone assays.

A common clinical problem is of the teenage boy with delayed puberty. The differential diagnosis between simple delayed puberty and permanent isolated gonadotrophin deficiency may be impossible. It is usually advisable to boost puberty artificially with testosterone to avoid psychological problems, and review the diagnosis later.

Investigation of endocrine function of the testes

A great deal can be learned about the endocrine function of the testes from a single measurement of the serum or plasma level of testosterone, plus the gonadotrophins LH and FSH. A grossly raised prolactin points to a prolactinoma which, though rare in men, is important to diagnose as early as possible since such tumours are often rapidly growing. If gynaecomastia is present, serum oestradiol and SHBG levels should be included in the assessment. Stimulation tests can be carried out at the level of the pituitary (with GnRH 10–100 μg iv) or the testes (with HCG 1500–5000 IU im), or oestrogen negative feedback can be assessed (with clomiphene citrate). These tests, especially the latter, are generally no more informative than basal hormone measurements.

Treatment

Male infertility

The principal treatable causes of male infertility are oligospermia due to varicocele, or exposure of testes to high temperature (the scrotum keeps the normal testes at about 32°C and prolonged high temperature impairs spermatogenesis). Sulphasalazine-induced infertility in ulcerative colitis (Table 18.15) can be treated by transfer to aminosalicylic acid. Gonadotrophin deficiency from any cause may lead to some permanent testicular damage. In most such cases, adequate spermatogenesis can be stimulated by administering purified FSH (Pergonal, 225 units thrice weekly) plus HCG (2000 units twice a week). An adequate trial of therapy is 3–6 months, the response being followed by semen analysis (count and motility). An alternative therapy, also expensive, is to administer GnRH by subcutaneous pump in pulsatile manner (15 μg every 90 minutes). Where gonadotrophin deficiency is caused by extratesticular androgens (as in congenital adrenal hyperplasia) the appropriate treatment is with replacement glucocorticoid therapy.

Androgen deficiency

When hypogonadotrophic, one option is to give HCG (1500–2000 IU twice a week, or 5000 IU once a week).

Fig. 18.34 Testicular dysfunction with androgen deficiency. Grossly eunochoidal 31-year-old man with Kallman's syndrome **A**. before and **B**. after two years of androgen replacement. **C**. A 21-year-old man with Klinefelter's syndrome. Note partial virilisation and minimal gynaecomastia.

Direct replacement is best made with testosterone. Implantation (600–800 mg every 4–6 months) of fused pellets is made, under local anaesthetic, subcutaneously in the lower abdominal wall. This provides steady release of testosterone, in contrast to marked peaks and troughs from depot testosterone injections of mixed esters in oil (Sustanon 250 mg) or oenanthate (Primoteston depot) every 2–3 weeks. Oral testosterone undecanoate (80 mg bd) is also effective and appears to be safe, but is expensive long-term therapy. When given for the first time to an adult who has never been through puberty, dosage should be cautious at first (e.g. 40 mg bd of testosterone undecanoate), to avoid triggering undue aggression.

THE OVARIES

ANATOMY AND PHYSIOLOGY

The ovaries consist of germ cells surrounded by granulosa cells (the homologue of the Sertoli cell); these are surrounded in turn by stromal cells of the theca interna.

As discussed above (p. 713), the ovaries are believed to have no role in the development of the internal or external genitalia in the embryo. These are determined by the presence or absence of testes, which depends in turn upon the presence of a Y chromosome. In contrast to the testes there is probably a little steroid secreted by the ovaries before birth, and this accounts for the finding of higher levels of LH and FSH in female than male fetuses in the second half of intra-uterine life. After birth and a transient surge in LH levels, the hypothalamic-pituitary ovarian axis becomes quiescent until puberty.

Changes during puberty

On average, puberty starts about two years earlier in girls than boys. The full complement of ovarian follicles (about half a million) is complete at birth, when all the primitive follicles have formed. Their number declines progressively thereafter, until exhaustion at the time of the menopause. There is evidence that crops of immature follicles advance to a certain stage and become atretic even before puberty. With the rise in FSH levels, these crops of follicles advance further and produce increasing amounts of oestrogen; at about 7 days before ovulation, one follicle becomes further advanced than the rest, progressively increasing in sensitivity to FSH (by increasing numbers of FSH receptors) and making progressively more oestradiol (Fig. 18.35A). This is believed to lead to suppression of FSH levels and atresia of the less advanced follicles in that cohort.

There is good evidence that the first cycles in girls are anovulatory, and they may be associated with erratic

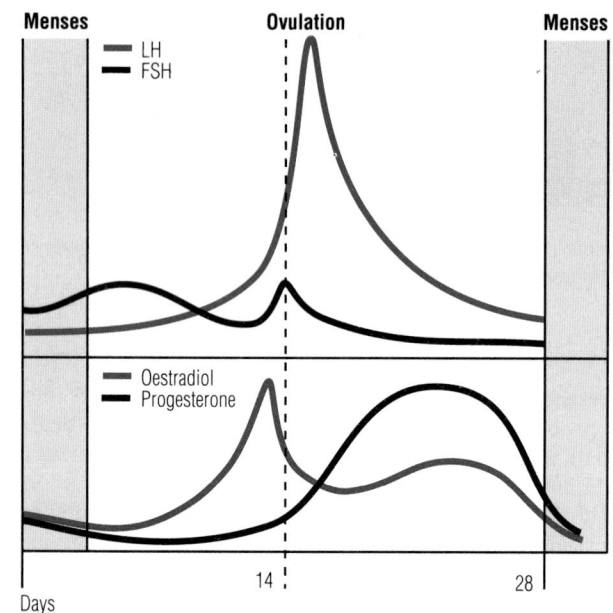

Fig. 18.35 The normal menstrual cycle. A. Diagram of the sequence of events of the normal menstrual cycle. (1) FSH leads to follicle maturation, and secretion of oestradiol which leads to proliferative endometrium and, with other factors, (2) feeds back on pituitary and hypothalamus. Mid-cycle positive feedback triggers LH surge (3) leading to follicle rupture and luteinisation. Corpus luteum (4) secretes progesterone and oestradiol, leading to a secretory endometrium. If conception occurs, implanted blastocyst secretes HCG, which maintains the corpus luteum and its secretions. **B.** Overall pattern of circulating hormone levels during a normal menstrual cycle.

'break-through' menstrual bleeding, due to oestrogenic stimulation of the endometrium. Eventually, however, conditions are right for the first ovulatory cycle.

Ovulation and the normal menstrual cycle

The biological purpose of ovulation is pregnancy. Menstruation may be thought of as biological failure, an indi-

cation that pregnancy with the last released ovum is impossible, and the starting point of the next cycle. The latter's purpose is once again to achieve release of a single fertilisable ovum and, simultaneously, to prepare the reproductive tract for successful pregnancy if fertilisation takes place.

The cohort of follicles destined to develop in a particular cycle have been selected, by a process quite unknown, two cycles earlier. The menstrual cycle, which in most women is surprisingly regular at about 28 days, depends upon inherent and interlocked cyclicity within the ovary, the hypothalamus and the pituitary gland. It is not surprising that defects in this complex system are common.

Figure 18.35B shows the stylised profile of hormone levels obtained if blood samples are taken at daily intervals throughout a normal cycle. These changes depend in part upon the inherent cyclicity referred to above, and in part upon two-way communication between the hypothalamus, pituitary gland and ovaries. Oestradiol exerts predominantly negative and intermittently positive feedback. When follicular oestradiol secretion rises, this appears to switch the pituitary gonadotrophs from an FSH- to a predominantly LH-secreting mode, and to reduce the pulse amplitude of GnRH secretion; meanwhile, the gonadotrophins become more sensitive to GnRH. The signal for the pre-ovulatory surge in LH secretion is believed to be a decline in oestradiol levels, together with the onset of progesterone secretion with attendant rise in GnRH amplitude. The mid-cycle LH surge, characterised by 24–48 hours of high peaks of LH secretion, is one of the turning points of the cycle. It arrives at the ovary precisely at the time when one follicle has reached a diameter of 2 cm, at which time its granulosa cells have proliferated and developed LH receptors sufficient to be induced to ovulate. The LH surge completes ovulation, while also inducing the granulosa cells to pass into their next endocrine state, namely to 'luteinise' and become the corpus luteum.

Pre-ovulatory steroid secretion, which is LH- and FSH-dependent, is mainly from the maturing follicle, and depends upon the two compartments of the follicle working in concert. The theca interna makes androstenedione and testosterone; the adjacent granulosa cells provide the last enzyme step (aromatase) necessary to convert these to oestrone and, more importantly, oestradiol (Fig. 18.26, p. 703). Post-ovulatory steroid secretion, which is still dependent upon low concentrations of LH, comes principally from the corpus luteum. This has formed from luteinised granulosa cells that have developed the capacity for de novo steroid synthesis and principally secretes progesterone, as well as oestradiol. It should be noted that plasma oestradiol levels fluctuate 10-fold and progesterone more than 20-fold during the normal menstrual cycle.

If pregnancy is to occur the uterine endometrium must first be prepared adequately. Firstly, proliferative phase development occurs due to the pre-ovulatory oestradiol surge; and secondly, post-ovulatory progesterone and oestradiol have to convert this to the receptive secretory phase endometrium. Mucus secretion from the cervix is only conducive to sperm penetration during the late secretory phase and mid-cycle; after this time, progesterone rapidly inhibits it. If fertilisation occurs, the blastocyst penetrates the endometrium and secretes its own LH-like hormone, HCG, which is absorbed into the circulation. HCG levels then rise sufficiently high to maintain the corpus luteum. In the absence of HCG, the corpus luteum atrophies, progesterone secretion declines, the spiral arteries of the endometrium collapse and the surface layers of endometrium die. The consequent bleeding is menstruation.

Secondary sexual changes during and after female puberty

Breast development is usually the earliest secondary sexual change in females, commencing at around 9–11 years. Primary changes are caused by the action of oestradiol on the duct epithelium; this in turn probably stimulates stromal fat development which accounts for most of the bulk of the breast. Progesterone also has an action on the oestrogen-primed breast epithelium, which is of importance in pregnancy in preparing for lactation. During the normal menstrual cycle, progesterone is responsible for the increase in breast volume (about 20%) during the luteal phase.

Oestradiol, and ovarian and adrenal androgens are responsible for stimulation of female pubic and axillary hair. Changes in uterine size (myometrial and endometrial) are caused by the joint effects of oestrogen and progestogen.

Oestradiol is principally responsible for the pubertal growth spurt by exerting both a direct effect on epiphyseal cartilage, and an indirect effect, by stimulating growth hormone and gonadotrophin secretion. The earlier time of puberty in women, and the potent effect of oestrogens on closing the epiphyseal plates of the long bones, lead to the shorter final stature. Oestradiol has a major effect in increasing endosteal new bone formation and skeletal mass, but it is less potent in this respect than testosterone. The increased muscle mass in males is probably also a factor in increasing the bone density (cortical and trabecular) in men (see also p. 733).

Age-related changes in ovarian function and the menopause

Contrary to popular belief, the menopause is not an abrupt process. It is preceded by hormone changes over ten years or more, that stem from the progressive depletion of follicles such that the cohort available to develop each month becomes progressively smaller. This is first evidenced by deeper troughs in oestradiol levels (especially early in the follicular phase) and higher peaks of FSH. The role in this of the ovarian peptide hormone inhibin, recently isolated from follicle fluid and characterised, is still speculative. Inhibin appears to act as a long-term regulatory growth factor, keeping gonadotrophs in a mode where they largely make LH. High FSH levels stimulate premature development of the next crop of follicles. Luteinisation without ovulation is commonplace; bleeding becomes erratic and the woman subfertile or infertile, long before the last menstrual period, which usually occurs at about 50 years of age.

The menopause (and often the pre-menopause) is commonly attended by frequent disabling and embarrassing hot flushes – due to central sympathetic nervous discharge related in some way to oestrogen deficiency. The timing of the flushes coincides with discharge of LH and FSH, but is not due to them. Vaginal dryness, lack of libido, breast atrophy, and urethritis are all common symptoms of post-menopausal oestrogen deficiency. The latter is also responsible for a rapid increase in the rate of bone mineral loss, which contributes to post-menopausal osteoporosis.

OVARIAN DYSFUNCTION: AMENORRHOEA AND OLIGOMENORRHOEA

Ovarian dysfunction may be associated with anything from regular menstrual cycles of normal length, through erratic and infrequent cycles (oligomenorrhoea) to absent periods (amenorrhoea). The presenting complaint may be of the menstrual disorder, infertility or accompanying problems such as breast discomfort, galactorrhoea or hirsutism. In general, the more severe the endocrine problem, the greater is the degree of menstrual disturbance.

Amenorrhoea or oligomenorrhoea may occur from the time of puberty (primary) or it may develop later (secondary). It is obviously always important to exclude pregnancy by a pregnancy test or ultrasound scan – the patients with erratic cycles who ovulate only occasionally can still conceive when they do so, in which case amenorrhoea persists! Especially in patients with primary amenorrhoea, it is important to try to determine whether the external and internal genitalia are those of a normal female.

Pituitary/hypothalamic causes

Gonadotrophin deficiency

Deficiency of gonadotrophin releasing hormone (GnRH) is most commonly secondary to weight loss. Many teenage girls are concerned about their weight, diet excessively and, as a consequence, develop amenorrhoea at a weight or lean body mass that varies between different individuals. This type of amenorrhoea is commonly seen in *anorexia nervosa*, a psychiatric disorder associated with abnormal weight loss, and a disordered perception of body image such that a woman states, and may believe, that she is of normal weight or even obese (p. 202). Weight loss is produced and maintained by a combination of dieting, obsessional exercise, and surreptitious vomiting or laxative abuse – the precise pattern varies from subject to subject. Circulating LH and FSH levels are low, as are those of oestradiol and progesterone. As a consequence there is, in addition to amenorrhoea, a degree of regression of secondary sexual characteristics towards a pre-pubertal state, with reduction in oestrogenisation of breasts and genital

18

tract. A variable degree of osteoporosis will occur in the long term. A similar state can result from the weight loss or starvation, or in athletes (especially long-distance runners) and ballet dancers: the periods usually, but not always, return if and when weight is regained.

Isolated gonadotrophin deficiency without weight loss (due almost certainly to GnRH deficiency), may occur as a lifelong selective hypothalamic defect in the female, as in the male. If associated with anosmia, it is called Kallman's syndrome (p. 716). It may also be seen in patients with craniopharyngioma, or after pituitary irradiation, in which case it is likely to be associated with other pituitary hormone deficiencies.

Prolactin excess

Prolactin excess from any cause is frequently associated with disordered ovarian function, with amenorrhoea occurring when the prolactin level rises to more than two or three times above normal. A classification of the causes of prolactin excess is given in Table 18.6 and the condition discussed on pages 686–88.

The mechanism whereby prolactin excess causes menstrual disturbance and amenorrhoea is still not completely understood; it is believed to exert a 'short loop feedback' effect at hypothalamic level, reducing the pulse frequency of GnRH secretion. Its effects can be overcome by gonadotrophin replacement or pump-induced GnRH administration, and so are probably not exerted on the gonads directly.

Ovarian causes

The ovarian causes of amenorrhoea and oligomenorrhoea are summarised in Table 18.17. In such cases, the circulating levels of LH and FSH are elevated.

Premature menopause

The menopause has been discussed above (p. 719), and a similar pattern may be seen at an early age (premature menopause), sometimes as early as the 20s, presumably as a consequence of starting with a greatly reduced number of ovarian follicles. Occasionally, the immune system may be implicated, with production of antibodies directed at one or more components of the ovary (p. 670). An identical syndrome often results from irradiation of the ovaries or administration of chemotherapeutic agents, usually directed against Hodgkin's lymphoma or other malignancies (p. 154).

Gonadal dysgenesis

An important group of ovarian causes of amenorrhoea comes under the general heading of *gonadal dysgenesis*. Here, the ovaries may either fail to develop or degenerate before puberty, because of an abnormal X chromosome complement which leads to follicular death.

Table 18.17 Ovarian causes of amenorrhoea or oligomenorrhoea

Failure of normal ovarian development
Pure XX gonadal dysgenesis
  Familial
  Sporadic
Turner's syndrome (XO)
Ovarian enzyme deficiencies (e.g. 17,20 desmolase)

Premature ovarian failure (follicular degeneration)
Idiopathic (low initial follicle number)
Autoimmune (antiovarian antibodies)
Infection (e.g. mumps, oöphoritis)
Radiotherapy
Cytotoxic drugs (e.g. for Hodgkin's disease, leukaemia)
Surgical/traumatic

Ovarian dysfunction
Polycystic ovary syndrome (uncertain if ovarian in origin)
Resistant ovary syndrome

Turner's syndrome

Turner's syndrome is the commonest form of gonadal dysgenesis; here, primary amenorrhoea is associated with short stature and a variable number of skeletal and somatic abnormalities (Table 18.18; see also Chapter 6, p. 90). The condition is most commonly caused by a 45X (termed XO) chromosome constitution, which has resulted from the loss of an X or Y chromosome before the first mitotic division of the fertilised ovum. The features of this syndrome result in part from the existence of only one X chromosome (without a Y), and in part from the resulting sex hormone deficiency from the time of puberty onwards.

Patients are phenotypic females with 'streak' gonads (the follicles degenerate in childhood), but normal female internal and external genitalia. Stature is almost invariably reduced, with final height seldom exceeding 5 ft (150 cm). The chest may be shield-shaped, with widely spaced nipples and underdeveloped breasts (these will, however, feminise with oestrogen administration). The facial appearance may be unusual, with a small 'button' nose and low hair-line posteriorly; there may be prominent epicanthic folds. Intra-uterine lymphoedema of the upper part of the body may lead to the development of a 'webbed' neck. Lymphoedema may also occur in the limbs (Bonnevie-Ullrich syndrome). Cardiovascular abnormalities include coarctation of the aorta, aortic stenosis or bicuspid aortic valve disease. Osteoporosis is common, and patients have an increased incidence of thyroid autoimmune disease. Renal abnormalities such as horseshoe kidney are common, occurring in 40% of cases.

Other forms of gonadal dysgenesis

Some patients with a classical 'Turner's' phenotype (Fig. 6.13) have a normal chromosome complement, but have part of an X chromosome missing. With XO/XY mosai-

Table 18.18 Clinical features of 45XO Turner's syndrome

Type	Feature
Sexual	Streak ovaries
	Sexual infantism
	Primary amenorrhoea
	High gonadotrophins
	Normal female genitalia
Skeletal	Short stature (100%)
	Characteristic facies – micrognathia, epicanthic folds, low-set ears, fish-like mouth, high arched palate
	Shield-like chest
	Wide carrying angle
	Short neck, low hairline
	Short metacarpals
	Scoliosis
	Localised areas of rarefaction
	Osteoporosis
Soft tissues	Lymphoedema
	Webbing of neck
Cardiovascular	Coarctation
	Bicuspid aortic valve
	Aortic stenosis
Renal	Rotation of kidney
	Duplex ureters etc.
	Hydronephrosis
Cutaneous	Small nipples
	Pigmented naevi
	Cheloid formation

cism and other variants, the patient normally has less severe skeletal abnormalities and may be of normal stature. Rare individuals have an apparently normal male genotype (46 XY), but normal female internal genitalia; in these instances, it is believed that the testes never develop (pure XY gonadal dysgenesis; see p. 723).

Conditions of uncertain aetiology

A number of conditions exist where the cause of the amenorrhoea or oligomenorrhoea is unknown. Prime among them is the so-called *Stein-Leventhal syndrome*, or *polycystic ovarian disease*. This was originally described in 1935 as hirsutism, obesity, and oligomenorrhoea associated with enlarged ovaries with a thickened and whitish-looking 'capsule' and multiple follicular cysts. This ovarian appearance is now believed to result from chronic bombardment of the ovaries by high levels of LH in an acyclical fashion. There is undoubtedly a sub-group that is obese, and here it is possible that increased production in adipose tissue of the oestrogen oestrone (from androstenedione) may trigger excessive pituitary LH secretion. Many cases are of normal weight, however, and the primary abnormality is not known for certain. It is likely that the cause varies from

hypothalamic, pituitary, ovarian and possibly even adrenal defects and that the ovarian histology is non-specific. In most cases, the high LH levels are associated with increased ovarian secretion of androstenedione, which is converted in peripheral tissues and red blood cells to testosterone. Plasma oestradiol is relatively constant at levels seen in the mid-follicular phase of the cycle; levels of sex hormone binding globulin (SHBG) are reduced, and so the unbound testosterone level is modestly raised. The LH:FSH ratio is also raised.

The extent of development of hirsutism and more marked virilisation (e.g. frontal balding) in this syndrome is very variable, and depends both on the hormone abnormality (which can be measured) and on the capacity of target tissues (in this example the hair follicles) to respond. Likewise, the ovulatory disturbance varies from slightly erratic cycles through to long-standing amenorrhoea (primary or secondary).

Treatment of amenorrhoea

The current treatment of patients with oligo- or amenorrhoea depends upon a number of factors, including the underlying cause, the age of the patient, and their requirements (for example for contraception, treatment of hirsutism or infertility). The treatment of prolactin excess is described on page 687. Restoring the prolactin level to normal is usually sufficient to restore normal ovulation and fertility; if the latter is not desired, then the oral contraceptive pill can be given safely with bromocriptine to a patient with suspected microprolactinoma.

With causes of amenorrhoea associated with gonadal dysgenesis or ovarian failure, attempts to restore ovarian function and fertility are generally unsuccessful. Sex hormone replacement is indicated in most cases, at least until the time of the menopause. This can be provided by low-dose oral contraceptive pills, most of which provide $30\,\mu g$ daily of ethinyl oestradiol, and a progestogen (21 days out of 28). Alternatively, the treatment can be tailored to the patient's perceived needs; a suitable regimen would include ethinyl oestradiol $10–20\,\mu g$ daily throughout, and a progestogen such as norethisterone acetate, $1–5\,mg$ daily for 7–12 days each month. The oestrogen can be given in a higher effective dose, for example to increase breast development. Where there is a history of deep vein thrombosis or hypertension, oestrogens can more safely be given as a subcutaneous implant in the lower abdominal wall of solid oestradiol (50 mg), periods being induced by cyclical administration of progestogen as above. A promising recent development is that of adhesive plastic patches containing oestradiol dissolved in ethanol (Estraderm), which are applied to the skin and from which the hormone is absorbed.

After the menopause, many women feel better on a continuing low-dose oestrogen replacement. Controversy continues on the relative merits and demerits of *hormone replacement therapy* (HRT). However, there is little doubt that it protects the bones against osteoporosis and the genital tract against atrophy, and that many women feel much better on it. The evidence of its effects on vascular disease is debatable; many feel that it is the (androgenic) progestogens, not the oestrogen, that are harmful. Growth of certain forms of breast and uterine cancer may be promoted by oestrogen but, at least in the latter case, this effect is prevented with a cyclical progestogen that leads to shedding of the endometrium.

Treatment of infertility

With *hyperprolactinaemia*, restoring the prolactin to normal usually restores both periods and fertility.

Gonadotrophin deficiency may be treated either by gonadotrophin administration, or by pulsatile administration of GnRH. The latter is intrinsically safer and apparently does not carry the risk of hyperstimulation of the ovaries. Gonadotrophin therapy consists usually of 3–7 days of injections of a preparation of human follicle stimulating hormone (FSH). The dose is titrated by measuring blood or urine oestrogens and by ovarian ultrasound scanning. When the right amount of follicular development has occurred, ovulation is induced by an injection of human chorionic gonadotrophin (HCG). This treatment is only given in specialised units with the appropriate backup, because of the risk of producing ovarian hyperstimulation, which is a potentially serious complication.

Polycystic ovaries. In the case of polycystic ovaries, treatment of the infertility is difficult and often unsatisfactory. About one-quarter of cases will ovulate on a low dose of glucocorticoid (such as prednisolone 7.5 mg daily). Clomiphene citrate (the anti-oestrogen) is often given, and induces ovulation in about half the cases. It is important to start with a low dose such as 50 mg daily for five days, again because patients may be very sensitive and develop multiple large follicular cysts. Some units are now treating patients by producing 'paradoxical' suppression of LH and FSH with a GnRH analogue, followed by conventional stimulation with FSH followed by HCG.

ENDOCRINOLOGY OF PREGNANCY

The earliest endocrine signal in pregnancy, which is of great importance, is the secretion of chorionic gonadotrophin (HCG) from the trophoblast. This occurs within a day or two of implantation, and is necessary to maintain the corpus luteum, which otherwise declines about 14 days after ovulation. HCG binds to LH receptors on the surface of corpus luteum cells and stimulates their continuing production of progesterone and oestradiol. These in turn sustain the endometrium to maintain its secretory (decidual) structure. As the fetus develops, the specialised placenta is formed. HCG secretion reaches a peak at around 12 weeks of fetal life and declines thereafter. By that time, the production of progesterone has been taken over by the (now large) placenta; the pregnancy from the second trimester onwards is no longer corpus luteum-dependent.

Other polypeptides unique to pregnancy are produced by the placenta; the most prominant of these is human placental lactogen (HPL, also called human chorionic somatomammotrophin), whose production reaches a peak late in pregnancy. It has an action similar to growth hormone, and is in part responsible for insulin-resistance and gestational diabetes.

The *feto-placental unit* assumes importance from the second trimester onwards, when the adrenal cortex develops and becomes responsive to ACTH. The fetal zone produces weak androgens, principally dehydro-epiandrosterone (DHEA) sulphate, using LDL cholesterol from the fetal liver as substrate. The placenta and the fetal liver both take part in its further metabolism. The liver contains the enzyme 16-α-hydroxylase, while the placenta contains aromatase and sulphatase enzymes; the net result is the conversion of DHEA sulphate to oestriol. The function of this weak oestrogen, produced in large amounts in pregnancy, is unknown. Absence of the enzyme sulphatase occurs in an X-linked disorder (sulphatase deficiency), which is not associated with any major problems during pregnancy or delivery, despite low oestriol levels. The condition is associated with icthyosis due to cholesterol sulphatase deficiency in the skin.

The placenta also secretes the active oestrogen oestradiol into the maternal circulation, and this is important in maintaining pregnancy. Progesterone is produced by placental enzyme action on cholesterol.

The *induction of labour* in women is poorly understood. In some species, such as the sheep, a rise in adrenal cortisol associated with a decline in progesterone is important, acting in conjunction with increased secretion of pituitary oxytocin. Certainly, glucocorticoids from the fetal adrenals are important in inducing fetal lung maturation; here, they act in concert with adrenaline, acting through its beta-2 receptor.

PREMENSTRUAL TENSION

Premenstrual tension is a common but rather poorly defined condition, in which a wide range of physical and emotional symptoms and signs are worst during the week or two preceding a menstrual period and generally improve with its onset. It is not primarily an endocrine disorder, but is probably best thought of as a cyclical disorder 'locked in' on the normal fluctuation in hormone levels that accompanies the menstrual cycle. Since most women experience some emotional and physical deterioration at this stage of the cycle it may, in many cases, be an exaggeration of the normal; in many women, however, it can be extremely disabling. Treatment may be directed at smoothing out or eliminating the normal hormone changes or at treating the symptoms.

DISORDERS OF SEX DIFFERENTIATION

The underlying mechanisms of primary sex differentiation are described on page 713. Where sex differentiation is evidently abnormal at birth, the problem is made particularly difficult by the urgency of determining the appropriate sex of rearing. Parents in particular are under great pressure to declare the sex of the infant at birth, and to stick to it. They require very sensitive handling. Most cases of abnormal sex differentiation are cases of pseudo- (rather than true) hermaphroditism.

MALE PSEUDOHERMAPHRODITISM

The male pseudohermaphrodite is a *genetically male* infant who does not have completely normal male sexual characteristics. In its mildest form, the infant has failure of development of the penile urethra (hypospadias); in its most severe form, the external genitalia appear to be those of a completely normal female. The causes of male pseudohermaphroditism are listed in Table 18.14 (p. 715).

Pure XY gonadal dysgenesis

In pure XY gonadal dysgenesis the individual is XY in sex chromosome constitution but the testes have never developed and so did not impose maleness on the 'background' female phenotype. Apart from the absence of gonads, the patient is a completely normal female. The major importance in recognising the condition, is that the gonadal remnants (streak gonads) are at risk of developing tumours (dysgerminomas) at, or after, the age of puberty. They should therefore be removed at that time. From puberty onwards, female sex hormone replacement should be given.

Testicular feminisation

Testicular feminisation occurs with a frequency of about 1 in 10 000 live births, and is inherited through an X-linked gene. XY individuals develop testes as normal, but are unable to respond to the androgen that these produce because they lack the androgen receptor. There are probably at least two distinct genetic defects responsible respectively for the complete and partial forms of the syndrome. In the complete form, the external genitalia are those of a normal female, but with a very short blind vagina. There is no development either at or after puberty of even the normal female amount of pubic and axillary hair. The testes are in the inguinal canal; indeed, presentation is often with inguinal herniae, each of which are found to contain a gonad.

The correct sex of rearing for individuals with either the partial or complete form of the syndrome is undoubtedly female. It is generally felt to be advisable to leave the testes *in situ* until breast development has taken place at the normal age of puberty. Feminisation of the breasts is usually excellent, under the influence of normal levels of testicular oestradiol (unopposed by androgen action). Circulating levels of LH and FSH are usually somewhat elevated, and testosterone levels in the high adult male range (after puberty). The gonads should be removed in early adult life, as there is considerable risk of development of tumours (dysgerminomas) within them.

5-α-reductase deficiency

5-α-reductase deficiency is inherited as an autosomal recessive disorder, and is therefore common where there has been intermarriage. It is very common, for example, in Salinas, in the Dominican Republic. The primary defect lies in the enzyme 5-α-reductase which is absent or of reduced activity. Production of 5-α-dihydrotestosterone (DHT) in androgen target tissues is reduced (Fig. 18.26, p. 703) and those effects that depend on DHT are therefore compromised. Females with the condition appear normal, but males have impairment of virilisation of the external genitalia. The phallus is small, and there is complete perineo-scrotal hypospadias, and incomplete fusion of the scrotum with a blind vaginal opening. The testes, epididymes, vasa and seminal vesicles are normal, while the prostate gland is, and remains, atrophic. Regardless of the sex of rearing, affected individuals generally insist that they are male, both at the time of puberty and beyond, and generally demonstrate male patterns of behaviour. After puberty, the voice deepens and normal male muscular development occurs but facial hair is absent or scanty. Some increase in hair development may be produced by injecting supra-normal doses of testosterone.

FEMALE PSEUDOHERMAPHRODITISM

In female pseudohermaphroditism, a *genetic female* is partially or completely virilised. The most likely cause is excess androgen secretion in utero, generally as a result of the action of increased ACTH upon the (abnormal) adrenal glands. The commonest defect is the autosomal recessive disorder 21-hydroxylase deficiency. The syndrome is described on page 707.

RARE DISORDERS OF STEROID BIOSYNTHESIS

The steroid pathway in adrenals, ovaries and testes are best thought of as a network, of which different pieces are missing in different tissues (Fig. 18.26, p. 703). Rare deficiencies of almost all the enzymes have been described, and the clinical picture can usually be understood by reference to these pathways and the normal physiology of the glands. Conditions that affect the testosterone pathway(s) lead to male pseudohermaphroditism; if they lie early on the pathway (which is shared with the adrenals) then adrenal insufficiency also occurs.

In addition to 21-hydroxylase deficiency (which is about five times commoner than the others put together), there are a number of other disorders of steroid biosynthesis which also lead to pseudohermaphroditism in affected females. These include 3-β-hydroxysteroid dehydrogenase deficiency, in which the weak Δ_5-androgens from the adrenals cause some virilisation of females (but males are inadequately virilised). Likewise, 11-hydroxylase deficiency is associated with a build-up of adrenal androgens; desoxycorticosterone is also overproduced, leading to hypertension.

DISORDERS OF MALE SECONDARY SEX DIFFERENTIATION

The physiological mechanisms that lead to male secondary sex differentiation are discussed above on pages 713–14.

Gynaecomastia

Gynaecomastia (breast development in the male) is extremely common; during puberty and in old age it may be regarded as physiological, resulting from a relative dominance of circulating oestradiol levels over testosterone. One-third of normal boys will develop a minor degree of breast enlargement and tenderness during puberty; this seldom requires any treatment and subsides spontaneously. However, gynaecomastia is also seen as a feature in a wide range of disorders (Table 18.19). These are generally associated with an increase in oestrogen production, and/or a decline in testosterone production. Some drugs cause gynaecomastia, the most notable being the aldosterone antagonist, spironolactone. This compound also binds to androgen receptors and is an anti-androgen. It may also inhibit the secretion of androgen, but not that of oestrogen. Digitoxin and the main metabolite of cannabis cause gynaecomastia because they have intrinsic oestrogenic activity.

Treatment may be directed at the underlying cause which, however, is often not apparent. Danazol, a synthetic androgen, has been used to treat the condition, as have anti-oestrogens such as tamoxifen. Hypogonadism should be treated with testosterone replacement; this is probably best given either as oral testosterone undecanoate or by implant, rather than by injection of testosterone esters (Sustanon or Primoteston). The latter lead to high peaks of testosterone and oestradiol levels after injection, and occasionally exacerbate or cause gynaecomastia.

Table 18.19 Causes and mechanisms of gynaecomastia

Cause	Low testosterone production	High oestrogen production	Direct oestrogenic effect	Direct anti-androgenic effect	Decreased androgen sensitivity	Increased oestrogen sensitivity
Physiological						
Neonatal	+	+	—	—	—	—
Pubertal*	+	+	—	—	—	—
Old age*	+	+	—	—	—	—
'Refeeding' (after starvation)	+	+	—	—	—	—
Pathological						
Hypogonadism	++	—	—	—	—	—
Steroid disorders						
17-ketosteroid reductase deficiency	+	+ (oestrone)	—	—	—	—
Testicular feminisation*	—	+	—	—	++	—
Cirrhosis**	+	+	—	—	—	—
Thyrotoxicosis*	+ (increased clearance)	+	—	—	—	—
Tumours*						
HCG-secreting	—	+	—	—	—	—
Leydig cell	+	++	—	—	—	—
Adrenal	+ (LH suppressed)	—	—	—	—	—
'Idiopathic'†	—	—	—	—	+?	+?
Pharmacological						
Spironolactone	+	+	—	++	—	—
Digitalis	—	—	+	—	—	—
Cannabis	—	—	+	—	—	—
Cyproterone acetate	+ (LH suppressed)	—	—	++	—	—
Oestrogen ingestion*	+ (LH suppressed)	—	++	—	—	—
Alcohol	+	—	—	—	—	—

* Associated with elevated SHBG levels, which may have moderate amplifying effect
× Fall in albumin selectively elevates free oestradiol
† Decreased androgen sensitivity and increased oestrogen sensitivity may be secondary to altered hormone production

Prostatic hyperplasia

Prostatic hyperplasia may be regarded as a later disorder of secondary sex differentiation. It results from increased androgen effect (via dihydrotestosterone and its hydroxylated metabolites) on the ventral lobe of the prostate, and causes urethral obstruction. It is usually treated by transurethral resection, although anti-androgenic progestogens have a significant effect in causing regression.

Prostatic cancer

Prostatic cancer is the commonest cancer in elderly males and is commonly androgen-dependent. A mainstay of treatment is thus suppression of androgen secretion and/or action. Surgery (subcapsular orchidectomy) is commonly used, as is medical therapy with the anti-androgenic progestogen, cyproterone acetate or gonadotrophin-releasing hormone analogues to cause down-regulation of LH and so testosterone secretion.

DISORDERS OF FEMALE SECONDARY SEX DIFFERENTIATION

Hirsutism in women is the obverse of gynaecomastia in men and is almost equally common. The term *virilisation* is reserved for androgenisation associated with very high levels of testosterone in, or approaching, the adult male range. Only 1–2% of women with hirsutism in Britain have frank virilisation. This may be due to ovarian or adrenal tumours, or to the so-called late onset form of congenital adrenal hyperplasia. Virilisation usually declares itself by a rapid development of hirsutism, with other signs such as frontal balding, clitoral enlargement, and deepening of the larynx.

Hirsutism

Hirsutism is conventionally subdivided into:

1. that due to *polycystic ovarian disease*, in which case menstruation is irregular or absent
2. '*idiopathic*' hirsutism, in which case the periods are regular. The latter was for long thought not to be due to androgen excess, but to increased target organ sensitivity.

It is evident from the wide variation between racial groups, and even within the same racial group, in the extent of facial and body hair in men, that the same genetic variability must also exist in women. Thus, some women with chronic anovulation, erratic cycles, polycystic ovaries and high levels of testosterone and androstenedione coming from the ovaries under the stimulation of LH show little or no hirsutism; while others, with a lesser endocrine defect, are severely hirsute. Furthermore, ultrasound scanning reveals that many women with 'idiopathic' hirsutism have polycystic ovaries. Another problem is to determine how much of the androgen excess is arising from the ovaries and how much from the adrenals. With the exception of 21-hydroxylase deficiency, the adrenals are probably usually the more minor source of excess androgens.

Prevention and treatment of hirsutism

Hirsutism develops over many years, and treatment should not be delayed until there is a serious clinical problem. Treatment is usually empirical, and may be hormonal or cosmetic; usually, both types of treatment are needed simultaneously.

Cosmetic treatment involves the use of creams, waxes (which root out the hairs), shaving, or electrolysis. The latter is usually reserved for strong terminal hairs on the face and breasts, or other psychologically important areas, and should only be carried out only by a trained electrologist. Contrary to popular belief, shaving does not make unwanted hair grow faster.

Hormonal treatment involves the use of adrenal and/or ovarian suppression and anti-androgens. Adrenal androgens can generally be suppressed with doses of glucocorticoid that are less than those required to suppress cortisol. Prednisolone (up to 7.5 mg daily) is usually used. In about one-third of cases with erratic cycles, ovulation becomes much more regular on this regime, and ovarian androgen production also declines. Ovarian suppression is achieved by using a low-dose 'pill' that does not contain a virilising androgen, e.g. Marvelon, which combines ethinyl oestradiol with dydrogesterone. Drugs that contain androgens, such as norgestrel, should be avoided. The available anti-androgens include cyproterone acetate, but its use for this purpose is not formally approved. It is probably more effective than a suitable contraceptive pill. Although spironolactone (100–200 mg daily) is sometimes remarkably effective, it can lead in some cases to menstrual disturbance. A recommendation has been issued by the Committee on Safety of Medicines that it should not now be used (for hypertension) because of doubts over its long-term safety.

Psychological support is of great importance and must include reassurance that the woman is not losing her femininity, or 'turning into a man'. Sometimes minimal hirsutism is a focus for an anxiety state; conversely, some women react by refusing to accept that there is a problem, and avoid even elementary cosmetic measures.

Management in pregnancy. The duration of drug therapy for hirsutism can be open-ended, and determined by the severity of the problem and the response; the patient with erratic cycles will simply have the same problem (no worse) when treatment is stopped. Where pregnancy is desired, a different strategy, designed to produce ovulation, is required. At its simplest, this involves low dose glucocorticoid therapy (if cycles are irregular) with or without clomiphene. In severe polycystic ovary disease, it may be necessary to induce ovulation with injections of FSH; this requires close monitoring of oestrogens and follicles on ultrasound and is a specialist procedure. Under no circumstances should cyproterone acetate be given on its own (i.e. without an oestrogen) to the pre-menopausal woman; there are serious consequences for sex differentiation in any male fetus if the woman conceives while on the drug.

SEX HORMONES AND BEHAVIOUR

Androgens, oestrogens and progestogens all affect the individual's behaviour either directly or indirectly. However, homosexuality, trans-sexualism and sexual deviation are not directly linked to androgen or oestrogen levels. It has been suggested that XYY men are more violent than normal men, in view of the finding of an increased number in penal institutions; however, the significance of this is uncertain.

Androgen-deficient men may develop protective mechanisms and become aggressive to compensate for the lack of physical development. If they are then abruptly put onto androgens at high doses, the aggression may become more overt. The transition to adult hormone levels (i.e. going through an endocrine adolescence, but very late) again requires medical guidance. Generally, hypogonadal men adapt very well to their new endocrine status and many go on to develop satisfactory heterosexual relationships.

FURTHER READING

Belchetz P E (ed) 1984 Management of pituitary disease. Chapman and Hall, London. *Comprehensive discussions of many aspects of pituitary disease.*

Edwards C R W (ed) 1986 Endocrinology. Integrated Clinical Science Series. Heinemann Medical, London. *A well-illustrated and clear account of the physiology and pathology of the endocrine system.*

Felig P, Baxter I D, Broadus A E, Frohman L A 1987 Endocrinology and metabolism, 2nd edn. McGraw Hill, New York. *A first class textbook of endocrinology and metabolism – highly recommended.*

Hadley Mac E 1988 Endocrinology, 2nd edn. Prentice Hall International, New York. *An excellent, up-to-date, single author text on endocrine biochemistry, physiology and pathophysiology.*

Knobil E, Neill J D (eds) 1988 The physiology of reproduction (2 vols). Raven Press, New York. *An enormous multi-author tome for the serious student who wishes to make an in-depth study of particular aspects of reproduction.*

Stanbury J B, Wynmgaarden D S, Frederikson, J L, Goldstein J L, Brown M S 1983 The metabolic basis of inherited disease, 5th edn. McGraw Hill, New York. *A valuable reference book on all inherited metabolic and endocrine disorders.*

Wilson J B, Foster D W 1985 Williams' textbook of endocrinology, 7th edn. W B Saunders, Philadelphia. *A comprehensive textbook – for long considered the 'bible' of basic and clinical endocrinoogy.*

Yen S S C, Jaffe R B (eds) 1986 Reproductive endocrinology, physiology, pathophysiology and clinical management, 2nd edn. W B Saunders, Philadelphia. *A good book, edited and largely written by two of the foremost reproductive endocrinologists in the US.*

Metabolic Bone Disease and Mineral Metabolism

Table 19.1 Distribution of body calcium

Compartment	Quantity/conc.
Whole body	
Skeleton	1 kg (25 mol)
Rapidly exchangeable-bone surface	8 g (200 mmol)
Extracellular fluid (ECF)	1 g (25 mmol)
Intracellular fluid (ICF)	1 g (25 mmol)
In plasma	
Free ionised Ca^{2+}	1.1 mmol/l
Protein-bound	
Albumin	0.75 mmol/l
Globulin	0.25 mmol/l
Ultrafiltrable bound (by bicarbonate citrate and phosphate)	0.3 mmol/l
Total in plasma	2.4 mmol/l

ANATOMY AND PHYSIOLOGY

The skeleton has three major functions:

1. it supports the soft tissue of the body
2. it encases and protects certain organs such as the central nervous system
3. it acts as an enormous chemical reservoir for various ions and minerals, in particular calcium, phosphorus, magnesium and sodium.

Although in health these functions are not in conflict, there are circumstances when the skeleton's contribution to chemical homeostasis under conditions of, for example, calcium deprivation, may lead to progressive demineralisation and compromise its mechanical functions.

Distribution of mineral

The adult human skeleton contains some 99% of total body calcium (Table 19.1), ranging from 1 to 2 kg (25–50 mol) depending on size, 88% of total body phosphorus, 80% of body carbonate, 50% of body magnesium and 35% of body sodium. Although calcium is distributed approximately equally between extracellular and intracellular fluid, the free calcium ion concentration in cell cytosol is approximately 10^{-7} to 10^{-6} molar, this being about three orders of magnitude less than the extracellular fluid free calcium ion concentration (10^{-3} molar, or 1 mM). Most of the intra-cellular calcium must therefore be sequestered in, or on, specific cell organelles. Calcium in blood plasma at 2.4 mM (Table 19.1) is present as free ions (1.1 mM), protein-bound to albumin (0.75 mM) and to globulin (0.25 mM) and ultrafiltrable bound, by carbonate, citrate and phosphate (total 0.3 mM). The biological functions of extracellular fluid calcium are thought to be effected by the ionised fraction only.

Inorganic phosphate in plasma is only slightly protein-bound (approximately 12%) the rest being present as $HPO_4^{2-}/H_2PO_4^-$ (in the ratio 4:1 at physiological pH), as well as in the form of sodium, calcium and magnesium phosphates. Most of the intracellular phosphate is co-valently bound to organic compounds or in the form of phospholipids. The free inorganic phosphate concentration in cells is probably less than 1 mM.

Bone composition

Bone consists of a calcified (mineralised) organic matrix. The organic matrix (osteoid) makes up about 30% of the total skeletal mass, and consists mainly of collagen and the recently identified, vitamin K-dependent protein osteocalcin, with small amounts of other proteins and lipids in addition. The mineral phase, which is deposited throughout the organic matrix, makes up the remaining 70% of skeletal mass and consists mainly of a complex crystalline salt of calcium and phosphate called hydroxyapatite $(Ca_{10}(PO_4)_6(OH)_2)$. There are also smaller amounts of amorphous acid phosphate, carbonate, sodium and magnesium.

Bone is a dynamic living tissue, with continuous modelling and remodelling by bone cells which allows the skeleton to grow and adapt itself to prevailing mechanical needs. The result is an organ that is, for its weight, extremely rigid and strong, without being brittle. The skeletal adaptation provides for appropriate strength only where it is needed, thus avoiding excess weight.

At least three distinct cell types contribute to these processes (Fig. 19.1).

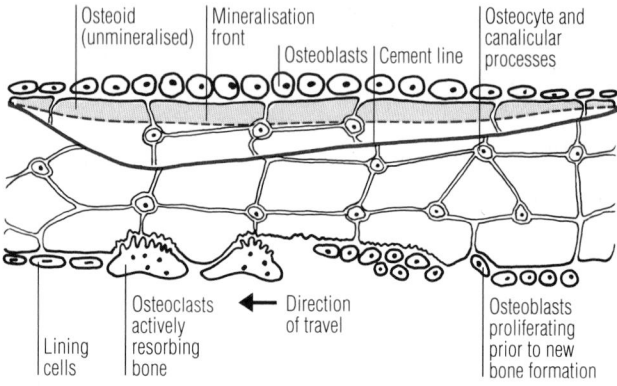

Fig. 19.1 Diagram of normal trabecular bone undergoing osteoclastic resorption followed by new bone formation by osteoblasts. The cement line is shown by a solid red line, and the mineralisation front by a broken red line. Unmineralised osteoid is shaded red.

The osteoblast

The osteoblast is derived from mesenchymal precursor cells and is the main bone-forming cell. It synthesises organic matrix (osteoid) and probably also controls the subsequent mineralisation of the matrix. It has plentiful mitochondria and an extensive Golgi apparatus, both features associated with rapid protein synthesis. It is rich in alkaline phosphatase and is the only important skeletal source of this enzyme. Osteoblasts, and probably also their precursors, possess specific receptors for parathyroid hormone (PTH) and 1,25-dihydroxyvitamin D $(1,25(OH)_2D$, calcitriol). As well as responding directly to these hormones, osteoblasts and their precursors may also act as intermediaries through communication with osteocytes and osteoclasts by means of locally produced cell regulating factors.

The osteocyte

Osteocytes are derived from osteoblasts that no longer have a major biosynthetic role and have become encased in bone, communicating with each other by extensions running through canaliculae in the bone. Their role is not fully defined, but they are likely to be involved in the movement of mineral in the vicinity of the osteocyte lacunae.

The osteoclast

Osteoclasts are the bone-resorbing cells. They are multinucleate and, when actively resorbing, have a deeply folded plasma membrane, creating a 'ruffled border' in close proximity to the bone surface. Osteoclasts are derived from cells of the monocyte and macrophage series. Although they are influenced by the calcium regulating hormones, PTH and $1,25(OH)_2D$, they do not apparently possess specific receptors for these hormones; it is therefore likely that hormonal control is exerted by way of communication with osteoblasts, or by effects of hormones on osteoclast precursors.

In addition to hormonal modulation by PTH and $1,25(OH)_2D$, osteoclasts may be influenced by other hormones, including calcitonin, thyroxine, glucocorticoids and the sex steroids. Furthermore, the functions of osteoblasts and osteoclasts are closely linked, such that an increase in the activity of one cell type is usually accompanied by a parallel increase in the activity of the other. This linkage, or coupling, is probably effected by locally produced regulators.

Bone growth, modelling and remodelling

The ordered processes of bone formation by osteoblasts and resorption by osteoclasts are continuous, and set the stage for growth and the achievement of adult bone architecture (modelling). During this phase, bone mass increases and net bone formation exceeds resorption. Once growth has ceased, coupled activity of osteoblasts and osteoclasts continues, although at a much slower rate, a process which allows alteration of bone architecture (without growth) in response to factors such as mechanical loading. As shown in Figure 19.2, skeletal mass peaks at about the age of 25, decreasing thereafter at a constant rate in males and with a transient acceleration after the

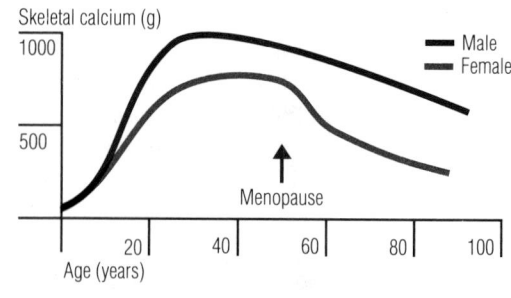

Fig. 19.2 Relationship between bone mass and age.

menopause in females. This progressive decrease indicates that, throughout most of adult life, net bone resorption just exceeds net formation. In some individuals, bone mass may decrease to the point where clinically important mechanical weakening arises (osteoporosis), leading to fractures that may be spontaneous or follow minimal trauma.

HORMONAL CONTROL OF BONE, CALCIUM AND PHOSPHORUS METABOLISM

The interrelationships between extracellular fluid calcium and inorganic phosphorus, and the skeletal reservoirs of these ions and their main entry and exit points (the intestine and the kidney respectively) are controlled by a hormonal system that is dominated by PTH and $1,25(OH)_2D$. The role of the third potential calcium regulating hormone, calcitonin, is more enigmatic. A schematic representation of calcium regulation by PTH and the vitamin D endocrine system is shown in Figure 19.3.

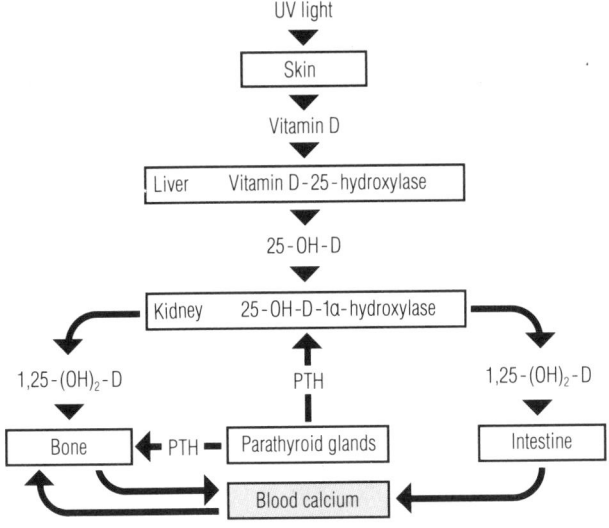

Fig. 19.3 Vitamin D metabolism and the hormonal regulation of calcium metabolism. PTH stimulates renal production of $1,25(OH)_2D$, and bone resorption.

Parathyroid hormone

Parathyroid hormone (PTH) is an 84 amino acid peptide hormone manufactured, stored and released by the chief cells of the parathyroid glands. Two intracellular precursors have been identified, pre-pro PTH being cleaved successively to yield pro-PTH and, finally, PTH 1–84 itself. The release of PTH is highly responsive to the prevailing ionised calcium concentration in the extracellular fluid, particularly in and around the range of physiological calcaemia. Thus, modest hypocalcaemia triggers a substantial PTH response and modest hypercalcaemia almost completely suppresses the secretion of biologically active PTH.

As shown in Figure 19.3, PTH forms part of a feedback loop that is well suited to maintaining calcium homeostasis. The actions of PTH itself are directed towards the elevation of blood and extracellular fluid (ECF) calcium concentration. These actions are:

1. to promote recruitment and activation of osteoclasts and so accelerate bone resorption (indirectly through osteoblasts)
2. to increase the renal tubular resorption of calcium
3. to decrease the renal tubular reabsorption of inorganic phosphate, thus promoting phosphaturia
4. to stimulate the production of $1,25(OH)_2D$, the hormonal form of vitamin D, thereby promoting intestinal calcium absorption.

1,25-dihydroxyvitamin D ($1,25(OH)_2D$, calcitriol)

The potent steroid hormone, 1,25-dihydroxyvitamin D, is produced almost uniquely in the kidney. It is the product of a series of chemical transformations that starts with the production of cholecalciferol (vitamin D_3) in the skin under the influence of ultraviolet light, or with the ingestion of ergocalciferol (vitamin D_2) added to the diet. Normally, very little comes from the latter source. Subsequently, the 25-hydroxylation of vitamin D in the liver and, finally, 1-hydroxylation of 25-hydroxyvitamin D in the kidney results in production of the active hormonal form of vitamin D, $1,25(OH)_2D_3$ (Fig. 19.3). Other hydroxylated metabolites of vitamin D are also produced by the kidney, but $1,25(OH)_2D$ is the only one with clearly defined biological actions. Like PTH, $1,25(OH)_2D$ is a calcaemic hormone; its known actions complement those of PTH. $1,25(OH)_2D$ has two major target organs, intestine and bone.

In the intestine, $1,25(OH)_2D$ increases the absorption of calcium and, to a lesser extent, phosphate by:

1. increasing the permeability of the brush border to calcium
2. promoting the synthesis of a high-affinity calcium-binding protein in the cell
3. accelerating active extrusion of calcium across the basolateral membrane.

In bone, the main action of $1,25(OH)_2D$ is to increase resorption. Indeed, on a molar basis, $1,25(OH)_2D$ is an even more potent stimulus to bone resorption than PTH. Because the terminally differentiated osteoclasts do not possess specific receptors for $1,25(OH)_2D$, the actions of the hormone may be to stimulate the differentiation of mononuclear cell precursors into mature multinucleate osteoclasts. In addition, osteoblasts (which do possess receptors for $1,25(OH)_2D$) can probably modulate the function of nearby osteoclasts, thus providing a link between the hormone and osteoclastic activity.

These actions of $1,25(OH)_2D$ favour elevation of the concentration of ionised calcium and inorganic phosphorus in blood. The extent to which bone formation, as well as resorption, is under the direct control of vitamin D metabolites is unclear, although indirectly, the vitamin D system certainly influences bone formation by controlling concentrations of calcium and phosphate in the extracellular fluid. Production of $1,25(OH)_2D$ is under tight control. In health, this control is dominated by PTH which, by stimulating 1α-hydroxylation in the kidney, increases the production of $1,25(OH)_2D$ (Fig. 19.3). Additional control is from ionised calcium and inorganic phosphate; hypocalcaemia (acting directly on the kidney and also indirectly via PTH) and hypophosphataemia both stimulate production of $1,25(OH)_2D$. Thus, as with PTH, the major modulators of $1,25(OH)_2D$ act in a fashion consistent with the known actions of the hormone, allowing the linked vitamin D and PTH endocrine systems to exert a high level of control over blood ionised calcium and inorganic phosphate concentrations (Fig. 19.3).

Other hormones

Although many other hormones have demonstrable effects on bone metabolism under appropriate circumstances, their physiological role is uncertain.

Calcitonin

Calcitonin is a 32 amino acid peptide hormone secreted by the C-cells of the thyroid gland. Its best defined actions are on bone, where it binds to specific receptors in osteoclasts leading to decreased resorptive activity. Not surprisingly, this effect is most striking where bone turnover is high, such as in growing bone or in Paget's disease (p. 744). Even when given in pharmacological doses, the influence of calcitonin on calcium and bone metabolism in the normal adult is subtle.

Sex steroids

The acceleration of bone loss after the menopause and its amelioration by oestrogen therapy, together with the high prevalance of osteoporosis in women with untreated primary or secondary hypogonadism, has long suggested that oestrogens exert an important influence on bone metabolism. This was thought to be indirect, but recently evidence has been presented for a direct effect, mediated by oestrogen receptors on osteoblasts.

Androgens are responsible for the attainment of higher peak bone mass in males (Fig. 19.2) directly, or indirectly by increasing muscle bulk and strength. Androgens and oestrogens also act on growth cartilage, in concert with growth hormone, promoting growth and, later, epiphyseal closure.

Glucocorticoids

In physiological amounts, glucocorticoids are important regulators of bone growth, probably by actions on both bone-forming and bone-resorbing cells. Pharmacological doses of these steroids decrease bone mass, leading to osteoporosis.

Thyroxine

About one-third of patients with thyrotoxicosis have mild hypercalcaemia, hypercalciuria, or both, and neglected thyrotoxicosis may lead to osteoporosis. Conversely, hypothyroidism is associated with low bone turnover which may be restored to normal by physiological doses of thyroxine.

Local modulation of bone, calcium and phosphorus metabolism

A variety of local factors contribute to the delicate balance that exists between the actions of the different types of bone cells, although many of these have not yet been fully characterised.

Prostaglandins

Local production of prostaglandins, such as PGE_2, may influence bone metabolism directly, or by promoting the synthesis of other locally acting factors such as epidermal growth factor and platelet-derived growth factor. Inhibitors of prostaglandin synthesis have occasionally been used successfully in patients with hypercalcaemia of malignancy (p. 738), but the normal skeleton is not perceptibly affected by these drugs.

Lymphokines

Interleukin-1 is a potent bone-resorbing agent derived from activated macrophages. Although its physiological role in bone is unclear, it has many interactions with other cytokines, such as gamma-interferon, all of which are consistent with local regulatory functions in bone. Tumour necrosis factors and transforming growth factor also have effects, and some or all may be involved in osteoblast/osteoclast coupling.

MAGNESIUM HOMEOSTASIS

Magnesium ions have a similar cellular/extracellular distribution to potassium, and parallel alterations in concentration of these cations are observed in a number of situations. However, the high content of magnesium found in bone results in important associations with calcium metabolism. In addition, magnesium is an effector of PTH secretion.

Hypomagnesaemia may occur with:

1. severe malnutrition
2. long-term intravenous feeding in the absence of magnesium supplements
3. certain long-term renal tubular disorders
4. chronic diuretic therapy
5. diabetes mellitus
6. alcoholism
7. following surgical correction of hyperparathyroidism
8. cytotoxic treatment with cisplatin.

Hypomagnesaemia is rarely severe but may, on occasions, give rise to symptoms and signs similar to hypocalcaemia, with tetany progressing to convulsions and cardiac arrhythmias, with or without associated hypocalcaemia. This may necessitate magnesium supplementation by oral magnesium salts (which, however, may cause diarrhoea) or parenteral magnesium sulphate. Coexisting hypocalcaemia is refractory until the hypomagnesaemia has been corrected; this is due to impaired secretion of PTH and also to target organ resistance to circulating PTH during hypomagnesaemia.

Hypermagnesaemia may complicate renal impairment. It results in gastrointestinal disturbance and may, if severe, cause central nervous system depression. It is rarely of clinical significance.

INVESTIGATION OF BONE DISEASE

The investigations that may be employed fall into five groups:

1. biochemical: blood and urine (Table 19.2)
2. radiographic
3. radionuclide studies
4. measurement of bone mass
5. histology.

Biochemistry

Blood calcium

Total calcium in plasma or serum is the usual measurement taken in clinical practice although, in some instances, direct measurement of the physiologically important ionised fraction is undertaken, using a calcium ion-selective electrode. The latter is likely to be employed with increasing frequency in the future, since it avoids the difficulties that may arise when abnormalities of plasma protein concentration or acid-base status alter the normal relationship between total and ionic calcium in blood. A reduced plasma protein concentration leads to a reduction in plasma total calcium concentration, even though free ionic calcium is normal. The error may be reduced by 'correction' of the observed calcium concentration, using the formula:

$$Ca \text{ (corrected)} = Ca^t + 0.02 \, (46 - alb)$$

where Ca^t is the observed concentration of total calcium in mmol/l and *alb* is the albumin concentration in gm/l. As pH falls, so does calcium binding to plasma proteins. Thus, during severe acidosis, plasma total calcium may be low, with a normal free ionic calcium concentration.

Increases in blood calcium usually reflect accelerated entry into the ECF, either as a result of rapid bone resorption (primary hyperparathyroidism, vitamin D intoxication, osteolytic metastases), or of increased intestinal absorption (high dietary calcium intake, primary hyperparathyroidism, vitamin D intoxication, or milk alkali

Table 19.2 Biochemical investigation of bone disease

Measurements	Associated disease
Blood plasma	
Urea, creatinine	Renal disease
Na^+, K^+, Cl^-, HCO_3^-	Acid-base disturbance
Calcium	Increased in primary hyperparathyroidism, malignant disease, granulomatous disease, vitamin D intoxication
	Decreased in renal disease, osteomalacia, hypoparathyroidism
Phosphate	Increased in renal disease
	Decreased in primary hyperparathyroidism, vitamin D deficiency, renal tubular disorders
Alkaline phosphatase	Increased in hyperparathyroidism, vitamin D deficiency, fracture, malignancy, Paget's disease
	Decreased in hypophosphatasia
Parathyroid hormone (PTH)	Increased in hyperparathyroidism and pseudohypoparathyroidism
	Decreased in hypoparathyroidism
25-hydroxyvitamin D	Vitamin D deficiency or intoxication
Urine	
Calcium	Hypercalciuria
	Familial hypocalciuric hypercalcaemia
Phosphate	Decreased tubular reabsorption in hyperparathyroidism
cAMP	Increased in hyperparathyroidism (provided kidneys normal)

syndrome), or both processes acting together.

Decreases in blood calcium are due to diminished bone resorption and/or diminished intestinal absorption of calcium. Important causes are hypoparathyroidism, vitamin D deficiency with calcium malabsorption, and severe renal disease.

Urine calcium

Urine calcium ranges from 2.5 to 7.5 mmol/24 h in adults and is increased in situations where calcium entry to the ECF is enhanced (leading to potential or actual hypercalcaemia), or where the renal tubular reabsorption of calcium is decreased ('renal leak' type of hypercalciuria), or both.

Plasma inorganic phosphate

Under physiological circumstances, plasma phosphate is determined by the level of renal tubular reabsorption of phosphate, a process that is itself modulated by the dietary intake of phosphate and by PTH. Tubular reabsorption of phosphate is decreased by PTH and increased by low dietary intake of phosphate. A low plasma phosphate is found in association with primary hyperparathyroidism, vitamin D deficiency, certain renal tubular disorders (p. 736) and prolonged dietary phosphate deprivation. Serum phosphate is elevated in patients with substantial impairment of renal function and reduction of glomerular filtration rate (GFR) and, occasionally, in patients with greatly accelerated tissue catabolism (e.g. rhabdomyolysis, tumour necrosis).

Alkaline phosphatase

The enzyme alkaline phosphatase is produced by osteoblasts, and its release into the circulation increases as osteoblast numbers and/or activity increases. This is seen in normal children; it is also seen in generalised disorders characterised by high bone turnover, such as hyperparathyroidism, and in focal lesions, such as healing fractures, Paget's disease, or bone metastases. Many other tissues also contain alkaline phosphatases which often differ slightly from one another (isoenzymes). To avoid diagnostic confusion, elevation of blood alkaline phosphatase must be interpreted in the clinical context and not in isolation. Measurement of specific isoenzymes is increasingly being undertaken to identify the tissue of origin.

Parathyroid hormone

Although measurement of PTH by radioimmunoassay is an important adjunct to the diagnosis of some metabolic bone disorders, interpretation of the results requires appreciation of the limitations of the methodology and of the relationships between PTH, calcium and the vitamin D endocrine system $(1,25(OH)_2D)$. PTH in plasma is present as intact PTH (84 amino acids) and also as several different peptide fragments, the latter reflecting catabolism of circulating PTH by liver, kidney and bone. Potential confusion arises because not all these fragments have biological activity, and different radioimmunoassays may detect the fragments in different proportions. However, with these provisos, elevated PTH is found in the plasma of most patients with primary hyperparathyroidism, virtually all patients with secondary hyperparathyroidism due to underlying renal or intestinal disease, and in all patients with target organ resistance to the action of PTH (pseudo-hypoparathyroidism). PTH is undetectable in patients with hypoparathyroidism.

25-hydroxyvitamin D

Although 25-hydroxyvitamin D (25(OH)D) is the pre-

cursor of the active hormonal form of vitamin D (Fig. 19.3), measurements of 25(OH)D are the best guide to vitamin D status. 25(OH)D in plasma shows a seasonal variation, being high in summer and lower in winter. This reflects dependence of cutaneous production of vitamin D on ultraviolet light. Plasma levels are lower in vitamin D deficiency, due to lack of sunlight exposure and poor diet, normal in patients with renal disease, and elevated in patients with vitamin D intoxication. Measurement of $1,25(OH)_2D$ (the active hormonal form of vitamin D) has little clinical application. Recent work shows that calcium deficiency augments vitamin D deficiency, since it leads to secondary hyperparathyroidism, and PTH apparently accelerates the hepatic degradation of 25(OH)D.

Urinary cyclic-AMP

Most of the cyclic-AMP (cAMP) in urine is generated by PTH action on the kidney; urinary cAMP therefore provides a good measure of a biological effect of circulating PTH and theoretically avoids the difficulties inherent in the radioimmunoassay of PTH. As expected, urinary cAMP is elevated in primary hyperparathyroidism (p. 739), secondary hyperparathyroidism due to intestinal disease, and is low in hypoparathyroid states (p. 742).

Radiography

By virtue of their ability to demonstrate the gross morphology of bone, plain radiographs are of great value in the diagnosis of localised disorders of bone, e.g. developmental abnormalities, fractures, tumours and infections. In addition, some diseases affecting the entire skeleton may also be diagnosed in this way. For example, severe osteoporosis may lead to radiologically evident fractures, and hyperparathyroidism may be associated with visible subperiosteal erosions in the hands and elsewhere (Fig. 19.4). In these instances, local abnormalities are acting as markers for generalised disease.

Radionuclide studies

Bone-seeking radio pharmaceuticals such as ^{99m}Tc methylene bisphosphonate may be given by intravenous injection, and the pattern of uptake assessed by external counting using a gamma camera. Uptake is largely determined by blood flow to bone and by the rate of bone turnover; the technique is therefore extremely good at detecting focal lesions, such as metastases, infections or

Fig. 19.4 X-ray showing subperiosteal erosions in the hands in a case of hyperparathyroidism.

subtle fractures, that may not be visible on conventional radiographs.

Measurement of bone mass

The increasing proportion of elderly people in populations worldwide inevitably leads to an increase in the incidence of age-related diseases such as osteoporosis. The ability to measure bone mass with precision and accuracy, and in a simple and safe manner, is central to the identification, assessment and monitoring of patients with osteoporosis. Conventional radiography is imprecise and crude for this purpose and has little to offer apart from identification of the complications of osteoporosis, such as crush fractures of the spine. However, photon-absorptiometry – in which attenuation by bone of a monoenergetic beam of gamma irradiation is measured – can be used to assess regional bone mass in, for example, the radius or the lumbar spine. Similar information can be obtained using a CT scanner. Both these techniques can offer fairly high precision and accuracy and their use is likely to increase in the future, particularly as useful treatments for osteoporosis are developed.

Histology

The technique of transiliac bone biopsy, whereby a cortex-to-cortex core of bone 5–8 mm in diameter is taken from the ilium under local anaesthetic, is increasingly employed in the diagnosis and assessment of generalised metabolic bone disease. Although invasive, with a skilled operator and appropriate precautions it is safe and generally well tolerated. The specimens are fixed, cut and stained undecalcified, and may yield useful information on the number and activity of osteoblasts and osteoclasts, and indicate whether organic matrix production is normal and whether it is being appropriately mineralised. A useful adjunct is the technique of tetracycline labelling. Here, tetracycline (300 mg of demeclocycline is sufficient) is given twice, with a 10-day interval between; the biopsy is performed four or more days after the second label is taken. The drug is taken up at the mineralisation front in bone, and can be detected in the biopsy specimen by fluorescence under ultraviolet light. Uptake is poor or absent in osteomalacia (p. 735) and enhanced in states of high bone turnover (e.g. hyperparathyroidism and thyrotoxicosis).

OSTEOPOROSIS

The term osteoporosis denotes loss of bone mass per unit volume; bone composition is normal. It becomes clinically important when bone is so weak that pathological fractures result. Most examples of osteoporosis arise as a result of the progresive decrease in bone mass with age (Fig. 19.2); since this occurs to a greater or lesser extent in all individuals, the distinction between pathology and the normal ageing process is blurred.

Pathological changes in bone mass

Bone mass is governed by the balance between bone formation and resorption. Positive, neutral and negative bone balance are found at different ages. Thus, in infancy and again in adolescence, bone formation clearly exceeds resorption; in early adult life, the processes are approximately equal; and later, a disparity in favour of resorption results in a slow decline in total bone mass. Whether or not this gives rise to clinical problems (fractures) depends to a large extent on the maximum bone mass achieved as an adult. This is greater in men than women and is also greater in blacks than whites.

Women are further disadvantaged by a more rapid decrease in bone mass in later adult life, and the net result is a much higher incidence of osteoporotic complications. On average, they also live for about five years longer than men. The reasons for the sex differences in rate of bone loss are probably multiple, but post-menopausal oestrogen deficiency is most strongly implicated. This condition may sensitise the skeleton to the bone-resorbing effects of PTH and possibly also impairs renal synthesis of $1,25(OH)_2D$. The resulting changes are subtle, but may lead to mild but chronic calcium malabsorption and consequent secondary hyperparathyroidism (pp. 735 and 741).

Idiopathic osteoporosis may occasionally occur in young people, especially during the adolescent growth spurt. It is usually self-limiting, but may be complicated by fractures.

Clinical features and investigation

Osteoporosis remains asymptomatic unless structural collapse or fracture of bone occurs. Damage is particularly likely to occur in the dorsal vertebrae, femoral neck and distal radius; precipitating trauma may be trivial.

There are usually no abnormalities on routine plasma biochemistry, except in those cases secondary to specific endocrine disorders (see below). In some patients, urinary calcium excretion may be elevated consistent with net bone resorption, and plasma calcium may be marginally elevated. This is particularly common when immobility is a contributory factor.

Radiology demonstrates decreased bone density due to loss of trabeculae, and reduced cortical thickness of long bones, although these changes are only evident in severe cases. The dorsal vertebrae may show the classical 'wedge collapse' of osteoporotic crush fracture and herniation of the disc into the centre of the vertebra to give a 'codfish' vertebra, and exaggeration of the normal curvature of the thoracic spine (Fig. 19.5). For detecting osteoporosis, measurements of bone mass by photon-absorptiometry, dual X-ray or CT scanning of the spine are much more sensitive and precise than are plain X-rays.

Normality of plasma calcium, phosphate and alkaline phosphatase helps to exclude osteomalacia but, in doubtful cases, further investigation may be necessary, including measurement of plasma 25-hydroxyvitamin D and transiliac bone biopsy.

In most instances, no specific underlying cause for os-

Fig. 19.5 X-ray of lateral thoracic spine of a 60-year-old woman with severe postmenopausal osteoporosis. Note gross loss of density, collapsed and 'cod fish' vertebrae, and kyphosis.

teoporosis will be found. However, careful consideration should be given to the causes outlined below, and further investigation initiated if the overall clinical picture so warrants.

Specific causes of osteoporosis

Osteoporosis is common in the elderly and it may be difficult to decide whether a vertebral collapse is due to osteoporosis or to another, coincidental, underlying disease such as secondary carcinoma. Cancer of the breast, lung, kidney and thyroid typically cause lytic lesions in bone. Prostatic cancer may also do so, though sclerosis is a more common complication. Breast cancer in particular has a predilection for secondary spread to the axial skeleton. Myeloma (Ch. 25, p. 1070) may be accompanied by generalised thinning of bones and/or focal lytic areas. Physical examination will usually detect a primary breast cancer, but further investigation may be needed to exclude other forms of cancer and myeloma.

Chronic liver disease (especially primary biliary cirrhosis) may give rise to a mixed picture of osteoporosis and osteomalacia (see below). Hereditary abnormalities in bone formation are discussed on page 745.

The conditions which may be complicated by significant osteoporosis are listed in Table 19.3.

Management

The prevention and treatment of osteoporosis is summarised in Summary 1.

Summary 1   Prevention and management of osteoporosis

Prevention	Treatment
Physical activity (youth and throughout adulthood)	Physical exercise
	Weight gain if underweight
Good diet (generous calcium intake and avoiding excess alcohol)	Oestrogen therapy
	Calcium supplements
Non-smoking	Stop smoking
Early and effective treatment of predisposing conditions:	Anabolic (androgenic) steroids
Hypogonadism/premature menopause	Symptomatic therapy, e.g. lumbar supports
Thyrotoxicosis	
Cushing's syndrome	Bisphosphonates or calcitonin
Diabetes mellitus	

Prevention

Prevention of the development of osteoporosis in individuals at risk is of the utmost importance. This is most obviously the case in females with primary or premature ovarian failure, and all such individuals should be treated with oestrogens. Progesterone supplements should also be given cyclically (p. 721) to avoid unopposed endometrial stimulation with its risk of neoplastic change. However, the use of prophylactic oestrogen supplements after the physiological menopause is more controversial. Oestrogen undoubtedly reduces the rate of bone loss after the menopause (and even increases bone mass in many patients); despite earlier concerns, this is probably not associated with an increased risk of vascular pathology, at least at low dosage. Appropriate exercise, e.g. regular swimming, should be encouraged in patients with relative immobility, and regular non-strenuous exercise in the elderly.

Treatment

The treatment of established osteoporosis is, unfortunately, often unsatisfactory. With the exception of oestrogens, no form of therapy has been shown to have a consistent effect in reversing bone changes, although retardation of bone loss may be possible. Dietary calcium should be generous (at least 25–50 mmol per day); if this is not achieved, the diet may be supplemented with calcium carbonate tablets. The evidence that calcium supplements are of benefit is conflicting, but the therapy is easy and does no harm. In selected patients, an argument may be

Table 19.3   Causes of generalised osteoporosis and their mechanisms*

Cause	Frequency of osteoporosis in the condition	Bone resorption	Bone formation	Plasma calcium	Comments
Corticosteroid excess	Common	↑	↓	Normal	Reduced intestinal calcium absorption Renal stones Not fully reversible
Early menopause	Common (if untreated)	↑	Normal	Normal	
Immobility	Common	Normal	↓	Normal	Increased urinary Ca^{2+} excretion Largely reversible
Multiple myeloma	Common	↑	↓	Normal or ↑	May be local lytic lesions as well Local osteoclast activating factor
Hypogonadism (primary or secondary)	Common (if untreated)	Normal	↓	Normal	Limits maximum adult bone mass
Thyrotoxicosis	Rare	↑	↑	Normal or ↑	Reversible
Diabetes mellitus	Rare	Normal	↓	Normal	Type I diabetes only
Pregnancy	Rare	↑	↓	Normal	

*Primary liver disease is omitted since this is associated with a combination of osteoporosis and osteomalacia.

made for oestrogen supplements, particularly where oestrogen deficiency has been present at an abnormally early stage in life.

Preparations of 'hydroxyapatite compound' are of no proven benefit, and anabolic steroids are of doubtful value. Other measures currently under investigation include the use of parathyroid hormone, calcitonin, bisphosphonate compounds and sodium fluoride. The last undoubtedly stimulates osteoblast function but, paradoxically, probably leads to bone that is structurally weak; the side-effects may also be troublesome.

RICKETS AND OSTEOMALACIA

Rickets and osteomalacia are conditions characterised by pathological defects in bone matrix mineralisation. Rickets refers specifically to osteomalacia where the defect occurs in *growing* bone. The aetiological factors are diverse, but the end result is an increased quantity of unmineralised bone matrix (osteoid). Histologically this is characterised by widened osteoid seams, morphologically flat 'inactive' osteoblasts, and absence of tetracycline uptake indicating impairment of mineralisation. The increase in osteoid must be distinguished from that seen in thyrotoxic bone disease, Paget's disease or hyperparathyroidism. In all these conditions, there is high bone turnover with 'hyperosteoidosis'; mineralisation of matrix is normal or enhanced.

Aetiology

The aetiology of osteomalacia (or rickets) is shown in Table

19.4. The conditions may arise in three distinct situations:

1. vitamin D deficiency or abnormal vitamin D metabolism
2. phosphate depletion
3. chronic metabolic acidosis.

Vitamin D deficiency is numerically by far the most important cause of osteomalacia (or rickets). It leads to combined deficiency of calcium and phosphorus. There is intestinal malabsorption of calcium, and to a lesser extent phosphorus as well. *Secondary hyperparathyroidism* results, and the ensuing phosphaturia accelerates the phosphate deficiency. Lack of vitamin D is often due to a combination of poor exposure to sunlight and dietary deficiency. The elderly population is particularly at risk. In the UK, there is a very high incidence of osteomalacia in the Asian immigrant population (p. 128). The reason for this is multifactorial and incompletely understood but dietary deficiency of vitamin D and calcium together with binding of calcium by the phytate contained in chapatti flour may contribute. In addition, deeply pigmented skin generates less vitamin D_3 in response to a given amount of ultraviolet exposure and this may be disadvantageous in temperate climates. Vitamin D deficiency may complicate fat malabsorption from any cause. Finally, calcium deficiency enhances the rate of degradation of 25(OH)D in the liver, further exacerbating the shortage of vitamin D and its metabolites.

Failure of 25-hydroxylation of vitamin D (p. 729, Fig. 19.3). This may be a feature of hepatocellular dysfunction. It may also result from hepatic enzyme induction consequent upon long-term anticonvulsant medication (leading to enhanced degradation).

19

Table 19.4 Causes of osteomalacia/rickets

Cause	Mechanism

Vitamin D deficiency	Defective intake/formation
	  Lack of solar exposure (D_3) and lack of dietary intake or fat malabsorption (D_2)
	  Severe chronic liver disease
	Increased/wasteful metabolism
	  Liver-enzyme-inducing drugs, e.g. phenytoin, phenobarbitone, carbamazepine, rifampicin
	Failure of activation, $25(OH)D \rightarrow 1,25(OH)_2D$
	  Chronic renal failure
	  Hereditary vitamin D-dependent rickets type I
	Target organ defect
	  Hereditary vitamin D-dependent rickets type II

Phosphate deficiency	Poor intake
	  Aluminium hydroxide – excess binding of dietary phosphate,
	Increased loss
	  X-linked hypophosphataemia (vitamin D-resistant rickets)
	  Fanconi's syndrome
	  Renal tubular acidosis
	  Ureterocolic anastamosis
	  Tumour-associated

Chronic metabolic acidosis	Renal tubular acidosis (may be phosphate depletion also) Ureterocolic anastamosis
Osteoblast/mineralisation defect	Hypophosphatasia Etidronate therapy Aluminium intoxication (in renal disease, see p. 808)

Reduced 1-hydroxylation of 25-hydroxyvitamin D by the kidney is a frequent accompaniment of chronic renal failure, and also occurs as a rare recessively inherited condition in which levels of the 1-hydroxylase enzyme are low (vitamin D-dependent rickets type I). Failure to hydroxylate 25-hydroxyvitamin D also occurs in hypoparathyroidism and pseudohypoparathyroidism. Another rare form is associated with an abnormality of the $1,25(OH)_2D$ receptor in target tissues (vitamin D-depen-dent rickets type II).

Phosphate depletion is a less common cause of rickets than vitamin D deficiency or altered metabolism. It arises as a result of a reduced maximal capacity for renal tubular phosphate reabsorption. This may either be inherited as an X-linked recessive characteristic (vitamin D-resistant rickets), or occur as part of Fanconi's syndrome – a more generalised hereditary or acquired renal tubular defect typified by aminoaciduria and glycosuria (p. 813). Rarely, excessive ingestion of antacids may restrict intestinal phosphate absorption to the point where clinically important phosphate depletion, and even osteomalacia or rickets, may appear.

Chronic metabolic acidosis, usually resulting from renal tubular disorders, may lead to rickets or osteomalacia. The bone lesions usually heal satisfactorily following treatment to correct the acidosis.

Clinical features

In children, failure of bone mineralisation gives rise to classical bone deformities which include widening of the metaphyses, prominence of costochondral junctions (so-called 'rickety rosary') and varus or valgus abnormalities of the knee joints. The bones are painful and statural growth is reduced. In adults, bone pain and tenderness are the most prominent features. A characteristic proximal myopathy may develop, and is more common in those cases that are due to vitamin D deficiency.

Investigation

Biochemical. In osteomalacia due to vitamin D deficiency or abnormal metabolism of vitamin D, biochemical investigations typically demonstrate a low normal plasma calcium (maintained by secondary hyperparathyroidism), a low plasma phosphate resulting from increased PTH-dependent phosphaturia, and a raised alkaline phosphatase indicating increased numbers of osteoblasts (Table 19.5). Vitamin D deficiency may be confirmed by measurement of 25-hydroxyvitamin D in plasma using a competitive protein-binding assay. X-linked hypophosphataemia, on the other hand, is characterised by normocalcaemia, hypophosphataemia and little or no alteration in plasma alkaline phosphatase level.

Radiological features of rickets include widening and irregularity of the metaphysis with an increased width of

Table 19.5 Plasma measurements in various causes of osteomalacia/rickets

Cause	Plasma measurements					
	Calcium	Phosphate	Alk. phos.	Urea	Creatinine	pH
Vitamin D deficiency	N or ↓	↓	↑	N	N	N
Familial hypophosphataemia	N	↓↓	N or ↑	N	N	N
Chronic renal failure	N or ↓	↑	N or ↑	↑	↑	N or ↓
Renal tubular acidosis	N or ↓	N or ↓	N or ↑	N	N	↓

the growth plate. In osteomalacia, the bones appear less dense than normal and the long bones may show localised areas of decalcification on the concave surface, referred to as pseudofractures or Looser's zones (Fig. 19.6). Decreased strength of bone may result in biconcave deformity of the vertebrae. In hypophosphataemic rickets, there may be a paradoxical apparent increase in bone density.

Histological. Occasionally a bone biopsy may be needed (following double tetracycline labelling) to confirm a diagnosis of osteomalacia, when biochemical investigations are equivocal. This is particularly the case in seeking possible treatable factors in elderly patients with decreased bone density.

Fig. 19.6 Radiological features of osteomalacia. Arrow indicates Looser's zone.

Treatment

Vitamin D deficiency is most conveniently treated by oral replacement of vitamin D_2 or vitamin D_3 in physiological quantities (500–1000 units per day). This can conveniently be given as combined calcium with vitamin D tablets. Alternatively, a single im dose of 150 000 IU of D_2 in oil is effective prophylaxis and treatment for at least six months. The possibility of intestinal malabsorption should be borne in mind, and appropriate investigation initiated if necessary. Osteomalacia associated with anticonvulsant therapy requires higher doses of vitamin D (3000–6000 units/day). Treatment of X-linked hypophosphataemia is generally unsatisfactory. The logical treatment is with oral phosphate supplements, but the doses needed are large and they may be poorly tolerated because of gastrointestinal side-effects. Oral phosphate works better when combined with pharmacological doses of vitamin D or (and probably best) in combination with $1,25(OH)_2D_3$. The management of renal tubular acidosis is dealt with in Chapter 21, pages 813–815.

HYPERCALCAEMIA

Elevation of total plasma calcium is usually associated with a concomitant increase in ionised calcium concentration.

Pathophysiology

A large number of conditions may be associated with hypercalcaemia (Table 19.6). Improvements in our understanding of vitamin D and parathyroid physiology enable reasonably accurate classification of the condition according to basic mechanisms. In Table 19.6 they are classified according to the level of $1,25(OH)_2D$. When this hormone is elevated, it may be presumed to be causing hypercalcaemia by stimulating intestinal absorption of calcium and bone resorption.

In *primary hyperparathyroidism*, PTH is elevated, usually as a result of a parathyroid adenoma, and stimulates osteoclastic bone resorption, tubular reabsorption of calcium and the activity of 1-hydroxylase in the proximal renal tubular cells. This in turn promotes conversion of $25(OH)D$ to $1,25(OH)_2D$, which acts on the upper small intestine to increase active calcium transport. Since PTH also enhances renal phosphate excretion, the serum phosphate level falls.

In *sarcoidosis*, and some other granulomatous diseases, macrophages in the diseased tissue make $1,25(OH)_2D$ outside the kidneys in amounts that are sufficient to produce hypercalcaemia. Calcium is absorbed by the intestine in increasing amounts, PTH is suppressed, and the normal feedback of the vitamin D-endocrine system is effectively sabotaged. The same mechanism occurs in some

Table 19.6 Causes of hypercalcaemia

Elevated levels of $1,25(OH)_2D$
With high levels of PTH
   Primary hyperparathyroidism – Adenoma
                                  – Hyperplasia
                                    – Carcinoma
   'Tertiary' hyperparathyroidism

With low levels of PTH
   Increased vitamin D intake
   Increased extrarenal synthesis of $1,25(OH)_2D$ – Lymphoma
                                             – Sarcoidosis
                                             – Tuberculosis
                                             – Glucocorticoid deficiency
                                                (Addison's disease)

Low or normal levels of $1,25(OH)_2D$
Tumour-induced
   Osteolytic bone lesions – Carcinoma (breast, oesophagus, lung, thyroid)
                                  – Multiple myelomatosis
   Circulating PTH-like peptide – Squamous carcinomas (lung
                                        and skin)
                                        – Renal carcinoma
                                        – Leukaemias
Milk alkali syndrome
Familial hypocalciuric hypercalcaemia

lymphomas and sarcomas.

Malignancy is an important cause of hypercalcaemia. There are several mechanisms.

1. Direct invasion of bone and production of local factors which either destroy bone directly or stimulate local osteoclasts to do so, leads to accelerated bone resorption. Breast cancer commonly causes hypercalcaemia by this mechanism. If calcium is elevated in a patient with breast cancer, it virtually always indicates that metastases are present.
2. Haematological malignancies may produce lymphokines which act as osteoclast-activating factors; included in this group is multiple myeloma, which may also cause a spurious elevation of (protein-bound) calcium, when the monoclonal immunoglobulin also binds calcium.
3. Some haematological malignancies can produce excessive amounts of $1,25(OH)_2D$ or bone-resorbing lymphokines, although this is uncommon.
4. Finally, some solid tumours (such as renal carcinomas and some squamous carcinomas) may cause hypercalcaemia by secreting PTH-related peptide (PTH-rp), a factor which activates bone resorption, and/or enhances renal tubular calcium reabsorption and the renal production of $1,25(OH)_2D$. This peptide has partial sequence homology with PTH (accounting for the hypercalcaemia) but is not detected by PTH immunoassays.

Clinical features

If the serum calcium concentration is only slightly raised, hypercalcaemia is generally asymptomatic. Severe hypercalcaemia, however, leads to a life-threatening acute illness; its treatment constitutes a medical emergency. The principle symptoms and signs are renal, gastrointestinal and neurological.

Renal. Thirst and polyuria are early symptoms which result from the production of a state of nephrogenic diabetes insipidus. The increased ionised calcium level impairs the ADH-mediated mechanism of water reabsorption in the distal nephron. There are also electrolyte abnormalities, notably enhanced sodium and potassium excretion, and collectively these lead to volume contraction, pre-renal reduction of glomerular filtration rate (Ch. 21, p. 787) and a further decrease in renal calcium excretion. The situation is compounded if the patient is ill and confined to bed, and so enters further negative skeletal calcium balance.

Gastrointestinal. In the gastrointestinal system, common early symptoms are anorexia and constipation. Later, particularly when pre-renal uraemia develops, the patient develops nausea and vomiting.

Neurological symptoms commonly include lassitude, anxiety and depression, or any psychosis to which that person may be otherwise predisposed. In severe hypercalcaemia (calcium levels above 4 mmol/l), confusion and drowsiness may be superseded by coma.

Regardless of cause, hypercalcaemia is liable to be com-

plicated by ectopic calcification. This is particularly likely if the hypercalcaemia is longstanding as in primary hyperparathyroidism or sarcoidosis. Those patients with malignancy rarely survive long enough for ectopic calcification to become a serious clinical problem. The renal tract is particularly susceptible, and renal stones or nephrocalcinosis (Fig. 19.7) commonly occur. Frequently, there is calcification of blood vessels, especially the media of arteries. Calcification bands on the medial or lateral edge

Fig. 19.7 Nephrocalcinosis in a patient with severe primary hyperparathyroidism.

of the cornea may be visible (band keratopathy) and conjunctival inflammation may develop if hypercalcaemia is severe. Acute pancreatitis is an important complication, particularly if other factors, such as high alcohol intake, are also operating.

Finally, the cardiovascular system is also susceptible through the increased incidence of hypertension associated with chronic hypercalcaemia. The ECG shows shortening of the QT interval.

Investigation

Potentially useful investigations in hypercalcaemia are listed in Table 19.7.

The *steroid suppression test* aims to identify those cases in which pharmacological doses of glucocorticoids reduce significantly the elevated plasma calcium. Hypercalcaemia due to elevated circulating $1,25(OH)_2D$ usually suppresses fully, and this is likely to be the case with underlying granulomatous disease (e.g. sarcoidosis, tuberculosis), some malignancies (e.g. leukaemia, lymphoma) and glucocorticoid deficiency (Addison's disease). In this test, prednisolone is given at 30 mg/day for 10 days, with

Table 19.7 Diagnostic yield in hypercalcaemia

Investigation	Potential information
Full blood count	Anaemia suggests non-parathyroid aetiology if renal function normal
ESR	Usually over 80 in myeloma
Plasma chloride	Upper normal in hyperparathyroidism
Plasma bicarbonate	Low normal in hyperparathyroidism
Creatinine	Significantly raised in the tertiary autonomous hyperparathyroidism of renal failure. Moderately raised in renal impairment secondary to hypercalcaemia
Plasma protein electrophoresis	Monoclonal band suggests myeloma
Bradshaw's test and urinary immunoelectrophoresis	Presence of light chains suggests myeloma
Plasma phosphate	Low normal in primary hyperparathyroidism unless renal function impaired
Plasma PTH	Upper normal or raised in hyperparathyroidism. Suppressed with other causes of hypercalcaemia
Steroid suppression test	Sarcoid hypercalcaemia always suppresses; hyperparathyroid never; malignant causes occasionally
24 h urine calcium	Decreased in familial hypocalciuric hypercalcaemia
Chest X-ray	Look for primary neoplasm; metastases; hilar lymphadenopathy suggesting sarcoid
Isotope bone scan	'Hot spots' suggest metastatic malignant disease
X-ray hands	Subperiosteal erosions suggest hyperparathyroidism

measurement of plasma calcium before, after 5 days and after 10 days of treatment.

Treatment

Asymptomatic hypercalcaemia requires no therapy except appropriate management of the underlying condition.

General measures

Symptomatic hypercalcaemia requires measures directed towards rehydration and appropriate sodium and potassium repletion. A forced saline diuresis (normal saline given iv at 4–6 l/day) substantially and immediately augments the urinary excretion of calcium; a further increase in calciuria may be induced by the addition of frusemide (20 mg/h), *provided that the saline infusion is fast enough to keep the patient volume-expanded.* With such treatment

alone, the plasma calcium will usually come down to safe levels (3.5 mmol/l or less).

Specific measures

Specific treatments depend upon the cause. Glucocorticoids are only effective for the hypercalcaemia of sarcoidosis, vitamin D intoxication and Addison's disease; for the first two, a high dose rapidly tapering down is used. Infusions of sodium phosphate (10 mmol/h for a maximum of 10 hours) are rapidly effective in the short term, particularly if initial plasma phosphate is low. However, sodium phosphate infusion is potentially dangerous, as it lowers calcium, principally by causing microscopic precipitation of calcium phosphate in soft tissues; this is particularly marked if initial plasma phosphate is high. Oral sodium phosphate therapy is safe provided renal function is good, but often causes diarrhoea. For hypercalcaemia due to increased bone resorption, calcitonin at high dose is effective but very short-lived.

The treatment of choice in hypercalcaemia of malignancy is now the bisphosphonate, pamidronate (aminohydroxy-propylidine 1,1 bisphosphonate, APD), which reliably restores calcium levels to normal within five days when infused at doses of 15 mg iv in saline over two hours daily for four days, or as a single dose of 60 mg over eight hours. Subsequent doses can be given prophylactically or when the calcium level rises again. The drug acts by inhibiting osteoclastic bone resorption. Mithramycin is a cytotoxic antibiotic that effectively lowers plasma calcium in most patients, but marrow and hepatic toxicity may preclude maintenance treatment. Both pamidronate and mithramycin have a delayed action (24–72 hours) and saline diuresis remains an important part of early management.

Summary 2   Treatment of severe hypercalcaemia

- Correct salt and water deficit with normal saline
- Begin forced saline diuresis + frusemide
- Give bisphosphonate, e.g. pamidronate (APD)
- Treat underlying cause if possible

SPECIFIC HYPERCALCAEMIC SYNDROMES

PRIMARY HYPERPARATHYROIDISM

Primary overactivity of one or more parathyroid glands is common, especially in elderly women. In the UK, routine measurement of serum calcium in the hospital population reveals an incidence of at least 1%. Of these, approximately three-quarters are associated with a single adenoma; in the others, there is either more than one adenoma, or four-gland hyperplasia. In about 1% of cases, a parathyroid carcinoma underlies the disease. Adenoma or hyperplasia may be associated with one of the syndromes (I or II) of multiple endocrine adenomatosis (p. 712).

Clinical features

The clinical features of primary hyperparathyroidism are variable. Patients commonly remain asymptomatic for long periods, and the finding of a mild elevation of serum calcium in an elderly asymptomatic patient requires no active intervention. In more severe cases, the symptoms may be those of *hypercalcaemia* (p. 738). Immobilisation is a potent precipitating factor, which may lead to a brisk rise in serum calcium.

Renal complications include renal calculi, which may present with renal colic and nephrocalcinosis (Fig. 19.7). This is particularly likely in warm climates, where insensible fluid and sodium loss are excessive and urine flow rate low. Hypertension is common, even in the absence of overt renal damage; there is debate as to whether it responds to surgical treatment of hyperparathyroidism.

Much more frequent is *bone disease*, which results from the development of increased bone turnover leading to high-turnover osteoporosis. As many as 10–15% of elderly patients with osteoporotic hip fractures may have primary hyperparathyroidism. Much less commonly, there may be osteitis fibrosa cystica, with the development of so-called 'brown tumours' of the mandible or long bones. Again, the finding of such a lesion is an indication to check the serum biochemistry. The typical radiological lesion is sub-periosteal erosion in the phalanges of the hands (Fig. 19.4).

Treatment

The severity of the hypercalcaemia should be assessed, as well as the occurrence of complications. In cases with severe clinical hypercalcaemia, emergency treatment should be initiated along the lines outlined on page 739. The only curative therapy is parathyroid surgery. Modern diagnostic techniques which may help to localise a tumour include technetium-thallium subtraction scanning of the neck, and (rarely) catheterisation of the veins draining from the neck, for measurement of PTH in blood from different sites. High resolution CT scanning and ultrasound may also be of value.

Surgery

Ultimately, treatment falls to the surgeon, whose expertise in identifying all four parathyroids will determine the success of the operation. Adenomas of the lower parathyroids (derived from the upper pair of branchial arches) are sometimes retrosternal, but can be located at surgery by pulling up the thymus gland, with which they are closely associated. All four glands should be biopsied, and adenomatous tissue removed. With four-gland hyperplasia, the safe course is probably to remove all four, and then to maintain the hypoparathyroid patient on $1,25(OH)_2D_3$ or $1(OH)D_3$ (alfacalcidol), a synthetic precursor of $1,25(OH)_2D_3$. Pre- and postoperative treatment with $1,25(OH)_2D_3$ or $1(OH)D_3$ may be helpful in preventing postoperative hypocalcaemia.

Other measures

In some patients, surgical cure is not achieved. Failure to remove enough parathyroid tissue may leave the patient with 'incurable' hyperparathyroidism. Some patients refuse surgery and, because primary hyperparathyroidism is principally a disease of the elderly, some will be deemed unfit for surgery. Conservative management of these patients may entail observation only, with monitoring of plasma calcium concentration and checking for complications. More active measures include the use of oral phosphate supplements or the bisphosphonate, pamidronate (p. 739). However, although both will alleviate hypercalciuria and hypercalcaemia in the short and medium term, surgery remains the preferred treatment in most younger and symptomatic older patients.

MISCELLANEOUS HYPERCALCAEMIC SYNDROMES

Milk alkali syndrome, now rarely seen, is associated with excessive ingestion of milk and alkali, particularly if taken in the form of calcium carbonate, to relieve dyspepsia. The hypercalcaemia is accompanied by metabolic alkalosis and is due to a combination of increased intestinal calcium absorption and decreased renal calcium excretion.

Addison's disease may present with hypercalcaemia through extra-renal production of $1,25(OH)_2D$. Glucocorticoid replacement leads to prompt response. In a patient with coincidental Addison's disease and hypoparathyroidism, the potential hypocalcaemia of the latter may be masked until glucocorticoids are given.

Thyrotoxicosis. Thyroid hormones increase bone turnover and, in excess, cause net efflux of calcium from bone. Some 30% of these patients display hypercalciuria and/or hypercalcaemia, although the latter is not severe. These abnormalities are corrected by treatment of the underlying thyrotoxicosis.

Familial hypocalciuric hypercalcaemia is a recently recognised syndrome that may be detected at any age. It is usually asymptomatic, and is not associated with renal damage (although it may cause pancreatitis). It is inherited as an autosomal dominant condition, and so can usually be excluded if both parents are available for blood sampling. It appears to be due to excessively avid renal tubular calcium reabsorption.

HYPOCALCAEMIA

Pathophysiology

The principle causes of hypocalcaemia are listed in Table 19.8. Since the major calcium-binding protein in plasma is albumin, hypoalbuminaemia is associated with a pro-

Table 19.8 Causes of hypocalcaemia

Cause	Comments
With low levels of PTH	
Hypoparathyroidism	Phosphate high
Post-surgical	Alkaline phosphatase and renal
Congenital	function normal
Idiopathic (autoimmune)	
With normal or high levels of PTH	
Rickets/osteomalacia	Phosphate low
Sunlight/dietary deficiency	Alkaline phosphatase high
Malabsorption	Calcium deficiency
Increased D metabolism	Drug-induced
Tumour-induced	
Chronic renal failure	Urea, creatinine, phosphate high
Pseudohypoparathyroidism	Phosphate high, somatic manifestations (type I only)

Table 19.9 Causes of secondary hyperparathyroidism

Cause	Example
Vitamin D deficiency	Lack of solar exposure
	Dietary deficiency
	Increased catabolism – drug-induced (e.g. anticonvulsants, rifampicin)
Dietary calcium deficiency	Low calcium intake
	High phytic acid intake (chapattis, wholemeal bread)
Gastrointestinal causes of low calcium or vitamin D intake	Gastric surgery
	Partial gastrectomy
	Gastroenterostomy
	Vagotomy and pyloroplasty
	Jejunal diverticulosis
	Crohn's disease
	Small bowel resection
Renal	Chronic renal failure
	Phosphate retention
	Reduced 1α-hydroxylation of 25(OH)D

portionate fall in plasma total calcium (see correction formula on p. 731), though not in ionised calcium. The ionised calcium concentration is affected by the blood pH, since the avidity of albumin for calcium falls at acid pH and rises with alkalosis. Hence, respiratory alkalosis due to overbreathing can lead to depression of ionic calcium and tetany. Rarely, infusion of citrate (e.g. in repeated blood transfusions) leads to a serious fall in ionised calcium by complexing the ion.

In *hypoparathyroidism* (p. 742) the major abnormalities result from failure of PTH-dependent renal synthesis of $1,25(OH)_2D$, leading to a reduction of intestinal calcium absorption. This is compounded by failure of osteoclastic bone resorption, by enhanced (inappropriate) urine calcium excretion and by hyperphosphataemia; all of these are due to loss of the normal effects of PTH on bone and kidney.

In *chronic renal failure* (CRF), several factors contribute to hypocalcaemia. These include phosphate retention, and loss of renal parenchyma with failure to produce normal amounts of $1,25(OH)_2D$. A rise in serum phosphate from any cause depresses the serum calcium, partly by leading to micro-precipitation of calcium phosphate in soft tissue. The associated bone disease is discussed on page 805. In CRF, metabolic acidosis is commonly present, and this diminishes the fall in ionised calcium. Tetany is rare in adults (but more common in children), at least until the acidosis is corrected. Hypocalcaemia in *vitamin D deficiency* is usually not severe, because secondary hyperparathyroidism enhances bone resorption and maintains the serum calcium level. The typical biochemical changes are borderline low serum calcium, a low phosphate, and elevated alkaline phosphatase level. If the parathyroid glands do not respond, or calcium intake is very low, hypocalcaemia may be more profound.

In CRF and vitamin D deficiency, and in other conditions (listed in Table 19.9), the parathyroid hypersecretion (secondary hyperparathyroidism) is an *appro-*

priate response to threatened or actual hypocalcaemia. In some patients, however, long-standing appropriate hypersecretion (secondary hyperparathyroidism) transforms to *inappropriate* autonomy and consequent hypercalcaemia. This is called tertiary hyperparathyroidism.

Pseudohypoparathyroidism is discussed on p. 742.

Clinical features

The clinical manifestations of hypocalcaemia are principally in the nervous system. Tetany, painful cramps and tingling in the extremities may occur, and muscle spasm may lead to a characteristic position of the hand, the so-called '*main d'accoucheur*'. These symptoms may be precipitated by exercise. Laryngeal spasm may lead to stridor and obstructed respiration. Hypocalcaemia lowers the epileptic seizure threshold, and fits may be the presenting symptom. The differential diagnosis is principally of tetany due to anxiety leading to hyperventilation and respiratory alkalosis, or hypokalaemic metabolic alkalosis. Hypocalcaemia, particularly when chronic, may present with psychiatric manifestations varying from general malaise to overt psychosis.

Differential diagnosis of hypocalcaemia

Correction for a low serum albumin concentration will allow the distinction between true (ionised) hypocalcaemia and the spurious fall due to hypoalbuminaemia. As with other calcium disorders, the combination of the clinical context and the routine biochemistry will usually establish the cause. Uraemia and elevated serum creatinine concentration point to chronic renal failure. *Hypoparathyroidism* and *pseudohypoparathyroidism* (p. 742) are associated with normal renal function with an elevated serum phosphate level. There may also be clinical pointers, e.g. recent thyroid or parathyroid surgery for the former, skeletal abnormalities for the latter.

Treatment

Hypocalcaemic tetany responds rapidly to the intravenous infusion of 10 ml of 10% calcium gluconate; the response, however, is short-lived. The underlying cause should be treated and, in the case of hypoparathyroidism, this has been greatly helped by the availability of $1,25(OH)_2D_3$ (calcitriol) or 1 hydroxyvitamin D_3 (alfacalcidol). The latter is then 25-hydroxylated in the liver to yield $1,25(OH)_2D_3$. By virtue of their high potency, rapid onset and short duration of action, these compounds have converted a very difficult therapeutic problem into an easy one. Hypocalcaemia in osteomalacia due to vitamin D deficiency is seldom marked; here, correct treatment is with vitamin D itself, rather than the active metabolite (p. 737).

SPECIFIC HYPOCALCAEMIC SYNDROMES

Hypoparathyroidism

There are three types of hypoparathyroidism:

1. post-surgical
2. idiopathic hypoparathyroidism
3. pseudohypoparathyroidism.

All are associated with hypocalcaemia (with or without symptoms and signs of hypocalcaemia) and with hyperphosphataemia in the absence of renal impairment.

Post-surgical hypoparathyroidism

Post-surgical hypoparathyroidism is the commonest cause of hypocalcaemia and follows thyroid or parathyroid surgery. Estimates of its frequency vary from 0.2% to 22%, depending on diagnostic criteria and the length of follow-up after surgery. Vascular or mechanical trauma to the parathyroid glands may contribute to the subsequent parathyroid insufficiency.

Idiopathic hypoparathyroidism

The condition of idiopathic hypoparathyroidism is most commonly acquired in adolescence or early adult life; it may be associated with auto-antibodies to parathyroid tissue, and with other organ-specific autoimmune diseases, such as Addison's disease and immune thyroiditis. Some cases are familial. An autoimmune aetiology has been postulated but not proven. Patients may suffer from widespread candida infections and dystrophic nails, alopecia, calcification in the basal ganglia and cataract, in addition to other symptoms and signs of hypocalcaemia.

PTH is undetectable despite hypocalcaemia, and the lack of its effect on the kidney is reflected by renal phosphate retention leading to hyperphosphataemia and low con-

version of 25(OH)D to $1,25(OH)_2D$. Administration of PTH corrects all the biochemical abnormalities, indicating that target organ responsiveness to PTH remains normal in this condition. However, long term treatment with PTH is impractical and management is with $1,25(OH)_2D_3$ or $1(OH)D_3$. Most cases respond well to 1–3 μg daily of either; there is, however, little margin for error and the dose should be titrated carefully against the serum calcium levels. Oral calcium supplements enhance the effect.

Pseudohypoparathyroidism

Pseudohypoparathyroidism is a rare disorder thought to be due to a defect in the PTH receptor or its coupling to adenylate cyclase. The clinical and biochemical features of hypoparathyroidism are associated with characteristic somatic manifestations; these include short stature, mental deficiency, and unusually short fourth and fifth metacarpals and metatarsals. There is a partial or complete failure of response (urinary cAMP or phosphaturia) to PTH, and high serum PTH levels. As with true hypoparathyroidism, $1,25(OH)_2D$ levels are low. Some patients have the somatic manifestations without the hypocalcaemia (pseudopseudohypoparathyroidism). In some cases, the biochemical changes are associated, paradoxically, with hyperparathyroid bone disease, possibly reflecting isolated renal resistance with normal skeletal responsiveness to PTH.

Hypomagnesaemia

Hypomagnesia is a rare but important cause of hypocalcaemia. It is refractory to calcium, but responds to magnesium therapy (p. 730).

PAGET'S DISEASE OF BONE

In 1879, Sir James Paget described a bone disease which he named 'osteitis deformans'. Although there have, in recent years, been important advances in uncovering the cause of the disease and in developing effective treatment, it remains something of an enigma.

Paget's disease is common and its frequency increases with age; as many as 4% of the population over the age of 40 may have evidence of the disease, although most have no associated symptoms. It is a chronic focal disease, which may affect virtually any bone in the body. It varies widely in extent, with individual patients having anything from one to 20 or 30 bones affected. Even in a patient with extensive disease, the structure of unaffected bones appears to be quite normal. In general, the axial bones and large long bones are more commonly affected than the small bones of the hands or feet, or the ribs. Within an individual, the distribution appears to be random. In most patients, the majority of affected bones are asymptomatic; this does not necessarily mean that they will always remain so.

Aetiology and pathophysiology

The primary disease process in Paget's disease appears to be in the osteoclasts of affected bone, and there is much circumstantial evidence pointing to a viral aetiology. These osteoclasts are abnormal both in structure and function; being larger than normal with more nuclei, and resorbing bone apparently without regard to normal anatomical restraints. Affected osteoclasts contain numerous cytoplasmic and nuclear particles thought to be viral nucleocapsids. Immunological and other evidence suggests that a virus similar to the measles virus may be responsible. Typically, the disease starts in one or more specific areas, e.g. epiphysis of a long bone, or skull base, and spreads through it with a lytic advancing edge at a rate of about 1 cm per year. In the skull, this gives rise to the picture of osteoporosis circumscripta, and in long bones to the 'blade of grass' appearance. This is the leading edge of 'vandal' osteoclasts which resorb bone in an uncontrolled way.

Residual osteoclasts in bone behind the leading edge of advancing disease remain abnormal in size and shape, and continue to resorb bone chaotically. Wherever it occurs, bone resorption is followed by bone formation which, after an initial lag, catches up and keeps pace with resorption. However, the new bone laid down follows the chaotic pattern of bone resorption, and the gross structure of the whole bone therefore becomes progressively distorted. Affected bones are greatly weakened and become expanded and bent – this is particularly so for the major long bones, such as tibia, femur, humerus and radius, which may develop partial fractures. The latter are unusual in extending from the inner cortex outwards, and being concentrated on the convexity of the bowing bone (Fig. 19.8). Vertebrae and the pelvis become distorted, and the skull thickens and its front and back sink, as the vertebral column selectively supports its centre. Secondary changes include osteoarthritis, e.g. of hips and knees.

Within one patient, the disease usually appears to be at the same stage of development at different sites, and unaffected bones remain so throughout the disease; this possibly reflects a single episode of widespread viral infection of blood-bone osteoclast precursors which were then carried into affected bones. Continuing viral replication within affected cells, combined with transfection by cell fusion (cell fusion being a normal property of the osteoclast), appears to explain why the disease is rampant in affected bones while initially unaffected bones generally seem to remain normal.

Clinical features

Since the natural time-course of Paget's disease is very long, and many patients have had it for 20 years or more before diagnosis, virtually nothing is known of the early clinical features of the disease, or whether there is an acute illness at the onset of the putative initial viral infection.

Many patients present fortuitously, either because a biochemical screen has revealed a high serum alkaline phosphatase level, or because an X-ray has revealed an affected bone. Bone pain is of at least four types:

1. a deep boring dull pain, probably due to increased vascularity, which is present at rest and not relieved by analgesics
2. a sharp pain, worse on movement or pressure, at the site of a partial or complete fracture
3. the pain of secondary osteoarthritis
4. pain due to pressure on nerve roots.

The patient may complain of deformity of an affected bone or bones, or enlargement and irregularity of the skull. There may be pressure effects, including cranial nerve lesions – of which tinnitus and deafness (nerve, as well as conductive) are very common – if the disease involves the skull. Occasionally, Paget's disease of the spine leads to paraparesis. Platybasia of the skull may lead to obstruction of the aqueduct and internal hydrocephalus.

Pagetic bone is highly vascular, and the patient is often aware of the warmth of an affected limb, especially of the tibia; the part is obviously hot to touch. Increased vascularity of the skull leads to prominence of the superficial temporal arteries and, occasionally, to distended external jugular veins. The cardiac output is modestly

Fig. 19.8 Gross expansion and deformity of right tibia in longstanding Paget's disease.

increased in extensive Paget's disease, as a result of vascular shunting of blood through diseased bone; this may occasionally lead to high output congestive cardiac failure. Patients with extensive Paget's disease commonly have generalised malaise and lethargy, which may improve with effective treatment.

An uncommon, but serious, complication of the condition is the development of bone sarcoma (usually osteogenic sarcoma), which is marked by expansion of the affected bone and further elevation of serum alkaline phosphatase activity. This complication may arise simultaneously at more than one Pagetic site and probably develops in less than 1% of cases.

Investigation

In general, bone resorption is reflected by increased excretion of collagen-derived hydroxyproline in urine (best measured as the fasting morning urine hydroxyproline/creatinine ratio). Bone formation is reflected by the level of serum alkaline phosphatase. These two markers, which together provide a measure of bone turnover rate, are a function both of the extent of skeletal involvement and of the disease activity within affected bones.

In addition to these measurements, a bone scan is performed using ^{99}Tc-labelled biphosphonate (Fig.19.9). This is followed by radiology of 'hot' bones. It is important to document the baseline state of disease before instituting therapy.

Fig. 19.9 Bone scan from a patient with extensive Paget's disease – in skull, several dorsal vertebrae, sternum, left humerus, and whole pelvis.

Treatment

Until the late 1960's, there was no effective treatment for Paget's disease. Although most patients have a mild condition which rarely kills, in some the disease is extremely disabling. Traditional criteria for instituting treatment, hitherto only for symptomatic disease, will change once an effective and simple treatment can be shown to arrest progress of the condition.

Calcitonin

Calcitonin given by repeated injection was the first treatment to have any beneficial effect, either on the deep-seated bone pain or on the course of the disease. The hormone acts by binding to surface receptors on osteoclasts and inhibiting their bone-resorbing function. There is an abrupt reduction in bone resorption, while bone formation continues; thus the onset of treatment in a severely affected patient with extensive disease leads to a transient fall in serum calcium concentration. Synthetic salmon, or human, calcitonin is given in doses of 50–100 IU by subcutaneous injection three times a week. The hydroxyproline and plasma alkaline phosphatase levels fall, but rarely dramatically, and an improvement in bone structure and recalcification of affected bone occurs. Unfortunately, 'escape' is commonly seen after about a year of treatment, usually as a result of antibody production. Side-effects are frequent and include flushing, palpitations, headache and malaise shortly after each injection. Calcitonin therapy is extremely expensive.

The bisphosphonates (diphosphonates)

The bisphosphonates are analogues of pyrophosphate that bind to hydroxyapatite, and are therefore taken up by newly laid down bone collagen matrix. *Etidronate*, the first bisphosphonate to be developed for clinical use, inhibits bone mineralisation as well as resorption, and tends to cause osteomalacia and pathological fracture. This drug is still generally available for oral use, though few specialist centres in the UK are now using it.

Pamidronate (aminohydroxypropylidene bisphosphonate, APD), as with other bisphosphonates, is poorly and erratically absorbed by mouth, and causes gastrointestinal side-effects when given by this route. Figure 19.10 illustrates the dramatic response to a short course of intravenous infusions of pamidronate in severe Paget's disease. Remineralisation of lytic Paget's disease may be evident radiologically as early as four months after the start of a three-month course of therapy and, in many cases, is followed by prolonged remission. In the early stages, pamidronate treatment is commonly followed by an increase in bone pain and by mild transient fever; however, this is quickly followed by symptomatic improvement, and reduction in bone pain. Similar responses can be achieved with some other bisphosphonates, such as dichloromethyline bisphosphonate (clodronate). These are now the preferred treatments for Paget's disease, although they are still not licensed as such. *Mithramycin*, although also quite effective, is much more toxic than pamidronate, and neither etidronate nor mithramycin can now be generally recommended for the treatment of Paget's disease.

A

B

Fig. 19.10   Response to pamidronate treatment in Paget's disease. A. Paget's disease in a 71-year-old woman before (left) and nine months after a course of iv pamidronate (right). Note restoration of bone in areas of osteolysis. Bone distortion remains. **B.** Decline in alkaline phosphatase level (normal less than 130 IU/l) and hydroxyproline/creatinine (HOP/Cr) ratio (normal less than 20 μmol/mmol) during and after a single course of 12 weekly 30 mg infusions of iv pamidronate (APD). Note decline in activity. Upper limit of normal indicated by red dotted line.

MISCELLANEOUS RARE BONE DISEASES

Hypophosphatasia

Hypophosphatasia is characterised by failure of mineralisation, possibly as a result of inhibition by increased concentrations of pyrophosphate. Its inheritance is autosomal recessive and it takes its name from the low levels of plasma alkaline phosphatase which are usually found. The pathogenesis is obscure. In the fully expressed severe form of the disease, a clinical picture similar to that of severe rickets is found, with abnormal dentition and premature fusion of the cranial sutures in addition. There is no specific therapy.

Osteogenesis imperfecta

Osteogenesis imperfecta, which is also termed fragilitas ossium or brittle bone syndrome, is a collection of rare inherited disorders in which there appear to be specific defects in the formation of type I collagen, the predominant collagen in mature bone. The disease occurs in two main forms:

1. a dominantly inherited variety, in which structural bone problems are not necessarily severe
2. a recessively inherited form with multiple fractures occurring in early life, sometimes at the time of birth.

In both forms there may be abnormalities of dentition and the sclerae may have a characteristic blue colour. The condition is caused by a subtle abnormality of collagen structure, the precise abnormality varying from family to family. There is some overlap with the syndrome of Ehlers-Danlos (p. 93).

Treatment is directed towards prevention of trauma and correction of post-traumatic deformity. There is a suspicion that some patients with osteoporosis and a strong family history of the disease may in fact have mild forms of osteogenesis imperfecta.

Osteopetrosis (marble bone disease, Albers-Schoenberg disease)

The term osteopetrosis describes a number of very rare conditions characterised by *increased* bone mass throughout the skeleton. Of these, a dominantly inherited and relatively mild form, and a recessively inherited severe form, are numerically the most important. The increase in bone mass is thought to be due to a defect in osteoclast activity. Radiological appearances are characteristic, with patchily increased bone density throughout the skeleton. In severe disease, encroachment of bone on the marrow or neural canals may lead to bone marrow failure with leucoerythroblastic anaemia (which may be total) and to cranial nerve palsies respectively. Hepatosplenomegaly may be evident, indicating extramedullary haemopoiesis. The dominantly inherited mild disease is usually symptomless, but classical radiological changes are found, with increased bone density and alternating dense and lucent bands in the vertebral column.

Severe osteopetrosis is, predictably, associated with a markedly positive calcium balance, and some benefit has been claimed for treatment of severe disease by calcium restriction. Treatment by marrow transplantation has been tried with some success; transplanted osteoclast precursors, formed in the bone marrow, are able to reestablish normal bone resorption.

FURTHER READING

Altmann P, Cunningham J 1987 Post Grad Med J. 63:77, London. *A review of the treatment of severe hypercalcaemia.*

Hamdy R C 1981 Paget's disease of bone: assessment and management. Endocrinology and management, Vol I. Praeger, New York. *A comprehensive and authoritative review of many aspects of Paget's disease.*

Manolages S C, Olefsky J M 1988 Metabolic bone and mineral disorders. Churchill Livingstone, Edinburgh. *A good review of important aspects of metabolic bone disorders.*

Mundy G R 1989 Calcium homeostasis: hypercalcaemia and hypocalcaemia. Martin Dunitz, London. *An excellent simple, but comprehensive and up-to-date account from an acknowledged expert in the field.*

Nordin B E C 1984 Metabolic bone and stone disease. Churchill Livingstone, Edinburgh. *A general review of metabolic bone disease.*

Riggs B, Melton L 1988 Osteoporosis: aetiology, diagnosis and management. Raven Press, New York. *A detailed and up-to-date account.*

Smith R 1987 Disorders of the skeleton. In: Weatherall D J, Ledingham J G G, Warrell D A (eds) Oxford textbook of medicine, 2nd edn., Oxford University Press, Oxford. *A general review of skeletal disorders.*

Woolf A D, Dixon A St J 1988 Osteoporosis: a clinical guide. Martin Dunitz, London. *A well-illustrated and authoritative account of many of the current issues relating to osteoporosis.*

Diabetes Mellitus and Diseases of Lipid and Intermediary Metabolism

INTERRELATIONSHIP OF CARBOHYDRATE, FAT AND PROTEIN METABOLISM

Metabolic homeostasis requires an appropriate substrate energy supply to all tissues in the basal state, when metabolic rate is increased (for example by exercise), and when food is unavailable during starvation. This is achieved by a complex interplay of factors, mediated mainly by hormones, which ensures storage of substrate in the fed state and its controlled release in the fasting state. This balance may become pathologically disturbed in the face of uncontrolled 'catabolic' breakdown of tissue fat and protein (for example due to trauma or sepsis), and reaches catastrophic proportions when catabolism is accelerated by insulin deficiency in insulin-dependent diabetes mellitus.

Metabolic control in the fed state

Food intake usually exceeds immediate metabolic requirements, and nutrients are stored for later use.

Carbohydrate is taken up by liver and adipose tissue for triglyceride synthesis, and by muscle for glycogen synthesis; amino acids enter liver and muscle and triglycerides enter adipose tissue under the influence of lipoprotein lipase (Fig. 20.1). These events are all promoted by insulin,

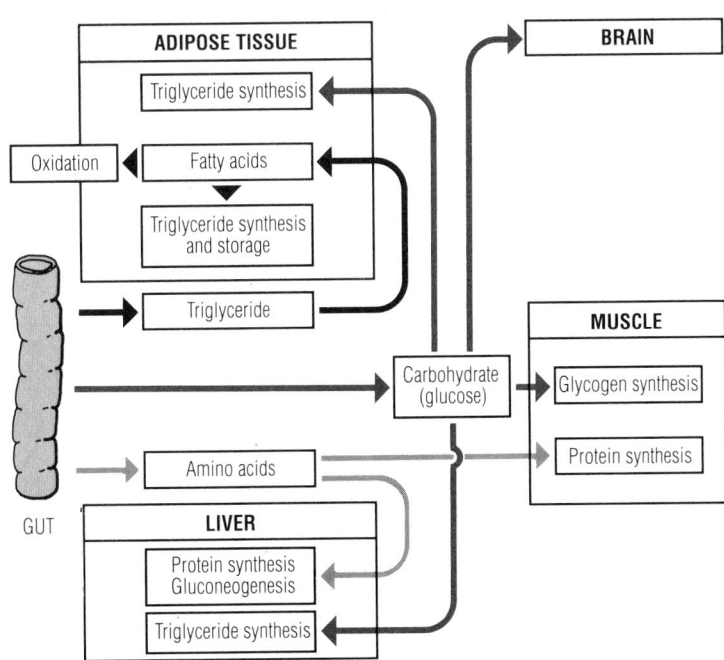

Fig. 20.1   The fate of ingested nutrients and their storage in the liver, brain, muscle and adipose tissues.

747

Diabetes and Lipid Metabolism

secreted in response to food ingestion (via enteroinsular mechanisms), as well as to the direct stimulatory effects of glucose and amino acids on the pancreatic beta cells.

The actions of insulin are invariably 'anabolic', i.e. it tends to prevent breakdown of stored triglycerides to free fatty acids and glycerol, and of protein to amino acids (Fig. 20.2). In addition, insulin acts on hepatic hexokinase and glycogen synthetase to promote glycogen storage (Fig. 20.2). Insulin has different actions at different plasma concentrations. For example, its hepatic effects in promoting glycogen storage are evident at relatively low concentrations, whereas its peripheral action in promoting glucose entry into cells only occurs at the higher levels present immediately after meals. In general, normal blood sugar levels and maintenance of a constant circulating energy supply are critically dependent on the effects of basal concentrations of insulin on hepatic metabolism.

Metabolic control in the fasting state

In the fasting state, mobilisation of stored energy depends initially on decreased insulin secretion, permitting the liver to release glucose from stored glycogen. This process is enhanced by glucagon, the actions of which predominate when insulin secretion is low. Although liver glycogen provides an easily mobilised store of energy, this is quantitatively very small compared to the calorific value of stored triglyceride. Prolonged starvation shifts the metabolic balance further towards catabolism under the influence of glucagon, catecholamines and corticosteroids (Fig. 20.3). The net result is increased lipolysis with a rise

in circulating free fatty acids, which are partially oxidised in the liver to the acidic ketone bodies, acetoacetate and 3-hydroxybutyrate. At the same time, the liver is presented with an increased supply of the gluconeogenic substrates, lactate, alanine and glycerol.

Lactate is produced by glycolysis of muscle glycogen and is converted back to glucose by hepatic gluconeogenesis before becoming available for muscle metabolism once again (the Cori cycle). Alanine is produced in the periphery by amination of pyruvate produced during glycolysis. Glycerol, the third and quantitatively least important gluconeogenic substrate, is produced by lipolysis of adipose tissue triglyceride. If food deprivation continues, ketone bodies become the main energy substrate for all tissues, although nervous tissue continues to need glucose for a period before 'keto-adaptation' occurs. Glucose is conserved for neural metabolism by inhibition of glucose metabolism in other tissues, probably due to the inhibitory effect of acetyl-CoA and citrate (metabolic products of free fatty acids and ketone bodies) on pyruvate oxidation and glycolysis (Fig. 20.4).

Control of ketogenesis

Ketone body production in the liver depends mainly on the rate of supply of free fatty acids, which depends in turn on the rate of lipolysis. Lipolysis is diminished by insulin and increased by glucagon; these two hormones thus exert indirect control over ketone body production. They also influence ketogenesis at the hepatic level, by indirect modulation of the rate at which fatty acyl-CoA derivatives

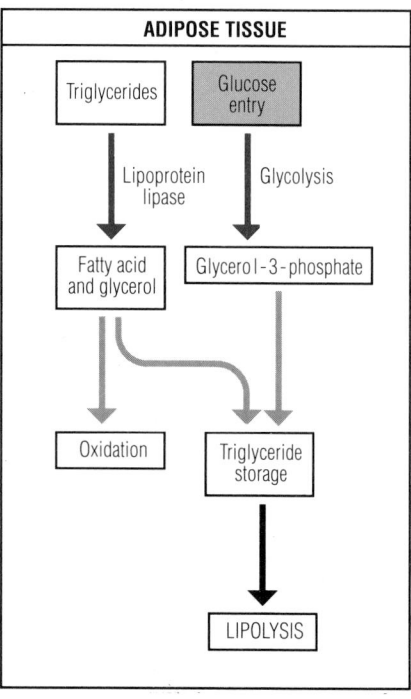

Fig. 20.2 The actions of insulin on intermediary metabolism in muscle, liver and adipose tissue. Insulin inhibits lipolysis and proteolysis and increases glycogen synthesis. Its actions are invariably anabolic.

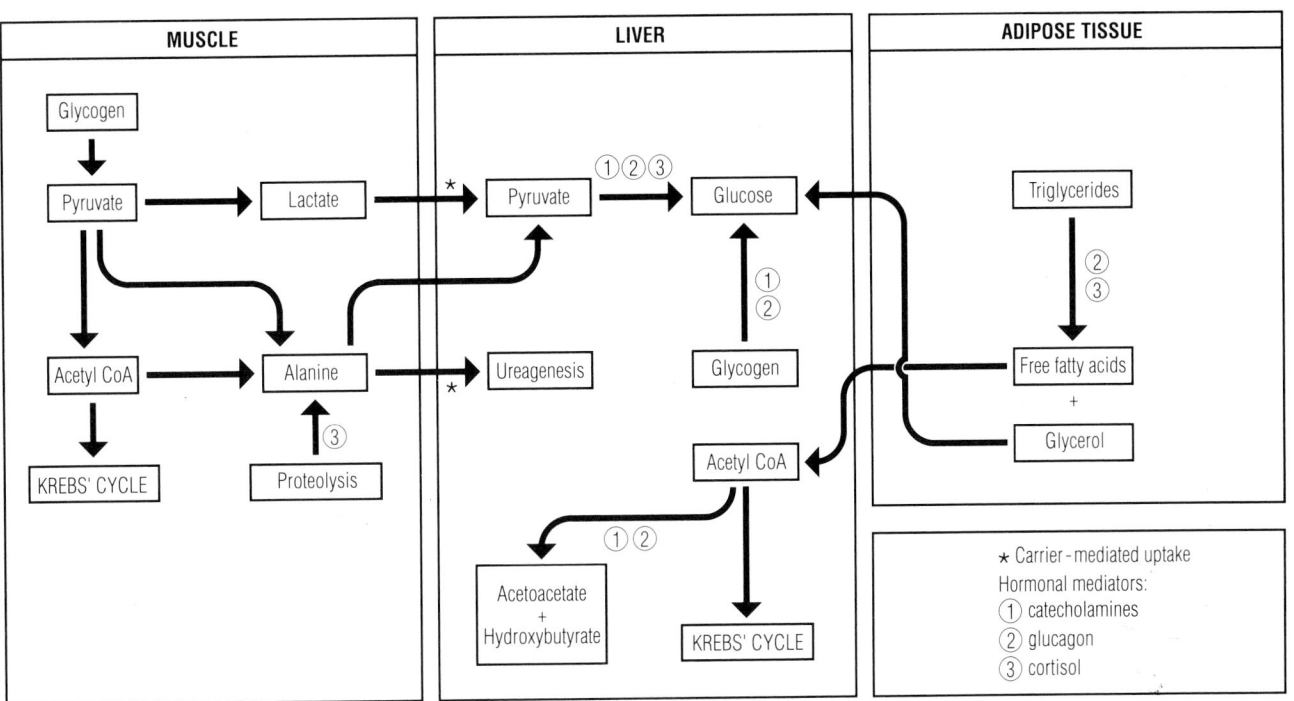

Fig. 20.3 The metabolic response to starvation. A controlled catabolic breakdown of triglyceride, glycogen and eventually protein occurs under the influence of catecholamines, glucagon and cortisol.

enter the mitochondria for ketone body production. This effect appears to be related to the rate of hepatic lipogenesis, which is increased by insulin and decreased by glucagon. Malonyl-CoA – an intermediate compound in hepatic lipogenesis – exerts an inhibitory effect on the enzyme carnitine acyl-transferase; the latter is an essential mediator of mitochondrial uptake of fatty acyl-CoA derivatives

(Fig. 20.5). Insulin and glucagon thus influence ketone body production not only by altering the supply of free fatty acids, but also by controlling subsequent hepatic metabolism. Feedback inhibition of lipogenesis (and thus malonyl-CoA formation) by fatty acyl-CoA derivatives constitutes a further important control on ketogenesis.

Control of energy supply in starvation

Stored energy is released during starvation in a controlled process dependent on glucagon, catecholamines, and cortisol on the one hand, and basal insulin secretion on the other. Muscle protein is preferentially preserved, possibly by inhibition of proteolysis by ketones. Since ketone bodies have a mild stimulatory effect on insulin secretion, this provides useful negative feedback control of peripheral lipolysis ensuring optimum utilisation of ketone bodies. Energy economy is also maintained by decreased formation of tri-iodothyronine (in favour of the metabolically inactive reverse tri-iodothyronine) from thyroxine in peripheral tissues, with a consequent lowering of the metabolic rate. Growth hormone tends to preserve tissue proteins by decreasing cellular glucose uptake and thus reducing the amount of pyruvate available for amination to alanine; muscle ketone metabolism is preferentially increased.

The effect of trauma and sepsis

These disturb the fine balance between anabolic and catabolic activity. Short-term starvation is also typically

Fig. 20.4 The regulation of peripheral glucose metabolism by free fatty acids and ketone bodies.

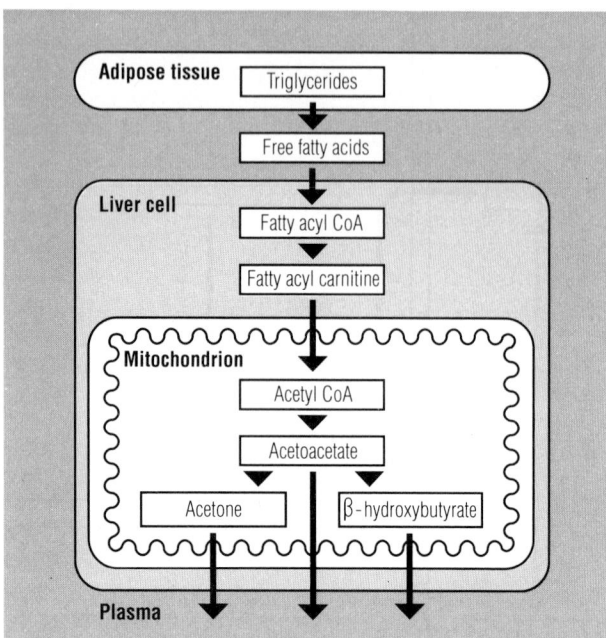

Fig. 20.5 Ketogenesis. Hepatic ketone body production depends on the rate of mitochondrial uptake of fatty acyl CoA derivatives under the influence of carnitine acyl transferase. This enzyme is inhibited by malonyl CoA, the production of which is increased by insulin and decreased by glucagon.

present, and this shifts the balance further in the direction of catabolism. Both catecholamine and cortisol secretion increase rapidly in the classical stress response, often with increased glucagon production and a degree of insulin resistance. The net result is increased gluconeogenic flux, peripheral lipolysis and net protein breakdown. The last is due initially to decreased protein synthesis, but proteolysis develops when severe physical stress and sepsis are present. Continued catabolism results in progressive loss of tissue protein (negative nitrogen balance), with impaired wound healing and resistance to infection.

Effect of insulin deficiency on the stress response

When insulin secretion is absent or severely reduced, an unrestrained catabolic response to stress occurs. This leads to peripheral fat and tissue breakdown, increased supply of gluconeogenic precursors, increased gluconeogenesis, decreased glucose uptake in peripheral tissues and, eventually, overproduction of ketone bodies with resultant acidosis. A similar situation may develop in individuals with partial insulin deficiency if insulin resistance is induced by severe physical stress.

DIABETES MELLITUS

Diabetes means passage of excess urine. The disease is characterised by chronic hyperglycaemia, caused by defec-

tive insulin secretion and/or insulin resistance. If not treated, diabetes may lead to acute hyperglycaemia and eventually, to ketoacidosis or non-ketotic hyperosmolar coma. Long-standing diabetes is accompanied by late complications, with a reduced life expectancy. The most important of these complications are arterial disease and diabetic microangiopathy.

Primary diabetes takes two forms:

1. insulin-dependent (IDDM)
2. non-insulin dependent (NIDDM).

The incidence of IDDM appears to be increasing in Northern Europe, and the incidence of NIDDM is increasing in all populations of the developed nations. The chronic nature of the disease, its wide range of disabling complications and its prevalence (affecting 30–50 million people) make diabetes a major drain on health resources. In 1984, estimates of direct health costs due to diabetes in the USA ranged from $7.4 to $12.0 billion, and the minimum estimate for the total economic impact of the disease was $14 billion. Comparable analyses are not available for the UK, but some 3–4% of all acute hospital beds are occupied by patients with diabetes.

Insulin secretion and the control of blood glucose

Insulin is synthesised in the beta cells of the pancreatic islets of Langerhans in the form of a prohormone termed proinsulin. Cleavage of this compound – in secretory granules within the beta cell – yields insulin and equimolar quantities of a connecting peptide (C-peptide) which is biologically inactive (Fig. 20.6). Measurements of C-peptide may be useful in documenting pathologically low insulin secretion, as in insulin-dependent diabetes mellitus or autonomous insulin production from islet cell tumours (p. 775). Secreted insulin reaches the liver via the portal circulation, and, as indicated in the section on metabolic interrelationships, the major effects of insulin are on hepatic metabolism.

The hepatic effects of insulin ensure that the blood glucose levels are tightly controlled in health between narrow extremes of approximately 3.0–8.0 mmol/l, with fasting levels averaging 3.0–6.5 mmol/l. This ensures an adequate glucose supply for the energy needs of the central nervous system which, unlike other tissues, is absolutely dependent on glucose metabolism. The exception is under conditions of prolonged starvation when some 'keto-adaptation' occurs.

Diagnostic criteria

The diagnosis of diabetes is straightforward because glucose is so closely regulated in healthy individuals. In the overnight-fasted state, glucose and insulin levels are virtually constant. Sensitive analytic methods show that levels of both oscillate with a cycle of around 13–15 minutes. This is interpreted as 'hunting' behaviour around a homeostatic set point. When food is taken, insulin levels jump 5–10-fold within a minute or so, sharply curbing the

Fig. 20.6 Micrographs showing insulin granules. A. Low power micrograph of two beta cells and the release of packaged insulin granules. **B.** High power micrograph of secreted insulin granules.

in method and interpretation caused endless controversy. In one famous study, the same series of test results was sent to leading diabetes specialists throughout the world for their comments. Diabetes was diagnosed in up to 30% of the test results by some specialists and in as little as 5% by others!

Patients should follow their normal diet for three days before taking the glucose tolerance test, and fast overnight before it is performed. Seventy-five grams of glucose are given dissolved in up to 200 ml of water, and blood glucose levels are measured before, and two hours after, the glucose is given. Intermediate samples are often taken at 30 and 60 minutes, but these are not necessary for the diagnosis (according to WHO criteria). Diabetes can be diagnosed on the basis of:

1. a fasting glucose above 6.7 mmol/l (venous whole blood) or 7.8 mmol/l (venous plasma)
2. a 2-hour glucose above 10 mmol/l (venous whole blood) or 11.1 mmol/l (venous plasma).

When the two-hour value is below 6.7 mmol/l (whole blood) or 7.8 mmol/l (plasma), the test is deemed normal; intermediate values of 6.7–10 and 7.8–11.1 mmol/l respectively are classified as 'impaired' glucose tolerance (IGT). The clinical implications and justification for this category are considered on page 755. For the moment, it is sufficient to bear in mind that IGT can only be diagnosed using a glucose tolerance test.

Although the glucose tolerance test is, by definition, the only way we have of diagnosing borderline diabetes, it is important to recognise its limitations. The outcome of the test can vary from one day to another in the same individual, even under standard conditions; the coefficient of variation of the 2-hour value is around 25%. In addition, the test is influenced by variables such as gastric emptying, time of day and diet over the previous days – glucose tolerance deteriorates on a low carbohydrate diet, for example.

Classification of diabetes

Diabetes is usually primary, but may be secondary to other diseases (Table 20.1). Primary diabetes is subdivided into insulin-dependent diabetes mellitus, also known as Type I diabetes, and non-insulin-dependent diabetes mellitus, also known as Type II diabetes. Many find this alternative nomenclature confusing, and some explanation is needed.

The terms *juvenile onset* and *maturity onset diabetes* were widely used in the past. However, this classifaction fell out of favour when some young patients were shown to have the 'mature' form of the disease, and vice-versa, making nonsense of the distinction.

Type I and *Type II diabetes* are terms introduced many years ago by Himsworth, who predicted (long before insulin assays were available) that the former resulted from insulin deficiency and the latter from insulin resistance. They were revived more recently when this prediction was seen to be broadly correct, and especially because Type I diabetes was found to be associated with certain HLA types

post-prandial rise in blood glucose levels. Peak levels rarely exceed 8 mmol/l after a normal meal, and the 97.5th percentile for a random blood glucose in a healthy young person is around 6.5 mmol/l.

The diagnosis of diabetes can be established by a fasting whole blood glucose value above 6.7 mmol/l, or a random value above 10 mmol/l. Note that the equivalent values for plasma glucose are 7.8 and 11.1 mmol/l (WHO criteria). The method of glucose measurement should be reliable, and it is prudent to obtain two abnormal values to minimise the possibility of laboratory error.

Glucose tolerance test

If the above criteria are followed, the *glucose tolerance test* is seldom needed in clinical practice, and is mainly reserved for borderline cases and to confirm the diagnosis of renal glycosuria. It does however have enormous importance as an epidemiological tool.

If the test is to be used, it is important for it to be performed and interpreted correctly. Hitherto, differences

Table 20.1 Classification of diabetes mellitus*

Primary

Insulin-dependent diabetes mellitus (IDDM)
Non-insulin-dependent diabetes mellitus (NIDDM)
  Non-obese
  Obese

Secondary

Malnutrition-related diabetes mellitus
Pancreatic disease
Other endocrine disease
Induced by drugs or chemicals
Abnormalities of insulin or its receptors
Genetic syndromes
Miscellaneous

* Adapted from WHO Study Group on Diabetes, 1985

Table 20.2 Comparison of IDDM and NIDDM

Feature	Insulin-dependent diabetes mellitus	Non-insulin-dependent diabetes mellitus
Epidemiology	Most common in Europeans	Most common in non-Europeans
Inheritance		
Chromosome 6	HLA-DR3 and/or DR4 in >90	Not associated
Chromosome 11	Associated with class 1 allele in hypervariable region adjacent to the insulin gene	No association (or weak)
Risk to siblings	6–7%	25%
Risk to offspring	3–5%	30%
Risk to identical co-twin	30–40%	>90%
Immunology Evidence of autoimmunity	Infiltration of islets Auto-antibodies to islets and to insulin Associations with other organ-specific autoimmune disorders Response to treatment with cyclosporin A	None of these
Metabolic	Near-total beta cell loss Insulin resistance not a major factor	Partial loss of beta cells Insulin resistance important in pathogenesis
	Always insulin-dependent	Sometimes need insulin
	Develop ketoacidosis (DKA)	Do not develop DKA but may develop hyperosmolar coma

and immune changes including the presence of islet cell antibodies (see p. 753). Tests for these are not readily available, however, and some have found the purely negative definition of Type II diabetes (i.e. by the absence of features associated with Type I) unsatisfactory.

The terms IDDM and NIDDM found favour with the WHO study group because they make no assumptions about aetiology, and are easy to apply in clinical studies. This would seem eminently sensible, except that many patients with NIDDM need or benefit from insulin therapy even though they may not 'depend' on it to the same extent as patients who are totally insulin-deficient. Indeed, there are about as many insulin-treated patients with Type II diabetes in the UK as there are with Type I. In practice, however, clinicians tend to use the terms IDDM and Type I diabetes synonymously, and tolerate the logical inconsistency of referring to insulin-treated patients with Type II diabetes as 'non-insulin-dependent'.

INSULIN-DEPENDENT DIABETES (IDDM)

Epidemiology

As mentioned above, the term IDDM is not in practice applied to all patients on insulin treatment, and of the 250 000 individuals treated with insulin in the UK about half would be considered to have 'non-insulin-dependent' diabetes. Provided one can avoid terminological confusion, the distinction between the two types of diabetes is quite straightforward and is summarised in Table 20.2.

Insulin-dependent diabetes is commonest in Caucasian populations. Within this overall pattern, however, there are considerable local variations which are not fully understood. They cannot with confidence be ascribed either to climatic or genetic influences.

The age of onset also shows a striking pattern (Fig. 20.7), with a sharp increase up to and around the age of puberty and a decline thereafter. Type I diabetes may present at any age, but some 50–60% of all cases present under the age of 20. The reasons for this pattern, which differs markedly from that for Type II diabetes (Fig. 20.7), are not clear.

Presentation is more common in the spring and autumn than in the summer, and it has been suggested that this might be related to the greater prevalence of viral infections at these times.

A further element in the puzzle is that there is evidence for a rising incidence of Type I diabetes in some parts of Northern Europe, although other areas report no such change. Evidence from the Netherlands and Scotland demonstrates a rise so rapid as to suggest a doubling within the course of a single generation. The speed of this process suggests involvement of an environmental agent, but the nature of this agent, whether viral or otherwise, remains obscure.

Aetiology and pathogenesis

Genetic susceptibility

Susceptibility to Type I diabetes is genetically determined, but only a proportion of susceptible individuals go on to develop the disease. The best evidence for this comes from the study of identical twins. The twin of a child with

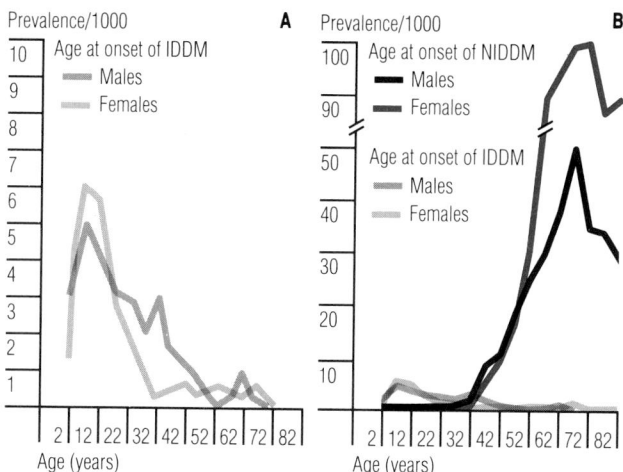

Fig. 20.7 The incidence of insulin-dependent (IDDM) and non-insulin-dependent diabetes (NIDDM) in Finland. IDDM (**A**) peaks around the time of puberty whereas the incidence of NIDDM increases with age (**B**). To demonstrate the relative incidence of the two forms of diabetes, the curves for IDDM are superimposed upon those for NIDDM in (**B**).

diabetes has a 30–50% chance of developing the disease, whereas the twin of an adult with Type II diabetes has a chance of at least 90% (Fig. 20.8). The implications of this observation are that the genetic contribution to Type I diabetes is less than that to Type II, and that some as yet unknown factor, probably environmental, is additionally involved in the pathogenesis of Type I diabetes. The child of an insulin-dependent diabetic patient has an increased chance of developing IDDM. Curiously, this risk is greater for a diabetic father (about one child in 20) than for a diabetic mother (about one in 40). The overall risk for a sibling of a child with IDDM is around 5%.

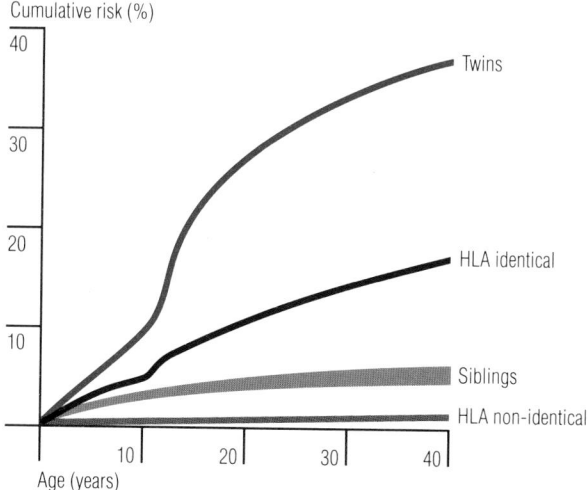

Fig. 20.8 Cumulative risk of developing diabetes in identical twins and siblings. About one in three identical twins will develop insulin-dependent diabetes, as against 5–8% of siblings. The risk for siblings is largely determined by HLA type. HLA identical siblings have a risk of 15–17%, while non-identical siblings have a risk indistinguishable from that of the general population.

Further evidence of the genetic contribution to susceptibility in Type I diabetes comes from analysis of HLA associations. At least 90% of diabetic children are positive for HLA-DR3 and/or DR4, as against about 50% of the background European population. Other reported HLA associations in the A and B regions are secondary to linkage disequilibrium (p. 95). The relative risk conferred by DR3 is estimated at 7, that of DR4 at 9, and that of DR3/DR4 at 14. Since this risk is additive, a model based on two susceptibility genes (one associated with DR3 and one with DR4) has been proposed. In contrast, individuals with HLA-DR2 have a considerably reduced risk (0.12) of developing diabetes. The reasons for this protective effect are unclear.

To complicate matters, there is evidence that the genetic contribution to Type I diabetes is not confined to the HLA region on the 6th chromosome. In particular, a polymorphous DNA region close to the insulin gene on the 11th chromosome has been reported, with short, intermediate and long insertions. Homozygosity of the short (Class I) allele is found in some 80% of IDDM, as against 40% of controls. The location of this region on the same part of the chromosome as the insulin gene appears to be fortuitous, since there is no known functional relationship between the two.

Immunological factors

There is now convincing evidence that autoimmune processes are involved in the pathogenesis of IDDM. Autopsies on young patients who have died soon after developing diabetes show extensive lymphocytic infiltration specific to the endocrine pancreas. After a longer duration of the disease, this inflammatory process can no longer be seen, but the islets are virtually depleted of beta cells. Many patients have increased numbers of circulating activated T lymphocytes at diagnosis, and auto-antibodies against islet cells are present in some 70% of newly-presenting young patients. Insulin auto-antibodies have also been described. Further, Type I diabetes is associated with HLA-DR3, which itself is associated with a number of organ-specific autoimmune diseases. This explains why autoimmune thyroid disease, pernicious anaemia and Addison's disease are more common in some patients and their families. While there are many pointers to disordered autoimmune processes in IDDM, this does not necessarily mean that they are direct causes of the disease; for example, the presence of auto-antibodies to insulin and islet cells might be secondary to an environmental insult such as viral infection.

Effects of immunosuppression

More direct proof that autoimmune processes are important in mediating beta cell damage has come from trials of immunosuppressive therapy in newly-presenting patients. Cyclosporin A was used in two large prospective randomised clinical trials, which demonstrated that C-peptide levels are better preserved, and insulin requirements lower, in treated patients. It was found that 20–30% of patients (compared with 10% of controls) could be managed without insulin at the end of one year. Unfortunately, the disease process relapses when immunosuppression is stopped; furthermore, the toxicity of the drugs currently available prohibits their introduction into clinical practice at our present level of knowledge and experience.

A further indication of the importance of autoimmune processes arose from the attempt to transplant pancreatic tissue between identical twins discordant for diabetes, without the use of immunosuppression. The transplanted tissue was not rejected, but an immune attack specific for the beta cells was observed, reenacting the original pathogenesis of diabetes in the transplant recipient, often many years after original onset of the disease.

Environmental factors

Evidence in favour of a viral aetiology includes the ability of viruses to induce diabetes in susceptible animal models, the increased incidence of diabetes in the spring and autumn when viral infections are prevalent, and anecdotal associations with illnesses such as mumps. Further evidence comes from the increased prevalence of diabetes (10–20%) in children with the congenital rubella syndrome, and from analysis of viral antibody titres at diagnosis; IgM antibodies to coxsackie B4 have been reported in 20–30% of new cases. However, in view of the long prodromal period (see below), it seems likely that Coxsackie viruses precipitate clinical onset in susceptible individuals with established subclinical beta cell damage, and do not initiate the actual disease process.

Indirect evidence that environmental factors are important comes from the study of identical twins (see above). Involvement of environmental factors is also suggested by the observation that the incidence of childhood diabetes is increasing in some parts of northern Europe. Type I diabetes was previously a lethal condition, but insulin treatment has meant that affected individuals now survive to have children of their own, thus increasing the proportion of susceptible individuals in the population as a whole. An increasing incidence of Type I diabetes might be expected on these grounds alone, but the speed of the increase is such as to suggest intervention of some as yet unknown environmental factor.

The prodromal phase

The clinical onset of childhood diabetes is typically, but not always, abrupt; in 50–60% of cases classic symptoms of thirst, polyuria and weight loss have been present for less than four weeks. However, evidence from studies in first degree relatives of children with diabetes indicates that there is a slow progressive process of beta cell damage (Fig. 20.9). The first evidence of this is usually the appearance of islet cell antibodies, and these have been described up to ten years before clinical onset of diabetes. Other autoantibodies have been described in this *prodromal period*, including antibodies directed against insulin. In time,

Fig. 20.9 Progressive beta cell loss preceding the onset of insulin-dependent diabetes extends over several years from the first appearance of circulating islet cell antibodies. At a later stage early abnormalities of insulin secretion and glucose homeostasis appear; these changes may represent the 'point of no return' in the development of diabetes.

abnormalities of insulin secretion appear, the most marked being loss of the first phase insulin response to intravenous glucose. At a later stage, borderline abnormalities of glucose tolerance may manifest, sometimes associated with non-specific symptoms; if one identical twin develops diabetes, comparison with the unaffected twin suggests a growth delay of at least 6 months.

Better understanding of this sequence may in time permit accurate prediction of diabetes in susceptible individuals. This in turn may make intervention, e.g. with more selective immunosuppressive therapy, a practical possibility.

NON-INSULIN-DEPENDENT DIABETES (NIDDM)

Epidemiology

In the United Kingdom, non-insulin-dependent diabetes affects 2% of the population, the incidence increasing with obesity and age. Clinically inapparent impairment of glucose tolerance may be present for many years before the clinical disease presents. The presentation may be precipitated by intercurrent illness, drugs such as steroids, or pregnancy.

Striking differences have been observed in the prevalence of non-insulin-dependent diabetes within populations of different ethnic backgrounds sharing the same environment. For example, diabetes is about five times more common among Asian immigrants in the UK than in the indigenous population, and about three times more common in Mexican Americans as among Americans of European origin. Studies of immigrants have suggested that the chances of developing NIDDM are from 2 to 20 times higher in well-fed populations than in lean populations of the same race.

Aetiology and pathogenesis

Genetic factors

The identical twin of a patient with NIDDM has an almost 100% chance of developing diabetes. Patients with

NIDDM also have a 20–30% chance of having an affected first-degree relative with NIDDM, whereas the rate for IDDM is from 12–15%. Both these observations suggest that the genetic contribution to NIDDM is considerably greater than that to IDDM. The precise nature of this contribution is poorly understood, mainly because we lack an effective genetic marker for the condition, but it seems almost certain that NIDDM is a polygenic disease, which overlaps with Type IV and V hyperlipidaemia. A distinct variant of NIDDM is known as 'maturity onset diabetes of the young' (MODY). This is characterised by autosomal dominant transmission, presentation in early adult life, moderate hyperglycaemia which does not require insulin treatment, and a relatively benign long-term course without major complications. Certain families, in which NIDDM presents in the classic manner in middle life, also show an autosomal dominant type of transmission; others, however, clearly do not. This almost certainly reflects genetic heterogeneity within NIDDM, as well as the variable contribution of environmental factors. In contrast to Type I diabetes, there are no HLA associations with Type II diabetes and no evidence of immune involvement in its pathogenesis.

Insulin secretion

Patients with Type II diabetes retain about 50% of their beta cell mass at autopsy. Circulating insulin levels are normal or raised when compared with those of normal subjects but, nonetheless, inappropriately low in terms of the prevailing hyperglycaemia. It is clear that abnormalities of insulin secretion and increased resistance of peripheral tissues to insulin both contribute to the development and progression of the disease.

In normal individuals, there is a biphasic response of insulin secretion following intravenous glucose. This is lost very early in the development of Type II (NIDDM) diabetes, and the secretion of insulin following oral glucose is both delayed and increased in amount. In NIDDM, beta cell loss occurs progressively; but in IDDM, the loss is much greater. The mechanism of the cell loss is poorly understood. Resistance to the action of insulin is present, particularly in those patients who are obese (who constitute the majority), although non-obese patients may also show insulin resistance. The mechanism of resistance is obscure. It may be partly related to hyperglycaemia itself, and may reverse with improved glycaemic control. The sequence of events is shown in Figure 20.10.

Impaired glucose tolerance

In Europeans, an oral glucose tolerance test shows a skew of 2-hour glucose levels towards higher values. Thus, the point on the curve judged to divide non-diabetic from diabetic will inevitably be arbitrary. A further problem is that the skewing increases with age, so that a population standard established for healthy young people would condemn a large proportion of older people to a diagnosis of diabetes. This proportion would rise as high as 40% in the UK if some suggested criteria were applied. Longi-

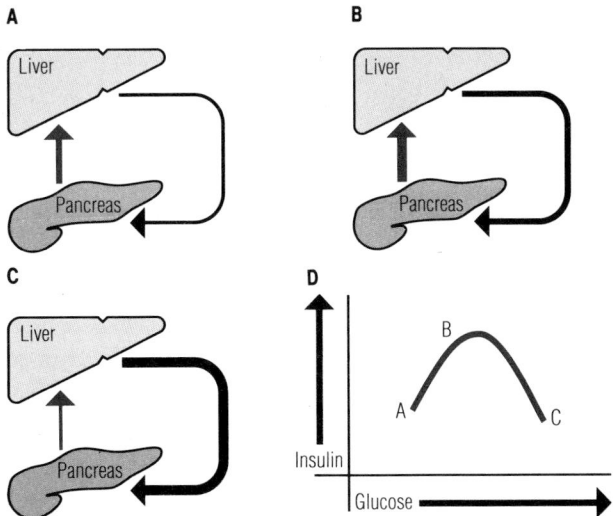

Fig. 20.10 Stages in the pathogenesis of non-insulin-dependent diabetes (NIDDM). A. (Normal) insulin secretion by the pancreas (red arrow) is closely and appropriately matched to hepatic glucose output (black arrow). **B.** (Early NIDDM) Hepatic and peripheral insulin resistance has risen. As a result hepatic glucose output has increased and peripheral glucose uptake is reduced. The pancreatic beta cells respond to the resulting hyperglycaemia by producing more insulin. Plasma insulin levels are therefore higher than in the non-diabetic, although low relative to the prevailing glucose level. **C.** (Late NIDDM) Pancreatic beta cell reserves are exhausted. As a result insulin secretion fades and hyperglycaemia becomes uncontrolled. **D.** Reciprocal changes in insulin and glucose in A, B and C can be summarised as a 'Starling curve of the pancreas'. Note that according to this model NIDDM is due to a combination of inadequate insulin secretion *and* hepatic and peripheral insulin resistance.

tudinal studies within a defined population have established two important points concerning those patients on the skewed portion of the curve:

1. Progression to diabetes is common but not inevitable, occurring in 2–4% of these individuals annually. Even so, a large proportion do not progress and some fall back within the normal range on re-testing.
2. This group has a substantially increased risk of atherosclerotic disease, but is spared the microvascular complications specific to diabetes.

For these reasons it was felt that a diagnostic category intermediate between diabetes and non-diabetes should be established (Fig. 20.11). This category of *impaired glucose tolerance* (IGT) seems justified on epidemiological grounds, and has the important clinical benefit of avoiding the insurance and social problems associated with a diagnosis of diabetes. It should be noted that the diagnosis can only be made on the basis of an oral glucose tolerance test, and that the group is almost certainly heterogeneous, e.g. some are obese, some have liver disease and others are on medication which affects glucose tolerance.

Management of an individual with IGT is directed towards the avoidance of diabetes and arterial disease. Healthy diet and maintenance of a lean weight are crucial to both objectives, and other atherosclerotic risk factors –

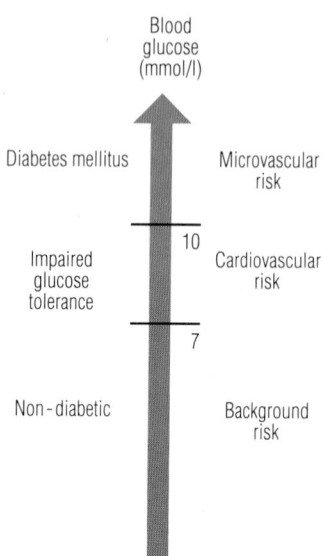

Fig. 20.11 Microvascular complications of diabetes. In population studies, these are associated with blood glucose levels >10 mmol/l (180 mg/dl) 2 hours after an oral glucose tolerance test. Those with 2 hour blood glucose values from 7 to 10 mmol/l have an increased risk of cardiovascular disease. These observations provide the rationale for the definitions of diabetes and impaired glucose tolerance chosen by the WHO.

smoking, hypertension and hyperlipidaemia – should be sought and treated. Long-term follow-up with regular blood glucose tests is also indicated.

Malnutrition-related diabetes

Tropical or malnutrition-related diabetes is a recently described condition. It occurs in developing equatorial countries, and is characterised by an onset before the age of 30 in patients who, at some stage, have had severe malnutrition. Fluctuating insulin dependence is typical, but ketoacidosis does not occur if insulin is withheld. Two types of disorder are described:

1. *Fibrocalculous pancreatic diabetes* is associated with exocrine pancreatic deficiency. Pathologically, there is pancreatic fibrosis which often leads to calcification, and stones are frequently found in the pancreatic duct. Recurrent abdominal pain occurs and 75% have radiological evidence of pancreatic calcification. Malnutrition is common in most populations in which this form of diabetes develops. The staple diet is based on cassava, and it has been suggested that cyanates, present in the cassava root, may be a contributory cause of the pancreatic damage.
2. *Protein-deficient pancreatic diabetes* seems to be caused directly by malnutrition. Unlike fibrocalculous pancreatic diabetes, there is no impairment of exocrine pancreatic function, and no evidence of pancreatic fibrosis, calcification or abdominal pain.

Insulin secretion is preserved (although impaired) in both forms of tropical diabetes, and is the likely explanation for the observed resistance to ketosis. Alternatively, mal-

nourished individuals may have so little stored fat that free fatty acids cannot be released in sufficient quantities to fuel the process of ketogenesis.

CLINICAL FEATURES AND INVESTIGATION OF DIABETES MELLITUS

Acute

In the young, the history is usually brief (under four weeks in about 50%), with the typical triad of primary symptoms: polyuria, thirst and weight loss. Increased urine production is caused by an osmotic diuresis produced when the renal threshold is exceeded and glucose enters the urine. Fluid and electrolyte losses stimulate thirst, sometimes intense. Fat and protein stores are broken down as a result of insulin deficiency, and this leads to weight loss and fatigue. If not recognised, the insulin lack leads to ketoacidosis which may then be the presenting feature.

Sub-acute

The onset may occur over several months, with thirst, polyuria and loss of weight, although less marked than in the acute form (which tends to affect younger patients). Other presenting symptoms may occur, such as fatigue, pruritis vulvae due to infection with *Candida albicans*, or blurring of vision caused by refractive errors.

Presentation with complications

The complications of diabetes (pp. 766–772) may also be the presenting feature. They include:

1. *infections*, e.g. staphylococcal skin infections including carbuncles and foot infections
2. *arterial disease*, causing myocardial infarction or peripheral vascular disease
3. *eye problems*, e.g. cataracts or retinopathy causing visual impairment, or those noticed by an optician
4. *neuropathy*, e.g. paraesthesia or ulceration of the feet.

Asymptomatic

Insurance or medical examination may reveal glycosuria or a raised blood glucose in asymptomatic individuals.

Physical examination

There may be no abnormal signs. Obvious weight loss may have occurred, and, in acute cases, there may be dehydration and the smell of ketones detected on the patient's breath. Evidence of complications (retinopathy, vascular disease, neuropathy and proteinuria) may be present, especially in older patients.

Investigation

In normal individuals, blood glucose levels are controlled within a narrow range. Variation from normality is there-

Summary 1 Presentations of diabetes

The patient may be symptomatic or asymptomatic

- Acute
  Thirst, polyuria and weight loss. Pruritus vulvae and visual blurring are common

- Sub-acute
  Symptoms as above, but insidious onset over many months
  Malaise and tiredness are common

- Delayed
  With complications such as skin infections, foot problems, impotence and retinopathy

fore easily detected. In *symptomatic* patients, elevated blood glucose indicates diabetes, although it is prudent to repeat the test to rule out laboratory error. In *asymptomatic* patients, or those with few symptoms, the diagnosis is made by two fasting venous blood glucose levels above 6.7 mmol/l (125 mg/dl), or two random values above 10 mmol/l (200 mg/dl). (Note that the equivalent venous plasma glucose levels are 7.8 and 11.1 mmol/l.)

If these three criteria are present, a glucose tolerance test (GTT) is unnecessary. There are occasional difficult cases (p. 751) where a GTT may be helpful.

Glycosuria is detected by means of enzymatic methods specific for glucose. Although not diagnostic of diabetes (since 1% of normal people have renal glycosuria), the finding indicates that further investigation is necessary, and the glucose tolerance test is helpful in ruling out diabetes for purposes such as insurance examinations.

Further tests are not needed to confirm the diagnosis, but other useful tests include examination of the urine for protein and ketones, blood urea and electrolytes, measurement of blood cholesterol and triglycerides carried out after blood glucose levels have returned to normal and a full blood count.

Other investigations to consider in diabetes mellitus include thyroid function and auto-antibody screening in the young, and chest X-ray, ECG and mid-stream urine in older patients.

BASIC PRINCIPLES OF TREATMENT OF DIABETES MELLITUS

Dietary modification is the basis of treatment. Without regulation of diet, control of the blood sugar is seldom obtained either with insulin or oral hypoglycaemics, particularly in obese patients. Insulin is always necessary if the patient has had an episode of ketoacidosis, and will usually be needed in patients presenting under 40 years of age. Oral hypoglycaemics should usually be avoided in younger patients and are contraindicated in pregnancy. Insulin is necessary in older patients when oral therapy fails.

In older patients, the first approach is by diet alone. A full assessment should be made of the patient's knowledge of his or her diet and compliance with it. The next form of treatment – oral hypoglycaemics – should only be introduced if satisfactory control is not achieved by diet, particularly in obese patients who are not losing weight. Obese patients are treated with biguanides, and non-obese patients with a sulphonylurea. *Primary failure* is defined as failure of these agents (alone or together) to achieve satisfactory control. *Secondary failure* is loss of control over a period of time following a good initial response. It is most important to recognise secondary failure early; one of the most common errors is to delay insulin treatment in a patient who really needs it.

The patient has to care for his or her diabetes, guided by professionals with specialised knowledge. Cooperation and understanding by the patient is the main determinant of good control of blood sugar. Such cooperation is obtained by the patient understanding the risks of diabetes and the benefits of control of blood glucose. The importance of controlling weight, of foot care, and the elimination of vascular risk factors (such as smoking) must be explained and understood.

Diabetes differs from most other chronic diseases in the extent of the demands it makes on the patient. These include unremitting attention to diet, energy expenditure and other factors (such as intercurrent illness) that will influence control, such as the performance of blood and urine tests and adjustment of the insulin dose. These skills need to be learned, and the modern emphasis is thus on training patients to take on responsibility for their own diabetes. It is clear that the routine hospital diabetic clinic is unsuited for this sort of educational function, and a number of new strategies have recently been tested. One very successful approach is the use of diabetes nurse specialists to take over many teaching and therapeutic functions previously reserved for doctors. A more recent development is the establishment of community-based diabetes day centres. These take over many of the routine educational and screening functions of the clinic, and, in the view of some optimists, may even supplant it entirely. Wherever these may be based, organised training programmes involving nurse specialists, dietitians and chiropodists as well as physicians, are now a recognised part of good modern diabetes care.

Summary 2 Management of NIDDM

- Weight reduction and exercise

- Diet should be calorie controlled; refined carbohydrate replaced with unrefined; fat intake restricted, with animal fats being replaced by vegetable fats

- Oral hypoglycaemics should only be introduced after an adequate trial of diet alone

- Many patients initially controlled on diet and oral agents will eventually need insulin

- Treatment should aim for weight control and fasting blood glucose levels below 7 mmol/l

- Reduce other cardiovascular risk factors such as hypertension, hyperlipidaemia and smoking

DIET

The diet for diabetics is no different from the normal healthy diet recommended for the rest of the population (Ch. 8). In former days, a low carbohydrate diet was recommended, with the consequence that the proportion of energy derived from fat was increased. This high-fat diet may even have increased the frequency of cardiovascular disease in the diabetic population. The assumption that a low-carbohydrate diet is good for diabetes is, in any case, probably unjustified; for example, glucose tolerance deteriorates in healthy subjects when carbohydrate is restricted in the days preceding the test. Modern diet treatment is based on an assessment of overall energy needs and the quality of food in the diet.

Calories

Caloric intake is calculated according to the needs of the patient, bearing in mind his work and weight. An obese patient is prescribed a reducing diet of between 1000 and 1600 kcal/day; a non-obese patient is recommended to take an isocaloric diet. Patients who have lost weight because of untreated diabetes and who are thin, are advised, temporarily, to eat a diet with excess calories.

Carbohydrate

Unrefined carbohydrate is preferable to simple sugars such as glucose. The carbohydrate in high-fibre foods is absorbed relatively slowly, preventing the rapid fluctuations in blood glucose which occur when refined sugars are eaten. In practice, this means that patients should take good plain food with plenty of bulk in it and should avoid the processed and packaged products of the modern food industry. The principle of delayed absorption has been used in therapy, both by addition of guar gum (a product of the Indian cluster bean which delays movement of carbohydrate from the gut) and by trials of acarbose, which inhibits enzyme systems responsible for transport of sugars across the intestinal mucosa. The carbohydrate content of the diet should provide 50–60% of the total calories.

Fat

Vegetable fat is preferred to animal fat, and the total contribution of fat to caloric intake should not exceed 30–35%. In the developed world, the standard diet is so rich in fat that this target is not easy to achieve.

Designing the dietary plan

The aim should be to modify the patient's eating habits while minimising disruption to life style; therefore, a detailed dietary and activity history should precede any dietary advice. For normal-weight patients, an isocaloric healthy eating plan should be advised, and the distribution of intake throughout the day should be matched to hypoglycaemic medication. This is particularly important for patients on insulin therapy, who require a reasonably constant carbohydrate intake at particular meal times, and who should also have small snacks at mid-morning, mid-afternoon and at bedtime in order to avoid unopposed insulin action. In general, the more flexible the insulin regimen, the more freedom the patient will have to vary insulin and food intake at a particular time of day; this is exemplified by newer routines of preprandial, short-acting insulin prescribed in combination with a single daily injection of long-acting background insulin.

Alcohol consumption

The dangers of excessive alcohol consumption should be stressed since its high calorific value may limit attempts at weight loss in overweight patients, while in insulin-treated patients it may predispose to hypoglycaemia through the inhibition of hepatic gluconeogenesis. The latter phenomenon becomes a very real danger in patients who consume alcohol on an empty stomach.

ORAL HYPOGLYCAEMICS

Oral hypoglycaemic therapy comprises two major classes of drug, namely sulphonylureas and biguanides.

Sulphonylureas

Sulphonylurea is a class of drug (chemically related to the sulphonamides) which was developed following the clinical observation that patients treated with modified sulphonamide agents developed hypoglycaemia. The mode of action is twofold. In the initial phase of therapy, the predominant effect is to increase insulin secretion from pancreatic beta cells, both basally and postprandially. With maintenance therapy, there appears to be an additional effect of increasing insulin sensitivity occurring at a post-receptor level. These agents, by definition, are only suitable for patients with residual insulin secretion and are, therefore, of no value in true insulin-dependent diabetics. Furthermore, they may prove suboptimal in non-insulin-dependent patients with severe intercurrent illness when temporary commencement of insulin may be required.

The currently available sulphonylureas and their equipotent doses are listed in Table 20.3. All may produce hypoglycaemia if the dose employed is excessive, or if

Table 20.3 Sulphonylurea agents

Drug	Action	Dose/24 h	Excretion
Gliclazide	10–12 h	40–320 mg	Hepatic and renal
Tolbutamide	6–8 h	1–2 g	Hepatic
Glibenclamide	12–20 h	2.5–20 mg	Hepatic and renal
Glibornuride	16 h	12.5–75 mg	Hepatic
Chlorpropamide	36–48 h	100–500 mg	Hepatic and renal

carbohydrate intake is inadequate. This risk is increased in patients with hepatic disease, because of impaired hepatic drug excretion compounded by possible reduction in glycogen reserve. Patients with renal impairment should be given a drug which is excreted by the liver, such as tolbutamide or glibornuride. Tolbutamide is the safest drug in the very elderly, because of its short duration of action. Chlorpropamide is still widely used, but has the disadvantage of a long duration of action and a wider range of side-effects, which include the idiosyncratic phenomenon of facial flushing after alcohol.

Adverse effects

Binding of sulphonylureas to albumin in the circulation may lead to mutual displacement by other drugs, such as oral anticoagulants. Cholestatic jaundice may also rarely occur. At high doses, chlorpropamide may produce dilutional hyponatraemia due to enhancement of the action of antidiuretic hormone.

Biguanides

Biguanides modify glycaemia by increasing peripheral glycolysis, decreasing hepatic glucose production and decreasing glucose absorption in the intestine. The only biguanide available in the UK is metformin; the previously prescribed agent, phenformin, has been withdrawn because of its predisposition to cause fatal lactic acidosis. There is no significant risk of lactic acidosis with metformin therapy, except in patients with hepatic, renal or advanced cardiovascular disease.

Biguanide drugs do not cause hypoglycaemia and, because insulin secretion is not stimulated, do not increase appetite. For this reason, they are particularly useful in overweight non-insulin-dependent patients in whom dietary measures alone have produced suboptimal results. Metformin may also be a useful addition to sulphonylurea therapy if the initially successful response to the latter decreases (so-called secondary sulphonylurea failure); this combination may postpone the need for commencement of insulin.

Adverse effects

The major side-effects with metformin therapy are gastrointestinal, particularly diarrhoea, and this limits the applicability of the drug.

INSULIN

Insulin is found in all vertebrates, and the central part of the molecule has remained remarkably constant over the course of evolution. Beef insulin was the mainstay of insulin therapy for many years. However, it has three amino acid differences from human insulin, and, as a result (also because of the relative impurity of earlier insulin preparations), insulin antibody formation was common. Porcine insulin differs in only one amino acid sequence

and is only slightly more antigenic than preparations of human insulin. In the 1970s, highly purified porcine insulin tended to supplant beef insulin in many countries; this, in turn, will almost certainly be replaced by human insulin by the early 1990s.

Human insulin is now produced biosynthetically by insertion of genetic material into *E. coli*. The original route of manufacture was by separate production of the alpha and beta chains and in vitro combination. More recently, the proinsulin molecule itself has been synthesised and insulin produced by cleavage of C-peptide. An alternative means of producing the molecule is by chemical modification of porcine insulin by substitution of threonine for alanine on position 30 of the beta chain.

Insulin preparations

Modern insulins are now very pure products without glucagon, proinsulin or other impurities. Insulin is prepared either as a clear solution (referred to as soluble, crystalline or regular insulin) or formulated with a retarding agent which gives the preparation a cloudy appearance. The most successful retarding agents have been protamine, which is extracted from fish sperm, and zinc. The protamine insulins are also known as isophane or NPH (neutral protamine hagedorn) insulins, and the zinc insulins as lente insulin.

Lente insulins are produced by crystallisation in the presence of an excess of zinc; depending upon the conditions employed, this results in the formation of large crystals known as crystalline zinc or ultralente, or of small crystals referred to as amorphous zinc or semilente. The mixture of these two varieties in a proportion of 70:30 produces the classical lente type of insulin. These insulins are available at a standard concentration of 100 units/ml in the UK and USA, and at concentrations of 40 or 80 units/ml in many other countries.

Protamine insulin is stable in mixtures with soluble insulin, and pre-mixed or combination insulins are available with the proportion of soluble insulin ranging from 10–50%. In contrast, the lente insulins contain zinc in excess and bind added soluble insulin, so that mixtures cannot be marketed. Soluble and lente insulins may, however, be mixed in the syringe, provided they are then injected without delay. When this is done, the soluble insulin should be taken into the syringe first to avoid unwitting addition of zinc to the soluble vial. Characteristics of the various human insulin formulations are summarised in Table 20.4.

Clinical use of insulin

The healthy adult pancreas stores some 200–250 units of insulin in the secretory granules of the beta cell and secretes some 30–40 units daily. This secretion is in two modes – a constant basal rate of secretion (overnight and between meals), and peaks of secretion (5–10-fold above basal levels) after food. This pattern is hard to imitate with injected insulin because insulin is given subcutaneously rather than into the pancreatic artery, and into the systemic rather than

Diabetes and Lipid Metabolism

Table 20.4 Human insulin preparations

Formulation	Manufacturer		
	Eli Lilly	Nordisk	Novo
Soluble	Humulin S	Velosulin*	Actrapid
Amorphous zinc	–	–	Semitard
Crystalline zinc	Humulin Zn	–	Ultratard
Amorphous/crystalline 30:70%	–	–	Monotard
Protamine (Isophane)	Humulin I	Insulatard*	Protaphane
Soluble/protamine (% soluble given in brackets)	Humulin M1 (10%)	–	–
	Humulin M2 (20%)	–	–
	Humulin M3 (30%)	Mixtard*	Actraphane
	Humulin M4 (40%)	–	–
	Humulin M5 (50%)	Initard*	–

* Also available as porcine insulin

portal circulation. Furthermore, absorption of subcutaneous insulin is often erratic, and circulating insulin concentrations of injected insulin inevitably peak and decline rather than producing a constant basal level.

Patients have to be taught how to inject themselves, and most of them are understandably apprehensive about doing so. Disposable needles (10–15 mm) are used, the length depending on how fat the patient is. The needle is inserted to its full depth at 90° to the skin. In most patients, the thighs and abdomen are the convenient sites; the arms should be avoided in beginners. Injection sites should be rotated since this prevents lipohypertrophy, and inspection of injection sites should be a routine part of clinical follow-up. Insulin absorption varies with subcutaneous blood flow, and is speeded by massage, exercise or warmth. It should be noted that insulin is absorbed more rapidly from the arm than from the abdomen, and more rapidly from the abdomen than from the leg.

Starting patients on insulin

Commencing insulin therapy is a major step in the life of the patient, and emotional support as well as careful training are essential. Routine hospital admission is not obligatory, and many centres have found the policy of starting patients at home with the assistance of a diabetes nurse specialist to be both successful and cost-effective.

An intermediate-duration insulin, given twice daily, is the usual starting regimen for young patients. Endogenous insulin secretion may sometimes recover in the first few months, and, if this happens, the insulin dose must be reduced and can occasionally be stopped. Failure to anticipate this may result in demoralising episodes of hypoglycaemia. Insulin requirements then rise steadily, and

patients are transferred to a twice-daily combination of soluble and intermediate insulin. As a rough guide, two-thirds of the total daily dose are given in the morning, and two-thirds of both morning and evening injections are given as intermediate insulin. However, it should be realised that the regimen has, in each case, to be tailored to the needs of the individual.

Insulin treatment is frequently used in the management of Type II diabetes, and the number of patients in this category probably equals the number of patients with Type I diabetes. There is less agreement as to the most appropriate regimen. Some doctors treat it in the same way as Type I diabetes, with two daily injections. An alternative approach is to aim for basal insulin supplementation on the grounds that many patients retain sufficient insulin secretion to respond adequately to meals once basal glucose levels have been normalised. Basal supplementation may be given as a single daily injection of a long-acting insulin, such as Ultratard, or as a bedtime injection of an intermediate insulin.

Intensified insulin therapy

Only a minority of patients with Type I diabetes are likely to achieve near-normal blood glucose control with conventional insulin therapy, and for this reason various approaches to intensified therapy have been tried. It is now appreciated that success does not depend simply upon the technique of insulin administration, but rather upon the knowledge and motivation of the patient. Once this is taken into account, it seems clear that multiple daily injections or continuous subcutaneous insulin infusion offer the prospect of improved control and a more flexible life style.

Pen injection devices have made multiple injection regimens more acceptable to patients. These regimens may be administered as a dose of soluble insulin before each main meal together with either a long-acting insulin at suppertime or an intermediate insulin with the bedtime snack. An alternative is the use of a small pump to deliver the basal insulin requirement by continuous subcutaneous insulin infusion (CSII). At meal times, the patient presses a button on a pump to deliver the dose. CSII gives a smoother blood glucose profile with less risk of hyper- and hypoglycaemia. Meal-times can be taken flexibly, which is helpful for busy people, and it is especially useful for the overnight period. The drawbacks of this approach include the problems of being attached to the pump, a risk of the flow of insulin being disrupted (causing ketoacidosis) and a risk of infection because of the permanently emplaced needle.

Social consequences

Patients starting on insulin are advised to tell their employers. Occupations unsuitable for insulin-treated patients include driving heavy goods vehicles, working with dangerous machinery or at heights. The police and armed forces do not accept diabetic patients. On starting insulin, patients should inform the driving licence authorities and their insurance companies.

Problems in insulin treatment

Local

Scarring and abscesses may occur at shallow injection sites, and advice on technique is necessary. *Lipoatrophy* is a form of allergic response now rarely seen with highly purified insulin. *Lipohypertrophy* is excess local fat due to excessive use of a single injection site. Local allergic responses may occur when insulin is first started, but these are uncommon with purified insulins and systemic allergy is very rare.

Systemic

Insulin resistance

Insulin resistance of a mild degree is common in over-weight patients, although daily requirement of more than 200 units is regarded as severe and is uncommon. The cause of this resistance is unknown. Some patients may gain weight when insulin is started, usually because the insulin dose and dietary calorie intake are not being regulated properly. Poor dietary compliance (often in late-onset diabetes), is the major problem, the insulin dose being increased to counter the resulting hyperglycaemia.

Hypoglycaemia

Hypoglycaemia is the commonest and most serious complication of insulin treatment. The majority of patients have occasional minor symptoms, if the insulin dosage is adequate to control the diabetes. About one-third will have at least one episode of coma, and a small proportion have recurrent and severe attacks. Those patients with NIDDM who are treated with insulin seldom suffer from the more severe manifestations of hypoglycaemia.

Clinical features. Typically, the symptoms occur over a few minutes. Usually the patient notices tremor and tachycardia, and starts to sweat. Vision may be blurred and motor co-ordination impaired, and there may be a sensation of hunger and faintness. Mental symptoms include confusion, irritability and abnormal behaviour, such as aggression. Patients on insulin for a long time may lose the premonitory symptoms, and the first manifestations are then behavioural changes which may lead rapidly to coma. The behavioural changes may be mistaken for inebriation and lead to arrest, although relatives often recognise the early signs. Some patients slip into coma without any warning.

Nocturnal hypoglycaemia causes nightmares, night-sweats, restlessness and morning headache. Convulsions may occur and be mistaken for epilepsy. Typically, the symptoms do not wake the patient. Neurological symptoms may be especially severe in older patients. Transient hemiparesis may occur which responds to intravenous glucose.

Aetiology. The cause of hypoglycaemia is a mismatch between the insulin requirements at a given time (which is related to basal insulin requirement and activity) and the dose injected. For this reason, the greatest risk is when the patient has missed a meal or a snack, or if there has been extra exertion. Alcohol may also precipitate hypoglycaemia. Other episodes occur without any obvious explanation. Insulin requirements increase in the early morning at 3–4 a.m., at a time when the previously injected insulin is declining. This results in morning hyperglycaemia, which can lead a patient to increase the insulin dose before bedtime, thus causing nocturnal hypoglycaemia.

The normal responses to counteract hypoglycaemia are often defective in diabetics, particularly if this is long-standing. The adrenalin response may be lacking as a consequence of autonomic neuropathy (p. 940), so the warning symptoms are missing. Only about two-thirds of diabetic patients retain these adrenergic symptoms after 10 years of treatment. For reasons which are not clear, the output of glucagon in response to hypoglycaemia gradually diminishes, even though there appears to be no other functional abnormality of pancreatic alpha cells.

Diagnosis. Clinical diagnosis of hypoglycaemia is usually simple, especially if the patient is known to be a diabetic. Presentation with behavioural or neurological symptoms, or in coma, can cause more difficulty. Patients should be encouraged to wear a bracelet or carry a card which identifies them as diabetic. A blood glucose confirms the diagnosis, but treatment should begin immediately (while waiting for the result) if hypoglycaemia is suspected. Laboratory blood glucose measurement is necessary to determine the low levels accurately.

Treatment. Treatment consists – initially – of *prevention* in the form of education in the use of insulin and the encouragement of patients to carry glucose tablets or sweets. In established hypoglycaemia, sugar drinks can be given, but confused or comatose patients should be treated with glucose intravenously (e.g. 50 ml of 50%). Glucagon (1 mg im) produces an effect almost as quickly, mobilizing glucose from hepatic glycogen. It is convenient and can be given at home by the family. In the elderly, neurological disturbance (especially coma) may take longer to recover. Following treatment, all patients should be encouraged to eat to replenish glucose stores, especially if they have been treated with glucagon. The cause of the episode should be determined.

ASSESSING CONTROL OF DIABETES

Diabetes would be easy to control if patients were able to sense changes in their blood glucose level. Unfortunately, many claim to feel perfectly well even when their mean glycaemia is well above the normal range. For this reason, they need a simple and accurate way of monitoring their control.

Urine testing

Urine dipstick tests are simple and specific for glucose, and they have replaced chemical tests of urinary reducing substances. The correlation between blood and urine glucose is not good, even though it is probably true that a patient who is not hypoglycaemic and has no glycosuria is probably well controlled. The poor correlation is due to two main factors. Firstly, urine tests give no indication of blood levels below the mean renal glucose threshold, which is about 10 mmol/l with a wide range (7–13 mmol). Secondly, changes in urine glucose lag behind changes in blood glucose, and reflect an average blood glucose level over a period of time. Dipstick tests are available for urine ketones, although routine measurement is rarely helpful. However, the tests may be useful in situations in which ketosis may occur, such as in infections.

Blood testing

Blood glucose is the best and most direct measure of control. A *fasting* glucose is useful in diagnosis of diabetes and in assessing patients with Type II diabetes (since this is related to overnight secretion of endogenous insulin), but has less value in Type I diabetes. With the advent of reliable tests on blood samples obtained by fingerprick and read on a visual chart or in a meter, patients can be taught to measure their own blood glucose and to keep account of a daily profile when necessary. This is of more value than a random glucose level. Blood is taken from the side of the finger pulp (not from the tip which is a sensory organ), using a modern lancet. Profiles are performed regularly, but not necessarily on a daily basis. These, and other items such as episodes of hypoglycaemia, are best noted in a special diary and brought to the clinic at each visit.

A more recent method of assessing overall glycaemic control is by measurement of glycosylated products circulating in the blood. Glucose may become attached to proteins by a non-enzymatic process, and the amount of this glycosylation is related to the blood glucose concentration over a period of time. The terminal valine on the haemoglobin beta chain is a site of glycosylation, and haemoglobin in this form can be measured by electrophoresis. About 5% of haemoglobin is glycosylated in the non-diabetic, but values above 10% (depending on the assay method) are found in poorly controlled diabetic patients. The test, therefore, summarises the changes in blood glucose levels over a period of several weeks, and this value (HbA_{1c}) is directly related to the mean blood glucose over this time. The measurement will be affected by a short red cell survival (for example due to haemoglobinopathy or marked renal impairment). HbA_{1c} gives an assessment of overall glycaemic control, but blood glucose testing (to determine the daily profile) is necessary before a change in treatment can be made.

DIABETIC METABOLIC EMERGENCIES

Diabetic ketoacidosis

As the name implies, diabetic ketoacidosis is a metabolic acidosis which develops in diabetic patients as a result of raised levels of circulating ketone bodies. No generally agreed quantitative definition exists, but, for purposes of clinical research, it has been defined as severe uncontrolled diabetes (requiring emergency treatment with insulin and intravenous fluids) where the total blood ketone concentration is greater than 5 mmol/l or, more pragmatically, arterial pH is below 7.2. Since marked insulin deficiency is a precondition of the development of ketoacidosis, it occurs only in patients with Type I diabetes.

In the pre-insulin era, the condition was known as 'diabetic coma', and physicians were obliged to stand by helplessly while their patients became unconscious and died. One physician provided the following description:

> *He finally collapses and is forced to bed, not to rest, but there to be tortured with a gruelling combat for breath. The food he has hitherto eaten nausea forces him to reject, the liquids he eagerly drinks he vomits. In his restlessness he throws off the clothes. Finally, beaten in his struggle for life, he falls back helpless, unconscious, with a pulse approaching 200, with a body temperature rapidly falling below normal, with so little liquid in the body that his muscles melt away before the touch, with the eyes as soft as jellyfish, with the skin parchment dry, with the cheeks now showing slow recovery of the circulation to pressure, with the pulse flickering, and with the blood pressure so low and the flow of blood so feeble that to get a specimen one may be forced to puncture the jugular, which in contrast to the other veins is large. In the brief space of hours the body has seemingly gone through months of the ravages of cancer, and death appears at hand.*

(Joslin, 1925)

Since insulin was introduced ketoacidosis is infrequently fatal, but it is also worth noting that the condition is almost always preventable since treatment is so simple in its early stages. Patients admitted to hospital fall into two main groups: those with previously undiagnosed diabetes and established diabetic patients undergoing the stress of intercurrent illness. In a surprising number of cases medical error is a factor. Undiagnosed patients have very often sought medical help with related symptoms days or even weeks before presentation in hospital. Established patients can almost always cope with minor illnesses without difficulty, provided they monitor themselves carefully and increase the dose of insulin. A common error is for insulin to be reduced in the presence of vomiting (the patient is afraid of going hypoglycaemic), and it is not uncommon for this to be done on the advice of a doctor. Interruption of insulin therapy is estimated to be a contributing factor in 25% of admissions with ketoacidosis.

Pathogenesis

Diabetic ketoacidosis develops when the balance between anabolic and catabolic activity is shifted towards uncontrolled catabolism as a result of insulin deficiency (Fig. 20.12). The consequences are a relatively unrestrained increase in hepatic gluconeogenesis and a parallel increase in peripheral lipolysis which leads to increased circulating free fatty acids and hepatic ketogenesis. As outlined in the preceding section on metabolic control in the fasting state, these processes are accelerated by catecholamines, glucagon and cortisol which are secreted in

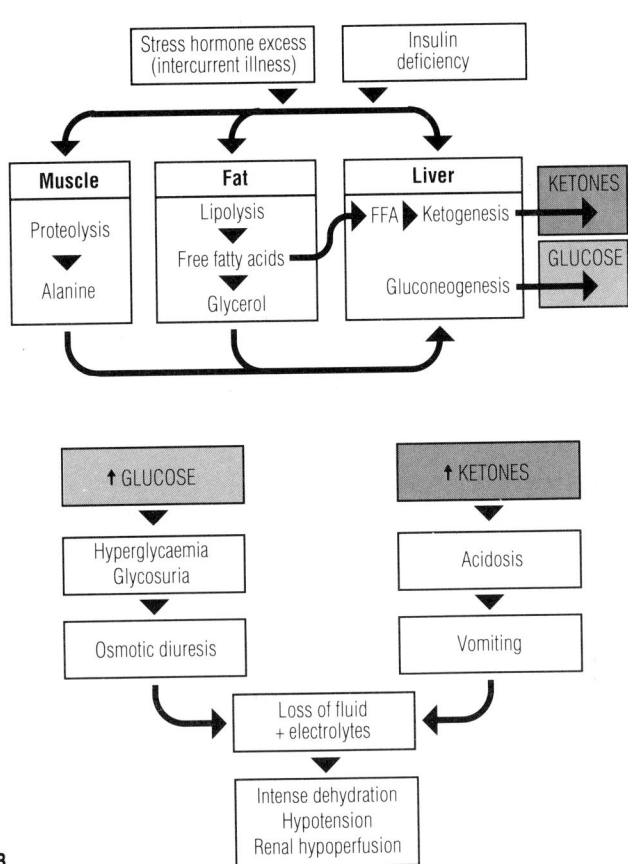

Fig. 20.12 Pathogenesis of diabetic ketoacidosis. A. Insulin deficiency leads to overproduction of glucose and ketones, especially if stress hormone release is also present. **B.** Dehydration results from the osmotic diuresis produced by hyperglycaemia, while vomiting secondary to metabolic acidosis causes further fluid loss.

increased quantities in response to the dehydration associated with uncontrolled diabetes and also as a result of any precipitating intercurrent illness.

Hyperglycaemia exceeding the renal threshold for glucose results in glycosuria and an osmotic diuresis with water depletion. The accelerated lipolysis (Fig. 20.12) increases free fatty acid supply to the liver, and their partial oxidation to the acidic ketone bodies, acetoacetate and 3-hydroxybutyrate, leads to a metabolic acidosis. The latter causes nausea and vomiting which further exacerbates the salt and water depletion, and urinary losses of potassium are substantial. Progressive dehydration results in a decreased circulating volume, reduced renal perfusion with prerenal uraemia and decreased peripheral perfusion which compounds the acidosis. Profound metabolic acidosis eventually disturbs cellular function, and cardiac function, in particular, may be compromised.

Clinical features

Patients present with profound dehydration, compensatory hyperventilation due to metabolic acidosis (Kussmaul respiration or air hunger), vomiting and –

sometimes – abdominal pain. Some disturbance of consciousness is common, but frank coma is comparatively unusual. The characteristic smell of ketones may be detected on the breath, and constitutes an important diagnostic sign. Core temperature may be decreased, despite intercurrent infections.

Diagnosis

Diagnosis is based on demonstration of hyperglycaemia in combination with acidosis and ketosis. Hyperglycaemia can be shown by stick testing, although it is always essential to send a sample to the laboratory for confirmation. Acidosis is proved by arterial blood gas measurement. The urine will be strongly positive for ketones on stick testing, and ketonaemia can be shown by centrifuging a sample of plasma and testing with a urine ketone stick.

The need for treatment is urgent, and intravenous fluids and insulin should be started as soon as the first blood sample is taken. Initial biochemistry will include a laboratory blood glucose, which in the case of ketoacidosis will normally be in excess of 20 mmol/l. Urea and electrolytes need to be measured frequently; the initial set of results will contain a mass of information. The *urea* may be raised, depending upon the degree of dehydration. The *venous bicarbonate* may be lowered in the presence of a metabolic acidosis. The *potassium* may be high, low or normal, but serves as a guide to the rate of potassium replacement. The *osmolality* may be measured directly or calculated from the formula:

$$\text{plasma osmolality} = 2(Na + K) + urea + glucose$$

Finally, the *anion gap* (Ch. 22) can be calculated from the following:

$$\text{anion gap} = (Na + K) - (Cl + HCO_3)$$

The normal anion gap is less than 17; values greater than this indicate the presence of an unmeasured anion in excess, such as lactate or ketones.

These investigations, together with the arterial gases, allow the biochemical disturbance to be assessed. Further investigations are directed towards identifying any condition (e.g. pneumonia or myocardial infarction) which might have precipitated the episode, and towards assessment of the general condition of the patient. A full blood count is taken. A neutrophil leucocytosis is often present, but this is non-specific and does not necessarily indicate the presence of infection. A chest X-ray may reveal an unsuspected pneumonia, and blood and urine cultures are taken. An ECG is performed and monitored during further therapy; T wave changes may provide the first warning of disturbed potassium balance.

Management

Typical water and electrolyte deficits are of the following order of magnitude:

Water	5–11 litres	Potassium	200–700 mmol/l
Sodium	300–700 mmol/l	Chloride	350–500 mmol/l

20

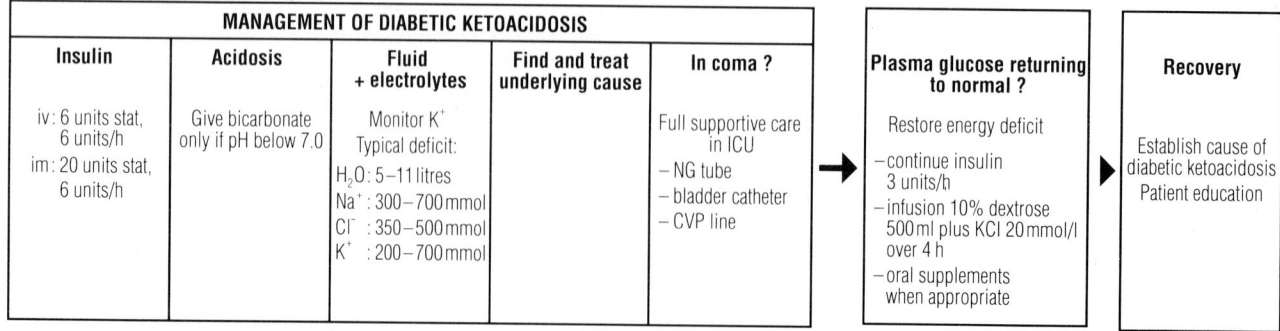

Fig. 20.13 Principles of management of diabetic ketoacidosis.

It is worth remembering that the patient is also fuel-depleted following this period of accelerated catabolism, and energy stores also need to be replenished. The principles of management (Fig. 20.13) are as discussed in detail below.

Fluid replacement

Normal saline is the standard fluid for rehydration, replacing deficits of chloride and sodium as well as water losses. If the patient is hypotensive, 1–2 litres of plasma or whole blood can be given to restore intravascular volume. Standard guides to fluid replacement are available, but should not be followed mindlessly. In particular, elderly patients may not tolerate a rate of fluid replacement appropriate to the young, and there is no point in forcing fluids through younger patients at the milder end of the clinical spectrum. With this proviso, severe cases need 1–2 litres over the first hour, a total of 3–4 litres over the first four hours and a total of 6–8 litres over the first 24 hours. It is good practice to change to dextrose solution as the blood glucose approaches normal (see below).

Potassium replacement

Although plasma potassium may be normal, high or low at presentation, it is important to appreciate that total body potassium is severely depleted. If potassium is not given early in treatment, hypokalaemia develops rapidly, partly because of dilution due to rapid expansion of the intravascular space, and partly because insulin treatment shifts potassium (together with glucose) into peripheral cells. A guideline for potassium replacement is given in Figure 20.14.

Restoration of acid-base balance

Insulin treatment rapidly halts ketogenesis, and fluid replacement flushes circulating ketones into the urine within a few hours. Under these circumstances, the normal compensatory mechanisms will rapidly correct the acid-base imbalance. The value (or risk) of alkali infusion has been debated for many years, and it has been pointed out that amounts normally given are derisory in terms of the total hydrogen ion excess and introduce an added risk of

hypokalaemia. It is, however, conventional to give bicarbonate to patients with a pH below 7.0; one suggested regimen is to give 100–150 ml of sodium bicarbonate 1.4%, and to repeat this half-hourly if necessary. In addition, 26 mmol of potassium should be given for every 100 ml of bicarbonate.

Insulin replacement

Traditional therapy was with a single large bolus of insulin, with half the dose given into a vein and half into muscle. Modern treatment is with a low-dose regimen, given either as an iv infusion or hourly im injections. The subcutaneous route is avoided because subcutaneous blood flow is reduced in shocked patients. The low-dose regimen lowers blood glucose by suppressing hepatic glucose production, whereas the high-dose regimen also promotes rapid entry of glucose and potassium into muscle cells. As might be expected, the high-dose regimen can lead to severe hypoglycaemia or hypokalaemia – complications largely avoided by the low-dose approach.

Energy replacement

It is helpful to replace saline with dextrose once blood glucose levels fall to around 10 mmol/l. This helps to replace the overall fluid deficit and permits continued insulin infusion without inducing hypoglycaemia.

Plasma K⁺ (mmol)	No K⁺ supplement — Check plasma levels frequently
6	
	KCl, 13 mmol/h
5	
	KCl, 20 mmol/h
4	
	KCl, 26 mmol/h
3	
	KCl, 39–50 mmol/h — Best given by iv infusion pump — Check plasma levels frequently

Fig. 20.14 A guide to potassium replacement during diabetic ketoacidosis.

> **Summary 3 Management of diabetic ketoacidosis**
> - Replace fluid losses – the average deficit is around 7 litres
> - Replace electrolytes; monitor potassium carefully
> - Restore acid-base balance – but bicarbonate infusion needed only in severe cases
> - Replace insulin deficiency – 4–6 units hourly is usually enough
> - Replace energy losses – dextrose infusion with insulin cover until the patient can eat
> - Look for the underlying cause – infection is a common precipitant

Seek the underlying cause

This, when present, is usually due to infection, although myocardial infarction and other underlying illnesses need to be considered in the elderly. Septicaemia, pneumonia or urinary tract infection may be present. Patients may present with hidden pus, e.g. a perinephric abscess. If infection is suspected, broad-spectrum antibiotics are started once the appropriate cultures have been taken.

Special problems in management

Difficulties in management arise in patients with profound ketoacidosis presenting relatively late. These include the following:

1. *Hypokalaemia* in the presence of acidosis implies profound total body potassium depletion. The danger is that further falls in plasma potassium will occur as the acidosis and hyperglycaemia are reversed. Potassium replacement and rehydration should take initial priority over insulin administration in these circumstances.
2. *Profound hypotension* ($\leq 90 \, mmHg$) due to salt and water depletion may be sufficient to severely compromise peripheral perfusion. This necessitates infusion of plasma expanders or blood to avoid renal tubular necrosis.
3. *Hypothermia* at the time of presentation is a poor prognostic sign; it is vital to avoid further falls in body temperature during the initial resuscitative phase of treatment.
4. *Coma* necessitates standard management of the unconscious patient, including airway maintenance and nasogastric intubation on free drainage to avoid aspiration of gastric contents.
5. *Cerebral oedema* has been described in children during the treatment of ketoacidosis and may be related to the relatively greater rise in osmolality in the central nervous system with profound dehydration, resulting in abnormal fluid shifts during therapy.

Post-resuscitative care

When glucose levels have stabilised and the patient is able to eat and drink normally, the drip can be taken down and soluble insulin given as three- or four-daily doses until maintenance insulin therapy can be restarted. Sliding scales are best avoided. The patient is still potassium-depleted, and the diet should contain adequate potassium, e.g. as orange juice. In the recovery period, the previously undiagnosed patient begins his or her education for a life with diabetes. However, if the patient has established diabetes it is important to enquire into the causes of the episode, whether it was due to physical illness or poor education. Diabetic ketoacidosis is a preventable condition.

Non-ketotic hyperosmolar coma

Non-ketotic hyperosmolar coma occurs when uncontrolled hyperglycaemia leads to dehydration, increased osmolality, and ultimately to coma, yet significant ketosis does not develop. As with ketoacidosis, there is no generally agreed definition, but the condition would typically present with a blood glucose in excess of 50 mmol/l and a plasma osmolality greater than 350 mosm/l. Non-ketotic coma and ketoacidosis represent two ends of a spectrum rather than two distinct entities. The non-ketotic state arises because sufficient endogenous insulin is secreted to inhibit peripheral lipolysis and hepatic ketogenesis. Ketogenesis is more sensitive to control by insulin than is hepatic glucose production. As a result hepatic glucose production is unrestrained, while ketone production is suppressed. Since residual insulin secretion is a factor in the pathogenesis of this condition, it can (and typically does) affect patients with NIDDM, and is not necessarily an indication for life-long insulin therapy. Patients present in middle or later life, often with previously undiagnosed or 'mild' diabetes. Common precipitating factors include consumption of glucose-rich fluids (e.g. Lucozade), concurrent medication such as thiazide diuretics or steroids, and intercurrent illness.

Clinical features

Patients present with profound dehydration and a decreased level of consciousness which is directly related to the elevation of plasma osmolality. The condition may be precipitated by intercurrent infection or, in older age groups, by vascular disease. The hyperviscosity consequent upon dehydration frequently leads to vascular occlusion in the cerebrovascular, coronary, gastrointestinal or peripheral arterial circulations.

Management

The principles of management do not differ from those for ketoacidosis, and successful outcome depends even more upon skillful rehydration, especially since many patients are elderly. Treatment with half-normal saline (0.45%) may be necessary if increasing hypernatraemia is noted during therapy. Despite these measures, fatalities are common and are usually related to vascular complications in the high-risk elderly patient.

Lactic acidosis

Lactic acidosis is a well-described complication of biguanide therapy, but is now rarely seen, since the withdrawal of phenformin. Occasional instances of lactic acidosis in patients taking metformin have been described, but have been associated with co-existent hepatic or renal disease.

The acidosis in these patients is severe and compounded by decreased hepatic lactate utilisation as a direct consequence of the fall in intracellular pH.

Treatment consists of sodium bicarbonate administration in large quantities, and it may be necessary to dialyse the patient to avoid sodium overload if cardiac or renal function are compromised.

COMPLICATIONS OF DIABETES

Diabetes is a major health problem in Western countries because it is common, and because it predisposes to many forms of tissue damage, collectively known as diabetic complications. The health impact of these complications is shown in Summary 4.

Disease of large vessels

Diabetes predisposes to atherosclerosis. The risk in differ-

Summary 4   Major clinical consequences arising from late complications of diabetes

Large vessel disease

Ischaemic heart disease is twice as common in men and three times as common in women.

– *Hypertension* is twice as common.

– *Stroke* is 2–6 times as common.

Peripheral vascular disease is much more common; diabetes accounts for about 45% of all non-traumatic amputations. Survival is worse following myocardial infarction, stroke or lower limb amputation.

Eye damage

The most common cause of *blind registration* in people of working age. Untreated diabetic proliferative retinopathy leads to blindness in 50% of eyes affected within 5 years.

Senile cataracts develop more rapidly.

Nephropathy

One in three patients diagnosed before the age of 30 develops diabetic nephropathy.

Persistent proteinuria, the hallmark of established nephropathy, progresses to end-stage renal failure within an average of 7–8 years.

Diabetes accounts for one in four of all cases of *end-stage renal disease* in the USA.

Nerve damage

One in three clinic attenders has clinical or subclinical nerve damage.

About 15% experience foot ulceration.

Impotence affects 50% of men over the age of 50.

Other problems

Neonatal death is twice as common in pregnancy in a diabetic woman.

5% of infants of diabetic mothers have congenital malformations, one in three of which is fatal.

Some infections are more likely, especially when the diabetes is poorly controlled.

---

ent countries follows that of the non-diabetic population. Coronary heart disease was the reported cause of death in 55% of diabetic patients in one large American series, roughly double the rate in the background population. The corresponding figures from a Japanese study were 10.7% for patients with diabetes and 5.4% for non-diabetics. The increased risk is greater in women than in men, cancelling out the relative protection that women enjoy against cardiovascular disease. The pathological findings do not differ, although atherosclerosis tends to be more severe and diffuse; this may be the reason that diabetic patients are less likely to survive a myocardial infarct. Since diabetic patients often have hyperlipidaemia, hypertension and obesity and may well be smokers, hyperglycaemia itself is often only one among several cardiovascular risk factors, although it has been shown to make a strong independent contribution. Since these risk factors are additive, treatment should aim to minimise them all, rather than focusing exclusively upon blood glucose levels.

Microvascular disease

Microvascular disease is a specific diabetic abnormality. The earliest structural abnormality is increased thickness of the basement membrane, and the corresponding pathophysiological change is increased permeability to fluid and molecules such as albumin. The small blood vessels – terminal arterioles, capillaries and venules – are affected throughout the body, but harmful consequences are largely confined to three specialised regions within the microcirculation: the retina, renal glomerulus and nerve sheath. Diabetic retinopathy, neuropathy and nephropathy usually appear before 10–20 years after diagnosis in the young (although never before the onset of puberty), but present earlier in older patients, possibly because unrecognised diabetes has been present for months or years prior to diagnosis.

Theories of pathogenesis

Although many metabolic pathways are disturbed in diabetes, resulting in altered levels of numerous metabolites and other substances in the blood and body tissues, glucose itself is the most likely initial mediator of tissue damage. This might occur by glycosylation of structural proteins, leading to breakdown of cross-linking cystine residues in the basement membrane, and increased permeability and infiltration by other substances.

An alternative hypothesis concerns the polyol pathway by which hexose sugars are reduced to their corresponding sugar alcohols; the rate-limiting enzyme is aldose reductase. This is present in high levels in the kidney, the retina and in nerves, but has a low affinity for glucose so that intracellular accumulation of sorbitol (the corresponding alcohol) only occurs when glucose levels are high, exceeding the capacity of the glycolytic pathway. Raised sorbitol levels cause osmotic changes within the cell, although the mechanism of cell damage is still somewhat conjectural. Inhibitors of aldose reductase are currently undergoing clinical trials in diabetic patients.

Another hypothesis is that vessel damage is secondary to altered haemodynamics. This includes increased plasma viscosity, altered levels of fibrinogen and clotting factors, increased platelet stickiness and reduced red cell deformability. The altered shear characteristics and haemostatic properties that result might be expected to distort and ultimately damage the endothelial lining of capillaries. The question remains unresolved at present; there is certainly a correlation between altered haemostasis and vascular disease, but it is unclear which, if either, comes first.

Relationship to diabetic control

Assessment of this relationship is unfortunately difficult because of the long gestation of complications (10–20 years), the difficulty of quantifying control over long periods (especially before the introduction of HbA_{1c}) and the difficulty of assessing the extent of diabetic tissue damage accurately in large groups of patients. Since really good control is uncommon, the comparison has usually been between varying levels of suboptimal control. Finally, some patients are more easy to control than others because, for example, of the persistence of endogenous insulin secretion. In view of these confounding variables, it is not surprising that retrospective or cross-sectional studies have often been hard to interpret, although most have suggested that those with the worst glycaemic control have the highest risk of developing complications.

Prospective randomised studies are therefore needed. These are easy to perform in animals, and provide unequivocal evidence of the benefits of good control. Studies of *primary prevention* (i.e. from the time of diagnosis in uncomplicated patients) are now under way in man, but face the considerable technical problems of following large numbers over many years and maintaining really good control over this period. An alternative is *secondary prevention*, i.e. attempting to halt or reverse established complications by imposing near-normoglycaemic control with insulin pumps. These studies have shown that there is an apparent 'point of no return', so that patients with proliferative retinopathy or persistent proteinuria do

not benefit. In contrast, good control is beneficial in those with background retinopathy (although there may be an early transient deterioration) or with microalbuminuria, although the benefit is not as rapid or as great as many had hoped.

One major limitation of research in this area is that it has concentrated upon the benefits of improved control upon microvascular disease in younger patients, whereas most diabetic patients are elderly and at greatest risk from arterial disease. There is, at present, little evidence that large vessel disease will benefit from improved glycaemic control, and it has even been suggested that high insulin levels in the systemic circulation (as found in insulin-treated patients and many patients with NIDDM and insulin resistance) may be a factor in the development of atheroma.

Diabetic retinopathy and other eye complications

The retinal circulation is extremely vulnerable to the microangiopathy caused by diabetes. The earliest change is an increase in thickness of the basement membrane, which is associated with increased capillary permeability. This change may be shown by fluorescein angiography (Fig. 20.15) in which a fluorescent dye is injected intravenously and can be shown passing through the retinal vessels and the changes recorded photographically. The increased permeability is demonstrated by leakage of the dye outside the vessels. With time, the vessel structure becomes disorganised and aneurysmal dilatation and occlusion occur. On ophthalmoscopy, the earliest abnormality is 'dot' haemorrhages which are microaneurysms of the capillaries, while 'blot' haemorrhages are due to

Fig. 20.15 Retinal angiogram of a Type I diabetic patient showing numerous microaneurysms and extensive capillary closure. (Photograph courtesy of Mr R Whitelocke)

Summary 5   Diabetic microangiopathy

Diabetes induces both structural (increased basement membrane thickness) and functional (increased permeability) changes in small blood vessels

Three specialised regions of the microcirculation are particularly at risk

- The retina – almost all patients with IDDM develop background retinopathy within 10–12 years; 30–50% progress to proliferative retinopathy and require laser therapy
- The renal glomerulus – increased permeability may lead to microalbuminuria; 30–40% develop frank proteinuria indicative of progressive nephropathy
- The nerve sheath – both microvascular and metabolic derangement contribute to diabetic neuropathy

bleeding into the deeper layers of the retina. Leakage of fluid from the capillaries leads to deposition of lipids and protein, causing so-called 'hard' exudates which are yellow-white and have a well-defined margin.

After 20 years of diabetes, the eyes of almost all diabetics show abnormalities on fluorescein angiography, but these changes are uncommon in young patients who have had diabetes for less than 10 years. Dot haemorrhages can usually be found on thorough ophthalmoscopy in patients after this period (Fig. 20.16). In older patients, retinopathy may sometimes be found at diagnosis or a short time after.

'Background' retinopathy such as that described above does not disturb vision, but, as time goes by, more serious retinopathic changes develop.

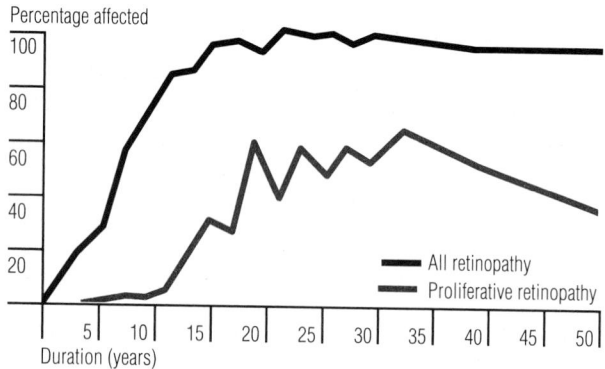

Fig. 20.16 Prevalence of retinopathy related to duration of disease in insulin-dependent diabetes. Almost all patients with IDDM develop evidence of background retinopathy within 10–15 years of onset, but only about half ever progress to proliferative retinopathy.

Proliferative retinopathy

The first indication of proliferative retinopathy is the appearance of what are called 'cotton-wool' spots – patches of retinal oedema which appear to develop on the basis of retinal ischaemia. They may also be seen in severe hypertensive retinopathy. Due to their indistinct margins and grey-white colour, they are sometimes called 'soft' exudates. The veins of the retina begin to form loops and have an irregular diameter; this is known as *venous beading*.

New vessels develop in the retina, probably in response to hypoxia. They lie on the retinal surface or extend to the vitreous and are unsupported and bleed easily. This leads to fibrosis and scarring. The haemorrhages may lie in front of the retina – recognised by a clear horizontal upper margin – and in the vitreous itself. A bleed into the vitreous causes complete or partial loss of vision in the affected eye. The patient may then describe a shadow affecting the field of vision. On examination, there is a grey, ill-defined opacity seen with the ophthalmoscope. The blood is slowly reabsorbed and vision then recovers partially, although further episodes are likely. The scarring and contracture of the retina also leads to loss of vision and retinal detachment may occur as the scars contract.

Maculopathy

Hard exudates are clustered around the macula, usually centrally and laterally in a circular formation. They cause loss of visual acuity by damaging the central retina and by associated oedema and ischaemia of the macula. The impaired acuity can usually be detected clinically and the exudates are often visible on ophthalmoscopy. Maculopathy may lead to blindness in the absence of new vessel formation, especially in older patients.

Cataracts

In diabetic patients, senile cataracts develop 10–15 years earlier than in the remainder of the population. Juvenile or 'snowflake' cataracts are rapidly progressive cataracts which are associated with very poorly controlled diabetes. They are much less common than senile cataracts.

Other eye complications

Transient deterioration of vision is a common feature of poorly controlled hyperglycaemia, and may persist for several weeks after a newly-diagnosed patient is stabilised. Acute changes in accommodation, presenting as intermittent blurring of vision, are features of swinging blood glucose levels. Transient diplopia is a common symptom of hypoglycaemia. Ocular palsies may occur, particularly in the older patient, and usually resolve spontaneously. The most common is a VIth nerve palsy, but palsies of IIIrd nerve also occur. A characteristic feature of these is that pupillary reflexes are preserved, owing to sparing of pupillomotor fibres. Rubeosis iridis may develop as a late change, and is due to neovascularisation of the pupil. Vessels appear in the pupil and can easily be seen. Secondary glaucoma may develop.

Management of the diabetic eye

There is no medical treatment which is specific for background retinopathy. Other risk factors for vascular disease are treated, i.e. patients are advised not to smoke and hypertension is controlled. Rapid progression of retinopathy may occur during pregnancy and in patients with nephropathy; these patients need careful monitoring. Patients with retinopathy should be examined regularly in the clinic, preferably in partnership with an ophthalmologist. An ophthalmologist's opinion is essential when unexplained visual deterioration occurs, or pre-proliferative or proliferative changes are present. Fluorescein angiography may be needed to demonstrate the extent of the retinopathy.

Maculopathy and proliferative retinopathy can be treated by photocoagulation of the retina with lasers. Effective early therapy of proliferative retinopathy reduces the risk of visual loss by about 50%.

Diabetic nephropathy

The kidney can be damaged by diabetes as a result of

glomerular disease, ischaemic renal lesions and infection of the urinary tract.

Diabetic glomerulosclerosis

Nephropathy secondary to glomerular disease affects 30–40% of patients who are diagnosed before the age of 30 (Fig. 20.17). It usually becomes clinically apparent 15–25 years from diagnosis and is the main cause of early death in young diabetics. Although older patients may develop nephropathy, the proportion is smaller.

Renal hypertrophy is an early functional abnormality associated with the raised glomerular filtration rate. It appears soon after diagnosis, and is related to poor glycaemic control. There is no structural change.

Thickening of the basement membrane of the glomerulus is the earliest structural lesion. There is disruption of the membrane proteins leading to a progressive leak of protein into the glomerular filtrate. This is shown by *microalbuminuria*, a term used to describe excretion of very small amounts of albumin which are only detectable by special techniques. With progression of membrane damage, frank proteinuria develops. Changes of diffuse and nodular glomerulosclerosis are seen histologically. Nodular change is the Kimmelstiel-Wilson lesion. Finally, the entire glomerulus is destroyed by hyaline material.

Microalbuminuria leads, at first, to intermittent proteinuria (detected on dipsticks) and then to persistent and increasingly heavy proteinuria. At first, the plasma creatinine is normal, but deterioration proceeds rapidly and terminal renal failure occurs on average in 8–10 years. The proteinuria may be sufficiently heavy as to induce nephrotic syndrome – albuminuria, peripheral oedema, hyperalbuminaemia and hypercholesterolaemia (p. 811). Patients in renal failure have a normochromic normocytic anaemia.

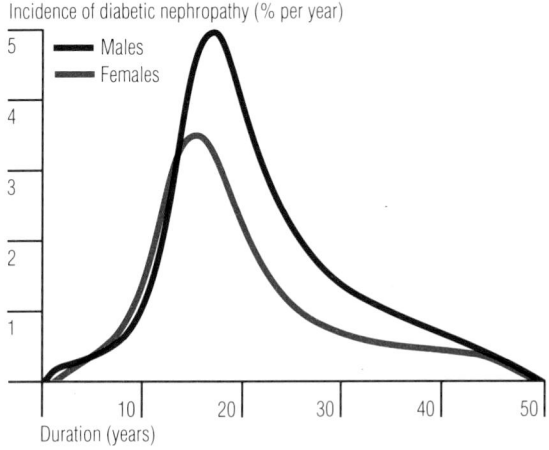

Incidence of diabetic nephropathy (% per year)

Fig. 20.17 Incidence of nephropathy in insulin-dependent diabetes. Some 30–40% of patients with IDDM develop diabetic nephropathy. This figure shows the onset of proteinuria, the first overt evidence of diabetic nephropathy, in relation to duration of diabetes. Peak incidence is from 15 to 20 years; those who survive 25 years or more without developing proteinuria are unlikely ever to do so.

Hypertension is common and may cause further kidney damage. The creatinine clearance falls, leading to a progressive rise in plasma creatinine and, eventually, end-stage renal failure.

Ischaemic renal lesions

Changes occur similar to those found in hypertension, but are not always related to the level of blood pressure. These changes are hypertrophy and hyalinisation of afferent and efferent arterioles.

Urinary tract infection

Infection may ascend from the bladder as a result of autonomic neuropathy, causing bladder and ureteric stasis. Damaged renal tissue is more easily infected. Interstitial changes which might be caused by pyelonephritis are often found at autopsy in diabetics. However, similar changes can be caused by ischaemia, and the frequency of pyelonephritic infection in diabetes is unclear. Pyelonephritis in diabetics can lead to renal papillary necrosis if not treated promptly. Although uncommon, this is a serious complication in which renal papillae are detached into the renal calyces.

Diagnosis and investigation

The earliest finding is proteinuria, which is also a sign of established disease. Although poor glycaemic control undoubtedly increases the risk of developing nephropathy, once established the disease, unfortunately, does not respond to improved diabetic control. Any hope of altering the progression of the disease depends on early diagnosis, since there are some indications that the early changes may respond to improved control. Screening for microalbuminuria is now commonly carried out in diabetic clinics.

If proteinuria is found, it usually indicates diabetic nephropathy, although not always. If the history is unusual (e.g. a history of pain or haematuria), or if there is no retinopathy (usually associated with diabetic nephropathy), other causes of renal disease should be considered. Under these circumstances, intravenous urography is useful to exclude structural lesions but is not without risk in diabetic patients, especially if the patients are dehydrated beforehand. Renal ultrasound is, therefore, widely used as an alternative. Rarely, renal biopsy may be necessary to exclude other forms of glomerular disease.

Other investigations include a 24-hour urine collection to measure protein loss and creatinine clearance; these serve as a baseline to judge future progress. The urine is always cultured, and the presence of white cells in the sterile urine should raise a suspicion of renal tuberculosis.

Management

Diabetic nephropathy is managed like other causes of renal failure (Ch. 21). However, there are a number of features specific to diabetic renal disease:

1. Sensitivity to insulin increases, and considerable reductions in dosage may be needed. Those oral hypoglycaemic agents which are excreted by the kidney (such as chlorpropamide) should be avoided.
2. Diabetic retinopathy may progress quickly; therefore, ophthalmic supervision should be more frequent.
3. Careful control of hypertension will decrease the rate of decline of renal function. The management of advanced renal failure is made more difficult due to the other complications of diabetes, such as vascular disease, neuropathy and blindness. Vascular shunts for dialysis tend to calcify rapidly, and chronic ambulatory peritoneal dialysis is thus often preferred. The failure rate of renal transplants in diabetics is higher than in non-diabetic renal failure. In some centres, a segmental pancreatic graft is performed at the time of renal transplantation. These have a lifespan of a year or more before they are destroyed by fibrosis, but may allow insulin to be stopped during this time.

Diabetic neuropathy

A variety of forms of diabetic neuropathy occur and the pathological processes causing the damage are not completely understood. Diffuse symmetrical neuropathy, which is the commonest form, is probably due to a metabolic cause. Schwann cell function may be disturbed by accumulation of fructose and sorbitol which are formed as a result of hyperglycaemia. Delayed nerve conduction velocity is an early functional change. Histologically, segmental demyelination occurs early as a result of damage to Schwann cells. At first, axons are intact and recovery can occur, but axonal degeneration later develops which cannot be reversed. Mononeuropathies are thought to be due to occlusion of the vasa nervorum.

The several distinct clinical syndromes are discussed below (see also p. 940).

Sensory polyneuropathy

Sensory polyneuropathy is a diffuse and symmetrical disorder of which the patient may at first be unaware. On examination, the early signs are loss of vibration, pain and temperature sensation in the feet. Deep pain is lost before pinprick sensation. Patients may later lose proprioception and touch, frequently falling when they are standing with their eyes shut or in the dark. Symmetrical loss of sensation may also occur in the hands. One of the commonest complications is tissue damage, especially in the feet, as a result of unnoticed injury (either mechanical or thermal). Pressure from shoes or a burn may lead to a blister which later becomes an ulcer. Occasionally diffuse and painful neuropathy occurs in which burning or crawling pains are experienced, typically in the feet, shins and front of the thighs. Usually the symptoms are worse at night; sleep is disturbed and even the bedclothes may produce severe pain. This syndrome occasionally occurs at the onset of diabetes, and then usually responds to meticulous control

of blood sugar. However, a chronic form may develop later in the disease and is sometimes unaffected by all forms of treatment, including strict diabetic control. On examination severe hyperaesthesia is present, but objective sensory loss may be subtle. Muscle wasting does not occur.

Diabetic amyotrophy

Diabetic amyotrophy is thought to be due to damage to motor roots (radiculopathy). It usually occurs in older patients and presents with an often painful and symmetrical wasting of the quadriceps muscles. There is marked proximal muscle wasting of the thighs, loss of knee jerks, and tenderness of the affected area, and, occasionally, the plantar responses become extensor. The protein content of the CSF is elevated. Onset of amyotrophy is often associated with poor diabetic control, and can be a presenting feature of diabetes. Importantly, it may improve with good control over time.

Peripheral and cranial nerve lesions

Individual peripheral nerves may be damaged, causing, sensory, motor or mixed symptoms and signs (mononeuritis multiplex). Multiple isolated lesions may occur, and the onset is usually abrupt. The most commonly involved nerves are those which are more likely to suffer pressure, such as the ulnar nerve at the elbow or the median nerve in the carpal tunnel. Recovery is usually slow and incomplete. The commonest cranial nerves to be affected are the IIIrd and VIth nerves causing external ocular pauses which usually resolve over time.

Autonomic neuropathy

Neuropathy of the sympathetic and parasympathetic systems is common and usually occurs in patients with evidence of neuropathy elsewhere. Although the autonomic neuropathy does not cause symptoms at first, its presence can be demonstrated by investigation. Later, severe symptoms occur.

Cardiovascular neuropathy

Vagal neuropathy leads to resting tachycardia. Early on it can be demonstrated by the loss of sinus arrhythmia. Later, the heart may become denervated. Reflex slowing of the heart during the Valsalva manoeuvre is impaired. Peripheral vasodilatation may lead to warm feet and a bounding pulse. Postural hypotension may be severe and is due to loss of sympathetic innervation of the peripheral arterioles.

Impotence

The first symptom of this common and distressing complication is incomplete erection and loss of ejaculation which may be retrograde into the bladder. In time, this may become total impotence. Impotence is not invariably due to autonomic neuropathy. Other contributory causes are anxiety, alcoholic excess, depression, medication (such as thiazides), gonadal failure (p. 715) and atheroma of the iliac vessels. Treatment is difficult and often unsuccessful. Sympathetic advice to both partners is essential and urological or psychiatric advice may be necessary.

Gastrointestinal neuropathy

Vagal damage may cause loss of gastric motility. This may not cause symptoms, but can lead to severe vomiting (for which metoclopramide may be helpful). Diarrhoea occurs typically at night and may be associated with urgency and even incontinence. The diarrhoea may be accompanied by steatorrhoea which is due to bacterial overgrowth (p. 587), and antibiotics may help by eliminating the bacterial flora.

Vesical neuropathy

There is loss of bladder tone, with incomplete emptying. Stasis in the bladder may lead to urinary infection. An atonic distended and painless bladder may result.

The diabetic foot

The management of established diabetes is directed towards prevention of tissue damage and the disability this may cause. Nowhere is this more true than in care of the feet. Simple preventive measures such as regular inspection, together with advice about shoes and foot care, would undoubtedly prevent many admissions to hospital. Apart from the lasting disability that results from an amputation or chronic ulceration, diabetic foot disease also puts a great strain upon hospital resources. It has been estimated that, in the UK, the average hospital stay for a person with a diabetic foot problem is three months, at a cost of some £14 000.

There are four major factors predisposing to foot problems in a patient with diabetes: peripheral vascular disease, neuropathy, infection and mechanical stress.

Peripheral vascular disease

Diabetes predisposes to atheroma. In the leg, diabetes is particularly associated with diffuse involvement of the distal vessels (i.e. below the popliteal fossa), although the iliac and femoral arteries are also more commonly affected than in non-diabetics. The other major factor in peripheral vascular disease is smoking cigarettes, providing yet another reason why people with diabetes should be encouraged not to smoke.

Clinical features

The clinical presentation is with claudication, rest pain, gangrene or ischaemic ulcers. On examination, the foot is cold with dependent rubor; the skin is thin with scaling or fissures and the nails may be dystrophic. If rubor is present, the skin will blanch on elevation, whereas redness due to inflammation will persist. The foot pulses are weak or

impalpable, and Doppler studies should be performed.

Doppler studies allow measurement of the ankle-brachial index – the ratio between supine systolic blood pressure in the posterior tibial and brachial arteries. Values below 0.9 are abnormal. Occlusion of digital vessels may result in gangrene of the toe which is typically dry and demarcates cleanly. In contrast, occlusion of more proximal vessels will, if untreated, result in progressive 'wet' gangrene requiring urgent amputation. Ischaemic ulcers are typically painful, with an irregular margin and slough formation, quite unlike the painless punched-out ulcers of neuropathy. The heel is a favoured site of ischaemic ulceration, and this may develop as a complication of bed rest if meticulous nursing care is not provided. The differences between an ischaemic and a neuropathic foot are outlined in Table 20.5.

Table 20.5 Differences between the neuropathic and ischaemic foot

	Neuropathic	Ischaemic
Symptoms	Usually painless	Rest pain Claudication
Signs	Warm, bounding pulses High arch and clawing of toes	Cold, pulseless Trophic changes Dependent rubor
Ulceration site	Plantar	Heels and toes

Management

Surgical assessment is always indicated. Arteriography may indicate a localised occlusion amenable to bypass surgery or angioplasty. Since diabetic patients tend to have diffuse disease, management often needs to be conservative with regular debridement of ulcers and antibiotic therapy at the earliest sign of infection. If amputation becomes necessary, it is usually best to opt for a major procedure immediately, rather than subject the patient to a series of debilitating minor procedures. The prognosis of diabetic patients requiring amputation for peripheral vascular disease is extremely poor. Bilateral amputations quite commonly become necessary, and 50% of patients undergoing an amputation die within 3 years.

Neuropathy

Some 30% of patients attending a diabetic clinic will have evidence, usually subclinical, of peripheral neuropathy. This predisposes to foot disease in a number of ways.

Clinical features

Sensory loss may lead to blistering and ulceration from ill-fitting shoes, or thermal injury (most often from a hot-water bottle). Denervation of a joint may lead to a Charcot arthropathy. Motor involvement leads to clawing of the foot due to denervation of the intrinsic muscles and unopposed action of the long extensor tendons. This, in turn, results in increased pressure under the ball of the foot and callus formation. The callus in turn acts as a foreign body, and the combination of anaesthesia with the pressure and shear involved in walking leads easily to ischaemia, necrosis and ulceration of the underlying tissue. For these reasons, neuropathic ulcers are typically painless, plantar and perforating.

Neuropathy also leads to vascular changes. Medial calcification of the small arteries in the foot is a distinctive feature, possibly related to sympathetic denervation. Flow is also affected, and the foot may be warm with bounding pulses due to arteriovenous shunting. The foot veins are often swollen, and the venous oxygen saturation is increased. Autonomic neuropathy may contribute to these changes, and impaired sweating leads to dry skin which fissures readily, providing entry for infection.

Diagnosis

On examination, the foot is usually warm and dry and appears well-nourished (Table 20.5). Clawing may be present, and callus formation should be sought. The foot pulses are usually easily palpable, and veins on the dorsum of the foot may be engorged. Perception of temperature, vibration and pain are impaired with the classic stocking distribution, while the ankle jerk is lost.

Infection

The foot is prone to infection in diabetes due to the combination of ischaemia, mechanical tissue damage and impaired resistance to infection. Once established, infection leads to swelling, local ischaemia and tissue necrosis – and may spread with startling rapidity.

Management

Acute spreading infection is a medical emergency, requiring hospital admission and intravenous antibiotic therapy. Infection by mixtures of organisms is common, and selective antibiotic therapy then simply favours the resistant strains. A further problem is that anaerobes colonise necrotic debris within the lesion. For these reasons, prolonged, broad-spectrum cover in high doses is necessary, and surgical drainage with excision of necrotic material should be undertaken wherever possible. Regular X-rays of the foot are needed as a guide to underlying bony involvement.

Mechanical stress

Mechanical stress to the foot may be exogenous (e.g. due to injury or unsuitable shoes) or endogenous, i.e. due to abnormal distribution of stress within the foot. The claw foot of neuropathy is one example of this, and the situation may also arise following surgery to the foot, or infection with resulting deformity. Assessment and anticipation of these problems in conjunction with a chiropodist, and the provision of surgical footwear when needed, are all part of good diabetes care.

Infection in diabetics

In the pre-insulin era, infection was a leading cause of death in diabetic patients, and tuberculosis was a frequent complication. These problems are still a major concern for diabetic patients in developing countries, but there is little or no evidence that well-controlled patients in more affluent parts of the world are at excess risk. Poorly controlled diabetes has been shown to impair the function of polymorphonuclear leucocytes, with reduced chemotaxis, phagocytosis and bactericidal activity.

Uncontrolled diabetes predisposes to infection, and infection leads to deteriorating control of diabetes. This is of particular significance in the pathogenesis of ketoacidosis, and insulin-treated patients must be warned of the need to continue or increase their insulin therapy in the face of infection, even if they feel nauseated and unable to eat. Non-insulin treated patients may need insulin cover for the same reasons. Diabetic complications may also predispose to infections in specific sites, e.g. ascending urinary tract infections (due to neuropathy and loss of bladder tone) and infections in the feet.

Infections common to diabetics

A number of rare opportunist infections occur almost exclusively in diabetic patients. These apart, the poorly controlled patient has an increased risk of genital candidiasis and staphylococcal skin infections, of staphylococcal and pneumococcal pneumonias, and of pyelonephritis and perinephric abscess (one-third of these occur in patients with diabetes). Urinary infections may rarely be complicated by papillary necrosis. Hidden pus warrants careful consideration in any patient who shows unexplained loss of control and failure to thrive.

Growth

Short stature was in the past a common complication of poorly controlled diabetes in childhood, but is now rare and seen only with fairly gross neglect. One common physical sign of childhood diabetes is minor non-progressive joint contracture in the hands. This is thought to be due to glycosylation of collagen around the joints and can be demonstrated by failure of the hand to flatten completely when pressed against a table, or when the hands are joined as if in prayer.

OTHER PROBLEMS IN DIABETIC MANAGEMENT

Surgery

Good management of a diabetic patient during surgery depends on a good liaison between physician, surgeon and anaesthetist. The aims should be:

1. to ensure the patient is fit for surgery
2. to achieve control of blood glucose before, during and after surgery.

Assessment

Assessment should include that of control, including the need for insulin in patients on other forms of therapy, and of complications. Ischaemic heart disease may complicate management, and proliferative retinopathy might, for example, predispose to a vitreous haemorrhage if intraocular pressure changes under anaesthesia. The feet should be checked with care since ischaemia or neuropathy may lead to ulceration during the period of enforced bed rest. If there is clear evidence of neuropathy in the feet, there is a high probability that autonomic neuropathy is also present, carrying an increased risk of cardiorespiratory arrest following induction of anaesthesia.

Control

Blood glucose is easy to control, provided frequent accurate measurement is available and the patient is closely supervised by someone with experience. The aim is to achieve stable control pre-operatively, to avoid the extremes of hypoglycaemia and hyperglycaemia during surgery, and to promote wound healing and minimise infection during the postoperative period by careful control of blood glucose levels.

Preoperatively the patient is admitted for 1–3 days, depending on the scale of the procedure; multiple injection regimens may be needed, with intermediate insulin given overnight to control fasting hyperglycaemia. The patient should, if possible, go first on the morning list. On the morning of surgery, subcutaneous insulin is omitted and the patient is started on intravenous dextrose and insulin. Insulin can be given via an intravenous pump, but, to avoid mishap, it is usually best to add the insulin directly to the dextrose solution. One standard regimen is 500 ml of dextrose 10% with 15 units of soluble human insulin and 10 mmol of KCl added, infused at a rate of 100 ml/hour. Blood glucose is measured before and after surgery, and at hourly intervals during lengthy procedures. Insulin-dependent patients requiring minor procedures can sometimes be managed more simply by measuring the blood glucose prior to surgery and omitting food and insulin on the morning of surgery. Non-insulin-dependent diabetics requiring minor procedures can also be managed by omit-

---

Summary 6   Diabetes and surgery

- No special treatment is necessary for patients with NIDDM undergoing minor surgery
- Patients on oral agents should have insulin cover for major surgery
- Long-acting insulins or sulphonylureas should be withdrawn at least 24 hours before elective surgery
- Combined glucose-insulin infusion is safe and effective during and after surgery in patients with IDDM, and patients with NIDDM having major procedures
- Regular blood glucose monitoring is essential
- Sliding scale administration of insulin is often unnecessary in the post-operative period

---

ting treatment. However, for major surgery, patients may require insulin cover as suggested above.

Post-operatively the infusion of dextrose, insulin and potassium can be continued until the patient has taken and retained his first meal. Thereafter, a regular multiple injection regimen can be started; a sliding scale approach should be avoided.

Pregnancy

There are two main categories of patient: those with established diabetes who become pregnant and those who develop diabetes in the course of pregnancy (gestational diabetes).

Pregnancy in the diabetic patient

Before insulin was introduced, diabetes was considered incompatible with successful pregnancy, and even in the 1950s, the perinatal mortality rate was around 30%. The rate has now fallen to around 5%, as against 1% in the general population. Despite this progress, congenital abnormalities (mostly affecting the heart and central nervous system) are 3–4 times more common in infants of diabetic mothers.

The outcome of a diabetic pregnancy is directly related to the degree of glycaemic control, and improved control is responsible for the improvement in perinatal mortality mentioned above. As a result, the traditional practice of admitting patients to hospital at 32 weeks for elective caesarian section at 36 weeks (chosen because it represented the optimum compromise between the risk of hyaline membrane disease and the risk of late intrauterine death) can now be abandoned. Instead, the patient has a reasonable expectation of a spontaneous vaginal delivery at term. However, this can only be achieved as the result of teamwork and planning on the part of the hospital, and of a disciplined effort on the part of the patient.

Glycaemic control

Glycaemic control should ideally be tightened prior to conception, since there is evidence that this reduces the rate of congenital malformation. The patient is then seen every 1–2 weeks throughout pregnancy by obstetrician and physician – preferably in a joint clinic. A multiple injection regimen and daily blood glucose monitoring at home are usually necessary; urine testing is completely unreliable since the renal threshold falls in pregnancy and insulin requirements often rise markedly as the pregnancy progresses, so that frequent adjustment is called for. Blood glucose levels of 5–7 mmol/l are aimed for and often achieved, although sometimes at the cost of hypoglycaemia in the mother. Fortunately, this is well tolerated by the fetus.

Complications

The obstetric problems which are associated with poor control of diabetes include pre-eclampsia, hydramnios and intrauterine death and macrosomia. Neonatal problems include delivery of an overweight, sluggish and plethoric child (happily a rare sight in modern units), and neonatal hypoglycaemia. This occurs because glucose can cross the placenta but not insulin. The consequence is hypersecretion of fetal insulin, leading to hypoglycaemia when maternal glucose is no longer available.

Gestational diabetes

This is a form of temporary diabetes, typically asymptomatic, which develops in the course of pregnancy. It is associated with obstetric problems, fetal macrosomia and an increased perinatal mortality rate. The glucose tolerance test normalises following delivery, but diabetes recurs with subsequent pregnancies and there is a high incidence of NIDDM later in life.

Diagnosis

There are no established criteria for the diagnosis of gestational diabetes, but most would agree that pregnant patients with impaired glucose tolerance on the WHO definition should be regarded as having gestational diabetes. Screening cannot usefully be based on urine tests, since the renal threshold falls during pregnancy, and the traditional obstetric criteria for ordering a glucose tolerance test are of little value. Many centres now screen blood glucose at intervals during pregnancy, and arrange for a glucose tolerance test if the random glucose value is above 6.4 mmol/l.

Treatment

Treatment is either with diet alone or diet with insulin, since oral agents are contraindicated in pregnancy. It is important to arrange for a further glucose tolerance test a few months following delivery since diabetes persists in a minority of patients.

Brittle diabetes

There is no precise definition for the term 'brittle diabetes', and indeed one physician has called it 'a term used by a doctor to describe a diabetic patient whom he or she finds impossible to control'! Since the expression is often used in a dismissive or pejorative sense and has no precise meaning it is better to talk of recurrent ketoacidosis and/or hypoglycaemia.

Recurrent ketoacidosis

Recurrent ketoacidosis is most common in adolescent patients and may be due to inadequate or inappropriate insulin regimens which cause unpredictable swings from hypo- to hyperglycaemia. In some instances, unstable control appears to result from excessive insulin action followed by rebound hyperglycaemia (the *Somogyi effect*), and this phenomenon has been attributed to the effects of counter-regulatory hormones on hepatic glucose release.

However, confirmation of this mechanism has not been achieved, and many doubt its existence.

Modern flexible insulin regimens have eliminated many of the problems of variable insulin deficiency associated with single injections of long-acting insulin. Despite this, some patients have persistently unstable diabetes, whether as a consequence of manipulation, psychological problems or some as yet unidentified neuroendocrine phenomenon. The problem is most frequently described in young female patients who may be overweight and, characteristically, have high insulin requirements. Menstrual disturbance is common but may be attributable to weight change and poor diabetic control rather than a primary disorder of hypothalamic-pituitary function. Careful attention to psychological factors as well as the diabetic condition is critical in these patients.

Recurrent hypoglycaemia

Long-standing insulin-dependent diabetes is associated with decreased glucagon secretion. Furthermore, autonomic neuropathy and decreased sympathoadrenal activation may limit catecholamine responsiveness to hypoglycaemia. These factors predispose the patient to unpredictable fluctuations in glycaemia. The problem may obviously be aggravated by variations in carbohydrate intake, whether consciously or resulting from variable gastric emptying associated with gastroparesis due to autonomic neuropathy (p. 940). Hypothyroidism, which frequently accompanies insulin-dependent diabetes, is an additional important predisposing cause of recurrent hypoglycaemia, and other endocrine disorders such as adrenal or pituitary failure should also be considered. Renal impairment, whether due to diabetic nephropathy or other causes, may present with episodes of hypoglycaemia due to decreased renal insulin clearance.

HYPOGLYCAEMIA

Blood glucose is normally maintained within strict limits despite feeding, fasting and exercise. This precise yet flexible control is made possible by the capacity of the liver to store carbohydrate as glycogen, and to release regulated quantities of glucose into the systemic circulation when food is not available. This function is under the direct control of insulin, although modulated in important respects by other hormones including glucagon, adrenaline and cortisol.

At constant blood glucose levels, such as those maintained during an overnight fast, glucose output by the liver equals uptake by peripheral tissues. The output is some 2 mg/min per kg bodyweight (or 200 g per 24 h in a 70 kg man), and much of this goes to the brain, which takes up around 100–120 g of glucose and oxidises it to carbon dioxide and water. This high energy requirement is needed to generate ATP which is used to maintain the potential difference across axonal membranes. Glucose entry and disposal in the brain is influenced by insulin, but not dependent upon it. In contrast, muscle and fat are facultative glucose users, capable of absorbing and storing large quantities in the postprandial state under the influence of insulin, but readily able to use other fuels such as circulating fatty acids. Under normal conditions, the brain derives 95% of its energy requirements from glucose, but during prolonged fasts can adapt to obtain most of its energy from circulating ketones.

Therefore, hypoglycaemia develops when the output of glucose from the liver falls below the rate of glucose uptake by peripheral tissues. The liver produces glucose either by mobilising stored glycogen or by gluconeogenesis. Both processes are inhibited at high insulin levels, and are sustained or enhanced by counter-regulatory hormones. Glycogen stores are depleted by fasting, malnutrition or acute and massive hepatocellular damage; gluconeogenesis is inhibited by alcohol, or limited by shortage of the necessary substrates, alanine, lactate or glycerol. Peripheral glucose uptake is increased by high levels of insulin (such as those stimulated by food intake) and by exercise.

Classification

Classification is based on clinical presentation, mechanism and cause, and corresponds to the steps on the diagnostic pathway one needs to follow in elucidating unexplained episodes of hypoglycaemia.

1. *Clinical presentation.* It is traditional to distinguish between *fasting* and *reactive* (postprandial) hypoglycaemia. Fasting hypoglycaemia (e.g. presenting before breakfast) always has a clear organic basis, whereas investigation of patients referred for possible reactive hypoglycaemia is often unfruitful.
2. *Mechanism.* The first step in establishing the mechanism of hypoglycaemia is to consider the role of insulin, whether endogenous or exogenous. When hypoglycaemia is produced by relative insulin excess, peripheral glucose uptake is accelerated and hepatic production is inhibited. Hepatic glycogen stores are intact and can be mobilised by injection of glucagon or adrenaline. In other situations, hypoglycaemia develops despite appropriate suppression of circulating insulin levels; alcohol-induced hypoglycaemia is an example of this. When insulin levels are low, the cause is usually compromised hepatic glucose output, although this may only become manifest under the stress of accelerated peripheral uptake, e.g. during exercise. In this type of hypoglycaemia, hepatic glycogen stores are depleted and glucagon injection is ineffective.
3. *Cause.* An aetiological classification is given in Table 20.6.

Insulinomas

Insulinomas are insulin-secreting tumours arising from pancreatic islet tissue. The classic presentation is with

Table 20.6 Causes of hypoglycaemia

Type	Cause
Insulinomas	Benign (85%)
	Malignant (15%)
	Pluriglandular syndrome (MEN 1)
Other tumours	Mesenchymal tumours
	Primary hepatic carcinoma
	Adrenal carcinoma
	Carcinoids
Endocrine	Pituitary insufficiency
	Isolated ACTH deficiency
	Addison's disease
	Hypothyroidism
Autoimmune	Autoimmune insulin syndrome
Hepatic/renal causes	Hepatocellular disease
	Congestive liver disease
	End-stage renal failure
Postprandial	Idiopathic
	Alcohol-induced
	Late dumping
Drug-induced	Insulin
	Sulphonylureas
	Alcohol
	Quinine
	Salicylates
Miscellaneous	Starvation
	Prolonged exercise
	Septicaemia
	Factitious hypoglycaemia

fasting hypoglycaemia, although early symptoms may develop in the late morning or afternoon. Diagnosis is often delayed because recurrent hypoglycaemia is one of the great masqueraders of medicine. Early symptoms include sweating, palpitations, weakness, diplopia or visual blurring, often progressing to mental confusion or odd behaviour. About 50% of patients present with loss of consciousness, sometimes with convulsions. Patients may seek psychiatric help because of bizarre behaviour, amnesia or automatism. Focal neurological manifestations, including transient hemiparesis, are also well-recognised.

Diagnosis

Whipple's triad of criteria are still used as the basis of diagnosis:

1. the symptoms are associated with fasting or exercise
2. hypoglycaemia is present while the symptoms are present
3. the symptoms are relieved by glucose.

Confirmation of the diagnosis is made by the demonstration that insulin levels fail to suppress in the presence of hypoglycaemia. The simplest way to do this is to measure glucose and insulin levels on three mornings after an overnight fast. If the fasting glucose is subnormal but the insulin is not, an insulinoma is likely, although other possibilities including *factitious hypoglycaemia* (surreptitious self-injection with insulin) need to be excluded. It is usual to go on to a supervised fast in hospital, with the aim of demonstrating Whipple's triad. It has been estimated that 95% of insulinomas will be picked up by this simple plan of investigation.

Abnormal insulin secretion may be demonstrated in a number of ways. The beta cell normally secretes about one molecule of proinsulin for every ten of insulin, but insulinoma tissue releases much more proinsulin into the circulation. Proinsulin assay is only available in a few specialised centres, however, and autonomous insulin secretion can be demonstrated by lack of the normal feedback suppression during hypoglycaemia. This may be shown by measurements during spontaneous hypoglycaemia or by the C-peptide suppression test. In this test, insulin is infused to induce hypoglycaemia, and circulating C-peptide levels are measured as an index of endogenous insulin secretion, which should be almost totally suppressed. The test is potentially hazardous, and should be reserved for more doubtful cases. The glucose tolerance test is often mildly abnormal, but this has no diagnostic value.

The main differential diagnosis, once hypoglycaemia has been demonstrated with elevated insulin levels, is factitious hypoglycaemia. A surprising number of such cases have been reported in the literature, mostly in individuals in some way associated with the medical profession or with access to insulin via a diabetic relative. Measurement of C-peptide during the C-peptide suppression test will identify those who are injecting insulin, since there is no C-peptide in pharmaceutical insulin.

Treatment

Surgical excision is the only effective cure. The majority of insulinomas can be felt at operation by a skilled surgeon, but localisation can be extremely difficult. It is therefore usual to perform CT scans and pancreatic angiography pre-operatively in an attempt to localise the tumour, and this may be supplemented by assaying the insulin content (or the ratio of insulin to glucagon) of blood sampled at different levels from the pancreatic vein. Medical treatment of the hypoglycaemia with diazoxide is useful in patients with malignant and inoperable tumours, in those patients where the tumour cannot be located, and in some elderly patients with mild symptoms, who would not tolerate surgery well.

Hypoglycaemia due to other tumours

Hypoglycaemia is a rare complication of other cancers. It may occur with retroperitoneal and thoracic sarcomas, lymphomas, hepatomas and adrenal carcinoma. It does not appear to be due to insulin, but elevated levels of somatomedin-like substances (which have an insulin-like action) have been found in some patients. Other tumour products which bind to the insulin receptor have been described. The attacks of hypoglycaemia occur spontaneously, or in the fasting state, and may be very severe. Plasma insulin is not raised as in insulinomas, and treatment with steroids, diazoxide or glucagon may be helpful if the tumour cannot be removed.

Endocrine causes

Hypoglycaemia, usually mild and asymptomatic, can arise in endocrine deficiency states, presumably because of impaired counter-regulation to the actions of insulin.

Autoimmune insulin syndrome

This is extremely rare but of considerable theoretical interest since hypoglycaemia is associated with antibodies to endogenous insulin. Most cases have occurred in Japanese patients treated with the antithyroid agent methimazole.

Hepatic and renal causes

Hypoglycaemia is uncommon except when extensive hepatocellular damage is present, as with acute toxic necrosis following poisoning with paracetamol or chloroform. Liver disease may however potentiate other factors predisposing to hypoglycaemia. Terminal renal disease may lead to severe hypoglycaemia, and reactive hypoglycaemia has been reported in patients dialysed against glucose-rich solutions.

Postprandial hypoglycaemia

A surprising number of people report the occasional feeling of faintness about the time that a meal is due, rapidly relieved by food. Some have the sensation so frequently that they adopt a regular eating pattern with snacks between main meals. For many years, it was assumed that people like this were suffering from postprandial or 'reactive' hypoglycaemia. It now seems clear that hypoglycaemia is rarely if ever responsible. The main difficulty

---

Summary 7   Diagnosis of insulinoma

The aim is to satisfy Whipple's triad:
– symptoms associated with fasting or exercise
– hypoglycaemia is confirmed while symptoms are present
– glucose relieves the symptoms

● Inappropriately elevated insulin (or proinsulin) levels should be present during hypoglycaemia

● Most patients can be identified by 3 fasting measures of blood glucose and insulin

● Controlled fast in hospital to confirm blood glucose and insulin levels

● In difficult cases insulin can be infused to produce hypoglycaemia; failure of suppression of endogenous C-peptide demonstrates autonomous insulin secretion

● Factitious (self-induced) hypoglycaemia is an important differential diagnosis arose from interpretation of the 5-hour glucose tolerance test which was introduced as the means of diagnosing the condition. This appeared to provide frequent confirmation since venous glucose levels tend to fall below the fasting level in the later stages of the test, and go under 3 mmol/l in about 25% of individuals. More critical evaluation showed that the equivalent of Whipple's triad was usually impossible to demonstrate. Patients with symptoms did not have low glucose values and vice-versa.

Measurement of arterial glucose levels explained much of this confusion by showing that the arteriovenous glucose difference is wide at this stage of the absorptive process due to rapid uptake of glucose by peripheral tissues. Arterial glucose levels (and hence the supply of glucose to the brain) remain quite normal, even though hypoglycaemia may be present on the efferent side of the circulation. If stringent criteria are applied, i.e. demonstration of hypoglycaemia in arterial or capillary blood (associated with symptoms which are relieved by intravenous glucose but not by saline), idiopathic postprandial hypoglycaemia becomes a rare and poorly understood entity. It would be premature to dismiss the symptom complex referred to above as in some way imaginary, but hypoglycaemia is unlikely to be the cause.

Secondary postprandial hypoglycaemia may develop in the presence of alcohol, which stimulates the beta cells to produce an enhanced insulin response to carbohydrate. Some people become mildly hypoglycaemic after drinking a gin and tonic! Postprandial hypoglycaemia has also been reported after gastric surgery, due to rapid gastric emptying and mismatching of food and insulin, and is referred to as 'late dumping' in the literature.

Drug-induced hypoglycaemia

Insulin, sulphonylurea agents and alcohol (see below) are the main causes of drug-induced hypoglycaemia. Quinine-induced hypoglycaemia is a recently recognised and sometimes fatal complication of the treatment of falciparum malaria. Salicylates (and alcohol) can cause severe hypoglycaemia if accidentally ingested by young children. Hypoglycaemia has been reported with many other drugs, but usually only when other predisposing factors are present.

Alcohol-induced hypoglycaemia

Alcohol-induced hypoglycaemia was first noticed in malnourished 'skid row' alcoholics, and most reported cases have been in this category, but sporadic heavy drinkers are also at risk. Patients present with coma and hypothermia, sometimes hours after alcohol ingestion. Hypoglycaemia is thought to arise from a combination of hepatic glycogen depletion, due to poor nutrition, and a direct inhibitory effect of alcohol upon hepatic gluconeogenesis; hypoglycaemia can be induced in fit young men by infusing ethanol after a 48-hour fast.

PLASMA LIPOPROTEINS AND NORMAL METABOLISM

The major lipids, *cholesterol* and *triglyceride*, are insoluble, and lipid transport between the gut, liver and peripheral tissues thus depends on complexing with phospholipid and specific proteins to form soluble lipoproteins (Fig. 20.18).

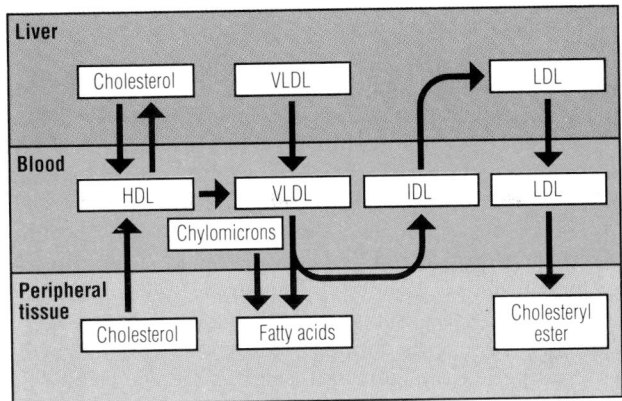

Fig. 20.18 Interrelationships of lipoprotein classes.

These have an inner core of cholesteryl ester and triglyceride, and an outer layer of phospholipid, cholesterol and protein. They vary in relative content of cholesterol and triglyceride. In general, lipoprotein density (determined by ultracentrifuge sedimentation rate) decreases as the triglyceride content increases, and the lipoproteins are classified accordingly. The proteins complexed with the lipid molecule are termed apoproteins and designated: A, B, CI, CII, CIII, D, E, and F (Table 20.7). These may determine the rate of metabolism of a given class of lipoprotein.

Chylomicrons are formed in the small intestine and serve to transport exogenous triglyceride to peripheral tissues.

Table 20.7 Classification of lipoproteins

	Ratio of triglyceride: cholesteryl ester in content of major lipoproteins	Major apoproteins
Chylomicrons	21:1	B, CI, CII, CIII
Very low density lipoprotein (VLDL)	3:1	B, CI, CII, CIII
Intermediate density lipoprotein (IDL)	2:3	B, E
Low density lipoprotein (LDL)	1:4.5	B
High density lipoprotein (HDL)	1:4.5	A

Endogenous triglyceride is transported from the liver to peripheral tissues in *very low density lipoproteins* (VLDL). Both endogenous and exogenous triglyceride are catabolised by lipoprotein lipase which is situated in the capillary endothelium of skeletal and adipose tissue; this yields *intermediate density lipoproteins* (IDL) which have a relatively higher cholesterol content and which are further metabolised in the liver to yield *low density lipoproteins* (LDL). LDL transports cholesteryl ester from the liver to the periphery where its cellular uptake depends on a specific receptor mechanism. The intravascular metabolism of VLDL provides essential apoproteins for *high density lipoprotein* (HDL).

The chylomicron and VLDL system is used to transport triglycerides (an important energy source, quantitatively) from the gut and liver, respectively, to the periphery for metabolism or storage. Cholesterol is carried to all tissues by the LDL system and is used in biosynthesis of cell membranes, vitamin D synthesis in the skin and steroid hormone synthesis in the adrenal glands.

The HDL system serves to esterify and transfer cholesterol from peripheral tissues to the liver, either directly or by transfer of cholesteryl ester (under the influence of lecithin cholesterol acyl transferase) to the VLDL pathway. Bile acids formed from cholesterol enter the enterohepatic circulation or are excreted in the faeces.

Measurement of plasma lipids

Total plasma cholesterol and triglyceride may be measured enzymatically (Table 20.8). The range of concentration varies considerably between different populations, e.g. the mean plasma cholesterol is lower in African and Asian populations than in the West. Levels also vary within a population according to the influence of factors such as diet, exercise, bodyweight and alcohol intake (Table 20.9). Sex differences also exist, and LDL cholesterol is higher in men than in premenopausal women, whereas HDL cholesterol is higher in women.

HYPERLIPIDAEMIA

Elevations of particular lipoprotein classes may arise as a result of hereditary defects in lipoprotein metabolism, or else may be secondary to specific diseases. Hyperlipidaemic states are usually classified (on the basis of the lipoprotein class or classes involved) into six categories, according to the Frederickson classification of hereditary hyperlipidaemia as extended by the WHO (Table 20.10). Specific diagnosis requires lipoprotein electrophoresis, but, for practical clinical purposes, measurement of total cholesterol, total triglyceride and perhaps HDL cholesterol is

Table 20.8 Reference range (fasting plasma sample)

Plasma lipid	Range
Total cholesterol	4.0–6.7 mmol/l
HDL cholesterol	0.9–1.4 mmol/l (men)
	1.2–1.7 mmol/l (women)
Triglycerides	0.8–2.0 mmol/l (men)
	0.6–1.5 mmol/l (women)

Table 20.9 Various factors influencing lipoprotein levels

	VLDL	LDL	HDL
Lifestyle			
Obesity	↑	↑	↓
High saturated fat intake		↑	
Polyunsaturated fat diet	↓	↓	
High fibre diet	↓	↓	
Alcohol	↑		↑
Exercise			↑
Disease state/drugs			
Hypothyroidism	↑*	↑	
Diabetes mellitus	↑		
Nephrotic syndrome	↑	↑	
Cholestatic liver disease, e.g. primary biliary cirrhosis		↑	
Myeloma	↑		
Oral contraceptives	↑*		
Thiazide diuretics	↑		
Alcohol	↑		

* Marginal effect

Table 20.10 Primary hyperlipidaemia

Type	Total plasma cholesterol	Total plasma triglyceride	Mechanism	Inheritance	Prevalence	Atherosclerosis risk
I	Normal	↑ (chylo)	Lipoprotein lipase deficiency or apo-CII deficiency	Autorecessive	Rare	No
IIa	↑ (LDL)	N	LDL receptor defect	Autodominant or polygenic	Common	Yes
IIb	↑ (LDL)	↑ (VLDL)	LDL receptor defect	Autodominant	Common	Yes
III	↑	↑ (IDL)	Apo-E abnormality	–	Rare	Yes
IV	Normal or slight ↑	↑ (VLDL)	Overproduction	Autodominant	Common	No
V	Normal or slight ↑	↑ (Chylo and VLDL)	Lipoprotein lipase deficiency or apo-CII deficiency	Autorecessive	Rare	No

all that is necessary. Additional information may be gained by the simple procedure of storing a fasting plasma specimen for 18 hours at 4°C. A floating layer of turbidity indicates chylomicronaemia, whereas uniform turbidity suggests VLDL or IDL excess.

Hereditary hypercholesterolaemia (Type IIa or IIb) is most commonly associated with an apparently polygenic inheritance. The autosomal dominant variety results in higher LDL levels and a dramatic increase in atherosclerosis; deaths from coronary artery disease occur in homozygotes before the age of 25. Heterozygotes also have reduced LDL cholesterol receptor numbers and a significant increase in coronary artery disease. The reduced incorporation of LDL cholesterol into cells results in a reduced negative feedback on hydroxymethyl glutaryl CoA reductase, causing increased intracellular cholesterol formation. A variable combination of Type IIa, IIb and IV hyperlipidaemia may be inherited as an autosomal dominant trait (familial combined hyperlipidaemia) and predisposes to atherosclerosis, even if only the Type IV abnormality is present.

Secondary abnormalities in plasma lipoproteins (Table 20.10) may arise in hypothyroidism, untreated diabetes mellitus, oral oestrogen or thiazide diuretic therapy, alcohol, the nephrotic syndrome and liver disease. These should all be considered in cases of lipid abnormality.

Marked hypertriglyceridaemia, whether primary or secondary, may precipitate acute abdominal pain which is usually due to acute pancreatitis.

Clinical features

The physical signs of hyperlipidaemia (Table 20.11) include:

1. *xanthelasmata* – subcutaneous cholesterol deposits at the inner margins of the eyelids
2. *tendon xanthomata* – subcutaneous cholesterol nodules mainly over elbows and patellar tendons
3. *eruptive xanthomata* – small subcutaneous deposits of triglyceride
4. *palmar xanthomata* – deposits in the palmar creases
5. *corneal arcus* – a white circle at the junction of the cornea and sclera
6. *lipaemia retinalis* – small retinal vessels appear paler.

The presence of xanthelasmata and corneal arcus suggests the possibility of hypercholesterolaemia, but may also be present in the absence of hyperlipidaemia. The other signs always indicate a lipid abnormality.

Hyperlipidaemia and vascular disease

Epidemiological studies indicate a definite relationship between the incidence of atherosclerosis and total plasma cholesterol, an association that depends on the cholesterol fraction in LDL. A simplistic view is that the mechanism is via increased entry of LDL and deposition of cholesteryl ester into established atherosclerotic plaques. LDL is implicated most strongly as a factor in patients with homo-

Table 20.11 Signs which are always indicative of lipid abnormality

Sign	Lipid abnormality
Tendon xanthomata	Hypercholesterolaemia
Palmar xanthomata	Type III (almost exclusively)
Eruptive xanthomata	Gross hypertriglyceridaemia
Lipaemia retinalis	Gross hypertriglyceridaemia

zygous Type IIa hyperlipoproteinaemia, who invariably suffer early coronary artery disease (usually in the third decade), and in heterozygotes, who have a much higher incidence of vascular disease than the general population. It is more difficult to quantitate the risk for patients with milder degrees of hypercholesterolaemia. Here it seems that the level of HDL, which has an inverse relationship with coronary heart disease, is a more important determinant. HDL levels are generally lower in obese patients, partly explaining the increased risk in this group, and also rise in response to regular exercise. There is no convincing evidence to date of a relationship between pure hypertriglyceridaemia and vascular disease, except in familial combined hyperlipoproteinaemia.

The risk of mild hypercholesterolaemia must be taken together with the presence or absence of other risk factors, including cigarette smoking, excess weight and hypertension. Cigarette smoking remains one of the single most important independent risk factors for the development of atherosclerosis.

Management

Who should be treated and what are the benefits?

Despite the association between LDL cholesterol and coronary artery disease, there is no conclusive proof that medical intervention to lower plasma cholesterol decreases the incidence of ischaemic heart disease, although the body of evidence tends to this conclusion. There is certainly no doubt that the severe hypercholesterolaemia associated with homozygous or heterozygous Type IIa warrants vigorous therapy. Milder hypercholesterolaemia, associated with polygenic inheritance, is more likely to indicate future problems in younger patients and those with a strong family history of vascular disease. On present evidence, an attempt should be made to lower cholesterol levels towards normal in patients under the age of 60, combined with an effort to eliminate other risk factors. On an empirical basis, it would seem prudent to increase plasma HDL levels if possible. Regular exercise is particularly important in this context, in addition to its other benefits in patients with established atherosclerotic disease. The current recommendation of the British Cardiac Society is that total cholesterol levels above 6.5 mmol/l should be treated, initially by diet, and with addition of drug therapy for levels remaining in excess of 7.8 mmol/l.

Hypertriglyceridaemia warrants therapy if it is associated with episodes of pancreatitis, or has resulted in widespread xanthomata. Present evidence does not justify treatment of mild hypertriglyceridaemia, except in the context of familial combined hyperlipidaemia in which the risk of ischaemic heart disease is raised. General advice should be given about achieving ideal body weight and avoidance of other risk factors.

Secondary hyperlipidaemia should be managed by treatment of the underlying abnormality whenever possible.

Treatment of hypercholesterolaemia

Diet is indicated in the first instance in treatment of hypercholesterolaemia. Fat is reduced because of the direct relationship between fat intake and dietary cholesterol, while the ratio of polyunsaturated to saturated fat is increased. These measures will produce a reduction of up to 10% in plasma LDL and are the mainstay of therapy in polygenic mild hypercholesterolaemia. In the autosomal dominant form, dietary measures alone are inadequate, and homozygotes are at sufficient risk to justify measures such as regular plasma exchange. Heterozygotes are treated with bile acid sequestrating compounds such as cholestyramine or colestipol (Table 20.12). These agents may cause gastrointestinal side-effects and should be introduced slowly. If cholesterol levels are not reduced satisfactorily by these measures, the isobutyric acid derivative bezafibrate, or nicotinic acid, may be added. These are well tolerated, although the bezafibrate-related drug, clofibrate, was associated with a slight increase in mortality from various non-atheromatous disorders in a large trial of its efficacy in preventing coronary disease. The recently developed HMG CoA reductase inhibitors provide an additional approach to the treatment of hypercholesterolaemia by inhibition of endogenous cholesterol synthesis. One example of this class of drug (simvastatin) is now available on general prescription in the UK and is likely to have an important role in the management of this condition, either in place of, or in addition to, cholestyramine if the latter is poorly tolerated.

Treatment of hypertriglyceridaemia

Diet treatment of hypertriglyceridaemia should aim at ideal body weight and reduction of dietary saturated fat. Severe degrees of hypertriglyceridaemia require treatment with bezafibrate or nicotinic acid (Table 20.12). Bezafibrate is particularly useful for Type III hyperlipidaemia. It is worth bearing in mind that hypertriglyceridaemia frequently indicates glucose intolerance.

PORPHYRIA

The term porphyria refers to a heterogeneous group of inborn errors of metabolism resulting in enzyme defects in the biosynthetic pathway of haem, and the accumulation of its precursors. Haem precursors, termed *porphyrinogens*, consist of four *cyclised* pyrrole rings and are further classified into uro-, copro- and protoporphyrinogens according to the distribution of acetyl, propionyl, methyl and urinyl substitutions around the porphyrin ring. Uro-, copro- and protoporphyrins are excreted in the urine if present in excess in blood. Porphyrinogens are colourless compounds which, when oxidised, yield highly coloured porphyrins; this is why dark urine may be found in some examples of acute porphyria.

HAEM SYNTHESIS

Porphyrin biosynthesis occurs in a variety of cell types, but predominantly in liver and bone marrow (Fig. 20.19). The initial step is the condensation of glycine and succinyl CoA to form delta-amino-laevulinic acid (d-ALA) under the influence of mitochondrial ALA synthase. The single pyrrole ring, porphobilinogen, is then formed in the cytosol from two molecules of d-ALA. Four molecules of porphobilinogen are cyclised under the influence of porphobilinogen deaminase to form the porphyrin ring structure. There follows a series of decarboxylation and mitochondrial oxidation reactions, eventually yielding protoporphyrin IX. The addition of ferrous iron, catalysed by ferrochelatase, is the final step in haem biosynthesis. The overall flux is controlled by a negative feedback effect of haem on d-ALA synthase.

Table 20.12 Some drugs used to treat hyperlipidaemia

Agent	Usual dose	Indications (types)	Side-effects	Contraindications and precautions
Nicotinic acid (Niacin)	1 g tds (9 g/day)	II, III, IV, V	Flushing, irritation of skin and eyes	Contraindicated in liver disease, peptic ulceration
Bezafibrate	200 mg tds or 400 mg nocte	III, IV	Abdominal discomfort, cholesterol cholelithiasis, myositis (rare)	Avoid in liver and kidney disease. Potentiates action of warfarin
Cholestyramine	8 g tds	II	Flatulence, bowel disturbance	Reduced drug absorption (e.g. digoxin, warfarin)
Simvastatin	10–40 mg nocte	II	Reversible increase in hepatic transaminases, gastrointestinal symptoms	Avoid concurrent use of bezafibrate Potentiates action of warfarin

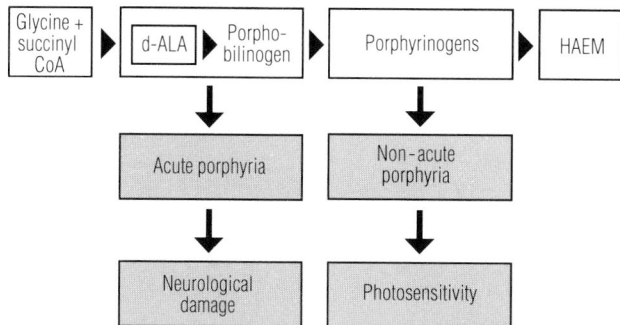

Fig. 20.19 Porphyrin metabolism. Increased d-ALA synthetase activity leads to increased porphryin production (porphyria). In acute porphyria, porphobilinogen metabolism is normal or reduced in contrast to non-acute porphyria in which it is increased.

CLASSIFICATION OF THE PORPHYRIAS

The porphyrias may be classified as hepatic or erythropoietic according to the main site of the biosynthetic defect and excess precursor formation. Alternatively, they may be classified as acute or non-acute, and this is clinically more useful (Table 20.13).

All porphyrias are associated with an increase in d-ALA synthase activity because of decreased negative feedback, usually enhanced by an environmental factor. This is accompanied by an increase in porphobilinogen (PBG) deaminase activity in the non-acute conditions, but a normal or reduced activity in the acute varieties. The net result in the acute conditions is an accumulation of d-ALA and porphobilinogen, which probably accounts for the neurological, psychiatric and acute gastrointestinal disturbances observed. In the non-acute conditions, specific uro- and coproporphyrins accumulate without porphobilinogen excess because the increased flux through the d-ALA synthase pathway is accompanied by increased PBG deaminase activity (Fig. 20.19).

Photosensitivity is a common feature of all types of porphyria with the exception of the acute intermittent variety. It is due to accumulation of porphyrin within the epidermis as a result of photo-oxidation of porphyrinogens.

Acute porphyrias

Acute porphyrias are all inherited as *Mendelian* dominant traits and are characterised by acute neurological and gas-

Table 20.13 Classification of porphyrias

Acute	Non-acute
Acute intermittent porphyria	Porphyria cutanea tarda (cutaneous hepatic porphyria)
Variegate porphyria	
Hereditary coproporphyria	Erythropoietic congenital porphyria protoporphyria

trointestinal symptoms usually followed by complete remission, although fatalities due to respiratory failure may occur. The episodes are rare before puberty, thus emphasising the important enhancing effect of sex steroids on ALA synthase activity. Acute attacks are precipitated by alcohol, sex steroids (e.g. oral contraceptives), and a variety of drugs – especially barbiturates and other lipid soluble enzyme-inducing drugs which increase ALA synthase activity.

Acute intermittent porphyria

Acute intermittent porphyria is due to a defect at the level of PBG deaminase. Most cases are clinically silent; women are more likely to manifest acute attacks. Abdominal pain and vomiting are the commonest presenting features (95%). Additional features include sinus tachycardia, hypertension and left ventricular failure (75%), sensorimotor peripheral neuropathy (50%), respiratory muscle paresis, coma and seizures. Psychiatric manifestations, which vary from depression to frank psychosis, may be present for the duration of the acute episode. Proteinuria and renal impairment may also occur.

The diagnosis may be suggested by a positive family history, or the passage of urine which turns red-brown on standing. Confirmation depends on colorimetric urine testing for excess porphobilinogen using Ehrlich's aldehyde reagent, which produces a pink colour insoluble in chloroform.

Variegate porphyria

The defect is at the level of protoporphyrinogen oxidase. Features are similar to those of acute intermittent porphyria, together with the cutaneous features of porphyria cutanea tarda (see below). The highest incidence is in South African whites.

Hereditary coproporphyria

The clinical features are similar to variegate porphyria. The defect lies at the level of coproporphyrinogen oxidase.

Management of acute porphyria

Prophylaxis in those at risk is of obvious importance. Suspected patients can be identified by urine testing (30% yield) and erythrocyte-enzyme assays. Those affected should avoid alcohol, barbiturates and oral contraceptives, and special observation during pregnancy is indicated.

In acute attacks, a high carbohydrate intake (e.g. 400 g/d iv) may be of benefit by depressing activity of ALA synthase. Inappropriate antidiuretic hormone secretion (p. 690) may be a complicating factor necessitating fluid restriction. Tachycardia and hypertension should be treated with beta blockade, and phenothiazines are indicated for psychiatric disturbances. Epileptic seizures should be managed with benzodiazepines; barbiturates are contraindicated. There is some evidence that intravenous haematin may limit acute attacks by reducing ALA synthase activity.

Non-acute porphyrias

Porphyria cutanea tarda

Porphyria cutanea tarda has a genetic element, but is predominently acquired. The condition is due to a defect in hepatic uroporphyrinogen decarboxylase and is characterised by bullae following sun exposure or minor trauma, which heal with scarring. The face, back of the neck, and backs of hands are the most commonly affected sites. There is also a diffuse thickening of the skin, which can resemble scleroderma, and hypertrichosis. Hepatomegaly can occur, particularly if alcohol intake has been high. Hepatic siderosis and diabetes mellitus may occur. Urinary uroporphyrin excretion is increased but porphobilinogen is normal. Treatment includes avoidance of alcohol, and venesection to achieve normal uroporphyrin levels in urine. Low-dose chloroquine, which increases urinary uroporphyrin excretion, may be useful.

Congenital porphyria

Congenital porphyria is a rare autosomal recessively inherited condition which presents early in childhood. It is due to a defect in uroporphyrinogen cosynthetase and is characterised by photosensitivity with bullous formation healing by scarring. Dystrophic nail changes and brown/pink tooth discolouration may also occur. A normochromic anaemia with normoblastic marrow hyperplasia and splenomegaly are usual features. Low-dose chloroquine may be of value in treatment.

Erythropoietic protoporphyria

Erythropoietic protoporphyria is an autosomal-dominant condition which is due to a defect in ferrochelatase activity. The condition presents in childhood with photosensitivity but often no rash, severe peripheral paraesthesia and hepatic dysfunction due to protoporphyrin deposition. The diagnosis is made by demonstrating characteristic erythrocyte fluorescence and elevated red cell protoporphyrin levels. Urinary and faecal protoporphyrin excretion may be increased. Treatment with oral beta carotene may protect against the photosensitivity, and bile salt sequestrating agents (e.g. cholestyramine) may protect the liver by interrupting the enterohepatic circulation of protoporphyrin.

INHERITED DISORDERS OF CARBOHYDRATE METABOLISM

Glycogen storage disease

Enzyme deficiencies and resulting disorders have been recognized for each of the steps in the pathways of glycogen synthesis and degradation, and all are inherited as autosomal recessive traits. The most usual consequence is accumulation of glycogen in liver and/or muscle, and hypoglycaemia due to failure to mobilize glucose when needed. Presentation is in early childhood with hepatomegaly, muscle weakness or cramps, congestive cardiac failure or hypoglycaemia. The main exception to this is Type V (McArdle) which presents in adult life. Some 12 variants have been recognised, but most are exceptionally rare. Among the more common are Types I and V.

Type I (Von Gierke)

Glucose-6-phosphatase deficiency presents in infancy with hepatomegaly, hypoglycaemia and lactic acidosis. The enzyme defect prevents mobilization of glucose after glucagon administration, and the diagnosis is confirmed by liver biopsy. Frequent glucose feeds, continued through the night by nasogastric tube, are needed to prevent hypoglycaemia. Some individuals survive into adult life, but the early mortality is high.

Type V (McArdle)

Muscle phosphorylase deficiency is a rare condition which presents in adult life with muscle cramps and myoglobinuria after exercise. Victims are easily fatigued and develop proximal muscle wasting. Despite its restrictions on activity, it is compatible with a normal lifespan.

Galactosaemia

Galactosaemia is a rare autosomal recessive condition resulting in deficiency of the liver enzyme galactose-1-phosphate uridyl transferase. Affected children are normal at birth, but develop symptoms soon after milk feeds are given, since the galactose contained in milk cannot be metabolised. If undetected, the condition progresses from diarrhoea and vomiting to hepatomegaly and jaundice. Death within a few weeks is common, while survivors develop cataracts, cirrhosis and mental retardation. On the other hand, prompt detection in the neonate and avoidance of galactose in the diet allows relatively normal development, although some degree of mental retardation may be present. Initial diagnosis is by detection of reducing substances in the urine; this is, therefore, positive on testing with Clinitest but negative to the enzyme-based stick tests (which are specific for glucose). Definitive diagnosis is based on assay of red cell galactose-1-phosphate uridyl transferase levels.

LYSOSOMAL STORAGE DISORDERS

Lysosomal storage disorders are a large group of inherited diseases in which there is an abnormal deposition of a substrate in vacuoles related to lysosomes as a result of an inborn gene defect of metabolism. These disorders include lipid-storage diseases, mucolipidoses, mucopolysaccharidoses and glycoprotein storage diseases. These diseases are autosomal recessive, except for Hunter's disease (type II) and Fabry's disease (p. 955), both of which are X-linked. The disorders are generally characterised by excessive deposition of substrate in brain, spleen, liver and bone; thus the main manifestations tend to be neurological and skeletal with hepatosplenomegaly.

A few of the most common disorders are briefly described below.

Gaucher's disease

In Gaucher's disease there is a deficiency of beta glucocerebrosidase, and, as a result, gangliosides accumulate in nervous tissue (in the childhood form – causing mental retardation and spasticity) or in the liver, spleen and bone (in the adult form). The adult form is more common and presents with hepatosplenomegaly, bony symptoms (including severe pain and deformity) and anaemia due to bone marrow infiltration. Typical Gaucher's cells can be recognised on liver or marrow biopsy. Splenectomy may be helpful.

Mucopolysaccharidoses

Mucopolysaccharidoses are a group of complex-carbohydrate storage disorders with abnormal accumulation in fibroblasts, chondrocytes and neural tissue. Common features include skeletal dysplasia, hepatosplenomegaly, coarse skin and corneal clouding. Gross mental retardation is present in the two best recognised (and, to some extent, overlapping) variants, Hurler's syndrome and Hunter's syndrome.

Fabry's disease

This is discussed in Chapter 23, page 955.

Tay-Sachs disease

This is discussed in Chapter 23, page 954.

FURTHER READING

Bliss M 1982 The discovery of insulin. Paul Harris, Edinburgh. *One of the best books of medical history ever written*

Keen H, Jarrett J 1982 Complications of diabetes, 2nd edn. Edward Arnold, London. *A particularly good account of the morphological changes*

Marble A, Krall L P, Bradley R F, Christlieb A R, Soeldner J S 1985 Joslin's diabetes mellitus, 12th edn. Lea and Febiger, Philadelphia. *A comprehensive textbook of diabetes*

Marks V, Rose F C 1981 Hypoglycaemia, 2nd edn. Blackwell, Oxford. *A compendious but readable textbook*

Renal and Urinary Disease

Table 21.1 Functions of the kidney

Excretion of products of metabolism	Regulation of homeostasis
Urea	Body water
Creatinine	Body sodium
Urate	Body potassium
Oxalate	Acid-base status
Sulphate	Calcium
Phosphate	Phosphate
Hydrogen ion	
'Uraemic toxins'	
Water of metabolism	
Excretion of substances ingested in excess of requirement	**Production of hormones**
Water	Renin
Sodium	Angiotensin
Potassium	Erythropoietin
Calcium	1,25–dihydroxyvitamin D
Phosphate	

The function of the kidney in health falls into three main areas (Table 21.1). These are:

1. excretion of waste products
2. maintenance of the constancy of the internal environment
3. biosynthesis of hormones.

The importance of these functions is vividly demonstrated in patients with kidney disease, in whom develop a wide variety of symptoms and signs associated with disordered metabolism. The sophistication of the various functions of the kidney is evident from the striking contrast between the limited efficacy of the various forms of artificial dialysis treatment, and the virtual normalisation of body function that attends reversal of kidney dysfunction or successful transplantation.

EPIDEMIOLOGICAL CONSIDERATIONS

Mortality figures from the WHO Statistics Annual 1975–1981 indicate that the death rate from renal and urinary diseases is about 60/million population per year in the UK. Renal failure and malignancy of the urinary tract account

for most of these cases. More recently it has been estimated that about 4000 people between the ages of 5 and 70 years develop terminal renal failure (end stage renal disease, ESRD) per annum in the UK. Of these, only about 50% are taken on to dialysis and transplantation programmes; by implication, the remaining 50% are thus allowed to die untreated. In December 1986, the number of patients in the UK receiving treatment for ESRD by means of dialysis or transplantation was 13 000, of whom 6600 had functioning transplants and the rest were undergoing some form of dialysis treatment (p. 809). Patients with the various forms of glomerulonephritis form the largest group receiving renal replacement therapy (RRT), followed by those with tubulointerstitial diseases (including pyelonephritis) and diabetic nephropathy. The incidence of end stage renal disease rises rapidly with age; its frequency is similar in males and females.

Urinary tract infection, though often not serious, is a considerable source of morbidity. It has been estimated that 1–2% of all general practice consultations are in relation to symptoms suggestive of urinary tract infection.

Women are most frequently affected, and prevalence studies have shown symptoms of dysuria in as many as 21% of females aged between 20 and 65 years. Demonstrable infection has a prevalence of 4% amongst females between the ages of 16 and 45 years, rising to 10% between the ages of 55 and 64 years and 15% above 65 years of age.

For some renal diseases, there are marked racial and regional differences in incidence. For example, ESRD resulting solely from severe hypertension is much commoner in blacks than in whites. Renal amyloid is an uncommon cause of ESRD in Western Europe and the USA, but in Israel, with its large population of Sephardic Jews, familial Mediterranean fever leading to amyloidosis accounts for 7% of patients reaching ESRD. In some parts of the world, endemic parasitic infection may be associated with an unusually high incidence of certain types of renal or urinary disease. Examples are: East Africa, where immune complex glomerulonephritis with nephrotic syndrome due to chronic infection with *Plasmodium malariae* is common (accounting for up to 2% of all hospital admissions); and Egypt and Sudan, where *Schistosoma haematobium* infection is associated with immune complex glomerulonephritis, obstructive uropathy and carcinoma of the bladder.

ANATOMY AND PHYSIOLOGY

THE KIDNEY AS AN ORGAN

In man, the kidneys are paired bean-shaped structures, measuring 10–12 cm in length, 5–6 cm in width and 3–4 cm in depth. The renal parenchyma consists of an outer cortex and inner medulla (Fig. 21.1A). The kidneys weigh about 150 g each, and are situated retroperitoneally on either side of the vertebral column, at the level of T12–L3, where they underlie the costo-vertebral angles posteriorly. The right kidney is about 1.5 cm lower than the left, and both move up and down about 3 cm during respiration. The functional unit of the kidney is the *nephron*. Each kidney contains about one million nephrons, each one made up of a glomerulus, a proximal tubule, a loop of Henle, a distal tubule and a collecting tubule (Fig. 21.1B).

Nerve supply. The renal capsule and ureters are innervated via the T10–T12 and L1 roots, and pain arising from the upper renal tract may be perceived over the corresponding dermatomes.

The blood supply is from the renal arteries, which may be single or multiple and which undergo a series of divisions within the kidney forming in succession *interlobar arteries* running radially as far as the corticomedullary junction, *arcuate arteries* running circumferentially along the corticomedullary junction and *interlobular arteries* running radially through the cortex towards the surface of the organ (Fig. 21.1B). Afferent arterioles arise from the interlobular arteries and supply the glomerular capillaries, which in turn drain into efferent arterioles. The subsequent movement of blood depends on the location of the glomeruli

within the kidney. Efferent arterioles from *outer cortical glomeruli* drain into a peritubular capillary network within the cortex, and thence into progressively larger and more proximal branches of the renal vein. In contrast, blood from *juxtamedullary glomeruli* passes into vasa recta in the medulla, where it maintains close proximity with the medullary portion of the tubules before turning back towards the area of cortex from which the vasa recta originated. The vasa recta have fenestrated walls which facilitate the movement of diffusable substances through the thin and thick limbs of Henle's loop.

Renal blood flow and glomerular filtration rate. Renal blood flow is high – about 25% of the resting cardiac output, or 1300 ml/min. This corresponds to a renal plasma flow of about 700 ml/min, of which 25% is ultrafiltered at the glomeruli, giving a glomerular filtration rate (GFR) of 120 ml/min (180 l/day).

Collection of urine. The collecting tubules merge in the inner medulla to form the papillary ducts of Bellini, which in turn empty at the apices of the papillae into the calyces. The calyces are lined by a transitional cell epithelium which is continuous with that of the renal pelvis, ureters and bladder. Urine is passed to the bladder by active peristalsis in the ureters, pending intermittent discharge to the exterior by the process of micturition.

MICROANATOMY AND PHYSIOLOGY

The glomerulus

Each glomerulus consists of vascular and epithelial elements and is made up of three basic cell types.

1. *Glomerular capillary endothelial cells.* These are unusual in that they are fenestrated with 500–1000 Å pores (Fig. 21.1E).
2. *Epithelial cells.* These are designated parietal or visceral depending on their location (Fig. 21.1E)
3. *Mesangial cells.* These specialised cells secrete the mesangial matrix of the glomeruli, and probably regulate the distribution of blood flow within the glomerulus. They are phagocytic, and are considered to be related to the macrophages of the reticuloendothelial system.

The basement membrane lies between the capillary endothelial and the visceral epithelial cells; this triad comprises the *glomerular sieve* across which glomerular filtration occurs.

The tubule

Throughout its length, the tubule is lined with epithelial cells which are cuboidal, except in the thin limb of Henle's loop where they are flat. A luminal brush border distinguishes the proximal tubular cells from those elsewhere in the tubule.

The anatomical arrangement of the different parts of the nephron and its blood supply is such that there is potential

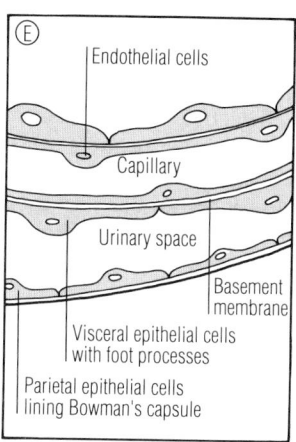

Fig. 21.1 Gross and microscopic anatomy of the kidney. A. Longitudinal section. **B.** Note that the loop of Henle dips deeply into the hypertonic medulla and, in the case of juxta-medullary nephrons (i.e. those with their glomeruli closest to the cortico-medullary junction area), the efferent arteriole is linked to the vasa recta, also dipping deeply into the medulla. **C.** A juxta medullary nephron is shown on the left, and a cortical nephron on the right. **D.** and **E.** Microanatomy of the renal glomerulus.

for events in a renal tubule to influence the behaviour of its own glomerulus. This phenomenon is called *tubuloglomerular feedback*. It is particularly evident at the *macula densa*, where each distal tubule is in close proximity to the afferent arteriole of its own glomerulus, forming the *juxta-glomerular apparatus* (JGA) from which renin is released.

Although the nephrons differ somewhat in their anatomical location within the kidney and in their structure and function, each nephron is capable of undertaking most, if not all, of the functions of the complete organ. These functions are centred on the need for *selective* excretion in a *regulated* manner. Each nephron achieves this by producing an ultrafiltrate of plasma and then modifying the composition of this ultrafiltrate to ensure reclamation of useful compounds and excretion of waste. These processes are conducted respectively in the glomerulus (formation of ultrafiltrate) and the tubules (modification of composition of the ultrafiltrate).

Formation of the glomerular filtrate

Hydrostatic, osmotic and electrostatic forces predominate in the formation of the glomerular filtrate (GF). The resistance to flow in the afferent and efferent arterioles is such that the hydrostatic pressure in the glomerular capillaries is much higher than in other capillary beds, approximating 40–60 mmHg. This favours the movement of water and other substances from the capillary lumen to the lower-pressure Bowman's space (Fig. 21.1D), and easily overcomes the opposing plasma osmotic pressure. Such movement requires passage across a functional 'sieve' which, as noted above, is made up of the capillary endothelial cells, the visceral epithelial cells of Bowman's capsule and the basement membrane between them. The effective pore size in the sieve is such that macromolecules are selectively retained within the capillaries, while water and other small and intermediate-sized molecules and ions pass through. Molecular charge is also important in determining movement across the sieve. The inner surface of the sieve is negatively charged and therefore repels anionic molecules such as albumin. The ease with which a substance will cross the glomerular sieve and so form a constituent of the glomerular filtrate thus depends on both its size and its charge. Plasma proteins are either too big (globulins) or both too big and unfavourably charged (albumin) to allow significant passage in the GF. However, immunoglobulin light chains (MW 22 kD) normally appear in the urine.

Approximately 180 litres of GF are formed each day in an average man. As the composition of the GF is very close to that of plasma from which the macromolecules have been removed, the daily GF contains enormous amounts of low and middle molecular weight plasma constituents (in addition to water). Many, but not all, of these must be reclaimed from the GF if rapid depletion is to be avoided.

Modification of GF by tubular action

As the GF passes along the renal tubule, its composition is progressively altered by two simultaneous processes:

1. *Tubular reabsorption*, i.e. the selective movement of substances from the tubular lumen across the tubular epithelium to the peritubular capillaries.
2. *Tubular secretion*, i.e. the selective secretion of other substances into the tubular lumen.

Both these processes may be passive or active and both change qualitatively and quantitatively along the length of the renal tubule. Important examples of tubular transport are given in Table 21.2 and an indication of their scale in quantitative terms in Table 21.3.

Selective filtration at the glomerulus, followed by tubular reabsorption and secretion, leads to the 'final urine'. Effective regulation of the processes of glomerular filtration, tubular reabsorption and tubular secretion ensures that the composition of the final urine is appropriate to the prevailing needs of the individual.

Table 21.2 Tubular transport

Substance	Reabsorbed	Secreted
Water	Yes	No
Sodium	Yes	No
Potassium	Yes (proximally)	Yes (distally)
Calcium	Yes	No
Phosphate	Yes	No
Hydrogen ion	No	Yes
Bicarbonate	Yes	No
Glucose	Yes	No
Amino acids	Yes	No

Table 21.3 Quantitative aspects of tubular transport

Substance	Filtered load (per 24 h)	Typical urinary excretion (per 24 h)	% reabsorbed
Water	180 l	0.75–2.5 l	98.6–99.6
Sodium	25 000 mmol	100–250 mmol	99.0–99.6
Potassium	720 mmol	60–120 mmol	83.0–92.0
Calcium	234 mmol	5 mmol	98
Bicarbonate	4300 mmol	5 mmol	99.9
Glucose	810 mmol	1 mmol	99.9

SPECIFIC HOMEOSTATIC FUNCTIONS

The specific homeostatic functions of the kidney are shown in Table 21.1.

Regulation of body water content

Body water, usually accounting for about 50% of adult body weight, is kept constant by a homeostatic system (see also Ch. 22) in which both thirst and the renal handling of water are closely linked to the osmolality of the extracellular fluid (ECF). An increase in ECF osmolality is detected by osmoreceptors in the hypothalamus, stimulating both thirst and the release of ADH from the posterior pituitary. ADH activates an adenylate cyclase in the distal part of the nephron, increasing its permeability to water. Water then moves from the tubular lumen to the hyperosmolar medullary interstitium, the result being to promote water conservation by the kidney (Fig. 21.2). In the absence of ADH, the distal nephron is relatively impermeable to water, and the reabsorption of Na^+ and Cl^- without water results in the formation of dilute urine.

In health, the kidney can adjust the rate of water excretion over an enormous range (0.5–25 l/day) in response to changing water intake and non-renal water losses. The lower limit is imposed by the need to excrete the daily load of 600–900 mosm of solute (made up largely of urea and sodium chloride), and the inability of the kidney to increase urine concentration above 1200 mosm/kg water. There is thus an obligatory water loss of 500–750 ml per day, the exact amount depending on dietary protein and sodium intake.

Abnormalities of body water content are described in Chapter 22.

Regulation of body sodium content

Body sodium content is governed by the balance between intake (from the diet) and output (mainly in the urine but also to a variable extent in sweat and faeces). As with water, sodium ingestion varies widely, and the kidney is capable of modifying its handling of sodium in such a way as to maintain the constancy of body sodium.

About 25 000 mmol of sodium is filtered at the glomeruli each day; to prevent overwhelming sodium depletion, the vast bulk of the filtered sodium must therefore be reabsorbed. To achieve a urinary sodium output of 100–250 mmol/day (the range typically seen in normal subjects eating a UK diet), 99% or more of the filtered sodium must be reabsorbed. When there is a need for extreme sodium conservation, as in subjects with a low sodium intake or who have become sodium-depleted as a result of non-renal sodium losses, tubular reabsorption can be increased further still, until a urinary sodium concentration as low as 1–2 mmol/l is reached.

Most (50–75%) of the filtered sodium is reabsorbed iso-osmotically with chloride and water in the proximal tubule, the remainder being reabsorbed in the ascending limb of Henle's loop and in the distal nephron (Fig. 21.2). The

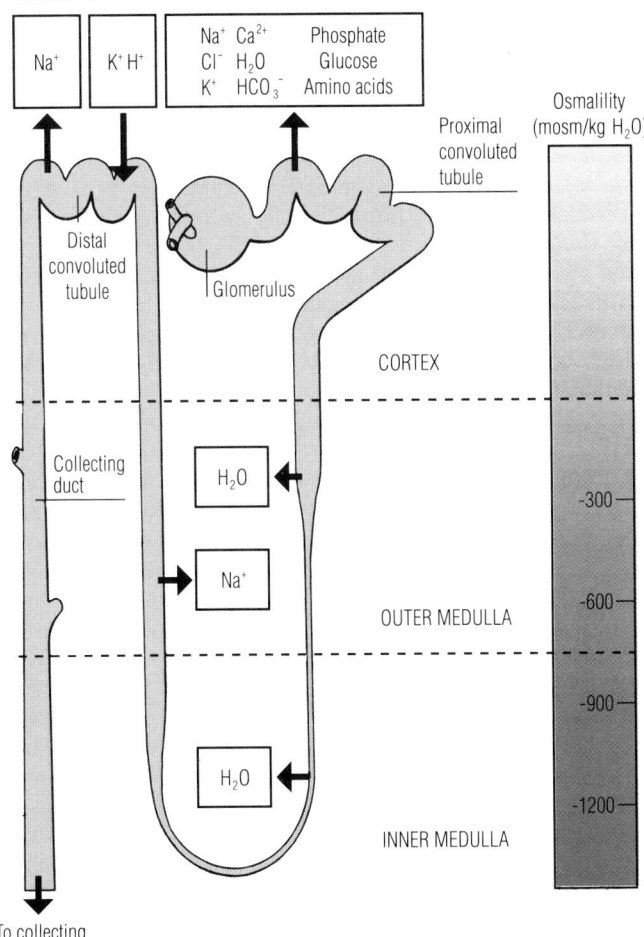

Na⁺ | K⁺ H⁺ | Na⁺ Ca²⁺ Phosphate
Cl⁻ H₂O Glucose
K⁺ HCO₃⁻ Amino acids

Proximal convoluted tubule

Osmalility (mosm/kg H₂O)

Distal convoluted tubule

Glomerulus

CORTEX

Collecting duct

H₂O

Na⁺

H₂O

-300

-600

-900

-1200

OUTER MEDULLA

INNER MEDULLA

To collecting system

Fig. 21.2 Modification of the glomerular filtrate by tubular action.

control of sodium reabsorption, and hence its excretion, is complex and incompletely understood, and is probably the result of a combination of hormonal (both systemic and local), neurogenic and vascular factors. Mineralocorticoids (predominantly aldosterone) are of great importance and act on the distal nephron to promote sodium reabsorption. These hormones are regulated in part by the activity of the renin-angiotensin system (itself influenced by the amount of sodium in the distal nephron in the vicinity of the macular densa) and in part by ACTH. In addition, the existence of a natriuretic hormone has been postulated and, recently, a potent peptide which promotes renal sodium excretion has been found in the atrium and chemically characterised. Designated *atrial natriuretic peptide* (ANP), its place in the overall scheme of renal sodium handling is still not clear, but it and other similar compounds may be of importance in the genesis of oedema-forming states (p. 842).

Regulation of body potassium content

As with sodium and water, the body content of potassium depends on the balance of intake (from the diet) and excretion, the latter being almost entirely renal. Potassium excretion by the kidney can also be varied over a wide

range (approximately 10–700 mmol/day). Typical dietary intake (and thus urinary excretion rate) in the developed countries is about 60–120 mmol/day.

The amount of potassium appearing in the GF is much lower than that of sodium because of its relatively low concentration in blood plasma – about 720 mmol/day assuming a GFR of 180 l/day and a plasma potassium concentration of 4 mmol/l ($180 \times 4 = 720$). About 75% of the filtered potassium is reabsorbed in the proximal tubule and further potassium reabsorption occurs along the ascending limb of Henle's loop (Fig. 21.2). Potassium secretion into the tubular fluid occurs in the distal nephron, and it is here that the excretion rate of potassium is regulated by a combination of factors of which the action of mineralocorticoids, especially aldosterone, is the most important. Aldosterone increases potassium secretion in the distal nephron, but this effect is not entirely subjugated to the control of aldosterone by body sodium. Potassium itself also influences aldosterone secretion; high plasma potassium concentration stimulates aldosterone secretion by the adrenal cortex directly, and also indirectly by augmenting potassium-dependent renin secretion. By this mechanism, potassium excess thus tends to correct itself. Additional control of potassium excretion is exerted by the prevailing requirements for sodium excretion and acid-base status (Ch. 22).

Regulation of acid-base status

In quantitative terms, by far the most important acidic product of metabolism is CO_2, derived mainly from aerobic respiration, but also from the hepatic metabolism of lactic acid, and the oxidation of free fatty acids (FFA) and ketone bodies. An adult produces some 15 000–20 000 mmol of CO_2 per day, and virtually all of this is eliminated via the lungs. However, in addition to CO_2, the body produces a much smaller amount of non-volatile acid, some of which (amounting to 50–100 mmol/day or approximately 1 mmol/kg body weight per day) can only be excreted by the kidney. This is the result of the metabolism of cystine- and methionine-containing proteins and also of the incomplete oxidation of fat, carbohydrate and protein; all of these processes yielding inorganic acids.

A helpful way to consider the role of the kidney in the maintenance of acid-base homeostasis is in terms of balance. The kidney generates and releases into the circulation an amount of bicarbonate that precisely balances the production of non-metabolisable, non-volatile acidic products of metabolism (i.e. 50–100 mmol of bicarbonate per day). To achieve this, a precisely equivalent amount of hydrogen ion (50–100 mmol/day) is excreted in the urine, the exact amount being regulated according to the prevailing production rate of non-volatile acids of metabolism.

The kidney achieves this balance in two ways (Fig. 21.3):

1. proximal 'reclamation' of filtered bicarbonate
2. urinary acidification in the distal nephron.

Proximal 'reclamation' of filtered bicarbonate. Bicarbonate ions in plasma are filtered at the glomerulus. The

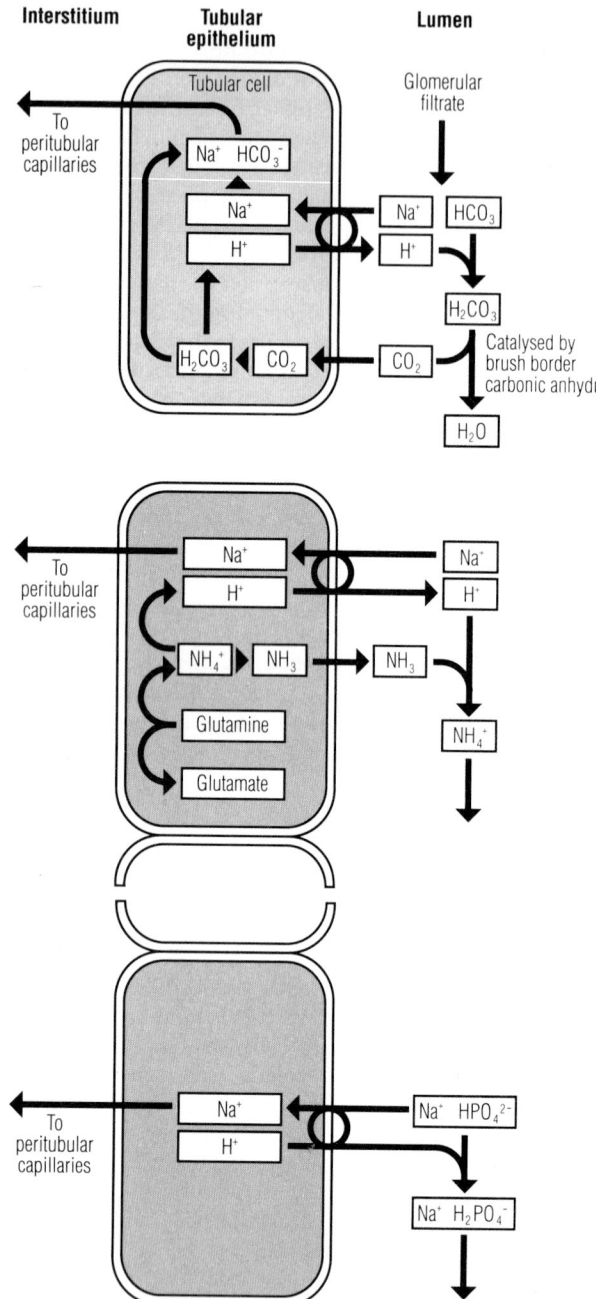

Fig. 21.3 Mechanisms of tubular action. Red = proximal tubular cell. Grey = distal tubular cells; the functions of the latter are separated for clarity.

blood. Between 80% and 90% of the bicarbonate reclamation occurs in the proximal tubule, and the rest in the distal tubule.

Urinary acidification in the distal nephron. The reclamation of the 10–20% of the filtered bicarbonate load that reaches the distal tubule is also dependent on active secretion of H^+ ions. Additional H^+ secreted is trapped in the tubular lumen by two urinary buffers, ammonia (NH_3) and phosphate, although the role of ammonia as a urinary buffer is becoming controversial. It has been thought that ammonia (produced from the deamination of glutamine by the tubular cells), acts as a proton acceptor in the tubular lumen, being converted to ammonium (NH_4^+) and trapping secreted H^+ in the lumen. Monohydrogen phosphate (HPO_4^{2-}), derived from the glomerular filtrate, accepts H^+ forming dihydrogen phosphate ($H_2PO_4^-$). These mechanisms allow substantial amounts of acid to be excreted in the urine, while at the same time limiting the resulting decrease in urinary pH.

Certain features of this classical description of distal acidification mechanisms may soon require revision, however. It is now clear that the bulk of renal NH_4^+ production occurs in the proximal tubular cells, and that NH_4^+ is then transported to distal sites. The pK of ammonia is 9.4, indicating that, at physiological pH, nearly all the ammonia is present as NH_4^+. Thus, the ammonia produced from glutamine in the proximal tubular cells is immediately converted to NH_4^+. The tubular cell membranes are relatively impermeable to NH_4^+, though permeable to ammonia, and so the NH_4^+ could only pass into the lumen by means of its equilibrium with ammonia (Fig. 21.3). Once in the tubular lumen, the ammonia can accept H^+ and thereby act as an urinary buffer. However, the generation of ammonia in this way also leads to the production of an equivalent amount of H^+. Thus, although the mechanism allows the buffering of urinary H^+ by ammonia, it cannot directly influence overall acid-base status.

The regulation of acid secretion is extremely complex. From the foregoing account, it is apparent that changes in the filtered load of bicarbonate and/or its reabsorption, alteration of the distal secretion of hydrogen ion or of the availability of the urinary buffers, ammonia and HPO_4^{2-}, can singly or in combination affect the return of bicarbonate ions to the renal venous blood.

Regulation of calcium and phosphorus metabolism

Calcium

Body calcium homeostasis is dependent on:

1. the movement of calcium between body fluids and the skeleton under the control of parathyroid hormone (PTH)
2. the intestinal absorption of dietary calcium, also under the control of PTH (acting indirectly via the vitamin D endocrine system)
3. the PTH-dependent regulation of the renal handling of calcium.

daily filtered load of bicarbonate is very large (about 4300 mmol/day) and, because its loss would rapidly lead to overwhelming bicarbonate depletion and acidosis, nearly all the filtered bicarbonate is reclaimed following titration in the tubular lumen by actively secreted H^+. The carbonic acid so formed is dehydrated to CO_2 and water (under the influence of brush border carbonic anhydrase). The CO_2 diffuses into the tubular cells and then combines with OH^- ions to form bicarbonate, before passing on to renal venous

Ultrafiltrable calcium in blood plasma amounts to about 1.3 mmol/l of the 2.4 mmol/l of calcium normally present in plasma. This means about 230 mmol of calcium appears in the GF each day. Of this, 50–60% is reabsorbed in the proximal tubule and the remainder in the thick ascending limb of Henle's loop, the distal convoluted tubule and the collecting tubule. In health, the reabsorption is almost complete, only some 5 mmol of the initial 230 mmol of filtered calcium appearing in the urine per day. The most important controlling influence on urinary calcium excretion is PTH, which increases tubular calcium reabsorption. Additional effects are exerted by the level of sodium excretion and acid-base status (both natriuresis and acidosis increase calciuria). Increases in the filtered load of calcium, such as occur in hypercalcaemic states, also increase the urinary output of calcium.

Phosphate

Renal phosphate handling is the major determinant of ECF phosphate concentration. The 80% of plasma phosphate that is not protein bound is filtered at the glomerulus and 80–90% of this is then reabsorbed by tubular transport. Most of the phosphate reabsorption occurs in the proximal tubule (70–80%), the remainder occurring in the distal convoluted and collecting tubules. The percentage of filtered phosphate that is reabsorbed can be varied over a wide range which, in health, is mainly in response to changes in dietary phosphate intake and PTH. The latter acts via cAMP to decrease tubular phosphate transport both in the proximal and distal nephron; PTH is thus a phosphaturic hormone.

THE ENDOCRINE FUNCTION OF THE KIDNEY

Hormone synthesis by the kidney. The hormones produced by the kidney are listed in Table 21.4. They may act locally in the kidney or on remote target tissues. In the cases of 1,25-dihydroxyvitamin D, renin and erythropoietin, the kidney is the sole, or major site of production.

Hormone metabolism by the kidney. Polypeptide hormones (PTH, insulin), steroid and thyroid hormones are subject to varying degrees of renal catabolism, which may be altered in the presence of kidney disease.

Hormones with major renal actions. The kidney is a target organ for many hormones (Table 21.4), all acting to influence the kidney's performance of its various homeostatic functions.

ASSESSMENT OF RENAL STRUCTURE AND FUNCTION

Examination of the urine

Quantity

Most normal adults in temperate climates pass between 750 and 2500 ml of urine per day. *Anuria* is the complete

Table 21.4 Hormones and the kidney

Hormone	Synthesised in kidney	Action on kidney
1,25-dihydroxyvitamin D	Yes	Increases tubular calcium reabsorption
Renin/angiotensin	Yes	Autoregulation and distribution of renal blood flow
Prostaglandins (PGE$_2$ and PGI$_2$)	Yes	Autoregulation and distribution of renal blood flow Increase renin release Influence water handling
Erythropoietin	Yes	None
Kallikrein	Yes	Autoregulation and distribution of renal blood flow Influences sodium and water handling
PTH	No	Increases phosphaturia Increases bicarbonaturia Increases tubular calcium reabsorption Increases synthesis of 1,25-dihydroxyvitamin D
Vasopressin	No	Increases antidiuresis
Aldosterone	No	Increases tubular Na$^+$ reabsorption Increases tubular K$^+$ and H$^+$ secretion
Catecholamines	No	Increase renin release
Atrial natriuretic peptide	No	Increases sodium excretion

absence of urine flow. *Oliguria* implies diminished urine flow and is present when the urine flow rate is less than the minimum required to allow excretion of a daily solute load (about 500 ml/day in an adult). *Polyuria* is a nebulous term, indicating passage of large volumes of urine, but implying nothing about the appropriateness (or otherwise) or cause of the high urine flow rate.

Specific gravity/osmolality

Measurement of the specific gravity and osmolality of the urine provide similar information and, in the absence of significant glycosuria, are functions of the urinary concentrations of sodium, chloride and urea. The range of specific gravity is 1.001–1.035 (equivalent to 50–1300 mosm/kg water). Even heavy protein excretion alters these figures only minimally.

pH

Urinary pH varies from 4 to 8 and may be measured

Renal and Urinary Disease

Table 21.5 Conditions associated with extremes of urinary pH

Acid	Alkaline
High protein diet	Vegetarian diet
Acid ingestion (ascorbic acid, ammonium chloride)	Alkali ingestion (sodium bicarbonate, potassium citrate)
Metabolic acidosis	Infection with urea-splitting organisms
Respiratory acidosis (acute)	Metabolic alkalosis
Water deprivation	Respiratory alkalosis (acute)
Potassium depletion	Renal tubular acidosis (type I)
Hyperaldosteronism	Water diuresis

using paper strips impregnated with an indicator or, more accurately, by means of a pH electrode. Conditions associated with extremes of urinary pH are shown in Table 21.5.

Glucose

The use of glucose-oxidase-impregnated dipsticks provides a simple and specific semi-quantitative test for glucose in urine. The commonest cause of abnormal glycosuria is elevation of the plasma glucose concentration to above 8.3–10 mmol/l, at which point the tubular reabsorptive capacity for glucose is exceeded. In addition, a number of rare disorders of tubular function may be associated with glycosuria at normal plasma glucose concentrations; these disorders are collectively designated *renal glycosuria*.

Protein

Most people excrete less than 150 mg of protein per day in the urine and, with the exception of orthostatic proteinuria (see below), levels above this imply disease of the kidney or urinary tract. Semi-quantitative testing is done using dipsticks (sensitive to 200–300 mg protein per l) or by the more cumbersome salicylsulphonic acid test (sensitive to 100–150 mg protein per l). The latter has the advantage of detecting Bence-Jones protein (immunoglobulin light chains). Additional information may be obtained from quantitative measurement of the protein content of timed urine collections. Variation in the albumin excretion rate below the threshold for detection by dipsticks can now be followed using sensitive specific assays for urinary albumin. This is increasingly employed to detect very early glomerular damage. For example, in diabetics, urinary albumin excretion above the normal range (i.e. exceeding 30–40 mg/day) predicts the later development of clinical diabetic nephropathy.

The protein excretion rate is generally increased in the upright posture and, on occasion, this may lead to abnormally high protein measurements in timed collections or spot measurements in normal ambulant subjects. This is termed *orthostatic proteinuria* and the diagnostic difficulty may be resolved by demonstrating that an early morning urine specimen is normal while a specimen taken later in the day with the subject ambulant contains excess protein.

The diagnostic implications of abnormal protein excretion depend on both its *magnitude* (Table 21.6) and, to a lesser extent, its *selectivity*. Heavy proteinuria is always of glomerular origin, and albumin predominates over larger molecular weight protein such as globulins. In *highly selective proteinuria*, only albumin is present in significant amounts, whereas, with non-selective proteinuria, the much larger globulins are present as well. Protein selectivity measurements are of little use in adults, but in children are helpful in predicting the nature and likely response to treatment of nephrotic syndrome (p. 811).

Table 21.6 Diagnostic implications of proteinuria

Degree of proteinuria	Diagnostic implications
Mild (up to 500 mg/day)	Fever Benign hypertensive nephrosclerosis Renal tumour Obstructive nephropathy Prerenal uraemia Tubulointerstitial nephropathy Chronic pyelonephritis Orthostatic proteinuria
Moderate (up to 3 g/day)	Urinary tract infection Chronic pyelonephritis Acute tubular necrosis Acute glomerulonephritis Chronic glomerulonephritis Obstructive nephropathy Accelerated phase hypertension Orthostatic proteinuria
Heavy (more than 3 g/day)	Pre-eclampsia Myeloma Acute glomerulonephritis Chronic glomerulonephritis All causes of nephrotic syndrome

Blood

Blood in the urine may lead to a visible red or brown discolouration or smoky appearance when present in quantities exceeding 0.5 ml/l. Potentially confusing appearances may be seen in haemoglobinuria (as a consequence of haemoglobinaemia), porphyria, and dye or drug ingestion (e.g. beetroot, rifampicin). Smaller amounts of blood, insufficient to lead to visible discolouration, may be detected by chemical tests for haemoglobin using dipsticks. A positive test for haemoglobin should always be followed by microscopic examination for red blood cells. This will distinguish haematuria from haemoglobinuria (in which no red cells will be seen). Careful assessment of red cell morphology using phase contrast microscopy may indicate whether they are derived from the renal parenchyma (dysmorphic red blood cells) or from the collecting system, ureters or bladder (normal red blood cells).

Culture

Although bladder urine should be sterile, voided urine is not and interpretation of bacteriological studies of the urine must take account of this. Contamination is minimised (though not eliminated) by use of the *midstream urine* (MSU) or *clean catch* technique, in which the initial part of the voided stream is discarded and the mid-portion of the stream collected in a sterile container. In the female, this should be preceded by cleaning of the external genitalia. The likelihood of significant infection is high if:

1. a pure growth of a single organism is obtained (multiple organisms often indicate contamination)
2. the number of bacteria exceeds 10^5/ml
3. leucocytes are present in the spun deposit of fresh urine (*pyuria*).

Deposit

The microscopic examination of a fresh unstained deposit of spun urine is an important part of the examination of any patient in whom disease of the urinary tract is suspected, and often yields important diagnostic information. A search is made for cells, casts and crystals (Table 21.7). Urinary casts consist of Tamm-Horsfall protein derived from the tubular epithelium, and are probably formed in the distal nephron. Hyaline casts contain no cellular elements or debris and may be seen in very small numbers in normal urine. Cellular casts, in which the Tamm-Horsfall matrix is studded with rbc's or wbc's are indicative of parenchymal renal disease. Granular casts are probably degenerate cellular casts and have a granular or grainy appearance. The number of cells and casts seen is usually expressed per high power field.

Measurement of GFR

The renal clearance of a substance is calculated from the formula:

$$\frac{UV}{P}$$

where U = urinary concentration, V = urine flow rate (usually expressed in ml/min) and P = plasma concentration. Calculation of GFR requires a test substance that is freely filtered at the glomerulus, but neither reabsorbed nor secreted by the tubules (Table 21.8). The polysaccharide, inulin, has ideal characteristics but the methodology is cumbersome, precluding its use in clinical practice. However, the renal handling of endogenously produced creatinine is similar to that of inulin and reliable estimates of GFR can generally be obtained from measurements of creatinine clearance. This requires only the measurement of plasma creatinine concentration in plasma and in a timed urine collection of known volume.

GFR can also be calculated simply from knowledge of the plasma creatinine concentrations and reference to 'normal values'. The formula for calculating creatinine clearance (UV/P) indicates that GFR is inversely related to plasma creatinine concentration (Fig. 21.4). Thus, assuming a constant production rate of creatinine, a halving of GFR will lead to a doubling of plasma creatinine concentration, a fourfold decrease in GFR to a fourfold increase in plasma creatinine concentration, and so on. This method is very useful for monitoring *changes* in GFR in the same subject, but substantial individual variations in muscle bulk (and hence creatinine production rate) necessitate the inclusion of several correction factors before reasonably accurate GFR estimates can be made. Never-

Table 21.7 The urinary sediment in various renal conditions

Condition	Rbc	Wbc	Rbc casts	Granular casts	Hyaline casts
Acute glomerulonephritis	4	0–4	1–4	1–3	1–3
Chronic glomerulonephritis	1–3	0–1	0–2	1–3	1–3
'Minimal change' nephrotic syndrome	0–1	0	0	0–1	0–3
Acute tubular necrosis	1–3	1–3	0–2	1–3	1–3
Prerenal uraemia	0–1	0–1	0	0–1	0–2
Acute pyelonephritis	0–2	4	0	1–2	1–2
Chronic pyelonephritis	0–1	0	0	0–1	0–1
Benign hypertensive nephrosclerosis	0–1	0	0	0–1	0–1
Accelerated phase hypertension	1–4	0–1	0–2	0–2	0–2
Pre-eclampsia	0–1	0–1	0	0–1	0–3
Urinary tuberculosis	0–4	2–4	0	0–2	0–2
Tumour	0–4	0–1	0	0	0–1

The numbers 0–4 refer to the extent of the abnormality in each case.

Table 21.8 Characteristics of compounds used to measure GFR

Characteristic	Ideal marker	Inulin	Creatinine	Urea
Freely filtered at glomerulus	Yes	Yes	Yes	Yes
Tubular reabsorption	No	No	No	Yes
Tubular secretion	No	No	Yes	No
Ease of assay	Easy	Difficult	Easy	Easy
Endogenously produced	Yes	No	Yes	Yes*

*but variable rate

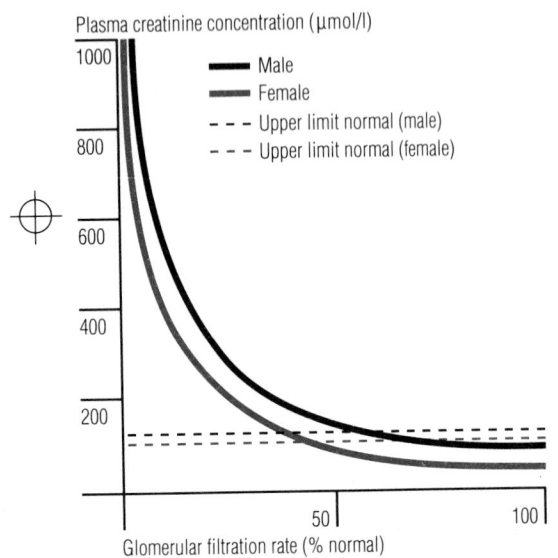

Fig. 21.4 Relationship between glomerular filtration rate (GFR) and plasma creatinine concentration. At relatively high levels of renal function, changes in GFR are associated with only very small changes in plasma creatinine concentration. However, at low levels of GFR, a relatively small change in GFR is associated with a very large change in plasma creatinine concentration.

Fig. 21.5 Changes in glomerular filtration rate with age.

theless, plasma creatinine measurement is one of the most frequently performed and useful tests of renal function.

Similar measurements can be made using urea instead of creatinine, but these are much less informative owing to wide fluctuations in urea production rate and substantial and variable tubular reabsorption of urea (Table 21.8).

Radionuclide methods

The GFR can be measured by injecting a radioactive substance that is handled by the kidney in the same way as inulin and then following its disappearance from plasma. ^{51}CrEDTA is a suitable radiopharmaceutical, and allows easy and reproducible calculation of GFR.

Range of GFR and effect of ageing

The GFR in a normal adult is about 120 ml/min (Fig. 21.5). In children over two years of age, GFR is closely related to body surface area and should be expressed in relation to this. GFR peaks between the ages of 20 and 30 years, subsequently decreasing by 1 ml/min per year, this decrease being paralleled by the slow decrease in muscle mass commensurate with ageing, such that plasma creatinine concentration changes little with advancing age. Appreciation of these age-related changes in GFR is important in clinical practice, particularly when considering dose modification of drugs prescribed to the elderly.

Measurement of renal plasma flow

The estimation of renal plasma flow requires a test sub-

stance that is both filtered at the glomerulus and rapidly secreted by the tubules such that none reaches renal venous blood. Para-aminohippuric acid has the required characteristics, but this measurement is almost never required in clinical practice; it remains important as a research tool however.

Imaging of the kidney and urinary tract

The principles of imaging are discussed in Chapter 2.

Plain radiographs

In many people, one or both kidneys may be visible on plain abdominal radiographs or plain nephrotomograms, giving information about the presence, location, size and shape of the kidneys, as well as revealing certain types of renal stone or other calcifications.

Intravenous urography (IVU)

The injection of organic iodine compounds that are excreted by the kidneys opacifies first the renal parenchyma (nephrogram), and later the collecting system (pyelogram), ureters and bladder. As well as providing important structural information, the IVU also demonstrates the presence or absence of excretory function (Fig. 21.6). The quality of images may be poor if excretion is slow, as in severe renal disease, but can be enhanced by the administration of large doses of contrast material and nephrotomography. Although the IVU is commonly employed and is often very useful, it is not entirely benign and carries a mortality of about one in 40 000 studies, with a substantial incidence of non-fatal adverse reactions to the injected contrast material.

Antegrade and retrograde urography

The morphology of the collecting system and ureters may not be demonstrated adequately by IVU if excretory function is poor. The direct introduction of contrast material into the kidney (antegrade pyelography) or lower ureter during cystoscopy (retrograde pyelography) may yield further information if these invasive procedures are

Fig. 21.6 Intravenous urogram showing obstructed right kidney. The IVU shows normal morphology on the left and dilatation of the pelvicalyceal system on the right, due to pelviureteric junction obstruction.

A

B

Fig. 21.7 Antegrade pyelograms showing obstruction of the right kidney due to a stricture in the lower part of the ureter. Contrast has been introduced directly into the dilated collecting system of the kidney via a percutaneously inserted catheter (**A**). The obstruction is shown in the lower ureter in **B**.

deemed appropriate (Fig. 21.7). Such investigations are most commonly used in the detailed assessment of patients with obstruction of the urinary tract.

Cystography

In cystography, the bladder is filled with contrast material via the urethra and radiographs taken before, during and after micturition, usually to see whether urine refluxes up the ureters. The investigation is invasive, carrying the risk of introducing infection. It is usually performed in children with urinary infections in whom reflux nephropathy is suspected.

Ultrasonography

Ultrasonography allows totally non-invasive evaluation of gross renal morphology and visualisation of adjacent tissues (Fig. 21.8). It is useful in the diagnosis of cystic diseases of the kidney, renal tumours and renal obstruction. Unlike the IVU, imaging by renal ultrasound does not depend on the presence of excretory function, and so non-functioning kidneys can be seen just as well as functioning ones. On the other hand, ultrasonography yields no information on the relative function of the kidneys.

Computerised tomography

Computerised tomography (CT) gives detailed structural information about the kidneys and surrounding tissues, the ureters and bladder. It is particularly useful in the assessment of the retroperitoneum in cases of obstruction.

Arteriography and venography

The arterial and venous vasculature of the kidney can be seen following direct injection of contrast material into the renal artery or vein respectively (Fig. 21.9). These procedures are invasive and are used when compromise of the renal blood supply, leading to hypertension or impairment of renal function, is suspected. Pathological circulation to a renal tumour can be demonstrated in this way, although the advent of good quality ultrasonography and CT has made most arteriography redundant, except when the tumour is to be embolised. Venography is performed in cases where ultrasonography and/or CT have failed adequately to exclude renal vein thrombosis.

795

Fig. 21.8 **Renal ultrasound examinations. A.** Longitudinal scan of a normal kidney. The characteristic renal outline can be seen with the echogenic centre area representing the normal pelvicalyceal system and its associated fat. The surrounding elliptical renal parenchyma produces low level echoes and appears much darker. **B.** A dilated and obstructed collecting system. The large echo-free (i.e. black) renal pelvis and widened upper ureter can be seen in the centre of the picture. **C.** In this kidney (18 cm in length), multiple cysts are seen as round, echo-free areas throughout the renal parenchyma: polycystic kidney disease.

Fig. 21.9 **Renal arteriograms. A.** Normal right kidney. **B.** Left renal artery stenosis.

Radionuclide studies

Radionuclide studies allow both structure and function to be evaluated and have the advantage of low associated radiation exposure compared with IVU. ^{99}TcDMSA (dimercaptosuccinic acid) is used to show gross renal morphology and either ^{99}TcDTPA (diethylenetriamine pentacetic acid) or ^{131}I hippuran renograms to investigate function. In isotope renography, simultaneous counting over both kidneys is done and analysis of the resulting renograms (Fig. 21.10) may indicate the relative contribution of the two kidneys to total function (divided renal function), delay in perfusion (suggestive of renal vascular disease), or a progressive increase in activity with time (suggestive of obstruction).

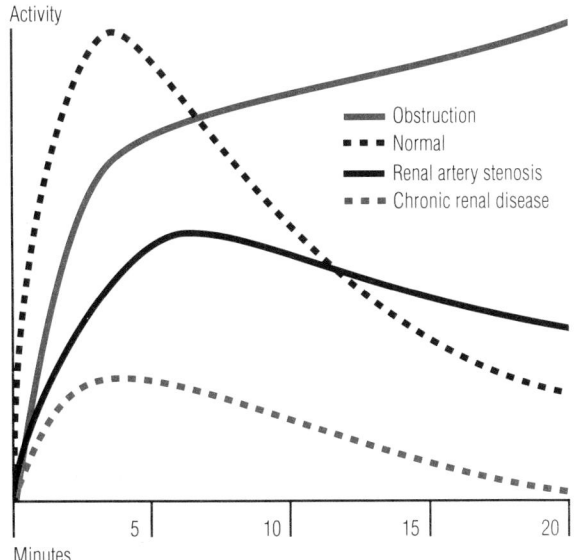

Fig. 21.10   DTPA isotope renograms typical of various conditions. In obstruction, the increase in activity up to twenty minutes results from the progressive accumulation of isotope within the obstructed collecting system. In renal artery stenosis, the arrival of the bolus of isotope is delayed, leading to a delayed peak and subsequently slow clearance. In chronic renal parenchymal disease, the arrival of the bolus is not delayed with respect to normal, but is of much reduced intensity, reflecting the low renal blood flow and low glomerular filtration rate.

Renal biopsy

The kidneys may be biopsied with relative safety using a cutting biopsy needle passed into the kidney through the renal angle under local anaesthetic. Preconditions that should be satisfied before biopsy is undertaken are:

1. an appropriate indication (Summary 1)
2. a cooperative patient
3. absence of bleeding disorder
4. prompt availability of blood for transfusion in the event of haemorrhage
5. prior knowledge of the position, size and function of both kidneys. A solitary functioning kidney should rarely be biopsied.

> **Summary 1   Utility of renal biopsy**
>
> *Often helpful*
> Acute renal failure of uncertain cause
> Rapidly progressive renal disease (especially if crescentic nephritis suspected)
> Collagen disease, e.g. SLE, polyarteritis
> Renal haematuria (cause unclear)
> Proteinuria (cause unclear)
> Nephrotic syndrome
> Transplant assessment
> Suspected amyloid
>
> *Sometimes helpful*
> Slowly progressive renal disease (with kidneys of normal size)
> Diabetic nephropathy
>
> *Not indicated*
> Suspected renal infection
> End stage renal disease, especially if kidneys are small
> Renal cystic disease

The procedure is carried out with the patient lying prone and may be aided by simultaneous localisation of both kidney and biopsy needle using ultrasonography. One or two small samples of renal cortex are taken, each containing 10–50 glomeruli, and used for light microscopy, electron microscopy and immunoperoxidase studies, allowing the presence and distribution of fibrin, complement, IgG, IgA and IgM to be defined.

The safety of renal biopsy is difficult to determine. Mortality appears to be in the region of 0.1% and serious morbidity, e.g. bleeding necessitating nephrectomy, occurs in about 0.25–0.5% of cases. Minor morbidity, such as significant pain or bleeding requiring transfusion, may arise in about 2% of cases.

MAJOR SYMPTOMS AND SIGNS OF RENAL AND URINARY DISEASE

The symptoms and signs associated with renal and urinary disease are diverse and often non-specific (Summary 2). In many patients, these features may remain subtle and nebulous, even when renal impairment is moderately severe, and this may lead to the patient seeking medical advice late in the course of the disease.

Haematuria

Haematuria may be macroscopic or microscopic, painful or painless, continuous or intermittent, persist throughout the act of micturition or be present only at the beginning or end of micturition. Haematuria due to renal parenchymal disease is usually continuous, painless and microscopic, although it may on occasion be macroscopic or intermittent. In contrast, haematuria arising from renal tumours is usually intermittent and painless and that from bladder tumours may be intermittent and sometimes painful.

Renal and Urinary Disease

Summary 3 Symptoms and signs of uraemic syndrome

Nervous system	Fatigue, malaise, depression, impaired thought, involuntary movements, nausea, fits, coma, pruritus, paraesthesiae, neuropathy
Cardio-pulmonary	Pericarditis, pleurisy, Kussmaul breathing, dyspnoea
Dermatological	Pruritus, purpura, pallor, pigmentation, urea frost
Gastrointestinal	Anorexia, nausea, vomiting, GI bleeding, constipation, diarrhoea, peptic ulceration, angiodysplasia, colitis, foetor
Haematological	Anaemia (normochromic, normocytic), bleeding (disordered platelet function)

Proteinuria

Protein does not discolour the urine, and is therefore usually noticed as a result of routine urine examination or following the development of associated symptoms of renal disease or, in the case of heavy proteinuria, the development of the nephrotic syndrome (p. 811).

Hypertension

Hypertension is much commoner in people with renal disease than in those without. As many as 80% of patients with abnormal renal function, or who are receiving renal replacement therapy by dialysis, will have experienced significant (and in many cases severe) hypertension at some stage during their illness. Conversely, there are occasions when severe hypertension may, by leading to vascular changes within the kidney, be the cause of renal disease.

Oedema

Renal disease may give rise to oedema as a consequence of inappropriate retention of sodium and water, leading to over-expansion of the ECF, or reduction in plasma oncotic pressure as a result of heavy urinary protein losses (nephrotic syndrome, see p. 811). In some cases, both these mechanisms are operative. Over-expansion of the ECF (in the absence of severe hypoalbuminaemia) may be accompanied by hypertension and expansion of the vascular compartment to the point where pulmonary oedema develops. This is particularly likely to occur in subjects with diminished cardiac reserve.

Uraemia

The *uraemic syndrome* is a group of symptoms and signs (Summary 3), some or all of which are found in patients with serious reduction of excretory capacity (i.e. of GFR), from any cause. The uraemic syndrome rarely manifests itself clinically until the GFR has fallen to 20% of normal or less. The pathogenesis and management of the uraemic syndrome is discussed on pages 804–811.

Renal pain

Renal pain is usually perceived in the loin or flank, although in the case of ureteric obstruction leading to renal pain,

Table 21.9 Causes of renal pain

Obstructive	Stone (kidney, ureter)
	Tumour
	Sloughed papilla
	Blood clot
	Pelviureteric obstruction
Non-obstructive	Renal swelling ± inflammation
	Acute pyelonephritis
	Renal vein thrombosis
	Renal cysts
	Renal tumour
	Acute nephritis (rare)
	Renal infarction
	Trauma

discomfort may be felt in the iliac fossa, testicle or labia, this depending partly on the level of the obstruction. The commonest, and most spectacular, cause of renal pain is acute obstruction by a stone; this is of fairly rapid onset and great severity. Other causes of renal pain are listed in Table 21.9.

Oliguria/anuria

Oliguria is the passage of less than 500 ml of urine/day; anuria means cessation of urine flow. The causes may conveniently be divided into:

1. *pre-renal*, where primary decrease in renal blood flow leads to compromise of function in an otherwise normal kidney

2. *renal*, i.e. intrinsic renal disease of any type

3. *post-renal*, due to mechanical obstruction, which may be at any point from the collecting system in the kidney

to the urethra. Acute obstruction to bladder outflow only results in impairment of renal function when the maximum bladder capacity is reached.

In general, the causes of anuria and oliguria are the same as those of acute renal failure (Table 21.13).

Polyuria

The causes of polyuria (increased urine flow) rate fall into three groups (Table 21.10). In some patients with diabetes insipidus, polyuria may be spectacular with daily urine output as great as 25 litres.

Table 21.10 Causes of polyuria

Excessive water intake	Abnormal tubular water handling
Psychogenic polydipsia	Pituitary diabetes insipidus
Beer drinking	Inherited nephrogenic diabetes insipidus (rare)
Osmotic diuresis	Acquired nephrogenic diabetes insipidus
Diabetes mellitus (glucose)*	Hypokalaemia
Chronic renal failure (urea)*	Hypercalcaemia
Diuretics (NaCl)*	Obstructive uropathy
	Tubulointerstitial diseases

* The respective osmotic diuretics are given in parentheses.

Frequency

Frequency of micturition may result from polyuria or decreased functional bladder capacity (Table 21.11).

Table 21.11 Causes of frequency and nocturia

Cause	Example
Infection*	Cystitis/urethritis/prostatitis Bacterial, including TB Fungal Parasitic (schistosomiasis)
Neoplasia*	Bladder tumour
Anatomical	Prostatic hypertrophy Urethral stricture
Neurological	Multiple sclerosis

* Often associated with dysuria also.

Nocturia

The absence of nocturia depends on the normal reduction in urine flow rate during the night and an adequate functional bladder capacity. Polyuria of any cause may thus result in nocturia, as may acute and chronic renal diseases, certain drugs such as corticosteroids and diuretics, and ingestion of large volumes of fluid late in the day; all of

these, in one way or another, interfere with the normal diurnal variation in urine flow rate.

Reduction of functional bladder capacity due to local factors (e.g. infection, contracted bladder, outflow obstruction, tumour) or remote ones (e.g. neurological diseases) will also result in nocturia, in this case not associated with polyuria.

Dysuria

Dysuria may be defined as pain immediately before, during or immediately after micturition. The discomfort is often perceived as a 'burning' or 'scalding' sensation from the urine, and may be associated with frequency, decreased functional bladder capacity, urgency or hesitancy of micturition. Infection and neoplasia are the main causes; these and other causes of dysuria may also be associated with frequency.

Urgency of micturition, incontinence and enuresis

Urgency is the inability to postpone micturition significantly beyond the moment when the desire to micturate is first perceived. It may lead to *urge incontinence* if the patient cannot get to an appropriate place to void quickly enough.

Incontinence is the involuntary passage of urine and may result from disorders of the bladder, its nerve supply or within the CNS (see also p. 836). Incontinence occurring exclusively at night is termed *enuresis* and may be primary (failure to attain nocturnal bladder control in childhood) or secondary (development of enuresis following previous nocturnal continence). The above conditions are discussed further on page 837.

MAJOR RENAL SYNDROMES

Each of the syndromes discussed below (and listed in Summary 4) has a variety of potential causes. Similarly, although some of these causes are usually associated with a particular renal syndrome, this is by no means always the case.

Summary 4 Major renal syndromes

- Acute renal failure (including acute tubular necrosis)
- Acute nephritic syndrome
- Rapidly progressive glomerulonephritis (RPGN)
- Chronic renal failure
- Nephrotic syndrome
- Recurrent haematuria
- Persistent, asymptomatic proteinuria and/or haematuria
- Renal tubular syndromes

ACUTE RENAL FAILURE

Acute renal failure (ARF) is the rapid deterioration of renal function over a period of hours or days. It is important to appreciate that, although oliguria and anuria are frequent accompaniments, this need not be the case; the cardinal index is a rapid decline in GFR, leading to nitrogen retention. This may arise de novo, or against a background of pre-existing stable chronic renal impairment (Table 21.12); and distinguishing between these two possibilities is an important part of the diagnostic process.

The causes of acute renal failure may be pre-renal, renal and post-renal (p. 798), and it is helpful to bear these categories in mind when assessing a patient with apparent acute renal failure (Table 21.13).

Pre-renal ARF

Pre-renal ARF is associated with a low cardiac output, intense renal vasoconstriction and reduced GFR with resulting oliguria, and avid salt and water retention. *The kidney is structurally normal but functionally compromised.* Removal of pre-renal factors leads to rapid and complete recovery of renal function. The necessary measures may include correction of hypovolaemia with blood or saline, treatment of sepsis or improvement of cardiac function (if possible). Adequate and prompt correction of any relevant pre-renal factors listed will lead to rapid improvement of renal function. However, if severe and/or prolonged, these factors may, by production of severe renal vasoconstriction, lead to ischaemic renal injury (*acute tubular necrosis*, ATN). Thus the identification and rapid correction of pre-renal factors is of paramount importance in the management of these patients. A very severe and intractable type of pre-renal ARF – the *hepatorenal syndrome* – is sometimes seen in patients with severe liver disease. The nature of the interaction between the liver and kidney is obscure. Renal recovery is unusual in the absence of hepatic recovery.

Renal ARF

In renal ARF, there are established structural abnormalities in the kidney. In some cases (e.g. post-infectious glomerulonephritis, acute tubulointerstitial nephropathy), the disease process may primarily involve the kidney with little evidence of disease elsewhere. Alternatively, there may be evidence of multisystem disease such as systemic lupus erythematosus, infective endocarditis, polyarteritis nodosa, Henoch-Schönlein purpura, or of nephrotoxic exposure.

The coexistence of any of the pre-renal factors (given in Table 21.13) raises the possibility of established ATN, and these factors should always be corrected as far as possible in the hope that progression from pre-renal ARF to ATN may be averted. The distinction between established ATN and pre-renal ARF in an oliguric patient is an important one, and, fortunately, is generally fairly straightforward. It may be made on the basis of one or more of the features

Table 21.12 Diagnostic features distinguishing between acute and chronic renal failure

Favour acute	Favour chronic
• Known recent onset	• History of nocturia
• Known precipitating factor(s)	• Pigmentation
• Near normal haematology	• Small kidneys
• Normal size kidneys (ultrasound, plain X-rays, IVU)	• Bone disease (radiographic or biochemical)
	• Normochromic anaemia

Table 21.13 Causes of acute renal failure

Pre-renal

Any cause of shock
    Hypovolaemia: haemorrhage, burns, salt and water depletion, perforated viscus, pancreatitis, post-operative (especially aortic, cardiac and biliary surgery)
Sepsis
Cardiogenic

Renal arterial or venous disease: renal artery stenosis, renal vein thrombosis

Inappropriate renal vasoconstriction, e.g. hepatorenal syndrome

Renal

Acute tubular necrosis following hypovolaemia or shock of any cause

Acute glomerulonephritis

Acute glomerulonephritis with multisystem disease, e.g. SLE, Henoch–Shönlein purpura, infective endocarditis

Disease of small/medium sized blood vessels, e.g. haemolytic uraemic syndrome, thrombotic thrombocytopenic purpura, disseminated intravascular coagulation, polyarteritis nodosa, systemic sclerosis, accelerated phase hypertension

Acute tubulointerstitial disease

Exogenous nephrotoxins, e.g. drugs, ethylene glycol, heavy metals, X-ray contrast media

Endogenous nephrotoxins, e.g. myoglobin, haemoglobin, bilirubin, uric acid, Bence-Jones protein

Post-renal

Any cause of obstruction
    Stone (bilateral or affecting solitary kidney)
    Ureteric obstruction by pelvic malignancy (cervix, bladder, prostate, rectum)
    Bladder outflow obstruction
    Retroperitoneal disease (lymphoma, aortic dissection, retroperitoneal fibrosis)

listed in Table 21.14. Renal hypoperfusion is the commonest cause of ATN, although in some cases the lesion appears to develop as a result of a combined insult due to hypoperfusion and exposure to a nephrotoxin (Table 21.13). The renal vasoconstriction may be very severe and in many cases seems out of proportion to accompanying

Table 21.14 Distinction between pre-renal and renal causes of acute renal failure in an oliguric patient

Feature	Favours pre-renal cause	Favours renal cause
Identifiable pre-renal factor, e.g. shock, hypovolaemia	Yes	No
Urine		
Protein	0–1	1–4
Red blood cells	0	1–3
White blood cells	0	1–3
Casts	0–1	1–3
Osmolality (mosm/kg/H_2O)	more than 500	less than 400
Sodium (mmol/1)	less than 20	more than 35
Urine/plasma urea ratio	more than 8	less than 3
Urine/plasma creatinine ratio	more than 40	less than 20
Fractional excretion of sodium*	less than 1%	more than 1%

* Fractional excretion of sodium is the percentage of the total filtered load of sodium that appears in the final urine (Table 21.3). The numbers 0–4 indicate the degree of urinary abnormality.

increases in systemic vascular resistance. Prevention of this 'inappropriately' severe renal vasoconstriction is a frequent therapeutic goal, but is difficult to achieve other than by avoiding or rapidly correcting shock states. The renal lesion is tubular necrosis with subsequent regeneration. The glomeruli are relatively spared. The process of repair may last from a few days to several weeks and generally leads eventually to complete or near complete recovery of renal function. If the ischaemic damage is very severe, however, varying degrees of cortical necrosis may occur and recovery of function is then limited or negligible. For reasons not fully understood, cortical necrosis is particularly likely to occur in relation to shock occurring during pregnancy, such as may arise following ante-partum haemorrhage.

Post-renal ARF

Important causes of post-renal ARF are given in Table 21.13. The syndrome of ARF will only develop if the obstruction is bilateral, or if it affects a solitary functioning kidney. Thus, obstruction of one ureter by a stone does not lead to ARF, whereas obstruction of both ureters by pelvic malignancy does. Early identification of post-renal factors in a patient with ARF is most important if therapy is to be appropriately directed and irreversible obstructive injury to the kidneys averted. Assessment may be aided by prior knowledge of the presence of one of the potentially obstructing lesions. Physical examination may reveal a pelvic mass or enlarged kidneys or bladder. Ultrasound examination of the kidneys is valuable, both to give a positive diagnosis of obstruction, and also to exclude obstruction as a likely factor in patients with ARF. In some cases, intravenous urography may be undertaken, but the pictures can be equivocal and delayed films (up to 24 hours following the injection) may be needed. Invasive imaging

of the urinary tract by antegrade or retrograde ureterography is rarely needed to make the diagnosis, but may, along with cystoscopy, be of help in the detailed assessment of the obstructed patient.

Management

Pre-renal ARF will, by definition, respond promptly to correction of the pre-renal factor(s).

Renal ARF may be of a type in which resolution usually occurs within days or weeks (e.g. ATN, post-infectious glomerulonephritis, some toxic nephropathies), or it may lead to irreversible renal failure (e.g. renal infarction, some types of acute glomerulonephritis and renal vasculitis). In some cases (e.g. renal vasculitis), resolution of the renal lesion may follow therapy with steroids, cytotoxic drugs or plasma exchange.

Post-renal ARF is treated by relief of the obstruction, usually by mechanical means (such as insertion of ureteric stent, percutaneous nephrostomy, removal of stone) pending further assessment of the feasibility of definitive relief of the obstructing lesion. In a few patients, non-mechanical measures, such as radiotherapy, anti-tumour chemotherapy or steroids, may obviate the need for mechanical relief of obstruction.

Regardless of the underlying cause, any patient with prolonged ARF will require energetic supportive measures. These may be conservative, or involve the use of dialysis.

Conservative

Fluid intake

Fluid intake must be adjusted to ensure that the patient is neither hypovolaemic nor overloaded. *Euvolaemia* is the objective, and careful clinical assessment of volume status is of the utmost importance (p. 842). The volume of fluid given will depend initially on the patient's state of hydration at presentation. If overloaded, the patient must be fluid restricted to the lowest attainable level; conversely, hypovolaemia must be corrected promptly by oral or intravenous fluids. Maintenance of euvolaemia requires careful assessment of external fluid losses, both measured (urine, faeces, nasogastric tube, fistula etc) and unmeasured (sweat, respiration), and appropriate replacement. Treatment is monitored by weighing the patient daily, with the objective of keeping the body weight near constant, and also by keeping accurate fluid balance charts.

Sodium intake

The hypovolaemic patient will require volume replacement with normal saline until euvolaemia is reached. From then on, sodium intake must be adjusted to balance sodium losses. These may be very small (less than 30 mmol/day) in an oliguric, afebrile patient, or very large (e.g. from the gastrointestinal tract). The external losses of sodium should be quantitated by measurement of the sodium concentration and volume of the fluid, although, in many cases, knowledge of where the fluid is coming from allows a reasonable estimate of its likely sodium concentration to be made (p. 846). Sodium intake is then adjusted to match the total sodium loss.

Potassium intake

The intake of potassium usually has to be reduced in an oliguric patient, typically to 30–40 mmol/day or less. The adequacy of potassium restriction may be monitored by serial measurements of plasma potassium concentration. Frequently, potassium restriction alone is insufficient to prevent hyperkalaemia; this progresses as a result of loss of potassium from the ICF due to accelerated tissue catabolism, and also by movement of potassium from the ICF to the ECF under the influence of developing renal acidosis. Sodium bicarbonate may be useful in this setting and, provided that its use is not precluded by body sodium and water overload, is often very effective. Cation exchange resins (e.g. Calcium Resonium) given orally or rectally may increase external potassium loss, and the combination of insulin and glucose can also be useful in the short term for management of hyperkalaemia (p. 851).

Protein and energy provision

Many patients with ARF have severe associated disease (such as shock, sepsis and trauma) so that the usual considerations regarding protein restriction in renal failure (p. 807) may not always apply to patients with ARF. The management of isolated ARF in an otherwise well and stable patient should include dietary protein restriction to about 0.6 g protein/kg bodyweight per day. This should be accompanied by generous energy provision from carbohydrate and fat, to a total of at least 30 kcal/kg bodyweight per day. This avoids the accelerated tissue catabolism that would be required to make up any shortfall in energy provision. In contrast, the patient with ARF and severe associated illness is likely to be in a hypercatabolic state and require as much as 50 kcal/kg bodyweight per day or more. Protein restriction has no place here; indeed, intake should be high (1.5 g/kg bodyweight per day).

Dialysis

Dialysis may be needed for one or more of the following indications:

1. uraemic syndrome (p. 804)
2. adverse biochemistry (urea levels greater than 40–45 mmol/l)
3. severe hypervolaemia with hypertension and/or pulmonary oedema
4. hyperkalaemia (potassium levels greater than 6.5 mmol/l)
5. severe symptomatic acidosis
6. the need to remove fluid to allow intensive feeding with high energy/high nitrogen diets or total parenteral nutrition (TPN). Such feeding usually requires an intake of at least 2500 ml/day.

Dialysis may be peritoneal or by haemodialysis (p. 809). *Peritoneal dialysis* has the advantage of simplicity, but may be difficult or impossible if there has been very recent abdominal surgery. *Haemodialysis* offers higher clearance of 'uraemic toxins' (p. 804), but requires partial anticoagulation of the patient and is more often associated with circulatory instability. Slow continuous haemodialysis is a recent development that has greatly improved the management of patients with ARF, especially those with multiple organ failure.

ACUTE NEPHRITIC SYNDROME

Acute nephritic syndrome is characterised by the abrupt appearance of blood and protein in the urine, in association with a decline in GFR, sodium and water retention and hypertension. The haematuria may be macroscopic or microscopic and the spun deposit of fresh urine contains red blood cells and casts which may be cellular, granular or both. The syndrome is often mild and transient, but may also be severe enough to present as acute renal failure. The renal lesion is usually acute glomerulonephritis, which may be primary or secondary (discussed on pp. 815 and 821), although a minority of patients will be found to have acute tubulointerstitial disease (p. 824). The causes of acute nephritic syndrome are listed in Table 21.15. The management of the diseases causing this syndrome is discussed on pp. 816–824.

Table 21.15 Causes of acute nephritic syndrome

Primary postinfectious	Secondary with underlying multisystem disease
Bacterial	SLE
Streptococci	Polyarteritis
Bacterial endocarditis	Wegener's granulomatosis
Ventriculo atrial shunt ('shunt nephritis')	Goodpasture's syndrome
Typhoid	Henoch–Schönlein purpura
Brucella	Haemolytic-uraemic syndrome
Meningococci	
Viral	**Other**
Cytomegalovirus	Idiopathic RPGN
Hepatitis virus	Acute tubulo-interstitial nephropathy
Epstein-Barr virus	
Parasitic	
Plasmodium falciparum	

RAPIDLY PROGRESSIVE GLOMERULONEPHRITIS

The pathological process of rapidly progressive glomerulonephritis (RPGN) often appears confined to the kidney (idiopathic RPGN) but may also be present on a background of a multisystem disease such as polyarteritis, Henoch-Schönlein purpura, systemic lupus erythematosus or infective endocarditis. There is usually a distinctive epithelial crescent within the glomerulus, leading to the alternative designation 'crescentic nephritis'. Fibrin deposition may be prominent. In this syndrome, renal function deteriorates progressively over days, weeks or months, usually with urine containing many casts, red blood cells and protein. The course is relentlessly downhill and, although some patients appear to respond to aggressive therapy with steroids, cytotoxic drugs, plasma exchange and in some cases antiplatelet and anticoagulant drugs, many progress to end stage renal disease and require dialysis. Diagnosis is based on renal biopsy. The individual diseases causing RPGN are discussed on pp. 816–822.

CHRONIC RENAL FAILURE

Aetiology

Chronic renal failure (CRF) may result from any cause of parenchymal renal disease, including unrelieved obstruction (Table 21.16).

Clinical features and investigation

Assessment of the patient with suspected CRF is shown in

Table 21.16 Causes of chronic renal failure

Vascular

Renal artery stenosis (only when bilateral or affecting solitary functioning kidney)

Hypertensive nephrosclerosis

Systemic sclerosis

Haemolytic uraemic syndrome/thrombotic thrombocytopenic purpura

Vasculitis (polyarteritis, Wegener's)

Glomerulopathy

All causes of primary glomerulopathy (except minimal change)

All causes of secondary glomerulopathy (with associated multisystem disease, e.g. SLE, Henoch–Schönlein purpura)

Toxic glomerulopathy (mercurial diuretics, gold, penicillamine, Bence-Jones protein in myeloma)

Tubulointerstitial nephropathy (TIN)

Idiopathic

Associated with multisystem disease (Sjögren's, sarcoidosis)

Associated with metabolic disorders (e.g. urate, nephrocalcinosis)

Toxic TIN, e.g. analgesic abuse

Infection and/or reflux

Chronic pyelonephritis

Renal tuberculosis

Cystic disease

Adult polycystic disease

Obstructive nephropathy

Diabetic nephropathy

Amyloid

Renal dysplasia, hypoplasia, agenesis

Table 21.17. In all cases, it is important to decide whether the renal impairment is indeed chronic or whether it is acute (Table 21.14). Chronic renal failure rarely has the potential to improve significantly (although appropriate treatment may slow or arrest progression), but many patients with ARF have potentially recoverable lesions. It follows that diagnosis of CRF does not usually require more than general information regarding the renal pathology. Thus, renal biopsies are seldom of value in patients with CRF. There are, however, certain factors that require careful consideration, and attention should be directed in particular to the following:

1. Is a pre-renal factor exacerbating the CRF? The most likely of these is salt and water depletion (which may itself be a consequence of a concomitant renal concentrating defect) and its correction may dramatically improve the level of renal function.
2. Has coexisting hypertension been controlled adequately?
3. Have post-renal factors been adequately excluded? The importance of this is clear – relief of an obstructing lesion is likely to halt progression of the CRF, and may lead to its partial reversal.

Advanced chronic renal failure is always associated with the development of the *uraemic syndrome*.

Table 21.17 Assessment of the patient who appears to have chronic renal failure

Clinical
Symptoms or signs of uraemia
Length of history
Family history of renal disease
Pointers to underlying multisystem disease (diabetes, SLE etc)
Symptoms and/or signs of obstruction
Palpably enlarged kidneys
Volume depletion or expansion
Blood pressure/signs of accelerated hypertension

Laboratory
Urine analysis – for blood/protein
           – microscopy of fresh spun deposit
           – culture
Assessment of GFR (plasma creatinine/clearance)
24 h protein excretion
Full blood count, ESR
Immunological studies (optional, depending on case), e.g. immunoglobulins, complement, immune complexes, auto-antibodies, ANCA
Infection – HBsAg and blood cultures (where appropriate)

Imaging
Plain abdominal X-ray with/without nephrotomography (renal size)
Ultrasound of kidneys (renal size, obstruction)
Radionuclide studies (level of renal function, obstruction)
IVU (renal size, gross morphology and function)
Hand X-rays (secondary hyperparathyroidism)

Histology
Renal biopsy – only if kidneys are not small and there is doubt over chronicity

Uraemia

The uraemic state eludes precise definition. A working description would be 'the constellation of symptoms, signs and altered body physiology and chemistry that arises when renal function is substantially impaired'. These features are listed in Summary 3 (p. 798). A large part of the state of uraemia results from toxic accumulation of waste products, but depletion of essential compounds and failure of biosynthetic functions of the kidney also contribute. Most organ systems are affected in one way or another. The conservative management of CRF is outlined in Table 21.18 (p. 807).

Uraemic toxins

There are many potential uraemic toxins. Urea is probably not an important toxin in clinical practice, although in vitro toxicity is demonstrable at appropriate concentrations. Other candidates are peptide hormones (parathyroid hormone, gastrin, glucagon and calcitonin), purine metabolites, aliphatic and aromatic amines, phenols and indols, all of which are demonstrably toxic in vitro. The demonstration of increased quantities of compounds of molecular weight 500–5000 daltons (so-called 'middle molecules') in uraemic patients has led to speculation that one or more of these may be involved. Both small molecules, such as urea, and middle molecules are removed by dialysis (p. 809), and this is associated with amelioration of the uraemic syndrome. However, evidence relating these compounds to clinical uraemia remains circumstantial and a causal link is still lacking.

Haematopoietic system in uraemia

Anaemia

The majority of patients with significant renal impairment have normochromic normocytic anaemia. The following contribute to the anaemia (see also Ch. 25, p. 1043):

1. decreased production of erythropoietin by the diseased kidney
2. direct marrow suppression by uraemic toxins
3. shortened red cell survival
4. increased blood loss.

Most patients approaching end stage renal disease or being treated by haemodialysis have haemoglobin concentrations in the region of 6–10 g/dl, although in those who have been nephrectomised, the anaemia is usually more severe. For reasons not yet understood, patients with polycystic kidney disease often continue to make erythropoietin. Such patients are rarely as anaemic and may have completely normal haemoglobin concentrations, even when on dialysis.

Haematinic deficiency may exacerbate the anaemia of chronic renal failure; iron and folate supply is often marginal in patients on restricted diets and, in addition, renal patients malabsorb iron and have increased iron needs as a result of mucosal bleeding.

Management. Evidence of iron and folate deficiency should be sought and treated if appropriate. Preliminary studies using regular injections of *synthetic human erythropoietin* have been very promising, and this approach is now being applied widely. Occasional, or even regular, blood transfusion is used in some patients. Symptoms (e.g. weakness, lethargy) and complications (angina, cardiac failure) of anaemia dictate the need for treatment; the absolute level of haemoglobulin is not, in isolation, a good indicator. Successful transplantation leads to rapid return of normal haematopoietic activity.

Bleeding

Bleeding in uraemia is mainly from capillaries and is due to abnormal platelet function (platelet numbers are usually normal in uraemia). Treatment of uraemia by dialysis improves, but does not normalise, the platelet defect. The bleeding tendency manifests itself clinically with cutaneous ecchymoses and mucosal oozing.

Cardiovascular system in uraemia

Pericardium

Haemorrhagic pericarditis is a frequent complication of terminal uraemia, but may also arise in the less uraemic patient approaching end stage renal disease or receiving dialysis treatment. Its occurrence is loosely related to the severity of uraemia, as judged by plasma urea concentration. The onset may be insidious or abrupt, the latter leading to severe pain or cardiac tamponade which may be fatal. Management is that of any pericardial effusion (p. 435) combined with intensive dialysis. Surgical relief of tamponade may be required but chronic constrictive pericarditis requiring pericardiectomy is very unusual.

Heart

Many patients with chronic renal failure, particularly those maintained for long periods on dialysis, appear to develop impaired cardiac function. Although this usually occurs as a consequence of hypertension or coronary artery disease, this is not always so. Chronic anaemia, volume overload, nutritional deficiency and uraemic toxins may all contribute to a uraemic cardiomyopathy. Rigorous control of intravascular volume and blood pressure (by dialysis and/or drugs) offers the best hope of prevention or amelioration of the condition. Symptomatic ischaemic heart disease and valve disease can be managed surgically if medication fails, without any great excess in morbidity or mortality.

Arteries

Chronically uraemic patients, whether treated by dialysis or not, have a greatly increased incidence of arterial disease. Uraemia is often accompanied by hyperlipidaemia, in which plasma triglycerides and very low density lipo-

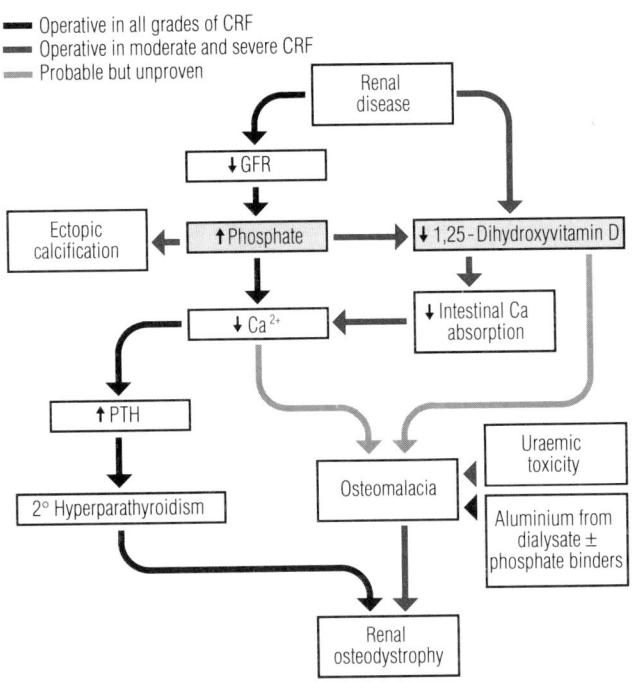

Legend:
- Operative in all grades of CRF
- Operative in moderate and severe CRF
- Probable but unproven

Fig. 21.11 Renal osteodystrophy. The process is dominated by a combination of phosphate retention (its consequences shown on the left side of the figure) and failure of the diseased kidney to synthesise 1,25 dihydroxyvitamin D (its consequences shown in the centre and right of the figure).

proteins are elevated and high density lipoproteins are reduced (p. 778). These abnormalities, in combination with hypertension, may account for the accelerated arterial disease that appears to be part of the uraemic state.

Skeletal and mineral metabolism in uraemia: renal osteodystrophy

Skeletal abnormalities are an invariable accompaniment of uraemia and comprise *hyperparathyroid bone disease, osteomalacia* and *osteosclerosis*. The pathogenesis of these conditions is dominated by two distinct processes, both leading to secondary hyperparathyroidism. These processes, phosphate retention and intestinal calcium malabsorption, are illustrated in Fig. 21.11.

Phosphate retention

Phosphate retention is a consequence of the decreasing filtered load of phosphate as glomerular filtration rate falls (p. 791). This causes a reciprocal fall in plasma calcium which, in turn, provokes increased release of parathyroid hormone (PTH). The result is normalisation of plasma calcium concentration and increased phosphaturia, such that plasma phosphate also returns to normal. Thus, with each decrement in glomerular filtration rate, a new steady state is reached with normal plasma concentrations of calcium and phosphate, but only at the expense of secondary hyperparathyroidism. The parathyroids compensate so well for the alterations in calcium and phosphorous

homeostasis as renal function declines, that overt hyperphosphataemia develops only when glomerular filtration rate falls to 25 ml/min or less. The price paid for this compensation is progressive PTH-mediated skeletal resorption.

Calcium malabsorption

Calcium malabsorption develops when renal damage has progressed to the point where the production of 1,25-dihydroxyvitamin D, the active hormonal form of vitamin D, from its precursor 25-hydroxyvitamin D (under the influence of 25-OHD-1α-hydroxylase) becomes significantly impaired (Fig. 21.12). Early in renal failure, plasma concentrations of 1,25-dihydroxyvitamin D are normal, probably because the accompanying hyperparathyroidism has the effect of stimulating the diseased kidney to maintain 1,25-dihydroxyvitamin D production (p. 737). In advanced renal failure (GFR less than 20 ml/min), 1,25-dihydroxyvitamin D concentration falls to low or undetectable levels. This is partly as a result of

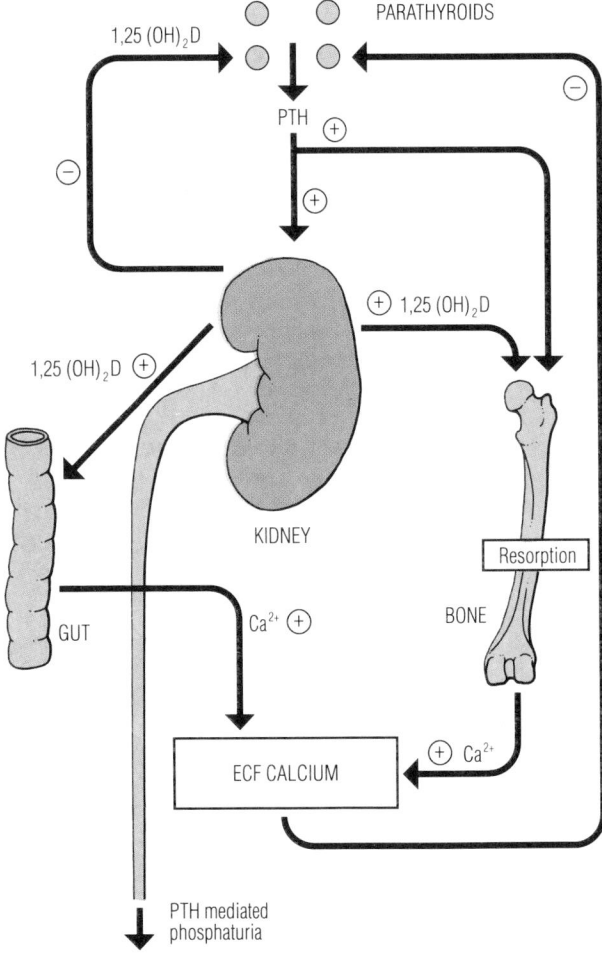

Fig. 21.12 Renal and hormonal control of calcium metabolism. PTH, secreted in response to decreasing ECF calcium, stimulates the production of 1,25(OH)₂D in the kidney. 1,25(OH)₂D in turn stimulates bone resorption and intestinal calcium absorption, and feeds back negatively to inhibit PTH secretion.

decreased renal mass and loss of the cells that contain 25-hydroxyvitamin D 1-α-hydroxylase (the proximal tubular cells), and partly as a result of the suppressive influence of hyperphosphataemia on the 1-α-hydroxylase enzyme. The consequent intestinal calcium malabsorption further exacerbates the secondary hyperparathyroidism.

The dominant skeletal lesion is thus that of *hyperparathyroid bone disease*, with increased numbers and activity of osteoclasts, accelerated bone resorption, a coupled increase in osteoblastic activity, high bone turn-over and variable degrees of peritrabecular fibrosis (osteitis fibrosa). These lesions can usually be reversed by therapy that alleviates the hyperparathyroidism (p. 808).

In addition, a proportion of patients show features of impaired mineralisation (osteomalacia), either in combination with hyperparathyroid bone disease, or in isolation. The pathogenesis of uraemic osteomalacia is less well understood than that of hyperparathyroidism, but it may be a direct consequence of 1,25-dihydroxyvitamin D lack, or a reflection of abnormal collagen synthesis or failure of transformation of calcium phosphate to hydroxyapatite in the presence of uraemia. Aluminium derived from dialysate or aluminium-containing phosphate binders may accumulate in the bone of some patients with uraemia and has been associated with severe and refractory osteomalacia (p. 808).

Although hyperparathyroidism and osteomalacia both lead to osteopenia, some patients show *regional osteosclerosis*, particularly involving the trabecular bone of the spine. Its pathogenesis is poorly understood but it usually develops on a background of severe hyperparathyroidism. *Soft tissue calcification*, generally vascular, subcutaneous or corneal, may occur, especially in patients with chronic elevation of plasma phosphate concentration. *Metabolic acidosis* – from which all uraemic patients suffer to some extent and which is buffered by skeletal alkali – contributes little to the development of renal osteodystrophy except when the acidosis is severe and prolonged.

Clinical features are usually subtle when hyperparathyroidism dominates the condition, but, in the presence of significant osteomalacia, bone pain, deformity and pathological fractures may occur. Radiological evidence of hyperparathyroidism (subperiosteal erosions affecting particularly the phalanges and spinal osteosclerosis – the *rugger jersey spine*) or osteomalacia (osteopenia, Looser zones, non-healing fractures) may be present. Plasma biochemistry shows normal or low calcium concentration, raised inorganic phosphate and, often, raised alkaline phosphatase reflecting increased osteoblastic activity. If measured, parathyroid hormone is high, 25-hydroxyvitamin D normal and 1,25-dihydroxyvitamin D low, indicating failure of renal bioactivation of vitamin D.

Gastrointestinal system and uraemia

Peptic ulcer disease is possibly more common in uraemic patients. Serum gastrin is elevated in uraemia, but basal and stimulated gastric acid secretion is elevated in only some patients. Haemorrhagic complications of peptic ulcer disease are more likely in uraemia because of the associated haemostatic defects (p. 804) and, in the case of haemodialysis patients, exposure to anticoagulants. Treatment is along conventional lines with antacids and H_2-receptor antagonists. Small and large bowel changes are usually mild and of little functional significance, except in near terminal uraemia when bleeding may be severe. Angiodysplasia (Ch. 16, p. 574) is relatively common in uraemia and accounts for bleeding in a number of cases.

Nervous system in uraemia

Uraemic encephalopathy (p. 968) is a syndrome of global CNS dysfunction, probably resulting from retained uraemic toxins. Its onset depends in part on the severity of uraemia (judged biochemically), but also on the rate of onset of uraemia, rapid onset being associated with earlier CNS decompensation. Higher mental functions are the first affected; poor concentration, apathy, insomnia and irritability occur frequently. Motor disturbances become evident later, leading to slurring of speech, tremors, asterixis (the 'uraemic flap'), myoclonus and even seizures. Nausea and vomiting are prominent in advanced uraemia and may respond to antiemetic drugs. 'Dialysis dementia' is a rare and often fatal complication of severe aluminium intoxication in uraemic patients.

Peripheral nervous system

Uraemic neuropathy is a frequent complication of terminal uraemia. Symptomatic neuropathy may also develop in patients in whom the initiation of dialysis treatment has been deferred for too long or who are under-dialysed; clinical and electrophysiological evidence of asymptomatic neuropathy is very common. The neuropathy is mixed sensory and motor and is an axonal degeneration. A variable degree of improvement follows treatment of the uraemia.

Metabolic and nutritional considerations in uraemia

Protein. A mixed picture with elements of both deficiency and toxicity develops. Protein restricted diets predispose to protein malnutrition, while accumulation of nitrogenous compounds, some of which may be 'uraemic toxins', results from impaired renal catabolism and excretion of waste. Additional problems may be present in specific diseases (e.g. massive protein losses in nephrotic syndrome).

Carbohydrate. As a group, uraemic patients are slightly hyperglycaemic compared with normals, both when fasted and following glucose challenge. Peripheral insulin resistance appears to be the major cause, and this may be further exacerbated by a tendency of uraemia per se to inhibit insulin secretion. Conversely, the renal catabolism of insulin is normally considerable and decreases as renal disease progresses. As a result, although uraemic patients have mild carbohydrate intolerance, overtly diabetic patients with nephropathy require less insulin as nephropathy progresses.

Lipids. Plasma triglycerides and very low density lipoproteins are increased and high density lipoproteins decreased in uraemia. All these changes potentially contribute to the observed increase in atherogenesis amongst uraemic patients.

Conservative management of chronic renal failure

This section deals with the clinical management of the patient who has severe impairment of renal function but who has not yet reached end stage renal disease and the need for renal replacement therapy. Because of the serious limitations of adaptive capacity in the diseased kidney, the central principles of conservative management are:

1. to minimise the functional stresses and strains imposed on the kidney, by attempting to define the appropriate intake of food, minerals and water in such a way as not to exceed the kidney's limits of adaptation
2. to identify and treat any coexisting factors that may further compromise renal function, e.g. hypertension, pre-renal factors, post-renal factors
3. to anticipate and, if possible, avoid future complications of uraemia, such as malnutrition, osteodystrophy, soft tissue calcification
4. to anticipate and prepare for the initiation of renal replacement therapy if needed.

Specific aspects of clinical management are as follows (and are summarised in Table 21.18).

Diet

Protein

Protein restriction is begun only when symptoms and/or signs of the uraemic syndrome become evident; this does not usually happen until glomerular filtration rate falls to 25 ml/min or less. Protein restriction decreases the rate of production of uraemic toxins and the acid products of metabolism, and is very effective in alleviating the uraemic syndrome (though it has no immediate effect on underlying renal function). In the UK, normal dietary protein intake is 70–140 g/day. This can be reduced in a stepwise fashion (as glomerular filtration rate decreases) to a lower limit of 25–30 g/day (0.5 g/kg bodyweight per day) without serious risk of nutritional deficiency, provided that it is accompanied by adequate energy intake in the form of carbohydrate and fat. At these very low protein intakes, it is important that the protein is of animal origin, in order to avoid selective deficiency of essential amino acids; these may only be present in small amounts in vegetable protein. The essential amino acids in animal protein are present in proportions that approximate to their minimum daily requirement in man.

Although it is conventional practice to restrict protein only for symptomatic treatment of the uraemic syndrome, there is convincing laboratory and some clinical evidence that much earlier protein restriction will retard, and in some cases halt, the progression of renal deterioration (p.

808). If this proves correct, protein restriction is likely to be employed earlier in the course of renal failure in the future.

Sodium

In many patients, urinary sodium excretion is reasonably well maintained even at very low levels of GFR. However, in the salt-consuming developed countries, sodium restriction often becomes necessary; the indications are hypertension or evidence of expansion of body sodium and water. The dietary intake may be set at about 60 mmol/day (moderate salt restriction), compared with the 100–250 mmol/day in a normal diet. More severe sodium restriction may be utilised, but renders the diet increasingly unpalatable. Fortunately, potent loop diuretics often obviate the need for unpleasantly low sodium diets. Conversely, there are cases where inappropriate salt losses through the diseased kidney may dictate a high dietary sodium intake in order to avoid sodium and water depletion and pre-renal exacerbation of the uraemic state. This is most likely to arise in diseases that predominantly affect the renal medulla, e.g. chronic pyelonephritis, polycystic kidney disease, obstructive nephropathy, papillary necrosis.

Table 21.18 Conservative management of the uraemic syndrome

Item	Comments
Identify and treat pre-renal factors	Many patients with CRF cannot conserve sodium/water.
Identify and treat post-renal factors	Exclude obstruction in all cases.
Restrict dietary protein	GFR usually less than 25 ml/min. Early restriction might protect remaining nephrons.
Adjust dietary sodium/potassium	Severe restriction unnecessary except in oliguria. Sodium supplementation needed in some cases.
Fluids	Aim for urine flow rate of 1500–2000 ml/day.
Prophylaxis or treatment of osteodystrophy	Restrict dietary phosphate. Give phosphate binders (calcium carbonate and/or aluminium hydroxide). Give calcium supplements. Consider vitamin D analogues (calcitrol, alfacalcidol, dihydrotachysterol).
Control blood pressure	Adjustment of body sodium/water by diet and diuretics. Beta-blockers, converting enzyme inhibitors, calcium antagonists if necessary.
Look out for deficiency of vitamins and minerals	Iron is the most likely to require supplementation.
Acidosis	Treat with sodium bicarbonate if a) severe and b) no contraindication.

Potassium

Even in advanced renal failure, the kidney is usually able to maintain adequate potassium excretion, provided that urine flow rate remains generous. Modest reduction of dietary potassium is required; 60–80 mmol/day is usually appropriate, compared with a typical 'normal' intake of 80–120 mmol/day. Severe hyperkalaemia may develop if there is oliguria, gross dietary indiscretion, acidosis (with shift of body potassium from ICF to ECF), or severe intercurrent illness with accelerated catabolism. Potassium-sparing diuretics (e.g. spironolactone, amiloride, triampterene) may impair potassium excretion severely in uraemia and should therefore be avoided. The treatment of hyperkalaemia is described on page 851, but, in patients with severely impaired renal function, a sudden rise in serum potassium may necessitate emergency dialysis.

Fluids

Fluid restriction is rarely necessary in a patient with chronic renal failure, unless oliguria or anuria supervene. On the contrary, it is important to ensure that the fluid intake is set at a level adequate to keep up with the relatively high obligatory urine flow rate in chronic renal failure, and thus prevent water depletion and pre-renal exacerbation of the renal disease. In practice, the fluid intake should be such as to maintain urine flow at around 1500–2000 ml/day, i.e. minimum daily fluid intake should be 2000–2500 ml. A minority of patients with more severe urinary concentrating defects will require larger amounts of fluid to maintain water balance.

Calcium, phosphorus and vitamin D

Chronic renal failure is associated with a tendency towards hyperphosphataemia, hypocalcaemia, hyperparathyroidism and, in its later stages, impaired production of 1,25-dihydroxyvitamin D and consequent intestinal calcium malabsorption (p. 805).

A number of therapeutic measures are employed.

1. Moderate dietary phosphate restriction.
2. Administration of oral 'phosphate-binders' with food. Aluminium hydroxide is routine, but fears of aluminium toxicity are leading to increased use of calcium carbonate and magnesium carbonate as phosphate binders.
3. Maintenance of a high oral calcium intake. Calcium carbonate is convenient here. Doses of 25–150 mmol/day (2.5–15 g/day) given with food will often control plasma inorganic phosphate adequately, and also increase vitamin-D-independent intestinal calcium absorption, thereby lessening hyperparathyroidism.
4. Use of potent analogues of vitamin D. The requirement is that they should bypass the vitamin D resistance of chronic renal failure, by not requiring renal 1-hydroxylation to achieve activity (Fig. 21.12). 1,25-dihydroxyvitamin D (calcitriol), 1-hydroxyvitamin D (alfacalcidiol) and dihydrotachysterol are all effective.

However because they also augment intestinal absorption of phosphate, they should not be given until plasma phosphate has been controlled as described above.

Other vitamins and minerals

Clinical deficiency is rare in the well-managed patient with chronic renal failure, although subtle deficiency states may be more common. Iron status in particular may be marginal, reflecting intestinal iron malabsorption and increased requirements due to blood tests and occult bleeding. Over-zealous and prolonged dietary protein restriction may lead to difficulties, but this usually reflects inappropriate persistence with conservative measures in a patient in whom dialysis treatment should have been started earlier.

Acidosis

In some patients, uraemic acidosis is sufficiently severe, even after appropriate dietary protein restriction, to warrant attempts to relieve it. This may be done with sodium bicarbonate, although the need for concomitant sodium restriction may preclude or limit its use. Potassium bicarbonate is never used in this setting for fear of causing hyperkalaemia.

Control of blood pressure

The control of blood pressure is discussed on page 827. Its importance cannot be over-emphasised.

Measures to halt or retard the progression of chronic renal failure

Progressive renal disease usually causes a decrease in the number of functioning nephrons; therefore it follows that each of the remaining nephrons must process an unusually large amount of water and solute. Adaptive changes in the residual nephrons are many, but there is good evidence that single nephron GFR (i.e. GFR per nephron) is increased in chronic renal disease and that this is associated with a raised hydrostatic pressure in the glomerular capillaries (glomerular hypertension). If sustained, this leads to glomerular sclerosis, loss of nephrons and progressive renal deterioration. In animals, this sequence of events can be prevented completely by dietary protein restriction and it is likely, though not yet proven, that the same holds for some types of chronic renal disease in man. Dietary phosphate restriction also confers benefit in animals and, experimentally, glomerular hypertension can be reduced by angiotensin-converting-enzyme inhibitors and also by aspirin, acting respectively on the renal production of angiotensin II and prostaglandin metabolism. At present, the clinical utility of these measures is not fully established. It is therefore not yet appropriate to implement them in all patients, although modest protein restriction (0.6–0.8 g/kg bodyweight per day) will certainly do no harm, and may be of benefit.

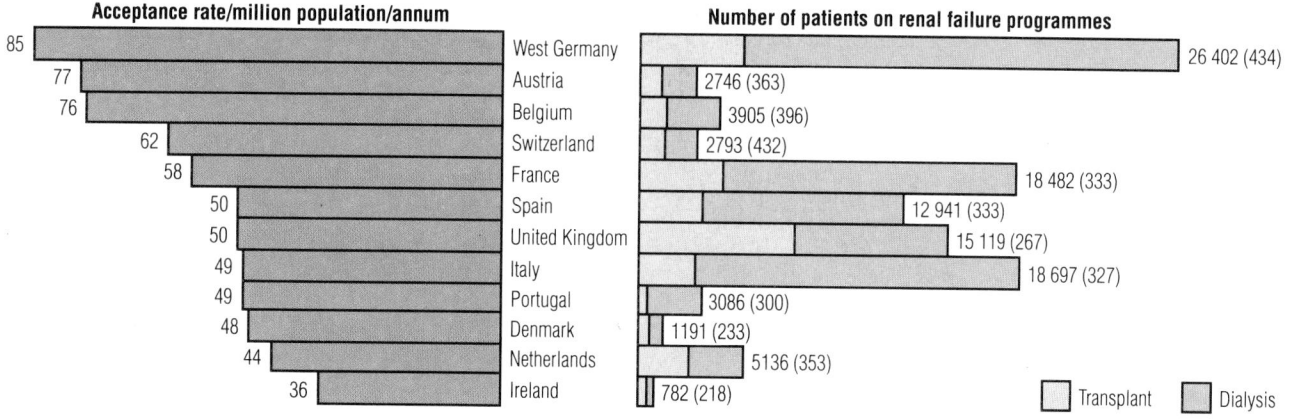

Fig. 21.13   Treatment of end-stage renal disease: international comparisons. On the left is shown the number of patients taken onto dialysis/transplant programmes during 1987 – the annual acceptance rate. On the right is a 'snapshot' indicating the total number of patients receiving treatment for renal failure, either by dialysis or renal transplantation, in December, 1987. The figures in parentheses are expressed per million population. (Source: Brunner F P, Fassbinder W, Broyer M et al. 1989 Combined report on regular dialysis and transplant in Europe XVIII, 1987. Nephrology, Dialysis and Transplantation 4 supp 2: 5–32.)

Renal replacement therapy for chronic renal failure

Renal replacement therapy (RRT) for chronic renal failure may be achieved by means of haemodialysis, peritoneal dialysis or renal transplantation. Most centres offering RRT integrate all three treatment modalities, with the aim of providing each patient with the most appropriate management.

The requirement for RRT

It is estimated that about 72 patients per million population (below the age of 70) reach end stage renal disease in the UK each year and will die if RRT is not provided. The UK currently treats only about 50 patients per million population, a figure substantially lower than in most developed countries (Fig. 21.13). Consequently, many people in the UK die from renal failure without receiving the benefits of RRT. The reasons for the shortfall are socio-political and economic, rather than technical.

Dialysis treatment

Dialysis involves placing a large volume of artificial fluid (dialysate) in very close proximity to a large volume of the patient's blood, separating the two with a semi-permeable membrane.

Haemodialysis

In haemodialysis, the membrane is synthetic and semi-permeable, and is arranged to form an 'artificial kidney' through which blood passes at about 250 ml/minute before being returned to the patient (Fig. 21.14). The chemical composition of the dialysate is similar to that of ECF. Urea and other waste products, which are present only in plasma,

diffuse down a concentration gradient across the membrane and into the dialysate. Changes in the composition of the dialysate and in the hydrostatic pressure gradient across the membrane allow 'tailoring' of the rate of removal of a variety of substances according to the patient's needs. Adequate access to the circulation is a prerequisite. This is obtained by percutaneous placement of large-bore central venous catheters (short-term treatment only), or by creation of an arteriovenous fistula at the wrist, thus increasing forearm blood flow and allowing large-bore needles to be placed in forearm veins (long-term treatment). Treatment is intermittent, typically three sessions of four hours each per week. In the UK, the majority of patients undergoing this form of treatment conduct their own treatment at home.

Fig. 21.14   Physical principles of haemodialysis.

Peritoneal dialysis

In peritoneal dialysis, the dialysate is fed into the peritoneal cavity via a flexible tube, and the peritoneum itself acts as a semi-permeable membrane. The dialysate is replaced with fresh fluid when chemical equilibrium is reached.

In the past this treatment was, like haemodialysis, given intermittently, typically as three sessions per week with each session comprising 20 exchanges of two litres each. Each session lasted about 20 hours. However, peritoneal dialysis now usually takes the form of continuous ambulatory peritoneal dialysis (CAPD) in which two-litre exchanges are performed three or four times per day. The technique is simple to learn and the vast majority of patients can carry out and supervise their own treatment at home.

Limitations of dialysis

Although dialysis can remove waste products, sodium, potassium and water reasonably well and thus control some aspects of the uraemic syndrome, it is very inferior to normal functioning kidneys for a number of reasons:

1. The *average* clearance of urea or creatinine achieved by intermittent haemodialysis (approximately 12 hours treatment per week) is only 6 ml/min and by CAPD about 7 ml/min, compared with 100–120 ml/min by normal kidneys.
2. The permeability characteristics of the artificial membrane in haemodialysis and, to a lesser extent, the peritoneum in peritoneal dialysis (CAPD) are inferior to those of the physiological glomerular sieve.
3. Dialysis has no equivalent of 'tubular action'; the dialysis membrane must therefore strike a compromise between being permeable enough to allow waste products to cross and not so permeable that excess loss of physiologically important compounds occurs. In practice, the membrane fails on both counts.
4. Dialysis has essentially no adaptive capability.
5. Endocrine functions of the kidney are not provided by dialysis. The anaemia (erythropoietin) and osteodystrophy (1,25-dihydroxyvitamin D) continue.

For these reasons most of the management considerations that apply to the non-dialysed patient with chronic renal failure also apply to the dialysed patient (Table 21.18).

Initiation of dialysis treatment

Because dialysis is inherently unnatural and invasive, its initiation should not be undertaken lightly. The optimum time to convert a patient with chronic renal failure from conservative management to dialysis is a finely judged clinical decision and is reached *just before* the development of uraemic complications (Table 21.19).

Renal transplantation

Successful renal transplantation is, compared to maintenance dialysis, a vastly superior form of treatment. There is little that normal native kidneys can do in the way of excretory, homeostatic or endocrine function that cannot be done equally well by a good transplanted kidney. This is reflected in the clinical outcome; it is apparent that many

Table 21.19 Indications for initiation of dialysis treatment

Suitability for long-term treatment and/or reversible cause of renal failure.

Uraemic syndrome

Neurological
  Coma, stupor, fatigue, abnormal mentation, fits, myoclonus, asterixis, peripheral neuropathy

Cardiovascular/pulmonary
  Pericarditis, pleurisy, volume overload unresponsive to conservative measures

Skin
  Pruritus

Gastrointestinal
  Anorexia, nausea, vomiting, unremitting diarrhoea

Metabolic
  Unremitting acidosis

Chemistry

Plasma urea more than 40 mmol/l on protein restricted diet

Plasma creatinine more than 1200 µmol/l

Creatinine clearance less than 5 ml/min

Hyperkalaemia unresponsive to conservative measures

transplanted patients are returned to a state of virtual normality. However, two problems continue to bedevil renal transplantation. These are inadequate supply of kidneys and graft rejection.

Kidneys are obtained from cadavers (usually with irreversible CNS injury due to trauma or stroke) or from fit, first degree relatives. ABO compatibility is essential and outcome is improved by good HLA matching. The transplanted kidney is placed in the left or right iliac fossa and anastamosed to the iliac vessels; the donor ureter is implanted into the recipient bladder. Immunosuppressive treatment is given routinely and comprises cyclosporin, often given with steroids and/or azathioprine. These drugs

Fig. 21.15 Patient and graft survival following renal transplantation. Dotted lines indicate treatment with cyclosporin A; solid lines with azathioprine. (Data from European Dialysis and Transplant Association Registry, 1987).

are toxic; this is particularly unfortunate with cyclosporin which, as well as being an excellent immunosuppressive agent, also has marked acute and chronic nephrotoxicity. About 80% of cadaveric grafts function for two years or more and, because most graft loss occurs early, the majority of this 80% will continue to do well thereafter (Fig. 21.15). Living related-donor transplants do even better. Most patients receiving kidney transplants are already being dialysed and can return to dialysis treatment if the transplant fails.

NEPHROTIC SYNDROME

Nephrotic syndrome is best defined as the presence of heavy proteinuria (usually greater than 3 g/day), hypo-albuminaemia, hyperlipidaemia and oedema. It is not helpful to pursue the definition beyond this semi-quantitative statement, because there is much interpatient variation in the clinical response to a given level of proteinuria.

Aetiology

Nephrotic range proteinuria, leading to the nephrotic syndrome, may result from a variety of different types of insult to the functional glomerular sieve (Table 21.20). The glomerular changes that result in nephrotic syndrome may reflect disturbances to the size selectivity or the charge selectivity (or both) of the glomerular sieve, such that substantial amounts of plasma proteins, particularly albumin, appear in the GF.

Table 21.20 Causes of nephrotic syndrome

Primary glomerular disease	Secondary glomerular disease
Minimal change GN	Infection (Infective endocarditis, visceral sepsis, quartan malaria, hepatitis B)
Membranous GN	
Focal segmental glomerulosclerosis	Neoplasia (carcinoma, lymphoma, leukaemia, myeloma)
Mesangiocapillary GN	Multisystem diseases (SLE, Henoch–Schönlein purpura, rheumatoid arthritis, amyloid, diabetes mellitus)
Drug/toxin-induced	
Gold	
Other heavy metals	
Penicillamine	
Intravenous drug abuse	

Pathophysiology

The amount of oedema is variable, but correlates better with the severity of hypoalbuminaemia than with the magnitude of proteinuria. The oedema is generalised and may be associated with pleural effusion and/or ascites, especially in children. The pathophysiological processes leading to oedema in the nephrotic syndrome are illustrated in Figure 21.16. This sequence predicts that the nephrotic patient has an expanded ECF, contracted vascular compartment, high plasma renin activity and aldosterone concentration,

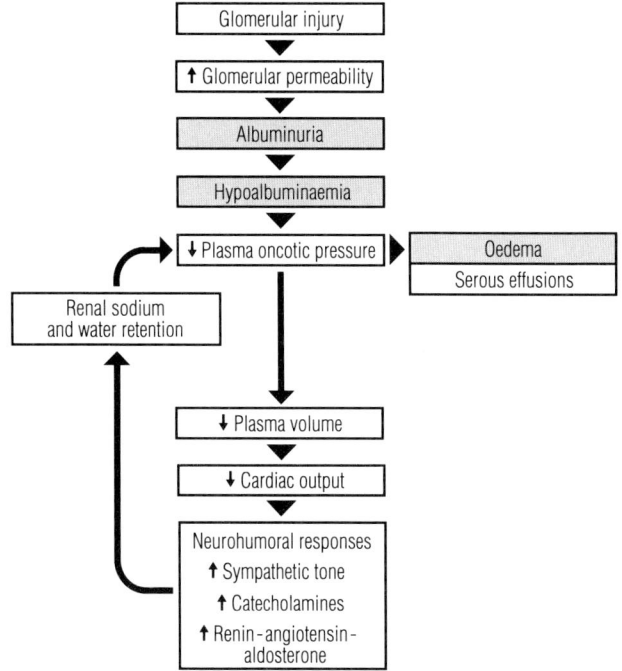

Fig. 21.16 Pathogenesis of oedema in nephrotic syndrome.

with avid renal sodium and water retention. This is indeed the case in many, though not all, nephrotic patients.

Investigation

In children, minimal change GN is the usual lesion. In such cases, the diagnosis can usually be made without recourse to renal biopsy. In a typical case, there is a normal GFR, an absence of significant numbers of red cells or casts in the urine and a highly selective urine protein excretion (p. 792). The abolition of proteinuria by steroid therapy is confirmatory. In children with disease which is steroid-resistant, or who have impaired GFR and/or red blood cells and casts in the urine, and in the majority of adults, identification of the renal lesion (Table 21.20) and appropriate management will usually necessitate renal biopsy.

Complications and treatment

The complications of the nephrotic syndrome are listed in Summary 5. They may be serious, and an important therapeutic objective is therefore the amelioration or elimination of the proteinuria. (The specific glomerulopathies causing nephrotic syndrome are discussed on pp. 816–823.) Often this is not possible, but certain general measures remain appropriate regardless of the underlying renal lesion (Table 21.21). Diuretics should be used judiciously and in conjunction with dietary sodium restriction. Although, in some cases, very large doses of a potent loop diuretic will be needed to effect a diuresis, these drugs carry the risk of inducing severe contraction of the vascular compartment (hypovolaemia) and may lead to pre-renal

---

Summary 5   Complications of nephrotic syndrome

- Massive oedema

- Effusions/ascites

- Hypovolaemia (reduced blood volume)

- Protein malnutrition – growth retardation
  - poor wound healing
  - osteoporosis

- Hyperlipidaemia – probable increased atherogenesis

- Hypercoagulability – renal vein thrombosis
  - stroke

- Susceptibility to infection (especially in children)

Table 22.21   General measures in the treatment of nephrotic syndrome

- High protein diet

- Dietary sodium restriction

- Water restriction (rarely necessary)

- Diuretic therapy

- Intravenous proteins (rarely necessary)

---

uraemia, shock and even acute renal failure in some cases. Severe hypovolaemia can be corrected temporarily by administration of colloid in the form of plasma proteins, a manœuvre that is also employed occasionally to initiate a diuresis. The use of the aldosterone antagonist, spironolactone, in these patients is both logical and useful. It has the advantage of rarely producing an unexpectedly rapid diuresis in sensitive patients and, in resistant cases, may potentiate the action of loop diuretics.

Protein malnutrition is a major hazard in patients with nephrotic syndrome, and encouragement should be given to maintain the highest possible protein intake, while also ensuring adequate energy provision to prevent further acceleration of protein catabolism. Despite these measures, growth retardation, poor wound healing and reduced immune competence are frequent. The hyperlipidaemia is refractory to dietary measures and lipid lowering agents have generally also been ineffective, although the new HMG-CoA reductase inhibitors are promising (p. 780). Thrombotic problems resulting from the hypercoagulable state that attends the nephrotic syndrome are probably commoner than generally appreciated (reaching nearly 50% in some series) and are almost certainly under-diagnosed. The hypercoagulability may be the result of urinary losses of antithrombin III. Thrombosis is particularly likely to involve the renal veins, leading to an abrupt decline in GFR that should not be misinterpreted as progression of the underlying nephropathy. Diagnosis of renal vein thrombosis in a nephrotic is important, because anticoagulation almost certainly reduces the risk of subsequent pulmonary embolism and may allow eventual recanalisation of the occluded vessel and improvement in GFR. Careful ultrasound or CT examination of the renal veins

may reveal the clot, but in some cases renal venography is required.

RECURRENT HAEMATURIA

Recurrent haematuria most frequently affects boys and young males. The syndrome is dominated by recurrent episodes of macroscopic haematuria, sometimes associated with loin pain and with a tendency to exacerbations following intercurrent viral upper respiratory infections or strenuous exercise. Microscopic haematuria usually persists between attacks and proteinuria is absent or modest (less than 1.5 g/24 hours).

In most cases, the renal pathology is characteristic, with florid mesangial deposition of IgA in the glomeruli; the nephropathy is then termed *IgA nephropathy* or *Berger's disease* (p. 820).

Investigation and treatment

Investigations should include measurement of GFR, examination of the urine and quantitation of protein output. An IVU should be performed in all cases. Children and young adults with a typical presentation can usually be spared cytoscopy, but middle-aged and elderly patients (in whom urological cancer becomes increasingly common) should undergo full urological assessment. Renal biopsy is needed to establish the diagnosis with certainty, especially if there is depression of the GFR, heavy proteinuria, hypertension, a low C3 complement, or a family history suggestive of hereditary nephritis (p. 820).

The course is often benign, although a proportion of patients go on to develop progressive renal disease. There is no specific treatment and management is therefore directed towards identifying and treating secondary hypertension and monitoring renal function.

PERSISTENT ASYMPTOMATIC PROTEINURIA AND/OR HAEMATURIA

The finding of abnormal proteinuria or microscopic haematuria in an apparently healthy person usually results from a routine medical examination for employment or insurance purposes, or is picked up incidentally during an unrelated illness. Table 21.22 lists the large number of conditions that may be associated with this syndrome.

Investigation

Inevitably, the question arises as to how far investigation should proceed in these otherwise healthy individuals. Assessment of renal structure and function by means of plasma biochemistry, creatinine clearance, 24-hour protein output, urine microscopy and culture, and either renal ultrasound or IVU should be undertaken in all cases. Dysmorphic red cells in the urine increase the probability of renal parenchymal disease rather than urological disease. Provided radiological investigation and GFR are normal, proteinuria is modest and the urinary sediment does not

Table 21.22 Causes of asymptomatic persisting proteinuria and/or haematuria in an apparently healthy person

Primary glomerular disease	Miscellaneous renal
Mesangial proliferative GN	Tubulointerstitial nephropathy
Mesangiocapillary GN	Cystic diseases of the kidney
Membranous GN	Renal tumours
Focal segmental glomerulosclerosis	Renal tuberculosis
IgA nephropathy (often causes intermittent gross haematuria)	
Multisystem disease	**Non-renal**
Henoch–Schönlein purpura	Urothelial tumours
SLE	Prostatic disease

show granular or cellular casts, it may be appropriate to adopt a 'wait-and-see' policy, only proceeding to invasive investigation, such as renal biopsy, if there is evidence of disease progression. However, early recourse to renal biopsy is usually justified in order to define prognosis or if there is suspicion that an active and progressive process may be present, particularly if this might be amenable to therapy.

RENAL TUBULAR SYNDROMES

Although most patients with renal disease will have evidence of disordered tubular function if a sufficiently diligent search is carried out, other manifestations of renal disease usually dominate the clinical picture. In a minority of patients, however, clinical disorders result directly from tubular dysfunction. In these cases, the disorder may be *inherited* with presentation generally in childhood, or *acquired*.

Renal glycosuria

Inheritance of renal glycosuria is autosomal recessive. The syndrome results from diminished proximal tubular glucose reabsorption, allowing glycosuria with normal blood glucose concentration. No clinical sequelae occur.

Aminoaciduria

The defects involved in aminoaciduria may be single or multiple. The most important is *cystinuria*, leading to recurrent cystine stone formation. Cystine solubility increases at alkaline pH and the disease is treated by a combination of high fluid intake and alkali ingestion. Penicillamine is also effective, although potentially toxic. Inheritance is autosomal recessive.

Phosphate transport defects

There are several types of phosphate transport defects, which result in inappropriate phosphaturia, hypo-

phosphataemia and rickets. Inheritance is usually X-linked (the disorder is known as *vitamin-D-resistant rickets* (VDRR) or *X-linked hypophosphataemic rickets*) but sporadic inherited cases also occur. Treatment usually takes the form of oral phosphate supplementation with pharmacological doses of vitamin D, or smaller doses of 1,25-dihydroxyvitamin D (calcitriol). The latter combination may be particularly effective in ameliorating the hypophosphataemia and healing rickets. A rare acquired form also exists, and is associated with certain mesenchymal tumours such as cavernous haemangioma, giant cell tumours of bone, and neurofibromata. In such cases of *oncogenous rickets*, the disordered phosphate metabolism may be corrected by removal of the tumour.

Multiple tubular defects (Fanconi's syndrome)

Patients with Fanconi's syndrome have abnormal urinary excretion of amino acids, phosphate, bicarbonate, glucose and small proteins. The classification of this disorder is complex, reflecting its many inherited and acquired causes. All are relatively uncommon; some of the more important acquired ones are shown in Table 21.23. The defects of phosphate reabsorption and proximal bicarbonate reclamation often lead to clinical disease – hypophosphataemic rickets and proximal 'Type II' RTA respectively. They require treatment with phosphate, 1,25-dihydroxyvitamin D, or alkali as appropriate (pp. 814 and 815).

Table 21.23 Causes of acquired Fanconi's syndrome

- Myeloma kidney
- Sjögren's syndrome
- Nephrotic syndrome
- Heavy metal poisoning
  Lead
  Mercury (organic and inorganic)
  Copper (Wilson's disease)
- Drugs
  Outdated tetracycline
  Salicylates
  Cisplatin

Renal tubular acidosis

Renal tubular acidosis (RTA) is metabolic acidosis of renal origin and is unrelated to the acidosis associated with severe impairment of GFR (uraemic acidosis). It is generally divided into three categories depending on the nature and site of the acidification disturbance (Table 21.24). Although the pathogenesis of the different types of renal tubular acidosis differs, all cause *hyperchloraemic metabolic acidosis* (low plasma bicarbonate, raised plasma chloride with normal anion gap) in contrast with the acidosis of uraemia (low bicarbonate, normal chloride and increased anion gap).

Table 21.24 Classification of renal acidosis

| | Renal tubular acidosis (RTA)* | | | Uraemic acidosis |
	Proximal RTA (type II)	Distal RTA with hypokalaemia (type I)	Distal RTA with hyperkalaemia (type IV)	
Defect	Decreased H$^+$secretion	Decreased H$^+$ secretion	Decreased H$^+$ and K$^+$secretion	Decreased nephron mass and decreased ammonia synthesis (controversial)
Acidosis				
Type	Hyperchloraemic	Hyperchloraemic	Hyperchloraemic	Normal plasma chloride
Anion gap	Normal	Normal	Normal	Increased
Severity	Moderate	Moderate or severe	Moderate	Usually moderate
Plasma K$^+$	Decreased	Decreased	Increased	Normal or increased
GFR	Usually normal	Normal or decreased	Usually decreased	Decreased
Treatment	Diuretics and alkali	Alkali	Mineralocorticoids	Protein restriction, sometimes alkali, dialysis

*Type III RTA (not shown) is a rare condition where a patient has manifestations of both type I and type II RTA.

Distal RTA (type I RTA)

The causes of distal RTA are listed in Table 21.25. There is selective impairment of the distal tubules' ability to secrete H$^+$, such that urinary pH cannot be lowered below 5.5. Other distal tubular functions are unimpaired. The resulting inability of the distal tubule to reclaim all of the 5–20% of filtered bicarbonate that normally escapes proximal reclamation leads to continuing bicarbonaturia,

Table 21.25 Causes and classification of distal renal tubular acidosis

With hypokalaemia (type I)

Inherited	**Associated with nephrocalcinosis**
Sickle cell anaemia	Primary hyperparathyroidism
Medullary cystic disease	Vitamin D toxicity

Autoimmune disease	**Tubulointestinal nephropathy secondary to:**
Cryoglobulinaemia	Obstruction
Sjögren's syndrome	Chronic pyelonephritis
Systemic lupus erythematosus	Renal transplantation
Chronic active liver disease	

Drugs
Amphotericin B
Analgesics (in analgesic nephropathy)

With hyperkalaemia (type IV)

Primary deficiency of mineralocorticoid	**Secondary deficiency of mineralocorticoid**
Isolated familial hypoaldosteronism (rare)	Hyporeninaemic hypoaldosteronism with underlying:
Generalised adrenocorticoid deficiency	Hypertensive nephrosclerosis
Addison's disease	Diabetic nephropathy
Adrenalectomy	Obstructive nephropathy
	Renal transplantation

Tubular resistance to mineralocorticoid
Some cases of chronic renal impairment
Spironolactone therapy

even in the presence of severe acidosis. It also limits the utility of urinary buffers such as HPO_4^{2-}, which require a low urinary pH if they are to act as efficient proton acceptors. Distal potassium ion secretion is unimpaired and is often enhanced by mild ECF volume contraction and secondary aldosteronism, leading to hyperchloraemia and hypokalaemia.

Diagnosis depends on demonstrating an inappropriately high urinary pH (> 5.5) during spontaneous or ammonium chloride-induced acidosis. Other diagnostic manœuvres are available, but are rarely needed in clinical practice.

Treatment takes the form of alkali given in amounts sufficient to restore plasma bicarbonate and chloride concentrations to normal. Severe hypokalaemia is often present and should be treated *before* administration of alkali, to avoid the further drop in plasma potassium that would follow correction of the acidosis. The amount of alkali required is small (1–3 mmol/kg bodyweight per day) because bicarbonaturia is not severe and does not increase as plasma bicarbonate concentration rises on treatment.

Proximal RTA (type II RTA)

Proximal RTA may occur in several rare inherited diseases but is more commonly acquired in association with myeloma, Sjögren's syndrome or toxic nephropathy (especially lead or mercury). There is a diminished capacity of the proximal tubule to reclaim filtered bicarbonate ions. The resulting bicarbonaturia leads to progressive metabolic acidosis and decreased plasma bicarbonate concentration, in turn lessening the filtered load of bicarbonate. This chain of events progresses until the filtered load of bicarbonate has fallen to the point where the abnormal proximal tubule can again reclaim a normal percentage of the filtered bicarbonate load. This creates a new steady state in which bicarbonate losses cease, but only at the expense of stable metabolic acidosis. Administration of sufficient bicarbonate to these patients will reverse the sequence of events described above.

Treatment comprises long-term administration of bicarbonate. Large amounts (10–30 mmol/kg per day) are needed because, as plasma bicarbonate rises, so the magnitude of the bicarbonaturia also increases. The bicarbonate requirement can often be reduced by concomitant therapy with a thiazide diuretic. Hypokalaemia is often worsened by therapy, but can be countered by giving some of the bicarbonate as potassium bicarbonate or by the use of potassium-sparing diuretics.

Distal RTA with hyperkalaemia (type IV RTA)

In type IV RTA, there is generalised impairment of distal tubular function, usually on a background of a mild or moderate reduction in GFR. Both H^+ and K^+ secretion in the distal tubule are impaired (Tables 21.24 and 21.25), resulting in hyperchloraemic metabolic acidosis accompanied by disproportionately severe hyperkalaemia. This is the commonest form of RTA and, although the acidosis is mild, the accompanying hyperkalaemia may be severe or even life-threatening.

Type IV RTA may result from the following:

1. *Primary lack of mineralocorticoid* due to adrenal disease in the presence of potentially normal distal tubular function (isolated hypoaldosteronism and Addison's disease).
2. *Disease of the juxtaglomerular apparatus* (JGA) leading to impaired production of renin and secondary hypoaldosteronism (hyporeninaemic hypoaldosteronism). This is associated particularly with hypertensive nephrosclerosis or diabetic nephropathy.
3. *Resistance of the distal tubule to mineralocorticoid action.* This is usually partial rather than complete, and may arise in some patients with chronic renal impairment. It is of course a direct (and deliberate) consequence of spironolactone therapy.

Treatment depends on the underlying abnormality. Deficiency of mineralocorticoid – whether isolated, part of Addison's disease, or secondary to hyporeninaemia – requires replacement with mineralocorticoid in the form of 9α-fludrocortisone. When there is renal resistance to mineralocorticoid, control may often be achieved with pharmacological doses of 9α-fludrocortisone.

Salt-losing nephropathy and nephrogenic diabetes insipidus

In adults, salt-losing nephropathy and nephrogenic diabetes insipidus (failure to conserve sodium and/or water) are nearly always acquired. They may result from almost any cause of renal disease, particularly those that predominantly affect the renal medulla, such as urinary obstruction, papillary necrosis, chronic pyelonephritis and tubulointerstitial diseases. Hypercalcaemia and hypokalaemia cause a functional nephrogenic diabetes insipidus, initially reversible on correction of the metabolic abnormality. The severity of the polyuria in these acquired tubular syndromes rarely approaches that of pituitary diabetes insipidus, but, in contrast, accompanying salt losses may be massive. The importance of inappropriate renal salt and water loss is their tendency to cause severe volume contraction and pre-renal uraemia; one should not be misled by the continuing production of large amounts of urine.

Management is usually straightforward. Underlying hypercalcaemia or hypokalaemia should be investigated and treated. In chronic renal disease, it is essential to ensure adequate intake of dietary salt and water, if necessary using salt tablets. This is especially important at times of intercurrent illness, when oral intake may fall. Some of these patients also have disordered renal acidification mechanisms (renal tubular acidosis) and it is then convenient to give the sodium supplementation as sodium bicarbonate.

PRIMARY GLOMERULAR DISEASE

IMMUNOLOGICAL AND OTHER MECHANISMS OF GLOMERULAR INJURY

Many glomerular diseases, whether occurring in isolation or as part of a multisystem disease, are associated with demonstrable immunological abnormalities. Although it is not always clear whether these are involved directly in the pathogenesis of the glomerular disease, much attention has been directed towards the identification of the immunological disturbances and their manipulation as part of treatment. The final common path of immunologically mediated glomerular injury is the activation of various inflammatory mediators, both cellular and soluble, which then inflict damage on the glomerulus, or less frequently on other tissue elements in the kidney (Fig. 21.17). It is likely that the production and activation of the mediators (Table 21.26) requires the presence of antigen-antibody complexes in the kidney and also of specific types of cell. Clearly, both the source of these immune complexes, the identification of their antigenic component(s), and the factors that control the behaviour of the involved cells are of great importance in the understanding

Fig. 21.17 Mechanisms of immunological glomerular injury.

Table 21.26 Initiators and mediators of glomerular injury

Cellular	Non-cellular
• Polymorphs	• Antibody
• Macrophages/monocytes	• Complement
• Lymphocytes (esp. T helper cells)	• Fibrinogen
• Platelets	• Histamine
	• Kinins
	• Prostaglandins
	• Some interleukins (esp. IL-1 and IL-2)
	• Tumour necrosis factor (TNF–alpha)
	• Free radicals

Table 21.28 Non-renal antigens linked with immune complex nephritis

Exogenous	Endogenous

• Bacterial
  Streptococcus
  Staphylococcus
  Meningococcus
  Treponema pallidum
	• DNA

	• Tumour specific
	• Rbc membrane

• Viral
  Hepatitis B
  Cytomegalovirus (CMV)
	• Thyroglobulin

	• IgG

• Parasitic
  Plasmodium malariae
  Schistosoma haematobium	

• Drugs Penicillin	
• Exogenous proteins Serum sickness	

of the diseases, and in the development of rational treatment.

Two general mechanisms of immunological injury to the glomerulus are proposed.

In situ complex formation. The antigens may be an intrinsic part of the glomerulus, or may be derived from other parts of the body and be deposited or 'planted' in the glomerulus. In either case, formation of an antigen-antibody complex may occur *in situ* if an appropriate antibody is generated (Fig. 21.17).

Circulating complexes. The second mechanism of injury involves the generation of antibody directed against an antigen derived from sources other than the kidney. In this case, the antigen might be endogenous or exogenous. When the resulting antigen-antibody complex gains access to, or is produced in, the circulation, it can be deposited in the kidneys and there activate mediators of inflammation. Antigens suspected of mediating human glomerular disease through this mechanism are listed in Table 21.28.

The production of glomerular injury is complex and probably depends on linked cellular and non-cellular mechanisms. Immunohistopathological study of renal tissue obtained from renal biopsies or at post-mortem sometimes reveals antibody (IgG, IgM or IgA) and complement components, the precise location and pattern of which can yield valuable diagnostic information. Furthermore, the common finding of monocytes/macrophages

Table 21.27 Involvement of immune complexes in pathogenesis of nephritis

Probable	Possible
• Post-infectious GN	• Henoch-Schönlein purpura
• Infective endocarditis	• IgA nephropathy (Berger's disease)
• Shunt nephritis	• Mesangiocapillary GN
• Quartan malaria	• Idiopathic rapidly progressive GN
• Syphilis	• Membranous GN
• Hepatitis B infection	• Focal segmental glomerulosclerosis
• Systemic lupus erythematosus	

(producers of TNF-alpha and interleukin-1) and T helper lymphocytes (producers of interleukin-2) suggests, but does not prove, a role for these cells and cytokines in pathogenesis. Similarly, in only a minority of cases has it been possible to identify the antigenic component of the immune complexes, and even in cases where this has been achieved with certainty, it is still not clear what triggers the sequence of events that leads ultimately to glomerular injury; many patients with circulating immune complexes do not develop nephritis. Examples of human nephritis in which immune complexes are thought to play a role are given in Table 21.27.

CLINICAL PRESENTATION OF GLOMERULAR DISEASE

The specific glomerular diseases described below may present as one of the following:

1. acute nephritic syndrome, with or without acute renal failure (p. 802)
2. rapidly progressive glomerulonephritis (p. 802)
3. chronic glomerulonephritis (p. 803)
4. nephrotic syndrome (p. 811)
5. hypertension (p. 826)
6. asymptomatic haematuria and/or proteinuria (p. 812)
7. recurrent macroscopic haematuria (p. 812)

Because some of these glomerular diseases may be part of a multisystem disease (e.g. systemic lupus erythematosus), problems unrelated to the kidney may dominate the clinical picture.

ACUTE POST-STREPTOCOCCAL GLOMERULONEPHRITIS

Acute post-streptococcal glomerulonephritis is most common in children of school age, though it may affect adults and, rarely, the very young. Males are more often affected. The preceding infection is usually in the upper respiratory tract, but can be in the skin or at other sites. There is usually a latency of 1–3 weeks. Group A, type 12, β-haemolytic streptococci are those most likely to cause acute glomerulonephritis.

Pathogenesis and pathology

Much circumstantial evidence points to a role for immune complexes, either circulating or formed in situ within the kidney, or both. Immune complexes are demonstrable in serum in most cases, and activation of serum complement is frequent. A diffuse generalised proliferative glomerulonephritis is present, often with an infiltrate of polymorphs. The tubules and interstitium are relatively spared. Immunofluorescence studies show granular deposits of C3 complement and IgG in the glomeruli.

Clinical features and diagnosis

The illness typically presents as an acute nephritic syndrome with oliguria, fluid retention, hypertension, proteinuria and haematuria. The degree of renal impairment is variable. In children, the illness is usually self-limiting, but adults show a greater propensity to develop severe renal impairment which may, in a minority of cases, be permanent.

The diagnosis is usually easy on clinical grounds alone. The urine is 'active' with red blood cells, cellular casts and protein. Evidence for preceding streptococcal infection is routinely sought by means of swabs of throat or any suspicious skin lesion, and serological tests for streptococcal infection such as the ASO titre and anti-DNase-B antibody. Hypocomplementaemia (low haemolytic complement and C3 with variable reduction of C2, C4 and C1q), probably due to alternative pathway activation (p. 101) and the presence of circulating immune complexes support the diagnosis. Renal biopsy is seldom required in children, although it may be in adults.

Treatment and prognosis

Anti-streptococcal antibiotics (penicillin or erythromycin) are generally given although there is no evidence that they influence the nephritis. In most cases, observation and general supportive measures are sufficient. In oliguric patients, fluid retention is controlled by appropriate restriction of dietary salt and water; protein and potassium are restricted if uraemia or hyperkalaemia threaten. Hypertension is best managed by avoiding or correcting over-expansion of the ECF, with the aid of loop diuretics if necessary. Careful control of blood pressure is particularly important in children, in whom hypertensive encephalopathy may develop when the blood pressure is only moderately elevated. Rarely, severe renal failure may require temporary dialysis treatment (p. 802) pending recovery of renal function. Long-term anti-streptococcal prophylaxis is not required.

Children have a better prognosis than adults. The early mortality is about 1% or less in children, but the minority in whom severe oliguria or proteinuria persist has a less favourable outcome. Long-term prognosis is uncertain, but it appears that a significant minority (up to 30%) may ultimately develop progressive renal disease, often 10 or more years later. Adults are more likely to show incomplete resolution after the initial attack and to progress thereafter to chronic renal failure.

GLOMERULONEPHRITIS IN ASSOCIATION WITH OTHER INFECTIONS

Pathology

The bacterial, viral or protozoan infections which may be complicated by glomerulonephritis are listed below in Summary 6.

Bacterial

The most important bacterial-associated glomerulonephritis is that seen in patients with infective endocarditis. These patients usually have only mild impairment of GFR, with microscopic haematuria, proteinuria and urinary casts, in association with clinical and laboratory manifestations of endocarditis. Rarely, the renal disturbance may dominate the clinical picture with the syndrome of rapidly progressive glomerulonephritis (RPGN) and renal failure. Circulating immune complexes are present and complement (C3 and C4) is reduced (classical pathway activation). Renal biopsy is only needed if the underlying diagnosis is in doubt or if renal impairment is severe and unremitting. A variety of renal lesions may be seen, but a focal proliferative GN is the commonest. Deposits of C3, IgG and IgM are conspicuous.

Other important chronic bacterial infections that may lead to GN include those arising on implanted devices (e.g. ventriculo-atrial shunts and synthetic vascular grafts) and in association with visceral abscesses.

Viral

The most important is chronic hepatitis B infection, which may lead to a variety of glomerular lesions, either in

Summary 6 Infections which may cause glomerulonephritis	
Bacterial	*Viral*
Group A, β-haemolytic streptococci	Hepatitis B
Other streptococci	Cytomegalovirus
Staphylococci	Epstein–Barr
Salmonella typhi	
Treponema pallidum	
Protozoan	
Plasmodium malariae	
Plasmodium falciparum	
Schistosoma haematobium	

isolation or in association with hepatic involvement, or a more generalised process such as systemic vasculitis or cryoglobulinaemia.

Parasitic

Plasmodium malariae and *Schistosoma haematobium* infection are important causes of nephrotic syndrome in endemic areas. This is particularly so in children, where they must be distinguished from idiopathic nephrotic syndrome due to minimal change disease.

Management

Removal of the offending antigen, if possible, may lead to resolution of the glomerulopathy, although this may be incomplete in some cases. Renal failure is managed along conventional lines. There is no evidence that other manoeuvres, such as immunosuppressive drugs or plasma exchange, are of benefit.

MEMBRANOUS GLOMERULONEPHRITIS

The majority of cases of membranous glomerulonephritis are idiopathic, but this lesion may also arise in a variety of underlying diseases (Table 21.29).

Table 21.29 Causes of membranous nephrophathy

Idiopathic	Drugs/toxins
Infections	Mercury
Malaria	Organic gold (in treatment of
Syphilis	rheumatoid arthritis)
Hepatitis B	Penicillamine
	Captopril
Neoplasia	
Lymphoma ⎫ rarely	**Multisystem disease**
Leukaemia ⎭	Systemic lupus erythematosus
Various carcinomas, especially of	Rheumatoid arthritis
the colon	

Pathogenesis and pathology

The pathogenesis is unknown. Renal biopsies show thickening of the glomerular basement membrane, with a spike and dome pattern visible using special stains. Diffuse deposits of IgG, IgM and C3 complement are present in glomerular capillary walls. The presence of immune complexes in serum is variable and their role in the pathogenesis unsubstantiated.

Clinical features and diagnosis

Most patients present with asymptomatic proteinuria or nephrotic syndrome. In adults, membranous glomerulonephritis is the commonest single cause of the nephrotic syndrome, and a significant minority of adults will have an underlying neoplasm, colonic carcinoma being the most common. Renal function is usually normal, or nearly so, at the time of presentation, but progression to chronic

renal failure is frequent, though difficult to predict. A proportion of patients, particularly those with underlying neoplasia, die of the non-renal cause of the disorder. Other complications, such as renal vein thrombosis and pulmonary emboli, are also a cause of morbidity and mortality. Hypertension becomes increasingly prevalent as the disease progresses.

The diagnosis rests on renal biopsy which should be carried out in adults and in those children whose nephrotic syndrome is resistant to corticosteroid drugs (see below).

Management

The nephrotic syndrome is managed conventionally (p. 811) and a watchful eye kept for renal vein thrombosis or pulmonary embolism, both of which are indications for anticoagulation. Treatment of the nephropathy is controversial. There is some evidence that regimens including chlorambucil and corticosteroids, given for six months improve the long-term outlook.

MINIMAL CHANGE NEPHROPATHY

Minimal change nephropathy (known in the past as 'lipoid nephrosis') is by far the commonest cause of childhood nephrotic syndrome. It is also an important cause of nephrotic syndrome in adults.

Pathogenesis and pathology

The pathogenesis and aetiology of the condition are unknown. There is some evidence of disordered T lymphocyte function, but the relevance of this to the pathogenesis is unproven. Of note, however, is the response of the lesion to steroids, alkylating agents and cyclosporin, all of which may interfere with T cell function. The glomeruli are normal by light microscopy; immunofluorescence is negative. Electron microscopy shows fusion of the epithelial cell foot processes, but this is also seen in many other glomerular diseases; it is of significance only when the glomeruli appear normal under light microscopy. These features in the presence of nephrotic syndrome favour a diagnosis of minimal change nephropathy.

Clinical features and diagnosis

Children and adults usually present with oedema and are found to have nephrotic syndrome. Hypertension is rare, and renal function is usually normal. Males predominate amongst young children, but, in adults, the sex incidence is approximately equal. Progression to chronic renal failure is exceedingly rare, although acute renal failure may supervene, particularly following excessive use of diuretics.

In adults, the diagnosis usually depends on renal biopsy. In children, however, the relative infrequency of other causes of nephrotic syndrome means that a more empirical diagnosis can often be reached, especially if the proteinuria is highly selective (p. 792). In all age groups, urinary cells and cellular casts are infrequent or absent.

Treatment and prognosis

In 80–90% of cases, the lesion responds to steroids given at moderate to high dose for 8 weeks, most patients showing a response in less than 4 weeks. Subsequent withdrawal of steroids may be followed by prolonged remission, or lead to relapse of the nephrotic syndrome necessitating a further course of steroid treatment. In steroid-resistant patients, or in those in whom remission can only be maintained by the use of unacceptably heavy exposure to steroids, cyclophosphamide or chlorambucil given for 8–10 weeks has led to prolonged remission or improved steroid responsiveness. Recent studies have suggested that the immunosuppressive agent, cyclosporin, is capable of inducing remissions in previously refractory patients.

The renal lesion virtually never progresses to chronic renal failure, and since the introduction of steroids and, more recently, cytotoxic therapy, the prognosis has been very good (Fig. 21.18), especially in children. Initial failure to respond to steroids heralds a less favourable outcome. Despite the benefits of these therapies, some of the small number of deaths are the result of complications of treatment, particularly infection.

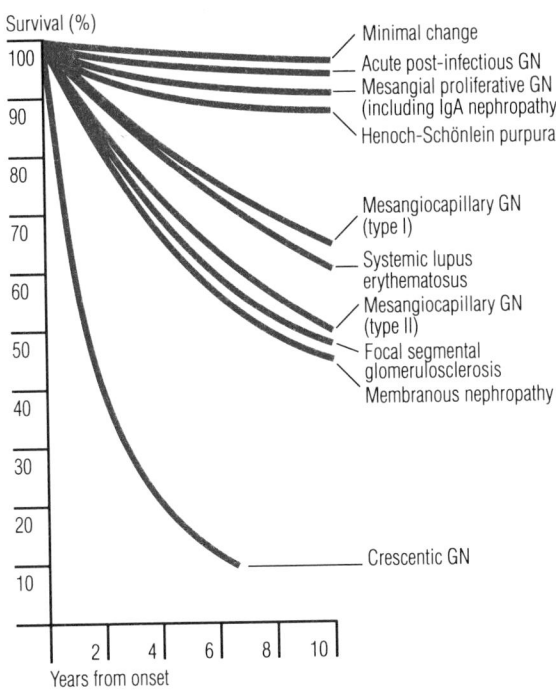

Fig. 21.18 Prognosis in various types of glomerulopathy.

FOCAL SEGMENTAL GLOMERULOSCLEROSIS

Focal segmental glomerulosclerosis (FSGS) is the second most common cause of nephrotic syndrome in children and, in contrast to minimal change GN, tends to progress to renal failure. Most cases are idiopathic, but some may be seen in association with underlying collagen vascular diseases.

Pathogenesis and pathology

The cause of FSGS is unknown. Although immune complexes may be found in as many as 70% of cases, there is no direct evidence of their involvement in the pathogenesis. The abnormal glomeruli are segmentally sclerosed, i.e. only a part of each glomerular tuft is affected. Early in the disease, only deep juxtamedullary glomeruli may be involved. IgM deposits are usually present, often with C3 complement also.

Clinical features, diagnosis and treatment

Children present with nephrotic syndrome and normal or near normal renal function. Amongst affected adults, a significant number present with asymptomatic proteinuria, hypertension and impairment of renal function.

The diagnosis invariably depends on renal biopsy. In early cases, there may be confusion with minimal change nephropathy unless the biopsy contains juxtamedullary glomeruli; these may be the only ones affected early in the course of FSGS. Proteinuria is usually non-selective and urine often contains red blood cells and casts, helping to distinguish it from minimal change nephropathy.

Some patients respond to steroids, but this is unpredictable. Cytotoxic drugs have been tried without established benefit.

MESANGIOCAPILLARY GLOMERULONEPHRITIS

Mesangiocapillary glomerulonephritis (MCGN) comprises at least two, and possibly three, distinct diseases, each with its own characteristic glomerular pathology. The types best characterised are designated type I and type II MCGN.

Pathogenesis and pathology

The pathogenesis is unknown and may well be different in the two types of MCGN. The glomerular pathology is characteristic. In *type I disease*, mesangial cell proliferation is marked and the glomerular basement membrane is intact, with subendothelial deposits easily visible on electron microscopy. *Type II disease* usually shows a lesser degree of mesangial cell proliferation and the electron-dense deposits appear to be intramembranous. IgG and complement are present, more consistently so, and in greater amounts, in type I MCGN. Persistent depression of plasma C3 complement is often found, particularly in patients with type II disease, and indicates complement activation by the alternative pathway. Circulating immune complexes are detectable in some patients.

Clinical features

Both types of MCGN may present with nephrotic syndrome, nephritic syndrome, hypertension or asymptomatic proteinuria/haematuria, and the majority of the presentations are in children or young adults. Slow progression to chronic renal failure is usual, though unpredictable. A minority of patients, usually with the type II variant, progress more rapidly and in a few patients, there is a fulminant course to end stage renal disease. It appears that those patients presenting with full blown nephrotic syndrome do worse than those with asymptomatic urinary abnormalities.

Diagnosis and treatment

The diagnosis depends on renal biopsy. The glomerular morphology of type I MCGN may be seen in patients with underlying SLE, hepatitis B infection and chronic bacterial infection (such as infective endocarditis) and steps should be taken to identify or exclude these conditions.

Steroids, with or without cytotoxic drugs, are probably not useful and may be harmful. Antiplatelet drugs and anticoagulants have also been tried and may be of benefit, but this remains to be confirmed.

IgA NEPHROPATHY (BERGER'S DISEASE)

Pathogenesis and pathology

In IgA nephropathy (Berger's disease), the glomeruli show extensive mesangial deposits of IgA, often accompanied by C3 complement. This pattern is also seen in patients with Henoch-Schönlein purpura. Diffuse mesangial proliferation with superimposed segmental lesions are seen on light microscopy.

Clinical features

This is predominantly a disease of young adult men, many of whom present with recurrent macroscopic haematuria sometimes accompanied by loin pain (p. 812). A degree of proteinuria is usual, and cellular casts in the urine confirm the glomerular origin of the red blood cells. Relapses may show a temporal relation with upper respiratory infections. The condition has had a benign reputation, but undoubtedly may progress to chronic renal failure, particularly if hypertension or heavy proteinuria is present early in the course. Occasionally, the disease may manifest itself with an acute nephritic syndrome.

Diagnosis and treatment

Although the clinical picture is often highly characteristic, renal biopsy is nearly always performed to establish the diagnosis with certainty. The IgA deposits that characterise the renal lesion are also evident in skin capillaries and this finding supports the diagnosis, even in the absence of renal biopsy. These patients should be spared fruitless and inappropriate urological investigation; a careful history and examination of the urinary deposit will usually indicate whether or not the haematuria is glomerular.

In many cases, the lesion is benign and observation only is required. No therapeutic intervention has been shown to alter the course of the progressive or relapsing disease.

IDIOPATHIC RAPIDLY PROGRESSIVE GLOMERULONEPHRITIS

Idiopathic rapidly progressive glomerulonephritis (idiopathic RPGN) is a serious condition which, as its name suggests, frequently progresses to renal failure.

Pathogenesis and pathology

There is little to suggest involvement of the immune system in this disease; neither circulating immune complexes nor glomerular deposits of immunoglobulin and C3 are evident in most cases. However apparently identical renal lesions can arise in patients with immunologically mediated disease, such as infective endocarditis or SLE. The pathological correlate of RPGN is the presence of glomerular crescents containing large amounts of fibrin.

Clinical features and diagnosis

The usual presentation is a sub-acute nephritic syndrome with malaise, hypertension, haematuria and proteinuria. Middle-aged and older adults predominate. Without treatment, the outlook is very poor.

RPGN should be suspected in any patient with apparent acute or sub-acute onset of renal impairment, particularly if the urine is 'active' with rbc's and cellular casts. Assessment of renal size will identify those patients with normal sized kidneys in whom chronic renal failure is unlikely. Renal biopsy is then required to establish the diagnosis.

Treatment

Empirical treatment with high doses of steroid drugs appears to be of some benefit, but these agents should not be given for more than four weeks unless there is clear evidence of a response. Plasma exchange and cytotoxic drugs have been tried and there are many anecdotal reports of success. Although this approach has yet to be subjected to controlled evaluation, standard therapy would comprise steroids at high dose, a cytotoxic drug such as cyclophosphamide or azathioprine (the latter possibly less effective) and intensive plasma exchange.

HEREDITARY NEPHRITIS (ALPORT'S SYNDROME)

Alport's syndrome is an inherited disorder that is characterised by progressive renal impairment and nerve deafness. Presentation is usually with microscopic or gross haematuria. Males tend to be more severely affected than females, particularly with regard to the nephropathy; and associated deafness is variable or even absent in some patients. The mode of inheritance is inconsistent, with some families showing a dominant, and others an X-linked pattern. The renal lesion is predominantly glomerular; although there are no specific features on light microscopy, electron microscopy reveals a thin, fragmented and sometimes split glomerular basement membrane. There is no known treatment.

RENAL INVOLVEMENT IN NON-RENAL AND MULTISYSTEM DISEASE

Involvement of the kidney occurs in many diseases. In most of these, the glomerulus is the site of damage, with a glomerulonephritis which may give rise to the syndromes of glomerular disease. The renal manifestations are of variable severity but, in some cases, may dominate the clinical picture.

SYSTEMIC LUPUS ERYTHEMATOSUS

Renal involvement in systemic lupus erythematosus (SLE) may manifest itself with haematuria/proteinuria, acute nephritic syndrome, nephrotic syndrome or chronic renal impairment. At least four glomerular lesions are described, all associated with deposition of complement and immunoglobulins within the glomeruli and with activation of complement and the presence of circulating immune complexes. The most benign lesion comprises deposition of Ig's and complement in an otherwise normal, or slightly abnormal, glomerulus. Focal and segmental proliferative glomerulonephritis and membranous glomerulonephritis both have an unpredictable prognosis, while diffuse proliferative glomerulonephritis with SLE progresses to renal failure in the majority of cases. In a few patients, tubulointerstitial involvement dominates, with demonstrable Ig and C3 deposition on the tubular basement membrane.

Treatment. The need to treat is dictated by evidence of progressive renal disease and/or the presence of a renal lesion that is likely to progress. Steroids, often in combination with cytotoxic drugs such as cyclophosphamide or azathioprine, are used, sometimes with plasma exchange. There is now accumulating evidence that regimens that include a cytotoxic drug, especially cyclophosphamide given intravenously, are more effective at preventing progression of nephropathy than are steroids alone.

POLYARTERITIS

Polyarteritis usually affects the middle-aged and elderly, with males predominating. Renal involvement is frequent and in some cases the disease may appear to be limited to the kidneys at the time of presentation. Patients with involvement of medium-sized vessels, so-called *polyarteritis nodosa* or *classical polyarteritis*, suffer the consequences of renal ischaemia with hypertension, renal infarction and renal failure. Diagnosis can be made by skin biopsy, by visceral arteriography which may show multiple small aneurysms in the kidney or other viscera, or by renal biopsy in which arteritic lesions may be seen.

Microscopic polyarteritis on the other hand usually presents with an acute or sub-acute nephritic syndrome, often with purpura, arthropathy and myopathy. Clinically it may resemble Henoch-Schönlein purpura. Renal biopsies show a florid necrotising glomerulonephritis. Anti-neutrophil cytoplasmic antibodies (ANCA) are often present in serum.

Treatment. Both types often respond to treatment with high dose steroids, and the addition of cyclophosphamide or azathioprine confers additional benefit. (Polyarteritis is discussed further in Ch. 24, p. 1023).

WEGENER'S GRANULOMATOSIS

Wegener's granulomatosis (see also Ch. 24, p. 1023) has features in common with microscopic polyarteritis, including the presence of ANCA, but may be distinguished by its propensity for involvement of the upper airways and lungs and by the granulomatous nature of the arteritic lesions. Renal biopsies show necrotising glomerulitis, which usually manifests itself clinically with an acute nephritic syndrome. The prognosis has improved greatly with the use of cyclophosphamide and steroids which control the disease in the majority of cases.

HENOCH-SCHÖNLEIN PURPURA

Henoch-Schönlein purpura is a condition of children and young adults who present with some or all of the following: glomerulonephritis, skin purpura, arthralgia/arthritis, abdominal pain. The renal lesion is a mesangial-proliferative GN with prominent IgA deposits. IgA is also deposited in skin and other tissues, in this respect resembling IgA nephropathy (Berger's disease). Disease activity is intermittent and tends to involve several organs at once. The glomerulonephritis is usually benign, especially in children, but may progress rapidly or slowly following a series of acute episodes with incomplete resolution. An immune complex aetiology is probable and no treatment is convincingly effective.

SYSTEMIC SCLEROSIS

Visceral involvement in systemic sclerosis frequently includes the kidneys, in which marked thickening of the walls of the medium-sized arteries occurs (see also p. 1021). The glomerular lesions are those of ischaemia and severe accelerated phase hypertension is a frequent complication. The aetiology is unknown and there is no effective treatment for the underlying condition. However, the advent of potent vasodilating drugs such as minoxidil and, more recently, of the angiotensin converting enzyme inhibitors, captopril and enalapril, allows effective blood pressure control in most of these patients. The result has been a greatly improved renal prognosis, although other manifestations of the disease, particularly cardiac ones, remain potentially lethal.

RHEUMATOID ARTHRITIS

Renal disease in patients with rheumatoid arthritis is usually the result of secondary amyloid (AA type) or of adverse reaction to anti-rheumatic drugs such as gold, penicillamine or non-steroidal anti-inflammatory agents.

Renal and Urinary Disease

However, a few patients, particularly those with wide-spread vasculitis, may develop glomerulonephritis or renal vasculitis. Steroids and cytotoxic drugs have been effective in some cases.

GOODPASTURE'S SYNDROME

The term Goodpasture's syndrome refers to a disease in which the following features are present: lung haemorrhage, glomerulonephritis and formation of antibody to glomerular basement membrane (anti-GBM antibody). Several other diseases, such as Wegener's granulomatosis, SLE and Legionnaire's disease, may have clinical features indistinguishable from Goodpasture's syndrome, but anti-GBM antibody is absent in these conditions.

The reason for the formation of anti-GBM antibody is unknown; it probably plays a central part in the pathogenesis of the disease, and renal biopsies show linear deposits of IgG and C3 complement along the glomerular capillary walls, accompanied by a proliferative GN, often with crescent formation. The anti-GBM antibody is also demonstrable in lung and deposits there probably mediate the lung haemorrhage.

The disease predominates in young male adults and there is considerable case to case variation. Either the pulmonary or the renal lesions may dominate the clinical picture.

Treatment centres around attempts to remove the offending antibody by means of plasma exchange, and to prevent its reappearance by the use of cytotoxic drugs. This approach, with dialysis support when needed, has greatly improved the outlook.

OTHER ACQUIRED COLLAGEN VASCULAR DISEASES

Mixed connective tissue disease (p. 511), essential mixed cryoglobulinaemia (p. 1092), sarcoidosis (p. 506) and Sjögren's syndrome (p. 990) may all be associated with glomerulonephritis, in addition to the more frequent association between Sjögren's syndrome and interstitial nephropathy (p. 824).

NEOPLASTIC DISEASE

Malignancy may disturb kidney function in a number of ways (Table 21.30). Both isolated solid tumours or diffuse neoplasms of lymphoid tissue may be involved. Tumour lysis syndrome results from the very rapid release of urate and phosphate from a tumour undergoing necrosis, and may lead to acute renal failure from acute uric acid nephropathy. The specific instance of multiple myeloma and the dysproteinaemias is discussed below.

DYSPROTEINAEMIA, MULTIPLE MYELOMA AND RENAL AMYLOID

Multiple myeloma and the other dysproteinaemias may all involve the kidneys and at least 50% of patients with

Table 21.30 Mechanisms of renal disturbance in malignant disease

Mechanism	Example
Obstruction	Carcinoma of prostate, bladder, cervix, rectum Para-aortic lymphadenopathy Intrarenal, e.g. urate, Bence-Jones proteinuria
Direct invasion of kidney	Leukaemia Hodgkin's disease and other lymphomas Myeloma
Secondary glomerulopathy Membranous nephropathy	Associated with carcinoma of lung, stomach, colon, breast, ovary
Minimal change glomerulopathy	Associated with Hodgkin's disease, lymphoma or leukaemia
Tumour-induced metabolic disturbance	Hypercalcaemia Urate nephropathy Syndrome of inappropriate ADH secretion (SIADHS)

multiple myeloma will ultimately die of renal failure. The most important renal manifestations are *amyloid* (p. 1092) and *myeloma kidney* (Table. 21.31).

Amyloid in patients with myeloma is of the AL type and its presence in the kidney (and an associated nephrotic syndrome) may antedate other clinical manifestations of myeloma. The nature of the renal lesion is essentially the same, whether the amyloid is associated with underlying multiple myeloma, unassociated with malignant disease, or secondary to a chronic inflammatory process, such as sepsis or rheumatoid arthritis (amyloid of AA type). There is no specific treatment for the renal lesion, which usually progresses inexorably, although it is possible that chemotherapy of the myeloma at an early stage of the disease may slow or halt the progression of the amyloid as well.

Table 21.31 Renal damage in multiple myeloma

- Bence–Jones proteinuria
- Myeloma kidney
- Hypercalcaemia
- Hyperuricaemia (especially at initiation of chemotherapy)
- Renal amyloid
- Dehydration ± X-ray contrast media (combination prone to induce acute renal failure)
- Plasma cell infiltration
- Glomerulonephritis (immunologically mediated)
- Hyperviscosity syndrome (e.g. in macroglobulinaemia) may cause papillary necrosis
- Obstruction (by stone or sloughed papillae)

822

Myeloma kidney is a tubulointerstitial nephropathy caused by nephrotoxic immunoglobulin light chains (Bence-Jones protein) in the glomerular filtrate. Recovery is unpredictable, and depends on successful treatment of the myeloma and reduction of the urinary Bence-Jones protein load. Even so, this lesion is often irreversible.

DIABETES MELLITUS

Renal involvement in diabetes becomes progressively more common with increasing duration of disease, such that after 20 years, some 30% of diabetics will have proteinuria or other evidence of nephropathy. The nephropathy is usually, though not always, associated with malignant vasculopathy and with other vascular complications of diabetes mellitus.

Glomerular changes predominate and are of two types:

1. *diffuse glomerulosclerosis*, in which there is thickening of the glomerular basement membrane, capillary wall and mesangium. This lesion is common, but is not specific for diabetes mellitus
2. *nodular glomerulosclerosis (Kimmelstiel-Wilson lesion)*, which is specific for diabetes mellitus but is present in only a minority of patients.

The pathogenesis of diabetic nephropathy is unknown but attention has focussed on two main possibilities:

1. *Genetic.* The renal lesion is a manifestation of a genetic defect that also leads to carbohydrate intolerance. Various observations make this unlikely, in particular the finding of diabetic nephropathy in some 'non-genetic' cases, e.g. following pancreatectomy.
2. *Acquired.* The renal lesion is acquired and is secondary to either lack of insulin, hyperglycaemia or both. This is now the favoured explanation, although the mechanism is unclear.

The disease generally passes through four recognisable phases:

1. hyperfiltration with supranormal GFR
2. microalbuminuria (but still dipstick-negative)
3. proteinuria (dipstick-positive)
4. heavy proteinuria (with nephrotic syndrome or renal failure).

Hypertension develops in virtually all these patients. Deterioration is inevitable, though its rate is unpredictable.

There is now, however, great interest in the possibility that reduction of the glomerular hypertension, that is known to coexist with hyperfiltration early in diabetes, may slow the development of nephropathy. In the short term, this can be achieved by means of protein restriction or use of angiotensin converting enzyme inhibitors (p. 808). Coexistent arterial hypertension accelerates progression; conversely, intensive anti-hypertensive therapy to the point of absolute normotension retards progression. There is no convincing evidence that good control of blood sugar either prevents the development of clinically significant nephropathy or slows progress. However, it is not yet clear whether this pessimistic view applies to the very tight control that is now available using insulin pumps. This question is unlikely to be resolved for 10–20 years, because of the long latent period between the onset of diabetes and the appearance of complications.

SICKLE CELL DISORDERS

The most important renal complications seen in sickle cell disorders (discussed in Ch. 25, p. 1054) are recurrent gross haematuria, papillary necrosis and glomerulonephritis.

INTRAVASCULAR COAGULATION

Several conditions may lead to intravascular coagulation (Ch. 25, p. 1099) and renal impairment, but these two features are especially characteristic in *haemolytic uraemic syndrome* (HUS) and *thrombotic thrombocytopenic purpura*. In both these conditions, there is evidence of micro-angiopathic haemolytic anaemia (MAHA) and thrombocytopenia. Although laboratory features are similar, haemolytic uraemic syndrome is mainly a disease of children with prominent renal involvement, whereas thrombotic thrombocytopenic purpura usually affects adults and renal disease is more variable. The aetiology is uncertain, although HUS appears to follow viral or bacterial infections in children and also has shown case clustering in schools or families. Recent evidence has implicated verucytotoxin producing *E. coli* infection: patients with HUS produce antibody to verucytotoxin and the toxin itself can produce similar angiopathic lesions in rabbits. A rare disease indistinguishable from haemolytic uraemic syndrome has been recognised following apparently normal pregnancy and also in women taking the contraceptive pill. Treatment of these conditions is difficult, and the best prospects are offered by a combination of antiplatelet drugs and infusions of fresh plasma.

GOUTY NEPHROPATHY

Man excretes urate/uric acid in amounts that are very high considering the low solubility of uric acid at acid pH. Three types of clinical problem may arise:

Uric acid stone formation (p. 831).

Acute uric acid nephropathy. This is due to massive deposition of uric acid crystals in the tubules, renal pelvis and ureters and arises as a complication of accelerated uric acid production during treatment of widespread malignancy, such as lymphoma or leukaemia (Ch. 25, p. 1073). The xanthine oxidase inhibitor, allopurinol, usually provides adequate prophylaxis.

Chronic urate (gouty) nephropathy. This is a common accompaniment of prolonged hyperuricaemia, itself strongly associated with clinical gout. The renal damage is mainly interstitial, although glomerular changes also occur. Sodium urate crystals may be demonstrable in renal tissue in some cases. Management is prophylactic using allopurinol to decrease plasma and urine urate levels. Established chronic urate nephropathy is irreversible, although progression may be halted or slowed by allopurinol therapy.

DISEASES OF THE RENAL INTERSTITIUM

Diseases of the renal interstitium are sometimes collectively termed 'tubulointerstitial disease' or 'interstitial nephropathy'.

Aetiology and pathology

These conditions have varied causes (Table 21.32). Pathologically the tubulointerstitial nephropathies are distinguished from the glomerulopathies by relative sparing of the glomeruli and prominent changes affecting the non-glomerular components of the renal parenchyma, i.e. the interstitium and tubules.

Table 21.32 Causes of tubulointerstitial disease

Cause	Acute	Chronic
Idiopathic	+	+
Drug hypersensitivity		
Penicillin	+	
Cephalosporins	+	
Sulphonamides	+	
Diuretics	+	
NSAIDs	+	
Toxin-induced		
Aminoglycoside antibiotics	+	
Analgesic abuse		+
Lithium		+
X-ray contrast media	+	
Heavy metals	+	+
Immunological disorders		
Sjögren's syndrome		+
SLE		+
Neoplasia		
Myeloma kidney	+	+
Leukaemic infiltration		+
Metabolic		
Hypercalcaemia	+	+
Hypokalaemia	+	+
Uric acid	+	+
Other		
Acute pyelonephritis	+	
Chronic pyelonephritis		+
Reflux		+
Obstruction	+	+
Sickle cell disorder		+

Table 21.33 Iatrogenic toxic nephropathy

Drug	Renal disturbance
Antibiotics	
Aminoglycosides (gentamicin, tobramycin, amikacin)	ARF with or without oliguria
Penicillins (methicillin, benzylpenicillin, ampicillin)	Acute interstitial nephropathy
Sulphonamides	Precipitation in tubules
Cephalosporins (especially cephaloridine)	ARF
Demeclocycline	Nephrogenic diabetes insipidus
Amphotericin B	Decreased renal blood flow; tubular toxicity
NSAIDs	Acute or chronic interstitial nephropathy
Penicillamine	Nephrotic syndrome
Organic gold	Nephrotic syndrome
Diuretics (thiazides, frusemide)	Interstitial nephropathy
Lithium carbonate	Tubular syndromes, chronic interstitial nephropathy
X-ray contrast media	ARF with or without oliguria

Acute tubulointerstitial nephropathy is characterised by prominent interstitial oedema with a heavy infiltrate of inflammatory cells, amongst which neutrophils, eosinophils or mononuclear cells may predominate.

In contrast, *chronic tubulointerstitial nephropathy* is associated with marked tubular atrophy, interstitial fibrosis and an infiltrate of mononuclear cells. Patients may present with acute renal failure (p. 800), chronic renal failure (p. 803) or a tubular syndrome (p. 813). Heavy proteinaemia (more than 3 g/day) is exceedingly uncommon. In general, although by no means always, tubulointerstitial diseases are less likely to be associated with oliguria or anuria and are more likely to give rise to one or more of the renal tubular syndromes than are the glomerulopathies.

Many nephrotoxins act primarily on the interstitial tissues. In some cases, toxicity may be confined to the kidney, while others may involve several organs. Drugs are an important cause of toxicity, antibiotic and anti-rheumatic agents being particularly important. The list given in Table 21.33 is far from exhaustive. *Analgesic nephropathy* is a tubulointerstitial disease that results from prolonged exposure to certain mild analgesics. Phenacetin (now withdrawn) was implicated, but there is also evidence that aspirin, and non-steroidal anti-inflammatory drugs may be involved in some cases. The disease eventually leads to ischaemic necrosis of the renal papillae and chronic renal failure; in the past, analgesic nephropathy was one of the major causes of end stage renal disease in a number of developed countries.

Conditions such as renal obstruction (p. 833), reflux

nephropathy and infection (p. 830) and multisystem diseases of the kidney (p. 821), may lead to severe interstitial damage. Obstruction (p. 833), reflux and infection (p. 830) are discussed in detail elsewhere, but nevertheless fall into the broad category of tubulointerstitial nephropathy.

Diagnosis and treatment

The frequency of drug-induced acute or chronic tubulo-interstitial nephropathy indicates that the diagnosis should be carefully considered in any patient presenting with an unexplained acute or chronic renal disturbance. A history of relevant drug exposure should be sought and, in many cases, a renal biopsy will be needed to define the renal lesion and the potential for recovery. In most cases, the treatment is expectant, with removal or avoidance of any relevant nephrotoxin if possible, and treatment of any underlying immunological disorder. Acute idiopathic cases and those associated with hypersensitivity reactions to drugs, such as penicillin, may benefit from a short course of steroids and generally have a good prognosis. Chronicity and the presence of marked tubular atrophy or interstitial fibrosis on biopsy are adverse features, although progression may be very slow.

CYSTIC DISEASES OF THE KIDNEY

Renal cysts are relatively common and vary greatly in significance. Table 21.34 gives a classification of the

Table 21.34 Cystic diseases of the kidney

Cystic disease	Clinical and pathological features
Polycystic kidney disease	
Adult polycystic kidney disease	Common. Dominant inheritance. Renal failure. Associated with hepatic cysts but no hepatic disease
Juvenile polycystic kidney disease	Rare. Recessive inheritance. Hepatic cysts, renal and hepatic failure
Simple cysts	
Single / Multiple	Common. Often asymptomatic
Neoplastic cysts	Renal cell tumour (hypernephroma)
Medullary cysts	
Medullary cystic disease	Usually dominant inheritance; presents in childhood. Progressive renal failure
Medullary sponge kidney	Tubular ectasia. Nephrocalcinosis. Recurrent urinary infections

important types, of which the three most deserving of attention are:
1. adult polycystic kidney disease
2. simple cysts (single or multiple)
3. neoplastic cysts.

Less common are medullary cystic disease (MCD) and juvenile nephronopthisis.

ADULT POLYCYSTIC KIDNEY DISEASE

Adult polycystic kidney disease is an important cause of renal failure, accounting for 5–10% of all cases of end stage renal disease. It is inherited as an autosomal dominant and the penetrance is 100%. Genetic counselling is therefore important. The gene has been localised to chromosome 16 close to the α-globin locus, enabling presymptomatic and prenatal diagnosis by DNA markers in some families.

Clinical features

Presentation may be with microscopic or macroscopic haematuria, hypertension, renal pain (associated with haemorrhage into a cyst or infection), chronic renal failure or identification of enlarged kidneys. Progressive enlargement of the cysts leading to impairment of renal function is the rule, about 10–20 years elapsing between presentation and end stage renal disease in most cases. About 30% of patients also have hepatic cysts; these are not associated with hepatic dysfunction. There appears to be an increased incidence of subarachnoid haemorrhage in patients with adult polycystic kidney disease, and 10–22% of patients may have intracranial aneurysms.

Diagnosis and treatment

Diagnosis is easy in advanced cases, where the enlarged kidneys may be palpated and their gross morphology assessed by renal ultrasound. However, in early cases, particularly in children and young adult relatives of affected patients presenting for screening, diagnosis may be extremely difficult. Good quality renal ultrasound offers the best combination of accuracy, sensitivity and acceptability to the patient, although the sensitivity of CT scanning may be slightly better than that of ultrasound. Renal biopsy is not appropriate in these patients.

Complications include hypertension, urinary infections and stone formation, and bleeding into cysts or the urine. Energetic treatment of these problems probably retards progression but, at present, there are no means of slowing or preventing the underlying process of cyst enlargement and renal damage.

SIMPLE CYSTS

Simple cysts may be single or multiple. If large enough, they may present with loin pain or a loin mass, but they are more frequently picked up incidentally during the course of renal imaging for other reasons.

NEOPLASTIC CYSTS

Some renal tumours may exhibit cyst formation and it is therefore most important to distinguish accurately between benign simple cysts and neoplastic cysts. This may often be achieved with acceptable certainty by means of careful imaging by ultrasound or computerised tomography; however, it may be necessary to aspirate the cysts percutaneously and perform cytological examination of the fluid or renal arteriography in doubtful cases.

JUVENILE POLYCYSTIC KIDNEY DISEASE

Juvenile polycystic kidney disease is an uncommon recessively inherited disorder also associated with hepatic fibrosis and cysts. Renal and/or hepatic failure develop early.

MEDULLARY CYSTIC DISEASE AND JUVENILE NEPHRONOPTHISIS

Medullary cystic disease (autosomal dominant) and juvenile nephronopthisis (autosomal recessive) are causes of renal failure in early adulthood and childhood respectively. The prominent tubulointerstitial involvement leads to urinary concentrating defects and other tubular syndromes. There is no specific treatment.

RENAL DISEASE AND HYPERTENSION

The kidney and blood pressure interact in a number of ways and the final common paths of these interactions are such that:

1. the kidney may cause hypertension
2. the kidney may be damaged by hypertension.

Raised blood pressure as a consequence of renal or renal vascular disease

Hypertension is much commoner in patients with renal diseases than in the population at large, and the incidence of hypertension in such patients increases as renal function declines. By the time that chronic renal failure occurs, at least 80% of patients will be, or will have been, hypertensive. Amongst these patients it is evident that those whose disease affects primarily the vascular elements (renal arterial disease, systemic sclerosis, polyarteritis nodosa) or glomeruli (all forms of glomerulonephritis) are more likely to become hypertensive than those whose disease affects mainly tubulointerstitial elements (pyelonephritis, tubulointerstitial nephropathy, obstructive injury).

It appears that two major processes, acting either in isolation or (probably more frequently) in concert, underlie the raised blood pressure in these patients. These are:

1. increases in body sodium and water content
2. inappropriately increased activity of the renin-angiotensin-aldosterone system.

Increased body sodium and water content. The most clear-cut example is the anephric patient receiving regular dialysis treatment. Here, the renin-angiotensin system is essentially non-functioning, and blood pressure is found to be closely related to the level of ECF expansion, rising as body sodium/water are allowed to increase and falling when sodium/water are removed by dialysis. Inhibition of the renin-angiotensin system by converting-enzyme inhibitors has only minor effects on blood pressure.

Increased activity of the renin-angiotensin-aldosterone system. In some patients in whom there is no evidence of excess body sodium and water, angiotensin-converting-enzyme inhibition dramatically reduces blood pressure, implying dependence of the elevated blood pressure on the renin-angiotensin-aldosterone system.

In practice, hypertension in most renal patients is probably a consequence of both the mechanisms outlined above. Impaired ability to excrete sodium/water in the patient with renal vascular or parenchymal disease favours ECF expansion and a rise in blood pressure. In a normal individual, this would trigger a pressure-induced natriuresis and neurohumoral responses (including decreased renin release and increased release of atrial natriuretic peptides), both of which favour natriuresis (Fig. 21.19). The abnormal kidney, however, may show a blunted natriuretic response and may also fail to demonstrate appropriate suppression of renin release under these circumstances. Thus, volume expansion develops, the renin-angiotensin-aldosterone system is unsuppressed and hypertension ensues.

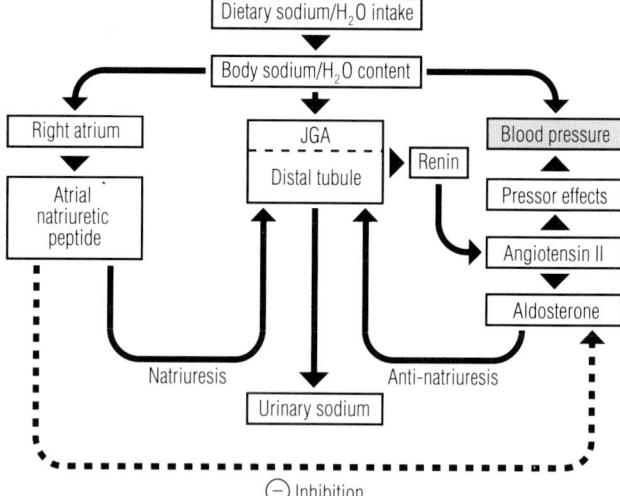

Fig. 21.19 Renal hypertension.

Renal damage as a consequence of raised blood pressure

The effect of raised blood pressure on the kidney depends on its severity, chronicity and whether or not the hypertension is in the *benign phase* or the *accelerated phase* (p. 438). It is doubtful whether hypertension in the benign phase poses a serious threat to renal function in the short or medium term, although there is some evidence that blacks may be more susceptible to renal damage in this setting. In contrast, the accelerated phase of hypertension is associated with florid changes in the renal circulation, with fibrinoid necrosis and very marked endothelial cell proliferation giving rise to the so-called 'onion peel' appearance of the small blood vessels. These lesions are remarkably similar to those seen in patients with systemic sclerosis (p. 821). Rapid progression to renal failure is the rule, unless the spiral of increasing blood pressure and increasingly severe glomerular ischaemia is interrupted by means of effective hypotensive treatment.

Management

Hypertension with underlying renal parenchymal disease

The aim of treatment is the normalisation of blood pressure, achieved in most cases by a combination of dietary manipulation and drugs. The following possibilities must be considered:

1. Is the patient fluid-overloaded? (Physical signs include raised JVP, peripheral oedema, pulmonary oedema.)
2. Is the patient in the benign or the accelerated phase of hypertension? (The signs are mainly in the optic fundi; grade III or grade IV changes indicate accelerated phase and the need for immediate treatment.)

Those patients in whom volume expansion is a major factor will respond well to a combination of dietary sodium restriction and a loop diuretic such as frusemide (thiazides do not work well in patients with significant impairment of renal function). It is important not to cause excessive reduction in body sodium/water; to do so would introduce a 'pre-renal factor' which could further compromise renal function.

Patients in whom there is no evidence of volume overload, or who have not responded adequately to therapeutic reduction of body sodium/water, will usually respond well to inhibition of the renin-angiotensin system, reflecting the overactivity of this system in the genesis of their hypertension. The renin-angiotensin system may be inhibited by beta-blocking drugs which reduce renin release from the juxta-glomerular apparatus (JGA), or by drugs that inhibit angiotensin-converting enzyme, such as captopril or enalapril.

There remains a group of patients whose response is inadequate, or who are unable to tolerate the above manoeuvres. The addition of calcium antagonists (e.g. nifedipine), vasodilating drugs (e.g. hydralazine or minoxidil), centrally acting drugs such as methyldopa, or peripheral adrenergic blocking drugs such as prazosin, will usually lead eventually to an acceptable and effective combination of hypotensive agents.

Hypertension with underlying renal vascular disease

Regardless of the site of the arterial lesion (renal artery, branches of the renal artery, arcuate or interlobular vessels, or arterioles), the result is reduced renal blood flow, reduced pulse pressure at the baroreceptor in the JGA, and consequently increased release of renin by the JGA. In these patients, overactivity of the renin-angiotensin system is usually the dominant factor. Body sodium/water status is variable and successful inhibition of the renin-angiotensin system with a beta-blocker or angiotensin-converting-enzyme inhibitor is likely to control blood pressure, if necessary with the help of a diuretic or additional hypotensive agents. Angiotensin-converting-enzyme inhibitors may cause a profound reduction in GFR in patients with critical renal artery stenosis, and are contraindicated if the stenosis is bilateral, or affects a solitary functioning kidney.

Disease of the renal artery

Disease of the renal artery poses a particular therapeutic problem because, in some cases, correction of the stenotic lesion will cure or ameliorate the hypertension and, if the stenotic lesion is severe, improve renal function. Stenosis of the renal artery is most often atheromatous and is therefore likely to be seen in middle-aged and elderly people with risk factors for arterial disease. A smaller number arise in young women in whom the pathology is fibromuscular hyperplasia of the renal artery. In both instances, the disease may be unilateral or bilateral.

Treatment, when indicated (see below), may be by open operation or balloon dilatation by the technique of percutaneous transluminal angioplasty. Two considerations may lead to a decision to undertake angioplasty or surgery for renal artery stenosis:

1. *The belief that correction of the lesion will cure or ameliorate the hypertension.* This is often very difficult to predict, but is more likely when the patient is young, when the hypertension is of very recent onset, when the disease is unilateral and confined to the renal artery, and when renal venous blood sampling shows plasma renin activity much higher on the affected side than elsewhere in the circulation.
2. *The hope that renal function can be improved by correction of the stenotic lesion.* This usually involves patients with bilateral atheromatous lesions in whom progression of the atheroma may lead to total occlusion, with a consequent catastrophic loss of renal function.

These decisions are rarely straightforward and, in general, with the better tolerated and more effective hypotensive drugs now available, there has been a swing away from 'curative' renal artery surgery as treatment for hypertension, although percutaneous transluminal angioplasty is increasingly used in carefully selected cases.

Unilateral renal disease and hypertension

In addition to unilateral renal artery stenosis, hypertension has been reported in association with unilateral renal emboli, renal tumours, unilateral hydronephrosis, unilateral trauma, renal vein thrombosis, unilateral chronic pyelonephritis, unilateral renal cysts and unilateral renal dysplasia. Nephrectomy may be considered in such cases, where the following indications may apply:

1. the kidney is dangerous, such as with renal tumour
2. the kidney is useless and there is a good chance of 'surgical cure' of hypertension, such as in dysplastic kidney, infarcted kidney or poorly functioning pyelonephritic kidney with good contralateral function.

URINARY TRACT INFECTION, PYELONEPHRITIS AND TUBERCULOSIS

URINARY TRACT INFECTION

Infection of the urinary tract is exceedingly common, but in the vast majority of cases it is mild and easily treated. Table 21.35 lists the most common infecting organisms. A working definition of urinary tract infection (UTI) is the presence, in an appropriately collected mid-stream specimen of urine (MSU), of more than 10^{-5} colony forming units per ml of urine. However, this is merely an arbitrary limit above which significant infection is likely and below which infection is less likely. Exceptions are frequent. The diagnosis is made more likely if there is accompanying pyuria (evident on microscopic examination of the urine) and much less likely if more than one organism is isolated. *Sterile pyuria* is defined as white cells in the urine in the absence of significant bacterial growth. The causes of sterile pyuria are shown in Summary 7. As UTI most frequently arises by means of ascending infection, faecal organisms predominate (Table 21.35). Important exceptions are *Staphylococcus aureus* and *M. tuberculosis*, both of which usually reach the kidney by the haematogenous route.

Table 21.35 Urinary pathogens

• *E. coli*	• *Staphylococci*
• *Enterococci*	• *Klebsiella*
• *Proteus*	• *Candida* (usually catheter associated)
• *Enterobacter*	
• *Pseudomonas*	• *Myobacterium tuberculosis*

Predisposing factors

A number of factors predispose to the development of UTI.

1. *Female sex.* The male urethra is longer than the female one and this, together with the antibacterial action of prostatic secretions, probably accounts for the substantially higher incidence of UTI in females of all ages as compared to males.
2. *Failure of complete bladder emptying.* The most import-

ant causes are outflow obstruction due to prostatic hypertrophy in males and neurological diseases leading to functional disturbances of micturition in either sex.

3. *Anatomical disorders of the bladder.* These may be congenital or acquired (e.g. bladder diverticulum(a), cystocoele).
4. *Vesicoureteric reflux.* Reflux of urine into the ureters or kidney during micturition is abnormal, and, as well as predisposing to UTI, also renders ascent of the infection to the kidney much more likely. It is commonest in children and its importance lies in its likely role in the aetiology of chronic pyelonephritis (p. 830).
5. *Pregnancy.* The ureters and renal pelves dilate during normal pregnancy and it is probable, though not proven, that this contributes to the substantially increased incidence of UTI seen in pregnant women. These infections are also more likely to be associated with pyelonephritis than in non-pregnant females.
6. *Diabetes mellitus.* Diabetics as a whole suffer more UTIs than non-diabetics. This increase is confined largely to those patients with long-standing disease and neuropathic bladder dysfunction. Young diabetics are not at risk of UTI.
7. *Tumours.* Urinary tract infection may be the first sign of an underlying bladder tumour.
8. *Stones.* The presence of stones anywhere in the urinary tract makes infection more likely and also renders it much harder to eliminate.
9. *Foreign body.* The commonest foreign body in the urinary tract is an indwelling bladder catheter, the insertion of which often introduces infection, and the presence of which makes existing infection virtually impossible to eliminate. Other foreign bodies, such as nephrostomy tubes and ureteric stents, also favour infection. However, in the short term, these are rarely dangerous provided that there is no obstruction to urine flow.

Summary 7 Causes of sterile pyuria

- Recently treated urinary infection
- Tuberculosis
- Acute interstitial nephritis
- Chronic interstitial nephritis (including analgesic nephropathy)
- Chronic pyelonephritis

Clinical features

The presentation of UTI depends on the location and type of infection, though the relationship between apparent location of infection based on symptoms (i.e. bladder or kidney) does not always correlate with definitively demonstrated site of infection.

Urethral syndrome. Urethral syndrome is the combination of dysuria, frequency, urgency and strangury without demonstrable UTI as defined above. Women are affected almost exclusively and the disorder is probably heterogeneous, resulting from mechanical factors (sexual intercourse), chemical irritation (toiletries) or atypical infection (chlamydia, viruses or bacteria in small numbers).

Cystitis. Symptoms are those of the urethral syndrome and range from trivial to severe. They are accompanied by pyuria and significant bacteriuria. The urine is usually cloudy and may be foul smelling. A variable degree of constitutional disturbance is usually present and, in a minority of cases, the infection may ascend leading to acute pyelonephritis (see below).

Asymptomatic bacteriuria. In adults, the incidental finding of significant bacteriuria is generally of little consequence, although pregnant women show a propensity for the asymptomatic bacteriuria to progress to cystitis and acute pyelonephritis. However, in children the position is less clear, in that a significant minority will prove to have associated abnormalities of the urinary tract. In both children and adults, spontaneous resolution is quite common and, with the exception of pregnant women and children with vesicoureteric reflux, antibiotic therapy is not of value.

Acute pyelonephritis. This usually results from ascending infection and may be preceded by a clinical episode of cystitis. Rarely, it may be acquired haematogenously. There is usually a substantial constitutional disturbance, with fever, rigors and malaise. Renal pain and tenderness is usual, though not invariable, and the infection may occasionally be very severe with bacteraemia, shock and even death. Two types of patient are at particular risk of overwhelming acute pyelonephritis. These are: diabetics, who may suffer papillary necrosis during the course of such an infection; and subjects with obstruction of the urinary tract and acute pyelonephritis above the obstruction (most commonly arising in association with renal or ureteric stones). The latter may develop severe and permanent renal damage over a very short period of time (hours or days), as well as being at high risk of bacteraemia.

Investigation

Investigation should focus on the isolation, identification and antibiotic sensitivity of the infecting organism. The fresh urine should be examined under the microscope for leucocytes and other formed elements. Patients with clinical evidence of acute pyelonephritis should have blood cultures. Additional investigations to be considered during or after treatment are intravenous urography (IVU) and cystourethroscopy.

Intravenous urography. This should be undertaken after the first infection in adult males and after the second or third in females, particularly if there was clinical evidence of pyelonephritis. Its purpose is to exclude the possibility of a functional or structural abnormality of the kidney or urinary tract.

Cystourethroscopy. In men, this will often be needed after even a single infection because of the rarity of UTI in the absence of significant prostatic or bladder disease.

Treatment

General measures. Fluid intake should be generous and achieve a urine flow rate of at least 100 ml/hour. Analgesics may be required.

Antibiotic therapy. This is often begun before the result of bacteriological investigations are available, though it may be modified subsequently if the bacteriological results so dictate. Conventionally, a course of 5 days is given for *clinical cystitis* but effective treatment may also comprise a large single dose of an appropriate antibiotic. The most frequently used agents are:

1. amoxycillin (250 mg tds for 5 days, or 3 g as a single dose by mouth)
2. trimethoprim (300 mg once daily for 5 days)
3. co-trimoxazole (960 mg or 2 tablets bd; or 2.88 g, 6 tablets as a single dose).

In complicated or severe infection, and where there is presumptive evidence of *acute pyelonephritis*, at least seven days of high dose chemotherapy should be given.

TUBERCULOSIS OF THE URINARY TRACT

Tuberculosis of the urinary tract almost always results from haematogenous spread, usually from a pulmonary focus, and involves one or both kidneys. A progressive interstitial nephropathy develops with extensive fibrosis and distortion of the gross anatomy of the kidney. Renal calcification is frequent, though not invariable. The disease spreads down the urinary tract, involving the renal pelves and ureters, and ureteric strictures frequently result. The bladder may be involved, leading to *tuberculous cystitis* and a contracted bladder, as may the epididymis, leading to tuberculous epididymitis. Renal damage is common, and may result from progressive destruction of parenchyma by the infection or from stricture formation leading to obstruction.

Clinical features and diagnosis

Unfortunately, some of these patients present with irreversible chronic renal failure. Others come to attention following painless haematuria, frequency or nocturia due to tuberculous cystitis, or with constitutional symptoms such as fever, malaise and weight loss. The urine shows a sterile pyuria and rbc's and casts are found frequently. The epididymis may be hardened and calcified and renal imaging often shows intrarenal calcifications with irregular loss of renal parenchyma and, in some cases, obstruction. Ultimately, the diagnosis depends on successful isolation of acid-fast bacilli from the urine. Early morning urine specimens are used, and at least three should be obtained and examined by microscopy and culture for six weeks before excluding active infection.

Treatment

Treatment is with antituberculous chemotherapy (p. 480). Careful assessment of the anatomy of the renal tract is essential to exclude obstruction, and follow-up IVUs should be performed during the first year to identify late stricture formation. Surgical reimplantation of the ureters may be needed in some cases, and severe contraction of the bladder may require an enlargement procedure (caeco-cystoplasty) or urinary diversion to alleviate frequency and protect against further renal damage.

CHRONIC PYELONEPHRITIS AND VESICOURETERIC REFLUX

Chronic pyelonephritis (CPN) is a diagnosis based on abnormalities of gross morphology of the kidney (either at post-mortem or by IVU or other form of imaging). The cardinal features of the condition are:

1. unilateral or bilateral parenchymal scars which give the kidney an irregular outline.
2. flattening of the renal papillae, giving a 'clubbed' appearance to the calyces. The parenchymal scars overlie the clubbed calyces.

Microscopically, there is severe interstitial fibrosis and scarring with tubular atrophy. The calyces and collecting system show mucosal thickening and inflammation. Glomerular lesions are variable.

Aetiology and pathogenesis

The aetiology of CPN is controversial. In the past, it was assumed that the scarring was the result of intermittent acute or chronic infection of the kidney. The main problem with this explanation is the absence of infection in many cases, and also the clear evidence that the disease may progress in the absence of persistent infection in the urine or in the kidney. It is now thought that a number of different factors, probably in association with transient infection in early life, may initiate and perpetuate the lesion that results in CPN. Of these, *vesicoureteric reflux* and *obstruction* are the two with the most clear-cut involvement, and it is therefore helpful to categorise CPN as follows:

CPN with vesicoureteric reflux. This association is far too frequent to be coincidental. It is likely that the repeated, and individually trivial, insults to the kidney following each episode of reflux (particularly in infancy, when the kidney is highly susceptible to damage) cause cumulative damage. It appears that reflux of *infected* urine is particularly harmful, but whether the injury is mechanical, chemical or immunological is unclear.

CPN with obstruction. Evidence of obstruction is found in a proportion of patients who satisfy the diagnostic criteria for CPN; some of these have functional and structural disorders of the bladder.

CPN in isolation. In a sizeable proportion of cases, reflux is absent, and there is no evidence of back pressure or obstruction. In these idiopathic cases of CPN, an explanation that is increasingly accepted is that reflux in early childhood (probably associated with urinary tract infection) and with resolution in adolescence, may be the underlying cause.

Clinical features, investigation and treatment

Many patients present for the first time with symptoms and signs of chronic renal failure or hypertension. In addition, severe reflux may give rise to renal pain or predispose to clinically evident attacks of acute pyelonephritis.

In addition to the general assessment of renal function, a search should be made for factors that might accelerate the progression of the disease, in particular obstruction, presence of stone and active urinary infection. Reflux may be documented by micturating cystography, but surgical correction is rarely warranted and does not appear to retard progression of the disease even though it may make control of infection easier.

The removal of a grossly infected, minimally functioning kidney may reduce the frequency and severity of infection and facilitate control of bladder pressure. As in all patients with renal disease, close attention to maintenance of appropriate fluid and electrolyte balance and control of blood pressure are essential.

NEPHROPATHY DUE TO PHYSICAL OR CHEMICAL AGENTS

Radiation nephritis

Radiation nephritis most often arises in the context of radiotherapy for tumours in or adjacent to the kidneys, such as ovarian or testicular cancer, lymphoma, neuroblastoma or Wilm's tumour. Pathological changes are widespread, and involve glomeruli, tubules, interstitium and vascular elements. There is no treatment other than general supportive measures and control of blood pressure. Dialysis and/or transplantation may be appropriate in some cases.

Nephropathy due to chemical toxins

The importance of chemical toxins as a cause of nephropathy is illustrated by studies showing that nephrotoxins are implicated in 20–25% of cases of acute renal failure. It is salutary to note that the vast majority of these cases are iatrogenic, with prescribed drugs identified as the offending agents. Chemical insult to the kidney may lead to any of the renal syndromes listed in Summary 4.

The nephrotoxicity of many of the agents discussed below is enhanced by concomitant volume contraction; identification and correction of this and other 'pre-renal factors' (Table 21.13) is thus of great importance when known nephrotoxins are being administered therapeutically.

Drug-induced nephrotoxicity (therapeutic)

Antibiotics are the major contributors, with those of the aminoglycoside group (gentamicin, tobramycin) prominent. Other frequently prescribed agents with nephrotoxic potential are non-steroidal anti-inflammatory drugs, penicillamine, gold and lithium. Withdrawal of the offending agent will often allow renal function to return to normal but, in some cases, renal damage is permanent (Table 21.33).

Nephrotoxicity resulting from drug abuse

In epidemiological terms, by far the most important example is analgesic nephropathy (p. 824) following habitual consumption of large amounts of certain proprietary analgesic mixtures. Phenacetin (now withdrawn), paracetamol, aspirin, and ibuprofen can be obtained over-the-counter without prescription. Of these, paracetamol is the least toxic.

Heroin abuse may lead to immune complex glomerulonephritis or acute myoglobinuric renal failure due to rhabdomyolysis.

Other environmental nephrotoxins

X-ray contrast media. The overall incidence of clinically significant contrast-induced nephropathy is very low, but amongst patients with established acute or chronic renal disease, diabetes, jaundice and those with multiple myeloma, the risks are much higher. In these groups, an important predisposing factor is volume contraction, which should be avoided or corrected prior to injection of X-ray contrast media. When adverse reactions do occur, they take the form of acute renal failure which usually recovers.

Mercury. Accidental industrial exposure or attempted suicide may lead to acute renal failure with good prospects for renal recovery. The consequences of chronic, low-level exposure to organic mercury compounds accumulating in the food chain are less clear-cut.

Lead. Interstitial nephropathy may result from chronic exposure to lead. Gout and superimposed urate nephropathy are frequently associated. Acute lead intoxication, although rare, may cause renal tubular dysfunction or acute tubular necrosis.

Organic solvents. Carbon tetrachloride is the nephrotoxic organic solvent most frequently encountered. Exposure may be deliberate or accidental, and lead to acute renal failure. Provided associated hepatic damage is not lethal, the renal lesion usually recovers. The renal sequelae of glue sniffing include proteinuria, haematuria and distal renal tubular necrosis.

Ethylene glycol (antifreeze) is occasionally used as a means of attempting suicide. As well as leading to fulminating metabolic acidosis, the metabolism of ethylene glycol to oxalic acid leads to acute renal failure with massive precipitation of oxalic acid crystals in the kidney.

Paraquat. Accidental or deliberate poisoning with paraquat frequently leads to acute renal failure. This may be reversible, but the associated pulmonary toxicity may prove fatal.

Paracetamol. Reversible acute renal failure may complicate attempted suicide with paracetamol, but hepatic toxicity usually dominates the clinical picture. Never-

theless, acute renal failure may occasionally occur in the absence of overt liver damage.

URINARY STONE

Urinary stone, or urolithiasis, and the dramatic symptoms that may be associated with it have been recorded for at least two millenia. The true incidence is difficult to assess, but it is likely that clinical stone events afflict about 1% of the population at some time during their lives. Men are affected with about four times the frequency of women and, in both sexes, stone formation tends to be recurrent and unpredictable, putting a substantial onus on doctors to devise effective means of prophylaxis.

Types of stone

Details of the major stone types are given in Table 21.36, from which it can be seen that the large majority of stones are made up of calcium oxalate or a mixture of calcium oxalate with hydroxapatite. Struvite stones (magnesium ammonium phosphate) usually contain calcium phosphate also and are invariably associated with infection. Uric acid stones and cystine stones are associated with elevated urinary excretion rates of these compounds.

Table 21.36 Types of urinary stone

Composition	Radio-opaque	Frequency (%)
Calcium oxalate	++	35
Calcium oxalate + hydroxyapatite	++	45
Calcium phosphate	++	1–3
Magnesium ammonium phosphate + calcium phosphate (struvite)	++	10
Uric acid	0	5
Cystine	+	1–2

Pathogenesis

Stone formation is frequent because of the precariously high urinary concentration of compounds of relatively low solubility. Certain protective mechanisms are built in, such that immediate precipitation is not an inevitable result of supersaturation. Inhibitors of crystal formation in urine are inorganic (magnesium, pyrophosphate, citrate) and organic (glycoseaminoglycans) and it is possible that the action of these is at least as important a determinant of stone formation as the absolute concentrations of, for example, calcium, phosphate and oxalate in the urine. Uric acid is of particular importance, in that it is not only itself capable of precipitating and forming stones, but also appears to interfere with the action of the organic inhibitors, thus predisposing also to non-uric acid stone formation.

Calcium

Amongst patients with calcium-containing stones, about 30% will have hypercalciuria (arbitrarily defined as more than 7.5 mmol/day in men and more than 6.5 mmol/day in women). A minority of these will also be hypercalcaemic because of underlying hyperparathyroidism, sarcoidosis, vitamin D intoxication, milk alkali syndrome, malignant disease or hyperthyroidism. In these cases, the objective is to treat the underlying metabolic abnormality, thereby resolving the hypercalciuria.

However, the vast majority of hypercalciuric stone formers will be found to be normocalcaemic and, provided that there is no identifiable cause for hyperabsorption of calcium by the intestine (e.g. mild vitamin D intoxication), or of renal tubular disorder leading to hypercalciuria (e.g. renal tubular acidosis, high salt intake, chronic frusemide therapy), they are designated as suffering from *idiopathic hypercalciuria*. Detailed investigation of these patients suggests that they fall into three main groups.

1. *renal hypercalciuria*, i.e. primary renal calcium leak with compensatory intestinal hyperabsorption of calcium
2. *absorptive hypercalciuria*, i.e. primary intestinal hyperabsorption of calcium with compensatory 'spillover' into the urine leading to hypercalciuria
3. *resorptive hypercalciuria*, i.e. primary acceleration of skeletal resorption with compensatory 'spillover' of calcium into the urine leading to hypercalciuria.

Oxalate

Reliable measurements of plasma and urinary oxalate are difficult, but it is now clear that there is a positive relationship between urinary oxalate excretion and the likelihood of calcium oxalate stone formation.

Uric acid

Hyperuricosuric individuals have a greatly increased incidence of uric acid stone formation and a moderately increased incidence of calcium oxalate stone formation. This association probably reflects interference by uric acid with the action of urinary inhibitors of crystal formation.

Cystine

Cystinuria is inherited as an autosomal recessive and is associated with elevated excretion of other dibasic amino acids. Cystine stone formation is the only important clinical sequela.

Clinical features

Presentation is usually with renal or ureteric colic, resulting from partial or complete obstruction to the flow of urine. The pain is usually intense and is nearly always accompanied by haematuria, which may be macroscopic. If the stone has obstructed a single functioning kidney, acute renal failure of post-renal type is inevitable.

However, less dramatic presentations are also common, with passage of tiny stones or gravel, usually with some associated discomfort. Symptoms may even be absent, or comprise merely dull back-ache which may lead to the erroneous diagnosis of a mechanical back lesion.

Fortunately, severe permanent renal damage is rare, and arises only when acute infection is present above an obstructing stone (leading to pyonephrosis) or following neglect of an obstructing stone.

Diagnosis and treatment

The diagnosis and treatment of urinary stone falls into an early phase of assessment and management of the immediate problems posed by the stone, and a late phase, concerned with the aetiology of the offending stone and the development of strategy to prevent future episodes.

Early

Diagnosis is usually easy and is often made on clinical grounds alone. Plain X-ray of the abdomen will reveal the majority of calcium-containing stones, but their location in relation to the kidney and ureter requires an IVU. The IVU will also allow identification of non-radio-opaque uric acid stones, and usually demonstrates the position of the stone and the consequent dilatation of the upper urinary tract above the level of obstruction. Ultrasound examination of the kidney may be helpful in identifying stones within the kidney. Urine should be examined for blood and cultured, and all urine passed should be strained in the hope of catching the stone which can then be analysed. Renal or ureteric colic requires strong analgesia – opiates should be given promptly and in adequate dosage. The role of 'antispasmodics' such as anticholinergic drugs is not clear, but inhibitors of prostaglandin synthesis (e.g. indomethacin) may be highly effective. A generous fluid intake is maintained and the patient mobilised as quickly as possible. These measures alone will allow spontaneous passage of the stone in many cases. Factors favouring spontaneous passage are small size (less than 5 mm), and location in the lower third of the ureter.

Active intervention is required for unremitting obstruction and pain, associated infection, a large stone that is unlikely to pass, and acute renal failure of post-renal type. Intervention may take the form of open surgery (nephrolithotomy or ureterolithotomy), endoscopic snaring from below during cystoscopy, or percutaneous removal from above via a nephrostomy. An important new development revolutionising the management of stone disease is external shock wave lithotripsy (ESWL). Here, appropriately directed ultrasound is used to shatter renal or ureteric stones in vivo, allowing spontaneous passage of the fragments.

Late

Once the acute event has resolved, steps must be taken to minimise the chances of recurrence. Analysis of the stone is desirable but not always possible. Routine metabolic tests to be undertaken in all cases are:

1. plasma calcium, phosphate, alkaline phosphatase, urea, urate, creatinine, electrolytes
2. 24-hour urine collection for simultaneous measurement of calcium, uric acid and creatinine, and nitroprusside test for cystine
3. if possible, measurement of 24-hour oxalate and citrate excretion.

Abnormalities in the initial screen may dictate measurement of serum parathyroid hormone, fasting urinary calcium excretion, tests of urinary acidification and plasma 25-hydroxyvitamin D concentrations to exclude vitamin D intoxication.

Depending on the results of the above assessment, the following specific measures should be taken (in addition to general advice to achieve fluid intake sufficient to maintain a urine output of at least two litres per day).

1. *Hypercalciuria with hypercalcaemia.* Treat underlying cause of hypercalcaemia.
2. *Idiopathic hypercalciuria.* Treat with thiazide diuretics to reduce urinary calcium excretion. In selected cases this may be combined with cellulose phosphate given orally (to decrease intestinal calcium absorption) or with allopurinol (to reduce urinary uric acid excretion).
3. *Calcium stones with no metabolic abnormality.* The patient should avoid excessive oxalate-rich foods (tea, coffee, nuts, spinach, rhubarb). Treatment with thiazide diuretics plus allopurinol (probably only justified if stones are recurrent). Oral potassium citrate also appears promising.
4. *Uric acid stones.* Allopurinol.
5. *Cystine stones.* Alkalinise urine with sodium or potassium bicarbonate. Maintain urine flow at 3 l/day minimum. Consider penicillamine if the above measures are ineffective.
6. *Struvite stones.* Surgical removal is the only effective treatment.
7. *Hyperoxaluria and hypocitraturia.* When documented, hyperoxaluria should be countered by a low oxalate diet and hypocitraturia should be treated with potassium citrate. However, these measurements are not routinely available.

Dietary calcium restriction is sometimes recommended in patients with calcium-containing stones. However, this therapeutic dogma is of unproven benefit and may in some cases be harmful. Decreased dietary calcium leads to increased absorption (and hence excretion) of oxalate and may thereby enhance, rather than reduce, calcium oxalate stone formation. In addition, prolonged restriction of dietary calcium may predispose to osteopenia, particularly in women. A sensible compromise is to limit calcium intake only when excessive, and not to attempt to reduce it below 25 mmol/day (1 g of elemental calcium per day) except in those subjects shown to have absorptive hypercalciuria.

URINARY TRACT OBSTRUCTION

Aetiology

Some of the main causes of urinary tract obstruction are given in Table 21.37. The clinical presentation is varied and depends on age at onset and the site, severity and rate of onset of obstruction.

Table 21.37 Causes of urinary tract obstruction

Level of obstruction	Pathophysiology
Any	Stone, sloughed papilla, blood clot, trauma
Renal parenchyma	Uric acid, Bence-Jones protein, cysts
Collecting system	Urothelial tumour, TB, pelviureteric obstruction (stricture, aberrant vessel, fibrous band)
Ureter	Retroperitoneal or pelvic malignancy (carcinoma of bladder, prostate, cervix, rectum, lymphoma), carcinoma of ureter, aortic aneurysm, idiopathic retroperitoneal fibrosis, TB, schistosomiasis, obstetric trauma
Bladder	Benign prostatic hypertrophy, carcinoma of prostate or bladder, neurogenic bladder, TB, foreign body, trauma
Urethra	Urethral valves, phimosis, stricture, meatal stenosis, trauma, foreign body

Clinical features

The following clinical features are of importance in the management of patients suspected of having an obstructing lesion.

1. *Pain.* Acute obstruction is usually associated with pain, regardless of the site of the lesion. In contrast, slowly progressive obstructions are likely to be pain-free and hence more likely to cause obstructive renal injury which may be severe and irreversible by the time the patient seeks help.
2. *Renal failure* resulting from obstruction implies that both kidneys are obstructed, or that a solitary functioning kidney is obstructed.
3. *Volume of urine.* The fact that a patient is passing normal volumes of urine does not exclude obstruction. While complete obstruction of the urinary tract of necessity causes anuria, the patient with partial obstruction will usually continue to pass normal, or even increased, volumes of urine. However, the continued passage of urine is at the expense of increasing and potentially damaging back pressure above the obstructing lesion.
4. *Renal impairment.* Because the early recognition and relief of obstruction is so important if unnecessary renal damage is to be avoided, the diagnosis must be considered in all patients presenting with acute or chronic renal impairment.
5. *Urinary infections* that are recurrent or difficult to

eradicate should raise the suspicion of an anatomical and possibly obstructing lesion.

Effects of obstruction on the kidney

The earliest functions to be compromised by progressive obstruction are urinary concentration and acidification, followed by a decrease in glomerular filtration rate. Relief of obstruction may sometimes be followed by temporary concentrating defects leading to inappropriate salt and water losses. More frequently this post-obstructive diuresis is short-lived, and reflects previous salt and water overload and the osmotic diuresis that results from high plasma urea concentration.

Diagnosis and treatment

Clinical assessment may reveal symptoms and signs that point to obstruction and may also indicate its likely site and aetiology. This is particularly so in patients with urethral disease or bladder outflow obstruction. Alternatively, the clinical picture may suggest a disorder known to be associated with urinary obstruction, for example carcinoma of the cervix or lymphoma in a patient with unexplained renal failure. Although the existence of obstruction is usually clear-cut, major problems arise in some cases. These fall into three groups.

Is the 'obstruction' significant? The finding of a dilated collecting system does not necessarily imply current obstruction, but may be an anatomical hangover from previous obstruction.

Extent of renal damage. Is renal function likely to improve following relief of the obstruction? This problem arises when, in the presence of clear-cut obstruction, it remains uncertain whether renal damage has progressed beyond the point where useful recovery of function is likely. A variety of non-invasive and invasive tests can be helpful, but in some cases, the answer is only obtained following a trial of palliative drainage by means of a nephrostomy tube.

Advanced malignancy. Should obstruction be relieved when it is the result of advanced malignancy? Malignant disease is an important cause of obstructive nephropathy (Table 21.37) and, in these patients, thought should be given to the likely prognosis of the tumour. If this is exceedingly poor, it may be kinder to allow the patient to die in uraemic coma, rather than as a result of uncontrolled pelvic malignancy.

Techniques used in the relief of obstruction include surgical bypass or urinary diversion through the skin, direct drainage from above via a nephrostomy tube, or internal stenting of an obstructing lesion.

NEOPLASIA IN THE KIDNEY AND URINARY TRACT

Cancers of the urogenital tract are common. The age-specific incidence rates for the UK are shown in Figure

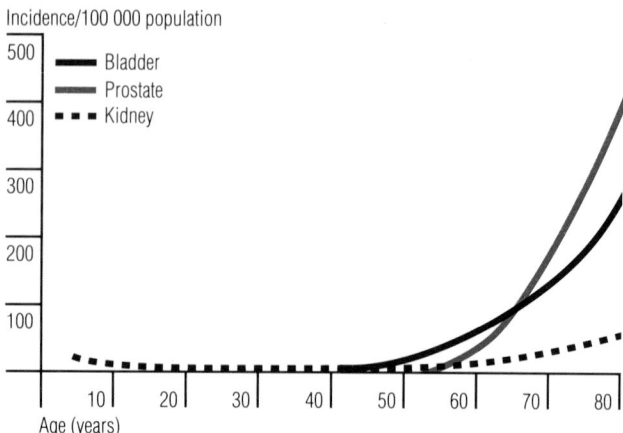

Fig. 21.20 **Age-adjusted incidence of urinary tract cancer in the UK in 1983.**

21.20. In the kidney, renal cell carcinoma is the commonest tumour (75% of cases) with transitional cell carcinoma accounting for 15% of cases. Carcinoma of the prostate is the third largest cause of death from cancer in males.

RENAL TUMOURS

Renal adenocarcinoma

Renal adenocarcinoma is three times commoner in men and may be related in part to cigarette smoking. It is also commoner in patients with von Hippel-Lindau syndrome (p. 908).

The tumour arises from the renal tubule cells. Lymphatic and haematogenous spread, and local spread through capsule mean that 30–40% of patients are inoperable when first seen.

Clinical features

Half of the patients have haematuria. Loin pain and an abdominal mass are frequently present. Presentation may also be with bone pain or cough and dyspnoea from metastases. Renal adenocarcinoma may also present with a variety of paraneoplastic symptoms including fever and night sweats, humoral hypercalcaemia, and polycythaemia due to excess erythropoietin production.

Investigation

Diagnosis can be difficult if the tumour is small. An IVU may show a space-occupying mass, but a negative X-ray does not exclude a small tumour. Ultrasound is more sensitive and CT scan is helpful in difficult cases. These techniques have reduced the need for renal angiography. The initial investigations should include chest X-ray, abdominal CT scan and isotope bone scan to exclude metastases.

Treatment and prognosis

Surgical resection offers the only hope of cure but over

30% of renal tumours are inoperable. Opinion is divided as to the extent of the operation. Lymph node dissection is usually carried out. Radiotherapy has a limited role, but is often used if extrarenal extension of the tumour is found at operation.

Chemotherapy is of little value. Alpha-interferon, interleukin-2 and vinblastine may cause regressions, and the tumour may spontaneously fluctuate in size. Although regression of metastases has been seen following removal of the primary, this is a rare event.

Of patients with small localised disease, 50% are alive at 10 years. Only 20% of patients with stage II disease (large tumours but no local or node spread) will be alive, and 5% of stage III cases (extracapsular spread). Cancer staging is discussed in Chapter 9, pages 147–148.

Nephroblastoma (Wilm's tumour)

Wilm's tumour is an embryonic renal tumour usually found in children, in whom it presents as an abdominal mass. Hypertension is common. Treatment is surgical with adjuvant chemotherapy and radiotherapy in many cases. The combined approach has led to major improvements in the prognosis of the neoplasm.

Transitional cell carcinoma of kidney

The main symptoms of transitional cell carcinoma of the kidney are haematuria and renal pain, often with unilateral obstruction. The IVU shows a filling defect in the collecting system and the kidney may be obstructed. Cytological examination of the urine reveals malignant cells in 50% of cases.

Treatment is by nephro-ureterectomy where possible. Because the whole urothelium is unstable, stump recurrences are quite common. Radiotherapy may slow local progression but is not curative.

Transitional cell carcinoma of the bladder

Transitional cell carcinoma of the bladder was shown to be more common in workers in the aniline dye industry. The carcinogen was identified as β-naphthylamine. The tumour is also more common in the rubber industry, and in cigarette smokers. Worldwide, the major predisposing cause is undoubtedly bladder schistosomiasis (p. 318).

Staging

The staging notation (Figure 21.21) is based on the mode of spread through the bladder wall.

Clinical features and investigation

The major symptom is haematuria which is usually painless. Urinary frequency, nocturia and back pain may all occur. Diagnosis is by cystoscopy. An IVU is essential to show renal anatomy, and simple renal function tests should be performed. Lymphography and CT scanning are increasingly used in staging.

Fig. 21.21 Staging of bladder cancer. (After: Blandy J P 1986 Operative urology. Blackwell Scientific, Oxford.) T1 tumours involve the bladder mucosa. T2 tumours involve the superficial muscle (dashed line), T3a extend into deeper muscle, and T3b involve the whole wall. T4a tumours invade the prostrate (or vagina), and T4b the rectum and pelvic wall.

Treatment

Small superficial lesions are treated transurethrally by cystodiathermy, and intravesical chemotherapy is being used increasingly. Up to 15% of such patients will develop more generalised intravesical recurrence requiring surgery.

For more advanced (T2–T3) tumours, treatment is with surgery or radical radiotherapy or a combination of the two approaches. Partial cystectomy may be possible in some cases, but in others, total cystectomy (with an ileal conduit for the ureters) may be needed. Recently, several studies have shown that radical radiotherapy produces results as good as radical cystectomy. Chemotherapy is increasingly used in advanced and metastatic disease, with long survival in a minority of patients. Cisplatin, adriamycin and methotrexate are the most useful agents.

Carcinoma of the prostate

The age-specific incidence of this very common cancer is shown in Figure 21.20. In the last 50 years, mortality from this disease has increased in the United Kingdom. Little is known of its aetiology. The tumour is nearly always an adenocarcinoma. The majority are well-differentiated cancers, anaplastic tumours being only 15% of the total. The tumour grows in the gland (T1/T2) and then invades the capsule (T3) and, finally, adjacent structures (T4). Spread is to regional lymph nodes and then to bone and lung.

Clinical features and diagnosis

The tumour is often asymptomatic and may be diagnosed on rectal examination for some other reason. The commonest local symptoms are related to bladder outflow obstruction or infection, but presentation with backache from metastases is also frequent.

A histological diagnosis may be obtained by biopsy, usually taken transrectally, or from curettings taken at transurethral prostatectomy. Further staging will include chest X-ray and bone scan. An IVU may show back pressure effects on the bladder and kidneys.

Treatment

For localised small tumours, both radical prostatectomy and radical radiotherapy have been used. The latter may employ external beam or interstitial implants using ^{123}I seeds. With radical treatment, 30–40% of patients will be alive at 10 years, the proportion falling if there is extra-capsular extension of the tumour.

The mainstay of treatment is hormone manipulation, using orchidectomy, stilboestrol, or the inhibitor of LH release, buserelin. For more advanced disease, radiotherapy may palliate both local symptoms and symptoms from bone metastases.

CONTINENCE AND INCONTINENCE

NORMAL MICTURITION

Functionally, micturition occurs in three phases:

1. bladder filling
2. postponement, comprising: perception of the need to void; movement to a suitable place to void; adoption of voiding posture
3. voiding of urine.

Thus, micturition may be disturbed by intrinsic diseases of the bladder or its outlet, disordered afferent or efferent nerve supply of the bladder, spinal cord lesions, intracranial disease, psychological disturbance or locomotor disturbance.

Neuropathic bladder is a widely used (and abused) term denoting no more than bladder dysfunction resulting from any type of neurological disturbance; it implies nothing about the nature of that neurological disturbance.

The detrusor muscle of the bladder (parasympathetic innervation) and the bladder outlet (sympathetic innervation) act in a co-ordinated fashion, such that outflow resistance is high and detrusor tone low during filling. When the bladder is full and voiding is appropriate, micturition is accomplished by simultaneous contraction of the detrusor (mediated by increased parasympathetic activity) and relaxation of the bladder outlet (mediated by decreased sympathetic and pelvic floor activity) (Fig. 21.22). This is co-ordinated by a micturition centre in the brain stem, which is itself subject to a degree of cortical control (Fig. 21.23).

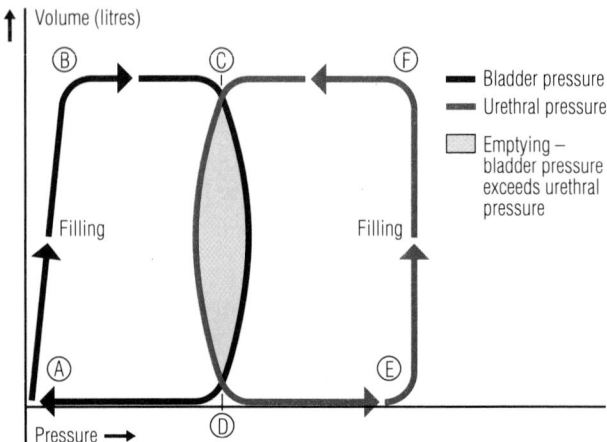

Fig. 21.22 The micturition cycle. Bladder emptying occurs at any time when bladder pressure is greater than urethral pressure (shaded area). During filling – (A) to (B) – bladder pressure rises little. Initiation of micturition at points (B) and (F) leads to a synchronous increase in bladder pressure and decrease in urethral pressure until, at (C), emptying begins. When emptying is complete (D), bladder and urethral pressures revert – points (A) and (E) – and filling resumes. (After Yeates W K in Hinman F (ed) 1983 Benign prostatic hypertrophy. Springer-Verlag, New York.)

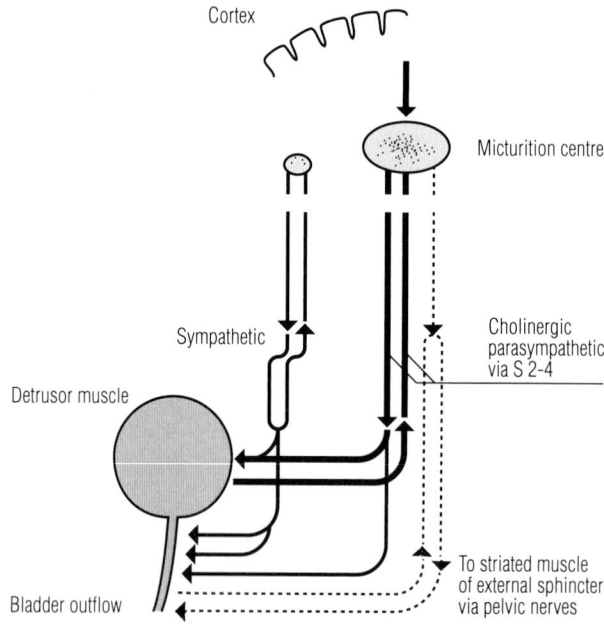

Fig. 21.23 Neurological control of micturition. The sympathetic efferent relaxes the detrusor muscle of the bladder and constricts the bladder outflow. The cholinergic efferent promotes contraction of the detrusor muscle. The pelvic nerve supply to the external sphincter stimulates further constriction of the bladder outflow. (After Yeates W K in Hinman F (ed) 1983 Benign prostatic hypertrophy. Springer-Verlag, New York.)

INCONTINENCE

Many of the causes of incontinence also result in a reduced functional bladder capacity which, of necessity, leads to frequency of micturition and/or nocturia (p. 799). The history and examination often yield a diagnosis but, in some cases, further investigations are needed to define the potential for pharmacological, urological or neurological treatment. Measurement of urine flow rate during the voiding phase is valuable in the assessment of bladder outflow obstruction. An IVU or ultrasound is often needed to determine the effects of the disordered bladder function on the upper urinary tract and kidneys. Residual urine after micturition can be demonstrated by IVU and/or ultrasound. Cine cystography shows the relevant anatomy during bladder filling and emptying, and may be combined with simultaneous pressure measurements to give a filling and voiding cystometrogram.

Stress incontinence

Stress incontinence is the involuntary passage of urine when intra-abdominal pressure is raised as in coughing, lifting, standing up etc. In the main, it is a disease of women, in whom pelvic floor laxity, often the result of pregnancy and/or childbirth, compromises the closure of the bladder outlet. There is no neurological defect. The dysfunction should be confirmed by performing a cine voiding cystometrogram.

Treatment with pelvic floor exercises may be effective, and some patients are improved by α-agonist drugs, such as phenylpropanolamine. However, surgical intervention is often needed and is usually effective.

Urge incontinence

In urge incontinence, the perception of the desire to void is followed within seconds or minutes by voiding, even though the patient attempts to delay it. Voiding is usually complete. This problem may reflect:

1. *increased afferent stimulation* from local pathology, e.g. infective cystitis, bladder tumour, bladder hypertrophy
2. *failure of central inhibition*, e.g. multiple sclerosis, cerebrovascular disease, cerebral tumour, spinal cord lesion
3. *cortical stimulation*, e.g. incontinence provoked by the sound of running water.

In many female cases there is no detectable organic cause of incontinence (idiopathic 'bladder instability'). Sacral reflexes are preserved, and so usually is sacral sensation and voluntary control of the anal sphincter. Instability of the detrusor muscle is usually demonstrable in the neuropathic group.

Treatment should be directed at the underlying pathology when feasible. Pharmacological attempts to decrease detrusor hyperexcitability using anticholinergic drugs (e.g. probantheline), tricyclic antidepressants or calcium channel blockers (e.g. nifedipine) are sometimes successful. In severe cases of neurological origin in women (particularly multiple sclerosis), the bladder activity may be greatly reduced by the injection of phenol into the pelvic autonomic nerves through the bladder base.

Reflex incontinence

Reflex incontinence is where voiding occurs periodically without advanced warning. The most important causes are spinal lesions above the level of the sacral outflow. Depending on the severity of the spinal lesion, neurological examination may show exaggerated sacral reflexes, a perianal sensory deficit and/or impairment of voluntary sphincter control. The interruption, not only of central inhibition but also of co-ordination, leads to detrusor hyperexcitability coupled with failure to relax the bladder outlet, a potentially dangerous combination that results in a high pressure bladder and risk of renal damage. Adequate decompression, by reduction of the resistance of the bladder outlet, is essential in these cases. Sometimes this can be achieved pharmacologically by α-adrenergic blocking drugs, such as phenoxybenzamine, or by endoscopic resection of the bladder neck and/or the external sphincter. The absence of bladder sensation, however, precludes the restoration of bladder control. In these circumstances, male patients nearly always require incontinence appliances. Female patients require continuous or intermittent catheterisation, and it is sometimes necessary to divert the urine by means of an ileal conduit.

Overflow incontinence

Overflow incontinence usually manifests itself with leakage of small amounts of urine, initially often at night only. The symptom is often quite subtle but it is important to recognise it because of the severe obstructive renal damage that usually ensues if the condition is neglected. The incontinence is always associated with a residual urine volume approaching that of the bladder capacity, usually resulting in a manifestly distended bladder. It is most often seen in a man with prostatic hypertrophy causing outflow obstruction. Other cases result from neurological lesions, either as an acute condition in spinal shock, or in sub-acute or chronic bladder dysfunction from prolapsed intervertebral disc, sacral plexus lesions or autonomic neuropathy (diabetes mellitus, tabes dorsalis), that decreases normal detrusor excitability. The urinary stream is slow.

Treatment is directed at correction of the mechanical outlet obstruction, e.g. by prostatectomy. In some neuropathic cases, α-blocking drugs (phenoxybenzamine, prazosin) or endoscopic resection or incision of the bladder neck or external sphincter, may improve matters by reducing outlet resistance. The outlook in those patients with local mechanical causes that increase bladder outlet resistance (e.g. prostatic hypertrophy) is usually excellent, whereas the prognosis in the long-standing neurogenic group is usually poor.

Enuresis

The term enuresis denotes bed-wetting in, or beginning in, childhood, though strictly it means merely the voiding of urine. Bed-wetting is universal in infancy, affects about

50% of children at age three and about 15% at age ten. It is commoner in children with psychological problems and amongst those with organic diseases of the kidney and/or urinary tract. Primary nocturnal enuresis (i.e. present from birth) does not usually require detailed investigation, provided that daytime micturition is normal, and there is no evidence of present or past infection or of urinary tract obstruction.

Treatment, in the absence of associated abnormalities of the urinary tract, may involve bladder training, with voluntary postponement of voiding by day, or alteration of sleep pattern by means of a bell set to sound when the child wets a sensor pad in bed. The tricyclic antidepressants (e.g. imipramine) are effective in many cases, probably by multiple actions on the depth of sleep and on the detrusor muscle. An alternative approach is to give the vasopressin analogue, desmopressin, intranasally last thing at night. This decreases urine output during the night and is successful in selected patients.

Incontinence in the elderly

The overall problem of incontinence in the elderly is considerable. It has been estimated to afflict 5–15% of the elderly in the general population and many more in institutions. The mechanism is often multifactorial, particularly neuropathic; however, in depressed or demented patients, it may include loss of the will to be continent and loss of appreciation of what is a socially acceptable micturition site.

Treatment is similar to that in younger patients, but therapeutic options may be constrained by drug side-effects or unacceptable risks of surgery. As a result, relatively more of the elderly will require palliation in the form of incontinence appliances, pads or indwelling catheters. The latter, though an easy option for the doctor and nursing staff, should be avoidable in most cases. More detailed discussion is given in Chapter 10.

PRESCRIBING IN PATIENTS WITH RENAL DISEASE

The extensive renal excretion of therapeutic agents and their metabolites means that the prescription of drugs to patients with renal disease must often be modified with regard to both the choice of drug and its schedule of administration. The main considerations (Table. 21.38) are:

1. decreased therapeutic efficacy
2. increased nephrotoxicity
3. decreased excretion of drug or metabolite.

Thus, some agents may have to be given in unusually large doses to patients with renal disease (e.g. diuretics) while others require dose reduction (e.g. digoxin) or, in some cases, should not be given at all if the risk of toxicity is too high.

Table 21.38 Therapeutic considerations in renal disease

Pharmacological consideration	Example
Decreased therapeutic efficacy	
Target organ resistance	Diuretics less effective in patients with renal disease
Failure of diseased kidney to bioactivate agent	Vitamin D not bioactivated to 1,25(OH)$_2$D in severe renal disease
Increased nephrotoxicity	X-ray contrast media, aminoglycoside antibiotics more nephrotoxic to previously damaged kidneys
Decreased excretion of drug or metabolite	Digoxin, many antibiotics

Body clearance

As applied to a particular drug, body clearance is the sum of the clearances (i.e. hepatic, renal, skeletal, muscle etc) of that agent in all organs contributing to its removal. When the kidney is the sole route of exit, the renal clearance approximates the body clearance, while in the case of the drug that is removed exclusively by hepatic metabolism, the hepatic clearance approximates the body clearance and the renal clearance is zero. The effect of decreasing GFR on body clearance of different types of drug is illustrated in Figure 21.24.

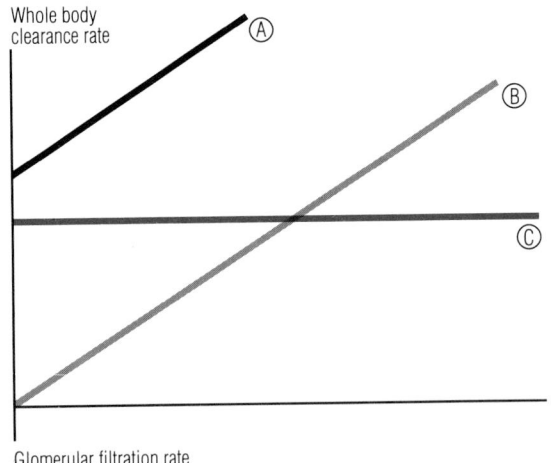

Fig. 21.24 Effect of changes of GFR on the elimination of different drugs. Drug (A) is cleared by both the kidney and the liver, and Drug (B) by the kidney alone. Drug (C) is cleared by the liver alone; its clearance rate is unaffected by changes in the glomerular filtration rate.

Principles of dose modification

The decision to decrease the dose of a drug is based on both its potential to accumulate in renal failure and the potential for toxicity if accumulation occurs. Drugs with a very high therapeutic index (e.g. penicillin) require dose modification only if very large doses are being given or if renal function is near zero. Conversely, drugs with a low therapeutic index (e.g. digoxin or aminoglycoside antibiotics) require dose modification even in the presence of slight impairment of renal function.

Depending on the pharmacokinetics of the drug, dose reduction may take the form of normal dose/increased dose interval, reduced dose/normal dose interval or a combination of the two. Appropriate modification can be aided by tables, nomograms and monitoring. In practice, tables and nomograms, used with an understanding of the relevant pharmacology, allow an educated guess of the correct dosage to be made; and subsequent monitoring of plasma concentrations of the drug helps to guide further dose adjustments.

FURTHER READING

Brenner B M, Coe F L, Rector F C 1987 Clinical nephrology. W B Saunders Company, Philadelphia. *Medium length text, with predominantly clinical emphasis. Well laid out and well referenced*

Brenner B M, Rector F C 1986 The kidney, 3rd edn. W B Saunders Company, Philadelphia. *Comprehensive and detailed text with extensive coverage of renal physiology and pathophysiology as well as of clinical nephrology. Extensively referenced*

Marsh F P 1985 Postgraduate nephrology. William Heineman, London. *Medium length, general text covering the whole field of nephrology*

Sweny P, Farrington K, Moorhead J F 1989 The kidney and its disorders. Blackwell Scientific Publications, Oxford. *Up-to-date, medium length textbook of nephrology.*

Salt and Water Metabolism and Acid-Base Balance

Fig. 22.2 The intra/extracellular ion distribution. Concentrations in mmol/l are shown in brackets. The solid arrows represent active transport mechanisms and the broken arrows passive diffusion, which depends on the electrochemical gradient.

WATER AND SODIUM HOMEOSTASIS

Total body water and sodium are maintained within narrow limits by a number of neural and hormonal homeostatic mechanisms which ensure that water and salt intake and excretion are equal. Disease states may perturb salt and water balance either by exerting direct effects on one or more of these homeostatic mechanisms or by altering water or sodium loss or intake. The distribution of water between intracellular fluid and extracellular fluid depends on the osmolality of the two compartments (Fig. 22.1). Sodium is quantitatively the most important extracellular cation and, as 80% of total sodium is present in the extracellular space due to active sodium-potassium exchange across cellular plasma membranes (Fig. 22.2), the extracellular osmolality approximates to the molar concentrations of sodium and its anion equivalents, chloride and bicarbonate. It follows that extracellular fluid volume

is largely dependent on the total body sodium. This applies to both intravascular and interstitial spaces, although the water distribution between these two components of extracellular space is further dependent on the osmotic effects of plasma proteins and on hydrostatic pressure. Net *sodium loss* will result in shrinkage of both interstitial and intravascular volumes but, since such losses are frequently accompanied by loss of water, the osmolar changes will be slight and marked changes in intracellular volume will not occur. Net *water loss* will, however, result in loss of water from all compartments as a result of free diffusion of water under the influence of extracellular osmolar changes.

Water homeostasis

Total body water is maintained primarily through the mechanism of action of *antidiuretic hormone* (ADH), also called *arginine vasopressin* (AVP) and by the sensation of thirst (Fig. 22.3).

Antidiuretic hormone

The net change in osmolality which follows any tendency to total body water deficit constitutes the most important

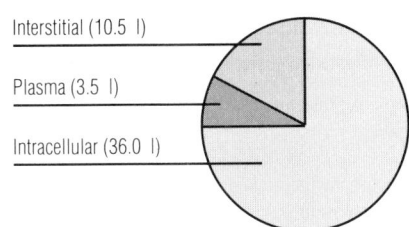

Fig. 22.1 The distribution of total body water. Osmolality is equal in all compartments.

Interstitial (10.5 l)

Plasma (3.5 l)

Intracellular (36.0 l)

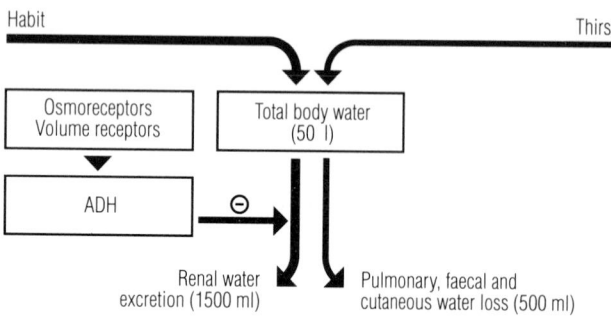

Fig. 22.3 Determinants of total body water balance. Water intake is initiated by habit and thirst. Total body water is maintained at a constant level by the thirst mechanism and by ADH modulation of renal water excretion; ⊖ denotes inhibition.

stimulus to the secretion of ADH by neurosecretory cells in the supra-optic and paraventricular nuclei of the hypothalamus. Sensitive receptors which mediate this phenomenon are localised primarily in the hypothalamus. These osmoreceptors are particularly sensitive to increased sodium concentrations, but less so to glucose or urea. Additional receptors, present in capacitance vessels near the heart and in the left atrium, mediate ADH release in response to vascular volume changes independently of changes in osmolality. This mechanism is less sensitive than that mediated by osmolar changes. Release of ADH may also be influenced by circulating angiotensin II, catecholamines and endogenous opiates.

ADH formed in the hypothalamus is transferred, in the form of secretory granules, along the axons of the neurosecretory cells to the posterior pituitary, where it is released into the circulation in response to stimulation of osmo- or volume receptors. The major sites of action of ADH are the distal tubules and collecting ducts of the kidney. Permeability to water is increased by a cyclic-AMP-mediated phosphorylation mechanism, and water reabsorption occurs by virtue of medullary hypertonicity achieved by means of the counter-current system.

In addition to its effect on the kidney, ADH has recently been shown to influence both glucose and urea production in the liver. The latter effect is of particular interest in view of the importance of urea in maintaining renal medullary hypertonicity.

The sensation of thirst

The sensation of thirst is predominantly mediated by hypothalamic osmoreceptors distinct from, but in close proximity to, those subserving ADH secretion. Some contribution to thirst may also come from vascular volume receptors. However, except in situations where water supplies are limited, much of the everyday fluid intake occurs out of habit or on a social basis. For this reason, urine flow rates are generally far in excess of, and urine osmolality lower than, the values found when a significant degree of renal concentration occurs due to the action of ADH.

Sodium homeostasis

Sodium is lost to the body in cutaneous sweat and, via the kidney, in the urine. The former source of loss cannot be regulated and is determined solely by environmental conditions. Maintenance of a constant total body sodium in the face of wide variations in sodium intake is therefore entirely dependent on appropriate variations in the rate of renal sodium excretion. This may be varied sufficiently to achieve a constant total body sodium when daily intake ranges from 20 to several hundred mmol. However, the mechanism of this phenomenon is incompletely understood. Changes in adrenal aldosterone production, dependent upon the renin-angiotensin system (p. 826), are undoubtedly important in the regulation of active sodium reabsorption in exchange for potassium and hydrogen ions in the distal tubule.

This mechanism alone cannot explain the observed capacity for variation of renal sodium excretion, however. It is probable that vascular receptors produce some of the effect by sensing changes in circulating volume; and there is now increasing evidence for a circulating peptide produced in the atrium which promotes renal sodium excretion. This is termed *atrial natriuretic peptide* (ANP). It would appear that secretion is stimulated by atrial stretch receptors activated by increases in blood volume due, for example, to increased sodium intake, congestive cardiac failure or renal failure. The precise mechanism of action of ANP is not known, but probably involves an increase in both renal blood flow and glomerular filtration rate together with inhibition of the renin-angiotensin-aldosterone system.

Clinical assessment of water and sodium balance

Derangements of sodium and water homeostasis are often obvious from the clinical history which may, for example, indicate abnormal losses of fluid and electrolytes from the gastrointestinal tract. Alternatively, symptoms of orthopnoea and oedema may suggest circulatory overload or heart failure.

Primary derangements in sodium balance alter the extracellular fluid volume and thus give rise to early alterations in circulating volume and consequent physical signs. Mild to moderate changes in water balance, on the other hand, are borne by intra- and extracellular compartments and are less obvious clinically. As a general principle, expansion

---

Summary 1 Indicators of disturbed water and sodium homeostasis

- Raised venous pressure
- Weight gain
- Oedema
- Chest radiography (information on cardiac status)
- Postural hypotension
- Weight loss
- Skin turgor and intra-ocular pressure (unreliable)
- Reduction in urine output (if profound salt and water depletion)

or contraction of the circulating volume may be determined by examination of the jugular venous pressure (low in sodium depletion, raised in sodium excess) and of the lying and standing blood pressure (postural drop in sodium depletion). However, venous pressure will also be raised in heart failure, and postural hypotension may be a feature of autonomic neuropathy, a condition most commonly secondary to diabetes mellitus, or to treatment with antihypertensive drugs. Peripheral oedema may also indicate a sodium retaining state (p. 848).

Estimating the state of hydration by clinical assessment of skin turgor or intra-ocular pressure is generally unreliable (although still widely practised). Daily weighing, on the other hand, provides a sensitive index of changes and is often used to monitor intensive diuretic therapy in hospitalised patients.

Further investigation of the patient's circulating volume and cardiac status may include measurement of central venous pressure (by means of a catheter placed in the superior vena cava), and chest radiography, which will demonstrate cardiac enlargement and pulmonary venous congestion in heart failure.

Profound sodium and water depletion results in a reduction in urine output. The distinction between this pre-renal oliguria and renal failure is discussed on page 849.

DISORDERS OF WATER HOMEOSTASIS

In some pathological conditions, dramatic changes in total body water may occur with little or no alteration in total body sodium or potassium; in others, water loss may be accompanied by significant losses of electrolytes. Even in the latter circumstance, however, the water deficit will usually be relatively greater than the sodium deficit, a fact with important implications for the interpretation of plasma sodium estimations (p. 849). The losses of potassium which may accompany water and sodium depletion in some situations are considered separately, as are those conditions in which changes in total body sodium occur in the absence of gross net changes in body water.

WATER DEPLETION

Water depletion may occur:

1. as a result of failure of renal concentrating capacity
2. by obligatory insensible water loss (through the skin, lungs and as concentrated urine) in situations when oral fluid intake is inadequate
3. via the kidney when osmotically active solutes are present in tubular fluid in increased quantity
4. via the gut
5. by increased pulmonary loss in acute respiratory disease.

Because water depletion is borne by both intra- and extracellular compartments, the physical signs of fluid depletion may not be marked and, in particular, signs of reduced circulating volume occur late. With a severe reduction in total body water, a decreased level of consciousness is common and may persist for a considerable time after the deficit has been corrected. Severe water depletion results in both extra- and intracellular hyper-osmolality (the rise in intracellular osmolality being highest in the central nervous system) and a tendency to intra-vascular thrombosis. Water depletion is accompanied by a rise in plasma sodium.

DIABETES INSIPIDUS

This condition arises when the kidneys lose, usually partially, the capacity to produce a concentrated urine. The classical presentation is with excessive thirst (polydipsia) and the passage of large volumes of dilute urine (polyuria). The length of history is usually short, although mild failure of concentrating capacity may be present for a considerable time prior to diagnosis.

Causes

Diabetes insipidus occurs as a result either of deficiency of ADH secretion or of failure of ADH action at renal tubular level. The important causes of the deficit, usually referred to as *cranial* or *neurogenic diabetes insipidus*, are listed in Table 22.1; postsurgical and so-called idiopathic causes

Table 22.1 Causes of diabetes insipidus

Cause	Example/comment
Cranial (neurogenic) diabetes insipidus	
Idiopathic	(Some autoimmune)
Familial	Autosomal dominant
	Autosomal recessive and including one or more of diabetes mellitus, optic atrophy, high tone deafness (DIDMOAD syndrome)
Postsurgical Traumatic	May be temporary
Tumours	Pituitary adenoma (rare)
	Craniopharyngioma
	Dysgerminoma ⎱ rare hypothalamic
	Teratoma ⎰ tumours
	Secondary carcinomas esp. lung, breast
Granulomata	Sarcoid
	TB
	Histiocytosis X
Infections	Meningitis/encephalitis
Vascular	e.g. Sheehan's syndrome – postpartum pituitary infarction (now rare)
Nephrogenic diabetes insipidus	
Familial	X-linked recessive
Hypercalcaemia	Malignancy, hyperparathyroidism
Hypokalaemia	Diuresis
Drug-induced	Lithium salts
	Demethylchlortetracycline

are by far the most common. There is now considerable evidence that a proportion of apparently idiopathic examples are in fact due to autoimmunity and fit into the spectrum of organ specific autoimmune diseases which includes autoimmune thyroiditis, adrenalitis, pernicious anaemia and some cases of diabetes mellitus. Pituitary adenomas rarely present with diabetes insipidus and, as a result of improvements in obstetric care, postpartum pituitary infarction is now rare. Diabetes insipidus secondary to pathological processes affecting the neurohypophysis but sparing the pituitary stalk and neurosecretory cells is frequently transient.

As adequate glucocorticoid is essential for water excretion, adrenocorticotrophic hormone (ACTH) deficiency may mask associated diabetes insipidus. The latter condition only becomes clinically evident when steroid replacement therapy is begun.

Failure of ADH action on renal tubules (*nephrogenic diabetes insipidus*) may occur as a primary inherited disorder, as a consequence of certain drugs, or secondary to hypercalcaemia or hypokalaemia (see Table 22.1). *Familial* nephrogenic diabetes insipidus is a rare X-linked recessive condition presenting in infancy. The underlying mechanism appears to be a defect either in the action of ADH on the renal tubule receptor, or in post receptor activity. The disease is fully expressed in males inheriting the affected X chromosome, but subclinical defects in renal concentrating capacity may be found in female carriers.

The common *drug-induced* causes of failure of renal concentrating ability include lithium salts (used to treat manic-depressive disorders) and the long-acting tetracycline, demethylchlortetracycline. This action of demethylchlortetracycline is used therapeutically to treat the syndrome of inappropriate secretion of antidiuretic hormone (SIADH) typically found in small cell lung cancer. These agents probably produce their effects by impairing ADH-induced cyclic-AMP formation in renal tubular cells.

Hypercalcaemia reduces renal concentrating capacity both by inhibiting chloride transport in the loop of Henle, with a consequent reduction in medullary hypertonicity, and by inhibiting the action of ADH on renal tubular cells. These effects may be marked in severe hypercalcaemia, and contribute to the vicious circle of dehydration and accelerating hypercalcaemia which may develop. Chronic *hypokalaemia* may produce the same effect, although usually to a lesser extent than is evident with hypercalcaemia.

Investigation of polyuria and polydipsia

The approach to this combination of symptoms is outlined in Figure 22.4. Prolonged water deprivation is usually unnecessary, it being sufficient to continue only until two-hourly measurements of osmolality have reached a maximum: a situation normally achieved within 8 hours. It is important that the patient is weighed at hourly intervals and that the test is discontinued if weight loss exceeds 3% of total body weight. The latter outcome is virtually

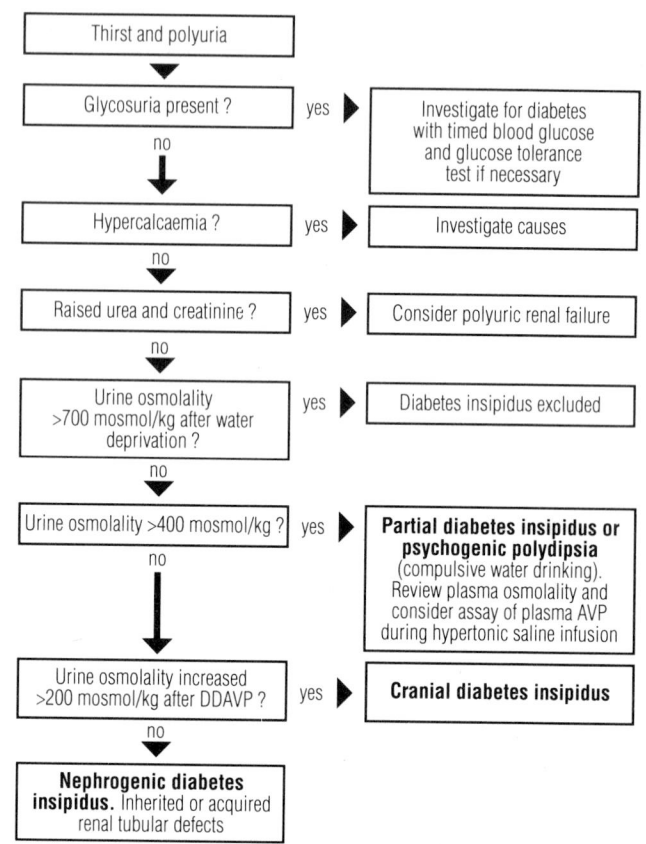

Fig. 22.4 The investigation of polyuria and polydipsia.

diagnostic of diabetes insipidus. Renal responsiveness to ADH is tested by means of an intranasal test dose (20–40 μg) of the synthetic ADH analogue, desmopressin (1-desamino-8-D-arginine vasopressin, DDAVP). The urine osmolality is measured in all specimens passed in the ensuing 9 hours.

The most difficult distinction to make is that between partial degrees of diabetes insipidus and compulsive water drinking. The latter condition, which represents an extreme of habit-mediated fluid consumption, results in renal medullary hypotonicity and a consequent secondary renal concentrating defect. Some assistance in diagnosis may be provided by the plasma osmolality (or plasma sodium) which is characteristically less than 290 mosm/kg at commencement of water deprivation in compulsive water drinkers (because of some degree of overhydration), but is frequently higher than normal in partial diabetes insipidus because of water depletion. When the history and preliminary investigations still fail to distinguish between these possibilities, there is a place for measurement of plasma ADH (by radioimmunoassay) in response to a continuous intravenous infusion of hypertonic saline. In this test, patients with compulsive water drinking show a normal rise in plasma ADH as plasma osmolality increases; whereas any rise in patients with partial degrees of cranial diabetes insipidus is demonstrably less. It is vital that fluid intake should be controlled when test doses of DDAVP are administered, because of the danger of water intoxication in patients with compulsive water drinking.

Treatment

Cranial diabetes insipidus is most conveniently treated with the synthetic ADH analogue, desmopressin (DDAVP). This agent has a greater weight for weight antidiuretic activity than ADH and lacks the latter's potentially hazardous vasopressor effects. It also has a prolonged half-life so that single doses act for up to 18 hours. For these reasons, it has replaced other vasopressin preparations such as aqueous vasopressin, lysine vasopressin preparations and pitressin tannate (no longer available in the UK). For maintenance therapy, desmopressin is administered intranasally in doses of 2.5–20 μg once or twice daily. In partial disease, a single nocturnal dose may be sufficient to alleviate symptoms. When intranasal administration is contra-indicated, desmopressin may be given intramuscularly once or twice daily (0.25–2.0 μg).

The aim of treatment is to replace antidiuretic activity partially with normal thirst mechanisms, thereby ensuring that fluid intake is adequate and that over-hydration and consequent intra- and extracellular dilution are avoided. Difficulties may arise with hypothalamic disorders which interfere with normal thirst mechanisms as well as ADH production. In these situations a fixed regimen of fluid intake and a carefully titrated dose schedule of desmopressin must be provided for the patient.

Chlorpropamide, a sulphonylurea oral hypoglycaemic agent, has been used to good effect in mild cranial diabetes insipidus. It acts by enhancing hypothalamic ADH release and may have a potentiating effect on the action of ADH on the renal tubule. Unfortunately, the possibility of hypoglycaemia limits its usefulness. The anticonvulsant carbamazepine may also enhance ADH release in mild disease. The efficacy and safety of desmopressin has reduced the use of these agents.

Nephrogenic diabetes insipidus, by definition unresponsive to desmopressin, is treated by means of thiazide diuretics and some limitation of sodium intake. The rationale behind this treatment is that the induced mild sodium depletion results in enhanced proximal renal tubular sodium and water re-absorption. Considerable amelioration of polyuria may be achieved by this regimen, which is fortunate as no other treatment is available.

Summary 2   Agents of choice in treatment of diabetes insipidus

Cranial
Desmopressin
Carbamazepine (mild cases)

Nephrogenic
Thiazide diuretics/limitation of sodium intake

OTHER CONDITIONS IN WHICH WATER DEPLETION PREDOMINATES

Because of the effectiveness of the renal mechanism of sodium conservation, water depletion may predominate in a number of conditions simultaneously threatening to deplete both body salt and body water.

1. It is most common in patients unable to maintain an adequate oral intake due either to upper gastro-intestinal obstruction or to a reduced level of consciousness. In this situation, continued obligatory insensible and renal loss of water results in slow, progressive intra- and extracellular dehydration. Urinary sodium loss is reduced to a minimum.

2. Obligatory gastrointestinal loss of water also occurs in response to a large solute load. This may be produced by the administration of hyperosmolar solutions via nasogastric tube to a partially conscious or paralysed patient.

3. Virtually pure water loss may also occur as exaggerated insensible loss, via the lungs, in acute respiratory disorders such as asthma.

4. Water depletion may be a feature of untreated diabetes mellitus, and is most likely to occur in the previously undiagnosed non-insulin-dependent diabetic who maintains a high intake of refined sugar (Ch. 20). A vicious circle of osmotic diuresis and rising extra- and intracellular osmolality may occur, particularly if an intercurrent illness is present. Some increased renal loss of sodium occurs but this is relatively less than the water deficit. In the absence of ketosis, vomiting and consequent marked salt depletion is uncommon.

Management

When oral fluid replacement is impractical, mild water depletion is treated by intravenous infusion of an iso-osmolar electrolyte-free solution (5% dextrose is the standard choice). However, this therapy is unsatisfactory if some degree of salt depletion has also occurred, and in this situation infusions of isotonic saline (0.9%) are usually employed. Provided cardiac and renal function are adequate, any excess sodium replacement will be excreted via the kidneys. Alternatively, combinations of dextrose and saline solutions may be used. Maintenance daily intravenous fluid replacement for an adult patient taking nothing by mouth would aim to provide approximately 2.0–2.5 l of water with 70 mmol of sodium and 60–80 mmol of potassium. This could be given as 2 l of 5% dextrose and 0.5 l of isotonic saline, with potassium chloride added in even distribution.

When water depletion has been sufficiently severe to elevate plasma osmolality markedly, there is a theoretical risk of cerebral oedema if water is rapidly replaced as 5% dextrose alone or in the form of hypotonic saline (e.g. half normal, 0.45%). For this reason, isotonic saline (0.9%) is often used to avoid an excessively rapid change in plasma osmolality. This policy may need to be modified, however,

Salt and Water Metabolism

if the plasma sodium concentration continues to increase during isotonic saline administration. This may arise as a result of persistent water losses and of continuing aldosterone-mediated renal sodium re-absorption (stimulated by hypovolaemia). Nonetheless, profound water depletion should be corrected slowly, although the rate of fluid administration must keep pace with continuing renal loss of water in conditions of osmotic diuresis.

WATER EXCESS

An excess of total body water arises when water intake exceeds renal and cutaneous losses. Water excess is unlikely in the presence of normal renal function, except in situations of increased water intake determined by psychological disturbance or, rarely, by hypothalamic disease. When water excretion is impaired, however, a rise in total body water is relatively common (Table 22.2), and is accompanied by a fall in plasma sodium (*dilutional hyponatraemia*).

The tendency to water excess in cardiac failure is usually compounded by diuretic therapy. This further impairs urinary dilution, and may result in stimulation of thirst as a result of increased activation of the renin-angiotensin system.

In the *syndrome of inappropriate secretion of antidiuretic hormone* (SIADH), ADH secretion occurs despite hypotonicity of extracellular fluid and in the absence of depletion of circulating volume. The common causes are listed in Table 22.3. In many of these situations, the severity of the relative water excess and its clinical consequences may be aggravated by inappropriate administration of intravenous fluids.

Clinical features and diagnosis

Mild degrees of water excess cause few symptoms and the clinical features of the underlying disease predominate. However, with severe water excess, as may occur in some cases of SIADH, the reduction in intracellular osmolality in the central nervous system may produce symptoms ranging in severity from general lassitude to decreased

Table 22.2 Causes of reduced water excretion

Cause	Mechanism
Renal impairment	
Liver cirrhosis (hypoalbuminaemia)	
Cardiac failure	Reduced glomerular filtration rate leads to reduced solute delivery to distal tubule
Nephrotic syndrome (hypoalbuminaemia)	
Glucocorticoid deficiency	
Inappropriate ADH secretion (SIADH)	Increased renal tubular re-absorption of water

Table 22.3 Causes of inappropriate ADH secretion (SIADH)

Source	Cause
Ectopic	Malignancies such as small cell bronchial carcinoma
Hypothalamic	Inflammatory lung diseases
	CNS infections
	Drugs Carbamazepine Chlorpropamide Tricyclics Phenothiazines Syntocinon Cytotoxic drugs Cyclophosphamide Vincristine
	Wasting diseases

levels of consciousness, coma and generalised convulsions.

The diagnosis of water excess is usually suggested in the course of routine investigation by the discovery of *hyponatraemia* in the absence of clinical or other evidence of volume depletion. Although sodium depleting states may also result in hyponatraemia, this is only the case if the losses are marked. However, hyponatraemia may occur without water excess when the contribution of glucose to plasma osmolality is increased in untreated diabetes mellitus. The potential rise in plasma osmolality results in a movement of water from the intracellular to extracellular spaces, and a consequent fall in plasma sodium. Furthermore, an apparent hyponatraemia (*pseudo hyponatraemia*) may be evident if marked hyperlipidaemia contributes significantly to plasma volume, thus reducing the water content per unit volume.

The assessment of the hyponatraemic patient is outlined in Figure 22.5. It will be noted that SIADH is characterised by hypotonicity of plasma (osmolality less than 280 mosm/kg) with inappropriate urinary concentration (more than 300 mosm/kg). This condition is associated with a normal or slightly increased circulating volume, so that activity of the renin-angiotensin-aldosterone axis is low and urine sodium excretion approximates to sodium intake. Measurements of plasma and urine osmolality in sodium-depleted patients (p. 849) may be similar to those in SIADH because of the hypovolaemic stimulus to ADH secretion. However, these patients will usually be distinguished by clinical evidence of sodium loss and consequent depletion of circulating volume. In addition, non-renal salt depleting conditions (e.g. gastrointestinal loss) will be associated with renal sodium conservation and a low urinary sodium excretion. In renal salt wasting conditions and in the sodium depletion of adrenal insufficiency, plasma osmolality, urine osmolality and urine sodium excretion may be indistinguishable from measurements in patients with SIADH. This latter point

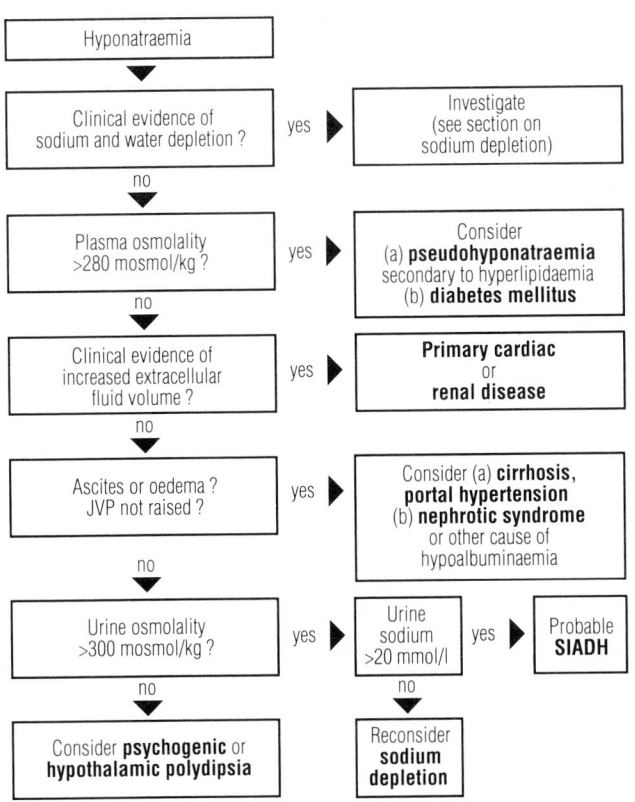

Fig. 22.5 The clinical and biochemical evaluation of hyponatraemia.

serves to emphasise the importance of *clinical* assessment of the extracellular fluid and circulating volumes in the hyponatraemic patient.

An approximate assessment of plasma osmolality may be made from the following calculation:

$$2\,Na^+ + 2\,K^+ + Glucose\,(mmol/l) + Urea\,(mmol/l)$$

where Na^+ and K^+ represent the millimolar concentrations of sodium and potassium and are doubled to account for their anion equivalents in plasma.

Precise measurements of osmolality in the laboratory depend on depression of freezing point techniques.

Management of relative water excess

Severe water intoxication with associated neurological problems requires emergency treatment in an attempt to correct profound hyponatraemia (usually less than 115 mmol/l). Hypertonic saline infusions ($2–5 \times$ isotonic; 1.8–4.5%) are temporarily effective, but carry the dangers of precipitating circulatory overload and of too rapid corrections of hypo-osmolality. Such measures should thus be employed with caution. Dexamethasone is frequently prescribed on an empirical basis to reduce cerebral oedema, but there is little evidence for its efficacy.

Intermediate degrees of water excess, are most often due to SIADH – are best managed by treatment of the underlying

cause. When this is impossible, modest water restriction (1000–1500 ml/day) is usually effective in elevating plasma sodium to safe levels. In some cases, however, increase in plasma osmolality can only be achieved by very strict limitations of water intake which the patient may find intolerable. In this situation, treatment with demethylchlortetracycline (demeclocycline), which reduces renal tubular responsiveness to ADH, is particularly useful. This long-acting tetracycline derivative exerts its full effect within a week of commencement of therapy. It is particularly useful in profound SIADH associated with carcinomas.

Mild degrees of water excess and consequent hyponatraemia (plasma sodium 125–135 mmol/l) do not require specific treatment.

DISORDERS OF SODIUM HOMEOSTASIS

There are many conditions associated with marked changes in total body sodium and thus extracellular fluid volume. Changes in total body water are also often present but are of secondary importance at the time of clinical presentation. Changes in plasma sodium concentration are not impressive unless the alteration in body sodium is marked, or is accompanied by decreased renal water excretion.

SODIUM EXCESS

This may occur iatrogenically as a result of massive sodium replacement with hypertonic saline infusions in hyponatraemic states. More commonly, however, sodium retention occurs as a result of *decreased glomerular filtration rate* in cardiac or renal failure, or under conditions of *increased mineralocorticoid activity* (Table 22.4). The latter arises as a primary phenomenon in Cushing's syndrome (mineralocorticoid effect of increased circulating glucocorticoids) and Conn's syndrome (increased aldosterone production from the adrenal zona glomerulosa due to tumour or hyperplasia). In these conditions, the blood pressure is usually elevated, plasma sodium concentrations are at the upper limit of normal, and plasma potassium is decreased.

Mineralocorticoid activity may be secondarily increased in any condition resulting in stimulation of the renin-

Table 22.4 Causes of sodium retention in disease

Decreased glomerular filtration rate	Secondary mineralocorticoid excess
Cardiac failure	Cardiac failure
Renal failure	Liver disease
	Nephrotic syndrome
Primary mineralocorticoid excess	
Cushing's syndrome	
Conn's syndrome	

angiotensin system. This so-called *secondary hyper-aldosteronism* occurs with the reduced renal perfusion in chronic cardiac failure, liver disease with portal hypertension, and various hypo-albuminaemic states (such as nephrotic syndrome), in which circulating volume is reduced, thereby stimulating the renin-angiotensin mechanism.

The sodium retention of Conn's and Cushing's syndromes does not result in oedema. The latter only arises if there is an associated increased intracapillary pressure (as in heart failure), or a reduced plasma oncotic pressure (in hypo-albuminaemia) (Table 22.5). Secondary hyper-aldosteronism is a contributory factor in the oedema which occurs in these conditions.

Table 22.5 Effects of increased mineralocorticoid activity

Cause of increased activity	Blood pressure	Oedema/ ascites	Plasma K$^+$
Primary			
Conn's syndrome	↑	–	↓
Cushing's syndrome (ectopic ACTH)	↑	–	↓
Secondary			
Cardiac failure	–	↑	↓
Portal hypertension	–	↑	↓
Nephrotic syndrome	–	↑	↓

Differential diagnosis of oedema

Oedema (or expansion of the interstitial fluid volume) is evident as subcutaneous swelling which predominates in dependent sites: feet and ankles in the upright posture; sacral region after prolonged recumbency.

Oedema may occur in a number of distinct conditions:

1. *Heart failure*, when it may reflect the generalised increase in intracapillary pressure. The diagnosis is confirmed by elevation of jugular venous pressure, cardiac enlargement, and clinical or radiological evidence of pulmonary venous congestion.
2. *Hypoalbuminaemic states* (e.g. nephrotic syndrome) in which plasma oncotic pressure is reduced.
3. *Peripheral venous insufficiency*, of which chronic ankle oedema is frequently a localised manifestation, particularly in association with varicose veins.
4. *Idiopathic oedema*, which may occur in women on an apparently cyclical basis, being worst premenstrually. It has been postulated that these individuals have increased capillary albumin leakage. However, it has also been suggested that, in a proportion of patients with idiopathic oedema, the primary abnormality is intermittent diuretic abuse with consequent secondary hyperaldosteronism.

SODIUM DEPLETION

A net sodium deficit may result from gastrointestinal or renal loss. The former, occurring as vomiting or diarrhoea, is usually obvious from the clinical history, whereas a diagnosis of renal salt loss is generally made only after investigation.

In the earliest stages, pure sodium deficiency may be associated with some suppression of ADH secretion because of the tendency to decreased extracellular osmolality. Eventually, however, the fall in total body sodium results in a decrease in extracellular fluid volume sufficient to stimulate ADH secretion (Fig. 22.3). Water excretion is further diminished by increased sodium re-absorption in the proximal tubules, with a consequent reduction in solute delivery to distal tubular diluting sites.

Clinical features

Sodium depletion is manifest clinically by signs of a reduction in extracellular fluid and circulating volumes. The most reliable indicators are postural hypotension and accompanying tachycardia. Skin turgor is an unreliable indicator of extracellular fluid volume because it is subjective and variable with age.

Upper gastrointestinal salt and water loss may be associated with metabolic alkalosis as a consequence of loss of gastric acid. Hydrogen ion depletion results in hypokalaemia (p. 850) and an increase in renal potassium excretion, because of decreased hydrogen ion availability for the shared renal tubular electrochemical exchange of potassium and hydrogen ions for sodium. Conversely, loss of bicarbonate-rich duodenal contents may result in metabolic acidosis.

Gastrointestinal sodium loss is distinguished from renal loss on the basis of the clinical history and by measurement of urinary sodium excretion, which is very low when there is a gastrointestinal cause. The causes of renal salt loss are given in Table 22.6. Sodium balance is particularly vulnerable in those forms of chronic renal disease which affect the medulla. Such patients lose the capacity to vary sodium excretion and are susceptible to dramatic salt depletion in the event of intercurrent gastrointestinal disturbance, with

Table 22.6 Causes of net renal sodium loss

Intrinsic renal disease
Recovery phase of acute tubular necrosis
Relief of longstanding urinary obstruction
Some forms of chronic nephropathy, particularly tubulo-interstitial disease

Mineralocorticoid deficiency
Adrenal failure
Isolated aldosterone deficiency

Diuretic therapy

a resultant further and rapid reduction in glomerular filtration rate. In different circumstances, however, these patients are in potential danger of sodium retention (p. 847).

As a consequence of the reduction in circulating volume which accompanies marked sodium depletion, there is a fall in glomerular filtration rate and thus a rise in both plasma urea and creatinine concentrations (Fig. 22.6). This is termed *pre-renal uraemia* (Ch. 21) and may, in some circumstances, prove difficult to distinguish from acute renal failure. In general, pre-renal states are associated with a disproportionate rise in the concentration of plasma urea compared to that of creatinine, and the haematocrit may also be raised to a degree consistent with haemoconcentration. However, other factors which affect plasma urea concentration, such as quantity of dietary protein or rate of body protein catabolism, may limit the usefulness of this comparison.

A low urinary sodium concentration distinguishes non-renal sodium depletion from acute renal failure (in which urine sodium concentration is normal or increased). In the diuretic phase of acute tubular necrosis, or after relief of urinary obstruction, the aetiology of the sodium loss is usually obvious. The possibility of adrenal insufficiency should be borne in mind in any patient who presents with evidence of unexplained salt depletion.

Management

Clinically obvious salt and water deficit almost always requires intravenous replacement. Isotonic saline (sodium chloride, 0.9%) is administered at a rate determined by the clinical severity of the case and on any continuing losses. Potassium supplements are required for gastrointestinal losses. If cardiac function is in doubt, the rate of saline replacement should be determined by careful and frequent clinical assessment of volume status and, if necessary, by direct measurement of central venous pressure. In situations where it proves impossible to distinguish definitely between salt depletion and established acute renal failure as the cause of the presenting oliguria and uraemia, it may be of benefit to administer 500 ml 0.9% saline rapidly and monitor urine output in response to this.

Salt depleting chronic renal disease may necessitate regular oral sodium supplements (Ch. 21).

Interpretation of plasma sodium concentrations

The plasma sodium concentration reflects the degree of dilution of extracellular sodium. It thus tells us a great deal about total body water but relatively little about total body sodium. We learn more about the latter from clinical examination, from such indirect indicators of glomerular filtration rate (dependent on circulating volume) as plasma urea and creatinine, and from urine sodium excretion rates (Table 22.7.)

Fig. 22.6 The renal consequences of sodium depletion. The percentage of increase in plasma urea exceeds that of creatinine by the mechanism shown, provided intrinsic renal function remains normal.

Table 22.7 Interpretation of the plasma sodium concentration

Diagnosis	Plasma Na$^+$	Plasma creatinine	Urine sodium (mmol/l)	Urine osmolality (mosm/kg)
SIADH	Low	↓	>20	>300
Adrenal failure	Low	↑	>20	>300
Renal failure	Low/normal	↑↑	>20	<300
Non-renal sodium loss	Low/normal	↑	<20	>300
Primary water deficit	High	N or ↑	>20	>300
Diabetes insipidus	High	N or ↑	<20	<300
Hyperosmolar diabetes mellitus	High	↑	Variable	>300

POTASSIUM HOMEOSTASIS

Potassium ions are predominantly intracellular, the concentration gradient depending on active Na$^+$/K$^+$ exchange across the plasma membrane (Fig. 22.2). The other major determinant of the distribution is pH. Alkalosis, associated with a fall in intracellular hydrogen ion concentration, results in a net flux of potassium into cells with a consequent fall in plasma potassium; acidosis has the reverse effect (Fig. 22.7). The mechanism of these changes is unknown but may be related to intracellular changes in hydrogen ion binding of negatively charged proteins. Cellular uptake of potassium is probably also partially insulin-dependent.

Maintenance of total body potassium depends on dietary

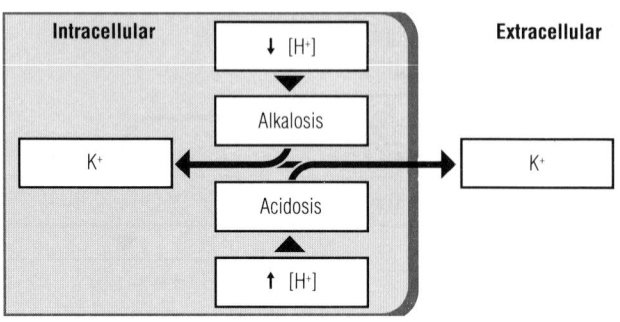

Fig. 22.7 The effect of acid-base changes on the distribution of potassium across cell membranes. The steady state distribution is altered by either acidosis or alkalosis in the directions shown.

intake (approximately 100 mmol per day in Western diets) and on control of renal potassium excretion. Potassium is actively re-absorbed in the proximal renal tubule. In the distal tubule, potassium excretion occurs by diffusion down its electrochemical gradient (Fig. 22.8). In the collecting ducts, passage of potassium into tubular fluid appears to be an active process shared with hydrogen ions, apparently in exchange for sodium ions in tubular fluid. This exchange is enhanced by increased concentrations of sodium in the tubular lumen and by aldosterone. Changes in intra- and extracellular pH alter concentrations of potassium in renal tubular cells and thus indirectly affect renal potassium excretion both by diffusion and in exchange for

Fig. 22.8 The influence of acid-base changes on intracellular potassium concentration and renal excretion in the distal renal tubule. Diffusion of potassium into the tubular lumen is increased by alkalosis and decreased by acidosis as a consequence of changes in potassium concentration in renal tubular cells.

sodium. Under conditions of high potassium intake, renal tubular potassium secretion is increased.

HYPOKALAEMIA

A significant reduction in plasma potassium usually indicates profound depletion of total body potassium but may occasionally be due to temporary shifts of potassium ions from the extra- to intracellular spaces. The important causes of hypokalaemia and the proposed underlying mechanisms are outlined in Table 22.8.

Clinical features

Non-specific symptoms of lethargy and weakness may accompany mild to moderate hypokalaemia (c. 2.8–3.5 mmol/l). Levels of potassium lower than this may give rise to marked muscular weakness, gut hypomotility, increased myocardial excitability and arrhythmias, and nephrogenic diabetes insipidus. A shift of hydrogen ions from extra- to

Table 22.8 Causes of hypokalaemia

Cause	Mechanism
Alkalosis	Intracellular shift of K^+ in exchange for H^+; increased renal excretion
Diuretics Diabetes mellitus	Increased renal excretion secondary to enhanced distal tubular sodium delivery and increased tubular flow
*Conn's syndrome	Increased aldosterone effect
*Cushing's syndrome (esp. ectopic ACTH from malignant source)	Mineralocorticoid effect of increased glucocorticoids
*Steroid therapy (esp. high dose hydrocortisone)	Mineralocorticoid effect of increased glucocorticoids
*Carbenoxolone therapy for peptic ulcer	Mineralocorticoid effect
*Congenital adrenal hyperplasia (11-hydroxylase deficiency)	Mineralocorticoid effect of deoxycorticosterone
Renal tubular acidosis (distal type)	Decreased Na^+/H^+ exchange in distal tubule (see Ch. 21)
Bartter's syndrome	Defective chloride absorption in loop of Henle with consequent solute loss and secondary hyperaldosteronism
Vomiting (esp. pyloric stenosis and bulimia nervosa)	Loss of gastric contents and effects of alkalosis
Secretory diarrhoea	Direct loss of potassium
Laxative abuse	Direct loss of potassium
Villous adenoma of rectum	Enhanced potassium loss from tumour cells
Hypokalaemic periodic paralysis	Intermittent shift of potassium into cells

* see Ch. 18

intracellular spaces is thought to be responsible for the *metabolic alkalosis* which accompanies most cases of hypokalaemia. This apparent hydrogen ion shift may be due to a relative failure of cell membrane proton pumps (H^+ extrusion). In addition, chronic hypokalaemia may reduce renal chloride conservation, with a consequent increased delivery of sodium to distal tubular sites. This promotes sodium exchange for hydrogen ions with accentuation of the alkalosis.

Investigation

In many instances, the mechanism of hypokalaemia is obvious from the history and clinical observations. When this is not the case, investigation is directed initially at distinguishing gastrointestinal from renal loss of potassium by means of total 24-hour urine potassium estimations. These are very low in all non-renal mechanisms of potassium loss, with the exception of repeated vomiting which is complicated by alkalosis. It may prove very difficult to diagnose surreptitious vomiting, or diuretic or laxative abuse. A finding of hypokalaemia with a *low* plasma bicarbonate always suggests the possibility of renal tubular acidosis and should prompt measurement of urinary pH (which will be inappropriately high in this condition). The rare combination of acidosis and hypokalaemia is also seen in the most severe examples of diabetic ketoacidosis, when potassium depletion is particularly marked.

Management

Hypokalaemia is usually corrected by oral potassium chloride in wax base (e.g. Slow K), unless potassium depletion is profound and life-threatening in which case potassium chloride is given intravenously. The rate of administration depends on any continuing losses, but it should rarely be necessary to exceed 30 mmol/hour even at the initiation of therapy. Plasma potassium concentrations should be monitored regularly.

HYPERKALAEMIA

Increases in plasma potassium usually arise against a background of decreased renal potassium excretion. Moderate increases are symptomless, but at levels exceeding 6.5 mmol/l, the risk of cardiac arrest increases, and severe hyperkalaemia constitutes a medical emergency. Aetiological factors and mechanisms are outlined in Table 22.9. The possibility of haemolysis of the sample causing artefactual hyperkalaemia should be considered in instances of isolated hyperkalaemia in the presence of normal renal function.

Management

Marked hyperkalaemia (more than 7 mmol/l) should be reduced as a matter of urgency because of the risk of cardiac arrest. Simultaneous intravenous administration of glucose (50 g) and insulin (15 units) is temporarily effective; and

Table 22.9 Causes of hyperkalaemia

Cause	Mechanism
Acute renal failure	Decreased excretion which may be compounded by acidosis, cell necrosis (esp. when infection present), transfusions of stored blood and potassium retaining diuretics
Acidosis	Shift of potassium from intra- to extracellular spaces
Cell necrosis (e.g. after cancer chemotherapy)	Release of cellular potassium
Type 4 renal tubular acidosis (see Ch. 21)	Impairment of K^+ secretion in the distal nephron caused by: (a) Decreased mineralocorticoid activity due to adrenal failure (b) Reduced activity of renin-angiotensin system ('hyporeninaemic hypoaldosteronism') e.g. in diabetic neuropathy (c) Angiotensin converting enzyme inhibitors (d) Potassium retaining diuretics i.e. direct inhibition of aldosterone action (spironolactone) or of Na^+/K^+ distal tubular exchange (amiloride, triamterene) (e) Tubular resistance to mineralocorticoid action

intravenous bicarbonate (50 mmol) will cause some shift of potassium from the extracellular to the intracellular compartment. (The associated sodium load may be poorly tolerated, however, and dialysis may be necessary.) Renal potassium losses may be increased by loop diuretics such as frusemide. Intravenous calcium salts afford some protection against the cardiac consequences of hyperkalaemia. Electrocardiographic monitoring is useful for acute assessment. Moderate hyperkalaemia is associated with peaking of T waves; more sinister changes include increasing width of QRS complexes. Longer-term control may be achieved by means of cation exchange resins (e.g. Resonium A-sodium, Calcium Resonium) which are given either orally or by retention enema.

The management of adrenal failure and hypoaldosteronism are considered in Chapter 18.

ACID-BASE HOMEOSTASIS

A large number of metabolic events are pH sensitive and maintenance of a stable acid base status is therefore of critical importance. In the healthy individual, extracellular pH is held within narrow limits (pH 7.38–7.42). Intracellular pH is generally lower than extracellular and varies both from one tissue to another and according to nutritional status and exercise state (mean range pH 6.7–7.3). Under normal circumstances, homeostatic mechanisms are generally concerned with the buffering and disposal of hydrogen ions generated by intracellular metabolic events, particularly aerobic respiration (CO_2 production), glycolysis (lactic acid production) and lipolysis (fatty acid and eventual ketoacid production, see Table 22.10).

The acceptance of hydrogen ions by intra- or extracellular buffer base constitutes the first line of defence against deviations from normal pH. Important buffer systems include bicarbonate/carbonic acid, red cell haemoglobin, phosphate and intracellular proteins. Exhaustion of buffer capacity is prevented by short- or long-term elimination of hydrogen ions or by regeneration of bicarbonate. This occurs through respiration (acid eliminated in the form of CO_2); metabolism (hepatic metabolism of lactic acid, tissue metabolism of ketone bodies and free fatty acid); and renal excretion (buffered by ammonia and phosphate).

Lactic acid metabolism provides an interesting example of immediate buffering with subsequent hydrogen ion consumption and bicarbonate regeneration. Lactic acid (pK 4.6) is fully dissociated in plasma, and protons are consumed by normal buffering mechanisms (e.g. bicarbonate). The subsequent hepatic metabolism of lactate ions to produce glucose requires the stoichiometric consumption of hydrogen ions with consequent formation of bicarbonate from carbon dioxide and hydroxyl ions.

Henderson-Hasselbalch equation

The equilibrium relationship between the protonated and anionic forms of a buffer pair such as bicarbonate/carbonic acid may be indicated as follows:

$$[H_2CO_3] \underset{K_2}{\overset{K_1}{\rightleftharpoons}} [H^+] + [HCO_3^-]$$

$$\frac{K_1}{K_2} = \frac{[H^+][HCO_3^-]}{H_2CO_3} = K \text{ (equilibrium constant)}$$

$$[H^+] = \frac{K[H_2CO_3]}{[HCO_3^-]}$$

$$pH = pK + \log \frac{[HCO_3^-]}{[H_2CO_3]} \text{ (proportional to } P_{CO_2})$$

This is the classical Henderson-Hasselbalch equation which can be applied to all physiological buffer systems. Reference to the above equation indicates the change in concentration of a given buffer component which is required for pH to remain constant following a primary alteration in acid-base status. Thus, metabolic production of acid which leads to an immediate fall in HCO_3^- will lead to a fall in pH unless P_{CO_2} also decreases by increased respiration. Increases in P_{CO_2} consequent upon respiratory failure necessitate a rise in HCO_3^- concentration (by increased renal conservation of bicarbonate) if pH changes

Table 22.10 Acid generation and elimination

Source	Acid	Elimination
Aerobic respiration	CO_2	Pulmonary
Glycolysis	Lactic acid	Hepatic metabolism to glucose or CO_2 (pulmonary elimination)
Lipolysis	Free fatty acids (FFA)	Oxidation to CO_2 (pulmonary elimination)
Hepatic metabolism	Ketone bodies	Oxidation to CO_2 (pulmonary elimination)
Dietary protein catabolism	Inorganic acids	Renal

are to be minimised. Similar arguments can be applied to situations in which primary increases in HCO_3^-, or decreases in P_{CO_2}, occur. Primary alterations in CO_2 are denoted as *respiratory acidosis or alkalosis* and primary changes in buffer base as *metabolic acidosis or alkalosis*. These terms apply regardless of whether or not appropriate compensatory mechanisms have been sufficient to maintain pH within the normal range (compensated metabolic or respiratory acidosis or alkalosis). Respiratory compensation is discussed in Chapter 14, p. 456; see also Fig. 14.7.

INVESTIGATION OF ACID-BASE STATUS

Blood gas analysis

Acid-base status is disturbed in a variety of clinical situations and is usually impossible to define precisely on clinical grounds alone. Measurements of arterial pH and P_{CO_2} are therefore frequently necessary in acutely ill patients. Blood gas analysers measure pH and P_{CO_2} directly by means of specific electrodes, and bicarbonate concentrations are automatically calculated using the Henderson-Hasselbalch equation. Values are usually also given for the so-called 'standard bicarbonate' which represents the theoretical bicarbonate concentrations at a P_{CO_2} of 5.3 kPa (40 mmHg), and thus purports to show the extent of a given acid-base disturbance attributable to metabolic

Table 22.11 Changes in P_{CO_2} and HCO_3 in acid-base disorders

	pH	P_{CO_2}	HCO_3^-
Metabolic acidosis	N or ↓	↓	↓↓
Metabolic alkalosis	N or ↑	slight ↑	↑↑
Respiratory acidosis	N or ↓	↑↑	↑
Respiratory alkalosis	N or ↑	↓↓	slight ↓

The primary derangements are denoted by double arrows.

causes alone. In practice, however, clinical assessment and measurements of pH, $P\text{CO}_2$, $P\text{O}_2$ and bicarbonate are sufficient for the accurate classification of pure or mixed (e.g. acute metabolic acidosis and chronic respiratory acidosis) acid-base disturbances (Table 22.11). Reliance on derived values for 'standard bicarbonate' (from blood samples) is not recommended, as they do not necessarily reflect *in vivo* buffering (by blood and tissue buffers) and may be grossly misleading.

Metabolic acidosis results in rapid respiratory compensation due to stimulation of carotid body, aortic and medullary chemoreceptors. *Metabolic alkalosis*, on the other hand, is less well compensated by respiratory mechanisms, probably because any decrease in ventilation is limited by hypoxic respiratory drive.

Chronic respiratory acidosis most commonly occurs as a result of chronic obstructive airways disease, and is partially compensated by a rise in plasma bicarbonate. This compensation occurs via increased hydrogen ion excretion and renal conservation of bicarbonate, a long-term effect occurring over two to three days and thus not evident in acute respiratory acidosis.

Difficulties in interpretation may arise with *mixed acid-base disturbances*. This is most commonly seen with the superimposition of metabolic acidosis on chronic respiratory acidosis. This combination results in a low pH (by definition), an elevated $P\text{CO}_2$ (inability to respond to acidotic respiratory drive), and a fall in previously elevated bicarbonate level. The clinical presentation, history and critical evaluation of pH, $P\text{CO}_2$ and bicarbonate will usually indicate the dual diagnosis, and a decreased $P\text{O}_2$ will provide additional evidence of the respiratory component.

The anion gap

Subtraction of the sum of plasma concentrations of the anions chloride and bicarbonate from the cations sodium and potassium normally yields a 'gap value' of 10–20 mmol/l, made up of negatively charged proteins, phosphate, sulphate, lactate and small quantities of keto-acids. Calculation of this *anion gap* in metabolic acidosis is useful for distinguishing those cases which are due to bicarbonate loss (e.g. pancreatic fistulae, renal tubular acidosis), in which the anion gap is normal, from those due to increases in endogenously produced acid (e.g. ketoacidosis, lactic acidosis and the acidosis of renal failure) in which the gap is increased. In the former cases, plasma chloride is increased (hyperchloraemic acidosis) to maintain electroneutrality.

ACID-BASE DISORDERS

Acid-base disorders include:

1. metabolic acidosis
2. metabolic alkalosis
3. respiratory acidosis
4. respiratory alkalosis.

Metabolic acidosis

The common causes of metabolic acidosis are listed in Table 22.12 and are subgrouped according to whether or not the anion gap is disturbed.

The increased respiratory drive resulting from severe metabolic acidosis is clinically recognisable as deep, sighing respiration (*Kussmaul respiration*). Respiratory compensation for metabolic acidosis is dependent on adequate respiratory reserve and therefore may not be possible if there is co-existing chronic respiratory disease. In many of the conditions listed in Table 22.12, accumulation of more than one acid may occur. If acidosis, from whatever cause, is severe, reduction in cardiac output may result in a superimposed lactic acidosis (Type A). This is due to peripheral glycolysis which occurs with tissue anoxia. Similarly, diabetic ketoacidosis is associated with salt and water depletion, and the resulting contraction in the circulating volume leads to increased peripheral glycolysis and lactic acid accumulation. The situation is further complicated because acidosis itself directly inhibits the glycolytic pathway in peripheral tissues (Fig. 22.9), and this effect tends to offset the increase in lactic acid production. However, acidosis directly inhibits hepatic gluconeogenic enzymes and, because lactate is an important gluconeogenic substrate, this may result in progressive lactic acid accumulation. Loss of the slight intracellular alkalinising effect of hepatic lactate metabolism further accentuates the effects of acidosis on hepatic lactate removal (Fig. 22.9).

The acidosis of renal failure has traditionally been attributed to decreased ammonia formation (from glutamine) in the diseased kidney, with consequent decreased buffering capacity in the urine. Decreased urinary buffer results in the minimum urinary pH being reached at a lower total hydrogen ion content, and thus leads to systemic acidosis. However, it has recently been pointed out that, because the metabolism of glutamine in renal tubular cells yields

Table 22.12 Causes of metabolic acidosis

Normal anion gap	Increased anion gap
Gut bicarbonate loss (e.g. pancreatic fistula)	Diabetic ketoacidosis
	Starvation ketoacidosis
Renal tubular acidosis (urine pH inappropriately high)	Lactic acidosis
Distal type (failure of proton secretion). Primary and secondary	Type A secondary to increased peripheral glycolysis in circulatory failure or hypoxia
Treatment with carbonic anhydrase inhibitors	Type B secondary to failure of lactate metabolism or to net lactate production in liver, e.g. biguanide drugs, ethanol, methanol, ethylene glycol, fructose, liver disease
Proximal type (bicarbonate wastage). Primary and secondary	
	Acidosis of renal failure
	Salicylate poisoning

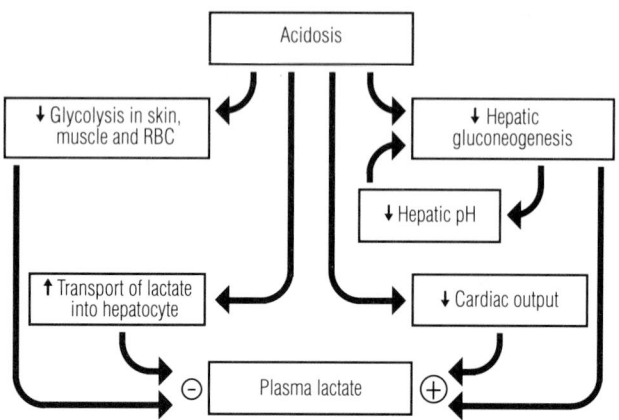

Fig. 22.9 The metabolic consequences of metabolic acidosis. Acidosis tends to decrease hepatic metabolism with resultant lactate and hydrogen ion accumulation. These effects are partially offset by a direct partial inhibition of glycolysis by acidosis and an increase in lactate transport into hepatocytes. ($-$) and ($+$) denote the potential changes in plasma lactate.

NH_4^+ rather than NH_3, this mechanism cannot be responsible for net hydrogen ion excretion by the kidney. The other route of glutamine metabolism is via urea formation in the liver. This mechanism results in net bicarbonate consumption and, since glutamine is diverted to hepatic metabolism when renal metabolism is impaired, it follows that the acidosis of renal failure may be primarily related to the acid-generating (i.e. bicarbonate-consuming) effect of hepatic ureagenesis (Fig. 22.10).

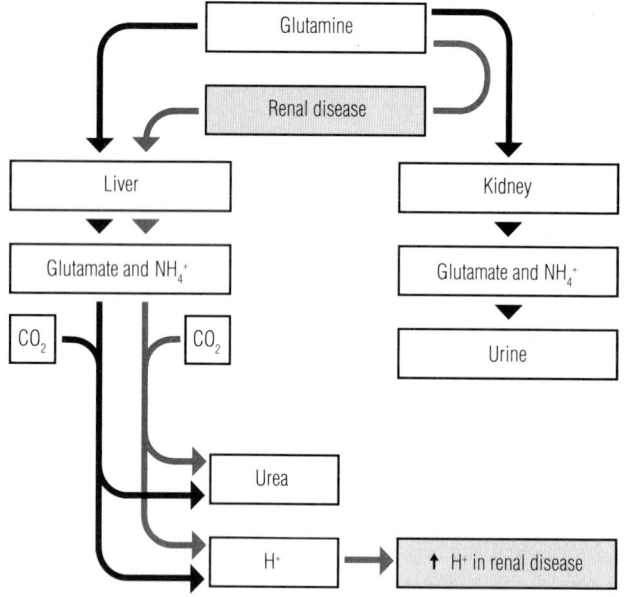

Fig. 22.10 Routes of glutamine metabolism in liver and kidney. Renal disease results in diversion of glutamine metabolism to the liver, with urea and hydrogen ion production.

Detailed consideration of renal tubular acidosis and salicylate poisoning are given in Chapter 21 and Chapter 4 respectively.

Metabolic alkalosis

Metabolic alkalosis results from direct loss of hydrogen ions or ingestion of bicarbonate (Table 22.13). Respiratory compensation is poor because hypoxia would be its direct consequence and possibly also because intracellular pH may increase relatively less than extracellular pH in some instances, leading to a lesser respiratory drive to compensate.

Table 22.13 Causes of metabolic alkalosis

Gastric acid loss (esp. pyloric stenosis)

Potassium deficit } leading to renal H^+ loss
Hyperaldosteronism

Ingestion of alkali or inappropriate intravenous administration

Respiratory acidosis

Carbon dioxide accumulation may occur as a result of disease affecting the respiratory centre, the chest wall, the muscles of respiration or the airways (Table 22.14; see also page 500, Table 14.31). The condition may be chronic (e.g. chronic obstructive airways disease) or acute (e.g. neuromuscular problems such as myasthenia); and there are marked differences in compensatory responses in the two situations because of the several days required for significant renal conservation of bicarbonate to occur. Thus, a new steady state of raised $P\text{CO}_2$ and bicarbonate with maintenance of normal pH is frequently seen in chronic lung disease. The latter situation is associated with some desensitisation to hypercapnic respiratory drive and increased importance of the hypoxic respiratory stimulus.

Table 22.14 Causes of respiratory acidosis

Pulmonary disease
Chronic airways obstruction
Acute severe asthma

Traumatic and mechanical problems
Flail chest
Gross obesity
Ankylosing spondylitis

Neuromuscular disease
Guillain-Barré syndrome
Myasthenia gravis
Poliomyelitis
Motor neurone disease
Respiratory centre depression by depressant drugs (e.g. opiates) or circulatory arrest

Respiratory alkalosis

An increase in ventilation and consequent fall in $P\text{co}_2$ usually arises as a primary event, as in hyperventilation due to anxiety or in hypoxic states (Table 22.15). When chronic hypoxia is the precipitating cause, some compensation may occur by means of increased renal bicarbonate excretion. In most instances, however, the fall in $P\text{co}_2$ is acute and pH rises rapidly.

Table 22.15   Causes of respiratory alkalosis

Stress hyperventilation

Hypoxic stimulus to ventilation
Alveolar disease
Right to left shunt
Altitude

Drug induced stimulus to ventilation
Salicylate poisoning

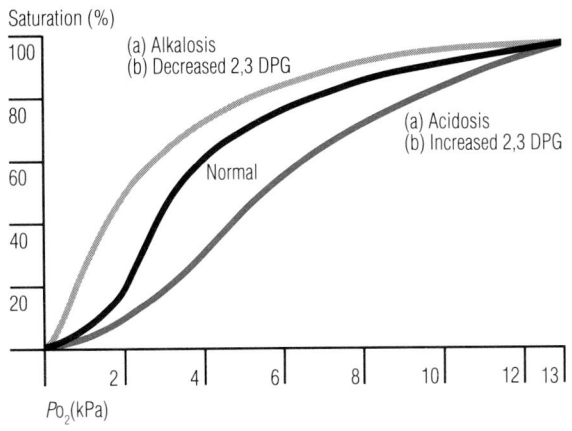

Fig. 22.12   The effects of (a) acid-base changes and (b) 2,3 DPG concentration on haemoglobin-oxygen dissociation. A shift to the right indicates increased oxygen delivery per unit fall in $P\text{o}_2$. A shift to the left indicates decreased oxygen delivery per unit fall in $P\text{o}_2$.

Clinical consequences of acidosis

The clinical consequences of acidosis are outlined in Figure 22.11.

Acidosis is associated with a shift to the right of the oxygen dissociation curve (Fig. 22.12), thus tending to improve oxygen delivery to the periphery (provided pulmonary function is adequate). This effect is reduced to some extent by the fall in 2,3 diphosphoglycerate (2,3 DPG) concentration in erythrocytes, which occurs over a period of days. This has important implications for the management of metabolic acidosis.

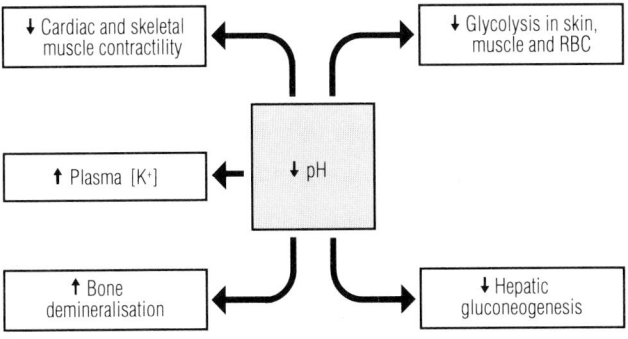

Fig. 22.11   The multiple effects of acidosis on heart, skin, red blood cells, liver and bone, and on plasma K^+ concentration.

Clinical consequences of alkalosis

In clinical terms, the most dramatic result of a rise in pH is a fall in ionised calcium resulting in tetany (carpopedal spasm). Milder symptoms, also suggesting a decreased ionised calcium, include peripheral and circumoral paraesthesia and are frequently found in patients with hyperventilation associated with stress.

Alkalosis has a hypokalaemic affect (p. 850) and also tends to increase peripheral glycolysis. In practice, however, raised lactic acid levels are not a feature of alkalotic conditions, with the possible exception of respiratory alkalosis accompanying liver failure, in which lactic acid metabolism is impaired.

Treatment of metabolic acid-base disturbances

Metabolic alkalosis rarely requires more than correction of salt, water and potassium depletion, and treatment of the underlying pathology. However, metabolic acidosis, particularly some forms of lactic acidosis, may require the administration of large quantities of sodium bicarbonate intravenously, in order to counteract the negative inotropic effect and inhibition of hepatic lactate metabolism. The sodium load, which inevitably accompanies bicarbonate administration, may necessitate dialysis, particularly if there is co-existing renal impairment.

Mild to moderate diabetic ketoacidosis (pH > 7.1) does not require alkali administration. In fact, such treatment may be potentially hazardous because of the risk of a leftward shift of the oxygen dissociation curve (Fig. 22.12) before peripheral perfusion has been improved by salt and water administration. This would exaggerate the adverse effects of lowered erythrocyte 2,3 DPG concentration on oxygen delivery. Restoration of circulating volume, lowering of blood sugar, and inhibition of lipolysis by insulin is followed by renal excretion and tissue metabolism of ketoacids (with net hydrogen ion consumption).

When administration of intravenous bicarbonate is necessary, it should be given in isotonic form (1.4%) if possible. The use of hypertonic solutions of bicarbonate (e.g. 8.4%, containing 1 mmol sodium/ml) is limited to the rapid administration of 50–100 mmol boluses in the management of cardiac arrest.

Renal tubular acidoses are treated by oral bicarbonate and/or potassium supplements (Ch. 21).

FURTHER READING

Arieff A I, De Fronzo R A (eds) 1985 Fluid, electrolytes and acid-base disorders, Vol I and II. Churchill Livingstone, Edinburgh. *A detailed treatment of this topic.*

Häussinger D (ed) 1988 pH homeostasis – mechanisms and control. Academic Press, London. *A collection of definitive accounts on pH regulation and the relationship between pH homeostasis and metabolic processes.*

Neurological Disease

23

sequence of development of the symptoms will usually give some idea as to the nature of the underlying pathology. Supplementary history from relatives or witnesses is essential in patients with episodes of impaired consciousness or impairment of higher mental function. The major neurological symptoms which should be covered by the history are listed in Table 23.1; and in each section of this chapter, the typical features of the history are discussed.

PRINCIPLES OF EXAMINATION

Neurological examination can be performed quickly and efficiently if a routine is adhered to (Table 23.2).

Level of consciousness

The neurological examination starts with an assessment of the level of consciousness. It is normal if there is no impairment at all. *Drowsy* patients tend to sleep if undisturbed, but can be woken and are able to hold a conversation and co-operate with the examination. *Stuporose* patients appear drowsy and may be restless, and may respond to shouted commands with groaning or single words and limb movements. In the *comatose* patient, the only response may be to painful stimuli, by withdrawal of the stimulated part or by a non-specific extensor posturing of the limbs, the so-called decerebrate response; in deep coma, there may be no response.

A practical approach to assessing the conscious level is the Glasgow coma scale (Table 23.3), which is increasingly being used. This scale has the advantages that it can be used by both medical and nursing staff and avoids the use of ambiguous terms, such as 'stuporose'.

Examination of the comatose patient

Detailed neurological examination in many patients permits an assessment of the site of the lesion. It is important to differentiate coma due to diffuse cerebral disease (either metabolic or inflammatory), from focal causes, either discrete brain stem lesions or focal cerebral hemisphere lesions associated with raised intracranial pressure

NEUROLOGICAL DIAGNOSIS

HISTORY-TAKING

Diagnosis in many patients with neurological disease depends entirely on the history; in patients with blackouts or headache, for example, there are usually no physical signs. Anatomical localisation of lesions can also often be correctly identified from the history, and the timing and

Table 23.1 Symptom review in neurological diagnosis

• Loss of consciousness	• Speech
• Higher mental functions	• Swallowing
• Headaches	• Limb weakness
• Vision	• Limb numbness and paraesthesiae
• Hearing	• Bladder and bowel control
• Dizziness	
• Unsteadiness	

Table 23.2   Neurological examination

1. Mental state
Level of consciousness
Orientation
Speech
General knowledge
Memory
Retention and recall
Reasoning and judgement
Reading, writing, calculation
Object recognition
Praxis
Perception
Mood and affect

2. Gait and station
Normal gait
Heel-toe walking
Romberg's test

3. Cranial nerves
I: Olfaction
II: Acuity, fields, colour vision, fundi
III, IV, VI: Eye movements,
              nystagmus, pupils
V: Facial and oral sensation.
    Masticatory muscles
VII: Facial muscles, taste
VIII: Hearing, Rinne and Weber tests
IX: Pharyngeal sensation, gag reflex
X: Speech, phonation, palatal
    movement, swallowing
XI: Sternomastoids, trapezii
XII: Tongue

4. Motor system
Posture, involuntary movements
Muscle bulk, fasciculation
Tone
Power
Coordination
Reflexes

5. Sensory system
Light touch, pin-prick, temperature,
vibration and position sense
Two-point discrimination
Stereognosis
Tactile localisation
Inattention

6. General
Bruits
Skull size and shape
Spinal deformity
Pes cavus
Neck rigidity
Skin changes

Table 23.3   Glasgow coma scale

Category	Score
Eye opening	
Spontaneous	4
To speech	3
To pain	2
None	1
Best verbal response	
Orientated	5
Confused	4
Inappropriate	3
Incomprehensible	2
None	1
Best motor response	
Obeying commands	5
Localising	4
Flexing	3
Extending	2
None	1

The scores applied to each category of the grading system are summed to give an overall
value, ranging from 3–14.

and secondary brain stem compression (Table 23.4). In all patients presenting in coma, a history from witnesses is crucial.

The first step in examining a patient in coma is to assess cardiorespiratory function.

When vital functions and the level of coma have been assessed, general examination may provide important clues. A rash may indicate meningococcal septicaemia with meningitis, purpura may indicate a bleeding disorder associated with a cerebral haemorrhage, and signs of portal hypertension raise the possibility of hepatic encephalopathy. The skull and scalp should be examined for head injury.

Neurological examination should include:

1. *Examination for neck stiffness*, indicating meningitis or subarachnoid haemorrhage. However, in deeply unconscious patients this nociceptive reflex may be absent.

2. *Examination of the fundi*, primarily to look for evidence of raised intracranial pressure. Comatose patients frequently have small pupils which should not be dilated with mydriatics. Normal pupillary responses and reflex eye movements indicate that coma is likely to be due to diffuse disease, rather than focal brain stem pathology.

3. *The pupils* are examined for equality of size and reaction to light. Cerebral hemisphere space-occupying lesions may cause herniation of the temporal lobe through the tentorium (coning); this frequently compresses the IIIrd cranial nerve, producing a large unreactive pupil, with downward, outward gaze of one eye and limitation of all reflex movement of the affected eye, except abduction. Pupillary constriction (pinpoint pupils) are often seen in acute pontine lesions and opiate overdose. Metabolic causes of coma tend to cause loss of reflex eye movements, but preservation of pupillary reflexes.

4. *Reflex eye movements* are examined by the doll's head manœuvre or by caloric testing (p. 869). An acute cerebral hemisphere lesion may produce conjugate deviation of the eyes towards the side of the lesion. Lesions within the brain stem may produce a variety of partial or complete gaze palsies and pupillary abnormalities. Lesions in the pons tend to produce conjugate gaze away from the side of the lesion. Pressure from above, arising from cerebral hemisphere disease, causes progressive loss of brain stem function, with gradual loss of pupil reflexes, reflex eye movements and other brain stem reflexes.

5. *Other brain stem reflexes* examined in comatose patients include the corneal reflexes (V), facial grimacing induced by pressure over the supraorbital nerve (V and VII), gag and coughing reflexes (IX and X), the rate, depth and pattern of breathing, and the tidal volume. Most irregular patterns of breathing suggest brain stem pathology. The exception is Cheyne-Stokes breathing, which is now recognised to occur both with brain stem lesions and with diffuse bilateral cerebral hemisphere disease.

6. *Examination of the limbs* in the comatose patient should include observation of any spontaneous movements and, in particular, any asymmetry, indicating a unilateral hemisphere or brain stem lesion. Muscle tone is usually not diagnostically helpful, although in patients with drug overdose or in metabolic causes of coma, the tone is usually flaccid. Tendon reflexes and plantar responses are often of localising value, but may be abnormal, and sometimes asymmetrical, with diffuse cerebral insults such as metabolic causes of coma (Table 23.4).

An attempt can thus be made to differentiate the three main types of lesion causing coma.

With *intrinsic brain stem lesions*, there are focal abnormalities in the brain stem reflexes, often with cranial nerve abnormalities, these signs being present from the time of the first examination and often persisting unchanged. In addition, there will be bilateral pyramidal tract signs in the limbs and there is likely to be an irregular breathing pattern.

In *brain stem compression* by lesions above the tentorium, brain stem signs appear in a progressive way. Early on, there is likely to be either a hemiparesis or asymmetrical bilateral pyramidal signs in the limbs. A unilateral IIIrd cranial nerve palsy may be an isolated early focal brain stem sign, due to compression of the nerve by herniation of the temporal lobe through the tentorium. Because pressure above the tentorium is raised, there may be papilloedema.

In *metabolic causes* of coma, pupillary and eye movement reflexes tend to be normal, although in deep metabolic coma, pupillary responses are preserved and reflex eye movements are lost. Pyramidal signs in the limbs are symmetrical. In overdose, particularly of opiates, breathing tends to be regular, but shallow.

Mental state examination

When it has been established that the conscious level is normal, the examination of the mental state may proceed. Full testing is a lengthy process, which includes tests of cognitive function and sometimes a formal psychiatric assessment (Ch. 11). The broad outlines of the functions forming the mental state are described here, followed by a suggested scheme of testing of cognitive function, the 'mini-mental state' examination, which takes only 5–10 minutes to perform.

Some cognitive functions are clearly localised in the brain, e.g. language and calculation in the dominant hemisphere, and focal impairment provides information of localising value. Other functions, such as memory, are less clearly lateralised, and others, such as reasoning ability, are so complex as to be of little localising value. However, it is usually possible to decide whether there is a focal or a global impairment of cognitive function, this being the diagnostically important conclusion.

Speech

Speech will already have been assessed to some extent during the history. There are three major abnormalities of speech.

Aphasia (dysphasia) is a difficulty with comprehension or expression of language, which results from a lesion of the dominant cerebral hemisphere. In all right-handed people and 90% of left-handed people this is the left hemisphere. In *motor* or *expressive aphasia*, there is no defect of comprehension of the spoken or written word and, through gesture or writing, the patient can demonstrate that he understands what is being said to him. In expressive aphasia, the patient cannot find the right words and has grammatical difficulty. In mild forms, the speech will be hesitant, with pauses due to difficulty in finding particular words (nominal aphasia). In severe cases, the patient may be speechless. Patients with expressive aphasia usually appear frustrated by the defect.

By contrast, in *receptive* or *sensory aphasia*, the patient does not fully comprehend spoken or written language. This results in an inability to understand what the examiner is saying and a failure to monitor his own speech. The speech is usually fluent and there is a tendency to talk in jargon.

Expressive aphasia is produced by lesions of Broca's area in the frontal lobe, and receptive aphasia is produced by lesions more posteriorly, in Wernicke's area in the anterior temporal lobe. In many patients, the lesion produces a *mixed aphasia*.

Dysarthria refers to a difficulty in articulation of speech. Any neuromuscular disorder affecting the control of the

Table 23.4 Causes of coma

Brain stem lesions
Tumour
Abscess
Infarction
Brain stem haemorrhage
Cerebellar haemorrhage
Thiamine deficiency (Wernicke-Korsakoff syndrome)
Brain stem encephalitis

particularly when complicated by hydrocephalus

Cerebral hemisphere lesions with secondary brain stem compression
Extradural haemorrhage
Subdural haemorrhage
Intracerebral haemorrhage
Abscess
Tumour
Large infarct
Cerebral venous sinus thrombosis

Diffuse neurological disease affecting cerebral hemispheres and brain stem
Encephalitis
Meningitis
Subarachnoid haemorrhage
Head injury
Hypertensive encephalopathy
Epilepsy
Encephalopathy in SLE

Metabolic disturbances
Drug overdose
Diabetes – hypoglycaemia
           ketoacidosis
           hyperosmolar coma
Hyponatraemia
Hypercalcaemia
Uraemia
Hepatic failure
Hypothyroidism
Hypoadrenalism
Hypopituitarism
Respiratory failure (CO_2 narcosis)
Severe heart failure
Hyperpyrexia
Hypothermia
Porphyria

Psychogenic coma

muscles involved in articulation may give rise to dysarthria.

Dysphonia refers to a defect in voice production. This may be due to disease directly affecting the vocal cords or ventilatory function.

Orientation and alertness

The patient should be orientated in time, place and person. He should be able to give the day, date, the name of the hospital and his home address. Alertness and attention may be simply tested by asking the patient to count backwards from 30; a time to do this exceeding 30 seconds is abnormal.

General knowledge

General knowledge is tested by asking general questions to which the patient can reasonably be expected to know the answers. However, the patient's general knowledge will depend much on his or her particular interests and previous academic achievements.

Memory

It is important to test both recent and remote memory. Recent memory is particularly affected in disease of the temporal lobes, and can be tested by asking the patient about events in his life over the last few days. Remote memory is tested by asking questions about the patient's childhood, where he used to live, his education, and previous employment. Impairment of remote memory occurs in more severe lesions of the temporal lobes.

Retention and recall

The patient's ability to comprehend new information and to recall it, both immediately and within a few minutes, is tested by asking him to remember a series of digits, being asked first to repeat the digit sequence forwards and then another sequence backwards. This test is supplemented by giving the patient an imaginary name and address and asking him to repeat it immediately and then again after several minutes. An alternative is to read a short story and then test the patient's ability to remember the salient points, both immediately and after an interval of a few minutes. Failure to perform these tests adequately again indicates impairment of temporal lobe function.

Reasoning

The patient should have some *insight* into his condition and the ways in which it affects him. *Judgement* refers to the patient's ability to form an acceptable opinion given a particular set of circumstances. For example, if the patient is asked what he would do if he saw a set of keys lying in the road, and he answers, 'Throw them in the dustbin', this would reasonably be considered to show poor judgement. *Abstraction* is tested by asking the patient the meaning of some proverbs. However, this is closely linked to academic achievement and, in some patients, a better test is to ask about similarities and differences between objects.

Impairment of insight, judgement and abstraction tend to occur together, and indicate disturbance of frontal lobe function.

Calculation

The ability to calculate depends on the integrity of the angular gyrus of the parietal lobe in the dominant hemisphere and is thus frequently disturbed in lesions producing aphasia. *Dyscalculia* – the inability to perform simple calculations – is assessed by asking the patient to serially deduct 7 from 100, noting the time taken and the number of mistakes, and by other simple tests of mathematical ability.

Reading

Comprehension of the written word is also a function of the dominant hemisphere. In the absence of aphasia, the patient is asked to read aloud. He is *dyslexic* if he is unable to read the words correctly or fails to understand what he has read.

Writing

As with calculation and reading, writing is also a function of the dominant hemisphere, particularly the region of the angular gyrus. *Dysgraphia* – the inability to write – is usually associated with aphasia.

Object recognition and agnosia

The inability to recognise objects in the absence of any defect of primary sensation, is termed *agnosia*. To test for *visual agnosia*, the patient is presented with simple objects and asked to name them; failure indicates a lesion of the visual association cortex in the posterior parietal region. With extensive lesions in this area, the patient may be unable to recognise familiar faces (*prosopagnosia*) or familiar places, and be unable to find his way about his own home (*topographagnosia*). Visual agnosia can be tested in the presence of expressive aphasia by asking the patient to match an object against a picture of a similar object. Visual agnosia includes finger agnosia, in which the patient is unable to correctly identify his own fingers and differentiate one from another. This is due to a lesion of the angular gyrus and is often associated with right/left disorientation, agraphia and acalculia (*Gerstmann's syndrome*).

Astereognosis, or tactile agnosia, is an inability to identify a simple object placed in the hand, with the eyes closed; this indicates a contralateral parietal lobe lesion. With severe parietal lobe lesions, the patient may completely ignore and fail to identify a limb or the whole of the contralateral side of the body (*autotophagnosia*). When the lesion involves the frontal, as well as the parietal, lobe, the patient may deny that any problem exists with the contralateral hemiplegic limbs (*anosognosia*).

Agnosia is more easily recognised with lesions of the

non-dominant hemisphere; with lesions in the dominant hemisphere, there is frequently associated aphasia which makes it difficult to detect agnosia.

Praxis

Praxis is the ability to perform a planned motor task and *apraxia* is the inability to do this in the absence of paralysis. Apraxia may be due to a lesion of the parietal lobe or the pre-motor frontal cortex, or to diffuse cortical disease. It is tested by asking the patient to perform simple tasks, such as combing his hair, using a pen or brushing his teeth. Constructional apraxia, which is more common with lesions of the non-dominant hemisphere, is the inability to construct shapes – by drawing or other means – either on request, or when asked to copy a particular design. It is usually tested by asking the patient to copy a drawing of a three-dimensional cube, or by asking him to draw a clock face or bicycle.

Perception

Disorders of perception are common in psychiatric disorders (p. 185), but also occur in organic brain disease. Visual, olfactory and auditory hallucinations are common in temporal lobe epilepsy. It is important to use the terms delusion, illusion and hallucination correctly. A *delusion* is a firmly held false belief. Delusions are common in normal people but tend to be more severe in patients with diffuse cerebral disease. An *illusion* is a false interpretation of a sensory perception. Again, illusions may occur in normal people, but also occur with acute organic brain syndromes. *Hallucinations* are false sensory perceptions which have no external stimulus. Hallucinations occur with temporoparietal lesions, most commonly in temporal lobe epilepsy and with acute organic brain syndromes. Prolonged hallucinations, usually auditory, occurring without impairment of consciousness, are suggestive of a schizo-affective disorder.

Mood

Abnormalities of mood are often obvious from the way in which the patient presents his history. Depression, elation, lability, irritability and anxiety are the main disorders. Many patients will attempt to conceal abnormalities and will need to be questioned directly, sometimes with additional history from relatives. Abnormalities of mood usually indicate psychiatric problems. Excessive lability of mood, however, suggests bilateral frontal disease.

Affect

Affect is the emotional response to a particular situation. A patient with hemiplegia who is euphoric can be said to have an inappropriate affect, suggesting a frontal lesion. It can be difficult to decide whether affect is appropriate or not, particularly in patients with long-standing disease who have come to terms with their disability.

Mini-mental state examination

The mini-mental state examination (MMSE) provides a rapid means of testing cognitive function (Table 23.5). Any abnormality detected using MMSE should prompt a more detailed psychological assessment. The MMSE can be applied to patients who are drowsy or stuporose but, if so, this must be recorded.

Table 23.5 Mini-mental state examination

Test	Max. score	Patient's score
Orientation		
What is the (year) (season) (date) (day) (month)?	5	( )
Where are you (country) (county) (town) (hospital) (ward)?	5	( )
Retention		
Name 3 objects, then ask patient to repeat these. Give 1 point for each correct answer. Then repeat them until patient learns all 3. Count the number of trials and record	3	( )
Calculation and attention		
Serial 7's. 1 point for each correct answer. Stop after 5 answers. If patient cannot, or will not, do this, ask him to spell 'world' backwards. Score 0–5 points	5	( )
Recall		
Ask patient to name the 3 objects learned earlier. Give 1 point for each correct answer	3	( )
'Language'		
Name a pencil and a watch (2 points). Repetition: ask patient to repeat a short sentence (0 or 1 point). 3-stage command: 'Take a piece of paper in your right hand, fold it in half and put it on the floor.' (3 points). Read and obey the following: 'Close your eyes' (0 or 1 point). Ask patient to write a sentence of his own choice. It must contain a subject and verb and make sense (0 or 1 point). Copying: ask patient to copy 2 intersecting pentagons (0 or 1 point)	9	( )
Total score	30	( )

Acute confusional states

Acutely confused patients are, to a variable extent, disorientated; their ability to concentrate and their memory are impaired, they have difficulty following even simple instructions, their attention is poor, and they are often drowsy. Acute confusional states are often associated with delirium, a state characterised by restlessness, agitation, irritability and, sometimes, frightening hallucinations.

Acute confusional states can occur with focal cerebral hemisphere lesions, but are more common with metabolic disturbances, which may eventually result in stupor and coma (Table 23.4), and with abrupt withdrawal of drugs, including barbiturates, alcohol and, occasionally, benzo-diazepines.

Confusion is a feature of dementia and some psychiatric diseases, particularly the psychoses. However, in contrast to other causes of acute confusional states, psychiatric disease and dementia do not cause drowsiness.

GAIT AND STATION

The ability to stand and walk depends on the integrity of many different neurological functions, both motor and sensory. These include:

1. position sense from muscles and joints in the limbs and also in the trunk and neck
2. sensory input from vision and from the labyrinths in the inner ear
3. motor functions, which include upper and lower motor neurones, the basal ganglia and cerebellum and, of course, the muscles and joints themselves.

Much can be learned from observing the gait carefully; certain types of gait disorder are easily recognised and provide immediate information about the causative lesion.

Station refers to the ability of the patient to stand and the posture of the stance. Examples of abnormalities include the stooped stance of a patient with Parkinson's disease, and the wide-based stance of a patient with cerebellar disease. It is relevant to observe how easily the patient is able to stand up, and whether assistance is required and, if so, how much. His ability to walk is then assessed. In patients whose gait appears normal, or only mildly abnormal, two further tests are useful.

Tandem gait. The patient is asked to walk heel-to-toe along a straight line (tandem gait). This is a fairly severe test of balance and coordination and, in the presence of normal power, failure usually indicates an impairment of cerebellar function, of vestibular function, or of postural sensation (sensory ataxia).

Romberg's test. If the tandem gait test is normal, the patient is asked to stand with his feet together and then to close his eyes (Romberg's test). An inability to maintain balance indicates either an impairment of postural sensation, or of vestibular function.

Some abnormalities of gait are easily recognised. For example, in a *spastic gait* the patient walks slowly, with obvious stiffness in the legs and, sometimes, with scissoring due to thigh adductor spasm. A hemiplegic gait is recognised by dragging, weakness and spasticity of one leg.

The patient with a *Parkinsonian gait* has a stooped posture and, when asked to walk, may have difficulty in initiating movement (start hesitation) and tends to take small shuffling steps, which quicken (the festinant gait).

With an *ataxic gait*, the patient is unsteady when standing and usually adopts a broad base; walking appears unsteady, with lurching from side to side, and the gait

resembles that of a drunkard. There may be associated nystagmus.

In a *steppage gait*, resulting from bilateral footdrop (as found for example in a peripheral neuropathy), the patient has to flex the leg at the hip more than usual in order to prevent catching his toes. The gait has the appearance of someone trying to step up and there is usually an associated stamping as each foot hits the ground, particularly when weakness is combined with severe proprioceptive loss.

A *waddling gait* is produced by proximal weakness at the hip girdle. There is an inability to tilt the pelvis normally when swinging each leg through to take the next step, and this is compensated for by exaggerated lateral movements of the trunk, producing a waddling movement.

In an *apraxic* gait, the patient is able to stand but is unable to perform the planned motor function involved in walking. If the patient can walk, the gait is usually small-paced and shuffling.

A *limping gait* is very common, the usual cause being some painful musculoskeletal, rather than neurological, condition affecting the leg.

CRANIAL NERVES

Olfactory nerve

Testing of olfactory function is particularly helpful in certain situations. In patients with frontal lobe tumours, e.g. olfactory groove meningiomas, there may be unilateral anosmia due to direct compression of the nerve. Bilateral anosmia or hyposmia is common following colds and with sinusitis. Impairment of smell is common in heavy smokers. Bilateral anosmia may also be produced by head injuries which damage the nerves as they pass through the cribriform plate; this is usually permanent. Smell is tested in each nostril separately. Test substances include camphor, peppermint, cloves, lavender and other distinctive strong-smelling substances, but not chemical irritants, such as ammonia, which stimulate trigeminal afferents.

Optic nerve

The assessment of optic nerve function includes measurement of visual acuity, colour vision, the visual fields, and examination of the fundi. The pupillary responses are mediated by the IIIrd nerve (p. 866); the optic nerve provides the afferent limb of the light reflex.

Visual acuity

Distant and near vision are examined. Distance vision is assessed using a Snellen chart. The patient is positioned six metres from the chart, and each eye is tested separately. If the patient has glasses, these should be worn. The patient is asked to read the smallest line that he can see, and the acuity is recorded as 6 (which is the numerator and is the maximum distance at which a subject with normal vision can clearly read the type) over the number of the smallest size of print which the patient can see. Normal vision is

6/6 and the largest letters on the chart have the number 60, this being the size which a person with normal vision can read at 60 metres. Since refractive error is common, acuity should be retested, using a pinhole, if abnormal. Near vision is tested using standard test types and, again, it is important to state whether glasses have been used.

Colour vision is dependent upon macular function. Colour desaturation, particularly to red, is the earliest and most sensitive indicator of impaired optic nerve function. Standard charts (Ishihara) for testing colour vision are available and should be used in patients suspected of having any lesion of the retina, optic nerve or optic chiasm, as long as acuity is not severely impaired.

Visual fields

A working knowledge of the neuroanatomy of the visual pathway is essential when examining the visual fields (Fig. 23.1). Light from the temporal half of the visual field is focused on the nasal half of the retina, and light from the nasal half of the visual field on the temporal half of the retina, with inversion of the images. There are no rods or cones over the optic nerve head, producing a blind spot in the visual field situated a few degrees lateral to central vision.

The optic nerve exits from the orbit through the optic foramen and, with the optic nerve from the other side, forms the optic chiasm. The fibres from the temporal halves of each retina pass through the chiasm, without decussating, into the optic tract on the same side. The nasal fibres decussate, the optic tract on each side therefore consisting of fibres from the nasal half of the contralateral retina and the temporal half of the ipsilateral retina. The fibres pass to the lateral geniculate body and thence, via the optic radiation, to the occipital cortex. The fibres concerned with pupillary reflexes pass from the lateral geniculate body to the pretectal nucleus in the mid-brain. The upper and lower fibres of the visual radiation pass through

the parietal and temporal lobe respectively before reaching the occipital cortex. Lesions at different points in the optic pathway produce characteristic visual field defects.

1. Complete destruction of one optic nerve results in blindness in that eye and loss of the direct pupillary light reflex.
2. A midline lesion of the optic chiasm produces a bitemporal hemianopia.
3. Lesions involving the optic chiasm and the optic tracts often produce incongruent field defects, with more marked involvement of one monocular field. Lesions involving the optic radiation or the occipital cortex are usually congruent and symmetrical.
4. An expanding pituitary tumour from below will produce an upper bitemporal quadrantanopia, due to the inversion of the image in the retina.
5. Pressure on the optic chiasm from above, usually due to a suprasellar meningioma, produces a lower bitemporal quadrantanopia.
6. A lesion involving the optic tract will produce a homonymous hemianopia.
7. A lesion in the parietal lobe involving the medial part of the optic radiation will result in a lower homonymous quadrantanopia.
8. A lesion in the temporal lobe involving the lateral fibres of the optic radiation will produce an upper homonymous quadrantanopia.
9. A lesion involving the whole of the optic radiation or the occipital cortex will produce a homonymous hemianopia.
10. A complete lesion of both occipital lobes will produce cortical blindness, but pupillary reflexes will be preserved.

The visual fields are tested by comparing the patient's visual field with that of the examiner. Each eye is tested separately. The peripheral field is tested using a white-headed pin of 5–10 mm diameter. The pin is brought into

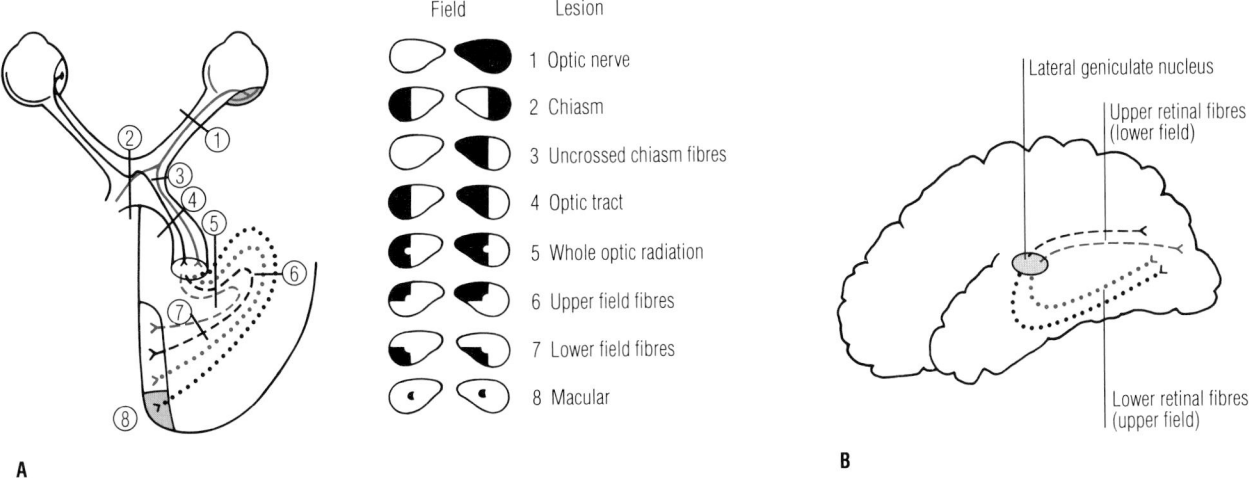

Fig. 23.1 Anatomy of the visual pathway. A. Lesions at points 1–8 produce the visual field defects shown. **B.** The arrangement of the visual radiation is shown in a lateral view. Lesions of the upper and medially situated part of the radiation in the parietal lobe produce a lower quadrantanopia, and lesions of the lower and laterally placed part of the radiation in the temporal lobe produce an upper quadrantanopia.

the visual field at about 45° in each quadrant. Any visual field loss can be mapped out by placing the pin within the area of loss and moving it from this position into the areas of normal vision. In this way, it is possible to detect all quadrantic and hemianopic defects and discrete areas of visual field loss (scotomas). The patient's blind spot, which represents a discrete scotoma, can be mapped out. A red pin is more sensitive for detecting central scotomas in which the only defect may be impairment of colour vision, e.g. as may be the case in optic neuritis.

Visual field defects can be fully documented by using a perimeter for the peripheral fields and a Bjerrum screen for testing the central fields.

Optic fundi

Examination of the optic fundi should include scrutiny of the blood vessels, retina and choroid and the optic discs. The anterior part of the eye can be examined using the 10 + lens on the ophthalmoscope.

Abnormalities of blood vessels

Hypertensive and sclerotic changes are the most commonly seen blood vessel abnormalities. Hypertensive changes are graded thus:

1. *Grade 1*. Arteriolar narrowing.
2. *Grade 2*. Narrowing with arteriovenous nipping where arteries cross veins.
3. *Grade 3*. Changes as for grade 2, together with haemorrhages and/or exudates.
4. *Grade 4*. Changes as for grade 3 with papilloedema.

Sclerotic changes in retinal arterioles are commonly associated with hypertension, but also occur in normotensive people and are increased in diabetes and hyperlipidaemias. The changes are narrowing, tortuosity and an increase in the light reflex (silver wiring).

Arterial emboli. Emboli, usually arising from atheromatous plaques in the carotid artery in the neck at the level of the bifurcation, are occasionally seen. They may be cholesterol emboli, which are highly refractile and often multiple, or platelet emboli which appear white. Small emboli may be asymptomatic, and usually move peripherally fairly rapidly. Larger emboli produce amaurotic attacks affecting part or the whole of vision of that eye.

Central retinal artery occlusion causes complete monocular blindness and is associated with a pale retina with very narrow pale vessels. The blood supply of the macular region is from the choroidal circulation, so this part of the retina has a pinker appearance, sometimes described as a cherry-red spot.

Venous occlusion. Thrombosis of the central retinal vein occurs in polycythaemia rubra vera but may occur spontaneously. Vision may be relatively well preserved; the ophthalmoscopic appearances are venous engorgement and multiple haemorrhages, together with swelling of the optic disc.

Other causes of retinal haemorrhage. Any cause of raised intracranial pressure will produce venous engorgement, which may produce retinal haemorrhages and papilloedema. In subarachnoid haemorrhage, subhyaloid haemorrhages may occur, which are large and well-defined and have a horizontal level in the upright posture. Bleeding disorders may produce retinal haemorrhages.

Abnormalities of the retina and choroid

Pigmentary degeneration of the retina. Retinitis pigmentosa is the most common type of pigmentary degeneration affecting the retina. It is hereditary in the great majority of cases, usually as an autosomal recessive trait although sometimes as an autosomal dominant or sex-linked recessive trait. Ophthalmoscopy shows a lace-like network of thin pigmented lines, sometimes with larger areas of confluent pigmentary change. Similar pigmentary changes may be seen in other conditions, including spinocerebellar degenerations (p. 923), Refsum's disease (p. 943), and mitochondrial cytopathy (p. 951).

Chorioretinitis. Inflammatory disease of the retina and underlying choroid may produce scarring, with pale areas where the retina has been destroyed, together with pigmentary change. Chorioretinitis may be caused by intra-uterine infection with toxoplasmosis or cytomegalovirus; syphilis may produce similar changes.

Optic discs

The normal optic disc has clearly defined margins and a central depression (optic cup) where the arteries and veins enter and leave the eye. In most people, venous pulsations can be seen in the large veins on the optic disc, but, when intracranial pressure rises, these pulsations disappear. The two main abnormalities of the optic disc are papilloedema and optic atrophy.

Papilloedema means oedema of the optic disc, caused either by local haemodynamic changes, raised intracranial pressure or inflammation of the optic disc (Table 23.6). Early changes include hyperaemia of the disc, and venous dilatation with absent venous pulsation. Swelling of the optic disc produces elevation and blurring of the disc margins. Small haemorrhages may appear at the disc margin. With more severe papilloedema, haemorrhages become larger, and the disc becomes further elevated and enlarged, giving rise to an enlarged blind spot in the visual field, usually detectable by confrontation. Folds may appear in the retina, together with white exudates with indistinct margins ('soft' exudates).

Indistinct optic disc margins are often present in hypermetropic people, but should not be confused with papilloedema. Occasionally, hyaline bodies are present on the optic nerve head; these may mimic papilloedema and are known as drusen. The other condition which is sometimes confused with papilloedema is the presence of myelinated nerve fibres spreading from the optic disc onto the surrounding retina.

Optic atrophy may result when papilloedema has been present for a prolonged period, whatever the cause, and it

Table 23.6 Causes of papilloedema

Raised intracranial pressure	Central retinal artery occlusion
Tumour	Occlusive
Abscess	Embolic
Hypertension	**Optic nerve tumours**
Hydrocephalus	Olioma
Venous sinus thrombosis	Meningioma
Meningitis	**Blood disease**
Encephalitis	Severe anaemia
Subarachnoid haemorrhage	Polycythaemia rubra vera
Intracerebral haemorrhage	DIC
CO_2 retention	Thrombocytopenic purpura
Venous obstruction	Leukaemia
Central retinal vein thrombosis	Sickle cell disease
Cavernous sinus thrombosis	**Toxic and deficiency**
Carotico-cavernous fistula (carotid	Methyl alcohol
aneurysm)	Uraemia
Thrombosis or obstruction of SVC	Arsenic
Orbital lesions, e.g. cellulitis, tumour,	B_1 deficiency
thyroid eye disease	B_{12} deficiency
Optic neuritis	**Raised CSF protein**
Isolated lesion	Guillain Barré syndrome
Multiple sclerosis	Spinal cord tumour
Meningitis, tuberculosis, syphilis	
Sarcoidosis	

Table 23.7 Causes of optic atrophy

Optic nerve compression	Tobacco
Pituitary tumour	Quinine
Carotid aneurysm	Lead and arsenic
Glaucoma	Anaemia
Optic nerve tumour	**Secondary to retinal disease**
Sphenoid meningioma	Senile macular degeneration
Olfactory groove meningioma	Retinitis pigmentosa
Optic neuritis	Severe chorioretinitis
Following long-standing	**Secondary to trauma**
papilloedema	Orbital fracture
Central retinal artery occlusion	**Hereditary**
Toxic/metabolic	Lever's optic atrophy
Diabetes	Hereditary ataxias
Methyl alcohol	Spinocerebellar degenerations

may also develop gradually in a number of other disease processes (Table 23.7). The appearance is a pale white optic disc, which is flat and has sharp margins.

IIIrd, IVth and VIth cranial nerves

Clinical anatomy

The *IIIrd nerve* contains motor fibres to the extraocular muscles (excluding lateral rectus and superior oblique), afferent proprioceptive fibres from these muscles, and motor parasympathetic fibres to the pupil which produce constriction.

The motor fibres arise from the IIIrd nerve nucleus in the mid-brain, ventral to the aqueduct. The nerve passes through the tegmentum of the mid-brain and on the medial aspect of the basis pedunculi, where it leaves the brain stem. At this point, it lies between the superior and posterior cerebellar arteries. It then passes forward over the free edge of the tentorium lateral to the posterior clinoid process and enters the lateral wall of the cavernous sinus. The nerve passes anteriorly in the lateral wall of the cavernous sinus to enter the orbit through the superior orbital fissure, where it divides into superior and inferior divisions.

The motor parasympathetic fibres to the pupil arise in the upper part of the oculomotor nucleus (Edinger-Westphal nucleus), pass through the mid-brain and reach the orbit together with the oculomotor motor fibres. Within the orbit, the parasympathetic fibres enter the ciliary ganglion; from here, the postganglionic fibres pass to the ciliary and sphincter pupillae muscles as the short ciliary nerves.

The *IVth nerve*, supplying superior oblique, has its nucleus ventral to the aqueduct at the level of the inferior colliculus. The nerve follows a similar course to the IIIrd nerve; it pierces the dura near the posterior clinoid process, and runs along the lateral wall of the cavernous sinus, entering the orbit through the superior orbital fissure.

The *VIth nerve*, supplying the lateral rectus muscle, arises from the nucleus in the upper pons, ventral to the floor of the fourth ventricle. The fibres pass forwards and downwards to emerge near the midline, in the sulcus between the pons and medulla. The nerve lies on the ventral surface of the pons, and enters the cavernous sinus below the posterior clinoid process. It passes through the sinus and enters the orbit through the superior orbital fissure.

The actions of the extraocular muscles are summarised in Figure 23.2. The oblique muscles are attached to the

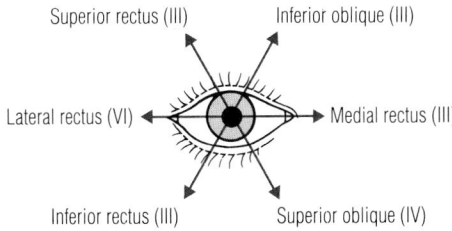

Fig. 23.2 Actions and innervation of the extraocular muscles.

eye behind the equator of the globe. Thus, superior oblique depresses the eye and inferior oblique elevates the eye during adduction. Elevation of the eyelid involves two muscles, the levator muscles supplied by the IIIrd nerve, and Muller's muscle supplied by the cervical sympathetic. Thus, any lesion affecting the superior division of the oculomotor nerve is likely to be associated with ptosis.

Pupillary reflexes

The anatomy of the light and near vision pupillary reflexes are shown in Figure 23.3.

Size. The pupils should be round and regular and equal in size. Mild degrees of inequality (anisocoria) can be normal, but a major difference in the size of the pupils is pathological.

Light reflex. The pupils are first tested to light, with observations of the direct response in the ipsilateral eye and the consensual response in the contralateral eye. Both should respond equally and briskly. Cataracts or corneal opacities will reduce the light stimulus. Degenerative disease of the retina results in a reduced afferent input, as may lesions of the optic nerve, chiasm or optic tracts. Local disease of the eye, such as iridocyclitis, may cause adhesions preventing pupillary constriction. A lesion of

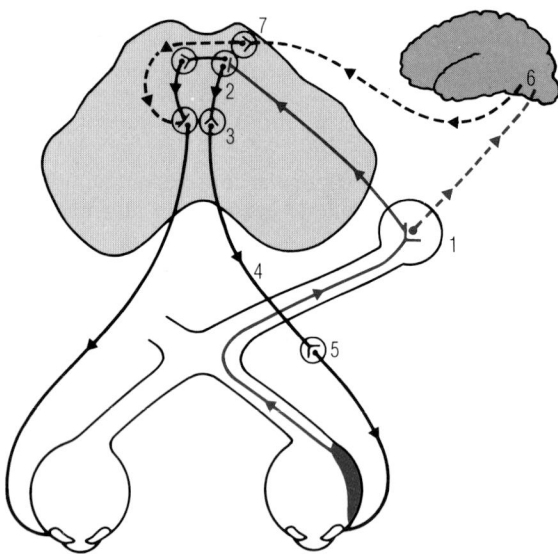

Fig. 23.3 Light and near vision pupillary reflexes. The afferent pathways to the brain stem for the light reflex is shown as a continuous red line and that to the occipital cortex for the near vision reflex is shown as a hatched red line. For the light reflex, fibres from the lateral geniculate nucleus (1) pass to the pretectal nucleus (2) in the midbrain. After synapsing, fibres pass to the ipsilateral and contralateral Edinger-Westphal nucleus (3), which is part of the oculomotor nuclear complex. From here, fibres travel in the IIIrd nerve (4) to the ciliary ganglion (5) and post-ganglionic fibres pass from here to innervate the iris and ciliary muscles. Afferent fibres for the near vision reflex pass to the occipital cortex (6); impulses are then relayed to the nucleus of the superior colliculus (7). From here, there are bilateral connections to the Edinger-Westphal nucleus (3). For clarity, only the contralateral connection is shown on the diagram.

the IIIrd nerve nucleus or IIIrd nerve, or of the ciliary ganglion or short ciliary nerves will also result in an impaired or absent pupillary reflex. By examining the direct and consensual light reflexes in the two eyes, it is possible to determine whether a pupillary abnormality is due to a lesion of the afferent or efferent limb of the reflex.

Near vision reflex. The near vision or convergence reflex is tested by asking the patient to fix his gaze on an object held at a comfortable distance from his eyes, and then to follow the object as it is brought nearer to him. The reflex depends on an intact visual pathway to the visual cortex, and from there to the pretectal area and on to the Edinger-Westphal nucleus. From here, the efferent limb of the reflex is the same as for the light reflex.

The *tonic pupil* (Holmes-Adie syndrome) is a large pupil which has a poor or absent response to light, but does show constriction on convergence. The response to near vision is usually slow, and the pupil then gradually reverts to its previous size. The tonic pupil usually affects one eye initially but may then become bilateral. It may be an isolated abnormality or occur in association with diminished or absent tendon reflexes. The lesion of the tonic pupil is thought to be in the ciliary ganglion, with defective reinnervation such that the majority of regenerated fibres are involved in the convergence reflex only.

The *Argyll-Robertson pupil* is usually associated with neurosyphilis. In contrast to a tonic pupil, the Argyll-Robertson pupil is often small and irregular. The response to light is reduced or absent and the pupil fails to dilate in the dark. The response to near vision is better than the response to light. The lesion producing the Argyll-Robertson pupil is probably immediately rostral to the Edinger-Westphal nucleus, affecting the light reflex but not the fibres serving the near vision reflex (which are located in a more ventral position).

Horner's syndrome is produced by a lesion of the cervical sympathetic fibres. It comprises miosis (whereby the pupil is smaller than the normal contralateral pupil), ptosis, apparent enophthalmos due to the ptosis, and loss of sweating on the ipsilateral side of the face.

The sympathetic fibres which supply the head pass from neurones in the lower brain stem, through the cervical cord and exit in the T1 and, to a lesser extent, C8 anterior spinal roots. They leave these roots via the white rami communicans and enter the cervical sympathetic ganglia. From the cervical ganglia, branches travel with the carotid artery into the head. A lesion affecting any part of this pathway will produce Horner's syndrome.

Examination of eye movements

The range of movement in each eye is assessed and the patient is asked to report any diplopia. In disturbances of conjugate gaze there will be no diplopia, but movement of both eyes will be incomplete in certain directions. Diplopia may be caused by lesions at the level of the nuclei in the brain stem supplying the extraocular muscles or their internuclear connections, or lesions affecting the peripheral nerves or the extraocular muscles themselves. The eye movements are routinely tested by asking the patient to look up, down, and to each side and then asking him to follow the examiner's finger moving laterally and medially, upwards and downwards. The eyes are also observed for nystagmus – an involuntary rhythmic movement of the eyes which may be present at rest or in certain directions of gaze, and which persists when the eyes are still.

Conjugate eye movements

Conjugate movements are both voluntary and reflex in nature. A disturbance of voluntary conjugate movement refers to an inability to gaze in a particular direction on command. A disturbance of reflex conjugate eye movement refers to an inability to follow a moving object presented to a conscious patient who understands the command. Reflex conjugate eye movements may also be tested in unconscious patients, by observing the eyes and moving the head in a horizontal or vertical plane. If the reflex eye movements are intact, this induces movements of the eyes known as *doll's eye movements*.

Destructive or irritative lesions involving supranuclear pathways to the eye movements may produce conjugate deviation of the eyes at rest. An acute destructive lesion in one frontal lobe causes conjugate deviation of the eyes towards the side of the lesion, whereas an irritative lesion leads to conjugate deviation of the eyes away from the side of the lesion. A destructive lesion involving supranuclear fibres below the decussation of the fibres in the upper part of the brain stem leads to conjugate deviation of the eyes away from the side of the lesion. An extensive lesion in the upper mid-brain may involve the supranuclear fibres bilaterally. This leads to severe impairment of involuntary eye movements, but the eyes remain conjugate and there is no diplopia. Reflex eye movements produced by head turning (doll's eye movements) or by vestibular (caloric) stimulation are normal.

Physiology of eye movements

Conjugate gaze is initiated from the paramedian pontine reticular formation, which is situated between the VIth and IVth nerve nuclei. This is thought to have inputs from a number of centres in the visual and frontal cortex, the vestibular system, and the cerebellum. Fibres from the paramedian pontine reticular formation pass to the nuclei controlling the extraocular muscles, the medial longitudinal fasciculus being one of the pathways. Reflex conjugate eye movements when following an object depend on visual perception; thus, visual acuity and all the structures on which this depends must be normal. From the primary visual area, fibres pass anteriorly to the association visual cortical areas in the occipital lobe. From here, corticotectal fibres concerned with upward gaze pass to the tectum in the mid-brain, and corticotegmental fibres concerned with horizontal gaze pass to the paramedian pontine reticular formation. Impairment of upward gaze may occur with lesions involving the corticotectal pathway; the causes include cerebral infarction, multiple sclerosis and, occasionally, a pineal tumour.

Doll's eye movements. The centres controlling eye movements receive a vestibular input which is responsible for the reflex conjugate doll's eye movements. In an unconscious patient, doll's eye movements depend on the vestibular apparatus and its brain stem connections with the centres for conjugate eye movements. The head is turned from side to side and, if intact, the reflex will induce lateral conjugate deviation of the eyes in the direction opposite to the direction of the head movement. Similar eye movements will be induced by flexion and extension of the neck. The absence of doll's eye movements indicates bilateral lesions of the brain stem connections and is usually associated with a very poor prognosis.

Eye movement disorders due to pontine lesions

Lesions in the pons are commonly associated with disorders of eye movements. The common abnormalities include involvement of the VIth nerve or its nucleus. This leads to paralysis of the lateral rectus and, if the lesion is at nuclear level, there may be conjugate gaze paralysis to the ipsilateral side. It is often associated with a facial nerve palsy, due to the proximity of the VIIth nerve nucleus. Lesions of the medial longitudinal fasciculus lead to paralysis of the ipsilateral medial rectus, producing defective adduction of the ipsilateral eye. On gaze to the contralateral side, there may be nystagmus, greater in the abducting eye (ataxic nystagmus). Pontine lesions affecting the medial longitudinal fasciculus may also produce skew deviation, in which one eye is elevated relative to the other eye. This usually leads to tilting of the head to compensate for the dysconjugate position of the eyes.

Paralysis of extraocular muscles

IIIrd nerve palsy leads to outward and, usually, slightly downward deviation of the eye on the affected side. If the pupillary constrictor fibres are also involved in the lesion, there will be dilatation of the pupil (internal ophthalmoplegia). Ptosis is also present.

VIth nerve palsy. A lesion of the VIth nerve produces paralysis of the lateral rectus muscle, leading to inward deviation of the affected eye at rest and an inability to abduct this eye.

IVth nerve palsy is difficult to detect and the changes induced by a complete IVth nerve palsy may be very mild. There is limitation of depression of the affected eye when adducted, and this leads to diplopia, with the false image being below and lateral to the true image. On covering the normal eye, the eye with the IVth nerve palsy deviates downwards and inwards. The head tends to be tilted towards the normal side.

Nystagmus may be congenital or may occur as a result of disturbances of visual acuity, vestibular function or cerebellar function; it may be drug-induced. Nystagmus is discussed in more detail on page 869.

23

Trigeminal nerve

Clinical anatomy

The anatomy of the trigeminal nerve is shown in Figure 23.4. Figure 23.6 shows the cutaneous territories of the divisions of the trigeminal nerve, and Table 23.13 lists the non-cutaneous innervation. The sensory root of the trigeminal nerve passes from the gasserian ganglion to enter the pons at the junction of the pons and the middle cerebellar peduncle. The main sensory nucleus subserves tactile sensation; fibres subserving pain and temperature sensation enter the spinal tract and nucleus, which extends downwards into the upper segments of the cervical spinal cord as low as C4. The fibres entering the spinal nucleus are arranged so that those from around the mouth enter the spinal nucleus in the medulla, and fibres from further out on the face enter the nucleus at progressively lower levels.

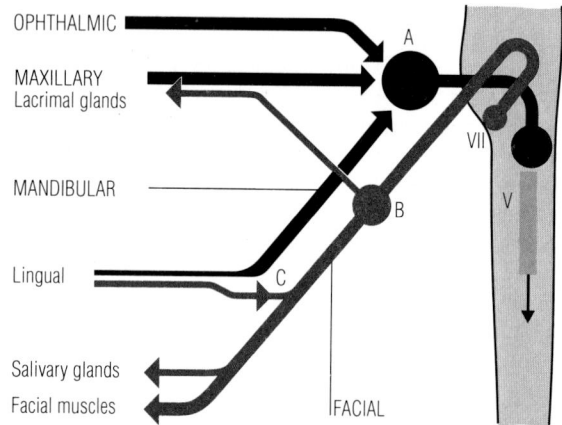

Fig. 23.4 Trigeminal (black) and facial (red) nerve anatomy. (A) Trigeminal (Gasserian) ganglion; (B) geniculate ganglion; (C) chorda tympani; (VII) VIIth nerve motor nucleus. Central connections of taste fibres from the tongue and secretomotor fibres are not shown; (V) main sensory nucleus of trigeminal nerve and spinal tract and nucleus of trigeminal nerve. See text for details.

Examination

The routine examination of the trigeminal nerve consists of assessment of both motor and sensory functions. The masseter and temporalis muscles are palpated with the jaw tightly clenched, and the pterygoids are tested by asking the patient to move the jaw laterally and resist pressure to maintain this posture. Sensation is tested to light touch and pinprick in all three divisions of the nerve, and the corneal reflex should also be tested. The afferent limb of this reflex is the ophthalmic division of the trigeminal nerve, and the efferent limb producing a blink response is the facial nerve. A small wisp of cotton-wool is gently stroked on the cornea. It is important that the patient is asked to look to one side, so that the approaching cotton-

wool is not seen, since the visual threat will produce a blink response. The reflex produces bilateral blinking; thus, if there is an ipsilateral VIIth nerve palsy, a blink will still occur on the contralateral side.

The jaw jerk should normally be present, but a brisk jaw jerk indicates bilateral upper motor neurone lesions.

VIIth cranial nerve

Clinical anatomy

The complex anatomy of the VIIth cranial nerve is shown in Figure 23.4. The functions of the facial nerve tested routinely are the power of the facial muscles and taste. The VIIth nerve has its nucleus in the lower part of the pons, the nerve emerging between the pons and the medulla just medial to the VIIIth nerve in the cerebello-pontine angle. It then enters the internal auditory canal, together with the VIIIth nerve, and passes to the geniculate ganglion. The main part of the facial nerve enters the facial canal, where it gives off the chorda tympani and a branch to the stapedius muscle, before leaving the skull through the stylomastoid foramen. The taste fibres from the anterior two-thirds of the tongue pass through the lingual nerve and then join the facial nerve via the chorda tympani. The cell bodies of these fibres are in the geniculate ganglion and, after joining the facial nerve, they enter the tractus solitarius and synapse with cells of the dorsal visceral grey nucleus. From here, there are projections to the thalamus and hypothalamus.

Examination

Severe facial weakness may be obvious at rest, with loss of the nasolabial fold, sagging of the lower eyelid and drooping of the side of the mouth. Partial weakness may not be obvious at rest. To test the facial muscles, the patient should be asked to close his eyes tightly and resist attempts to open the eyelids. He should be asked to grimace, hold his lips together tightly, and blow out his cheeks.

With an upper motor neurone lesion, the lower facial muscles are much weaker than the upper facial muscles. This is because there are bilateral cortico-bulbar projections to the neurons of the VIIth nerve nucleus supplying the upper facial muscles, while that to the neurones supplying the lower facial muscles is unilateral. In lower motor neurone lesions, all the muscles are usually equally affected. If the nerve is affected distal to the stylomastoid foramen, there is paralysis of the facial muscles but preservation of taste. A lesion of the nerve proximal to the point where the chorda tympani joins it will involve taste on the same side of the anterior two-thirds of the tongue. An injury of the facial nerve in the facial canal proximal to the origin of the nerve to the stapedius muscle will also produce an abnormal loudness of sound in the ear on the same side (hyperacusis). A lesion of the facial nerve proximal to the geniculate ganglion will additionally produce absence of lachrymation on the same side, due to involvement of the greater superficial petrosal nerve.

Finally, damage to the facial nerve in the pons is often associated with a VIth nerve palsy producing weakness of abduction of the eye.

To test taste, four solutions – sweet, salt, sour and bitter – are applied carefully on each side of the tongue.

VIIIth cranial nerve

Clinical anatomy

The VIIIth cranial nerve comprises the cochlear and vestibular nerves. The cochlear nerve passes from the inner ear through the internal auditory canal and enters the upper medulla at the level of the inferior cerebellar peduncle. Within the medulla, the auditory fibres reach the dorsal and ventral cochlear nuclei, where they synapse; fibres from these nuclei cross the midline as the trapezoid body, and enter the lateral lemniscus on the opposite side. They terminate in the inferior colliculus and the further projection is thence to the medial geniculate body and the auditory radiation to the temporal cortex. There are bilateral connections in the cochlear nuclei and at sites above this level, so that unilateral lesions of the temporal cortex and the brain stem do not produce deafness. Unilateral lesions of the cochlear nucleus or the VIIIth nerve will produce unilateral deafness.

Examination of hearing

The ability to hear a watch ticking a few inches from the ear indicates normal hearing; alternatively, the examiner whispers numbers at a slight distance from the ear, with the contralateral ear occluded, and asks the patient to repeat what he has said. In most instances, this assessment of hearing is adequate, but audiometry may be required in some patients.

In *Rinne's test*, air and bone conduction are tested using a 128 cycles per second tuning fork. Air conduction should be better than bone conduction, and this is tested firstly by placing the tuning fork in front of the ear and secondly, by placing the base of the tuning fork on the mastoid process. If the latter is heard more loudly than the former, it indicates a conductive deafness due to disease of the middle ear. In nerve deafness, both air and bone conduction are diminished compared with the other side, but air conduction should still be better than bone conduction.

In *Weber's test*, the tuning fork is placed on the middle of the forehead and the patient is asked whether the sound is heard in the middle or off to one side. In conductive deafness, the sound is lateralised towards the affected side, whereas, in disease of the cochlea or nerve deafness, the sound is lateralised towards the unaffected side.

Vestibular division

The vestibular division of the nerve carries fibres from the vestibular apparatus, comprising the saccule, utricle and three semicircular canals. The cell bodies of these fibres lie within the internal auditory meatus, and the centrally directed axons of the cell bodies pass to the upper medulla, together with the auditory division of the eighth nerve, and then pass to the flocculo-nodular lobe of the cerebellum and the four vestibular nuclei. All four vestibular nuclei have connections with the cerebellum and with the medial longitudinal fasciculus, by which they are connected with the IIIrd, IVth and VIth cranial nerves. The cortical projections from the vestibular nuclei are diffuse and poorly understood.

Vertigo

The major symptom of vestibular disease is vertigo. This can be defined as a false sense of rotary movement, either of the patient himself or the world surrounding him. It is associated with sympathetic overactivity, producing nausea, vomiting, tachycardia and, sometimes, diarrhoea. When it is severe, balance will be impaired and the patient will be unable to walk (p. 881).

Nystagmus

Nystagmus is a rhythmical, involuntary, oscillatory movement of the eyes, which may be present in any direction of gaze. It may be produced by lesions affecting the labyrinth in the ear, the central vestibular connections in the brain stem (it is a very common sign in a whole range of diseases affecting the brain stem), and the cerebellum or its connections in the brain stem. In addition, it may be drug-induced (e.g. by anticonvulsants such as phenytoin), it may be caused by lifelong, very poor visual acuity (amblyopic nystagmus) or it may, occasionally, be a congenital abnormality. The oscillatory movement of nystagmus usually consists of a rapid jerking component, followed by a slower movement in the opposite direction. The direction of nystagmus may be horizontal, vertical or rotatory. Vertical and rotatory nystagmus are always central in origin, while horizontal nystagmus may be peripheral or central in origin. Nystagmus of peripheral origin is often associated with vertigo, whereas nystagmus due to central lesions is usually present without this symptom.

Tests of vestibular function

Vertigo is often accompanied by nystagmus, due to an abnormal stimulus arising in one labyrinth or to acute loss of function in one labyrinth. The slow phase of the nystagmus is induced by vestibular stimulation; it is in the direction of the movement of the endolymph and has a fast phase of recovery. Vestibular nystagmus is increased on turning the head or the eyes in the direction of the fast phase. Vestibular nystagmus can be induced either by sudden head movements (of which the most reliable technique is the use of a rotating chair), or by *caloric testing*, which is simpler to perform. The labyrinth is stimulated by irrigating each external auditory meatus with water, first at 30°C and then at 44°C. For most purposes, only the cold water test is necessary. The test is performed with the patient lying on his back with the head held flexed to about 30° above the horizontal. Nystagmus is induced by the cold water and normally persists for about two minutes. The response is absent if there is total destruction of the vestibular apparatus or vestibular division of the VIIIth nerve; less severe degrees of damage produce impairment, rather than absence, of the response. If the vestibular lesion is irritative and nystagmus is already present, it will increase with caloric testing.

IXth cranial nerve

Of the many functions of the glossopharyngeal nerve, sensation of the posterior third of the tongue and the pharyngeal wall is the only one tested routinely. As well as supplying sensation to this area, the nerve also supplies motor fibres to the stylopharyngeus muscle, secretor-motor fibres to the parotid gland, and taste to the posterior third of the tongue. The nerve passes between the internal jugular vein and the internal carotid artery, enters the skull through the jugular foramen and joins the medulla between the inferior olive and the inferior cerebellar peduncle.

Light touch of the posterior third of the tongue and the pharyngeal wall can be tested using an orange stick. All but the lightest stimuli in this area will produce a gag reflex. This consists of elevation of the palate, retraction of the tongue and contraction of the pharyngeal muscles. The afferent limb of this reflex is the glossopharyngeal nerve, and the efferent limb is the vagus nerve. The gag reflex is more likely to be absent with lesions of the glossopharyngeal nerve than of the vagus.

Xth cranial nerve

As well as supplying general visceral efferent preganglionic fibres to the thoracic and abdominal viscera and visceral afferents, the vagus nerve supplies motor fibres to the intrinsic muscles of the larynx, the cricothyroid muscle and the pharyngeal musculature; it also supplies sensation to the pharyngeal wall, the epiglottis, the base of the tongue and the larynx, and a small sensory branch to the external auditory meatus.

The nerve rises from the dorsal nucleus and the nucleus ambiguus in the medulla. It exits from the medulla between the inferior olive and the restiform body, passes through the jugular foramen, and then enters the carotid sheath and passes down through the neck and into the thorax. The recurrent laryngeal nerve winds around the subclavian artery on the right side, before ascending between the oesophagus and the trachea to enter the larynx. On the left, the recurrent laryngeal nerve winds around the arch of the aorta and ascends to the larynx.

Examination

Articulation of speech, the ability to phonate, palatal movement and swallowing are the principal clinical tests of vagal function.

Dysarthria may occur with impairment of vagal function, but may also occur in edentulous people or those with poorly fitted dentures. Other causes include facial weak-

ness, weakness of the tongue, or impaired coordination of movement due to a pyramidal, extrapyramidal, or cerebellar defect. Some causes of dysarthria produce characteristic speech abnormalities:

1. Edentulous people have difficulty in pronouncing the consonants 's', 'th' and 't'.
2. Patients with a VIIth nerve palsy have particular difficulty with lip movements and, thus, most difficulty in pronouncing the consonants 'b' and 'p'.
3. Weakness of the tongue leads to difficulty in the pronunciation of the consonants 'd' and 't'.
4. Palatal paralysis causes a nasal quality to the voice, and difficulty in pronouncing the consonants 'k', 'q' and 'ch'. This is more marked if the paralysis is bilateral.
5. Cerebellar lesions produce so-called scanning speech, which has an interrupted quality.
6. Bilateral upper motor neurone lesions induce speech which is slow, spastic and sometimes grunting.
7. Extrapyramidal disease causes dysarthria which is slurring and is often associated with dysphonia. The speech may peter out in mid-sentence and there may be difficulty in initiating speech.

Soft palate. Movement of the soft palate is tested by asking the patient to say 'ah'. This produces palatal elevation and the uvula should remain in the midline as the palate rises. A palatal paralysis on one side will produce deviation of the uvula towards the normal side.

Laryngeal function is tested by listening to the voice. This may be hoarse or husky and of low volume. The ability to sing is lost in either unilateral or bilateral vocal cord paralysis.

Swallowing is tested by asking the patient to drink some water. Regurgitation of liquid through the nose indicates palatal weakness and the patient with dysphagia may cough as fluid spills into the trachea.

XIth cranial nerve

The XIth cranial nerve supplies the sternomastoid and trapezius muscles. The motor cells lie in the upper five cervical segments, the nerve passing upwards through the foramen magnum and into the posterior fossa, where it joins the bulbar accessory nerve which is part of the vagus nerve. Together, they leave the skull through the jugular foramen with the glossopharyngeal and vagus nerves. The spinal accessory fibres then descend in the neck to supply the sternomastoid and trapezius muscles. The sternomastoid muscles contract together to flex the neck, and each one acts to turn the head towards the opposite side. The patient's ability to turn the head against resistance is tested and the sternomastoid can be both seen and palpated. The trapezius is tested by asking the patient to shrug his shoulders against resistance.

XIIth cranial nerve

The hypoglossal nucleus lies in the dorsal part of the medulla. The nerve leaves the medulla between the pyramid and the inferior olive, and passes out of the posterior fossa through the anterior condylar foramen. It then passes anteriorly through the neck and reaches the tongue.

To test the tongue, the patient is first asked to open his mouth and the tongue is examined lying at rest in the floor of the mouth. The bulk of the tongue is assessed. Wasting and fasciculation indicate a lower motor neurone lesion. Tremor in the tongue can be difficult to distinguish from fasciculation. Protrusion of the tongue should be in the midline. A weakness on one side will lead to the tongue being protruded towards the weak side. Lower motor neurone lesions produce ipsilateral wasting of the tongue with weakness. Only occasionally, with an acute severe upper motor neurone lesion, there is deviation to the opposite side.

THE MOTOR SYSTEM

The motor unit – consisting of an anterior horn cell or motor neurone of a cranial nucleus, the peripheral axon and the muscle it supplies – is influenced by activity in the cortex, via the corticospinal tracts, the cerebellum, the basal ganglia, the vestibular system and afferent information, largely postural sensation. The routine examination of the motor system allows the identification of dysfunction of one or more of these centres influencing movement.

Motor system lesions

Muscle disease

Disease of the muscles themselves produces weakness. In many acquired muscle diseases, weakness is mainly in the large proximal hip and shoulder girdle muscles, and is often accompanied by wasting. Tendon reflexes are preserved and plantar responses are flexor. Muscle tone is reduced, in proportion to the degree of muscular wasting and weakness.

Lower motor neurone lesions

Lesions of the anterior horn cell or the lower motor neurone at any point will lead to denervation of the muscle supplied. This produces muscle wasting, fasciculation, a reduction in muscle tone and depressed or absent tendon reflexes.

Cortex and corticospinal (pyramidal) tract lesions

Lesions of the cortex or corticospinal tract lead to an increase in tone without muscle wasting, except after long periods, as a result of disuse. There is no fasciculation. The distribution of weakness with pyramidal lesions is characteristic. In the upper limbs, the flexor muscles remain stronger than the extensors and, in the leg, the extensors remain stronger than the flexors. The tendon reflexes are brisk and the plantar response is extensor.

Cerebellum

Cerebellar disease produces incoordination. There is often a tremor which develops on action, and this may involve the trunk as well as the limbs. Head tremor is called *titubation*. Speech may be involved, typically producing a scanning dysarthria. Muscle tone is normal, or sometimes reduced, and reflexes may be sluggish. Cerebellar lesions do not lead to weakness, though incoordination may cause disabling loss of function (p. 923).

Basal ganglia

The term *extrapyramidal disease* is loosely used to refer to disease of the basal ganglia; this causes a number of motor abnormalities, including a rest tremor (which often disappears or is reduced with purposeful movement), and other involuntary movements including chorea, athetosis, dystonia and ballismus. Basal ganglia lesions may also lead to akinesia (poverty of movement), difficulty in initiating movements, and rigidity in the muscles, with a characteristic irregular increase in tone, producing 'cogwheeling' (p. 914). The tendon reflexes in extrapyramidal disease are usually normal.

Examination of the motor system

The motor system is examined in the following order.

1. *Posture and involuntary movements*

Inspection of the patient may reveal a number of abnormalities of posture which are helpful in diagnosis. For example, the patient with a hemiplegia whose affected arm is held flexed, or the patient with Parkinson's disease with mask-like facies and a flexed posture of the trunk. The opportunity is also taken to observe the patient for involuntary movements at rest. These are common in extrapyramidal disease.

2. *Muscle bulk*

The bulk of the muscles in the limbs and on the trunk is assessed. Wasted muscles should be carefully examined for fasciculation.

3. *Muscle tone*

With complete relaxation, there should be little resistance to passive movement of limbs. With pyramidal tract lesions, there is a spastic increase in tone, which is usually a constant resistance to movement. However, with rapid passive movement the clasp-knife phenomenon may be elicited, in which there is an increase in tone followed by a sudden decrease. Sudden passive movement about a joint may elicit clonus, which reflects a disinhibited stretch reflex. This is most easily obtained at the ankle in the calf muscles, though it may be present in any spastic muscle group. In extrapyramidal disease, the increase in tone is intermittent and feels like a ratchet (cogwheel rigidity). Tone may be reduced in a severe neuropathy or myopathy leading to marked muscle wasting, and also, occasionally, in cerebellar disease.

Neurological Disease

23

4. Power

Power should be tested with attention to the segmental innervation of the muscles being tested. It is usual to do this in the order set out in Table 23.8. Those shown in bold type are the movements routinely tested. Power of trunk flexion and extension should be tested as well as muscles in the limbs.

It is useful to grade power in each muscle group. A number of scales have been suggested. In the United Kingdom, the most widely used scale is that of the Medical Research Council:

Table 23.8 Innervation of muscle groups*

Muscle/muscle group	Segmental/nerve innervation	
Neck flexors	C1–6	
Neck extensors	C1–T1	
Diaphragm	C3, 4, 5	
Rhomboid	C4, 5	
Serratus anterior	C4, 5, 6	
Supraspinatus	C4, 5, 6	
Infraspinatus	C4, 5, 6	
Pectoralis major	C5, 6, 7, 8, T1	
Latissimus dorsi	C6, 7, 8	
Deltoid	C5, 6	
Biceps/brachialis	C5, 6	
Triceps	C6, 7, 8	Radial
Brachioradialis	C5, 6	Radial
Supinator	C5, 6, 7	Radial
Pronator teres	C6, 7	Median
Wrist extensors	C5, 6, 7, 8	Radial
Wrist flexors – carpi radialis	C6, 7	Median
carpi ulnaris	C7, 8, T1	Ulnar
Finger extensors	C6, 7, 8	Radial
Finger flexors	C7, 8, T1	Median
Extensor pollicis longus and brevis	C7, 8	Radial
Abductor pollicis brevis	C8, T1	Median
Abductor pollicis longus	C7, 8	Radial
Opponens pollicis	C8, T1	Median
Interossei	C8, T1	Ulnar
Hypothenar muscles	C8, T1	Ulnar
Upper abdominal	T6–9	
Lower abdominal	T10–L1	
Iliopsoas	L1, 2, 3	
Adductors of hip	L2, 3, 4	
Abductors of hip	L4, 5, S1	
Extensors of hip	L5, S1, 2	
Knee flexion	L4, 5, S1, 2	
Knee extension	L2, 3, 4	
Dorsiflexion of foot	L4, 5	
Plantarflexion of foot	S1, 2	
Toe extension	L5, S1	
Extensor hallucis longus	L5	
Extensor digitorum brevis	S1	
Toe flexion	S1, 2	
Inversion of foot	L4, 5	
Eversion of foot	L5, S1	

* Those shown in bold type are those routinely tested

Grade 0 – no movement at all
Grade 1 – flicker of movement
Grade 2 – movement with gravity eliminated
Grade 3 – movement against gravity
Grade 4 – movement against resistance. This covers a wide range of power and is usually subdivided in grades 4−, 4 and 4+.
Grade 5 – normal power.

5. Co-ordination

Tests of co-ordination are of little value if marked weakness is present. In the upper limbs, the finger-nose test assesses the presence of an action tremor, and co-ordination is further tested by rapid repetitive movements, such as tapping the back of one hand with the other, and fine finger movements, such as touching each finger in turn with the thumb of the same hand. Physiological tremor is a fine tremor of the outstretched hands and fingers which does not impair coordination to any significant degree. Inco-ordination due to an action tremor on finger-nose testing is termed *past-pointing* or *dysmetria*, and is seen in cerebellar disease. Impairment of rapid repetitive movements is *dys-diadochokinesis*. Further tests of co-ordination in the upper limbs are writing and use of a knife and fork. In the legs, the heel-shin test is the equivalent of the finger-nose test, and foot-tapping on the examiner's hand is a test of rapid repetitive movement.

6. Reflexes

The main reflexes tested are listed in Table 23.9. In routine practice, it is usually necessary only to test the jaw jerk, the tendon reflexes, the plantar reflexes and the abdominal reflexes. The reflexes may be absent in peripheral neuropathy. They may be reduced in cerebellar disease or, in the case of a corticospinal tract lesion, be increased and

Table 23.9 Segmental reflex levels

Reflex	Level
Glabellar	Corticopontine
Snout	Corticopontine
Sucking	Frontal
Palmomental	Frontal
Grasp	Frontal
Jaw	Pons
Biceps	C5, 6
Supinator	C5, 6
Triceps	C7, 8
Finger	C7, 8, T1
Abdominal – upper	T9, 10
lower	T11, 12
Knee	L2, 3, 4
Ankle	S1
Plantar	Corticospinal tract (afferent L5, S1)
Cremasteric	L1, 2
Anal	S3, 4, 5

872

Table 23.10 Motor system examination

Deficit	Muscle bulk	Fascicula-tion	Tremor	Tone	Power	Coordination	Reflexes	Plantars	Gait
Lower motor neurone (including anterior horn cell)	Reduced	Usually	—	Reduced	Reduced	Impaired with severe weakness	Reduced or absent	Flexor	Steppage
Upper motor	Normal	—	—	Increased (spastic)	Usually reduced	Sometimes impaired	Increased	Extensor	Spastic or hemiplegic
Extrapyramidal	Normal	—	+ (At rest)	Increased (cogwheel)	Normal	Impaired (slow)	Normal	Flexor	Stooped hypokinetic
Cerebellar	Normal	—	+ (On action)	Normal or reduced	Normal	Impaired	Normal or reduced	Flexor	Ataxic
Myopathy	Wasting proximally	—	—	Reduced	Proximal weakness	Impaired in proportion to weakness	Normal or reduced	Flexor	Waddling

accompanied by an extensor plantar response.

The *abdominal reflexes* may be absent with a cortico-spinal tract lesion. They are otherwise usually present in the young, but may disappear with age and obesity.

The *glabellar reflex* is performed by tapping the forehead between the eyebrows with a finger, from behind the patient so that the finger cannot be seen. This is positive if there is persistent closing of the eyes, the reflex indicating damage of the frontopontine pathways to the facial nerve nucleus. It is an early sign in Parkinson's disease and it is also seen in dementia, with cerebral atrophy and with frontal lobe tumours.

The *snout reflex* is elicited by tapping the nose and is positive if this induces excessive grimacing of the face. Like the glabellar reflex, it indicates frontal lobe disease. The *sucking reflex* is also a frontal lobe sign. It is positive when stroking of the lip produces pouting and sucking movements of the lips. It is a normal reflex in young babies but usually disappears within the first 18 months of life. It is seen with diffuse lesions affecting the frontal lobes. The *chewing reflex* also indicates diffuse frontal disease. A tongue depressor is placed in the mouth, and this provokes reflex chewing movements. The *grasp reflex* also indicates frontal lobe disease. The patient's palm is stroked and this elicits reflex grasping which becomes stronger if attempts to remove the fingers from the grasp are made. Sometimes stroking of the dorsum of the patient's fingers of the same hand will inhibit the reflex and allow release of the examiner's fingers from the grasp. These reflexes, indicating frontal lobe damage, are collectively known as the *primitive reflexes*.

Table 23.10 summarises the main findings on examination of the motor system with various types of neurological deficit.

SENSORY SYSTEM

Primary sensations

The primary sensations tested are light touch, pin-prick, temperature, vibration and joint position sense. A working knowledge of peripheral nerve and dermatomal anatomy is essential (Fig. 23.5). Light touch is tested with a wisp of cotton-wool; pin-prick with a disposable pin, not a hypodermic needle. Temperature sensation is tested with tubes filled with hot or cold water, vibration with a 128 cycles per second tuning fork and joint position should be tested initially in the distal interphalangeal joints of the fingers and toes.

Body charts are useful to record the sensory abnormalities.

Sensory system lesions

Sensory tract lesions

Lesions of the spinal cord and lesions rostral to this may affect the sensory tracts in a differential way. For example, in cervical spinal cord compression from a prolapsed disc, it is common to find that loss of postural and vibration sense (dorsal columns) is more marked than pin-prick and temperature sensation, whereas, with an intramedullary lesion of the spinal cord involving decussating spinothalamic tract fibres, there will be a dissociated impairment of pain and temperature at the level of the lesion.

Cortical sensation

More complex types of sensory disturbance occur with lesions affecting the parietal lobe.

Two-point discrimination, the ability to detect two separate stimuli closely applied on the finger, is normally 3–5 mm on the finger pulps. Parietal lesions impair discrimination. Sensory extinction of one of a pair of simultaneously applied stimuli on each side of the body is also a feature of parietal lobe lesions. The patient is asked to close his eyes, and the examiner then touches one side of the body with a pin and asks the patient to report on which side the stimulus was felt. The patient with a parietal lobe lesion will be able to correctly identify a single right-sided or left-sided stimulus, but, with paired stimuli, will only report feeling the pin on the side contralateral to the normal parietal lobe.

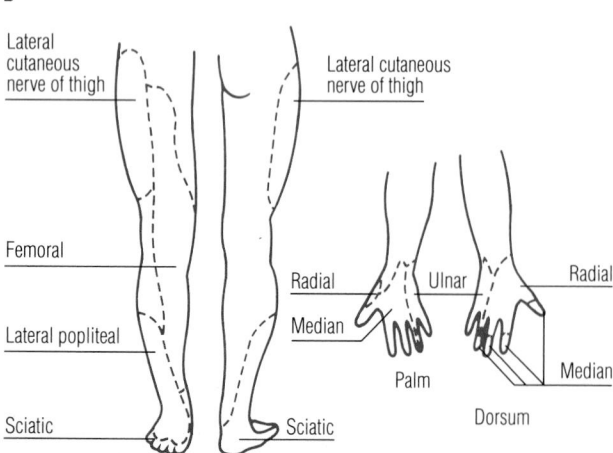

Fig. 23.5 Peripheral nerve and dermatomal anatomy. A. Dermatomal fields. **B.** Sensory territories of selected peripheral nerves of clinical importance.

Graphaesthesia is the ability to identify figures or letters drawn on the palm of the hand with an orange stick, with the eyes closed. This ability may be lost in the hand contralateral to a parietal lobe lesion.

Stereognosis is the ability to manipulate objects within the hand and correctly identify them. Coins are usually used for this purpose. A contralateral parietal lobe lesion may lead to astereognosis.

Tactile localisation refers to the ability to identify the part of the body touched briefly by the examiner. The patient is asked to localise the point touched by the examiner by placing his own finger on the same spot. Again, this is impaired with a contralateral parietal lobe lesion.

Identification of body parts is another function which is impaired with a parietal lobe lesion. Such a patient is unable to correctly identify his different fingers and show them to the examiner. With severe lesions, this agnosia of parts of the body may lead to denial of the existence of part of the body or even the whole of one side of the body. Some patterns of sensory deficit are included in Table 23.11.

LESIONS OF THE LOBES OF THE BRAIN

Localised lesions of the different lobes of the brain produce readily recognisable clinical syndromes. The lesions most often producing focal deficits are tumours and areas of infarction.

Frontal lobe

Lesions of the frontal lobe commonly produce a contralateral hemiparesis due to involvement of the motor area and upper part of the corticospinal tract. However, a hemiparesis is not invariable with frontal lobe lesions. Involvement of Broca's area will produce an expressive aphasia. Mental changes are common with frontal lobe lesions. There is often some degree of intellectual impairment, consisting of poor attention span, some loss of retention and recall, impairment of judgement and loss of insight. Mood changes are prominent, with periods of euphoria or depression. The affect is typically fatuous or frivolous, and behaviour may become disinhibited; these effects together may lead to considerable social disruption. Bladder and bowel control may be lost, leading to incontinence, sometimes with an inappropriate lack of concern. Fits are common with frontal lobe lesions.

Parietal lobe

Abnormalities of cortical sensation are prominent (see above). Impairment of tasks involving visuospatial skills and apraxia is common. Topographagnosia refers to the difficulty experienced by patients, particularly those with non-dominant parietal lobe lesions, in finding their way in familiar places. Prosopagnosia refers to the inability to recognise familiar faces. Apraxia leads to serious practical problems, such as an inability to dress and perform other simple tasks, for example eating and shaving. Involvement of the visual radiation produces a lower homonymous quadrantanopia.

Table 23.11   Common patterns of neurological deficit

- **Muscle disease**
  Usually proximal wasting and weakness
  Reduced or absent reflexes if wasting severe
  Plantars flexor. No sensory deficit
  No bladder or bowel involvement

- **Peripheral nerve**
  Mononeuritis: motor (LMN) and/or sensory loss in distribution of a single peripheral nerve

  Mononeuritis multiplex: asymmetrical, patchy motor and/or sensory deficit attributable to multiple peripheral nerve lesions

  Polyneuropathy: symmetrical motor (LMN) and/or sensory deficit most marked distally. Usually legs more affected than arms. Reflexes variably absent, depending on type and extent of neuropathy

- **Roots**
  Motor (LMN) and/or sensory loss in a root distribution
  Tendon reflex absent if it affects appropriate root

- **Cauda equina**
  Multiple lumbosacral root lesions. Often asymmetrical
  Bladder and bowel involvement common
  Absent reflexes at affected root levels

- **Motor neurone disease**
  Combination of LMN and UMN signs, widespread wasting, fasciculation and weakness, with brisk reflexes in wasted muscles
  Affects limbs and cranial nerve innervated muscles
  Fasciculation of tongue an important diagnostic sign
  Plantars often extensor

- **Spinal cord**
  May be root signs at level of lesion
  UMN (pyramidal tract) weakness below level of lesion
  Extensor plantars and brisk reflexes below lesion
  Abdominal reflexes reduced or absent
  May be sensory level on trunk – this may be at or below the level of the lesion
  Sensory loss in limbs may be of dorsal column (DC) or spinothalamic (ST) type, or affect all modalities
  Intrinsic cord lesions more likely to cause ST loss
  Compressive cord lesions more likely to cause DC loss
  Bladder and bowel involvement very common and may be the major early symptom.

- **Brain stem**
  Cranial nerve lesions at the level of the brain stem lesion
  UMN signs in brain stem below level of lesion, and in limbs
  Limb signs often bilateral
  Sensory impairment variable – often contralateral ST loss
  Bulbar (medulla) involvement common – dysarthria, dysphagia, impaired breathing
  Variable bladder and bowel involvement
  Cerebellar signs very common
  Impairment of consciousness common with acute lesions, unless ventrally placed
  Mass lesions may be associated with hydrocephalus due to aqueduct obstruction

- **Cerebellum**
  Ataxia of trunk with midline lesions
  Ipsilateral ataxia of limbs and nystagmus with cerebellar hemisphere lesions

- **Extrapyramidal**
  Akinesia
  Abnormal posture
  Rest tremor
  Cogwheel rigidity

- **Cerebral hemisphere**
  Hemiparesis, dysphasia, sensory loss, visual loss (hemi- or quadrantanopia) and other specific features, depending on lobe affected
  May be raised intracranial pressure, sometimes with false localising signs (e.g. IIIrd nerve palsy)

- **Diffuse cerebral**
  Dementia, with or without physical signs, depending on cause

- **Expanding pituitary lesions**
  Bitemporal visual field loss, usually asymmetrical
  Hypopituitarism – usually partial
  Sometimes optic atrophy
  Sometimes ocular movement palsies

Temporal lobe

A lesion involving Wernicke's area, which lies in the anterior part of the temporal lobe, produces a receptive aphasia. In addition, temporal lobe lesions produce memory impairment. Involvement of the visual radiation leads to an upper homonymous quadrantanopia.

Occipital lobe

A lesion involving the visual cortex will produce a hemianopic visual field defect. Lesions more anterior in the occipital lobe, in the visual association areas, may lead to visual agnosia and agnosia for colours. Fits are com-monest with frontal and temporal lobe lesions, less common with parietal lesions, and least common with occipital lesions.

HEADACHE

Headache is one of the commonest symptoms in medicine (Table 23.12). It usually does not indicate serious intra-cranial disease and it frequently accompanies systemic ill-nesses as a non-specific symptom. In the great majority of patients presenting with headache, there are no abnormal

Table 23.12　Causes of headache

Tension headache	**Post-ictal headache**
Without any demonstrable underlying structural abnormality	**Post-concussional headache**
Headache associated with cervical spine disease	**Diseases of the skull and sinuses**
	Sinusitis
Diseases affecting blood vessels	Fractures
Intracranial	Mastoiditis
Intracerebral haemorrhage	Paget's disease
Cerebral thrombosis	Tumours of bone
Cerebral embolism	**Ear disease**
Berry aneurysm	Acute otitis media
Arteriovenous malformation	Chronic suppurative otitis media
Cortical thrombophlebitis	**Diseases of the eyes and orbits**
Hypertensive encephalopathy	Glaucoma
Extracranial	Iritis
Migraine	Orbital tumour
Giant cell arteritis	**Toxic and metabolic causes**
Raised intracranial pressure	Infections with fever
Tumours	Hypercapnia
Abscess	Hypoxia
Encephalitis	Hypoglycaemia
Hydrocephalus	Alcoholic hangover
Benign intracranial hypertension	**Haematological disease**
Pituitary tumours	Anaemia
Acute trauma with oedema	Polycythaemia
Subdural haematoma	**Coital cephalgia**
Meningeal irritation	**Psychogenic headache**
Meningitis	
Subarachnoid haemorrhage	

physical signs, so that the diagnosis depends entirely upon an accurate history.

Aetiology

A number of intracranial and extracranial structures may give rise to headache. It may be due to referred pain from the muscles and joints of the cervical spine, and disease of the sinuses, temporomandibular joints, teeth, ears and eyes may all produce headache, rather than local pain, and may on occasions cause diagnostic difficulties. Raised and reduced intracranial pressure can both cause headache. Intracerebral arteries innervated by the trigeminal nerve are sensitive to stretch and pressure, and the leptomeninges are also very sensitive to distortion and inflammation. Subarachnoid haemorrhage and meningitis usually produce severe headache. Spasm, dilatation or inflammation of branches of the external carotid artery may lead to headache. A number of metabolic disturbances such as hypoglycaemia and hypercapnia are associated with headache; in these, the mechanisms of pain are largely unknown.

Taking a history

When taking a history of headache, a structured approach along the following lines is suggested:

1. When did the headaches start?
2. How often do the headaches occur? Are they continuous or episodic?
3. How long does each headache last?
4. How severe is the headache and how does it affect daily activities including work and sleep?
5. Where is the headache felt? Is it localised or generalised?
6. Are there associated symptoms, particularly any visual or gastrointestinal symptoms?
7. What has been the effect of treatment already tried?

TENSION HEADACHES AND HEADACHES ASSOCIATED WITH CERVICAL ARTHRITIS

Tension headaches

Tension headaches are by far the commonest type of headache. Pain is usually described as continuous, occurring every day with a tendency to worsen during the day. They rarely disturb sleep, and patients are usually able to continue their activities. There are no specific associated symptoms and analgesics have limited or no effect. Periods of relaxation, such as holidays, often have a beneficial effect. The headaches are generalised, occipital or frontal, are often described as a dull ache, a band around the head or a pressure feeling, and may be associated with pain and stiffness in the neck. There may be a history of domestic or work stress or anxiety. Neurological examination is normal, but there may be tenderness of the neck muscles.

The basis for the pain of tension headache is uncertain. The frequent occurrence of muscular tenderness suggests that undue sustained contraction plays a part. Treatment with analgesics is not usually successful. Explanation, reassurance and instruction in techniques of relaxation by a physiotherapist is often all that is required, though some tension headaches prove extremely refractory to treatment.

Cervical osteoarthritis

Headaches associated with cervical osteoarthritis are very similar, although neck symptoms are more prominent and neck movements are limited and painful. Disease of the joints of the cervical spine probably causes referred headache, and there is often associated muscle spasm. Physical measures are usually more helpful than analgesics, although NSAIDs may be useful in some patients.

MIGRAINE

Migraine affects up to about 5% of the population and is more common in women. It may start in childhood, adolescence or early adult life; it rarely starts after the age of 35.

Clinical features

In children the development of obvious migraine attacks may be preceded by episodic vomiting associated with abdominal pain (bilious attacks), headache often being a relatively minor symptom at this stage. Migraine is defined as episodic headache usually lasting 6–24 hours, and which is associated with transient visual and/or gastrointestinal disturbances. Headache is often preceded by a visual aura of teichopsia (flashing moving dots) or fortification spectra (zig-zag scintillating lines partly obscuring vision), scotomas (discrete areas of loss of vision), blurring of vision or hemianopic obscurations. Photophobia and phonophobia are common. Additional prodromal symptoms include hemiparaesthesia, occasionally mild unilateral weakness and dysphasia, but these are present in only a small minority of patients. The prodromal disturbances last for 5–30 minutes and are followed by the headache. This is unilateral or generalised, some patients always experiencing pain on the same side. It is often severe, leading to prostration, and is described as throbbing or continuous in nature. In some instances, it is relieved by sleeping, in others by vomiting. Nausea and vomiting are experienced by the majority of patients in some attacks at least.

Provoking factors include fatigue, alcohol, menstruation and hunger. In some patients, there is a history suggesting food allergy and migraine appears to be induced by dietary factors; the common provoking foods are chocolate, cheese, shellfish and red wine.

Rare forms of migraine

Hemiplegic migraine. This is a rare form of migraine, in which a profound hemiplegia, sometimes with dysphasia and hemianopia, precedes the development of headache by 30–60 minutes. The weakness and other focal deficits usually resolve quickly; occasionally, however, they may improve only gradually and, very occasionally, a permanent deficit may result. Hemiplegic migraine sometimes occurs as a familial condition, in which case only this type of migraine occurs.

Basilar migraine. This is an unusual form of migraine, in which brain stem disturbances are common, including impairment of consciousness, vertigo, dysarthria, diplopia and limb weakness.

Ophthalmoplegic migraine. In this very rare condition headache is followed by transient unilateral ophthalmoplegia with ptosis, which may last for several days.

Pathophysiology

The pathophysiology of migraine remains controversial. Migraine was generally considered to have a vascular basis, the prodromal visual and other symptoms of neurological deficit being the result of vasospasm affecting intracerebral and meningeal vessels. However, it has been proposed that the primary event in migraine is neuronal, the vascular changes being secondary.

Treatment

Acute attacks

Most patients will experience attacks less frequently than once a month. In these patients, vigorous early treatment of the acute attack with an adequate dose of an analgesic, such as aspirin, paracetamol or dihydrocodeine, together with an anti-emetic, such as metaclopramide, domperidone or prochlorperazine, is frequently all that is necessary. Emphasis should be placed on early treatment. Many patients will have up to 30 minutes of prodromal symptoms before the onset of headache. Many patients are helped by lying in a darkened room, others by sleeping.

Identification and avoidance of provoking factors is an important and often neglected aspect of treatment.

Ergotamine is an effective drug in migraine, but is frequently associated with side-effects of nausea and vomiting. Usually, the drug is not necessary; however, in a few patients, relief of headache can only be achieved with ergotamine, which can be taken either orally or by suppository. Regular frequent use of ergotamine can induce headaches and, rarely, cause peripheral ischaemia and gangrene.

Frequent attacks

Patients with frequent attacks should be considered for prophylactic therapy. The three drugs most frequently used are clonidine, propranolol and pizotifen, although many patients will not respond to any of these. Methysergide should only be prescribed when all other treatment has failed and when migraine is disabling, because the drug has serious unwanted effects, including retroperitoneal fibrosis.

MIXED HEADACHE

Patients who have migraine seem more prone than average to develop tension headaches; the result being a confusing presentation of the two different kinds of headache. Often, it is found that all the headaches are being inappropriately treated as if they were migraine, when the majority of the headache is tension headache.

Some persistent, benign headaches defy diagnosis and treatment, and some of these undoubtedly have a psychological basis. Such patients are often extensively investigated without a cause becoming apparent. Their headaches are often of several years duration and are resistant to all treatment.

INTRACEREBRAL BLOOD VESSELS AND HEADACHE

A number of diseases affecting the cerebral circulation may cause headache. The most dramatic is subarachnoid haemorrhage, most commonly caused by rupture of a berry aneurysm (p. 901). Headache is abrupt in onset, usually very severe and often associated with vomiting and impairment of consciousness. Any headache of instantaneous onset should raise the possibility of an aneurysm. Small leaks from aneurysms, causing headache alone, are common in the weeks or months before a larger, more severe bleed. In some instances, enlargement of an aneurysm, rather than rupture, may cause headache, and this type of headache is usually not so severe. Haemorrhage within the brain substance itself may occur in arteriovenous malformations or with hypertension, but many occur as apparently spontaneous events without any underlying hypertension or demonstrable vascular pathology. Bleeding causes an acute rise in intracranial pressure which usually causes severe headache. Cerebral thrombosis or embolism is usually painless, but a small number of patients with thrombotic stroke will complain of headache, which can be transiently severe.

Hypertensive encephalopathy (p. 902) may cause headache, but this is usually overshadowed by fits and impairment of consciousness.

Giant cell (temporal) arteritis is a cause of severe headache in the elderly (p. 1024).

OTHER INTRACRANIAL CAUSES OF HEADACHE

With the exception of those due to diseases of the cerebral circulation, most intracranial causes of headache do so by raising intracranial pressure. Expanding pituitary tumours cause pain by local pressure in the pituitary fossa. Headache immediately following cranial trauma is very common (p. 919) and a minority of patients will continue to complain of post-concussional headaches for months, or even years, after head injury. The mechanism of such headaches is unknown. Suggestions of a relationship with impending litigation in some patients may hold some truth, but for the majority this is not the case.

Meningeal irritation

Headache with meningeal irritation is usually associated with neck stiffness. Meningitis and subarachnoid haemorrhage are the main causes. Localised disease involving the meninges, such as meningioma, focal metastatic tumour deposits and subdural haematoma, may each cause headache which may be felt as localised or generalised pain.

Post-ictal headache

Epileptic convulsions are often followed by headache. This usually lasts for less than 24 hours, but may be severe. There is often post-ictal drowsiness, confusion and fever; in addition, the CSF cell count and protein level may both be slightly elevated. This means that, unless a clear history of a fit is obtained from a relative or friend, the situation can be diagnostically difficult and, in particular, meningitis should be considered.

Other causes of headache

Table 23.12 lists a number of other focal conditions which may present with headache, rather than pain localised to the region of pathology. Some metabolic and haematological disturbances are particularly associated with headache, including infections (associated with fever), hypoglycaemia, hypoxia, hypercapnia and alcoholic hangover headache. Anaemia is commonly associated with headache, as is polycythaemia. Coital cephalgia is a rare condition, seen mainly in men, in which headache, often of abrupt onset, occurs during or just after intercourse. It

may be severe, and the clinical picture may resemble that of subarachnoid haemorrhage (which, of course, may also be provoked by intercourse). Patients require careful assessment, and it is better in doubtful cases to examine a normal CSF than to miss a subarachnoid haemorrhage. Headache as a symptom of psychiatric disease is extremely common.

FACIAL PAIN

Facial pain has numerous causes and, as with headache, the majority of patients with pain in the face have no signs. The presence of trigeminal sensory loss or other abnormal physical signs suggests a structural cause. A working knowledge of the cutaneous and non-cutaneous innervation of the trigeminal nerve is necessary (Fig. 23.6 and Table 23.13), and a recognition that pain may be referred onto the face from diseases affecting deeper structures.

It is clinically useful to classify the causes of facial pain according to the site of the lesion, these being the local causes (Table 23.14), lesions between the cavernous sinus and the pons (Table 23.15) and central lesions (Table 23.16). The facial neuralgias (Table 23.17) cause the greatest diagnostic difficulty. Most lesions which involve the trigeminal nerve produce sensory impairment and, sometimes, paraesthesia rather than pain.

Table 23.13 Non-cutaneous trigeminal innervation

Division	Structures innervated
Ophthalmic	Eye, including cornea Mucosa of frontal sinus and upper part of nose
Maxillary	Lateral wall and floor of nasal cavity Upper jaw and teeth Roof of mouth Mucosa of maxillary sinus
Mandibular	Anterior wall of external auditory meatus Temporo-mandibular joint Lower jaw and teeth Floor of mouth Anterior two-thirds of tongue

Table 23.14 Disease of local structures causing facial pain

Teeth Impacted wisdom teeth Dental abscess	**Salivary glands** Infection, e.g. mumps Inflammation due to duct obstruction
Sinusitis	Granuloma, e.g. sarcoidosis Tumour, e.g. lymphoma, primary tumour
Giant cell arteritis	
Migrainous neuralgia	**Eye**
Temporo-mandibular joint disease	Glaucoma Iritis
Nasopharynx Tumour	Optic neuritis

Table 23.15   Lesions causing facial pain between cavernous sinus and pons

Root	Basal meninges
Trigeminal neuralgia	Granuloma, e.g. TB, sarcoid, syphilis
Cerebellopontine angle tumour	Tumour, e.g. lymphoma, carcinoma
Acoustic neuroma	**Ganglion**
Meningioma	Herpes zoster
	Middle fossa fracture

Table 23.16   Central lesions causing facial pain

- Thalamic infarcts
- Brain stem glioma
- Posterior inferior cerebellar artery thrombosis (Wallenberg syndrome)
- Syringomyelia/syringobulbia
- Tabes dorsalis

Table 23.17   The facial neuralgias

- Trigeminal neuralgia
- Post-herpetic neuralgia
- Migrainous neuralgia (cluster headache)
- Atypical (psychogenic) facial pain

TRIGEMINAL NEURALGIA

Trigeminal neuralgia (tic douloureux) is a severe paroxysmal pain with a lancinating shock-like quality. It occurs in women more than men with a ratio of 3:1, with onset usually over the age of 50, though it may occur much earlier than this. It is sometimes seen in association with multiple sclerosis, but it may occur in young people without any associated disease.

Pathology

The cause of the condition is uncertain. The fact that there is no detectable trigeminal sensory impairment on routine testing indicates that the lesion must be minimal. In patients with intractable trigeminal neuralgia coming to operation, it has been observed that, in the posterior fossa, the superior cerebellar artery may be unusually tortuous, producing compression of the trigeminal root. Histologically, minor degenerative changes are seen both in the trigeminal ganglion and in trigeminal root fibres.

Clinical features

Trigeminal neuralgia nearly always occurs in a maxillary or mandibular distribution, and ophthalmic division pain is rare. It is always unilateral at any time, though later development on the contralateral side is described. The commonest sites are shown in Figure 23.7. Pain either originates in the region of the upper lip and radiates upwards over the cheek towards the eye, or originates from the angle of the mouth and radiates backwards and upwards towards the ear. Occasionally, pain is migratory, occurring in different sites in different bouts of pain. Between the paroxysms of pain, which last from 10 to 60 seconds, there is usually no pain, although patients with long-standing trigeminal neuralgia may describe a dull background ache. Paroxysms of pain may become so frequent that the pain may be described by the patient as continuous; careful enquiry on this point is therefore essential. There is always triggering of the pain in trigeminal neuralgia. Innocuous cutaneous stimuli in the upper lip or at the angle of the mouth, any movement of the face or jaw, eating or drinking, may all provoke the pain. This usually occurs in bouts of weeks or months with long periods of freedom from pain of up to several years. In long-standing trigeminal neuralgia, there may be no remission. Neurological examination reveals no abnormal physical signs, although the pain can often be provoked by cutaneous stimulation or by asking the patient to open the mouth. Many patients will be loath to speak, eat or drink during a bout of severe pain.

Treatment

Carbamazepine

The introduction of carbamazepine in the 1960s transformed the treatment of trigeminal neuralgia, and many

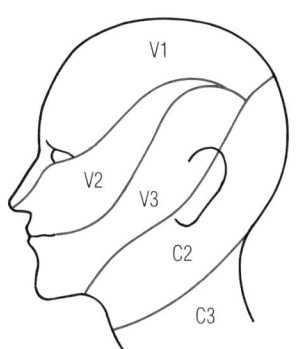

Fig. 23.6   Cutaneous fields of the three trigeminal divisions (V1, V2, V3) and two upper cervical dermatomes (C2, C3).

Fig. 23.7   Trigeminal neuralgia. The two most common sites of origin and radiation of pain are shown; mouth-ear zone and nose-orbit. The pain usually starts in the region of the encircled area and radiates in the directions shown.

patients have their pain satisfactorily controlled for many years with this drug.

Carbamazepine treatment may be effective for many years. In some patients, however, although the pain is controlled, side-effects from the drug are intolerable; these include drowsiness, unsteadiness of gait, nausea and vomiting. If pain becomes unresponsive to carbamazepine, it is worthwhile trying phenytoin, but frequently surgical treatment will need to be considered. Of the treatments currently available, the best is probably thermocoagulation gangliolysis. This involves making a controlled radio-frequency heat lesion to the peripheral branch of the trigeminal nerve in the territory of which the pain is felt. It is a relatively innocuous procedure, and one which can be repeated if necessary. More than 90% of patients with trigeminal neuralgia respond to this treatment and there is a low incidence of complications.

Other approaches

Prior to the introduction of carbamazepine, there was reliance on a variety of neurolytic and surgical ablative procedures of the trigeminal system. These were associated with loss of facial sensation, including sensation to the cornea. This may, in turn, lead to keratitis and loss of vision. Numbness on the face is a particularly unpleasant symptom.

A number of newer surgical techniques are now used which usually produce analgesia without anaesthesia; the feature common to most of these procedures is that they produce minor damage to the trigeminal nerve, either in the region of the ganglion or in the root. The reasons why such treatment is effective are not clear, and raise interesting questions about the pathogenesis of the neuralgia.

Other alternative procedures are the injection of glycerol around the trigeminal ganglion, or cryotherapy to produce freezing lesions of the branches of the peripheral nerve in the territory of the pain. A surgical approach to the trigeminal root through a posterior fossa craniotomy is based on the finding in many patients with trigeminal neuralgia of an ectatic artery or vein pressing on the trigeminal root.

POST-HERPETIC NEURALGIA

Shingles affecting the trigeminal nerve nearly always involves only the ophthalmic division (p. 863). Herpes zoster ophthalmicus is a disease of middle and old age, and is rarely seen in people under 55. There is usually acute shingles and obvious scarring within the ophthalmic nerve territory. The acute zoster infection produces damage in the nerve, causing numbness and hyperaesthesia. The pain is usually continuous, and has a burning or stinging quality. There may be superimposed lancinating pains which, in contrast to the pain in trigeminal neuralgia, often disturbs patients during the night. It is frequently associated with some permanent loss of scalp hair and the eyebrow within the affected area.

Treatment

Post-herpetic neuralgia is extremely difficult to treat. Local measures, such as cold, sometimes heat, vibration, ultrasound and acupuncture may all have some limited symptomatic effect. Simple analgesics have little effect, and a number of psychotropic drugs have been used, again with limited success. Opiate analgesics often only partly relieve the pain and lead to addiction. Buprenorphine, taken sublingually, is sometimes useful.

There is no convincing evidence that local or systemic corticosteroid treatment decreases the incidence of post-herpetic neuralgia, although acute neuralgia may be lessened. Systemic steroid treatment has the potential risk of disseminated infection. Idoxuridine applied locally to the rash may hasten recovery, but has no effect on the incidence of post-herpetic neuralgia. Systemic acyclovir does not lessen the incidence of post-herpetic neuralgia and ablative surgical treatment also has little to offer.

MIGRAINOUS NEURALGIA (CLUSTER HEADACHE)

Migrainous neuralgia (cluster headache) is usually considered as a migraine variant. The cause and underlying pathology of the condition are unknown. The condition occurs much more frequently in men than women, with a ratio of around 7:1.

Clinical features

Migrainous neuralgia is characterised by bouts of daily pain occurring for a few weeks or months at a time, with long periods of complete freedom from pain between these bouts. This pattern of the pain has given rise to the alternative name of cluster headache.

The pain is always unilateral and it is centred on the eye and the upper part of the cheek. It may be very severe and, characteristically, occurs once a day, waking the patient from sleep in the early hours.

Each episode of pain lasts from 20–60 minutes and there

Summary 1   Facial pain

- Disease of deep structures innervated by the trigeminal nerve may produce pain referred onto the face.
- Trigeminal neuralgia is a paroxysmal, lancinating pain, lasting less than a minute, in maxillary or mandibular division territory, which is triggered by cutaneous or oral stimuli.
- Post-herpetic neuralgia nearly always affects the ophthalmic division. It is usually a continuous pain, with cutaneous hyperaesthesia.
- Migrainous neuralgia (cluster headache) is much more common in men. The pain is in the eye and on the cheek, lasts 20–30 minutes, often occurs at night and is very severe.
- Atypical facial pain may be bilateral and often extends outside trigeminal territory. It is continuous, and is often associated with depression. Treatment of the depression usually relieves the pain.

may be associated unilateral facial flushing, nasal secretion on the affected side and profuse watering of the eye with conjunctival hyperaemia. Occasionally, an ipsilateral Horner's syndrome will develop. This is usually transient, but may persist and become permanent. Alcohol provokes attacks during a cluster.

Examination between the bouts of pain is usually normal though there may be a Horner's syndrome.

Treatment

Treatment for migraine is usually ineffective for this type of pain. Drugs are useless once the pain has started, since, by the time the drug is absorbed from the gut, the pain will have come to an end. Prophylactic treatment is thus necessary and, in most cases, is successfully achieved with ergotamine. This drug may be taken orally, sublingually, by inhalation, by suppository, or by subcutaneous injection. It is usual to advise oral or sublingual treatment in the first instance, and the patient is instructed to take 2 mg a few hours before the pain is due. In some patients, parenteral ergotamine is more effective. The drug should be stopped periodically to see whether a spontaneous remission has occurred. Most clusters of this type of headache last for less than three months. Occasionally, the pain will not respond to ergotamine by any route. A number of other treatments have been advocated, and may be successful in occasional patients. These include oxygen inhalation at the time of the pain, lithium and corticosteroids.

ATYPICAL (PSYCHOGENIC) FACIAL PAIN

Pain in the face is a surprisingly common symptom of psychological disturbance, usually depression. It is much more common in women, and the onset is usually in middle-age. Differentiation of this type of facial pain from organic causes can be extremely difficult. The pain is usually unilateral and is often confined to a trigeminal distribution. In patients in whom the pain is bilateral and clearly extends outside trigeminal territory, the diagnosis is made more easily. The pain is usually described as being continuous and severe, and may have lasted months or even years. Many patients will attribute the pain to minor dental surgery and some will have had repeated dental procedures. The pain often has a burning quality and may involve the tongue and other intra-oral structures. There is, in some patients, an obvious associated depression and the response to a tricyclic antidepressant drug is usually good.

DIZZINESS

The word 'dizziness' may be used variously by patients to refer to feelings of disequilibrium, rotational vertigo, light-headedness, faintness, unsteadiness, loss of balance, impairment of consciousness, confusion and even weakness of the legs. It is essential to distinguish symptoms indicative of a vestibular disturbance from those attributable to disturbances of other neurological functions. Dizziness is difficult to define but 'an hallucination of movement' or 'a disagreeable sensation of instability' are descriptive definitions which avoid aetiological or pathological connotation. *Vertigo* refers to a particularly severe dizziness in which there is a sensation of gross rotational movement.

A wide range of pathological processes may lead to dizziness (Table 23.18). Diagnostically, it is most helpful to determine the circumstances in which the symptoms of dizziness developed, its duration and the presence or absence of associated symptoms, either cochlear, cardiovascular or neurological.

Dizziness is extremely common. It has been estimated that about 30% of people have experienced the symptom by the age of 65. Coordination of posture, motor acts and gaze is dependent upon input from the vestibular system, proprioceptive afferent information from the limbs and trunk, and the visual system, to the brain stem, which also receives modulating inputs from the cerebral cortex, basal ganglia, cerebellum and reticular formation.

The *vestibular system* refers to the vestibular end organs in each inner ear, and their connections in the brain stem. There is a continuous input from each labyrinth (vestibular tonus). Changes of head posture increase the input from one side and decrease it from the contralateral side, and cause corrective eye movements via pathways subserving the vestibulo-ocular reflex (VOR). Any pathological process which upsets the balance of the vestibular inputs may lead to a sensation of dizziness. This may be mild, and reported as light-headedness or a 'swimming sensation'. It may be sufficient to cause some unsteadiness of gait, or be so severe as to cause an inability to stand and walk without assistance. This degree of dizziness is often associated with nausea and vomiting.

Table 23.18 Causes of dizziness

Otological	Cardiovascular
Labyrinthitis	Syncope
Benign positional vertigo	Postural hypotension
Meniere's disease	Dysrhythmias with reduced cardiac
Post-traumatic vestibular damage	output
Vascular occlusion affecting labyrinth	Aortic stenosis
Ototoxic drugs	Hypertrophic cardiomyopathy
Neurological	**Haematological**
Multiple sclerosis	Anaemia
Vertebrobasilar insufficiency, PICA	Polycythaemia
syndrome	**Metabolic**
Migraine	Hypoglycaemia
Infection: geniculate herpes, syphilis,	Hyperventilation
TB	
Acoustic neuroma	**Ocular**
Temporal lobe epilepsy	Impaired visual acuity
Brain stem tumours	Diplopia

Clinical features and diagnosis

An acute brief episode of dizziness is usually due to a peripheral labyrinthine disturbance, although central lesions, such as temporal lobe epilepsy and, very occasionally, vertebrobasilar insufficiency, can produce this isolated symptom. Meniere's disease may, in the early stages, cause episodes of dizziness lasting less than a minute, but episodes lasting one or two days are more usual in later attacks. Dizziness from vestibular neuronitis may be severe for several days. Central lesions causing vestibular disturbances as the only symptom usually lead to dizziness of gradual onset, which is less severe than that caused by peripheral lesions. Acute severe vertigo may occur with central vascular lesions, e.g. posterior inferior cerebellar artery thrombosis or vertebral artery occlusion, but there are always associated neurological symptoms and signs.

Dizziness is a common symptom in anxious patients, sometimes associated with over-breathing, and in patients with depression.

Central vs peripheral lesions

Flow charts are useful in the diagnosis of dizziness (Fig. 23.8). Having established that the patient's complaint is a symptom of a vestibular disturbance, the next important clinical distinction to make is whether the symptom is due to a central or peripheral lesion.

Peripheral

Associated deafness, tinnitus or pain in the ear, particularly when unilateral, suggests a peripheral disturbance. A very gradually progressive unilateral deafness associated with dizziness raises the possibility of an acoustic neuroma. If, in addition to a sensory neural deafness, there is a cerebello-pontine angle syndrome – comprising an ipsilateral lower motor neurone facial weakness, trigeminal hypoaesthesia and ipsilateral limb ataxia – an acoustic neuroma is by far the likeliest diagnosis, although other tumours such as meningiomas may also produce this syndrome. An abrupt mild deafness or tinnitus with acute severe vertigo suggests a viral labyrinthitis or an acute vascular occlusion affecting the inner ear. Intermittent episodes of tinnitus, deafness, dizziness and pain in the ear are characteristic of Meniere's disease (p. 884).

Central

With the exception of acoustic neuromas, the presence of associated neurological symptoms usually indicates that the cause of dizziness is a central lesion. Many brain stem lesions may affect the vestibular nuclei and pathways, and these pathologies will tend to produce symptoms and signs in other systems, including the cranial nerve nuclei, pyramidal and sensory tracts together with cerebellar deficits.

The aura of temporal lobe epilepsy may include dizziness, but there will be other symptoms (p. 838), the most important being impairment of consciousness.

Other causes of dizziness

Any cardiac disease leading to a low cardiac output, whether chronically, exacerbated by exertion (as in aortic

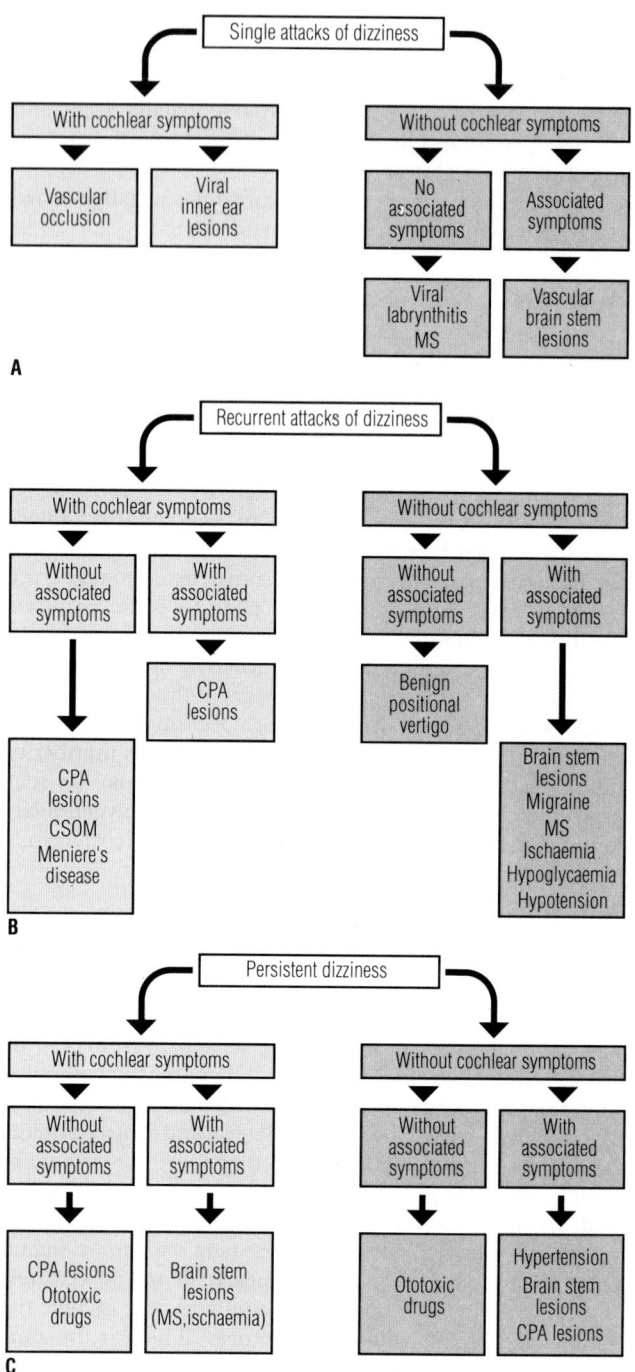

Fig. 23.8 Diagnostic flow diagrams for dizziness and associated symptoms.
CPA = cerebello-pontine angle; CSOM = chronic suppurative otitis media; MS = multiple sclerosis.

stenosis), or as a result of dysrhythmia, may cause dizziness. Dizziness is a common first symptom in a vaso-vagal fainting attack, but, again, is not the only symptom.

Other important causes of dizziness include ototoxic drugs, such as the aminoglycosides, or treatment with tranquillisers, antidepressants, or neuroleptic drugs. A previous history of ear disease may also be relevant. Impaired visual acuity or eye movement disorders causing diplopia or oscillopsia may all cause patients to complain of dizziness rather than a visual symptom.

Examination

The examination is often normal, particularly in younger patients. General examination, including lying and standing blood pressure, are as important as the neurological examination. Some patients have mild disturbances of gait and nystagmus. Clinical testing of hearing is an important part of the neurological examination.

Romberg's test

In Romberg's test, in a patient with an acute peripheral vestibular lesion, there will be a tendency for the patient to fall towards the affected side. Patients with non-organic illnesses tend to fall backwards in Romberg's test, without immediate appropriate attempts to correct their posture; however, they will usually avoid injury by acrobatic manoeuvres to maintain balance at the last moment.

Vestibulo-ocular testing

Examination of the eye movements (vestibulo-ocular testing) should first establish that there is a full range of movement in each eye and that gaze remains conjugate. Slow following eye movements (pursuit) and rapid eye movements (saccadic) should be normal.

Nystagmus (p. 869) is the most important vestibulo-ocular reflex. A unilateral vestibular disturbance upsets the balance of impulses from each labyrinth tending to cause deviation of the eyes towards the side of the lesion. This is balanced by a rapid saccadic movement of the eyes towards the opposite side. Nystagmus, described in the direction of the fast component, is away from the side of the lesion. Mild nystagmus of this sort may be seen only with caloric or rotational stimulation.

Routine testing for nystagmus is relatively crude and is greatly helped by electronystagmography, a technique in which electrodes are placed on each side of the eye with a remote ground electrode, measuring potential differences between the cornea and retina. When the eye moves towards an electrode, a positive potential is recorded. In a peripheral vestibular lesion, spontaneous nystagmus at 30° of lateral gaze occurs only in one direction, the eyes always remain conjugate and the nystagmus is increased by removing fixation using Frenzel's glasses. The nystagmus is most marked with acute lesions, and the central nervous system compensates over a period of weeks so that nystagmus (and dizziness) tends to improve. In central vestibular lesions, compensation tends not to occur, the nystagmus may occur in more than one direction of gaze, the eye movements are sometimes dysconjugate, and removal of fixation has little effect.

Caloric testing (p. 869) is an easily performed and reliable measure of vestibulo-ocular reflexes. If the response to caloric testing is reduced on one side, there is said to be canal paresis, which indicates a peripheral lesion (labyrinth, nerve or vestibular nucleus). A directional preponderance refers to an increase in the nystagmus in one direction. This occurs when there is an imbalance of the peripheral vestibular inputs or a central imbalance. In some patients, there will be a mixture of these abnormalities.

Optokinetic nystagmus is the normal reflex oscillation of the eyes induced by movements of the subject's surroundings. It is disturbed in central vestibular lesions, but not with peripheral lesions.

Testing for positionally induced nystagmus is particularly helpful when there is a history of dizziness provoked by certain positions of the head, usually lying down or extending the neck to look upwards. Placing the patient's head in the position which induces dizziness may also induce nystagmus. A better test is the Hallpike manoeuvre, in which the patient's head is rapidly lowered from a sitting position backwards and over the end of the bed with head turned either to the right or the left. In benign positional vertigo (see below) of peripheral origin, nystagmus is provoked with a latent period of 2–20 seconds, disappears (adapts) within one minute, is associated with vertigo and fatigues with repeated testing; the fast phase of the nystagmus is towards the lower ear with the head in this posture. Positional nystagmus may sometimes be a feature of central vestibular lesions, but the Hallpike manoeuvre in these patients characteristically provokes nystagmus without vertigo. There is no latent period, nor any fatiguability, on repeated testing. The direction of the saccadic phase of nystagmus is variable.

Hearing

Cochlear function is routinely tested as described on page 869, supplemented by audiometry.

Aetiology

There are a number of common causes of dizziness.

Acute labyrinthitis

The usual history in acute labyrinthitis is vertigo of abrupt onset, occurring first thing on waking in the morning. It may be severe for one to three days, is minimised by keeping the head still and is provoked by any head movement. It is often associated with nausea and vomiting. There is gradual resolution of the symptoms over a few weeks, although mild symptoms may be provoked by sudden head movement for up to several months later. Examination during the acute stage may reveal nystagmus, either spontaneously present on forward gaze or only on lateral gaze. Later, nystagmus will be absent, but caloric testing shows a unilateral canal paresis. The audiogram is normal. Complete resolution of symptoms eventually occurs in the great majority of patients, although mild symptoms may persist for months.

Up to half of patients with acute labyrinthitis will have had a cold or other viral infection shortly before the onset

Summary 2 Dizziness

- In the majority of patients presenting with dizziness, the cause is a peripheral labyrinthine disturbance or syncope.

- Acute episodes of dizziness with nausea and vomiting, but without other neurological symptoms, are nearly always due to a peripheral labyrinthine disturbance.

- Episodes of vertebrobasilar ischaemia may produce dizziness, but almost always with other neurological symptoms.

- Peripheral labyrinthine disturbances are much more likely to be associated with tinnitus and/or deafness than central lesions.

- When there is doubt whether dizziness is due to a peripheral or central lesion, caloric testing is useful; a canal paresis indicates a peripheral lesion.

- Long-term use of vestibular sedative drugs, such as prochlorperazine or cinnarizine, is rarely necessary.

- When dizziness occurs in association with other neurological symptoms and signs, the patient should be referred for a neurological opinion.

of the symptoms; it is thus often regarded as a viral or post-viral syndrome. Treatment for a few days is often necessary during the acute stage. The vestibular sedatives, cinnarizine or prochlorperazine, are effective.

Benign positional vertigo

Benign positional vertigo is produced by certain head postures, most commonly lying down with the head turned on one side or extending the neck. Vertebrobasilar ischaemia is often invoked as the cause of such vertigo, but this is probably very unusual (see below) and making a diagnosis of vertebrobasilar ischaemia on the basis of vertigo as the only symptom is rarely justified. Vertigo, often positional, is a common symptom following head injury.

The labyrinth is the likely site of the lesion. The Hallpike manœuvre is particularly helpful in eliciting nystagmus in this condition, which has the features of a peripheral lesion. A vestibular sedative, such as cinnarazine, is occasionally necessary when symptoms are severe or persistent.

Meniere's disease

Meniere's disease results from endolymphatic hydrops (increased pressure in the membranous labyrinth) and is of unknown cause. It is characterised clinically by attacks of severe vertigo occurring several times in a few weeks, followed by long periods of remission of months or years. The onset of Meniere's disease is usually between 40 and 60 years of age and the condition is more common in men. It is always initially unilateral, although, in about 25% of patients, the other ear is later affected.

Each attack is usually preceded by a sensation of pressure in the ear. The subsequent onset of vertigo may be severe and is associated with nausea, vomiting, deafness and tinnitus. Between attacks, the tinnitus and deafness persist and gradually worsen. Recurrent attacks lead to increasing deafness; when hearing is completely lost, the attacks of vertigo cease.

Audiometry shows a sensorineural deafness, and caloric testing an ipsilateral canal paresis. During a bout of attacks, a vestibular sedative, such as cinnarazine, may be helpful. In very severe cases, surgical measures to destroy the labyrinth can be considered, but should not be contemplated if there is deafness in the other ear. Surgical procedures which ablate the labyrinth, but preserve residual cochlear function, are now increasingly used.

Vertebrobasilar ischaemia

Vertigo is a common symptom of vertebrobasilar ischaemia, but the diagnosis must rest on a description of attacks, which also include one or more of the following symptoms: diplopia, bilateral visual obscurations, bilateral facial numbness or paraesthesiae (commonly circumoral), bilateral facial weakness, dysarthria, dysphagia, dysphonia, weakness or sensory loss in the limbs, and impairment of consciousness (p. 894).

Ototoxic drugs

Many drugs are potentially ototoxic, and some cause permanent vestibular damage, particularly streptomycin and gentamicin.

Multiple sclerosis

Plaques of demyelination in the brain stem quite frequently cause dizziness (p. 952).

Acoustic neuroma

Acoustic neuromas do not usually cause major vestibular involvement; when it does occur, vertigo is usually mild (p. 906).

Geniculate herpes zoster (Ramsay Hunt syndrome)

Geniculate herpes zoster is a rare condition, but important to recognise. It is due to involvement of the geniculate ganglion by *Herpes zoster* and there is often involvement of neighbouring nerves. Severe earache is the first symptom, and a discrete vesicular rash develops within 1–3 days of the onset of pain. The rash is present on the tympanic membrane and external auditory meatus, and spreads onto the concha. It is occasionally also present on the palate and pharynx. The rash is often discrete, with only a few visible vesicles spreading onto the concha. There is a lower motor neurone facial palsy, which may be the only neurological abnormality; however, dizziness is common, together with some impairment of hearing, and, very occasionally, there is involvement of the glossopharyngeal and vagus nerves. Adequate analgesia is essential for this extremely painful condition. Like other forms of shingles, it tends to affect an older age group, and, occasionally, can produce a very severe illness, with meningitis and an acute confusional state.

SYNCOPE AND EPILEPSY

The term 'blackout' means different things to different people and it is important to establish in what sense the patient is using the word. If the patient is describing disturbed consciousness, his recollection of events is bound to be incomplete, and a detailed independent account of the episode is invaluable.

The great majority of patients presenting to their doctors with blackouts will have no physical signs. The diagnosis rests entirely on a meticulous history.

Differential diagnosis of epilepsy and syncope

Syncope is defined as loss of consciousness due to transient impairment of cerebral blood flow.

Epilepsy is a paroxysmal, abnormal cerebral electrical discharge associated with a clinical change; this may take a wide variety of different forms, but usually includes some impairment of consciousness.

Features which help in distinguishing epilepsy from syncope – the commonest clinical differential diagnostic problem – include the following:

The time of day and circumstances of the attack

Attacks during the night, while the patient is recumbent in bed, are not likely to be syncopal. Nocturnal attacks which the patient cannot remember, but which wake other members of the family, are likely to be fits. Syncopal attacks may occur during the night on getting up, often during micturition.

Events causing squeamishness, or bad news, may provoke syncope. Patients with photosensitive epilepsy may have a history of attacks provoked by watching television (usually when sitting too close), or flickering lights.

Posture

Standing for long periods, particularly in hot surroundings, often provokes syncope.

Warning of the attack

Loss of consciousness in syncope is nearly always preceded by a period of malaise with dizziness, nausea, visual blurring and dimming, and a feeling of impending loss of consciousness. Many patients will have discovered that lying down promptly during this prodromal phase will prevent loss of consciousness.

Period of unconsciousness and post-ictal state

Syncope usually causes brief loss of consciousness of less than a minute. Exceptions are usually due to attempts by onlookers to sit the patient up. This merely intensifies the period of unconsciousness and may, on occasions, provoke a secondary hypoxic convulsion. Such attacks are then often mislabelled as being epileptic. Minor fits may cause a period of absence which may be momentary (see below) and which may appear to witnesses as absentmindedness, rather than impairment of consciousness. Convulsions are associated with loss of consciousness of more than one minute (and sometimes up to 10 or 15 minutes), followed by a period of post-ictal drowsiness and confusion; this is often accompanied by irritability and, sometimes, aggressive, irrational behaviour if the patient is disturbed. Patients recovering from syncope are orientated and rational.

Appearance during the period of unconsciousness

A history from witnesses of convulsive tonic or tonic clonic movements of the limbs, with facial grimacing, jaw clenching, tongue biting and grunting noises and irregular breathing, clearly indicate a fit. A patient who lies limp while unconscious, appears pale and sweaty, whose pulse is difficult to feel and who rapidly regains consciousness, is likely to have had a syncopal attack. Nevertheless, patients with fits may also appear pale and sweaty and tonic clonic movements may be discrete or absent. The differential diagnosis can sometimes be impossible from the accounts given by some patients and witnesses of their attacks.

Incontinence

Incontinence of urine, and, sometimes, faeces is relatively common in epilepsy, and urinary incontinence occasionally occurs in syncope.

SYNCOPE

Syncope is very common. In a healthy young adult, a blood pressure of less than 50 mmHg will reduce cerebral blood flow sufficient to cause loss of consciousness (Table 23.19). The conditions most commonly leading to syncope are discussed below.

Table 23.19 Causes of syncope

- Vasovagal attacks
- Cardiogenic syncope
- Cough, sneeze and micturition syncope
- Breath-holding attacks
- Orthostatic hypotension
- Carotid sinus sensitivity

Vasovagal syncope

Vagal overactivity produces a bradycardia and a fall in blood pressure, which is associated with peripheral vasodilatation. Such attacks are often reflex in nature and provoked by emotional or painful circumstances. Vasovagal faints often occur in adolescents and young adults who are otherwise entirely healthy and, occasionally, children of less than 10 years are prone to fainting. Faints are more common soon after getting up. They are always postural, the symptoms starting while standing or sitting. They are more frequent in women than men, may be associated with menstruation or intercurrent febrile illness, and are more frequent after sleep deprivation and prolonged fasting.

Cardiogenic syncope

Heart disease may cause syncope in three main ways:

1. by acute dysrhythmias, as in supraventricular tachycardia or heart block
2. by obstruction to flow, as in aortic stenosis
3. in low output states, as with a pericardial effusion.

These conditions are discussed in more detail in Chapter 13. Cardiac causes of syncope are particularly important in the older population. Syncope on exertion suggests the possibility of cardiac disease.

Cough, micturition and sneeze syncope

Prolonged bouts of coughing raise intrathoracic pressure, impair venous return to the heart, and cause syncope. Sneezing occasionally induces syncope, probably by a vagal reflex mechanism. Coughing or sneezing in patients with cerebellar tonsillar herniation through the foramen magnum (Arnold-Chiari malformation) may provoke syncope, the mechanism of which is uncertain. Fainting may occur during micturition in men, particularly during the night, due to a postural fall in the blood pressure, reflex vagal activity stimulated by a full bladder, and reduced venous return caused by straining.

Breath-holding attacks

These usually occur in very young children as a reaction to emotional stress. They are sometimes seen with prolonged crying. There is prolonged breath-holding, leading to cyanosis and, eventually, loss of consciousness. Attacks usually start before the age of 18 months and stop by the age of 5 years. In severe prolonged attacks, secondary hypoxic convulsions may be induced and the child is frequently mislabelled as epileptic.

Orthostatic hypotension

The term orthostatic hypotension refers to a fall in blood pressure on standing. Hypotension may be sufficiently profound to cause a loss of consciousness. There are numerous causes (Table 23.20).

Postural hypotension may be a result of impaired sympathetic activity, as occurs in some neuropathies (diabetes being the commonest), and in central autonomic failure; the latter may occur as an isolated phenomenon, as part of the Shy-Drager syndrome associated with Parkinsonism or as part of a multiple systems atrophy (p. 916).

Many drugs, in addition to hypotensive agents, can lower blood pressure sufficiently for loss of consciousness to occur. Corticosteroid deficiency, which may be due to Addison's disease, abrupt withdrawal of administered steroid or hypopituitarism, leads to hypotension exacerbated by standing.

Chronic idiopathic orthostatic hypotension is a rare condition, in which there is no cardiovascular sympathetic response to a fall in blood pressure induced by standing. Tachycardia, vasoconstriction and sweating (the normal responses to hypotension) are all absent.

Table 23.20 Causes of orthostatic hypotension

Venous pooling	**Reduced muscle and vascular tone**
Prolonged standing	Prolonged bed rest
Severe varicose veins	
	Fluid depletion
Impaired vasomotor activity	
Peripheral neuropathy	**Drugs**
Diabetes	Hypotensive therapy
Guillain-Barré syndrome	Tranquillisers
Surgical sympathectomy	Phenothiazines
Spinal cord lesions	Levodopa
Syringomyelia	
Tabes dorsalis	**Steroid deficiency**
Familial dysautonomia	Hypopituitarism
Shy-Drager syndrome	Addison's disease
	Chronic idiopathic orthostatic hypotension

Carotid sinus sensitivity

Carotid sinus sensitivity is the result of atherosclerotic disease affecting the carotid artery at its bifurcation in the neck. It is usually seen in middle-aged or elderly people in the setting of widespread vascular disease. Mild pressure over the sinus, such as that which might be caused by a tight shirt-collar, combined with head turning, causes an excessive bradycardia, hypotension and, occasionally, transient asystole which may last 10–15 seconds (Ch. 13).

Summary 3   Differential diagnosis of syncope and epilepsy

- Always try to obtain an eye-witness account of an episode of loss of consciousness; do not diagnose epilepsy on insufficient grounds.

- Syncope is usually postural, with prodromal symptoms before loss of consciousness. Fits often occur without any warning.

- Loss of consciousness in syncope usually lasts less than a minute, in contrast to most fits.

- Confusion, headache and drowsiness are common after fits, but not after syncope.

- Excessive alcohol – either binge drinking or chronic alcoholism – is a common cause of isolated fits.

- The inter-ictal EEG may be normal in epilepsy. The diagnosis of epilepsy is essentially clinical and does not depend on the EEG.

EPILEPSY

A number of terms are used to describe the clinical and associated electrical abnormalities of epilepsy. Epileptic attacks, fits, seizures and convulsions all refer to the same phenomenon – a paroxysmal electrical discharge affecting a group of neurones, starting in one part of the brain, but often spreading to become a generalised abnormality.

Paroxysmal activity of the sort seen in fits may occur intermittently without any clinical abnormality, but the incidental finding of such activity on an EEG does not necessarily imply a diagnosis of epilepsy. The diagnosis of a fit or fits is essentially a clinical one.

Classification

Fits are clinically and electrically heterogeneous. Aetiological classifications (Table 23.22) are useful reminders of the many causes of fits but must be supplemented with a classification of the type of fit (Table 23.21). Fits are always disturbing events, but there is a great difference to the patient in the impact of, for example, an absence attack of petit mal and a generalised tonic clonic convulsion. It is thus helpful to qualify a diagnosis of epilepsy with a statement about the type of attack or attacks suffered by a particular patient.

Table 23.21 Types of fit – WHO classification

Generalised seizures
Absence attacks
    Petit mal – 3 Hz spike and wave
    Atypical absences
Myoclonic seizures
    Myoclonic jerks, single or multiple
    Clonic seizures
Tonic-clonic seizures
    Grand mal, major fits
Tonic seizures
Atonic or akinetic seizures

Partial seizures
Simple, without impairment of consciousness
    Motor, sensory, aphasic, cognitive, affective, amnesic, illusional, olfactory, psychic. Includes Jacksonian, temporal lobe, psychomotor epilepsy
Complex partial seizures (temporal lobe epilepsy) with impairment of consciousness
    Simple partial onset, followed by impairment of consciousness
    Impairment of consciousness from the onset
Partial seizures, either simple or complex, evolving into generalised tonic-clonic seizures
Generalised tonic-clonic seizures, with EEG but not clinical evidence of focal onset

Hysterical seizures

Pathophysiology

Partial seizures

In focal epilepsy (partial seizures), paroxysmal discharges develop in one part of the cerebral hemispheres, the temporal lobe being the most common site. If it remains focal, such activity will produce a minor fit in which the type of symptom experienced depends on the region of the brain involved; there may or may not be impairment of con-

sciousness. In many minor temporal lobe attacks, the impairment of consciousness takes the form of brief lapses of awareness without obvious loss of consciousness observable by witnesses of the attack. In focal motor fits that remain focal, there may be no impairment of awareness or consciousness, so that the patient will be in a position to provide a complete account of events. However, focal epileptic activity may become generalised, in which case there is loss of consciousness and, usually, clinical evidence of a convulsion. Many patients will have both focal attacks and fits which are preceded by symptoms of the focal electrical disturbance.

Generalised seizures

In the other main neurophysiological category of epilepsy, paroxysmal discharges are generated in deep sites at the hypothalamic, thalamic or upper brain stem level, and rapidly spread to both hemispheres simultaneously to produce generalised epileptic discharges. This type of abnormality is present in many patients with so-called idiopathic or constitutional epilepsy, and is also responsible for petit mal attacks.

Aetiology

The many causes of fits are listed in Table 23.22. It is important to recognise that a particular cause of fits may produce fits of different kinds. Thus, perinatal anoxia, for example, may cause either generalised or partial seizures.

Table 23.22 Causes of fits

Idiopathic/constitutional	**Infection**
Hereditary and familial	Febrile convulsions
Petit mal	Viral encephalitis
Some patients with temporal lobe	Bacterial meningitis
epilepsy	Tuberculous meningitis
Aminoacidurias	Cerebral abscess
Trisomy D	Cysticercosis
Lipidoses	Neurosyphilis
	Echinococcus
Developmental defects	Toxocariasis
Phakomatoses	Toxoplasmosis
Intrauterine rubella, CMV,	
toxoplasma	**Inflammatory**
Irradiation	SLE/PAN/multiple sclerosis
Birth trauma	**Metabolic**
Perinatal anoxia	Uraemia/water intoxication/
Cerebral contusion	hyponatraemia/hypoglycaemia/
Cerebral haemorrhage and	hypomagnesaemia
thrombosis	
	Toxic
Anoxia in infancy and childhood	Alcohol/drugs, e.g. barbiturates,
	amphetamines, lignocaine, tricyclic
Tumours	antidepressants, phenothiazines,
Primary and secondary	Lead
Vascular	**Degenerative**
Mature infarcts/arteriovenous	Alzheimer's disease/Creutzfeld-
malformations	Jacob disease/Huntington's disease

Idiopathic or constitutional epilepsy is a term used to refer to patients with recurrent fits in whom no cause can be identified. This forms by far the largest group of epileptic patients. Patients probably include those who have had intra-uterine, birth and neonatal insults. In some patients, there is a strong family history; this is often the case with petit mal and in some patients with temporal lobe epilepsy. In the majority of idiopathic epileptics, however, there is no family history and, in most cases, no predisposing factors can be identified.

Of the many causes of acquired fits (Table 23.23), hereditary factors deserve special mention. Apart from the rare degenerative disorders which may cause epilepsy (see below and Table 23.24), genetic factors are also important in febrile convulsions and petit mal. In the latter, the typical EEG abnormality has been found in nearly 50% of siblings whether or not they have clinical fits.

Factors provoking fits

Some agents may cause fits in people not normally prone to having fits, e.g. alcohol (both bingeing and abrupt withdrawal, p. 972) and drug abuse (particularly with barbiturates and amphetamines). In epileptics, sleep deprivation is a common provocative factor. In some patients, there is a clear relationship between fits and stressful life events. Some patients have fits only, or mainly, at night, the epileptic threshold being reduced during sleep. In some women with epilepsy, their fits tend to occur just before or during menstruation (catamenial epilepsy).

Photosensitivity is important in a relatively small proportion of epileptics, particularly those with petit mal and myoclonic epilepsy. Rarely, fits can be induced by music, looking at certain patterns, and reading.

Types of fit

Tonic clonic fits (grand mal epilepsy, major fits)

In tonic clonic fits (grand mal epilepsy, major fits), there is abrupt loss of consciousness associated initially with a *tonic phase*, in which there is sustained muscular contraction affecting all muscles, including respiratory, facial and jaw muscles. Breathing may cease and the patient becomes cyanosed. It is during this phase that the tongue may be bitten and incontinence occurs. After a short period (usually less than 30 seconds) a *clonic phase* supervenes, in which there are repeated violent jerking movements of the trunk and limbs. Self-inflicted injury is common during this phase, which may last for several minutes. On cessation of the fit, consciousness is slowly regained, passing through a stuporose phase. There is often post-ictal confusion, irritability and headache; irrational behaviour may occur during this stage, of which the patient is later amnesic.

Many patients will have a few seconds warning of a fit. The symptoms are often non-specific, and include malaise, dizziness and a feeling of detachment. Patients who come to recognise these symptoms may have time to sit or lie down before losing consciousness. However, others will have no such prodrome.

Management. A patient having a fit should be turned onto his side to prevent the tongue obstructing the airway, and self-injury should be prevented as far as possible. It is a mistake to attempt to force open the mouth. The vast majority of fits are single, self-limiting events. It is unnecessary to admit known epileptics to hospital after a single fit.

Partial seizures (minor epilepsy)

Focal epileptic discharges may arise in any part of the cerebral hemispheres, causing partial seizures. *Focal motor* fits characteristically cause convulsive twitching of one side of the body, starting in the face, arm or leg and gradually spreading (Jacksonian epilepsy). *Focal sensory* fits arising in the post-central gyrus cause a similar march of sensory symptoms. *Versive fits*, in which the eyes and the head are turned to one side, are produced by contralateral posterior frontal epileptic activity.

Temporal lobe epilepsy

Temporal lobe epileptic attacks are by far the commonest type of partial seizure. These may occur as a *simple* type of partial attack without loss of consciousness (psychomotor fits) with aphasia or cognitive, affective, amnesic, olfactory, illusional or psychic symptoms; or they may be *complex* partial seizures, in which the symptoms are followed by a period of impaired consciousness. However, it is clinically useful to use the term 'temporal lobe' epilepsy to refer to both simple and complex partial fits.

In temporal lobe attacks, the patient appears vacant and this may be associated with inability to talk, though simple commands may be obeyed. Olfactory, epigastric and psychic phenomena, such as déjà-vu and jamais-vu, are very common. During an attack, repetitive motor behaviours may occur; lip-smacking, chewing and grimacing movements are the commonest. In simple attacks, at least partial awareness is preserved, while, in complex partial seizures, the patient will be amnesic for part of the attack and may not afterwards realise that anything has happened. Like other partial seizures, minor temporal lobe fits may progress to a generalised convulsion.

Petit mal

Petit mal refers to brief (10–15 second) absence attacks associated with a generalised 3-second spike-and-wave discharge on the EEG. The fits always start in childhood, and consist of a brief cessation of activity associated with a blank staring look and, occasionally, nodding of the head, fluttering of the eyelids and (very occasionally) small convulsive movements of the limbs. Objects may be dropped, but postural control is maintained if the child is sitting or standing. It is common for petit mal to continue into adolescence, but only occasionally into adult life. About 50% of children with petit mal will later develop grand mal fits.

Febrile convulsions

In young children, sudden rises in body temperature may provoke convulsions. Such fits are usually generalised and brief; they occur between the ages of 6 months and 5 years, and only occur with fever. There is a small increased risk of later development of epilepsy in children who have had febrile fits.

Rarer types of fit

Many other, rarer types of fit are described (Table 23.23). These include *atypical absences* which appear exactly like petit mal but which are associated with different EEG abnormalities and are often seen in association with mental retardation and cerebral atrophy (Lennox Gastaut syndrome).

In *infantile spasms*, there is sudden brief head nodding (salaam attacks). These develop within the first year of life and are usually associated with regression and failure of development. Such attacks may be refractory to treatment.

In *tonic fits*, there is maintained dystonic posturing of the limbs and sometimes the trunk, not followed by a clonic phase.

Myoclonic jerks are single, sometimes repetitive, sudden convulsive movements of the limbs and trunk; they are usually seen in patients who have, or later develop, idiopathic epilepsy. Single myoclonic jerks occur in some normal people when drifting off to sleep, but are of no pathological significance.

Table 23.23   Rarer types of epilepsy

Atypical absences
Clinically the same as petit mal; slower EEG, other abnormalities and often associated mental retardation and atrophy (Lennox-Gastaut syndrome); seizures hard to control

Tonic seizures
Tonic posturing only

Infantile spasms
Brief sudden head flexion – 'salaam' attacks often with failure of development and regression. Onset at 3–9 months

Myoclonic epilepsy
Mostly children with idiopathic epilepsy; attacks early in the morning
Photosensitive myoclonus and epilepsy
Hereditary myoclonic epilepsies – generalised seizures and myoclonus with degenerative disease, e.g. Lafora body disease: children/adolescents with myoclonus, major seizures and dementia. Death occurs within a few years. Intracellular inclusion bodies present
Gangliosidoses.

Hysterical seizures

It can be difficult to determine clinically whether or not attacks are organic or hysterical in nature. Most patients who have hysterical attacks also suffer organic seizures. EEG monitoring during an attack may be helpful, but, in some instances, continuous 24-hour recording with simultaneous video recording is necessary to establish the organic or hysterical nature of the attacks.

Investigation

A diagnosis of epilepsy cannot be made from an EEG, but an abnormal EEG showing clear epileptic activity supports the clinical diagnosis. An EEG should be done in a patient presenting with a first fit. Where alcohol or drug abuse is suspected as the underlying cause, the EEG is likely to be normal. The investigation is of most value when there is a history of focal onset and the presence of abnormal physical signs suggests a structural abnormality. Further investigation with a CT scan is then indicated, but, in general, CT scans are of limited value in epilepsy.

Meningovascular syphilis is now uncommon and a WR is rarely of value. Lumbar puncture is of very limited value. In children in whom a metabolic disturbance is suspected, special investigation is necessary, as is the case with the phakomatoses and lipidoses.

Treatment

Principles of medical treatment

A single fit in an adult is rarely an indication to start anticonvulsant treatment. Exceptions are patients with a clear history of focal seizures, in whom an underlying structural cause is likely, and patients who have abnormal physical signs following a fit, indicating a hemisphere lesion. Otherwise, most neurologists would wait until two or three fits have occurred within a period of two years or less before starting treatment.

Patients with fits clearly related to alcohol withdrawal (p. 972) should not be given anticonvulsants.

Having decided that treatment is necessary, the choice of drug will depend on the type of seizure, the age of the patient, the possibility of pregnancy, interaction with other medication and the likelihood of producing unacceptable side-effects. It is best to use a single drug, starting at a dose which will avoid excessive side-effects and increasing to a therapeutic level. Monitoring of blood levels of anticonvulsants is indicated, both to ensure therapeutic levels in patients who continue to have fits on treatment or if symptoms and signs of toxicity develop. Blood levels of the shorter-acting anticonvulsants, such as valproate and clonazepam, are of little value.

Follow-up is important to monitor the efficacy of treatment and the occurrence of drug side-effects. Patients must understand the details of their treatment. A card carried by the patient with drug information can be invaluable in an acute situation. Periodic review of the continuing need for treatment is necessary. In patients with adult onset of relatively infrequent fits, it is reasonable to consider gradual withdrawal of treatment when they have been free from fits for two years.

Choice of drug

For petit mal, ethosuximide is the drug of choice, though

Table 23.24 Anticonvulsant drugs in adults

Drug	Average dose	Unwanted effects	Comment
Phenytoin	250–400 mg od	Sedation, ataxia, dizziness, intellectual impairment, hirsutism, seborrhoeic skin thickening, gum hypertrophy	Avoid in pregnancy
Carbamazepine	300–800 mg per day, as bd dosage	Sedation, ataxia, nausea and vomiting. Rarely, bone marrow suppression and hepatotoxicity. Skin rash	Safe in pregnancy
Phenobarbitone	30–90 mg per day, as bd dosage	Sedation, intellectual impairment	Safe in pregnancy
Clonazepam	1.5–6.0 mg per day, as tds dosage	Sedation with initial treatment	? Safe in pregnancy
Primidone	250–750 mg per day, as bd dosage	Sedation. As for phenobarbitone. May be better tolerated than phenobarbitone	Avoid in pregnancy
Valproate	600–1500 mg per day, as tds dosage	Occasional sedation, nausea and vomiting	Least sedating A/C drug. No liver enzyme induction. Avoid in pregnancy
Ethosuximide	250–750 mg per day, as tds dosage	Occasional sedation	Of greatest value in children and adolescents, with little effect in adults

alternatives in resistant cases are valproate and clonazepam (Table 23.24). For tonic clonic seizures, or for partial seizures alone, several drugs are appropriate. Carbamazepine is now probably the drug of choice, mainly due to its low incidence of long-term side-effects, both in children and adults. Phenytoin and phenobarbitone are alternatives. For tonic clonic seizures associated with petit mal, valproate is probably better than carbamazepine, phenytoin or phenobarbitone, but, as with other forms of epilepsy, there is considerable individual variation. Infantile spasms are usually refractory to all treatment, but ACTH and nitrazepam have been effective in some cases.

All major anticonvulsant drugs (apart from valproate) induce liver enzymes, and this is important with concurrent drug therapy including the oral contraceptive pill. Valproate, like phenytoin, is potentially teratogenic and for women in whom pregnancy is a possibility, carbamazepine or phenobarbitone are the safest drugs.

Serial epilepsy and status epilepticus

A succession of convulsions in a single day constitutes *serial epilepsy*. When fits follow each other without consciousness being regained, this is known as *status epilepticus*. Urgent treatment is necessary to stop the fits, since continuing epileptic activity leads eventually to exhaustion and cerebral damage. Initial treatment with a slow bolus of intravenous diazepam (10–30 mg) may terminate status, but its anticonvulsant action is short-lived. Further doses are likely to produce increasing sedation and the need for ventilation. A continuous infusion of diazepam may occasionally be successful. A slow bolus of clonazepam (0.5–1.5 mg) is often more effective than diazepam, due to its longer duration of action.

Chlormethiazole, given as a ready-made 8.4% solution at a rate of 20–60 ml per hour, is the treatment of choice in status, having a good therapeutic ratio. The drug has a short half-life, so that if an excessive dose is given, causing respiratory depression, the effect is short-lived. If this is ineffective, an alternative is an infusion of pentothal which is very long-lasting and which may take several days to clear from the body after stopping the drug, particularly in obese patients. When all else fails, paraldehyde (10 ml) by intramuscular injection of 5 ml into each buttock, followed at 4-hourly intervals by single 5 ml doses up to a total of 30 ml, is sometimes effective.

It is unwise to paralyse and ventilate patients in status epilepticus unless continuous EEG monitoring is available; removal of the observable manifestations of convulsive cerebral activity by paralysing the patient leaves no indication of whether the anticonvulsant treatment is being effective or not.

Partial seizures may also occur continuously (*epilepsy partialis continua*). In focal motor epilepsy, this takes the form of continuous jerking of one side, or part of one side, of the body. In psychomotor (temporal lobe) status, the patient is confused and disorientated, will appear detached and may not respond to questions, but will be conscious. An EEG is invaluable in identifying the cause of the confusion; in general the EEG is the most valuable test in confused patients without localising neurological signs.

Surgical treatment

Since epilepsy may be a symptom of a progressive cerebral lesion, surgical treatment may become part of overall therapy, but may not abolish fits. In a selected group of patients with intractable temporal lobe epilepsy, in whom it can be shown that epileptic discharges arise entirely unilaterally, a temporal lobectomy may produce a marked improvement. Histological examination of the resected temporal lobe often reveals no abnormality, but mesial temporal sclerosis and, occasionally, small benign tumours have been found.

Prognosis

With the exception of patients with progressive structural or metabolic cerebral disease, in childhood or adult life, the overall prognosis is relatively good. In one large series, 20 years after the time of initial diagnosis, about 50% of patients were free from fits and off anticonvulsant treatment; a further 20% continued to take anticonvulsants and were fit-free; and fits continued in about 30% of patients who remained on treatment. Fits are less likely to remit in patients with mental retardation, abnormal neurological signs, clustering of fits, and complex partial and grand mal seizures.

Psychiatric and social factors

In the majority of patients, the timing of fits is unpredictable and there is no, or only the briefest, warning of an impending attack. This alone may lead to social withdrawal and avoidance of public places. Patients are limited in their choice of work and may feel victimised by employers unwilling to continue their employment. There is still considerable social stigma attached to epilepsy, and this may cause difficulties in personal relationships. Psychotic disorders may develop in a few patients with complex partial seizures.

Few restrictions need to be imposed on the majority of patients. However, the law concerning epilepsy and driving is understandably cautious. A distinction is made between nocturnal and daytime fits. Patients who have had only nocturnal fits for a period of at least three years may hold a licence; patients who have had a single daytime fit may not drive for one year; in all other cases, where there have been two or more fits, the licence will be withdrawn and will not be reinstated until a period of at least two years fit-free has elapsed. Holders of Heavy Goods Vehicle licences who have fits will have their licence permanently removed. Discussion of the law and driving is an issue that often threatens the relationship between doctor and patient. It is the doctor's duty to inform the patient that he should not drive after a fit and that he should seek the advice of the licensing authorities.

NARCOLEPSY

In narcolepsy, episodes of sleep occur during the day with a prodrome of an irresistible desire to sleep. The attacks occur in inappropriate circumstances and can usually be distinguished from normal daytime post-prandial drowsiness. Narcolepsy is associated with an abnormal EEG pattern of rapid eye movement (REM) sleep, REM sleep occurring quickly during the daytime sleeping episodes. There are three associated clinical phenomena in narcolepsy.

1. *Cataplexy* is an abrupt reduction in muscle tone leading to collapse to the ground, induced by emotion, often laughter and loud noises. Consciousness is preserved and recovery usually occurs within a few minutes.

2. *Sleep paralysis* describes episodes of complete paralysis (without respiratory involvement) which occurs transiently on waking. It is usually short-lived, a few minutes at most.

3. *Hypnagogic hallucinations* are a feature in some patients. These are vivid, sometimes frightening hallucinations which occur as the patient is falling asleep.

Narcolepsy and the related symptoms are thought to be due to the abnormalities of monoaminergic pathways in the brain stem reticular-activating formation, and there is a very strong association with HLA-DR2. There is often a family history of the condition. Combination treatment with a tricyclic antidepressant and amphetamine is usually effective.

CEREBROVASCULAR DISEASE

The term cerebrovascular disease embraces:

1. disease of the cerebral arteries (atheroma being by far the commonest cause) and of the major neck vessels supplying the brain
2. disease of the heart, which may adversely affect the blood supply to the brain by changes in blood pressure and as a source of emboli
3. disorders of the blood, which may lead to impaired clotting, causing haemorrhage, hyperviscosity or hypercoagulable states, which increase the tendency to cerebral thrombosis.

Thus, in a patient presenting with a stroke, particularly younger patients, the diagnostic net must be cast wide.

Definitions

Stroke

A stroke is an acute event, in which a neurological deficit appears over minutes or a few hours, sometimes in a stepwise fashion, persists for more than 24 hours, and is presumed to be due to an impairment of the blood supply to one part of the brain. Recovery is variable, but can eventually be complete. Stroke may be due to focal cerebral infarction, spontaneous intracerebral haemorrhage, or to subarachnoid haemorrhage. Although subarachnoid haemorrhage is one type of stroke, the clinical presentation of subarachnoid haemorrhage and other types of stroke are typically quite different and usually easily distinguishable. The term 'cerebrovascular accident' has found widespread usage, but 'stroke' is preferable, not least because it is a term understood and used by both doctors and patients.

Epidemiology

Stroke is the third commonest cause of death in the UK. It has an incidence of 1–2 per 1000 population per year,

Neurological Disease

but is much higher than this in older age groups. The incidence in men is slightly higher than in women at all ages. Stroke has a prevalence of around 5 per 1000 population. It has been estimated that about 80% of strokes are due to cerebral infarction, 10% to spontaneous intracerebral haemorrhage and 10% to subarachnoid haemorrhage.

While transient ischaemic attacks (see below) are probably mainly due to emboli, the proportion of strokes which are embolic rather than thrombotic in situ remains uncertain.

Transient ischaemic attack

The term transient ischaemic attack (TIA) refers to an episode of an acute neurological deficit, of presumed vascular origin, which resolves completely within 24 hours. The resolution of symptoms and signs does not necessarily mean that infarction has not occurred; indeed, small infarcts may be identified on CT scans in patients with TIA.

Anatomy and physiology

Cerebral circulation

Figure 23.9 shows the origins of the great vessels from the aortic arch, the circle of Willis and its branches, and the areas of the brain supplied by the major intracerebral arteries. There are four branches from the terminal part of the internal carotid artery: the anterior and middle cerebrals, the anterior choroidal and the posterior communicating artery. A number of small branches are given off within the cavernous sinus. The most important of these is the

ophthalmic artery, which passes anteriorly into the orbit where it divides, the central retinal artery being one of the branches. The other branches form anastamotic connections with branches of the external carotid artery. These anastamoses are a source of an important collateral circulation, which may develop after occlusion of the internal carotid artery in the neck.

The vertebral arteries arise from the subclavian artery. The arteries join to form the basilar artery at the level of the lower pons. In addition to the terminal branches shown in Figure 23.9, the vertebral arteries give off the anterior and posterior spinal arteries.

Autoregulation

Cerebral blood flow (CBF) is maintained in the normal subject despite a wide range of blood pressures. A fall in blood pressure causes cerebral vasodilatation, and a rise produces vasoconstriction. Above a certain level, however, this autoregulation ceases and, with high enough pressures, cerebral oedema develops, eventually resulting in hypertensive encephalopathy (p. 902).

A rise in haematocrit reduces cerebral blood flow to an extent appropriate for the increase in oxygen carrying capacity, but above a packed-cell volume (PCV) of 55, the increased blood viscosity is associated with an increased risk of cerebral arterial thrombosis.

Causes of cerebrovascular disease

Atheroma

Of all the causes of cerebrovascular disease listed in Table 23.25, atheroma is by far the most important, and patients often have evidence of peripheral or coronary vascular

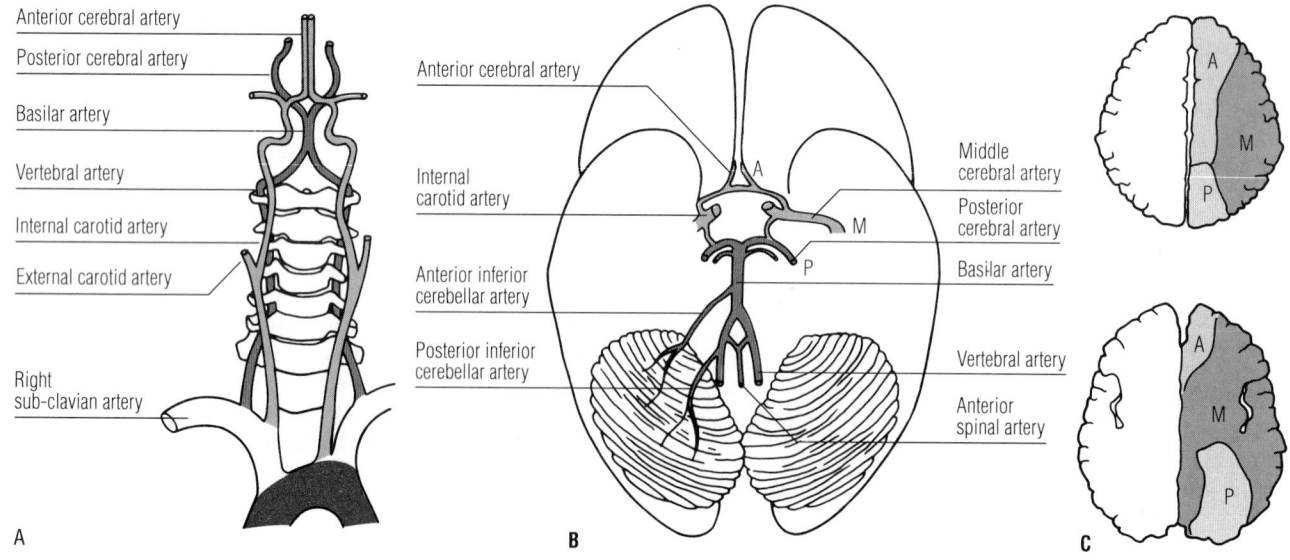

Fig. 23.9 The cerebral arterial supply. A. The origins of carotid (pale red) and vertebral (dark red) arteries are shown, as is their relationship to the cervical spine. **B.** The major branches of the circle of Willis at the base of the brain are shown. **C.** The distribution of the anterior (A), middle (M) and posterior (P) cerebral arteries are shown. In the upper diagram they are at a level above the bodies of the lateral ventricles and in the lower diagram, at the level of the internal capsule.

Table 23.25 Causes of cerebrovascular disease

Atheroma	
Hypertension	
Congenital	Aneurysms Fibromuscular dysplasia
Trauma	Injuries to the neck, e.g. whiplash, blow on the neck, cervical manipulation, angiography
Dissection	Cystic medial necrosis, atheroma, fibromuscular dysplasia, arteritis, pseudoxanthoma elasticum
Arteritis	SLE, PAN, giant cell arteritis, Wegener's, Behçet's, sarcoid
Infection	Secondary to bacterial, mycobacterial, or fungal infection, and syphilis Tonsilitis, pharyngitis, cervical lymphadenitis
Irradiation of the neck	
Malignant disease with direct arterial wall invasion	
Haematological disease	Polycythaemia rubra vera Idiopathic thrombocytopenic purpura (ITP) Leukaemia Sickle cell disease Severe anaemia Myeloma Waldenström's macroglobulinaemia
Prolonged hypotension	Infarction in watershed areas Infarction in territory of pre-existing vessel atheroma

disease. The coexistence of cerebral and peripheral vascular disease is emphasised by the fact that a patient presenting with a first stroke is as likely to have a myocardial infarction in future as a further stroke. Atheroma tends to be most marked at branch points in the major vessels and in the carotid syphon. In relation to the cerebral circulation, the origins of the arteries from the aorta, brachiocephalic trunk and subclavian artery, the carotid bifurcation, the basilar artery and the origins of the anterior, middle and posterior cerebral arteries are all sites for atheroma formation.

Atheroma may cause stenosis or complete obstruction, but thrombus commonly forms on atheromatous plaques in the absence of any haemodynamically significant stenosis. Fragments of thrombus may then break off and become lodged in a smaller artery distally. Partial obstruction or rapid lysis may lead to prompt restoration of the circulation producing the clinical picture of a TIA, but infarction results if the circulation is interrupted for more than a few minutes. Alternatively, thrombus forming on an atheromatous plaque causing stenosis may lead to complete obstruction in situ. The presence of bruits in the neck and supraclavicular fossa indicates arterial stenosis, but partial stenosis may occur without thrombo-embolism or any significant haemodynamic effects. The natural history of asymptomatic carotid bruits is still controversial, but recent studies suggest that it is more benign than previously thought.

Other causes of cerebral embolism

There are numerous other causes of cerebral embolism apart from atheroma in the great vessels (Table 23.26). Emboli or local occlusion of the intracerebral vessels may each present with either a TIA or a stroke; it is often impossible to distinguish between local thrombosis and embolism.

Table 23.26 Causes of cerebral embolism

Atheromatous disease affecting large neck and intracranial vessels		
Large aneurysms of arteries, with mural thrombus		
Cardiac		
Endocarditis of mitral or aortic valve		
Left atrium	– Mural thrombosis with AF – Myxoma	
Left ventricle	– Mural thrombus after myocardial infarction – Mural thrombus with cardiomyopathy	
Cardiac surgery	– Air embolism	
Paradoxical embolism	– Patent foramen ovale – ASD	
Prosthetic aortic or mitral valve thrombus		
Marantic endocarditis		

Risk factors

The most important risk factor for stroke (Table 23.27) is hypertension. Recent studies have clearly shown that both smoking and alcohol are risk factors.

Table 23.27 Risk factors for TIA and stroke

• Hypertension	• Previous TIA

• Cardiac disease
  Ischaemic heart disease
  Causes of embolism
  (Table 23.26)
	• Cervical bruit
	• Hyperlipidaemia
	• Raised haematocrit
	• Raised plasma fibrinogen

• Peripheral vascular disease	• Alcohol
• Diabetes	• Oral contraceptive pill, particularly
• Smoking	in smokers

TRANSIENT ISCHAEMIC ATTACKS

Transient ischaemic attacks (TIA) are generally considered to be due to embolism and this seems the most likely explanation, particularly when repeated stereotyped episodes occur. The proportion of TIA caused by emboli arising from the heart has probably been overestimated in the past; a recent estimate is 5–10%.

Clinical features

Carotid territory TIA

Transient ischaemia in the carotid territory usually produces a contralateral hemiparesis (with or without hemisensory or hemianopic disturbance), and dysphasia if the dominant hemisphere is affected. Attacks last from a few minutes to several hours; by definition, all symptoms and signs have resolved within 24 hours. Amaurosis fugax is the term used to describe transient monocular blindness. It is most often caused by embolism of the retinal circulation, but similar transient loss of vision may occasionally occur in glaucoma, or with papilloedema, retrobulbar neuritis, orbital tumours, retinal haemorrhage and retinal detachment.

Vertebrobasilar TIA

In the vertebrobasilar territory, TIA may cause vertigo, diplopia, visual blurring or loss (due to occipital cortical ischaemia), facial paraesthesiae and numbness (often circumoral and bilateral), facial weakness, dysarthria, dysphagia and dysphonia, nausea and vomiting, ataxia, hemiparesis or tetraparesis, and hemisensory or four-limb sensory impairment. There is frequently impairment or loss of consciousness. It is an error to make a diagnosis of vertebrobasilar TIA on the basis of dizziness alone, in the absence of other symptoms suggesting a brain stem lesion. Isolated dizziness on head movement is most likely due to a peripheral vestibular lesion. On rare occasions, with vertebral artery stenosis, neck movement (particularly extension), may further impair blood flow by cervical compression, leading to a vertebrobasilar TIA.

Subclavian steal syndrome

Subclavian steal syndrome is rare and is due to subclavian stenosis proximal to the origin of the vertebral artery. During exercise of the arm, there is peripheral vasodilatation and blood flows retrogradely from the vertebral artery into the subclavian artery, causing vertebrobasilar ischaemia. There is usually a substantial reduction in blood pressure on the side of the subclavian stenosis, and a palpable difference between the pulses in the two arms.

Examination

It is rare to witness a TIA, and patients seen between attacks will have no neurological signs, apart from, occasionally, a cervical bruit. General examination is directed towards identifying associated factors such as hypertension, peripheral vascular disease and cardiac abnormalities. During an attack of amaurosis fugax, emboli can occasionally be seen in the retinal arterioles; platelet emboli are white, cholesterol emboli are yellowish.

Investigation

Investigations for TIA and stroke are listed in Table 23.28. CT scanning is of little value in patients with TIA. However, in a patient with a potential cardiac source of emboli, CT scanning may show evidence of previous silent cerebral infarction which, particularly if bilateral, increases the likelihood of TIA being embolic. The indication for angiography is considered below.

Table 23.28 Investigation of TIA and stroke

- Full blood count, ESR
- Urea and electrolytes, MSU
- Glucose tolerance test
- Chest X-ray
- ECG
- In selected patients, CT scan, echocardiography, angiography

Treatment and prognosis

Further TIA may be prevented by identifying and minimising the risk factors for stroke. The risk of further stroke is about 5% per annum, and that of fatal myocardial infarction, of the same order. Only recently has the relatively low incidence of further stroke after TIA been fully recognised. The benefit of potentially hazardous surgical procedures needs to be compared with this relatively benign natural history.

Hypertension remains the major risk factor for stroke and, if persistent, requires treatment. Diabetes should be controlled, smoking stopped, and weight reduced if necessary. There is no firm evidence that treatment of hyperlipidaemia decreases the risk of further stroke, but gross familial hyperlipidaemia in young patients must be treated.

Anticoagulants

The use of anticoagulants for prevention of TIA has been shown to be of no value and is potentially dangerous. However, when a continuing cardiac cause of emboli can be identified, anticoagulant therapy is indicated. Prosthetic valves remain the main indication. Atrial fibrillation on its own is not sufficient ground for starting anticoagulants, but documentation of a changing rhythm may be, since emboli are then more likely to be released, particularly when atrial fibrillation reverts to sinus rhythm. Patients with acute myocardial infarction and mural thrombus causing emboli should be anticoagulated for six months. It is best to do a CT scan before starting warfarin after a TIA thought to be due to an embolus from the heart. A normal neurological examination does not exclude the possibility of a small area of infarction, and if this is present anticoagulation therapy may exacerbate the situation by turning an ischaemic cerebral infarct into a haemorrhagic infarct (p. 900).

Surgery

Carotid endarterectomy has not been shown to improve the prognosis in TIA and has associated morbidity and mortality. Many surgeons have now abandoned the operation. Similarly, external carotid internal carotid by-pass to overcome stenosis or occlusion does not offer long-term benefit to the great majority of patients with TIA. Given the lack of clear indication for these two operations, there is no need for carotid angiography, which carries its own morbidity. The non-invasive test of carotid ultrasound

Fig. 23.10 Acute cerebral infarction. **A.** There is an extensive right cerebral hemisphere infarct in this patient, scanned 24 hours after the onset of a complete left hemiparesis with left hemisensory loss and a left homonymous hemianopia. An ill-defined area of low attenuation, occupying most of the right hemisphere, is not causing midline shift, but there is obliteration of the overlying sulci, indicating cerebral oedema. **B.** Acute left occipital infarction, showing some mass effect.

can be used to provide diagnostic information about the anatomy of the carotid bifurcation.

Anti-platelet therapy

Drugs reducing platelet aggregation in vitro include sulphinpyrazone, dipyridamole and aspirin. Of these, only aspirin (150–300 mg daily) has a proven preventive action in vivo; it reduces the incidence of non-fatal stroke and myocardial infarction by about 25% and of all vascular deaths by about 15%.

STROKES DUE TO CEREBRAL INFARCTION

The causes of cerebral infarction are the same as for TIA, but it is generally considered that fewer strokes than TIA have an embolic basis. Most cerebral infarcts swell during the first few days after the acute event with surrounding oedema (Fig. 23.10). Large infarcts may exert considerable mass effect, sometimes causing life-threatening herniation at the tentorium. Cerebral oedema is usually at its most severe at 4–7 days after infarction and then gradually resolves over 2–4 weeks (Fig. 23.11).

There is always a possibility that an ischaemic infarct may become haemorrhagic. This is most likely if the infarct is due to an embolus which is then cleared at an early stage,

Fig. 23.11 **A mature cerebral infarct, in the distribution of the right middle cerebral artery.** The infarct has a lower attenuation than adjacent normal brain, there is no mass effect, and there is a clear line of demarcation between infarct and normal brain.

allowing blood under arterial pressure to enter the fresh infarct. An infarct may also become haemorrhagic due to the collateral blood supply at the boundaries of the infarct.

Clinical features

The cardinal clinical feature of a stroke is its abrupt onset. Occasionally, there is a slow worsening over hours, or a stepwise deterioration in function over a day or two (stroke in evolution). Strokes vary enormously in both their severity and the combination of symptoms and signs. When occlusion of a major cerebral artery occurs, the extent of infarction will depend on the degree of collateral blood supply. For example, occlusion of the internal carotid artery, either at the carotid bifurcation or in the syphon (the two common sites for atheroma formation in the carotid), may cause no deficit at all if the circle of Willis is complete and flow through the other carotid and vertebrals is sufficient.

Major cerebral vessel occlusion syndromes

Middle cerebral artery occlusion

Middle cerebral artery and internal carotid artery occlusion may be indistinguishable clinically, and the extent of infarction after either is very variable. Preceding amaurosis fugax may indicate either internal carotid artery occlusion or embolic occlusion of the middle cerebral artery. The middle cerebral artery is also the most frequent vessel occluded by emboli from the heart. However, the majority of middle cerebral artery territory strokes are probably due to thrombosis of the main trunk of the middle cerebral artery or its branches.

The usual deficit after middle cerebral artery occlusion is a contralateral hemiparesis, affecting the arm more than the leg, due to infarction of the internal capsule. When the dominant hemisphere is affected, dysphasia is usually expressive more than receptive. Contralateral homonymous hemianopia and a mild contralateral hemisensory loss may also be present.

Anterior cerebral artery occlusion

Unilateral occlusion of the anterior cerebral artery results in contralateral hemiparesis and hemisensory loss, in which the leg is often more severely affected than the arm. Occlusion of the recurrent artery of Heubner, supplying the anterior limb of the internal capsule, causes contralateral facial weakness and a monoparesis of the contralateral upper limb. After anterior cerebral artery occlusion in the dominant hemisphere, there may be an expressive dysphasia; and, in either hemisphere, there may be marked motor dyspraxia, causing particular difficulty in walking.

Anterior choroidal artery occlusion

The anterior choroidal artery arises either from the terminal carotid or from the proximal part of the middle cerebral artery and is very variable in size and importance. It may supply the optic tract, the middle third of the cerebral peduncle, the lateral geniculate nucleus and the internal capsule, as well as the choroid plexus in the lateral ventricle. Occlusion of this vessel alone may produce a deficit indistinguishable from middle cerebral artery occlusion.

Infarction of the brain stem and cerebellum

Ischaemic lesions in the posterior circulation, due to vertebral, basilar, or branch artery occlusions, are very variable in extent. There are many described discrete syndromes but, in clinical practice, the deficit in a particular patient usually does not correspond exactly to one of these. It is usually sufficient to recognise the major area of infarction within the brain stem.

Infarction of the medulla

Hemiparesis, tetraparesis or triparesis with lower cranial nerve palsies may occur after vertebral artery occlusion, together with disturbances of breathing and cardiovascular control due to involvement of the medullary reticular formation. Respiratory irregularities, apnoea, hypotension or hypertension, and a number of cardiac arrhythmias may result.

Posterior inferior cerebellar artery occlusion (Wallenberg syndrome, lateral medullary infarction)

The posterior inferior cerebellar artery (PICA) occlusion syndrome is as often due to vertebral occlusion as to occlusion of the PICA. The clinical syndrome is striking, and occurs sufficiently frequently to be recognisable as a separate entity. Reference to the anatomy of the medulla provides an understanding of the deficit produced (Fig. 23.12). Symptoms usually consist of ipsilateral facial paraesthesiae or pain due to involvement of the spinal nucleus and tract of the trigeminal nerve, severe vertigo and vomiting due to involvement of the vestibular nucleus and its medullary connections, dysphagia, dysphonia, ataxia and contralateral limb sensory impairment.

Examination reveals an ipsilateral Horner's syndrome from involvement of descending sympathetic fibres in the medullary reticular formation, horizontal nystagmus towards the side of the cerebellar lesion, ipsilateral trigeminal pain and temperature sensory impairment. There is also, occasionally, an ipsilateral lower motor neurone facial palsy, ipsilateral palatal, vocal cord, pharyngeal and lingual palsies (which may cause severe dysphagia), ipsilateral limb ataxia, and, sometimes, ataxia of gait. In addition, there is a contralateral spinothalamic limb and trunk sensory impairment. Rarely, there is a contralateral hemiparesis, but this only occurs with extensive infarcts.

Pontine infarction

Pontine infarction, due to basilar artery thrombosis, is often fatal. The signs are coma, quadriplegia, multiple cranial

Sympathetic fibres	Ipsilateral Horner's syndrome
Vagal nucleus	Dysphagia, dysphonia
Vestibular nucleus	Vertigo
Hypoglossal nucleus	Ipsilateral tongue palsy
Spinal nucleus of trigeminal nerve	Ipsilateral pain and temperature facial sensory loss
Ventral spinocerebellar tract	Ipsilateral limb cerebellar ataxia
Lateral spinothalamic tract	Contralateral limb and trunk pain and temperature loss

Fig. 23.12 Lateral medullary syndrome (Wallenberg syndrome), due to occlusion of either posterior inferior cerebellar artery or vertebral artery. The red area shows the usual extent of infarction. The structures affected and the symptoms and signs which result are shown.

nerve signs (usually involving gaze palsies), nystagmus, facial paralysis and cardiorespiratory abnormalities. Bilateral infarction of the basis pontis, with relative sparing of the more dorsal parts of the pons, results in quadriplegia and, often, anarthria, and jaw, facial, palatal and tongue paralysis with preservation of consciousness. This is the so-called 'locked-in' syndrome, in which patients are only able to communicate with movement of the eyes.

Paramedian infarction of the pons causes patchy damage, involving the pyramidal tracts, pontine cranial nerve nuclei and fibres passing to the middle cerebellar peduncle.

In lateral infarction of the pons, the trigeminal nucleus, medial lemniscus and the middle cerebellar peduncle are mainly affected, with some involvement of the pyramidal tract to the legs more than to the arms.

In tegmental infarction of the pons, the trigeminal, abducens and facial nuclei, together with the medial longitudinal fasciculus and superior cerebellar peduncle, are affected; this causes a variety of conjugate gaze palsies, ipsilateral trigeminal, abducens and facial lower motor neurone lesions, and ipsilateral cerebellar signs.

Midbrain infarction

Midbrain infarction occurring alone is unusual. Syndromes of ipsilateral third nerve palsy with contralateral hemiparesis (Weber's syndrome) and ipsilateral third nerve palsy with contralateral cerebellar signs (syndrome of Benedikt) are described, but are rare. Superior cerebellar artery thrombosis causing infarction of the midbrain-pontine junction leads to an ipsilateral Horner's syndrome, ipsilateral nystagmus and cerebellar signs, ipsilateral lower motor neurone facial weakness, contralateral spinothalamic sensory loss in the limbs, and, sometimes, Parkinsonian signs from involvement of connections to the substantia nigra.

Cerebellar infarction

Pure cerebellar infarction probably occurs only rarely; most infarcts also involve the brain stem, although cerebellar signs predominate.

Posterior cerebral artery occlusion

The posterior cerebral arteries supply the upper part of the midbrain, the cerebral peduncles, parts of the thalamus and the subthalamic nuclei, as well as the occipital lobes. Thus, although homonymous visual field defects predominate in posterior cerebral artery occlusion, hemiparesis, sensory disturbances and, occasionally, hemiballismus (p. 918) may also occur. In addition to the primary visual cortex, the more anteriorly placed association cortex may also be damaged. Patients with extensive lesions here may deny being blind (Anton's syndrome); they will describe objects incorrectly and may wrongly be thought to be confused. Posterior cerebral artery occlusion may lead to infarction as anteriorly as the angular gyrus; this causes Gerstmann's syndrome, which comprises right-left disorientation, finger agnosia, dyscalculia, dyslexia and dysgraphia.

Thalamic pain is a rare consequence of stroke. It arises from infarction of the lateral part of the thalamus. Thalamic stroke causes contralateral sensory loss, often with only a mild hemiparesis. The pain may come on weeks or months later and is usually continuous, severe and chronic; it has a burning quality, often with associated cutaneous hyperaesthesiae. Treatment with antidepressants, benzo-

---

Summary 4   Stroke

- Cerebral infarction causes about four times as many strokes as cerebral haemorrhage.

- Probably only a small minority of cerebral infarcts are caused by emboli from the heart. Very few patients require anticoagulants to prevent further strokes.

- Primary intracerebral haemorrhage may cause strokes which are clinically indistinguishable from cerebral infarction, but impairment of conscious level and signs of raised intracranial pressure are more common with large haemorrhages.

- Secondary prevention of cerebral infarction includes treatment of hypertension, diabetes and severe hyperlipidaemia if present, weight loss, cessation of smoking and low-dose aspirin.

- Unusual causes of stroke are more common in younger patients.

diazepines or anticonvulsants is occasionally successful. Thalamic electrical stimulation may give partial relief.

Lacunar infarcts

Lacunar infarction refers to small deep infarcts in the region of the internal capsule, the basal ganglia and the thalamus (Fig. 23.13). These are often multiple. The deficit from such strokes is usually mild. Lacunar infarction is most common in hypertension but also occurs in normotensive subjects. Lacunae are thought to be caused by occlusion of small branch arteries, or by microaneurysm formation (Charcot-Bouchard aneurysms) followed by rupture, producing a small haematoma which resolves leaving an area of infarction. The common lacunar syndromes are listed in Table 23.29.

Fig. 23.13 CT scan showing bilateral small lacunar infarcts in the internal capsule.

Table 23.29 Common lacunar syndromes

Type	Clinical features	Lesion
Pure motor stroke	Partial hemiparesis	Internal capsule
Pure sensory stroke	Partial hemisensory impairment	Internal capsule
Hemiparesis with ataxia	Partial hemiparesis Ataxia of cerebellar type Dysarthria	Internal capsule or pons

Diffuse small vessel disease

The third, least common pattern of ischaemic cerebrovascular disease is diffuse small vessel disease. It is more frequent in hypertensive patients. The typical presentation is difficulty in walking and dementia, which is usually progressive. There is sometimes urinary incontinence. Examination reveals intellectual impairment, often with prominent primitive reflexes, and bilateral pyramidal tract signs which affect the cranial nerve nuclei as well as the limbs. There is a brisk jaw jerk, dysarthria (of spastic type), and dysphagia (the lower cranial nerve signs constituting a pseudo-bulbar palsy). The signs in the limbs are often asymmetrical, with little or no sensory impairment. The gait is characteristically small-paced, unsteady and slow, the so-called 'marche à petit pas'. It can mimic a Parkinsonian gait.

CT scanning (Fig. 23.14) shows a variable degree of cortical atrophy and a characteristic diffuse periventricular low attenuation indicating deep white matter loss (sometimes known as Binswanger's disease).

Fig. 23.14 Diffuse small vessel disease. These four scans show cerebral atrophy, with well-marked low attenuation diffusely in the subcortical white matter surrounding the ventricles. (Reproduced by permission of Dr J Stevens and Dr A Valentine.)

Multi-infarct dementia

Patients presenting with a history of progressive dementia are sometimes found to have multiple cerebral infarcts of differing size. They usually have physical signs corresponding to some, if not all, of the lesions (Fig. 23.15).

Fig. 23.15 Multiple bilateral cerebral infarcts in a middle-aged man with a history of coronary artery and peripheral vascular disease.

Other patterns of cerebrovascular disease

Cerebral infarction may rarely result from vasospasm in migraine. It is advisable to avoid ergotamine in patients with migraine in whom symptoms and signs of neurological deficit occur.

Prolonged severe hypotension (e.g. after cardiac arrest) may lead to focal cerebral infarction even with normal cerebral vessels, although diffuse cortical damage is more common. Patients with pre-existing cerebral arterial narrowing are particularly at risk.

Watershed infarction most commonly affects the boundary parieto-occipital area between anterior, middle and posterior cerebral artery territories.

Investigation

Basic investigation of cerebral infarction is essentially the same as for TIA. In elderly patients, investigation may be inappropriate.

CT scan. Not all patients with strokes require a CT scan, the indications for which are:

1. *Young patients.* Although there may be a history of a single clinical event, a higher proportion of strokes in young people are caused by embolism; CT scanning may reveal previous clinically silent infarcts.
2. *Uncertain diagnosis of infarction.* Haemorrhage, tumour, subdural haematoma or cerebral abscess may mimic a stroke.
3. *Inadequate history.*
4. *Suspected hydrocephalus.* Strokes in the vertebrobasilar territory in which there is subsequent deterioration in conscious level suggests the development of hydrocephalus.
5. To help distinguish primary intracerebral haemorrhage from subarachnoid haemorrhage.
6. *Continuing clinical deterioration* following an apparent stroke.

It is important to recognise that acute infarcts may not cause CT scan abnormalities for 1–2 days; cerebral oedema, maximal within the first week of infarction, may give rise to appearances mimicking a tumour.

Angiography has a significant morbidity and is necessary in very few patients. It may be indicated in young patients with stroke in whom a congenital vascular anomaly is suspected; in addition, it will occasionally confirm a diagnosis of cerebral embolism. The indications for angiography after intracerebral haemorrhage and subarachnoid haemorrhage are considered below.

Examination of the CSF is usually unhelpful and can be dangerous. Positive syphilitic serology is an indication for examination of the CSF, but this can be done as a planned later investigation.

Differential diagnosis of cerebral infarction

The abrupt onset of a neurological deficit, often with a distribution corresponding to a single vessel territory, and with a tendency to slowly improve, usually leaves little doubt about the diagnosis of a stroke. Other diagnoses should be considered when the history is atypical, inadequate or unreliable. These include:

1. chronic subdural haematoma, sometimes bilateral
2. cerebral abscess
3. encephalitis (particularly due to Herpes simplex)
4. cerebral tumour.

Other conditions may occasionally produce stroke-like presentations, including demyelinating disease, cerebral venous thrombosis and acute hypoglycaemia.

Complications of cerebral infarction

The complications of cerebral infarction are listed in Table 23.30. Death from the stroke itself usually occurs within the first two weeks. Pneumonia is an early and sometimes fatal complication. Incontinence, a poor prognostic feature, is associated with recurrent urinary tract infections.

Table 23.30 Complications of cerebral infarction

Neuropsychiatric	Renal and metabolic
Cerebral oedema (early)	Urinary infection
Epilepsy (late)	Renal failure
Spasticity	Dehydration
Contractures, frozen shoulder,	Electrolyte abnormalities
shoulder subluxation	SIADH (early)
Depression	Hyperglycaemia/diabetes (early)
Incontinence	
	Skin
Respiratory and cardiovascular	Pressure sores
Neurogenic pulmonary oedema	
(early)	**General**
Cardiac arrhythmias (early)	Weight loss
Pneumonia	Weight gain
DVT	Malnutrition
Pulmonary embolism	Dependent oedema

Treatment

Acute treatment

Many medical treatments, including anticoagulants, putative cerebral vasodilators, haemodilution, dextran, hyperbaric oxygen, hypercapnia and hypocapnia, have been advocated as measures which may improve the prognosis of acute cerebral infarction. However, none has been proven to be of benefit in adequate clinical trials.

Dexamethasone. There is some evidence that reducing cerebral oedema with dexamethasone may enable some patients to survive. However, life-threatening cerebral oedema is associated with large infarcts, so that the quality of survival in the few patients who may be saved in this way is poor.

Anticoagulation. There is no place for routine anticoagulation in stroke, except in patients in whom a cardiac source for emboli is certain, or strongly suspected. It is common in patients presenting with stroke to see atrial fibrillation, but this is not sufficient ground for recommending anticoagulation.

For patients with a cerebral infarct who have a cardiac lesion likely to be the source of an embolus, the timing of anticoagulation is problematical. Immediate anticoagulation carries a risk of turning a soft cerebral infarct into a haemorrhagic one, but, against this, is the possibility of further cerebral embolism. This issue has not yet been the subject of a proper clinical trial. A reasonable course is to wait 10 days after the onset of the stroke before starting oral anticoagulation. The duration of anticoagulant therapy will vary, from a few weeks after an embolus from a mural thrombus, to lifelong treatment for an embolus due to rheumatic mitral or aortic valve disease.

Cerebral emboli occurring during the course of acute bacterial endocarditis or subacute endocarditis are usually considered to be a contraindication to anticoagulants; this is because of the high risk of haemorrhage from mycotic aneurysms, which are formed from spread of infection from the embolus into the vessel wall.

Hypotensive treatment. Many patients presenting with stroke have transient high blood pressures on admission. However, a sustained diastolic pressure of 110 mmHg or more is an indication for hypotensive treatment.

Surgery. At present, there is no clear evidence that carotid endarterectomy or other surgical procedures are beneficial in the treatment of stroke.

Rehabilitation

The mainstay of treatment after strokes from all causes is rehabilitation. This involves nursing and medical staff, physiotherapists, occupational therapists and speech therapists. Even in patients with considerable residual deficit, return home is often possible with sufficient support.

Secondary prevention

As for TIA, secondary prevention after stroke involves minimising exposure to risk factors.

Prognosis

Most patients show some recovery after cerebral infarction, but this is very variable and difficult to predict. In general, the more severe the initial deficit, the less complete will be the eventual recovery. Certain features are of poor prognostic significance; these include impaired consciousness, incontinence and sustained lateral deviation of gaze. About 20% of all patients with strokes due to cerebral infarction die within the first month, and the long-term death rate is about 5–10% per annum. These late deaths are as likely to be due to myocardial infarction as to further stroke.

STROKES DUE TO PRIMARY INTRACEREBRAL HAEMORRHAGE

Aetiology

The causes of spontaneous intracerebral haemorrhage are listed in Table 23.31. Haemorrhage is most commonly due to hypertension or intracerebral extension of bleeding from a berry aneurysm. Subarachnoid haemorrhage is considered separately below. Cerebral infarction is at least four times as common as haemorrhage as the cause of stroke. Although haemorrhage without hypertension occurs, haemorrhage with hypertension is much more common. Many cerebral haemorrhages are thought to arise from Charcot-Bouchard microaneurysms, situated deep in the cerebral hemispheres, cerebellar hemispheres and pons. Haemorrhage situated superficially in the cerebral hemi-

Table 23.31 Causes of spontaneous intracerebral haemorrhage

- **Hypertension**
- **Cerebrovascular disease without hypertension**
- **Subarachnoid haemorrhage**
- **Arteriovenous malformations** (alone, or as part of Sturge-Weber syndrome*)
- Other cerebrovascular disease: Mycotic aneurysms
  Cortical thrombophlebitis
  Capillary haemangiomas
  Haemorrhagic telangiectasia**
  Cavernous haemangiomas
  Haemangioblastomas***
  Congophilic (amyloid) angiopathy

- Cerebral tumours
- Haematological disease: Thrombocytopenia from any cause
  Haemophilia
  Sickle cell disease
  Iatrogenic – anticoagulants
  – cytotoxic drugs

Common causes are shown in bold type.
* Sturge-Weber syndrome – AVM with ipsilateral trigeminal cutaneous capillary angioma ('port-wine' stain).
** Osler-Rendu-Weber syndrome – haemorrhagic telangiectasia in brain and retina
*** Von Hippel-Lindau disease – CNS haemangioblastomas, particularly in cerebellum, brain stem and spinal cord, with retinal haemangioblastomas, renal or pancreatic cysts, hypernephroma and adrenal tumours.

spheres is more likely to be due to one of the less common causes of haemorrhage.

Surrounding oedema develops within a few hours of cerebral haemorrhage; this exacerbates the space-occupying effect, which is much greater with haemorrhage than with infarction. Extension of a cerebral haemorrhage into the lateral ventricle carries a worse prognosis.

Clinical features

The clinical presentation of cerebral hemisphere haemorrhage is often indistinguishable from cerebral infarction. However, because intracranial pressure is more likely to be raised with haemorrhage, severe headache, vomiting and impairment of consciousness are more common with haemorrhage. The presence of meningism indicates blood in the subarachnoid space, and therefore haemorrhage extending either from an intracerebral haemorrhage or from a primary subarachnoid source.

Haemorrhage in the cerebellum produces a typical presentation of ataxia, headache and vomiting, often with vertigo. This is followed by progressive impairment of the conscious level, resulting both from brain stem compression directly due to the haematoma, and from hydrocephalus due to obstruction of CSF flow through the aqueduct of Sylvius (Fig. 23.28). It is important to recognise this, since the results of surgical removal of such haemorrhages are often good, and failure to relieve hydrocephalus may be fatal.

Pontine haemorrhage usually causes rapid loss of consciousness, a quadriplegia, multiple brain stem signs, and is usually fatal.

The recovery from spontaneous intracerebral haemorrhage (excluding subarachnoid haemorrhage), is not as good as from infarction. Mortality during the first few weeks is considerably greater than for infarction.

Investigation

Patients with a stroke and meningism should have a CT scan. Other patients, without meningism but with impairment of consciousness, should also have a scan, since some will be found to have had a haemorrhage. The CT scan is helpful in defining the exact site of a haemorrhage, and contrast enhanced scans may demonstrate an arteriovenous malformation or a tumour.

Angiography is only an appropriate investigation if aneurysm, arteriovenous malformation or some other cerebral vascular abnormality is suspected.

Treatment

Treatment is essentially supportive in the acute stage. Surgical evacuation of large cerebral hemisphere haematomas is sometimes undertaken in patients whose condition is deteriorating. Evacuation of cerebellar haematomas with progressive hydrocephalus is essential. Dexamethasone may reduce cerebral oedema. However, as with infarction, its benefit has not been proven in controlled trials, and one

may be saving the lives of those destined to be the most severely disabled in the long term.

Subarachnoid haemorrhage

The majority of spontaneous subarachnoid haemorrhages are caused by berry aneurysms which develop at proximal branch points in the major cerebral vessels at the base of the brain. The common sites are the bifurcation of the middle cerebral artery, the terminal carotid, the anterior cerebral artery and the posterior communicating artery. Basilar artery aneurysms are uncommon. Aneurysms are sometimes multiple. Although mainly congenital, aneurysms may develop as a result of degenerative and hypertensive changes. Subarachnoid haemorrhage can occur at any age, but is a particularly important cause of death and disability in the 20–40 year age group. In a minority of cases, the other causes listed in Table 23.31 may be responsible. In about 10% of patients, no cause for the haemorrhage is found.

Clinical features

The typical history of subarachnoid haemorrhage is severe headache of abrupt onset accompanied by neck pain and stiffness, and vomiting. Drowsiness is common, and there is often confusion and impairment of consciousness. Some patients will be deeply unconscious at presentation. In such patients, neck stiffness may be absent.

Focal hemisphere signs may be present, due either to intracerebral bleeding or to vasospasm, which may affect the aneurysm bearing vessel or other vessels. A third cranial nerve palsy (due to direct compression) occurs commonly with posterior communicating artery aneurysms and, less commonly, with carotid and middle cerebral artery aneurysms.

There may be papilloedema and subhyaloid haemorrhages, seen only in subarachnoid haemorrhage.

Investigation

If the patient is conscious, without focal hemisphere signs, a lumbar puncture is performed to establish the diagnosis. If done within eight hours of the haemorrhage, the CSF may not contain blood, though the pressure is usually raised. Xanthochromia – the yellowish discolouration of the supernatant CSF in a spun sample, due to haemoglobin breakdown products – does not develop for at least 24 hours. The CSF in subarachnoid haemorrhage is often obviously uniformly blood-stained. Cell counts of CSF in three separate bottles distinguishes a traumatic tap from true subarachnoid haemorrhage.

It is potentially hazardous to perform a lumbar puncture in an unconscious patient or one with focal hemisphere signs. In each case, it is likely that there is an intracerebral haematoma, with an increased supratentorial intracranial pressure. CT scanning demonstrates even quite small quantities of subarachnoid blood (Fig. 23.16), and also intracerebral blood if present.

23.16 Extensive subarachnoid haemorrhage from an anterior communicating artery aneurysm. In these unenhanced scans, blood (showing as a dense white image) is present in the interhemispheric fissure anteriorly, the Sylvian fissures, the IIIrd ventricle, the body of the right lateral ventricle and the posterior parts of both lateral ventricles.

Angiography is contraindicated in stuporose or comatose patients, but should be done at an early stage if the patient is fit enough, because of risk of re-bleeding (maximal between 7 and 14 days). Many of those not fit enough initially will improve over a few days, and angiography can then be undertaken with reasonable safety (Fig. 23.17).

Patients may deteriorate after subarachnoid haemorrhage, due to re-bleeding, vasospasm, or hydrocephalus. CT scanning will often identify the cause.

Treatment and prognosis

Many aneurysms are accessible to surgical treatment by clipping. However, many, perhaps 30–40% of all patients with subarachnoid haemorrhage from aneurysms, do not survive for more than a few hours, and some will never reach hospital alive. A further 30% of patients die within the first month; the remainder survive with a re-bleed risk of about 2% per annum, unless the aneurysm can be successfully clipped.

Arteriovenous malformations

Arteriovenous malformations (AVM) tend to bleed from the venous side. Haemorrhage terminates at an earlier stage, probably because the pressure is lower, and the clinical effects are often less severe than bleeding from aneurysms. There can be episodes of bleeding over a period of many years, causing a relatively mild neurological deficit. Epilepsy is common with AVM. The diagnosis can be made on an enhanced CT scan, but the definitive test is an angiogram (Fig. 23.18). Many AVM, due to their deep situation and extent, are best left alone. Others are amenable to partial, or sometimes total, excision. Embolisation of feeding vessels offers an alternative method of treatment but, as with surgery, this often carries an unacceptable risk of producing a major deficit due to infarction of surrounding normal brain.

Hypertensive encephalopathy

The encephalopathy resulting from severe hypertension is characterised by coma, fits and a very high blood pressure, in excess of 220/130 mmHg. Papilloedema is invariably present. There is cerebral oedema and multiple small cerebral haemorrhages.

Reduction of the blood pressure is essential (Ch. 13) and recovery is often surprisingly rapid and complete. Gradual reduction of the blood pressure over a few hours is preferable to an abrupt lowering, which is more likely to lead to ischaemia and infarction.

Fig. 23.17 Left carotid angiogram showing an anterior cerebral artery aneurysm.

Fig. 23.18 Arteriovenous malformation. A. CT scans showing an acute left frontal cerebral haemorrhage, with surrounding oedema. **B.** Left carotid angiogram in the same patient, showing an extensive arteriovenous malformation.

DEMENTIA

Dementia means a progressive impairment of cognitive function. This is usually global, affecting all higher cerebral functions, but it may be relatively selective, particularly in the early stages. A number of important psychiatric diseases may mimic dementia (Ch. 11), the condition most often leading to diagnostic difficulty being depression.

Causes of dementia

A diagnosis of dementia should always lead to a search for a potentially treatable cause (Table 23.32). A useful general clinical rule is that patients have an organic basis for their dementia if they also have abnormal neurological signs. However, in Alzheimer's disease (the commonest cause of dementia), mental symptoms and signs invariably precede the physical signs, usually by months or years.

It is probably best to consider dementia as a whole, rather than subdivide the condition into senile and presenile on the basis of age. The younger the patient, the less likely it is that Alzheimer's disease is the cause.

Table 23.32 Causes of dementia

Cause	Examples
Degenerative	Alzheimer's disease Pick's disease Huntington's chorea Multisystem atrophy Steele-Richardson syndrome Friedreich's ataxia and other spinocerebellar degenerations Some patients with Parkinson's disease
Vascular	Multiple cerebral infarcts Diffuse small vessel disease
Toxic	Alcohol/lead/carbon monoxide poisoning/Wilson's disease
Drugs	Hypnotics, tranquillisers, barbiturates, neuroleptics
Trauma	Head injury, including subdural haematoma
Neoplastic	Frontal tumours, multiple metastases Posterior fossa tumour with hydrocephalus
Hydrocephalus	Tumour Normal pressure hydrocephalus
Infection	TB meningitis, syphilis, encephalitis, toxoplasmosis, SSPE, PML, AIDS-related dementia, kuru, CJD
Inflammatory	MS, SLE, sarcoidosis
Metabolic	Hypothyroidism, uraemia, hepatic failure, B_{12} deficiency, prolonged hypoglycaemia, prolonged hypoxia, respiratory failure, low output cardiac failure
'Pseudodementia'	Depression

SSPE = subacute sclerosing parencephalitis; PML = progressive multifocal leucoencephalopathy; CJD = Creutzfeld-Jakob disease.

Investigation of dementia

All younger demented patients should have a CT scan. Table 23.33 lists the investigations which should be undertaken in a demented patient without physical signs. Pointers to an underlying cause from history or examination will permit a more selective approach to investigation in some patients.

Table 23.33 Investigation of dementia

● Full blood count, ESR	● Glucose
● Renal function	● Chest X-ray, ECG
● Liver function	● Skull X-ray
● Thyroid function	● CT scan
● Calcium	● EEG
● Toxicology	● CSF (selected patients)
● Treponemal infection	

ALZHEIMER'S DISEASE

The great majority of patients over the age of 60 with progressive dementia have Alzheimer's disease. It has been estimated that approximately 7–8% of all people over the age of 65 have this disease (Summary 5).

Aetiology

Alois Alzheimer described the histological abnormalities in the atrophied brains of patients dying with dementia, and these changes remain the defining characteristics of the condition; however, none of the histological changes is, in itself, unique to Alzheimer's disease. In addition to atrophy and reduced numbers of cortical neurones in all areas, many surviving neurones contain neurofibrillary tangles. Senile plaques (amyloid plaques) – structures of about 50 microns diameter – are invariably present. Both changes are found to some extent in the brains of elderly non-demented patients, so may be considered normal ageing changes. With the growth of our understanding of brain histochemistry, a number of theories based on altered chemistry have been proposed. Much attention has focussed recently on the degenerative changes in the wide cortical cholinergic projection from the nucleus basalis of Meynert, deep in the frontal lobe.

Occasional families are found in which Alzheimer's disease is clearly inherited as an autosomal dominant trait.

Clinical features

Loss of recent memory with a complaint of forgetfulness is the most common presenting symptom. Loss of interest in life and personality change, sometimes with antisocial and disinhibited behaviour, are also common early symptoms. Dysphasia, dyslexia, dysgraphia and dyscalculia are sometimes focally impaired out of proportion to other deficits. Dyspraxic symptoms, such as topographagnosia (inability to find one's way about in familiar surroundings) and dressing apraxia, are frequent. Loss of bladder and bowel sphincter control may be an early or late feature. Sleep disturbance is common. Wandering may become a serious problem. Increasing confusion and complete social disintegration eventually occur. The most common physical complaint in Alzheimer's disease is unsteadiness of gait. The gait may appear ataxic or Parkinsonian, and a combination of cerebellar, extrapyramidal and pyramidal signs may be found later in the disease.

The course of Alzheimer's disease is very variable, average survival being between 5 and 7 years.

Summary 5   Dementia

- Alzheimer's disease (AD) is the commonest cause of dementia in people over 60 years of age.

- In the elderly, depression may closely mimic dementia.

- AD nearly always presents at over 55 years of age.

- Dementia in younger patients must always be thoroughly investigated, including CT scanning.

- Dementia with abnormal neurological signs as an early feature is unlikely to be AD.

Investigation and treatment

There is no single diagnostic test for Alzheimer's disease. The finding of diffuse cerebral atrophy on CT scanning (Fig. 23.29) and exclusion of other treatable causes of dementia usually leaves little doubt about the diagnosis.

Treatment is largely supportive. The disease imposes huge strains on the spouse and family of the patient. Inevitably, many patients eventually require institutional care.

PICK'S DISEASE

Pick's disease is rare. It consists of dementia with selective impairment of speech function associated with focal atrophy of frontal and temporal lobes. It is frequently inherited as an autosomal dominant condition.

HUNTINGTON'S CHOREA

Huntington's chorea is a dominantly inherited condition consisting of chorea and progressive dementia of unknown cause. It is not common, with an estimated prevalence of 1 in 20 000.

Clinical features

The onset of symptoms is gradual, usually between 30 and 50 years, beginning either with chorea or early symptoms of dementia, often taking the form of a change in personality. Chorea gradually becomes more marked, and eventually interferes with all voluntary movements. A feature of the early stages of the dementia of Huntington's chorea is some retention of insight which, associated with a knowledge of the family history, can lead to severe depression, and sometimes suicide. The average duration of the disease from onset of symptoms to death is about 15 years. In the advanced stages, there is increasing dementia, akinesia and rigidity.

Treatment

Treatment is purely symptomatic. Neuroleptic drugs such as chlorpromazine, perphenazine, pimozide or haloperidol may help the chorea to some extent. Genetic counselling is vital. The children of a parent with Huntington's chorea have a 1 in 2 risk of developing the disease, and their children have a 1 in 4 risk. A recent advance has been the identification of a gene marker for Huntington's chorea, which should permit identification of those carrying the abnormal gene.

CEREBRAL TUMOURS

Primary cerebral tumours account for about 10% of all tumours, and about a quarter of all intracranial tumours are metastatic. Some are much more common than others (Table 23.34 and Fig. 23.19).

Table 23.34 Classification of cerebral tumours

Tumour	Origin	Site	Age
Astrocytoma grades I–IV	Astrocytes	Mainly cerebral hemisphere. Also cerebellum and optic nerves	20 years or more, occasionally in children
Oligodendroglioma	Oligodendrocytes	Cerebral hemisphere	20 years or more
Ependymoma	Ependyma	Ventricles	Mainly children
Microglioma	Reticulum cells	Cerebral hemisphere	Adults
Medulloblastoma	Neurones	IVth ventricle and cerebellum	Children
Ganglioneuroma	Neurones	IVth ventricle	Mainly children
Primary lymphoma	Lymphoid	Hemisphere or cerebellum	Mainly adults, particularly in HIV infection
Pinealoma	Pineal	Pineal gland	Mainly children
Haemangioblastoma	Uncertain	Cerebellum	Children and young adults
Pituitary adenomas	Adenohypophyseal cells	Pituitary gland	Mainly adults
Craniopharyngioma	Epithelial cell rests in Rathke's pouch	Hypothalamus	Children and adults
Chordoma	Notochord remnants	Clivus and pituitary fossa	Young adults
Meningioma	Arachnoid	Any site of meninges	Adults (40–50 years)
Schwannoma	Schwann cells	VIIIth nerve	Mainly adults
Glomus tumour	?Nodose ganglion of vagus	Jugular foramen	Adults
Cholesteatoma	Uncertain	Cerebello-pontine angle/petrous temporal bone	Adults
Skull tumours Osteoma Osteosarcoma Myeloma Metastatic carcinoma		Any part of skull	Mainly adults
Metastases	Lung, breast, kidney, colon, thyroid, etc.	Hemisphere or cerebellum	Mainly adults

There are considerable differences between tumours in children and adults. In children, the great majority of tumours arise in the posterior fossa, whereas in adults, the majority are supratentorial. Gliomas and meningiomas are rare in children.

Clinical features

Cerebral tumours present in four main ways:

1. with symptoms and signs of focal neurological deficit
2. with epilepsy, either focal or generalised (when supratentorial)
3. with symptoms and signs of raised intracranial pressure
4. with endocrinological effects (pituitary tumours).

Cerebral hemisphere tumours

A tumour arising in one cerebral hemisphere will eventually cause symptoms and signs of focal neurological deficit, the nature of these depending upon the lobe of origin. Surrounding cerebral oedema often leads to focal deficit, which is greater than that caused by the tumour itself. Epilepsy is a common manifestation, whereas headache is a very variable symptom. Local invasion of the meninges by

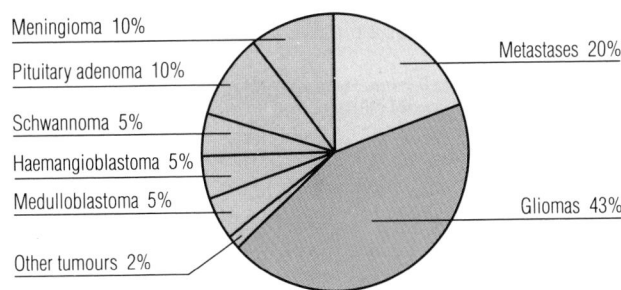

Fig. 23.19 Relative frequencies of cerebral tumours.

tumour may cause localised headache. A large hemisphere tumour may cause hydrocephalus, and this may occasionally be accompanied by an abrupt clinical deterioration. In general, the deficit produced by tumours is contralateral to the lesion, but a swollen hemisphere may compress the contralateral cerebral peduncle against the free edge of the tentorium, causing a hemiparesis ipsilateral to the tumour. The ipsilateral IIIrd nerve may be compressed. These signs of tentorial coning occur as a late feature of a cerebral hemisphere tumour.

Papilloedema may, or may not, accompany raised intracranial pressure and, when present, is often more marked on the ipsilateral side.

Neurological Disease

Posterior fossa tumours

Tumours arising in the cerebellum cause gait ataxia if situated medially in the vermis, or of the ipsilateral limbs if situated in one cerebellar hemisphere. Later, compression of the brain stem produces local effects and involvement of the long tracts. Tumours within the brain stem itself (usually gliomas) are rare. Midbrain and pontine tumours lead to ocular gaze palsies, internuclear palsies and upper cranial nerve palsies, and long tract signs. Lower cranial nerve palsies occur with intrinsic medullary tumours, but are commoner in involvement by extrinsic tumours, such as glomus tumour or meningeal infiltration by carcinoma or lymphoma.

Enlarging posterior fossa tumours of any type may obstruct the aqueduct of Sylvius and cause hydrocephalus, with abrupt clinical deterioration. Coning at the foramen magnum may occur with large posterior fossa tumours. The cerebellar tonsils are pushed downwards through the foramen magnum, with accompanying compression of the medulla.

Pituitary tumours

Pituitary tumours rarely increase intracranial pressure, but may cause headache due to expansion within the pituitary fossa. Pituitary adenomas may be secretory, presenting with endocrine effects (Ch. 18). Pituitary tumours which expand out of the pituitary fossa, impinge on the optic chiasm (Fig. 23.20). The characteristic visual field defect is a bitemporal hemipanopia, but temporal field loss in one eye only may occur. Occasionally, pituitary tumours expand laterally into the cavernous sinus, involving the oculomotor and trigeminal nerves. Craniopharyngiomas may impinge on the optic chiasm, producing visual field loss identical to that of a pituitary tumour.

Fig. 23.20 Magnetic resonance scan, showing a large pituitary tumour in sagittal section. The tumour, an adenoma, has extended upwards, out of the pituitary fossa, and is compressing the optic chiasm. (Reproduced by permission of Dr J Stevens and Dr A Valentine.)

Cerebello-pontine angle tumours

The commonest cerebello-pontine angle (CPA) tumour is the acoustic neuroma (Fig. 23.21), but meningiomas also occur at this site as, less frequently, do other tumours, such as epidermoids. An enlarging extrinsic CPA mass produces progressive deafness (VIIIth nerve), facial sensory loss (trigeminal nerve), facial weakness (facial nerve) and then ipsilateral cerebellar signs. Eventually, brain stem compression leads to brain stem and long tract symptoms and signs, and hydrocephalus develops.

Investigation

Clinical suspicion of cerebral tumour comes from a history of insidious onset and gradual progression. The absence of

Fig. 23.21 Acoustic neuroma. A. Unenhanced scan of the posterior fossa. A mass can just be seen on the right side, causing mild brain stem compression. **B.** After contrast enhancement, the tumour is easily seen. These appearances are typical of an acoustic neuroma. Tumours of this size frequently produce cerebellar and long tract signs, and an obstructive hydrocephalus.

neurological signs does not exclude a cerebral tumour. Raised intracranial pressure may give rise to subtle intellectual impairments, and careful assessment of the mental state is an important part of the examination.

Skull X-ray. The skull X-ray is of limited value but may be diagnostic in pituitary tumours, in which the pituitary fossa is often enlarged, or in CPA tumours in which views of the internal auditory meati may demonstrate unilateral enlargement due to bony erosion from an acoustic neuroma. In meningiomas, the skull vault overlying the tumour may become thickened (hyperostosis) and the impression of large draining veins may be apparent. Chronically raised intracranial pressure causes erosion of the skull vault giving rise to a 'copper beaten' appearance, and there may also be erosion of the posterior clinoid processes. In adults, in whom the pineal may become calcified, shift from the midline by an expanding hemisphere tumour may be seen. Certain tumours – particularly oligodendrogliomas and slowly growing astrocytomas – may become calcified, and this is sometimes visible as speckled calcification on a plain skull X-ray.

CT scanning, with and without intravenous contrast enhancement, is the definitive investigation in patients suspected of having a cerebral tumour (Figs 23.21–23.24). Early gliomas and small tumours, particularly in the posterior fossa, may be missed on CT scans. NMR scanning may demonstrate these lesions.

Angiography. Although vascular tumours such as meningiomas can usually be confidently identified on CT scans, neurosurgeons often require detailed information about blood supply only obtainable from angiography.

Individual cerebral tumours

Astrocytomas

Astrocytomas are the commonest primary malignant cerebral tumours. They are of variable malignancy, grade I being the least and grade IV being the most malignant. Grade IV astrocytomas are known as *glioblastoma multiforme* (Fig. 23.22). Survival times of 20–30 years are possible with a grade I astrocytoma, while only about one patient in five will survive longer than one year with a glioblastoma multiforme.

In adults, the great majority of astrocytomas arise in the cerebral hemispheres, brain stem astrocytomas being rare. A relatively benign form of astrocytoma occasionally occurs in the cerebellum in adults.

In children, cerebellar gliomas are often cystic, and long survivals have been reported after resection of these tumours. The optic nerve and hypothalamus are other preferential sites of astrocytoma formation in children.

Most astrocytomas remain unilateral in the cerebral hemisphere, but some grow through the corpus callosum to the contralateral hemisphere. These tend to be the histologically more malignant tumours.

Slowly growing tumours are associated with less surrounding oedema than rapidly growing tumours. Partial relief of oedema with dexamethasone may produce con-

Fig. 23.22 Astrocytoma. A. A highly malignant astrocytoma, grade IV (glioblastoma multiforme), showing marked mass effect and irregular contrast enhancement. **B.** An astrocytoma, grade II histologically, in the anterior part of the right temporal lobe. This tumour is cystic; there is some associated oedema and ring enhancement around the cystic part of the tumour shown in the right-hand scan.

siderable clinical improvement, but the effect is usually short-lived.

Oligodendrogliomas

Oligodendrogliomas are slowly growing tumours, often partly calcified, arising in the cerebral hemispheres in adults. They carry a relatively good prognosis.

Ependymomas

Ependymomas arise from the ependymal cells lining the IVth and lateral ventricles. They usually present in childhood or adolescence, and tend to run a fairly malignant course. Spread of these tumours may occur via the CSF; thus, wide dissemination sometimes results.

Medulloblastoma

Medulloblastoma is the commonest CNS tumour in children. The tumour arises in the roof of the IVth ventricle, causing ataxia, local brain stem signs, long tract signs and, eventually, hydrocephalus. They are of variable malignancy, but almost always fatal within three years.

Microglioma

Microgliomas are rare tumours which only arise in the cerebral hemispheres in adults. They are diffusely spreading, highly malignant tumours, resistant to all treatment.

Meningioma

Meningiomas arise from the arachnoid and are benign tumours. The most common sites are the parasagittal region arising from the falx, the meninges of the convexity over the hemispheres, the olfactory groove, and the wing of the sphenoid (Fig. 23.23). They are more common in women, and tend to present over the age of 40 years. Involvement of bone is common in meningioma, with erosion and hyperostosis. These slowly growing tumours are extremely vascular and often calcify. Surgical resection may be technically difficult and the tumours tend to regrow if incompletely removed. Occasionally, malignant change to meningosarcoma occurs.

Fig. 23.23   An enhanced scan showing a right-sided parasagittal meningioma, arising from the falx. This tumour had produced a slowly progressive left hemiparesis developing over five years.

Pituitary tumours

The endocrinological aspects of pituitary tumours are discussed in Chapter 18. Prolactinomas are associated with weight gain, amenorrhoea and galactorrhoea. Growth-hormone-secreting tumours produce gigantism in childhood and acromegaly in adults. ACTH-secreting tumours cause Cushing's syndrome. Symptoms and signs of hypopituitarism are frequent.

Schwannoma

Schwannomas arise from the Schwann cells of the peripheral nerves and nerve roots. Within the cranium, acoustic neuromas are by far the commonest of these tumours (p. 906), but Schwannomas may occasionally arise on other cranial nerves.

Less common primary cerebral tumours

Pinealomas are rare tumours seen mainly in children. They affect the dorsal midbrain, causing a characteristic failure of upward gaze, pupillary abnormalities and, sometimes, other ocular palsies.

Ganglioneuromas are uncommon tumours of relatively low malignancy. They occur in children and arise from the floor of the IIIrd ventricle.

Haemangioblastomas arise in the cerebellum in children or young adults. They may be either solitary tumours, or occur as part of the rare Von Hippel-Lindau syndrome (haemangioblastoma in CNS and retina, with renal or pancreatic cysts, hypernephroma and adrenal tumours). Haemangioblastomas are often cystic, with a vascular enhancing area of solid tissue seen on CT scanning. They present with ataxia and then symptoms of brain stem compression and hydrocephalus. Occasionally, they secrete erythropoietin, causing polycythaemia. Many are amenable to surgery.

Chordomas arise from the primitive notochord structures, the sella and clivus. They cause multiple lower cranial nerve palsies and sometimes invade the brain stem.

Craniopharyngiomas arise from epithelial cells in the pituitary stalk. They are slowly growing and often calcify. They cause optic chiasmal compression and compression of the IIIrd ventricle, leading to hydrocephalus.

Glomus jugulare tumours are highly vascular tumours, the precise cellular origin of which is uncertain. They may arise from the nodose ganglion of the vagus nerve. They give rise to the characteristic jugular foramen syndrome, which includes IXth, Xth, XIth and XIIth cranial nerve palsies on one side, accompanied by an ipsilateral Horner's syndrome, due to involvement of the cervical sympathetic fibres travelling with the carotid artery. Extension into the petrous temporal bone and middle ear causes conductive deafness, and the tumour is often visible through the tympanic membrane. With intracranial extension, brain stem and cerebellar compression may occur. Occasionally, these tumours extend into the upper part of the neck, where they may form a visible mass. Bruits over these vascular tumours are common.

Cholesteatomas within the petrous temporal bone probably arise from epithelial elements. Their relationship to middle ear disease remains uncertain. They usually present as a CPA syndrome and may involve the middle ear, producing conductive deafness.

Choroid plexus papillomas are benign tumours which

arise from the choroid plexus in the IVth or lateral ventricles, and usually present before the age of 10 years. They cause hydrocephalus and, sometimes, symptoms attributable to excess secretion of CSF. Very occasionally, these tumours are malignant.

Colloid cysts arise in young adults in the anterior end of the IIIrd ventricle. They cause recurrent symptoms by intermittent blockage of the CSF circulation at the foramen of Munro, causing loss of consciousness, sometimes with respiratory irregularities and decerebrate posturing. Death may occur in such a hydrocephalic attack.

Cerebral and cerebellar metastases

Although metastases commonly cause symptoms, many clinically silent metastases are found at post-mortem. Many are multiple (Fig. 23.24) and the cerebellum seems to be a preferential site for metastases. The commonest primary tumours are bronchus, breast, kidney, colon and thyroid; leukaemia and lymphoma are also common tumours, leading to intracranial metastases. Secondary spread may also occur to other intracranial structures, particularly the meninges, producing a malignant meningitis.

The neurological non-metastatic effects of systemic malignancy are considered on page 970.

Differential diagnosis

The differential diagnosis of cerebral hemisphere tumours is wide, and includes cerebral abscess, tuberculoma, chronic subdural haematoma, vascular disease and, occasionally, encephalitis. In the posterior fossa, demyelinating disease needs to be considered, together with structural abnormalities such as an Arnold-Chiari malformation (p. 933).

Treatment

The urgency of treatment of cerebral tumours depends on whether there is raised intracranial pressure, due either to the mass effect of the tumour itself, or to associated hydrocephalus.

Fits require anticonvulsants but sometimes prove particularly resistant to therapy. Raised intracranial pressure leading to impairment of consciousness is an indication for urgent treatment to reduce cerebral oedema. Dexamethasone (10 mg immediately, followed by 4 mg 4-hourly) is usually effective, an alternative being mannitol (200 mg of a 20% solution given intravenously over 15–30 minutes). Dexamethasone is used pre- and postoperatively to protect against the development of excessive cerebral oedema induced by surgery.

Surgery

Whenever possible, the aim of treatment for benign cerebral tumours is complete surgical resection. However, inaccessibility and potential damage to normal tissue often

Fig. 23.24 A series of enhanced CT scans, all from the same patient, showing multiple metastases in the cerebellum and cerebral hemispheres. The lesions appear as ring shadows and are of different sizes. There is hydrocephalus, resulting from the mass effect of the multiple metastases in the cerebellum, obstructing CSF flow into the IVth ventricle.

dictates a less ambitious surgical approach. Some benign tumours may recur, but very slowly, and many patients with residual meningioma tissue will have no further problems after the main bulk of the tumour has been resected.

The role of surgery for malignant primary cerebral tumours remains uncertain. Biopsy of the tumour to establish the diagnosis and plan further treatment is often advisable. Hydrocephalus should be relieved as soon as possible by ventriculoperitoneal shunting.

While malignant primary cerebral tumours are not curable by surgery, removal of a large part of a tumour

Summary 6 Presentation and investigation of cerebral tumours

- Cerebral hemisphere tumours may present with epilepsy, progressive focal neurological deficit, or signs of raised intracranial pressure (ICP).

- Posterior fossa tumours often present with ataxia, with or without focal brain stem and long tract signs. Raised ICP is common with larger lesions, due to hydrocephalus.

- Raised ICP may not be associated with either symptoms or papilloedema.

- Pituitary tumours present with a variety of endocrine effects and, characteristically, a bitemporal hemianopia.

- Cerebellopontine angle tumours present with unilateral deafness (VIII), facial sensory loss or pain (V), facial weakness (VII), and later, ataxia and long tract signs due to brain stem and cerebellar compression; eventually, hydrocephalus occurs.

- If a cerebral tumour is suspected, a CT scan is the investigation of choice

- Lumbar puncture should never be done if a focal cerebral lesion or raised ICP is suspected.

- Cerebral metastases are single or multiple and may be indistinguishable on CT from primary tumours.

- Stroke, cerebral abscess, tuberculoma or chronic subdural haematoma may mimic cerebral tumour.

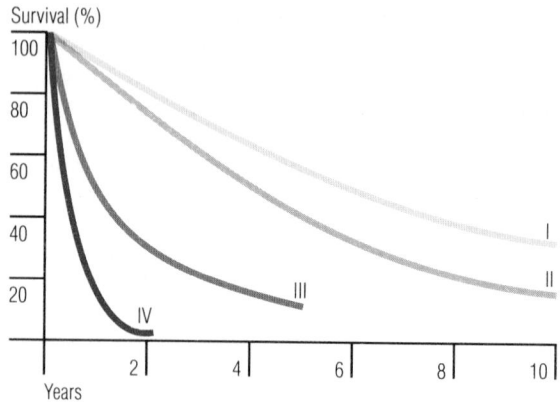

Fig. 23.25 Survival curves for astrocytoma grades I to IV.

may produce improvement and relieve the effects of raised intracranial pressure. Surgery is not without risk of damaging normal cerebral tissue. The usual practice with probable malignant primary cerebral tumours presenting with epilepsy and/or a mild neurological deficit, is to delay craniotomy and biopsy until a significant neurological deficit develops. In most cases, a definite early diagnosis is unlikely to lead to any change in management.

Metastases, both cerebral hemisphere and cerebellar, are often separable from surrounding brain tissue and can, occasionally, be completely surgically removed.

Radiotherapy

The role of radiotherapy in the management of malignant gliomas remains controversial. Recent studies have shown very limited benefit in any type of adult glioma, and the morbidity of the treatment has to be weighed against the marginal benefits from radiotherapy. This treatment is particularly upsetting in older patients, producing headache, nausea, vomiting, malaise and, sometimes, exacerbation of the neurological deficit. At the start of treatment, there is often an increase in cerebral oedema, necessitating the use of large doses of dexamethasone.

Radiotherapy is usually advised for the more malignant histological types of astrocytoma (grades III and IV) but not for astrocytomas grades I and II. The effect in glioblastoma multiforme (grade IV) is, however, disappointing, and the prognosis is probably not significantly altered (20% survival at one year). For grade II astrocytoma, the prognosis is marginally improved by radiotherapy.

The overall prognosis for astrocytomas grade I–III is about 50% survival at 5 years (Fig. 23.25). However, some low-grade tumours remain clinically static for many years. Survival for 20–30 years is possible with such tumours.

Whole neuraxis radiotherapy for childhood medulloblastoma improves the prognosis, though overall survival rates are poor (between 1–3 years).

Ependymomas are variably radiosensitive. Radiotherapy is usually recommended after surgery for pituitary adenomas and craniopharyngiomas.

Multiple metastases are often palliated with a combination of radiotherapy and dexamethasone.

Chemotherapy

The role of chemotherapy for primary cerebral tumours remains uncertain. Cis-platinum is the most frequently used agent. Intracerebral and meningeal leukaemia and lymphoma are often treated with a combination of radiotherapy and intrathecal methotrexate (p. 1080).

BENIGN INTRACRANIAL HYPERTENSION (PSEUDOTUMOUR CEREBRI)

Benign intracranial hypertension (BIH) is also known as pseudotumour cerebri, since it may mimic a cerebral tumour. There is raised intracranial pressure without a demonstrable mass or hydrocephalus.

Aetiology and pathology

The cause of BIH is unknown. There is a strong association with obesity and an empty sella. Occasionally, there is a history of a preceding episode of dural sinus thrombosis. Hypovitaminosis A in children may cause BIH, and the prescription of certain antibiotics (including tetracycline and nitrofurantoin) and, occasionally, corticosteroids may precede the development of the condition.

Cerebral blood volume is increased in BIH and a disorder of autoregulation has been proposed. There is no evidence that vasogenic oedema occurs in BIH, and the syndrome is probably not due to overproduction of CSF. Reduced absorption of CSF has been demonstrated, but it is not clear why hydrocephalus does not develop if this is the major abnormality.

Clinical features and investigation

BIH is a rare condition most commonly affecting young women. There is headache, with associated malaise and nausea. Visual obscurations are frequent, resulting from papilloedema. Visual acuity may be impaired when papilloedema is severe, with enlarged blind spots and, sometimes, constriction of the visual fields. Reduced colour vision is common. About a third of patients develop diplopia, due to an associated VIth nerve palsy. Many patients are grossly obese.

Patients require a CT scan to investigate a possible mass lesion. The CT scan is either normal or shows small ventricles. When CT scan has excluded a mass lesion, lumbar puncture is safe and the diagnosis is confirmed if an opening pressure of more than 200–250 mmHg is recorded. The CSF is normal.

Treatment and prognosis

The most important complication of BIH is permanent loss of vision. To prevent this, treatment is directed at reducing intracranial pressure, achieved by repeated lumbar puncture, with removal of 20–30 ml of CSF several times a week. This treatment may induce a remission. Some patients respond to a few weeks of high doses of prednisolone. Diuretics and carbonic anhydrase inhibitors (acetazolamide) may reduce the pressure in some patients. In obese patients, there is often a reduction in pressure with weight loss. In a few patients resistant to all other treatment, lumboperitoneal shunting may be necessary, or optic nerve sheath decompression to protect vision.

Spontaneous remission usually occurs after a few months or years, but a small proportion of patients develop recurrent symptoms.

HYDROCEPHALUS

Hydrocephalus means an excess of cerebrospinal fluid within the ventricles and has many causes (Table 23.35). CSF is secreted by the choroid plexus in the lateral, IIIrd and IVth ventricles (Fig. 23.26). It passes from the IIIrd ventricle into the IVth ventricle via the cerebral aqueduct, and from the IVth ventricle into the subarachnoid space through the foramina of Magendi and Lushka in the roof of the ventricle. The CSF then circulates through the subarachnoid spaces around the surface of the brain and spinal cord. Most CSF is absorbed through the arachnoid villi into the dural sinuses, although some is absorbed through the veins of the arachnoid. When there is obstruction to the flow of CSF, and CSF pressure rises, fluid may be forced through the ependymal lining of the ventricles directly into the brain substance. This oedema, most evident in the periventricular white matter of the lateral

Table 23.35 Causes of hydrocephalus

Cerebral dysgenesis	**Impaired CSF absorption**
	Subarachnoid haemorrhage
Obstruction to flow of CSF	Meningitis
At level of third ventricle	
Hemisphere tumour	**Excess production of CSF**
Tumour involving third ventricle	Choroid plexus papilloma
At level of aqueduct	
Aqueduct stenosis	**Secondary to cerebral atrophy**
Posterior fossa tumour	
At level of fourth ventricle	**Unknown cause**
Atresia of exit foraminae	Includes normal pressure
Dandy-Walker syndrome	hydrocephalus
Arnold-Chiari malformation	

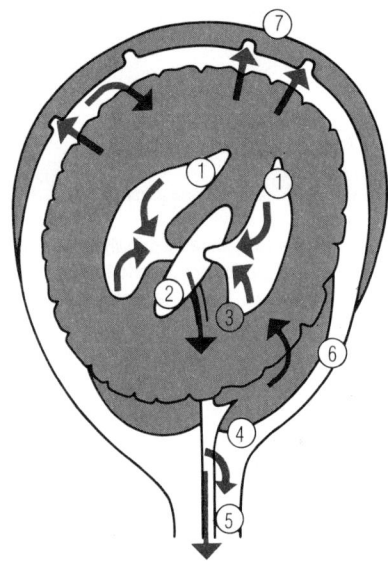

Fig. 23.26 The normal production and flow of CSF. CSF is secreted by the choroid plexuses in the lateral, IIIrd and IVth ventricles. It flows from the lateral ventricles (1), into the IIIrd ventricle (2), through the cerebral aqueduct (3), into the IVth ventricle (4). From the IVth ventricle, CSF passes downwards into the central canal of the spinal cord, and through the foramina of Magendi and Lushka out into the subarachnoid space (5). CSF flows over the whole surface of the brain in the subarachnoid space (6) and is reabsorbed into the dural sinuses (7) via the arachnoid granulations.

ventricles on CT scanning (Fig. 23.27), is characteristic of acute obstructive hydrocephalus.

Causes of hydrocephalus

The causes of hydrocephalus are listed in Table 23.35.

Cerebral dysgenesis

Maldevelopment or absence of any part of the brain will lead to a compensatory excess of CSF.

Obstruction to flow of CSF

This may occur within the ventricular system (non-com-

Fig. 23.27 Acute hydrocephalus, showing grossly dilated lateral ventricles, with periventricular lucency, particularly anteriorly, indicating peri-ventricular white matter oedema. From a patient with obstruction at the level of the IIIrd ventricle.

Fig. 23.28 CT scans from a patient with an acute cerebellar haemorrhage. Blood has a high attenuation and appears as a white mass in the cerebellum. The haemorrhage and surrounding oedema are obstructing the cerebral aqueduct, causing acute hydrocephalus, with well-marked periventricular lucencies.

municating' hydrocephalus) or within the subarachnoid space as a result of failure of absorption or flow through the subarachnoid space (communicating hydrocephalus). A large cerebral hemisphere lesion may compress the IIIrd ventricle and obstruct the flow of CSF, producing hydrocephalus in one, or both, lateral ventricles. Very often, a mass lesion in one hemisphere will produce compression of the ipsilateral lateral ventricle and an obstructive hydrocephalus of the contralateral lateral ventricle. Any mass lesion in the posterior fossa may obstruct the flow through the cerebral aqueduct, causing enlargement of the lateral and IIIrd ventricles (Fig. 23.28).

Impaired CSF absorption

Dilatation of the lateral IIIrd and IVth ventricles indicates a communicating hydrocephalus and may result from impairment of reabsorption of CSF. However, in many cases of communicating hydrocephalus, the CSF pressure is found to be normal (normal pressure hydrocephalus, see p. 914). Communicating hydrocephalus may occur in acute meningitis, and is seen particularly with tuberculous meningitis. It may also occur after subarachnoid haemorrhage, and in diseases in which the CSF protein remains greatly elevated over long periods of time.

Excess production of CSF

This occurs very rarely and usually indicates a papilloma of the choroid plexus.

Atrophic

Any acquired disease leading to loss of brain volume will result in a compensatory hydrocephalus. By far the commonest cause is the atrophy associated with Alzheimer's disease (pre-senile dementia). In this disease, there is both ventricular dilatation and cortical atrophy, giving characteristic CT scan appearances in most cases (Fig. 23.29). Diagnostic difficulties arise when the degree of ventricular enlargement is out of proportion to the extent of cortical atrophy, raising the possibility of an obstructive hydrocephalus.

INFANTILE HYDROCEPHALUS

Most infants with hydrocephalus appear normal at birth.

Aetiology

Occasionally, hydrocephalus leading to enlargement of the head may be present in utero and cause birth difficulties. About half of those affected have associated malformations of the brain. Congenital cerebral aqueduct stenosis, atresia

Fig. 23.29 Generalised cerebral atrophy, from a patient with Alzheimer's disease. Note the cortical atrophy, with widened sulci, and the ventricular dilatation.

of the exit foramina of the IVth ventricle and the Dandy-Walker syndrome are the commonest abnormalities. In the *Dandy-Walker syndrome* there is atresia of the foramen of Magendie, with a failure of development of the vermis of the cerebellum, and a grossly enlarged IVth ventricle, which occupies most of the posterior fossa. In the *Arnold-Chiari malformation*, there is elongation of the medulla with herniation of the cerebellar tonsils through the foramen magnum, associated with obstruction of the outflow of CSF from the IVth ventricle (see also p. 933). Very occasionally, a posterior fossa tumour in infancy may be the cause of hydrocephalus.

Trauma leading to subarachnoid haemorrhage and sub-

sequent hydrocephalus is probably a fairly common cause of infantile hydrocephalus, as is meningitis. In many children, however, the cause of the hydrocephalus cannot be identified with certainty.

Clinical features, investigation and treatment

Progressive enlargement of the head is the earliest clinical feature, with delayed developmental milestones, mental retardation, fits, spastic weakness in the limbs (particularly in the legs), optic atrophy and limitation of upward gaze. The condition is often fatal if untreated, but, occasionally, children may survive with a state of arrested hydrocephalus

Fig 23.30 Normal pressure hydrocephalus. There is gross enlargement of the entire ventricular system. This patient has been treated with a ventriculo-peritoneal shunt; the shunt tube can be seen in the right lateral ventricle.

into adult life. They are almost invariably physically and mentally retarded.

Investigation of infantile hydrocephalus includes the sequential measurement of head circumference. In suspected cases, investigations include skull X-rays (which show cranial enlargement and separation of the sutures), CT scanning and, in selected cases, contrast radiology.

Treatment is with a shunt, which usually arrests further hydrocephalus and neurological deficit.

NORMAL PRESSURE HYDROCEPHALUS

The term normal pressure hydrocephalus refers to the presence of ventricular enlargement affecting all the ventricles without cortical atrophy (Fig. 23.30), and with normal CSF pressure (as measured at lumbar puncture).

Clinical features, investigation and treatment

Patients present in adult life with dementia, and, usually, an associated physical neurological deficit, comprising cerebellar ataxia of gait, pyramidal signs in the limbs and incontinence of urine. In patients with pre-senile dementia, but without physical abnormalities, diagnostic difficulties may arise in distinguishing normal pressure hydrocephalus from Alzheimer's disease (p. 904). There may be similar difficulties distinguishing normal pressure hydrocephalus from diffuse small vessel cerebrovascular disease (p. 898).

The pathogenesis of normal pressure hydrocephalus is unknown in most patients. A single measurement of CSF pressure at lumbar puncture is likely to be normal, but monitoring of intracranial pressure over 24–48 hours reveals intermittent periods of raised pressure.

In patients shown to have periods of sustained increased intracranial pressure, the results of ventriculoperitoneal shunting are fair; about half of the patients show some improvement both in intellectual and physical deficits. Occasionally, this improvement is dramatic and occurs within days of shunting.

EXTRAPYRAMIDAL DISEASE

The term extrapyramidal disease is used to refer to disorders produced by lesions affecting the basal ganglia. Diseases of the extrapyramidal system may be divided into:

1. the *akinetic-rigid syndromes*, such as Parkinson's disease, which lead to a poverty of movement associated with an increase in tone
2. the *dyskinesias*, which produce involuntary movements.

Major symptoms of extrapyramidal disease

Akinesia means a loss or poverty of movement and is usually the most striking and disabling feature of Par-

kinson's disease. The terms bradykinesia, hypokinesia and akinesia are used interchangeably.

Rigidity refers to the increase in tone in the limbs and trunk which frequently accompanies akinesia. It is typically of a cogwheeling type, and may be increased in a limb by asking the patient to perform a repetitive movement, such as turning the head from side to side (reinforcement, or synkinesis).

Dyskinesia includes a number of different types of involuntary movement. *Tremor* is a rhythmical movement of variable amplitude and frequency. The main causes are noted in Table 23.37 (p. 917). *Chorea* refers to irregular jerky movements of variable amplitude usually involving all limbs, the trunk and sometimes the facial muscles, though not simultaneously. In its mild forms, chorea may be a discrete physical sign mimicking fidgeting movements. In its severe form, e.g. as in Huntington's chorea (p. 904), it is readily recognisable. The causes of chorea are listed in Table 23.38.

Dystonia refers to the adoption of an abnormal posture of any part of the body of variable duration. Dystonia is often not static, but associated with slow writhing movements of the affected part (athetosis). The term dystonia is now preferred to describe such dynamic abnormal movements in the setting of an abnormal posture. The causes of dystonia are listed in Table 23.39.

Myoclonus is a rapid jerking movement, usually of large amplitude, affecting one or several limbs and the trunk. It may occur as a single involuntary movement, or may be repetitive. The causes of myoclonus are listed in Table 23.40.

Tics are rapid repetitive, sometimes semi-purposeful movements, which may look like myoclonic jerks. Unlike other involuntary movements, it is usually possible for patients to voluntarily control tics, but this leads to increasing anxiety and, eventually, resumption of the tic.

PARKINSON'S DISEASE

Parkinson's disease is an akinetic-rigid syndrome affecting about 1 in 1000 adults and about 1 in 200 over the age of 65. First described as the 'shaking palsy' by James Parkinson in 1817, this is a slowly progressive condition in which there is akinesia, a rest tremor, cogwheel rigidity and postural abnormalities. Several other disease processes may produce an identical akinetic-rigid clinical presentation; Parkinsonism is the term used to refer to such patients. The causes of Parkinsonism are listed in Table 23.36.

Table 23.36 Akinetic-rigid syndromes

Parkinson's disease	Parkinsonism with other neurological features
Pure Parkinsonism	
Post-encephalitic Parkinsonism	Wilson's disease
Neuroleptic drugs	Huntington's chorea
MPTP toxicity	Cerebral palsy
Cerebral anoxia	Progressive supranuclear palsy
	Multiple system atrophy

Aetiology

The cause of Parkinson's disease is unknown. Pathology shows degeneration of the substantia nigra and other brain stem pigmented nuclei. It is currently thought that about 85% of substantia nigra neurones must be lost, with a corresponding decrease in dopamine, before symptoms and signs of Parkinson's disease develop. The search for possible environmental factors has increased following the recent discovery that a synthetic opiate analogue, MPTP, mistakenly synthesised by opiate addicts a few years ago, can cause an illness identical to Parkinson's disease.

Clinical features

The mean age of onset of Parkinson's disease is 55 years. Tremor is the most common early symptom. Akinesia is often not noticed by the patient in the early stages, but may be commented on by relatives.

Tremor. This is initially only present at rest, disappearing transiently on voluntary action. It is a slow (4–6 Hz) tremor, and usually affects the hands first, producing a typical pill-rolling tremor. It may involve the whole limb, the legs and sometimes the trunk. It is exacerbated by stress and anxiety and is worse in company. The tremor is often also present on maintained posture, and may thus cause increasing difficulty with everyday tasks, such as eating and drinking. The increase in tone causing rigidity is usually of cogwheeling type.

Akinesia is frequently the most disabling feature of Parkinson's disease. There is slowness and difficulty in initiating movement which affects all voluntary activity.

Postural abnormalities are common in Parkinson's disease, a stooped flexed posture being typical. There is loss of postural control leading to falls, both standing and while walking.

The abnormalities of motor control outlined above combine to produce all the clinical features of Parkinson's disease. These include the abnormal posture, with facial masking, dribbling of saliva due to reduced swallowing, dysphonia, dysphagia and dysarthria. The combination of dysphonia and dysarthria produces the typical quiet monotonous speech with a tendency to peter out with continued effort. Difficulty initiating movement leads to pausing before walking (start hesitation), and sudden freezing when attempting to change direction. Difficulty in stopping walking, once started, may lead to festination.

Physical signs reflect the extrapyramidal abnormalities. There is an increased incidence of dementia in patients with Parkinson's disease.

Natural history

The course of Parkinson's disease is very variable. Quality of survival has undoubtedly been improved by levodopa treatment, but the drug has probably not greatly altered average survival, which is in the region of 10 years from the onset of symptoms.

With initial treatment at the time of diagnosis, about one-third of patients with Parkinson's disease improve markedly, one-third show some improvement and one-third show no significant improvement in terms of regaining function. When there are no signs of improvement at all, the diagnosis should be reassessed and one of the causes of Parkinsonism should be considered (Table 23.36). As a rule, Parkinsonism which is not Parkinson's disease does not respond to drug treatment.

Treatment

The pharmacological approach to treatment recognises both that there is a deficiency of dopamine in the corpus striatum and that a balance exists between dopaminergic and cholinergic activity. Side-effects of the anticholinergic drugs used include blurred vision due to impairment of accommodation (these drugs should not be used in glaucoma), a dry mouth, constipation and urinary hesitancy. Injudicious use in men with prostatic enlargement may precipitate urinary retention. The cerebral side-effects of these drugs include mental agitation, a toxic confusional state, psychosis and occasionally fits, although fits are unusual at lower doses of the drugs normally used.

Levodopa. The introduction of levodopa revolutionised the treatment of Parkinson's disease. The drug exerts its greatest effect on akinesia. It is now given in combination with an extracerebral decarboxylase inhibitor, either as Sinemet (levodopa plus carbidopa) or Madopar (levodopa plus benserazide), which prevents systemic metabolism of levodopa, thereby promoting higher CNS levels. Much smaller doses of levodopa can thus be given, leading to a reduction in the systemic side-effects of the drug which include nausea and vomiting, postural hypotension and cardiac arrhythmias. Nausea and vomiting can be further reduced by taking levodopa after food. The drug may produce agitation, poor concentration, hallucinations and

---

Summary 7 Treatment of Parkinson's disease

- When symptoms and disability are mild, in the early stages, drug treatment may not be required.
- If tremor is the main problem, start with an anticholinergic drug, unless contraindicated (glaucoma, prostatic hypertrophy).
- If akinesia is the main problem, start dopamine with a decarboxylase inhibitor.
- Aim to alleviate, rather than abolish, the symptoms and signs.
- Be aware of the major side-effects of the drugs, which become much more common in the later stages of the disease.
- Intolerance to the drugs, particularly dopamine, is common later in the disease, and often necessitates reduction of dose and sometimes withdrawal.
- Dose-related motor oscillations may be reduced in some patients by giving divided doses more frequently.
- In later stages, motor oscillations are frequently not related to dosage.
- Selegiline is useful in some patients with the on-off phenomenon.

a frank psychosis. These effects frequently limit or prevent the use of the drug and are more common in elderly patients, and in those with long-standing Parkinson's disease or coexistent dementia. Excessive levodopa treatment often leads to dyskinetic movements.

Anticholinergic drugs have most effect on tremor and relatively little on the akinesia in Parkinson's disease. Anticholinergics are useful, but are now usually given in conjunction with levodopa therapy.

Amantadine, which increases synthesis and release of dopamine, has a weak anti-Parkinsonian effect and is occasionally helpful when there is intolerance to anticholinergic or levodopa therapy.

In the early stages, Parkinson's disease does not merit drug treatment. If tremor is the major disability, without symptomatic akinesia, either benzhexol (2 mg three times a day) or orphenadrine (50 mg three times a day) are recommended. Amantadine (100 mg twice a day) is an alternative.

When akinesia is severe enough to lead to disability, Sinemet or Madopar (62.5 mg of either three times a day after meals) should be started. The dose can be gradually increased. Common dose-limiting side-effects are nausea or mental changes. In patients intolerant of therapeutic doses of levodopa, bromocriptine (a dopamine receptor agonist) can be tried. It is not superior to levodopa in its therapeutic effects and causes all the same side-effects. It is rarely used as initial therapy, but, occasionally, patients intolerant of levodopa may show a better response to bromocriptine.

Levels of dopamine may be increased by the selective monoamine oxidase B inhibitor, selegiline. This drug has an effect in some patients with long-standing Parkinson's disease who develop the *on-off phenomenon*, in which, unrelated to timing of dosage of levodopa, there is an abrupt onset of severe akinesia which lasts for up to two hours, followed by an equally abrupt restoration of mobility.

In long-standing Parkinson's disease there is often decreasing responsiveness and increasing intolerance to treatment. However, many patients do relatively well and eventually die of causes unrelated to Parkinson's disease.

OTHER AKINETIC-RIGID SYNDROMES

Encephalitis lethargica (post-encephalitic Parkinsonism)

Encephalitis lethargica is now a very rare illness. It is a Parkinsonian syndrome which may occasionally result following encephalitis. The great flu epidemics of the 1920s resulted in many cases of encephalitis lethargica. All the features of Parkinson's disease may be present, but there is a limited response to drug treatment.

Multiple systems atrophy

The term multiple systems atrophy (MSA) is now used to refer to three overlapping degenerative conditions in which Parkinsonism is an important feature.

Progressive autonomic failure

In progressive autonomic failure (*Shy-Drager syndrome*), there are degenerative changes in the basal ganglia, cerebellum, brain stem and the intermediolateral column of the spinal cord (producing sympathetic dysfunction). Patients often present initially with a syndrome indistinguishable from Parkinson's disease, although tremor is uncommon. Incontinence and impotence are early symptoms and, later, an obvious widespread autonomic disturbance develops, with postural hypotension, failure of sweating and respiratory problems, including sleep apnoea.

Olivopontocerebellar degeneration

In olivopontocerebellar degeneration, there are severe degenerative changes in the cerebellum, pons and medulla. Clinically, a progressive cerebellar, limb and gait ataxia, with dysarthria and nystagmus, overshadows Parkinsonism. Pyramidal signs are also present.

Strionigral degeneration

In strionigral degeneration, there are extensive degenerative changes in the basal ganglia. This is the akinetic syndrome most likely to be confused with Parkinson's disease. As with progressive autonomic failure and olivopontocerebellar degeneration, there is little or no response of the Parkinsonism to levodopa therapy.

All three syndromes comprising MSA are essentially untreatable. Syndromes are relentlessly progressive and death usually occurs within five years of onset.

Steele-Richardson-Olszewski syndrome (Progressive supranuclear palsy)

Steele-Richardson-Olszewski syndrome is characterised by Parkinsonism without tremor, and a progressive supranuclear ocular (gaze) palsy, widespread pyramidal signs and, sometimes, dementia. Patients present with difficulty in walking or visual symptoms, particularly with reading or looking downwards. The syndrome is rarely helped by levodopa or other drug treatment.

Cerebral anoxia

Diffuse cerebral anoxia (usually resulting from cardiorespiratory arrest) occasionally leads to Parkinsonism, due to bilateral basal ganglia infarction with relative preservation of other parts of the CNS. In younger people, carbon monoxide poisoning and severe hypotension with hypoxia in opiate overdosage are the usual causes of this syndrome. The Parkinsonism is unresponsive to drug treatment and is sometimes progressive.

Wilson's disease (hepatolenticular degeneration)

Behavioural changes and dyskinesias are the common neurological manifestations of Wilson's disease in childhood, but Parkinsonism, often with dyskinesias, is the more common adolescent and early adult presentation (p. 650). Presentation of Wilson's disease in adult life is almost invariably with the neurological manifestations, and patients may present as late as the fifth decade. Although the basal ganglia bear the brunt of neurological damage in Wilson's disease, copper deposition in the CNS is widespread, with dementia developing in untreated patients. Wilson's disease must be considered in any child or young adult presenting with an extrapyramidal syndrome. Copper deposition in Descemet's membrane at the margin of the cornea may produce a Kayser-Fleischer ring. Copper deposition in the lens may cause a cataract, and deposits in the nail beds a bluish discolouration.

DYSKINESIAS

The dyskinesias include tremor, chorea, hemiballismus, dystonia and myoclonus.

Tremor

Tremor (see also p. 914) may be classified as:

1. *postural* tremor when it is maximal with maintained posture
2. *rest* tremor, the type characteristic of extrapyramidal diseases
3. *action* tremor, due to diseases affecting the cerebellum directly or its connections in the brain stem (Table 23.37).

Normal physiological tremor may be exaggerated by anxiety and is also enhanced in thyrotoxicosis, by sympathomimetic drugs and by alcohol.

Table 23.37 Causes of tremor

Tremor	Cause
Postural tremor	
Exaggerated physiological tremor	Anxiety
	Alcohol
	Thyrotoxicosis
	Drugs – some tricyclic
	antidepressants
	Lithium
	Sympathomimetics, e.g.
	bronchodilators
Benign essential tremor	Uncertain
Severe cerebellar disease (rubral tremor)	
Rest tremor	Parkinson's disease
	Causes of Parkinsonism (Table 23.36)
Action tremor	Cerebellar and brain stem disease
	MS
	Infarction or haemorrhage
	Tumours
	Hereditary ataxias and
	spinocerebellar degenerations
Benign essential tremor	Uncertain

Essential tremor

Essential tremor (also known as benign essential tremor, familial tremor and senile tremor) is the commonest of the dyskinesias. It is usually mild. The cause remains uncertain. It is a postural tremor which is also present on action but which is not exacerbated by action. This differentiates it from cerebellar or Parkinsonian tremor. There are no other neurological abnormalities.

Emotional circumstances increase the tremor, and unlike other forms of tremor, small amounts of alcohol have a therapeutic effect. There is a positive family history in at least 50% of cases, and the condition is thought to be dominantly inherited with variable penetrance.

Beta-receptor-blockers, such as propranolol, help about one-third of patients. Judicious use of alcohol can be recommended in certain patients, and benzodiazepines are occasionally helpful.

Asterixis

The term asterixis is used to refer to the flapping tremor seen in the severe metabolic disturbances of respiratory, renal and hepatic failure. It is a postural tremor, and is best seen in the outstretched hands.

Chorea

Chorea (see also p. 914) has a number of causes, listed in Table 23.38.

Huntington's chorea

Huntington's chorea is discussed on page 904.

Sydenham's chorea

Sydenham's chorea, a complication of rheumatic fever first described by Thomas Sydenham in the 17th century, is now rare. The onset is usually gradual, most cases occurring between 7 and 12 years of age. In only 30% of cases is there a clear preceding history of a streptococcal infection with rheumatic fever.

More widespread cerebral disturbance occurs in some patients, who may develop a confusional state or behavioural changes. The pathogenesis of these neurological

Table 23.38 Causes of chorea

Sydenham's chorea	**With systemic disease**
Chorea gravidarum	Thyrotoxicosis
Chorea with oral contraceptive pill	Polycythaemia rubra vera
	Encephalitis lethargica
Huntington's disease	SLE
	Hypocalcaemia
Drug-induced	Hypernatraemia
Neuroleptic drugs	
Phenytoin	**Hemiballismus or hemichorea**
Alcohol	Infarction
	Tumour
	Trauma

917

complications of streptococcal infection is uncertain, but immune complex deposition is likely.

Chorea is of variable severity. All the neurological manifestations resolve gradually over one to six months. Symptomatic treatment with neuroleptics, such as chlorpromazine or tetrabenazine, may be necessary. A history of Sydenham's chorea predisposes to the later development of chorea gravidarum, or chorea with the oral contraceptive pill or other drugs, such as phenytoin.

Hemiballismus

Hemiballismus, or hemichorea, is a dramatic type of involuntary movement in which there are large amplitude throwing movements of the limbs on one side. It usually occurs acutely in elderly patients, and is the result of infarction involving the contralateral subthalamic nucleus. It very occasionally occurs with a tumour or after head injury. Hemiballismus is usually an isolated abnormality, but may be accompanied by a hemiparesis or hemisensory impairment. It usually spontaneously resolves within a few months, but symptomatic treatment with neuroleptic drugs is necessary when the movements are severe.

Dystonia

The causes of dystonia are listed in Table 23.39. Acute drug-induced dystonia is the most common type; it is usually mild and reversible on stopping the offending drug.

Spasmodic torticollis

Spasmodic torticollis may occur as an isolated phenomenon or as part of a generalised dystonia. There is involuntary turning of the head to one side, which may be a maintained

Table 23.39 Causes of dystonia

Focal dystonia
Writer's cramp
Spasmodic torticollis
Cranial dystonia
Hemiplegic dystonia, due to, e.g. strokes, tumours, encephalitis, trauma

Generalised dystonia
Drug-induced acute and tardive dystonias
  Anti-emetics; prochlorperazine, metaclopromide
  Neuroleptics
  Levodopa and dopamine agonists
Torsion dystonia
Dystonia with other cerebral diseases
  Hereditary – Gangliosidoses
           Metachromatic leucodystrophy
           Wilson's disease
           Huntington's disease
           Homocystinuria
  Acquired – Cerebral palsy
           Encephalitis lethargica
           Mitochondrial cytopathy

posture or a rhythmical movement, and there is frequently associated extension of the neck (retrocollis). Onset is usually in adult life without obvious provocation, although occasionally there is a history of trauma to the neck. It may last a few weeks or months, remit and not recur. However, recurrent episodes are common, and in some patients there is no remission.

Treatment is difficult. Neuroleptic drugs may help, but may eventually induce extrapyramidal disease. A combination of diazepam and benzhexol can be effective and is safe if long-term treatment becomes necessary. Surgical denervation of the neck muscles is rarely successful.

Torsion dystonia (dystonia musculorum deformans)

Torsion dystonia is a rare and disabling generalised dystonia of unknown cause. When it presents in childhood, there is often a family history, or examination of other family members may reveal milder forms of the condition. Inheritance as an autosomal dominant or recessive trait has been reported. The disease tends to be more severe in children than in the adult-onset group. Typically, dystonic posturing of the trunk and limbs is provoked or exacerbated by voluntary actions.

Large doses of benzhexol (up to 120 mg a day), sometimes combined with diazepam, offer the best chance of improvement. Attempts at stereotaxic surgery may have to be considered, but bilateral thalamotomy necessarily carries substantial risks.

Cranial dystonia

Cranial dystonia includes: *blepharospasm*, an involuntary closure of the eyelids due to spasm of the orbicularis oculi muscles; and *oromandibular dystonia*, which refers to involuntary dystonic movements of the tongue, jaw and face which may seriously interfere with speech and eating. The cause of these dystonias is unknown. Cranial dystonia usually starts in middle-age and does not remit.

Treatment, as in other dystonias, is unsatisfactory. Neuroleptic drugs are sometimes helpful and the best combination is high-dose benzhexol and diazepam. Recent reports suggest that injection of botulinum toxin into the orbicularis oculi muscles may relieve blepharospasm for up to three months. Wider application of this technique may prove to be appropriate in other types of dystonia, such as torticollis.

Writer's cramp

Some cases of writer's cramp are undoubtedly psychogenic, but the condition is widely regarded as being a focal dystonia with an organic basis, albeit of unknown nature. It almost always occurs as an isolated abnormality. Observation of the patient writing demonstrates the problem. The pen is usually gripped awkwardly and/or too tightly with an abnormal posture of the hand and arm and sometimes also of the trunk and head. Writing is slow and laborious, and becomes increasingly illegible with continued effort. The condition may also affect other repetitive, fine manipulative tasks; for example it is common for musicians to present with a similar difficulty in playing their instruments.

Myoclonus

The causes of myoclonus are listed in Table 23.40. Myoclonus may be divided into two major categories, generalised and focal or segmental myoclonus.

Generalised myoclonus may be divided into three subgroups:

1. *Essential myoclonus* refers to myoclonus which is not associated with any other neurological abnormality. It is often familial and runs a benign course.
2. *Myoclonic encephalopathies* are generalised progressive or static encephalopathies in which myoclonus is a frequent or recognised feature.
3. *Myoclonus associated with epilepsy.* (See page 888.)

Focal myoclonus is rare. Lesions of the cortex or cerebral hemisphere may occasionally be the cause. Hemifacial spasm sometimes takes the form of myoclonic jerking, but a more continuous, less myoclonic, type of involuntary muscular contraction is more usual. The pathophysiology in hemifacial spasm remains unknown. In some cases, a peripheral nerve basis is suggested by the occasional occurrence of hemifacial spasm with posterior fossa compressive tumours, and following Bell's palsy.

Palatal myoclonus is indicative of a brain stem lesion involving olivodentatorubral pathways. Myoclonus occurs very rarely with spinal cord lesions.

Drug-induced extrapyramidal disease

Chlorpromazine and related drugs (the neuroleptics) may produce a number of extrapyramidal side-effects including Parkinsonism, acute dyskinesias, tremor, and tardive dyskinesia. The anti-emetics, metaclopramide and prochlorperazine, also have neuroleptic properties, and may produce acute and chronic extrapyramidal syndromes. Most tremors and dystonias resolve on withdrawing the offending drug, and involuntary movements can often be acutely stopped by intravenous anticholinergic drugs, such as benztropine. Tardive dyskinesias are the exception. Excessive levodopa therapy is a common cause of dyskinesia and dystonia in patients with Parkinson's disease.

Tardive dyskinesia

Tardive dyskinesia is the most serious side-effect of neuroleptic treatment; it requires at least six months of continuous neuroleptic administration. The usual manifestations are orofacial dyskinesias with a variety of chewing, pouting and lip-smacking movements, combined with a discrete dystonia, or choreiform limb movements and, sometimes, rocking trunk movements. Occasionally, the dyskinesias may be incapacitating. Withdrawing the drug

Table 23.40 Causes of myoclonus

Type of myoclonus	Cause
Generalised myoclonus	
Essential familial myoclonus	
Myoclonic encephalopathies	Degenerative cerebral diseases, e.g. gangliosidoses, Lafora body disease, hereditary ataxia
	Encephalitis lethargica
	Subacute sclerosing panencephalitis
	Creutzfeldt-Jacob disease
	Metabolic – uraemia, hypocalcaemia, hepatic failure, hyponatraemia, respiratory failure (CO_2 narcosis) alcohol withdrawal
	Post-traumatic myoclonus
	Post-anoxic myoclonus
Myoclonus with epilepsy	
Focal myoclonus	Cortical or cerebral hemisphere lesions
	Brain stem degeneration or infarction
	Spinal myoclonus

responsible leads to gradual improvement in about half the patients, with resolution over a period of up to three years. However, in other patients, there is no improvement and in a small minority the dyskinesia is progressive and resistant to all treatment, despite stopping the neuroleptic drug.

The frequent prescription of drugs with neuroleptic properties, such as prochlorperazine and metaclopramide, emphasises the need to take a careful and detailed drug history in all patients presenting with symptoms and signs of extrapyramidal disease.

HEAD INJURY

In the UK, approximately 5000 people die each year as a result of head injury and many others survive, but with some disability. Road traffic accidents are the commonest single cause, and alcohol can be implicated both in many of these and in other causes of severe head injuries. Fracture of the skull occurs in only a small proportion of head injuries. Its absence does not imply a mild head injury, but the presence of a skull fracture is associated with a greatly increased incidence of intracranial haemorrhage.

Effects of head injury

Immediate

Severe blows to the head cause shearing forces within the brain, causing both diffuse axonal injury, particularly to the white matter, and also focal areas of damage in the cortex and deeper parts of the brain. Haematomas may develop deep within the hemispheres, often distant from the site of impact. The inferior surfaces of the frontal and temporal lobes are particularly common sites of haematoma formation, because of their rough bony surfaces. Lacerations of the cortex may be produced by depressed skull fractures.

Secondary

Haematoma formation

Haematomas may form at the time of the head injury, but often develop during the first 24 hours after injury and sometimes over longer periods. Their maximum effect on cerebral function may occur at much longer intervals, the most extreme example being chronic subdural haematomas.

Intracerebral haematomas may be multiple and are of very variable size (Fig. 23.31). Oedema developing around haematomas will further contribute to a rise in intracranial pressure. Extradural haematomas (Fig. 23.32) develop within hours of head injury in which the skull vault is fractured. On arrival at hospital, the patient may be alert and orientated, but the conscious level then rapidly deteriorates. Extradural haematomas may be fatal, or lead to permanent brain damage, unless promptly treated. Large acute subdural haematomas may produce similar effects, but are less likely than extradural haematomas to lead to a rapid early deterioration of cerebral function.

Cerebral oedema and raised intracranial pressure

Cerebral oedema may result from diffuse cerebral injury without haematoma formation; it also develops around haematomas. The effect is a rise in intracranial pressure which may be life-threatening.

Infection

There is a risk of meningitis or cerebral abscess with any penetrating injury of the skull. Leakage of CSF through the nose (rhinorrhoea) or the ear (otorrhoea) indicates a basal skull fracture and the potential for development of meningitis. Fractures involving the nasal sinuses may also lead to infection.

Extracranial factors complicating the effects of head injury

A compromised airway, chest injury or infection and, rarely, the adult respiratory distress syndrome, may all lead to hypoxia. Together with hypotension, usually the result of bleeding in the abdomen or associated with other injury, hypoxia intensifies cerebral ischaemia.

Management

Early management

The first consideration in the management of head injury is resuscitation (Ch. 15). The airway must be cleared. Intu-

Fig. 23.31 Multiple, bilateral intracerebral haematomas in a young man with a severe closed head injury. In the right hemisphere, there is massive oedema, causing midline shift and obstruction of CSF flow, leading to hydrocephalus of the left lateral ventricle.

bation and artificial ventilation may be necessary. Shock in head-injured patients is almost always the result of other major injury, and requires immediate correction.

Having resuscitated the patient, an initial neurological examination is undertaken. This includes a thorough examination of the skull and scalp, determining any CSF leaks, and assessing the conscious level; it is particularly

Fig. 23.32 Right-sided extradural haematoma, associated with a skull fracture. There is acute severe cerebral compression. (Reproduced by permission of Dr J Stevens and Dr A Valentine)

important to monitor subsequent improvement or deterioration. The Glasgow coma scale (p. 858) provides a simple means of assessment.

Neck injuries are a common accompaniment of head injury. The neck must therefore be handled with care until cervical spine X-rays have excluded major bony injury.

Controversy surrounds the necessity for skull X-rays in mild head injury. Definite indications are a history of loss of consciousness at any time, the presence of scalp bruising or swelling, any neurological signs, a CSF leak or evidence of a penetrating injury. The absence of a skull fracture does not exclude serious intracranial problems in an individual patient, but for patients with a fracture whose conscious level is impaired, there is a 1 in 4 risk of intracranial haemorrhage. This compares with a 1 in 30 risk of haemorrhage in patients with a fracture but with a normal conscious level; a 1 in 120 chance in patients without a skull fracture, but with impairment of conscious level; and a 1 in 6000 chance in patients without skull fracture or impairment of conscious level.

It is important to know what the conscious level was immediately after the head injury; a history of a lucid interval of consciousness suggests the possibility of an extradural haemorrhage, for which urgent CT scanning and treatment is necessary.

Neurological referral

Many patients with minor head injury can be rapidly discharged if there is no history of loss of consciousness, no evidence of skull fracture and no abnormal neurological signs. Any patient in whom there has been loss of consciousness for any period must be admitted and observed for 24 hours. Neurosurgical referral in obvious severe head injury is clearly essential. Neurosurgical advice should also be sought for any patient who has suffered a period of unconsciousness lasting for more than an hour, who has abnormal neurological signs persisting for more than a few hours, or who has a skull fracture. Referral is particularly important if there is a basal skull fracture, a compound depressed fracture, or if there is evidence of a penetrating injury.

Treatment of intracranial haematomas

Extradural haematomas often increase in size during the first few hours after head injury, and prompt evacuation is crucial. Acute subdural haemorrhage is less common, and deterioration in the hours following head injury is not characteristic of this type of bleeding. Large subdural collections need to be evacuated.

Large intracerebral haematomas are evacuated, particularly if associated with neurological deterioration or a very poor initial neurological state. Multiple small haematomas are best managed conservatively.

CSF leaks usually resolve within a few days and surgical treatment is not necessary. Prophylactic antibiotics should be given.

Depressed skull fractures alone do not necessarily require treatment, but if there is cortical damage, reduction is necessary, and open fractures require surgical closure of the dura and skin.

Cerebral oedema frequently develops after major brain injury, compounding the neurological deficit. Mannitol and frusemide are effective in reducing this, but the use of dexamethasone in the treatment of cerebral oedema resulting from head injury is controversial. Artificial ventilation is often necessary in severe head injury, and ventilation is sometimes used electively to reduce arterial CO_2 levels in order to reduce intracranial pressure. Whether or not this alters the outcome of brain damage due to head injury is uncertain.

Late complications of head injury

Persistent physical neurological deficit is the rule after severe head injury. In addition to hemiparesis or quadraparesis, dysphasia and visual field defects are common. Cranial nerves are commonly affected (e.g. diplopia is a common and troublesome post-head-injury symptom). Cerebellar deficits are fairly common. Brain injury may eventually lead to focal or generalised cerebral atrophy, as well as hydrocephalus. Epilepsy usually develops later, sometimes years after the injury.

Chronic subdural haematoma

Chronic subdural haematoma is more common in older patients. In at least 50% of cases there is no history of any preceding head injury, and in others, the injury recalled is usually trivial and not associated with loss of consciousness or other immediate neurological sequelae. Degradation of the subdural blood produces smaller molecules with

Fig. 23.33 Chronic bilateral subdural haematomas. On the left hemisphere, there is a clear line of demarcation between compressed brain and the subdural collection. The attenuation of the subdural is mainly low, indicating that it is chronic, but there is fresh blood, producing a fluid level in the posterior part of the subdural. There is a smaller right chronic subdural haematoma.

greater osmotic effect, and the subdural haematoma increases in size over weeks or months, changing into a straw-coloured fluid. This may present with hemisphere symptoms and signs, together with symptoms and signs of raised intracranial pressure. A mild hemiparesis with intellectual deterioration and a fluctuating level of consciousness is the classical, but by no means the only, presentation of chronic subdural haematoma. Papilloedema is often present. Chronic subdural haematomas are bilateral in a proportion of cases (Fig. 23.33).

The differential diagnosis includes cerebral tumour or abscess, and chronic subdural haematoma is often misdiagnosed as cerebrovascular disease. Treatment by drainage of the haematoma through burr holes often produces a marked improvement, regardless of the age of the patient.

Boxing encephalopathy

A combination of progressive cognitive impairment, dysarthria, ataxia, extrapyramidal and pyramidal signs may develop in some boxers. This 'punch drunk' syndrome is the result of repeated blows to the head, and a similar syndrome may result from repeated minor head injury in other sports, e.g. rugby football or diving. The cerebral damage is irreversible. CT scans usually show diffuse atrophy.

Psychological effects of head injury

Amnesia for events after the injury (post-traumatic amnesia) is always longer than that before the event (pre-traumatic or retrograde amnesia). The period of post-traumatic amnesia is related to the severity of the head injury. Some intellectual impairment after severe head injury is inevitable. Most improvement occurs within the first few months, but can occur for up to two years. Increasingly, multidisciplinary rehabilitation units are adapting to the needs of increasing numbers of head-injured patients, many of whom are young.

CEREBRAL PALSY

The term cerebral palsy refers to a variety of neurological deficits, mainly affecting motor function, which arise as a result of prenatal insult, birth injury or some illness in early infancy. Implicit in the diagnosis is the assumption that the deficit is static, but it is usually impossible in early life to establish the extent of the cerebral injury, which only becomes fully manifest in late childhood. In addition to motor deficits, intellectual impairment and behavioural problems are common. The majority of children with cerebral palsy survive into adult life.

Incidence and aetiology

The incidence of cerebral palsy varies from country to country, but is of the order of 2–5 per 1000 live-born children surviving to school age.

Table 23.41 summarises the many factors known to be important in the development of cerebral palsy.

Major types of cerebral palsy

The classification of the cerebral palsies is descriptive, and is based on the major motor deficit (Table 23.42).

Spastic hemiplegia. This is the commonest type of cerebral palsy, in which, in addition to the hemiplegia, there may be a hemisensory and hemianopic visual field defect, and sometimes dysphasia. There are often bilateral lesions, and up to half these children have learning difficulties. Some have associated choreoathetosis and many develop epilepsy.

Spastic paraplegia. Spastic paraplegia causes difficulty in walking, and the legs often do not develop properly and become shortened. The upper limbs are relatively spared, although the reflexes are brisk, and there is sometimes clumsiness of the hands. Learning difficulties, fits, and squints are all common.

Table 23.41   Factors important in causation of cerebral palsy

Antenatal
Developmental abnormalities
Infections, e.g. CMV, rubella, toxoplasma, syphilis
Hypoxia, e.g. placenta praevia, placental haemorrhage, maternal hypotension
Pre-eclamptic toxaemia
Irradiation
Maternal age <20 or >35
Twins

Natal

Trauma
Breech delivery
Prolonged or precipitous delivery

Intracerebral haemorrhage
Subdural haemorrhage
Intraventricular haemorrhage
Subarachnoid haemorrhage

Prematurity
Post-maturity

Post-natal in pre-term infants
Cerebral ischaemia
Cerebral haemorrhage
Hypoxia secondary to respiratory distress syndrome
Acidosis
Hypothermia
Hypoglycaemia

Post-natal in children with normal CNS at birth
Encephalitis
Meningitis
Hypoxia, e.g. during cardiac surgery
Kernicterus
Trauma, including non-accidental injury

Tetraplegia. This is the result of extensive bilateral cortical damage, which leads to mental retardation and, often, visual and sensory deficits, in addition to a spastic tetraplegia. The visual defect may be cortical in origin, or due to optic nerve atrophy. Squints are common, as is epilepsy. The bilateral upper motor neurone deficit leads to a pseudobulbar palsy. Many children do not survive for more than a few years.

Choreoathetosis and dystonia. Choreoathetoid movements in this type of cerebral palsy may not develop for some months post-natally. The early brief choreiform movements may be subtle, and athetosis may not develop until the child is about two years old. The involuntary movements often lead to dysarthria, but these children are usually of normal intelligence. In the past, kernicterus was

Table 23.42   Classification of cerebral palsy

Spasticity	Cerebellar ataxia
Hemiplegia	
Paraplegia (diplegia)	**Mixed syndromes**
Tetraplegia	

Involuntary movements
Choreoathetosis
Dystonia

a common cause of this type of palsy.

Ataxia. A form of pure cerebellar ataxia, thought to be usually due to maldevelopment of the cerebellum, is occasionally seen; it is often associated with mental retardation.

Mixed syndromes. Children with mixed deficits are common, the most frequent being a combination of a spastic paraplegia and ataxia. There is often associated hydrocephalus, possibly the result of intraventricular haemorrhage pre-natally, or birth trauma.

Treatment

The full extent of disability in children with cerebral palsy may not be evident for some years, and it is important from an early stage to recognise potentially treatable additional deficits such as squints, epilepsy and deafness. Physiotherapy has a large role to play, but contractures and other deformities inevitably develop in some children and may require surgical treatment. Dislocation of the hip is common in spastic legs. The combined efforts of therapists from various disciplines are necessary, together with family counselling and social support. Many children require special education. Specially adapted equipment, such as typewriters and communicators, may be needed, to enable the child with severe disability but normal intelligence to communicate. Lack of mobility is a major problem, threatening to deprive children of many educational and recreational opportunities, and special wheelchairs may be needed. Many less severely affected patients with cerebral palsy are able to lead reasonably independent lives.

CEREBELLAR ATAXIAS

Impairment of cerebellar function is common in neurological disease (Tables 23.43 and 23.44 and Summary 8). The cerebellum is responsible for monitoring afferent activity and influencing the cerebral cortical control of movement. Afferents to the cerebellum arise from muscle and joint receptors via fibres travelling in the spinocerebellar tracts; there is also some input from cutaneous afferents, the vestibular system and some visual afferents. For clinical purposes, the cerebellum may be divided into the two hemispheres and the midline vermis. Lesions of one hemisphere produce ipsilateral limb incoordination (ataxia), hypotonia and, sometimes, nystagmus. Vermis lesions cause disturbance of control of truncal movement, leading to the characteristic wide-based unsteady gait.

Limb or gait ataxia may also be caused by weakness or sensory impairment, particularly proprioceptive loss.

Hereditary ataxias, spinocerebellar degenerations and hereditary spastic paraparesis

The neurological deficit in cerebellar ataxias ranges from a pure cerebellar ataxia (as in autosomal dominant inherited, late-onset cerebellar ataxia), through mixed syndromes, involving spinal as well as cerebellar features (*spinocerebellar degenerations*), to a pure spastic paraplegia. There are often other neurological and non-neurological associated features (Table 23.43).

The hereditary ataxias

Most hereditary ataxias are rare; many are of concern principally to the paediatric neurologist, as those affected usually fail to survive into adult life.

Early-onset hereditary ataxias

Friedreich's ataxia, an autosomal recessive condition, is much the most common type of hereditary ataxia. Progressive ataxia of gait and limbs usually develops in childhood and always before the age of 25 years, and is associated with dysarthria, nystagmus, a spastic paraparesis and extensor plantars, but with areflexia due to an axonal sensory neuropathy. A cardiomyopathy is present in about two-thirds of patients, and diabetes in about 10%; some patients are of low intelligence. The ataxia is relentlessly progressive and death usually occurs during the fourth decade from cardiac failure. A similar, but more benign, autosomal recessive condition (also arising in childhood), occurs, in which there is no evidence of neuropathy.

Ataxia telangiectasia – an autosomal recessive syndrome of progressive cerebellar ataxia with onset in childhood – is associated with conjunctival and cutaneous telangiectasia.

Late onset hereditary ataxias

A number of hereditary ataxias do not develop until the patient is more than 20 years of age. It is clinically useful to consider these cases as a single group (Table 23.43). A pure cerebellar ataxia of onset at over 50 years is occasionally seen. In all patients with dominantly-inherited, late-onset ataxias, the major feature is a slowly progressive gait and limb ataxia, with dysarthria and nystagmus.

Cerebellar ataxia also occurs as a minor feature of many other inherited metabolic defects, most of which produce widespread neurological deficits (Table 23.43).

Acquired ataxias

Mild unsteadiness of gait is extremely common in elderly patients and is often multifactorial in origin. A degree of cerebellar degeneration is common in old age. Iatrogenic, drug-induced ataxia is also common, particularly in the elderly, the offending drugs including phenytoin, carbamazepine, and benzodiazepines. An acute reversible ataxia is produced by alcohol, but chronic alcohol abuse may lead to a predominantly midline vermis degeneration which is largely irreversible (p. 973). Cerebellar involvement is common in MS. Mild ataxia is quite common in hypothyroidism and may occasionally be the presenting factor. Cerebellar tumours and some paraneoplastic syndromes can cause ataxia. Pyogenic abscesses and tuberculomas occasionally develop in the cerebellum. Encephalitis may produce a cerebellar ataxia, particularly in children, in whom a pure syndrome of cerebellar ataxia is now recognised. Other causes of ataxia in childhood are listed in Table 23.44.

Ataxia arising as a result of foramen magnum and posterior fossa congenital malformations, particularly Arnold-Chiari type I malformations (p. 933), may present in adult life, without any neurological deficit in early life.

Table 23.43 Hereditary ataxias and spinocerebellar degenerations

Early-onset ataxia
Friedreich's ataxia
Ataxia with retained tendon reflexes
Ataxia telangiectasia
Ataxia with other features including myoclonus, pigmentary retinopathy, optic atrophy, mental retardation, deafness, extrapyramidal signs

Inherited metabolic defects producing ataxia as a minor feature
Metachromatic leucodystrophy (p. 954)
Refsum's disease (p. 943)
Mitochondrial cytopathy (p. 951)
Wilson's disease (p. 916)
Disorders of sphingolipid metabolism (p. 954)
Abetalipoproteinaemia
Hexosaminidase deficiencies (e.g. Tay-Sachs disease, p. 954)
Adrenoleucodystrophy (p. 955)

Late-onset ataxia (more than 20 years)
Autosomal dominant ataxia with ophthalmoplegia/optic atrophy/dementia/extrapyramidal features
Autosomal dominant ataxia with pigmentary retinopathy with or without ophthalmoplegia/extrapyramidal features
Autosomal dominant ataxia with myoclonus and deafness
Pure autosomal dominant ataxia

Table 23.44 Causes of cerebellar ataxia in children

Congenital malformations	Infectious
Cerebellar agenesis/hypoplasia	Secondary to bacterial meningitis
Dandy-Walker syndrome*	Secondary to encephalitis
Arnold-Chiari malformation**	
	Hydrocephalus*
Hereditary ataxias	
See Table 23.44	**Tumours**
	Medulloblastoma
Trauma	Astrocytoma
Birth trauma*	Haemangioblastoma
Head injury in childhood*	

* May persist into adult life. ** May present in adult life

Summary 8 Acquired cerebellar disease

- Senile degenerative cerebellar ataxia
- Drug-induced ataxia, e.g. anticonvulsants, benzodiazepines
- Multiple sclerosis
- Toxic – alcoholic acute ataxia and chronic cerebellar degeneration
- Neoplastic – primary, secondary and paraneoplastic
- Metabolic – hypothyroidism
- Infective – abscess, tuberculoma, encephalitis

DISEASES OF THE SPINAL CORD

Anatomy and physiology

The spinal cord extends from the foramen magnum to the level of the lower border of the first lumbar vertebra. The essential features of spinal cord lesions are bilateral symptoms and/or signs, together with impairment of bladder and bowel control, impairment of sexual function in men and, sometimes, a sensory level on the trunk. Partial spinal cord lesions do not produce all these effects; when the signs are unilateral, they may be difficult to distinguish from lesions at higher levels in the nervous system.

The major motor pathways in the spinal cord are the *corticospinal tracts*. These decussate at the level of the lower medulla and descend in the anterolateral columns of the spinal cord, ending on anterior horn cells.

The two major sensory pathways are the dorsal columns and the spinothalamic tracts. *Dorsal column* fibres convey joint position and vibration sensation and some touch. *Spinothalamic tract* fibres convey information about pain, temperature and some touch. Some spinal cord lesions produce selective sensory tract damage, giving rise to dissociated sensory loss on the trunk and in the limbs. A sensory level on the trunk is a hallmark of spinal cord disturbances, but is present only in a minority of lesions. The sensory level is often several segments below the actual level of the lesion in the spinal cord.

The abdominal reflexes are occasionally helpful in determining the level of a thoracic cord lesion. However, the abdominal reflexes are lost with increasing age and are absent in obese patients. The segmental level of the upper abdominal reflexes is T9, and of the lower T11.

It is often not possible to localise the precise level of a spinal cord disturbance on clinical grounds; in most instances, special investigation will therefore be necessary. Compressive lesions of the spinal cord may be complicated by disturbances of blood supply which cause additional damage to the cord.

Any acute spinal cord lesion may give rise to a flaccid paraplegia with areflexia and non-reactive plantar responses, rather than a spastic paraparesis. It can be difficult to distinguish a spinal cord lesion from a peripheral lesion causing widespread weakness, such as an acute Guillain-Barré syndrome. However, the involvement of the bladder and the presence of a sensory level will clearly indicate that the lesion is within the spinal cord in most cases.

Clinical differentiation of extradural, intradural, extra-medullary and intramedullary lesions, is often not possible. Some intramedullary lesions, such as syringomyelia, give rise to a highly characteristic evolution of symptoms and signs.

Patterns of spinal cord deficit

Cervical lesions

The two commonest causes of cervical cord lesions are demyelinating disease and cervical spondylosis. Degenerative change is usually most pronounced in the mid-cervical region at C5–6, and the myelopathy which may be associated with cervical spondylosis is often maximal at this level. Any cervical cord lesion may produce a combination of root signs (leading to lower motor neurone signs in the upper limbs), radicular sensory impairment, and a spastic paraparesis.

A lesion at C5 or 6 results in sluggish or absent biceps and supinator reflexes with brisk reflexes below this, including the triceps jerk and lower limb reflexes. The occurrence of a finger jerk when eliciting the biceps or supinator reflexes is referred to as an *inverted supinator reflex*.

Cervical cord compression may give rise to dorsal column sensory impairment in the legs, while intrinsic lesions tend to produce spinothalamic disturbances more often than compressive lesions.

Bladder symptoms usually consist of urgency and frequency, eventually with incontinence. Acute cervical cord lesions may result in retention with overflow. Impotence in males is common in cervical cord disturbances.

Lesions at C3 or above affect the phrenic nerve outflow and cause respiratory paralysis.

Many cervical lesions produce minor symptoms in the upper limbs, such as reflex asymmetry, but the major problem is a spastic paraparesis. Careful examination of the upper limbs is essential in all patients presenting with a paraparesis, since there may be signs helpful in localising the lesion to the cervical region.

Thoracic cord lesions

Thoracic cord lesions cause a spastic paraparesis, with bladder, bowel and sexual impairment, and sensory loss as with cervical lesions. A sensory level on the trunk is particularly helpful in establishing the level of the lesion but, as mentioned above, a level on the trunk may be caused by a lesion in the cervical region.

Brown-Séquard syndrome

The clinical features of hemisection of the spinal cord were first described by Brown-Séquard (Fig. 23.34). This syndrome may be produced by compression and may also occur with inflammatory disease of the spinal cord and, occasionally, with vascular lesions. There is ipsilateral sensory loss over one or several segments at the level of the lesion, and also ipsilateral dorsal column sensory impairment. Ipsilateral pyramidal signs occur and, sometimes, bilateral pyramidal signs, but these are always worse on the ipsilateral side; there is also contralateral spinothalamic sensory impairment. Bladder and bowel involvement is variable.

Conus medullaris

Lesions at the conus produce a mixture of upper and lower motor neurone lumbosacral root signs, and are usually

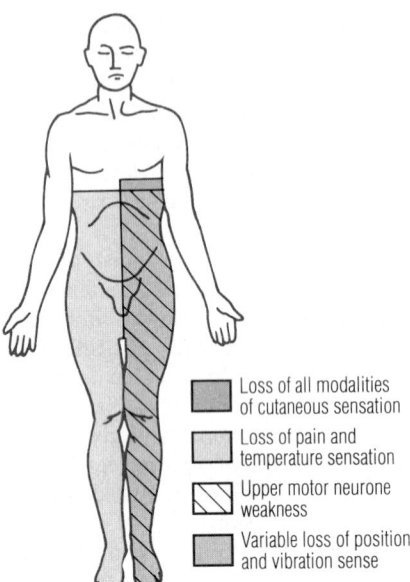

▨	Loss of all modalities of cutaneous sensation
☐	Loss of pain and temperature sensation
▨	Upper motor neurone weakness
▨	Variable loss of position and vibration sense

Fig. 23.34   The features of hemisection of the spinal cord, the Brown-Séquard syndrome. In addition to the signs shown, there is sometimes border zone hyperaesthesia, either at the upper limit of the contralateral spinothalamic sensory loss, or the ipsilateral root sensory loss, or both.

Table 23.45   Causes of acute or subacute paraplegia

Trauma to a previously normal spine

Vertebral disease	**Infection**
Metastatic carcinoma	Epidural abscess
Cervical spondylosis*	TB abscess
Dorsal disc prolapse*	Syphilitic myelitis*
Paget's disease	HIV infection
Rheumatoid arthritis*	Vascular myelopathy
Pott's disease of spine*	
	Vascular
Tumours	Anterior spinal artery occlusion
Extradural or intradural carcinoma, lymphoma, myeloma, leukaemia	Infarction secondary to hypotension
Dorsal meningioma*	Embolic infarction
Neurofibroma*	Infarction secondary to aortic dissection
	Arteriovenous malformation: infarction or haemorrhage
Haematological disease	Primary intramedullary haemorrhage
Any cause of thrombocytopenia	Vasculitis – PAN
Other clotting disorders ⎫ Epidural or	**Inflammatory**
Leukaemia ⎬ intra- medullary	Myelitis of unknown cause
Anticoagulant ⎭ haemorrhage	Myelitis with multiple sclerosis
treatment	SLE
	Sarcoidosis*

* May also cause chronic progressive paraplegia

Table 23.46   Causes of chronic progressive paraplegia

• Causes marked * from Table 23.45	• Subacute combined degeneration of the cord

• Tumours
  Glioma
  Ependymoma
  Chordoma
  Lipoma
	• Hereditary spastic paraplegia

	• Radiation myelopathy
	• Arachnoiditis

• Syringomyelia
  With Arnold-Chiari malformation
  With tumour
	• Ankylosing spondylitis

	• Tropical spastic paraparesis

caused by a tumour, such as an ependymoma or Schwannoma. The bladder disturbance is usually retention and overflow in a large atonic bladder.

Investigation and management of paraplegia

It is essential in any patient presenting with a spinal cord syndrome – particularly when of acute or subacute onset – to exclude spinal cord compression (Summary 9), as this is potentially surgically remediable. Complete loss of bladder function for more than 24 hours cannot be reversed, even if a compressive lesion is relieved, though there may be partial recovery of complete motor and sensory deficits after this time. Table 23.45 lists the many causes of acute and subacute spinal cord lesions and Table 23.46, the causes of chronic progressive paraplegia.

Summary 9   Spinal cord compression

• Progressive weakness of the legs and bladder symptoms should be considered to be due to spinal cord compression until proved otherwise.

• Total loss of bladder control for more than 24 hours, due to spinal cord compression, is likely to be permanent, even if the compression is subsequently relieved.

• Urgency of investigation of cord compression will depend on the speed of progression of symptoms, but is always urgent when bladder function is threatened.

• Minimum investigation includes chest X-ray, plain X-rays of the spine, full blood count and ESR and then a myelogram.

• Investigation of suspected cord compression should always be performed in close consultation with a neurosurgeon.

Initial investigations include a chest X-ray, which may demonstrate a primary carcinoma or metastases. Plain X-rays of the cervical and thoracic spines may show spondylotic change or lytic change or collapse of a vertebra. Plain CT scans of the spine may be helpful, but most patients presenting with an acute or subacute paraplegia will require a myelogram. If there is spinal block, a lumbar puncture may occasionally lead to an abrupt deterioration and myelography should be performed in consultation with a neurosurgeon.

Myelography is the definitive test in establishing spinal cord compression, and is sometimes combined with CT scanning. In patients in whom no structural lesion is demonstrated, examination of the CSF is particularly important. A raised lymphocyte count and protein content suggest an inflammatory cord lesion.

Treatment of spinal cord compression depends on the severity of the deficit and the cause. Where there is substantial loss of cord function, and in particular when there is bladder or bowel disturbance, surgical decompression is usually necessary. In the case of destructive malignant disease, decompression may have to be combined with procedures to stabilise the spine. With less severe deficit, a combination of radiotherapy and dexamethasone may produce improvement. However, operation is often required in order to establish a histological diagnosis.

CAUSES OF SPINAL CORD LESIONS

Spinal cord injury

A substantial number of spinal cord injuries are the result of road traffic accidents and sports injuries. Initially, a spinal cord injury may not be suspected, particularly when there is associated head injury. All patients with severe head injury require cervical spine X-rays to investigate an associated spinal injury. If X-rays of the cervical spine show no bony displacement or fracture, the patient can be managed conservatively. If X-rays demonstrate a fracture or displacement indicating instability, great care is necessary with movement of the patient. Surgical reduction of fractures may be necessary, but many patients are treated with traction in the hope that some neurological recovery will occur.

In the elderly with associated cervical spondylosis, spinal cord injury is likely to occur with relatively minor trauma. Hyperextension injuries lead to contusion of the cord in a canal narrowed by spondylotic change. When examining a patient suspected of having a cervical spine injury, it is important not to move the neck excessively. Neck X-rays must be obtained urgently and neurosurgical advice taken. The management of severe paraplegia due to spinal cord injury is best undertaken in spinal injury units. The condition often results in permanent paralysis.

Spinal cord injury in the dorsal region is less common than in the cervical region.

Degenerative cervical spine disease

Degenerative cervical spine disease may present with local neck pain, symptoms and signs of a radiculopathy, or evidence of a myelopathy.

Neck pain due to a cervical degenerative arthritis is an extremely common problem in middle-aged and elderly people, but in the majority of cases there is no associated neurological deficit.

Cervical radiculopathy is caused by narrowing of the exit foraminae by osteophyte encroachment combined with disc degeneration and loss of disc space height. The most common level for cervical radiculopathy in degenerative cervical spine disease is at C5 and C6. This causes pain which radiates over the shoulder and into the upper arm and, sometimes, diffusely throughout the arm. Signs include wasting, weakness and sometimes fasciculation in deltoid, spinati and biceps, with loss of the biceps and supinator reflexes and sometimes sensory impairment in a root distribution. If there are no signs of an associated myelopathy, it is best to treat initially with a firm cervical

collar by day, and a soft cervical collar at night. Root pain often settles within a few weeks with this treatment and motor signs may also sometimes improve. In a few patients, with evidence of a persistent or progressive radiculopathy, investigation with myelography may be necessary, followed by surgical treatment to decompress the root.

Myelopathy. In patients with a myelopathy, with progressive paraparesis, myelography is necessary (Fig. 23.35). With a disc prolapse, surgery is by an anterior

Fig. 23.35 Cervical myelopathy. A. Cervical myelogram, in a man aged 60 years, with a progressive spastic paraparesis. The column of contrast material is visible behind the vertebral bodies. The cervical canal is narrow, with maximal compression at the level of the C4/5 disc. Disc space narrowing and osteophyte formation is seen at several levels. **B.** CT scanning in the same patient, immediately following the myelogram, shows marked flattening of the cervical cord at C4/5.

approach in which the degenerative disc material is removed and a bone graft inserted (Cloward procedure). For diffuse cervical canal stenosis, which usually occurs in old people, it is often not possible to perform the Cloward procedure at multiple levels and, when indicated, a posterior decompression is preferred.

Thoracic disc

Prolapse of a thoracic disc is relatively rare. It may present as a progressive paraparesis. Following myelography decompression is necessary, usually via an anterior approach.

Paget's disease

Paget's disease occasionally produces localised vertebral involvement in one or several adjacent vertebrae in the thoracic region which can cause compression. Surgical decompression is followed by treatment with calcitonin.

Pott's disease of the spine

Tuberculosis affecting the spine usually occurs in the thoracic region of children or young adults. A single vertebra, or several adjacent vertebrae, may be affected and the onset is insidious. The first symptom is usually back pain and this is sometimes severe. With gradual destruction of one or more vertebrae, a kyphosis may develop. Infection by tuberculosis starts in an adjacent disc and then involves the vertebral body. This leads to collapse of the vertebra, with eventual wedge collapse of one or several adjacent vertebrae and the development of a paravertebral cold abscess. A slowly progressive paraparesis is the usual neurological presentation. X-rays demonstrate rarefaction of the bones and loss of disc space height. The differential diagnosis includes pyogenic infection (which may produce similar X-ray changes) and malignancy.

When Pott's disease of the spine is not associated with neurological involvement, anti-tuberculous drugs are usually all that is required. When there is neurological involvement, decompression may be necessary, followed by anti-tuberculous chemotherapy.

Rheumatoid arthritis

Rheumatoid arthritis (Ch. 24) may produce diffuse cervical arthritis, but the characteristic lesion is atlanto-axial subluxation. Narrowing of the upper cervical canal is produced by subluxation of the odontoid process. This may present as a chronic progressive tetraparesis. Occipital neuralgia, due to compression of the upper cervical sensory roots (C2), is a common early symptom. Occasionally, the onset of symptoms is abrupt and provoked by minor head trauma. There may also be symptoms of brain stem dysfunction – dysarthria and dysphagia being the commonest – due to compression of the anterior spinal artery or vertebral arteries by upward displacement of the odontoid process.

The upper cervical region is sometimes difficult to

visualise by myelography, and CT myelography is usually the most helpful investigation (Fig. 23.36). Elderly, very

Fig. 23.36 CT myelogram of upper cervical region in a patient with rheumatoid arthritis. There is atlanto-axial subluxation, with upward and posterior displacement of the odontoid (arrowed), which is causing compression at the cervico-medullary junction.

Fig. 23.37 (left) Cervical myelogram, showing complete block to flow of contrast at C4/5, associated with extensive vertebral bony destruction at this level. The spinal cord is compressed by a large extradural mass. This was metastatic carcinoma of the lung.

Fig. 23.38 (right) Myelogram showing the mid-thoracic region, in an elderly woman presenting with a slowly progressive spastic paraparesis and a sensory level on the trunk at T10. A large rounded mass is compressing the spinal cord. At operation a meningioma was removed.

disabled patients with atlanto-axial subluxation may be managed conservatively with a firm cervical collar, but if there is evidence of a progressive myelopathy, operative treatment is usually recommended. This involves removal of the odontoid process and posterior stabilisation of the upper cervical spine.

Metastases

Metastatic deposits of cancer or lymphoma are common causes of acute or subacute paraplegia. Compression of the cord usually results from extradural deposits, and there is often associated vertebral collapse (Fig. 23.37). Surgical treatment followed by radiotherapy is usually required. In some cases of relatively mild cord compression, urgent radiotherapy is performed with careful neurological observation.

Primary spinal cord tumours

Meningiomas occasionally occur in the thoracic region, usually in middle-aged or elderly women (Fig. 23.38). They present with a gradually progressive paraparesis. The results of surgical removal are usually good.

Neurofibromas may develop on spinal roots at any level (Fig. 23.39). These gradually enlarge, producing bony erosion of the exit foraminae and then spread into the spinal canal, compressing the theca and spinal cord. The history is usually of a gradually progressive paraparesis or tetraparesis. Plain X-rays of the spine will often suggest the diagnosis of neurofibromatosis, showing extensive bony erosion (Fig. 23.39A).

Intramedullary tumours are rare. They include gliomas, which usually occur in the cervical region in young adults. Some are amenable to partial surgical resection. When an intrinsic tumour causes enlargement of the cord, bony decompression of the spinal canal by laminectomy may be helpful. Some spinal cord gliomas are radiosensitive, so that prolonged survival, with slow progression, can occur; other tumours, however, run a much more aggressive course.

Ependymomas may arise at any level of the spinal cord and are often associated with cysts. Although these tumours are histologically benign, they are often difficult to remove surgically.

A *lipoma* may occur anywhere in the cervical or thoracic spinal cord, as well as the cauda equina where they are associated with spina bifida and spinal dysraphism. When they cause neurological deficit, partial surgical resection is usually necessary.

Fig. 23.39 Cervical neurofibroma. A. Plain oblique view of the cervical spine in a woman of 63 years with a spastic tetraparesis. A grossly enlarged exit foramen is present at C3/4. **B.** and **C.** Cervical myelograms in the same patient. In (B) with contrast injected in the lumbar region, there is a block to flow at C4. In (C), with contrast injected above the lesion at C2, the upper border of the rounded neurofibroma is shown.

Chordomas are rare tumours, derived from remnants of the embryonic notochord. In the head, they arise in the region of the clivus, and in the spinal canal, usually in the sacrococcygeal area.

Myelitis

Acute inflammation of the spinal cord may occur at any level and is usually of unknown cause. In some patients, there is a history of preceding viral infection, and myelitis commonly occurs as part of MS. There is usually a history of weakness and sensory loss in the legs progressing over a few days, sometimes leading to a severe paraparesis with a clear sensory level on the trunk. A Brown-Séquard syndrome may result from myelitis. Bladder and bowel involvement are common, and back pain at the level of the lesion is also a common feature.

Investigation and treatment

Many patients will require myelography to exclude spinal cord compression. The CSF shows a raised lymphocyte count and protein level. Treatment is with steroids or ACTH. In myelitis due to MS, there is usually partial recovery of function. In idiopathic myelitis, when severe paralysis occurs, many patients are left with a severe residual deficit.

Epidural abscess

Epidural abscesses are usually pyogenic and most often due to staphylococcal infection, usually blood-borne from another site of infection. The history is of a rapidly progressive paraparesis with local back pain and tenderness, and there is often fever. Urgent surgical decompression and antibiotic treatment are necessary.

Vascular disease

Vascular disease affecting the spinal cord is relatively uncommon, although some of the neurological deficit seen with compressive lesions may be due in part to interruption of the blood supply to the cord. Anterior spinal artery occlusion produces an acute paraparesis, often with predominantly spinothalamic sensory impairment. Recovery from this is variable. Generalised hypotension, embolism, and dissection of the aorta can all impair spinal cord blood supply.

Arteriovenous malformations are the commonest cause of vascular lesions of the spinal cord. These usually present acutely due to infarction or haemorrhage, but there is sometimes a stepwise or gradually progressive paraparesis. The diagnosis may be apparent at myelography and is then confirmed by spinal angiography (Fig. 23.40). Some are amenable to surgical treatment.

Vasculitis occasionally leads to acute spinal cord lesions; this occurs most commonly in polyarteritis nodosa.

Fig. 23.40 Spinal angiogram, showing an arteriovenous malformation.

Syringomyelia

In syringomyelia, a large fluid-filled cavity develops within the spinal cord; it is in communication with the central canal and contains CSF. Syrinxes may be long cysts extending over the whole length of the spinal cord, but are often more localised. They are most common in the cervical region, where they are often associated with Arnold-Chiari malformations (p. 933). Syrinxes may also be associated with spinal cord tumours and can occur as a late sequel of trauma. The pathogenesis of most syrinxes remains uncertain. However the fact that there is a frequent association with Arnold-Chiari malformations suggests that partial obstruction to the flow of cerebrospinal fluid from the foramina in the roof of the IVth ventricle may play some part.

Clinical features

The clinical presentation of a syrinx is characteristic of an intrinsic cord lesion. The developing cyst impinges upon anterior horn cells, and produces unilateral or bilateral (often asymmetrical) wasting, affecting particularly the small hand muscles, but eventually also other muscles in the upper limbs. Interruption of the decussating spinothalamic fibres centrally in the spinal cord leads to a

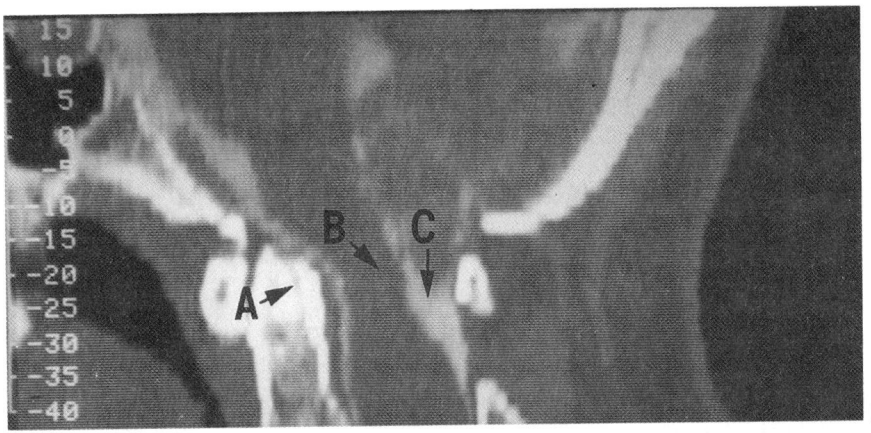

Fig. 23.41 CT myelogram showing syringomyelia. A. A transverse scan at the level of the odontoid. **B** is a computer reformat showing the odontoid (A), the spinal cord (B) anteriorly and the cerebellar tonsils (C) in an abnormally low position posteriorly. This confirms the Arnold-Chiari malformation and shows a grossly expanded upper cervical spinal cord.

dissociated sensory impairment in the upper limbs involving pain and temperature sensation, with preservation of other modalities. Since the spinothalamic fibres from the lower limbs have decussated lower down in the cord and their fibres lie laterally in the spinothalamic tracts, there is no impairment of spinothalamic sensation in the lower limbs. Eventually, the corticospinal tracts become involved, producing a spastic paraparesis; a late feature is involvement of dorsal column sensation (joint position and vibration sensation).

The dissociated sensory impairment in the hands leads to painless traumatic lesions of the fingers. The upper limb reflexes are usually absent. In the legs, a mild paraparesis develops. Syringomyelia is usually slowly progressive and the chronic loss of pain sensation may lead to the development of Charcot joints in the hand, elbow or, occasionally, shoulder joints.

Occasionally, cervical syrinxes may extend into the brain stem (syringobulbia), affecting the lower cranial nerve nuclei producing dysphagia and dysarthria. There may be sensory loss on the face of spinothalamic type, due to the involvement of the spinal nucleus and tract of the trigeminal nerve.

Investigation

Myelography usually shows an expanded cord in the region of the syrinx (Fig. 23.41) and delayed CT scanning after myelography may demonstrate contrast medium within the syrinx itself. NMR scanning also demonstrates syrinxes clearly (Fig. 23.42).

Treatment and prognosis

When there is an associated Arnold-Chiari malformation, foramen magnum decompression may arrest the further progression of the syrinx in some but not all patients. The more recent operation of syringoperitoneal shunting is now preferred by some neurosurgeons.

The prognosis is variable. In some patients the neurological deficit arrests after a time, while in others there is relentless progression.

Subacute combined degeneration of the cord

Long-standing B_{12} deficiency in pernicious anaemia may lead to degeneration of the lateral and posterior columns of the spinal cord, together with a peripheral neuropathy. This produces the clinical syndrome known as subacute combined degeneration of the cord. There may be an

Fig. 23.42 NMR scan of a patient with an extensive mid- and lower-cervical syrinx. This is associated with cerebellar ectopia (arrow). (Arnold-Chiari type I malformation).

associated mild dementia and optic atrophy. Patients with subacute combined degeneration are usually middle-aged or elderly. Paraesthesiae or pain in the hands and feet are frequent presenting complaints; there are often few signs in the early stages, but a progressive paraparesis soon develops.

Only some patients are anaemic; a normal haemoglobin does not exclude this diagnosis, but a macrocytosis is invariably present (Ch. 25). Treatment with parenteral B_{12} is usually beneficial, but an established severe paraparesis and peripheral neuropathy may not respond well.

Radiation myelopathy

Occasionally, damage of the cervical spinal cord occurs following radiotherapy to the neck for conditions such as Hodgkin's disease. Symptoms of a progressive myelopathy usually develop between six months and five years after radiotherapy. The myelopathy may be mild, but in some cases it is steadily progressive and leads to a severe deficit.

Sarcoidosis

Sarcoidosis has many neurological manifestations (p. 967) and is an occasional cause of myelopathy.

Hereditary spastic paraplegia

Hereditary spastic paraplegia – of dominant inheritance often with variable penetrance – takes the form of a slowly progressive paraplegia without sensory deficit. Bladder and bowel involvement is often a late feature and may be absent. Onset is usually in the second or third decade. Paraparesis associated with the spinocerebellar degenerations is considered on page 923.

Tropical spastic paraparesis

A slowly progressive paraparesis is seen in the tropics and migrants from these countries. There is sometimes an associated mild peripheral neuropathy. The condition was previously known as Jamaican neuropathy, but the spinal cord disturbance tends to dominate the clinical picture. Occasionally other lesions such as optic atrophy and ataxia are present. The paraparesis is usually slowly progressive and may remain mild. It has recently been suggested that HTLV I infection may be the cause.

DEVELOPMENTAL ANOMALIES AFFECTING THE SPINAL CORD

Spina bifida

Spina bifida refers to defective fusion of the vertebral arches.

Aetiology

The cause of spina bifida in the majority of patients is unknown, but there is an association with trisomy 13 or 18 in a few infants. The condition is commoner in girls. There has been a decrease in incidence of spina bifida in recent years, the reason for which is uncertain. Nutritional factors have been proposed; in particular deficiency of folic acid early in pregnancy has been suggested as a possible cause, although this remains unproven.

Clinical features

Defective fusion of the vertebral arches is most common in the lumbar region. It is extremely common in a single lumbar vertebra and is an incidental radiological finding of no significance in many normal people. However, when the defect of the vertebral arches extends over several segments, there may be associated abnormalities. These include:

1. a tuft of hair overlying the defect
2. a low, tethered spinal cord extending below the lower border of L1
3. a dermal sinus extending towards the spinal canal
4. intraspinal lipoma
5. sometimes, diastematomyelia (splitting of the spinal cord).

Neurological problems associated with this type of bony abnormality are collectively known as *spina bifida occulta*. However, an extensive bony abnormality may be present without any neurological deficit.

Spina bifida cystica

Spina bifida cystica refers to a more severe defect, in which the meninges prolapse through the bony defect of the vertebral arches. The meninges may prolapse without including neural tissue (a *meningocele*), or may include neural elements (a *meningomyelocele*). In its most severe form, spina bifida leads to a wide-open defect without covering of the cauda equina; this is known as *rhachischisis*. With meningocele and meningomyelocele, there is nearly always an associated Arnold-Chiari type II malformation (see below), with hydrocephalus and a kyphosis.

Treatment. Meningoceles require closure, but following this, some infants develop hydrocephalus and will require shunting. Spina bifida cystica is associated with obvious cauda equina problems at birth with paralysis of the legs. The decision whether to treat some of these infants or not remains controversial. If nothing is done, death from meningitis is almost inevitable. Treatment consists of closure of the defect and shunting for hydrocephalus. With these measures many of these children will survive. However, most will be severely handicapped and will require further operations later for contractures and other problems resulting from their severe neurological deficit.

Spina bifida occulta

Spina bifida occulta may present in childhood, adolescence or in adult life. Many of these patients have a partial cauda equina syndrome. There is often a long-standing history of bladder difficulties with enuresis, frequency and, sometimes, incontinence during the day. The signs of cauda equina deficit in the legs may be relatively mild or be fairly obvious, with underdeveloped, short legs and muscle wasting.

Investigation and treatment. Patients whose symptoms (particularly bladder symptoms) are progressing, warrant investigation with myelography. This may demonstrate a low tethered cord, some degree of spinal dysraphism and, occasionally, a lipoma or haemangioma. Surgical intervention seldom produces improvement; the aim of operative treatment is to prevent further progression. This may be achieved when a lipoma or haemangioma is present, and in some cases of spinal dysraphism, but release of a tethered cord alone does not usually produce any benefit.

Arnold-Chiari malformations

Arnold-Chiari malformations are of two types.

In *type I malformations*, there is cerebellar tonsilar herniation through the foramen magnum, often associated with syringomyelia (Fig. 23.41). Most patients present in adult life, either with symptoms and signs attributable to the syringomyelia, or with ataxia, lower cranial nerve palsies, nystagmus and a mild spastic tetraparesis. Treatment is initially by foramen magnum decompression, and sometimes later shunting of the syrinx.

In *type II malformations*, there is herniation of the cerebellar vermis as well as of the tonsils, and of the lower part of the brain stem through the foramen magnum. There is associated hydrocephalus, and as mentioned above, there is a strong association of the type II malformation with meningomyeloceles. The type II malformation usually presents in infancy with dysphagia causing feeding difficulties. There may be associated platybasia, an upward displacement of the skull base. The treatment is to shunt the hydrocephalus and perform a foramen magnum decompression.

Dandy-Walker syndrome

Dandy-Walker syndrome is a severe congenital abnormality in which there is hypoplasia of the vermis of the cerebellum, with massive cystic dilatation of the IVth ventricle and expansion of the posterior fossa; there is secondary hydrocephalus. This malformation is often associated with other major brain and spinal cord malformations. The abnormality is usually obvious at birth, though it occasionally presents later in childhood, with ataxia. Shunting of the hydrocephalus is necessary, sometimes together with posterior fossa surgery.

Klippel-Feil deformity

The Klippel-Feil deformity consists of fusion of two or more cervical vertebrae, sometimes involving most of the cervical spine. There may be abnormal and unstable joints in the cervical spine. The neck is short and the posterior hairline is low. There is often associated platybasia and other abnormalities of the petrous temporal bone, which

lead to conductive deafness in some patients. There is also an association with syringomyelia. Often, the presence of incomplete decussation of the pyramidal tracts produces the curious physical sign of mirror movements. Patients with the Klippel-Feil deformity may present with a gradually progressive tetraparesis or a cervical radiculopathy but, occasionally, with a sudden onset of tetraplegia following minor neck trauma, as a result of instability in the cervical spine. They may also present with symptoms and signs of syringomyelia.

DISEASES AFFECTING SPINAL ROOTS

Anatomy and physiology

Dorsal and ventral spinal roots are given off by every segment of the spinal cord; thus, there are 8 cervical, 12 thoracic, 5 lumbar, 5 sacral and 1 coccygeal pair(s). The dorsal and ventral roots join in the intervertebral foramina. The lumbar and sacral roots pass downwards, below the lower end of the spinal cord, which terminates at the lower border of the L1 vertebral body (conus medullaris); the lower lumbosacral roots form the cauda equina below this level. The sympathetic outflow from the spinal cord travels in the T1 to L1 roots; the caudal parasympathetic outflow is localised to the S2-S4 roots.

An important part of the blood supply to two watershed regions of the spinal cord enters via roots, one in the lower cervical region, one at the thoraco-lumbar junction, the artery of Adamkiewicz. Interruption of the arteries travelling on these roots may critically impair the blood supply of the cord, causing infarction.

Effects of root lesions

The clinical effects of root lesions may be both negative and positive. Negative effects include segmental wasting and weakness, sometimes with reflex loss if an appropriate root is affected, and a dermatomal sensory impairment. Positive effects are sensory – root pain which may or may not be clearly localised, paraesthesiae and hyperaesthesiae. Root pain due to structural lesions which tether the root and inhibit movement may be exacerbated by spinal movement and by manoeuvres which increase intraspinal pressure, such as coughing, sneezing and straining.

The commonest cause of root lesions is degenerative spine disease affecting the lower cervical and lumbar regions.

Cervical spondylosis

Spondylosis is the term loosely used to describe the degenerative changes which occur very frequently in the cervical and lumbar regions (Ch. 24). The spinal canal is narrowed by these degenerative changes which, in the cervical spine, are usually most marked at C4–5, C5–6, and C6–7.

Clinical features

Cervical spondylosis presents in three ways:

1. with local pain related to the degenerative changes, but without neurological involvement
2. with root compression, either motor, sensory, or both
3. with spinal cord compression.

Root or cord compression may develop gradually over long periods of time, or may present acutely, usually as the result of a disc prolapse.

If a root is compressed by the disc protrusion, pain and paraesthesiae in a radicular distribution are usually the first symptoms, sometimes followed by motor symptoms and signs appropriate to the root involved. Acute disc protrusions may also cause symptoms and signs of cord compression.

Diagnosis

In many patients, the signs indicating a root (rather than a peripheral nerve or brachial plexus) basis for the symptoms are not clear-cut. Investigation with EMG and nerve conduction studies is often helpful. Other investigations include X-rays of the cervical spine with oblique views to show the intervertebral foramina.

Although root pain is usually due to a disc protrusion, there are a number of other causes including compression in malignant vertebral body collapse, and other spinal tumours. Malignant invasion of the brachial plexus must also be considered (p. 943).

Treatment

In patients with minor symptoms of cervical root compression, a period of rest in a firm cervical collar, together with analgesia, will often help the pain and aid the spontaneous resolution of the signs over several weeks. Continuing severe pain, the failure of signs (particularly motor) to improve, or progression of signs, are indications to investigate further with myelography. Myelography is also indicated if there are signs of cord compression (p. 926). A disc causing continuing pain and neurological deficit may be surgically removed via facetectomy or foraminotomy from a posterior approach, or anteriorly through the disc with vertebral body fusion, using a bone graft (Cloward's procedure).

Lumbar spondylosis

Low back pain is experienced by virtually all adults at some time (Ch. 24). The cause of pain in most patients with back pain cannot be identified with confidence. Pain radiating down one leg is not always due to root compression; musculoskeletal pain may radiate in a similar way. The two roots most commonly compressed by prolapsed lumbar discs are the L5 root (by a prolapsed L4–5 disc), and the S1 root (by an L5–S1 prolapse). L5 root pain is felt on the lateral aspect of the leg and dorsum of the foot, while S1 pain tends to radiate down the back of the leg to the sole

of the foot. However, many patients are unable to clearly localise their pain. With L5 root compression, there is partial weakness of dorsiflexion and eversion of the foot. As extensor hallucis longus is supplied by L5 alone, it is relatively weaker, and this is of help in distinguishing a root lesion from a peroneal nerve lesion. Sensory loss will be within an L5 distribution. With S1 lesions, it is difficult to detect minor degrees of weakness of gastrocnemius soleus because of its strength. However, there may be reduction or loss of the ankle jerk and, on sensory testing, impairment of sensation on the lateral border of the foot, and on the sole. In either L5 or S1 lesions due to compression by a disc, the tethering of the root by the disc may cause a positive root stretch test; straight leg raising is the standard test for this.

Back, and/or leg pain with focal neurological signs may settle with a period of bed rest, and traction is sometimes helpful. However, the continuing presence of focal signs is an indication for investigation with myelography, with a view to decompressive surgery.

Lumbar canal stenosis

The combination of a congenitally narrow lumbar canal with subsequent degenerative change leads to canal stenosis. This may cause low back pain, together with focal signs, sometimes indicating a lesion of more than one root. The syndrome of cauda equina claudication is almost always associated with lumbar canal stenosis; its symptoms are thought to be due to impairment of the blood supply of the roots of the cauda equina, secondary to the canal stenosis.

The history is pain, numbness, paraesthesiae or weakness in the legs or buttocks, provoked by exertion and relieved by resting; there is often more rapid resolution of the symptoms when the lumbar spine is flexed, i.e. in a sitting posture. The symptoms may mimic vascular claudication in the legs, but the symptoms of numbness and paraesthesiae (when present) are a helpful clue to the diagnosis. There may be no abnormal neurological signs at rest, but sometimes, immediately after exertion, focal signs may develop. Foot pulses are normal. Myelography confirms the stenosis, which is often most pronounced at several disc levels, presenting a formidable surgical challenge.

Cauda equina lesions

Lesions of the cauda equina usually cause bilateral leg symptoms and signs, together with bladder and rectal involvement. The bladder symptoms comprise reduced sensation, both of bladder filling and of urethral sensation, with difficulty voiding, a poor stream, and incomplete emptying. Eventually, painless retention with overflow incontinence develops. Constipation and faecal soiling may occur.

It is essential to examine sensation on the buttocks and perineum in any patient with unexplained loss of bladder or rectal sphincter control. The development of bladder symptoms is an indication for urgent myelography.

Other lesions occasionally affecting the cauda equina include neurofibromas, Schwannomas, lipomas, meningiomas and ependymomas. Spina bifida is considered on page 932.

Thoracic disc prolapse

Thoracic disc prolapse is relatively rare. It usually causes cord compression rather than root symptoms. The diagnosis is confirmed by myelography. Surgical treatment is hazardous, and a lateral or anterior approach is necessary.

MOTOR NEURONE DISEASES

Motor neurone disease (MND) is a progressive degenerative disease of unknown cause which affects upper and lower motor neurones in the brain and spinal cord. It is rare, with a prevalence of about 4–5 per 100 000, and usually affects middle-aged or elderly people. The disease is usually rapidly progressive, with death within 3–4 years of onset of symptoms. A much more benign type of motor neurone disease with an hereditary basis, termed *spinal muscular atrophy*, affects adolescents and young adults.

MOTOR NEURONE DISEASE (MND)

Pathology

The pathology of MND is degeneration of anterior horn cells in the spinal cord, and lower motor neurones in the cranial nerves; the upper cranial nerves controlling eye movements, and the motor neurones to the bladder and bowel sphincters are spared. Cortical upper motor neurones supplying both cranial nerves and spinal motor neurones also degenerate, leading to the characteristic combination of widespread upper and lower motor neurone signs. In the great majority of patients, there is no intellectual impairment. Sensory tracts and nuclei remain normal.

Aetiology

In a very small number of cases, there is a family history. HLA typing shows no consistent trends. The pathology is not inflammatory, and there is no other evidence indicating an immune mechanism. Searches for toxic factors have been fruitless.

Clinical features

Motor neurone disease may present with almost any combination of upper and lower motor neurone symptoms and signs, and is often asymmetrical in the early stages. As the disease progresses, however, a common pattern emerges.

Patients present with bulbar problems or limb symptoms or a combination of both. Early bulbar symptoms are dys-arthria and dysphonia, dysphagia and difficulty in chewing, with nasal regurgitation of fluids. There may be recurrent chest infections, and respiratory muscle weakness may cause dyspnoea. In the limbs, the common presentations are weakness of a hand or whole arm, often with wasting which the patient has noticed, or, in the leg, progressive foot drop. Cramps are common.

Examination often reveals wasting, fasciculation and weakness in the muscles innervated by the cranial nerve nuclei. A particularly important sign is fasciculation in a wasted tongue. In the limbs, a combination of fasciculation and weakness, with brisk reflexes in wasted muscles, in the absence of any sensory abnormality, is strongly suggestive of MND.

Differential diagnosis

In many patients, a confident diagnosis can be made at the initial presentation, but in some, particularly those without cranial nerve signs, diagnostic difficulties may arise. A progressive bulbar palsy without limb signs may resemble myasthenia gravis. Multiple bilateral cerebral hemisphere infarcts or diffuse subcortical small vessel disease can produce bulbar problems similar to those of MND. When there are no cranial nerve signs, a cervical lesion producing a combination of motor root signs in the upper limbs with myelopathic upper motor neurone signs in both upper and lower limbs must be considered. This is the presentation of the *amyotrophic lateral sclerosis* variant of MND. Any sensory deficit or the presence of bladder symptoms suggests that the diagnosis is not MND. When limb signs are entirely lower motor neurone, a pure motor neuropathy is a possibility. In cases with predominantly proximal weakness and wasting, diabetic amyotrophy may be considered, and in occasional patients with signs confined to the legs, a cauda equina lesion may require exclusion.

Summary 10   Diagnosis of motor neurone disease (MND)

● Never make a diagnosis of motor neurone disease (MND) in the presence of sensory loss or bladder symptoms.

● Upper motor neurone (UMN) and lower motor neurone (LMN) signs in the upper and lower limbs may be produced by a combination of cervical and lumbar spondylosis.

● Do not make a definite diagnosis of MND until there are UMN and LMN signs in the same muscle groups in the limbs, and similar signs affecting cranial nerve-innervated muscles.

● If there is any doubt that a spinal cord lesion is present, myelography is essential.

Investigation

The diagnosis of MND is essentially a clinical one. Needle EMG shows denervation but not its cause. Surface EMG of all the limbs is often the more helpful test, in that it may demonstrate widespread denervation even in the absence of physical signs. Muscle biopsy is seldom necessary.

Prognosis and treatment

There is relentless progression. In older patients, and particularly those presenting with limb, rather than bulbar problems, the disease may last for 5–10 years from onset of symptoms to death. In others, death may result in less than a year. A few patients become demented. There may be emotional lability.

There is no cure for MND, which is invariably fatal. Only supportive measures can be provided. For patients with dysarthria and dysphonia, a range of communicators is now available. In the earlier stages, these symptoms, together with dysphagia, may be considerably ameliorated by speech therapy. Dysphagia requires careful attention to consistency of the food. Thin liquids and solids often lead to choking, while a blended diet may cause fewer problems. Nonetheless, eating usually imposes increasingly severe problems. A nasogastric tube or gastrostomy may be helpful in many patients. Dribbling of saliva may be helped by oral atropine or a tricyclic antidepressant, the latter also sometimes having a beneficial effect on mood. Progressive respiratory paralysis with aspiration pneumonia is the usual cause of death. Some patients with troublesome nocturnal dyspnoea and sleep disturbance are helped by a cuirass, but artificial ventilation via an endotracheal tube merely prolongs suffering.

Most patients become immobile and eventually require full nursing care. Patients remain alert to the end, and drug treatment to alleviate distress is often indicated.

HEREDITARY SPINAL MUSCULAR ATROPHY

Several rare disorders are described, but the two commonest are Werdnig-Hoffman disease and the Kugelberg-Welander syndrome.

Werdnig-Hoffman disease

Werdnig-Hoffman disease is an autosomal recessive condition presenting either neonatally as a floppy baby, or with progressive weakness and wasting within the first year of life, due to widespread lower motor neurone degeneration. Death occurs within the first four years of life.

Kugelberg-Welander syndrome

Kugelberg-Welander syndrome is a progressive spinal muscular atrophy of either autosomal dominant or recessive inheritance. The disease sometimes affects children over the age of two, but onset is usually in adolescence or early adult life, when there is degeneration of lower motor neurones, with relative sparing of cranial nerve nuclei. Kugelberg-Welander syndrome often presents with a predominantly proximal weakness, which may give a similar picture to a limb girdle dystrophy. This form of spinal muscular atrophy is relatively benign, but most patients eventually become disabled.

DISEASES OF PERIPHERAL NERVES AND PLEXUSES

PERIPHERAL NEUROPATHY

Peripheral nerves contain motor, sensory and autonomic fibres, with their cell bodies in the anterior horn, dorsal root ganglia, and autonomic ganglia respectively. Nerve fascicles are surrounded by connective tissue, the perineurium, which forms a blood-nerve barrier maintaining a special environment in the endoneurium, the intrafascicular compartment in which the fibres lie. Myelinated nerve fibres are of varying size, the largest in diameter conducting at velocities of up to 70 metres per second, the smallest at about 5 metres per second. Unmyelinated axons conduct at less than 1 metre per second. The Schwann cells provide axons with a certain amount of physical support, form the myelin of myelinated fibres and probably act in a nutritional capacity to axons. Most of the synthesis in nerve fibres occurs in the cell bodies, with subsequent transport down axons.

Pathophysiology

The principal pathology in diseases affecting peripheral nerves is either axonal degeneration or demyelination. *Axonal degeneration* may take the form of a neuronopathy, in which the cell body and whole axon are affected, or an axonopathy, in which the part of the axon furthest from the cell body is first affected. In *demyelinating neuropathies*, the primary pathological process is demyelination. This may lead to conduction block with consequent loss of function. Severe demyelination may lead to secondary axonal degeneration.

Regeneration in axonal neuropathies may occur after a period of Wallerian degeneration. Regeneration proceeds at only 1–2 mm per day. Remyelination in demyelinating neuropathies initially leads to short internodes and thin myelin sheaths, causing greatly reduced conduction velocities. A severely reduced nerve conduction velocity on electrophysiological testing indicates a demyelinating neuropathy; this may be generalised, e.g. as in Guillain-Barré syndrome (acute inflammatory polyneuropathy), or focal, as in an entrapment neuropathy such as the carpal tunnel syndrome.

The fibres in peripheral nerves are occasionally damaged by diseases which primarily affect the connective tissue, particularly the blood vessels of the nerve. Examples are the neuropathies due to vasculitis seen in polyarteritis nodosa, or SLE.

Clinical classification

Neuropathies may be divided into:

1. *Mononeuropathy*, when a single nerve is involved
2. *Multiple mononeuropathy* (mononeuritis multiplex or multifocal neuropathy), in which more than one, and sometimes many, individual nerves are affected in a

patchy distribution. Multifocal neuropathy is typical of some diseases (Table 23.47).

3. *Polyneuropathy*, in which there is a diffuse symmetrical involvement of the peripheral nerves. Some diseases, notably diabetes, may also produce a multifocal neuropathy. Some polyneuropathies (e.g. Guillain-Barré syndrome), also affect the spinal roots, and in such cases the terms *polyradiculoneuropathy* or *polyradiculopathy* are more accurate.

Table 23.47 Causes of mononeuritis multiplex (multifocal neuropathy)

- Diabetes
- Connective tissue disease, e.g. SLE, RA, PAN
- Inflammatory, e.g. sarcoid
- Infective, e.g. leprosy, Herpes zoster (usually a mononeuritis)
- Familial disposition to entrapment neuropathy (tomaculous neuropathy)
- Other physical injury, e.g. radiotherapy, electrical injury, thermal injury, ischaemia
- Neoplastic, e.g. carcinomatous or lymphomatous infiltration, neurofibromatosis, malignant nerve tumours, related to paraproteinaemia

Clinical features

Neuropathies may affect motor and sensory fibres or each differentially. Autonomic involvement is prominent in certain neuropathies, the commonest being diabetes.

Motor nerve involvement

The major symptom of motor nerve involvement is weakness. Examination reveals wasting and weakness, which, in the case of mononeuropathies, is appropriate to the distribution of a particular nerve; in the case of polyneuropathy, it is usually most marked distally in the limbs. Most peripheral neuropathies involve the lower limbs before the upper limbs. Occasionally, a predominantly proximal weakness may result from peripheral neuropathy, e.g. as in Guillain-Barré syndrome. Fasciculation is sometimes seen in peripheral neuropathy, usually in patients with rapidly progressive denervation. Tendon reflexes are often absent, usually more as a result of sensory loss than of motor impairment. Loss of the ankle jerks is common in normal elderly people.

Sensory nerve involvement

Sensory involvement includes the negative symptom of numbness and the positive symptoms of paraesthesiae and pain. Some neuropathies differentially affect large and small fibres. Neuropathies selectively affecting large fibres (e.g. uraemic neuropathy) impair touch, pressure, two-point discrimination and joint position sense, leaving pain and temperature sensation unaffected. Neuropathies selectively affecting small fibres (e.g. small fibre diabetic neuropathy or amyloid neuropathy) produce loss of pain and temperature sensation with relative preservation of other modalities. All the tendon reflexes may be present in this situation, since these depend on large fibre function. Substantial loss of pain and temperature sensation may lead to neuropathic feet ulcers.

In mononeuropathy, sensory impairment is within the distribution of a single nerve. In polyneuropathy, a stocking and glove, distal sensory impairment is typical.

Autonomic involvement

A severe type of burning pain (*causalgia*) occurs after injury to major limb peripheral nerves – such as the median, ulnar and sciatic nerves – and occasionally with injury to smaller nerves. Causalgia is often associated with evidence of local or regional reflex sympathetic disturbance, including vascular and sweating changes, together with trophic changes in the skin and nails. Causalgia may be partly or completely relieved by sympathetic blockade, indicating the role of sympathetic activity in maintaining such pain. Similar burning pain, together with sympathetic changes, is sometimes a feature of polyneuropathy, must notably alcoholic neuropathy.

In a minority of patients, autonomic involvement is sufficiently severe to cause symptoms. Loss of blood pressure control leads to syncope. There may be impairment of sweating, sometimes severe enough to cause hyperpyrexia in hot weather; impairment of bladder and bowel sphincter function may lead to incontinence.

Diagnosis and investigation

In cases where the history and examination leave doubt about the presence of a neuropathy, motor and sensory nerve conduction studies are valuable. Demyelinating neuropathies lead to severe slowing of conduction, while in axonal neuropathies, the degree of slowing is much less. Denervation of muscle is more common in axonal neuropathies in the early stages, and reduced motor and sensory compound action potential amplitudes are features

---

Summary 11 Peripheral neuropathy

- Peripheral neuropathy is classified clinically into mononeuropathy (mononeuritis), mononeuritis multiplex (multifocal neuropathy) and polyneuropathy.
- Polyneuropathies may be motor or sensory, but are usually mixed (sensorimotor).
- The clinical type of the neuropathy may be helpful in identifying the cause.
- In polyneuropathies, legs are affected before the arms.
- Tendon reflexes may be partly preserved in a polyneuropathy in the early stages, or when the neuropathy predominantly affects the legs, or is predominantly motor rather than sensory.
- Autonomic involvement characteristically occurs with some neuropathies.
- Some neuropathies (e.g. Guillain-Barré) may affect respiratory function.

of both motor and sensory neuropathies.

Small fibre neuropathies pose particular diagnostic difficulties in that, with large fibre preservation, tendon reflexes are not lost and sensory loss is selective and often discrete. Recording of thermal thresholds for warming and cooling offers a simple way of assessing small fibre sensory function.

Nerve biopsy is only occasionally helpful in establishing the cause of a neuropathy. It is most often useful in patients with multifocal neuropathy, in those suspected of having amyloid, and in a number of the rare inherited metabolic disorders which lead to abnormal depositions in peripheral nerves, such as metachromatic leucodystrophy.

Mononeuropathy

The more common entrapment neuropathies are described below and Table 23.48 lists the main features of a number of less common traumatic mononeuropathies. Brief periods of nerve compression cause focal demyelination, leading to conduction block, but without loss of axonal continuity (*neurapraxia*). Remyelination will restore both conduction and function over days or weeks. With more severe compression, which often occurs over a longer period, axonal interruption may result; this leads to Wallerian degeneration of the axons distal to the site of compression, but with continuity of the connective tissue elements of the nerve. Axonal regeneration and remyelination with relief of compression occur over a much longer period after such injury, but good restoration of function is possible. With severe, penetrating injuries causing division of the nerve, connective tissue continuity is also lost, and regeneration is always incomplete, even with the most careful surgical apposition of nerve ends.

Median nerve

Carpal tunnel syndrome

Compression of the median nerve at the wrist beneath the flexor retinaculum gives rise to the carpal tunnel syndrome. This is most common in middle-aged women, and more likely to occur after wrist fracture, in pregnancy, in rheumatoid arthritis with involvement of the wrist joint, in myxoedema and in acromegaly. The median nerve may also be damaged by penetrating trauma at the wrist. Symptoms may be provoked by occupational use of the hands.

The symptoms of carpal tunnel syndrome are pain, numbness and paraesthesiae in the hand. The symptoms are often diffuse, affecting the whole hand. Pain may radiate

Table 23.48 Causes and features of individual nerve lesions (See also Figure 23.5)

Nerve (root)	Site and cause of lesion	Clinical features
Axillary (C5, 6)	Brachial plexus. Crutches. Sleeping partner's head – 'honeymoon palsy'	Paralysis of shoulder abduction, deltoid
Musculocutaneous (C5, 6)	Humeral fracture with brachial plexus injury	Paralysis of biceps, brachialis. Sensory loss on lateral aspect of forearm
Femoral (L2–4)	Fracture pelvis or femur Dislocation of hip Hip operations Psoas abscess or psoas haematoma in haemophilia	Paralysis of iliacus, quadriceps, sartorius. Sensory loss over anterolateral thigh and saphenous distribution. Absent knee jerk
Lateral cutaneous nerve of thigh (L2,3)	Pressure of inguinal ligament Obesity. 'Meralgia paraesthetica'	Sensory loss over anterolateral thigh. Often with burning pain and paraesthesiae
Obturator (L2, 4)	Neoplastic or radiotherapy damage in pelvis. Fetal head pressure, or forceps injury	Weakness of hip adductors. Sensory loss lower medial thigh
Sciatic (L4, 5, S1–3)	Pelvic mass. Fracture/dislocation of femur Penetrating trauma Baker's cyst in popliteal fossa Pressure palsy in drug addicts and alcoholics	Paralysis of all lower leg and foot muscles. Absent ankle jerk. Sensory loss of whole foot, extending up lateral aspect of lower leg. Often painful
Peroneal (L4, 5, S1, 2)	Compression at neck of fibula: squatting, sitting cross-legged, pressure under anaesthesia Fibular fracture	Foot-drop and weakness of eversion. Sensory loss over lateral aspect of lower leg and dorsum of foot
Tibial (L4, 5, S1–3)	Trauma in thigh and popliteal fossa Distal injury in tarsal tunnel	Paralysis of plantar flexion and inversion. Sensory loss on sole. Pain common. In tarsal tunnel syndrome, paralysis of medial foot muscles and sensory loss on sole
Sural (L5, S1–2)	Pressure in lower calf and at ankle, e.g. from tight boots	Sensory loss over lateral border of foot
(Median, ulnar and radial nerves: see text)		

through the forearm and, occasionally, may involve the whole arm. Typically, pain is most troublesome at night or first thing in the morning. Sensory symptoms are more common than motor symptoms, but some patients notice weakness of the thumb. On examination, there is weakness of abductor pollicis brevis (APB), with or without wasting, and also weakness of opponens. There is sensory impairment in a median distribution (Fig. 23.5). The Tinel sign is positive when gentle tapping over the carpal tunnel causes paraesthesiae in part of the cutaneous distribution of the nerve.

In mild cases, a wrist splint to reduce movement at the wrist may help, and an injection of hydrocortisone into the carpal tunnel may give temporary relief. In cases where there is sensory loss or weakness, surgical decompression of the carpal tunnel is required. Mild carpal tunnel syndrome symptoms often resolve spontaneously.

Proximal lesions

More proximal injuries of the median nerve are unusual. A lesion at the elbow causes weakness of the long finger flexors (except the ulnar half of flexor digitorum profundus), together with weakness of flexor carpi radialis, pronator teres, most of the thenar muscles and the two radial lumbricals. There is weakness of flexion of the index and middle fingers and distal phalanx of the thumb, in addition to weakness of APB and opponens. Sensory loss is the same as in carpal tunnel syndrome.

Ulnar nerve

Ulnar nerve lesions usually follow entrapment at the elbow. Above the elbow, the nerve gives rise to branches supplying the medial part of the deep finger flexors and flexor carpi ulnaris. In the forearm, the nerve gives off the dorsal branch which supplies the skin over the medial part of the dorsal aspect of the hand, the medial one-and-a-half digits, and the medial part of the palm over the hypothenar eminence (Fig. 23.5B). The deep branch of the nerve supplies the hypothenar muscles, the interossei, adductor pollicis, the third and fourth lumbricals and part of flexor pollicis brevis.

Sensory symptoms from ulnar nerve lesions include pain, paraesthesiae and numbness in the hand; as with carpal tunnel syndrome, these symptoms may not be confined to the anatomical distribution of the nerve. Weakness is often asymptomatic.

A lesion of the nerve in the region of the elbow may lead to palpable thickening of the nerve in the ulnar groove. The muscles in the forearm are spared. In the hand, there is wasting of the first dorsal interosseus and abductor digiti minimi, and wasting of the other interossei, causing guttering between the metacarpals with weakness of finger abduction. In severe lesions, a claw-hand posture develops. This is due to paralysis of the interossei and medial two lumbricals, which normally flex the fingers at the metacarpophalangeal joints, and extend the fingers at the interphalangeal joints. In claw-hand, there is extension at the

metacarpophalangeal joints due to the unopposed action of the long extensors of the fingers, and flexion at the interphalangeal joints due to the action of the flexor digitorum superficialis. The posture mainly affects the little and ring fingers, since, although all the interossei are weak, the radial lumbricals supplied by the median nerve prevent extension of the lateral metacarpophalangeal joints.

Lesions of the ulnar nerve above the elbow produce weakness of finger flexion and flexor carpi ulnaris. Lesions at the wrist and in the hand spare the dorsal branch, so that sensation on the dorsum of the hand and fingers is preserved. Lesions at the wrist involve the superficial branch, so that sensory loss occurs on the medial palm and palmar aspects of the ring and little fingers; lesions within the hand usually spare this branch.

Radial nerve

The radial nerve lies on the posterior surface of the humerus in the radial groove, and supplies triceps in the upper arm and the skin on the back of the upper arm. In the forearm, the nerve gives branches to brachioradialis, and extensor carpi radialis longus and brevis. The deep branch supplies supinator, extensor digitorum, extensor carpi ulnaris and extensor digiti minimi. The extension of the deep branch is the posterior interosseous nerve, which supplies abductor pollicis longus, extensor pollicis longus and brevis, and extensor indicis. The terminal superficial radial nerve innervates the skin over the lateral part of the dorsum of the hand and of the thumb, index and middle fingers.

When the radial nerve is injured in the axilla or in fractures of the humerus, there is paralysis of all these muscles, including triceps. 'Saturday night palsy' is a neurapraxia in which the nerve is damaged in the upper arm when compressed over the arm of a chair, the result of going to sleep in this position when drunk. Triceps is spared, but there is weakness of all other muscles supplied by the nerve, producing a wrist-drop, together with sensory loss over the dorsum of the hand. Recovery takes place over several weeks; function in the hand is improved by a splint to correct the wrist-drop.

Mononeuritis multiplex (multifocal neuropathy)

By comparison with polyneuropathy, mononeuritis multiplex has relatively few causes (Table 23.47). Biopsy of an affected sensory nerve may reveal specific pathological changes much more often than in polyneuropathy.

Polyneuropathy

The many possible causes of polyneuropathy are shown in Table 23.49. Despite extensive investigation, the cause of some neuropathies is never established. In such cases, it is particularly important to examine family members, both clinically and electrophysiologically, as this may establish the diagnosis of an hereditary neuropathy.

Neurological Disease

Table 23.49 Causes of polyneuropathy

Metabolic	Toxic
Diabetes	Alcohol
Uraemia	Lead
Myxoedema	Arsenic
Amyloid	Gold
Ischaemia	Mercury
Inflammatory	Thallium
Acute inflammatory polyneuropathy:	Triorthocresyl phosphate (TOCP)
Guillain-Barré syndrome	Insecticides
Chronic relapsing inflammatory	Acrylamide
polyneuropathy (CRIP)	N-hexane
Chronic progressive inflammatory	**Drugs**
polyneuropathy (CPIP)	Isoniazid
Serum sickness	Nitrofurantoin
Sarcoidosis	Vincristine
SLE	Metronidazole
PAN	Disulphiram
Nutritional	Clioquinol
Beri-beri (thiamine deficiency)	Dapsone
Pellagra (niacin deficiency)	Sulphonamide
B_{12} deficiency	Emetine
Burning feet syndrome	Phenytoin
Sprue	Pyridoxine
Malabsorption	Griseofulvin
Neoplastic	Cisplatinum
Non-metastatic	Perhexiline
Myeloma	Tricylic antidepressants
Paraproteinaemia	**Hereditary**
Macroglobulinaemia	HMSN type I
Infections	HMSN type II
Leprosy	HMSN type III
Diphtheria	Hereditary sensory neuropathy
Measles	Friedreich's ataxia
Mumps	Familial dysautonomia (Riley-Day)
Infectious mononucleosis	Porphyria
Brucellosis	Metachromatic leucodystrophy
HIV	Fabry's disease – angiokeratoma corporis diffusum

COMMON CAUSES OF NEUROPATHY

Endocrine and metabolic neuropathies

Diabetic neuropathy

Diabetes is the commonest cause of neuropathy in the UK.

Mononeuropathy and multifocal neuropathy

Entrapment neuropathies, e.g. carpal tunnel syndrome, are much more likely to develop in diabetes. In addition, peripheral nerves may be affected by the small vessel disease of diabetes. This microangiopathic pathology underlies the IIIrd cranial nerve palsy, which typically produces an ophthalmoplegia but spares the pupil. This is because the fibres to the pupil are distributed in the peripheral parts of the nerve, and the ischaemia produced by small vessel occlusion affects predominantly central parts of the nerve. Other cranial nerves may be affected. A multifocal neuropathy in the limbs is occasionally seen, and is presumed to have a microangiopathic basis.

Diabetic amyotrophy

Diabetic amyotrophy is a proximal multifocal neuropathy which affects the femoral nerve and, to a lesser extent, other nerves supplying proximal muscles in the leg. It occurs in middle-aged or elderly diabetics, commonly in those with poor diabetic control. The condition is usually unilateral. The first symptom is pain in the thigh lasting for weeks or months. Weakness rapidly develops; this is most marked for hip flexion and knee extension, but usually also involves other muscles at the hip and the hamstrings. Distal power is normal. The knee jerk is absent. Recovery begins within weeks or months and is usually good.

Polyneuropathy

Polyneuropathy is the commonest type of diabetic neuropathy. It is a sensory motor neuropathy, but in many patients, it remains predominantly sensory. Numbness and paraesthesiae are the main symptoms, occasionally with hyperaesthesiae on the soles of the feet. Pain, either a continuous aching or burning, or shock-like stabbing pains, may occur. The onset is usually insidious over weeks or months.

A much rarer type of painful polyneuropathy affects predominantly the small myelinated and unmyelinated fibres, leading to impaired pain and temperature sensation. Tendon reflexes, which depend on large fibre afferents, are preserved. Patients with this type of neuropathy complain of severe pain in the feet, often associated with hyperaesthesia. Another type of acute peripheral polyneuropathy in diabetes affects all fibre types. The onset is preceded by rapid weight loss. This neuropathy, which is very painful, resolves after nine months to a year in most patients.

Autonomic neuropathy

An autonomic neuropathy is common in diabetes and is nearly always seen in association with the sensory motor polyneuropathy. The pupils may be affected, with reduced response to light. There may be dysphagia if the oesophagus is involved. Gastric atony causes vomiting, and denervation of the lower bowel leads to diarrhoea. Postural hypotension with syncope is the commonest early symptom. Diagnostically, postural hypotension and the absence of the normal cardiac beat-to-beat interval variation are useful observations. Erectile impotence, retrograde ejaculation, retention of urine, and incontinence may all be troublesome features.

Treatment

The mainstay of treatment of diabetic neuropathy is good control of the diabetes (Ch. 20). This particularly helps the mononeuritis and multifocal neuropathies. Symptomatic treatment for neuropathic pain is often unsatisfactory. Simple analgesics, anticonvulsants and benzodiazepines may all occasionally help.

Treatment of autonomic neuropathy is always difficult. Usually, the most troublesome symptom is postural hypotension. Tight stockings to prevent venous pooling in the legs rarely have a major effect. The blood pressure tends to be at its lowest in the morning and rises gradually during the day. Patients with autonomic failure tend to lose excess sodium and water during the night. This can be counteracted to some extent by sleeping with the head of the bed raised. This lowers the recumbent blood pressure, leading to renin release and a reduction in the nocturnal sodium and water loss.

Fludrocortisone, which causes sodium and water retention, is also effective. A dose of 0.1–0.2 mg daily is usually sufficient, but excessive sodium and water retention, particularly in elderly patients, may lead to heart failure. Pressor drugs are seldom useful.

Other endocrine and metabolic neuropathies

Uraemic neuropathy is described on page 968. Myxoedema causes an axonal, predominantly sensory polyneuropathy, but this is a much less common manifestation than either the proximal myopathy (p. 950) or cerebellar ataxia (p. 924) that occur in hypothyroidism. Amyloid, of either the hereditary or acquired type, may cause a peripheral sensory motor neuropathy, which particularly affects small fibres and is characteristically painful. A helpful diagnostic sign in this type of neuropathy is palpable thickening of the peripheral nerves. Long-standing lower limb ischaemia may lead to peripheral nerve damage, giving rise to signs of a peripheral polyneuropathy in the legs.

Inflammatory polyneuropathies

Guillain-Barré syndrome

Guillain-Barré syndrome (acute inflammatory polyneuropathy) is an acute, demyelinating, predominantly motor polyradiculoneuropathy which affects people of all ages.

Aetiology

In some (but not all) patients there is a preceding history of a viral illness, often an upper respiratory infection. A number of specific preceding infections have been identified, including enterovirus and mycoplasma infections. It is thought that preceding infection or some other immune stimulus may trigger a mainly cell-mediated process causing demyelination of spinal roots and peripheral nerves. There is little evidence that circulating antibodies are involved in this process.

Clinical features

Maximum weakness usually occurs between 10 and 14 days after the onset of the neuropathy. Occasionally, profound paralysis may develop within 24 hours. The first symptoms are usually sensory, with distal paraesthesiae, numbness and sometimes pain. Cranial nerve involvement occurs in 30–40% of patients, with bilateral facial weakness being the common manifestation. Bulbar weakness predisposes to aspiration pneumonia. The autonomic nervous system is sometimes involved, causing lability of blood pressure and arrythmias. Bladder dysfunction is rare. The CSF protein is sometimes raised to very high levels, causing impaired reabsorption in the arachnoid granulations, leading to papilloedema.

Examination reveals weakness, with variable cranial nerve involvement. There is no wasting, as the neuropathy is acute in onset. Reflexes are nearly always all absent. Despite prominent sensory symptoms, objective signs of sensory loss are slight. Occasionally, there is an ascending dense sensory loss affecting first the limbs and then the trunk.

Investigation

The CSF is under normal pressure and shows a normal cell count, or slight pleocytosis of lymphocytes, and a markedly elevated protein of between 1 and 10 g/l. Demyelination quickly spreads distally and, by the time electrodiagnostic tests are done, there is usually some slowing of conduction, which later may become severe. The vital capacity must be measured regularly.

Differential diagnosis

The diagnosis is obvious in the majority of cases. Acute cervical spinal cord lesions, acute myasethenia gravis, and poliomyelitis all require consideration. In acute poliomyelitis, weakness is often asymmetrical and, in contrast to Guillain-Barré syndrome, the CSF always shows a raised cell count of 10–200 cells/mm³.

Treatment and prognosis

With supportive treatment alone, 85–90% of all patients with Guillain-Barré syndrome recover completely over several months. Others are left with some residual deficit, usually mild. A few patients show a slowly progressive course (*chronic progressive inflammatory polyneuropathy*) but may respond to corticosteroid and other anti-inflammatory treatment and, occasionally, to plasma exchange. A variant of this chronic demyelinating neuropathy is one showing a relapsing course (*chronic relapsing inflammatory polyneuropathy*), which may respond to similar treatment.

There is no evidence that corticosteroids or other anti-inflammatory drugs improve the outcome in acute inflammatory polyneuropathy. However, plasma exchange improves the prognosis if used early in patients who are rapidly deteriorating and severely affected.

Even those patients who require ventilatory support may make a complete recovery. The best prognostic guide is the compound motor action potential which, if reduced to 20% or less of normal, is associated with a poor prognosis.

Miller Fisher syndrome

Miller Fisher syndrome is a variant of acute inflammatory polyneuropathy, in which there is an ophthalmoplegia, probably of peripheral origin, due to demyelination of any or all of the IIIrd, IVth and VIth cranial nerves, together with ataxia and areflexia, with little or no weakness in the limbs. The prognosis is good; no treatment has been found to have an effect.

Nutritional neuropathies

The neurological consequences of B_{12} deficiency are discussed on page 931. In addition, a number of other nutritional deficiencies may cause polyneuropathies which are characteristically painful. The burning feet syndrome, described in Japanese prisoners of war, was probably the result of multiple nutritional deficits. Peripheral neuropathy – one of the neurological manifestations of pellagra due to niacin deficiency – is a sensory motor polyneuropathy in which severe burning of the feet with tenderness and hyperaesthesia of the lower legs and feet is prominent. A painful neuropathy also occurs in beriberi due to thiamine deficiency.

Neoplastic neuropathies

The neoplastic neuropathies are described on page 970.

Paraproteinaemia neuropathy

Myeloma and other malignancies, such as some types of lymphoma and Waldenström's macroglobulinaemia, which produce a monoclonal gammopathy may be associated with a demyelinating neuropathy. In addition, a benign IgM gammopathy associated with a chronic, slowly progressive demyelinating neuropathy is now recognised; there is evidence that the neuropathy is caused by the abnormal IgM. Some patients respond to immunosuppression or plasma exchange.

Infective neuropathies

Worldwide, leprosy (p. 277) is the most frequent infective cause of peripheral neuropathy. It produces a multifocal neuropathy and there is marked nerve thickening.

Both brucellosis and infectious mononucleosis are rarely associated with an acute, predominantly motor, polyneuropathy, similar to acute inflammatory polyneuropathy. The neuropathy occurring with infectious mononucleosis may respond to steroid treatment. A mononeuritis or multifocal neuropathy may also develop with either of these infections. Mumps and measles are very rarely complicated by a transient polyneuropathy.

Diphtheria (p. 266) may cause a profound demyelinating peripheral neuropathy, due to the action of the exotoxin. The first symptom is palatal weakness, usually occurring about two weeks after pharyngeal infection. Weakness of the external ocular muscles may develop after about four weeks, and a generalised polyneuropathy after about seven or eight weeks. This may include respiratory weakness, for which ventilation is necessary. Remyelination with gradual recovery occurs over several months, but the commonly associated myocarditis may prove fatal.

Neuropathies occurring with HIV infection are considered on page 965.

Toxic neuropathies

Alcoholic neuropathy, described on page 973, is easily the most important of the toxic neuropathies.

Other toxic causes of neuropathy are listed in Table 23.49. These produce axonal neuropathies and many cause widespread central nervous system damage in addition.

Drug-induced neuropathy

Certain drugs almost inevitably cause a neuropathy if given in sufficiently large dosages for long enough. Examples include vincristine and metronidazole. Other drugs show a strong tendency to produce neuropathy but depend on host susceptibility. For example, isoniazid neuropathy (preventable with small doses of pyridoxine) is much more likely to develop in patients whose liver is only capable of slow acetylation of the drug.

Hereditary neuropathies

HMSN types I and II (peroneal muscular atrophy and Charcot-Marie-Tooth disease)

Peroneal muscular atrophy and Charcot-Marie-Tooth disease are the commonest of the hereditary neuropathies. They have recently been subdivided into hereditary motor and sensory neuropathy (HMSN) types I and II, on the basis of motor nerve conduction velocity.

Type I HMSN tends to present in the first decade of life, with difficulty walking and pes cavus or equinovarus foot deformity. Associated kyphoscoliosis is common. There is severe distal wasting in the legs and, later, in the upper limbs. The wasting in the legs sometimes spares the upper part of the thighs, producing the so-called 'inverted champagne bottle legs'; however, a diffuse pattern of wasting in the legs is more common. In the upper limbs, in addition to wasting, weakness and generalised areflexia, there is frequently tremor and a cerebellar type of ataxia. Peripheral nerves are sometimes thickened. Nerve conduction velocity is reduced to less than 38 m/s, and is often severely slowed, indicating a severe demyelinating type of neuropathy.

HMSN type II is of later onset, with a peak onset in the second decade but with many cases presenting much later than this. It is primarily an axonal neuropathy. Weakness and wasting are less marked than in type I, and tend to be confined to the lower limbs. Foot and spinal deformity are less common than in type I and there is no palpable nerve thickening. The tendon reflexes are absent in the legs, but are often preserved in the arms. Motor conduction velocities are reduced, but not below 38 m/s.

In both types of HMSN, the inheritance is usually auto-somal dominant, although sporadic cases occur of both types and a few cases probably have an autosomal recessive mode of inheritance. In both types, men tend to be more severely affected than women.

HMSN type III (Dejerine-Sottas disease)

Dejerine-Sottas disease – a very rare condition of auto-somal recessive inheritance – is a severe demyelinating neuropathy of onset in childhood, with ataxia. Nerve hypertrophy is a striking feature.

Hereditary sensory neuropathy

A purely sensory neuropathy of either dominant or recessive inheritance affects particularly pain and temperature sensation (small fibres), leading to neuropathic ulceration of the feet, and Charcot joints.

Porphyria

An axonal neuropathy may develop in attacks of acute intermittent porphyria (p. 781). The neuropathy is unusual in distribution, in that a predominantly proximal weakness may develop together with a proximally distributed sensory impairment.

Refsum's disease

Refsum's disease is a condition with autosomal inheritance which results from defective metabolism of the long-chain aliphatic alcohol, phytol. Metabolism cannot proceed past the stage of phytanic acid due to deficiency of the enzyme, phytanic acid alpha hydroxylase. Phytanic acid thus collects throughout the body and affects the nervous system, producing a demyelinating sensory motor polyneuropathy, cerebellar ataxia, sensory neural deafness, retinal pigmentary degeneration and anosmia. A cardiomyopathy is also common. Presentation is usually in the second decade but, occasionally, patients may present much later.

Phytol is derived from chlorophyll in the diet and the condition may be alleviated by a chlorophyll-free diet.

DISEASES AFFECTING BRACHIAL AND LUMBOSACRAL PLEXUSES

Brachial plexus lesions

The brachial plexus is a relatively infrequent site of peripheral nerve damage.

Trauma

Lesions involving the upper part of the brachial plexus (C5 and C6, upper trunk) result from downward traction of the arm or forceful downward trauma on the shoulder. Severe trauma may avulse the C5 and C6 roots completely, causing extensive proximal weakness at the shoulder and sensory loss involving the outer aspect of the arm and the thumb, index and middle fingers. Trauma causing damage to the lower part of the plexus (C8 and T1) usually occurs with upward traction on the arm. There is paralysis of the small hand muscles and weakness of wrist and finger flexors, with sensory loss on the medial aspect of the arm and the little and ring fingers. Horner's syndrome is often present.

Birth injuries exemplify these two types of damage. In Erb's palsy, due to excessive traction on the head or a breech delivery, there is an upper brachial plexus lesion in which paralysis of abduction occurs with the arm internally rotated at the shoulder, the elbow extended, and the forearm pronated in the 'waiter's tip' posture. In Klumpke's paralysis, due to traction with the arm abducted and extended, a lower brachial plexus lesion occurs.

In adult life, trauma to the brachial plexus most commonly occurs as a result of motor-cycle accidents.

Cervical rib

Cervical rib refers either to a bony rib or a fibrous band arising from the seventh cervical vertebra and attached anteriorly to the first rib. The C8 and T1 roots and the subclavian artery may be distorted as they pass over the cervical rib. Symptoms arise in adult life and may be either vascular or neurological, but rarely both together. Neurological symptoms are pain in the arm along the medial border and on the ulnar aspect of the hand, with weakness of grip. Very often symptoms are provoked by carrying heavy objects. Examination shows wasting and weakness of the small hand muscles and the medial finger and wrist flexors, with sensory loss affecting the little and ring fingers extending along the ulnar border of the forearm. Vascular symptoms comprise ischaemia in the hand, sometimes embolic symptoms and Raynaud's phenomenon. Treatment is surgical resection of the rib or band.

Neuralgic amyotrophy

Neuralgic amyotrophy, also called cryptogenic brachial plexus neuropathy, is an acute patchy lesion of the brachial plexus, usually involving mainly C5 and C6 innervated muscles. Occasionally, the condition may follow immunisations or be associated with a connective tissue disorder. The first symptom is severe pain around one shoulder. Weakness develops within a few days of onset of the pain, and most often affects the deltoid, spinati and serratus anterior, less commonly biceps and triceps, and rarely forearm and hand muscles. There is sometimes sensory loss, but this is usually mild. Demyelination is the likely underlying pathology. The prognosis is good.

Malignant invasion of the brachial plexus

The commonest tumours invading the brachial plexus are carcinoma of the lung and breast. Lymphoma, spreading from cervical glands, is occasionally responsible. Virtually complete brachial plexus lesions may be seen with malignant invasion, and pain is a common and usually very troublesome symptom.

Benign nerve tumours, such as neurofibromas, occasionally arise in the brachial plexus; very occasionally, primary malignant tumours involve the plexus.

Radiation brachial plexus lesions

Radiation may cause delayed damage to the brachial plexus, and considerable diagnostic difficulties arise when it is difficult to distinguish malignant invasion from radiation damage. Radiation lesions usually develop several years after treatment.

Lumbosacral plexus lesions

A wide variety of lesions may affect the lumbosacral plexus. The main diagnostic problem lies in confirming that the lesion is of the lumbosacral plexus, rather than an intraspinal lesion causing a lumbosacral radiculopathy. The two commonest lumbar root lesions due to discs are at L5 and S1 (p. 934). Lumbosacral plexus lesions will often affect root levels higher than L5 and the presentation of an atypical lumbar radiculopathy syndrome should always therefore raise the possibility of a plexus lesion. The commonest cause is malignant invasion from carcinoma of the cervix, rectum, uterus, bladder, prostate and, occasionally, lymphoma. As with malignant invasion of the brachial plexus, pain is a prominent symptom, with progressive wasting and weakness, and sensory impairment. The lumbosacral plexus may be involved in pelvic fractures. The fetal head is occasionally responsible for damage during parturition.

Neurophysiological investigation is often helpful in demonstrating that the extent of denervation is greater than would be found with a single root. CT scanning offers the best single radiological means of visualising the posterior pelvic region if a lumbosacral plexus lesion is suspected.

MUSCLE DISEASE

The term *myopathy* refers to any condition which primarily affects muscle physiology, structure or biochemistry. The functional unit of muscle is the motor unit, which comprises a variable number of muscle fibres all innervated by a single anterior horn cell via a motor axon. Muscle fibres are of three types, subdivided on the basis of histology and enzyme content (Fig. 23.43).

1. *Type I* fibres are smaller than type II and contain larger numbers of mitochondria and oxidative enzymes, and a larger amount of fat. They are relatively slow contracting and relaxing, and are important in postural control.

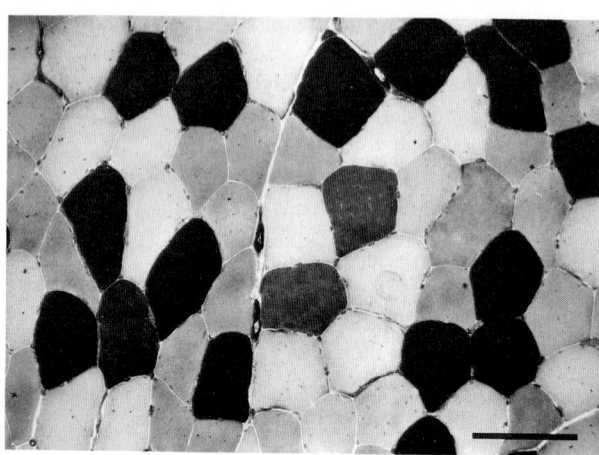

Fig. 23.43 Transverse frozen section through a biopsy sample of human vastus lateralis, stained for myosin ATPase. The black fibres are type I, the intermediate staining fibres type IIb, and the remainder of varying paler shades type IIa. Scale bar = 100 μm. (Photomicrograph by courtesy of Dr D N Landon.)

2. *Type II* fibres have a higher content of glycogen and certain enzymes, including phosphorylase, necessary for anaerobic metabolism. These fibres are rapidly contracting, so-called *fast twitch* muscle fibres. Type II fibres are further subdivided into *types IIa* and *IIb* on the basis of oxidative enzyme content.

Histochemical and biochemical techniques are increasingly used in the recognition and diagnosis of metabolic defects which affect muscle function.

Clinical features

The major categories of muscle disease are:

1. the dystrophies (hereditary)
2. the myotonic disorders (hereditary)
3. inflammatory muscle disease
4. the myasthenic syndromes
5. a number of endocrine and metabolic disorders (some hereditary).

Symptoms

The main symptoms of muscle disease are weakness, wasting (often a symptom as well as a sign), pain and fatiguability. Less common symptoms are cramps and muscle twitching.

Weakness. The distribution of wasting and weakness is characteristic for many myopathies, particularly the dystrophies. The time course of development of weakness is also diagnostically helpful.

Muscle pain. Pain is particularly a symptom of inflammatory muscle disease and may be present at rest as well as on exertion. Metabolic disorders often lead to exertional pain. Other muscle diseases are less likely to cause pain.

Fatiguability. Fatiguability is a leading symptom of the myasthenic syndromes. Continuing use of a muscle leads to rapidly progressive weakness which is relieved by a period of rest. An acute fatiguability of this sort may be less noticeable than a gradual weakness towards the end of the day, which also occurs in the myasthenic syndromes.

Cramps. Cramps usually occur at night and are only rarely a symptom of myopathy. They may be relieved by a small dose of quinine sulphate.

Other important points in the history are details of any current or past systemic illnesses which may be associated with myopathy, and – in view of the many inherited disorders of muscle – a family history.

Signs

Wasting and weakness are the major signs of muscle disease. The distribution is characteristic for the various dystrophies. Most acquired myopathies have a proximal limb girdle type of distribution. Muscle hypertrophy is an occasional feature of muscle disease. Muscle tone is usually reduced in wasted muscles, though this is not specific for muscle disease. Myotonia is a delayed muscular relaxation following voluntary contraction seen in dystrophia myotonica and myotonia congenita. Tenderness of the muscles is usually seen only in inflammatory disorders.

Tendon reflexes are preserved in myopathies until wasting is severe. In some dystrophies, reflexes in affected muscle groups are absent from an early stage.

Investigation

Nerve conduction tests and electromyography (EMG) will distinguish neurogenic and myopathic electrical changes, and are the most reliable quick methods of identifying the underlying cause of wasting and weakness when there is clinical doubt.

Diseased muscle fibres tend to release the enzyme, creatine kinase (CK). In Duchenne dystrophy and polymyositis, very high serum levels may be found; in other myopathies, the CK may be raised to a lesser degree. However, it is important to recognise that any generalised denervating process may cause a modest rise in CK; motor neurone disease is the commonest cause of this. Other enzymes, including aminotransferases and aldolase, are also released from diseased muscles, but are not specific for muscle.

Tests of thyroid and adrenal function are appropriate in some patients, while in those with the periodic paralyses, investigation of potassium levels and balance may be necessary. The complex mitochondrial myopathies and the glycogen storage diseases require special investigation.

Muscle biopsy is only occasionally needed to settle diagnostic doubt as to whether a myopathy is present, since it is usually possible to answer this question on the basis of physical examination, EMG and biochemical findings. A combination of histology and histochemistry in muscle biopsy now permits characterisation of the disease process in many patients with muscle disease.

THE MUSCULAR DYSTROPHIES

The muscular dystrophies are classified according to the mode of inheritance (Table 23.50). The Duchenne type is the commonest of all the dystrophies; the rest are much rarer. The symptoms, signs and rate of progression are extremely variable in the different dystrophies. Skeletal deformities and contractures are common in some types.

Table 23.50 Classification of the muscular dystrophies

X-linked	Autosomal dominant
Duchenne	Facioscapulohumeral
Becker	Scapuloperoneal
Autosomal recessive	Oculopharyngeal
Limb-girdle	Ocular
Childhood dystrophy	

Duchenne muscular dystrophy

Duchenne muscular dystrophy (DMD) has an incidence of 13–33 per 100 000 live births.

Clinical features

It usually presents in the third year of life with weakness of the pelvic girdle muscles, leading to delay and difficulty in walking, falls, difficulty in rising from the floor and climbing stairs. Hypertrophy of the calf muscles and, sometimes, the deltoids occurs. This is probably a true hypertrophy resulting from relative sparing of these muscles. Exaggeration of the normal lumbar lordosis develops, together with an equinovarus deformity due to weakness of the tibialis anterior and peroneal muscles, with relative sparing of the calf muscles; this leads to a tendency to walk on tiptoe. When rising from the floor, a characteristic method of climbing up the legs is adopted (Gowers' sign). Contractures at the knees and elbows are common. The condition is relentlessly progressive, so that most boys are in a wheelchair by 10 years of age, and have died before the age of 20. Cardiac failure, due to cardiac muscle involvement, and respiratory failure are the commonest causes of death. Some boys with DMD are of low intelligence. Diagnosis of DMD over the age of three is usually not difficult on clinical grounds, though diagnosis in the early stages can be difficult. The condition must always be suspected in boys with delayed walking past the age of 18 months. The CK is raised from birth.

Genetics of DMD

Much recent research has been devoted to the genetics of DMD and the gene has been localised on the short arm of the X chromosome, in a region designated Xp21. With a number of DNA probes (p. 84), it is now possible to identify the gene in carriers and affected fetuses. However, accuracy of identification depends on the availability of DNA samples from many members of a particular family because, in DMD, different mutations may occur over a long stretch of the gene. A number of cases of DMD result from spontaneous mutations in maternal ovarian cells, the exact proportion of all cases of DMD being uncertain. Thus, the risk of the sister of a DMD boy being a carrier of the abnormal gene is less than the 50:50 expected if half the mother's X chromosomes carry the DMD gene inherited from her mother. The identification of carriers does enable the incidence of DMD to be reduced in families with a known history of the condition, but not when DMD occurs as a result of spontaneous mutation. Affected boys can be identified in utero and aborted, but this tends to lead to an increased number of female children, many of whom will be carriers of the DMD gene.

Other dystrophies

Becker dystrophy

Becker dystrophy is an X-linked dystrophy similar in its distribution of weakness to DMD, but more benign. Onset of symptoms occurs between 5 and 25 years, with inability to walk occurring about 20 years after the onset of symptoms. Muscle hypertrophy is a common prelude to development of weakness. Cardiac muscle is not involved in this type of dystrophy. As Becker patients survive into adult life, they may pass on the abnormal gene to their daughters, who may then have affected sons.

Limb girdle dystrophy

Limb girdle dystrophy – an autosomal recessively inherited condition – begins in the second or third decade of life and affects the sexes equally. Initially, the onset of weakness may be in either the shoulder girdle or pelvic girdle muscles. Severe disability usually results within 20 years of onset, though benign forms do occur. Wasting and weakness may become widespread in the limbs, and the condition can be confused with spinal muscular atrophy (p. 936).

Childhood dystrophy

The term childhood dystrophy refers to dystrophy in children of autosomal recessive inheritance. Occasionally, a Duchenne-like dystrophy is seen in girls, often when the parents are consanguinous. The disease is more benign than DMD in boys.

Congenital muscular dystrophy is a rare condition presenting at birth with severe generalised hypotonia, and then progressive wasting and weakness. The condition mimics the infantile form of anterior horn cell degeneration, Werdnig-Hoffman disease. The prognosis is very poor.

Facioscapulohumeral dystrophy

Facioscapulohumeral dystrophy is an autosomal dominant condition affecting boys and girls with onset during childhood or early adult life. Facial muscle weakness leads to a typical drooping appearance around the mouth, with difficulty closing the eyes. Weakness around the scapula causes winging and riding up of the scapulae on the chest wall on abducting the arms. There is associated wasting of pectoralis major and other shoulder girdle muscles. Later, weakness of the anterolateral muscles in the lower legs develops, causing foot drop and weakness of eversion. Other muscles in the legs are sometimes affected. There is no cardiac muscle involvement and many patients have a normal lifespan.

Scapuloperoneal dystrophy

Scapuloperoneal dystrophy is rare, and is probably an autosomal dominantly inherited condition. It causes weakness of the scapular muscles, biceps and pectoralis, and also of tibialis anterior and the peroneal muscles. It may be of late onset in middle-age and is benign. Spinal muscular atrophy (p. 936) may present with a similar distribution of weakness.

Oculopharyngeal dystrophy

An autosomal dominant condition, oculopharyngeal dystrophy usually starts in middle-age, with slowly progressive ptosis, external ophthalmoplegia and dysphagia due to pharyngeal muscle involvement. The facial, neck and shoulder girdle muscles are sometimes affected. The prognosis is good, though dysphagia may become severe.

Ocular dystrophy

Ocular dystrophy is usually of earlier onset than oculopharyngeal dystrophy, but is exactly similar in its distribution of weakness except for the absence of pharyngeal involvement.

MYOTONIC DISEASES

Myotonia – the continuing contraction of a muscle after voluntary contraction ceases – is usually seen as a feature of dystrophia myotonica but also occurs in the rarer myotonia congenita.

Dystrophia myotonica

Dystrophia myotonica is an autosomal dominant condition, and the gene locus is now known to be on chromosome 19. The features are initially a distal muscle dystrophy with myotonia, with later involvement of proximal muscles, causing respiratory failure, facial muscle weakness and ptosis. Other features of the condition are low intelligence or progressive dementia, cataracts, frontal balding in males, cardiomyopathy, diabetes and gonadal atrophy. Dysphagia is common due to dystrophic change and incoordination of contraction caused by the myotonia. Occasionally, external ophthalmoplegia occurs. Somnolence is common.

The condition usually presents in the third and fourth decades. The degree of myotonia is variable. Most men are infertile. Survival is usually not beyond middle-age.

Myotonia may be helped by procainamide (250–500 mg tds) or phenytoin (300 mg daily), but these drugs should only be given when myotonia impairs functional ability.

Myotonia congenita (Thomsen's disease)

Myotonia congenita is a dominantly inherited condition in which myotonia is present from birth, when it may cause feeding difficulties. There is no dystrophy; indeed, in some children there is muscular hypertrophy. Myotonia tends to improve with age. It is usually worst at rest and in the cold, and is relieved to some extent by exercise.

MYASTHENIA GRAVIS

Myasthenia gravis (MG) is a disease characterised by fatiguable weakness of striated muscle. This may be localised or generalised and is due to a defect of transmission at the neuromuscular junction. Women are affected twice as often as men, with the onset usually in early adult life. However, it may appear at any age. Neonatal MG, which occurs in 1 in 8 babies born to mothers with MG, resolves over a few weeks.

There is an association of MG with the presence of a thymoma in older patients. Such tumours may be benign or malignant. MG also shows a strong association with thyrotoxicosis and associations also exist with diabetes mellitus, rheumatoid arthritis and SLE, suggesting an auto-immune basis. There are antibodies to acetylcholine receptor and, while the titre of antibody does not correlate well with disease severity, the presence of a raised titre of acetylcholine receptor antibody is a useful diagnostic test.

Apart from thymoma, thymic histology is often abnormal in MG, showing hyperplasia. This does not usually cause gross thymic enlargement.

Clinical features

The commonest initial presentation is weakness, often affecting only the external ocular muscles, and usually with ptosis (ocular myasthenia). However, any muscle may be involved, including bulbar and neck muscles, respiratory, shoulder girdle and pelvic girdle muscles. MG may be very localised at the onset but usually becomes generalised with time. There is a tendency for the condition to relapse and remit, and intercurrent illness, particularly infection, may provoke severe exacerbations.

Initially, diplopia may only be noticeable at the end of the day. Ptosis is common. Bulbar weakness causes difficulty in chewing, weakness of the facial muscles, dysarthria, palatal weakness leading to regurgitation of fluids, and dysphagia and dysphonia. Neck weakness is common when there is bulbar weakness. In the limbs, symptomatic weakness is usually proximal and affects shoulder girdle more than pelvic girdle muscles.

The hallmark of myasthenic weakness is fatiguability, and this must therefore be tested in the physical examination. Ptosis tends to appear more rapidly on sustained upward gaze. Eye movements should be tested with maintained gaze in different directions, and the patient questioned for the appearance of diplopia. Repetitive counting may reveal bulbar weakness. In the limbs, power is tested before and after repetitive proximal limb movements.

In early MG, muscle bulk is normal. However, in advanced MG, permanent, often non-fatiguable, weakness with wasting sometimes develops, the so-called *myasthenic myopathy*. Even in wasted, weak muscles reflexes are present and may be brisk.

Diagnosis

The diagnosis can usually be made with confidence on clinical grounds, but can be confirmed or established in cases of doubt by the intravenous edrophonium (Tensilon) test. This anticholinesterase drug has a duration of action of only a few minutes. A test dose of 1–2 mg is given to ensure no major adverse effects, followed by 5–10 mg as an intravenous bolus. Myasthenic weakness is usually improved with this drug, but the success of the tests depends on timing and a certain degree of clinical expertise. Eye movements in ocular MG may appear not to be improved even when this is the correct diagnosis, since the improvement may be limited.

EMG can be helpful, showing a decremental response to supramaximal repetitive stimulation of a muscle nerve. Acetylcholine receptor antibody titres are raised in about 90% of patients with MG. A frontal and lateral chest X-ray should be done to investigate the possibility of thymic enlargement, and a thoracic CT scan may also be helpful. There is a strong association of thymoma with striated muscle antibody.

Treatment

Initial treatment is with the long-acting anticholinesterase, pyridostigmine, a usual starting dose being 60 mg three or four times a day. Atropine is given if muscarinic side-effects are troublesome. Larger doses of pyridostigmine are given if there is deterioration. Large doses of pyridostigmine (more than 12–15 60 mg tablets daily) are capable of producing a cholinergic block at the neuromuscular junction; this leads to weakness which may be indistinguishable from myasthenic weakness. When there is uncertainty as to whether weakness is due to a cholinergic or myasthenic crisis, a test dose of Tensilon should be given, with an anaesthetist and full resuscitation equipment on hand.

Thymectomy in MG is likely to benefit a majority of patients if it is undertaken relatively early in the course of the disease. It is nearly always done in patients suspected of having a thymoma, the exceptions being old age and other associated illness. Thymectomy may produce a long period of remission, particularly in younger patients.

Immunosuppression with prednisolone and azathioprine is beneficial in patients with a limited response to pyridostigmine. The use of these drugs at an early stage of the disease remains controversial. Many patients are maintained in reasonable health for long periods with a

23

combination of these drugs.

Plasma exchange improves weakness in MG, probably by removing circulating acetyl choline receptor antibody. It is extremely helpful as an immediate life-saving measure in severe MG with respiratory involvement.

A number of drugs with membrane stabilising properties may profoundly worsen the weakness of MG. These drugs include suxamethonium (the initial diagnosis of MG may be made after prolonged paralysis with this anaesthetic drug), beta-blockers, the aminoglycoside antibiotics and anticonvulsant drugs.

Prognosis

The prognosis is variable. Some patients, young or old, run a progressive downhill course despite all treatments, and die within a few years. Others remit for variable periods. The prognosis is much worse for patients with a thymoma (usually patients in the older age group).

LAMBERT-EATON MYASTHENIC SYNDROME

In Lambert-Eaton myasthenic syndrome (LEMS), the defect at the neuromuscular junction is pre-junctional, due to failure of release of acetylcholine. Typical fatiguable weakness develops proximally in the limbs and trunk, and there is occasionally ptosis. Bulbar muscles are unaffected. In some patients, there is no clear history of fatiguable weakness. In contrast to MG, tendon reflexes are usually absent, but can be reinforced by a brief maintained isometric contraction. This is the so-called *post-tetanic potentiation*, a useful sign in diagnosis.

Autonomic symptoms, due to failure of acetylcholine release in the parasympathetic nervous system, are common, and include a dry mouth, sphincter dysfunction and erectile impotence.

About half the cases of LEMS arise in patients with small cell cancer of the lung, while half are not associated with any disease. Both types appear to have an autoimmune basis and may be helped by prednisolone and azathioprine. Guanidine and 3,4-aminopyridine have both been used to increase release of acetylcholine at the neuromuscular junction.

BOTULISM

The exotoxin of *Clostridium botulinum* binds irreversibly to the presynaptic terminals of nerves whose impulse transmission is mediated by acetylcholine. Those include neuromuscular junctions, autonomic ganglia and parasympathetic nerve terminals. The toxin acts by preventing release of acetylcholine. Antitoxin has no effect once the toxin has become bound, but recovery of transmission is achieved by terminal axonal sprouting and formation of new synaptic contacts. Botulism results from eating food contaminated with *Clostridium botulinum*, which produces the toxin under anaerobic conditions. The toxin is neutralised within 60 seconds by heating to above 85° and botulism thus usually results from eating home-made food preserves, small outbreaks being the rule. It is a rare disease in the UK, but is more frequent in other parts of the world where preparation of uncooked food preserves is common.

Clinical features

The first symptoms, which occur 12–72 hours after ingestion, are a dry mouth, abdominal distension with constipation, hesitancy of micturition, blurred vision (due to failure of accommodation), nausea and vomiting. Weakness of cranial nerve innervated muscles occurs early, so that diplopia is often the first symptom of weakness. Widespread weakness, including respiratory paralysis, then develops.

Diagnosis and treatment

The symptoms and signs of autonomic cholinergic dysfunction distinguish botulism from Guillain-Barré syndrome, MG and diphtheria. EMG may also be helpful. Sensory action potentials and conduction velocities are normal, and there is a reduced compound motor action potential to stimulation of motor nerves. However, as with LEMS, in which a similar pre-junctional defect occurs, tetanic stimulation of the nerve gives rise to an increase in the amplitude of the muscle action potential (post-tetanic potentiation). Injection of the patient's serum into mice will reproduce the weakness.

Treatment involves intensive supportive measures with ventilation in many patients. Botulinum antitoxin is given to neutralise any remaining circulating unbound toxin, and benzyl penicillin to destroy any *Clostridium botulinum* in the gut. With these measures, the mortality is low.

INFLAMMATORY MUSCLE DISEASE

Inflammatory diseases of muscle may be divided into those in which a causative infective organism can be identified, and those in which the cause is unknown (Table 23.51).

Infective causes

Bacterial myositis

In the UK, clostridial myositis develops in dirty wounds with anaerobic conditions. *Clostridium welchii* produces a toxin and enzymes which cause necrosis of muscle with inflammation and haemorrhage. Urgent treatment with surgical debridement and penicillin is necessary.

In tropical countries, acute suppurative tropical myositis is relatively common (it is rarely seen in temperate zones). The initiating lesion may be a penetrating injury or crush injury, or it may be secondary to a staphylococcal arthritis. *Staphylococcus* is the usual infecting organism. Proximal lower limb muscles are usually most affected.

Viral myositis

A number of viruses regularly produce myositis. Myalgia with a bad cold (adenovirus or rhinovirus) is a non-specific

Muscle disease

23

Table 23.51 Inflammatory myopathies

Infective

Bacterial	– Clostridial myositis (gas gangrene)
	Stapylococcal myositis
Viral	– Post-viral myalgia
	Influenza myositis
	Coxsackie A & B
	Echo
Parasitic	– Cysticercosis
	Trichinosis
	Toxoplasmosis
	Trypanosomiasis

Unknown cause – Polymyositis
Dermatomyositis
Polymyositis with connective tissue disease
Sarcoidosis
Other granulomatous myositis
Eosinophilic polymyositis

effect. A more severe polymyalgia may arise after influenza infections. It affects the thigh or calf muscles, which may swell, and the CK is raised.

Two of the Coxsackie viruses occasionally cause myositis. Bornholm disease and epidemic myositis affecting muscles in the trunk, particularly the chest, is now known to be caused by Coxsackie B5. Polymyositis with myoglobinuria may be caused by Coxsackie B6. Other viruses, notably the echoviruses, have occasionally been associated with myositis.

Parasitic myositis

Myositis may occur as part of a number of parasitic infections, none of them common in the UK.

In *cysticercosis*, ingested larvae spread from the gut to all parts of the body. Their presence in muscles and the nervous system may be asymptomatic at the time of infestation. In the muscles, an acute painful myositis may result or, as the encysted larvae gradually enlarge, a diffuse hypertrophic myopathy may occur. In the brain, epilepsy may result.

In *trichinosis*, larvae of the nematode *Trichinella spiralis*, eaten in inadequately cooked pork, spread widely via the blood, including to muscles. There, they cause an acute, painful myositis, together with conjunctivitis, periorbital oedema and, often, a generalised rash.

Toxoplasma gondii occasionally causes a myositis. Collections of parasites (pseudocysts) are found in the muscles.

Trypanosomiasis causes an acute polymyositis, often with encephalomyelitis and myocarditis. The treatment of all these diseases is considered in Chapter 12.

Myositis of unknown cause

Polymyositis refers to a group of conditions the cardinal feature of which is a myopathy, usually proximal in distribution, and of acute, subacute or chronic presentation, in which the CK is variably raised, myopathic changes are present on EMG, and muscle biopsy shows an inflammatory infiltrate with varying degrees of muscle necrosis.

Polymyositis

The typical presentation of polymyositis is with a history of several weeks' progressive, painful, proximal upper and lower limb weakness. Dysphagia and other bulbar involvement is common, together with respiratory muscle weakness. In addition to muscle pain, arthralgia is common, and general malaise and fever are also frequent.

There is little wasting if the onset is acute. Muscles are often tender. Although any striated muscle may be involved, the eye muscles are only rarely affected. The ESR is often, and the CK invariably, raised in acute or subacute polymyositis. EMG shows myopathic changes. Muscle biopsy shows an inflammatory infiltrate with perivascular lymphocytes and plasma cells and a variable degree of necrosis and phagocytosis of muscle fibres.

Treatment. As soon as the diagnosis is established, treatment with corticosteroids should be started, usually prednisolone at a dose of 60–80 mg daily. Azathioprine or cyclophosphamide are usually also prescribed for their steroid-sparing effect. Most patients begin to improve within two to three weeks, and for most, polymyositis without associated disease runs a course of a few months to two years. Serial measurements of strength and serum CK are the best indices by which treatment is monitored. Sometimes polymyositis becomes chronic, requiring continuing immunosuppressive treatment. Plasma exchange has been used, without clear evidence of benefit. In patients failing to respond to other treatment and severely affected, total body irradiation has occasionally produced improvement. Patients with respiratory muscle involvement sometimes require assisted ventilation.

Polymyositis with associated disease

Polymyositis is frequently seen in association with other diseases, e.g. the collagen disorders, particularly SLE and scleroderma. Raynaud's phenomenon is common. In dermatomyositis, skin changes comprise periorbital oedema, with heliotrope erythema around the eyes, and an erythematous, sometimes scaling and, occasionally, weeping rash, most marked over the face, forehead, neck, elbows, knuckles, upper chest, back and knees. There may be associated ulceration in the mouth and pharynx. Dermatomyositis occurs both in children and adults. In the latter, particularly men of more than 40 years, there is a high incidence (around 50%) of underlying cancer. In patients with pure polymyositis, the increase in cancer is much less. Sarcoidosis may cause a proximal myopathy, usually subacute in onset, in which typical non-caseating granulomas are found on muscle biopsy. Other conditions which occasionally produce an inflammatory proximal myopathy are polyarteritis nodosa and Wegener's granulomatosis. In eosinophilic polymyositis, muscle involvement is only one part of a multisystem disease associated with eosinophilia, which includes heart and lung involvement, peripheral neuropathy, encephalopathy, skin changes and hypergammaglobulinaemia.

Prognosis of polymyositis and related disorders

The prognosis for polymyositis not associated with other disease at presentation is good. Childhood, adolescent and early adult dermatomyositis similarly has a good prognosis. However, in later-onset dermatomyositis, particularly in men, the prognosis is poor, due to the 50% incidence of underlying cancer. The outlook is also worse for polymyositis associated with collagen disease. The prognosis for polymyositis with sarcoidosis is variable.

ENDOCRINE MYOPATHIES

Thyroid disease

In some patients with uncontrolled thyrotoxicosis, a symptomatic proximal myopathy develops, and mild degrees of asymptomatic proximal weakness can be demonstrated in many thyrotoxic patients. This resolves with treatment of the thyrotoxicosis. About 5% of all patients with MG also have thyrotoxicosis.

A normokalaemic periodic paralysis is occasionally seen in thyrotoxicosis (see below).

Hypothyroidism is occasionally associated with a proximal myopathy, typically leading to pain in the muscles after exertion.

Myopathy with adrenal and pituitary disease

In Cushing's syndrome, there is usually some evidence of a proximal myopathy with wasting and weakness. Steroids given therapeutically for any reason may lead to a similar proximal myopathy. The rate at which this appears in different people is extremely variable.

Patients who have had adrenalectomy for Cushing's disease may develop a proximal myopathy, thought to be caused by raised levels of circulating corticotrophin. In acromegaly and pituitary gigantism, generalised weakness, particularly proximally, is common. In Addison's disease and hypopituitarism, weakness is a leading symptom, usually secondary to salt and water abnormalities.

Parathyroid disease

In hyperparathyroidism, a painful proximal myopathy may develop. A particularly painful myopathy characteristically occurs in osteomalacia, often without much wasting or weakness.

TOXIC MYOPATHIES

Various drugs may cause a myopathy, of which the most important are the corticosteroids. Steroid myopathy is usually reversible if the drug is withdrawn. Other drugs which occasionally cause myopathy include vincristine, chloroquine, and amiodarone, all of which also cause a neuropathy. Emetine and epsilon aminocaproic acid also cause a myopathy. Penicillamine leads to the development of a myasthenic syndrome indistinguishable from MG. This is sometimes reversible on withdrawal of the drug, but in many patients it is permanent.

Alcohol may produce an acute myopathy with myoglobinuria, usually following an alcoholic binge. Many cases of reported chronic alcoholic myopathy probably have a neuropathic rather than a myopathic basis (p. 973).

An acute reaction to halothane anaesthesia, malignant hyperpyrexia, is now known to have a muscular basis, though the mechanism remains unclear. The condition is familial and is rare. Dantrolene has been used to prevent the reaction but, if suspected from a family history, it is best to use alternative anaesthetic agents.

METABOLIC MYOPATHIES

Glycogen storage diseases of muscle

The most important of the glycogen storage diseases of muscle is *McArdle's disease*, due to deficiency of myophosphorylase in muscle leading to impaired utilisation of muscle glucose. The disease presents with muscle pain and stiffness which is made worse by exertion. The condition usually comes on in early adult life and, although usually non-progressive, some patients develop increasing wasting and weakness.

Many other biochemical abnormalities affecting muscle glucose utilisation have been described, most leading to multiple system disorders and disability and death in children. Acid maltase deficiency is one important exception, which may present with a limb girdle dystrophic picture. The specific underlying metabolic defect is suspected when biopsy shows characteristic glycogen-containing vacuoles. None of the glycogen storage diseases affecting muscle is yet treatable.

The periodic paralyses

The periodic paralyses are dominantly inherited conditions in which episodic weakness is associated with a change in plasma and muscle potassium concentrations. There are two major types: the commoner hypokalaemic periodic paralysis and the less severe hyperkalaemic variety.

In the *hypokalaemic type*, episodes of weakness are provoked by exertion, but usually occur on the following day during a period of rest. In some patients, attacks are provoked by large carbohydrate meals. Each attack may last several hours. During the episodes of weakness, plasma potassium is below 3.0 mmol/l, with some accumulation of potassium within muscle cells. Acetazolamide or a thiazide diuretic usually prevents attacks, and some patients respond to oral potassium. The disease usually starts in the second or third decade, and attacks tend to gradually improve during adult life.

In the *hyperkalaemic* variety, attacks of generalised weakness lasting about 30 minutes are also provoked by exertion, but the weakness immediately follows the exercise. During the attack, the plasma potassium concentration increases. Acetazolamide helps this type of attack.

Mitochondrial myopathies (cytopathies)

The mitochondrial myopathies are rare, and their numerous clinical manifestations have only recently been recognised. Since tissues and organs other than muscle, notably the CNS, may also be affected, producing multisystem diseases, the broader term *mitochondrial cytopathy* is now used. Some of the disorders are confined to muscle, but clinical syndromes also include dementia, fits, ataxia, stroke-like episodes, extrapyramidal syndromes, deafness and peripheral neuropathy without clinically obvious myopathy. A number of underlying mitochondrial defects are responsible for these myopathies and multisystem diseases. In muscle biopsies, the common feature is the so-called *ragged red fibre*, in which there are accumulations of abnormal mitochondria at the periphery of the muscle fibres. Ultrastructurally, mitochondria are abnormal in size and shape, and often contain paracrystalline inclusions. These mitochondrial abnormalities, however, are not always present.

At least 25 different biochemical abnormalities have now been described.

DEMYELINATING DISEASES

Demyelinating disease refers to a group of central nervous system disorders in which the primary pathological process is demyelination without axonal degeneration. By far the most important of these is multiple sclerosis (MS). Demyelination is also the result of a number of rare inherited disorders of sphingolipid metabolism; these include the leucodystrophies and some lipid storage diseases.

MULTIPLE SCLEROSIS

Multiple sclerosis is a disease of unknown cause, in which discrete areas of demyelination develop at many sites in the brain and spinal cord. Lesions develop in different sites at different times, usually with some capacity for regeneration and restoration of function; this leads, in many patients, to a characteristic relapsing and remitting history. In other patients, a slowly progressive deficit occurs. Although demyelination is the primary pathology in MS, extensive areas of demyelination are associated with axonal loss and, in most patients, there is a slowly cumulative neurological deficit.

Epidemiology

The prevalence of MS shows a strong geographical variation, being essentially a disease of temperate climates. Even within the UK there are considerable variations in prevalence, e.g. around 30 per 10 000 in Shetland and Orkney, compared with 6 per 10 000 in England.

Multiple sclerosis is very rare in childhood and uncommon in early adolescence. There is an increasing incidence with age, peaking at about 30 years. It is uncommon over the age of 50. Often, in late presentations, it is possible to obtain a history of a previous minor neurological episode in earlier life which was likely to have been due to MS. This emphasises the relatively benign course of the disease in some patients. Slightly more women than men are affected by MS.

Aetiology

There have been many hypotheses about the cause of MS. Acute demyelination is an inflammatory process and the most favoured explanation, at present, is that acute demyelination is the result of an abnormal immune response to an antigen, perhaps of viral origin. A contributory role has been suggested for other environmental factors, including diet, but none has been substantiated. Genetic factors may be important in some instances, as there is an association of MS with HLA-A3 and DR2 antigens. There is no clear mode of inheritance, however. Studies of migrants show that, if migration occurs before the age of 15, the risk of developing MS becomes that of the country to which the patient has migrated. This evidence emphasises the importance of an environmental factor or factors.

Pathology

Acute demyelination occurs in discrete areas known as plaques, which may be single or multiple. The lesions may occur anywhere in central white matter, but common sites are the optic nerve, the brain stem and cerebellum, the periventricular regions and the cervical spinal cord. Later, glial scarring results in the whitish appearance of the chronic plaque. Some remyelination may be possible, but this is limited. Resolution of oedema in and around plaques reverses conduction block and improves function. Even without symptoms or signs, slowing of conduction can often be demonstrated in visual, auditory and somatosensory pathways by electrophysiological testing.

Clinical features

Since plaques may occur at any site in central white matter, the clinical manifestations of MS are extremely variable. However, early in the disease a number of presentations are characteristic.

Optic neuritis

Inflammation of the optic nerve may be symptomatic or asymptomatic. When it affects the optic nerve head, it is sometimes termed *papillitis*; when inflammation occurs in the optic nerve further away from the eye, it may be called *retrobulbar neuritis*.

Neurological Disease

Symptoms. In acute optic neuritis, (which is nearly always unilateral), there is dimming of vision, blurring, loss of acuity and reduced colour vision. These symptoms usually progress over hours or a few days. Rarely, vision may be lost altogether. Patients may be aware of the central or paracentral scotoma characteristic of this condition. Pain in and around the eye, particularly with movement of the eye, is common. The symptoms may be mild and transient, lasting only a few days, and may not cause patients to present to their doctors.

Signs. Examination during acute symptomatic optic neuritis will usually show impaired visual acuity, but formal visual field mapping may be necessary to detect small scotomas. The pupillary reaction to light shone in the affected eye will be sluggish in both the affected and unaffected eyes; a brisker response is obtained in both eyes when the same light is shone into the unaffected eye, indicating an afferent pupillary defect. On fundoscopy, there may be no abnormality if inflammation is located proximally in the optic nerve, but with inflammation near to the optic nerve head, there may be papilloedema.

Optic neuritis usually resolves within a few weeks, frequently without residual symptoms. However, a degree of optic atrophy is often detectable as pallor of the optic disc, a useful diagnostic sign in MS. Some patients will be aware of continuing impairment of visual acuity and colour vision and, rarely, there is severe visual impairment after a single episode.

Repeated acute episodes of optic neuritis during the course of MS are common. Sometimes, a slowly progressive visual impairment results from indolent optic neuritis. Other rare causes of optic neuritis include sarcoidosis, syphilis, Herpes zoster and SLE. About 30% of patients presenting with optic neuritis have no other evidence of MS, and do not develop the disease.

Cervical cord

Involvement of the cervical spinal cord is very common early in the course of MS, presenting with motor, sensory, or bladder, bowel and sexual disturbances. Symptoms may be unilateral, but pyramidal signs are usually bilateral. Although there are usually no symptoms in the upper limbs in the early stages, brisk reflexes are often found.

Sensory symptoms include tingling paraesthesiae and numbness. Examination reveals disturbance of dorsal column function (impaired joint position and vibration sensation) and, less often, of spinothalamic sensation. A common early manifestation of MS is the L'Hermitte symptom, in which the patient notices tingling paraesthesiae in the legs and sometimes trunk and upper limbs on flexing the neck. This is probably due to mechanical sensitivity of dorsal column fibres in an area in, or surrounding, a plaque of demyelination. It may occasionally occur after cervical cord trauma, with cervical tumours and in subacute combined degeneration due to B_{12} deficiency.

Bladder disturbances are common in MS and may occasionally be the presenting complaint. Urgency and frequency of micturition, then incontinence, are charac-

teristic. Constipation is the main bowel disturbance early in MS, but sometimes urgency of defaecation with soiling occurs. Erectile impotence and ejaculatory failure are common symptoms.

Brain stem and cerebellum

Visual disturbances other than optic neuritis are frequent, and include diplopia due either to VIth nerve palsy or an internuclear ophthalmoplegia (INO). In INO, due to a lesion of the medial longitudinal fasciculus, eye movements are dysconjugate on lateral gaze; thus, on right lateral gaze there is incomplete adduction of the left eye, and there may be associated nystagmus, which is of greater amplitude in the abducting right eye, so-called ataxic nystagmus. Nystagmus without any ocular palsy is a common manifestation of brain stem demyelination, and may be horizontal, vertical or rotatory.

Vertigo is a fairly common early symptom of MS, due to plaque formation involving the vestibular nuclear complex. Ataxia involving limbs and/or trunk is also frequent early in the disease, and is due to plaque formation within the cerebellum or affecting its connections in the brain stem. Long motor and sensory tracts may also be involved in the brain stem; this produces symptoms and signs similar to those of cervical cord demyelination.

Later features

Depression in long-standing MS is common, and requires vigorous treatment. Widespread cerebral hemisphere demyelination leads to intellectual impairment. Often, there is a predominantly frontal impairment, producing disinhibition and other frontal features (p. 874).

Brain stem demyelination leads to complex ocular palsies, ataxia and long tract signs. Trigeminal neuralgia shows an assocation with MS, and there is also an increased incidence of atypical neuralgic pains in a trigeminal distribution. Rubral tremor is a particularly disabling type of cerebellar tremor; it is postural and of large amplitude, preventing purposeful actions in the arms. Myokymia

---

Summary 12 Multiple sclerosis (MS)

- Multiple sclerosis is the commonest progressive disabling neurological disease affecting young adults in the UK.

- Common sites of symptomatic demyelination are the optic nerves, cervical cord, brain stem, cerebellum and, usually later in the course of the disease, the cerebral hemispheres.

- MS may run a relapsing-remitting or chronic progressive course. The former is more likely to occur with younger age of onset.

- Prognosis is better with young onset and a relapsing-remitting course, but is very variable.

- Corticosteroids may shorten relapse, but immunosuppressive treatment has no effect on the long-term course of the disease.

- There is no clear-cut evidence that dietary restrictions or supplements, or hyperbaric oxygen, alter the course of the disease.

refers to a continuous rippling twitching of the facial muscles on one side. It is probably due to irritation of the facial nucleus. Progressive bulbar involvement producing dysarthria, dysphagia, and dysphonia indicates a particularly poor prognosis. Lower motor neurones are rarely affected in MS.

Other factors

Patients with MS frequently remark that their symptoms are worse in hot weather, after a hot bath, during fever or after exertion, all of which raise body temperature. Conduction in demyelinated axons is blocked by small rises in body temperature.

There is probably no increased risk of relapse during pregnancy but there is in the puerperium.

Course and prognosis

Multiple sclerosis can be a remarkably benign disease with long periods of remission and relatively little neurological deficit. However, in most patients an increasing neurological deficit accumulates. The end stage of MS is characterised by dementia, quadriplegia, incontinence, blindness, pressure sores and recurrent respiratory and urinary tract infections.

In about three-quarters of patients, the disease has a relapsing and remitting course, and, in the remainder, a chronic progressive course. In about 20% of patients there is no significant disability after five years, and the average life expectancy overall from the onset of symptoms is 20–30 years. In about 5% of patients, the disease is rapidly progressive and fatal within five years. Poor prognostic factors are an older age at onset, the development of dementia, and the early development of ataxia.

Diagnosis

In many patients the diagnosis is straightforward and established on clinical evidence of more than one lesion in the nervous system, together with a characteristic relapsing and remitting history. The finding of optic atrophy in a patient presenting with a brain stem or cervical cord lesion is particularly helpful diagnostically.

Evoked potentials. Evoked potentials, either visual, auditory or somatosensory from the limbs, are sensitive measures of damage in these sensory pathways. Visual evoked potentials are recorded from the scalp over the occipital cortex. A flash or regular pattern reversal stimulus produces a small visual evoked potential, which can be averaged. The latency is prolonged if there has been significant demyelination at any time in the past. Similar information can be obtained concerning brain stem auditory pathways and large fibre, dorsal column somatosensory pathways from the limbs. The evoked potentials are often delayed in the absence of any present or past symptoms.

CSF protein content may be raised. The IgG fraction of this may be greater than 10%, and CSF electrophoresis

Fig. 23.44 Magnetic resonance scan in multiple sclerosis. Multiple areas of abnormal signal, here shown in white, are visible in the cerebral hemisphere white matter, particularly adjacent to the lateral ventricles.

may show discrete bands in the gamma 4 and gamma 5 regions (*oligoclonal bands*). These immunoglobulins are synthesised locally within the CNS. Oligoclonal bands are not unique to MS, and occur occasionally in other conditions, including neurosyphilis and neurosarcoidosis. However, the finding of oligoclonal bands in the clinical setting of suspected MS lends support to this diagnosis.

CT scans are usually normal in the early stages. Large areas of acute demyelination may be seen, and chronic plaques, particularly in the periventricular regions, give rise to discrete abnormalities. *NMR scanning* provides a much more sensitive means of imaging the white matter (Fig. 23.44).

Treatment

There is no specific treatment for MS. Corticosteroids may promote remission in relapse, probably by reducing inflammation and oedema in acute plaques. Steroids have no effect on the outcome of a particular relapse and do not protect against further relapse. Long-term immunosuppression with cytotoxic agents is of no proven benefit.

Dietary restrictions or supplements are frequently recommended, but there is no evidence of efficacy for any of these. Hyperbaric oxygen has also had a vogue in recent years. Carefully controlled clinical trials have not shown any benefit.

The treatment of MS remains symptomatic and supportive. Physiotherapy and occupational therapy have a large role to play. Spasticity may be relieved by anti-spastic drugs, such as baclofen and dantrolene, but these may exacerbate weakness.

Urinary urgency and frequency are often partly relieved by anticholinergics. Other patients will require urinary devices, such as sheaths and pads, and some patients eventually need permanent catheterisation An alternative, increasingly used and suitable for many patients, is intermittent self-catheterisation.

Counselling in MS

Multiple sclerosis is a common neurological disorder, and patients with a wide variety of symptoms think – often incorrectly – they have MS. The lay view of MS and its prognosis is often more gloomy than the reality. In patients with a single neurological episode possibly due to MS, it is usually ill-advised to discuss the possibility of MS unless directly asked by the patient. When the diagnosis is definite, however, it is nearly always best to inform the patient. Time must be set aside to discuss the disease, its effects and its prognosis with the patient and relatives. Open discussion and allaying fears, which are often misguided or ill-founded, is usually helpful.

OTHER ACQUIRED DEMYELINATING DISEASE

Post-viral and post-vaccinial encephalomyelitis

In post-viral and post-vaccinial encephalomyelitis, widespread acute inflammation with demyelination in the brain and spinal cord follows a viral illness – either one of the exanthemata or an intercurrent viral infection. Occasionally, a similar disease follows smallpox vaccination and other inoculations, particularly rabies. Because of the frequency of the exanthemata in childhood, children are affected by this type of encephalomyelitis more often than adults. Occasionally, there is no preceding history of infection or inoculation.

The illness is characterised by subacute onset of malaise, headache, vomiting, drowsiness, convulsions and fever, together with focal symptoms and signs. A hemiparesis, brain stem and cerebellar signs, and evidence of a myelitis are the principal focal features. Occasionally, optic neuritis occurs. Coma and death may ensue, but the majority of patients recover, some with residual intellectual and physical deficit, including epilepsy.

Occasionally, recurrent episodes occur. Rarely, an initial severe episode of MS presents in this way.

The acute illness resembles an encephalitis due to direct viral infection and, clinically, it can be impossible to distinguish the two (p. 962).

Acute haemorrhagic leucoencephalopathy, in which there are accompanying multiple areas of haemorrhage, probably represents a particularly severe form of encephalomyelitis.

The demyelinating conditions of central pontine myelinolyis and Marchiafava-Bignami disease are discussed on pages 973–74.

Disorders of sphingolipid metabolism

A large number of rare disorders of myelin metabolism exist. These fall into two broad groups, the leucodystrophies and the lipid storage diseases (Table 23.52). Demyelination is the feature common to both groups of disorders. They are primarily of relevance to paediatric practice. Most lead to progressive mental deterioration and a multiplicity of neurological signs, often including spasticity in the limbs, fits, ataxia and optic atrophy. Death within months or a year or two occurs in many of these disorders; metachromatic leucodystrophy, adrenoleucodystrophy and Fabry's disease are exceptions. There is no specific therapy for these conditions.

Metachromatic leucodystrophy

Metachromatic leucodystrophy is an autosomal recessive condition, due to deficiency of aryl sulphatase A, in which there is tissue accumulation of metachromatic lipids in the white matter of the central nervous system and in

Table 23.52 Disorders of sphingolipid metabolism

Disease	Biochemical defect	Clinical features
The leucodystrophies		
Metachromatic leucodystrophy	Aryl sulphatase A deficiency	See text
Adrenoleucodystrophy	Unknown	See text
Globoid cell leucodystrophy	Galactocerebroside β-galactosidase deficiency	Onset in infancy Irritability, motor regression, nystagmus, spasticity or hypotonia, optic atrophy, fits. Death within 1 year
Lipid storage diseases		
Gangliosidoses, e.g. Tay-Sachs disease	β-acetyl hexosaminidase deficiency causing accumulation of GM2 ganglioside	Motor regression in infancy. Optic atrophy. Death within 2 years
Gaucher's disease	Glucocerebrosidase deficiency	Progressive neurological deterioration after birth. Death within 1 year
Niemann-Pick disease	Sphingomyelinase deficiency	Onset at 6 months. Progressive mental and neurological deterioration. May survive many years
Fabry's disease	Ceramide trihexosidase deficiency	See text

peripheral nerves. The effects are widespread, with onset of symptoms usually in early childhood, but sometimes as late as adolescence. There is weakness, ataxia, dementia and fits. Examination shows signs of peripheral neuropathy, in addition to pyramidal weakness, ataxia and dementia, and there is often optic atrophy. The diagnosis is made by assay of the enzyme in leucocytes, and metachromatic material can be seen on rectal or peripheral nerve biopsy.

Adrenoleucodystrophy

Adrenoleucodystrophy is a sex-linked disorder of unknown biochemical basis. It presents in boys, during childhood, with progressive dementia, ataxia, spasticity, a peripheral neuropathy and signs of hypoadrenalism.

Fabry's disease (angiokeratoma corporis diffusum)

Fabry's disease (angiokeratoma corporis diffusum) is caused by deficiency of ceramide trihexosidase, which leads to accumulation of trihexose ceramide in blood vessel walls and smooth muscle cells throughout the body. The presentation in late childhood or early adolescence includes renal failure, skin lesions, a painful peripheral neuropathy, cardiac failure, ataxia and cerebrovascular occlusions causing hemiparesis, brain stem and cerebellar signs.

BACTERIAL INFECTIONS OF THE NERVOUS SYSTEM

ACUTE BACTERIAL MENINGITIS

Bacterial meningitis is infection of the leptomeninges and the cerebrospinal fluid (CSF) which diffusely affects the whole meninges and subarachnoid space and, sometimes, also the ventricles (ventriculitis). The three bacteria most commonly causing meningitis, *Neisseria meningitidis*, *Haemophilus influenzae* and *Streptococcus pneumoniae* gain access to the meninges and subarachnoid space via the bloodstream from the nasopharynx, through the walls of the intracranial venous sinuses. Once in the CSF, bacteria rapidly multiply. Other bacteria may also cause meningitis (Table 23.53; see also Ch. 12); any bacterium causing septicaemia may enter the CSF and cause meningitis. Haematogenous spread may also occur from infective endocarditis, osteomyelitis and pyelonephritis.

Mechanisms of infection

Direct infection occurs from penetrating trauma, including compound skull fractures, and gunshot wounds. Fractures of the skull with CSF leaks are common causes of meningitis. Septic foci closely adjacent to the meninges (and thus potential causes of meningitis) include sinusitis, middle ear and mastoid infection, and osteomyelitis of the skull bones. Lymphatic spread of infection to the spinal cord occurs from retropharyngeal, retroperitoneal and psoas abscesses.

Table 23.53 Treatment of bacterial meningitis in adults

Organism	Treatment
Neisseria meningitidis	Benzyl penicillin (4 megaunits, 4-hourly) or chloramphenicol (20 mg/kg, 6-hourly) in hypersensitivity to penicillin
Streptococcus pneumoniae	Benzyl penicillin or chloramphenicol, doses as for *N. meningitidis*
Haemophilus influenzae	Cefuroxime (3 g, 8-hourly) or chloramphenicol (20 mg/kg, 6-hourly) or ampicillin (2 g, 6-hourly for 2 days, then 1 g, 6-hourly) or co-trimoxazole (160 mg trimethoprim and 800 mg sulphamethoxazole, 12-hourly)
Staphylococcus aureus *Staphylococcus epidermidis*	Flucloxacillin (3 g, 6-hourly) or vancomycin (500 mg, 6-hourly) or gentamicin (5 mg/kg/day*) in penicillin hypersensitivity
Pseudomonas aeruginosa	Piperacillin (4 g, 6-hourly) with tobramycin (3–5 mg/kg/day) or Ticarcillin (5 g, 6-hourly) with gentamicin (5 mg/kg per day*)

* Gentamicin blood levels necessary

Congenital abnormalities, particularly meningomyeloceles, provide a further route of infection.

Despite the most careful aseptic precautions, meningitis still remains a serious complication of neurosurgical procedures. Shunts are particularly likely to lead to infection. Very occasionally, meningitis occurs after lumbar puncture. As part of their general increased susceptibility to infection, diabetics are more prone to develop meningitis. Finally, meningitis is a much more common illness in immunocompromised patients. These include the very young and elderly, patients treated with corticosteroids for any reason, patients undergoing organ transplantation, patients with malignant disease (particularly Hodgkin's lymphoma) and patients with HIV infection.

Complications of meningitis

Meningitis may be complicated by *ventriculitis* or *intracerebral abscess*. There may be obstruction of flow of CSF through the foramina between the ventricles and the cerebral aqueduct, causing *hydrocephalus*. Purulent exudate may cause reduced reabsorption of CSF in the arachnoid granulations, also leading to hydrocephalus; and septic thrombosis of the venous sinuses can occur, leading to an increase in intracranial pressure with a communicating hydrocephalus. The purulent exudate in the basal meninges may affect the cranial nerves and arteries which cross the subarachnoid space; *cranial nerve palsies* are thus common complications of bacterial meningitis. The IIIrd and VIth cranial nerves may also be affected by direct pressure from downward displacement of an oedematous brain with raised intracranial pressure. The major arteries at the base of the brain may, occasionally, become occluded by the purulent arteritis, leading to major *strokes*, affecting either the cerebral hemispheres or brain stem. Cortical veins may also become occluded, and this may lead to areas of infarction.

Infection may also spread into the subdural space, causing a *subdural empyema*. Localised *epidural abscesses* may occur over the cerebral hemispheres and epidural abscesses may develop secondary to meningitis in the spinal cord, leading to spinal cord compression.

Late sequelae of acute bacterial meningitis include persistent cranial nerve palsies, though the palsies seen acutely usually improve to some extent. *Deafness*, due to VIIIth nerve damage, is often bilateral, severe and permanent. This has been estimated to occur in 5–40% of all patients. In young children, diffuse cerebral damage with *mental retardation* often results from acute meningitis, particularly with *Haemophilus influenzae* infection.

Clinical features

In adults, the main symptoms of meningitis are headache, vomiting, irritability, photophobia and drowsiness. Fits are usually a later symptom. In meningococcal meningitis, the progression of symptoms may be extremely rapid, the patient presenting in coma within hours of the onset of symptoms.

The signs are fever, neck stiffness, drowsiness, stupor or coma; sometimes, there is neurological deficit – cranial nerve palsies, hemiparesis or other focal signs – which result from occlusion of the basal cerebral arteries. Focal deficit is more common in advanced, untreated cases of meningitis. Neck stiffness may be mild or absent in the young, the elderly and in deeply comatose patients. Meningeal irritation may cause a positive Kernig's sign, and Brudzinski's sign, in which neck flexion causes flexion of the legs. Later, there may be a posture of extension of the neck and spine. The typical rash of meningococcal septicaemia may be present (p. 230).

In neonates and young children, the symptoms and signs of meningitis may be minimal. Fits are a much more common presenting feature in the young, and irritability, fever and drowsiness may be the only signs, without neck stiffness. Likewise, in the elderly, there may be few signs and, in some cases, a much more insidious onset.

Differential diagnosis

The commonest alternative cause of severe headache, neck stiffness, vomiting, with or without focal signs, is subarachnoid haemorrhage. This is usually but not always of abrupt onset. CT scanning is helpful in demonstrating subarachnoid blood in such cases. Aseptic viral meningitis is the other main differential diagnosis. Other types of meningitis may cause an identical presentation to acute bacterial meningitis. The onset of tuberculous meningitis can be acute, but is more often subacute and may be very insidious. In immunocompromised patients, fungal (cryptococcal or candida) or amoebic meningitis must be considered and an India ink stain of the CSF performed. The opisthotonos of tetanus may mimic meningeal irritation. In children, acute fever is fairly often associated with neck stiffness as a non-specific sign.

Investigation

Examination of the CSF is diagnostic but lumbar puncture can be a dangerous procedure in certain instances, e.g. in the presence of a developing cerebral abscess complicating the meningitis. Intracranial pressure is nearly always raised in meningitis, but, in the presence of papilloedema, focal signs or coma, it is safest to perform a CT scan to exclude hydrocephalus or a focal mass lesion prior to performing lumbar puncture. When scanning is not available, clearly a risk must be taken and the CSF examined.

At lumbar puncture, the opening pressure should be measured before samples are taken for a Gram stain, culture, cell count, protein and glucose estimation. Typical findings in acute bacterial meningitis are a neutrophil count of more than $1000/mm^3$, a glucose which is less than 40% of the blood glucose or below 1.7 mmol/l, and a considerably raised protein concentration. Blood cultures, and any other relevant cultures, from suspected foci of infection should be taken. However, it cannot be over-emphasised that prompt treatment of acute meningitis is essential for survival and prevention of complications. Meningococcal meningitis may be fatal within 24 hours. In immunocompromised patients, unusual pathogens must be looked for, such as *Listeria monocytogenes*, tuberculosis, amoeba and fungal infections, particularly *Cryptococcus*.

Findings similar to those of acute bacterial meningitis may be found in viral meningitis. The pleocytosis in the CSF usually comprises lymphocytes but can be due to neutrophils, and the CSF glucose is occasionally low. CSF glucose may also be low in malignant meningitis, subarachnoid haemorrhage, tuberculous meningitis and

---

Summary 13 Lumbar puncture in meningitis

- Lumbar puncture (LP) is safe in patients with meningitis without focal signs and whose conscious level is no worse than drowsy.

- If there are focal signs or the patient is in coma, a complication of meningitis (e.g. cerebral abscess, hydrocephalus), may have supervened. There is a risk of coning with LP. Get a CT scan.

- If in doubt, ask for neurological advice before doing a LP.

- Minimum examination of the CSF in suspected meningitis includes cell count, protein, glucose, Gram stain, and Z–N stain.

- In any patient who may be immunocompromised, ask for special microbiological CSF tests for fungal, Listerial, amoebic and other rare organisms.

- Tuberculous meningitis rarely causes a white cell count of more than $1000/mm^3$, and a Z–N stain may be negative. If there is strong clinical evidence, treat for TB.

- Never give intrathecal antibiotics.

malignant hypertension.

Failure of the patient's clinical state to improve within 24–36 hours of starting antibiotic treatment is an indication for further CSF examination. This is particularly important when there is microbiological doubt about the causative organism. A rise in cell count in the second CSF, with a persistently low glucose, implies an inadequate antibiotic treatment which must therefore be changed. With correct treatment, the cell count rapidly falls.

If signs indicate a spinal cord lesion in a patient with meningitis, a spinal epidural abscess should be suspected and, in consultation with a neurosurgeon, myelography should be urgently performed.

Treatment

Antibiotics

Antibiotic treatment must be started immediately the CSF has been taken. In rare instances where there is likely to be delay in performing a lumbar puncture, treatment must be started blind. Table 23.53 sets out the antibiotics used for different organisms; these are usually given intravenously. Chloramphenicol should not be used in neonates, due to bone marrow and renal toxicity occurring as a result of inadequate metabolism by the liver. Chloramphenicol is effective against the rarer *Listeria monocytogenes*.

For patients suspected of being immunosuppressed and who may thus be infected with one of the less common bacteria, an initial broad-spectrum antibiotic combination is given, such as gentamicin and cefuroxime.

Bacterial culture is usually available within 24 hours, by which time some clinical improvement should have occurred. If not, the CSF must be re-examined.

High-dose intravenous antibiotics should always be continued for at least a week. As meningeal inflammation decreases, the blood-brain barrier is gradually restored, allowing less of the drug to gain access to the infected meninges. An identified focus of infection, e.g. sinusitis or suppurative otitis media, is an indication for a longer period of treatment, during which time the focus must be treated on its own merits. Immunosuppressed patients also require longer periods of treatment.

Intrathecal penicillin makes no difference to outcome and is potentially dangerous. Large doses cause an encephalopathy with fits, which is usually fatal.

Fits

Fits are common, particularly in children with meningitis. Treatment of status epilepticus or serial epilepsy is as described on page 890. Regular oral anticonvulsant treatment should be started in all patients having fits, but it is not necessary to give an anticonvulsant prophylactically if there have been no fits. Oral treatment can be given via a nasogastric tube, but phenytoin may also be given by slow intravenous injection, and phenobarbitone by intramuscular injection. Loading doses are necessary, followed by regular maintenance doses. Phenytoin competes with chloramphenicol for glucuronation in the liver and so increases levels of this antibiotic.

Raised intracranial pressure and hydrocephalus

Generalised cerebral oedema may produce life-threatening rises in intracranial pressure. This is treated urgently with mannitol and then dexamethasone. Hydrocephalus may develop after an interval of several days; in such cases, there is typically clinical improvement after initiation of treatment, followed by a deterioration. The diagnosis is established by a CT scan. Some patients with progressive hydrocephalus will require treatment with a ventricular drain.

Cerebral abscess

Despite adequate treatment, some patients will develop cerebral abscesses. The development of fits and focal signs also raises the possibility of venous sinus thrombosis (p. 959). Clinical deterioration, with or without focal signs or fits, is an indication for an urgent CT scan. If the CT scan is normal, the CSF must be re-examined.

Prevention

Treatment of close contacts (family, medical and nursing staff) of patients with *Streptococci pneumoniae* meningitis is not necessary, but it is recommended with *Haemophilus influenzae* or *Neisseria meningitidis*. Rifampicin (600 mg bd for adults or 20 mg/kg per day for children for 2 days) is effective prophylaxis for both bacteria.

Vaccines for *Neisseria meningitidis* may be used in family members when the meningococcus occurs in small epidemics, and for contacts at particular risk, such as the immunocompromised, the very young and the elderly.

Prognosis

Overall mortality for the three common pathogens ranges from as low as 3% for *Haemophilus influenzae* to as high as 60% for *Streptococcus pneumoniae*. In the very young and the elderly, mortality is higher.

INTRACRANIAL ABSCESS

Intracranial abscesses are most commonly intracerebral, but pus may collect in the subdural space (subdural empyema) or in the extradural space. Subdural empyema or intracerebral abscesses may extend to the meninges and cause meningitis, or, conversely, infection may spread from the meninges. Intracerebral abscesses may rupture into the ventricles, causing a ventriculitis.

An intracerebral abscess starts as an area of cerebritis which then develops into a pus-filled cavity surrounded by a wall of variable thickness, and, outside this, cerebral oedema. The oedema is often extensive and, together with the abscess itself, leads to increased intracranial pressure and mass effect on surrounding structures. Some abscesses are single, others multilocular or multiple (Fig. 23.45).

Fig. 23.45 Cerebral abscess. Enhanced CT scan of a patient with a multiloculated left frontal acute pyogenic abscess. Note the typical ring enhancing lesion, with massive surrounding cerebral oedema, causing midline shift. There is also a small subdural collection of pus (subdural empyema). The intracranial abscesses in this twenty-one-year-old man were secondary to frontal sinusitis.

Aetiology

Cerebral abscesses. Excluding cerebral abscesses occurring in AIDS (which are usually multiple and are most often caused by *Toxoplasma gondii*, p. 966), about 60% of intracerebral abscesses are caused by middle ear infection and are situated in the temporal lobe or cerebellum. About 20% are secondary to frontal sinusitis, which results in frontal lobe abscess; approximately 10% are due to bacteraemia or septicaemia from the lung (abscess, empyema or bronchiectasis), the heart (infective endocarditis), dental sepsis, or some other peripheral site, with penetrating skull trauma accounting for a small proportion of cases; and, in about 10% of cerebral abscess, no source for the infection is found. Cerebral abscess is more likely to occur in patients with debilitating illness and in the immunocompromised.

Subdural empyema usually results from frontal sinusitis or penetrating injury, and sometimes middle ear infection. In infants, it is commonly secondary to meningitis. In adults it is occasionally secondary to septicaemia. Extradural abscess has similar causes and may, in addition, be secondary to osteomyelitis of the skull, now a rare condition.

Bacteriology

In contrast to meningitis, intracranial abscesses are often due to mixed infection. The organisms most frequently causing abscesses are *Strep. viridans*, *Staph. aureus*, *Klebsiella*, and, occasionally, other Gram-negative bacteria. Infection with one of these is frequently associated with an anaerobe, either anaerobic streptococcus or bacterioides. In immunocompromised patients, a wide range of bacteria may be responsible, together with occasional amoebic or fungal abscesses.

Clinical features

Intracerebral abscess. An acute pyogenic abscess is likely to cause symptoms which progress quickly over days rather than weeks. Multiple abscesses may cause a plethora of symptoms and signs. A combination of headache, rapidly progressive neurological deficit and symptoms of raised intracranial pressure, with or without fever, and a deteriorating conscious level, suggests the possibility of an intracerebral abscess. Fits are also very common.

Fever is very variable in cerebral abscess. Meningism is quite common. A careful search for a systemic source of infection must be made in every case of suspected abscess.

Subdural empyema. Patients with subdural empyema are usually very ill. The pus spreads rapidly over the surface of the hemisphere, producing hemiparesis, raised intracranial pressure, fits and meningism.

Extradural abscess. Extradural abscesses are often well localised and may present less acutely. They usually cause localised, severe headache and are associated with sinusitis, mastoiditis or penetrating trauma.

Investigation

The most important immediate investigation is a CT scan. Most acute pyogenic abscesses are rounded lesions of low attenuation with ring enhancement and much surrounding oedema, producing mass effect (Fig. 23.45). However, these appearances are not specific to abscess and may occur with tumours. In the earlier stage of spreading cerebritis, there is no ring enhancement.

Plain radiology should include skull X-rays, to look particularly for evidence of sinusitis or mastoiditis and middle ear infection, and a chest X-ray. Culture of any possible source of infection, together with blood cultures, should be done. Lumbar puncture is contraindicated.

Treatment

Rapidly rising intracranial pressure is usually the life-threatening factor in pyogenic intracerebral abscess, and urgent drainage of the pus is necessary. Although Gram stain of the aspirated pus may give some guide to antibiotic treatment, initial treatment must be guaranteed to be effective against a wide range of organisms. A combination of benzyl penicillin, cefuroxime, gentamicin and metranidazole is reasonable, until bacterial results are available.

All patients with supratentorial abscess, with or without fits at presentation, should be given an anticonvulsant, because of the high incidence of fits. Cerebral oedema may require treatment either with mannitol or dexamethasone, and ventilation is sometimes necessary.

Some abscesses only need to be drained on one occasion, but others may need several evacuations. Serial CT scanning permits frequent monitoring of abscess size. Surgical treatment for supratentorial abscesses is usually limited to regular aspiration. Eventual healing with antibiotic treatment is often good, with little or no neurological deficit. In cerebellar abscess, many surgeons will attempt complete excision, both because of the dangers of hydrocephalus and because it is possible to excise sizeable lesions with relatively little risk of producing neurological deficit. Subdural empyema and extradural abscesses require surgical drainage and high doses of intravenous antibiotics.

Prognosis

The prognosis is related to the clinical state at the time of presentation. The overall mortality of intracerebral abscess is in the region of 10%. In survivors, lasting neurological deficit is often not severe. Persistent fits are a problem in 30–50% of patients with supratentorial abscess.

CORTICAL VENOUS THROMBOPHLEBITIS AND VENOUS SINUS THROMBOSIS

Thrombosis of cortical veins and thrombosis of the dural venous sinuses are relatively rare. Thrombosis of the dural sinuses is nearly always preceded by cortical vein thrombosis. The exception to this is cavernous sinus thrombosis.

Aetiology

The causes of cortical thrombophlebitis and dural venous thrombosis are listed in Table 23.54. The commonest

Table 23.54 Causes of cortical vein and dural sinus thrombosis

- Infection, of scalp, skull, sinuses, face, middle ear, mastoiditis. Also secondary to meningitis and septicaemia
- Post-partum (days or weeks following delivery)
- Dehydration, e.g. dysentery, cholera
- Diabetes mellitus
- Trauma (open or closed head injury)
- Catheterisation of jugular veins
- Blood dyscrasias, particularly leukaemia
- Post-operative hypercoagulability
- Severe heart failure
- Tumour invasion of sinuses
- Rare non-metastatic effect of malignant disease
- Contraceptive pill, particularly in smokers

causes are infection and the hypercoagulable state which occurs post-partum.

Clinical features

There is an acute or subacute onset of severe headache, fits, hemiparesis, drowsiness and then a progressive impairment of conscious level due to cerebral oedema, together with an increase in intracranial pressure. Focal signs, such as aphasia or hemianopia, sometimes occur. A low-grade fever is often present, even in patients without a primary infective cause.

Investigation

Skull X-ray may reveal evidence of sinus or middle ear infection. CT scans may show patchy or confluent areas of cerebral cortical oedema, sometimes with haemorrhage. In cases of doubt, cerebral angiography may reveal reduced or absent filling of one of the dural sinuses. Lumbar puncture should not be done in the presence of severe cerebral oedema, as judged from the CT scan. The CSF is under raised pressure and may be normal or, frequently, lightly bloodstained.

Treatment

Fits must be urgently controlled, and raised intracranial pressure is treated with dexamethasone. In patients with an infective cause, appropriate antibiotics should be given. Anticoagulants should not be given because of the danger of exacerbating or causing cerebral haemorrhage. The prognosis is good, with resolution of all symptoms and signs in the majority.

CAVERNOUS SINUS THROMBOSIS

Cavernous sinus thrombosis is usually secondary to infective lesions originating on the face or to sinusitis of the frontal sphenoidal or ethmoidal sinuses. Untreated unilateral thrombosis often spreads to become bilateral within a few days.

Clinical features

The onset of the illness is with fever, then headache, severe malaise, pain in the eye and diplopia, and, eventually, loss of visual acuity in the affected eye. There is sometimes also nausea and vomiting. Examination reveals orbital oedema, sometimes with proptosis, normal or impaired visual acuity, and there may be papilloedema. There is a partial or complete ophthalmoplegia with ptosis. The pupil is not spared. The trigeminal nerve is sometimes involved, leading to sensory impairment on the face and cornea.

Differential diagnosis

Caroticocavernous fistula, either due to rupture of an intracavernous carotid aneurysm or occurring secondary to head injury, may produce a similar clinical picture. However, the degree of proptosis is often greater with a caroticocavernous fistula and the proptosis is pulsatile. There is usually a loud bruit in the region of the eye which may be altered by ipsilateral carotid artery compression.

Investigation and treatment

Venography by injection of contrast into the frontal vein demonstrates non-filling of the thrombosed cavernous sinus.

Treatment is with high-dose intravenous antibiotics and fluids, and sometimes by surgical treatment of associated sinusitis.

TUBERCULOUS MENINGITIS

Tuberculous meningitis (TBM) is now an uncommon condition in the UK but is still a major problem in developing countries. In the past, the peak incidence was in children but, nowadays, a larger proportion of patients with tuberculous meningitis are adults.

Pathology

Tuberculous meningitis is nearly always due to infection with *Mycobacterium tuberculosis* and only rarely with the atypical mycobacteria. Infection reaches the meninges via haematogenous spread during miliary infection. A granulomatous inflammation develops, particularly affecting the basal meninges, where it involves the large arteries and the cranial nerves. The optic chiasm may also be affected, leading to a variety of visual field defects. Reabsorption of CSF may be impaired by granulomatous inflammation, leading to hydrocephalus, and hydrocephalus may also be caused by obstruction of CSF outflow from the fourth ventricle.

Granulomatous inflammation over the cerebral hemispheres may lead to cortical infarction. Fits are common in TBM. Tuberculomas may develop deep within the brain, behaving as tumours. Generalised cerebral oedema with raised intracranial pressure is common.

Tuberculous meningitis frequently leads to spinal arachnoiditis, which may cause root or cord lesions. These are often transient, but severe cord lesions with complete spinal block (as demonstrated at myelography) may develop.

Clinical features

Tuberculous meningitis usually presents subacutely. There is often a prodrome of general malaise, without specific symptoms, of up to six weeks, followed by headache, lethargy and vomiting. Examination may reveal no focal abnormal neurological signs, and even meningism may be mild or absent in the early stages. A low-grade fever is usual, but may be intermittent.

Focal signs include cranial nerve palsies in about a quarter of patients. These may occur as single or multiple palsies, those most commonly affected being the IIIrd, IVth, VIth, IInd, VIIth and VIIIth nerves. Fits, which may be focal or generalised, occur in about a quarter of patients. Raised intracranial pressure, due to generalised cerebral oedema or hydrocephalus, produces papilloedema. Hemiparesis, dysphasia or hemianopia may be caused by cortical infarction, major vessel occlusion at the base of the brain, or the development of a tuberculoma (Fig. 23.46). Many patients are drowsy or stuporose at the time of presentation, but coma during the course of TBM indicates a poor prognosis; only about 50% of patients surviving from this state. Finally, inappropriate ADH secretion may develop.

Investigation

The most important investigation is examination of the CSF. This is safe in patients without signs of raised intracranial pressure or focal signs (excluding cranial nerve palsies). In any patient suspected of having TBM with papilloedema or focal hemisphere signs, a CT scan should be done prior to lumbar puncture to exclude hydrocephalus or tuberculoma. Obtaining CSF for diagnostic purposes in these patients should be done after consultation with a neurosurgeon. Likewise, in patients with signs of a myel-

Fig. 23.46 Large left frontal tuberculoma. Unenhanced (upper) and contrast enhanced (lower) scans show appearances indistinguishable from an acute pyogenic cerebral abscess with mass effect, substantial cerebral oedema and ring enhancement. Although the tuberculoma in this patient was solitary, they are frequently smaller and multiple.

opathy, spinal block and the possibility of exacerbating the cord lesion by lumbar puncture must be considered. Again, close collaboration with a neurosurgeon is necessary.

The CSF in TBM usually contains 50–500 cells/mm³ and only rarely more than 1000/mm³. In the early stages, these are mainly neutrophils; later, lymphocytes predominate. The protein is raised, sometimes to very high levels. The glucose is nearly always low. This is helpful in differentiating aseptic meningitis due to tuberculosis, from viral meningitis. Ziehl-Neelsen staining of the CSF is not infrequently negative, even when tubercle bacilli are later cultured. A lengthy and careful search of a stained centrifuged deposit of CSF is necessary.

Differential diagnosis

Viral meningitis is excluded if the CSF glucose is low; however, malignant meningitis, whether carcinomatous, leukaemic or lymphomatous, may cause a similar picture.

Fungal meningitis may also cause a similar clinical presentation and CSF findings. India ink staining is useful. Meningovascular syphilis and sarcoidosis are two rare causes of aseptic meningitis.

Treatment

It is important in tuberculous meningitis to start treatment as soon as possible. Even with prompt chemotherapy, complications such as hydrocephalus, cerebral infarction, development of tuberculomas, and cranial nerve palsies, are common. Drugs normally given (Table 23.55) are ison-

iazid, rifampicin, pyrazinamide and, sometimes ethambutol.

Streptomycin is not commonly used; if it is used, there is no advantage in giving the drug intrathecally. Penetration of cycloserine, ethionamide and pyrazinamide, is better than that of the other antituberculous drugs, but this is not an important factor when the meninges are inflamed. Second line drugs are used only when sensitivities from culture indicate their use.

Clinical improvement in TBM is slow. Clinical deterioration suggests the possibility of hydrocephalus, and the diagnosis is confirmed by CT scanning. Persistence of fever after three weeks is cause for concern, and the CSF should be re-examined after obtaining a CT scan, if possible. A minimum of 18 months of treatment is necessary and two years is recommended by most authorities.

Anticonvulsants are often needed but should not be given unless fits occur.

Tuberculomas (Fig. 23.46) may arise during the course of treatment even when the organism is sensitive to the drugs being given. They may be solitary or multiple. Most resolve with continued medical treatment, but larger lesions may have to be surgically drained.

The place of corticosteroids in treatment remains controversial. Claims have been made for lessening of the basal and spinal arachnoiditis with prevention of hydrocephalus, cranial nerve palsies, strokes and spinal cord syndromes, but none of these claims has been substantiated by careful clinical trial. Steroids are often given when one of these complications arises, or in very sick patients, but there is as yet no clear indication for such treatment.

Prognosis

The mortality of TBM in the UK is still high (15–30%) and, in developing countries, is much higher. Adverse factors affecting prognosis are coma at presentation, pregnancy and an age of less than 2 years or more than 65 years. Persistent problems in survivors include major cranial nerve palsies causing blindness, squints and deafness; strokes causing hemiparesis, dysphasia, and other focal hemisphere signs; and a paraparesis from spinal arachnoiditis. In a small proportion of patients, hydrocephalus develops as a late complication, sometimes years after successful treatment.

VIRAL INFECTIONS OF THE NERVOUS SYSTEM

Viral infection of the nervous system produces illness by two mechanisms – either direct invasion, or as a postinfectious illness, in which initial infection leads to an immunological reaction which itself causes damage at a short interval after infection. This damage is usually predominantly demyelination, and it is likely that viruses cause some type of sensitisation to CNS myelin. The clinical spectrum of viral diseases comprises meningitis, encephalitis and myelitis, occurring either alone or, quite frequently, in combination. In addition, it has recently

Table 23.55 Treatment of tuberculous meningitis

Drug	Dose	Major side-effects
Isoniazid	300 mg/day	Peripheral polyneuropathy, preventable with pyridoxine 20 mg daily Hepatitis
Rifampicin	10 mg/kg per day, up to maximum of 600 mg/day	Hepatitis
Ethambutol	15 mg/kg per day	Optic neuritis with doses of 25 mg/kg per day or more. Nausea, vomiting
Streptomycin	30–40 mg/kg per day, up to 1 g	Ototoxicity, either vestibular or cochlear. Skin rash. Lower doses necessary with renal impairment
Cycloserine	500 mg–1 g/day. Maintenance not more than 500 mg/day	Convulsions, drowsiness, headache, dysarthria, vertigo, confusion, psychosis. All may occur with large doses
Pyrazinamide	20–35 mg/kg per day and not more than 3 g/day	Hepatic: raised enzymes, jaundice, hepatosplenomegaly. Gout, sideroblastic anaemia, arthralgia, nausea and vomiting, fever, urticaria

been recognised that some progressive fatal encephalitides may be the result of persistent viral infection. These include subacute sclerosing panencephalitis, progressive multifocal leucoencephalopathy and Creutzfeld-Jakob disease.

Viruses

Some viruses are very selective in the regions and cell types within the nervous system which they affect. For example, the polio virus affects predominantly anterior horn cells, while others may produce a wide variety of illnesses; Coxsackie, for example, may cause either meningitis or a diffuse encephalitis.

Viral meningitis is most often caused by Coxsackie, Echo, measles, mumps, Herpes simplex, Herpes zoster, adenoviruses and EB virus. Direct HIV infection must now be added to this list, and is of increasing importance.

The viruses causing encephalitis vary in different parts of the world. In the UK, mumps, Echo, Coxsackie, measles, Herpes simplex, Herpes zoster, EB virus and adenoviruses are the commonest causes, in this order of frequency. HIV is now also recognised to produce encephalitis. In Asia, Japanese B virus is the commonest cause of encephalitis, while in North America, Herpes simplex is the leading pathogen.

Myelitis is caused by Coxsackie, Echo, Herpes zoster, EB virus and, occasionally, polio and rabies viruses. Immediate identification of the virus causing many presumed viral meningitides and encephalitides is often difficult, retrospective diagnosis often resting on the result of antibody titres in paired sera. In post-infectious encephalomyelitis, diagnosis often depends entirely on serological testing, except when the cause is one of the exanthemata. The common causes of post-infectious encephalomyelitis are measles, varicella, vaccinia, mumps, rubella, influenza and, occasionally, rabies vaccine.

Pathology of viral infection

Most viruses reach the nervous system via blood spread from the initial site of infection, often the respiratory or gastrointestinal tracts. Some viruses spread centripetally via the nerves, for example the Herpes viruses, which may lie dormant in sensory ganglia for many years. It is not clear why some viruses remain confined to the meninges and others invade the brain or spinal cord, nor why some viruses show such a predilection for certain sites in the nervous system.

Within the brain and spinal cord, viruses lead to destruction of neurones, followed by phagocytosis, demyelination, vascular inflammatory change with perivascular lymphocytic cuffing, diffuse inflammatory change with a predominantly lymphocytic infiltrate, and a variable amount of oedema. Oedema may cause life-threatening rises in intracranial pressure. These pathological changes occur both in direct viral invasion and in post-infectious encephalomyelitis, but, in the latter, demyelination in association with oedema is the predominant pathological change.

VIRAL MENINGITIS

Clinical features and investigation

In a minority of cases of viral meningitis there is a history suggesting viral infection. The meningitis may be of acute or subacute onset, with headache, fever, neck stiffness, nausea and vomiting, and diagnosis is not usually difficult. It is indistinguishable clinically from bacterial meningitis.

The crucial investigation is examination and subsequent culture of the CSF. The pressure is usually raised, with a pleocytosis up to several $1000/mm^3$; this is usually of lymphocytes but sometimes predominantly polymorphs. The protein is increased but, in contrast to bacterial meningitis, the glucose is only very occasionally low. No organisms are seen on Gram staining. These changes may be seen in other causes of aseptic meningitis, including partly-treated bacterial meningitis.

The blood count may show a lymphocytosis, and antibody titres on acute and convalescent sera may enable a retrospective aetiological diagnosis to be made.

Treatment and prognosis

Treatment is symptomatic in the majority of cases. Herpes simplex or Herpes zoster meningitis is treated with a five-day course of intravenous acyclovir. A history of steroid or other immunosuppressive treatment, or of systemic disease likely to produce an immunocompromised host, should lead to a search for unusual pathogens.

The prognosis of viral meningitis is excellent. However, HIV infection is an exception to this (p. 966) and Herpes simplex meningitis is sometimes recurrent.

VIRAL ENCEPHALITIS

Clinical features

As with meningitis, there is usually no prodromal illness in viral encephalitis. The symptoms and signs are drowsiness, headaches, nausea and vomiting, confusion, fits and, sometimes, focal signs. Occasionally, a predominantly brain stem encephalitis occurs. In severe cases, stupor and coma develop. A low-grade fever is usual. Raised intracranial pressure due to oedema is common. An associated meningitis may cause neck stiffness. The onset can be rapid, with coma developing within 12–24 hours, but the onset usually occurs over 24–72 hours.

In Herpes simplex encephalitis, focal temporal lobe lesions are common, in the setting of a diffuse encephalitis. This may be apparent both clinically with dysphasia, a visual field defect or temporal lobe epilepsy, and on investigation with EEG or CT scan. However, other viruses may cause a similar clinical picture.

The *differential diagnosis* of viral encephalitis includes other infections, particularly cerebral abscess, cerebral malaria (p. 299), metabolic encephalopathies (p. 968), cerebral tumours, and occasionally the presentation may mimic subdural haematoma or stroke.

Investigation

It is wise to do a CT scan before examining the CSF if there is an impaired conscious level, signs of raised intracranial pressure or focal signs. Scanning may demonstrate an abscess. Focal low density in one or both temporal lobes suggests Herpes simplex infection. Often, there is no abnormality on the CT scan, or else diffuse cerebral oedema.

The CSF usually shows a modest rise in the cell count, usually lymphocytes; the protein is raised with a normal glucose, and the pressure is increased.

The EEG in encephalitis usually shows diffuse changes of encephalopathy, sometimes with focal features.

Treatment and prognosis

Treatment is largely supportive. Acyclovir is beneficial in Herpes simplex and Herpes zoster encephalitis, and it is reasonable practice to give a course of intravenous acyclovir to all patients with encephalitis in whom Herpes simplex may be the cause.

Commonly, it is not clinically possible to differentiate direct viral infection from postinfectious encephalomyelitis, unless there is a clear preceding history of an identifiable viral illness, or a preceding vaccination or immunisation.

The position of steroid treatment in postinfectious viral encephalitis is uncertain. A reasonable approach is to reserve steroids for very sick patients with encephalitis, and to give steroid with acyclovir.

The prognosis of known causes of encephalitis is very variable. Rabies encephalitis is always fatal. Mortality rates for other viruses include 40–75% for Herpes simplex, 10–20% for measles, and less than 1% for mumps. There may be permanent deficit after severe encephalitis due to any virus, whether direct viral or postinfectious. Physical deficits such as hemiparesis are less common than intellectual impairment and behavioural disturbances.

POLIOMYELITIS

Poliomyelitis remains a major health problem in developing countries and sporadic cases of polio are still seen in the UK. Following a viraemia, the virus spreads to the meninges and gains access to the CNS, where it shows an extraordinary tropism for anterior horn cells in the spinal cord and brain stem, with inflammation and cell destruction.

Clinical features

Only in 1% of those infected with the virus does a paralytic illness occur. The onset of this is three to four days after the initial febrile illness has resolved. However, the minor illness may be very mild in adults and may pass unnoticed. Predisposing factors to the development of the paralytic form of the illness are a history of recent tonsillectomy, recent inoculation and pregnancy. The site and severity of the paralysis is probably partly determined by physical exertion during the period between the minor illness and the onset of the paralysis (major illness).

The major illness is heralded by fever and neck stiffness, and then paralysis with myalgia develops. In the spinal form there is involvement of spinal anterior horn cells only, and there is often temporary bladder paralysis.

In the bulbar form, there is paralysis of the muscles supplied by the IXth, Xth and XIIth cranial nerves, causing pharyngeal, laryngeal, and lingual paralysis. Vasomotor centres in the brain stem are also involved, causing tachycardia and lability of the blood pressure. In the bulbospinal form, there is a mixture of bulbar and spinal paralysis.

Respiratory paralysis may result either from the spinal form, with paralysis of the diaphragm, intercostal and abdominal muscles, or from bulbar paralysis, which is usually complicated by a pharyngeal paralysis leading to severe dysphagia. Paralysis is generally worse in adults than in children, with less capacity for recovery.

Differential diagnosis

Diagnosis of polio in epidemics is not difficult, but the diagnosis in isolated cases is often not suspected until paralysis develops. Occasionally, other viruses may lead to temporary paralysis, including Coxsackie, Echo and arboviruses. Differential diagnosis from Guillain-Barré syndrome is occasionally a problem, but the CSF in Guillain-Barré shows no increase in cell count, and the presence of sensory symptoms and signs in this syndrome usually leaves no doubt about the diagnosis.

Investigation and treatment

The CSF in poliomyelitis shows normal or slightly increased pressure, a pleocytosis of 10–200 cells/mm³ (initially polymorphs changing to lymphocytes within 24–36 hours), a moderate increase in protein and a normal glucose. Virus may be isolated from a throat swab for a few days only, but is present in the stool for many months.

Treatment may be prophylactic if the minor illness can be recognised (in epidemics), by advising strict rest in order to reduce the risk of severe paralysis. Analgesia is often needed for the severe myalgia, and ventilation for respiratory paralysis. Regular measurement of vital capacity is essential. Pneumonia is a common complication. Many patients are left with severe paralysis and require the full resources of rehabilitation. Patients with severe respiratory paralysis require long-term respiratory support.

UNUSUAL VIRAL INFECTIONS OF THE CNS

Subacute sclerosing panencephalitis

Subacute sclerosing panencephalitis (SSPE) is subacute encephalitis occurring in children, due to persistent infection with measles virus. It is more common when there is a history of infection at an early age, often less than two years. After a latent period of months or, in some cases several years, there is an insidious onset of intellectual decline, behavioural change (particularly apathy), then ataxia, myoclonic jerking and, often, a hemiparesis or tetraparesis. Other features include a retinitis and choroiditis, papilloedema, optic atrophy and cortical blindness. The disease is relentlessly progressive and death usually occurs within two years of onset.

CT scans in SSPE show patchy, low-density lesions in the cerebral hemisphere white matter, and progressive cerebral and cerebellar atrophy.

There is no effective treatment.

Progressive multifocal leucoencephalopathy

Progressive multifocal leucoencephalopathy (PML) is an illness occurring only in immunocompromised patients, particularly those with lymphoma. It is now also being increasingly seen in AIDS. The causative viruses are the JC and SV40 Papovaviruses. Oligodendrocytes are preferentially affected, producing widespread demyelination, spreading from many different foci in the white matter. Patients present with progressive dementia, and focal signs including hemiparesis, hemianopia, dysphasia and ataxia. The disease is progressive and death usually occurs within a few months.

CT scans in PML show multiple low-density lesions, with atrophy in the later stages. The CSF is normal. Treatment with cytosine arabinoside may slow the progress of the disease in some patients, but a fatal outcome is inevitable.

Creutzfeld-Jakob disease

Creutzfeld-Jakob disease (CJD) is a very rare disease which has been shown to be transmissible and which is thought to be due either to a viral infection or infection with a virus sub-particle (prion). There is a family history in about 6% of cases. The pathology is a progressive neuronal loss without inflammation. In man, CJD has been transmitted to children in growth hormone made from pituitary extracts and in corneal grafts. The transmissible agent is apparently resistant to both heat and formalin.

The clinical features of CJD include myoclonus, ataxia, extrapyramidal rigidity, dementia, hemiparesis, aphasia and fits. The onset may be gradual or subacute. In the early stages, the differential diagnosis includes PML or cerebral tumour. CT scans eventually show atrophy but may be surprisingly normal early in the disease. There is no treatment.

SYPHILIS

The major features of syphilis infection are described in Chapter 12. *Treponema pallidum* may invade the CNS weeks or months after the initial infection, but only causes a meningitic illness in about a quarter of these cases. Occasionally, the meningitis is severe, with transient cranial nerve palsies and convulsions; usually, however, it is mild or even asymptomatic.

All the clinical manifestations of late or tertiary syphilis have a chronic meningitis as the underlying pathological process. This process leads to arterial involvement (syphilitic arteritis), affecting meningeal and parenchymal vessels. Tertiary syphilis may present as:

1. chronic meningovascular syphilis
2. parenchymatous involvement as general paralysis of the insane (GPI) or tabes dorsalis. Syphilitic amyotrophy is a rare form of parenchymatous involvement.

Diagnostic tests

Details of the serological tests for syphilis are discussed in Chapter 12. In active neurosyphilis of any type, the CSF is always abnormal, showing a raised cell count with positive antibody tests (VDRL, TPHA, FTA and TPI). The protein content is also usually raised, and there is evidence of local synthesis of IgG, with oligoclonal bands on electrophoresis. Difficulty arises when positive antibody tests are found, without a rise in the cell count, in a patient with a neurological presentation not typical for one of the syndromes of neurosyphilis. Under these circumstances, it is important to give a full course of antibiotic treatment and to re-examine the CSF six months later.

Meningovascular syphilis

In meningovascular syphilis, there is a combination of chronic basal granulomatous meningitis and syphilitic arteritis.

The condition presents within 10–12 years of primary infection, either with a generalised illness, including headache, neck stiffness, convulsions, and confusion or psychosis, usually without fever, or with focal neurological symptoms, often cranial nerve palsies and, sometimes, strokes affecting either the hemispheres or brain stem. Optic atrophy is a common feature. Although meningovascular syphilis is relatively uncommon, it is important to recognise since it usually responds well to treatment in the earlier stages.

Syphilitic gumma

Gummas are large granulomatous lesions arising in the meninges with central necrosis. They usually remain superficial over the hemisphere, and present with fits, hemiparesis, dysphasia and other focal deficit. Gummas occasionally occur in the spinal meninges and cause cord compression.

Parenchymatous syphilis

In all three forms of parenchymatous syphilis – general paralysis of the insane (GPI), tabes dorsalis and syphilitic amyotrophy – the pathology is a meningoencephalomyelitis. The meninges show changes of chronic granulomatous with confusion and delirium. Death may occur from ventricular tachycardia.

Hypomagnesaemia

Hypomagnesaemia usually occurs with severe vomiting or diarrhoea, particularly if fluid replacement is given without adequate magnesium. It is commonly associated with hypocalcaemia. Symptoms of hypomagnesaemia include irritability, confusion, muscle twitching, hallucinations, myoclonus, chorea, coma and fits. Hypermagnesaemia is rare, but may occur in renal failure due to administration of magnesium salts, usually inadvertently in the form of antacids. Magnesium is important in acetylcholine release at the neuromuscular junction, and hypermagnesaemia results in generalised weakness, lethargy, coma and death from respiratory paralysis.

Hypercalcaemia

The neurological symptoms of hypercalcaemia (p. 737) are agitation, confusion, hallucinations and, sometimes, delirium and fits. Papilloedema is occasionally a feature.

Hypocalcaemia

In chronic hypocalcaemia (p. 741), mental blunting is the rule and patients are often thought to be demented or retarded. Other features are fits and raised intracranial pressure. Tetany, which may be symptomatic, can be demonstrated as a positive Chvostek sign. Cataracts and basal ganglia calcification occur in long-standing hypocalcaemia.

Porphyria

Of the two types of porphyria (p. 780), erythropoietic and hepatic, only the latter (acute intermittent porphyria) is associated with neurological consequences. Aminolaevulinic acid (ALA) binds to GABA receptor sites in the central nervous system and the neurological complications of porphyria are thought to be due in part to facilitation by ALA of transmission at GABA receptors.

In acute intermittent porphyria, mental changes are prominent, with agitation, mania, tremor, delirium, hallucination, fits and eventually coma. Strokes and retinal ischaemia may occur, and are thought to be due to cerebral arterial spasm. A polyneuropathy in the limbs may also occur, as may multiple cranial neuropathies, together with brain stem signs, in particular ocular movement abnormalities. These neurological manifestations are usually preceded and accompanied by abdominal symptoms.

NEUROLOGICAL MANIFESTATIONS OF ENDOCRINE DISEASE

Diabetes

Peripheral neuropathy (p. 936) and coma due to hypoglycaemia are common problems. Uncontrolled hyperglycaemia (Ch. 20) also causes coma. Diabetes is a major

predisposing cause of atheromatous vascular disease and therefore of cerebral infarction.

Hyperthyroidism

The general neurological effects of hyperthyroidism (p. 696) include anxiety and tremor. Proximal myopathy is common in untreated thyrotoxicosis (p. 697). Chorea is a rare sign of hyperthyroidism. Dysthyroid eye disease may occur while the hyperthyroid patient is thyrotoxic or euthyroid. In some cases, the symptoms arise only after a euthyroid state has been achieved with treatment; in other patients, the eye disease arises in the absence of any preceding toxicity. In dysthyroid eye disease, there is an enlargement of the external ocular muscles due to a lymphocytic infiltration, with oedema. The eye muscles can become enormously swollen (Fig. 23.47), causing impaired venous drainage from the orbit; this leads to papilloedema and reduced visual acuity. The pathogenesis of these changes remains uncertain (p. 697).

The first symptom of the exophthalmic ophthalmoplegia is diplopia. The changes may be asymmetrical in the early stages. Examination reveals unilateral or bilateral proptosis, an ophthalmoplegia which usually affects all movements with sparing of downward gaze and lid retraction; corneal ulceration may also occur.

Treatment is urgent in patients with reduced visual acuity or papilloedema. Oral steroids usually relieve orbital pressure, with rapid recession of the exophthalmos. Failure to respond to steroids requires surgical decompression. Tarsorrhaphy may be necessary to protect the cornea.

Dysthyroid eye disease usually runs a course of 1–2

Fig. 23.47 Coronal CT scan in a patient with dysthyroid eye disease. There was marked proptosis, bilateral papilloedema, and severe ophthalmoplegia. The scan shows gross enlargement of the extraocular muscles.

years. Surgical measures to correct residual squint should be reserved until this stage.

Hypothyroidism

The neurological manifestations of myxoedema include mental slowing and, sometimes, dementia. Alternatively, behavioural disturbances, psychosis and even mania may result ('myxoedema madness'). A predominantly sensory polyneuropathy is associated with hypothyroidism. Occasionally, patients with myxoedema present with ataxia of gait without other obvious abnormal signs. A proximal myopathy can be a feature.

Apart from the mental slowing, a common neurological complication of hypothyroidism is unilateral or bilateral carpal tunnel syndrome, due to compression of the median nerve by myxoedematous tissue.

Cushing's syndrome

Mental changes in Cushing's syndrome can take the form of a mild euphoria associated with an increase in appetite or, occasionally, psychotic illnesses. A proximal myopathy is inevitable with large doses of steroids taken over a period of months but the tendency to develop this complication is extremely variable.

Hypoadrenalism

In Addison's disease, hypoadrenalism causes hyponatraemia, hyperkalaemia and, often, hypotension; together, these factors cause lethargy and weakness. In severe Addisonian crises, coma develops and fits may occur.

NEUROLOGICAL MANIFESTATIONS OF MALIGNANCY

About 20% of all malignancies are associated with some type of neurological involvement. Metastatic spread may occur to the brain, spinal cord substance, epidural space or vertebral body. Direct invasion of the brachial or lumbosacral plexus is common with breast and pelvic tumours. Occasionally, individual peripheral nerves may be directly infiltrated.

A number of tumours are also capable of producing remote neurological effects without direct invasion of the nervous system – the so-called non-metastatic or paraneoplastic effects of malignancy. Neurological problems may also result directly from treatment, e.g. the peripheral neuropathy due to vincristine. Opportunistic infection of the nervous system is an important problem following immunosuppressive therapy.

Cancer

Metastatic spread of cancer to the brain or spinal cord is particularly common with primaries in breast, lung, bowel, skin, kidney and testes. Direct invasion of the meninges (malignant meningitis) is relatively unusual.

The two commonest non-metastatic effects of cancer are a predominantly sensory polyneuropathy and a cerebellar ataxia. Cancer of the lung is by far the commonest primary associated with these non-metastatic effects. A proximal myopathy has been described, sometimes associated with an elevated CPK. There is an increased incidence of inflammatory polymyositis associated with cancer, but it still remains relatively uncommon. The incidence of underlying cancer in patients presenting with polymyositis (p. 1022) has been greatly overestimated in the past, except in the case of adult onset dermatomyositis. A rapidly progressive encephalomyelitis has been described as a non-metastatic complication of carcinoma, but is very rare. Finally, the Lambert-Eaton myasthenic syndrome (p. 943) is occasionally seen with small cell carcinoma of the lung. This condition, due to a failure of acetylcholine release at the neuromuscular junction, is characterised by a progressive proximal myopathy, sometimes with fatiguability mimicking myasthenia gravis.

Lymphoma

Lymphomas rarely metastasise to cause intracerebral mass lesions, but malignant meningitis is not uncommon. Localised masses of lymphoma tissue present occasionally in the nasopharynx, and invade either upwards to involve the lower cranial nerves, or within the orbit, causing a progressive ophthalmoplegia, proptosis and, eventually, visual loss. The spinal cord may be compressed by epidural collections of lymphomatous tissue.

Non-metastatic neurological complications are more common with lymphoma than with cancer, except perhaps cancer of the lung. A degenerative cerebellar ataxia occurs, together with a variety of different types of polyneuropathy. An encephalitic illness is also described with lymphoma. Opportunistic nervous system infection is particularly likely to occur with this malignancy.

Although not exclusive to lymphomas, the condition of progressive multifocal leucoencephalopathy occurs most frequently with this type of tumour. It is thought to be caused by a papovavirus, which leads to progressive massive areas of demyelination (p. 964).

Leukaemia

By far the most common form of neurological involvement in leukaemia (Ch. 25) is a malignant meningitis; this often occurs at a time of systemic remission. It is thought that small numbers of leukaemic cells which are relatively immune to the effects of systemic chemotherapy cross the blood-brain barrier during periods of systemic relapse. These cells are then able to proliferate later, causing a malignant meningitis. The frequent development of CNS relapse in leukaemia led to the early adoption of prophylactic therapy. This is standard in younger patients to avoid CNS relapse. Malignant meningitis is occasionally complicated by hydrocephalus, due to a reduced capacity for reabsorption of CSF.

As in lymphoma, opportunistic infection is very common

in leukaemia; progressive multifocal leucoencephalopathy is an occasional development.

Myeloma

Spinal cord compression resulting from vertebral collapse is particularly common in myeloma. Surgical decompression is complicated by the special difficulties of spinal stabilisation when several adjacent vertebral bodies are involved. A painful neuropathy may be a non-metastatic complication; it may occur with solitary plasmacytoma or with multiple myeloma and, in contrast to other non-metastatic neuropathies, may show some improvement with tumour treatment. Occasionally, myeloma neuropathy is complicated by the development of amyloid, which is an independent cause of peripheral neuropathy (p. 941).

Large quantities of paraprotein occasionally lead to a hyperviscosity syndrome with the development of multiple cerebral infarcts, a situation not unlike that seen with polycythaemia rubra vera. Finally, severe hypercalcaemia is common with myeloma, and may cause neurological symptoms (p. 969).

Radiation damage to the nervous system

Radiotherapy can cause neurological damage. Treatment of malignant invasion of the brachial or lumbosacral plexuses seems particularly likely to cause damage, with symptoms of progressive, often painful, plexopathy starting 1–5 years after radiotherapy. Radiation to the spinal cord may rarely produce an acute myelopathy, which usually resolves slowly after radiotherapy is stopped. A delayed, slowly progressive, radiation myelopathy with onset 1–5 years after radiotherapy is more common.

In children with acute leukaemia treated prophylactically, the somnolence syndrome, consisting of drowsiness, lethargy, irritability and anorexia is common. It resolves after radiotherapy is stopped. The question of whether radiotherapy produces permanent intellectual damage in children remains controversial. There is some evidence that this may occur in adults.

ALCOHOL AND THE NERVOUS SYSTEM

Alcohol causes a wide range of neurological effects, both acute and chronic.

Acute intoxication and coma

Alcohol is absorbed rapidly from the gut and easily crosses the blood-brain barrier. The cerebral effect of alcohol taken acutely is due to a direct inhibitory effect on membranes, which leads to a reduction in neurone excitability. In non-alcoholics, blood ethanol concentrations of 30–70 mg/100 ml will affect coordination, sensory perception and intel-

lectual functions. Drunkenness is associated with levels of between 50 and 150 mg/100 ml. The effects of acute intoxication are well known. A feeling of well-being and relaxation is associated with loss of inhibition, loss of judgement and an inability to sustain or follow critical argument. Mood changes depend to a large extent on personality and pre-existing mood. There may be excitement, depression or paranoia. Memory for events during the period of intoxication is usually impaired and, with very high levels of alcohol, there may be amnesic periods of several hours or longer. These are sometimes known as alcoholic blackouts, though there is no loss of consciousness. The effects of acute intoxication are associated with dysarthria, ataxia and increased sympathetic activity, producing flushing, pupillary dilatation and tachycardia; the respiratory rate is often increased. With increasing levels of alcohol, disorientation is followed by stupor and then coma, with a reduced respiratory rate. Death may occur due to the direct toxic effects of very large amounts of alcohol; more commonly, vomiting leading to aspiration pneumonia is the cause of death. In certain susceptible people, hypoglycaemia occurs, particularly when alcohol has been taken without food.

In chronic alcoholism, tolerance to ethanol develops, so that at levels well in excess of 100 mg/100 ml there may be no apparent impairment of intellectual or motor function.

Alcoholic coma is rare; disorientation and stupor are more common. Patients should be allowed to rest, and many will sleep. On the day following acute alcohol excess, there is dehydration, sometimes tremulousness, headache, malaise and nausea.

Many patients in coma also abuse other drugs; the combination of alcohol and barbiturate is particularly dangerous. The association of alcoholism and cranial trauma leads to an excess of subdural haematomas in this group.

Delirium tremens

Delirium tremens is an acute psychosis seen in chronic alcoholics during alcohol withdrawal. The effects are probably due to withdrawal of sedation, and release of autonomic activity and neuronal irritability.

There is a change in personality, the patient becoming withdrawn, restless, irritable, anorexic and sleepless; there are often frightening hallucinations, which tend to be visual more than auditory. Disorientation, dysarthria and progressive clouding of consciousness also occur. Fits occur 12–48 hours after alcohol withdrawal and, when present, always precede the period of delirium. Death occasionally occurs from ventricular tachycardia secondary to hypokalaemia.

The mainstay of treatment is sedation, and the drug of choice is chlormethiazole, given either orally or as a continuous intravenous infusion. In severe refractory cases, it may be necessary to use paraldehyde. It is necessary to correct fluid and electrolyte imbalance, ensure adequate nutrition at an early stage, and to give thiamine to prevent the development of a Wernicke-Korsakoff syndrome (see below).

Alcoholic fits

Alcoholic fits, sometimes known as 'rum fits', are a common complication of alcoholism, and they may also be seen in non-alcoholics after a single acute excess of alcohol. Fits occur 12–48 hours after alcohol withdrawal, and nearly always take the form of generalised convulsions. Fits rarely occur during a period of drinking; if they do, it is usually related to a rapidly falling blood alcohol level. The majority of patients with alcohol withdrawal fits have not had previous fits, and the subsequent EEG is normal.

Alcoholic dementia and cerebral degeneration

Chronic alcoholism may cause a slowly progressive dementia associated with generalised cerebral atrophy. There is often associated depression. Dementia in alcoholics may also be due to repeated head injuries, undetected subdural haematoma, insidious hepatic encephalopathy and chronic fits.

In the early stages, some degree of dementia may be reversible if the patient abstains completely from alcohol. Depressed patients should respond to antidepressant drugs. Many patients, however, continue to drink.

In some alcoholics, without any clinical evidence of dementia or other brain damage but with cerebral atrophy on CT scanning, the CT scan appearances improve with abstinence from alcohol. This improvement occurs slowly over a period of 6 months to 3 years. Similar, partly reversible cerebral atrophy has also been observed in anorexia nervosa, kwashiorkor and in patients treated with corticosteroids.

Wernicke-Korsakoff syndrome

In 1881, Karl Wernicke described three patients with confusion, ataxia and ophthalmoplegia with nystagmus. All were dead within two weeks of the onset of the illness. Independently, Sergei Sergeyevich Korsakoff described 20 chronic alcoholics with severe impairment of short-term memory associated with disinhibition, leading to a confabulatory dementia. Most patients also had a peripheral neuropathy, and this led Korsakoff to describe the syndrome as psychosis polyneuritica. It was not until some years later that the close association of the two conditions was recognised, and it is now clinically useful to consider them together as the Wernicke-Korsakoff syndrome.

Aetiology

The syndrome does not only occur in alcoholics. It is due to thiamine deficiency, and may therefore be seen in severe starvation, malnutrition, intravenous feeding without vitamin supplementation, occasionally in hyperemasis gravidarum and in vomiting due to high gastrointestinal obstruction.

Clinical features

The clinical features of the syndrome initially include a triad of ophthalmoplegia, ataxia and confusion. The ophthalmoplegia and ataxia may precede the mental symptoms by several days. In the early stages, the mental changes are dominated by confusion and restlessness, followed by drowsiness, disorientation and then coma. The Korsakoff confabulatory dementia often only becomes evident after treatment. The eye signs consist of nystagmus, VIth and IIIrd nerve palsies, gaze palsies and, occasionally, ptosis.

Hypothermia due to hypothalamic involvement may occur, and sudden death is a feature of the syndrome.

The confabulatory dementia is selective, in that the ability for retention and recall and short-term memory are severely impaired, while other intellectual functions are relatively well preserved. A peripheral neuropathy is present in up to 80% of patients with Wernicke-Korsakoff syndrome.

The pathology of the syndrome includes punctate haemorrhages and non-haemorrhagic areas of necrosis in periventricular sites around the third and fourth ventricles.

Diagnosis and treatment

The diagnosis of Wernicke-Korsakoff syndrome is essentially clinical. A high index of suspicion is needed. There may be associated alcohol withdrawal and acute delirium tremens in the early stages, and making a definite diagnosis of the Wernicke-Korsakoff syndrome can be difficult. Thiamine should be given to all alcoholics who present acutely with problems associated with alcohol withdrawal.

Biochemical abnormalities in Wernicke-Korsakoff syndrome include a raised blood pyruvate level and a reduced red cell transketolase, and these may be of retrospective diagnostic value.

The response to thiamine of the ocular signs in Wernicke-Korsakoff syndrome is often dramatic, occurring within 24–48 hours. The ataxia shows some recovery, and the confusion and restlessness also improve fairly rapidly. In contrast, the Korsakoff confabulatory dementia shows a limited response to treatment.

Despite early recognition and prompt treatment, about 20% of patients die during the first few days.

Hepatic encephalopathy

From a neurological point of view, three types of hepatic encephalopathy (Ch. 17) are recognised:

1. acute coma associated with fulminating hepatic failure
2. reversible hepatic encephalopathy in cirrhotics with a recognisable precipitating cause
3. hepatocerebral degeneration syndrome, which is a consequence of the portosystemic shunting of long-standing liver disease. This is a slowly progressive condition and responds poorly to treatment.

The neurohistopathological abnormalities are minimal in acute fulminant hepatic failure. However, in chronic hepatic encephalopathy, there is neuronal loss, diffuse gliosis and many astrocytes containing enlarged irregular nuclei, with astrocytic proliferation.

Clinical features

Acute fulminant hepatic failure is accompanied by confusion, delirium, stupor and then coma. Eye movements become disconjugate and tone is increased in the limbs with brisk reflexes; eventually, with deepening coma, decerebrate posturing, loss of tendon reflexes, fits and then death occur.

In *reversible chronic hepatic encephalopathy* a hallmark of the condition is a fluctuating level of consciousness with confusion. Euphoria may be present and, characteristically, there is marked intellectual impairment in a patient who is alert and may have no other abnormal neurological signs. Constructional apraxia, which can be measured serially from day to day, is a useful index of improvement or deterioration. With worsening encephalopathy, drowsiness, dysarthria, asterixis, myoclonic jerks, fits, choreoathetosis and extrapyramidal rigidity, together with pyramidal signs, appear. Recovery from a deeply comatose state is unusual, since this reflects severe hepatic dysfunction.

In the *hepato-cerebral degeneration syndrome*, there is a progressive dementia, extrapyramidal rigidity, asterixis and pyramidal signs in the limbs. The neurological deficit may remain stable for many months before deteriorating.

Investigation and treatment

The most helpful neurological investigation in hepatic encephalopathy is the EEG. This shows progressive slowing of activity, loss of the normal alpha rhythm, paroxysmal slow waves, and, in many patients, triphasic waves. The value of the EEG is that the sequence of changes in a particular patient is a reliable index of the severity of the encephalopathy, and that the EEG changes may precede any obvious change in the clinical state.

The treatment of hepatic encephalopathy is that of the hepatic failure (Ch. 17). There are suggestions that large doses of L-dopa or bromocriptine may partially reverse the encephalopathy, associated with an improvement in the EEG.

Cerebellar degeneration

Cerebellar degeneration is a fairly common consequence of chronic alcoholism, and is probably due to a combination of nutritional deficiency and alcohol toxicity. There is marked atrophy of the upper part of the vermis, but the cerebellar hemispheres are relatively spared. This leads to ataxia which is most marked for the trunk, leading to gait ataxia. Nystagmus is uncommon. A fairly acute form of cerebellar syndrome may respond well to abstinence, but recovery from chronic cerebellar degeneration is limited.

Peripheral neuropathy

Signs of a peripheral neuropathy may be present in up to

10% of all chronic alcoholics, in most cases it is mild and asymptomatic. The neuropathy is usually, but not exclusively, seen in malnourished patients. In well-nourished alcoholics, the neuropathy tends to be less painful than that occurring in malnourished patients. In the early stages, the neuropathy is predominantly sensory and, characteristically, there is severe burning pain with paraesthesiae and hyperaesthesia of the feet and lower legs. The hands are usually affected later, and distal wasting and weakness develops. Some patients may be unable to walk because of pain and hyperaesthesia. Treatment is abstinence from alcohol and an adequate diet. Pain responds poorly to analgesics, and symptoms improve slowly over several months. Patients find they can relieve their severe symptoms with alcohol and many therefore return to excessive drinking.

Alcoholic amblyopia

Impairment of vision in one or both eyes due to an optic neuropathy may occasionally occur in chronic alcoholics. At one time it was thought that the combination of heavy smoking and alcohol was responsible, but the condition is also seen in alcoholics who do not smoke. Fundoscopy shows optic atrophy.

The pathology of the condition is a loss of ganglion cells in the retina and necrosis of central parts of the optic nerve and chiasm.

Alcoholic myopathy

Rarely, an acute destructive alcoholic myopathy occurs, and the consequent myoglobinuria can cause acute renal failure.

A chronic, predominantly proximal, alcoholic myopathy has also been described.

Central pontine myelinolysis

Central pontine myelinolysis is a rare condition. It is usually seen in chronic alcoholics, but there is also an association with hyponatraemia, particularly in children, liver disease being the major cause. The pathology is a massive, progressive demyelination affecting the basis pontis and involving pontocerebellar fibres, long tracts and myelinated fibres in the pontine nuclei. The clinical features are confusion and cranial nerve palsies, particularly affecting the IVth, Vth and VIth nerves, with gaze palsies and bulbar signs; there are pyramidal signs in the limbs, occasionally cerebellar signs and, often, disturbances of vasomotor control with hypotension.

The differential diagnosis includes vascular lesions affecting the pons, multiple sclerosis and brain stem encephalitis.

In 75% of cases, death occurs within one month, but occasionally it runs a chronic course over several months, sometimes with a partial recovery. There is no specific treatment.

23

Marchiafava-Bignami disease

The rare Marchiafava-Bignami disease was originally described in heavy Chianti drinkers in Italy, but is now known to occur with other types of alcohol abuse as well. It consists of a massive central demyelination affecting the corpus callosum, with neuronal necrosis and extensive degeneration in the cerebral cortex. It is almost invariably fatal, within weeks or months.

FURTHER READING

Asbury A K, McKhann G M, McDonald W I (eds) 1986 Diseases of the nervous system. Clinical neurobiology. Vols 1 and 2. W B Saunders, Philadelphia, and Heinemann Medical Books, London. *A large two-volume work which deals with the scientific basis of clinical neurology. Highly recommended for the inquisitive student.*

Harrison M J G 1987 Neurological skills. Butterworths, London. *About half of this short book deals with a very practical approach to history-taking and examination; the remainder is concerned with common neurological symptoms and brief descriptions of selected common diseases affecting the nervous system.*

Lindsay K W, Bone I, Callander R 1986 Neurology and neurosurgery illustrated. Churchill Livingstone, Edinburgh. *The richly illustrated text covers all the common neurological and neurosurgical disorders.*

MRC memo 45 1976 Aids to the investigation of peripheral nerve injuries. HMSO, London. *An invaluable slim volume showing the details of the peripheral motor and sensory systems, with photographs demonstrating the correct technique for examining individual muscles and muscle groups.*

Patten J 1978 Neurological differential diagnosis. Harold Stacke Ltd, London and Springer-Verlag, New York. *Another very well-illustrated volume, which deals particularly well with applied anatomy and physiology and the neurological deficits caused by lesions at different sites in the nervous system.*

Weatherall D J, Ledingham J G G, Warrell D A (eds) 1988 Neurology. In: The Oxford Textbook of medicine Vol. 2, 2nd edn. Oxford University Press, Oxford. *A multi-author text containing more detail than is needed for the clinical student, but most sections are very well-written, and references to original papers are provided for each subsection.*

Musculoskeletal and Connective Tissue Disease

Fig. 24.1 Schematic cross-section (A) and X-rays of normal synovial joints (B and C)

The rheumatic diseases encompass a broad range of disorders, from musculoligamentous lesions to systemic connective tissue disease. Many of these share the same symptoms and signs, particularly at the onset, but a single condition may show considerable clinical variation. Rheumatic diseases may cause widespread involvement of other systems; similarly, many multisystem diseases may have joint involvement as part of the disorder.

In the United Kingdom each year, an estimated 20 million people experience some form of rheumatic complaint and eight million seek help from their general practitioner. At least half a million people have rheumatoid arthritis (RA) and around five million are affected by osteoarthritis (OA). There are 500 000 patients with gout and about the same number with ankylosing spondylitis; while low back pain and soft tissue rheumatic disorders together account for over 50% of the rheumatic causes of working days lost annually in the United Kingdom (amounting in total to around 88 million days). These are consequently important causes of morbidity. Only one person in 50 will escape some form of rheumatic complaint in their lifetime. By recognising arthritis early, much can be done to help these patients.

STRUCTURE AND FUNCTION OF JOINTS

Synovial joints have a capsule to which or through which the tendons of muscles are inserted (Fig. 24.1). The capsule is continuous with the periosteum covering the bone. The non-articular surfaces within the joint are covered by synovial tissue. Articular cartilage lies on subchondral bone. Additional 'spacers' may be present in the form of fibrocartilage (e.g. knee menisci) or fat pads covered by synovium. Muscles acting across joints have an important function in maintaining joint stability.

Joint capsule

In most joints, the capsule is composed of bundles of collagenous fibres arranged somewhat irregularly, in contrast to their more regular arrangement in tendons and many ligaments. These bundles tend to spiral, thus making them sensitive to tension in most positions that the joint adopts. Change in tension stimulates proprioceptive nerve endings in the capsule and ligaments. Most ligaments have both mechanical and proprioceptive functions.

Synovial tissue

The synovial membrane is a specialised connective tissue lining the capsule of diarthrodial joints, bursae and tendon sheaths. Its main function is to produce synovial fluid, which has useful biomechanical properties and, in addition, provides nutrition for articular cartilage.

Important differences between joint tissue and other tissues include the lack of epithelial tissue in every part of the joint, the marked vascularity of the synovium and the complete avascularity of articular cartilage. This may explain why it is that in rheumatoid arthritis, a disease with systemic manifestations, the major site of injury is the joint itself.

The normal synovium – glistening, slightly pebbly and with multiple redundant folds in its gross appearance – has only three or four cell layers lining its surface. It is customary to divide the synovial lining cells into:

1. *Type A*, which are macrophage-like and have a primarily phagocytic function
2. *Type B*, which are secretory and similar to fibroblasts, with a large amount of endoplasmic reticulum.

It is likely that intimal synoviocytes belong to a single cell type, which assumes the A or B form according to local environmental conditions.

Neither the structure of the synovium nor the composition of the synovial fluid suggests that there is a major barrier to fluid movement between the synovial capillaries and the synovial cavity. Furthermore, fenestrated capillaries have been described in the superficial part of synovium, and this type of capillary is usually found in tissues where there is a relatively high fluid and plasma protein flux between blood and tissues.

Synovial fluid

The normal joint contains only a small volume of synovial fluid, such that fluid clinically evident always indicates an abnormality. Normal synovial fluid is essentially a dialysate of blood plasma with the addition of hyaluronic acid, which is secreted by synovial lining cells and imparts to the fluid its stickiness and high viscosity. Both the concentration of hyaluronic acid (normally about 3.5 g/l of fluid) and its

molecular weight are reduced in conditions of inflammatory synovitis, particularly rheumatoid arthritis, with a resulting decrease in fluid viscosity. Most of the protein (60–75%) in synovial fluid is albumin; the larger globulin molecules are present in relatively lower concentrations. Plasma proteins of high molecular weight are present in small amounts in normal synovial fluid. When the synovium becomes inflamed, the protein content of the synovial fluid increases and the quantity of large molecular weight proteins is greater than in normal fluid.

The functions of synovial fluid are lubrication (in association with articular cartilage) and nutrition of cartilage cells.

Articular (hyaline) cartilage

Like other connective tissues, hyaline cartilage consists of three components:

1. *Cells*. The cells are chondrocytes, and they synthesise the other components.
2. *The matrix*, which consists of proteoglycans linked to hyaluronate to form large aggregates.
3. *The fibres*, consisting of collagen which binds the cartilage to bone and entraps the proteoglycan aggregates. Because proteoglycans absorb water, they swell to distend the collagen network and give cartilage elastic properties.

Joint sensation

Synovial membrane is relatively insensitive to pain but, in contrast, capsule, ligaments and periosteum have a rich sensory supply and these tissues are probably the main source of pain in arthritis. With advanced joint damage, sensory fibres from bone are also stimulated, due to the release of chemical mediators.

CLINICAL ASSESSMENT

Rheumatoid arthritis (RA) and osteoarthritis (OA) are the commonest causes of joint disease and their differentiation is usually simple. The differentiation of RA from the less common causes of inflammatory arthritis is sometimes more difficult. In arriving at a diagnosis, the information obtained from a detailed history and careful clinical examination must be collated with the radiological and laboratory findings. In addition, it should be remembered that often no single physical sign, laboratory test or radiological appearance is unique for a particular disease.

HISTORY

General

Age, sex and race

Age and sex are of some diagnostic value. Systemic lupus erythematosus (SLE), rheumatoid arthritis and Reiter's syndrome predominately affect the young and middle-aged, while polymyalgia rheumatica and giant cell arteritis tend to affect the elderly. Rheumatoid arthritis and systemic lupus erythematosus are more common in females, whilst ankylosing spondylitis, Reiter's syndrome and polyarteritis nodosa are more common in males. Gout is more common in men, the sex ratio being 20:1 and the mean age of onset 40 years; in women, the onset of gout is postmenopausal.

There is a higher incidence of systemic lupus erythematosus in female American blacks than in black males and Caucasians, and familial Mediterranean fever is common in Sephardic Jews.

Occupation

Repeated minor trauma resulting from occupational factors, unaccustomed exercise, leisure activities or changes in lifestyle may lead to arthropathy or soft tissue inflammation involving tendons, bursae or ligaments. Osteo-arthritis may be causally related to minor trauma, as in the proximal interphalangeal joints in wicket-keepers' hands, or to a specific toxic agent, as in saturnine gout (lead), acrosteolysis (polyvinyl chloride) or avascular necrosis of the femoral head (nitrogen in deep sea divers). In rheumatoid and osteoarthritis, the dominant hand may be preferentially, or more severely, affected. The effect of the disease on occupation may be very serious, for example rheumatoid arthritis may totally disable a manual worker.

Family history

A genetic factor is present in some rheumatic diseases, e.g. ankylosing spondylitis, gout, psoriasis and haemophilia. First-degree relatives of patients with RA have an increased incidence of RA, as well as other autoimmune diseases, such as myxoedema and pernicious anaemia. There is an association between rheumatoid arthritis and histocompatibility antigens DRW4 and DR4. Most patients with ankylosing spondylitis have the histocompatibility antigen B27. There may be familial associations with ulcerative colitis, Crohn's disease and systemic lupus erythematosus.

Social history

A detailed assessment of the patient's functional capacity, both at home and at work, is important. The patient's ability and independence in dressing, washing, bathing, using a lavatory, cooking and feeding should be assessed, and the layout of domestic facilities, stairs and steps considered. Practical details of the patient's occupation, mode of transport to work, and leisure pursuits are also important, as is the involvement of friends, family, community and social services. In addition, the patient's cooperation, motivation and goals must be assessed.

Drug history

The introduction or withdrawal of many drugs may exacerbate existing rheumatic conditions or precipitate them.

Attention must be paid to the dosage and duration of steroid therapy, as this can cause vertebral crush fractures and, less commonly, avascular necrosis of bone. Exacerbation of symptoms is common if steroids are withdrawn too quickly. Details of previous drug therapy, the response to these agents and any adverse effects associated with them should be noted.

Gout and SLE may be precipitated by drugs in susceptible individuals (Table 24.1).

Table 24.1 Drugs precipitating gout and lupus syndrome

Gout	Lupus syndrome
Thiazide diuretics	Hydralazine
Aspirin (low dosage)	Procainamide
Allopurinol/uricosuric agents (initial therapy)	Phenytoin
	Isoniazid
Cytotoxic therapy for malignancy or polycythaemia	Oral contraceptives (may exacerbate pre-existing SLE)
	Penicillamine

Previous medical history

Inquiry should be made about similar illnesses in the past and their response to treatment (e.g. salicylates in rheumatic fever, colchicine in gout), as well as results of investigations, such as blood tests and radiographs performed during these illnesses. Previous aches and pains, rashes, venereal diseases or other recent infections may have a bearing on the present illness. When attacks or exacerbations of symptoms are intermittent, their periodicity should be established. For example, attacks of intermittent hydrarthrosis occur at regular intervals, whereas in palindromic rheumatism (p. 984), attacks occur at irregular intervals.

Prodromal illness

A recent history of streptococcal sore throat is usual in rheumatic fever, and non-specific rashes or upper respiratory tract infection commonly precede viral arthritis. Previous episodes of diarrhoea, iritis or urethritis may indicate Reiter's sydrome or arthropathy complicating inflammatory bowel disease.

Constitutional symptoms

The constitutional symptoms are usually nonspecific. Low-grade fever, fatigability, lethargy and night sweats are common in the connective tissue diseases and inflammatory joint disease, but are absent in osteoarthritis. These symptoms may be present in acute rheumatoid arthritis, as well as in patients with an underlying malignancy. A swinging fever characteristically occurs in Still's disease, and also in connective tissue diseases such as polyarteritis. A persistent low-grade fever may accompany tuberculous arthritis.

History of presenting complaint

It should be clearly established which joints are the most

troublesome and whether the patient is affected by pain, stiffness, impaired function or immobility.

Pain is the chief symptom and major cause of disability in most rheumatic diseases. Its site, nature, duration, aggravating and relieving factors, radiation and relation to any specific incident must be determined. Some causes of pain have characteristic features: the pain of malignancy is constant, persists at night and is usually unrelieved by rest; that due to ankylosing spondylitis may be relieved by exercise; pain from the hip may often radiate to the knee.

Stiffness may be particularly marked in the mornings, or after immobility. The former is typical of RA and is a useful guide to disease activity.

The nature of onset of joint symptoms must be noted: e.g. whether this is acute and abrupt (as in infection or crystal synovitis) or chronic and insidious (as in RA and OA). RA may be of acute onset in the elderly. It should also be determined whether the progression of symptoms is episodic (as in gout) or migratory (as in rheumatic fever); and the number and order in which joints are involved. Many rheumatic diseases have characteristic patterns of joint involvement, for example:

1. *monoarticular* as in infective and crystal arthritis
2. *oligo-* or *pauciarticular* (four joints or less) as in juvenile arthritis
3. *polyarticular* as in RA and SLE.

Problem identification

It is necessary at the beginning to identify the major clinical problems. Once the doctor has established the reason for the consultation, then the site and principal symptoms can be clearly identified. In particular, symptoms arising from the joints should be differentiated from those due to bursitis, tendinitis, myalgia, vascular insufficiency, peripheral neuropathy or radicular or spinal compression. In peripheral arthritis, pain is usually maximal over the joint; in soft tissue rheumatism (including low back pain), it is less easy to localise.

PHYSICAL EXAMINATION

Many rheumatic complaints are part of a multisystem disorder and, even if the history is devoid of extra-articular symptoms, a complete physical examination is necessary. Special attention must be paid to those organs which are most frequently involved in rheumatic conditions, such as the skin and mucus membranes, the eyes, and the gastrointestinal and genitourinary systems.

The patient's posture in bed may indicate 'protection' of affected joints from movement or undue pressure. Pallor, suggesting anaemia, may be related to disease activity or drugs. Mouth ulcers may be a manifestation of disease, for example Behçet's (painful) or Reiter's syndrome (painless). These conditions are often associated with genital ulcers or circinate balanitis and, in Reiter's syndrome, plaque-like lesions on the glans penis. Ulcers in the mouth and throat may also be caused by infection secondary to the

neutropenia of Felty's syndrome or drug-therapy, particularly the use of gold and immunosuppressive agents. Leg ulcers are a feature of Felty's syndrome (p. 990). Dryness of the conjunctiva and mucus membranes, as a result of reduced lacrimal and salivary gland secretions, occurs in the sicca syndrome (p. 990). Splenomegaly and hepatomegaly are found in Still's disease, Felty's syndrome and systemic lupus erythematosus.

Abnormalities of the skin and its appendages may be associated with joint disease (Table 24.2). The eyes are commonly involved in connective tissue disorders, and symptoms may antedate those due to joint disease (Table 24.3).

Table 24.2 Dermatological signs in joint disease

Rash
Localised
   Butterfly rash and light-sensitive rash in SLE
   Psoriatic plaques
Generalised
   Macular rash in Still's disease
   Drug rash
   Erythema marginatum in rheumatic fever

Ulcers
Leg ulcers in Felty's syndrome and rheumatoid vasculitis
Ischaemic ulcers of fingertips in systemic sclerosis

Infarction
Nail fold infarcts in RA, SLE and vasculitis

Nodules
Sited over pressure areas and tendons in RA
Tophi in gout

Nails
Pitting and onycholysis in psoriasis

Hair
Alopecia or loss of frontal hair in SLE

Table 24.3 Ophthalmic complications of joint disease

Disease	Structure(s) affected
Gonococcal arthritis	Conjunctiva
Sicca syndromes (e.g. Sjögren's syndrome)	Lacrimal gland and conjunctiva
Rheumatoid arthritis	Sclera and episclera
Ankylosing spondylitis, Reiter's	Iris, uveal tract
Behçet's syndrome	Iris
Vasculitis in SLE	Retina
Drug treatment of joint disease	Cataract (e.g. due to steroids in children) Retinopathy (e.g. due to chloroquine)

Musculoskeletal system

Clinical assessment of the musculoskeletal system involves inspection, palpation and assessment of function based on the range of joint movement. Most joints and muscle groups are paired and can therefore be compared. Inflamed joints are painful and must be examined gently. Symptoms arise from the structures that surround joints, such as tendons and muscles, as frequently they do from the joints themselves.

Type and distribution of joint involvement. Many rheumatic diseases have characteristic patterns of joint involvement (Table 24.4). However, clinical variants are not uncommon and the pattern may be atypical in the early stages of disease.

Table 24.4   Patterns of polyarticular disease

Peripheral (small joints of hands, feet and wrists)

Symmetrical
  Rheumatoid arthritis

Asymmetrical
  Psoriatic arthritis
  Osteoarthritis
  Gout

Central (sacroiliac joints, spine, lower limb joints)

Ankylosing spondylitis, enteropathic arthritis, Reiter's syndrome etc.

In the hand (Fig. 24.2), RA usually affects the metacarpal phalangeal (MCP) and proximal interphalangeal (PIP) joints, while sparing the distal interphalangeal (DIP) joints. In contrast, primary osteoarthritis involves the PIP and DIP joints as well as the first carpometacarpal joints and tends to spare the MCP joints.

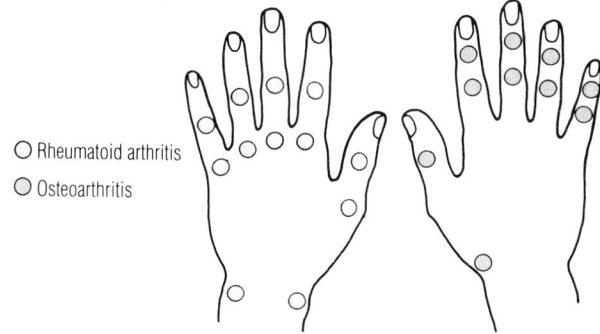

○ Rheumatoid arthritis
○ Osteoarthritis

Fig. 24.2   Joints of the hands involved in rheumatoid arthritis and osteoarthritis. Note how OA affects the carpometacarpal joint of the thumb, and RA affects the wrist.

Joint swelling may be caused by fluid, subcutaneous tissue, synovial or bony overgrowth (for example, Heberden's nodes in osteoarthritis). Fluid may result from effusion within either a joint or bursa. It is often tense but, when present in small amounts, may be squeezed from one side of the joint to the other. Subcutaneous tissue is often warm and tender indicating acute disease, commonly septic arthritis, gout or tendinitis. Pitting oedema of tissues overlying a joint is also a sign of acute inflammation and may occur in early rheumatoid arthritis.

Synovial or *capsular thickening* is confined to the anatomical boundaries of the joint. It feels doughy and can

best be felt by pinching the soft tissues gently and rolling the synovium over the joint.

Deformity is usually a feature of established disease and has many causes (Table 24.5). It may limit both function and movement and should be accurately described.

Table 24.5   Factors contributing to joint deformity

- Synovial hypertrophy
- Bony or cartilaginous overgrowth
- Urate deposits
- Joint subluxation/dislocation
- Bone absorption/misalignment
- Muscle contracture
- Tendon rupture

Tenderness may be localised when caused by meniscal tears, inflamed Heberden's nodes and bony spurs. Synovial inflammation, however, is diffusely tender over the joint surface and its severity is a useful parameter in the assessment of disease activity.

Range of movement. The movement of an individual joint is determined by its anatomical configuration. Active movement may be limited by damage to the articular surfaces, muscle weakness and tendon involvement. Passive movement may produce pain or discomfort, resulting in reflex spasm or voluntary contraction of muscles which reduces the actual range of movement. When the active and passive ranges are not equal, the passive is usually the greater and is a more reliable indicator of the actual range of movement. Reproducible measurements may be made with a goniometer. This is useful for the knee and elbow and for assessing the results of surgery, but is of limited value in reflecting moderate changes in synovial activity in peripheral joints, with the exception of finger joint motion.

The range of movement may be increased in hypermobility syndromes, such as Ehler's-Danlos and Marfan's (p. 93).

During movement, crepitus may be felt. This is a sensation of creaking or grinding which is a sign of damage to the bearing surfaces. Characteristically, this is coarse in osteoarthritis and fine in rheumatoid arthritis. Crepitus may also arise from tendon sheaths.

Instability is usually caused by a combination of ligament laxity, rupture or joint displacement. The knee and ankle joints should be tested with the patient bearing weight, as well as on the examination couch.

Gait should be observed with the patient wearing shoes. The patient's ability to rise from a chair, bend and undress will provide valuable clues in diagnosis.

Muscle power. The muscles should be evaluated for both atrophy and weakness. In patients with joint disease, these usually involve muscles adjacent to the affected joints. Generalised atrophy and weakness reflect primary muscle disorders. Muscle tenderness is uncommon, except in patients with inflammatory muscle disease.

INVESTIGATION

Selected laboratory tests complement the clinical assessment of patients with rheumatic diseases. There are few specific and reliable tests in rheumatology, so results should not unduly influence clinical judgement.

An inflexible interpretation of results may lead to diagnostic error.

Haematological and immunological investigations

Haemoglobin

A moderate anaemia is the commonest systemic manifestation of inflammatory joint disease, and its severity reflects the activity of the disease (Table 24.6). Though the anaemia is often hypochromic and sometimes microcytic, it generally reflects the inability of the reticuloendothelial cells to release sequestered iron, and only occasionally a genuine iron deficiency. In RA, iron deficiency due to gastrointestinal blood loss is the cause of anaemia in less than 2% of patients. The principal practical problem is to differentiate this cause of anaemia from the anaemia of chronic disease.

The avid retention of iron by the reticuloendothelial system and synovial membrane is reflected by a rise in both serum ferritin concentration and normal iron stores within the bone marrow. In this situation, measurement of serum iron and transferrin is often unreliable: the serum iron level may fall, as it is no longer released, and transferrin synthesis by the liver may be depressed, causing a slow fall in the total iron-binding capacity (the anaemia of chronic disease, see p. 1061).

Serum ferritin concentrations fluctuate during episodes of inflammation, the percentage change within the individual, rather than the absolute concentration, reflecting the degree of inflammation. Consequently, serial measurements of serum ferritin concentration can be used to monitor inflammatory activity. An initial high concentration in patients presenting with early RA has been suggested as being an indicator of severe disease.

Macrocytic anaemia is five times more common in rheumatoid patients than in the general population. There is reduced folate release from red blood cells (the body's main store of folate), and an increased uptake by proliferating

Table 24.6 Anaemia in rheumatoid arthritis

Measurement	Typical value in RA	
Haemoglobin	Males	12.5 g/dl
	Females	11.0 g/dl
Mean corpuscular haemoglobin concentration	28–32.0 g/dl (normal 32–36 g/dl)	
Serum iron	Low	
Transferrin	Normal or low	
Ferritin	Lower limit of normal (without iron deficiency); low with iron deficiency	
Serum folate	Low	
Red blood cell folate	Occasionally low	
Bone marrow	Normoblastic; very occasionally megaloblastic	

synovial tissue. Megaloblastic marrow appearances are unusual; rarely, macrocytosis may be caused by haemolysis, systemic lupus erythematosus or an idiosyncratic drug reaction (e.g. aspirin or mefenamic acid).

White cell count

A raised white cell count, of 12 000–20 000/mm³ with a neutrophilia, occurs in infective arthritis, acute gout, juvenile chronic polyarthritis and in rheumatoid patients receiving corticosteroids. Higher counts of 30 000/mm³ or more, with or without eosinophilia, may be a feature of polyarteritis nodosa (PAN). Eosinophilia also occurs in rheumatoid patients as a result of gold sensitivity and, rarely, in association with nodular, vasculitic, erosive and strongly seropositive disease. Rheumatoid arthritis with splenomegaly and neutropenia is referred to as *Felty's syndrome*; anaemia and a slight thrombocytopenia are common accompaniments. Drug sensitivity, e.g. to gold or penicillamine, may cause a pure agranulocytosis, whereas cytotoxic drugs tend to cause a more general depression of the white cell count. Leucopenia is a feature of SLE, although counts of under 2×10^{-9}/l are infrequent, and the response to infection is usually preserved.

Platelets

Thrombocytosis is found in approximately one-third of patients with RA, and has been observed to correlate directly with disease activity.

Thrombocytopenia occurs in SLE and may be sufficiently low to cause purpura. More commonly, thrombocytopenia is related to therapy with antirheumatoid drugs, such as penicillamine, gold and cytotoxic agents. Regular platelet counts are necessary when these agents are used.

Erythrocyte sedimentation rate

The erythrocyte sedimentation rate (ESR) is a non-specific indicator of inflammation and is rarely of diagnostic value. Although normal values rise slowly with age, a practical upper limit for men aged 20 to 50 years is 15 mm/hour (25 for women) and for older men, 20 mm/hour (30 for women). In *rheumatoid arthritis* the ESR is measured to follow the course of disease. However, patients with long-standing disease and hyperglobulinaemia may have persistently raised values – over 50 mm in the first hour. Conversely, patients with progressive erosive disease may have only a mildly elevated ESR. Similarly, in other inflammatory arthritides, normal values do not exclude active disease. In *polymyalgia rheumatica* (PMR) an ESR of over 50 mm in the first hour is usual and alerts the clinician to the possibility of this disease in patients with rheumatic symptoms but minimal joint signs. A normal ESR can occur even in active PMR.

Viscosity

Plasma viscosity has replaced the ESR in some laboratories, as the test can be automated and the results are not influenced by age, sex or haematocrit. Both measurements are mainly dependent upon changes in fibrinogen and other globulins. However, the values of one test cannot be used to predict the value of the other.

Acute-phase proteins

The acute-phase proteins, which include C-reactive proteins (CRP), fibrinogen, haptoglobin, caeruloplasmin and alpha₁-antitrypsin, are raised in 'active' inflammatory joint disease. In RA patients, measurement of both CRP and ESR may be more helpful than either alone in assessing disease activity. As acute-phase proteins are single proteins, measurement is less influenced by anaemia, changes in size and shape of red cells, serum immunoglobulins and cholesterol concentrations. In some centres, all are measured to give a corporate picture of disease activity in RA. All fall sooner than the ESR in response to treatment, and are particularly useful in penicillamine or gold therapy.

Rheumatoid factors

Rheumatoid factors (RF) are autoantibodies directed against antigenic determinants on the Fc fragment of immunoglobulin G (IgG). While rheumatoid factor may also belong to immunoglobulin classes IgG and IgA, the standard tests measure IgM rheumatoid factor. The commonly used tests are those in which indicator cells (sheep red cells) or particles (latex), coated with IgG, are agglutinated (Fig. 24.3). The latex test is more widely used and is cheaper than the more specific but time-consuming sheep cell agglutination test (SCAT). Patients whose sera cause agglutination at levels selected to exclude most non-rheumatoid subjects (usually 1:20 in the latex test or 1:32 in the SCAT), are termed seropositive.

Although RF is found in up to 80% of patients with RA, its presence is by no means diagnostic: it is also present in other connective tissue diseases (Table 24.7), chronic infections, other immunological disorders, and in 4% of the general population. The incidence in the general population increases with age (25% over the age of 75 years) and is higher in relatives of people with positive tests, whether or not they have RA. Recent work suggests that a common factor may be a defect in glycosylation of the IgG molecule, leading to a reduction of terminal galactose and an increase of N-acetyl glucosamine. This has revived interest in the idea that mycobacteria or streptococci (which also express this sugar) may be involved in the aetiology of RA. This defect in galactosylation appears to be related to disease activity, becoming less marked with disease remission.

In early rheumatoid arthritis, RF may be absent. Indeed, it commonly takes up to six months from the onset of symptoms before RF is detectable. The role of IgM rheumatoid factor is not entirely clear, but evidence suggests that it is capable of fixing complement and it may facilitate the phagocytosis of immune complexes by neutrophils in the synovial fluid. High RF titres tend to occur in RA patients with nodules and/or vasculitis and severe erosive disease. It is very unusual for seronegative patients to develop nodules or vasculitis. However, RF in the individual patient is not an accurate guide to disease severity. IgG rheumatoid factor may have a more significant role in causing inflammation within the joint, since it is responsible for a major part of complement fixation and activation. IgG rheumatoid factor, being both antigen and antibody within the same molecule, can self-associate to form immune complexes capable of binding IgM, RF and complement.

Lupus erythematosus cells and antinuclear antibodies

The basis of the tests for lupus erythematosus (LE) cells and antinuclear antibodies is described on page 1016. Table 24.7 shows the incidence of antinuclear antibodies in connective tissue disease. Antinuclear antibodies include antibodies binding to a wide range of structures, including DNA, RNA, histones etc.

Table 24.7 Seropositivity and antinuclear antibodies in connective tissue disease

Disease	IgM rheumatoid factor (%)	Antinuclear antibodies (%)
Rheumatoid arthritis	70	20–30
Sjøgren's syndrome	90	60–80
Systemic lupus erythematosus		90–100
Systemic sclerosis	30	70
Dermatomyositis		30
Polyarteritis nodosa		10–20
Juvenile chronic arthritis	10	30
Other diseases		
Chronic hepatitis		65
Fibrosing alveolitis	15	30
Sarcoidosis		–

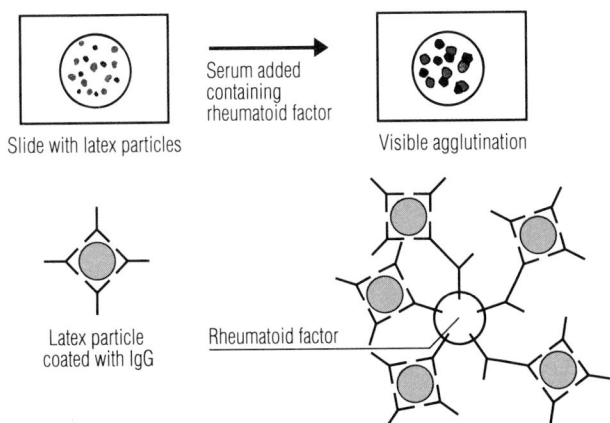

Slide with latex particles   Serum added containing rheumatoid factor   Visible agglutination

Latex particle coated with IgG   Rheumatoid factor

Fig. 24.3 The RA latex test. Latex beads passively coated with human IgG are cross-linked by rheumatoid factor to produce visible flocculation.

Connective Tissue Disease

Serum complement

The complement system consists of a number of plasma proteins which are activated sequentially by certain stimuli. The serum complement level (total haemolytic complement, C3 or C4) is a useful investigation in SLE. Low complement levels in the presence of a high DNA-binding titre are diagnostic of active SLE. Serial measurements of complement are useful in following the clinical course of lupus, as the level drops by about 50% before, and remains low during, an exacerbation. Particularly low levels of complement components, especially C3 and C4, are strongly indicative of active lupus nephritis, as a result of complement being continuously consumed by the immune complexes deposited in the glomeruli.

Individuals with a genetic deficiency of C2 appear to have an excessive incidence of SLE.

Biochemical investigations

Biochemical screening results are frequently abnormal in connective tissue diseases but, apart from a markedly raised serum urate in gout, have little diagnostic value. Tests of renal function are essential, since the kidney is frequently affected by glomerulonephritis in SLE and may be affected by amyloid in RA and ankylosing spondylitis.

Synovial fluid examination

Synovial fluid examination is critically important if septic arthritis is a possibility. The appearance, cell count, Gram stain and culture all contribute to the diagnosis. For other rheumatic conditions, results must be interpreted in the light of biochemical and other laboratory features because considerable overlapping of diagnostic groups can occur.

Skill in joint aspiration is easily acquired and it is a virtually painless procedure; indeed, removal of fluid often relieves pain. It is important not to introduce infection and scrupulous attention to asepsis is therefore required. The need for local anaesthetic depends on the doctor's skills and the joint to be aspirated. Fluid for a differential cell count should be placed in anticoagulant, and is best examined within a few hours; fluid for culture and for crystal examination should be placed in a sterile container without anticoagulant or preservative and, if necessary, can be kept overnight in a refrigerator.

Examination of the synovial fluid identifies urate and calcium pyrophosphate crystals by using the effect of polarising light to demonstrate the differences in crystal lattice structure of the compounds. When viewed under the compensated polarised light microscope, urate crystals show strong negative birefringence and calcium pyrophosphate shows weak positive birefringence. Their differences are summarised in Figure 24.4.

A drop of aspirated synovial fluid is placed on a microscope slide with a cover slip. Any clot in the aspirate should also be examined because the crystals can often be seen within it. The fluid in the needle of an apparently unsuccessful aspiration is often sufficient. Both intracellular

Urate Size: 2-10 μm Birefringence: strongly negative

Pyrophosphate Size: 1-10 μm Birefringence: weakly positive

Fig. 24.4 Identification of joint crystals by polarised light microscopy.

(within polymorphonuclear leucocytes) and extracellular crystals with specific birefringence will be found in positive cases.

Synovial biopsy

Tissue may be obtained by open surgery, arthroscopy or needle biopsy. Needle biopsy has the disadvantage of possible sampling error. Synovial biopsy is indicated in monoarthritis, when the diagnosis is in doubt.

Specific histological features are found in tuberculosis, amyloid and Whipple's disease. Occasionally, urate or pyrophosphate crystals will be identified.

Radiological investigations

X-rays of clinically involved joints are often helpful in the investigation of rheumatic disease, and complement the clinical findings. X-rays of the hands and feet are the most valuable films, for the bones and joints of the hands and wrist are involved in many types of arthritis, the connective tissue diseases and some metabolic disorders. X-rays may demonstrate diagnostic features despite the absence of symptoms and signs in these joints; this is particularly so in RA, juvenile arthritis and psoriatic arthropathy.

Radiological changes in rheumatoid arthritis

The radiological changes seen in rheumatoid arthritis are illustrated in Figure 24.5. They are as follows:

1. *Soft tissue changes.* An increase in soft tissue shadows due to an effusion. It should alert one to look for small bone changes.
2. *Juxta-articular osteoporosis.* Rarefaction of bone due to decreased use caused by pain.
3. *Uniform narrowing of joint spaces.* This implies loss of cartilage.
4. *Erosions at margins of joints* (near origin of synovium and capsule). This is the most definitive radiological change and implies removal of bone substance.

In most patients, it takes at least three months for bone changes to appear (e.g. cartilage thinning or bone erosion). Occasionally, these may not be evident for six months or longer; it is unusual to see them within weeks of clinical onset.

Radiology is helpful in the diagnosis of conditions mimicking rheumatoid arthritis. In the case of gout, tophi may erode bone outside the joint capsule (unusual in rheu-

Fig. 24.5 Rheumatoid arthritis of the wrist and hands: progressive radiological changes over a five year period.

matoid arthritis) and frequently tophi have greater density than surrounding soft tissue. In degenerative arthritis, reactive bone formation is prominent and distal interphalangeal joint involvement is common, whereas osteopenia around joints, and metacarpophalangeal joint damage is rare. It should be remembered that degenerative changes in joints are a feature of ageing and should not be used indiscriminately to explain musculoskeletal symptoms in the elderly.

Chondrocalcinosis (Fig. 24.6) is a radiological finding characteristic of 'pseudogout' or calcium pyrophosphate arthropathy (p. 1014). This disorder is characterised by attacks of acute arthritis and the findings of crystals in the synovial fluid. Calcification involves fibrocartilage, particularly the menisci of the knee, the triangular cartilage of the wrist, the symphysis pubis and the intervertebral discs. Calcification also appears in the hyaline articular cartilage of synovial joints.

DIFFERENTIAL DIAGNOSIS OF POLYARTHRITIS

Chronic rheumatic disorders, with their characteristic deformities and clinical, radiological and serological abnormalities, do not usually pose problems in differential diagnosis. However, an acute polyarthritis may be the presenting feature of many rheumatic diseases (Table 24.8) and, at this early stage, diagnosis may be difficult: there is wide variation in the severity of acute attacks and the number of joints involved, and the pattern may change with recurrent attacks of the same illness.

It must be stressed that an acute polyarticular presentation is not the only mode of onset in the diseases listed in Table 24.8, and the list itself is by no means exhaustive.

A practical approach to differentiate diagnosis is to separate rheumatoid arthritis from the rest. Evidence must be sought for features supporting a diagnosis of rheumatoid arthritis, or for features suggesting an alternative diagnosis.

General points that may help in the differential diagnosis of polyarthritis are given in Table 24.9.

Certain types of arthritis tend to be commoner in particular sexes and age groups (Table 24.10). Determining

A

Triangular ligament

Deposition

Meniscus

Articular cartilage

B

Fig. 24.6 Chondrocalcinosis. A. Common radiological sites for pyrophosphate deposition (knee, symphysis pubis and wrist). B. Chondrocalcinosis in the knee joint. Calcification is present in the menisci and the joint shows degenerative changes.

24

Table 24.8 Diseases that may present as acute polyarthritis

- Rheumatoid arthritis and palindromic rheumatism
- Adult and childhood Still's disease (juvenile chronic arthritis)
- Rheumatic fever
- Systemic lupus erythematosus
- Infections – viral (rubella), rarely pyogenic and tuberculous
- Reiter's disease
- Seronegative arthritides, e.g. psoriatic arthritis
- Gonococcal arthritis
- Gout and pyrophosphate arthropathy
- Serum sickness
- Acute sarcoidosis with erythema nodosum
- Familial Mediterranean fever
- Henoch-Schönlein purpura
- Type II hyperlipoproteinaemia
- Leukaemia

Table 24.9 Clinical clues in the differential diagnosis of polyarthritis

- Family history – of gout and familial Mediterranean fever
- Similar episodes in the past, and response to treatment, e.g. salicylates in rheumatic fever and colchicine in gout
- Genitourinary symptoms suggest Reiter's syndrome; in homosexual males, suspect gonococcal arthritis
- Symptoms of inflammatory bowel disease suggest enteropathic arthritis
- Immunosuppressive therapy, e.g. corticosteroids may predispose to septic arthritis
- A history of photosensitivity, Raynaud's phenomenon or recurrent abortions suggest SLE

Table 24.10 Types of arthritis according to age and sex

Age/sex	Type of arthritis
Child	Juvenile arthritis, viral infection, rheumatic fever
Adolescent	Traumatic synovitis, ankylosing spondylitis, infectious mononucleosis
Adult	Reiter's syndrome, rheumatoid arthritis
Elderly	Degenerative joint disease, pyrophosphate arthropathy (pseudogout)
Female	Rheumatoid arthritis, systemic lupus erythematosus
Male	Gout, Reiter's syndrome

Table 24.11 The balance between joint and systemic symptoms* in acute polyarthritis

Conditions in which joint disease predominates
Acute onset RA
Rheumatic fever
Reiter's syndrome
Gonococcal arthritis
Gout and pseudogout (pyrophosphate arthritis)

Conditions in which systemic disease predominates
SLE
Still's disease – adult and juvenile systemic type
Acute sarcoidosis with erythema nodosum
Polyarteritis nodosa

*Systemic features include fever, rash, lymphadenopathy and hepatosplenomegaly

the balance of joint and systemic symptoms may also be helpful in diagnosis (Table 24.11).

The combination of symptoms in well-recognised clinical syndromes can help in the diagnosis, for example, Reiter's syndrome presents as a classic triad of acute polyarthritis, urethritis and conjunctivitis. The major clinical features of rheumatic fever are carditis, chorea, arthritis, subcutaneous nodules and erythema marginatum.

Patterns of arthritis and progression

In addition to the anatomical distribution (Table 24.4) of joint involvement, the temporal pattern and progression of polyarthritis is helpful in arriving at a probable diagnosis.

Temporal patterns

Migratory pattern. Joints that were initially inflamed remit, while other joints simultaneously become acutely inflamed. Although occasionally seen in rheumatoid arthritis and systemic lupus erythematosus, this pattern is more common in acute rheumatic fever, post-viral arthritis, gonococcal arthritis and meningococcal septicaemia.

Additive pattern. Here, features tend to accumulate during the disease while the original features persist. This pattern is non-specific and is seen in rheumatoid arthritis, SLE and post-rubella arthritis.

Palindromic or intermittent pattern. This describes those conditions associated with recurrent attacks of synovitis which remit completely without sequelae. Short episodes (two to three days) are seen in rheumatoid arthritis and gout, and may occur in sarcoidosis and familial Mediterranean fever (FMF). Longer episodes (seven to ten days) occur in the peripheral synovitis of spondylitis, the arthropathy of inflammatory bowel disease, Behçet's syndrome and also in FMF.

Concerning progression, polyarthritis may be transient, e.g. in viral infections; recurrent, as in palindromic rheumatism; or it may develop into a chronic disorder, e.g. in rheumatoid arthritis.

Palindromic rheumatism is a descriptive term for acute episodes of joint pain, swelling, redness, tenderness and stiffness recurring at irregular intervals, developing spontaneously and lasting a few hours. Up to one-third of cases subsequently develop rheumatoid arthritis.

RHEUMATOID ARTHRITIS

Epidemiology

Rheumatoid arthritis is a generalised or systemic chronic inflammatory condition of unknown aetiology whose distinctive features include a persistent and symmetrical peripheral inflammatory arthritis. Rheumatoid arthritis remains the major disease against which other forms of arthritis are compared, because it is the most common (2–3% of the population) and the most disabling of the inflammatory arthritides. There is a female preponderance of three to one and 70% of cases begin between the ages of 25 and 59, although it can begin at any age (Fig. 24.7). The contraceptive pill may protect against development of the disease. The onset appears more common in winter.

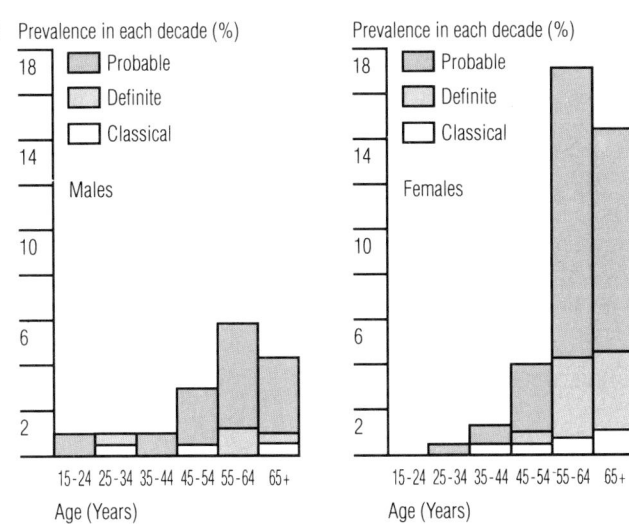

Fig. 24.7 Epidemiology of rheumatoid arthritis. A. Estimates of prevalence of rheumatoid arthritis (probable and definite) in different countries derived from surveys conducted at similar times. **B.** Prevalences of rheumatoid arthritis in the UK 1954–62 using American Rheumatism Association criteria. (After Lawrence JS, 1977).

Aetiology

The aetiology of rheumatoid arthritis remains unknown. Of interest is its relatively recent development as a major disease (the first description only appeared in the middle of the 19th century), the high risk conferred by HLA D4, and its high prevalence in women.

From experimental models in animals, two main hypotheses have been proposed which may not be mutually exclusive.

1. *Infection.* This hypothesis proposes that RA is caused by infectious agents such as bacteria, mycoplasma or viruses.
2. *Autoimmune.* It may be that the disease is the expression of disordered immunity leading to an autoimmune attack on the body's own constituents. The current suggestions are autoimmunity to type II collagen or to IgG.

In addition, it is clear that the development of chronic arthritis in animals is dependent in part at least on genetic factors.

A major difficulty in attributing an aetiological role to any agent isolated from synovial tissues is to exclude secondary contaminants. Although mycoplasma and diphtheroids have been demonstrated in synovium, as have antibodies to peptidoglycans (a constituent of bacterial cell walls), it seems unlikely that these are causative agents. Attempts to demonstrate viruses in tissues have generally been unsuccessful. Recent interest in the Epstein-Barr virus has been stimulated by the finding of an antibody in rheumatoid sera which cross-reacts with a nuclear antigen extracted from Epstein-Barr virus infected lymphocytes.

Genetic factors

Genetic studies of the distribution of RA in families and in mono- and dizygotic twins show that there is a small but definite contribution of genetic factors to the disease. In twin studies, there is around 48% concordance of the disease in identical twins and around 10% in non-identical twins. This familial aggregation is most marked in severe, erosive forms of RA. Recent studies have shown an association between HLA-D4, HLA-DR4, and seropositive disease. In 70% of cases, patients with RA are positive to these antigens and an individual with one of these antigens is 6–12 times more likely to develop the disease. Genetic factors probably interact with unknown environmental agents in causing the disease.

Pathology

In the rheumatoid synovial membrane there is a marked increase of macrophage-like cells (type A cells, see p. 976) and the synovium becomes oedematous, thickened and vascular, with surface deposition of fibrin. The synovium is also infiltrated by lymphocytes, predominately of the T cell population and, in particular, of the helper class. Lymphoid follicles can form and plasma cells are present.

Connective Tissue Disease

Active inflammation of the synovium is also associated with inflammatory changes in the synovial fluid, which contains large numbers of granulocytes (these are not present in the synovium).

The inflamed synovium produces a chronic inflammatory *pannus* which grows from the joint margins to cover the articular cartilage and leads to cartilage and bone destruction. This bone damage usually first appears as a marginal erosion at the site of synovial proliferation, where bone is unprotected by hyaline cartilage. Subsequent bone destruction leads to subluxation and deformity.

Pathological effects of RA are also found in the lymph nodes (which may show reactive hyperplasia), blood vessels (which may show vasculitis) and in nodules. Only the nodules are pathognomonic of RA. They are seen at sites of pressure, such as the extensor surface of the forearm. Palisaded tissue macrophages (histiocytes) surround a central area of hyaline necrosis. Around the histiocytes are scattered lymphocytes and the occasional plasma cell.

Pathogenesis

The major events in the pathogenesis of rheumatoid arthritis are shown in Figure 24.8. The inflamed synovial membrane produces large quantities of immunoglobulin, mainly as rheumatoid factors. The cellular basis for production of rheumatoid factors is well-established, although the factors which initiate this process are unknown. Rheumatoid factors, like other immunoglobulins, are products of plasma cells.

Lymphokines. The inflamed synovium also contains activated T lymphocytes; these produce lymphokines which can be found in synovial fluid. Lymphokines have a number of properties; they can activate additional T lymphocytes, act as helper factors for B cell proliferation,

stimulate fibroblasts to produce collagen and stimulate macrophages. Activated macrophages produce prostaglandins and other inflammatory mediators and enzymes, in particular collagenase, interleukin 1 (IL-1) and tumour necrosis factor (TNF), which may play a part in destruction of bone and cartilage.

Interleukin 1 and TNF have potent effects on the synovial fibroblast and chondrocyte functions, that may involve stimulation of prostaglandin and collagenase production as well as modulation of the synthesis of proteoglycans, collagen and fibronectin. In organ culture, both IL-1 and TNF cause cartilage cells to resorb matrix. In addition, macrophage-derived IL-1 can act on osteoblasts to generate osteoclast activation. It also induces the acute-phase response and fever and may potentiate chronic inflammation by induction of lymphocyte growth factors such as interleukin 2 and its receptor.

Rheumatoid factors. Immunological abnormalities in the serum of patients include hypergammaglobulinaemia and the presence of rheumatoid factors. IgG rheumatoid factor, in particular, readily undergoes self-association through its binding affinity for its own Fc determinants, forming immune complexes. These complexes have been detected in the synovial membrane, synovial fluid, serum and surrounding blood vessels; they are phagocytosed by neutrophils, monocytes and macrophages, with the release of a number of inflammatory mediators and enzymes. In addition, immune complexes containing rheumatoid factor can activate the complement cascade, which generates inflammatory and chemotactic factors with further accumulation of inflammatory cells. High titres of rheumatoid factors, both IgG and IgM, correlate closely with the presence of severe erosive joint disease, nodules, vasculitis and extra-articular complications of RA.

Inflammatory mediators. Local release of inflammatory mediators leads to increasing exudation of high molecular weight proteins such as fibrinogen. This results in local fibrin deposition, with activation of the fibrinolytic system and release of further inflammatory and destructive enzymes. Local fibrin deposition may be a further immunological stimulus to the cellular phase of the inflammatory response.

Enzymes. Local destruction of bone and cartilage is brought about by local enzyme release. These include neutral proteinases such as collagenase, elastase and cathepsins secreted by the macrophages, and lysosomal enzymes secreted by the leucocytes.

Clinical features

Disease onset

Rheumatoid arthritis is a variable disease that takes many different forms, so that few cases are exactly alike. In most cases, RA begins insidiously or subacutely, and this pattern may be associated with a worse prognosis. In 10–20% of patients, the onset is very sudden and may be associated with systemic symptoms, including fever. Many patients describe prodromal symptoms such as aches and pains in

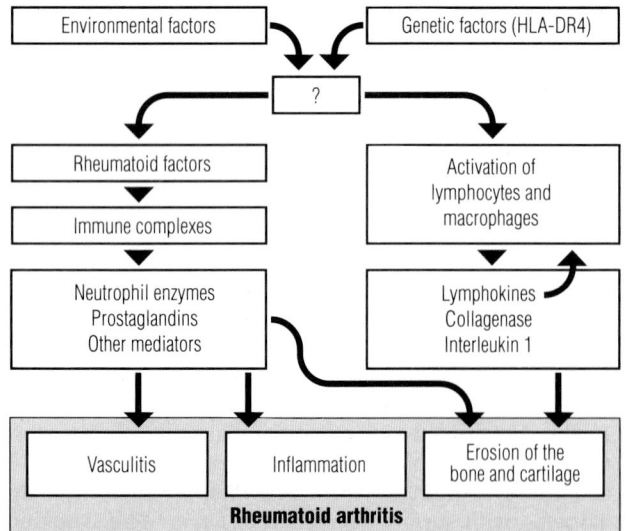

Fig. 24.8 A schematic representation of the major events thought to be involved in the immunopathogenesis of rheumatoid arthritis.

Fig. 24.9 Rheumatoid arthritis in the hands, illustrating ulnar deviation, metacarpal phalangeal swelling and swan-neck deformity.

a variety of joints. Carpal tunnel syndrome or episodic arthritis (palindromic rheumatism) may antedate acute symptoms by months or years. Many patients date the onset of their symptoms to episodes of infection, physical or mental stress and trauma; whether these are relevant or coincidental is not known.

Articular features

The characteristic pattern of joint involvement at onset – occurring in 65% of cases – is symmetrical and peripheral, involving the wrists, metacarpophalangeal and proximal interphalangeal joints of the hands and the corresponding joints of the feet. Large joints are involved in 30% of cases, and both large and small joints in 5%. In a few patients, involvement of a single joint may occur, the disease remaining localised to that joint and then spreading slowly. Joint pain and swelling, and stiffness on waking in the morning and after periods of rest, are the main symptoms. Stiffness may be related to fluid retention in the peri-articular tissues; it is the hallmark of inflammatory activity and also a valuable semi-quantitative measure of the activity of the inflammatory process.

In the early stages of RA, the inflammatory changes may not be localised to the joints. Tender swelling of the entire hands or forearms, or swollen feet and ankles may be the earliest findings. As joint destruction progresses, the anatomical changes themselves produce increasing functional disability. The distinctive features of RA are the symmetry, the prominent signs of inflammation and, to a lesser degree, the location. The most commonly affected joints (in order of decreasing frequency) seem to be proximal interphalangeal, metacarpophalangeal, metatarsophalangeal, wrists, knees and ankles. Any joint can be affected. Persistent inflammation leads to destruction of cartilage and bone, stretching and rupture of tendons and, eventually, to subluxation and dislocation of the joints themselves; this results in the characteristic rheumatoid deformities of the peripheral joints (Fig. 24.9).

Hands and wrists

The typical patient shows fusiform inflammatory swellings, often with a dusky cyanosis over the inflamed joints. Later, there may be marked synovial hypertrophy on the dorsum of the wrist with involvement of the extensor tendon sheath, which may cause rupture of the tendons. In the palmar aspect of the wrist, synovial hypertrophy may lead to the carpal tunnel syndrome. The ulnar head may be prominent and extremely tender. Early synovial swelling of the wrist is highly characteristic and is a valuable sign in distinguishing inflammatory from degenerative disease. Wasting of the dorsal interosseous muscles is often marked, and rheumatoid arthritis is the commonest cause of wasting of the small muscles of the hand.

Synovial infiltration of flexor tendon sheaths often causes a trigger finger. Palmar erythema is common. Other mild vasomotor disturbances are frequent in rheumatoid arthritis. Typical Raynaud's phenomenon may occur, but if it is severe in the presence of only mild arthritis, then one should consider the diagnosis of scleroderma.

Deformity of the hands takes the form of ulnar deviation of the fingers, the button-hole or boutonniere deformity and the swan-neck deformity (Fig. 24.9). Involvement of the distal interphalangeal joint is rare. Anterior subluxation of the wrist may occur.

Knee joint

Involvement of the knee joint accounts for a great deal of disability. Synovial hypertrophy and effusion are often marked, and the bursae in the popliteal fossa may be swollen and may communicate with the joint cavity. These enlarged bursae are called Baker's cysts and may sometimes rupture. Quadriceps wasting is often marked, even in the early stages of the disease. Flexion contractures may develop, and these are especially important because of the disability that they produce. Both the cruciate and lateral ligaments may be destroyed, resulting in gross joint instability and valgus or varus deformity.

Rupture of the joint or a Baker's cyst, as a consequence of the high intra-articular pressure developed during exercise, causes acute pain in the knee radiating into the calf, which becomes swollen and tender on pressure. This may lead to a misdiagnosis of deep vein thrombosis, but an arthrogram will demonstrate the lesion.

Cervical spine

The upper cervical discs are frequently involved in rheumatoid arthritis, in contrast to lower cervical involvement in osteoarthritis (p. 1003). The cervical vertebrae may become subluxed and this may cause serious neurological involvement.

The atlantoaxial articulations and their associated ligaments are frequently involved. This is detected by taking lateral radiographs in both flexion and extension, where separation between the odontoid process and the first cervical vertebra exceeds the normal 2–3 mm. Patients with this involvement often complain of pain radiating along the distribution of the first and second cervical nerves. Pain commences in the cervical spine and radiates upwards over the occiput and vertex to the forehead. Symptomatic relief may be found with a well-fitting cervical collar.

Atlantoaxial dislocation may cause vertebrobasilar insufficiency or may produce neurological signs by direct pressure on the cord. However, neurological sequelae are less common than might be expected. The abnormality is present in 25% of patients requiring joint reconstructive surgery, and it is important that anaesthetists are aware of the potential dangers of neck manipulation.

Involvement of other joints

Pain in the forefoot is commonly due to downward metatarsal head subluxation. The patient complains of a feeling of 'walking on pebbles', and the metatarsal heads are readily palpable on the sole of the foot. The most common deformities are subluxation of the metatarsophalangeal joints with the toes displaced upwards, together with fixed flexion deformities of the interphalangeal joints.

The hip joint is less commonly involved than the knee or metatarsophalangeal joints, but when it occurs, it causes serious disability. The femoral head may penetrate the acetabulum (protrusio acetabuli) and the femoral head may collapse. This is often referred to as *aseptic necrosis* and is more common in corticosteroid-treated patients.

Extra-articular manifestations

Although articular symptoms and signs often dominate the clinical picture, rheumatoid arthritis is a systemic disease; some 75% of patients have two or more extra-articular features at some stage (Summary 1). It is important to look for them because signs of systemic involvement occur in patients with more active disease, and warrant a more aggressive therapeutic approach. Systemic features also increase the likelihood that there will be premature death from rheumatoid arthritis.

Active rheumatoid arthritis is associated with a number

Summary 1 Extra-articular manifestations of rheumatoid arthritis	
Common	*Uncommon*
● Fever, weight loss, malaise	● Hearing impairment
● Anaemia	● Myositis
● Osteoporosis	● Episcleritis
● Lymphadenopathy	● Systemic vasculitis
● Infection	● Pericarditis
● Depression	● Pulmonary fibrosis
● Muscle wasting	● Pulmonary nodules
● Peripheral oedema	● Splenomegaly
● Nodules	● Amyloidosis
● Tendinitis and bursitis	
● Scleritis	
● Keratoconjunctivitis sicca	
● Carpal tunnel syndrome	
● Nail fold vasculitis	
● Peripheral neuropathy	
● Pleural effusion	

---

of systemic features including low-grade fever, anorexia, weight loss and malaise. Being underweight early in the disease indicates a more severe disease process. Weight loss is often accompanied by malaise and generalised muscle wasting; the latter may be so marked as to suggest a neuropathy and is particularly found around active joints. Wasting of the intrinsic muscles of the hand is a common and characteristic finding. A low-grade fever is common and may rarely precede the arthropathy.

Anaemia

Anaemia is the commonest extra-articular manifestation of rheumatoid arthritis and is present in about two-thirds of patients with active disease. Usually, it resembles the anaemia of chronic disease (p. 1061), and the severity varies with the activity of the rheumatoid arthritis. However, iron deficiency anaemia and macrocytic anaemia also occur (p. 1034).

Osteoporosis

Spontaneous fractures occurring in the long bones, neck of the femur and the pelvis are well-recognised in patients with rheumatoid arthritis (whether or not they are receiving corticosteroid therapy). It is important to recognise these fractures, as it is tempting to accept an increase of pain in the region of a diseased hip joint as being due to an exacerbation of arthritis.

Osteoporosis occurs early in active rheumatoid arthritis, and rarefaction of the bones in the neighbourhood of an affected joint is one of the first radiological signs of the disease. Osteoporosis of the spine, and even of the whole skeleton, occurs, due in part to immobility and disuse, and in some cases as a result of corticosteroid therapy.

Lymph node enlargement

Generalised lymphadenopathy is a common feature of Still's disease, but is rare in adult arthritis. Some patients, particularly those with seropositive rheumatoid arthritis, develop marked enlargement of nodes proximal to the inflamed joint. Biopsy shows large germinal centres and, occasionally, hyperplasia is so marked as to resemble giant follicular lymphoma.

Infection

An increased frequency of infection in patients with rheumatoid arthritis was noted even before steroids were introduced, and there has probably been a further increase in infection since the introduction of steroids and immunosuppressive agents. It has been estimated that deaths from infections occur at eight to ten times the rate for the normal population. It appears that the patient with severe chronic seropositive rheumatoid arthritis, or the neutropenic patient with Felty's syndrome, is particularly susceptible to infection.

Periarticular manifestations

Subcutaneous rheumatoid nodules

Rheumatoid nodules occur in approximately 25% of patients at some time in the course of their disease. These nodules are pathognomonic of the disease, are found in patients with high titres of rheumatoid factor and indicate severe, potentially more destructive, disease. The nodules are a few centimetres in diameter and are not tender upon palpation. Normally, they are subcutaneous, but can be intracutaneous or attached to periosteum. They vary in size and number with the activity of the disease. They are found along the extensor surfaces of the forearms, but also occur over pressure areas or may be related to tendons. The nodules can ulcerate and can be painful over the ischial tuberosities and on the feet. Excision is rarely helpful since they reform.

Tendons and bursae

Rheumatoid synovitis can extend to the synovial sheaths of tendons and bursae, particularly in the hands, where pressure from the granulation tissue may contribute to extensor tendon rupture. In addition, nodules can form in the tendons and can impact in the flexor tendon sheaths of the fingers to produce triggering. Local steroid injection will often relieve this condition.

When the ulnar styloids become unduly prominent, because of erosions and/or dorsal subluxation at the inferior radio-ulnar joint, there may be progressive rupture of the extensor tendons, starting from the ulnar side.

Some bursae become inflamed in almost all cases of rheumatoid arthritis and, since there are more than 150 bursae, there are numerous ways bursitis can present. The following are common:

1. *Olecranon bursitis* is a common problem; rarely it becomes infected.
2. *Prepatella bursitis* (housemaid's knee); this is uncommon in rheumatoid arthritis.
3. *Subacromial bursitis*, which is a common cause of shoulder pain.
4. *Trochanteric bursitis*, this may cause pain down the antero-lateral aspect of the thigh.

Myositis

Muscle wasting is very common in rheumatoid arthritis, mainly due to disuse associated with painful joints. It is possible that the disease affects muscle cell metabolism. In addition, ischaemic atrophy can result from vasculitis and, very rarely, true polymyositis can occur. In the latter, the patient develops marked weakness associated with typical muscle histology, electromyogram changes and elevated serum enzymes, as in idiopathic polymyositis (p. 1022).

Corticosteroid therapy causes proximal myopathy. The severity correlates with dosage, and significant myopathy is uncommon in patients taking less than 10 mg prednisolone, or its equivalent, daily. Chloroquine can also cause a myopathy associated with characteristic vacuolation of muscle fibres. Rarely, penicillamine therapy may lead to polymyositis.

Skeletal muscle biopsies from patients with severe rheumatoid arthritis often contain small lymphocytic nodules. These are non-specific, normally do not produce symptoms and have been described in a variety of connective tissue disorders.

Oedema

Recurrent oedema of the lower limbs is commonly found in association with rheumatoid arthritis. In some cases it develops around an acutely inflamed ankle joint. In many instances there is no clearly defined cause.

Organ involvement

Heart

Cardiac involvement takes the form of pericarditis and effusion, rheumatoid granulomata, myocarditis and coronary arteritis.

In patients with rheumatoid arthritis, clinical evidence of pericarditis is not common, but at post-mortem it is found to be present in about 40%. Clinical evidence of pericarditis is found in 10% of patients admitted to hospital and, using echocardiography, subclinical pericardial effusions can be detected in one-third. Effusions are usually small and posterior. The pericardial fluid is an exudate characterised by very low levels of glucose and complement. Gammaglobulin and lactate dehydrogenase levels are increased.

Rheumatoid granulomata can occur in any layer of the heart or in the valves. They are found in 1–3% of post-mortem studies. The valve lesions are usually mild and of no haemodynamic significance. The valves are thickened, with distorted, shrunken cusps; occasionally, nodules can be seen on them, although usually these are only revealed on histological examination.

Non-specific interstitial myocarditis and endocarditis occasionally occur, presumably secondary to vasculitis; they can be associated with patchy valvular fibrosis. Coronary arteritis is rare, and is usually part of a generalised vasculitis. Diagnosis is made at post-mortem and there is rarely a history of ischaemic symptoms during life.

Lungs

Pulmonary lesions complicating rheumatoid arthritis have been described with increasing frequency in recent years. The main syndromes are shown in Table 24.12.

Pleural effusion. Typically, pleural effusion is unilateral and occurs in seropositive males over 45 years of age. It may precede the arthritis and, unlike most other extra-articular lesions, can occur early in the disease. The effusion can be chronic and be associated with considerable pleural thickening.

Rheumatoid nodules. These are usually symptomless and solitary, and are found, by chance, on a routine chest X-ray. Like pleural effusions and pericarditis, with which they can be associated, they are commoner in males with seropositive nodular disease. Rarely, they can precede the arthritis, but even at that stage the patient is usually seropositive. The nodules are often subpleural and may be multiple and recurrent. The histology resembles subcutaneous nodules. They may disappear, may remain unchanged for years, or rarely, cavitate, become infected or even rupture. Biopsy is sometimes necessary to exclude tuberculosis, fungal infection, or malignancy.

Fibrosing alveolitis. This condition may occur in isolation (Ch. 14, p. 517) or be associated with a variety of disorders, including rheumatoid arthritis. Fibrous tissue proliferates round small bronchioles and in the alveolar walls, impairing gas exchange. There is also a chronic inflammatory infiltration of the interstitial spaces.

Obliterative bronchiolitis. Recently, an association has been suggested between this condition and rheumatoid disease. The illness is characterised by a rapid onset of breathlessness, progressing over a few months to complete incapacity or death. Lung function tests show gross reduction in vital capacity, with severe hyperinflation. The chest radiograph is virtually normal. Obliterative bronchiolitis has been reported following inhalation of chemical fumes in adults but is otherwise only rarely diagnosed.

Table 24.12 Pulmonary complications of rheumatoid arthritis

- Infection
- Pleural effusion
- Rheumatoid nodules or granulomata
- Fibrosing alveolitis
- Rheumatoid pneumoconiosis (Caplan's syndrome)
- Pulmonary hypertension
- Empyema
- Obliterative bronchiolitis

The condition may also be associated with penicillamine therapy.

Nervous system

Both the peripheral and the central nervous system can be involved in rheumatoid arthritis. CNS involvement may occur due to cervical cord and vertebral artery compression (p. 928); while peripheral neuropathy may be:

1. due to entrapment
2. symmetrical – either sensory or sensory and motor
3. due to mononeuritis multiplex.

Entrapment neuropathies develop where the nerve is enclosed by a tight soft tissue band, or where a nerve passes over a bony area close to the skin. The usual presentation is an insidious onset of pain and paraesthesiae in the distribution of a peripheral nerve; weakness is sometimes the main problem. The median nerve at the wrist, the ulnar nerve at the elbow, the tibial nerve at the ankle and the lateral popliteal nerve at the head of the fibula are the most common sites.

Sensory, or *mixed motor and sensory peripheral neuropathies* present with a glove and stocking distribution. The cause is probably a vasculitis of the vasa nervorum. A sensory neuropathy is most common and is benign; a mixed neuropathy occurs with systemic vasculitis.

Mononeuritis multiplex is caused by vascular lesions in several different peripheral nerve trunks. The sites of involvement are similar to the entrapment neuropathies.

The neurological consequences of cervical subluxation are unpredictable, but survival tables suggest that they do not, in themselves, significantly shorten life expectancy in rheumatoid disease.

Splenomegaly

Splenomegaly occurs in about 5% of patients with rheumatoid arthritis, but only 1% develop leucopenia as well. Felty's syndrome is the association of rheumatoid arthritis, lymphadenopathy, splenomegaly, anaemia, thrombocytopenia and neutropenia. Patients have severe rheumatoid arthritis, usually with high titres of rheumatoid factor, LE cells and antinuclear antibody. Leg ulcers are also common.

Skin

Skin complications are common. The elderly rheumatoid patient has thin fragile skin often made worse by corticosteroid therapy. Ulceration frequently occurs, particularly on the legs where it may be due to trauma (often minimal), stasis and poor venous return due to inactivity, Felty's syndrome or vasculitis.

Rheumatoid nodules can also ulcerate, particularly over pressure points such as the elbow and sacrum.

Sjøgren's syndrome

Sjøgren's syndrome is the association of keratoconjunctivitis sicca and/or xerostomia with rheumatoid arthritis or another connective tissue disorder. The lacrimal glands are infiltrated by chronic inflammatory cells, producing acinary atrophy and fibrosis, and a reduction of tear and saliva secretion. The same pathological process may affect other exocrine glands, such as bronchial, pancreatic and vaginal glands. Patients may have a high incidence of adverse drug reactions, particularly to antibiotics and gold therapy, and have an increased risk of developing lymphomas.

Gastrointestinal tract

Most of the gastrointestinal symptoms in rheumatoid arthritis are related to drug therapy. However, vasculitis can cause ischaemic colitis and infarction, and amyloidosis can result in malabsorption. Apart from amyloidosis, no histological abnormality is found on jejunal biopsy, although malabsorption can be demonstrated in up to one-quarter of patients with active arthritis.

Gastrointestinal ulceration and haemorrhage frequently occur from the ingestion of aspirin and other non-steroidal anti-inflammatory drugs. The development of gastric mucosal damage with these drugs is multifactorial. The impairment of mucosal prostaglandin production may be one important factor in affecting the vascular and/or sensory functions in the gastric mucosa. This leads to mucosal ischaemia, stimulation of acid and pepsin production, mast cell degranulation, and increased membrane permeability. Increased permeability and haemorrhage may occur from the small intestine as well.

Kidney

Although infections are common in patients with rheumatoid arthritis, the urinary tract is seldom affected. However, structural changes are commonly found in the kidney at autopsy. These changes usually consist of non-specific interstitial nephritis, with or without papillary necrosis. It is difficult to assess the role of drug therapy in these changes. It is currently thought that phenacetin (no longer available in the UK) and its metabolites produce direct oxidative damage to the renal papillary cells and that phenacetin abuse can cause papillary necrosis. Salicylates and NSAIDs potentiate this damage, by inhibiting the synthesis of renal prostaglandins and reducing medullary blood flow. They also inhibit glucose-6-phosphate dehydrogenase, an enzyme which may be important in defence against oxidative damage. There is no evidence that the replacement of phenacetin by paracetamol in analgesic mixtures reduces the incidence of analgesic nephropathy, but paracetamol alone is probably not nephrotoxic. NSAIDs can cause an acute or chronic tubulo-interstitial nephropathy. All patients receiving drug treatment for rheumatoid arthritis should have their renal function intermittently assessed. D-penicillamine can cause proteinuria and nephrotic syndrome due to the development of an immune-complex nephritis. Gold salts can produce similar changes. With gold, proteinuria may present at any time or with any dose, and a clear association has been described between the presence of the B cell auto-antigens HLA-

DR3 and/or HLA-B8 and the development of proteinuria.

Drug-induced proteinuria may persist or initially increase after stopping therapy, before decreasing gradually and resolving completely in more than 80% of cases by two years. In those with persistent proteinuria, moderate impairment of renal function may occur, but this has not been shown to progress to chronic renal failure. Proteinuria in rheumatoid arthritis may also be caused by amyloidosis.

Amyloidosis

Rheumatoid arthritis is the commonest cause of amyloidosis in the Western world. It is found in 20–60% of cases at post-mortem, but is rarely evident during life, when it is usually manifested by proteinuria. Renal amyloidosis is rarely associated with hypertension. Involvement of the gastrointestinal tract can result in malabsorption or intractable bloody diarrhoea. The liver, spleen, or kidney can be infiltrated but are seldom greatly enlarged.

Arteritis

Approximately 25% of patients with RA have been found to have vasculitis at post-mortem examination. Arteritis may conveniently be considered in three categories:

1. *Obliterative endarteritis* of small end-arteries, such as the anterior ciliary arteries and those in the nail folds, obstruction of which produces minute ischaemic areas. These changes are not usually significant in the nail-bed, but are of great significance in the eye (see below).
2. *Necrotising arteritis* of large arteries, e.g. mesenteric or major limb vessels, leads to peripheral gangrene, mesenteric occlusion, or cerebrovascular accident.
3. *Subacute inflammatory arteritis* of small and medium-sized arteries, such as those of the vasa nervorum and muscle. The larger the vessel affected, the more severe is the histological abnormality. Thus, the nail-fold lesions result from intimal hyperplasia, but when the medium-sized arteries are involved, there is a much more active process with fragmentation of the elastic lamina and cellular infiltration. These destructive changes, which may lead to gross necrosis of the arterial wall, can be indistinguishable from polyarteritis nodosa; unlike the latter, however, they tend to spare the kidneys and only rarely lead to hypertension. In peripheral nerves, a mononeuritis multiplex can result.

The eye

Rheumatoid arthritis and other rheumatic diseases frequently involve the eye. Keratoconjunctivitis sicca, scleritis, and uveitis are the commonest manifestations. In RA, 11% of patients have keratoconjunctivitis sicca, and 0.5% develop scleritis with a marked predilection for severe cases with a bad prognosis. Uveitis is a complication of juvenile chronic arthritis.

A large number of drugs used for the treatment of the

rheumatic diseases can themselves cause eye lesions. Drugs that can cause ocular damage include chloroquine, mepacrine, allopurinol, indomethacin and ibuprofen. These complications should always be remembered, as their onset may be insidious and the consequences far-reaching.

In summary, although rheumatoid arthritis is chiefly a disease of joints, there are often major systemic manifestations. Indeed, these features may impose a prognosis far more serious than that of the patient's joint disability. Extra-articular features, particularly vasculitis, are more commonly observed in patients with subcutaneous nodules and high titres of rheumatoid factor. It has been found that mortality is higher when two or more extra-articular lesions are present, providing these features signify continuing activity of rheumatoid disease and are not merely secondary to corticosteroid treatment or burnt-out articular disease. The presence of such extra-articular features indicates that aggressive therapy should be started at an early stage. In the vast majority of patients, complete or adequate control of the disease can be achieved.

Principles of management

The progressive destructive inflammatory process in rheumatoid arthritis may cause not only crippling deformity, but systemic illness and changes outside the joints that may prove fatal. In its early stages, before joint destruction and deformity have occurred, it can be a reversible disease.

It is important to remember that drug treatment is just one component in the total management of arthritic patients (Summary 2). Management must also include advice about rest and exercises, splintage, the provision of appliances designed to reduce dependence upon others, and advice about employment.

It is essential to set guidelines, but these should be constantly reviewed. The general principle of drug therapy is to use the least number of agents in the lowest effective dosage. Drug regimes must be tailored to the needs of the individual patients; indications for a particular drug will vary throughout the course of the disease.

Rheumatoid arthritis is often badly treated; patients are kept on anti-inflammatory drugs alone for long periods, in the face of obvious deterioration, or corticosteroids are given early with considerable immediate effect but at the cost of complications later on. There is an understandable tendency to gradually increase the dose of drugs to alleviate

the patient's symptoms. This is dangerous, however, and often unnecessary.

The inflammatory process can usually be suppressed, with symptomatic improvement, better function, less stiffness and considerable pain relief, but the disease cannot be cured. Hence, adequate patient education is required from the outset, stressing the importance of controlling the disease, to help give the patient realistic expectations.

The aims of treatment are to reduce inflammation, maintain function and prevent deformities. The need to tailor the dose of any drug to suit each patient cannot be over-emphasised. Aspirin has the advantage over other drugs in this regard, in that plasma salicylate levels can be readily measured. Sometimes, because only partial suppression of the disease is possible, the development of joint deformity may occur, and early local treatment is required. Adequate suppression of chronic inflammation allows secondary manifestations, such as anaemia, to revert to normal.

Physiotherapy and occupational therapy

The physiotherapist can help in relieving musculoskeletal symptoms of pain and stiffness, improve joint movement and muscle power and re-educate function of the joints. Heat, ice, wax baths and other local external applications may relieve symptoms and aid relaxation. Patients are also instructed to exercise at home to maintain joint movement and muscle power in order to prevent deformities. Hydrotherapy has an important role, allowing muscles to relax and joints to move freely in a warm environment. It is particularly useful for painful hips and backs.

Splints may be used to rest joints, to prevent deformity or to aid power and functions of a limb. Splints are useful in active disease as rest is an important part of treatment, but daily exercises to maintain joint motion and muscle bulk are necessary. In chronic disease, wrist splints may aid power when finger movement is impaired by pain and deformity, or inflammation at the wrist; and back splints for the knee may prevent flexion contractures. Orthoses are more permanent appliances used to prevent instability and movement, and require fitting to each patient. They include spinal supports and braces, and T-straps to control ankle instability.

A variety of simple aids and appliances may transform the lives of disabled patients, as joint deformity may prevent normal function. Occupational therapists assess the difficulty encountered in daily tasks and advise about aids to daily living such as toilet seat raises, long-handled combs and handles for taps. These and similar appliances can often allow independent living. A home visit is often helpful.

Drug therapy

The increasing number of drugs available for the treatment of rheumatic disease requires a detailed knowledge of drug metabolism, drug interaction and drug dosage. The drugs used can be classified into seven groups (Table 24.13). Alteration in disease activity in response to a drug treat-

---

Summary 2 Principles of management of rheumatoid arthritis	
Medication	Splinting
Anti-inflammatory	Graduated exercise
Simple analgesia	
Immunosuppressive	Explanation and reassurance
Gold, penicillamine	Other physical treatment
Intra-articular radioactivity	Physiotherapy
	Home appliances

Table 24.13 Drugs used in rheumatoid arthritis

Type of drug	Example
Simple analgesics	Paracetamol
Analgesics with minor anti-inflammatory properties	Propionic acid derivatives
Analgesics with major anti-inflammatory properties	Indomethacin Aspirin
Pure anti-inflammatory drugs	Corticosteroids
Compounds with more specific action in rheumatoid arthritis	Gold Penicillamine
Anti-inflammatory immunosuppressives	Azathioprine
Intra-articular radioactive colloids	

ment can be assessed by a number of subjective and objective parameters (Table 24.14). This is particularly important in drug trials, because changes tend to be subtle rather than dramatic. Pain, however, remains the parameter which correlates best with the overall assessment of a change in disease activity.

Table 24.14 Assessment of disease activity

- Assessment of pain
- Measurement of joint tenderness
- Measurement of grip strength
- Measurement of joint size
- Assessment of joint stiffness
- Functional evaluation
- Aspirin or paracetamol consumption
- Patient's drug preference
- Radioactive technetium bone scans
- Laboratory correlates (ESR, acute phase proteins)

Simple and opioid analgesics

Simple analgesics such as paracetamol and weak opioid analgesics such as dihydrocodeine, dextropropoxyphene, and pentazocine have no anti-inflammatory activity and should not normally be used alone in an inflammatory arthropathy. They can be useful in alleviating the pain in degenerative joint disease and occasionally to supplement an anti-inflammatory agent in rheumatoid arthritis.

Non-steroidal anti-inflammatory drugs

The class of non-steroidal anti-inflammatory drugs (NSAIDs) encompasses both aspirin and its derivative, indomethacin, and the more recently introduced propionic acid derivatives. These drugs must be given in full dosage to achieve a continuing anti-inflammatory effect, lower dosage merely producing analgesia.

There is little to choose between the non-steroidal anti-inflammatory analgesics in terms of pain relief, nor is it likely that using them in combination will provide any more relief than using them singly. Because of the increasing

evidence of pharmacokinetic interaction between these drugs, pain should, whenever possible, be controlled with a single drug.

Aspirin (acetylsalicylic acid)

Aspirin has analgesic and anti-inflammatory properties, but it requires blood levels of 250–300 mg/l for adequate anti-inflammatory effect; this requires a daily dose of 3–6 g. As the therapeutic level is near toxic levels, salicylism (tinnitus, deafness, nausea and vomiting) may occur. An adequate trial of several weeks at therapeutic dosage should be tried before the drug is rejected. Often, patients have tried a variety of drugs at low dosage, when the full dose of any one would have been effective. However, nearly one-third of patients find full doses unacceptable because of dyspepsia, although this can often be relieved by using other salicylate formulations such as enteric coated aspirin.

Gastric bleeding is a frequent complication of aspirin therapy, and 70–80% of patients will lose 2–10 ml of blood per day. Ten per cent will lose less than 2 ml of blood per day and 10% will lose much more and are liable to develop iron-deficiency anaemia and acute gastrointestinal haemorrhage. There appears to be no relationship between dyspepsia and blood loss. Taking aspirin with food diminishes the dyspepsia but does not affect blood loss, whereas taking the drug with antacids causes a reduction in both dyspepsia and blood loss but may also prevent aspirin absorption. There are a variety of different drug formulations, designed to try to minimise side-effects.

The content of standard aspirin BP tablets is 300 mg. These are seldom used, however, because they consistently cause gastric mucosal injury. Soluble aspirin is better tolerated, as are enteric-coated preparations. Aspirin has been combined with other substances, such as aluminium oxide and glycine; these have the advantage of containing 500 mg and 600 mg of aspirin respectively, which reduces the number of tablets required. The paracetamol ester of aspirin, benorylate, causes less gastrointestinal bleeding. It is given as a suspension, and can be added to drinks such as tea or coffee. Because of its long duration of action, it only has to be given twice a day.

Indomethacin

Indomethacin is a potent anti-inflammatory agent. It is an indolylacetic acid and can be considered as equal in efficacy to aspirin. In certain experimental systems, indomethacin is found to be a potent inhibitor of the enzyme prostaglandin synthetase.

This drug has been found to be particularly useful in reducing morning stiffness when given at a dosage of 50–100 mg at night. The daily dose is up to 150 mg and the main restrictions on the drug are its side-effects, which occur in 10–20% of patients. The two common problems are gastric irritation and ulceration (even when given as a suppository) and cerebral symptoms. These include headaches, muzziness and dizziness and seem to be dose-related. Other infrequent side-effects include leucopenia, thrombocytopenia, skin rashes, oedema and hypertension.

Other non-steroidal drugs

The common adverse effects of aspirin and indomethacin have led to the production of a wide range of drugs, many of which are derivatives of propionic acid. The major advantage of these compounds is a reduction in adverse effects rather than an improvement in efficacy. They also have advantages over aspirin in the smaller number of tablets required and often, using drugs such as benorylate and naproxen, less frequent administration is needed. When NSAIDs have been compared in controlled studies, no significant differences have been found in terms of pain relief or the patient's assessment of efficacy. If a patient finds one drug ineffective or it causes adverse effects, an alternative member of the group is worth a trial. Some of the drugs in current use are:

1. *Ibuprofen.* The drug is well tolerated, and doses above 1200 mg are often required.
2. *Naproxen.* Although at first claimed to have no gastrointestinal complications, reports of gastrointestinal haemorrhage have occurred.
3. *Ketoprofen.* Trials suggest that this drug appears to be effective and well tolerated.

All anti-inflammatory drugs can cause gastrointestinal bleeding, partly by a local action on the stomach and partly by a systemic effect, since when given by suppositories they can still cause bleeding.

More specific anti-rheumatic drugs

If an adequate trial of treatment with a combination of physical therapy and anti-inflammatory drugs fails to reduce inflammation, then treatment with gold salts, chloroquine, sulphasalazine or penicillamine should be considered. The aim is to initiate disease-suppressing treatment before irreversible joint destruction has occurred. Of the three, gold salts are particularly popular and effective, although their adverse effects have led to periods when their use has fallen into disfavour. None of these drugs has a short-term effect in relieving symptoms; however, they suppress the underlying disease process in a proportion of patients when given over a period of months. They have considerable potential toxicity and major side-effects include renal and haematological toxicity.

Sulphasalazine

Sulphasalazine, an acid azo compound of sulphapyridine and 5-aminosalicylic acid, is an effective antirheumatoid agent. Its mode of action is unknown, but sulphapyridine appears to be the active moiety. It is as well tolerated as gold or penicillamine over 2–5 year periods, and has fewer serious adverse effects; its principal problem is the symptom complex of nausea, dyspepsia and depression encountered early in treatment.

Gold salts

Gold salts have been used in the treatment of rheumatoid

arthritis for over 50 years. In the UK, the gold preparation sodium aurothiomalate has been used for longer than any other. It is given by weekly intramuscular injections of 50 mg, after a 10 mg test dose, either until a total dose of 1 g has been given or disease remission has occurred. It does not produce a disease-suppressing effect before two to three months of treatment. After remission, gold is continued indefinitely with a monthly maintenance regime. About one in three patients develop toxic adverse effects, which include rashes, stomatitis, thrombocytopenia, leucopenia and, occasionally, bone marrow aplasia, glomerulonephritis and pneumonitis. Regular monitoring of platelet and white cell counts, and of urine for proteinuria, is essential in patients receiving therapy.

Auranofin is an orally active gold preparation; it has a lower incidence of adverse effects compared to intramuscular gold. The most common reaction is diarrhoea or loose stools.

D-penicillamine

D-penicillamine is a sulphur-containing amino acid related to cysteine. It was first used in the treatment of rheumatoid arthritis in 1970 and has similar indications and incidence of adverse effects to those of gold therapy. Loss of taste is an early adverse effect, but this usually disappears if the drug is continued. Myasthenia gravis and a drug-induced lupus syndrome rarely occur as complications.

Chloroquine and hydroxychloroquine

The antimalarial drugs chloroquine and hydroxychloroquine also have antirheumatic properties. The main factor limiting their use is ophthalmic complications; progressive accumulation of the drug in the retina can lead to blindness. The risk of retinal toxicity is minimised if the daily drug dosage is kept at or below 250 mg of chloroquine phosphate or 400 mg of hydroxychloroquine.

Corticosteroids

Corticosteroids are undoubtedly the most powerful agents in suppressing the inflammation of arthritis, but there is little evidence that they affect the ultimate course of rheumatoid disease, including joint destruction. Because of their many adverse effects, e.g. osteoporosis, adrenal suppression and susceptibility to infections, it is important that they should be given only after NSAIDs have had an adequate trial. Although it is clear that most patients with early rheumatoid arthritis are as well-controlled symptomatically and objectively on aspirin, steroids are useful in the presence of systemic disease, e.g. vasculitis, and are valuable in a patient severely incapacitated by acute disease when there is an urgent need for symptomatic relief. Incapacitating morning stiffness is also relieved, and the elderly rheumatoid may be kept independent on a small dose of prednisolone. Corticosteroids are also used in intractable iritis, common in juvenile arthritics or in Reiter's syndrome. There are no categorical rules as to its use, but it should be remembered that most patients who begin steroid treatment remain on it more or less permanently, although repeated attempts should be made to wean patients from the drug.

Intra-articular therapy

Corticosteroids can also be given as an intra-articular injection, usually after the aspiration of fluid; 12.5–50 mg of hydrocortisone acetate is commonly used, depending on the size of the joint. Its local effect in preventing recurrent effusion and pain may be dramatic. Repeated injections may result in joint destruction resembling a neuropathic joint, and for this reason it is often recommended that weight-bearing should be reduced immediately after an injection. Stringent aseptic precautions are required to minimise the risk of septic arthritis. Although most peripheral joints can be so treated, this therapy should only be considered when one or possibly two joints are actively inflamed, while others are under good control from general treatment. The major contraindication to intrasynovial steroid administration is the presence of infection; this procedure should, therefore, never be performed without a definite diagnosis and previous synovial fluid examination. An injection of corticosteroid can relieve the symptoms of carpal tunnel compression and localised areas of tenosynovitis, although injections directly into a tendon can lead to rupture.

Immunosuppressive drugs

The use of immunosuppressive drugs in the treatment of rheumatoid arthritis has attracted much interest, but they are mainly reserved for the treatment of severe rheumatoid arthritis and its complications and for use in patients who have not responded to gold and pencillamine. Azathioprine and cyclophosphamide are the drugs most commonly used. Methotrexate is widely used in N. America and its use is becoming more frequent in the UK; it is commonly given once a week. A drug-induced pneumonitis is an occasional severe complication. The problem of long-term treatment and hepatotoxicity still requires resolution.

The general principle governing the use of available drugs is to use the least number of drugs in the lowest *effective* dose, to suppress the inflammatory response. The drug regime must be tailored to the needs of the individual patient. The flow chart shown in Figure 24.10 (for clarity rather incomplete), can only give guidelines, because the indications for a particular drug vary thoughout the course of the disease, which is often unpredictable.

Patient support

Rheumatoid arthritis is not a disease the patient should contend with alone. Not only is a comprehensive programme of management required, but also considerable understanding by patients of their own part in it. Patients

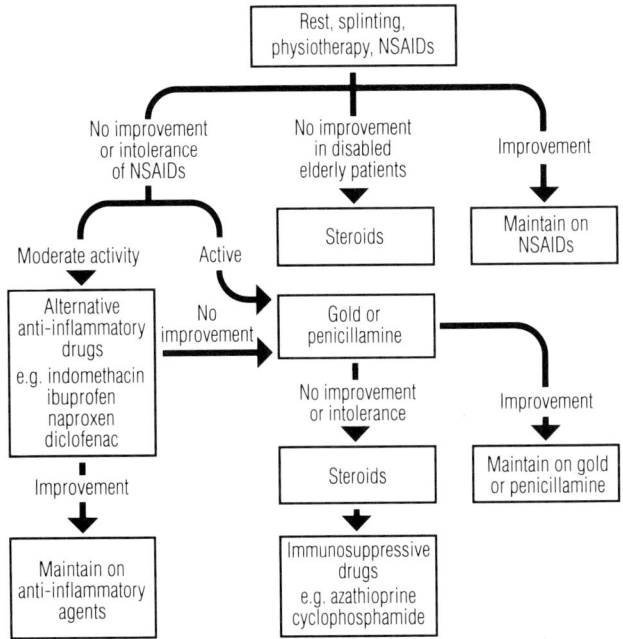

Fig. 24.10 A flow chart of the treatment regimes for rheumatoid arthritis.

with any chronic disease must know something of their disability, how to control it, how to live with and adapt to it. In the UK, explanatory handbooks for patients can be obtained without charge from the Arthritis and Rheumatism Council, 41 Eagle Street, London, WC1R 4AR.

Surgery

Combined clinics with physician and orthopaedic surgeon are now common in most rheumatology centres, surgical treatment being an important stage in a patient's continuing therapy and management. This team approach allows surgery to be carried out at the optimum time, rather than only when patients become seriously disabled from joint damage and wasted muscles.

Surgery has two main objectives, depending on the stage of the disease: prophylactic, designed to prevent joint damage and deformity; and reconstructive, aimed at restoration of function and stability and the correction of deformity. The severity and extent of tissue destruction determines the choice of operation. Certain procedures are appropriate in certain disease stages (Table 24.15).

Table 24.15 Indications for surgery in rheumatoid arthritis

Stage of disease	Surgical procedure
Proliferation of synovium	Synovectomy and debridement
Destruction of tendon	Tendon reconstruction
Moderate to advanced destruction and deformity	Interposition arthroplasty Total joint replacement or excision arthroplasty.

Excision of inflamed synovium will often relieve pain and swelling although, contrary to earlier expectations, it does not halt the progress of the disease. Persistent synovitis of the wrist and extensor-tendon sheath of the hand commonly leads to rupture of the tendons, which can be prevented by synovectomy and excision of the ulnar head. If the tendons rupture, suture or transfer of a slip of adjacent tendon corrects 'dropped fingers'.

The reconstructive surgical procedures used include arthroplasty (provision of a new joint), arthrodesis, osteotomy, tendon repair and transplantation. Joint replacements are most successful in the hip, and usually both acetabular and femoral components are replaced. Complications of joint arthroplasty include thromboembolic episodes, infection, loosening and even fracture of the implant, wear and heterotopic bone formation.

For the most satisfactory results, careful selection is essential. Consideration must be given to the overall disease state, the patient's general health and motivation and how he will respond to supportive physiotherapy and occupational therapy. Any surgical programme must include a detailed assessment of the patient's needs and of the likely improvement in function following surgery.

Prognosis

The course of rheumatoid arthritis is variable and it is often not possible to predict at onset those patients who will develop severe disease. In general, 25% remain fit for all normal activities, 40% have moderate impairment of function, 25% are quite badly disabled and 10% become wheelchair patients.

A poor prognosis is indicated by high titres of rheumatoid factor, early appearance of erosions, rheumatoid nodules, systemic manifestations and the presence of HLA DR4. Patients who have remissions generally do better than those with continuous disease, and explosive onset is often associated with a good outcome.

SERONEGATIVE SPONDYLARTHRITIDES

The seronegative spondylarthritides (spondyl: joint of the backbone) are a group of disorders characterised by a consistent absence of rheumatoid factors in the serum, by involvement of the sacro-iliac joints and by peripheral inflammatory arthritis. These conditions are, as a group, clinically distinguishable from rheumatoid arthritis (Table 24.16). Clinical evidence of overlap exists between the various seronegative spondylarthritides (Summary 3). Thus a patient with psoriatic arthropathy may develop uveitis or sacroiliitis, and a patient with inflammatory bowel disease may develop ankylosing spondylitis or mouth ulcers. Pathological changes are concentrated at sites of insertion of ligaments or tendons (enthesopathy) rather than the synovium, and changes may also be seen in the eye, aortic valve and skin. There is a tendency to familial aggregation and the disorders are linked as a group

Table 24.16 Comparison of seronegative spondylarthritis and seropositive rheumatoid arthritis

Feature	Seronegative	Seropositive
Peripheral arthritis	Asymmetrical	Symmetrical
Spinal involvement	Ankylosis	Cervical subluxation
Cartilaginous joints	Commonly affected (especially SI joints)	Rarely affected
Tissue typing	HLA-B27	No association known (HLA/D4/DR)
Eye involvement	Anterior uveitis, conjunctivitis	Scleritis, keratoconjunctivitis sicca
Skin involvement	Epidermal dysmaturation (psoriasis keratoderma blenorrhagica), mucosal ulceration, erythema nodosum	Cutaneous nodules, vasculitis
Heart involvement	Fibrosis of aortic root, aortic regurgitation, conduction defects	Pericarditis
Pulmonary involvement	Chest wall ankylosis	Alveolitis, nodules, effusions
Gastrointestinal involvement	Ulceration of small or large intestine	Drug-induced symptoms
Genitourinary involvement	Urethritis/prostatitis, genital ulceration	

by association with histocompatability antigen HLA-B27. This association ranges from 50% for psoriatic and enteropathic spondylitis to over 95% for ankylosing spondylitis.

The concept of seronegative spondylarthritis is useful in a clinical context for a number of reasons:

1. the prognosis is better than for rheumatoid arthritis
2. a knowledge of the clinical associations can allow an earlier diagnosis to be made
3. physical management differs from that of rheumatoid arthritis
4. awareness of sacro-iliitis in this group can avoid the error of labelling back pain as lumbar disc disease
5. awareness of the frequency of familial associations may help the patient or undiagnosed relative.

In the differential diagnosis of arthritis, seronegativity is of wider importance than these spondylarthritic conditions and includes all forms of inflammatory polyarthritis in which the rheumatoid factor is absent. For this reason, the term seronegative *spondyl*arthritis should only be applied when there is spinal involvement.

Radiological examination of the affected joints aids diagnosis because bony ankylosis, marginal periostitis, and asymmetrical involvement are found more often in the seronegative group. These differences suggest separate underlying pathological processes between the two groups.

Summary 3 Conditions that overlap to form the seronegative spondylarthritides, and their common features

The seronegative spondylarthritides

- Ankylosing spondylitis
- Psoriatic arthritis
- Enteropathic arthritis (associated with ulcerative colitis, Crohn's disease and Whipple's disease)
- Reiter's syndrome/reactive arthropathy
- Behçet's syndrome

Common features

- Negative tests from rheumatoid factor
- Absence of rheumatoid nodules
- Inflammatory peripheral arthritis
- Radiological sacroiliitis
- Evidence of clinical overlap between members of the group
- Tendency to familial aggregation

Fig. 24.11 Ankylosing spondylitis. A. Prevalence of ankylosing spondylitis and HLA-B27 in different parts of the world. (After Lawrence JS, 1977). **B.** X-ray of the spine in severe ankylosing spondylitis; there are extensive syndesmophytes ('bamboo spine') and the sacroiliac joints are fused.

Pathogenesis

The pathogenesis of these disorders is poorly understood, even in those conditions where the infective agent (e.g. *Yersinia*, *Shigella* or *Salmonella* infection) is known.

Hereditary factors play an important role. Individuals with HLA-B27 have a 1–2% chance of developing disease, whereas the risk for HLA-B27-positive relatives of HLA-B27-positive patients with ankylosing spondylitis is about 10%. The offspring of an individual with HLA-B27 have a 50% chance of carrying the same antigen. Approximately 10–20% of HLA-B27-positive individuals develop Reiter's syndrome after exposure to *Shigella* or other infectious agents. The explanation for the link between HLA-B27 and the spondylarthropathies remains unknown. Three hypothesis have been put forward:

1. HLA-B27 acts as a receptor site for an infective agent
2. HLA-B27 is a marker for an immune response gene that determines susceptibility to an environmental cause
3. HLA-B27 may induce tolerance to foreign antigens with which it cross-reacts.

ANKYLOSING SPONDYLITIS

Epidemiology

Although Hippocrates described a condition identical to the modern disease, it was not until the separate description by Bechterew, Strumpell and Marie at the end of the 19th century that the disease was widely recognised.

Ankylosing spondylitis occurs in both sexes but is usually milder, and therefore less frequently diagnosed, in women. Recent estimates of the sex ratio suggest that it is three times more common in men. Clinical features of ankylosing spondylitis are seen in 0.5% of males. The prevalence in different ethnic groups is related to the frequency of HLA-B27 in these populations (Fig. 24.11A).

Ankylosing spondylitis is uncommon in African blacks and in the Japanese, who have a low frequency of B27, while the North American Haida Indians have a high frequency of both HLA-B27 and ankylosing spondylitis. An abnormal response to bacteria, such as *Klebsiella*, which carry an antigen that mimics B27, has been suggested as the underlying cause of ankylosing spondylitis.

Pathology

The early histological changes in the synovial joints resemble rheumatoid arthritis, but with less prominent lesions of the surface layers. However, the most important effects are in the cartilaginous joints. Bony ankylosis is more frequent and the sacroiliac joints often become fused. The apophyseal joints are involved and the discs show replacement of the nucleus pulposus, the annulus fibrosus and parts of the vertebral body by vascular fibrous tissue without any evidence of marked inflammatory changes. In the spine, the lesion is in the ligamentous attachment to bone (the enthesis) and this is characteristic of the disorder.

The disease is characterised by bilateral sacroiliitis. The sacroiliac joint is a composition joint with the lower half to two-thirds a synovial joint, and the upper part ligamentous. Early inflammatory changes occur in the synovial joint.

As the disease extends up to the intervertebral joints, there is 'squaring' of the vertebral bodies radiologically (Fig. 24.11B) and calcification of the annulus fibrosus giving the characteristic syndesmophytes which fuse to form the classic 'bamboo spine'. This is caused by inflammation of the anterior corners of the vertebrae which extends into the outer layers of the annulus fibrosus.

Calcification of the inter-vertebral ligaments occurs. At this stage, there is osteoporosis of the vertebra, and fractures of the spine after minor trauma can occur. Other cartilaginous joints, such as the sternomanubrial joint and symphysis pubis, can be affected with erosions and bony ankylosis.

Clinical features

The disease most commonly begins between 16 and 40 years of age.

Articular features

Back pain is the usual presenting symptom. Its onset is gradual and is often accompanied by constitutional disturbances. The pain usually disturbs sleep and is associated with morning stiffness and stiffness after immobility. In the late stages of the disease, there may be reduction in spinal pain as the axial skeleton becomes ankylosed. Involvement of the costovertebral joints may result in chest pain and, later, decreased chest expansion. Symptoms improve with exercise.

Diagnosis is often delayed, symptoms being ascribed to lumbar disc disease. In spondylitis, spinal mobility is limited in all directions in contrast to disc prolapse, when lateral flexion is usually normal. The lumbar spine becomes flattened and the normal lordosis is lost. Sacro-iliac tenderness may be present. In an advanced case, the diagnosis is easy, as posture, gait and limitation of back movements are typical. However, only a few patients exhibit marked

kyphosis and spinal rigidity.

Peripheral joints are involved in about a quarter of patients, and involvement of the hip is important because of the functional implications. Sometimes, pain and tenderness at the site of tendinous insertions can be a prominent feature, with the back, pelvic brim and ischial tuberosities being characteristic sites. Several joints are involved, usually the large joints of the lower limb.

Extra-articular features

Although primarily an articular disease of the axial and peripheral skeleton, other organs may be involved (Summary 4).

Iritis may be a presenting feature; it occurs in 25% of cases and can cause blindness. Aortitis and myocarditis are causes of death, as is uraemia from amyloidosis. Spinal cord or cauda equina compression may occur because of atlanto-axial subluxation or fracture of a rigid spine. Patients with severe ankylosing spondylitis may exhibit chronic fibrotic changes in the upper lung that resemble tuberculosis.

Summary 4   Extra-articular features of ankylosing spondylitis

- Malaise and weight loss
- Iritis
- Apical pulmonary fibrosis
- Amyloidosis
- Cardiac involvement
  Aortic regurgitation
  Conduction defects
- Neurological features
  Spinal fractures
  Cauda equina syndrome

Investigation

The ESR is often elevated in active phases of the disease. There is little correlation with disease severity. Tissue typing for HLA-B27 is both expensive and unnecessary, as diagnosis can be made on the clinical findings and X-rays. Raised IgA levels are associated with activity.

Anterio-posterior views of the sacro-iliac joints and lateral X-rays of the lumbar spine should be obtained. Both may be normal in early disease. The earliest changes are of sclerosis and erosions in the sacro-iliac joints, usually bilateral. Later, complete fusion may occur. The changes should be distinguished from *osteitis condensans ilii*, which is an asymptomatic and benign abnormality found in women, and also from infection of sacro-iliac joints, e.g. brucellosis.

Early changes in the lumbar spine are erosions of the edges of the vertebral bodies with squaring of the vertebrae and syndesmophyte formation (Fig. 24.11B). In the most severe cases, ossification of the anterior longitudinal ligaments and apophyseal joints occur with production of a 'bamboo spine'.

Treatment

A long-term programme of active mobilisation in combination with anti-inflammatory drug therapy are the mainstays of treatment. Indomethacin is usually effective. The aim is to ease pain and stiffness, to keep deformity to a minimum and to maintain spinal mobility as much as possible. In contrast to the patient with rheumatoid arthritis, who is put to bed during an exacerbation, the patient with ankylosing spondylitis stiffens with bed rest and should be encouraged to remain active. Lumbar supports should not be prescribed. The patient must understand that the purpose of anti-inflammatory drugs is to reduce pain and stiffness so that an active exercise programme can be followed. Phenylbutazone can still be prescribed for ankylosing spondylitis and sulphasalazine can help the peripheral synovitis.

Advice should be given about posture. A firm bed with one pillow is appropriate at night. The patient should be taught exercises which can be performed daily at home and these should include spine extension and breathing exercises. Support groups and group physiotherapy sessions may help in providing advice and support in carrying out exercises.

Surgical intervention is most often carried out for hip involvement. Rarely, spinal osteotomy is used for severe spinal curvature. If there is severe neck restriction, the occupational therapist can advise about appropriate wing mirrors for the car.

Genetic counselling

Most patients with ankylosing spondylitis are HLA-B27-positive, and 50% of their offspring will carry this antigen. If HLA-B27-positive, a son or daughter has a 33% chance of developing ankylosing spondylitis. Parents should be advised that if the child develops symptoms such as swollen joints or painful eyes, they should seek medical advice.

Prognosis

With suitable treatment, the prognosis is excellent and 85% of patients never lose a day's work. After the early, painful phase, the back may be stiff but disability is minimal unless hip involvement is present. The objectives of treatment are to relieve pain, decrease inflammation and maintain good posture and function. About 5% of patients have an unfavourable course from the outset. Why some patients do well and others poorly remains unknown.

PSORIATIC ARTHRITIS

Psoriasis and rheumatoid arthritis each occur in about 2% of the population. Hence, there can be a coincidental association of these conditions. However, the arthropathy which develops most commonly in psoriasis is distinct. It affects the sexes equally. Arthritis occurs in about 10% of patients with psoriasis, particularly in those with nail involvement. The skin changes involved in psoriatic arthritis are described on p. 1123.

Clinical features

The onset of arthritis usually follows a long history of psoriasis and can be acute, insidious, monoarticular or polyarticular. Occasionally it precedes the skin lesions. There does not appear to be a correlation between the severity of the skin lesions and the development of the arthropathy, although the joint lesions are usually associated with involvement of the nails. This can be seen as pitting, thickening of the nail plates, discolouration and ridging, with splitting of the nail.

The severity and ultimate deformity caused by the disease is usually less than that due to rheumatoid arthritis, and remissions are more frequent. There may be some synchrony of activity of joint and skin manifestations. Different types of psoriatic arthropathy are recognised:

1. *Asymmetric oligoarthritis*, which involves one or two joints of fingers or toes, but can affect large joints.
2. *Symmetrical polyarthritis*, which resembles rheumatoid arthritis.
3. *Arthritis mutilans*, the most severe form of destructive arthritis.
4. *Psoriatic spondylitis* in which radiological sacroiliitis occurs in 20% of cases.
5. *Psoriatic nail disease* and *distal interphalangeal joint involvement*.

The histological synovial changes resemble rheumatoid arthritis, but the joints involved and the pattern of destruction are different. While any joint can be affected, the most characteristic are the distal interphalangeal joints of the hands and feet.

Investigation

Radiological features of psoriatic arthritis are erosions in the distal interphalangeal joints with ankylosis, reabsorption of the terminal phalanges, and marginal bone overgrowths at the tendon insertions. When this last feature is associated with osteolysis of the middle phalanx the radiological 'pencil in cup' deformity appears. If osteolysis progresses to 'telescoping' of the phalanges, the condition is known as *arthritis mutilans* (Fig. 24.12).

Sacro-iliitis is found in up to 30% of cases in which erosions, sclerosis and ankylosis may occur. Unlike ankylosing spondylitis, the involvement is usually asymmetrical. It is particularly common in patients with the severe arthritis mutilans form of disease. Paravertebral calcification and occasional large syndesmophytes may be seen. However, the incidence of typical ankylosing spondylitis is also higher in psoriatics and relatives than might be expected in the general population. Hyperuricaemia can occur in up to 20% of all psoriatics and the arthropathy should not therefore be confused with gout.

Fig. 24.12 Psoriatic arthropathy, with extensive involvement of the distal interphalangeal joints.

Treatment and prognosis

The treatment of the peripheral arthritis is similar to that of rheumatoid arthritis. Gold therapy may be required for the more severe cases. Spinal disease is treated in the same way as ankylosing spondylitis.

In most cases, the prognosis is good end joint function is barely impaired; but deformity and disability occurs in patients with arthritis mutilans.

REITER'S SYNDROME

Reiter's syndrome was described several times before 1916, when Hans Reiter described the case of a Prussian cavalry officer serving on the Balkan Front who developed an acute febrile illness characterised by arthritis, urethritis and conjunctivitis. The attack followed an episode of bloody diarrhoea. Although the venereal form of the disease is commoner in the UK, the post-dysenteric form predominates in Europe. The incidence in patients with dysentery is approximately 0.24%, and 0.8% of patients with non-specific urethritis develop Reiter's disease. The disease may be defined as an episode of arthropathy within one month of urethritis or cervicitis.

Aetiology

The disease follows an infection of either the bowel or lower genital tract. In the dysenteric form, several organisms have been implicated, chiefly *Shigella flexneri*, *Salmonella typhimurium* and *Yersinia enterolitica* but, in many cases, no causal agent has been found. *Salmonella* and *Yersinia* are also associated with 'reactive arthritis' without concomitant urethritis and conjunctivitis. Reactive arthritis is an arthritis occurring as a result of an infection elsewhere in the body, but that is not caused by a direct infection of the joint.

In the urogenital form, there is evidence that *Chlamydia* may be responsible for at least some of the cases. There is a genetic predisposition to the disease, since 60–90% of patients have the tissue antigen HLA-B27. A family study performed in England showed an increased prevalence of sacro-iliitis, spondylitis and psoriasis in relatives of patients with Reiter's syndrome.

Clinical features

The diagnostic triad in Reiter's syndrome is urethritis, conjunctivitis and arthritis. One of this triad may be absent, and it should be noted that urethritis can occur even in the post-dysenteric form of the disease. Most cases of Reiter's syndrome occur in the age range 16–35 years, and the male to female ratio is 20:1. However, urethritis is often clinically inapparent in females, and women presenting with an inflammatory arthritis in association with the HLA-B27 antigen may have Reiter's syndrome. Post-dysenteric Reiter's syndrome has an equal sex distribution.

Urethritis is usually the first feature to appear, and occurs up to one month after sexual exposure. It is often mild but, rarely, there is a blood-stained discharge. The complaint of dysuria is almost invariable and there is frequency and suprapubic discomfort due to bladder involvement and prostatitis. Usually there are no urinary sequelae, but cases of hydronephrosis may occur as a late complication of fibrosis of the bladder.

Mucocutaneous lesions in the glans penis are characteristic. Superficial ulcers often coalesce to form circinate patches. Involvement of the mucous membranes of the mouth is found in ten per cent of patients. The lesions are often painless and subside spontaneously.

The typical cutaneous lesion of Reiter's disease is *keratoderma blenorrhagica*. Initially a red macular eruption, it becomes hyperkeratotic and histologically identical to pustular psoriasis. This can occur anywhere on the body, but is most characteristically seen on the palms of the hands and soles of the feet. The crust is eventually shed leaving no scar.

Sterile conjunctivitis is the most common form of eye involvement and is usually mild. Occasionally, ocular involvement may be very severe, with almost all parts of the eye being involved, although the disease has a predilection for the conjunctiva and anterior uveal tract. Frequently, there are transient abnormalities of cardiac conduction which may progress to complete heart block. Pericarditis and aortic valve lesions also occur. Transient pulmonary shadowing has been described.

The *arthritis* varies in severity from a mild, transient synovitis to a chronic destructive arthritis. It tends to involve large weight-bearing joints and although it may on occasion be monarticular, this is uncommon; it is usually asymmetrical, involving fingers and toes. In a typical case, arthritis may last for weeks or months, although in a few cases permanent joint damage may result. A feature of the condition is its liability to recurrences. Over 60% of cases have two attacks or more. Symptom-free intervals of 10 years or more are not uncommon, but in a small number, no clear-cut remission occurs.

Investigation

The ESR is elevated, sometimes markedly in the acute phase. Radiological examination in the early weeks may reveal no abnormality or only juxta-articular osteoporosis. Periostitis is a characteristic finding, especially in the metatarsals and in the phalanges of the feet. The new bone formation has an exuberant, fluffy appearance. Plantar spurs occur in 20–45% of cases (Fig. 24.13). Unilateral or bilateral changes are seen in the sacroiliac joints, the frequency increasing to 50% after five years, and changes of ankylosing spondylitis may be seen in the spine.

The skin lesions and the arthropathy may resemble psoriasis. There have been cases when apparently typical Reiter's disease has progressed to typical psoriatic arthropathy. The link is emphasised by family studies where, among the male relatives of patients with Reiter's disease, the prevalence of psoriasis is 13%.

Treatment and prognosis

For most patients, a NSAID is useful. Methotrexate or azathioprine should be considered for severe intractable disease. Uveitis should be evaluated by an ophthalmologist if it does not respond rapidly to steroid eye-drops.

Spouses are often concerned that they may catch the disease from the patient. This does not occur. Most patients with Reiter's syndrome do not seem to have sexually acquired disease.

Fig. 24.13   Reiter's disease; X-ray showing plantar spur.

Tetracycline is effective in the treatment of non-specific urethritis, but has no effect on the other manifestations of the disease.

Reiter's syndrome was, at one time, considered to be a self-limiting condition. It is now known to be a persistent disease in many patients; about 80% of patients have evidence of disease activity when they are examined after five years.

ENTEROPATHIC ARTHROPATHIES

The term enteropathic arthropathy means arthropathy associated with bowel disease (usually ulcerative colitis and Crohn's disease). There are two main clinical patterns:

1. an episodic synovitis mainly involving weight-bearing joints
2. sacro-iliitis.

About 50% of individuals with both inflammatory bowel disease and ankylosing spondylitis are HLA-B27-positive, a percentage which is lower than that found in patients with primary ankylosing spondylitis.

Synovitis occurs in 12% of patients with ulcerative colitis and 21% of those with Crohn's disease. The synovitis correlates with exacerbations of ulcerative colitis and is more likely when the bowel disease is extensive or when complications such as perianal suppuration occur. A total proctocolectomy abolishes the synovitis completely. In Crohn's disease, surgery seldom offers a radical cure, but synovitis tends to correlate with bowel activity. In both cases, the synovium shows non-specific inflammatory changes and, irrespective of the number of recurrences of the condition, progression to radiological joint destruction does not occur.

Radiologically typical ankylosing spondylitis or sacro-iliitis occurs in 17% of cases of inflammatory bowel disease. This frequently antedates the bowel symptoms and the progress of the two manifestations are not synchronous. In ulcerative colitis, radical excision of the colon does not provide a cure for the spondylitis. The involvement of the peripheral joints may lead to confusion with enteropathic synovitis; however, the presence of sacro-iliac and spinal disease, the lack of association of joint and bowel symptoms, and the presence of radiological changes in the involved joints all help in differentiation.

Family studies show an increased evidence of sacroiliitis and ankylosing spondylitis in relatives. This lends weight to the view that the spondylitis is an hereditary accompaniment, rather than a complication, of the disease.

WHIPPLE'S DISEASE

Whipple's disease is a rare condition. The finding of bacilli-form bodies on electron microscopy and the good response to long-term antibiotic therapy suggest that it has an infectious aetiology.

An episodic arthritis is a common presentation, and may precede the gut symptoms by several years. The pattern of joint disease is similar to that seen in intestinal inflammatory disease, but the absence of overt gut symptoms should alert one to the possibility of Whipple's disease.

Prolonged antibiotic therapy leads to improvement. It is usual to give tetracycline 1 g daily for 12 months, following an initial 10 days' treatment with parenteral penicillin and streptomycin.

BEHÇET'S SYNDROME

Behçet's syndrome was first described in Turkey and is common in Eastern Mediterranean countries and Japan, though rare in England. It is of unknown aetiology and is characterised by the triad of aphthous-type oral and genital ulceration and iritis. Other features that commonly occur include thrombophlebitis, erythema nodosum, pustules and folliculitis. Some patients show the phenomenon of postule formation where the skin is subjected to trivial injury, e.g. venepuncture. Large vessel thrombosis and bowel disease resembling ulcerative colitis can occur. The central nervous system can be involved, with meningo-encephalitis, cranial nerve palsies, hemiparesis and transient episodes resembling strokes. The vascular involvement of the eye is one of the most serious aspects of Behçets syndrome, with blindness being a frequent outcome.

Arthritis occurs in 60% of cases, affecting mainly the weight-bearing joints, and the course tends to be chronic. The inclusion of Behçet's syndrome in the seronegative group is somewhat speculative. There is association with HLA-B5 but not HLA-B27, and eye disease is particularly associated with HLA-B51. Some HLA DR loci appear to determine the organs involved in Behçet's disease. Immunological abnormalities have been described, such as circulating immune complexes, and there is some evidence that Behçet's syndrome has an underlying viral aetiology, but the pathogenesis remains uncertain.

Acute episodes, especially those involving the eye, usually require high-dose corticosteroid therapy. Colchicine is useful for some aspects of the disease, especially the orogenital ulceration. Cyclosporin A has shown promise, particularly for controlling the eye disease.

OSTEOARTHRITIS

Osteoarthritis is defined pathologically and radiologically by reduced joint space secondary to loss of cartilage, by sclerosis of subchondral bone and by osteophyte formation. The term primary osteoarthritis is used to distinguish cases with no apparent cause from secondary osteoarthritis, when a number of localised or generalised pre-existing disorders are present (Table 24.17).

Table 24.17 Secondary causes of osteoarthritis

• Previous inflammatory arthritis	• Congenital dislocation of hip
• Previous joint infections	• Perthe's disease
• Avascular necrosis	• Acromegaly
• Intra-articular fracture	• Ochronosis
• Joint dysplasias	• Haemochromatosis

Epidemiology

Radiographic evidence of osteoarthritis is found in 35% of people under 30 years of age, and in 85% of 80-year-olds (Fig. 24.14). Osteoarthritis of the hip is more common in men under 35 years of age, but in later years it is more common and more severe in women. Although radiographic evidence of osteoarthritis appears to have an equal sex ratio, symptoms are three times more common in women. There is a marked familial tendency, particularly in association with Heberden's nodes, and the geographical distribution of joint involvement varies. Certain occupations have a high frequency of osteoarthritis; for example coal miners develop osteoarthritis of the spine and knees.

Aetiology

A number of processes are involved in the development of osteoarthritis:

1. failure of bone and cartilage remodelling
2. inflammation

3. deposits of apatite and calcium pyrophosphate are common, but how they affect the joint remains unknown
4. alterations of the complex reflex neurological and muscle function around a joint, resulting in an impaired shock-absorbing capacity
5. enzymic destruction of cartilage.

Fig. 24.14 Age and sex distribution of generalised osteo-arthritis (GOA) in the UK in patients with, and without Heberden's nodes. (After Lawrence JS, 1977).

Pathology

The early stages of osteoarthritis include an increase in proteoglycan turnover, a change in proteoglycan composition and an increase of type II collagen production. The relationship of these changes to ageing is uncertain.

Cartilage shows thinning, erosions, fibrillation, clefts and loss of joint surface congruity with areas of chondrocyte loss. Subchondral bone becomes sclerotic with increased vascularity and bone distant from the joint undergoes remodelling. Proliferation of the cartilage produces osteophytes, which is usually a late phenomenon. In the later stages, cysts are formed in the underlying subchondral bone, and the articular surface may collapse.

A mild synovitis may be seen, and the synovial fluid may contain apatite and pyrophosphate crystals.

Clinical features

The main initial symptom of osteoarthritis is pain made worse by movement and eased by rest. Stiffness may be present after inactivity, but morning stiffness is not a feature. As the joint deteriorates with loss of joint movement and joint instability, the pain becomes more pronounced, and is present at rest and in the night. Only about a third of patients with radiological osteoarthritis have symptoms, and the cause of pain is not understood, as there are no pain receptors in cartilage. Pain may also arise from the ligaments or bursae around the joint.

Examination shows deformity and bony enlargement of the joint, with occasional synovial thickening and effusion.

There is coarse crepitus on joint movement. The pattern of joint involvement varies, but those most commonly affected include the first metacarpophalangeal joint, the first metatarsophalangeal joint and the distal interphalangeal joint of the hands (Fig. 24.2). The hip and knee are affected less frequently and the shoulder and ankle are seldom involved. In the spine, the apophyseal joints around C5–C7 and L3–L5 are commonly involved.

The pattern of joint involvement varies, and several subgroups can be distinguished. Osteoarthritis is not a single static condition but a family of conditions, with widely different pathogenetic factors. Generalised osteoarthritis affects several joints and there are usually Heberden's nodes present. 'Inflammatory' osteoarthritis affects particularly the interphalangeal joints, and is associated with cartilage erosion. Hip arthritis can be confined to one area of the hip, particularly the superior pole or the medial pole, or may involve the entire joint. Similarly, there are different patterns of knee involvement. Lateral compartment changes seldom occur without medial compartment changes. Predominate patello-femoral disease is a feature of pyrophosphate arthropathy (p. 1014).

There are many ways to classify osteoarthritis, but the most important considerations are the patient's symptoms and joint function.

Investigations and differential diagnosis

All blood tests are normal in uncomplicated osteoarthritis. If the radiological abnormalities are minor, other causes for the patients' symptoms should be considered. These include:

1. *Rheumatoid arthritis* can be distinguished from osteoarthritis as the pattern of joint involvement differs and there is juxta-articular osteoporosis as well as associated clinical features. Other causes of seronegative arthritis can similarly be recognised.
2. *Avascular necrosis* can be differentiated from osteoarthritis by the sudden onset of symptoms.
3. In *calcium pyrophosphate* disease, the pattern of joint involvement is different, with more knee, shoulder, wrist and hip disease. In this condition, there may be asymptomatic chondrocalcinosis or, at the other extreme, there is a chronic destructive arthritis (p. 1014).

Treatment

The natural history of osteoarthritis is poorly documented. There is evidence that the process may stop, or even improve, in some patients, and in those that have progressive disease, severe joint failure tends to occur in a weight-bearing joint in a minority of patients.

Generalised osteoarthritis tends to progress slowly, and prognosis with respect to preservation of joint function is excellent. Patients should be reassured that they do not have a relentlessly progressive disease such as rheumatoid arthritis. Hand function may be improved by simple exercise routines and wax baths. Pain relief can be achieved with analgesics such as paracetamol. NSAIDs have more side-effects, but may be necessary when pain is severe.

Osteoarthritis in a weight-bearing joint may be helped by physiotherapy. This may restore the function of wasted muscles, improve mobility and compensate for some instability. Splints may support unstable joints, and walking aids may be helpful. Intra-articular steroid injections and aspiration of joints may help in restoration of function if there are effusions and inflammatory changes.

Surgery

Surgery is indicated if pain and loss of function have failed to respond to conservative measures. Surgical procedures include removal of loose bodies, osteotomy to relieve pain and arthrodesis and arthroplasty (joint replacement). The low friction hip arthroplasty is the most successful form of joint replacement, but there are many surgical procedures which can help the arthritic patient (Table 24.18). Proper assessment is the key to a successful outcome and surgery should only be carried out when there is a clear indication that function will be improved. Joint replacement will continue to develop. There is still much basic research to be done into biomechanics of joints under normal conditions and after prosthetic replacement, and on the problems of lubrication.

Table 24.18 Some surgical procedures in arthritis

● Synovectomy/debridement	● Arthrodesis
● Arthroplasty	● Tendon repairs
● Osteotomy	● Nerve decompression

INFECTIVE ARTHRITIS

Arthritis may arise from direct infection of joints by microorganisms, or as a reaction to a preceding infection. Infection must be considered in all cases of acute arthritis, particularly when only one joint is affected. Delay in treatment may lead to permanent joint damage or septicaemia.

BACTERIAL INFECTIONS

Most cases of bacterial arthritis result from haematogenous spread; much less frequently, infection results from joint aspiration or injection, or spread from osteomyelitis. The most frequent organisms are *Staphylococcus aureus, Streptococcus pyogenes, Diplococcus pneumoniae* and *Neisseria gonorrhoeae*. Certain organisms appear to exhibit a tropism for joints: for instance, septic arthritis complicates about 1% of pneumococcal and salmonella infections when treatment is delayed, whereas about 80% of patients with gonococcal septicaemia develop arthritis. The frequency with which different organisms are associated with septic arthritis is partly age-dependent. The organisms which cause septic arthritis in young children are usually not the same as those causing it in adults.

Septic arthritis may occur at any age, but is particularly common under the age of 15 years and in the elderly. Other predisposing factors include debilitating disease, hypogammaglobulinaemia, corticosteroid and immunosuppressive therapy, and rheumatoid arthritis.

Clinical features

Usually, a single joint is involved and there is marked inflammation with severe pain, tenderness, erythema and swelling. There may be minimal signs of inflammation in patients receiving corticosteroids or with a debilitating illness. In an infant, there may also be little systemic illness and the child may present with sudden refusal to move a limb.

An infected joint is commonly associated with a fever, often accompanied by rigors, and the patient looks ill. When the organism is the gonococcus, a migratory polyarthritis may precede localisation in a single joint. 10–20% of staphylococcal infections and 75–85% of gonococcal infections involve two or more joints. More than one joint may also be involved in immunosuppressed and debilitated patients. The identification of a septic joint in rheumatoid arthritis can prove difficult, but must be considered whenever there is increase in pain, swelling or other evidence of inflammation in one or a limited number of joints. The development of low-grade infection in prosthetic joints is an increasing problem, and recognition may take several months. Organisms of low virulence, especially *Staphylococcus albus*, predominate.

Diagnosis

Diagnosis of septic arthritis depends on demonstrating the organism in joint fluid or tissue, and synovial fluid and blood should be sent for culture. In addition to routine aerobic and anaerobic cultures, special media are needed for the isolation of *N. gonorrhoeae*, and additional culture of sputum, urine and cervical mucus may prove helpful in special circumstances.

Although osteomyelitis usually results in sterile joint effusions, it can lead to septic arthritis. Osteomyelitis should be considered if the site of maximal tenderness extends beyond the joint. If there is any doubt about the bone adjacent to an infected joint, an isotope scan will demonstrate bone involvement.

The condition known as *transient synovitis of the hip* can prove a difficult differential diagnosis. No definite cause has been established for this disorder and it may represent a number of conditions. It affects children between the ages of two and 12 years, who present with pain, a low-grade fever and slight elevation of the ESR. It is safest to treat this as an infection until the diagnosis of septic arthritis has been excluded.

Treatment

Antibiotics should be started as soon as specimens have been sent to the laboratory. Changes in therapy can be made once the sensitivities of the infecting organism are known. Therapy should be administered intravenously for up to two weeks. Drug concentrations within the joint are adequate when antibiotics are given systemically, and intra-articular therapy is not required. The joint should be splinted in a suitable position to relieve pain until the inflammation has subsided.

Synovial fluid should be aspirated when it reaccumulates, since the presence of purulent material may inhibit the action of antibiotics. Gross joint destruction and the presence of contiguous osteomyelitis are indications for surgical drainage, as is failure of response to drug therapy within 72 hours. Once the acute inflammation has subsided, passive, then active exercises can be given. Weight-bearing can be resumed when signs of inflammation have subsided.

Specific bacterial arthritides

Gonococcal arthritis

Gonococcal arthritis is most common in females and homosexual males, in whom the primary infection is often asymptomatic.

Clinical features. The most common pattern of joint involvement is a migratory polyarthritis associated with tenosynovitis, with the synovitis localising in one or two joints. Joint symptoms occur within three weeks of infection and are accompanied by fever and rigors. There is a tendency for the small joints of the upper limbs, e.g. the finger joints, to be involved, rather than larger joints; however, the knee is also frequently affected. A sparse erythematous skin rash, which may be macular, vesicular or pustular, occurs in one-third of cases and is found adjacent to involved joints. It appears before, or within a few days of, the arthritis and may be painful at the outset.

Diagnosis. The gonococcus is difficult to grow, and repeated blood and synovial fluid cultures may be required to confirm the diagnosis. The organism is identified in joint fluid in only 25% of patients.

There should be little difficulty in distinguishing between Reiter's disease and gonococcal arthritis. There is an 80% female preponderance of gonococcal arthritis, compared with a high proportion of males with Reiter's disease. In gonococcal arthritis, pyrexia is more common, the upper limb joints are involved more frequently, and the arthritis is less symmetrical than in Reiter's disease. Reiter's disease is associated with the tissue antigen B27; gonococcal arthritis is not.

Treatment. Penicillin is still the drug of choice and benzylpenicillin is given intravenously until there is a clinical response. Penicillinase-producing strains of gonococci are resistant to penicillin and cephaloridine. For such patients spectinomycin or cephoxitin is the treatment of choice.

Meningococcal arthritis

Meningococcal infection is complicated by arthritis in 5–10% of patients. Characteristically, it affects large joints, and sometimes flits from one to another. The onset is a few days after the beginning of the illness. Once on therapy, resolution occurs in one to four weeks.

Tuberculous arthritis

Tuberculosis should be considered in the differential diagnosis of chronic joint disease. It is most common in immigrant children and in the middle-aged or elderly. Only about 1% of all patients with tuberculosis have skeletal involvement; of these, approximately 50% have spinal disease, 30% infection of hips or knees, and 20% arthritis of other joints, particularly the sacro-iliac joints. Involvement of the knee is more common in adults, and the spine and hips in children. About half the patients do not have pulmonary disease. It is assumed that haematogenous dissemination infects subchrondral bone adjacent to a joint or to a spinal intervertebral disc. The resulting osteomyelitis may remain dormant for years before there is reactivation. Alcoholism and chronic debilitating disease may predispose to reactivation.

When the vertebral column is involved, dissection along fascial planes may cause a psoas abscess. Spread of infection to involve adjacent vertebrae may lead to wedging and kyphosis. The anterior portions of the vertebrae between the sixth thoracic and fifth lumbar level are usually involved. Bone biopsy may be necessary to confirm the diagnosis.

Peripheral joint involvement is usually monoarticular and destruction of cartilage occurs later than in pyogenic arthritis. The usual organism is *Mycobacterium tuberculosis* but atypical organisms (e.g. *M. kansasii*, *M. trivale*) have been isolated from infected joints, and the bovine strain has been implicated in carpal tunnel infection.

Diagnosis and treatment. The diagnosis is made by biopsy and culture of the synovium, since the bacilli are rarely grown from synovial fluid. Treatment is with antituberculous therapy (p. 480).

Syphilitic arthritis

Direct invasion of the synovium by *Treponum pallidum* is uncommon. A migratory polyarthritis occurs infrequently during the secondary stage of acquired syphilis and may resemble rheumatic fever.

Congenital syphilis may cause:

1. acute epiphysitis or osteochondritis, most commonly of the humerus and usually in the first weeks of life
2. 'Clutton's joints', painless bilateral swelling of the knees between the ages of 8 and 16 years
3. rarely, a neuropathic arthropathy secondary to tabes dorsalis (Charcot's joint).

FUNGAL INFECTIONS

Fungal infections of joints are rare. Culture of pus, synovial fluid or biopsy material permits diagnosis. Surgical drainage and excision of necrotic tissue may facilitate recovery.

Actinomycosis commonly affects the mandible, but

involvement of vertebrae occasionally occurs from local spread. Bone abscesses develop. Blastomycosis, cocci-diomycosis, histoplasmosis and sporotrichosis can all affect the joints.

ARTHRITIS IN VIRAL DISEASE

Several viral infections may be accompanied or followed by an arthropathy (Summary 5). Joint symptoms may coincide with, follow, or even precede the onset of other signs and symptoms; they are usually mild and tend to resolve spontaneously in a few weeks. In contrast to bacterial infections, viral arthropathies are usually polyarticular. It is thought that the synovitis results from immune complex deposition. Only in rubella arthritis has the virus been isolated from an affected joint, but in arthritis caused by infection with hepatitis B and adenovirus, low serum levels of C3, C4 and CH50 have been observed, which return to normal during convalescence; immune complexes have also been detected in both serum and synovial fluid. A viral arthritis should be suspected if the patient has a low white count with a relative lymphocytosis.

Summary 5 Viral causes of arthritis

- Rubella and rubella vaccination
- Infectious hepatitis
- Mumps
- Infectious mononucleosis
- Adenovirus infections
- Arbovirus infections
- Chickenpox

Viral causes of arthritis

Rubella

The highest incidence of rubella is in adolescent females, the disease being less frequent in childhood. Joint symptoms may accompany, precede or follow the rash, which may be so faint or transient that it is easily missed. Awareness of a rubella epidemic or contact in the family, the rash, and occipital lymphadenopathy aid diagnosis.

The arthritis involves the metacarpophalangeal (MCP) or proximal interphalangeal (PIP) joints (85%), elbows, wrists and knees, in a symmetrical fashion. Morning stiffness, painful tenosynovitis, the occasional occurrence of carpal tunnel syndrome and a positive latex test for rheumatoid factor (RF) may make the resemblance to rheumatoid arthritis even more striking, and differentiation between the two conditions in the early stages is not always possible on clinical grounds alone. The ESR is usually normal or slightly elevated. Rubella antibodies may be demonstrable in high titre.

Complete resolution of the arthritis occurs within a few weeks to a few months. Only in rare cases are symptoms so severe that a short course of corticosteroids is required. Arthralgia may persist for several months.

Rubella vaccination

Rubella vaccination produces musculoskeletal symptoms in up to 20% of cases. An arthritis similar to that associated with the natural infection occurs two to four weeks after vaccination and lasts for a few days, although it can persist for several weeks. Occasionally, synovitis continues for months. Joint pain affecting the arms or legs 2–10 weeks after rubella vaccination is caused by radiculoneuritis, and may be associated with paraesthesia.

Infectious hepatitis

During the early incubation period of viral hepatitis, some patients may experience joint symptoms; these may be mild and transient (usually type A infections) or acute and prolonged (usually type B). It is rare before adolescence.

There is bilateral and symmetrical involvement of the PIP joints and the spine is occasionally involved. Other symptoms are a rapid onset of morning stiffness, and warm, red and tender joints with slight effusions, associated with fever, anorexia, malaise and an occasional urticarial rash. The arthritis usually resolves with the appearance of jaundice. Joint disturbances can also be prominent in anicteric cases.

The diagnosis should be considered in those exposed to a risk of hepatitis and substantiated by appropriate liver function tests and hepatitis serology.

Mumps

Arthritis caused by mumps is most common in male teenagers. Overall, less than 1% of those affected by mumps develop arthritis, usually 1–4 weeks after the start of the illness. It is usually migratory and asymmetrical, involving large joints. When the pattern of joint movement is accompanied by pericarditis, it can resemble rheumatic fever. During an epidemic, children may have an arthritis but no parotitis. The presence of rising antibody titres to mumps virus helps to confirm the diagnosis.

Chickenpox

Chickenpox may be complicated by bacterial arthritis with spread from infectious scabs. A transient, acute arthritis may occur at the time of the rash.

Adenoviral arthritis

The arthritis associated with adenovirus infections usually occurs in children. It begins with fever, coryza and pharyngitis, followed by a macular erythematous rash and symmetrical arthritis.

Infectious mononucleosis

In infectious mononucleosis, widespread lymphadenopathy, splenomegaly, rash, fever and transient arthritis or arthralgia may mimic both rheumatic fever and systemic juvenile chronic arthritis. However, the skin lesions tend to be larger and raised and do not recur as often as those of juvenile arthritis. The presence of mononuclear cells in the blood, and a positive monospot, confirms the diagnosis. This is a disorder of adolescents. In children, cytomegalovirus can cause a similar picture.

Arboviruses

Viral infections endemic to certain parts of the world can give rise to illnesses with prominent musculoarticular symptoms. The Ross River virus, a group A arbovirus found in Australia, causes a macular rash and fever, and a polyarthritis usually involving the small joints of the hands. Dengue fever, of South and South-East Asia, can cause a haemorrhagic rash, fever and severe joint and muscle pains. Both these illnesses are self-limiting. Arboviruses are discussed further in Chapter 12, page 247.

Infective endocarditis

Joint manifestations are present in about half the patients with infective endocarditis. Large joint involvement is usual, and symptoms vary from mild arthralgia to an acute, red, swollen painful joint. The combination of fever, arthritis and cardiac murmur may initially suggest rheumatic fever. Other features, such as splinter haemorrhages, microscopic haematuria or splenomegaly, may help in diagnosis, which is confirmed by positive blood cultures.

Lyme arthritis

This was first described in Old Lyme, Connecticut (USA) in 1972. Symptoms include a recurrent asymmetrical arthritis involving a few large joints. The arthritis follows 1–24 weeks after an erythematous rash, erythema chronicum migrans. The causative agent is a tick-borne spirochaete, *Borrelia burgdorferi*, which is transmitted by *Ixodes dammini* or related ixodid ticks. Penicillin or tetracycline therapy given at the time of the rash may shorten the early illness and prevent arthritis. Later stages respond to high dose intravenous penicillin.

Lyme disease usually begins in summer with erythema chronicum migrans; this is the unique clinical marker which begins as a red macule or papule which expands to form a large annular lesion. Skin involvement is often accompanied by fever, headache and regional lymphadenopathy, and migratory musculoskeletal pain and arthritis. Meningeal irritation and cardiac involvement may follow.

Rheumatic manifestations of HIV infections

Increasingly, HIV-infected individuals are presenting to rheumatologists, and, in some, rheumatic symptoms are the first manifestation of infection. Patients may present with Reiter's syndrome, or an acute oligoarthritis, which predominantly affects lower limb joints, in the absence of clinical features of Reiter's syndrome.

Other rheumatic syndromes which have been associated with HIV infection incude myositis, vasculitis and lupus-like illness with low-titre antinuclear antibodies. It is difficult to attribute these clinical features exclusively to HIV infection, as many patients are likely to be exposed to other infections. At present, there have been no reports of rheumatic complications in haemophiliacs who have become infected with HIV.

CHILDHOOD ARTHRITIS

There are a number of causes of arthritis in children and the diagnosis can be difficult. The commonest cause used to be rheumatic fever but there has been a marked reduction in its incidence in the past 40 years. However, an increasing number of other conditions are recognised where there is a combination of arthritis and systemic features. Because of differences in prognosis and management, it is important to distinguish between them; the pattern of joint involvement and the accompanying systemic features help in this differentiation. Conditions to consider are shown in Summary 6. Children seem to suffer less discomfort from arthritis than adults. Arthritis may be first suggested by joint swelling, or by a limp or guarding of the joints.

Summary 6   Differential diagnosis of arthritis in children

- Joint infections (bacterial, tuberculous)
- Virus infections (rubella and mumps in particular)
- Juvenile chronic arthritis (JCA)
  Still's disease (systemic JCA)
  Pauciarticular JCA
  Polyarticular-onset JCA
- Still's disease in young adults
- Rheumatic fever
- Henoch-Schönlein purpura
- Leukaemia and haemorrhagic disease
- Trauma and synovitis

JUVENILE CHRONIC ARTHRITIS

Juvenile chronic arthritis (JCA) is a generic term covering several overlapping patterns of disease (Summary 6).

Systemic JCA (Still's disease)

The most common age of onset of systemic JCA is under five years, when boys are affected as frequently as girls; but the disease can present later in childhood, and even in adult life (see below). With later presentation, girls are affected more commonly than boys.

Clinical features

Fever and rash are the main clinical features. The fever is characteristic and is present in most children with JCA. It differs from that of rheumatic fever in that the temperature may be normal or subnormal in the morning, and the child may then appear to be reasonably well. By the late afternoon, however, a temperature of up to 40°C may be recorded and the child looks ill. Salicylates usually control the fever. When high fever precedes arthritis, diagnosis can prove difficult and is often aided by the appearance of the rash.

About 40% of children develop a rash which is evanescent, often appearing when the temperature is high. It is usually pink, macular, discrete and non-pruritic, and affects the trunk and limbs, although it can be widespread and involve face, palms and soles.

Generalised lymph node enlargement may be marked, so that the clinician may suspect leukaemia or lymphoma, but histology shows reactive hyperplasia and the nodes regress as the disease subsides. Enlargement of the mesenteric glands may cause abdominal pain. Splenomegaly is moderate. If it persists, the complication of amyloidosis should be considered.

Initially, there may be no joint symptoms, minor arthralgia or definite arthritis. Ultimately, however, most patients develop arthritis affecting the knees, wrists and ankles. Flexor tendon involvement of the hands is common. Involvement of the cervical spine occurs and leads to pain and limitation of movement (Fig. 24.15).

Pericarditis is detected in 7% of patients, but is found in approximately 45% of necropsies. This condition is therefore underdiagnosed in life, as in adult rheumatoid arthritis. Myocarditis may also occur.

Subcutaneous nodules are less common in children than in adults. Interestingly, their histology resembles that of the nodules of rheumatic fever.

Differential diagnosis

The diagnosis remains clinical. Infective causes of fever and arthritis must be excluded. In the first few days, it can be difficult to distinguish systemic juvenile chronic arthritis from a viral infection, but the persistent spiking fever and recurrent maculopapular eruptions, together with a rising white blood count, are helpful. The doctor should be aware of the risks of infection where there is a single involved joint. In the past, the most difficult differential diagnosis was rheumatic fever, but this is now rare.

Pauciarticular JCA

In pauciarticular JCA, four or less joints are involved in the first three months, and this is by far the commonest mode of presentation. The knee, ankle and elbow are most commonly affected, although involvement of a single finger or toe is also common. There are probably several different patterns of illness, the most common being that seen in younger children. Here, the most serious complication is chronic iridocyclitis, which is either present at the onset or develops within the next year. The iridocyclitis affects both sexes and is associated with antinuclear antibody in the serum. The danger to these children is therefore not from joint involvement, which is usually mild, but from serious eye involvement. Slit lamp examination is therefore mandatory in all children diagnosed as having JCA. The high incidence of an HLA-D determinant, DW5, is further evidence that this is a specific subgroup. Children that present in their teens often have the early features of ankylosing spondylitis.

Polyarticular-onset JCA

Polyarthritis (defined as involvement of five or more joints) can develop at any time in childhood. Females and older children are predominantly affected. Patients are usually seronegative; however, 10% have persistent IgM rheumatoid factor, tend to be older (over 10 years) and have a slightly different prognosis and distribution of joint involvement. They often progress to severe RA.

Clinical features

The disease may begin acutely or insidiously. The most commonly involved joints are the knees, the wrists and the ankles, with relative sparing of the metatarsophalangeal joints. There is flexor tenosynovitis of the hands, neck involvement is seen early and lymphadenopathy may be present. Although there may be an occasional spike of fever, the marked spiking of systemic illness is absent. When IgM rheumatoid factor is present, joint involvement has a clinical appearance and course indistinguishable from adult rheumatoid arthritis – that is, polyarticular, peripheral and symmetrical. Large joints may be involved,

Fig. 24.15 Juvenile arthritis; X-ray of cervical spine showing fusion of upper two cervical vertebrae.

but usually in association with small joint involvement. Systemic features are similar to those of the adult disease: nodules occur and the prognosis is poor.

Treatment of JCA

The ultimate prognosis is favourable. Around 80% are able to lead useful independent lives, although one-third may require anti-inflammatory drugs to control pain, and up to 10% die from infection or chronic renal disease secondary to amyloidosis.

The aim of treatment is to achieve a state in which the child lives at home with minimal residual joint deformity. A successful outcome depends on two main factors: support from the child's family who must understand the aims of treatment; and liaison between the general practitioner and hospital, social and educational services. Drugs form only part of the treatment.

Daily exercises are important. Bed rest is indicated only in children with severe systemic features because it can result in muscle wasting and joint ankylosis. Weight-bearing is restricted only if there is severe pain or a flexion deformity which requires serial splinting. Hip and knee flexion is discouraged by daily periods of lying prone. Night splints are used during the acute phase, to rest the joints in a good position.

Aspirin usually controls the fever and is the drug of choice. It is given at approximately 90 mg/kg of body weight per day in divided doses. This produces a blood salicylate level of about 25 mg/100 ml. Young children rarely complain of tinnitus or deafness and it is important to monitor the blood level and look for signs of toxicity (overbreathing, drowsiness or vomiting). In view of the association with Reye's syndrome, a NSAID such as naprosyn is often used. If the disease progresses, gold or penicillamine can be given. There are few indications for using corticosteroids; they do not influence the ultimate prognosis or prevent complications, and can cause alarming iatrogenic effects which cannot be justified in a disease with a good prognosis. They are, however, indicated in severe systemic disease, chronic iridocyclitis that does not respond to local steroids, and progressive disease that is resistant to other drugs. Alternate day dosage is preferred; this allows for some skeletal growth and does not suppress growth spurts, sexual maturation or reaction to stress. Surgery is restricted to synovectomy in children old enough to cooperate with postoperative physiotherapy. Correction of joint deformities, or joint replacement, is carried out in adolescence or adult life after growth has ceased.

ADULT STILL'S DISEASE

Adult Still's disease is a distinct entity, almost exclusively affecting young adult females. Characteristically, it is a flitting polyarthritis with a similar distribution to that encountered in the childhood variety. Systemic features are also similar. The fever, which usually responds to salicylates, may sometimes be prolonged, requiring treatment with corticosteroids. A meticulous search for sources of sepsis must be made before embarking on steroid therapy. Recurrences are frequent. Usually, the arthritis resolves without residua and crippling deformity is very rare. Synovial histology is non-specific and rheumatoid factor tests are negative.

RHEUMATIC FEVER

Rheumatic fever was at one time the commonest cause of acute polyarthritis in childhood, but has been declining in incidence for many years. It is seldom seen before 4 years of age; the peak age for first attacks is around 6 years and they are rare after 15 years. The sexes are equally affected. Rheumatic fever starts one to five weeks after a throat infection with a group A β-haemolytic streptococcus.

Clinical features

Articular symptoms

Arthritis is the most common major manifestation and is usually the presenting symptom. Joint involvement may vary from arthralgia, where patients have acutely painful and tender joints with little objective signs of inflammation, to an acute arthritis with effusion and involvement of pericapsular structures. The overlying skin is hot and red. Carditis is frequent and severe in the younger child, while arthritis is frequent and severe in the adolescent and adult.

The onset of arthritis is typically acute and polyarticular, affecting mainly the knees (75%) and ankles (50%), and occasionally the wrists and elbows. In contrast to RA, involvement of the small joints of the hands (8%) and feet (15%) is uncommon. The older the child, the smaller the joints involved. Historically, the arthritis of rheumatic fever was described as 'migratory' or 'flitting', conveying the erroneous impression that, as the inflammation flits from one joint to another, the joint involved earlier may revert to normal. In practice, particularly if untreated, many joints may remain actively involved at the same time, and give the appearance of a symmetrical polyarthritis.

Symptoms of a throat infection may be so mild as to have passed unnoticed. A preceding streptococcal infection can be demonstrated by a rising antistreptolysin 0 titre (greater than 250 units for adults; greater than 333 for children), and lack of evidence of recent streptococcal infection makes the diagnosis less likely. A leucocytosis is common, and a raised ESR is invariable unless cardiac failure is present.

Systemic symptoms

Systemic symptoms are prominent but non-specific. Fever usually starts at the onset of joint involvement, is usually high (up to 40°C) and sustained. It is accompanied by sweating, anorexia, malaise and vomiting, all of which could also result from salicylate therapy. When abdominal pain occurs with nausea and vomiting, it is usually caused by mesenteric adenitis and may simulate an acute abdomen. The subcutaneous nodules of rheumatic fever, like those of RA, occur at pressure points – elbows, knees and the soles of the feet – but (unlike RA) they occur early in the course of the disease, are smaller and more numerous, and tend to last for a shorter period. Histologically, they are distinguishable from those of seropositive rheumatoid arthritis by the lack of necrosis and palisade layer. Nodules are more numerous in patients with rheumatic carditis.

Erythema marginatum

Erythema marginatum is strongly suggestive of, but not entirely specific for, rheumatic fever and occurs in only a small proportion of patients. It is a fleeting, non-pruritic, pink or red, macular or papular rash which extends centrifugally (in contrast to fixed drug eruptions) to become circinate or leaf-like while fading at the centre. It occurs most frequently in children, in association with carditis and subcutaneous nodules, and is most apparent at the height of the fever. It mainly affects the trunk, and less frequently the proximal parts of the limbs, but never the face. (Note that in SLE and adult Still's disease, the face is involved.)

The appearance of signs and symptoms and ECG evidence suggestive of carditis (p. 427) in the presence of a rash and fever are strongly suggestive of rheumatic fever. The difficulty in establishing a diagnosis has led to the development of diagnostic criteria (Table 24.19).

Table 24.19 Criteria for diagnosis of rheumatic fever*

Major manifestations	Minor manifestations
• Carditis	• Fever
• Polyarthritis	• Arthralgia
• Chorea	• Previous rheumatic fever or rheumatic heart disease
• Erythema marginatum	• Elevated ESR or CRP
• Subcutaneous nodules	• Prolonged PR interval

* These criteria are a revised version of the Jones critiera. Diagnosis is based on one major and two minor criteria plus supporting evidence of preceding streptococcal infection.

Treatment

Complete bed-rest is important to minimise cardiac work and rest painful joints. Penicillin should be given to eradicate any streptococci. Fever and joint pain can be controlled with salicylates. Although the initial response to salicylates (in adequate dosage) and corticosteroids can be equally dramatic in RA and Still's disease, the response to salicylate in rheumatic fever seems to be more complete and longer lasting. With clinical improvement, all but pencillin should be withdrawn slowly and activities gradually increased. In severe carditis, steroids will often prevent or resolve cardiac failure. Neither steroids nor salicylates have any other effect on the disease, on the likelihood of recurrences, or on the final cardiac state.

ANAPHYLACTOID (HENOCH-SCHÖNLEIN) PURPURA

Anaphylactoid purpura is due to a widespread vasculitis involving arterioles and small capillaries. It can occur at any age, but primarily in children, especially boys. The disease occurs most often in the spring, and usually follows an upper respiratory tract infection. The onset is acute, with fever, headache and rash. Initially, macules or urticarial papules occur on the buttocks and the extensor aspects of the limbs. These become flat, purpuric, and may coalesce or even ulcerate. Localised oedema of the face, scalp, hands and feet occurs; in young children, it can mimic arthritis. Haemorrhage into the gut wall can cause colic, melaena or haematemesis.

Usually the joint involvement is mild, consisting of transient, non-migratory synovitis with synovial swelling, pain and stiffness, typically affecting more than one joint. The ankles, knees, hips, wrists and elbows are usually affected, with a tendency to lower limb involvement. The synovial fluid is inflammatory in character. Joint destruction does not occur.

A mild focal glomerulonephritis (p. 821), producing proteinuria and microscopic haematuria, occurs in 50% of cases. Occasionally, it progresses to the nephrotic syndrome and, very rarely, to renal failure. Renal biopsy shows deposits of IgA and C3, suggesting an immune complex aetiology, probably following viral or bacterial infection. The disease usually settles in 4–6 weeks without sequelae, but may recur.

CRYSTAL SYNOVITIS

The association between crystals and joint disease has been recognised since the 17th century, when Leeuwenhoek identified crystals in patients with gout. In the 19th century, Garrod suspected a relationship between urate crystals and symptoms, and in the latter part of that century Swiss workers Hiss and Freudeiler described the inflammatory response that occurs after an injection of urate crystals. These studies were forgotten, however, and it was only in the 1960s that the importance of crystal-induced inflammation was realised; the mechanisms were partly elucidated only recently.

GOUT

Gout is the principle clinical manifestation of sustained hyperuricaemia. Clinical features include acute arthritis (tenosynovitis, bursitis), tophaceous deposits, renal disease and urolithiasis.

Epidemiology

Gout occurs mainly in developed countries, with a prevalence in the UK and USA of 0.3%. The prevalence of hyperuricaemia is about 5%. Men are ten times more likely to have gout than women. At puberty, male blood uric acid levels rise and remain higher than those of females until the menopause, when female uric acid levels also rise. Gout is very uncommon before puberty, when it usually suggests an enzyme defect.

Serum uric acid concentrations are related to a number of demographic factors, the most important being age, sex, body bulk and genetic constitution (Fig. 24.16). Values are higher in urban than in rural communities and are positively correlated with social class, weight and a high protein diet. Values are distributed in a population as a continuous variable, with a skew towards the higher values. Hyperuricaemia can be defined as the mean plus two standard deviations, which gives values of above 0.42 mmol/litre in adult males and above 0.36 mmol/litre in adult females.

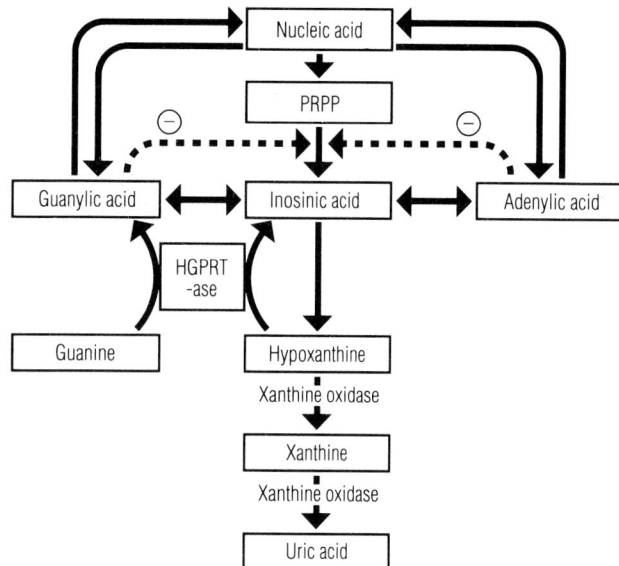

Fig. 24.17 A simplified diagram of some of the metabolic pathways involved in the formation of uric acid. PRPP = phosphoribosyl pyrophosphate. HGPRT-ase = hypoxanthine-guanine-phosphoribosyl transferase.

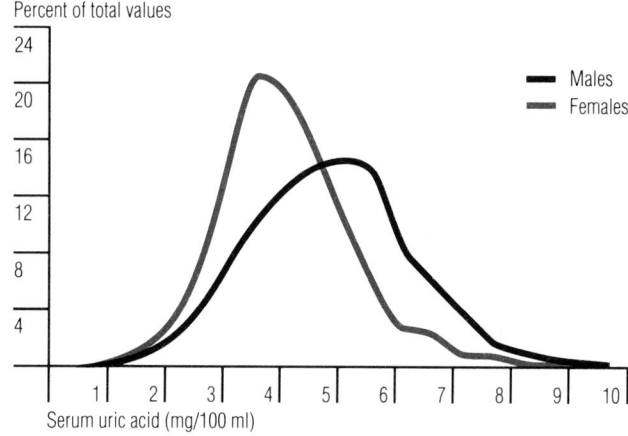

A Serum uric acid (mg/100 ml)

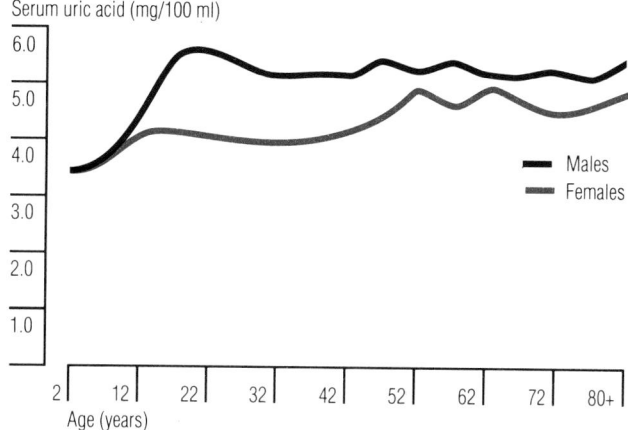

B Age (years)

Fig. 24.16 Age and sex distribution of serum uric acid levels. A. Distribution of serum uric acid levels by age in males and females after the age of six. B. The mean serum uric acid levels in males and females for different age groups.

Uric acid production and disposal

Uric acid is derived from the breakdown of purine bases (Fig. 24.17). These are the products of essential nucleotides which are synthesised in the liver. Adenine and guanine are re-utilised. About 60% of uric acid is replaced daily; the quantity produced is directly proportional to body size. Less than 10% comes from preformed dietary nucleotides.

Seventy-five per cent of uric acid is excreted in the kidneys and the remainder is lost in the gut. The uric acid is freely filtered at the glomerulus and 90% is then resorbed. Renal handling of uric acid involves glomerular filtration, proximal tubular reabsorption, tubular secretion, and post-secretory reabsorption. The paradoxical effects of high and low dose aspirin on uric acid excretion can be explained by differential effects on active secretion and reabsorption.

Uric acid circulates as monosodium urate, but is found mainly as the free acid in the urine. In hyperuricaemia, urate is usually present in the blood as a supersaturated solution. Lowering of the pH lessens the solubility and increases the likelihood of crystal formation. A number of laboratories use a colorimetric assay to measure uric acid, but some drugs and reducing substances can interfere to give falsely high values. A more specific enzymatic (uricase) spectrophometric assay is available.

Causes of hyperuricaemia

Diuretic drugs are the main cause of hyperuricaemia, accounting for some 60% of cases, but clinical gout is an uncommon association. Hyperuricaemia occurs with renal failure, but here too gout is surprisingly rare. Other genetic and environmental factors lead to hyperuricaemia by decreasing the excretion, or by increasing the production, of uric acid (Table 24.20). There are many biochemical or physiological derangements that may cause hyperuricaemia in an individual patient. In the majority, however,

Connective Tissue Disease

Table 24.20   Causes of hyperuricaemia

Increased production of uric acid

Increased purine synthesis
  Hypoxanthine guanine phosphoribosyl transferase deficiency
  Phosphoribosyl pyrophosphate synthetase overactivity

Increased turnover of preformed purines
  Lymphoproliferative and myeloproliferative disorders
  Secondary polycythaemia
  Chronic haemolytic anaemia
  Severe psoriasis
  Carcinomatosis

Decreased renal excretion of uric acid

Chronic renal disease

Drug administration
  Diuretics
  Salicylates (low dosage)
  Pyrazinamide

Reduction in fractional urate clearance
  Increased levels of organic acids (exercise, starvation, alcohol, ketoacidosis)
  Hypertension
  Hyperparathyroidism
  Hypothyroidism

although there is often a family history, no definite cause can be found.

The typical gouty patient is obese, eats well and drinks more alcohol than average. Dietary purines have only a modest effect on plasma urate levels and avoidance will lead to a fall of uric acid of some 1 mg/100 ml. Short-term alteration in diet, such as starvation and ingestion of large amounts of alcohol, may cause hyperuricaemia by reducing renal clearance of uric acid due to increased lactic acid production, which competes with uric acid excretion in the kidney.

In only 10-15% of patients is gout due to overproduction of uric acid. These patients can be detected by measuring the excretion of uric acid on a 70 g protein, purine-free diet. Overproducers excrete more than 3.6 mmol/24 hours (600 mg/24 hours).

Gout and hyperuricaemia are often associated with obesity, type IV hyperlipoproteinaemia, impaired glucose tolerance, hypertension and ischaemic heart disease.

Hyperuricaemia may occur when large quantities of nucleoprotein are broken down during treatment of leukaemia or lymphoma, and prophylactic therapy is sometimes given to avoid the risk of urate nephropathy (Ch. 21, p. 823).

Enzyme defects may, rarely, cause overproduction of uric acid. Hypoxanthine-guanine phosphoribosyl transferase deficiency is associated with accelerated purine synthesis, childhood gout and renal stones. Complete deficiency is a rare, X-linked, inborn error of metabolism in which gout is associated with spasticity, a variable degree of mental deficiency and a compulsive self-mutilation (the Lesch-Nyhan syndrome).

Phosphoribosyl pyrophosphate synthetase overactivity is another X-linked inborn error of metabolism associated with gout and increased purine synthesis.

Many drugs affect renal elimination of uric acid. For example, aspirin reduces clearance at low doses but is uricosuric at high doses. Other drugs reducing clearance include diuretics (except amiloride and spironolactone), pyrazinamide and ethambutol. Lead also reduces clearance, and causes saturnine gout.

Pathology

Prolonged hyperuricaemia leads to the formation of small crystal aggregates. These accumulate in the synovium and at external sites, such as the ear, cartilage and olecranon, and may eventually become visible tophi. Crystal deposition may proceed over several years without symptoms. Uric acid and urate deposition in the kidney can lead to a variety of pathological effects, including interstitial nephritis, renal stones and acute tubular damage (Ch. 21, p. 823).

Joint inflammation is the result of uptake of crystals by polymorphonuclear leucocytes. When crystals are phagocytosed they enter an endocyte vacuole (phagosome). Fusion with lysosomes occurs and these contain hydrolytic digestive enzymes. There is interaction between the crystals and the phospholipid of the lysosomal membrane, possibly due to the weak acidic groups on the surface of the crystal forming hydrogen bonds. Disruption of the membrane follows, with release of lysosomal enzymes and the crystal. Phagocytosis of urates leads to increased production of lactic acid which causes further precipitation of crystals.

Crystal ingestion stimulates the production of a chemotactic factor producing further recruitment of leucocytes. Hageman factor is activated and this leads to a series of further reactions releasing chemical mediators of inflammation, including kinins. Colchicine has been shown *in vitro* to stabilise the lysosomal membrane, block the release of chemotactic factor and hinder the assembly of intracellular microtubules involved in lysosomal release. These factors are less pronounced in pyrophosphate arthropathy; this is consistent with the relative ineffectiveness of colchicine in this condition.

Clinical features

Classical gout is easily diagnosed. As stated above, the typical patient is obese, young or middle-aged and drinks more alcohol than average. He is usually male, and wakes in the early hours of the morning with severe pain, usually in the big toe. On average, three out of four attacks affect the big toe and one attack in 10 affects more than one joint. Several factors may provoke an attack (Table 24.21).

The affected joint is usually red, swollen and warm. The overlying skin is often shiny, with periarticular oedema, and there is often fever. The joint is extremely painful and tender. Untreated, the attack lasts days or weeks before subsiding spontaneously. Patients may have just one attack,

Table 24.21 Factors provoking an acute attack of gout

- Joint trauma
- Unusual physical exercise
- Alcohol
- High protein diet or starvation
- Surgery
- Drugs
    Diuretics
    Initiation of uricosuric or allopurinol therapy
- Severe incidental illness

or may have recurrences at monthly or yearly intervals. Recurrent attacks may merge into each other, leading to destruction of cartilage, bony erosion (Fig. 24.18) and disability. No synovial joint is immune from gout, but feet, ankles, knees, wrists and fingers are the most susceptible. Bursitis, especially of the elbow, may occur.

Polyarthritis as an initial manifestation of gout is unusual, but when it occurs, it can mimic RA. Similarly, about 5% of patients with pyrophosphate arthropathy have multiple joint involvement with subacute attacks lasting from four weeks to several months. In gout, non-specific symptoms of inflammation, such as morning stiffness and fatigue, are common, and signs include synovial thickening, limitation of joint movement because of inflam-

Fig. 24.18 Gout; X-ray of proximal interphalangeal joint showing erosion with no surrounding osteoporosis.

mation and/or flexion contractures, and elevated ESR. Such cases are often initially diagnosed as RA and, since about 10% have rheumatoid factor present in low titre, diagnosis can prove difficult. The diagnosis of crystal synovitis should be considered in patients whose joints are inflamed sequentially (rather than together as in RA), and when osteophytes are present; diagnosis is proven by the demonstration of crystals in the joint fluid.

Tophi. Recurrent acute attacks of gout leads to asymmetrical, hard swellings, and tophaceous deposits may also occur in periarticular tissues, the cartilage of the ear, bursae and tendon sheaths. Tophi of the elbow may be confused with rheumatoid nodules; they may also arise within Heberden's nodes and may be misdiagnosed. Tophi may also occur at atypical sites (e.g. fingertips), especially in elderly patients receiving diuretics.

Renal calculi. A history suggestive of renal calculi is present in up to 10% of gout patients; this is higher in hot climates. Uric acid calculi may be radiolucent (composed of uric acid alone) or radio-opaque (combined with calcium salts). They are produced by dehydration and excessive purine ingestion, or may be associated with defects in tubular reabsorption of uric acid, or the use of uricosuric drugs. All patients should be instructed in the necessity for a high fluid intake.

Diagnosis and investigation

A number of conditions should be considered in the differential diagnosis of acute and chronic gouty arthritis (Table 24.22). Joint aspiration, serum uric acid measurement and X-rays may be necessary to make the diagnosis, but biopsy will only rarely be performed.

In all cases of suspected gout, details of previous rheumatic symptoms and those of urinary tract calculi should be elicited. The patient's family history should be recorded and serum uric acid measurements made. Synovial fluid should be examined under polarising light for monosodium urate crystals, and possible causes of secondary hyperuricaemia should be investigated.

Serum uric acid measurements. A high serum level of uric acid with a typical history is almost diagnostic of gout. However, a raised serum uric acid alone does not justify the diagnosis of gout, because of the many factors which

Table 24.22 Differential diagnosis of gout

Acute arthritis

Infective arthritis
Another crystal arthritis, e.g. pseudogout due to pyrophosphate crystals, or apatite arthritis
Traumatic arthritis
Rheumatoid arthritis
Seronegative arthritis

Chronic arthritis

Nodular rheumatoid arthritis
Osteoarthritis with Heberden's and Bouchard's nodes
Xanthomatosis

raise the serum level. Although it is usual for the serum uric acid to be elevated in gout, this is not always the case. The plasma urate may be normal because the patient has taken uricosuric anti-inflammatory treatment (salicylates or azapropazone) or because of a recent change in lifestyle.

Polarised light microscopy. Diagnosis can only be made with certainty by demonstrating crystals in joint fluid taken during an attack. In gout, the synovial fluid is turbid, and although other inflammatory joint conditions and sepsis can have similar appearances, the diagnosis is made by the presence of monosodium urate crystals. A wet film should be examined under a compensated polarising microscope. In practice, urate and calcium pyrophosphate are the only two crystals of significance to be identified in synovial fluid. Other crystals which may be seen are cholesterol, and corticosteroid esters after intra-articular therapy. Urates and calcium pyrophosphate can be accurately identified using polarising light, due to differences in their crystal lattice structure. Urate crystals show strong negative birefringence and calcium pyrophosphate weak positive birefringence, when viewed under the compensated polarised light microscope (Fig. 24.4).

Treatment

The treatment of gout has three main aims: to reduce acute synovitis, prevent further crystal formation and identify associated disease.

Reduction of acute synovitis

The first line of treatment of acute synovitis is with a NSAID. Indomethacin is the drug of choice, at a dose of 50 mg four-hourly until the attack subsides. Other anti-inflammatory drugs can be used; azapropazone (standard dose 600 mg twice daily) is both uricosuric and anti-inflammatory.

Colchicine is effective, but has to be taken every two hours until control is achieved. Main side-effects include nausea, vomiting, intestinal colic and diarrhoea. These develop at the time of clinical improvement. Intravenous colchicine is effective, but is not generally used because of the small risk of serious toxicity. If long-term management is to be instituted, then allopurinol or uricosuric drugs should not be started for several weeks, as they may prolong the acute attack or trigger further episodes. Salicylates and diuretics should also be avoided.

Prevention of crystal formation

A single attack of gout does not justify preventive drug treatment. Obese patients should lose weight, alcohol should be reduced and the need for diuretics causing hyperuricaemia should be reconsidered. Indications for long-term therapy include recurrent attacks, tophaceous gout, and renal disease. During the reduction of plasma urate, there is a risk of provoking acute gouty arthritis and therefore prophylactic anti-inflammatory drugs or colchicine should be prescribed concomitantly for the first three months. Successful lowering of plasma urate abol-

ishes the risk of gout and tophi will eventually disappear. If the underlying cause of hyperuricaemia cannot be modified, indefinite hypouricaemic therapy is required. Treatment is aimed at keeping the serum uric acid level below the solubility level (0.45 mmol/l).

Uricosuric drugs (probenecid and sulphinpyrazone) act by blocking the renal tubular transport of uric acid which allows the filtered load to be excreted. Side-effects are uncommon, but include nephrotic syndrome and skin rashes. These drugs are less effective than allopurinol in severe disease, and often ineffective in patients with renal failure. They are best avoided in patients with urolithiasis or purine overproduction, because they do not reduce the risk of nephropathy or stone, and are best reserved for under-excretors of uric acid.

Allopurinol, a xanthine oxidase inhibitor, reduces the oxidation of hypoxanthine to xanthine, and of xanthine to uric acid (Fig. 24.17). The more soluble xanthine is excreted. Indications for this drug include extensive tophaceous gout, renal impairment, hyperuricaemia due to antimitotic drug therapy and intolerance or failure of response to uricosuric therapy. Side-effects are few, and include dyspepsia and skin rash. Therapy is usually for life.

Asymptomatic hyperuricaemia

Provided blood pressure, weight and renal function remain normal no therapy is required for asymptomatic hyperuricaemia. Some authorities recommend treatment if the serum uric acid is consistently above 9 mg/100 ml.

PYROPHOSPHATE ARTHROPATHY (CALCIUM PYROPHOSPHATE DIHYDRATE DEPOSITION DISEASE)

Crystals of calcium pyrophosphate dihydrate were first found by chance in joint fluid from patients with acute arthritis by McCarty and Hollander in 1961. At about the same time, Zitnan and Sit'aj from Czechoslovakia described a 'new' rheumatic disorder which they called 'chondrocalcinosis articularis'. These patients had articular calcification, and developed an acute inflammatory arthritis which usually started in the third or fourth decade. Repeated episodes led to degenerative changes. These authors were describing the same clinical syndrome; *pyrophosphate arthropathy* is now used to describe the clinical presentation of acute and chronic arthritis, whereas *chondrocalcinosis* refers to the radiological appearance due to the deposition of calcium pyrophosphate crystals in cartilage. Fibrocartilage is most commonly involved, especially the menisci of the knee, but articular hyaline cartilage also calcifies as do other articular structures, including ligaments and joint capsules. This leads to a degenerative arthropathy which usually affects old people, but can occur earlier in life if there is a strong family history.

Aetiology

The pathogenesis of both the chronic crystal deposition

and acute arthritis (*pseudogout*) are improperly understood. Acute attacks of arthritis are precipitated by shedding of crystals from preformed deposits in cartilage into the joint cavity. The mechanism leading to the formation of these deposits is unknown. Present evidence suggests a local articular, rather than a systemic metabolic, disturbance of pyrophosphate metabolism.

A large number of other conditions have been associated with calcium pyrophosphate deposition, including diabetes mellitus, hypertension, hypothyroidism and hyperuricaemia. Not all are necessarily of aetiological significance, because patients are often elderly and multiple diseases might be expected to be present. However, 7% of patients prove to have hyperparathyroidism, and pyrophosphate deposition also occurs in haemochromatosis and Wilson's disease.

Clinical features and diagnosis

Pyrophosphate arthropathy may present as an acute arthritis affecting particularly the knees and wrists, which resolves within 1–4 weeks. Trauma, surgery or medical illnesses may precipitate an attack. Less frequently, rheumatoid arthritis may be mimicked as there may be multiple joint involvement and associated joint inflammation.

Pyrophosphate deposition may present as asymptomatic chrondrocalcinosis and is a common finding in the elderly. Common sites of chrondrocalcinosis include pubic symphysis, triangular ligament of the wrist and knee menisci. Deposition may also be seen with severe generalised osteoarthritis. There may, or may not, be inflammatory exacerbations. The knees are most frequently affected, and hips, shoulders, elbows, ankles and wrists may also be involved.

The diagnosis is made on the basis of clinical features, chondrocalcinosis on X-ray and demonstration of crystals by polarising microscopy of synovial fluid from an involved joint (Fig. 24.4).

Treatment

Primary metabolic disorders should be identified and treated appropriately. Treatment of an acute attack of pyrophosphate arthropathy is similar to that for acute gout, although drugs are less effective; joint aspiration together with the injection of corticosteroid gives relief.

Unfortunately, there is no effective means of preventing further attacks of pyrophosphate arthropathy, although colchicine may sometimes prove helpful. Management is that of osteoarthritis, with analgesics, physiotherapy and local measures when appropriate.

SYSTEMIC LUPUS ERYTHEMATOSUS

Systemic lupus erythematosus (SLE) is a disease of unknown aetiology, which affects predominantly young women, and has a marked tendency to exacerbation and remission. The diverse clinical features reflect the multisystem involvement which is characteristic of the disease.

SLE represents a spectrum of disease which at one end can be entirely cutaneous. The skin changes of lupus were first recognised in the nineteenth century, and in 1872, Kaposi emphasised the serious systemic aspects of the disease. As is often the case with a 'new' disease, the first review in 1935 by Baehr, Klemperer and Schifrin described fatal cases. With the discovery of the LE cell in 1948 by Hargraves, Richmond and Morton, and the description of various antinuclear antibodies by Kunkel et al in 1960, it became possible to develop sensitive diagnositic criteria. It then became apparent that the disease was neither particularly rare, nor inexorably fatal.

Currently, there is much interest in the possibility that the disease may arise from an interaction of genetic factors and viral infection. The high prevalence of SLE in women of reproductive age suggests that female hormones may modify the immune response. There are a number of haematological and serological abnormalities, of which the key one is the formation of antinuclear antibodies. The use of DNA-antibody and complement estimations has improved the clinical management of SLE patients and led to a greater understanding of their role in immune-complex-mediated tissue damage.

Epidemiology

The prevalence of SLE appears to vary from country to country; in the UK, it is about one per 10 000 of the population. Females are affected 6–9 times more frequently than males, and the disease is especially common during the childbearing years. Blacks and Chinese are particularly susceptible; in the USA one in 250 blacks of childbearing age may be affected.

There is an increased prevalence of SLE in the families of patients with the disease, and the incidence of antinuclear antibodies, hypergammaglobulinaemia and false positive serological tests for syphilis are also increased in healthy members of these families. There may therefore be a genetically determined susceptibility to the development of SLE in appropriate environmental circumstances in some individuals. A null or absent allele for C4 on the sixth chromosome has been noted in family studies, and twin studies show a greater than 60% concordance of SLE in monozygotic twins.

Pathology

Many of the histological changes are non-specific. Two findings suggestive of SLE are the periarteriolar or onion-skin fibrosis in the spleen, and the haematoxylin body – the tissue counterpart of the LE cell. There is usually widespread small and medium vessel vasculitis, portions of the walls of which may become necrotic and be found to contain fibrinoid deposits. These deposits contain immune complexes consisting chiefly of DNA, anti-DNA antibody and complement components.

Immunological features of SLE

LE cells

The LE cell factor is an IgG antibody to native DNA histone. LE cell formation is an *in vitro* event, although the haemotoxylin body in tissue sections is a related phenomenon. The LE cell test is best performed in two stages. Firstly, the antibody is incubated with a source of dead cell nuclei which allows it to bind to the nucleoprotein. Secondly, living polymorphs are added; in the presence of complement, these phagocytose the nuclei with fixed antibody. Lysosomal enzymes react on the nucleus causing denaturation of proteins, with swelling, loss of chromatin pattern and change in staining properties. The preparation is then stained, and examined under the microscope, where the LE cells are seen as polymorphs containing a large, homogenous purplish-staining inclusion.

The test is positive in up to 75% of SLE patients. Positive, though weak, reactions are found in a number of other conditions, particularly rheumatoid arthritis, Sjøgren's disease, chronic active hepatitis and other connective tissue diseases. This test is time-consuming and is more specific, but less sensitive, than that for antinuclear antibodies (ANAs).

Antinuclear antibodies

Antinuclear antibodies (ANAs) are a constant feature of SLE and are directed at different antigenic components. The demonstration of ANAs, by immunofluorescence, provides the most widely used screening test for SLE. The test is very sensitive but is negative in about 5% of patients (uraemia may render an ANA result negative). However, positive tests are found in many other conditions. A frozen tissue section is incubated with the test serum to allow antibodies to fix, washed thoroughly to remove any unfixed antibodies and then stained with a fluorescent antibody to human globulin. This will bind to any fixed antibody. The tissue is then examined using an ultraviolet microscope. Sometimes, the pattern of nuclear staining gives a clue to the antigen involved (e.g. chromatin pattern staining is associated with antibody to nucleoprotein) and carry some diagnostic significance; for example the rim (or ring) staining patterns represent antibodies to double-stranded DNA and are thus more specific for SLE.

In 1957, a number of groups reported findings of antibodies against native (double-stranded) DNA in the serum of patients with SLE. It later became apparent that the antibodies were a heterogenous group, binding to a variety of sites on the DNA molecule. Antibodies against native DNA were found to be almost always specific for SLE. The measurement of DNA antibodies by immunoassay has proved a major advance in the management of SLE. Problems remain in standardisation of the DNA and in the exclusion of denatured DNA fragments or strands. In the majority of patients with SLE, fluctuations in DNA-binding parallel clinical activity. It may rise before a clinical exacerbation becomes apparent. In diseases such as Sjøgren's syndrome, rheumatoid arthritis and sclero-

derma, where positive ANA tests are common, DNA antibodies are usually absent or in low titre. The methods used to detect these antibodies include:

1. *Farr technique (DNA-binding test)*. The serum containing antibodies is mixed with a preparation of radiolabelled DNA, and the immune complexes so formed precipitated with 50% ammonium sulphate. The radioactivity in supernate and precipitate is then measured, and a formula used to calculate the DNA-binding value (expressed as a percentage). ELISA anti-DNA antibody assays are now widely available and distinguish IgG, IgM and IgA isotypes.
2. *Counter-immune electrophoresis*. This is a sensitive and rapid test for precipitating antibodies to DNA. It is not quantitative.
3. *Crithidia-immunofluorescence test*. Trypanosomes have nuclei which do not contain nucleohistone and also have a large kinetoplast containing a high concentration of ds-DNA. This has been found useful in the diagnosis of SLE. Species of *Crithidia* which are not pathogenic for man are grown easily in rats. A film of these, treated with a serum containing DNA antibodies and then stained with fluorosceinated anti-human gammaglobulin, gives a strong staining of the kinetoplasts. This is a reliable screening test for antibodies to ds-DNA.

RNA antibodies

Antibodies to both single-stranded and double-stranded RNA can be detected in SLE by a variety of techniques. The occurrence of antibodies to double-stranded RNA is interesting, as human RNA is single-stranded with the exception of small helical regions on transfer RNA. Some viral RNA, on the other hand, is double-stranded and this finding has stimulated speculation on the possibility of a viral aetiology in this disorder.

Serological tests for syphilis

False positive tests for syphilis are found in up to one-third of SLE patients. Rarely, a positive TPI test occurs; this is probably caused by antibody reacting against the DNA in the treponeme.

Other auto-antibodies in SLE

Table 24.23 demonstrates the wide variety of antibodies that occur, the pattern varying from patient to patient. They appear to reflect a general immunological disturbance, which results in an exaggerated production of humoral antibodies. Sometimes, the antibodies precede the clinical manifestations of SLE by years. They only rarely give rise to clinical abnormalities, although antibodies to platelets, red cells, leucocytes and clotting factors may cause haematological disorders. Patients may also have serum antibodies which are apparently lymphocytotoxic.

Clinical subsets of SLE have been defined by antibody typing, as certain antibodies appear to be associated with

Table 24.23 Immunological features in SLE

Antinuclear antibodies

Anti-DNA histone (LE cell)
Anti-DNA (double-stranded)
Anti-DNA (single-stranded)
Anti-RNA
Anti-nucleoprotein (soluble or particulate)
Antinuclear glycoprotein (Sm antigen)
Anti-extractable nuclear antigen (ENA)

Other antibodies

Anti-cytoplasmic antibodies (mitochondrial and microsomal)
Rheumatoid factors (IgG and IgM – 33% of cases)
Cryoglobulins
Lymphocytotoxic antibodies
Anti-phospholipid (cardiolipin, lupus anticoagulant)
Organ-specific auto-antibodies
Elevated titres of anti-viral antibodies (e.g. measles)
Antibodies against: red cells
        lymphocytes
        leucocytes
        platelets

Low complement level (C3, C4)

specific clinical features. Anti-Ro antibodies are associated with the development of congenital heart block in the offspring of SLE patients. Anti-phospholipid (cardiolipin) antibodies are responsible for the false positive VDRL and the circulating lupus anticoagulant, and are associated with an increased thrombotic tendency and a high incidence of recurrent abortion. Patients with raised serum anti-cardiolipin may also have thrombocytopenia, livedo reticularis, neurological disorders other than stroke, and aortic and mitral valve disease. Although the anti-phospholipid syndrome may be related to SLE and other autoimmune diseases, it may also exist as a distinct entity.

Serum complement

The serum complement level (either total haemolytic complement, or C3 or C4) is a useful investigation in SLE. Low complement levels in the presence of a high DNA binding titre is diagnostic of active SLE. Serial measurements of complement are useful in following the clinical course, as the level drops about 50% before, and remains low during, an exacerbation. Particularly low levels of complement components, especially C3 and C4, are strongly indicative of active lupus nephritis, during which complement is continuously consumed by the immune complexes deposited in the glomeruli.

Individuals with a genetic deficiency of C2 appear to have an increased incidence of SLE. SLE is not associated with any particular HLA antigen, but associations have been described with HLA-B8, DR2 and DR3.

Aetiology

The aetiology of SLE is unknown. There is some evidence for a viral aetiology, including the following:

1. Inclusion bodies with some resemblance to viral material have been found in SLE, although this is not a consistent or specific finding.
2. Antibodies to some viruses are raised, although this parallels the general hyperglobulinaemia.
3. Antinuclear antibodies may represent a response to viral material.
4. Murine viral antigens have been shown on human SLE lymphocytes.
5. In animal models, oncorna viruses have been implicated as causative agents.
6. Antibodies to oncorna viruses will stain the renal deposits of human SLE in a fluorescent antibody test.

Animal models

A strain of mice known as New Zealand Black/New Zealand White Fl hybrid develop a lupus-like disease. They develop antinuclear antibodies, some of which are directed against ds-DNA, develop an immune complex nephritis and die of progressive renal failure. In addition, there is lymphadenopathy, splenomegaly, leucopenia and changes resembling Sjøgren's syndrome. The immune complexes in the kidney can be shown to contain DNA and various oncorna virus antigens. NZB/NZW Fl mice, like many other mouse strains, show persistent infection with an oncorna virus, which is transmitted vertically. The aetiological importance of this virus infection in murine lupus is still not fully established, since many strains of mice who carry oncorna viruses do not get lupus though they may develop leukaemia. All these findings point to a viral aetiology, but no oncorna virus has been isolated in human SLE. The disease is more severe in females, and can be partially reversed by testosterone. Immunosuppression selective for T cells (such as with cyclosporin A) also reduces severity.

Pathogenesis

There is considerable evidence that the lesions of SLE are due to immune complexes causing local damage. Immune complexes can be detected free in the serum, and precipitated in the kidneys on the mesangium and glomerular basement membrane. These would be expected to fix complement, and complement breakdown products (e.g. C3d) are present in the serum. Patients possessing anti-DNA antibodies and entering a relapse will have free circulating DNA, and must therefore go through a stage where immune complexes form. At this stage, the serum complement levels fall. DNA itself will bind to glomerular basement membrane, and this membrane-bound DNA can react with antibody and complement to give a nephrotoxic type of damage.

Clinical features

The clinical features of SLE are extremely variable both in nature and severity. An exacerbation may be precipitated by exposure to sunlight, an infection, drugs or pregnancy. Common initial features are general malaise, with fever, fatigue and loss of weight. SLE presents in the majority of patients with articular or cutaneous features.

Table 24.24 shows the relative incidence of some of the major clinical features.

Table 24.24 Relative incidence of the major clinical manifestations of SLE*

Manifestations	Incidence (%)
Musculoarticular	95
Cutaneous	81
Fever	77
Neuropsychiatric	59
Renal	53
Pulmonary	48
Cardiac	38

* After Estes D and Christian CL 1971 Medicine 50; 85.

Musculoskeletal features

The commonest musculoskeletal complaint is of joint or muscle pains, occasionally presenting years before other features become obvious; the pain often appears out of proportion to the degree of synovitis. The small joints are most commonly involved and the arthritis is symmetrical. Erosions are rare. Occasionally, a patient develops a deforming arthritis, as a result of capsular and ligamentous laxity. Tendon involvement may be prominent, leading in some cases to flexion contractures at the forearm and wrist. Haemolytic complement activity may be decreased in synovial effusion fluid as in rheumatoid arthritis, suggesting the presence of immune complexes in affected joints. A proximal myopathy occurs in 5% of patients; this differs from steroid myopathy in that the shoulder girdle is more commonly involved and the serum muscle enzymes are usually elevated. True myositis occurs in 5% of SLE patients. Aseptic necrosis affecting the weight-bearing joints occurs in patients who have been receiving high doses of corticosteroids for long-standing SLE.

Skin manifestations

The skin lesions appear most often on sun-exposed areas. The classical eruption is the 'butterfly' rash, an erythematous eruption over the nose, spreading to the cheeks. It occurs in less than half of all patients. Discoid lupus erythematosus is characterised by erythema, scaling and scarring, and keratin plugging of hair follicles is often a feature. Telangiectasia and minute areas of purpura may be seen on the atrophic scars. The scalp is frequently involved in patients with cutaneous LE, producing patches of permanent alopecia. Photosensitivity is particuarly common in patients with anti-Ro. Livedo reticularis, a reticular blotchy pattern especially common on the lower extremities, is often associated with anticardiolipin

antibodies. Diffuse alopecia occurs in about 60% of patients and is an important sign of active systemic disease. The hair tends to regrow when the disease enters a remission. Erythema, telangiectasia and capillary infarcts in the proximal nail folds are often seen. Chilblain-like purplish-red swellings on the digits, and vasculitic lesions which can ulcerate, also reflect involvement of the cutaneous vasculature.

Skin biopsy can be helpful in diagnosis; immunoglobulin and complement being demonstrated at the dermal epidermal junction both in discoid lesions and generally in SLE, including unaffected skin.

Purpura may occur, usually associated with thrombocytopenia. Mucosal ulcers, affecting mouth and genitalia, occur in active SLE but settle in remission, unlike skin lesions which may persist.

Cardiovascular features

Pericarditis frequently occurs during acute exacerbations of the disease and is best detected by echocardiography. Myocardial disease is common in SLE, and may lead to arrythmias and, uncommonly, to cardiac failure. Hypertension occurs following severe renal involvement. A non-infective endocarditis occurs (Libman-Sacks endocarditis); this most commonly affects the mitral valve and is usually clinically insignificant. Murmurs are frequently heard in SLE, often in the absence of any anatomical proof of endocarditis, and are an unreliable guide to its diagnosis.

A vasculitis may produce scleritis, myocardial infarction, Raynaud's phenomenon, digital ulceration and atrophic skin changes, bowel perforation and chronic leg ulceration. Thrombophlebitis also occurs, and may be recurrent or migratory.

Respiratory system

Pleurisy is common and usually bilateral, and pleuritic pain may remain a problem long after all other evidence of disease activity has regressed. LE cells may be present in pleural fluid and complement levels decreased. Recurrent pneumonitis may occur, with scanty physical signs but with radiological evidence of patchy, plate-like atelectasis or diffuse basal infiltration. Loss of lung volume from vascular damage leads to gradual elevation of both hemidiaphragms and restrictive lung defects. The diaphragm may also be affected by a myopathy. Acute pulmonary lesions are responsive to steroid therapy. Bacterial pneumonia is common. Pulmonary function tests may be abnormal in the absence of clinical symptoms.

Renal system

Sixty per cent of patients have renal involvement, and its extent and severity significantly affect the patient's prognosis. According to current concepts of immune complex disease, renal involvement probably occurs transiently in the majority of cases. Mesangial deposition of immunoglobulin may be a reversible change. Diffuse proliferative glomerulonephritis often leads to nephrotic syndrome, hypertension and uraemia and the mortality is greater than 60% at three years. Patients with the membranous form of nephritis almost all develop the nephrotic syndrome, but hypertension and uraemia are less frequent.

Nervous system

The importance of neuropsychiatric involvement in SLE has recently become apparent, because of both its prevalence and its association with a poorer prognosis than renal disease. The commonest abnormalities are disorders of mental function and seizures; other manifestations include cranial nerve palsies, chorea, tremor, headache.

In the absence of frank psychosis, patients with SLE may have personality problems and difficulties in holding down a job or maintaining personal relationships; marital breakdown is quite common. Corticosteroid therapy is sometimes blamed for the psychotic changes, but they also occur in patients not on treatment and may improve when the activity of SLE is controlled by steroids. Very large doses, up to 100 mg/day, are sometimes needed to control CNS involvement.

CNS involvement is most frequent in well-established cases of lupus, and 50% of patients with renal involvement also have some CNS abnormality. The CNS symptoms are likely to be the result of small vessel vasculitis in the CNS. Immunoglobulin deposits in the choroid plexus and depression of CSF complement (C4) levels have been reported. Peripheral neuropathy may occur and is probably due to vasculitis.

Haematological features

Neutropenia and/or absolute lymphocytopenia is a frequent finding. An autoimmune haemolytic anaemia may antedate the other manifestations of the disease by many years. This responds well to corticosteroids but not to splenectomy. The normochromic anaemia of chronic disease, and the hypochromic anaemia that may accompany drug therapy or bleeding from vasculitis lesions, are more frequent causes of anaemia in SLE than are immune mechanisms.

A low platelet count, with or without demonstrable platelet antibodies, is common and may be sufficiently low to cause all the signs and symptoms of idiopathic thrombocytopenic purpura. Response to splenectomy is good. Lymphadenopathy is common; the pathological changes are those of reactive hyperplasia. Splenomegaly is rarely gross.

Bacterial infection occurs frequently in SLE, and infections with opportunistic organisms are more common in patients on suppressive therapy.

Syndromes related to SLE

Discoid lupus erythematosus

Discoid lupus erythematosus is a chronic skin disease characterised by erythema, scaling, plugging of the seb-

aceous glands and scarring, often on the cheeks and bridge of the nose. There may be marked alopecia. It is generally benign, but a small proportion of patients do develop systemic disease. A variety of serological abnormalities may be found in otherwise healthy discoid patients, for instance antinuclear antibody may be positive.

Mixed connective tissue disease

In a small group of patients, the features of SLE, myositis and systemic sclerosis occur in sequence or concurrently. The original description was of a good prognosis and a low incidence of renal disease. The term 'mixed connective tissue disease' has been proposed for this group. The sera of these patients do not have anti-DNA antibodies, but show both a strongly positive 'speckled' pattern of ANA tests, and antibodies to extractable nuclear antigen, an RNA protein. Whether or not it is clinically useful to so define a group of patients remains a subject of debate.

Drug-induced lupus

A large number of drugs (Table 24.25) may, in certain individuals, give rise to a syndrome closely resembling SLE, with rashes, fever arthritis, polyserositis and pulmonary manifestations. Steroids are occasionally required to suppress symptoms, even after discontinuing the drug. Drug-induced lupus was first recognised in 1954, when $10-20\%$ of patients taking hydrallazine for hypertension developed a syndrome which resembled SLE. Circulating antinuclear antibodies developed in the majority. In drug-induced lupus, anti-DNA antibodies are usually present in low titre, and renal disease is absent in the majority of cases. Furthermore, the disease is usually reversible on stopping the drugs, though up to 70% of patients with hydrallazine-induced lupus have a more prolonged course.

Table 24.25 Possible causes of drug-induced lupus syndrome

● Hydrallazine	● Sulphonamides
● Procainamide	● Isoniazid
● Penicillamine	● Oral contraceptives
● Hydantoins + carbamazepine	● Chlorpromazine

Treatment

The high incidence of emotional and neuropsychiatric problems, together with the unpredictability of the disease, call for particularly sympathetic care of patients with SLE. There is no evidence that treatment during periods of remission alters the long-term prognosis, and it is usual policy not to treat patients in remission with normal complement levels.

Chloroquine salts should be considered before corticosteroids in patients where the skin and joint manifestations predominate, although many of the joint symptoms respond to salicylates alone. The possibility of retinal damage by chloroquine must be borne in mind. Local application of steroids can be helpful for rashes. Effective sun screens should be used routinely on light-exposed skin.

Measures designed to help prevent a relapse include the avoidance of sunlight and all non-essential drugs, and prompt treatment of infections. Regular measurement of anti-DNA antibodies will often show a rise preceding clinical relapse.

In the management of active SLE, prednisone dosage should be the lowest sufficient to control symptoms and signs. Some features, such as pericarditis or haemolytic anaemia, respond well to corticosteroids. Others, particularly CNS manifestations, are difficult to manage. It is now realised that the steroid dose may be fairly rapidly reduced once the acute episode is over, and most patients are maintained on dosages of 10 mg daily or less. Lowered serum complement levels have serious implications and, in a patient previously known to have had normal complement levels, it is justifiable to assume that this finding represents renal involvement and to treat accordingly. There is limited evidence that immunosuppressive drugs, such as azathioprine or cyclophosphamide, are of value. Most controlled studies have been of patients with renal lupus, where it appears that the combination of prednisone with an immunosuppressive drug is superior to the use of either drug alone.

Prognosis

Unless there is severe renal or CNS involvement, the outlook in SLE is now much improved. This is due to the detection of milder cases with more sensitive diagnostic tests, and to improved management. The estimated five year survival is now over 90%. There is no contraindication to pregnancy in a patient who is in reasonable remission and who has good renal function.

For those with renal disease, however, the prognosis is less good; the outlook for diffuse proliferative nephritis is poor, with a five year survival of around 50%. Causes of death in SLE include renal failure and sepsis. There is an increased mortality from the complications of atherosclerosis in later years; corticosteroids probably predispose to atheroma.

Pregnancy in SLE

Fertility is normal, except when there is severe renal involvement or when high-dose steroid therapy causes amenorrhoea. Recurrent abortion can occur before or during the clinical course of SLE; this may be due to the presence of anticardiolipin antibodies. Although remission of the disease occurs in 30% of patients, an exacerbation may occur at any time during pregnancy. A post-partum deterioration is common, and may occur very early after delivery. Patients with active renal disease have a much worse prognosis; they seldom become pregnant and the fetal mortality is around 30%. Increasing proteinuria and hypertension may mimic pre-eclamptic toxaemia.

Neonatal SLE is uncommon; it may be associated with a lupus rash, anaemia, thrombocytopenia, splenomegaly and cardiac conduction abnormalities.

SYSTEMIC SCLEROSIS

Systemic sclerosis is an uncommon multisystem disorder caused by fibrosis of connective tissue throughout the body. Systemic sclerosis is distributed widely, both geographically and racially. It is three times more common in women than men, and its peak age of onset is between the third and fifth decades. *Scleroderma* is the name used for the fibrosis and hardening of the skin but, occasionally, patients have limited or absent skin involvement.

Aetiology and pathology

There are familial cases reported suggesting that genetic and environmental factors may be important in the aetiology of systemic sclerosis. Chromosomal abnormalities have been reported, and there are weak associations with HLA antigens DR3 and DR5.

There is extensive deposition of collagen in the skin, internal organs and blood vessels. The sequential changes of inflammation, fibrosis and atrophy are most frequent in the skin, but occur to a lesser extent in the gut, heart, lungs and kidneys.

The widespread vascular changes involve both small and medium-sized arteries as well as arterioles and capillaries, and the relationship between the fibrosis and vascular abnormalities remains to be determined. The characteristic changes include concentric proliferation and thickening of the intima, with fibrosis of the adventitia. The capillary abnormalities can be seen at the nailfold. Raynaud's phenomenon occurs in up to 90% of patients.

Classification of scleroderma

Scleroderma-like changes occur in diseases other than systemic sclerosis, e.g. carcinoid syndrome, and systemic sclerosis varies from a mild, limited disease with a good prognosis to a severe disease with diffuse skin involvement and a high risk of renal disease.

The *CRST syndrome* is a benign variant associated with calcinosis (C), Raynaud's phenomenon (R), sclerodactyly of the fingers (S), telangiectasiae (T) and sometimes also oesophageal involvement.

Localised forms of scleroderma include *morphoea* where there are discrete cutaneous plaques of induration, sometimes yellowish in colour and often with violaceous borders; and linear scleroderma, where a band of fibrosis may involve subcutaneous tissue, muscle and even bone (Table 24.26). These localised forms are rarely associated with systemic disease and are usually self-limiting.

Sclerodema is a painless self-limiting oedema of the face, neck and upper trunk which occurs in children.

Eosinophilic fasciitis is a rare disorder associated with acute swelling and thickening of forearm and legs, often

Table 24.26 Classification of scleroderma

Classification	Example
Localised	Morphoea Linear scleroderma
Generalised	With diffuse visceral involvement CRST syndrome Overlap with other connective tissue disease
Chemical or drug-induced scleroderma	Polyvinylchloride Bleomycin
Diseases with skin changes mimicking scleroderma	Sclerodema
Eosinophilic fasciitis	

following trauma or unaccustomed exercise. There is eosinophilia, a high ESR associated with a typical histological appearance. This condition responds to corticosteroids.

Clinical features

Skin involvement

There are three stages in evolution of the skin disease. Firstly, there is an oedematous phase associated with bilateral painless oedema of hands, legs and face. This is followed by thickening and tightening of the skin affecting the fingers, face and hands and spreading sometimes to involve the limbs and trunk. Finally, atrophy occurs and limb contractures can occur, often with areas of hyperpigmentation, vitiligo and alopecia. The face becomes pinched, microstomia develops, and telangiectasiae are seen on face, lips, mouth, palms and nail folds. There is intracutaneous and subcutaneous calcification which affects the fingertips and may also affect the forearm; this may ulcerate.

Raynaud's phenomenon is a common early feature of systemic sclerosis and may precede cutaneous changes by many years. Raynaud's occurs in many connective tissue disorders, and the risk of patients with Raynaud's developing systemic sclerosis is less than 2% in females and about 6% in males. In severe disease, there may be ischaemic changes of the fingertips and gangrene may develop.

Musculoskeletal involvement

Tendon involvement leads to friction rubs and flexion contractures. Arthralgia and arthritis are often early features of systemic sclerosis; the arthritis can be erosive and progressive. Muscle weakness and wasting is common, and muscle biopsy shows deposition of collagen and myofibrillar degeneration; florid inflammation is uncommon.

Gastrointestinal involvement

After the skin, the gut is the most common organ to be involved, and this can lead to severe morbidity and death.

The oesophagus is frequently affected, and barium swallow shows decreased or absent peristalsis with oesophageal dilatation. The commonest clinical complaint is of dysphagia for solid foods and heartburn, but the patient can be asymptomatic. The small bowel is involved in about 50% of patients, causing symptoms from intestinal stasis or malabsorption. These include abdominal pain, distension, diarrhoea and weight loss. The characteristic radiological changes of dilatation and barium flocculation are seen most frequently in the duodenum and proximal jejunum. Large bowel involvement is fairly common but usually asymptomatic; wide-mouthed colonic diverticulae are characteristic in the condition.

Other clinical features

Cardiac abnormalities include those secondary to hypertension. Other abnormalities include conduction defects, pericarditis and cardiomyopathy; these are often asymptomatic. Renal involvement is the major cause of death in systemic sclerosis, the onset being acute or chronic. Chronic renal failure is associated with proteinuria and hypertension. Acute renal disease presents with malignant hypertension, rapid renal failure and microangiopathic haemolytic anaemia. Pulmonary complications, which occur in 50% of patients, include interstitial fibrosis, pleurisy and pulmonary hypertension.

Antinuclear antibodies are positive in about 70% of patients; a nucleolar or speckled pattern of fluorescence is characteristic. Anti-centromere antibodies occur in patients with the CRST syndrome. Anti-Scl-70 antibodies are present in 20% of scleroderma patients. The antigen has recently been identified as a topoisomerase enzyme.

Treatment

No treatment has been shown to alter the long-term progression of systemic sclerosis. The natural tendency of the disease is towards skin softening, which complicates the assessment of new treatments. D-penicillamine may have some therapeutic effect, and is commonly used.

Oesophagitis due to oesophageal involvement responds to antacids and H_2-antagonists. Strictures of the gastro-oesophageal junction may require surgery or dilatation. In patients with hypertension, control of blood pressure improves survival. Raynaud's phenomenon may be particularly troublesome. Patients should be told to avoid both smoking and exposure to cold, as lowering of the hand or body temperature may precipitate vasospasm. Nifedipine can be helpful, as can thymoxamine. Prostaglandin infusions can improve peripheral blood supply in severe Raynaud's.

DERMATOMYOSITIS AND POLYMYOSITIS

Polymyositis is an inflammatory disease of muscle which may occur either alone or in association with another connective tissue disease. It is characterised by symmetrical proximal muscle weakness, and when associated with a rash, the term *dermatomyositis* is used. Polymyositis is less common than SLE, and of similar frequency to systemic sclerosis. Both dermatomyositis and polymyositis may occur in childhood and there is an association with underlying malignancy in a minority of cases. Peak ages of onset are in childhood and in the fifth and sixth decades.

Aetiology

The aetiology of polymyositis is unknown. Several viruses, including rubella, influenza and coxsackie can cause acute myositis, and cellular immunological mechanisms are implicated in causation. Cytotoxic lymphocytes from patients have been shown to kill muscle cells. An underlying malignancy may be present in adults with dermatomyositis, and treatment of the cancer can lead to resolution of the skin and muscle changes. There is a weak association with HLA-B8 and DR3. A number of autoantibodies have been detected including Jo-1; sera with anti-Jo-1 activity bind histidyl-t-RNA and block its aminoacylation. Jo-1 is associated with myositis and pulmonary involvement.

Clinical features

The hallmark of polymyositis is progressive proximal muscle weakness, often insidious in onset. In severe acute forms, there is muscle pain and tenderness, but there is usually little pain. Typical presenting features are difficulty in climbing stairs and weakness of the neck muscles. There may be dysphagia and weakness of the respiratory muscles and, with progressive disease, muscle wasting and muscle contractures. Arthralgia occurs in about 25% of patients but is usually mild.

Cutaneous features include oedema and erythema and a characteristic rash causing a lilac (heliotrope) discolouration of the eyelids and periorbital oedema. A scaly erythematous rash involves the dorsum of the hands, knuckles and extensor surfaces of other joints. Longstanding disease is associated with skin deposits of calcium, which can present as nodules that may ulcerate. Calcinosis of subcutaneous tissue and fascial planes between muscles can occur, particularly in children. Vasculitis may involve the skin and internal organs, especially the gastrointestinal tract. Involvement of cardiac muscle can cause arrythmias and congestive cardiac failure. Pulmonary problems can be severe. Weakness of the respiratory muscles may result in breathlessness and ventilatory failure. Weakness of upper airway musculature combined with disordered swallowing predispose to aspiration, and impaired cough predisposes to pneumonia. Fibrosing alveolitis may also occur.

An underlying malignancy is present in up to 20% of adults, particularly with dermatomyositis. The commonest neoplasms are carcinoma of the bronchus, breast, stomach and ovary.

Investigation

The most important investigations are serum muscle enzyme measurements, electromyography (EMG) and muscle biopsy. Any one of these investigations may be normal, even during active disease. The creatine phosphokinase (CPK) is usually the most sensitive muscle enzyme to measure, and may be used in following the course of the disease. Serial measurement of muscle strength can also be useful in assessing progress.

EMG abnormalities are well-described and are useful in establishing the diagnosis and in distinguishing between myositis and steroid myopathy. Muscle biopsy changes include necrosis, muscle fibre regeneration and lymphocytic infiltration.

A search for underlying cancer should be made in adults over the age of 50 with dermatomyositis. The skin and muscle disease may, however, appear 1–2 years before the cancer is apparent.

Treatment

Corticosteroids usually control the disease, and are given initially in dosages of 40–60 mg of prednisolone daily. Immunosuppressive therapy with azathioprine, methotrexate or cyclophosphamide is frequently used, particularly if the disease is difficult to control with steroids. Treatment may be required for years.

VASCULITIS

The vasculitides are characterised by inflammation of blood vessels. Many classifications have proved unsatisfactory because of the variety of clinical syndromes; they are now commonly classified on the basis of vessel size and histology (Table 24.27).

Giant cell arteritis is common in the elderly, but many

Table 24.27 Classification of vasculitis

Systemic necrotising arteritis

Of the polyarteritis nodosa type
  Polyarteritis nodosa
  Arteritis of connective tissue disease
  Kawasaki's disease
With granulomatosis
  Churg-Strauss syndrome
  Wegener's granulomatosis

Hypersensitivity or small vessel vasculitis

Henoch-Schönlein purpura
Vasculitis of connective tissue disease

Giant cell or large artery arteritis

Giant cell arteritis
Takayasu's arteritis

of the other vasculitides are uncommon; the most frequent are those associated with the connective tissue diseases and drug hypersensitivity. Biopsy is central to the diagnosis, and the changes reflect a spectrum ranging from pure arteritis without granuloma formation to pure granulomatosis without vasculitis. Thus, polyarteritis nodosa and the arteritis of rheumatoid arthritis are at one end of the spectrum, while rheumatoid nodules and midline granulomata are at the other.

POLYARTERITIS NODOSA

Polyarteritis nodosa is a systemic necrotising arteritis which may be associated with a variety of cutaneous as well as systemic features (p. 1132). The disease affects men more frequently than women.

Pathology

Muscular arteries throughout the body are affected, particularly in the kidneys, heart, gastrointestinal tract and peripheral nervous system. All layers of the vessel wall are affected, and acute vasculitis is associated with fibrinoid necrosis and an inflammatory infiltrate of predominantly polymorphonuclear leucocytes. Multiple aneurysm formation is common. Chronicity of the lesion leads to fibrosis and narrowing of the vessel lumen with thrombosis.

The vascular lesions may be due to local deposition of immune complexes, and a similar disorder can be produced in animals by intravenous immunisation. Some cases may be associated with hepatitis B infection.

Clinical features and diagnosis

The clinical features of polyarteritis are listed in Table 24.28. Systemic features include fever, myalgia and weight loss, and these may be the presenting complaint. Cutaneous features include peripheral gangrene, rashes and livedo reticularis. The commonest neurological manifestation is mononeuritis multiplex. Renal involvement is common, the clinical features include haematuria, loin pain, acute and chronic renal failure and hypertension. Abdominal pain is a common presenting symptom and may reflect severe arteritic involvement. Articular features are usually mild.

The diagnosis is made on the basis of typical multisystem disease features. There is frequently anaemia, leucocytosis

Table 24.28 Relative incidence of features of polyarteritis

Clinical feature	Incidence (%)
Systemic symptoms (fever, weight loss)	80
Renal	75
Arthritis/myalgia	60
Cutaneous	55
Neurological	50
Abdominal	45

and a raised ESR. Angiography may demonstrate microaneurysms, especially in renal arteries and the coeliac axis. Arteritis can also be detected in about 50% of renal biopsies, and rectal or sural nerve biopsies may also be diagnostic.

Treatment

Untreated the prognosis is poor. Prompt treatment with corticosteroids and immunosuppressive drugs is associated with an improved prognosis. The prognosis improves markedly after the first three months, and the majority of patients do not have further attacks after the first year.

KAWASAKI'S DISEASE

Kawasaki's disease (mucocutaneous lymph node syndrome; see also p. 1116) is a rare acute systemic illness of infants and children, characterised by fever, exanthematous rash, mucous membrane involvement, conjunctival congestion and cervical lymphadenopathy. There is a necrotising arteritis, and coronary arteritis can be detected angiographically in up to 60% of cases. The disease is usually self-limiting, although sudden death may be caused by acute myocardial ischaemia resulting from coronary artery occlusion, myocarditis or aneurysm rupture.

CHURG-STRAUSS DISEASE

Churg and Strauss described a vasculitic syndrome that differed from polyarteritis nodosa in that pulmonary vessels were frequently affected. Patients have a history of allergy, and asthma develops in adult life. The high frequency of pulmonary symptoms, peripheral eosinophilia and the absence or mildness of the renal disease help to distinguish the disease from polyarteritis nodosa (p. 503).

WEGENER'S GRANULOMATOSIS

Wegener's granulomatosis (see also pages 512 and 821) is often classified separately from the other systemic arteritides, because of the severity of pulmonary, sinus and nasopharyngeal symptoms in this condition. However, vasculitis is a common feature and the range of the vessels involved is similar to that seen in Churg-Strauss syndrome.

Clinical features and diagnosis

Both granulomatous and necrosing arteritis may be detected in biopsies, particularly of the nasopharynx and lung. The major difference between Wegener's granulomatosis and Churg-Strauss syndrome is the lack of blood or tissue eosinophilia, or a history of allergy or asthma, in patients with Wegener's granulomatosis.

Vascular lesions or granulomata may affect any part of the upper respiratory tract and oral mucosa. Gingivitis and stomatitis are common, and destructive ulceration of the oropharynx can occur. The disorder usually presents with a purulent or bloody nasal discharge and sinusitis. Saddle-nose deformity is common, and is due to destruction of nasal cartilage by granulomata. The other lesions are very similar to those seen in polyarteritis nodosa. Local granulomatous lesions may involve the orbit of the eye, causing proptosis, uveitis or keratitis.

Radiological abnormalities are commonly seen in the lung and facial bones. Pulmonary nodules or infiltrates which are frequently bilateral may progress to cavitation.

Treatment

Wegener's granulomatosis is fatal if untreated. Cyclophosphamide is started as soon as the diagnosis is made, usually in combination with corticosteroids. The disease is very responsive to therapy, which should be continued for at least one year.

SMALL VESSEL VASCULITIS

Small vessel vasculitis is a feature of a number of different disorders including the connective tissue diseases. A number of distinct clinical syndromes are characterised by small vessel vasculitis including Henoch-Schönlein purpura and cryoglobulinaemic vasculitis.

A characteristic feature of small vessel vasculitis is a non-thrombocytopenic purpura which is caused by inflammation of small cutaneous capillaries, particularly in dependent parts of the body. Disease features include purpura, haematuria, polyarthritis, abdominal pain and peripheral neuropathy. The progress of this type of vasculitis is influenced by the underlying disease process but, often, these vasculitides are self-limiting.

GIANT CELL ARTERITIS AND POLYMYALGIA RHEUMATICA

Giant cell arteritis is a panarteritis predominantly affecting elderly patients. It is often associated with polymyalgia rheumatica. Although almost any large artery may be involved, the majority of clinical signs and symptoms result from involvement of the carotid artery or its branches.

Both polymyalgia rheumatica and giant cell arteritis are more common in the elderly, and both conditions are more common in women. The incidence is probably about one in 10 000. Giant cell arteritis and polymyalgia are well-recognised in the UK and in Scandinavia. In the USA, most reports derive from Northern states, few cases are reported from Southern states or in blacks, but the diseases are recognisable worldwide.

Aetiology and pathology

The aetiology of polymyalgia and temporal arteritis is unknown. The constitutional features suggest a viral infection, and many patients notice a distinct prodromal illness resembling influenza. There is little evidence of primary muscle disease in polymyalgia. Muscle biopsy shows only mild atrophic changes and the EMG is normal. Muscle enzymes, aldolase and creatine phosphokinase are normal and rather non-specific changes have been found on histochemical study of biopsy specimens.

Giant cell arteritis affects large and medium-sized arteries and involvement is patchy, 'skip lesions' often being found. The arteritis is a panarteritis with giant cell granuloma formation, often in close relationship to a disrupted internal elastic lamina. The gross features are not characteristic. The vessels are enlarged and nodular, having little or no lumen due to marked intimal proliferation. The adventitia is invaded by mononuclear cells, often with cuffing of the vasa vasorum. Giant cells may be seen close to the internal elastic lamina, often with elastic fragments in their cytoplasm. At first, the most severe changes are centred on the internal elastic lamina, which becomes swollen and fragmented. A definite progression of changes can be demonstrated, from the active infiltrative phase to the scarred artery with little cellular infiltrate.

There may be widespread vasculitis, with involvement of the aorta and its branches, the abdominal vessels and the heart. The pulmonary and renal vessels and the small arterioles are generally not involved, and this may be useful in differentiating between this condition and polyarteritis nodosa.

Clinical features

Giant cell arteritis

Some patients have symptoms suggestive of arteritis. Headache is common and may be either a non-specific tension type, or well-localised, severe, continuous, and with associated scalp tenderness. There can be pain in the face on chewing, due to claudication from facial artery involvement. Tingling in the tongue, and loss of taste and pain in the mouth and throat can also occur, presumably due to vascular insufficiency. Infarctions of the skin can occur, sometimes as a presenting feature, producing bizarre ulcers on the face and scalp.

The great danger, particularly but not exclusively in patients with symptoms of arteritis, is sudden irreversible blindness. This may be preceded by transient visual disturbances, e.g. field defects. Blindness results from ischaemic optic neuritis caused by arteritis of the posterior ciliary and branches of the ophthalmic arteries. The ocular complications usually occur within weeks or months of the onset of systemic manifestations of the disease. If temporal arteritis is suspected, steroid therapy, in adequate dosage, should be started immediately before further investigation of the patient in order to protect sight. The blindness is irreversible and is often bilateral, and loss of sight in the second eye may follow within hours of the first.

Arteritis can involve the carotid, vertebral, meningeal and, rarely, the intracerebral vessels, leading to hemiplegia, epilepsy or focal vertebral or occipital lobe lesions. Dementia, hallucinations or even coma can follow intracerebral arteritis. Aortic involvement can lead to an aortic arch syndrome. Aortic aneurysm is rare, probably because of the protective role of intimal proliferation. Congestive cardiac failure and myocardial infarction can follow coronary arteritis.

The amount of constitutional upset is variable, but lassitude, arthralgia, anorexia, weight loss, a low-grade fever and depression are all common. A transient synovitis can occur, particularly in the knee and often with an effusion. The systemic features can be vague and easily overlooked; conversely, they can be striking.

Polymyalgia rheumatica

Approximately 50% of patients have features of polymyalgia rheumatica. The initial symptoms of polymyalgia rheumatica may be sudden, with pain and severe stiffness of proximal muscles and periarticular tissues. The shoulder girdle is usually involved first, later the buttocks and thighs and occasionally the chest wall and forearms also became involved. Stiffness is usually the predominant feature; this is particularly severe after rest, and may prevent the patient getting out of bed in the morning. The muscular pain is often diffuse, and worse after resting. The musculoskeletal symptoms are almost always bilateral and there is tenderness of muscle and periarticular structures.

There is often little to find on examination of patients with polymyalgia rheumatica, although anaemia and obvious weight loss are quite frequent. The muscles may be tender, and stiffness may limit joint range, but there is no muscle weakness. Classically, when the temporal artery is involved, the vessel is thickened, tender and red, with absent pulsation, but usually the signs are limited to diminished or absent pulsation, perhaps with tenderness of the scalp. Tenderness in areas distant from arteries may be present even when the vessels are clinically normal. There may be synovitis, particularly in the knees. Bruits are often present over large arteries and there may be tenderness, particularly over the subclavian; these are presumably due to arteritis as they disappear with treatment.

Investigation

Investigations in polymyalgia and giant cell arteritis are essentially normal apart from a high ESR and increases in the acute phase proteins. The ESR is usually at least 70 mm/h and is often over 100 mm/h, particularly if arteritis is present: this provides a useful means of monitoring treatment. Some elevation of the ESR may occur in otherwise healthy elderly people, and a normal ESR does not exclude the diagnosis.

Anaemia, usually of a mild hypochromic type, is common and resolves without specific treatment, but a marked normocytic anaemia occasionally occurs and may be responsible for presenting symptoms. Protein electrophoresis may show a non-specific rise in alpha$_2$-globulin with less frequent elevations of alpha$_1$-globulin and gammaglobulins. Immunoglobulins IgG and IgM are frequently elevated in untreated disease. Rheumatoid factor may be present in low titre in about 5% of patients, as with the normal population.

Abnormalities of thyroid and liver function have been described. Raised serum values for alkaline phosphatase are found in 20% of patients with polymyalgia rheumatica and increased 5-nucleotidase and/or mitochondrial antibodies in 50% of patients. Liver biopsy specimens are reported to show portal and intralobular inflammation, with focal liver cell necrosis and small epithelioid cell granulomas.

Temporal artery biopsy is the most important procedure to aid diagnosis but, in view of the patchy nature of the arteritis, a negative biopsy does not exclude the disease. Biopsy can be performed as an outpatient procedure under local anaesthetic. Since the arterial pulsation is frequently diminished or absent, identification at biopsy can be difficult. Temporal arteriography is not helpful in diagnosis or as an aid to biopsy site. Steroids reduce the inflammatory infiltrate within days, so temporal artery biopsy should be carried out before treatment is started if possible, but if there is any delay, then steroids should be started immediately, in order to prevent visual complications.

Diagnosis

The diagnosis of polymyalgia rheumatica is initially one of exclusion. The differential diagnosis (Table 24.29) in elderly patients with muscle pain, stiffness and a raised ESR is wide because the prodromal phases of several serious conditions can mimic it. In practice, non-specific clinical features and the frequent absence of physical signs makes diagnosis difficult. A careful history and physical examination are necessary, as the sites of acute arteritis are frequently transient and the previous history of headaches, scalp tenderness, jaw claudication and prominent scalp vessels may not at first be mentioned by the patient.

Table 24.29 Differential diagnosis of polymyalgia rheumatica

● Neoplasm	● Lymphoma
● Connective tissue disease	● Polymyositis
● Multiple myeloma	● Dermatomyositis
● Leukaemia	● Myopathy

Treatment

Most of the symptoms of polymyalgia rheumatica are improved with salicylates or other anti-inflammatory agents. However, these drugs do not control the underlying arteritis or stop the development of vascular complications. Corticosteroids dramatically relieve myalgic symptoms and suppress the arteritis, and because of the difficulty in establishing the presence of vasculitis, it is usually advocated that corticosteroids be used in almost every case of polymyalgia.

It is rarely necessary to exceed 20 mg of prednisolone to control the myalgic symptoms, the ESR being used to titrate the dosage. In proven arteritis, doses exceeding 60 mg of prednisolone may be required to suppress disease. The dramatic response to steroid therapy supports the diagnosis. The constitutional symptoms – muscle pain and stiffness – disappear within days, although the ESR falls more slowly. Patients must be reviewed regularly for exacerbations of the disease or for the development of arteritis and the steroid dosage adjusted accordingly. Once there is no clinical evidence of disease activity, the steroids can be gradually discontinued, but recurrences are common, sometimes many years later.

TAKAYASU'S ARTERITIS

Takayasu's arteritis is a large vessel arteritis in which giant cells are rarely detected. It is a rare disease, predominantly of young women. Features include systemic symptoms, with weight loss and fever. The arteritis involves the aortic arch and its branches, and the inflammation results in stenosis, which may be demonstrated angiographically. Features of arterial stenosis include dizziness, fainting, exertional dyspnoea and reduced or absent peripheral pulses. The acute symptoms may respond to steroid therapy, but vascular reconstruction may be helpful in later stages of the disease (p. 447).

LOW BACK PAIN

Although back pain results in the loss of millions of working days each year, most individuals recover without medical attention. Of the small proportion of people who consult a general practitioner, only a very small proportion ultimately undergo surgery.

Anatomy and biomechanics

The spine is a weight-bearing structure. Movement occurs at the apophyseal joints, which are synovial, and at the intervertebral discs. These structures are closely related, and disease or deformity of one often affects the other. In the lumbar spine, the apophyseal joints resemble a mortise and tenon arrangement, which provides strength at the expense of mobility. There is very little rotation and flexion is 45° (Fig. 24.19).

Lumbar disc lesions usually cause root syndromes, because the spinal cord ends at L2. The lumbar nerve root exits high in its foramen, and is usually above a prolapsing disc which compresses the nerve root passing to the interspace immediately below.

Pain fibres are present within the spinal ligaments, in the apophyseal joint capsules, in the periosteum at the fascial and tendon attachments and in blood vessels, but only in the outer layers of the intervertebral discs. Pain is produced by pressure on these structures from disc protrusions, osteophytes or trauma. The healthy nucleus pulposus behaves like a gel, and distributes pressure equally in all directions. With age, this property declines, and localised points of high pressure develop. The pressures within the discs are increased most by lifting whilst bending forwards or sitting.

Fig. 24.19 **Diagram showing the position of the nerve roots and spinal nerve in relation to skeletal structures. A.** Lateral aspect of the lumbar spine. **B.** Superior aspect of a cervical vertebra. The precise position of the union of the ventral and dorsal nerve roots, to form the spinal nerve, in the intervertebral foramen is a little variable. Dotted lines indicate the usual sites of disc herniation.

Pathology

Disc protrusions usually occur postero-laterally, because here the annulus fibrosus is no longer reinforced by the posterior longitudinal ligament. Occasionally, pain is produced when there is a tear in the annulus but no protrusion. Disc lesions heal by fibrosis but there is always a risk of recurrence. Degenerative changes are present in the intervertebral discs of all subjects by middle-age. These are more marked, and occur earlier, after disc prolapse. There is a direct relationship between the degree of disc degeneration, osteophyte formation on the margins of vertebral bodies and apophyseal joint changes, suggesting that disc degeneration is the primary event leading to degenerative spondylosis.

Aetiology

The mechanical and non-mechanical causes of backache are listed in Table 24.30. A detailed history and examination, with the appropriate laboratory studies, usually identifies non-mechanical causes (Table 24.32). The age groups at particular risk are listed in Table 24.31. In general practice, it is people between the ages of 50 and 60 that attend most commonly with low back pain.

Table 24.30 Causes of backache

Cause	Example
Mechanical	Prolapsed intervertebral disc
	Apophyseal osteoarthritis
	Ankylosing hyperostosis
	Spinal stenosis
	Spondylolisthesis and other congenital abnormalities
	Scheuermann's osteochondritis
	Fractures
	Non-specific
Inflammatory	Ankylosing spondylitis and related seronegative spondylarthritides
	Rheumatoid arthritis
	Infection
Neoplastic	Bone – primary or secondary
	Spinal tumours
Metabolic	Osteoporosis
	Osteomalacia
	Ochronosis
	Chondrocalcinosis
Paget's disease	
Referred	Pelvic/abdominal disease
	Posture
Depression	

Table 24.31 Causes of low back pain related to specific age groups

Age group (years)	Cause of pain
Children	Osteochondritis (Scheuermann's disease)
	Scoliosis – primary or secondary
15–30	Ankylosing spondylitis
	Prolapsed intervertebral disc and fractures
	Spondylolisthesis
	Postural pain from pregnancy
30–50	Degenerative joint disease
	Prolapsed intervertebral disc
	Malignancy
50 and over	Degenerative joint disease
	Osteoporosis
	Paget's disease
	Malignancy

Clinical features

The clinical features in low back pain are listed in Table 24.32.

History

Mechanical and inflammatory back pain must be differentiated: the former is exacerbated by movement and improved by rest, while the latter is associated with stiff-

Table 24.32 Clinical features of low back pain

Feature	History	Examination
Mechanical	Precipitating strain	Asymmetrical restriction of movement and of straight leg raise
	Previous episodes	
	Unilateral leg/buttock pain	
	Worse on movement and coughing	Uniradicular signs
	Eased by rest	
Systemic disease	Constant or progressive	Features of ill health
	Worse on rest or at night	Rigid lumbar spine
	Morning stiffness	Symmetrical restriction of movement and straight leg raise
	Bilateral or alternating pain	
	Systemic illness	Multiradicular signs
	Diffuse pain and tenderness	Other neurological signs
		Wasting of paraspinal muscles
		High ESR
Non-specific	Postural factors	Normal movement
	Depression	Local tenderness
	Gynaecological symptoms	
	Diffuse pain	

ness after rest. These distinctions are not absolute, since inflammation involves some local swelling (i.e. mechanical change) and trauma generates some inflammation.

Back pain also occurs when bone is affected by tumour, infection or metabolic disease. The patient experiences unremitting pain, which is worse at night and exacerbated by movement.

Examination

The way in which a patient moves should be noted. Painful conditions can cause scoliosis through a protective muscle spasm. Sometimes this is only present on forward flexion, whereas secondary scoliosis (e.g. that caused by unequal leg length) disappears on flexion. Inflammatory conditions cause flattening of the lumbar lordosis. Patients with degenerative disease and disc lesions typically have restricted back movements, but with limitation of lateral flexion to one side; whereas, in ankylosing spondylitis, there is bilateral limitation of lateral flexion.

Neurological examination identifies nerve root irritation. Straight-leg raising is performed with the patient supine. The sciatic nerve is stretched by raising the straight leg until this becomes painful; a restriction to 45° or less indicates significant root irritation. The femoral stretch test is often misinterpreted. Root irritation is present if pain is produced in the anterior thigh on flexing the knee, with the patient *prone*.

Investigation

Radiology

Plain radiographs of the lumbar spine are of little diagnostic help. Radiographs are normal in 25% of patients with disc prolapse confirmed at operation, in early ankylosing spondylitis and early metastases. Bone density appears unchanged until 50% of the mineral has disappeared. In contrast, marked degenerative and disc space changes can be present in the absence of any symptoms or can easily be falsely interpreted as the cause of symptoms. In localised *bone* disease, isotope scanning is often helpful.

Radiculography

Radiculography has largely replaced myelography in the investigation of back pain, and may be indicated in severe or progressive disc lesions. Water-soluble radio-opaque contrast is introduced into the subarachnoid space and outlines the nerve roots. Other techniques occasionally used include:

1. *epidural myelography*, where the contrast is injected into the extradural space, but interpretation can be difficult
2. *discography*, where contrast is injected directly into the disc which may reproduce the patient's symptoms and be helpful in the presence of multiple protrusions
3. *venography*, which examines the vertebral venous system. Disc protrusion may be recognised from obstructed veins
4. *CT scans*. Recently these have been increasingly used and may supersede radiculography.

Laboratory investigations

Only simple screening tests are usually required (Table 24.33). The ESR is the most useful.

Prolapsed intervertebral disc

Only a few patients with back pain have a disc prolapse and the condition is often diagnosed erroneously. The diagnosis is *unlikely* if there is:

1. no evidence of nerve root compression
2. more than one root involved

3. bilateral and symmetrical nerve involvement
4. diffuse pain and tenderness
5. unremitting pain, worse on resting at night.

The leg symptoms and signs are the result of pressure on the dura mater and nerve roots. Straining or sneezing exacerbate disc pain by raising pressure within the spinal canal. A central protrusion may cause cauda equina compression, with saddle-shaped sacral anaesthesia, flaccid paralysis of the legs and sphincter involvement (usually urinary retention). This constitutes a surgical emergency. The presenting symptoms may be no more than impairment of urethral sensation. Early surgical exploration is indicated to preserve sphincter control (p. 934).

Back pain or sciatica is very occasionally caused by a cauda equina tumour. Diagnosis is difficult, but bladder or bowel symptoms, impotence, and wasting of the legs require urgent investigation.

Treatment

The causes of back pain are not well understood and treatment is largely empirical. Prophylactic exercises, advice on future activities and general back care should form the basis of treatment. However, for more severe back pain, treatment may include bed rest, traction, manipulation, the wearing of a surgical corset and surgery.

Mechanical back pain

Complete prolonged bed rest, and analgesics, successfully treat most cases of mechanical back pain. The mattress should be firm (boards can be placed underneath), and muscle relaxants may help. If the pain persists, or neurological signs or symptoms progress, continuous lumbar traction should be added for at least two weeks. After a period of immobilisation, exercises are started gradually. Isometric exercises (sometimes combined with traction), give better results than active mobilising exercises (which increase the load on the lumbar spine). A surgical corset may be useful if there is residual pain.

Table 24.33 Radiological and laboratory findings in back pain

Cause of back pain	Radiological features	ESR	Calcium	Phosphate	Alk. Phos.
Mechanical	Normal or degenerative changes	N	N	N	N
Inflammatory	Sacro-iliitis Osteomyelitis Psoas abscess	↑	N	N	N
Neoplastic	Osteolytic or sclerotic deposits Vertebral collapse	↑	N or ↑	N	↑
Osteoporosis	Reduced bone density Vertebral collapse	N	N	N	N
Osteomalacia	Osteoid seams Reduced bone density	N	↓ or N	↓	↑
Paget's disease	Sclerosis and expansion of bone	N	N	N	↑↑

Traction. Although symptoms are often relieved during traction, there is no evidence that it improves the rate of recovery. Patients with root pain, who find that it is relieved by lying down, benefit most from traction. It is seldom effective in chronic back pain or severe sciatica with neurological signs.

Manipulation can help in both acute and chronic low back pain. Unfortunately, one cannot identify in advance those patients who will respond. Trials suggest that manipulation gives significant immediate benefit but, after 1–2 weeks, manipulated and non-manipulated groups of patients show equal improvement. Manipulation should be restricted to mechanical back pain without neurological involvement or any spinal instability.

Lumbar supports probably act not so much by immobilising the spine as by raising the intra-abdominal pressure, so that some body load is transmitted through the abdomen, rather than through the spine. They can be helpful if:

1. the patient remains ambulant
2. heat and intermittent traction are ineffective
3. manipulation is contraindicated
4. bed rest has not relieved pain
5. back pain recurs in spite of prophylactic exercises and back care.

The spinal support should be worn continuously during the acute episode, and then during the day for several weeks. However, it is important to avoid dependence, and trunk muscle bulk must be maintained during immobilisation by static and then active exercises. Prophylactic use during hard physical work and long car journeys is recommended.

Epidural injections of local anaesthetic and steroid may reduce pain and allow a patient to return to work earlier. The main indications are chronic sciatica, and sciatica with root interruption. This presents as severe pain unrelieved by rest. It improves spontaneously after several days, but an epidural injection can give immediate relief. The benefit may result from the anti-inflammatory action of the steroid, or by the large volume of fluid freeing adhesions around nerve roots.

Chemonucleolysis. An injection of chymopapain into the nucleus pulposus leads to a reduction in disc size and results in improvement in 80% of selected patients.

Surgical treatment is seldom necessary, unless severe pain either persists in spite of adequate treatment or recurs often, or if neurological signs are progressing. Laminectomy is successful in 80% of selected patients.

General rehabilitation. Patients should be encouraged to resume normal activities, and advised on lifting and bending, exercises, weight control, posture, beds, chairs and the correct height for work surfaces. Prolonged sitting without lumbar support (e.g. by a small cushion or bedrest), stooping and carrying should be avoided. Patients with recurrent pain may have to accept some limitations on their previous activities.

Chronic low back pain. Despite treatment, less than 50% of patients with low back pain of over six months' duration ever return to full employment. A rehabilitation unit may be beneficial; confidence may be increased through a progressive exercise regimen and advice given on employment. Caution and restraint are required when contemplating back surgery.

Other causes of back pain

Degenerative disease of the lumbar spine is accompanied by central low back pain and buttock or thigh pain. Neurological signs are uncommon. Many patients respond to heat and mobilising exercises, while others benefit from gentle manipulation. Surgery is rarely required.

Paget's disease is a common radiographic finding, but not always the cause of symptoms (p. 742).

Metabolic bone disease (Ch. 19). In osteoporosis and osteomalacia, sudden pain may result from compression fractures of the vertebral bodies or from microfractures not visible on the radiograph. Nerve root and cord compression are uncommon, even when there is gross deformity of the spine. Chondrocalcinosis and ochronosis also cause premature disc degeneration and back pain. Patients with any of these conditions should be encouraged to be mobile, since immobility aggravates bone loss.

Short leg syndrome. Differences in leg length of greater than 12.5 mm may lead to the gradual onset of backache (usually in middle-age), which may be initiated by minor trauma. Provided there are no structural changes, correction of discrepancies of greater than 12.5 mm should relieve or prevent pain.

Infections of the spine are uncommon. Early diagnosis can be difficult, as backache may develop insidiously with few signs of systemic illness. Tuberculosis of the spine is increasing in incidence, particularly in immigrants. It affects the anterior border of the vertebral body, producing collapse and possible destruction of the disc. Spinal cord compression (Pott's paraplegia) or a cold abscess 'pointing' into the loin or iliac fossa may develop. In one-half of patients, there is tuberculous infection elsewhere in the body. Both tuberculosis and brucellosis may produce unilateral sacroiliitis.

Congenital abnormalities are usually identified radiologically. Common abnormalities include spondylolisthesis, spondylolysis, transitional vertebrae, spina bifida and abnormalities of the posterior articular facets. *Spondylolisthesis,* in which there is forward subluxation of the body of one vertebra onto the one below, usually occurs at L5–S1 in athletic adolescent boys. It is usually secondary to *spondylolysis* (a bony defect of the neural arch), which is symptomless by itself. Approximately 70% of patients with spondylolisthesis have back pain, but only 10% have sciatica. Pain usually responds to conservative treatment, including the use of a corset.

Sprung back. Tears in ligaments or paraspinal muscles cause acute localised pain and tenderness. Pain is often exacerbated by lifting or by a period of inactivity and may radiate to the buttocks. There are no articular or dural signs.

Neoplastic disease. Persistent pain, particularly at night, with associated tenderness should always be investigated. A bone scan may confirm the presence of metastases before there are any radiological changes. Vertebral collapse may precipitate root pain, and intraspinal tumours may mimic prolapsed disc. However, there are a number of distinguishing features: no response to treatment, progressing neurological signs, sphincter disturbance, multiple root involvement, nocturnal pain and pain unrelated to exercise, presence of an upper motor neurone lesion and signs of ill health. Bony metastases are much commoner than primary intraspinal tumours of the vertebral column, particularly from carcinomas of the breast, bronchus, kidney and thyroid (all osteolytic), or of the prostate (osteosclerotic). Primary bone tumours are rare.

Spinal stenosis. Variations in the size and shape of the spinal canal are common. Narrowing can result in pressure on the spinal cord or on nerve roots, or can leave less space to accommodate a prolapse or osteophytes.

Scheurmann's osteochondritis occurs in adolescent males and causes a dull ache in the lower thoracic region. Radiographs are diagnostic. They show fragmentation of the vertebral epiphysial end-plates and, later on, narrowing of the disc space and wedging of the vertebrae, producing a smooth kyphosis. The cause is unknown.

Ankylosing hyperostosis. In this syndrome, bony spurs usually form on the antero-lateral aspect of several dorso-lumbar vertebral bodies and fuse to form bridges. There is progressive stiffening of the spine but little pain or disability.

Psychological factors are important in chronic back pain. Such pain is common in patients who are unhappy at work or at home. In many of these patients, no overt psychiatric symptoms are present, and they may prove very difficult to treat.

Compensation neurosis. Some patients develop symptoms following an accident that are totally resistant to treatment, and which may remain even after the claim has been settled.

SOFT TISSUE RHEUMATISM

Lesions of tendons and their sheaths, fasciae, bursae, joint capsules and the tenoperiosteal junction (the enthesis) cause much morbidity and loss in productivity. They constitute a significant proportion of the workload of general practices and hospital accident, orthopaedic and rheumatology departments. As biopsy and surgery are rarely employed in their diagnosis and treatment, histological data are scanty and their pathologies are poorly understood. While there are adequate anatomical and clinical features to allow identification of individual conditions, diagnosis is often imprecise and management remains largely empirical.

Any or all of these lesions may occur in association with overt systemic disease, as, for example, in inflammatory arthritis or infection. A large proportion, however, occur in the absence of systemic disease. In these circumstances, local causes, such as chronic repetitive low-grade trauma, or excessive and unaccustomed use either at work or at play, may be responsible. These factors may also cause partial interruption of the blood supply, resulting in incomplete attempts at healing and degeneration; this renders these structures more vulnerable in the middle-aged and elderly, in whom these lesions predominate.

Classification

There is no universally accepted classification of soft tissue rheumatic lesions. The following is practical and problem-orientated, and divides the conditions into generalised and localised.

Generalised soft tissue lesions

The generalised soft tissue lesions are listed in Table 24.34. They may result from underlying disease, and most of the primary conditions can be diagnosed by careful clinical and laboratory assessment. These conditions will not be discussed here; polymyalgia rheumatica has been considered previously.

The diagnosis of *psychogenic rheumatism* must be made with caution and after exclusion of other disease. Chronic pain may itself lead to psychological problems. Psychiatric symptoms are not usually present in rheumatic disorders, but are common in patients who are unhappy at work or at home. Several features suggest a psychological illness, including written lists of symptoms, inconsistent or negative physical findings on repeated examinations and inappropriate concern with serious future disability.

Table 24.34 Generalised soft tissue lesions

With evidence of inflammation

Polymyalgia rheumatica and cranial arteritis
Prodrome of inflammatory arthropathies and connective tissue diseases
Viral and bacterial infections

Without inflammation

Hypothyroidism
Drug-related painful states associated with steroid withdrawal, chronic barbiturate abuse and the contraceptive pill
Dyskinetic phase of Parkinson's disease
Chronic brucellosis, Bornholm's disease
Associated with malignancy, e.g. myeloma, carcinoma
Osteomalacia
Fibrositis

Associated with weakness

Prodrome of polymyositis or dermatomyositis
Carcinomatous neuromyopathy (some forms)
Hypokalaemic states

Psychogenic rheumatism

Localised soft tissue lesions

The major structures involved in localised soft tissue lesions and the associated lesions are listed in Table 24.35. Examination should permit accurate localisation of the anatomical structure involved. Figure 24.20 shows common sites of soft tissue lesions.

Table 24.35 Localised soft tissue lesions

Structure	Lesion
Tendons and tendon sheaths	Rupture, degeneration tendinitis, peritendinitis, tenosynovitis, ganglia
Bursae	Bursitis – acute or chronic
Tenoperiosteal junction	Enthesopathies, apophysitis
Fasciae	Fasciitis, Dupuytren's contracture
Ligaments	Sprain, strain, tear

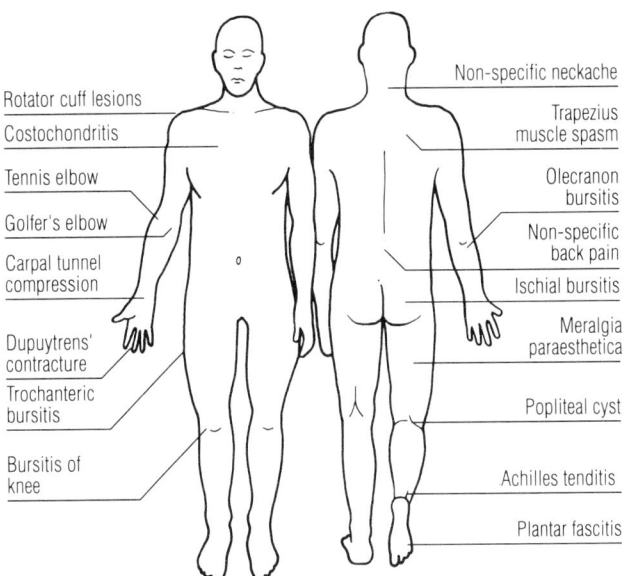

Fig. 24.20 Common sites of soft tissue lesions.

The painful shoulder

More than 90% of lesions causing a painful shoulder result from extracapsular soft tissue lesions (Summary 7). Trauma is often slight or unnoticed. Night pain and inability to lie on the affected shoulder are common to all the lesions, but careful clinical assessment with particular attention to the presence of a painful arc, location of tenderness and manœuvres that increase pain (Table 24.36) usually permit accurate diagnosis. Bony crepitus, when present, is of limited diagnostic value.

Rotator cuff tendinitis

While any of the tendons of the rotator cuff may be affected by tendinitis, it most commonly affects the supraspinatus

Summary 7 The painful shoulder

Rotator cuff lesions

Tendinitis – supraspinatus
          – acute calcific supraspinatus
          – infraspinatus and subscapularis
Rupture – partial
          – complete

Bicipital syndromes

Tenosynovitis of long head
Rupture of long head

Subacromial bursitis

Usually secondary to adjacent pathology

Frozen shoulder (adhesive capsulitis)

Shoulder-hand syndrome and referred pain

portion of the cuff close to its insertion to the humeral head. Overuse, with resultant wear and tear and relative avascularity, may be important in inducing tendon degeneration. The lesion often remains asymptomatic, but can manifest itself as pain and limitation of active (and sometimes passive) movement, especially abduction. A painful arc on abduction and tenderness over the tendon insertion may be noted.

Calcific supraspinatus tendinitis

Some cases of supraspinatus tendinitis are associated with calcific deposits visible on X-ray (Fig. 24.21). The exact mechanism responsible for the deposition of the calcium hydroxyapatite crystals in the tendon is unclear. The deposits may remain asymptomatic, or produce chronic

Fig. 24.21 X-ray of shoulder showing calcification of supraspinatus tendon.

symptoms with nagging discomfort in the region of the affected tendon. The crystal may also be extravasated into the subacromial bursa, causing acute bursitis with intense shoulder pain, loss of movement, severe tenderness, swelling and muscle spasm. Fever, sweating and other systemic symptoms may be present, mimicking gout or septic arthritis.

Infraspinatus and subscapularis lesions

Infraspinatus and subscapularis lesions are less common and seldom calcify. While the symptoms are usually similar to those of supraspinatus tendinitis, pain induced by resisted external or internal rotation (Table 24.36) usually allows the correct diagnosis to be made.

Table 24.36 Clinical features of some extracapsular shoulder lesions

Lesion	Painful arc	Pain increased by
Supraspinatus tendinitis, calcific deposit or incomplete tear	Yes	Resisted abduction
Infraspinatus tendinitis	Yes	Resisted external rotation
Acromioclavicular joint disease	Yes. Pain begins later in abduction (not below 90°) and increases as full elevation is reached	Local palpation Resisted adduction
Subscapularis	No	Resisted internal rotation
Bicipital tendinitis	No	Resisted flexion and supination of the elbow Tender bicipital groove

Rupture of the rotator cuff

Rupture of the rotator cuff is most common in patients over the age of 50 years, and almost always begins in the supraspinatus tendon. It probably follows long-standing tendon degeneration. Partial tears are more usual and are a cause of the painful arc syndrome, although they may also be asymptomatic. Complete tears are associated with marked weakness and inability to initiate active abduction; passive movement is full. Pain can be severe and there may be a history of injury. Partial tears may be difficult to differentiate from tendinitis and local anaesthetic infiltration, and contrast arthrography may be necessary. Atrophy of supra- and infraspinatus muscles often follows.

Bicipital syndromes

Tendinitis of the long head of the biceps is less common than are rotator cuff lesions, but may lead to rupture of the tendon.

Subacromial bursitis

Subacromial bursitis is almost always secondary to tendinitis or another adjacent lesion.

Frozen shoulder (adhesive capsulitis)

Frozen shoulder may occur spontaneously but can follow other rotator cuff lesions or trauma. In addition, conditions that produce pain (e.g. the referred pain of myocardial infarction) or immobility (e.g. stroke or polymyalgia rheumatica) of the shoulder or arm can predispose to the development of a frozen shoulder. Severe night pain and pain on all movement develops and lasts for 4–12 weeks. Severe restriction of all active and passive movements is noted, lasting 6–18 months, before improving to near normal. Early arthrography may reveal a small, shrunken, thickened capsule.

Patients with even minor degrees of frozen shoulder may develop a secondary reflex sympathetic dystrophy syndrome – the shoulder-hand syndrome. The symptom complex is characterised by an immobile painful shoulder associated with a swollen, painful, cold and dystrophic-looking hand. The lesion may progress until the patient is left with a painful, tender and useless hand.

The painful elbow

Pain round the elbow is commonly caused by soft tissue lesions (Summary 8), but care must be taken to exclude referred pain from the cervical spine, brachial plexus, shoulder and wrist.

Humeral epicondylitis

In humeral epicondylitis, lateral involvement (tennis elbow) is much more common than medial involvement (golfer's elbow). In spite of their sporting connotations, both occur more frequently in those performing repetitive movements with their arms, such as operating machinery, using a screwdriver or doing housework.

In tennis elbow, there is pain over the lateral aspect of the elbow with localised tenderness near the lateral epicondyle. Resisted dorsiflexion of the wrist exacerbates the pain and there is a reduction in grip strength. Thermography usually shows a discrete 'hot spot' on the side of the elbow.

Summary 8   The painful elbow

Humeral epicondylitis

Lateral – tennis elbow
Medial – golfer's elbow

Olecranon bursitis

Traumatic – student's elbow
Secondary to inflammatory joint disease

Friction neuritis of ulnar nerve

In golfer's elbow, there is a tender spot at the medial epicondyle and pain is induced by flexing the wrist against resistance, with the elbow fully extended. An enthesopathy has recently been suggested as a unifying pathological basis for lesions, including humeral epicondylitis and shoulder tendinitis, but many other histological changes have also been reported.

Olecranon bursitis (miner's elbow)

The superficial bursa over the olecranon process is commonly involved in rheumatoid arthritis (with nodule formation) or gout, but can also be affected by trauma or infection. In the acute stage, it distends with fluid, with prominent signs of acute inflammation. If it becomes chronic, the wall can be greatly thickened. As the posterior wall of the bursa is so close to the periosteum of the olecranon, pain can be felt down the border of the ulna.

The painful wrist and hand

Both seropositive and seronegative arthritides have a predilection for inflammatory involvement of the synovial structures of the tendons and joints in the wrist and hand (Summary 9). Tenosynovitis denotes an inflammation of the synovial lining of the tendon sheath usually accompanied by inflammation of the contained tendon. The clinical manifestations are pain, tenderness and swelling, with 'crepitus' that is palpable when the tendon moves within the inflamed sheath.

Stenosing tenosynovitis

Stenosing tenosynovitis is primarily a disorder of fibrosis of the tendon sheaths with intrathecal narrowing of the lumen, especially involving sites near bony prominences where tendons pass through fibrous rings. This more commonly affects the flexor than extensor tendons in the hand. If a fibrous nodule develops in the flexor tendons, a 'trigger finger' can result, which further limits function. The finger often locks in flexion. Extension can be forced with difficulty and is often painful. Palpation during muscle action may reveal a mobile nodule within a tendon sheath of a finger or palm.

De Quervain's tenosynovitis

De Quervain's tenosynovitis is a common lesion. It is caused by repeated minor trauma, and results from

---

Summary 9   The painful wrist and hand

- Stenosing digital tenosynovitis
- Tenosynovitis – De Quervain's and others
- Dupuytren's contracture
- Rupture of tendons
- Ganglion
- Median nerve compression – carpal tunnel syndrome

---

involvement of the tendon sheaths of the abductor pollicis longus and extensor pollicis brevis. The patient complains of pain on using the thumb or wrist. Tenderness is maximal in the 'snuffbox' area between the two tendons, and there is often a visible tender swelling about the radial styloid. Pain can be elicited by forced ulnar deviation after placing the patient's thumb in the palm (Finkelstein's sign).

Acute frictional tenosynovitis

Acute frictional tenosynovitis occurs after unusually active use of the wrist over a period of days or weeks. Pain is felt at the back of the wrist and lower forearm, and affects the extensor tendons of the wrist and thumb. A characteristic fine crepitation, caused by the fibrin-covered tendon gliding within the inflamed paratendon, is felt if the examiner's hand is placed over the swollen wrist while the patient extends and flexes the affected wrist and digits.

Dupuytren's contracture

The condition of Dupuytren's contracture, of unknown aetiology, produces progressive thickening of the palmar fascia and causes flexion contracture predominantly affecting the ring and little fingers. It is commonly bilateral and can also involve the plantar fascia. The palm of the hand becomes indurated, and lines of fibrosis, with nodules and skin puckering, run along the tendons causing progressive fixed flexion of the metacarpophalangeal and proximal interphalangeal joints.

The rate of progression is variable. Surgical fasciectomy should be performed when disability is severe, and should be considered before amputation becomes the only alternative.

Ganglia

Ganglia are tense uni- or multilocular cystic swellings that develop in relation to a joint capsule or tendon sheath, and contain a clear jelly-like substance. They vary in size and can be so tense that they may be mistaken for a bony swelling. They are sometimes provoked by injury or arthritis but often occur spontaneously.

Entrapment neuropathy (carpal tunnel syndrome)

Nerve compression can occur at any site where a peripheral nerve passes though an opening in fibrous tissue or an osseofibrous canal. If the clinical diagnosis is in doubt, it may be confirmed by electromyography (EMG).

Entrapment of the median nerve in the carpal tunnel at the wrist is the commonest entrapment lesion. It is more common in females. Most cases are idiopathic or caused by unaccustomed repetitive use, but carpal tunnel compression may be associated with rheumatoid arthritis, myxoedema, acromegaly, pregnancy and the contraceptive pill. Fracture, deformity or dislocation of the carpal bones can cause similar problems. Early symptoms include painful tingling in the wrist and hands, mainly affecting the thumb, index and middle fingers, but often symptoms are poorly localised. The pain may occasionally extend up the arm well above the wrist and often interferes with sleep. Patients try to obtain relief by hanging the affected limb out of the bed. Later, weakness (first in the abductor pollicis brevis) develops. Diminution of sensation to touch and pinprick, usually over the palmar aspects of the distal phalanges of the index and middle fingers, may be found. Untreated, wasting of the muscles of the thenar eminence develops. EMG is helpful where the clinical diagnosis is in doubt. A delay in motor or sensory conduction velocity across the wrist confirms the diagnosis, although no electrical abnormality may be detected in early cases.

The painful knee

Tendons, ligaments and bursae are the soft tissue structures around the knee from which pain may originate. The conditions affecting this region are listed in Summary 10. When assessing the knee, the clinical history is more valuable than the findings of clinical examination. The patient's account of the symptoms and their onset will usually make it possible to decide which structures in the knee have been damaged and how seriously.

Patellar tendinitis

The ligamentum patellae may become painful and tender at its attachment to the upper or lower pole of the patella or at its distal attachment to the tibia. Prolonged and heavy exercise, such as jogging, predisposes to this condition which usually occurs in adults. Steroid injections may be effective but should be used cautiously; surgical exploration is occasionally necessary.

Osgood-Schlatter disease

Apophysitis of the tibial tubercle at the insertion of the patellar tendon occurs predominantly in adolescent children and is another common cause of pain in front of

---

Summary 10   The painful knee

- Patellar tendinitis
- Rupture of quadriceps apparatus
- Apophysitis of tibial tubercle – Osgood-Schlatter disease
- Bursitis
  Prepatellar
  Infrapatellar
  Popliteal cysts – semimembranous
                    – Baker's cyst
  Anserine
- Infrapatellar fat pad lesions
- Medial and lateral ligament injuries
- Tendon lesions
- Anterior tibial syndrome

---

the knee. The condition is more common in boys, and symptoms include localised tenderness and swelling at this site. Pain can be reproduced by resisted knee extension, and radiographs may be abnormal and show an isolated spicule of bone at the site of the swelling. Most patients improve spontaneously but, sometimes, the pain may persist for several years, and injection, plaster immobilisation or even excision of the bony spicule may then be required. A similar, but rare, condition can occur at the lower pole of the patella (*Sinding-Larsen disease*).

Bursitis

Some bursae are in direct contact with the knee joint while others are separate. Like bursae elsewhere, acute or chronic inflammation, infection and involvement in systemic diseases, such as gout and arthritis, can occur.

Acute bursitis is characterised by classical signs of acute inflammation with intense localised tenderness and marked restriction of movement. Chronic bursitis may follow acute episodes but is much more commonly associated with repeated trauma. The bursal lining becomes thickened and cells degenerate; adhesions, villi and calcaneous deposits eventually develop. The degree of inflammation, muscle weakness and wasting and limitation of movement can vary widely, making diagnosis difficult.

Prepatellar bursitis (housemaid's knee). Here, the bursa is subcutaneous, and inflammation usually results from repeated kneeling, but can follow a fall onto the patella. Infection of the prepatellar bursa gives a characteristic red, shiny appearance over the knee, and is often mistaken for an infected knee joint. When chronic, fibrous bodies and fibrous bands form in the thickened enlarged bursa.

Infrapatellar bursitis. This small, deep bursa occupies the space between the upper part of the tibial tuberosity and ligamentum patellae, separated from the synovium by a fat pad. When inflamed, the fluid obliterates the depression on each side of the ligament, the fluctuant swelling being most marked when the knee is actively extended.

Popliteal cysts (Baker's cysts). Synovial cysts in the popliteal fossa are usually referred to as Baker's cysts. They may arise from the semi-membranous bursa when they communicate with the knee joint, or from a posterior rupture of the knee joint capsule. Cysts are common in children and are of no serious significance although, in young adults, there may be quite severe pain after exercise. The most common course is gradual resolution. If the cyst does not resolve, it may extend into the calf or burst, with fluid tracking down the fascial planes of the calf, mimicking an acute deep venous thrombosis. Arthrography of the knee joint establishes the diagnosis but must be performed early after the onset of symptoms, as the leak may seal off after a few days.

Anserine bursitis (that is related to pes anserinus). The tendons of sartorius, gracilis and semitendinosus all cross the lower medial side of the femur and attach by a common tendon. The anserine bursa lies beneath this tendon. Pain is felt diffusely on the medial aspect of the knee, but tenderness can usually be localised to the area of the bursa.

Knee range is normal, but contracting the hamstrings induces pain. The bursa is often inflamed in elderly obese women with a valgus deformity, and is also a common source of pain in inexperienced joggers, often being mistaken for joint injury.

Ligament injuries

If a patient has injured the knee in such a way that the structures on the medial side have been stressed, damage to the medial ligament must be suspected. Clinical examination may reveal tenderness localised to the attachment of the ligament to the femur or tibia. The diagnosis can be confirmed by stressing the medial ligament; this will reproduce the pain or demonstrate ligament laxity.

Tendinitis

The popliteus tendon runs through the knee joint from the lateral femoral condyle, between the lateral meniscus and the capsule, to the back of the tibia. Inflammation may cause lateral knee pain.

The biceps tendon is attached to the head of the fibula, and inflammation will cause pain around the tendon insertion, felt particularly when the knee is flexed against resistance and the area pressed firmly.

Pain in the back of the knee may arise from a hamstring injury. The pain usually develops acutely after sudden activity without adequate warming-up.

Anterior tibial syndrome

The anterior tibial syndrome condition consists of severe pain in the anterior aspect of the leg, associated with foot drop, occurring after exercise and relieved by rest. It is thought to be the result of a tight fascia compressing the muscles in the anterior tibial compartment of the leg. There are many predisposing factors, of which exercise is the commonest. Surgery gives relief.

The painful heel

Pain can arise from either the posterior or plantar aspects of the heel (Summary 11). Most lesions occur in people who walk or stand a great deal and are particularly common in athletes. Whatever the cause, the pain tends to be aggravated by walking and relieved by rest. Accurate localisation of tenderness is important in diagnosis.

Pain behind the heel

Tendon rupture

Complete or partial tendon rupture may occur after vigorous activity. In the young, the musculotendinous junction tends to be the site of rupture, while in the old, the tendon itself is at risk. Complete rupture is easily recognised by loss of anatomical continuity and function. Partial rupture is more difficult to diagnose. Initially, swell-

---

Summary 11   The painful heel

Pain behind the heel	*Pain under the heel*
Achilles tendon lesions	Plantar fasciitis
Rupture – partial/total	Calcaneal apophysitis and spurs
Central core degeneration	Tender heel pad
Ossification	
Peritendinitis (Achilles	
tendinitis)	
Bursitis	
Subachilles (retrocalcaneal)	
Subcutaneous (postcalcaneal)	
Retrocalcaneal apophysitis	
(Sever's disease)	

---

ing and marked tenderness is noted just above the tendon insertion, with exquisite pain on movement. Later, a more irregular swelling due to fibrous tissue develops, with continuing pain on movement.

Central core degeneration of the Achilles tendon

Central core degeneration of the Achilles tendon must be differentiated from the more common peritendinous lesion, as tendon rupture is much more likely and local steroid injections are contraindicated. Onset is less dramatic than partial rupture, but other clinical findings can be similar.

Pain gradually increases as the day progresses. Careful examination also reveals a localised tender nodule or thickening, 3–6 cm above the insertion to the calcaneum.

Peritendinitis (Achilles tendinitis)

Peritendinitis is the common cause of chronic, persistent and often annoying pain at the back of the heel. It occurs most commonly, but by no means exclusively, in athletes, especially long-distance runners. In the acute stage, there is diffuse swelling and tenderness on both sides of the tendon, sometimes accompanied by crepitus. Later, signs become less obvious, but pain and tenderness recur with exercise. The symptoms usually develop gradually, distinguishing the condition from rupture of the tendon, and occasionally the tendon may calcify. Inflammation of the peroneal tendons behind the lateral malleolus causes pain when the muscle is contracted, as when walking over rough ground. If this tendinitis is chronic, rheumatoid arthritis should be considered.

Bursitis

Subachilles (retrocalcaneal) bursitis may also cause pain at the lower end of the Achilles tendon. Physical examination reveals the bulging tender bursa on either side of the Achilles tendon with normal ankle joint movement. Dorsiflexion of the foot aggravates the pain by compressing the bursa. Frequently, the patient can recall a traumatic incident.

Subcutaneous (postcalcaneal) bursitis

A more superficial bursitis can develop over the tendon attachment as a result of poorly fitting shoes; here, the swelling is lower down, large and fluctuant. Inflammatory changes in the overlying skin are common.

Retrocalcaneal apophysitis (Sever's disease)

The insertion of the Achilles tendon into the calcaneum can become inflamed, resulting in symptoms of pain and tenderness behind the heel. This usually occurs in boys aged between 9 and 15 years.

Pain under the heel

Plantar fasciitis

In weight-bearing, stress is placed on the long plantar ligament and fascia which support the longitudinal arch of the foot. An enthesopathy can develop at the point of attachment of the ligament to the heel. Pain and tenderness may be confined to the point of attachment but can be much more widespread; it is always aggravated on walking. The presence of a calcaneal spur on the X-ray is not necessarily significant, as it is also commonly seen on films of asymptomatic heels. Plantar fasciitis may be associated with the seronegative arthritides, such as Reiter's syndrome and ankylosing spondylitis.

Tender heel pad

The condition of tender heel pad causes pain in the hind part of the heel on standing or walking. The tough fibro-fatty pad beneath the prominent weight-bearing part of the calcaneus is tender to finger palpation. The area of tenderness is well localised and may be a result of simple contusion; in most cases, there is no history of trauma and, in these patients, the tenderness may result from obesity combined with excessive walking in unsatisfactory footwear, or from mild inflammation of uncertain origin.

The painful foot

The major causes of painful feet are listed in Summary 12.

'Flat feet'

'Flat feet' rarely cause symptoms in the young. In adolescents they may be part of a general postural defect. At this age, especially in boys, spasmodic flat foot is caused by peroneo-extensor spasm. The foot is rigid and painful and symptoms are worse on walking. Flat foot usually leads to osteoarthritis of the midtarsal joint in later life.

'Spring' ligament

The 'spring' or plantar calcaneonavicular ligament supports the talonavicular joint from below; it may be strained, leading to deep-seated pain on weight-bearing.

Summary 12   The painful foot

- Anterior flat foot – dropped transverse arch
- Injuries to the spring ligament
- Plantar digital neuritis – Morton's metatarsalgia
- Tarsal tunnel syndrome
- Plantar warts and callosities
- Hallux valgus (bunion)
- Dorsal exostoses with bursae

Metatarsalgia

Patients with anatomical abnormalities of the feet, such as claw-toes or equinus deformity, are liable to develop pain in the metatarsal heads on walking. Metatarsalgia, or pain around the metatarsal heads, is not itself a diagnosis. Between the metatarsal heads and the skin lie the flexor tendons and their sheaths and, in the case of the great toe, the sesamoids in the flexor hallucis brevis. Inflammatory joint disease can cause inflammation of the tendon sheaths and causes generalised pain.

Hallux valgus

Hallux valgus (bunion) is an example of an adventitious bursa resulting from prolonged pressure over a bony prominence as a result of valgus deformity of the hallux. It is frequently inflamed. Initially, treatment consists of padding to reduce pressure and advice on suitable footwear. If these measures prove unhelpful, surgical treatment may be necessary.

Tibialis anterior and posterior

Pain in the mid-foot may arise around the insertion of the tibialis anterior after strenuous walking. Pain on the medial side of the foot, at the point of insertion of the tibialis posterior tendon on the navicular, is more common; it is particularly severe if the patient has an accessory navicular bone.

Dorsal exostoses

Some patients develop a bony prominence on the dorsum of the foot at the joint between the navicular and the cuneiform bone. Excessive friction may lead to the formation of a bursa.

Entrapment syndromes in the foot

Tarsal tunnel syndrome. Compression of the posterior tibial nerve under the flexor retinaculum below the medial malleolus can lead to burning pain under the medial side of the longitudinal arch of the foot.

Morton's metatarsalgia (plantar digital neuritis). In this condition, patients complain of a sharp pain in the forefoot shooting through to the toes, usually the third and fourth. There may be tingling, or even numbness, in the adjacent sides of the third and fourth toes. The pain is localised between the metatarsal heads, and the transverse metatarsal compression may produce a palpable click. The condition is caused by interstitial fibrosis compressing the digital nerve just before it divides into its two terminal branches. In the early stages, well-fitting shoes, with or without a metatarsal bar, give relief. Excision of the thickened tissue effects a cure.

Other common entrapment syndromes in the lower limb

Lateral popliteal nerve lesions

The lateral popliteal branch of the sciatic nerve lies superficially against the head and neck of the fibula, where it is susceptible to compression, especially when sitting with legs crossed, kneeling or wearing knee pads. Anaesthesia and periods of unconsciousness present particular risks. The symptoms are pain and tingling in the lateral aspect of the leg and dorsum of the foot, associated with weakness of dorsiflexion and eversion of the foot. Wasting of tibialis anterior, peronel and extensor digitorum brevis can occur. The high-stepping gait is typical. Electromyography can confirm the diagnosis.

Lateral femoral cutaneous nerve entrapment (meralgia paraesthetica)

The lateral cutaneous branch of the femoral nerve traverses a tunnel formed by the lateral attachment of the inguinal ligament as it runs towards the anterior superior iliac spine. Entrapment produces paraesthesia and burning pain over the lateral thigh with reduced sensation. Local trauma, obesity or pressure from tight garments are known predisposing factors.

Treatment of patients with soft tissue rheumatism

One feature common to all of the soft tissue rheumatism syndromes is a tendency to spontaneous remission. Many of the syndromes take weeks to improve, and few persist with significant symptoms beyond six months. A clear diagnosis therefore allows the physician to reassure the patient that arthritis is not present and that the prognosis is good. However, failure to resolve is often due to further injury. Few of the conditions require complete rest; most respond to selective rest of the involved region.

Immobilisation

Tenosynovitis around the wrist may respond to immobilisation in a light forearm splint, maintaining the wrist in a position of optimum function (10–15° extension), and

median nerve compression may respond to night-splinting alone. The acutely painful shoulder also benefits from rest, mobility being maintained by pendular exercises. Physiotherapy in the acute stages only exacerbates the condition. Rest is essential for the painful heel and foot. Raising the heel of the shoe reduces tension on the Achilles tendon, and Elastoplast strapping will help immobilise the ankle. If there is flattening of the medial arch of the foot, then physiotherapy and an arch support may be helpful.

Drug therapy

The short-term use of NSAIDs may be necessary. Their immediate use is beneficial in limiting the pain and swelling of soft tissue trauma. Many soft tissue lesions respond to a local injection with steroid and anaesthetic. Some experience in the various techniques is necessary before reasonable success can be obtained.

The choice of steroid and local anaesthetic varies between physicians but, for most purposes, the shorter-acting hydrocortisone acetate is suitable. The longer-acting steroids, methyl prednisolone acetate and triamcinolone hexacetonide, may cause skin atrophy when used for superficial lesions such as tennis elbow. After injection, there may be an increase in symptoms for up to 48 hours and patients should be warned of this possibility. About 80% of patients gain symptomatic benefit from these injections. It is important not to inject the tendoachilles itself, as this may predispose to rupture. In spite of decades of use of ultrasound in treating a wide spectrum of musculoskeletal disorders, its effectiveness remains unproven. Persistent lesions may require further injections, and if conservative measures fail, surgery may be required.

About seven people in every hundred who visit their general practitioner seek help with symptoms arising from the soft tissues. The loss of work resulting from these symptoms is of the order of 11 million days annually. However, the great bulk of soft tissue lesions are, as discussed above, eminently manageable.

FURTHER READING

Dixon A St J (ed) 1979 Soft tissue rheumatism clinics in rheumatic diseases, Vol 5. W B Saunders, London. *A good review of soft tissue rheumatism*

Ebringer A, Shipley M (ed) 1988 Pathogenesis of ankylosing spondylitis and rheumatoid arthritis. British Journal of Rheumatology (Suppl Issue 11). *A good review of the pathophysiology of these two diseases*

Hughes G R V 1987 Connective tissue diseases. Blackwell Scientific Publications. *An excellent introduction to these disorders, including current ideas on pathogenesis and treatment*

Lawrence J S 1977 Rheumatism in populations. Heinemann, London. *An epidemiological account of the rheumatic diseases*

Moll J M H, Bird H A, Rushton A (ed) 1986 Therapeutics in rheumatology. Chapman and Hall, London. *A good introduction to the drugs used in treatment and the management of rheumatic disorders*

Haematological Disorders

HAEMOPOIESIS

Haemopoiesis is the process by which blood cells are derived from multipotential stem cells.

Ontogeny of haemopoiesis

In the human embryo, nucleated erythrocytes develop in the extra-embryonic membranes and synthesise specific embryonic haemoglobins. In the sixth week of gestation, erythropoiesis transfers to the fetal liver and the embryonic haemoglobins ($\alpha_2\varepsilon_2$, $\zeta_2\varepsilon_2$ are replaced by fetal haemoglobin ($\alpha_2\gamma_2$). Bone marrow haemopoiesis is established between the 11th and 22nd week of gestation and probably arises by stem cell migration into the developing marrow stroma. Hepatic haemopoiesis declines in the third trimester and ceases soon after birth. Finally, at about the time of birth, fetal haemoglobin is replaced by adult haemoglobin (HbA, $\alpha_2\beta_2$), a switch accompanied by other changes in the red cell including a decrease in cell size and a large rise in carbonic anhydrase-I content.

These sequential changes in haemoglobin synthesis during development represent the orderly activation of the globin genes from the 5′ to 3′ end of the globin gene clusters (Fig. 25.1). The δ gene is never fully expressed and HbA$_2$ ($\alpha_2\delta_2$) represents only 2% of adult haemoglobins. The molecular mechanism of Hb gene switching is incompletely understood, but may be related to changes in gene methylation.

At birth, most of the bone marrow cavity is haemopoietically active but, during the first decade, this active red marrow is replaced by inactive fatty yellow marrow. In adults, red marrow and hence haemopoiesis is restricted to the upper ends of the femora and humeri, the vertebrae, ribs, sternum, clavicles, scapulae, skull and pelvis.

Committed granulocytic and monocytic progenitor cells can be detected early in fetal life, but there is very limited granulocyte and monocyte production until the end of gestation. Lymphoid cells first appear during the first trimester and, by the second trimester, the majority of leucocytes in the blood are phenotypically mature T and B lymphocytes. However, full functional integrity of the immune system is not achieved until after birth.

Haemopoietic differentiation

The mature elements of the blood probably all arise from a multipotent haemopoietic stem cell. Such cells may self-replicate (and so replenish the stem cell pool) or, alternatively, may proliferate and enter the differentiation pathway (Fig. 25.2). With each division there is increasing

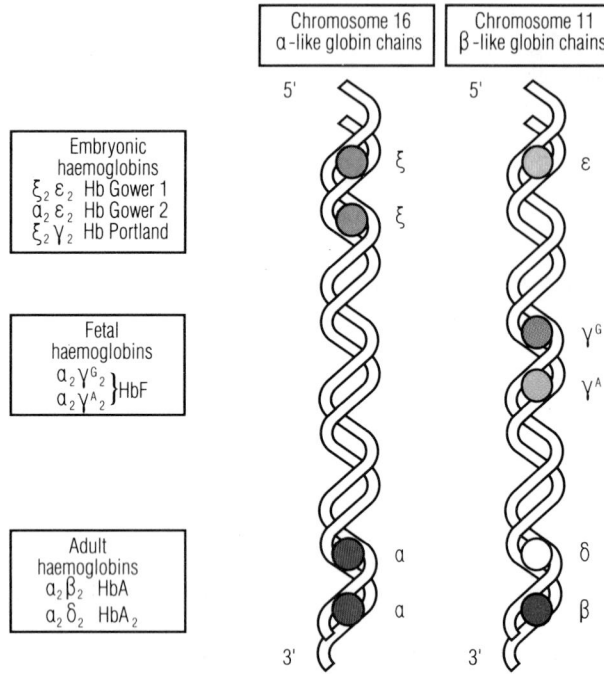

Embryonic
haemoglobins
$\xi_2 \varepsilon_2$ Hb Gower 1
$\alpha_2 \varepsilon_2$ Hb Gower 2
$\xi_2 \gamma_2$ Hb Portland

Fetal
haemoglobins
$\left.\begin{array}{c}\alpha_2 \gamma^G{}_2 \\ \alpha_2 \gamma^A{}_2\end{array}\right\}$HbF

Adult
haemoglobins
$\alpha_2 \beta_2$ HbA
$\alpha_2 \delta_2$ HbA$_2$

Fig. 25.1 Diagrammatic representation of the α-like globin gene cluster and β-like globin gene cluster on chromosomes 16 and 11 respectively. Hb switching during ontogeny represents the orderly expression of the globin genes from the 5′ to 3′ end of the globin gene clusters.

loss of multipotentiality and the stem cells thus become committed to one or more lineages. The initial loss of lineage potential seems to be random, but monocytes and neutrophils (though not eosinophils) appear to be closely related, as are red cells and megakaryocytes. Committed myeloid progenitor cells do not self-replicate, so their proliferation will ultimately lead to the production of functional end cells. Progenitor cells have the appearance of

undifferentiated blast cells and many doubling divisions occur in this blast cell pool. In the final five or six division stages of the differentiation pathway, the cells progressively acquire the morphological features and functional attributes of the mature cell. These recognisable precursor and end cells account for more than 95% of the normal marrow cells.

Myeloid end cells do not divide and have a limited lifespan. The steady state is maintained by a continuous influx of stem cells and progenitor cells into the precursor cell pool, together with their amplification due to doubling divisions. Mature lymphoid cells, on the other hand, are capable of clonal expansion or, alternatively, of transition to a resting 'memory cell' which is able to divide at a later date when appropriately stimulated. It is this feature of the lymphoid system that underlies the nature of the immune response.

Regulation of haemopoiesis

The regulation of haemopoiesis is only partially understood. The proliferation and self renewal of multipotential stem cells appears to be dependent on intimate contact with a complex cellular microenvironment.

Erythropoiesis

Progenitor cells committed to erythropoiesis divide and differentiate in the presence of growth factors referred to as *burst promoting activity* (BPA). BPA – which includes interleukin 3 (IL-3) and granulocyte macrophage colony stimulating factor (GM-CSF) – is produced by a variety of cell types, including T cells and monocytes. It is likely that these cells provide a permissive environment rather than play a regulatory role, but inhibitory T cells, monocytes and *natural killer cells* may have some regulatory activity by inhibiting haemopoiesis at this level, par-

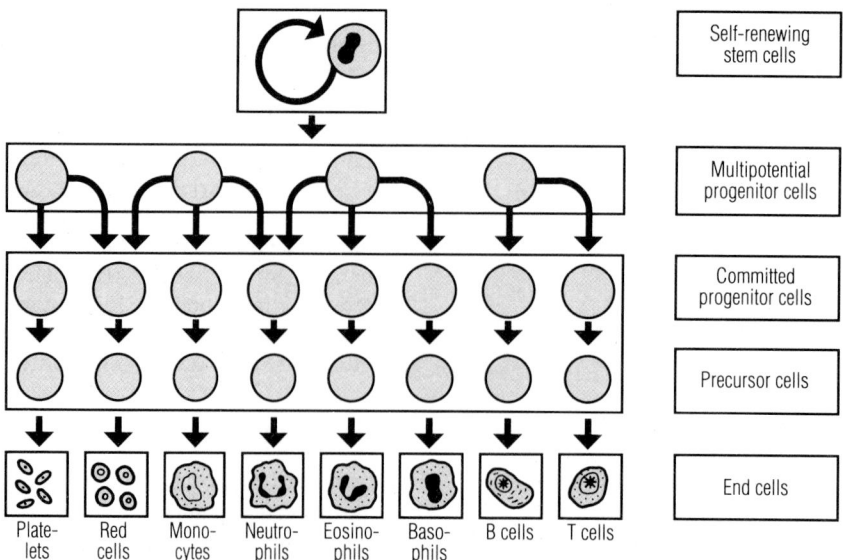

Self-renewing
stem cells

Multipotential
progenitor cells

Committed
progenitor cells

Precursor cells

End cells

Plate-lets · Red cells · Mono-cytes · Neutro-phils · Eosino-phils · Baso-phils · B cells · T cells

Fig. 25.2 Diagrammatic representation of the differentiation of haemopoietic stem cells.

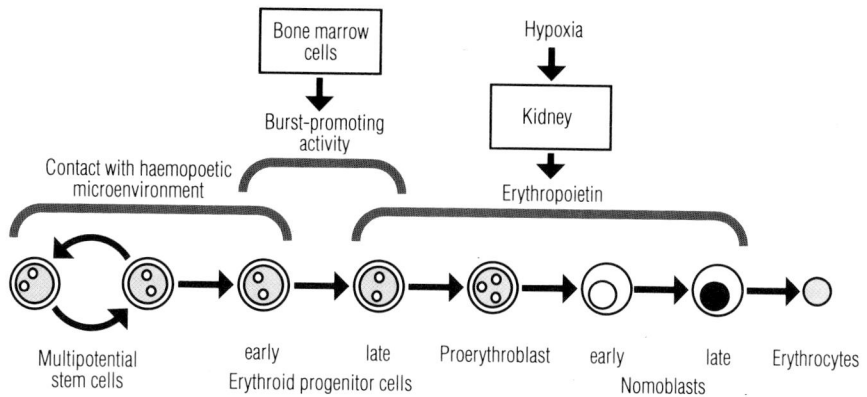

Fig. 25.3 Diagrammatic representation of the regulation of erythropoiesis.

ticularly in pathological states. The fine control of erythropoiesis is regulated by erythropoietin, a hormone probably released directly from the kidney in response to hypoxia (Fig. 25.3). Erythropoietin is produced by peri-tubular adventitial cells. The sensing of hypoxia by these cells involves a haem protein. A small amount of erythropoietin is also produced from non-renal sources, probably the liver and spleen.

Granulopoiesis

The regulation of granulopoiesis is less well understood. In response to an inflammatory stimulus, granulocytes can be rapidly mobilised from a marginated cell pool. Further demands for granulocytes are met by increased bone marrow turnover and release. This appears to be controlled by local release in the bone marrow of a family of growth factors functionally defined as *colony stimulating activity* (CSA), which includes granulocyte colony stimulating factor (G-CSF) and granulocyte monocyte colony stimulating factor (GM-CSF). Monocytes, endothelial cells, and T cells can all produce such factors, but the mechanism by which they are activated by a peripheral stimulus is not known. A series of complex feedback loops involving prostaglandins, lactoferrin, transferrin and acid isoferritins have been proposed from *in vitro* studies, but their *in vivo* significance is not clear.

FUNCTION OF HAEMOPOIETIC CELLS

Red cells and haemoglobin

Erythrocytes package haemoglobin for the delivery of oxygen from the lungs to the tissues; carbon dioxide is carried by red cells in the reverse direction. Haemoglobins have a molecular weight of approximately 65 000. Each molecule consists of two α-like and two β-like polypeptide chains, with a haem group attached to each chain within a hydrophobic pocket. The tetramer is held together pre-

dominantly by bonds between the α and β chains rather than between the like chains (e.g. α-α and β-β). Because these bonds are not irreversible, the molecule exists in equilibrium between two configurations, one with a low, and one a high affinity for oxygen. Binding of oxygen to a haem group destabilises the low affinity form, thus increasing the oxygen affinity of the molecule. Due to this cooperative binding, a sigmoid oxygen dissociation curve is produced (Fig. 25.4). In the lungs, P_{O_2} is approximately 14 kPa and the haemoglobin is nearly fully saturated. In the tissues, where the P_{O_2} is about 5.4 kPa the haemoglobin saturation is about 70%. If tissue oxygen consumption rises, a small fall in tissue P_{O_2} will bring about a large further release of oxygen because these values of P_{O_2} correspond to the steep part of the oxygen dissociation curve. Various other factors also influence oxygen dissociation. A fall in pH or a rise in P_{CO_2} decreases the oxygen affinity (moves dissociation curve to right) by strengthening salt linkages between the globin chains found only in the deoxy-configuration. This tends to increase oxygen delivery to the tissues where the pH is lower and the P_{CO_2} higher than in the lungs. A rise in temperature, e.g. during heavy exercise, also decreases the oxygen affinity. Haemoglobin's

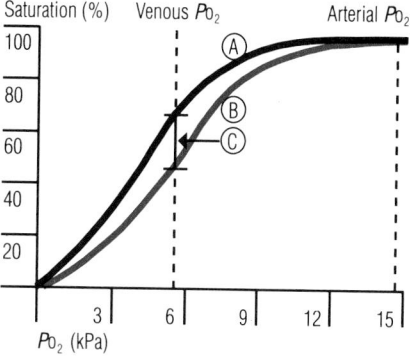

Fig. 25.4 The sigmoid nature of the oxygen dissociation curve. (A) represents the normal steady state. (B) represents the shift of the curve to the right seen with increased pH, increased P_{CO_2} or increased 2,3-DPG. At a given venous P_{O_2} this results in a larger amount of oxygen (marked C) being given to the tissues.

affinity for oxygen is also modulated by 2,3-diphosphoglycerate (2,3-DPG). When the haemoglobin molecule moves from the deoxy- to the oxy- form, there is a rotation of one α-β dimer around the contact point between that α-chain and the other β chain which brings the two β chains closer together (Fig. 25.5). 2,3-DPG binds to haemoglobin in the space between the β chains thus preventing this rotation, stabilising the deoxy- form and reducing the molecule's oxygen affinity.

2,3-DPG is an intermediate on the glycolytic pathway (Fig. 25.6) and is present in relatively high concentrations within the red cell (its molar concentration is similar to that of haemoglobin). Hypoxia within the red cell tends to increase 2,3-DPG levels in two ways. Firstly, the increased quantity of deoxygenated haemoglobin means that more 2,3-DPG is bound, thereby reducing product inhibition of DPG mutase. Secondly, deoxyhaemoglobin is a weaker acid than its oxygenated form, so that hypoxia leads to a rise in internal red cell pH. This increases 2,3-DPG levels both by stimulating glycolysis in general and by inhibiting DPG phosphatase. With an anaemia of 7.5 g/dl, the rise in 2,3-DPG levels is sufficient to move the oxygen dissociation curve to the right and increase oxygen delivery by about 25%. If, however, the hypoxia is sufficiently severe to cause acidosis within the red cell, 2,3-DPG levels will tend to be depressed. Fortunately, this effect on oxygen affinity is balanced by the direct effect of H^+ on oxygen affinity (*Bohr shift*). This is of considerable importance in patients with a severe acidosis treated with bicarbonate. Sudden correction will immediately negate the Bohr shift and move the dissociation curve to the left; while the compensatory rise in 2,3-DPG will take many hours to occur. During this interim period, tissue oxygenation will be further impaired.

Some of the carbon dioxide released from the tissues diffuses into the red cells and is rapidly hydrated to carbonic acid (H_2CO_3) because of the high levels of carbonic anhydrase. The $H_2CO_3^-$ dissociates to H^+ and HCO_3^- and the H^+ is buffered predominantly by deoxy-haemoglobin while the HCO_3^- re-enters the plasma. In the lungs, this process is reversed with the resultant CO_2 released into the alveoli.

The normal red cell mass is 25–35 ml/kg in men, and 20–30 ml/kg in women. The more readily measured haemoglobin concentration has a wide normal range which changes with age and sexual development (Table 25.1).

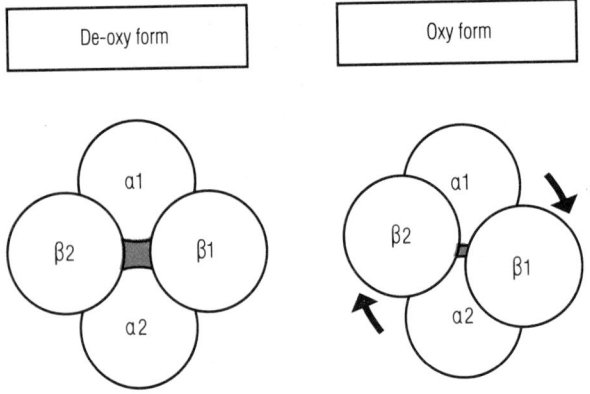

Fig. 25.5 Diagrammatic representation of the change in configuration of the haemoglobin molecule associated with oxygenation. Oxygenation is accompanied by a rotation of the α_1-β_1 dimer about the contact point between α_1 and β_2, thus closing up the pocket in which 2,3-DPG binds. Insertion of 2,3-DPG into this pocket stabilises the deoxy configuration.

Table 25.1 Changes in haemoglobin concentration with age

Age	Haemoglobin concentration (g/dl)
First 3 days of life	13–21
First month thereafter	10–18
1–12 months	10–13.5
1–12 years	11.5–15.5
Adult males	13.0–18.0
Adult females	12.0–16.0

Leucocytes

Neutrophils

Neutrophils are mobile phagocytic cells able to recognise, phagocytose and then kill micro-organisms opsonised by IgG or C3b. They also migrate to non-infective sites of tissue damage, where they contribute to the inflammatory process. The neutrophil count is high in the first weeks of life but thereafter remains between 2.5 and 7.5×10^9/l.

Eosinophils

Eosinophils are phagocytes particularly effective in the elimination of parasites. They also participate in hypersensitivity reactions, especially in the skin, lungs and gut. The normal eosinophil count is less than 0.4×10^9/l.

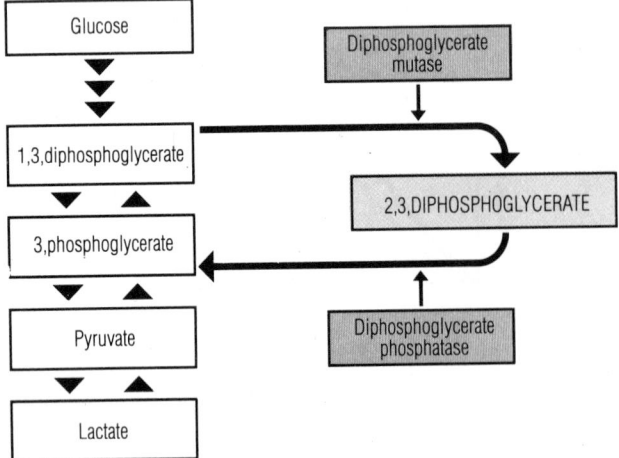

Fig. 25.6 The production of 2,3-diphosphoglycerate.

Basophils

Basophils are involved in the pathogenesis of immediate hypersensitivity. When IgE is bound to their surface, they release histamine, which causes increased vascular permeability and smooth muscle contraction. The normal count is less than $0.1 \times 10^9/l$.

Monocytes

Monocytes are phagocytic cells which remove micro-organisms, damaged cells and cell fragments. They also have a central role in the generation of the immune response, through presentation of the antigen to lymphocytes, regulation of many T and B cell functions, and cytotoxic activity towards antibody coated cells. The monocyte count can be relatively high in the neonate (up to $4 \times 10^9/l$) but falls rapidly during early childhood. By four years of age, the normal adult values of $0.2-0.8 \times 10^9/l$ are attained.

Lymphocytes

Lymphocytes in the blood consist of many functionally discrete populations.

Thymus-dependent T cells are the major population of lymphocytes in the blood, accounting for approximately 70% of all lymphocytes. Two-thirds of T cells express the CD4 antigen on the cell surface and one-third the CD8 antigen. CD4+ cells are predominantly involved in interactions with other cells in association with class II HLA antigens, and serve to initiate and regulate the immune response (helper/inducer cells). The CD8+ population includes cells with cytotoxic activity which is usually specific for antigen recognised in association with class I HLA antigens; and also cells which suppress the immune response. The extent of overlap between these T cell populations is not clear.

B cells – which account for only 5–10% of peripheral blood lymphocytes – have the potential to synthesise and secrete antibody and express surface immunoglobulin. Several heavy chain isotypes may be expressed, but only one light chain is expressed by a single cell.

The remaining 10–25% of peripheral blood lymphocytes are *non-T, non-B lymphocytes*. Some of these cells (natural killer cells) have a large granular appearance and non-MHC-restricted cytotoxic activity.

Neonates and young children have a high lymphocyte count, but this falls at puberty to the normal adult range of $1.5-4.5 \times 10^9/l$.

CLASSIFICATION AND CAUSES OF ANAEMIA

Anaemia occurs when the haemoglobin concentration [Hb] falls below the normal range, taking into account the age and sex of the individual concerned. It must also be remembered that [Hb] may be altered when living at high altitudes (which elevates the normal range), and in states such as pregnancy and splenomegaly, which lead to an increased plasma volume so that a normal red cell mass is maintained at lower haemoglobin concentrations.

True anaemia arises when there is an imbalance between red cell production and red cell destruction (Fig. 25.7). Increased red cell destruction can be compensated for in part by increased marrow production, so that chronic anaemia only occurs when red cell survival is less than half normal. Many causes of anaemia have multiple mechanisms. In thalassaemia, for example, both ineffective erythropoiesis and haemolysis occur.

From the practical standpoint, the classification of anaemia is based on routine haematological investigation – viz. automated cell counter analysis – considered in the context of the clinical history and examination. The automated counters measure the haemoglobin concentration, red cell count and mean cell size (MCV). The mean cell haemoglobin (MCH) and mean cell haemoglobin concentration (MCHC) are derived from these parameters and provide limited additional information. The counters also produce a white cell count (nucleated red cells, which may be prevalent in some haemolytic states, are counted as white cells) and may also produce an automatic platelet count. The most sophisticated machines are able to perform a white cell differential count. The anaemias are initially characterised in terms of the red cell size (Table 25.2). The precise cause of the anaemia can often be surmised from the combination of automated counter analysis and clinical situation, while examination of the blood film

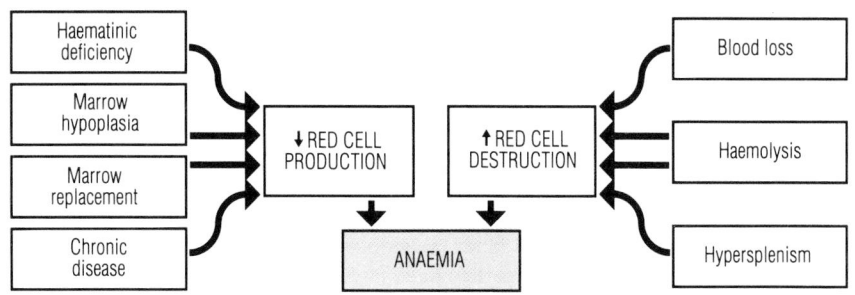

Fig. 25.7 The aetiology of anaemia.

Table 25.2 Classification of anaemia according to the MCV

Type of anaemia	Cause	Features on blood film
Microcytic	Iron deficiency	Marked anisocytosis and poikilocytosis Pencil cells
	Thalassaemia	Target cells Nucleated red cells Reticulocytes
	Chronic disease	May be neutrophilia Target cells – liver disease Burr cells – renal failure
Normocytic	Acute haemorrhage	Reticulocytosis
	Haemolysis	Reticulocytosis
	Marrow hypoproduction	Pancytopenia May be abnormal cells, e.g. leukaemia
	Chronic disease	
	Combination iron and folate deficiency	Microcytes and oval macrocytes
Macrocytic	Megaloblastic change	Prominent oval macrocytes Pancytopenia Multisegmented polymorphs
	Reticulocytosis (haemorrhage, haemolysis)	Polychromasia and reticulocytosis
	Alcohol	
	Liver disease	Target cells
	Myxoedema (rare)	
	Aplastic anaemia (rare)	Pancytopenia
	Leukaemia and related disorders (rare)	Abnormal cells Normoblasts and myeloid precursor cells in blood (leukoerythroblastic)

provides further clues as to aetiology. Further specific investigations are individually planned, depending on the results of these screening tests.

IRON DEFICIENCY ANAEMIA

Pathophysiology

Iron deficiency is the commonest form of anaemia and is particularly prevalent in underprivileged communities. The daily intake of iron is closely related to the calorific value of the diet, so that individuals with poor diets (especially menstruating women) are particularly at risk. Even in Western societies, it would appear that over 5% of such women have iron deficiency anaemia. Others at risk include: premature babies, as they have low iron stores

and a milk diet which is relatively low in iron content; children during rapid growth periods; and women during pregnancy and lactation, when iron requirements are high.

The average Western diet contains 10–15 mg of iron per day and about 10% of this is absorbed. In iron deficiency, absorption is increased and may be as high as 30% of the total ingested. Iron enters the mucosal cells of the upper small intestine and is bound to apoferritin for transport across to the inner membrane of the mucosal cell, where it is given up to plasma transferrin. The level of transferrin saturation thus regulates absorption. Transferrin transports iron to the bone marrow where it is incorporated into haemoglobin. Iron is taken up by the reticulo-endothelial (RE) system and other tissues, where some is bound to enzymes and myoglobin but most is stored as ferritin and haemosiderin. Iron is lost from the body in sweat, urine, desquamated cells and in breast milk, but most of the iron released from effete red cells is recycled. Any bleeding is a major source of iron loss; menstruating women, for example, are only in marginal iron balance.

When iron loss exceeds iron absorption, the iron stores become depleted and the transferrin saturation in the blood then falls. When this drops to below around 10%, abnormal, iron deficient, erythropoiesis occurs. The first event is a fall in the MCV with signs of abnormal erythropoiesis on the blood film such as variation in size (poikilocytosis) and shape (anisocytosis). As the iron deficiency progresses, microcytic anaemia develops, the anisocytosis and poikilocytosis becomes more marked and very narrow elliptocytes known as pencil cells may be seen. In more severe cases, target cells may also be detected. The red cells are hypochromic in appearance, but this is more a reflection of their small size than poor haemoglobinisation, as the MCHC only falls below the normal range when the anaemia is severe.

Clinical features

Iron deficiency anaemia leads to the gradual onset of the symptoms of anaemia, with lethargy, weakness, dizziness and palpitations particularly on exertion. In addition, the hair and nails may become brittle and the nails spoon-shaped (koilonychia). Pruritus vulvae may occur and, in severe cases, cerebral irritability and even cerebral oedema may arise. Very rarely, a post cricoid web develops which initially causes dysphagia for solids but not liquids.

Aetiology and investigation

The aetiology of iron deficiency is illustrated in Fig. 25.8. Nearly one-half of patients who have had a partial gastrectomy develop iron deficiency if not given iron supplements, due primarily to rapid gastrojejunal transit. Achlorhydria may also cause iron deficiency as hydrochloric acid is important for the absorption of iron contained in foodstuffs. The cause of iron deficiency must always be established and particular attention paid to possible gastrointestinal bleeding. Malignancies of the gas-

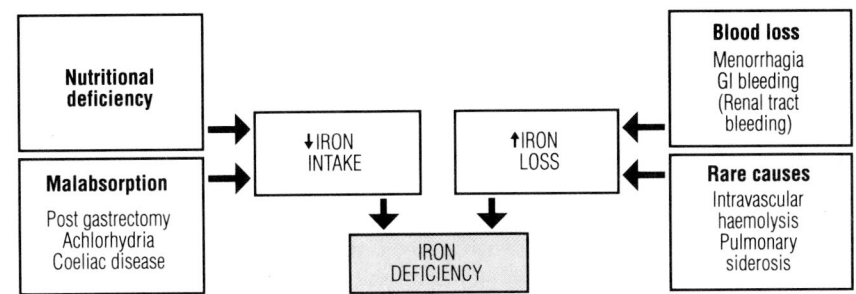

Fig. 25.8 The aetiology of iron deficiency.

trointestinal tract may present with iron deficiency anaemia in the absence of any other symptoms.

Diagnosis

The diagnosis of iron deficiency anaemia is suggested by the finding of microcytosis on the automated counter print-out and associated changes on the blood film (p. 1044), and is confirmed by finding a low serum iron and high/normal total iron binding capacity (TIBC). The percentage TIBC saturation is less than 10%. In the anaemia of chronic disease (p. 1061) – which may also be microcytic – the serum iron is also low, but the TIBC is reduced and the percentage saturation is thus usually above 10%. In thalassaemia, the percentage saturation is high due to ineffective erythropoiesis, haemolysis and transfusion. Where difficulties occur in interpreting serum iron and TIBC values, the measurement of serum ferritin may be useful. This is usually below $40\,\mu g/l$ in iron deficiency (normal range 15–300 $\mu g/l$), but may be higher if there is coexistent inflammatory disease. A bone marrow examination gives definitive evidence of the status of the iron stores, as there is no Prussian Blue-stainable iron in marrow fragments in iron deficiency anaemia.

Treatment

The treatment of iron deficiency requires identification and correction of its cause where possible. The iron deficiency anaemia itself is usually correctable with oral iron supplements. Ferrous sulphate (200 mg tds) is cheap and usually well tolerated. If gastric intolerance occurs, reduction of the dosage to 200 mg once or twice per day will usually be acceptable and provide sufficient iron. Therapy should be continued until the anaemia has resolved, and then for a further three months to replete the iron stores. Parenteral iron is only necessary if oral preparations cannot be tolerated, or if inadequate iron is absorbed by that route. The response to parenteral iron is no faster than that to oral iron. Intramuscular iron is usually given as an iron-sorbitol-citric acid complex (Jectofer). Iron dextran can be given intravenously to correct the iron deficiency in a single infusion, but this therapy can be hazardous and is not generally advisable.

THE MEGALOBLASTIC ANAEMIAS

The megaloblastic anaemias are caused by impaired DNA synthesis and are almost always due to a deficiency of either B_{12} or folate. These anaemias are characterised by the abnormal morphology (megaloblastosis) of all cell lines within the bone marrow and blood. While the precise biochemical mechanism of megaloblastic change is unknown, it is clear that DNA replication is blocked whilst synthesis of cytoplasmic RNA and protein continues. The production of mature end cells is thus reduced and many precursor cells die within the marrow (ineffective haemopoiesis).

Clinical features

The onset of megaloblastic anaemia is usually insidious and the disease can be very advanced before presentation. The patients have symptoms of anaemia and may, as well as being pale, have a slight yellow tinge due to the haemolytic component of the ineffective erythropoiesis. The tongue may be red and sore, and slight splenomegaly may be present. In severe cases, there may also be a low grade pyrexia together with infections and purpura secondary to pancytopenia. In the elderly, the gradual onset of anaemia may produce heart failure. In megaloblastic anaemia secondary to B_{12} deficiency, there may be neurological symptoms and other signs including optic atrophy, peripheral neuropathy, subacute combined degeneration of the cord and dementia. Due to considerable individual variation in the susceptibiity of the nervous system to B_{12} deficiency, severe neurological sequelae can occur even with relatively minor anaemia.

Haematological features

The automated counter printout shows a macrocytic anaemia with a subpopulation of very large, oval macrocytes usually visible on the film. Excessive alcohol intake and liver disease are also frequently associated with a macrocytic anaemia, as is a reticulocytosis; but the blood film will often resolve any diagnostic difficulties. In megaloblastic anaemia, the white cells and platelets are also affected and the counts may be low. This may also be the case in liver disease with hypersplenism but, in megaloblastic change, the neutrophils are typically multisegmented, some with five or six lobes. In very severe anaemia, nucleated red cells may appear in the blood and have the appearance of megaloblasts.

The definitive diagnosis of megaloblastic anaemia is made by examination of the bone marrow. In the red cell series, the nucleus looks 'open' with delayed maturation relative to the haemoglobinising cytoplasm; the white cell series is also abnormal with giant metamyelocytes present. It is often said that the bone marrow should be examined in all cases of macrocytic anaemia but this is not necessary.

Aetiology and investigation

Megaloblastic change may be due to either B_{12} or folate deficiency and very rarely to other inherited and acquired anaemias. In patients with *macrocytic* anaemia, samples for serum B_{12} and red cell folate (red cell folate is less affected by recent diet than serum folate) should be taken immediately; and liver function tests and plasma thyroxine should also be measured. Where examination of the patient and blood film suggest megaloblastic change, therapy with B_{12} and folate should be started immediately, as delay could result in the development of neurological problems. Bone marrow examination can usually be restricted to those patients where there is considerable initial uncertainty about the diagnosis, or where a rapid response to therapy is not achieved. Further investigation will then depend on whether the cause of the megaloblastic anaemia is deficiency of B_{12} or folate.

B_{12} DEFICIENCY

Animal products are the main source of B_{12} in the diet. Ingested B_{12} binds to intrinsic factor (IF) secreted by the gastric parietal cells, and the B_{12}-IF complex is then absorbed in the terminal ileum. Large stores of B_{12} are contained in the liver so that B_{12} deficiency takes three or four years to develop in the face of normal requirements. The normal serum B_{12} level is 150–950 pg/ml and may be measured by bioassay or radioimmunoassay. The major function of B_{12} is as a cofactor in the methylation of homocysteine to methionine. Methionine is then oxidized to

formate which is used in purine synthesis, conversion of deoxyuridine to thymidine and in the formation of folate polyglutamate (the major red cell form of folate). In B_{12} deficiency, red cell folate levels are also low, although serum folate is normal or high.

Aetiology

The causes of B_{12} deficiency are shown in Fig. 25.9. Nutritional deficiency occurs predominantly in vegans and chronic alcoholics. Intrinsic factor (IF) deficiency occurs following gastric surgery and in pernicious anaemia – a relatively common condition (6000 cases/year in the UK) which occurs mainly in the elderly. In pernicious anaemia, there is an autoimmune-mediated atrophic gastritis resulting in achlorhydria and inability to produce IF. It may be associated with other autoimmune diseases such as myxoedema, diabetes mellitus and vitiligo. There may be a family history of other autoimmune disorders and sometimes a history of premature greying of the hair. The disease is more common in individuals with blood group A.

Malabsorption of B_{12} due to terminal ileal disease occurs most commonly in Crohn's disease, when there is often concomitant iron and folate deficiency. Pancreatic failure may also cause B_{12} malabsorption, probably by reducing the pH and Ca^{2+} concentration of the terminal ileal fluid to below the optimum for absorption. A variety of drugs have been reported as inhibiting B_{12} absorption, including the biguanides and high dose potassium supplements. Bacterial overgrowth, such as occurs with intestinal 'blind loops' (p. 587), may consume ingested B_{12}. The Scandinavian fish tapeworm is a more exotic cause of such intestinal competition.

Diagnosis

The diagnosis of the cause of B_{12} deficiency is made by the *Schilling test*, in which the fasting patient is given a loading dose of parenteral vitamin B_{12} to saturate both plasma and liver binding sites, and is then given oral radioactive B_{12}. Any absorbed B_{12} is excreted in the urine. In patients with normal absorption, 10% or more of the administered radioactivity appears in the urine over the next 24 hours. If there is less than this, B_{12} malabsorption is present and

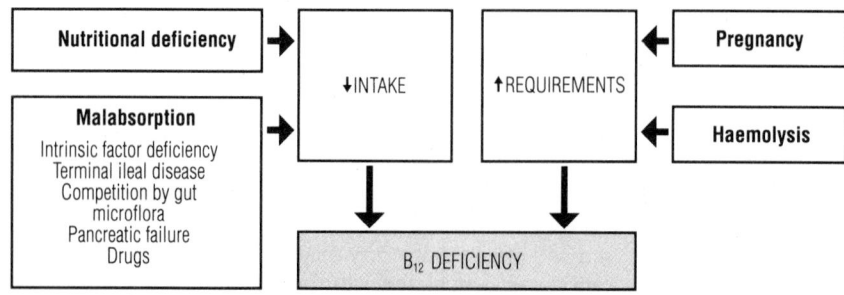

Fig. 25.9 The aetiology of vitamin B_{12} deficiency.

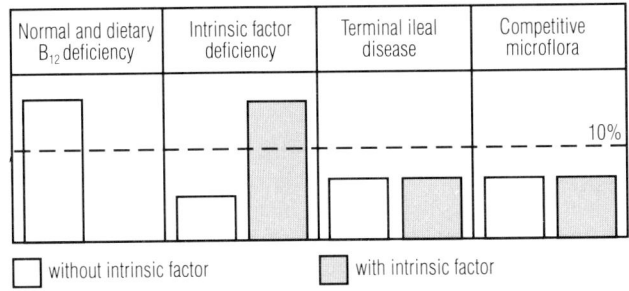

Normal and dietary B₁₂ deficiency	Intrinsic factor deficiency	Terminal ileal disease	Competitive microflora

□ without intrinsic factor   ■ with intrinsic factor

Fig. 25.10 The Schilling test. The urinary excretion of orally administered radioactively labelled vitamin B₁₂ is measured. Low levels are excreted if there is malabsorption of B₁₂ for any reason. If malabsorption is due to pernicious anaemia (intrinsic factor deficiency), there is correction with simultaneous oral administration of intrinsic factor. This correction does not occur when the cause of malabsorption is terminal ileal disease or competitive gut microflora.

the second part of the Schilling test is performed. In this case, the radioactive B₁₂ is given together with IF, and IF deficiency is indicated if the malabsorption corrects (Fig. 25.10). Parts I and II of the Schilling test can be done simultaneously if two different cobalamin isotopes are used – one to label free B₁₂ and one to label B₁₂ complexed to IF.

The diagnosis of pernicious anaemia is confirmed by the presence in the serum of autoantibodies to both parietal cells (in over 90% of patients with pernicious anaemia, but also in 15–20% of normal elderly people) and intrinsic factor (in over 50% of patients). Histamine-fast achlorhydria and a raised serum gastrin are also present, but rarely need to be measured.

Treatment

B₁₂ deficiency is treated with hydroxycobalamin supplements. These may be given orally in patients with a dietary deficiency (5–10 μg/day), but must be given intramuscularly when malabsorption is present. It is usual to give five or six loading doses of 1000 μg over a period of one to two weeks, followed by 1000 μg every three months. A brisk reticulocyte response is usually seen after one week, although this may be delayed if the patient has other coexistent disease such as alcoholism. Hypokalaemia and gout may develop during treatment of severe megaloblastic anaemia, and diuretics must be used cautiously if there is heart failure. Therapy with B₁₂ may also precipitate incipient iron deficiency. Blood transfusion is rarely necessary and is best avoided.

FOLIC ACID DEFICIENCY

Folic acid is the parent compound of the folates, which facilitate the transfer of one-carbon units necessary in the synthesis of purine and pyrimidine bases. Folates are found in fresh fruit and vegetables, liver and kidney, and are destroyed by thorough cooking. Folate is absorbed in the upper small intestine and stored in a number of tissues, but particularly the liver. These stores provide about four months' supply of folate in the absence of further intake.

Aetiology

The aetiology of folate deficiency is illustrated in Fig. 25.11. Dietary deficiency is seen particularly in milk-fed premature babies, the elderly (especially if living alone), and in chronic alcoholics. As coeliac disease and tropical sprue primarily affect the jejunum, folate deficiency is also very common in these diseases. They are also often associated with iron deficiency and the combined deficiency may result in normocytic indices on the automated printout. Examination of the blood film may reveal evidence of both iron deficiency and macrocytosis (dimorphic picture). Megaloblastic change is still apparent on bone marrow examination and pancytopenia and multisegmented polymorphs may be seen in the blood. Folate deficiency is also common (though less so than B₁₂ deficiency) after gastrectomy; both decreased dietary intake and rapid gastro-jejunal transit may contribute to its development. Drugs such as phenytoin may inhibit folate

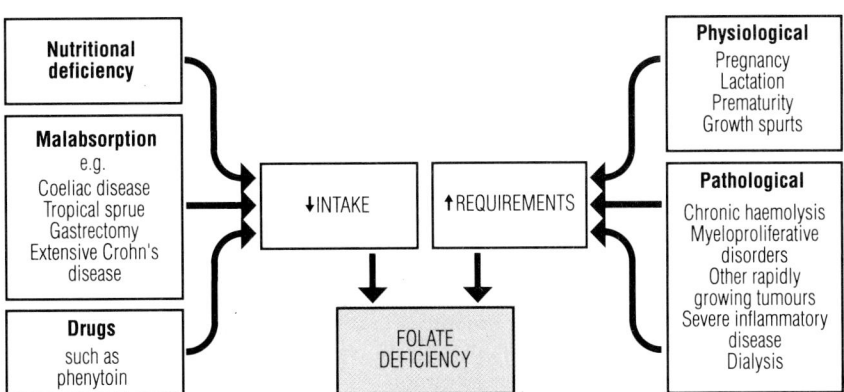

Fig. 25.11 Aetiology of folate deficiency.

25

absorption, probably through a direct effect on the enterocyte brush border. Other drugs may interfere with folate utilisation, giving rise to megaloblastic anaemia in the presence of normal folate levels. These include the antifolate cytotoxic drugs (e.g. methotrexate), trimethoprim and anticonvulsants (e.g. phenytoin and phenobarbitone). Alcohol may also interfere with folate utilisation and this may account in part for the macrocytosis seen with excess consumption.

Treatment

The underlying cause of folate deficiency must be found and treated. The deficiency is treated with oral folic acid supplements (5–15 mg/day) which is usually adequate, even in malabsorption states. Folic acid is also given prophylactically to pregnant women, premature babies, patients receiving dialysis and in severe chronic haemolytic states. Folic acid should not be given alone in megaloblastic anaemia until B_{12} deficiency has been excluded, since folate administration may precipitate neurological changes in B_{12} deficiency.

THE HYPOPLASTIC ANAEMIAS

The hypoplastic or aplastic anaemias are a group of disorders in which there is anaemia due to decrease in erythropoietic marrow. Although there is usually pancytopenia with reduction of all marrow elements, selective cytopenias do occur.

CONGENITAL/INHERITED HYPOPLASTIC ANAEMIAS

Congenital forms of hypoplastic anaemia occur in childhood. In *Fanconi's anaemia* (an autosomal recessive condition), pancytopenia usually develops between five and ten years of age. Many of the children also suffer from other congenital abnormalities, including skeletal malformations (especially affecting the radii and thumbs), renal anomalies, microcephaly, and congenital heart disease. This type of aplastic anaemia is characterised by a high red cell MCV, increased levels of HbF, a high ESR and a high incidence (5–10%) of transformation to acute leukaemia. Without successful bone marrow transplantation, the disease is invariably fatal.

Pure red cell aplasia (*Diamond-Blackfan syndrome*) may also be inherited, although the pattern of inheritance is not clear. Again, other congenital abnormalities may be present but are not as common as in Fanconi's anaemia. The anaemia usually appears in the first few weeks of life, although the diagnosis may be made considerably later. Steroids induce remissions in many patients but the majority become transfusion dependent.

Other familial and congenital hypoplastic states have also been described but are far less common.

ACQUIRED HYPOPLASTIC ANAEMIAS

Aetiology

The causes of the chronic acquired aplastic anaemias are shown in Table 25.3. Most cases are idiopathic in origin. It has been suggested that, in many such cases, there is an immunological suppression of haemopoiesis, possibly mediated by gamma-interferon production; but definite proof is lacking.

Transient episodes of marrow hypoplasia also occur, particularly following infections and idiosyncratic drug reactions. For example, very transient selective erythroid hypoplasia accompanies parvovirus infections. In normal individuals, this results in a transient reticulocytopenia; but in patients with haemolytic disease, there can be a dramatic fall in the haemoglobin level. Chronic pure red cell aplasia also occurs in adults, associated in nearly half the cases with a benign thymoma.

Table 25.3 Aetiology of chronic acquired aplastic anaemia

- Idiopathic
- Drugs
  Cytotoxic drugs
  Idiosyncratic reaction to drugs (including choramphenicol, phenylbutazone and thiouracils)
- Irradiation
- Chemicals, e.g. benzene
- Associated with infections, particularly viral hepatitis
- Associated with autoimmune disease
- Associated with pregnancy
- Paroxysmal nocturnal haemoglobinuria

Clinical features

Patients with chronic aplastic anaemia present with insidious onset of the symptoms of anaemia, infections secondary to the granulocytopenia, and bleeding due to thrombocytopenia. Examination may reveal signs of the above, but is otherwise usually normal. Splenomegaly, which occurs in less than 10% of cases, always suggests that the

Table 25.4 Differential diagnosis of pancytopenia

- Aplastic anaemia
- Bone marrow replacement
  Leukaemias, lymphomas and myeloma
  Non-haematological malignancies
  Fibrosis
  Osteoporosis (rare)
  Gaucher's disease (rare)
- Hypersplenism
- Immune destruction (rare cause of pancytopenia)

pancytopenia may be due to another cause.

The differential diagnosis of pancytopenia is shown in Table 25.4. In the marrow replacement states, the anaemia is often leucoerythroblastic, i.e. with nucleated red cells and granulocyte precursor cells in the blood.

Laboratory features

The anaemia of aplastic anaemia is usually normocytic but may be slightly macrocytic. There is an absolute reticulocytopenia. HbF levels may be modestly increased. Granulocytopenia and monocytopenia are present but the lymphocyte count may initially be near normal. The platelets are generally reduced. Severe aplastic anaemia is considered to be present when the reticulocyte level is below $20 \times 10^9/l$, the granulocytes below $0.5 \times 10^9/l$ and the platelets less than $20 \times 10^9/l$. The diagnosis of aplastic anaemia is made by examination of a large sized bone marrow biopsy (preferably from two sites). Fat spaces predominate and there is markedly reduced haemopoiesis. Islands of haemopoiesis may be found and can be particularly confusing on a small biopsy specimen.

Management

Support

The successful management of aplastic anaemia is dependent on aggressive supportive care. Infections must be actively sought, recognised early and treated with intravenous antibiotics. In patients with a neutrophil count below $0.5 \times 10^9/l$, it is usual to give prophylactic oral antifungal agents such as nystatin or amphotericin. Some centres also give prophylactic oral cotrimoxazole, but this is controversial. Isolation facilities are advisable for severely neutropenic inpatients, but this alone is not an indication for hospitalisation. Therapy should be started empirically in patients with significant fever (above 38°C) sustained for two hours (less if clinical signs or symptoms are present). If there is a fever, the antibiotics must be broad spectrum and cover Gram-negative organisms including the coliforms and pseudomonas. A combination of an aminoglycoside plus a ureido penicillin, or an aminoglycoside plus a third generation cephalosporin or quinolone (e.g. ciprofloxacin), are usually used. Before initiating such therapy, a throat swab, sputum (if available), midstream specimen of urine, swabs from intravenous catheter sites, and blood taken from both a peripheral site and from any central intravenous lines, should be sent to microbiology for culture. The antibiotics can be rationalised later, if and when an organism is isolated and the sensitivities determined. A serum sample should be saved for possible viral antibody titres at a later date. A chest X-ray should be performed.

In patients who fail to respond to broad spectrum antibiotics within five days, an opportunistic infection with fungus or pneumocystis should be suspected. Bronchoscopy may be considered. Intravenous amphotericin therapy is used for suspected fungal infection, while

---

> **Summary 1 Management of hypoplastic anaemia**
>
> *Supportive*
>
> Early treatment of infection with intravenous antibiotics (initially broad-spectrum, rationalised later)
> Prophylatic oral anti-fungal agents
> (Isolation facilities, if severely neutropenic)
> Red cell transfusion
> Platelet transfusion
> (Granulocyte transfusion)
>
> *Specific therapy*
>
> Androgen therapy (oxymethalone)
> Intensive immunosuppression
> Bone marrow transplantation

pneumocystis infection may respond to high-dose cotrimoxazole therapy.

Red cell transfusions should be given as required and leucocyte-poor red cells used if sensitisation to white cell antigens occurs. Although repeated transfusions do increase the risks of graft rejection in patients who are later treated by bone marrow transplantation, it is more important to keep the patient in a good general condition.

Platelet transfusions are given to all patients with thrombocytopenia and evidence of bleeding. The use of platelets prophylactically in aplastic anaemia is limited by the chronic nature of the disease and the sensitisation that may occur to HLA and platelet-specific antigens. Granulocyte transfusions are not given prophylactically, and their use is limited to the treatment of life-threatening infections in severely neutropenic patients who are not responding to broad spectrum antibiotic therapy. Even in this situation, their value is unproven.

Specific therapy

The traditional therapy for aplastic anaemia is *androgen therapy*, continued for at least 3–6 months. Oxymethalone is used, as it is less virilising than the testosterone derivatives. Proof of efficacy is lacking, however, and in severe cases, many centres initiate more aggressive treatment strategies such as intensive immunosuppression or bone marrow transplantation early in the course of the disease.

Intensive immunosuppression usually consists of high dose methyl prednisone and/or a course of anti-lymphocyte serum. In some series, up to half the patients show a significant response, although there is considerable variation in the response to different batches of anti-lymphocyte globulin. This type of therapy is intensive, and requires inpatient support similar to that required for transplantation. In the patients who do respond, the response is usually only partial and completely normal haemopoiesis is not re-established.

Bone marrow transplantation is currently only available to those individuals under 40 years of age with an HLA identical sibling. Patients are usually prepared for transplantation with cyclophosphamide (50 mg/kg) on four successive days. In multiply-transfused patients, some centres use total nodal irradiation to reduce the risk of graft rejection, but similar results can be achieved with cyclosporin A. The marrow inoculum required for transplantation in aplastic anaemia is probably higher than that for acute leukaemia, and at least 2×10^8 cells/kg should be given. The development of graft versus host disease (GVHD) can be minimised by administration of methotrexate or cyclosporin A. More recently, the removal of mature T cells from the marrow inoculum has been shown to be very effective in reducing GVHD; but there is some concern that there may be increased graft rejection, particularly in multiply-transfused aplastic patients.

Complications of bone marrow transplantation

Graft versus host disease is an ill understood immunological reaction of mature donor lymphoid cells against host tissue. The acute form arises coincident with, or shortly after, haemopoietic regeneration, and manifests as a maculopapular rash involving the hands and feet, hepatocellular liver toxicity and diarrhoea. In its severest forms, there can be erythroderma (p.1132), widespread bullae and then desquamation and torrential diarrhoea. Acute GVHD is treated with a course of high dose methylprednisone. Severe cases may respond but the mortality is appreciable. Chronic GVHD develops several months after transplantation and is not necessarily preceded by the acute form. It takes the form of sclerodermatous skin changes and obstructive liver disease which can be debilitating and refractory to treatment. Immunosuppressive agents, such as azathioprine, are usually tried in this situation.

Immediately following preparative chemo/radiotherapy the patients with aplastic anaemia become even more pancytopenic. The risks of bacterial and fungal infection are thus very high in the 2–3 week period before graft regeneration occurs. These risks decline somewhat after graft-take, but the patient remains immunosuppressed for many months, and opportunistic viral and fungal infections may still occur. Pneumocystis pneumonia is a particular problem in some centres and may be fatal; prophylactic septrin is given to reduce this. Cytomegalovirus infections may also be fatal, especially if there is coincident GVHD.

However, over half the patients survive transplantation for aplastic anaemia and obtain haematological normality. In some centres, the success rate is in excess of 70%.

HAEMOLYTIC ANAEMIAS

The aetiology of haemolysis (excessive destruction of red cells) is given in Table 25.5.

Clinical and laboratory features

Patients with acute haemolysis develop profound symptoms of anaemia. However, in the chronic haemolytic states

Table 25.5 Aetiology of haemolysis

Congenital

Defects of haemoglobin synthesis and structure
   Thalassaemia
   Sickle cell disease
   Unstable haemoglobins (rare)

Membrane defects
   Hereditary spherocytosis
   Hereditary elliptocytosis

Red cell enzyme defects
   G6PD deficiency
   Pyruvate kinase deficiency (rare)

Acquired (non-immune)
(see p. 1059, Table 25.8)

Acquired (immune)
(see p. 1058, Summary 3)

quite severe anaemia can be tolerated with symptoms only arising on exercise. The patient is jaundiced but this is often mild and easily missed. The urine is dark (especially after standing), due to the oxidisation of urobilinogen to urobilin. The spleen tends to be enlarged to a degree dependent on the underlying cause of the haemolysis. Leg ulcers, usually over the lateral malleolus, occur in the congenital haemolytic anaemias, particularly sickle cell disease.

The presence of haemolysis is usually established in the laboratory by a raised level of unconjugated bilirubin and reticulocytosis. Examination for urine haemosiderinuria is particularly useful in low grade chronic haemolysis. Red cell survival studies with ^{51}Cr-labelled red cells are rarely required, but may be useful when combined with surface counting to estimate the role of the spleen in the haemolysis. The normal $t_{\frac{1}{2}}$ of ^{51}Cr-labelled red cells is 25–35 days. The marrow can compensate for a $t_{\frac{1}{2}}$ reduced to about 15 days, but below this anaemia occurs.

Investigation

Investigation of a patient with haemolysis begins with a very thorough history. This will often indicate whether a haemolytic anaemia is familial or congenital. Particular attention must be paid to coexistent systemic disease and drug ingestion, both of which may be associated with haemolytic anaemia. Examination of the peripheral blood film may show red cell changes indicative of the underlying cause (Table 25.5). White cell abnormalities – such as the atypical mononuclear cells of infectious mononucleosis, or the lymphocytosis of chronic lymphocytic leukaemia – may also indicate the cause of haemolysis. In those patients in whom an acquired haemolysis is suspected, the initial investigation is the direct antiglobulin test to determine whether this has an immune aetiology.

DEFECTS OF HAEMOGLOBIN SYNTHESIS AND STRUCTURE I: THE THALASSAEMIAS

Defects of haemoglobin synthesis and structure are one of the major congenital causes of haemolysis. The major examples are the thalassaemias and sickle cell disease.

The thalassaemias are inherited disorders in which there is a reduced synthesis of one or more globin chains. This results in unbalanced globin chain synthesis, globin precipitation, ineffective haemopoiesis and haemolysis. The α-thalassaemias are mainly found in the Far East, Middle East and Africa, while the β-thalassaemias are particularly prevalent in the Mediterranean. Thalassaemic genes are found in all racial groups.

The primary defect occurs either in the DNA sequences coding for the globin chains or in the intervening sequences between these coding regions. Chromosome 16 contains two genes coding for α chains, and there is a single gene coding for the β globin chain on chromosome 11 (Fig. 25.1, p. 1040). In the α-thalassaemias, the α genes are usually deleted, but such whole gene deletions are rare in the β-thalassaemias. In these cases, small aberrations in the gene may lead to decreased or absent transcription of the gene and intervening sequences, or they may prevent processing of the nuclear RNA to cytoplasmic RNA (during which the intervening sequences are removed). Rarely, cytoplasmic RNA is produced but cannot be translated into protein, e.g. where point mutations have introduced a stop sequence. A thalassaemic β gene may thus produce no β globin (β^0 gene) or low levels of β globin (β^+ gene).

β-THALASSAEMIAS

Clinical features

Clinically, the β-thalassaemias fall into three broad categories – thalassaemia minor (trait), intermedia and major. Individuals with thalassaemia trait are heterozygous for the thalassaemic gene and are usually fit and well: however, anaemia may develop during pregnancy, or in association with infections. In thalassaemia major, both β genes are abnormal so that the α:β chain synthesis imbalance is sufficient to cause a severe anaemia developing several months after birth. At birth, most of the haemoglobin is HbF ($\alpha_2\gamma_2$) and haemoglobin levels are normal. After birth α chain production continues, but γ chain synthesis diminishes to be replaced (in normal individuals) by β chain synthesis. In thalassaemia major, there is synthesis of α chains, but little or no β chain production. The result is a gradual onset of severe anaemia. Infants with thalassaemia major become listless, have a poor appetite and fail to thrive. Mental development is normal but walking is frequently delayed, and untreated children are grossly incapacitated and fail to develop. Expansion of the marrow cavities of the skull and facial bones results in a typical *mongoloid facies*, with frontal bossing of the skull and a 'hair on end' appearance on skull X-ray. Hepatomegaly and marked splenomegaly occur, and leg ulcers are frequent. Without transfusions, these children die in childhood or adolescence, usually from high output cardiac failure. Sexual maturity is not attained.

In thalassaemia intermedia, both β genes are affected but the clinical course is less severe, with haemoglobin levels typically in the range 6–9 g/dl. The molecular basis of β-thalassaemia intermedia is varied and includes:

1. homozygosity for mild β^+ thalassaemic genes
2. combinations of β^+ thalassaemia genes and δβ thalassaemia genes, in which there is decreased δ and β globin production but raised production of γ chains
3. homozygotes with β-thalassaemia in whom there is a genetic predisposition to high HbF production.
4. The combination of β-thalassaemia with α-thalassaemia trait, which also results in less chain imbalance and decreased severity of the disease.

Growth is not retarded and diagnosis is frequently delayed for several years until an intercurrent infection precipitates an acute fall in haemoglobin. These patients frequently survive into adulthood without transfusion and achieve normal sexual maturity, but pigment gallstones and leg ulceration are often a major problem.

Laboratory features

The thumbprint of thalassaemic genes is the appearance of microcytic red cells in the peripheral blood. In the β-thalassaemia traits, the haemoglobin concentration is normal or slightly reduced. The diagnosis is made by exclusion of iron deficiency and the anaemia of chronic disease, and the demonstration of a raised HbA_2 in a blood haemolysate. Levels of HbA_2 ($\alpha_2\delta_2$) are typically in the range 4–6% (normal 1.5–3%). In patients with homozygous β-thalassaemia, there is marked anaemia to a degree dependent on the nature of the underlying genetic defect. Poikilocytes and target cells are seen in the blood as well as polychromasia, and nucleated red blood cells are also present in the most severe cases. Haemoglobin electrophoresis usually shows HbF to be the major component. The level of HbA_2 is very variable. HbA is present in β^+ cases (Fig. 25.12).

In very difficult diagnostic cases – usually β-thalassaemia traits with microcytosis but a normal HbA_2 – the thalassaemic defect can be demonstrated by showing imbalance of α and β globin synthesis in reticulocytes, following pulse labelling with radioactive leucine.

Management

Patients with thalassaemia minor require no specific therapy, but the nature of the genetic defect should be thoroughly explained. In thalassaemia major, the backbone of therapy is blood transfusion. This is administered once every four to six weeks from the time of diagnosis, in an attempt to provide sufficient blood to maintain a normal

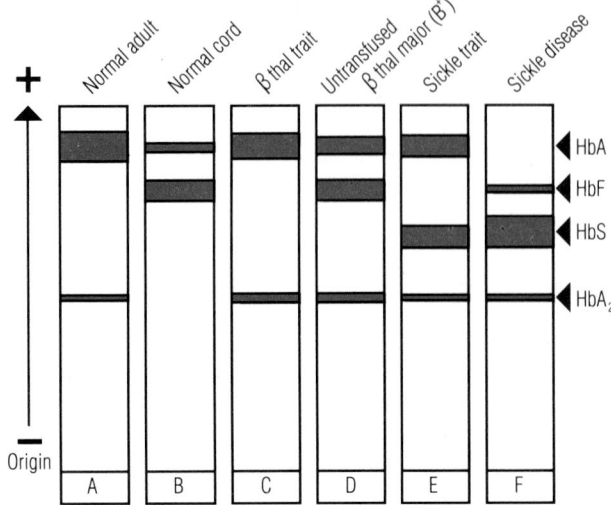

Fig. 25.12 Diagrammatic representation of haemoglobin electrophoresis at pH 8.9. HbD migrates in the same position as HbS, and HbC and HbE in the same position as HbA₂.

[Hb]. Such regimes enable a young child to grow satisfactorily and live a relatively normal life. Unfortunately, repeated blood transfusions result in iron overload and iron accumulates in many tissues. Although much remains within the reticuloendothelial system, some enters and damages parenchymal tissues and multiple organ failure develops – most notably in the liver, the endocrine glands and the heart. Thus, if left untreated, the child who initially grew well, ceases to do so and does not attain sexual maturity. Instead, he dies in adolescence as a result of cardiomyopathy secondary to iron toxicity. Serum ferritin levels provide information about the kinetics of iron accumulation, but the absolute levels do not correlate very closely with tissue toxicity.

The problems of iron overload can be reduced by regular administration of an iron chelator – generally desferrioxamine given subcutaneously (approximately 60 mg/kg/day) by infusion pump over eight hours, five or six days a week. Ideally, the individual dose should be adjusted in accordance with iron balance studies. Oral vitamin C is also sometimes given to improve iron excretion. Children given desferrioxamine from the age of 2–3 years have grown well and developed sexually; but the ultimate life expectancy of these young adults is not yet known. There is, moreover, the major problem with subcutaneous desferrioxamine of being attached to a pump for a quarter of one's life. Compliance is often poor and constant encouragement for the patients and family is required. Orally active iron chelators are being developed and offer hope for the future.

Hypersplenism frequently exacerbates the anaemia of thalassaemia, and splenectomy is therefore indicated if the transfusion requirements progressively increase or other cytopenias develop. Anti-pneumococcal vaccine may be of value if given before splenectomy, and oral penicillin V should certainly be given as prophylaxis against pneumococcal infections.

Antenatal diagnosis

Antenatal diagnosis of thalassaemia with abortion of affected fetuses is acceptable in some communities, and appropriate facilities are available in specialist centres. Prenatal diagnosis begins with screening of all pregnant women attending their first antenatal clinic. In thalassaemia trait, the MCV is low and the MCHC is normal; the MCH is a product of these measurements and is therefore a useful screening index. Patients with MCH values below 27 pg should have haemoglobin electrophoresis performed to look for a raised HbA₂. The iron status should also be determined, as patients with β-thalassaemia trait and iron deficiency may have a normal HbA₂. If the mother is found to have thalassaemia trait, the father should also be screened. Where both parents have the trait and the fetus is therefore at risk, prenatal diagnosis can be offered after both full discussion of the implications of the disease and consideration of the ethical issues involved. Prenatal diagnosis can be performed in the second trimester of pregnancy through globin chain synthesis studies on fetal blood obtained by fetoscopy. Diagnosis may also be made by DNA analysis of first trimester chorionic biopsy specimens. This has the great advantage of being possible earlier in gestation, but is expensive and not yet widely available.

α-THALASSAEMIAS

The α-thalassaemias have a wide spectrum of clinical manifestations, partly because there are four genes coding for α globin. The commonest genetic abnormality is a complete deletion of one or more genes.

1. Where only one gene is defective, the condition is often clinically silent, with a normal [Hb] and only a slight reduction in the MCV.
2. In the α-thalassaemia trait, there are usually two genes involved. Here, the [Hb] tends to be in the low/normal range, and microcytosis, poikilocytosis and some target cells are present in the blood. Supravital staining of the red cells may reveal inclusion bodies, which are precipitates of β chain tetramers known as HbH. HbA₂ levels are not raised. In newborn infants with α-thalassaemia trait, approximately 5% of the haemoglobin is in the form of γ chain tetramers known as Hb Barts.
3. The more severe form of this disorder (Haemoglobin H disease) is frequently due to the presence of three abnormal α genes. The patient usually has a mild anaemia, which may drop rapidly with intercurrent infections or during pregnancy. The blood film shows the typical changes of thalassaemia and 5–20% of the total Hb is HbH. HbA₂ is not raised. Patients with HbH disease tend to become folate-deficient and should be given prophylactic supplements. Intercurrent infections should be treated vigorously.
4. If all four α chains are deficient, there is no α chain

synthesis and no production of HbF, HbA or HbA$_2$. The fetus dies *in utero* of hydrops fetalis and examination of the blood shows that about 80% of the haemoglobin is Hb Barts (γ_4), with small amounts of HbH (β_4) and small amounts of the embryonic haemoglobin Hb Portland ($\varepsilon_2\gamma_2$).

OTHER FORMS OF THALASSAEMIA

Haemoglobin Constant Spring is a variant of the normal α globin, in which a mutation in the normal terminating codon results in elongation of the α chain by 31 amino acid residues. Synthesis of this globin is reduced, resulting in an α-thalassaemic syndrome with an abnormal band on starch gel electrophoresis running just behind HbA$_2$.

Alpha-thalassaemic genes may be associated with β-thalassaemic genes or abnormal chain variants. In general, this results in a reduction in severity of the underlying β-thalassaemic disease. Thus, a combination of β-thalassaemic genes that might otherwise be expected to cause thalassaemia major, may give rise to thalassaemia intermedia if there is concomitant α-thalassaemia. In sickle cell disorders, the presence of α-thalassaemia genes tends to reduce the MCHC with a lower absolute concentration of HbS. The effects of heterozygosity on β-thalassaemia and HbS are variable. If there is HbS/β^0, no HbA is produced and sickling may occur. With HbS/β^+ however, up to 30% of the Hb may be HbA and the situation is less serious.

The β-thalassaemic syndromes sometimes involve δ chain production, in which case no increase in HbA$_2$ occurs. In Hb Lepore there is low production of a hybrid formed from a part of the δ and part of the β chain, giving another form of thalassaemic syndrome with an abnormal haemoglobin on electrophoresis. When there is a major deletion in both the β and δ chain genes, γ gene expression remains high, giving rise to one of the forms of *hereditary persistence of fetal haemoglobin* (HPFH). The heterozygous form of this disorder should be distinguished from the variety of conditions in which reactivation of HbF production occurs (Table 25.6). In the marrow expansion states, the [HbF] is usually less than 3% and is often only detected as a rise in the number of red cells containing HbF (F-cells).

DEFECTS OF HAEMOGLOBIN SYNTHESIS AND STRUCTURE II: SICKLING DISORDERS

The sickle cell gene has a single base substitution which results in a change of valine for glutamine in the sixth amino acid position of the β chain. In the deoxygenated form, HbS forms non-hydrophobic bonds with adjacent HbS molecules, resulting in fibril formation and the appearance of distorted sickle-shaped cells. Initially, this process is reversible when the haemoglobin becomes oxygenated, but eventually the red cell membrane becomes damaged and leads to the formation of irreversibly sickled cells. The sickle gene originates primarily in areas where the malarial parasite (*Plasmodium falciparum*) is endemic, and owes its prevalence to the selective advantage conferred by the sickle cell trait on young children infected with this organism (Fig. 25.13).

SICKLE CELL TRAIT

In sickle cell trait (heterozygous state), at least 50% of the haemoglobin is HbA. The concentration of HbS is relatively low, so that sickling only occurs under anoxic conditions such as occur with non-pressurised air travel, poor anaesthetics, or (rarely) in conditions of marked acidosis and dehydration as may occur with severe infections. Individuals with sickle cell trait are not anaemic and are also otherwise asymptomatic. However, the sickle cell screening test – in which an HbS haemolysate precipitates and becomes cloudy at pH 7.1 – is positive. Haemoglobin electrophoresis reveals 35–50% HbS, which runs as a slow band at alkaline pH (Fig. 25.12), with the remainder nearly all HbA. [HbA$_2$] and [HbF] are not raised.

Table 25.6   Causes of a raised [HbF]

- β-thalassaemia major
- Hereditary persistence of HbF
- Marrow expansion states
  Pregnancy
  Recovery from hypoplasia
- Abnormal erythroid clone
  Chronic myeloproliferative diseases, especially juvenile chronic myeloid leukaemia
  Acute leukaemia
  (Paroxysmal nocturnal haemoglobinuria)
- Other
  Some cases of acquired aplastic anaemia
  (Occasionally in myeloma)

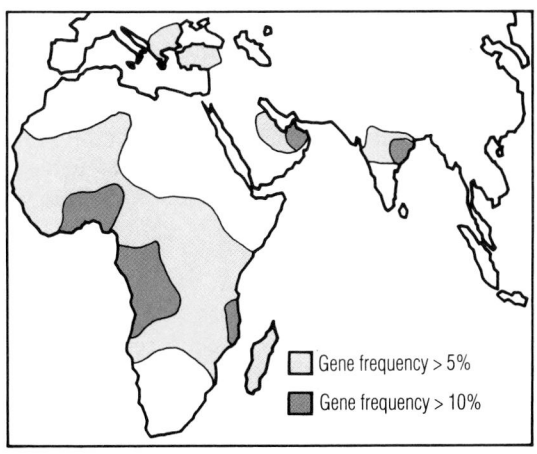

Gene frequency > 5%
Gene frequency > 10%

Fig. 25.13   Geographical incidence of the sickle cell gene.

SICKLE CELL DISEASE

Clinical features

Symptoms occur from the second half of the first year of life onwards, as the HbF levels fall. The major problems caused by sickling in young infants are haemolytic anaemias and dactylitis. Later, the main problem is the occurrence of painful vasocclusive crises caused by the sickled cells. These crises are frequently provoked by minor infections or dehydration.

The pain may be mild or so agonising as to require large doses of opiate analgesics. Fever and malaise are common, making it difficult to determine whether there is an underlying infection. Pain may arise in the limbs, back, abdomen or trunk. In childhood, splenic infarcts are frequent, leading to splenic atrophy and functional hyposplenism. Aseptic necrosis of the femoral head is a common and disabling complication.

Small vessel occlusions in the retinae lead to ischaemia and vascular proliferation, with visual impairment and a high risk of vitreous haemorrhage and retinal detachment. Retinopathy is particularly common in sickling disorders with a high [Hb], such as HbS/C disease. Haematuria occurs frequently due to papillary necrosis, but even in patients without such overt renal episodes, there is an acquired tubular reabsorption defect with inability to produce a concentrated urine. Priapism may occur due to sickling in the corpora cavernosa. This is extremely painful and, unless decompressed rapidly, results in impotence.

The anaemia of sickle cell disease may be exacerbated by episodes of erythroid hypoplasia (aplastic crises) precipitated by parvovirus infections, acute splenic and rarely hepatic sequestration of red cells, or folate deficiency. The chronic haemolytic anaemia frequently leads to ankle ulceration and the development of gallstones.

Patients with sickle cell disease also have an increased risk of infection, which is only partly explained by splenic atrophy. Fulminating pneumococcal infections may occur, and there is an unusually high incidence of Salmonella osteomyelitis which, initially, can be difficult to differentiate from a vasocclusive infarction.

Acute pulmonary episodes are the most common, and also potentially most dangerous, complications of sickle cell disease. The pulmonary lesions may be infective, ischaemic or a combination of the two. Minor lung changes can progress rapidly with development of widespread intra-alveolar consolidation and respiratory failure within hours.

Laboratory features

Haematological investigations in sickle cell disease reveal a mild to moderate normocytic anaemia. Anisocytosis, poikilocytosis and sickled cells can be seen on the blood film while, in older children and adults, target cells and Howell Jolly bodies are also seen as a result of the hyposplenic state. The sickle screening test is positive and haemoglobin electrophoresis shows the haemoglobin composition to be as described on page 1053 (see also Fig. 25.12).

Management

Appropriate measures should be taken to try and avoid sickling crises. Thus, patients should avoid severe cold and dehydration, and infections must be treated early and aggressively. Prophylactic penicillin V should be given to all children in view of the hyposplenism, with some centres recommending continued use throughout life. Hypoxia with anaesthesia or unpressurised air travel must be avoided. In patients with very frequent and severe sickling episodes, a hypertransfusion regime can be instituted to replace HbS with HbA. This is mainly of value as a relatively short term measure prior to surgery (particularly ophthalmic surgery), and in the management of major complications.

It is essential to keep the patient undergoing a sickle crisis warm, hydrated and well oxygenated. Large quantities of opiate analgesics are often required. Possible infections must be investigated and treated appropriately. It is common practice to give all patients with sickle crises a course of ampicillin after appropriate cultures have been taken, though proof of beneficial effect is lacking. Where a pulmonary infection is suspected, broad spectrum cover – such as that obtained with a combination of cephalosporin and erythromycin – should be given. If a sickle-lung syndrome develops, regular blood gases should be performed and the patient ventilated early if hypoxia develops.

Contraception

Double barrier techniques, such as the cap and spermicidal foam and pessaries, are safe and effective if used correctly. The intrauterine contraceptive device (IUCD) and low dose contraceptive pill are used in some circumstances, but there is little firm data on their safety in sickle cell disease.

Management of pregnancy

Folate supplements should be given but there is otherwise little agreement as to the correct management of sickle cell disease during pregnancy. Many centres institute a 3–4 weekly transfusion regime during the last trimester, with the aim of achieving normal haemoglobin levels with 70–80% HbA at the expected time of delivery. If there is a history of first or second trimester abortions, transfusion is started as soon as possible in the pregnancy. Other specialists, however, feel that transfusion during pregnancy is unnecessary.

SICKLE CELL GENES IN ASSOCIATION WITH OTHER ABNORMAL Hb GENES

Sickle cell genes frequently interact with thalassaemic genes. In α-thalassaemia, the severity of sickle cell disease in β^s (sickle gene) homozygotes is often reduced, possibly a result of the slightly decreased concentration of HbS in the red cells.

If a heterozygote β^s interacts with a β-thalassaemia gene, the HbS level is higher than in a usual HbS trait leading to clinical symptoms. If the thalassaemia gene is a β^0 gene, a severe sickle cell syndrome may arise.

Interaction of β^s with an hereditary persistence of fetal haemoglobin (HPFH) (Table 25.6) results in virtually no normal β chain production. However, although the level of HbS may be as high as 80%, the high levels of HbF present reduce the risks of sickling. Other forms of 'high F gene' exist and may also reduce the sickling tendency.

The sickle gene may also interact with other β gene haemoglobinopathies. Thus, HbS/C disease, for example, results in a moderate or reasonably mild anaemia. The blood film shows sickle cells and many target cells, and haemoglobin electrophoresis shows that approximately half is HbS and half HbC, the latter running behind HbS in the same position as HbA_2 (Fig. 25.12). The clinical picture is very varied, but ocular complications are particularly common (although usually less severe than in sickle cell disease). In contrast to adult sickle cell disease, splenomegaly is often present.

OTHER HAEMOGLOBINOPATHIES CAUSING HAEMOLYSIS

HbC

HbC is very common in West Africa, particularly Ghana. The heterozygous state is symptomless and the haemoglobin concentration normal. In the homozygous state, however, the [Hb] may be slightly reduced, the spleen is usually large, gallstones may develop and ocular lesions are frequent.

HbD

HbD is found in many ethnic groups. It migrates with HbS on standard agar gels at pH 8.6 but not at acid pH. The heterozygous state is asymptomatic, with a mild anaemia occurring in the homozygous state. An asymptomatic patient with apparent homozygosity for HbS may in fact be HbS/D.

HbE

HbE is found predominantly in South-East Asia. It migrates on standard agar gels with HbC and HbA_2. The trait (heterozygous state) is symptomless; with a mild microcytic haemolytic anaemia in the homozygous state.

Unstable haemoglobins and methaemoglobinaemia

A variety of unstable haemoglobins have been described which tend to precipitate and cause a haemolytic anaemia.

Heinz bodies are seen within erythrocytes on a reticulocyte stain. Some forms of autosomal dominant congenital methaemoglobinaemia are due to aminoacid substitutions in the region of the haem pocket of globin. The patient is cyanosed and may have a mild haemolytic state.

CONGENITAL RED CELL MEMBRANE DEFECTS

Haemolysis can be due to congenital red cell membrane defects, the commonest of which are hereditary spherocytosis and hereditary elliptocytosis.

Hereditary spherocytosis

The commonest membrane defect is hereditary spherocytosis, an autosomal condition affecting one in 5000 individuals. The abnormality usually resides in the spectrin molecule of the cytoskeleton. Clinically, the disease is very varied. Haemolysis may be well compensated with no anaemia, or anaemia may be severe. There may also be acute exacerbations of anaemia, such as haemolytic crises associated with intercurrent infections and aplastic crises associated with parvovirus infections or folate deficiency. The spleen is usually palpable and not tender, but may become so during haemolytic crises. There is usually mild jaundice but, in the neonate, it may be sufficiently severe to cause kernicterus. Gallstones may arise in late childhood and adult life.

There is usually a mild normocytic anaemia, but during crises the [Hb] may fall below 8 g/dl. The blood film reveals spherocytes and a reticulocytosis. The diagnosis is confirmed by demonstration of increased red cell osmotic fragility (Fig. 25.14), and by exclusion of other causes of spherocytosis such as autoimmune haemolysis. Family studies may also prove useful.

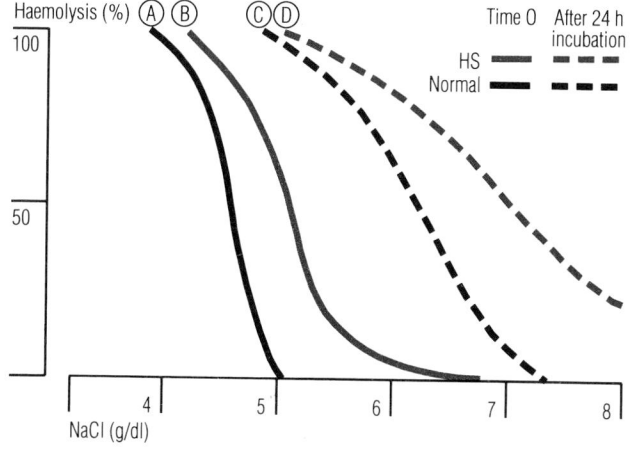

Fig. 25.14 Osmotic fragility curves showing lysis of red cells at low salt concentrations. (A) represents the normal curve and (C) represents normal cells pre-incubated for 24 hours at 37°C. (B) and (D) represent fresh and pre-incubated hereditary spherocytic cells respectively.

Children, non-splenectomised adults and pregnant women should receive folate supplements. Transfusion may be required for aplastic crises. Splenectomy reduces the haemolysis, prevents acute haemolytic crises and reduces the incidence of pigment gallstone formation; but this is usually delayed until adolescence because of the risks of post-splenectomy infections. If splenectomy is to be performed, gallstones should first be looked for using ultrasound and a simultaneous cholecystectomy considered. Following splenectomy, prophylactic penicillin should be given.

Hereditary elliptocytosis

Hereditary elliptocytosis is an autosomal dominant condition in which an abnormality of the cytoskeleton results in oval red blood cells. The osmotic fragility is normal. In some (usually mild) cases, the inheritance is linked to the rhesus genes.

Most patients are asymptomatic but a small proportion have the signs and symptoms of chronic haemolysis which may necessitate splenectomy.

Other hereditary red cell membrane defects

These include: hereditary stomatocytosis, in which the red cells have a slit-like central pallor resembling a mouth; hereditary pyropoikilocytosis in which there is marked haemolysis and *in vitro* fragmentation of red cells upon gentle heating; and hereditary acanthocytosis. This last condition is inherited in an autosomal recessive manner and is associated with abeta-lipoproteinaemia, malabsorption, retinitis pigmentosa and diffuse nervous system abnormalities.

CONGENITAL RED CELL ENZYME DEFECTS

The glycolytic enzymes in the erythrocyte generate two mols of ATP for each mol of glucose metabolised (Fig. 25.15). ATP is required for transmembrane ion transport and for the maintenance of the shape and flexibility of the red cell. NADH is also produced by the glycolytic pathway and is required for the maintenance of haem iron in the ferrous state. NADPH – produced by the hexose monophosphate shunt – is necessary for the reduction of glutathione which protects the red cell from oxidant stress. 2,3-DPG is derived as an offshoot of the glycolytic pathway and is important for its modulating effects on haemoglobin-oxygen affinity. The tricarboxylic cycle, protein synthesis, and nucleic acid synthesis do not occur in the erythrocyte.

Glucose-6-phosphate dehydrogenase deficiency

Glucose-6-phosphate dehydrogenase (G6PD) deficiency is the commonest inherited disease in the world. G6PD is the first enzyme in the hexose monophosphate shunt, so

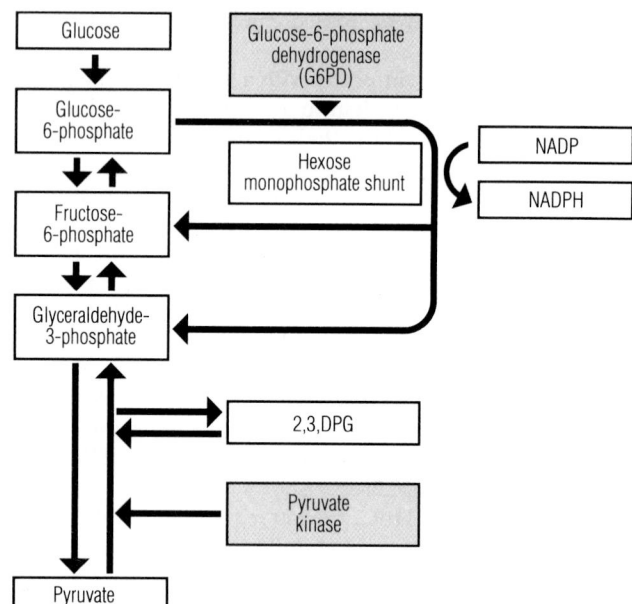

Fig. 25.15 Simplified scheme of glycolysis and the hexose monophosphate shunt.

that deficiency leads to a fall in NADPH and increased sensitivity of the erythrocytes to oxidant stress. The G6PD enzyme is coded on the X chromosome, so that disease due to deficiency of this enzyme mainly affects males. Female heterozygotes (carriers) have just over 50% of normal levels overall, but within individual red cells the G6PD levels are either completely normal or grossly deficient so that clinical disease may also occasionally occur in females. Many isoenzymes of G6PD have been described. The predominant isoenzyme – found in Caucasians and 60% of blacks – is designated B+. A normal African variant found in 25% of blacks is designated A+. Other isoenzymes, however, lead to G6PD deficiency. In the African A- variant, G6PD is produced in normal quantities and initially has full functional activity. However, the enzyme is unstable, so that the G6PD activity of an erythrocyte declines with time. In Mediterranean-Oriental type G6PD deficiency, the enzyme usually has low or absent functional activity from the beginning. Many different variants of this isoenzyme have been described.

Clinical features

The clinical spectrum of G6PD deficiency is wide (Summary 2). The commonest presentation is that of an *acute haemolytic episode*, precipitated by infection, acute illness or drugs. Many drugs have been implicated in causing acute haemolysis in G6PD deficiency, but only a few commonly used drugs consistently have this effect (Table 25.7). In the African-type G6PD deficiency (A-), the haemolysis leads to a brisk reticulocytosis and – as the reticulocytes have adequate levels of G6PD – is thus self-limiting. However, in G6PD deficiency variants where

Table 25.7 Drugs which may precipitate acute haemolysis in G6PD deficiency

Type of drug	Example
Analgesics	Aspirin
Antibiotics	Sulphonamides
	Nitrofurantoin
	Chloramphenicol
	Quinolones
	Para-aminosalicylic acid
Anti-malarials	Quinine
	Chloroquine
	Primaquine
Anti-leprotics	Dapsone
Miscellaneous	Vitamin K
	Vitamin C

reticulocyte G6PD levels are low, the intravascular haemolysis may be sufficiently severe to cause collapse and death. *Favism* is the condition when acute haemolysis is precipitated in G6PD deficiency following exposure to broad beans, either as lightly cooked food or as pollen. It is mostly confined to the Mediterranean variants of G6PD deficiency and mainly affects young children. The *chronic haemolytic anaemia* of G6PD deficiency is rare but has been described with many different variants. The anaemia is usually mild. *Neonatal haemolysis* occurs mainly in Mediterranean and Oriental variants, and is an important differential diagnosis of immune haemolysis of the newborn in these areas. Even female heterozygotes may become jaundiced. The administration of vitamin K may precipitate or exacerbate some cases.

Summary 2 Clinical presentations of G6PD deficiency

- Stress-induced acute haemolysis
- Drug-induced acute haemolysis
- Favism
- Chronic congenital haemolytic anaemia
- Neonatal jaundice

Laboratory features

During haemolytic episodes there is a non-spherocytic anaemia with anisocytosis. Vital staining of the blood film reveals a reticulocytosis and many Heinz bodies (precipitated haemoglobin). Erythrocyte G6PD levels can be measured in a commercially available enzyme kit, but it must be borne in mind that in the Negro type of G6PD deficiency, the level may rise into the female heterozygote range during acute episodes with a reticulocytosis. In these circumstances, definitive assays should be delayed until the convalescent period.

Treatment

Patients with G6PD deficiency should receive prompt therapy of all infections and avoid drugs known to precipitate haemolysis. Blood transfusion is occasionally required for severe episodes of haemolysis, and exchange tranfusion may be needed in cases of neonatal jaundice.

Pyruvate kinase deficiency

Pyruvate kinase (PK) deficiency is rare compared to G6PD deficiency. It is generally an autosomal recessive condition (although occasionally heterozygotes may have minor haemolysis), and is most common in Caucasians. PK deficiency results in the reduced generation of ATP and NADH and inability of the cells to maintain electrolyte balance. Haemolysis is extravascular, with removal of defective cells by the reticulo-endothelial system.

Clinical and laboratory features

There is a congenital non-spherocytic anaemia of very variable severity. Severe anaemia is partially ameliorated by the high 2,3-DPG levels present (distal block) which help maintain tissue oxygenation (p. 1042, Fig. 25.6). The anaemia is often exacerbated by infections. Splenomegaly is common and severe cases may require regular transfusions.

Examination of the blood film reveals poikilocytosis and reticulocytosis. The diagnosis is confirmed by measurement of erythrocyte PK enzyme activity.

General approach to erythrocyte enzymopathies

When haemolysis due to an enzyme defect is suspected, the G6PD level should be measured first, as this is much the most common enzymopathy. If this is normal, PK activity should be measured. Many other enzyme deficiencies have been reported, but these are extremely rare and few laboratories have facilities to measure other enzymes or intermediate metabolites. The approach at this stage is thus largely empirical. The family and clinical history may provide clues, and measurement of 2,3-DPG levels may help localise a defect in the Emden-Myerhof pathway. The level is usually raised in anaemia but tends to be still higher than expected in blocks distal to 3-phosphoglycerate, and lower than expected in blocks proximal to 1,3-diphosphoglycerate. In defects of glutathione metabolism, Heinz bodies are usually prominent in the red cells.

AUTOIMMUNE HAEMOLYTIC ANAEMIAS

Autoimmune haemolytic anaemias (AIHA) are generally categorised according to whether the anti-red cell antibody is cold or warm. Warm antibodies react with red cells at 37°C, tend to be IgG and usually destroy red cells by means of opsonisation and extravascular clearance in the reticuloendothelial system. IgG antibodies are 'incomplete' antibodies and thus do not agglutinate cells in saline; hence, the addition of albumin or anti-human gamma-globulin (direct antiglobulin test = DAT; see p. 1063, Fig. 25.19) is required.

Cold antibodies are usually IgM complete antibodies which agglutinate cells in saline at room temperature. The thermal amplitude of such antibodies is very variable and many with low thermal amplitude have no clinical significance although they do make crossmatching more difficult.

Aetiology

AIHA is most commonly idiopathic in origin (Summary 3). Cold antibodies are most common although they frequently cause little problem. Anti-red cell antibodies may occur secondary to malignancies, especially the low grade lymphoproliferative disorders such as chronic lymphocytic leukaemia. The warm antibodies produced in such circumstances are polyclonal, do not originate from the malignant clone, and are indicative of the overall immune dysregulation that occurs in these conditions. However, when cold antibodies are produced in lymphoma they are frequently monoclonal. AIHA can occur in association with all the autoimmune diseases but is most common in systemic lupus erythematosus when it may occasionally be the presenting feature. Viral infections frequently predate warm antibody AIHA in children and young adults. Infectious mononucleosis may lead to production of cold antibodies with *i* blood group specificity and mycoplasma pneumoniae with *I* specificity.

Drugs may cause AIHA by several mechanisms.

1. Certain drugs, such as methyldopa, L-dopa and mefanamic acid, induce the production of auto-antibodies directed against red cell antigens. With chronic methyldopa use, up to 20% of patients acquire a positive direct antiglobulin test, although haemolytic anaemia occurs in less than 1%. If haemolysis does occur, it usually ceases within two weeks of stopping the drug, although the DAT may remain positive for several years. In this case, the antibody is usually a warm IgG reactive with the rhesus antigen system.

Summary 3   Aetiology of autoimmune haemolytic anaemia

- Idiopathic

- Secondary
  Neoplasms, especially lymphoproliferative disorders
  Autoimmune disorders
  Infections
  Drugs – Induction of 'true autoantibodies'
    – Drugs acting as haptens on red cell surface
    – Passive absorption of drug antibody complex onto erythrocyte

- Complication of blood transfusion (transient)

- Immune haemolytic disease of the newborn

The mechanism of autoantibody production is not clear.

2. Some drugs cause haemolysis by acting as a hapten. The drug which most frequently causes haemolysis by this mechanism is high dose parenteral penicillin. It is absorbed onto the red cell and in that form stimulates antibody production. IgM antibodies are frequently produced without clinical effect, but if IgG antibodies are produced, haemolysis may be severe.

3. Immune complex-mediated haemolysis is rare but has been reported with a wide range of drugs. In these cases, the patient has usually received the drug before and has become sensitised to it. On rechallenge, immune complexes containing the drug are formed, bind to the red cells and precipitate complement-mediated intravascular haemolysis.

Immune haemolysis may complicate blood transfusion, and this and haemolytic disease of the newborn are discussed on pages 1066–68.

Clinical features

Warm antibodies do not generally cause complement activation and intravascular haemolysis. Instead, the red cells are opsonised and removed in the reticulo-endothelial system, resulting in anaemia which may be either acute and severe or a mild chronic disorder. Occasionally, AIHA may be complicated by immune thrombocytopenia and, in these cases, bruising and petechial haemorrhages may occur.

Cold antibodies may be asymptomatic or, alternatively, give rise to cold haemagglutinin disease (CHAD). The idiopathic form occurs mainly in the elderly. On exposure to the cold, acute episodes of haemolysis may occur and peripheral cyanosis and Raynaud's phenomenon are also frequent. In between episodes, the haemoglobin may be normal or only slightly reduced. Rarely, there is a chronic severe anaemia which is refractory to treatment. Infection-induced cold haemolysis is usually characterised by acute onset of anaemia, jaundice and haemoglobinuria which subsides after several weeks.

Paroxysmal cold haemoglobinuria (PCH) is a very rare form of cold antibody haemolysis, in which the antibody is a cold IgG specific for the P blood group system. It may be idiopathic or post infective, particularly following syphilis. The degree of cold exposure required to precipitate attacks is very variable.

Laboratory features

The anaemia is usually slightly macrocytic due to the reticulocytosis. If haemolysis is severe, nucleated red cells may be seen in the blood. Spherocytes are frequently seen and the osmotic fragility may be increased, although usually to a lesser extent than in hereditary spherocytosis. Red cell aggregates are commonly found on the blood film, particularly with cold antibodies. The ESR is usually markedly raised.

Hyperbilirubinaemia is present and reflects in part the severity of the haemolysis. Haemoglobinuria occurs with acute intravascular haemolysis, and haemosiderinuria with chronic intravascular haemolysis (p. 1050).

The diagnosis of AIHA is made by demonstrating the presence of a red cell auto-antibody. With warm antibodies (active at 37°C in DAT), this is usually IgG and only occasionally IgA or IgM. Cold antibodies are usually IgM and agglutinate at room temperature (less so at 37°C). The DAT is usually positive with anti-C3d, and in some cases only C3d can be demonstrated on the cell surface.

Management

Warm antibody haemolysis

In primary (idiopathic) cases, remission induction is attempted with a course of high dose steroids (prednisone 1 mg/kg per day), which is then tailed off gradually according to the response. Blood transfusion may be necessary, and this causes considerable difficulties with the cross-match. Splenectomy is usually tried if steroids fail; and immunosuppression with azathioprine, chlorambucil or cyclophosphamide may prove effective in splenectomy resistant cases. In cases of chronic haemolysis, folic acid supplements should be given.

In secondary AIHA, appropriate treatment of the underlying disease will often terminate the haemolytic process. Drugs suspected of causing haemolysis should be withdrawn. Spontaneous remissions may occur, particularly in post-infective AIHA in children.

Cold antibody haemolysis

If the haemolysis is mild and well compensated, no specific therapy is required but the patient must avoid exposure to cold. During acute episodes (especially following infections), confinement to a very warm room may be necessary; and if transfusion is required, washed cells should be given (reduced complement) through a blood warmer. Steroids and splenectomy rarely help in cold haemagglutinin disease: if the haemolysis is chronic and severe, chlorambucil or cyclophosphamide should be tried.

ACQUIRED NON-IMMUNE HAEMOLYTIC ANAEMIAS

The aetiology of acquired non-immune haemolytic anaemias are shown in Table 25.8.

Hypersplenism

Hypersplenism is defined as a peripheral blood cytopenia which can be cured by splenectomy. The spleen is usually enlarged (splenomegaly), the causes of which are shown in Table 25.9.

The mechanism of hypersplenism is multifactorial and includes both pooling of cells within the spleen and rapid

Table 25.8 Aetiology of acquired non-immune haemolytic anaemias

Hypersplenism

Toxic states
Infections, e.g. malaria
Uraemia
Drugs
Chemicals, e.g. lead poisoning
Venoms, e.g. cobra bites

Microangiopathic haemolytic anaemias
Disseminated intravascular coagulation (DIC)
Haemolytic uraemic syndrome (HUS) and thrombotic thrombocytopenic purpura (TTP)
Malignant hypertension

Trauma to red cells
Cardiac prostheses
March haemoglobinuria
Burns

Acquired red cell membrane defects
Paroxysmal nocturnal haemoglobinura (PNH)
Liver disease
Vitamin E deficiency, especially in premature babies

destruction of cells within the spleen. The plasma volume is usually increased in splenomegaly and a dilutional factor contributes to any anaemia. Assessment of hypersplenism can be difficult. The diagnosis is usually suggested by the finding of a peripheral blood cytopenia, an active cellular marrow and splenomegaly. However, if there is an underlying haematological disease such as a haemolytic anaemia, it can be difficult to separate out the effects of this from the hypersplenism. In some cases, radioactive isotope studies may be of value. Using ^{51}Cr labelled red cells, a shortened red cell survival can be demonstrated, and surface counting can then be performed over the spleen.

Table 25.9 Causes of splenomegaly

Primary haematological disorders
Haemolytic anaemias, especially if severe and chronic

Lymphoproliferative disorders

Myeloproliferative disorders

Non-haematological disorders
Congestive splenomegaly
    Portal hypertension
    Hepatic or portal vein thrombosis
    Chronic congestive cardiac failure

Infections
    Bacterial, e.g. septicaemia, typhoid, tuberculosis
    Viral, e.g. hepatitis, infectious mononucleosis
    Tropical, e.g. malaria, kala-azar

Collagen vascular diseases

Metabolic 'storage diseases'

Sarcoidosis

In hypersplenic states with pooling of red cells, there is a long equilibration time before steady state counts are achieved. In extravascular haemolytic anaemias, the role of the spleen in red cell destruction can be partly assessed by comparison of the spleen and liver uptake of ^{51}Cr labelled red cells over a period of ten days. If this ratio is greater than four, it suggests that considerable splenic destruction is occurring, and that splenectomy may be clinically beneficial.

Blood changes following splenectomy

If hypersplenism was present, the cytopenias should resolve following splenectomy. A number of other changes in the blood also occur (Table 25.10). It must be noted that these changes also occur in other hyposplenic states (Table 25.11).

Table 25.10 Blood changes post splenectomy

Blood cell type	Change
Red cells	Howell-Jolly bodies (nuclear remnants)
	Siderocytes
	Target cells
	Normoblasts
Leucocytes	Neutrophil leucocytosis (usually transient)
	Myelocytes appear in the blood during infections
Platelets	Thrombocytosis (usually transient)

Table 25.11 Causes of hyposplenism

- Splenectomy
- Sickle cell disease
- Coeliac disease
- Congenital absence (rare)
- Systemic lupus erythematosus (rare)
- Senile atrophy (rare)

Microangiopathic haemolytic anaemias

The microangiopathic haemolytic anaemias include disseminated intravascular coagulation, haemolytic uraemic syndrome and thrombotic thrombocytopenic purpura. These are discussed on pages 1097–1100.

Trauma to red cells

Trauma to red cells may occur in a number of situations, including cardiac prostheses, march haemoglobinuria and burns.

Cardiac prostheses. Trauma to red cells due to cardiac prostheses occurs predominantly with prostheses on the left side of the heart where systolic pressures are high. It is particularly common with faulty valves through which there is regurgitation. The anaemia is usually mild, and red cell fragments (schistocytes) are seen on the blood film. The platelet count may also be low.

March haemoglobinuria. In march haemoglobinuria, red cells are ruptured in the small vessels of the feet in some otherwise healthy individuals when they engage in long marches or runs. It may be sufficiently severe to cause frank haemoglobinuria, nausea and abdominal cramps. The condition may be eased by use of specially padded footwear. A similar condition may occur in the hands of karate participants.

Paroxysmal nocturnal haemoglobinuria

Paroxysmal nocturnal haemoglobinuria (PNH) is a rare multipotential-stem-cell disorder in which an affected clone gives rise to abnormal red cells, leucocytes and platelets. Why the PNH clone should obtain a selective advantage over normal haemopoietic clones is not known. The membranes of these cells are deficient in those proteins normally anchored to the cell membrane through a phosphatidyl inositol linkage. As these include complement deactivating factors, the cells are very sensitive to complement lysis activated by the alternative pathway. There is a high incidence of aplastic anaemia and acute leukaemia reflecting the aberrant nature of the stem cell.

Clinical features

This disorder usually presents in adults and is more common in women. The clinical manifestations are wide (Summary 4) and paroxysmal haemolysis and haemoglobinuria during sleep is reported in only 25% of patients. Severe bouts may be associated with jaundice and low back pain.

Chronic low grade intravascular haemolysis is more common than the severe form and usually leads to iron deficiency. Mild neutropenia and thrombocytopenia are also common, and occasionally severe aplastic anaemia may arise or be the presenting feature. The thromboses that occur are usually venous, though occasionally arterial. The sites of thromboses are often atypical and include the hepatic veins and cerebral sinuses.

Diagnosis and treatment

Non-immune intravascular haemolysis should always raise the suspicion of PNH, but haemosiderinuria may be the

---

Summary 4 Clinical features of PNH

- Paroxysmal nocturnal haemoglobinuria
- Chronic haemolysis
- Mild cytopenias
- Severe aplastic anaemia
- Thromboses
- Leukaemic transformation

only evidence of haemolysis. Iron deficiency and cytopenias are frequent. The neutrophil alkaline phosphatase score is usually low in PNH (unless aplastic anaemia occurs) and is a useful diagnostic indicator. The definitive diagnostic test is the *Ham's test*, in which PNH (but not normal) red cells lyse during a one hour 37°C incubation with normal sera, but do not lyse if complement is first removed from the sera by inactivation at 56°C.

There is no specific therapy for PNH and treatment is supportive. Initiation of iron therapy for haemolysis may cause a reticulocytosis and a temporary exacerbation of the haemolytic process.

ANAEMIA OF CHRONIC DISEASE

The anaemia of chronic disease is multifactorial. Haematinic deficiency, poor iron utilisation, relative erythroid hypoplasia and a slightly decreased red cell survival may all contribute to the anaemia, while other factors may also contribute in specific diseases.

The anaemia is usually mild or moderate and may be microcytic or normocytic. The serum iron is usually low, but the total iron binding capacity is also reduced, giving a percentage saturation greater than 10%. Marrow iron is present and the serum ferritin is normal or raised. There may be a leucocytosis and the blood film may show features specific to the underlying disease process. Several chronic diseases merit special attention.

Renal failure

The anaemia may be severe in chronic renal failure. Retained toxic metabolites may directly suppress erythropoiesis, but the major cause of anaemia is decreased production of erythropoietin. This is largely due to destruction of erythropoietin-producing tissue, but is also a result of the acidosis and raised phosphate levels (including 2,3-DPG) that occur in renal failure. This results in a rightward shift in the oxygen dissociation curve and a corresponding reduction in tissue hypoxia. Red cell survival is also frequently shortened and, in severe renal failure, there may be a microangiopathic haemolysis. The anaemia of chronic renal failure may also be caused in part by any underlying disease, such as chronic infection or a collagen vascular disease.

Examination of the blood in renal failure reveals a normocytic anaemia with crenated cells and often also red cell fragments.

Despite the multifactorial nature of the anaemia of chronic renal failure, a normal haemoglobin can be obtained in most patients by the administration of erythropoietin.

Liver disease

In liver disease, there is a mild anaemia which may be normocytic but is frequently macrocytic. Target cells are usually seen on the blood film. There may be a slight reticulocytosis, as mild haemolysis occurs as well as decreased erythropoiesis. Excessive bouts of alcohol intake in patients with chronic liver disease can produce frank haemolysis associated with abdominal pain, jaundice and hyperlipidaemia (Zieve's syndrome). The anaemia of liver disease may be further exacerbated by the complications of that disease, i.e. hypersplenism and blood loss.

Malignant disease

The anaemia of non-haematological malignancy is multifactorial, and that which may occur in carcinoma of the bronchus is shown as an example in Fig. 25.16.

BLOOD TRANSFUSION

Donors

All blood products should ideally be obtained from volunteer donors to reduce both the expense and the risks of

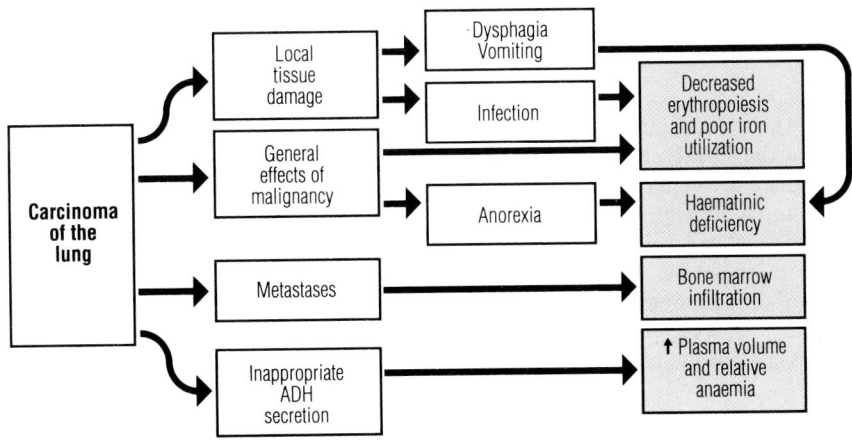

Fig. 25.16 Development of anaemia in carcinoma of the bronchus showing the multiple mechanisms involved.

infection transmission. The risks to the donor are very small, consisting mainly of bruising at venepuncture (and rarely arterial puncture) sites. The commonly used criteria for the acceptability of donors is shown in Table 25.12.

Table 25.12   Criteria for the acceptability of blood donors in the United Kingdom

- Aged 18–65 years

- Good general health and 'feeling well'

- [Hb] greater than 13.1 g/dl (men)
      greater than 12.5 g/dl (women)

- Not pregnant at present or in the last year

- Not suffered from:
Cancer	ever
Syphilis	ever
Brucellosis	ever
Malaria	in last three years
Infectious mononucleosis	in last two years
Hepatitis/jaundice	in last one year

- Not had:
Transfusion of blood or blood products in last six months	
Surgery in last six months	
Acupuncture in last three months	Small risk of viral infection, especially hepatitis
Tattoos in last six months	
Ears pierced in last six months	
Close contact with hepatitis/jaundice in last six months	

- Not:
Practising homosexuals	
Users of intravenous drugs	High risk groups for AIDS
Born in Haiti, Zaire or Congo	
Sexual partners of the above three groups	

- Not travelled to tropical country in last three months

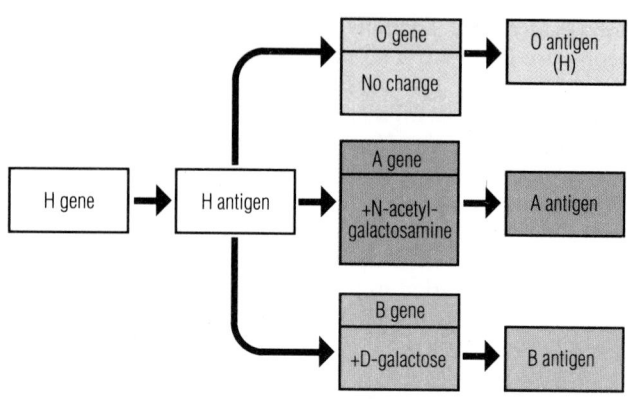

Fig. 25.17   The ABO antigen system.

Table 25.13   Incidence (%) of ABO blood groups in various racial groups

Blood Group	Caucasians	Asians & Indians	African Blacks
A	36	24	21
B	14	24	29
AB	3	9	5
O	47	33	43

Table 25.14   ABO genotype, phenotype and naturally occurring antibodies

Genotype	Phenotype	Antibodies
AA	A	Anti-B
AO	A	Anti-B
BB	B	Anti-A
BO	B	Anti-A
OO	O	Anti-A + Anti-B

Red cell antigens and antibodies

All blood is classified according to its ABO and rhesus antigen phenotype.

ABO system

There are three alternative genes which act on the product of the H gene to produce the O (H), A and B antigens (Fig. 25.17). The approximate incidence of the ABO antigens in various racial groups is shown in Table 25.13. At approximately six months of age, so-called *naturally occurring antibodies* arise to the ABO system as shown in Table 25.14. These antibodies probably arise as cross-reactions to antigens on gut flora. They are IgM antibodies which will agglutinate red cells in the cold in saline (*complete antibodies*).

Subgroups of A are recognised. Thus, approximately 80% of Caucasians are A1 and 20% are A2; other subgroups of A also occur but are very rare. A2 behaves like a weak A1, but qualitative antigenic differences are present as some A2 individuals can produce anti-A1 antibodies.

Rhesus system

The rhesus system is composed of three closely linked allelic genes, one group of three being inherited from each parent. The common genotypes in the UK are shown in Table 25.15. The D antigen is clinically most important and approximately 85% of Caucasian individuals are D⁺. In Chinese populations, nearly 100% are D⁺ and in Negroes the incidence is approximately 95%. For general blood transfusion purposes, a recipient is called Rh-negative if he or she is d/d, but a Rh-negative donor is defined as cde/cde. Some patients have an abnormal D antigen (Dᵘ) which may type very weakly, or even as d.

Naturally occurring antibodies to the rhesus system do not occur. However, antibody formation occurs following

Table 25.15 Incidence of rhesus genotypes

Genotype		Incidence	
CDe/cde	D	31%	85%
CDe/CDe		16%	
CDE/cde		13%	
CDe/cDE		13%	
cde/cde	d	15%	15%

sensitisation during pregnancy or after mismatched transfusion. The antibodies formed are warm reacting IgG antibodies that do not agglutinate in saline (*incomplete antibodies*). They can be detected on addition of albumin (which reduces the repulsive electrostatic charge on red cells) or by using anti-immunoglobulin as a cross-linking reagent. Anti-Rh antibodies are most important in the context of immune haemolytic disease of the newborn (p. 1067).

Other antigen systems

Many other red cell antigen systems have been described but are not routinely typed. However, preformed antibodies to these antigens will be detected in a cross-match and can then be identified with panels of *typing cells*.

Blood grouping and cross-matching

ABO typing is performed by adding known anti-A and anti-B sera to a red cell suspension at room temperature, and then looking for agglutination (Fig. 25.18). The serum is also typed against known red cells as a back check. Rhesus typing with anti-D cannot be performed in saline at room temperature, but must be carried out at 37°C in the presence of albumin or anti-human globulin in an *indirect antiglobulin test* (Fig. 25.19). At least two anti-D reagents should be used.

When the patient's ABO and rhesus group have been determined, a cross-match between the potential donor cells and the recipient serum is performed. A control is also performed using the recipient's own cells and serum

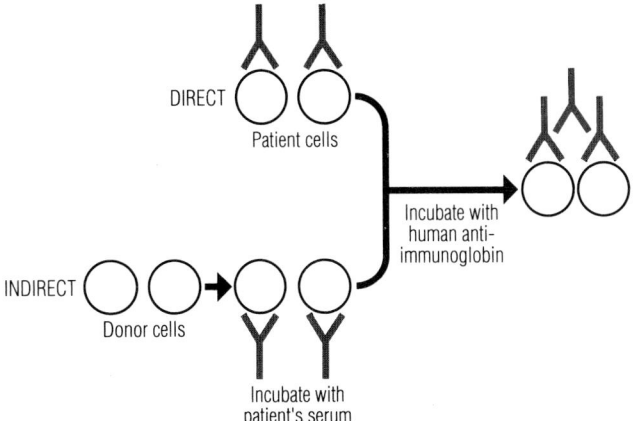

Fig. 25.19 Diagrammatic representation of the direct and indirect antiglobulin test. Human anti-immunoglobulin is shown in red.

to check for autoagglutinins. The cross-match should be performed both in saline at room temperature to detect cold complete antibodies, and in albumin at 37°C to detect warm incomplete antibodies. An indirect antiglobulin test at 37°C is also performed and is generally the most sensitive test available.

A variety of techniques have been developed to speed up the cross-match which, traditionally, takes one and a half hours. These include centrifugation of cells and serum, and use of low ionic strength saline. In low ionic solutions, red cells have less mutually repulsive electrostatic charge and agglutination is apparent within 10–20 minutes in positive samples.

An alternative approach is to perform an antibody screen on the serum of all potential recipients, using two batches of carefully selected target cells. If any antibodies are found, they must be identified, appropriate antigen-negative blood found and a full cross-match performed. If no antibodies are found, cross-matching is only performed in surgical cases, such as cardiac surgery or a Wertheim's hysterectomy, in which there is a very high chance of blood being used. Blood is not cross-matched in surgical cases where blood is not usually required. If blood is then required urgently, group matched blood is issued after a 5–10 minute rapid (spun) cross-match. In some American centres, group matched blood is issued to pre-screened recipients without any attempt at a cross-match.

Use of blood, blood products and substitutes

Whole blood

Whole blood should only be used in circumstances such as acute haemorrhage, where there is a need to restore the intravascular volume as well as the oxygen carrying capacity of the blood (Table 25.16). For exchange transfusions in neonates, the blood should be less than 48 hours old and CMV negative.

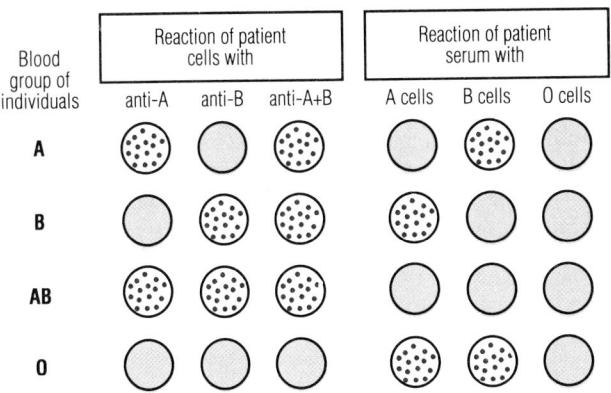

Fig. 25.18 ABO file grouping.

The table illustrated shows:

Blood group of individuals	Reaction of patient cells with			Reaction of patient serum with		
	anti-A	anti-B	anti-A+B	A cells	B cells	O cells
A	+	−	+	−	+	−
B	−	+	+	+	−	−
AB	+	+	+	−	−	−
O	−	−	−	+	+	−

Table 25.16   Indications for the use of whole blood

- Acute blood loss
- Exchange transfusions
  Sickle cell disease
  Haemolytic disease of the newborn
- Priming extracorporeal circulations
  Heart-lung machines
  Some dialysis equipment

Red cell concentrates

It is essential that packed cells are used for patients with anaemia but without hypovolaemia. Otherwise the national blood transfusion service would be unable to obtain enough plasma to provide the required amounts of plasma products (Table 25.17). It should also be noted that the majority of patients with anaemia due to haematinic deficiency do not require transfusion, unless very ill, pregnant, or being prepared for surgery.

Table 25.17   Blood products and substitutes

Cellular products
Whole blood
Packed red cells
Washed red cells
Filtered blood
Frozen red cells

Red cell substitutes
Platelet concentrates
Granulocyte concentrates

Plasma products
Fresh frozen plasma
Plasma protein fraction
Freeze–dried, salt–poor albumin

Artificial plasma expanders

Clotting factors
Cryoprecipitate
Factor VIII concentrates
Factor IX concentrates
Freeze – dried fibrinogen

Washed red cells

Red cells washed three times in saline contain few white cells and platelets, and reactions to platelet and leucocyte antigens in patients with preformed antibodies are thus reduced. In general, the use of washed cells for this purpose is now replaced by use of filtered blood. As the plasma is removed, reactions to plasma products – especially IgA – are avoided. Washed blood must be used within 12 hours of washing.

Filtered blood

Modern filters effectively remove over 95% of leucocytes, and filtered blood is thus very useful in patients with anti-leucocyte antibodies causing febrile reactions. Unfortunately, the filters are expensive.

Frozen red cells

Frozen red cells (after thawing and washing) are free of leucocytes and were used in the past in multiply-transfused sensitised patients. However, filtered blood is now generally used and red cell cryopreservation is mainly of value for the indefinite storage of blood with rare phenotypes.

Red cell substitutes

Emulsions of perfluorocarbons can be used to transport oxygen and carbon dioxide in the blood. However, they have a short half-life in the circulation and require the patient to inhale 50% oxygen to be effective. Their use is therefore limited to the management of individuals with religious objections to blood products, and perhaps also as a reserve for the treatment of large numbers of casualties after a major disaster.

Platelet concentrates

Platelet concentrates can be obtained from donor units of blood by centrifugation, or in larger quantities using cell separators. As platelet concentrates are invariably contaminated with red cells, ABO and rhesus compatibility between donor and recipient should be maintained. Platelets are best stored at room temperature, preferably with constant agitation, and should be used as soon as possible (and not at all after 3–4 days from collection). Platelets stored at 4°C survive less well but have greater initial activity in the recipient. Attempts to cryopreserve platelets are in progress. The use of platelet concentrates is discussed on p. 1049.

Granulocyte concentrates

'Buffy coats' are available from donor units but the number of granulocytes obtained is too small to be of value. Larger numbers can be obtained by use of cell separators, but proof of their efficacy in the treatment of sepsis in neutropenic patients is lacking.

Fresh frozen plasma

Fresh frozen plasma (FFP) contains the plasma proteins including labile clotting factors. The uses of FFP are confined to those shown in Table 25.18, as it is essential that fresh plasma is used primarily for the production of other plasma products. It should not be used as a plasma expander.

Plasma protein fraction

Plasma protein fraction is the solution remaining after removal from plasma of cryoprecipitate, fibrinogen and immunoglobulins. It is largely composed of albumin. The

Table 25.18 Indications for use of fresh frozen plasma

Acquired coagulation disorders
Liver disease
Over anticoagulation with oral anticoagulants
Following massive transfusion with stored blood (if indicated by clotting screen)

Congenital coagulation disorders
Factor XI deficiency
Minor bleeds in von Willebrand's disease (cryoprecipitate usually used)
Factor V deficiency
Factor VII deficiency
Factor X deficiency
Factor XIII deficiency

Thrombotic thrombocytopenic purpura

Angioneurotic oedema (FFP provides C1 esterase inhibitor)

solution is heat-treated to destroy hepatitis and CMV viruses and is used as a volume expander when red cells are not required, and for replacement therapy in hypo-albuminic states.

Freeze-dried salt-poor albumin

Freeze-dried, salt-poor albumin is of limited use but may be of value in some patients with nephrotic syndrome or liver disease.

Artificial plasma expanders

Hydroxethyl starch is a very useful and safe plasma expander. High molecular weight dextrans are also used, but anaphylactic reactions occasionally occur and there may also be occasional interference with subsequent cross-matching (rouleaux formation). Gelatin solutions are also safe but only remain in the circulation for a relatively short period.

Cryoprecipitate

When fresh frozen plasma is just thawed to between 4°C and 8°C, a white gelatinous material remains as cryo-precipitate which can be removed and refrozen. This substance enters solution when thawed at 37°C. Cryo-precipitate contains approximately 50% of the original factor VIII present, including von Willebrand factor. It also contains high levels of fibrinogen but no factor IX. It is used as replacement therapy in factor VIII deficiency states including classical haemophilia, von Willebrand's disease, disseminated intravascular coagulation and (occasionally) following massive transfusions.

Factor VIII concentrates

Highly concentrated factor VIII preparations are available in freeze dried forms. They are less bulky than cryo-precipitate, can be stored at 4°C, and contain less fibrino-gen than cryoprecipitate, all of which properties make them

suitable for major bleeds. However, because they are produced from pooled plasma collections, they inevitably contain non-A non-B hepatitis, and also often human immune deficiency virus (HIV). Heat treatment appears to eliminate HIV and reduce (but not totally eliminate) hepatitis viruses. The process reduces the functional factor VIII content and is therefore very expensive.

Porcine and bovine factor VIII concentrates are occasionally useful in patients who have developed anti-factor VIII antibodies.

Genetically engineered factor VIII has now been produced and should become commercially available in the near future. These products will have the advantage of being virus-free.

Factor IX concentrates

Factor IX concentrates are used in the treatment of congenital factor IX deficiency not responding to fresh frozen plasma, and also occasionally in liver disease. These preparations also contain factors II, VII (depending on the method of preparation), and X. Activated clotting factors may also be present. Although their presence makes the concentrate potentially thrombogenic, they also provide a way to bypass the factor VIII requirement in haemo-philiacs with anti-factor VIII antibodies. Special 'activated' factor IX concentrates are available for this purpose, but must be used with great caution. These products should now be heat-treated to inactivate HIV.

Freeze-dried fibrinogen

Freeze-dried fibrinogen is available for use in congenital fibrinogen deficiency and dysfibrinogenaemia, but cryo-precipitate usually contains adequate fibrinogen.

Complications of blood transfusion

The complications of blood transfusion are shown in Table 25.19.

Table 25.19 Complications of blood transfusion

- Haemolytic reactions
      Serological – immediate
                      – delayed
                      – sensitisation
      Thermal   – faulty blood warmers
- Febrile reactions
- Infections
- Circulatory overload
- Thrombophlebitis at transfusion site
- Transfusion siderosis
- Air embolism (with use of central lines)
- Ion toxicity (e.g. citrate and potassium)
- Special problems associated with massive transfusion

Haematological Disorders

Serological reactions

If blood has been incorrectly cross-matched (or not cross-matched), or if (more commonly) there has been a clerical error and the patient has antibodies in the serum to antigens expressed on the donor red cells, then rapid complement-dependent lysis of the transfused cells may occur. Very rarely, immediate haemolysis may also be due to high titre anti-A or anti-B IgG antibodies in the donor blood, when group O blood is given to A or B recipients. Symptoms may arise within minutes or up to several hours after the transfusion has started, and include fever and rigors, headache, lumbar back pain, abdominal discomfort and vomiting, and chest pain. In severe cases, the patient becomes shocked and then suffers acute renal failure and disseminated intravascular coagulation (DIC). When an immediate serological reaction is suspected, the transfusion must be stopped immediately and appropriate action taken (Table 25.20).

Serological reactions may also be delayed. This occurs when an antibody to donor red cells, which was not present in the patient's serum at the time of transfusion, develops rapidly afterwards. This is almost invariably a secondary antibody response in previously transfused individuals. Haemolysis usually occurs between one and two weeks after transfusion.

It should also be noted that a transfusion may produce sensitisation to donor red cells. Although this may not cause haemolysis, future transfusions may be compromised and there may be a risk in young women of haemolytic disease of the newborn.

Febrile reactions

In multiply-transfused patients, febrile reactions frequently accompany transfusion due to the development of antibodies to leucocyte and platelet antigens. The fever usually comes on several hours after starting the transfusion and may last for up to 12 hours. Filtered blood, slow rate of transfusion, and intravenous chlorpheniramine or hydrocortisone will reduce this problem.

Infections

Blood rarely becomes contaminated with bacteria but the organisms which are able to grow at 4°C (such as pseudomonas and coliforms) produce bacteraemic shock and can be rapidly fatal. Many viruses can be transmitted by blood transfusion. Blood donations are screened for hepatitis B, but transmission of non-A non-B hepatitis may occur with multiple transfusions. CMV transmission may occur as the virus can be dormant in leucocytes. In immunocompromised patients without anti-CMV antibodies, and in neonates, blood from CMV-negative donors should be given. There is an extremely small risk of HIV transmission from blood donated in the UK, and this risk is further reduced by screening the donated blood for anti-HIV antibodies. Infectious mononucleosis may occasionally be transmitted. Other contaminating organisms include brucellosis, malaria, trypanosomes, leishmania and

Table 25.20 Plan of action for a suspected immediate haemolytic transfusion reaction

1. STOP TRANSFUSION
2. Maintain venous access (give saline initially)
3. Check names, groups and numbers on the blood pack and blood transfusion report forms
4. Return blood pack to laboratory with:
   Clotted blood sample
   – re-check group of patient and donor pack
   – perform a direct antiglobulin test
   – repeat cross-match and identify any antibodies
   Heparinised blood sample
   – check for free Hb in plasma
   Citrated sample
   – check clotting screen
   Sequestrene sample
   – check [Hb] and platelet count
5. Give intravenous hydrocortisone and chlorpheniramine
6. Maintain venous return if shock develops – give saline, plasma and whole blood if necessary
7. Maintain urine output by using intravenous diuretics *after* establishment of adequate venous return
8. Replenish clotting factors and platelets if DIC develops

filaria. Syphilis can be transmitted by blood transfusion, but this is rare as all blood is pre-screened for antibodies to *Treponema pallidum* and positive units discarded.

Transfusion siderosis

Each unit of blood contains about 0.25 g of iron and so, with frequent transfusions, iron overload with parenchymal tissue damage may occur. Serious problems arise after about 30 g of iron accumulation. When repeated transfusion is anticipated, desferrioxamine therapy must therefore be considered.

Ion toxicity

Blood is stored in citrate which can chelate calcium and can sometimes cause tetany. However, as citrate is rapidly metabolised in the liver, citrate toxicity only occurs in severe liver disease and during rapid and massive blood transfusion.

During blood storage, the $[K^+]$ in the plasma rises by about 1 mmol/day due to leakage from red cells. After transfusion, the red cells rapidly remove this excess K^+, so that problems only arise in patients who already have a raised plasma $[K^+]$, or with massive transfusions, especially exchange transfusion in neonates. Stored blood also contains high levels of NH_4^+ and should therefore be avoided in liver disease.

Problems of massive transfusion

Large volume blood transfusions given over a short period

of time may be associated with special problems. Where stored blood has been used, there is a theoretical risk of toxicity from citrate, hydrogen ions (acidosis) and potassium ions, but these problems are in fact rare. Dilution of platelets and clotting factors does occur, however, and must be corrected by replacement therapy after appropriate assays. If stored blood is given rapidly the patient may become hypothermic if a blood warmer is not used.

IMMUNE HAEMOLYTIC DISEASE OF THE NEWBORN

Aetiology

In immune haemolytic disease of the newborn (HDN), IgG antibodies produced by the mother against fetal red cell antigens cross the placenta and produce haemolysis in the fetus (Fig. 25.20). In 90% of cases, the antibodies are directed to antigens of the rhesus group and severe disease is mainly caused by anti-D antibodies. Other antibodies causing occasional problems are shown in Table 25.21. In the UK, 85% of the population are Rh-positive (D+) and 13% of UK marriages are between a dd (D−) woman and a D+ man. Three in four of their children will be D+. Sensitisation of the mother requires passage of a considerable quantity (approximately 0.5 ml) of fetal cells into the maternal circulation and this usually happens at birth. Firstborn children are therefore rarely affected. However, the mother is now primed, and can produce a secondary antibody response to the small quantity of fetal red cells that enter the maternal circulation during a subsequent normal pregnancy. Group O mothers are less frequently sensitised if the fetus is Group A or, to a lesser extent, Group B – presumably because the fetal cells are rapidly

Table 25.21 Antibodies causing haemolytic disease of the newborn*

Anti-rhesus (in order of incidence)
Anti-D
Anti-C + D
Anti-E
(Anti-C) (often severe)
(Anti-D + E)
(Anti-C + E)
(Anti-e)

Anti-Kell

Anti-Duffy

Anti-Kidd

Anti-A + Anti-B

* Brackets indicate rarity

cleared from the maternal circulation by naturally occurring anti-A and anti-B antibodies. It should also be noted that rhesus sensitisation can occur with antepartum haemorrhages, obstetric manipulations, Rh-positive blood transfusions and other blood products.

ABO incompatibility is a rare cause of HDN, as most individuals produce only IgM antibodies which do not cross the placenta. Only occasional Group O women will produce high titre IgG anti-A or anti-B when carrying an A+ or B+ fetus. It should be noted in these cases that, at birth, the cord cells often give a negative DAT (probably due to the low ABO antigen density on cord cells), and this may make the diagnosis very difficult.

Clinical features

The affected fetus becomes anaemic, and produces a reticulocytosis and many nucleated red cells in the peripheral blood (erythroblastosis fetalis). As the anaemia progresses, cardiac failure develops with scalp oedema, pericardial effusions and ascites (hydrops). Hyperbilirubinaemia is not a problem *in utero* because of placental clearance but, after birth, haemolysis continues until all the maternal antibody has been used up, and severe jaundice may develop quickly. High levels of unconjugated bilirubin can cause severe damage to the central nervous system, especially in premature infants.

Approach to the monitoring of pregnancy in Rh-negative women

All pregnant women should have a red cell group performed at the booking clinic at 12 weeks gestation. The serum should also be screened against a cell panel at this stage to look for antibodies which, if found, must then be identified. This should not be restricted to Rh-negative women (cde/cde) as anti-c antibodies, as well as other rarer antibodies, would then be missed. In the case of Rh-negative women, it is also usual to genotype the father to determine whether he is Rh-positive and whether he is DD or Dd. Antibody screening should ideally be repeated

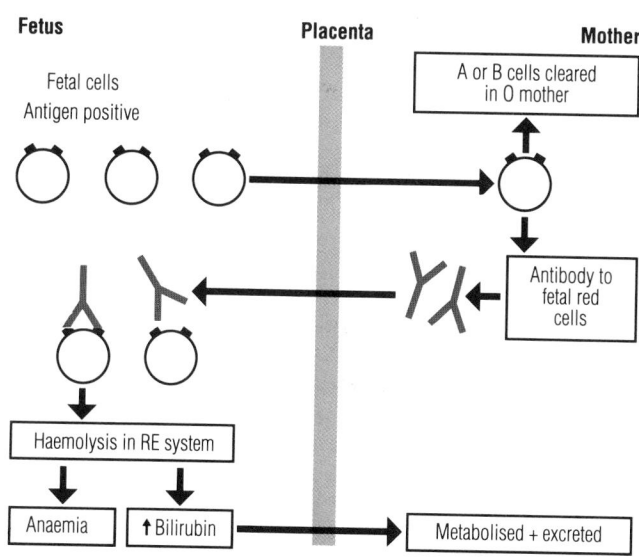

Fig. 25.20 Diagrammatic representation of the pre-natal mechanism of haemolytic disease of the newborn (HDN).

in Rh-negative women at 24 weeks, 34 weeks and at delivery if it is a first pregnancy, and even more frequently in later pregnancies. If an antibody screen is positive, it should be repeated at four-weekly intervals throughout the second trimester and at two-weekly intervals during the last trimester. Rising levels of antibody indicate an affected fetus, and amniocentesis should be performed if the anti-D titre is greater than 1:16 (4 μg/ml). If high levels of antibody are present before amniocentesis is feasible, then the fetus should be monitored by ultrasound for evidence of hydrops. It must be noted that the level of maternal antibody correlates rather poorly with the severity of HDN, and amniocentesis should therefore be performed whenever doubt arises. In these circumstances, the previous obstetric history must be taken into account. In first-affected fetuses, it is likely that the disease will be mild; whereas the disease is more likely to be severe in subsequent pregnancies, with a five-fold greater mortality. If a mother has had a previous severely affected fetus, she should be monitored by ultrasound from 16 weeks gestation and by amniocentesis from 25 weeks gestation, even if the antibody titres are low.

The purpose of amniocentesis is to measure the bile pigment levels in the fetal blood. This is measured spectrophotometrically by absorption at 450 nm. The value obtained must be plotted on a graph of optical density of the amniotic fluid versus gestation, and interpretation is made using well standardised criteria (Fig. 25.21). If a value is obtained in zone A, the fetus is severely affected and at high risk of death. Therapeutic intervention is therefore necessary. If in zone B, great vigilance is required and amniocentesis should be repeated after two weeks.

Fig. 25.21 Chart of optical density of the amniotic fluid versus gestation, showing ranges of risk. (A) Fetus at high risk. (B) Fetus at risk. (C) Fetus at low risk.

Treatment of HDN

Antenatal

Intra-uterine transfusions can be given to severely affected fetuses. This can be given by the intraperitoneal route from 24 weeks of gestation onwards, or by injection (fetoscopic or ultrasound-guided) into an umbilical blood vessel from 16 weeks onwards. The blood given is washed O Rh-negative (cde/cde) and is cross-matched with the mother's serum. It should also be from an anti-CMV negative individual.

Maternal plasmapheresis is sometimes used in cases with high antibody titres early in pregnancy, in an attempt to reduce the severity of the haemolysis. To be effective, very large exchanges are required three or four days a week from about 10 weeks gestation onwards. The plasma replacement should be from Rh-negative donors to prevent contamination with Rh-positive red cell stroma.

The mainstay of management remains the induction of premature labour. In most severely affected fetuses, this is done at 32 weeks, and at later dates in less severely affected fetuses. Measurement of lecithin:sphingomyelin ratios in the amniotic fluid at the time of amniocentesis provide some indication of lung maturity, and may assist in the decision of when to induce labour.

Postnatal

Exchange transfusion should be performed immediately after birth in severely anaemic or hydropic infants. The best indicator of severity at birth is the cord blood haemoglobin concentration – values below 12.5 g/dl are indicative of the need for exchange. The bilirubin level is less valuable but a value above 70 μmol/l probably indicates the need for exchange. At a later stage, bilirubin estimations are paramount and exchanges must be performed to keep this well below an accepted value, i.e. below 240 μmol/l for infants delivered between 30–31 weeks; below 290 μmol/l for infants delivered between 31–34 weeks; and below 350 μmol/l for 'older' infants. These values should be lowered if the infant is clinically unwell. In exchange transfusion, fresh blood collected into citrate phosphate dextrose is used. The blood should be O-negative, compatible with both the mother's and infant's serum, and CMV-negative. Usually a two volume exchange (1 vol = wt(kg) × 90 ml) is performed; this removes antibody coated red cells which would eventually be destroyed, removes unbound antibody and reduces the bilirubin level.

In mildly affected infants, phototherapy may augment bilirubin breakdown and avoid the necessity for exchange tranfusion.

Prevention of HDN

Rh-negative women should not be given Rh-positive blood or blood products.

At childbirth, Rh-negative women should be given intramuscular anti-D within 72 hours of delivery of an Rh-positive child, in order to neutralise any fetal cells in the circulation and prevent sensitisation. The dose of 100 μg usually given should be sufficient to neutralise approximately 4 ml of fetal blood. A Kleihauer test should be performed on the mother's blood (fetal cells stain darkly, adult cells very weakly) and, if fetal cells are detected at a frequency of more than 1 in 600, further anti-D should be given. Anti-D should also be given to Rh-negative women for threatened abortions, abortions, haemorrhages and obstetric manoeuvres. Fifty micrograms is given before the twentieth week of pregnancy, and after this, $100\,\mu$g. The antibody only crosses the placenta slowly and the fetus is not harmed.

Despite such measures, nearly 1% of women still become sensitised during their first pregnancy. It has therefore recently been recommended that all Rh-negative women with a potential Rh-positive child should receive $100\,\mu$g of anti-D at 28 weeks and 34 weeks gestation, to minimise sensitisation from silent fetal to maternal blood transfer *in utero*.

NON-MALIGNANT LEUCOCYTE ABNORMALITIES

Leucocyte abnormalities can be considered as qualitative or quantitative.

The causes of a raised leucocyte component in the peripheral blood are shown in Table 25.22. Infection is the commonest cause and the response usually varies both with different organisms, and at different phases of the disease.

Thus, acute pyogenic infections cause an initial neutrophilia, but may give rise to monocytosis in the recovery period. Parasitic infections typically give rise to eosinophilia, and viral infections to lymphocytosis, although considerable variation to this general rule may occur. The reactive lymphocytes may appear atypical, and this is particularly prominent in infectious mononucleosis. Neutrophilia also occurs in response to all forms of tissue injury or inflammation, whereas eosinophilia is usually associated with inflammation which has an allergic basis. Basophilia is only rarely a reactive condition, and always suggests an underlying myeloproliferative disorder.

The causes of a decreased neutrophil or lymphocyte count are shown in Table 25.23. The minor components of the leucocyte population may also decrease, but this is not usually detected on a routine differential count. Although the cytopenias must be due to either decreased production or increased loss/destruction, it is difficult to classify the causes in this way as some are multifactorial (e.g. neutropenia in acute infections) and the mechanism is not always well understood (e.g. lymphopenia in advanced Hodgkin's disease). Qualitative lymphocyte abnormalities are discussed in Chapter 7.

Functional abnormalities of phagocytes also occur and may be primary or secondary (Table 25.24). The primary

Table 25.22 Causes of raised leucocyte counts in the peripheral blood

Cause	Neutrophils	Eosinophils	Basophils	Monocytes	Lymphocytes
Infections	Pyogenic organisms Some viruses Spirochaetes Rickettsia	Parasites Mycobacteria Occasional bacteria	Occasional chronic infections	Convalescent phase from acute infections Protozoa Some viruses Mycobacteria Occasional chronic infections	Viruses Pertussis Mycobacteria Spirochaetes Occasional chronic infections
Non-specific tissue injury/inflammation	Often marked	–	–	–	–
Connective tissue disease	Often marked	Moderate Especially polyarteritis nodosa, ulcerative colitis	–	Often marked	Often marked
Skin diseases	Moderate	Often marked	–	–	–
Allergic conditions	Moderate	Often marked	–	–	–
Severe metabolic disorders	Often marked	–	–	–	–
Hyposplenism	Often marked	Moderate	–	Moderate	Moderate
Miscellaneous	–	Pulmonary eosinophilia Loeffler's endocarditis	Myxoedema	–	Thyroid disease
Non-haematological malignancies	Often marked	Moderate	–	–	Moderate
Myeloproliferative disorders	Often marked	Often marked	Often marked	Often marked	–
Lymphoproliferative disorders	–	–	–	–	Often marked

Table 25.23 Causes of low leucocyte count in the peripheral blood

Neutrophils	Lymphocytes
Marrow aplasia	Severe marrow aplasia
Marrow infiltration	Severe marrow infiltration
Megaloblastic anaemia	Severe megaloblastic anaemia
Cyclical neutropenia	
Congenital agranulocytosis (Kostman's syndrome)	
	Congenital immunodeficiency disorders
Some acute infections	Rarely in acute infections
Typhoid, brucella, miliary TB	
Protozoa	
Fungi	
Rickettsia	
Viral	
HIV infection	**HIV infection**
Collagen disorders	**Collagen disorders**
	Lymphomas
Exposure to high dose irradiation	**Exposure to irradiation**
Immune destruction	Immune destruction
Idiopathic	
Associated with drugs	
Hypersplenism	Hypersplenism
	Intestinal loss due to lymphatic obstruction

Bold type Indicates that the relevant cytopenia is common in that condition; it does *not* mean that the particular condition is a common cause of the cytopenia.

abnormalities include:

1. *Chediak-Higashi syndrome*, a rare autosomal recessive disorder in which there is oculocutaneous albinism, neurological deficit, a bleeding tendency and frequent pyogenic infections. Inclusion bodies are visible in the leucocytes.
2. *Chronic granulomatous disease*, which is usually X-linked but may be autosomal recessive. There is an absence of cytochrome b or some other component of the oxidase system, such that phagocytosis does not lead to a respiratory burst with ultimate free radical production and bacterial killing. It presents with chronic and recurrent infections during infancy, with abscess and granuloma formation.

The secondary causes of abnormal neutrophil function are extensive, but their true significance *in vivo* is not clear.

HAEMATOLOGICAL MALIGNANCY

The nature and aetiology of haematological malignancies has been more extensively studied than in other tumours, largely because of the ease with which single cell suspensions can be obtained from blood, marrow and lymph nodes. However, the insights gained from these studies can probably be applied to many other types of neoplasia.

Pathogenesis

Nearly all haematological malignancies examined have been shown to be clonal in origin. The B cell malignancies express light chain restricted surface immunoglobulin (if the cells are sufficiently mature to express surface immunoglobulin), and nearly all cases show a clonal rearrangement of the immunoglobulin genes. Similarly, T cell malignancies have been shown to have clonal rearrangements of the T cell antigen-receptor genes. Some of these malignancies – and also the myeloid leukaemias – may have clonal chromosomal abnormalities, such as alterations in chromosome number or chromosome translocations. Other myeloid leukaemias have been shown to be clonal by studies in women heterozygous for glucose-6-phosphate dehydrogenase (G6PD) isoenzymes. (G6PD is coded on the X-chromosome and, as one X-chromosome is inactivated in each cell early in embryogenesis, a clonal population expresses only one G6PD isoenzyme.)

The phenotype of malignant cells is almost always similar to that of their normal counterparts. The phenotype of blast cells in acute myeloid leukaemia (AML) is thus identical to that of a rare population of normal primitive cells, although the Auer rods sometimes seen in AML cells are not seen in normal adult cells. No leukaemia-specific surface antigens have been defined (but see p. 1072). Thus, for example, the common acute lymphoblastic leukaemia (ALL) antigen, which is expressed on the cells in most cases of ALL, has been shown to be a normal early lymphoid differentiation antigen.

Blast cells in acute leukaemia are not completely homo-primitive phenotype than the main cell population. In chronic granulocytic leukaemia (CGL), G6PD isoenzyme studies have shown that, although the majority of malignant cells are late granulocytic cells, the clonal disorder also affects red cells, platelets and some B lymphocytes. The 'leukaemic hit' must therefore have occurred at the

Table 25.24 Aetiology of phagocytic functional abnormalities

Abnormal phagocytic function	Disorder	
	Primary	Secondary
Movement	Lazy leucocyte syndrome	Renal failure Diabetes Malnutrition
Recognition		Immunoglobulin and complement (opsonins) deficiency
Phagocytosis	Chediak-Higashi syndrome	Severe malnutrition Vitamin E deficiency
Killing	Chronic granulomatous disease	Severe iron deficiency Post-irradiation

Summary 5   Features of haematological malignancies

- Clonal
- Malignant cells have normal counterparts
- Malignant populations have stem cells more primitive than the majority of the malignant population
- The level of 'differentiation block' may change
- Growth is not autonomous
- The growth rate is not necessarily higher than in normal cellular counterparts
- Growth rates are not always constant

multipotential stem cell level. Similar findings have been reported in cases of adult AML. The oncogenic event occurs at a multipotential stem cell level but the malignant cells are still able to differentiate in part down all the myeloid pathways. A 'differentiation block' is, however, present at the myeloblast stage and these cells therefore accumulate. This level of differentiation block may change over time and the blastic transformation that occurs in CGL probably represents such a process.

In vitro studies have demonstrated that leukaemic cell growth is not autonomous. In polycythaemia rubra vera (PRV), the erythroid progenitors will (like their normal counterparts) only grow in the presence of erythropoeitin, although their sensitivity to erythropoeitin is considerably greater. In AML and CGL the concentrations of colony stimulating factors required for *in vitro* growth are very similar to normal cell requirements. The process of malignant transformation is clearly extremely subtle.

The growth rate of leukaemic cells is also thought to be about the same as (or even slower than) that of normal cells, so that the expansion of the leukaemic mass is not due to accelerated growth. In the chronic leukaemias, it is likely that there is instead an alteration in the balance between stem cell self-renewal and commitment/differentiation. Initially, a malignant clone with a slightly higher self-renewal rate will produce fewer end cells, but eventually it will produce an exponentially increasing population of end cells. A similar process may occur in the acute leukaemias, but here, cell population growth is also affected by the differentiation block, which reduces the cell death rate associated with terminal differentiation.

It should be noted that the growth rate in the haematological malignancies is not necessarily constant over time. In multiple myeloma, for example, treatment will often induce a plateau phase during which the tumour is kinetically quiescent and resistant to further chemotherapy. If chemotherapy is stopped at this stage the plateau phase is often maintained for many months.

Aetiology

The aetiological factors associated with haematological malignancies have been widely studied (Summary 6).

Hereditary/congenital factors

Familial tendencies to acquire haematological malignancies are weak, with the exception of identical twins. Here, if one twin develops acute leukaemia, the risk of the remaining twin is reported to be 25%, although most of this high risk is accounted for by twins presenting with leukaemia in the first eighteen months of life. There are in addition a variety of congenital disorders – such as Down's syndrome, Bloom's syndrome and Fanconi's anaemia – in which the incidence of leukaemia is markedly increased.

Ionising radiation and drugs

Exposure to excessive ionising radiation increases the risk of all haematological malignancies except chronic lymphocytic leukaemia. Many drugs have also been proposed as carcinogens, but the data is only firm for benzene. Both ionising radiation and benzene directly damage DNA.

Gross chromosomal abnormalities

Gross chromosomal abnormalities – such as additional chromosomes, deletions or major translocations – can be detected in many cases of leukaemia or lymphoma and certain of these have prognostic significance. Thus, acute lymphoblastic leukaemia patients with a 4:11 translocation have a very poor prognosis; whereas patients with hyperdiploid (more than 50 chromosomes) blast cells respond very well to treatment.

Proto-oncogenes

At a finer level, great interest has recently been focussed on proto-oncogene expression in malignant cells. In any one case of leukaemia or lymphoma, there may be high levels of multiple proto-oncogene mRNA and this may be indicative of a multistep oncogenic process in which more than one oncogene is involved. This finding must be viewed with some caution, however, because the normal levels of gene expression in cells of the same lineage at the same stage of differentiation have not yet been determined. The cellular myc gene is highly expressed in many haematological malignancies as compared to resting lymphocytes or mature myeloid cells, but c-myc expression is also high in normal primitive myeloid cells and in mitogen activated lymphoblasts. It thus appears that c-myc expression is a

Summary 6   Aetiological factors in haemotological malignancies

- Familial and congenital associations
- Ionising irradiation
- Chemical carcinogens
- Chromosome abnormalities including expression of proto-oncogenes
- Viruses – HTLV I
             – EBV

frequent feature of the proliferating cells rather than a primary oncogenic process. Of particular interest, is the anatomical siting of certain proto-oncogenes in relation to common translocations in the haematological malignancies. In Burkitt's lymphoma, for example, the majority of patients have a translocation of the long arm of chromosome 8 to the long arm of chromosome 14, close to the region coding for immunoglobulin heavy chains. The break point on chromosome 8 is close to the 8q 24 band, which is the site of the c-myc oncogene. It is possible that the high c-myc expression found in this tumour is due to the ectopic siting of the c-myc oncogene either in proximity to a different promotor, or beyond the influence of a local suppressing sequence.

In other situations, the aberrant location of a proto-oncogene can lead to production of an abnormal mRNA species and protein product. Thus, in the Philadelphia (Ph') chromosome – which is present in most cases of chronic granulocytic leukaemia – there is a translocation between chromosome 9 and chromosome 22. The site of the translocation on chromosome 9 is within the c-ableson sequence, at a splicing site between the 5' and 3' end of this gene. In the Philadelphia chromosome, a region of chromosome 22 known as the *breakpoint cluster region* (*bcr*) becomes joined to the 3' end of c-abl, leading to the production of a unique fusion gene product in relatively large quantities (Fig. 25.22). This suggests that tumour specific antigens may be present after all in some human tumours, although the protein levels may be too low to be detected by routine immunofluorescent techniques.

The precise functions of most oncogene products are still unknown, but many of the proto-oncogenes studied to date have been found to code for tyrosine kinases or growth factor receptors, and are therefore likely to be important metabolic regulatory proteins.

In addition to the possible role of structural abnormalities in, or ectopic siting of, proto-oncogenes in malignant tranformation, there may be further gene sequences which normally suppress proto-oncogene expression. Such genes have been called *anti-oncogenes*, and mutations in these genes might also give rise to malignant change. However, while there is considerable evidence for this in neuroblastomas, there is no evidence to date for such a process in the haematological malignancies.

Viruses

Although many malignancies in the animal kingdom can be transmitted by retroviruses containing sequences similar to cellular proto-oncogenes, this has not been described in man. *Human T cell lymphotrophic virus I* (HTLV I) is a retrovirus and is undoubtedly associated with certain T cell leukaemia/lymphomas, but it does not contain a gene sequence with a normal cellular counterpart. The precise mechanism of oncogenesis is not known, but may involve an indirect increase in growth factor (interleukin-2) receptor expression. It is important to note that the vast majority of patients infected with HTLV I do not develop lymphoproliferative diseases. HTLV I neoplasms nonetheless comprise a large proportion of the haematological malignancies in South-West Japan and the Caribbean basin, although they represent a very small proportion of such cases in most other parts of the world.

The other virus implicated in haematological malignancy is the *Epstein Barr virus*, which is associated with Burkitt's lymphoma. The mechanism of transformation, which occurs in small numbers of individuals (mainly in areas of Africa), is again obscure.

Finally, it should be noted that there are a few rare instances where relapse has occurred in donor cells in patients given ablative radiotherapy and allogeneic marrow transplants for treatment of acute myeloid leukaemia, suggesting the possibility of a transmissible agent. Overall, however, the evidence to date does not suggest that viruses are a major cause of haematological malignancies in most geographical areas.

Fig. 25.22 Diagrammatic representation of c-abl gene. A. In the normal gene there is variable spacing to give 4 species of mRNA. **B.** In the Philadelphia (Ph') chromosome the bcr from chromosome 22 joins the 3' end of the c-abl gene to give a novel hybrid gene.

MYELOPROLIFERATIVE DISORDERS

The myeloproliferative disorders are defined as neoplastic proliferations of the myeloid stem cell and its progeny. This is a simplification in that the multipotential stem cell may also be involved in the malignant process with additional involvement of the lymphocyte series. Although the level of leukaemic transformation is at the most primitive stem cell level, the individual disease entities are recognised by the predominant cell type accumulating in the blood and marrow (Fig. 25.23). Intermediate states and transitions between one entity and another may occur.

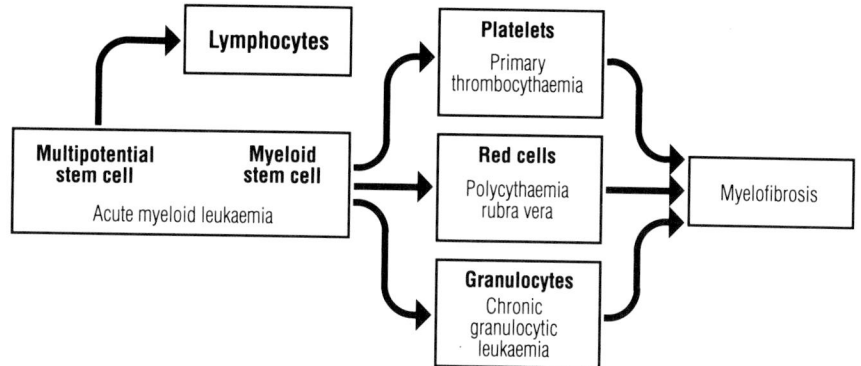

Fig. 25.23 The myeloproliferative disorders.

Acute myeloid leukaemia is clearly a myeloproliferative disorder although it is common to consider only the chronic proliferations under this heading. Fibrosis frequently occurs as a reaction to the malignant proliferation, especially if there is a prominent megakaryocytic element. Occasionally, marked fibrosis is the presenting feature and is then known as primary myelofibrosis; it is, nonetheless, a secondary process.

CHRONIC GRANULOCYTIC LEUKAEMIA

Chronic granulocytic leukaemia (CGL) is a disorder of the multipotent stem cell in which the myeloid progenitor cell compartment – and subsequently the maturing granulocytic cell compartment – becomes grossly expanded. The erythroid, megakaryocytic and B lymphoid cells are also part of the malignant clone; their accumulation is not usually prominent, although polycythaemia and thrombocytosis may occur. Over 90% of cases have the Philadelphia chromosome, in which there is a translocation from the long arm of chromosome 22 to the long arm of chromosome 9 with the resultant production of an abnormal c-abl gene product (p. 1072). Even in cases of apparent Philadelphia-negative CGL, detailed molecular analysis has often shown a translocation involving the c-abl-bcr gene regions. The mechanism by which the c-abl product is associated with malignant transformation is not known.

Clinical features of chronic phase CGL

CGL occurs predominantly in those over 30 years of age, although childhood variants do occur (p. 1074). Males and females are equally affected and the annual incidence in the UK is approximately one in 100 000. CGL is initially an indolent disease that can, in the chronic phase, be readily controlled by chemotherapy, but transformation to an *accelerated phase* is almost invariable. Typically, there is slow onset of symptoms of anaemia, often accompanied by weight loss. Infections and bleeding are rare at presentation. The spleen is almost always palpable and may become enormous. Splenic pain due to infarction may arise. Lymphadenopathy does not generally occur.

Haematological features of the chronic phase

The most striking peripheral blood abnormality is the rise in white cell count; there is an increase in neutrophils, basophils and eosinophils. Many precursor cells, particularly myelocytes, are present and up to 5% of the circulating leucocytes may be blast cells. The haemoglobin tends to fall as the white cell count rises, although, occasionally, it may be high at presentation. The platelet count is variable. The bone marrow shows myeloid hyperplasia and sometimes an increase in reticulin.

Differential diagnosis

The main differential diagnosis of CGL is that of reactive leucocytosis due to infection or inflammation. A *leukaemoid reaction* (a non-neoplastic leucocytosis of marked degree) can usually be distinguished from CGL, as splenomegaly is not common in the former, and eosinophilia and basophilia are not usually a component of the leucocytosis. The neutrophil alkaline phosphatase (NAP) level (detected by cytochemical staining) is typically very low in CGL and high in reactive leucocytoses. The final arbiter in difficult cases is the demonstration of the Philadelphia chromosome in CGL (p. 1072).

Chronic myelomonocytic leukaemia with a high count may also cause confusion but, in this condition, monocytes are plentiful and eosinophils and basophils are not usually increased (p. 1081). Primary myelofibrosis may also be associated with an initial leucocytosis but, in this disease, there are also usually red cell changes attributable to marrow fibrosis, the NAP score is raised, and the Philadelphia chromosome is absent.

Management of chronic phase CGL

Therapy is essentially palliative for most patients. Blood transfusions should be given as necessary and any infections treated vigorously. Allopurinol is often given to prevent secondary gout, especially if there is hyperuricaemia. Chemotherapy is given in an attempt to normalise the blood count and shrink the spleen. This undoubtedly improves the quality of life but does not delay acute transformation. Alkylating agents (e.g. busulphan) are usually given as a small daily dose (2–6 mg/day) either alone, or in combination with anti-metabolites such as 6-thioguanine. Larger doses of busulphan can be given at less frequent intervals, but there is the risk of causing severe long lasting aplasia. Hydroxyurea is a useful alternative to busulphan, and has the advantage that its effects are readily reversible. Occasionally, a very high leucocyte count at presentation can lead to hyperviscosity and thrombotic events such as confusion and priapism. Should hyperviscosity occur, or if the leucocyte count is over $200 \times 10^9/l$, leucopheresis is advisable until the chemotherapy has decreased the rate of white cell production.

Attempts have been made to eliminate the Philadelphia-positive clone during the chronic phase by using intensive acute leukaemia regimens, but these have almost invariably proved ineffective. For younger patients who have an HLA identical sibling, massive chemo/radiotherapy and allogeneic bone marrow transplantation during the chronic phase is probably the treatment of choice. The immediate mortality is less than 30% and many patients will have prolonged disease-free survival. It is, as yet, premature to consider these patients cured.

Clinical features of acute transformation

Acute transformation of CGL may take the form of increasing myelofibrosis or transition to an acute leukaemia. On average it occurs within three years of onset, although there is considerable individual variation. Many clinical events may herald transformation, including increasing anaemia, fever, increasing spleen size and bone pain. A patient is considered to have entered an accelerated phase when the therapy (which was previously effective) can no longer control the symptoms, signs and haematological features of the disease. In a myelofibrotic transformation, there is progressive anaemia, thrombocytopenia and possibly even neutropenia. The spleen enlarges markedly and may cause severe discomfort. In blastic transformation, the features are those of marrow failure as they are with other types of acute leukaemia (p. 1077).

Haematological features of acute transformation

Acute transformation may be heralded by a fall in the haemoglobin, platelet count, or by a rise in the white cell count while still on therapy. There may be a rise in the basophil and blast cell count and in the NAP score. In a myelofibrotic transformation, the blood picture is similar to that seen in any case of marrow fibrosis, with leuco-erythroblastic anaemia (primitive red and white cell precursors in the blood) and marked poikilocytosis with tear-drop forms.

In a blastic crisis, blast cells predominate in the blood and marrow. In about 80% of cases, these are myeloblasts; but in the remaining 20% of cases they are pre-B lymphoblasts, which express the common acute lymphoblastic leukaemia antigen (CALLA). This illustrates the fact that CGL involves a multipotent stem cell with both myeloid and lymphoid potential.

At the time of accelerated phase or blast crisis, cytogenetic analysis frequently reveals clonal abnormalities additional to the Philadelphia chromosome.

Treatment of the acute phase

In a myelofibrotic transformation, transfusion should be given for symptomatic anaemia. Splenectomy should be considered for spleen pain, or if splenic pooling in a big spleen is considered to contribute to the anaemia or other cytopenia. Local irradiation may ease splenic pain, but it rarely causes a long-lasting reduction of spleen size.

In blastic transformation, acute leukaemia therapy of appropriate type is given (p. 1079). Remissions in which there is return of chronic phase CGL may be achieved, but they are usually of brief duration.

Allogeneic transplantation in acute phase CGL has not been very successful.

Chronic myeloproliferative disorders in childhood

Diseases resembling CGL may occur (rarely) in infancy and childhood. So-called *juvenile CGL* presents in infancy with anaemia, infection, facial rashes, lymphadenopathy and hepatosplenomegaly. The white cell count is elevated with a prominent monocytosis. The HbF is markedly raised in most cases. The disease is rapidly progressive, with death usually due to marrow failure rather than transformation to acute leukaemia. Therapy is currently unsatisfactory.

A variant form of juvenile CGL which occurs in infancy is the myeloproliferative disease associated with monosomy 7 in the malignant clone. The HbF level is not markedly raised in this condition. The prognosis is again very poor.

Adult-type CGL with a Philadelphia chromosome occasionally occurs in older children and has a natural history similar to that seen in adults.

POLYCYTHAEMIA RUBRA VERA

Polycythaemia refers to an increase in the red cell mass. If due to a malignant myeloproliferative disorder, it is known as *polycythaemia rubra vera* (PRV); if due to a raised level of erythropoietin, it is known as *secondary polycythaemia*. A raised haemoglobin concentration may also occur due to a decreased plasma volume without an increase in the red cell mass; this is known as *pseudopolycythaemia* or *stress polycythaemia* (Fig. 25.24).

Polycythaemia rubra vera is a malignant disorder of the multipotential haemopoietic stem cell, with predominant expansion of the mature erythroid cell population. The erythroid progenitors have increased sensitivity to erythropoietin, although the mechanism of this change in responsiveness is not known. There is often also an increase in

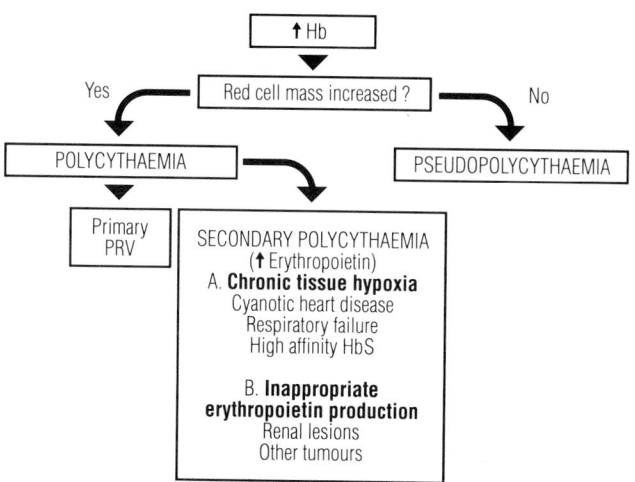

Fig. 25.24 Approach to the diagnosis of a raised haemoglobin (Hb) level.

granulocytic cells and platelets, in keeping with the stem cell nature of this disease.

Clinical features

PRV is largely a disease of the middle-aged and elderly. It has been reported slightly more often in males than females.

The symptoms and signs of the disease are shown in Table 25.25, but it should be noted that symptoms may be minimal. Splenomegaly is present in 75% of cases: the diagnostic difficulties mainly arise in those patients without splenomegaly. The major symptoms and causes of death are due to the hyperviscosity associated with a raised haematocrit (Fig. 25.25A). Despite the elevated [Hb], blood flow and oxygen delivery is actually reduced to critical organs, particularly the brain (Fig. 25.25B). Pruritus is common and may in part be related to basophil production; iron deficiency may exacerbate this complaint. Peptic ulceration is very common. This is mainly due to hyperviscosity but may be exacerbated by excessive histamine release from basophils. Gastrointestinal bleeding from gastric erosions is not infrequent, and may be partially due to abnormalities of platelet function.

Table 25.25 Clinical features of polycythaemia rubra vera

Cause	Effect
Haemopoietic proliferation	Gout
	Hepatosplenomegaly
	Splenomegaly
Increased haematocrit	Hypertension
	Cerebral ischaemia
	Myocardial ischaemia
	Other thrombotic events
Multifactorial	Pruritus
	Peptic ulceration
	Bleeding

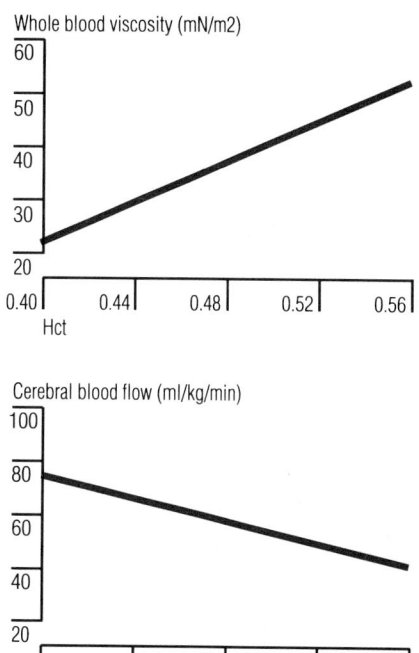

Fig. 25.25 Relationship of blood viscosity and cerebral blood flow to the haematocrit (Hct). As the haematocrit rises, there is a marked rise in viscosity and fall in blood flow.

Haematological features

Haematological investigations show that the [Hb] and rbc are usually raised but, if iron deficiency occurs, the [Hb] may fall to within the normal range. The red cells are then microcytic and the red cell count remains high. The neutrophil count is modestly raised in three-quarters of patients and the platelet count in about one-half. The increased neutrophil production gives rise to a raised B_{12} level, secondary to an increased B_{12} binding protein release. The NAP score is usually raised (unlike the situation in CGL). The bone marrow shows gross erythroid hyperplasia. Some fibrosis may be apparent. Chromosome analysis is usually normal at presentation.

Diagnosis

The first step in diagnosis is to demonstrate the presence of a raised red cell mass. The patient's red cells are labelled with ^{51}Cr, the total radioactivity bound to the red cells measured, and the red cells reinjected. Samples are taken after equilibration and the red cell mass calculated using the expression:

$$\text{Red cell mass} = \frac{\text{Total counts/min injected}}{\text{Counts/min per ml of sample}} \times \text{haematocrit}$$

The result is expressed in ml/kg body weight.

The next stage is to exclude secondary polycythaemia. The Pa_{O_2} should be measured and a renal ultrasound performed. Polycystic kidneys and even hydronephrosis can cause a rise in erythropoietin, although polycythaemia of renal origin usually indicates a renal tumour. Other investigations to exclude an underlying cause of polycythaemia should be performed if the clinical situation merits it. If there is no splenomegaly and no raised white cell or platelet count, particular care must be taken to exclude a secondary cause. An Hb-oxygen dissociation curve is essential (especially in younger patients) to exclude the possibility of a high affinity haemoglobin. This is an inherited abnormality which gives rise to tissue hypoxia in the presence of a normal Pa_{O_2}.

It might be thought that measurement of erythropoietin levels would readily differentiate between primary and secondary polycythaemia, but the results of erythropoietin assays are not always discriminatory. The criteria adopted for the diagnosis of PRV by the National (USA) PRV Study Group are shown in Table 25.26.

Those patients with a raised red cell mass and normal Pa_{O_2} who do not have splenomegaly or two category C features should be referred to as having *idiopathic erythrocytosis*. Although most such patients will develop a myeloproliferative disorder, this is not invariable, and they should not therefore receive cytoreductive therapy at this stage.

Table 25.26 National (USA) PRV Study Group criteria for the diagnosis of polycythaemia rubra vera

A	↑Red cell mass Normal O_2 saturation
B	Splenomegaly
C	↑Platelets ↑Leucocytes (more than 12×10^9/l) ↑AP score ↑B_{12} (more than 900 pg/ml)

PRV is diagnosed if both A and B group symptoms are present; or if group A symptoms are present with any two symptoms from group C.

Treatment

Support measures should include allopurinol for the prevention of secondary gout, especially if the uric acid level is high or if cytoreductive therapy is to be commenced. Antihistamines may help pruritus, and the symptom often improves with control of the disorder.

Once the diagnosis of PRV has been made, venesection should be commenced. Approximately one unit of blood should be removed every second day until a normal haematocrit is obtained. Younger patients may tolerate more intensive initial venesection, while the converse applies in the elderly. Regular venesection alone can also be used to maintain the haematocrit below 0.46–0.48. Venesection may cause a thrombocytosis, and cytoreductive therapy must be instituted if platelet levels rise above 800×10^9/l, as this may exacerbate the thrombotic tendency of PRV.

Cytoreductive therapy is usually with radioactive ^{32}P or

an alkylating agent such as busulphan. ^{32}P (3–8 mCi) is given as a single iv bolus, and results in suppression of haemopoiesis with minimal systemic disturbance. The injection of ^{32}P can be repeated if necessary, but only after an interval of several months as the full effects of ^{32}P may take this long to be seen. It is usual to discontinue ^{32}P when a total dose of 30 mCi has been given.

Busulphan can be used as an alternative to ^{32}P given (as in CGL) as either a small daily dose, or intermittently in higher dose. Care must be taken to avoid prolonged hypoplasia.

Prognosis

Untreated, the median survival is only two years, most deaths being due to strokes and myocardial infarctions. With adequate therapy, however, the median survival is over 13 years. About 10% of cases transform to a myelofibrotic state and a similar number transform to an acute leukaemia (usually myeloid). Leukaemic transformation is higher in patients receiving cytoreductive therapy, particularly with ^{32}P.

Treatment of other forms of polycythaemia

The problems of hyperviscosity in other forms of polycythaemia are similar to PRV. Patients with idiopathic erythrocytosis and pseudopolycythaemia should be venesected to achieve a haematocrit below 0.48. In secondary polycythaemia, the situation is more complex as erythrocytosis is secondary to hypoxia. Nonetheless, the increased oxygen carrying capacity of the erythrocytosis is often more than offset by the decreased blood flow to critical organs and, in patients with neurological symptoms, a trial of venesection is worthwhile. It can be very difficult to maintain a lowered haematocrit.

ESSENTIAL THROMBOCYTHAEMIA

Essential thrombocythaemia (ET) is a myeloproliferative disorder in which there is a predominant proliferation of the megakaryocyte series. It occurs predominantly in the middle-aged and elderly. The clinical features are shown in Table 25.27. Splenomegaly may be present but is frequently absent due to repeated infarction.

The [Hb] is often reduced, especially if there is iron deficiency. The red cells frequently display the features of hyposplenism. The white cell count is often modestly

Table 25.27 Clinical features of essential thrombocythaemia

Cause	Effect
Myeloproliferation	Anaemia Splenomegaly (frequently absent)
High/abnormal platelets	Arterial and venous thromboses Haemorrhage
Multifactorial	Peptic ulceration

raised and the NAP score increased. The platelet count is usually in excess of $1000 \times 10^9/l$. The bone marrow is hypercellular, with a marked proliferation of megakaryocytes; myelofibrosis is often present.

Diagnosis

The diagnosis of ET can be difficult, especially when the thrombocytosis is modest and there is no splenomegaly. Causes of secondary thrombocytosis must be excluded (p. 1101) and platelet function tests may be helpful, as there is often an aggregation defect in ET.

Treatment

Patients with a raised platelet count and a thrombotic history should be treated with anti-platelet aggregating agents, such as aspirin and dipyridimole. Cytoreductive therapy with busulphan or ^{32}P should be given to reduce the platelet count to below $500 \times 10^9/l$. Many patients survive for more than 10 years with appropriate therapy, but transformation to acute leukaemia or, more commonly, myelofibrosis may occur.

PRIMARY MYELOFIBROSIS

Primary myelofibrosis is a misnomer, in that it is a reaction to an underlying myeloproliferative disorder (although this primary cause may be occult).

The disease mainly affects the middle-aged and elderly, and presents with anaemia due to marrow failure and massive splenomegaly. The blood film reveals a leuco-erythroblastic anaemia. A bone marrow aspirate is usually dry and a trephine biopsy shows extensive fibrosis. The diagnosis is not usually difficult, but it should be remembered that infections (particularly tuberculosis) can cause extensive marrow fibrosis.

Treatment is largely supportive, with regular transfusions. Splenectomy may be indicated if the large spleen is causing local symptoms, if there is an excessive transfusion requirement, or if there is marked granulocytopenia or thrombocytopenia.

The median survival is approximately five years. Progression to acute leukaemia occurs in 5–10% of cases.

ACUTE LEUKAEMIA

In acute leukaemia, there is accumulation in the blood and marrow of primitive haemopoietic cells (blast cells). Untreated, the course is rapidly progressive in the large majority of patients. The disease is rare, with an annual incidence of 3.5 per 100 000, although in children, acute leukaemia – particularly acute lymphoblastic leukaemia – is the commonest form of malignancy.

Acute leukaemia is divided into:

1. acute lymphoblastic leukaemia (ALL)

2. acute non-lymphoblastic leukaemia (ANLL), which is also called acute myeloid leukaemia (AML).

Each broad category can be further divided using morphological, cytochemical, immunological and genetic criteria.

Clinical features

Acute leukaemia typically presents with the features of marrow failure – anaemia, infection and bleeding. The latter may be particularly severe in promyelocytic variants of AML, where disseminated intravascular coagulation is a common complication. Onset is nearly always rapid in ALL, but there may be a preceding myelodysplastic phase in AML, with variable cytopenias lasting months or even years. In ALL, there is no such pre-leukaemia phase, although occasional cases present with an *aplastic* picture; the malignant proliferation then becomes apparent during the ensuing three months.

Hepatosplenomegaly is common in acute leukaemia, and lymphadenopathy is often present in ALL. Bone and joint pain may occur, particularly in ALL. Infiltration of soft tissues such as skin, gums and perineum may occur, and usually indicates a monocytic type of AML. Central nervous system disease is rare at presentation although it is a common site of relapse in ALL. A wide range of metabolic disturbances may also be present at diagnosis, including hyperuricaemia, hyponatraemia and hypokalaemia. These changes may all be exacerbated by treatment.

ACUTE MYELOID LEUKAEMIA

The annual incidence of acute myeloid leukaemia (AML) is approximately 2.2 per 100 000. Although the disease does occur in children and young adults, it is more common in the middle-aged and elderly (Fig. 25.26).

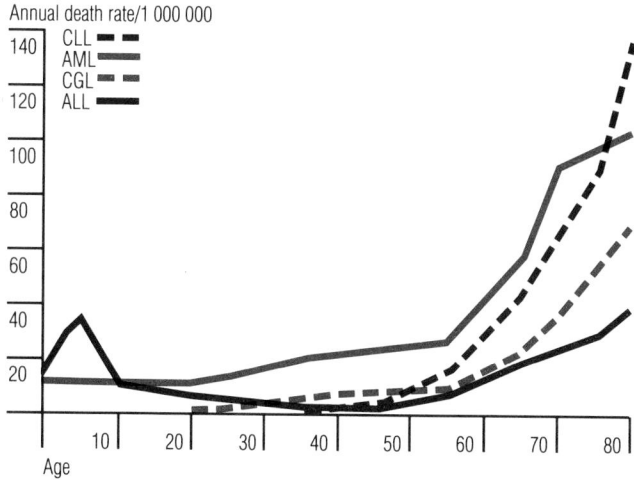

Fig. 25.26 Annual death rate for different types of leukaemia at different ages.

Diagnosis

The blood count typically reveals a normocytic or macrocytic anaemia, often with marked anisocytosis and poikilocytosis on the blood film. The platelet count is usually reduced, and the white count is usually – although not invariably – raised, with myeloblasts the predominant cells. Neutrophils are usually reduced in number and may appear dysplastic. There are relatively few intermediate myelocytes in the blood (unlike the situation in CGL).

The bone marrow is hypercellular but may produce a dry tap. The majority of cells are myeloblasts (over 30% required for diagnosis) and the remaining haemopoietic cells may show marked dysplastic changes. In some cases, pathognomonic rods (Aver rods) are seen in the myeloid cells.

Classification

Most cases of AML can be readily identified using morphological criteria, although some cases may be difficult to distinguish from ALL (especially the L2 subtype). The diagnosis of AML can be supported by cytochemical, immunological and genetic studies where appropriate (Table 25.28).

The subdivisions of AML are based on the nature of any differentiation that is present, using morphological and cytochemical criteria (Table 25.29).

Chromosome analysis

Chromosomal abnormalities are seen in about 50% of cases, using Giemsa banding analysis. As a group, these patients tend to have a worse prognosis. Trisomy 8, loss of the Y chromosome and monosomy 7 are the most common defects found. Specific translocations are also seen. A chromosome 8:21 translocation is associated with some M2 leukaemias and perhaps also with an improved prognosis; while a 15:17 translocation occurs in many cases of M3 leukaemia. More recently, high resolution banding analysis has been performed in AML, and abnormalities detected in over 80% of cases.

Treatment

The treatment strategy for AML is outlined in Figure 25.27. The *induction therapy* used in AML is very intensive as it is necessary to induce a hypoplastic marrow in order to achieve remission. The most effective drugs used are the anthracyclines and antimetabolites, and a typical induction regime is illustrated in Figure 25.28. Intensive blood product, antibiotic and psychological support is required during the hypoplastic period (p. 1049). In cases of M3 leukaemia, low dose heparin therapy is probably advisable, to reduce the risks of disseminated intravascular haemolysis associated with tumour lysis.

Remission is obtained in about 70% of younger patients,

Table 25.28 Differentiation between myeloblasts and lymphoblasts

	Myeloblasts	Lymphoblasts
Morphology		
Cell size	Moderate to large	Small to moderate
Cytoplasm	Moderate to abundant	Scanty to moderate
Granules in cytoplasm	Often in some cells	Rare
Auer rods	May be present	Absent
Nucleoli	Often more than two	One or two
Cytochemistry		
Perioxidase/Sudan black	+	−
PAS	−	+
Immunology		
Nuclear terminal deoxynucleotidyl tranferase (Tdt)	Occasionally +	+
CD10 antigen (CALLA)	−	+
CD19 antigen (pan-B)	−	+ (common ALL and null ALL)
CD7 antigen (pan-T)	− (rarely +)	+ (T-ALL)
CD33	+	−
HLA-DR	+	+ (− in T-ALL)
Genetics		
Immunoglobulin light chain gene rearrangement	−	+ (common ALL and null ALL)
T cell receptor gene rearrangement	−	+ (T-ALL)

Table 25.29 Subdivisions of acute myeloid leukaemia

M1 **AML without maturation:** The myeloid nature of the cells is illustrated by finding more than 3% peroxidase or Sudan Black positive blasts; or by the presence of blasts with occasional granules or Auer rods.

M2 **AML with maturation:** Evidence of maturation at, or beyond, the promyelocyte stage.

M3 **Promyelocytic leukaemia:** Majority of cells promyelocytes. Note that leukaemic promyelocytes may be hypergranular.

M4 **Myelomonocytic leukaemia:** Granulocytic and monocytic differentiation both present. Monocytic cells more than 20% of blood or marrow. Granulocytic cells more than 20% of marrow. Demonstration of fluoride sensitive non-specific esterase staining aids the diagnosis of monocytic cells.

M5 **Monocytic leukaemia:**
   a) Poorly differentiated monoblasts
   b) Monoblasts, promonocytes and monocytes. Granulocytic cells less than 20% of marrow.

M6 **Erythroleukaemia:** Erythropoietic component exceeds 50% or 30% if associated with severe dyserythropoiesis. Myeloblasts must still constitute more than 30% of marrow cells.

M7 **Megakaryocytic leukaemia:** Identification of megakaryoblasts aided by electron microscopic demonstration of platelet specific peroxidase or platelet specific surface antigens. This disease often presents as acute myelofibrosis in which the blasts are few in number in the marrow.

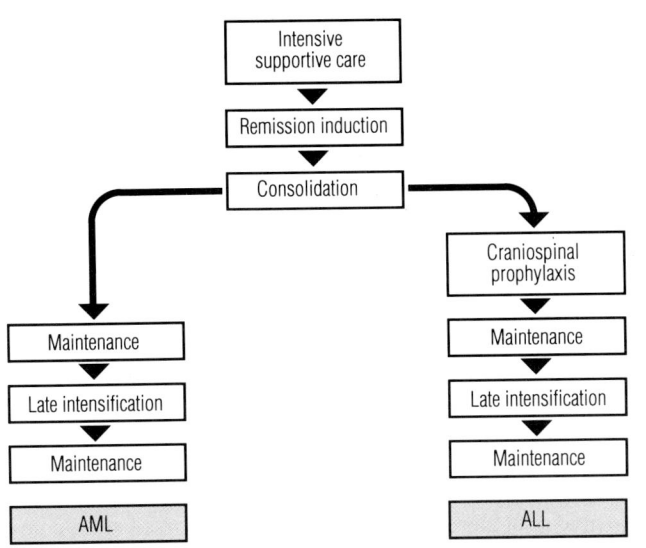

Fig. 25.27 Schematic representation of the treatment of acute leukaemia.

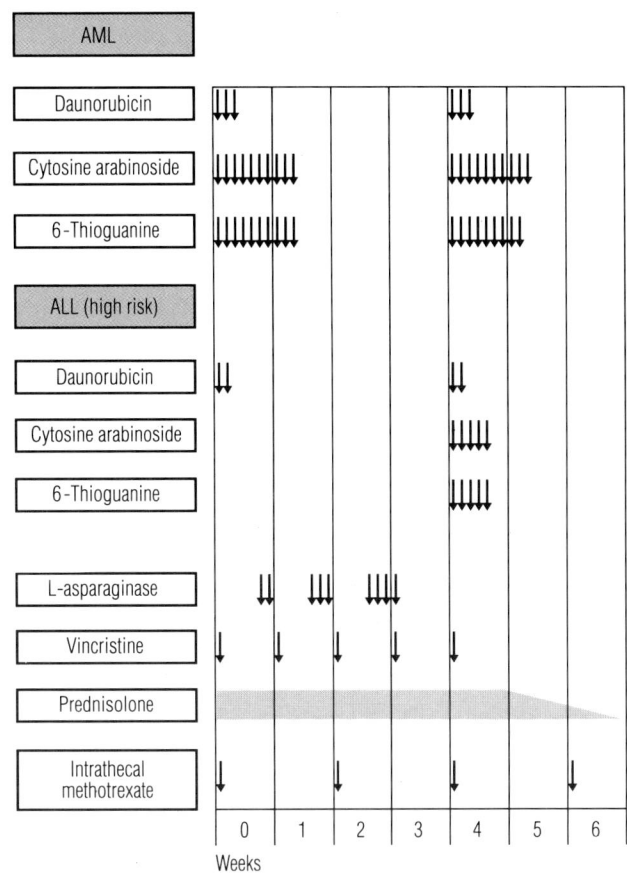

Fig. 25.28 Typical drug regimens used for induction therapy in acute myeloid leukaemia and high risk acute lymphoblastic leukaemia.

although this may take several induction courses. Once remission has been obtained, it is usual to give several further courses of induction type therapy; this is referred to as *consolidation*. Cycles of less intensive therapy (which exclude an anthracycline because it causes cumulative cardiotoxicity) are then given as *maintenance therapy* for one to two years, although the evidence showing the benefits of maintenance therapy is slight. Current studies in AML are investigating either more intensive maintenance therapy or the use of a course of *late intensification* therapy similar to the induction regime.

Bone marrow transplantation is an alternative form of late intensification therapy, available for young patients who have an HLA matched sibling donor (only a minority of patients with AML). The cytoreductive therapy usually given is a combination of cyclophosphamide and total body irradiation. This is the treatment of choice in patients below 30 years of age, but in the 30–40 year old age group the benefits are presently marginal. This situation might change, if early deaths due to graft versus host disease (GVHD) fall without a rise in graft failure or leukaemia recurrence. High dose chemo/radiotherapy with autologous marrow rescue has been used as a form of late intensification therapy, with promising preliminary results. It has certain advantages over allogeneic marrow grafting, in that every patient is his own donor and much older patients can be considered due to the absence of GVHD. The main disadvantages are the possibility of re-infusing untreated leukaemic cells with the marrow innoculum, and the absence of any graft versus leukaemia effect.

In patients who relapse, a second remission can sometimes be obtained; the chances are good in patients who relapse after ceasing chemotherapy. However, second remissions are almost invariably short-lived unless an allogeneic transplant can be performed. The results of transplantation at this stage are less good than in first remission.

Prognosis

The complete remission rate is close to 70% and, although most patients relapse on conventional therapy, approximately 25% of complete responders will still be alive after five years. Recipients of allogeneic grafts have an overall long-term (five year) survival of approximately 50%, this figure being somewhat higher in the under 25's. Half of the deaths are due to transplant related complications, and half to leukaemic relapse.

Various factors influence response and survival on conventional therapy. On the more intensive regimes, children fare better than adults; and monocytic variants probably do less well than the non-monocytic variants. There is a higher early death rate in M3 leukaemia, due to haemorrhage; but in those achieving complete remission the survival may be longer than in other types of AML. The presence of nuclear terminal deoxynucleotidyl transferase (Tdt) or chromosomal abnormalities are thought to be poor prognostic indicators.

ACUTE LYMPHOBLASTIC LEUKAEMIA

The annual incidence of ALL in the UK is approximately 1.3 per 100 000. The incidence peaks in mid-childhood, falls in adolescence and then rises steadily with age (Fig. 25.26). There is a slight excess in males.

Diagnosis

The haematological findings are similar to those found in AML (p. 1078), except that the anaemia is nearly always normocytic; myelodysplastic features are not seen; and lymphoblasts predominate in the marrow and usually also the blood.

Classification

The morphological, cytochemical, immunological and genetic features of malignant lymphoblasts are shown in Table 25.28. ALL has been subdivided into three morphological variants (L1-L3) by the French-American-British (FAB) Co-operative Group, although this is of limited value in determining prognosis and therapy (Table 25.30). ALL may also be classified on immunological and genetic criteria (Table 25.31).

Chromosome analysis

Cytogenetic abnormalities are detected in about two-thirds of cases by routine banding techniques. Both numerical and structural changes are seen. Unlike AML, hyperdiploidy (less than 50 chromosomes present) is not infrequent, and may be associated with a good prognosis. The Philadelphia chromosome (9:22 translocation) is present in 5% of childhood ALL and approximately 20% of adult cases. These patients have a poor prognosis. Other

specific translocations also occur, for example an 8.14 translocation is found in most cases of L3 leukaemia (as well as in Burkitt's lymphoma).

Treatment

The treatment strategy in ALL is shown in Figure 25.27. In the early 1970s, remission was *induced* with vincristine and prednisone; both drugs have specificity for lymphoblasts and do not cause severe haematological suppression. Since then, regimens have become more intensive, and the differences from induction regimens used in AML are less marked (Fig. 25.28). With modern anthracycline-containing regimens, over 95% of children and over 85% of adults with ALL obtain remission. Most induction regimens also contain L-asparaginase (Fig. 25.28).

Once remission is obtained, it is now common practice to give a further intensive *consolidation* course before commencing *maintenance* therapy. Maintenance is less intensive than induction therapy, and cyclical combinations of 6-mercaptopurine, methotrexate, vincristine and prednisone are usually given. Unlike the situation in AML, there is reasonable evidence that maintenance should be given for at least two years in ALL. In many centres, a further ablative therapy course is given after about six months; this is known as *late intensification*, and appears to be particularly valuable in high risk cases.

Craniospinal prophylaxis must also be given during remission, to prevent relapse in this 'privileged site'. It is usual to give 18 Gy in 10 daily fractions to the cranium, and repeated injections of intrathecal methotrexate or cytosine arabinoside to treat the spinal compartment. Testicular

Table 25.30 Subdivisions of acute lymphoblastic leukaemia based on morphology

Feature	L1	L2	L3
Cell size	Small	Small to moderate Heterogeneous	Moderate Homogeneous
Amount of cytoplasm	Scanty	Scanty to moderate Heterogeneous	Moderate Homogeneous
Cytoplasmic basophilia	Minor	Minor to moderate	Marked
Cytoplasmic vacuolation	Minor	Minor	Marked
Nuclear irregularity	Unusual	Frequent	Unusual
Discernability of nucleoli	Often difficult (usually small)	Easy (often large)	Prominent
Nuclear chromatin pattern	Homogeneous	Heterogeneous	Homogeneous

Table 25.31 Subcategories of acute lymphoblastic leukaemia based on lineage and differentiation stage

Cell lineage	Differentiation stage	Alternative name	Incidence in children	Incidence in adults
B lineage	Very early	Null cell ALL	12%	38%
	Early	Common ALL	75%	50%
	Late	B cell ALL	<1%	2%
T lineage	Very early and early	T cell ALL	12%	10%

irradiation has also been used as prophylaxis against relapse at this site (10% of relapses in boys); but this has made little impact on survival and causes hypogonadism and infertility.

The role of allogeneic bone marrow transplantation in ALL is still not fully defined. It is not justified in the large majority of children in first remission, because recent intensive regimes are so effective even in high risk cases. It may have a role in first remission adults. Once a relapse has occurred, bone marrow transplantation in second remission is probably the treatment of choice if the patient is below 40 years of age and a matched donor is available.

Prognosis

Nearly all patients with ALL achieve remission, but relapse is still a major problem. The factors influencing survival are shown in Table 25.32. The immunological phenotype is clearly related to prognosis, with common ALL doing well and T- or B-ALL badly; but phenotyping probably provides little additional prognostic information, beyond that obtained from the age, sex and presenting white cell count. Many regimens identify the high risk group at presentation and more intensive therapy is then given. With some regimens, this has removed the survival difference between the good and poor risk cases, both groups having a projected five year survival in excess of 60%. Death

Table 25.32   Factors at presentation of acute lymphoblastic leukaemia indicative of a poor prognosis

- High peripheral white count
- Age less than two years or over 10 years
- Male sex
- Certain chromosomal abnormalities (p. 1080)
- Morphological L3, and possibly L2, subtype
- Immunological
    Null ALL
    T cell ALL
    B-cell ALL

usually follows once relapse occurs, but second remissions may be protracted, especially if relapse occurs late after stopping therapy. Allogeneic bone marrow transplantation may cure some patients in second remission, but the relapse rate is high; long-term survival is probably less than 30%.

MYELODYSPLASIA

Myelodysplasia refers to an acquired state of haemopoietic dysfunction, in which there is cytopenia (involving one or more cell lines) without evidence of peripheral destruction and a cellular marrow. Haemopoiesis is ineffective, and morphological abnormalities are prominent in blood and marrow. Anaemia is common and there is frequently a mild to moderate macrocytosis, anisocytosis and poikilocytosis. The neutrophil count is often low, and the neutrophils exhibit abnormalities of granulation. The platelet count may also be reduced. A monocytosis may occur in some cases. The bone marrow shows dysplastic changes in one or more cell lines, the blast cell count may be raised, and an iron stain may reveal ringed sideroblasts. Clonal chromosomal abnormalities are detected in 50–60% of cases, and many other cases also undoubtedly represent a clonal expansion. The myelodysplastic syndromes (MDS) have been subdivided by the French-American-British (FAB) Group and are shown in Table 25.33. It should be noted that while this terminology refers to 'refractory anaemia', it does in fact include 'refractory neutropenia or thrombocytopenia' due to ineffective production. Also, although chronic myelomonocytic leukaemia is included in the MDS, and although anaemia is almost invariable in this condition, the white cell count may be raised suggestive of a myeloproliferative disorder.

Clinical features

The MDS are a group of diseases that occur predominantly in the elderly, but can arise at any stage of adult life. Patients usually present with symptoms attributable to the

Table 25.33   FAB classification of the myelodysplastic syndromes

Syndrome	Blasts in marrow	Blasts in blood	Auer rods	Monocytes $> 1 \times 10^9/l$ in blood	Ringed sideroblasts $> 15\%$ of nucleated bone marrow cells
Refractory anaemia (RA)	<5%	<1%	−	−	−
Acquired idiopathic sideroblastic anaemia (AISA)	<5%	<1%	−	−	+
Refractory anaemia with excess blasts (RAEB)	5–20%	<5%	−	−	±
Refractory anaemia with excess blasts in transformation (RAEBT)	21–30%	>5%	+	±	±
Chronic myelomonocytic leukaemia (CML)	<20%	<5%	−	+	±

cytopenias. Fever not related to infection, bone pain and splenomegaly occasionally occur.

The MDS clearly represent a spectrum of disorders, from mild marrow dysfunction to almost frank leukaemia. Many cases of refractory anaemia with ringed sideroblasts and normal white count and platelets remain stable for many years; whereas refractory anaemia with excess blasts can be difficult to differentiate from acute leukaemia at presentation, and usually progresses rapidly. The features suggestive of a poor prognosis are the involvement of more than one cell lineage and a high blast cell count; but, even in these cases, the term 'pre-leukaemia' is best avoided. This is because the term can only be used with certainty in retrospect, and because many of the deaths in severe MDS arise from worsening cytopenias, rather than from blastic transformation to frank acute leukaemia.

Treatment

The conventional approach to the management of the MDS is to provide supportive therapy, only instituting acute leukaemia therapy when leukaemic progression occurs. The response to treatment at this later stage is not good, and it may therefore be appropriate to institute more aggressive therapy earlier in young patients with MDS who exhibit poor prognostic features. It has been suggested that a variety of agents such as low dose cytosine arabinoside and retinoic acid, which can induce differentiation in leukaemic cells *in vitro*, may have a role in the management of the MDS. Controlled trials will be required to establish this.

MALIGNANT LYMPHOPROLIFERATIVE DISORDERS

The malignant lymphoproliferative disorders represent a spectrum of neoplastic proliferations of the lymphoid series and other cells (such as histiocytes), which comprise the normal lymphoreticular system. The lymphoid leu-

kaemias – both acute and chronic – are usually considered as distinct from the lymphomas, which preferentially involve nodes and spleen. Overlap is frequent, however.

Lymphocyte proliferation is the normal response of the lymphoid system to antigenic or inflammatory challenge and, although this is usually self-limiting, diagnostic confusion between reactive and neoplastic nodes can arise. Features of a node biopsy suggesting malignancy include: effacement of the normal node architecture; extension beyond the usual confines of the node; and the presence of a uniform population of cells. This latter feature is often absent, however, partly because the malignant clone may be represented by cells at more than one stage of differentiation, and partly because a marked reactive proliferation may also occur in the same node.

It is possible on clinical, morphological and immunological criteria to define distinct entities within the spectrum of the lymphoproliferative disorders, but it is difficult in some cases to relate a malignant proliferation to the differentiation level of its normal cell counterpart. The cell lineage of some lymphomas (particularly Hodgkin's disease) is uncertain as, in contrast to the myeloid system, the morphology of the lymphoid cells reflects the proliferative status of the cell as much as its stage of differentiation. A blast cell may be a very primitive cell or an activated mature lymphocyte, and an apparently mature lymphocyte may in fact be a resting virgin lymphocyte. Figures 25.29 and 25.30 outline B and T cell differentiation pathways, and give an approximation of the corresponding malignancies.

HODGKIN'S DISEASE

Hodgkin's disease (HD) is a clinically and histologically distinct malignant lymphoma, although the cell of origin is uncertain. Some cases appear to be of B cell origin, although it is possible that the disease is in fact heterogeneous in origin. Much of this confusion arises because the malignant HD cells are relatively rare in affected tissues and are not readily purified.

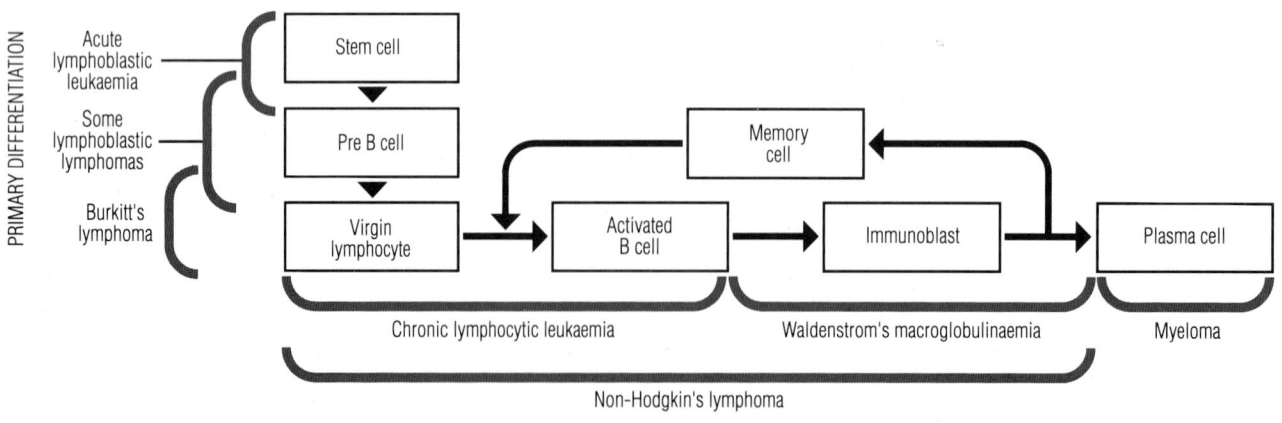

Fig. 25.29 B cell-lymphoproliferative diseases and their putative relationships to normal B lymphocytes.

Fig. 25.30 T cell-lymphoproliferative diseases and their putative relationships to normal T lymphocytes. The HTLV 1 associated malignancies typically have a helper inducer phenotype (CD4+) but have suppressor function *in vitro*.

Clinical features

The annual incidence of HD in the UK is approximately 3 per 100 000. It is uncommon in childhood, with peak incidence in early adulthood and again in the elderly. The clinical manifestations of HD are protean, but patients most commonly present with lymphadenopathy, especially in the cervical region. When more than one region is involved, the areas are usually contiguous, consistent with the view that spread is predominantly through the lymphatics. The lymph nodes may or may not be tender, and may initially fluctuate in size. Alcohol-related pain in the nodes may occur but is rare. Hepatosplenomegaly occurs with more advanced disease, and there can be infiltration of almost all organs. Systemic symptoms are frequent, especially in disseminated disease, although some patients with extensive tumour bulk feel well. Intense generalised itching (pruritis) is common. Anaemia occurs in about 35% of patients, and is correlated with advanced disease rather than marrow infiltration, which is found in less than 10% of cases. Neutrophilia is common and eosinophilia occurs in 15% of patients. Lymphopenia is frequent in disseminated disease but, even in patients with normal lymphocyte numbers, there is often a functional T cell deficit the cause of which is not fully understood. Clinical depression of cell mediated immunity is most clearly manifest as *Herpes zoster* infection.

Histological classification

The diagnosis of HD is made from histological diagnosis of affected tissue, usually lymph node. The malignant Reed Sternberg cells and their mononuclear counterparts are present in variable (often small) numbers in an appropriate reactive background of lymphocytes, eosinophils and fibrous tissue. The Reed Sternberg cell is classically a large binucleate cell with vesicular nuclei and prominent

eosinophilic nucleoli. These cells may appear to be in lacunae, especially if fibrosis is present. The classification of HD is shown in Table 25.34 and is primarily dependent on the composition of the reactive elements. In the original classification by Lukes and Butler, nodular sclerosis (subdivision of node by fibrous tissue and presence of lacunar cells) was not subdivided, but this broad category accounts for over 70% of cases. Nowadays, subdivision of nodular sclerosis into high and low grade is made, with reference to the reactive cellular elements. The presence of easily recognised areas of lymphocyte depletion or of numerous pleomorphic Hodgkin's cells is indicative of high grade (grade II) nodular sclerosis. Lymphocyte depleted HD is rare (less than 5% of cases) and has a very poor prognosis.

Table 25.34 Histological classification of Hodgkin's disease and relation to prognosis

Lymphocyte predominant Nodular sclerosis – low grade	Good prognosis
Nodular sclerosis – high grade Mixed cellularity Lymphocyte depleted	Poor prognosis

Staging

Accurate staging provides important prognostic information and dictates the appropriate treatment strategy. The Ann Arbor staging system is usually used (Table 25.35). A thorough history and examination is required, involving chest X-ray, liver function tests and good quality imaging of the abdomen such as ultrasound and computerised tomography, or nuclear magnetic resonance scanning. With the increasing availability of these techniques, lymphangiography is performed less often, although the latter will demonstrate abnormal node architecture in relatively small nodes and, as the contrast material persists in the nodes, it can facilitate follow-up assessments. In an attempt to define the extent of intra-abdominal spread, staging laparotomy and splenectomy

Table 25.35 The Ann Arbor staging system

Stage I	Single lymph node region involved, sometimes with local spread to extralymphatic tissue (**IE**).
Stage II	Involvement of two or more node regions on the same side of the diaphragm, sometimes with local spread to extralymphatic tissue (**IIE**).
Stage III	Involvement of nodes on both sides of the diaphragm. (The spleen is considered as a 'node'.)
Stage IV	Diffuse or disseminated involvement of one or more extralymphatic organs.

Each stage is also divided into A or B according to absence or presence of systemic symptoms; these include a sustained fever (>38°C), weight loss (more than 10% of body weight in six months) and night sweats, but not pruritus.

were introduced, but these are now performed infrequently in many centres. They are not indicated in cases where evidence of advanced disease is already proven and where the staging laparotomy will not dictate a possible change of therapy. It could also be argued that detailed staging now adds little to overall survival in any circumstance. This is because most patients with occult intra-abdominal disease who are treated inappropriately with radiotherapy to the lymph nodes above the diaphragm, can later be rescued with chemotherapy when intra-abdominal relapse occurs.

Summary 7	Treatment of Hodgkin's disease according to stage
IA IB IIA	Radiotherapy
IIB IIIA	Radiotherapy or chemotherapy
IIIB IVA IVB	Chemotherapy

Treatment

Localised disease (stages IA and IIA, Table 25.36) without symptoms is conventionally treated by radiotherapy alone (Summary 7). It is usual to irradiate all node areas above or below the diaphragm, according to the site of the disease. These extended fields are known as *mantle fields* and *inverted Y fields* (Fig. 25.31). It may be acceptable to irradiate only the involved nodal areas, but there is then a higher relapse rate in adjacent node regions. These nodes are, however, amenable to further radiotherapy, and the more localised therapy has fewer side effects. The overall relapse rate following a mantle field for supradiaphragmatic disease is high (approximately 40%). Although most relapses are not in the irradiated field, it is usual to give chemotherapy as well when there is a large mediastinal mass. Some centres give adjuvant chemotherapy for many cases of localised disease. This minimises relapse but does not necessarily improve survival, as chemotherapy salvage is highly effective.

Patients with stage IIB disease have a very high relapse rate following radiotherapy, and are therefore usually treated by chemotherapy. This is particularly appropriate in centres which do not perform a staging laparotomy, since the probability of intra-abdominal disease is high. Stage IIIA disease can be effectively treated by total nodal irradiation (mantle and inverted Y) but, again, some centres prefer to use chemotherapy rather than employ such extended radiation fields. If the patient relapses soon after total nodal irradiation has been given, it is very difficult to treat with chemotherapy because of lasting myelosuppression caused by the radiotherapy.

All patients with stage IIIB and IV disease must be treated with chemotherapy. The standard treatment has been 6–8 monthly cycles of 'MOPP' (mustine, vincristine, procarbazine, prednisone) combination therapy, or minor modifications of this. There is no value in protracted maintenance therapy. More recently, apparently non-cross-resistant drugs have been added to MOPP either as alternating cycles (alternating regimens) or in combination with these drugs (hybrid regimens). These regimens are probably more efficacious but are also more toxic. In some centres, radiotherapy to sites of previous bulk disease is also given following chemotherapy, but its value is unproven.

Relapse of local disease may be amenable to further radiotherapy if tissue limits have not been reached in that region. Alternatively, chemotherapy can be used. If relapse occurs many months after stopping therapy in those patients who received initial chemotherapy, it is often possible to induce a further remission with the same drugs. If the patient is resistant to primary therapy, or if relapse has

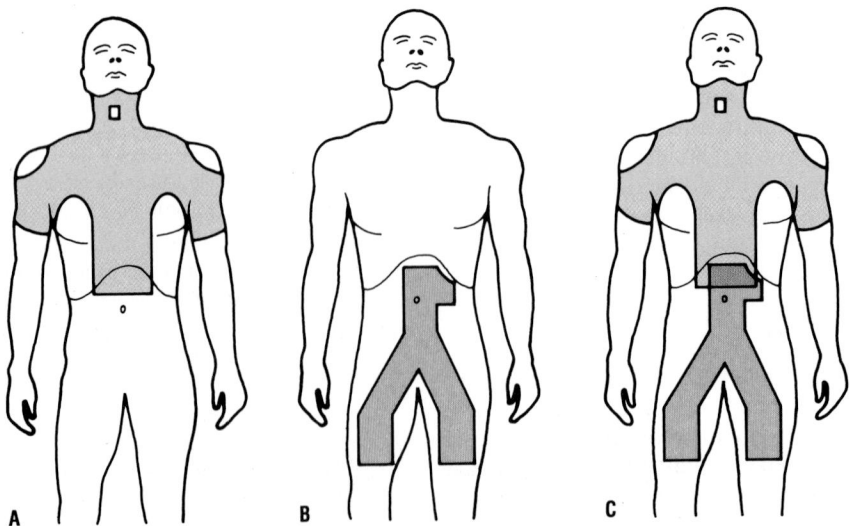

Fig. 25.31   Irradiation fields used in the treatment of Hodgkin's disease. (A) Mantle field. (B) Inverted Y field. (C) Total nodal irradiation.

Table 25.36 Prognosis in Hodgkin's disease

Stage	Symptoms	% total cases	Histological grade	CR rate (%)	Five year survival (%)
I	A	20%	I	99	92
			II	98	83
	B	very rare			
II	A	21%	I	96	94
			II	90	77
	B	7%	I	74	78
			II	55	70
III	A	17%	I	85	80
			II	70	71
	B	13%	I	69	77
			II	60	55
IV	A	6%	I	62	74
			II	44	56
	B	14%	I	61	64
			II	43	46

(Based on data from over 2000 cases entered into the British National Lymphoma Investigation)
Histological grade I = good prognosis, and grade II = poor prognosis. See Table 25.34.

occurred soon after stopping the initial drugs, then a so-called non-cross-resistant regimen such as ABVD (adriamycin, bleomycin, vinblastine, dacarbazine) should be tried. The clinical situation is very difficult in patients relapsing soon after alternating or hybrid regimens.

Prognosis

The overall 10 year survival in HD is approximately 60%, but both the complete remission (CR) rate and the long-term survival is influenced by the stage and histological grade of the disease (Table 25.36). Age is also very important, with patients over 50 years faring much worse. Most relapses occur in the first few years, although late relapses do occasionally occur.

NON-HODGKIN'S LYMPHOMAS

Non-Hodgkin's lymphomas (NHL) are more common than Hodgkin's disease; the annual incidence in the UK being approximately 4 per 100 000. Although there is a small peri-adolescent peak, they are most common in the elderly.

Clinical features

Most patients have lymphadenopathy at presentation but, unlike the situation in Hodgkin's disease, the spread is not contiguous and disseminated disease at presentation is common. Patients with histologically low grade disease are frequently asymptomatic; whereas patients with high grade disease tend to have symptoms of fever, anorexia and weight loss. A multiplicity of local symptoms can arise from nodal pressure or extranodal disease. These include:

obstruction of the superior vena cava; abdominal distension and back pain due to enlarged para-aortic nodes; bone pain from erosion or metastases in bone; chylous ascites and chylothorax from rupture of lymphatic channels; and cutaneous, pulmonary and hepatic infiltration. Non-Hodgkin's lymphomas can also arise as primary tumours of the gastrointestinal tract, brain, thyroid, bone, orbit and testis and are discussed in these chapters. Anaemia may arise from marrow infiltration, hypersplenism or from auto-immune haemolysis; this is particularly common in the low grade lymphomas. Low levels of paraprotein are often present in the low grade lymphomas, although hyper-gammaglobulinaemia in NHL is usually polyclonal.

Histological classification

There are many classifications of NHL, all of which have their advocates. The working formulation shown in Table 25.37 has the advantage of simplicity, being based largely on cell size and shape and the presence of malignant follicles. It is also particularly useful in translating from one classification to another. The working formulation considers lymphomas in three prognostic categories but, in practice, they are usually divided into two categories (low and high grade) as shown in Table 25.37.

The great majority (70%) of non-Hodgkin's lymphomas are tumours of the follicular centre cell (centrocytes and centroblasts). These cells appear either as small cells with a cleaved nucleus (centrocyte) or as larger cells with less marked nuclear cleavage (centroblasts). In these follicular centre cell lymphomas, the tumour may make large follicles (follicular appearance) or the node may be diffusely replaced by sheets of tumour cells (diffuse appearance).

Table 25.37 Classification of non-Hodgkin's lymphomas

Grade	Working formulation	
Low grade	Small lymphocytic cell Follicular small cleaved cell (centrocytic) Follicular mixed small cleaved and large cells (centrocytic/centroblastic)	commonly referred to as **low grade**
Intermediate grade	Follicular large cell (centroblastic) Diffuse small cleaved cell (centrocytic)	
High grade	Diffuse mixed small and large cell (centrocytic/centroblastic) Diffuse large cell (centroblastic) Diffuse large cell (immunoblastic) Lymphoblastic – convoluted – non-convoluted Small non-cleaved cell	commonly referred to as **high grade**
Miscellaneous	Including Mycosis fungoides and composite lymphomas	

Summary 8 Therapeutic strategies in non-Hodgkin's lymphomas

Low grade	
Stages I & II (excluding gut)	Local radiotherapy if symptomatic
Stages III & IV	Single agent chemotherapy with/without radiotherapy if symptomatic
High grade	
Stage I	Local radiotherapy/combination chemotherapy
Stage II	Combination chemotherapy
Stage III	Combination chemotherapy
Stage IV	Combination chemotherapy

There is not always a clear dividing line between the two, and different lymph nodes may show both diffuse and follicular change in the same patient. As the follicular lymphoma progresses, it may also change to a diffuse appearance.

The lymphomas may also be classified according to their cell of origin. The follicular centrocytic/centroblastic lymphomas are B cell tumours, as are many of the diffuse lymphomas. A significant porportion of the diffuse large cell and lymphoblastic lymphomas are of T cell origin, as are the cutaneous T cell lymphomas such as Mycosis fungoides. T cell lymphoblastic lymphomas and some mature T cell lymphomas have a very poor prognosis, but it is not yet clear that all patients with T cell lymphomas fare badly. A very small proportion of diffuse large cell lymphomas may be of true histiocytic origin.

Staging

The Ann Arbor staging system is used in NHL, but is less useful than in HD as most cases of low grade disease (Table 25.37) are already stage IV at presentation. Marrow infiltration is particularly common in these cases. Accurate staging is important if patients are involved in clinical trials, since stage may affect prognosis; but invasive investigations, particularly laparotomy, are rarely justified.

Treatment

There has been a paucity of controlled clinical trials in NHL and, in many circumstances, the optimal therapy has not been defined. In general terms, the low grade lymphomas only require treatment if they are symptomatic or have a critical organ dysfunction. If the disease appears localised to one or two node regions, then local radio-

therapy is probably the treatment of choice (Summary 8). If the disease is generalised, systemic chemotherapy is usually given, with or without radiotherapy to any particularly troublesome node region. Single agent therapy such as chlorambucil (5–10 mg/day) is usually sufficient to induce a response. Most patients obtain a good response (Table 25.38) but relapse frequently occurs. Once a good response has been achieved, therapy can be discontinued and the patient carefully followed up.

In the high grade lymphomas, intensive therapy should be instituted immediately. The patients are already symptomatic or will soon become so. In rare circumstances, a high grade lymphoma is truly stage I and, in these circumstances, full dose local radiotherapy is usually curative. However, this approach necessitates a staging laparotomy; many centres desist from this investigation and give chemotherapy as in all other stages of the disease. The CHOP regimen (cyclophosphamide, doxorubicin, vincristine, prednisone) has been standard therapy for high grade NHL but, in recent years, attempts have been made to improve results by adding further drugs to this regimen, e.g. bleomycin and methotrexate; by using alternating regi-

Table 25.38 Prognosis in the non-Hodgkin's lymphomas

Histological grade	Stage	Complete remission rate (%)	Five year survival (%)
Low grade	I & II	85	80
	III & IV	60	65
High grade	I	95	75 (90% in large cell lymphomas)
	IIA	70	60
	IIB	50	40
	IIIA	70	60
	IIIB	45	40
	IVA	50	35
	IVB	30	25

Figures given are approximate values obtained from the British National Lymphomas Investigation data bank.

mens of CHOP and other potentially non-cross-resistant regimens; or by using hybrid regimens in which two different drug combinations are combined into a single drug cycle. Preliminary results with these more intensive regimens are encouraging, but none have yet been proved to be superior to CHOP. Most treatments are continued for about three months after complete remission is obtained, and there is no benefit from protracted maintenance therapy. In patients with lymphoblastic lymphomas or small non-cleaved cell lymphomas, the risk of relapse in the central nervous system is high and CNS prophylaxis is therefore essential.

It should be noted that some low grade lymphomas do behave in a very aggressive manner either at presentation or during the course of the disease. These patients can be recognised clinically and should receive combination chemotherapy. Progression to a more aggressive course may not indicate a change in histology, but about 25% of low grade lymphomas do transform to high grade histology.

Prognosis

The complete remission and five year survival rates are dependent on the histological grade and stage (Table 25.38). In the low grade lymphomas, relapse and a continuing death rate are the rule; whereas in the high grade lymphomas, about two-thirds of patients who obtain a complete remission are probably cured. By 10 years, therefore, the overall survival of the low grade and high grade lymphomas are identical (Fig. 25.32).

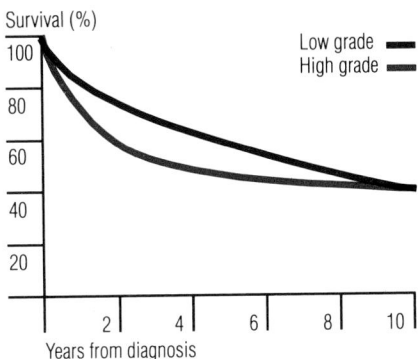

Fig. 25.32 Comparison of survival with low and high grade non-Hodgkin's lymphoma. The initial death rate is high with high grade tumours, but the curve then flattens with 40% of patients cured. A steady, slower, death rate occurs with low grade tumours, with no evidence of cure.

Cutaneous T cell lymphomas

Many mature T cell tumours involve the skin; the major example is mycosis fungoides and its leukaemic counterpart, the Sézary syndrome, both of which occur most commonly in middle-aged males. In both cases, the malignant cell is a CD4+ mature T cell which frequently has a highly convoluted and bizarre morphological appearance. These *Sézary cells* are not pathognomonic of a lymphoma, and may be seen in significant numbers in the blood in light-sensitive eczemas. As mycosis fungoides often begins as an eczematous reaction, precise definition of when the disorder should be considered malignant is difficult; however, demonstration of clonality by T cell receptor gene rearrangement may be of value. In the later stages of Mycosis fungoides, the skin lesions form plaques, tumours and fungating ulcers. Erythroderma (p. 1132) may occur which is often highly pruritic. In the Sézary syndrome, there is leukaemia, generalised lymphadenopathy and hepatosplenomegaly in addition to skin infiltration (usually erythroderma).

Lesions of mycosis fungoides can be treated with topical steroids, topical cytotoxic agents, PUVA (p. 1124) or radiotherapy. When visceral involvement is present, systemic cytotoxic therapy is required, although the responses are often of brief duration. The median survival of Mycosis fungoides is five years but is much less if there is a leukaemic element.

Adult T cell lymphoma/leukaemia

This entity is rare in the UK but is common in South-West Japan and the Caribbean basin. It is of particular interest because it is caused by the human T cell lymphotropic virus (HTLV I). The infectivity of this virus is low, and only a small proportion of patients who have been infected with HTLV I develop T cell lymphomas. These lymphomas involve phenotypic CD4+ cells and behave in a very aggressive manner. Widespread visceral involvement with a leukaemic element is usual, and cranial involvement and hypercalcaemia are common. The response to chemotherapy is usually poor.

Angio-immunoblastic lymphadenopathy

Angio-immunoblastic lymphadenopathy is a name given to a spectrum of disorders characterised clinically by lymphadenopathy, hepatosplenomegaly and hypergammaglobulinaemia. The patient is often febrile and autoimmune haemolytic anaemia is common. Histologically, the node is infiltrated by a mixed proliferation of immunoblasts, plasma cells, lymphocytes, eosinophils and small blood vessels. In some cases, this is a self-limiting condition often responsive to steroids. In other cases, a lymphoma develops; many of these cases are T cell lymphomas.

Histiocytic medullary reticulosis

This is a rare malignant proliferation of monocytic/histiocytic cells that usually presents with fever and pancytopenia. The histiocytes in the marrow exhibit haemophagocytosis. The disease responds poorly to chemotherapy and is rapidly fatal. This condition may be difficult to differentiate from virus-induced histiocytosis which is a potentially self-limiting disorder.

Histiocytosis X

Histiocytosis X refers to a spectrum of disorders of uncertain aetiology (Table 25.39); these are distinct from the monocytic leukaemias and the rare 'true histiocytic' lymphomas. The lesions are characterised by variable proliferation of histiocytes, with formation of giant cells and granuloma, and infiltration by eosinophils, foam cells and fibrosis.

Table 25.39   Classification and treatment of histiocytosis X

Classification	Symptoms	Treatment and prognosis
Unifocal eosinophilic granuloma	Usually single destructive bone lesions	Curable by curettage and radiotherapy
Multifocal eosinophilic granuloma (Hand-Schuller-Christian disease)	Multiple osseous and extra osseous lesions Triad of bone lesions, exophthalmos, diabetes insipidus occurs in 25%	Local lesions treated by curettage and radiotherapy Permanent remissions rare
Letterer-Siwe syndrome	Bone lesions, skin infiltration, lymphadenopathy and hepatosplenomegaly	Partial response to cytotoxic drugs Usually fatal

Childhood lymphomas

The malignant cells in childhood lymphomas usually have an immature phenotype, with T cell-lymphoblastic lymphomas and small non-cleaved cell lymphomas predominating. The small non-cleaved lymphomas may be associated with Epstein Barr virus (EBV) infection (Burkitt's lymphoma). With recent intensive therapy, it appears that many of the Burkitt's lymphomas are curable, but reports of high cure rates in the T lymphoblastic lymphomas have not been universally upheld. Hodgkin's disease may also occur in childhood.

CHRONIC LYMPHOCYTIC LEUKAEMIA

The annual incidence of chronic lymphocytic leukaemia (CLL) in the UK is approximately 2.0 per 100 000. It does not occur in children and is rare in young adults, but the incidence rises steeply with advanced age. It is nearly twice as common in males as females.

Clinical and laboratory features

CLL usually presents with lymphadenopathy with or without splenomegaly. Some early cases are discovered on an incidental blood count. As the disease progresses, there is insidious development of anaemia. Occasionally, the onset of anaemia may be rapid and of severe degree. This usually indicates the development of autoimmune haemolytic anaemia. There is also an increased incidence of

bacterial and, to a lesser extent, viral infections.

Laboratory investigations show that the lymphocyte count is very variable, from just above normal up to $300 \times 10^9/l$. Most are small, mature lymphocytes and a variable number are larger cells with a nucleolus but still a mature nuclear chromatin pattern (prolymphocytes). Smudge cells are also numerous on the blood film.

In over 95% of cases, the lymphocytes are B cells which express low levels of light chain restricted surface immunoglobulin. They also express pan-B antigens detectable by monoclonal antibodies and the CD5 antigen – a pan-T antigen expressed on cells transiently during B cell differentiation. CLL cells also express receptors that cause them to form rosettes with mouse red cells. Surface marker analysis with demonstration of light chain restriction may be particularly helpful in making the diagnosis of CLL when the lymphocyte count is only marginally raised.

Biopsy of affected nodes (which is seldom necessary to make the diagnosis), shows a low grade diffuse lymphocytic lymphoma, with cells identical to those in the blood.

Hypogammaglobulinaemia due to suppression of normal immunoglobulin production occurs at some stage of the disease in about one-third of cases; paraproteins (usually IgM) occur in about 5% of cases.

Treatment

As with the low grade lymphomas, treatment is only indicated if the patient is symptomatic or has critical organ dysfunction. Initial treatment is usally with chlorambucil (2–10 mg/day). In good responders, it is often possible to stop therapy as it is not necessary or feasible to strive for a complete remission. Steroids are of value if the patient has thrombocytopenia or an autoimmune haemolytic anaemia. As the disease progresses, resistance to chemotherapy occurs with an increasing lymphocyte count, lymphadenopathy, hepatosplenomegaly and bone marrow failure. In such patients, combination chemotherapy will frequently bring the disease under control, but this is usually only temporary. In some patients, progression is associated with increasing numbers of prolymphocytes in the blood; rarely, there is transformation to a histologically aggressive lymphoma (Richter's syndrome).

Prognosis

The median survival is approximately five years, but patients presenting with advanced disease have a much shorter survival. Poor prognostic features at presentation include large numbers of prolymphocytes on the blood film, massive splenomegaly and marrow failure.

Prolymphocytic leukaemia

Prolymphocytic leukaemia (PLL) is a variant of CLL in which the majority of peripheral blood cells are prolymphocytes. In most cases, these are B cells but a significant proportion of cases are of mature T cell origin. In PLL, the leucocyte count tends to be high and massive splenomegaly is common, often with little lymphadenopathy. The prognosis is poor compared to typical CLL.

Hairy cell leukaemia

This is a chronic B cell lymphoproliferative disorder in which the malignant cells have a typical 'hairy appearance' with multiple fine cytoplasmic projections. Pancytopenia and splenomegaly are usual, and lymphadenopathy is uncommon. There is often fibrosis of the marrow with a dry tap. Therapy is not usually required unless there is marked neutropenia. Splenectomy may be of value, and good responses may be obtained with α-interferon or deoxycoformycin therapy. The median survival is in the order of five years.

T cell chronic lymphocytic leukaemia

T cell chronic lymphocytic leukaemia encompasses several rare entities with distinct natural histories. CD4+ proliferations generally have an aggressive natural history, whereas the CD8+ proliferations are comparatively benign. The cells in CD8+ T cell CLL are usually large granular lymphocytes, the lymphocyte count is only moderately raised and, although the marrow infiltration is usually not total, very severe red cell aplasia or neutropenia may occur. The precise pathogenesis of these cytopenias is not clear. The disease may remain stable for many years and a complete remission is often obtained with single agent cytotoxic therapy. T cell CLL has been associated with rheumatoid arthritis.

TUMOURS OF IMMUNOGLOBULIN-PRODUCING CELLS

This term refers to monoclonal proliferations of B cells at a relatively late stage of differentiation. The cells are usually secreting immunoglobulin, in which case the abnormal proliferation is accompanied by an abnormal band on serum protein electrophoresis. The monoclonal immunoglobulin is called a paraprotein.

Multiple myeloma

Multiple myeloma is a malignant B cell proliferation in the bone marrow, in which the predominant cell type is the plasma cell. This disease occurs predominantly in the elderly, and the annual incidence is approximately 3 per 100 000.

Clinical and laboratory features

The development of the symptoms and signs of multiple myeloma is shown in Figure 25.33.

Direct effects of plasma cell proliferation

The proliferation of plasma cells within the marrow leads to *skeletal destruction*. The bone destruction may be due to the release of an osteoclast activating factor (OAF) by the plasma cells, rather than to a direct expansion of the plasma cells within the bones. Widespread osteoporosis and lytic lesions without osteoblastic reaction (no sclerosis and normal alkaline phosphatase) occur in most cases. Multiple lytic lesions of the skull and crush fractures of the spine are particularly common. Hypercalcaemia in association with bone resorption occurs in 30% of cases at some stage of the disease, not infrequently at presentation. This gives rise to thirst, polyuria, and dehydration, constipation and abdominal pains, lethargy, confusion and coma.

The plasma cell proliferation frequently causes a *mild to moderate anaemia*. This is in part due to replacement of the marrow space by tumour, but the proliferation may also suppress haemopoiesis. Neutropenia and thrombocytopenia are rarely severe at presentation, but may become so following chemotherapy or with very advanced disease. The cytopenias may also be exaggerated by the increase in plasma volume that may accompany paraproteinaemia.

Plasma protein abnormalities

Paraproteins do not usually cause symptoms, but when in sufficient quantity they may cause *hyperviscosity* with lethargy, confusion, loss of vision and coma. This is particularly likely to occur with IgA paraproteins, since the IgA molecules have a tendency to polymerise thus greatly increasing their intrinsic viscosity. Paraproteins may cause a haemorrhagic tendency mainly through non-specific coating and interference with platelet function. Some paraproteins are also cryoglobulins (p. 1092) and may give rise

Fig. 25.33   Development of symptoms and signs in multiple myeloma.

to Raynaud's phenomena.

More importantly, myeloma is accompanied by suppression of normal immunoglobulin production (*hypogammaglobulinaemia*) and infection is thus a major cause of morbidity and mortality. The mechanism of suppression of normal antibody production is obscure, but it is severe and usually persists even in patients whose paraprotein disappears on treatment.

Multifactorial

Renal dysfunction commonly occurs at presentation or with advancing disease. There are multiple causes, including light chain precipitation in the renal tubules and amyloid deposition in the glomeruli. Hypercalcaemia causes impaired glomerular function and a failure of renal tubular function, resulting in an inability to concentrate the urine. As a result, many patients are dehydrated at presentation; the pre-renal element in the renal failure must be recognised and treated by salt and water replacement. Other causes of renal damage include hyperuricaemia with tubular deposition of urate, and myeloma infiltration of the kidney.

Myeloma deposits extruding from bone (particularly collapsed vertebrae) may cause cord compression or root lesions. Cranial nerve lesions due to compression occur rarely. Peripheral neuropathies may also arise as a non-metastatic manifestation of malignancy.

Investigation

Mild anaemia is common, leucopenia and thrombocytopenia less so unless as a result of treatment. Plasma cells are only rarely seen in the peripheral blood. If a paraprotein is present, rouleaux formation and a high ESR are usually found. Bone marrow examination usually shows a plasmacytosis (more than 10%), but the disease can be 'patchy' and the sample not fully representative. The plasma cells often have an abnormal appearance with a centrally placed nucleus, which is often binucleate or trinucleate. The total serum gammaglobulin level is usually increased due to the paraprotein, and the serum albumin often reduced. Plasma protein electrophoresis reveals a narrow monoclonal band in over 75% of cases (Fig. 25.34). The incidence of the different types of immunoglobulin production in myeloma is shown in Table 25.40. Light chains are rapidly metabolised and often do not give rise to a serum paraprotein. They can nearly always be detected by immunoelectrophoresis of the urine; free light chains can also be detected in the urine of many patients who have a paraprotein composed of intact immunoglobulin – so-called Bence-Jones proteinuria.

Serum B_2 microglobulin (a protein molecule associated with Class I HLA antigens) levels are usually raised and give an indication of the myeloma mass.

The investigation of the patient with suspected myeloma should also include a skeletal survey, and estimation of urea, creatinine and electrolytes, calcium, phosphate and uric acid.

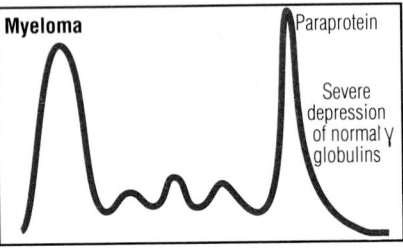

Fig. 25.34 Densitometry traces of serum protein electrophoresis from a normal individual and a patient with multiple myeloma.

Table 25.40 Approximate incidence of different types of immunoglobulin production in myeloma

Immunoglobulin	Incidence (%)
IgG	55 (IgG + urinary light chain in 35%)
IgA	20 (IgA + urinary light chain in 15%)
Light chain only	20
IgD	2
IgE	
IgM	} Very rare
Non-secretory	

Diagnostic criteria

The three major diagnostic criteria for myeloma are:

1. Bone marrow plasmacytosis (greater than 20%, but lower level acceptable if proven to be monoclonal).
2. Lytic lesions on X-ray (severe osteoporosis acceptable if marrow plasmacytosis greater than 30%).
3. Paraprotein in blood or urine.

At least two of these criteria should be present for a definitive diagnosis, as each feature alone can be due to other diseases (Table 25.41). Where there is doubt, it is often advisable to wait and reassess later.

Treatment

Most patients are symptomatic at presentation and merit immediate therapy. Occasionally, patients are found who are asymptomatic and do not have advanced bone disease, a high level of paraprotein or organ dysfunction. Treatment can be delayed in these patients.

Table 25.41 Differential diagnosis of myeloma

Symptom	Differential diagnosis
Paraproteinaemia	Benign monoclonal gammopathies Idiopathic – malignant lymphoproliferative disorders Reactive – infections autoimmune disease Liver disease non-lymphoid tumours
Bone marrow plasmacytosis	Chronic infections Chronic inflammatory disorders Liver disease Other tumours
Lytic lesions	Multiple metastases 'Spotty osteoporosis' Multiple eosinophilic granulomas Hyperparathyroidism Primary amyloid Hydatid disease Fibrous dysplasia

Supportive therapy

Immediate therapy is supportive. Pain must be controlled and, if there are fractures, this may require continuous infusion of opiates. Local radiotherapy is often strikingly effective in the relief of bone pain. Vertebral collapse and spinal pain must be treated promptly, as there is a risk of cord compression resulting in paraplegia. Radiotherapy is the treatment of choice. Careful attention must be paid to the fluid status; in patients with renal dysfunction or hypercalcaemia, a high fluid intake is essential. Prompt rehydration will often prevent permanent renal damage. In some patients with renal tubular damage, there is a chronic inability to conserve fluid and the weight and standing and lying blood pressures must be carefully followed in these patients. Hypercalcaemia is treated in the usual way with fluids, loop diuretics and steroids (p. 739). Infections are common and must be treated vigorously. The hyperviscosity syndrome will respond temporarily to plasma exchange.

Specific therapy

Standard specific therapy for myeloma is with the alkylating agent melphalan, approximately $7 \, mg/m^2$ daily for four days every three weeks, providing renal function is normal. Intermediate dose prednisone ($60 \, mg/m^2$ per day) is usually given in addition over the treatment days, but is of limited value in the absence of bone pain or hypercalcaemia. Approximately 50% of patients have a good initial response on this type of regimen, with a decrease in myeloma mass and fall of paraprotein to a stable plateau level. Disappearance of paraprotein with normalisation of the marrow is rare (5% of cases). In the plateau phase, the tumour is kinetically quiescent and therapy can be discontinued until progression occurs. In patients who become resistant to melphalan, second line therapies are available; these include drugs such as anthracyclines, nitrosoureas, vinca alkaloids and very high dose steroids. The side-effects of these regimens are usually much greater than with melphalan with (or without) prednisone, and the duration of response is usually short.

At the present time, very intensive therapy is being explored in younger patients, in an attempt to improve the complete remission rate and, hopefully, long-term survival. Very high dose melphalan is being tried as initial therapy, while cyclophosphamide, total body irradiation and allogeneic transplantation has been used in some patients under 45 years of age. Preliminary results with such approaches are encouraging, although very few patients are young enough to be considered for allogeneic transplant.

Prognosis

The overall survival is poor, with a median survival of approximately two years (marginally better in younger patients), although occasional long-term survivors do occur. It is possible to categorise patients at diagnosis into good, intermediate and poor prognostic groups on the basis of the [Hb], urea (post hydration) and the performance status (Table 25.42). The $\beta_2 M$ microglobulin level is also a valuable prognostic indicator. Good prognosis patients have a two year survival of about 75%, and poor prognosis patients about 10%.

Table 25.42 Prognostic categories in myeloma

Prognosis	Criteria
Good	Post hydration urea less than 8 mmol/l [Hb] greater than 10 g/dl No or few symptoms
Intermediate	Patient in neither good nor poor prognostic categories
Poor	Post hydration urea greater than 10 mmol/l and restricted activity; or [Hb] less than 7.5 g/dl and restricted activity

Plasmacytomas

Plasmacytomas are collections of plasma cells at a single site. They are usually part of a more generalised myeloma, but isolated tumours do occur without evidence of widespread disease. Many of the latter patients will go on to develop myeloma. Full dose radiotherapy should be given to solitary plasmacytomas, followed by chemotherapy if there is persistence of paraproteinaemia (usually only at low levels). Careful long-term follow-up is required.

Waldenstrom's macroglobulinaemia

This is a rare, low grade, B cell malignancy presenting in the elderly as a lymphoma or chronic leukaemia. Biopsy of affected tissue shows a diffuse lymphocytic lymphoma with plasmacytoid differentiation. Similar cells are seen in the marrow and in the blood. The hallmark of this disease is the production of large quantities of IgM paraprotein leading to symptoms of hyperviscosity, haemorrhagic tendencies and cold sensitivity (cryoglobulins in 30%). Weight loss, lymphadenopathy and hepatosplenomegaly are all common, but lytic bone lesions and renal failure are rare (unlike the situation in myeloma).

No therapy is necessary in asymptomatic patients, although they must be followed up carefully. When symptoms arise, therapy with alkylating agents such as chlorambucil will often produce a satisfactory response, though not a complete remission. Hyperviscosity syndrome may respond to plasmapheresis while the disease is being brought under control with chemotherapy. The median survival is about five years.

Cryoglobulinaemia

Cryoglobulins are immunoglobulins which precipitate when cooled. They may be monoclonal, polyclonal or mixed. The monoclonal cryoglobulins are usually indicative of a lymphoproliferative disease and the polyclonal varieties are often reactive and transient. A mixed monoclonal and polyclonal cryoglobulin is not infrequently associated with autoimmune disease. Clinically, their presence may give rise to Raynaud's phenomena, acrocyanosis, vascular purpura, arthralgia and – in the most severe cases – renal failure, hepatic failure and isolated neurological lesions.

The blood film typically shows marked agglutination of red cells, and the ESR may be spuriously low at room temperature although normal if performed at 37°C.

The mainstay of treatment is avoidance of cold and treatment of any underlying conditions such as a lymphoma. Plasmapheresis may have a role if there are severe symptoms.

Heavy chain disease

Heavy chain disease (HCD) refers to rare B cell proliferations in which there is secretion of heavy chains uncoupled to light chains. Serum electrophoresis usually shows hypogammaglobulinaemia without a clear monoclonal band. Immunoelectrophoresis is therefore required to demonstrate the abnormal heavy chain unassociated with light chain. Immunoelectrophoresis of the urine is often helpful.

Alpha-HCD occurs mainly in the Mediterranean countries, Asia and South America. It typically presents with abdominal pain, malabsorption and clubbing. Lymphadenopathy and hepatosplenomegaly are not usually present and (because of the malabsorption) coeliac disease is often suspected. In the early phases, the mucosa is infiltrated with polyclonal plasma cells and lymphocytes, and the disease is called immune proliferative disease of the small intestine. Later, a frankly invasive lymphoma develops. The production of α chains diminishes as the lymphoma progresses. The disease may respond to tetracycline in its early stages, but the established lymphoma is not very responsive to treatment.

Gamma-HCD mainly occurs in the elderly, and presents with weakness, fever, palatal oedema, lymphadenopathy and hepatosplenomegaly. The marrow is usually infiltrated with lymphocytic cells, and pancytopenia is common. The course is variable but death occurs in most cases.

Mu-HCD is rare and is usually associated with typical chronic lymphocytic leukaemia in which the plasma contains μ heavy chains.

AMYLOIDOSIS

Amyloidosis is a generic term for a group of conditions in which there is waxy infiltration of the tissues, the amyloid infiltrate staining pink with haematoxylin and eosin stain, and green with Congo red. The amyloid material is birefringent and is composed of fibrils formed into β-pleated sheets. These infiltrates ultimately damage normal tissue by means of pressure, atrophy and hypoxia.

Classification

The amyloidoses are best classified on an aetiological basis (Summary 9). The amyloid associated with immunoglobulin-producing tumours includes what was formerly known as *primary amyloid*, as well as that associated with myeloma. The primary amyloid is best thought of as early myeloma without lytic bone lesions. A monoclonal band on serum electrophoresis is present at diagnosis or appears during the course of the disease in nearly all cases. The amyloid deposits in this type of amyloidosis are made up of intact immunoglobulin light chains or parts of the variable domains; it is clear that certain myeloma proteins are more amyloidogenic than others. In reactive systemic amyloidoses – which typically occur in association with chronic infections (e.g. bronchiectasis), chronic inflammatory disorders (e.g. rheumatoid arthritis) or neoplastic disorders – it is thought that the amyloid is primarily composed of an acute phase reactant protein.

The heredofamilial amyloidoses include familial Mediterranean fever and Portuguese nephropathy. The amyloid seen around some endocrine tumours is thought to be composed of hormone precursors. Finally, amyloid occurs in many tissues in the elderly, especially brain and heart. It is usually asymptomatic.

Summary 9 Aetiological classification of amyloidosis

- Amyloid associated with immunoglobulin-producing tumours
- Reactive systemic amyloidosis
- Heredofamilial amyloidosis
- Local amyloid associated with endocrine tumours
- Amyloid of ageing

Clinical features

Amyloid can cause diverse organ dysfunction but the features shown in Table 25.43 should always raise the possibility of amyloidosis. It appears that renal amyloid is more prominent in the reactive amyloidosis, with cardiac and gut amyloid predominating in those associated with immunoglobulin producing tumours; but the overlap is wide.

Table 25.43 Clinical features suggestive of amyloidosis

- Nephrotic syndrome and renal failure
- Peripheral neuropathy with or without a carpal tunnel syndrome
- Restrictive cardiomyopathy
- Malabsorption and protein losing enteropathy
- Polyarthropathy
- Skin nodules, infiltrates and periorbital purpura
- Macroglossia

Diagnosis

The diagnosis is made by histological inspection of infiltrated tissues. Where tissue is not readily accessible, a renal or rectal biopsy often gives the diagnosis. Appropriate tests should also be performed to exclude myeloma, even when the patient has another chronic disorder.

Treatment and prognosis

This is primarily supportive, with specific treatment of any underlying disease. Care should be taken with the administration of diuretics or digitalis, as these can precipitate severe hypotension or dysrhythmias respectively.

The median survival of patients with myeloma and amyloid is probably less than two years, but is nearly 10 years with the reactive systemic amyloidoses.

NORMAL HAEMOSTASIS

The haemostatic processes involve a complex sequence of interacting events which serve both to protect the integrity of the vascular system and to re-establish patency of small segments which become occluded (Fig. 25.35). There is initial vasoconstriction at the site of injury, but this is transient and not a major component of the haemostatic mechanism. The major component of haemostasis is the formation of a platelet plug followed by the laying down and cross-binding of fibrin.

Platelets

Injury exposes collagen and the subendothelial basement membranes. Circulating platelets adhere to these structures, aided by fibronectin and high molecular weight mul-

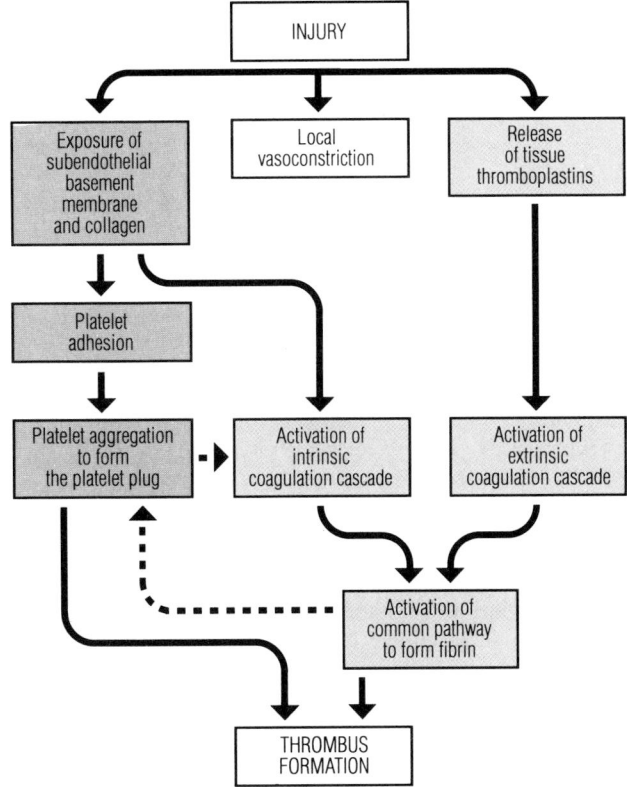

Fig. 25.35 The mechanisms of haemostasis. The process of platelet aggregation and activation is shown in grey; and the formation of fibrin in red.

timers of factor VIII complex (factor VIII/von Willebrand factor = fVIIIvWF, p. 1094) which coat the surface of the platelets. Following the adhesion of a single layer of platelets to the damaged vascular endothelium, further platelets stick to one another, aggregate, become activated, and ultimately form a platelet plug. The aggregation is mediated via a large range of factors which are produced at the site of injury and react with receptors on the platelet surface. Many of these factors – such as ADP, serotonin and thromboxane A_2 – are themselves released by activated platelets (Fig. 25.36), producing a positive feedback loop. ADP is also released from damaged red cells at the site of injury. Thrombin is a potent aggregatory agent, so the activation of the common pathway in the coagulation cascade (p. 1095) further stimulates the formation of a platelet plug.

The process of platelet aggregation and activation is mediated by two separate biochemical pathways.

1. Ligands such as ADP, or collagen in low doses, bind to specific receptors. This leads to activation of membrane phospholipases with the release of arachidonic acid from the platelet membrane phospholipids. A proportion of arachidonic acid is then converted to the cyclic endoperoxides, and then to thromboxane A_2 (TXA_2). TXA_2 is biologically highly active, and mediates a rise in intracellular $[Ca^{2+}]$ and platelet

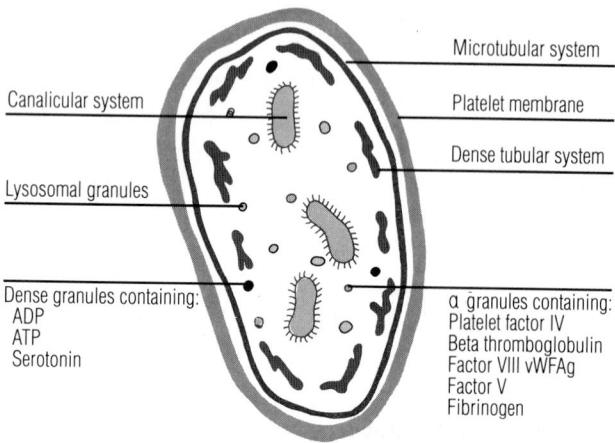

Fig. 25.36 Diagrammatic cross-sectional view of a platelet.

granule release (Fig. 25.37) which promotes further platelet aggregation.

2. Thrombin and high doses of collagen bring about a rise in intracellular [Ca²⁺] and degranulation by a mechanism distinct from that of arachidonic acid metabolism and TXA₂ generation.

Platelet activation and aggregation also has a role in the coagulation cascade that becomes activated at the site of injury. Factors VIIIvWF, V and fibrinogen are stored in granules and are released on activation; but more importantly, the platelet undergoes a configurational change during the activation process, such that phospholipid micelles on the platelet surface become available to facilitate the action of factors VIII and V. Activated platelets may also actually trigger the coagulation cascade by directly activating factors IX and X.

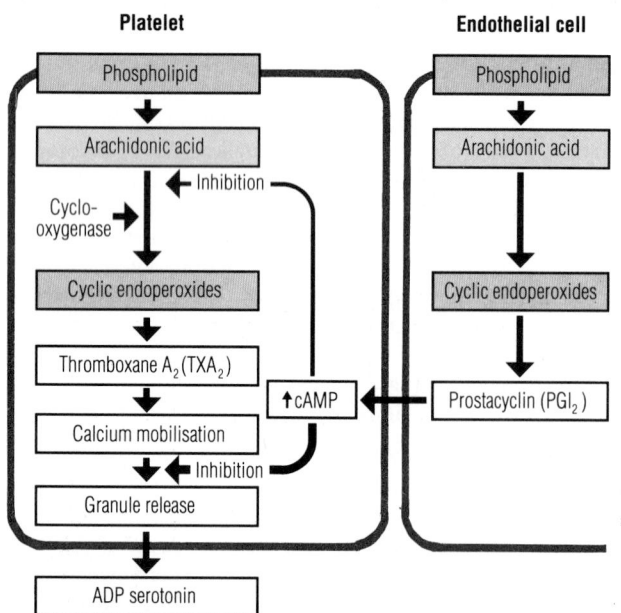

Fig. 25.37 Arachidonic acid metabolism in platelets and endothelial cells.

The coagulation cascade

Intrinsic coagulation cascade

Exposure of negatively charged endothelial surfaces following injury or damage leads to the adsorption of both factor XII and high molecular weight kininogen (Fig. 25.38). Prekallikrein and factor XI then bind to the high molecular weight kininogen, with activation of factor XI by factor XII. There follows a series of amplification reactions, during which an inert precursor is converted to an active serine protease with ultimate formation of fibrin. Factor XI activates factor IX which in turn activates factor X at the site of tissue injury. This reaction requires calcium ions, a platelet or phospholipid surface and factor VIII as a cofactor.

The factor VIII molecule is a complex structure. The component with procoagulant activity is referred to as factor VIIIC (antibodies to this moiety detect factor VIIICAg). Factor VIIIC has a molecular weight of approximately 220 000 and is synthesised in the spleen, other parts of the reticulo-endothelial system, and the kidney. The factor VIIIC moiety then binds to factor VIIIvWF (Fig. 25.39). This is synthesised in vascular endothelial cells and (to a much lesser extent) in megakaryocytes. The VIIIvWF protein consists of subunits

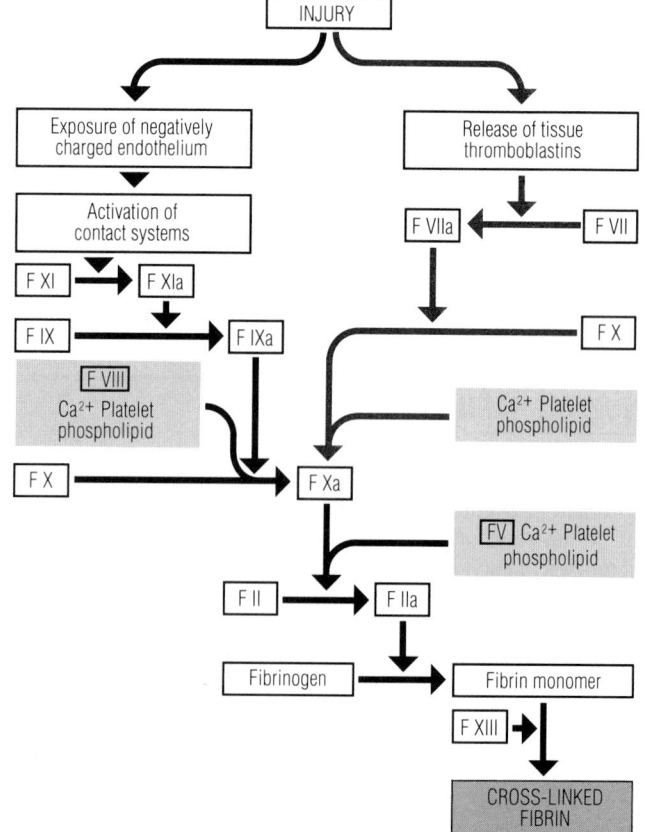

Fig. 25.38 The coagulation cascade. The extrinsic pathway is shown in red.

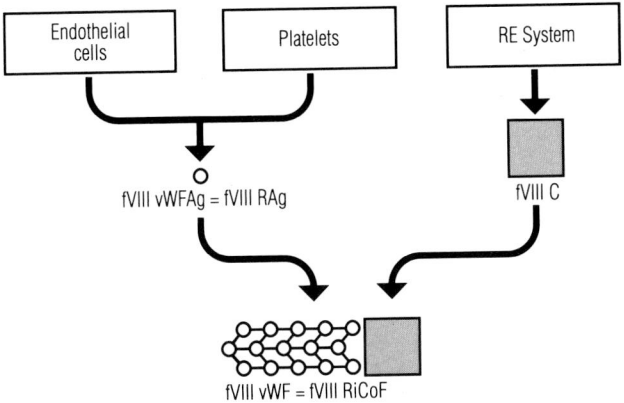

Fig. 25.39 Schematic representation of the production and structure of factor VIII.

with a molecular weight of 200 000–240 000 which can be detected immunologically as factor VIIIvWFAg – previously called factor VIII related antigen (factor VIIIRag). This rapidly forms dimers and subsequently large multimers with a range of molecular weights up to 20×10^6. These high molecular weight multimers are required for functional activity, both to prolong the half-life of factor VIIIC and to participate in platelet adhesion to the damaged vessel wall. Ristocetin induced platelet aggregation is dependent on the high molecular weight factor VIII multimers, and this test is therefore used to measure factor VIIIvWF, also known as ristocetin cofactor (VIII-RiCoF).

Extrinsic coagulation cascade

Trauma produces release of tissue thromboplastins. These bind to and activate factor VII, which then cleaves factor X to produce factor Xa. As with the intrinsic system, this reaction requires calcium ions and phospholipid.

The common pathway

Factor Xa, generated via the extrinsic and intrinsic cascades, converts prothrombin (factor II) to the serine protease thrombin (factor IIa). The reaction again requires calcium ions and phospholipid, and is accelerated by factor V which serves as a cofactor. Thrombin then digests fibrinogen to form fibrin, which is readily converted to fibrin polymers. The digestion of fibrin (and fibrinogen) is associated with release of fibrinopeptides (fibrin degradation products). The loose fibrin polymer is stabilised by a cross-linking reaction employing factor XIII as a catalyst.

Haemostatic inhibitory systems

A complex system of physiological inhibitors and feedback control mechanisms exists to control and limit excessive or inappropriate activation of the haemostatic system and thus help maintain vascular patency.

Endothelial cell inhibitors

Vascular endothelial cells synthesise prostacyclin from arachidonic acid (Fig. 25.37). Prostacyclin causes vasodilation and potent inhibition of platelet adhesion and aggregation. It is released in increased quantities when the vessel wall is stressed or injured, and binds locally to specific platelet membrane receptors which mediate activation of adenylate cyclase and a consequent rise in cyclic-AMP. This blocks aggregation through inhibition of platelet arachidonic acid metabolism and calcium flux. Endothelial cells also synthesise plasminogen activator, and a heparin-like anticoagulant.

Coagulation inhibitors

A natural system of coagulation inhibitors exists to limit the activity of the coagulation cascade. Antithrombin III is the major inhibitor of thrombin (factor IIa) and also inhibits factors IXa, Xa and XIa. Other plasma thrombin inhibitors include α_2-macroglobulin and α_2-antitrypsin. Protein C is a vitamin K dependent protein which inactivates factors V and VIII; and protein S – also a vitamin K dependent protein – serves as a cofactor for protein C activity.

The fibrinolytic system

The fibrinolytic system is activated simultaneously with the intrinsic coagulation system via the contact factor system of factor XII kallikrein and kinin (Fig. 25.40). The inactive circulating pro-enzyme, plasminogen, is converted to the active serine protease plasmin, which hydrolyses fibrin into soluble fibrin degradation products and also inactivates factors V and VIII.

Plasminogen can also be activated by tissue plasminogen activator (tPA) released from endothelial cells and from

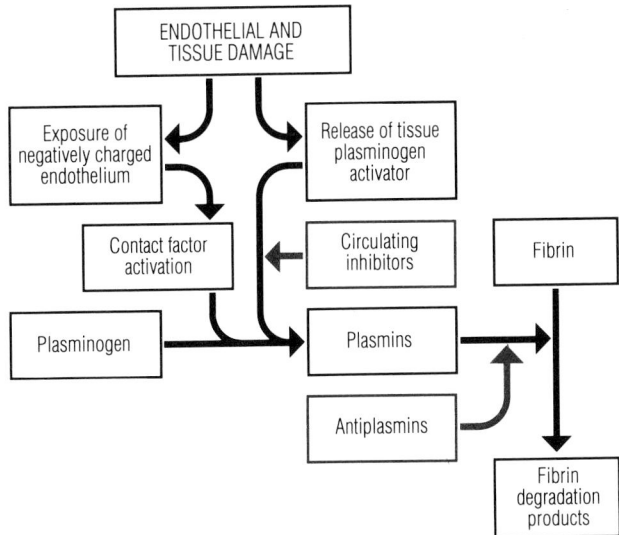

Fig. 25.40 The fibrinolytic system.

traumatised tissues. Several factors ensure that plasminogen conversion to plasmin is largely restricted to the site of trauma and thrombus formation.

1. Tissue plasminogen activators are inactivated by circulating inhibitors and are also degraded in the liver.
2. The affinity of tPA for plasminogen is greatly increased when the tPA is bound to a fibrin complex.
3. Any circulating plasmin is rapidly bound to α_2-antiplasmin, which has far less affinity for plasmin bound to fibrin.

DIAGNOSIS OF DISORDERED HAEMOSTASIS

History and examination

A detailed history and examination is of paramount importance and will often indicate the cause of bleeding (Fig. 25.41). Firstly, it must be determined whether bleeding is a localised problem, such as a gastric ulcer, or a generalised bleeding tendency (although it must be remembered that minor defects in haemostasis may only be brought to light by specific injuries). Secondly, the type of bleeding should be ascertained: purpura and mucosal bleeding usually suggest a platelet disorder, whilst confluent skin bruises and haemarthroses are more indicative of disorders of coagulation. The length of the bleeding history and the age of onset must be noted and a family history taken. It is often informative to ask specific questions, e.g., 'has any member of the family had excessive bleeding after dental extractions?'. Attention must be paid to any previous medical history of the current illness, and a careful examination should be performed. A detailed drug history is essential.

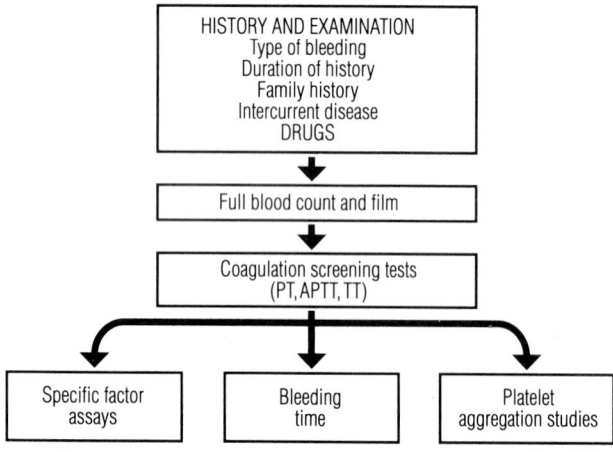

Fig. 25.41 Approach to investigation of a patient with a bleeding disorder.

Screening tests

The first step is to perform a full blood count and to examine the blood film. This will detect anaemia and thrombocytopenia (the commonest platelet defect), and the morphology of the platelets should also be noted. Occasionally, the blood film also reveals the cause of bleeding, such as disseminated intravascular coagulation or acute leukaemia. The second phase is to perform the coagulation screening tests – the prothrombin time (PT), activated partial thromboplastin time (APTT) and the thrombin time (TT).

Prothrombin time

The prothrombin time (PT) examines the extrinsic and common pathways. Citrated plasma is recalcified, excess tissue thromboplastin is added, and time to clot formation measured. The normal range is 10–14 seconds and prolongation of more than two seconds compared to control is suggestive of defective factors VII, X, V or II or the presence of an inhibitor to these factors. The PT is relatively insensitive to the level of fibrinogen.

Activated partial thromboplastin time

The activated partial thromboplastin time (APTT) screens the intrinsic coagulation cascade and the common pathway. Platelet-poor plasma is incubated with kaolin to provide *contact activation* in the presence of added phospholipid, and the clotting time after recalcification is noted. The normal range is approximately 38–45 seconds but this varies between laboratories. An abnormal result indicates deficiencies or inhibitors to one or more of factors XII, XI, IX, VIII, X, V, II or I (i.e. not factor VII).

Thrombin time

The thrombin time (TT) is performed by adding thrombin to plasma, thus bypassing the extrinsic and intrinsic systems, and measuring the time to clot formation. It is a measure of thrombin-fibrinogen reaction, and is particularly useful for detecting inhibitors such as fibrin degradation products or heparin. The results of screening tests in several clinical conditions are shown in Table 25.44.

Table 25.44 Results of coagulation screening tests in different clinical conditions (N = normal)

Clinical condition	Platelet count	PT	APPT	TT
Haemophilia A	N	N	↑	N
Von Willebrand's disease	N	N	↑	N
Factor VII deficiency	N	↑	N	N
Liver disease	N or ↓	↑	↑	N or ↑
Disseminated intravascular coagulation	↓	↑	↑	↑↑
Warfarin	N	↑	↑	N
Heparin	N	↑	↑	↑

Further tests

Where an abnormality is detected in the intrinsic or extrinsic coagulation cascade, the test is repeated using a 50/50 mixture of the patient's plasma and normal plasma. If this corrects the test, there is a deficiency in one or more of the factors assayed by the test. If full correction does not occur, then this implies the presence of a coagulation inhibitor.

Specific factors can be measured functionally by the use of mixtures of the patient's serum with serum known to be deficient in a single factor. Thus, if a prolonged APTT is obtained which is corrected by normal plasma but not by plasma from a patient with factor IX deficiency, then this implies that the patient is also deficient in factor IX. Some factors can also be measured immunologically, and the measurement of factor VIIIvWFAg is often of value in differentiating between haemophilia and von Willebrand's disease. The functional activity of factor VIIIvWF is determined by ristocetin platelet aggregation studies.

When a bleeding disorder is strongly suspected and the platelet count and clotting screen are normal, a template bleeding time should be done; if prolonged (normal bleeding time is less than 10 min), this is indicative of a vessel wall or platelet defect. The latter includes von Willebrand's disease in which the platelet/vessel wall interaction is defective; the bleeding time may be abnormal in mild von Willebrand's disease when the APTT is within the normal range.

Platelet aggregation studies are performed both to help detect the rare congenital platelet abnormalities and to determine the level of fVIIIvWF (ristocetin cofactor). Platelet aggregation is based on the fact that platelet rich plasma is turbid but clears as platelets aggregate; this is measured by increased light transmission.

PLATELET DISORDERS I: THROMBOCYTOPENIA

Thrombocytopenia is the commonest disorder of platelets and may be due to either decreased production or increased destruction (Table 25.45). The two mechanisms can usually be differentiated by bone marrow examination: megakaryocyte numbers are decreased in production thrombocytopenias, and increased where there is excessive platelet destruction. In some circumstances (e.g. severe infection), both mechanisms may be operative.

PRODUCTION THROMBOCYTOPENIAS

Production thrombocytopenias may be congenital or acquired. There are a number of rare congenital disorders in which thrombocytopenia occurs, or where there are normal numbers of qualitatively defective platelets. Several of these rare disorders have a storage pool defect such that there are defective platelet nucleotide stores resulting in defective aggregation at sites of vascular injury. *In vitro*, this is manifest as loss of the secondary aggregation wave to ADP.

Table 25.45 Causes of thrombocytopenia

Decreased production of platelets

Congenital

Acquired
  Marrow hypoplasia
  Marrow replacement
  Megaloblastic anaemia
  Specific platelet suppression by drugs
  Occasional viral infections

Increased destruction of platelets

Immune thrombocytopenia
  Idiopathic
  Viral infections (including HIV)
  Associated with drugs
  Isoimmune neonatal thrombocytopenia
  Post transfusion purpura

Microangiopathic platelet destruction
  Disseminated intravascular coagulation
  Haemolytic uraemic syndrome
  Thrombotic thrombocytopenic purpura

Severe sepsis

Massive transfusions

The acquired production thrombocytopenias may be due to:

1. generalised marrow hypoproduction as in aplastic anaemia
2. megaloblastic anaemia
3. less commonly, a megakaryocyte specific suppression. This may occur with chronic alcohol ingestion and (rarely) with some drugs such as the thiazide diuretics.

INCREASED PLATELET DESTRUCTION I: IMMUNE THROMBOCYTOPENIC PURPURA

The commonest cause of thrombocytopenia is immune destruction. In many children, immune thrombocytopenic purpura (ITP) follows a recent viral infection, while in some adults there is an underlying predisposing cause, such as a collagen vascular disease or a lymphoproliferative disorder. In many cases, however, there is no relevant preceding history, i.e. they are idiopathic. Whatever the aetiology, the mechanism of platelet destruction is similar, namely opsonisation of platelets by platelet specific autoantibodies, leading to phagocytosis of the platelets by the reticulo-endothelial system. It should be noted that it is not possible to identify platelet associated antibodies in every case. This may reflect lack of sensitivity of the test used, but should always alert one to alternative diagnoses.

Clinical and laboratory features

The peak incidence in childhood is between the ages of two and five years, at a time when they are most at risk for the common exanthemata. In both children and adults there is sudden onset of purpura, easy bruising and frequently also epistaxis. Gastrointestinal bleeding occurs occasionally, but clinically significant intracerebral bleeding is rare. Fatalities in children are extremely unusual even with very low platelet counts. The exception is babies born to mothers with ITP, who become affected owing to transplacental passage of antibody. If severely affected, such babies are at risk, during delivery and in the early neonatal period, of cerebral haemorrhage and even death.

The haemoglobin and white cell count are usually normal, although atypical lymphocytes may be seen on the blood film if there has been a recent viral infection. Very occasionally, the haemoglobin is reduced either due to blood loss or concomitant immune haemolysis. The platelet count is variably reduced, but in the presence of purpura is usually less than $50 \times 10^9/l$. Some of the platelets may appear large.

Treatment

Childhood

ITP in childhood is usually self-limiting, and treatment is rarely necessary even with a very low platelet count. Occasionally, bleeding may be troublesome and prednisone should be given (approximately 1 mg/kg and reduced as quickly as possible). Rarely, the disease becomes chronic and splenectomy may be considered; this is seldom justifiable, however, as the benefits must be balanced against the operative risks and problems of post-splenectomy infection. It must be remembered that late spontaneous remissions in children do occur.

Adults

In adults, it is usual to give a trial of corticosteroids if the platelet count is very low. However, the response is often suboptimal or the dose of steroids necessary is high with unacceptable side-effects. Splenectomy is then beneficial in 50-75% of cases. This may reduce antibody levels and, more importantly, removes a major site of reticuloendothelial platelet destruction. In splenectomy-resistant patients, immunosuppression with azathioprine, cyclophosphamide or chlorambucil may be of value. Vinca alkaloids may also be effective. Temporary respite can often be achieved by intravenous infusion of large doses of immunoglobulin preparations, which result in reticuloendothelial blockade. This is extremely expensive, but may be warranted in a life-threatening situation. In Rh-positive individuals, an injection of anti-D immunoglobulin will often produce similar reticulo-endothelial blockade; unfortunately, anti-D is in short supply.

At birth

The neonate born to a mother with ITP merits further consideration. The neonate is usually only severely affected if the mother has severe ITP but this is not invariable. Particular attention must be paid to women with ITP who have had a successful splenectomy; their platelet count may be normal but their babies severely affected. If the mother has a low platelet count, a course of steroids or intravenous immunoglobulin should probably be given several days before delivery (if this can be anticipated). The birth should be as atraumatic as possible, and protracted labours must be avoided. At birth, the baby's platelet count must be checked and monitored daily for several days, as late falls are not infrequent. If the thrombocytopenia is very severe in the neonate, it is probably wise to give a short course of steroids and to minimise bouts of crying (which increase intracerebral pressure). Some centres would consider exchange transfusion to reduce the antibody titre.

Drug-induced immune thrombocytopenia

Drugs may induce immune thrombocytopenia by serving as haptens, with subsequent absorption of immune complexes onto the platelets. Quinidine may produce thrombocytopenia by this mechanism. Alternatively, the drug may interact with a platelet protein, with the production of specific drug-platelet protein antibody. When drug-induced thrombocytopenia occurs, it is usually reversible within several days of stopping the offending drug.

Isoimmune neonatal thrombocytopenia

The mechanism of isoimmune neonatal thrombocytopenia is similar to that of isoimmune neonatal haemolysis and usually occurs when the mother (but not the baby) lacks the platelet A1 antigen present in 98% of the population. Treatment of the infant is usually not necessary, but in extreme situations maternal (PLA-1 negative) platelets should be given.

Post transfusion purpura

This is an unusual cause of thrombocytopenia which occurs in PLA-1-negative individuals about one week after a transfusion of blood containing PLA-1 positive platelets. The antibodies formed to the PLA-1 antigen bind to autologous platelets, probably as preformed immune complexes, and cause thrombocytopenia.

INCREASED PLATELET DESTRUCTION II: MICROANGIOPATHIC DESTRUCTION

Microangiopathic platelet destruction occurs in the presence of extensive small vessel disease. As blood passes through the damaged vessels, the platelets are removed and the red cells subjected to extreme shearing stresses, resulting in a concomitant haemolytic anaemia. Thus, the blood film typically shows red cell fragmentation and polychromasia (reticulocytosis), as well as thrombocytopenia.

Haemolytic uraemic syndrome/thrombotic thrombocytopenic purpura

Haemolytic uraemic syndrome and thrombotic thrombocytopenic purpura are related syndromes whose aetiology is poorly understood. In many cases, there appears to be breakdown in the normal platelet/vessel wall interaction, with excessive adhesion of platelets to intact endothelium.

Clinical features

Haemolytic uraemic syndrome (HUS) usually presents in young children with the triad of haemolytic anaemia, purpura and acute renal failure. Thrombotic thrombocytopenic purpura (TTP) occurs predominantly in young adults (18–40 years). There is haemolytic anaemia, purpura, hepatic damage and neurological impairment which – in the acute form – may cause clouding of consciousness and coma. Digital ischaemia and small vessel infarcts may occur. Renal function is initially well preserved. TTP may also become chronic or undergo multiple relapses.

The mortality in HUS with good supportive care is below 10%, and in TTP about 10–25%.

Laboratory features

In the appropriate clinical setting, the finding of a microangiopathic blood film is highly suggestive of the diagnosis. At least in the early stages, the clotting screen is virtually normal, thus differentiating this cause of thrombocytopenia from disseminated intravascular coagulation. The hydroxybutyrate dehydrogenase level (HBD) is raised as a component of the haemolysis and this parameter is often valuable in assessing daily progress.

Treatment

Vigorous medical support for organ failure is paramount. Early dialysis in HUS is indicated. Large quantities of fresh frozen plasma appear to be beneficial in many cases and this usually requires daily plasma exchange. The mechanism of action is unclear.

Disseminated intravascular coagulation

In disseminated intravascular coagulation (DIC), there is widespread deposition of fibrin and platelets within the microcirculation with consumption of coagulation factors and platelets (Fig. 25.42). The presence of fibrin degradation products exacerbates the bleeding tendency, by inhibiting the polymerisation of fibrin.

Clinical features

The causes of DIC are varied (Table 25.46) but sepsis is the most common cause. Precipitating factors include the release of procoagulant materials from damaged leukocytes and endothelial cells, and widespread activation of the contact factor system. In severe cases, there is widespread bruising and oozing from mucous membranes and venepuncture sites; but DIC is more often subclinical and merely a laboratory finding. Although small vessel occlusions do occur, clinically apparent thromboses are not commonly detected.

Table 25.46 Causes of disseminated intravascular coagulation

Sepsis
Gram-negative septicaemia
Meningococcal septicaemia

Shock
Hypovolaemia
Anaphylactic

Obstetric complications
Amniotic fluid embolism
Intra-uterine death
Abruptio placentae

Tissue factor release
Severe trauma
Burns
Promyelocytic leukaemia
Haemolytic transfusion reactions
Acute pancreatitis

Laboratory features

Thrombocytopenia and a normocytic anaemia with red cell fragmentation are seen, although the latter may not be noticed in mild cases. There is prolongation of the PT, APPT and TT, the last being most affected, especially in mild cases. Fibrin degradation products (FDPs) – produced by the proteolytic action of plasma on fibrin and fibrinogen – are found in raised amounts in the serum, although it must be remembered that serum FDPs are also raised after major trauma or surgery and in renal failure without DIC. The measurement of FDPs is therefore not the primary screening test for DIC and is only indicated if the TT is significantly prolonged.

Treatment

The underlying cause of DIC should be treated vigorously, and full supportive measures given. Hypoxia and hypovolaemia must be corrected, and platelets and clotting factors replaced as necessary; this usually requires both

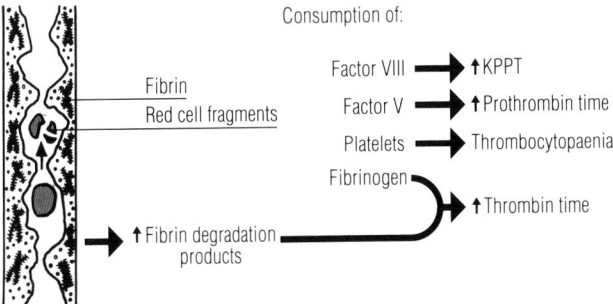

Fig. 25.42 The pathogenesis of disseminated intravascular coagulation.

fresh frozen plasma and factor VIII concentrates. Although there was a vogue at one time for the use of heparin in DIC, to try and break the vicious cycle of thrombosis and haemorrhage, such treatment is dangerous and now has few advocates. Low dose heparin may have a role, however, in the prevention of DIC during induction therapy for acute promyelocytic leukaemia.

Other causes of microangiopathic thrombocytopenia

Microangiopathic haemolytic anaemia and/or thrombocytopenia may also occur in malignant hypertension, pre-eclampsia and in association with giant haemangiomas.

QUALITATIVE PLATELET ABNORMALITIES

There are several rare congenital disorders in which platelet function is abnormal (Table 25.47) as well as the more common von Willebrand's disease.

Qualitative platelet abnormalities may also be acquired in a variety of systemic disorders (particularly uraemia and liver disease), and the platelet defect may contribute to any bleeding diathesis in these conditions. Platelet function may also be abnormal in the myeloproliferative diseases due to both the production of abnormal platelets from a malignant stem cell, and to a poorly understood failure to produce normal high molecular weight multimers of factor VIII. Platelets may also function poorly in the presence of paraproteinaemia due to non-specific protein coating of the platelets.

The commonest acquired platelet abnormality, however, is due to the ingestion of aspirin and other anti-platelet drugs (p. 1106).

PLATELET DISORDERS II: THROMBOCYTOSIS

The aetiology of thrombocytosis is shown in Summary 10. The myeloproliferative disorders may give rise to very elevated platelet counts, especially in essential thrombocythaemia. If the platelet count is only moderately raised, it may be difficult to differentiate primary from secondary causes (p. 1076). The platelet count rarely exceeds $1500 \times 10^9/l$ in secondary thrombocytosis, but may do so following splenectomy. Here, the platelet count rises within hours or days and usually declines to the high normal range in the ensuing weeks, although the thrombocytosis is occasionally persistent. The thrombocytosis post-splenectomy is accompanied by a modest leukocytosis (usually transient) and the permanent appearance of abnormal shaped red cells, spherocytes, target cells and Howell-Jolly bodies. Probably the commonest cause of secondary thrombocytosis is in response to the stress of major surgery. Other forms of stress such as exercise may also cause the platelet count to rise. Both bleeding and haemolysis may stimulate a thrombocytosis, and this may be more marked if there is concomitant iron deficiency. This may imply that the physiological stimuli for increased red cell production cross-react with megakaryopoiesis, but the detailed mech-

Table 25.47 Congenital primary platelet disorders

Syndrome	Inheritance	Platelet count	Platelet aggregation	Other features
Fanconi's anaemia	Autosomal recessive	↓	Normal	Multiple skeletal/organ abnormalities (p. 1048)
Amegakaryocytic thrombocytopenia	Variable	↓	Normal	Absent radii and skeletal abnormalities in some cases
Wiskott-Aldrich syndrome	X-linked	↓	Reduction in secondary aggregation wave (storage pool defect)	Eczema Immunodeficiency
May-Hegglin syndrome	Autosomal dominant	↓ (variable) Giant size	Normal	Inclusion bodies in leucocytes
Bernard-Soulier syndrome	Autosomal recessive	Normal or ↓ Giant size	↓ aggregation to ristocetin	
Glanzmann's thrombasthenia	Autosomal recessive	Normal	↓ aggregation to ADP, adrenaline and collagen. Normal aggregation to ristocetin	
Grey platelet syndrome		Slightly ↓		Myelofibrosis may occur
Chediak–Higashi syndrome	Autosomal recessive	Normal	Reduction in secondary aggregation wave to ADP (storage pool defect)	Oculocutaneous albinism, phagocytic defect. Neurological impairment
Hermansky-Pudlak syndrome	Autosomal recessive	Normal	Reduction in secondary aggregation wave to ADP (storage pool defect)	Albinism

anisms are not understood. All forms of inflammation can cause a rise in the platelet count, but it appears to be particularly common in the inflammatory bowel disorders and in sarcoidosis. The neoplasms most often associated with thrombocytosis are lymphomas and gut carcinoma.

Clinical features

Patients with primary thrombocytosis may present with bleeding or thrombotic problems (p. 1076). Thrombotic phenomena attributable to a secondary thrombocytosis are unusual, and rarely require treatment. In patients with thrombocytosis in whom thrombotic events have occurred, treatment with anti-platelet agents is advisable.

HEREDITARY COAGULATION DISORDERS

HAEMOPHILIA A

Haemophilia A (classical haemophilia) is an X-linked recessive disorder which affects males and is transmitted by female carriers. The incidence in the UK is approximately 12 per 100 000. There is low or absent factor VIIIC but factor VIIIvWFAg and factor VIIIvWf are normal (pp. 1094–95).

Clinical features

The clinical severity of haemophilia A is very variable and is dependent on the level of factor VIIIC (Table 25.48). In the absence of trauma or surgery in the first few months of life, the disease does not usually present until the child starts to crawl or walk. In mild cases the diagnosis may be

Table 25.48   Severity of haemophilia A

Clinical manifestations	Factor VIIIC levels (% of normal)
Severe	less than 1%
Moderate	1–5%
Mild	over 5%

further delayed. There is easy bruising, soft tissue muscle bleeding and haemarthrosis often appearing spontaneously and not related to obvious trauma. The repeated joint bleeds may lead ultimately to restriction of movement and deformity. Less commonly, there is retroperitoneal haemorrhage, spontaneous haematuria and pseudotumour formation in the long bones or pelvis, secondary to recurrent subperiosteal haemorrhage and new bone formation. Severe psychological and family problems may also arise as a result of the chronic disease and its treatment.

Diagnosis

The diagnosis is suspected from the history and the finding of a prolonged APTT, and proven by demonstration of a low factor VIIIC level in a specific assay.

Assessment of the ratio of factor VIIIC:VIIIvWFAg can be used in about 80% of cases to identify female carriers. Daughters of haemophiliacs are of course obligate carriers (p. 88). Prenatal diagnosis is available for male fetuses of known carriers by analysis of factor VIIIC levels in the fetal blood or by analysis of DNA from chorionic villus samples.

Treatment

Bleeding episodes require prompt treatment by factor VIII replacement, given either as cryoprecipitate or freeze-dried factor VIII concentrate. Approximately 0.5 units are required per kg body weight to raise the factor VIII level by 1%. Thus, if a level of 100% is required in a severe 70 kg haemophiliac, then a dose of approximately 3500 units should be given. Each bag of cryoprecipitate contains 70–120 units. It also contains high levels of fibrinogen and the development of hyperfibrinogenaemia can therefore limit its continued use after major surgery or trauma. The injections are repeated to maintain a trough level above 20% for minor bleeds, and above 60% for major trauma or surgery. The half-life of injected factor VIII is approximately 12 hours and so it is usual to give twice daily factor VIII during an acute episode. The dose and frequency of administration can be modified according to pre- and post-injection factor VIIIC levels. Some patients keep a stock of factor VIII at home and will inject themselves at the first sign of a bleed, thereby often averting a severe problem. In very severe cases, prophylactic factor VIII injected by the patient at home twice a week may markedly reduce the frequency of haemorrhagic incidents.

Bleeding episodes (especially into joints) are very painful and adequate analgesia must be given, often with opiates. During acute bleeds, rest is required followed by gradual mobilisation. The optimal management of haemophilia requires a team approach, with interested haematologists, physiotherapists and orthopaedic surgeons working together to minimise permanent joint damage.

Oral anti-fibrinolytics (e.g. tranexamic acid) may aid haemostasis, and are particularly useful in mild haemophiliacs after dental procedures. For minor procedures in very mild haemophiliacs, DDAVP (1-deamino-8-D-arginine vasopressin) may circumvent the need for factor VIII, as it may lead to a temporary rise in autologous factor VIII production.

Complications of therapy

Inhibitory antibodies develop in some severe haemophiliacs after factor VIII administration, and these make treatment extremely difficult. Should this occur, massive doses of factor VIII may temporarily swamp an inhibitor, or factor IX concentrate containing some factor IXa may be used to circumvent the need for factor VIII. Although the latter approach carries some risk of precipitating thrombosis, it is probably small with modern material. In life-threatening situations, purified porcine factor VIII can be given as the antibodies do not usually cross-react with the pig protein. However, anti-porcine antibodies tend to form rapidly, and limit recurrent use. In desperate situations, immunosuppression and even plasmapheresis may have a role in reducing the inhibitor level.

Transmission of viral infections – especially HIV – is a serious complication of factor VIII concentrate administration, and many severe haemophiliacs are now HIV antibody positive. There are some differences in the natural history of HIV infection in haemophiliacs compared to other patient groups, with Kaposi's sarcoma rarely occurring. The proportion of HIV antibody patients who will progress to the acquired immunodeficiency syndrome is not yet clear. The risk of HIV transmission has been greatly reduced by heat treatment of factor VIII. Non-A non-B hepatitis occurred in 90–100% 'virgin' haemophiliacs (who had not previously received factor VIII) following concentrate administration. Wet heat treatment of factor VIII probably reduces this to 10–20%, but the pooled concentrate should nevertheless be avoided, and cryoprecipitate given, to mild virgin haemophiliacs who will need little factor VIII.

The treatment of haemophilia may contribute to psychological trauma, with 'needle phobias' in children and narcotic analgesic abuse in adults being uncommon, but severe, problems.

VON WILLEBRAND'S DISEASE

Von Willebrand's disease is a syndrome, rather than a single disease entity, which is usually transmitted as an autosomal dominant condition. The incidence is greater than that for haemophilia A. In the commonest variety, there is deficiency of factor VIIIvWFAg, with consequent low factor VIIIvWF activity as measured by ristocetin aggregation. Factor VIIIC levels are also low, as the half-life of factor VIIIC is reduced when not bound to the vWFAg. In some other variants, the factor VIIIvWFAg is quantitatively normal, but is unable to form high molecular weight multimers so that factor VIIIvWF activity is reduced. The factor VIIIC may be normal or reduced. In almost all forms of von Willebrand's disease, the bleeding time is prolonged.

Clinical features

Bleeding is generally less severe than in haemophilia A, with skin and mucus membrane bleeding predominating. Many cases only become apparent after dental extractions.

Diagnosis

The bleeding time is usually prolonged and is the best indicator of clinical severity. Factor VIIIvWF is reduced, as is the factor VIIIvWFAg in most cases. The factor VIIIC level is more variable, but is usually low and thus causes a prolonged APTT with a normal PT. However, it must be noted that factor VIII levels rise as acute phase reactants, and one set of normal factor VIII parameters does not exclude von Willebrand's disease.

Treatment

Minor bleeding or dental episodes can often be contained by use of DDAVP and tranexamic acid, although DDAVP is ineffective in variants where factor VIIIvWFAg is qualitatively abnormal and unable to form high molecular weight multimers. In more serious circumstances, factor VIIIvWFAg replacement should be given in the form of fresh frozen plasma or cryoprecipitate. This produces a disproportionate and prolonged rise in factor VIIIC levels compared to haemophilia A.

OTHER CONGENITAL COAGULATION FACTOR ABNORMALITIES

Other congenital coagulation factor abnormalities are summarised in Table 25.49.

ACQUIRED COAGULATION DISORDERS

The causes of acquired coagulation disorders are outlined in Figure 25.43.

Table 25.49 Less common congenital coagulation factor deficiencies

Abnormal factor	Inheritance	Bleeding disorder
Factor IX (Haemophilia B or Christmas disease)	X-linked	Severe
Factor XI	Autosomal recessive	Mild
Factor VII	Autosomal recessive	Severe
Factor XII	Autosomal recessive	Very mild
Factor V	Autosomal recessive	Mild
Factor XIII	Variable	Mild
Fibrinogen		
Afibrinogenaemia	Autosomal recessive	Surprisingly mild
Dysfibrinogenaemia	Autosomal recessive	Mild

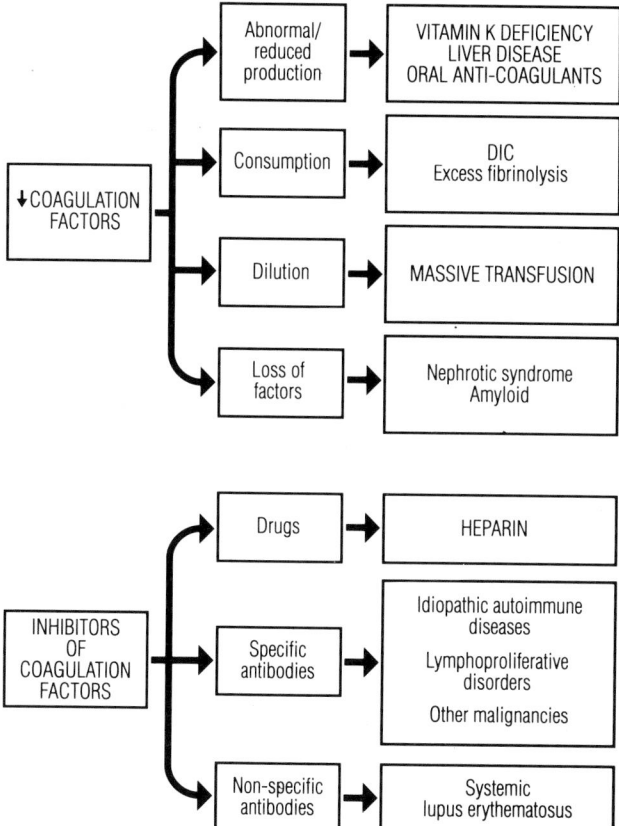

Fig. 25.43 Acquired coagulation disorders and their causes. Capital letters indicate the commoner causes.

Vitamin K deficiency

Vitamin K is a fat-soluble vitamin which carboxylates the glutamic acid residues on factors II, VII, IX and X. This enables them to bind to phospholipid in the presence of calcium and thus rapidly activate the next part of the cascade. Vitamin K deficiency may arise readily in newborn infants, in malabsorption states and also in patients with marginal stores who are severely ill and receive protracted broad spectrum antibiotic therapy. In addition, oral anti-coagulants of the warfarin and phenindione family lead to increased accumulation of phylloquinone epoxide (an inactive product of vitamin K_1), with a consequent net reduction in carboxylation of factors II, VII, IX and X.

Vitamin K deficiency leads to a bruising tendency, with a prolonged PT and APTT but a normal TT. It is reversible following vitamin K administration, although its effects take several hours to appear.

Liver disease

The aetiology of the bleeding tendency in liver disease is multifactorial (p. 628). There is decreased production of the vitamin K dependent factors, followed by decreased factor V production and (in some cases) the production of decreased or abnormal fibrinogen (dysfibrinogenaemia). If there is biliary disease, the clotting factor deficiencies may be exacerbated by malabsorption of vitamin K. This, together with the presence of ill-defined inhibitors, accounts for the difficulty in correcting the coagulation defects with fresh frozen plasma. The liver is the major site of degradation of activated factors, and hepatic insufficiency may therefore lead to disseminated intra-vascular coagulation and excessive fibrinolysis. There may also be hypersplenism and thrombocytopenia associated with the liver disease, and qualitative platelet defects have been reported. Excessive alcohol may also directly suppress platelet production.

In liver disease the PT and APTT are frequently prolonged. Prolongation of the TT – indicating hypo/dysfibrinogenaemia or disseminated intravascular coagulation (DIC) – is less common. A five-day course of vitamin K should be given if there are bleeding problems, although the benefit is marginal. Fresh frozen plasma can be given if clinically required, although the clinical and laboratory response is often poor. Platelets should be given to bleeding thrombocytopenic patients.

Disseminated intravascular coagulation and fibrinolysis

Disseminated intravascular coagulation (DIC) is discussed on page 1099. Very rarely, excess fibrinolysis occurs without DIC, due to high levels of plasminogen activator. This may follow major trauma, extensive surgery and carcinoma (especially prostate) in which there is excessive release of tPA; some snake venoms; and in severe liver disease in which there is failure to inactivate tPA. Generalised fibrinolysis is also produced by streptokinase therapy.

Acquired inhibitors

Specific anti-factor VIIIC antibodies may arise in severe haemophiliacs following factor VIII therapy. They may also arise in other individuals, often in association with autoimmune disease (such as rheumatoid arthritis, lymphoproliferative disease and other malignancies); but they are also frequently idiopathic in origin. Less commonly, antibodies to other clotting factors may also develop.

Anti-factor VIII antibodies may be produced in systemic lupus erythematosus, but more commonly there is a non-specific *lupus anticoagulant*, which inhibits the coagulation reactions that occur on phospholipid surfaces. There is prolongation of the APTT, which becomes disproportionately longer upon dilution of the thromboplastin. Patients with lupus anticoagulants do not bleed, but may have thromboses and spontaneous abortions. Many are asymptomatic.

ANTICOAGULANTS AND ANTITHROMBOTIC DRUGS

This group of drugs includes both inhibitors of platelets and the coagulation cascade, and activators of fibrinolysis.

HEPARIN

Mechanism of action

The heparins are a group of negatively charged polysaccharide sulphates which combine with antithrombin III, thereby increasing its activity against the activated serine proteases – thrombin and factors XI, IX, X and XIII. The effect is almost immediate. Heparin may also have some effects on platelets but these are of lesser importance.

Indications

The indications for the use of heparin are outlined in Table 25.50. Intravenous heparin helps prevent pulmonary embolism in patients with popliteal femoral and iliac vein thromboses. Its value in more superficial, or calf vein, thromboses is less certain, but it is usually given if the patient has significant symptoms. Heparin is also frequently used to prevent the development of thromboembolism in high risk situations, e.g. following major gynaecological or abdominothoracic surgery. The low dose subcutaneous heparin given in these circumstances has some anti-thrombotic effect, but does not in general cause post-operative haemorrhage.

Table 25.50 Indications for the use of heparin

- Treatment of deep vein thrombosis
- Treatment of pulmonary embolism
- Treatment of acute arterial occlusions
- During cardiac bypass surgery
- Thromboembolic prophylaxis

Administration

Full dose heparin is given as a loading dose of 5000–10 000 units, followed by a continuous infusion of 25 000–40 000 units/day depending on patient size and laboratory tests. Heparin affects all the routine coagulation tests, but none are entirely satisfactory for control of heparin therapy. The APTT is usually used and should be 1.5–2.5 times the normal control. The thrombin time (plus correction with protamine) is a quicker test and is used by some laboratories. Heparin assays are available but are not widely used. Following a thromboembolic episode, heparin should be given for 5–7 days.

Low dose subcutaneous heparin is usually given into the abdominal wall or thigh in a dose of 5000 units bd. Laboratory control is not necessary.

Complications

If bleeding occurs, the heparin should be reversed with protamine sulphate and the response monitored by laboratory tests such as the APTT or TT. Heparin may cause hypersensitivity reactions and acute thrombocytopenia, but this is rare before seven days of therapy. In those few patients receiving heparin for protracted periods, alopecia and osteoporosis may occur.

The most common complication is haemorrhage, and full anticoagulation should therefore be undertaken with great caution in patients with an active – or potentially active – bleeding site, severe hypertension, liver disease, haemorrhagic tendency of any form, or immediately following surgery (especially to the eye or central nervous system).

ORAL ANTICOAGULANTS

Mechanism of action

Bishydroxycoumarin (warfarin) and phenindione (dindevan) interfere with vitamin K metabolism by augmenting the formation of the inactive phylloquinone epoxide. This leads to the formation of factors II, VII, IX and X in which the glutamic residues have not been carboxylated. These *acarboxy factors* cannot interact with calcium and phospholipids and cannot therefore participate in the rapid clotting cascade.

Indications

The indications for use of oral anticoagulants (Table 25.51)

Table 25.51 Indications for use of oral anticoagulants

- Pulmonary embolism (following heparin therapy)
- Deep vein thrombosis (following heparin therapy)
- Prosthetic heart valves
- Rheumatic heart disease
- Following myocardial infarction

are still controversial in many circumstances due to conflicting trial results. This particularly applies to their use following myocardial infarction. An isolated deep vein thrombosis or pulmonary embolus merits four weeks therapy, although a second episode should be treated for three months. Recurrent pulmonary embolism is an indication for lifelong therapy.

Administration

Following a thrombotic episode, anticoagulation is usually started with intravenous heparin which is commonly given for five days. Oral anticoagulants are also started at the same time – their maximum effect taking five days to develop. A loading dose of warfarin (10 mg/day for three days, or similar regimen) is given, and the dose adjusted thereafter according to the results of a PT. The therapeutic range is an *international normalised ratio* (INR = ratio of patient's PT to control PT, with allowance made for different batches of prothrombin) of 2–4, depending upon the indication for anticoagulation. When blood is taken from a patient also receiving heparin, the heparin in the sample must first be neutralised with protamine sulphate if the APTT is greater than 2.5 times control. The half-life of warfarin is 30–60 hours, so daily administration gives rise to fairly stable steady state levels. Once good control has been achieved, monthly checks on the PT are usually acceptable. Drugs which inhibit liver enzyme degradation of oral anticoagulants – such as cimetidine and sulphonamides (including co-trimoxazole) – will also potentiate the anticoagulant effect. By contrast, barbiturates and rifampicin (which induce liver enzymes) will decrease the activity of oral anticoagulants. Broad spectrum antibiotics, which interfere with vitamin K biosynthesis by intestinal flora, will augment the action of oral anticoagulants; and cholestyramine reduces their effect by preventing anticoagulant absorption. The list of possible drug interactions is enormous and only some of the more common are shown in Table 25.52. It is essential to use a reference source of drug interactions when changing concurrent drug therapy, and the PT must be monitored frequently in these circumstances.

Complications

The major complication of anticoagulation is bleeding. As with heparin, some patients are at particular risk (p. 1104), but haemorrhagic disaster can occur in any patient and diligent control is therefore essential at all times. Most importantly, patients should not receive long-term therapy unless it is absolutely necessary. If the PT is found to be between 4.5 and 7 (INR), warfarin should be withheld for one or two days, and then restarted at a lower dose. If the PT is greater than 7, either vitamin K (1 mg iv) should be given or fresh frozen plasma (FFP) infused. FFP should be given immediately if there is any sign of bleeding. Additional (but rare) side effects of warfarin include skin rashes, diarrhoea, jaundice and alopecia.

Table 25.52 Drugs modulating warfarin activity

Type of drug	Drugs potentiating warfarin activity	Drugs diminishing warfarin activity
Gut	Cimetidine (moderate) Liquid paraffin (minor)	Cholestyramine (minor)
Circulation	Sulphinpyrazone (marked) Clofibrate (moderate) Amiodarone (moderate) Dipyridamole(minor)	
CNS		Carbamazepine (minor) Primidone (minor) Barbiturates (minor)
Endocrine	Thyroxine (moderate) Anabolic steroids (moderate) Steroids (minor)	Oral contraceptives (minor)
Anti-inflammatory	Salicylates (moderate) Phenylbutazone (moderate) Mefenamic acid (moderate) Azapropazone (moderate)	
Antibiotics	Cotrimoxazole (moderate) Metronidazole (moderate) Erythromycin (minor)	Rifampicin (minor)

ANTICOAGULATION IN PREGNANCY

Pregnancy is itself a prothrombotic state, due to both local pressure on the venous system from an enlarged uterus, and also an increase in coagulability and decrease in fibrinolysis. Thromboembolic disease occurs in approximately two per 1000 pregnancies. Other pregnant women require prophylactic anticoagulation because of previous thromboses, or high risk situations such as prosthetic heart valves.

Warfarin crosses the placenta and may cause chondrodysplasia punctata and abnormal development of the brain and face. The risk is greatest in the first three months, but is still present in the second trimester. Heparin should therefore be used instead as it does not cross the placenta. For an acute thromboembolism in the first trimester, full intravenous heparinisation should be given, followed by subcutaneous heparin (10 000 units bd). Some clinicians change to warfarin for the second trimester, but this still carries some risk of fetal malformation. In the third trimester, subcutaneous heparin should again be used, as warfarinisation may cause serious bleeding in both mother and baby at the time of delivery. Warfarin can be started 10 days after delivery, even in mothers who are breast-feeding.

Unfortunately, subcutaneous heparin is not as effective as full dose intravenous heparin or oral warfarin, and is probably not therefore acceptable for the safety of mothers with the most high risk prosthetic heart valves. A difficult compromise must be achieved after detailed discussion with the parents, if the pregnancy is to continue.

Some women become pregnant whilst taking warfarin and may not report it to their doctor until the pregnancy is well advanced into the first trimester. Clearly, all fertile women should be warned about the problems of pregnancy when warfarinisation is commenced.

ANTI-PLATELET AGENTS

Mechanism of action

The mechanisms of action of the more commonly used anti-platelet agents are shown in Table 25.53. The inhibition of platelet cyclo-oxygenase by aspirin is irreversible, and the effects of a single dose will last several days until new platelets are produced. Aspirin also inhibits endothelial cyclo-oxygenase which blocks prostacyclin production, a potent natural anti-platelet agent. Endothelial cells (unlike platelets) are nucleated, and continue to synthesise cyclo-oxygenase; as a result, the aspirin effect is short-lived. Thus, in theory, the maximal anti-platelet effect of aspirin may be achieved simply by a twice-weekly regimen, although most trial evidence is based on daily doses. Sulphinpyrazone similarly blocks cyclo-oxygenase, but its effect is reversible. Dipyridamole reversibly suppresses platelet cyclic AMP levels with consequent inhibition of agonist mediated rises in intracellular calcium ions.

Table 25.53 Drugs interfering with platelet function

Drug	Mechanism of action
Aspirin	Irreversible acetylation of platelet cyclo-oxygenase with blockade of platelet prostaglandin production
Sulphinpyrazone (Anturan)	Competitive inhibitor of cyclo-oxygenase
Dipyridamole (Persantin)	Reversible inhibition of platelet phosphodiesterase

Indications

Some of the possible indications for anti-platelet agents are shown in Table 25.54, although it must be noted that the data from clinical trials is not conclusive in all circumstances, particularly in the last three indications listed.

Table 25.54 Possible indications for the use of anti-platelet agents

- Cerebrovascular transient ischaemic attacks
- Prethrombotic states in which there is thrombocytosis or increased platelet aggregation
- Acute myocardial infarction
- Maintenance of A-V shunts
- Valvular disease of the heart
- Prevention of deep vein thromboses after surgery

Administration and complications

There is no universally accepted optimum regimen. Aspirin (300 mg daily) with or without dipyridamole (50–200 mg qds – higher doses may not be tolerated) is widely used. Anti-platelet agents do increase the bleeding time, but this alone causes few problems. Aspirin may, however, lead to gastric erosions and major bleeding from this site. Dipyridamole causes migrainous type headaches in many patients at the start of therapy, although these usually subside within a few weeks.

INTRAVASCULAR FIBRINOLYTIC THERAPY

Mechanisms of action

Streptokinase (which is derived from β haemolytic streptococci) combines with plasminogen and leads to the formation of the fibrinolytic compound plasmin. *Urokinase* (which is isolated from human urine) has a similar mechanism of action. It is a less toxic, naturally occurring compound, but is very expensive to purify. More recently, the naturally occurring *tissue plasminogen activators* (tPAs) have been produced by recombinant DNA technology, and it is hoped that the activity of these substances will be more restricted to the site of thrombus formation than is the case with streptokinase and urokinase.

Indications

The indications for use of intravascular fibrinolytic agents are shown in Table 25.55. Fibrinolytic therapy has been most commonly used in severe pulmonary embolism that does not merit immediate surgery – a fine distinction that accounts in part for the rarity of its use. Some centres have also used streptokinase in extensive deep vein thromboses; if given early, it is probably superior to heparin in preventing clot extension and preserving valvular competence. Fibrinolytic therapy may also be of value in acute thromboembolic phenomena in the limbs. Recently, streptokinase has been shown to reduce the mortality after myocardial infarction (p. 410).

Table 25.55 Indications for use of intravascular fibrinolytic agents

- Pulmonary embolism (acute massive)
- Major deep vein thrombosis
- Acute arterial thrombo-embolism
- Acute myocardial infarction (within 6–12 hours)
- Unblocking indwelling central venous catheters and arteriovenous shunts

Administration

Streptokinase is antigenic and most patients have circulating antibodies due to previous streptococcal infections. These must first be neutralised by a loading dose, which is then followed by continuous infusion for 3–7 days.

There is no consensus as to the optimum dosage schedule, although after myocardial infarction a single infusion dose has been shown to be effective. Fibrinolytic therapy reduces the fibrinogen level, markedly prolongs the thrombin time, and causes a rise in serum fibrin degradation products; this data is of little help, however, in monitoring the dosage. Ideally, streptokinase is infused locally – i.e. using a pulmonary artery catheter for pulmonary embolism – in the hope that this will reduce systemic fibrinolysis to some extent. Systemic fibrinolysis may prove to be much less of a problem with the human tissue plasminogen activators, and these compounds can be given into peripheral veins.

Complications

Streptokinase therapy is potentially hazardous. Bleeding, especially from drip sites, is very common and can be fatal. All patients receiving streptokinase should therefore have blood cross-matched and available. Fevers and other allergic phenomena are not infrequent, and it is common practice to give prophylactic steroids.

The recombinant tPAs may prove to be safer and enable the use of fibrinolytic therapy to increase dramatically.

Oral fibrinolytic agents

A variety of oral drugs such as the biguanides (e.g. metformin) and anabolic steroids (e.g. stanozolol) increase fibrinolytic activity, and may have occasional value in patients with recurrent venous and arterial thromboses who are on oral anticoagulants. These agents do, however, have major potential side effects, e.g. hypoglycaemia and masculinisation, unrelated to their fibrinolytic function.

PRETHROMBOTIC STATES

A *prethrombotic state* is any situation in which there is an increased risk of thrombo-embolism. Possible causes with examples are shown in Table 25.56.

The full investigation of a potential prethrombotic state is both extremely time-consuming and expensive. All patients presenting with a thrombo-embolic episode should be thoroughly examined to exclude local causes of circulatory stasis, and systemic diseases associated with hypercoagulability. A full blood count should be performed to exclude polycythaemia or thrombocytosis. Further studies (Table 25.57) are only cost effective in selected cases. The criteria for selection of patients (Table 25.58) are designed primarily to allow detection of the hereditary prethrombotic states.

Interpretation of the laboratory investigations for a prethrombotic state is not always easy. Firstly, raised clotting factors or increased levels of activated factors may be secondary to a recent (possibly subclinical) thrombosis, rather than the cause of a prethrombotic state. Similarly, increased levels of platelet release products, such as platelet

Table 25.56 Possible causes of a prethrombotic state

Mechanism	Example
Circulatory stasis	
Immobilisation	Prolonged bed rest
Mechanical obstruction	Pelvic tumours
Increased Hct	Polycythaemia
Greatly increased WBC	Chronic granulocytic leukaemia
Increased plasma viscosity	Myeloma
Abnormalities of platelet/vessel wall interaction	
Thrombocytosis	Essential thrombocythaemia
Increased platelet aggregability	Diabetes
Decreased vessel wall prostacyclin production	Thrombotic thrombocytopenic purpura
Coagulation abnormalities	
Clotting factors	Increased levels of VIIIC and VIIC associated with risk of coronary death
	Antithrombin III deficiency
	Lupus anticoagulant
Coagulation inhibitors	Protein C deficiency
	Protein S deficiency
Fibrinolytic abnormalities	
Plasminogen activators	Found in some patients with
Inhibitors of plasminogen	thrombotic episodes (significance
Increased anti plasmin	uncertain)

Table 25.57 Investigation of a prethrombotic state

- Full blood count
- Liver function tests
- Analysis of plasma lipids
- Protein electrophoresis to exclude hypergammaglobulinaemia
- Coagulation screen with particular attention to abnormalities due to dysfibrinogenaemia, or a lupus anticoagulant
- Euglobin clot lysis time as an index of the fibrinolytic pathway
- Antithrombin III levels
- Protein C levels (also Protein S levels if available)
- Platelet aggregometry to detect hyperaggregable platelets
  or
- Measurement of platelet release products (PF4, β-TG) within the plasma

Table 25.58 Possible criteria for the selection of patients for detailed investigation of a prethrombotic state

- Patient with DVT in whom there is a positive family history
- Thrombosis in unusual site, e.g. mesenteric vein
- DVT or pulmonary embolism in early pregnancy
- Recurrence of DVT while on oral anticoagulants
- Recurrent DVT in a patient under 35 years of age

factor 4 (PF4) or β-thromboglobulin (β-TG), within the serum, may reflect ongoing thrombosis rather than a primary platelet/vessel wall abnormality. Secondly, many patients requiring investigation will already be taking oral anticoagulants; determining deficiencies of vitamin K dependent proteins such as antithrombin III and protein C is then very difficult.

Antithrombin III deficiency

Anti-thrombin III (AT-III) deficiency may be either congenital or acquired.

Congenital

This is an autosomal dominant condition in which there is decreased synthesis of AT-III or synthesis in part of a dysfunctional molecule. The incidence is estimated to be 20–50 per 100 000. Affected individuals have functional AT-III levels of 40–70% (normal range 70–130%).

The disease typically presents with venous thromboses in early adulthood. Thromboses are particularly common after starting the contraceptive pill, during pregnancy or following surgery. Heparin is usually given in the short term, but is less effective here than in other situations, as AT-III is required as a cofactor for heparin and warfarin resistance may be a clinical indicator of AT-III deficiency. The administration of heparin also actually causes the AT-III level to fall further. For these reasons, fresh frozen plasma (or AT-III concentrates if available) should also be given in the acute stages. Long-term oral anticoagulants do reduce the incidence of recurrent thromboses and increase the circulatory levels of AT-III.

Acquired

As noted above, AT-III levels fall with the contraceptive pill, during surgery and after major surgery or trauma and this may contribute to the prethrombotic state in these situations. AT-III levels may also fall with severe proteinuria, thereby contributing to the documented thrombotic tendency in the nephrotic syndrome. AT-III

synthesis is reduced in liver disease, but bleeding (rather than thrombosis) is usually the problem in this situation.

Protein C and protein S deficiency

Protein C deficiency is an autosomal dominant condition, with an incidence probably similar to that of AT-III deficiency. The clinical course is also similar. Extensive skin necrosis has been noted in some patients following the initiation of anticoagulants.

Protein S deficiency (autosomal dominant) is probably less common, but may still account for up to 10% of thromboses in the high risk categories shown in Table 25.58.

Lupus anticoagulant

The lupus anticoagulant is associated with an increased incidence of thrombosis, although it is detected by the prolongation of the APTT. It is discussed on page 1104.

FURTHER READING

Chanarin I (ed) 1989 Laboratory haematology. Churchill Livingstone, Edinburgh. *An up-to-date account of haematological laboratory techniques, by multiple experts in the field.*

Dacie J V, Lewis S M 1984 Practical haematology. Churchill Livingstone, Edinburgh. *The classical reference work for laboratory methodology.*

Hoffbrand A V, Pettit J E (eds) 1988 Clinical haematology. Gower Medical Publishing, London. *An illustrated guide to haematology with excellent photomicrography.*

Hardisty J, Weatherall D 1982 Blood and its disorders. Blackwell Scientific Publications, Oxford. *A comprehensive haematological reference work.*

Hush J, Marden V J, Salzman E W 1987 Hemostasis and thrombosis: basic principles and clinical procedures. J B Lippincott Co., Philadelphia. *A comprehensive reference work on haemostasis and thrombosis.*

Kay L, Huehns E R 1986 Clinical blood transfusion. Churchill Livingstone, Edinburgh. *A simple guide to blood transfusion theory and practice.*

APPENDIX: NORMAL HAEMATOLOGICAL VALUES

The following are guidelines only – ranges may vary with the methods of assay used.

Measurement	Range	Units	Measurement	Range	Units
Red cell count	M 4.5–6.5	10^{12}/l	Monocytes	0.2–0.8	10^9/l
	F 3.8–5.8	10^{12}/l	Eosinophils	<0.4	10^9/l
Haemoglobin	M 13.0–18.0	g/dl	Basophils	<0.1	10^9/l
	F 11.5–16.5	g/dl	Platelet count	150–400	10^9/l
PCV	M 0.4–0.5	ratio	Serum iron	12–32	mmol/l
	F 0.35–0.47	ratio	TIBC	45–72	mmol/l
MCV	78–96	fl.	B_{12}	150–900	ng/l
MCH	27–32	pg.	Serum folate	3–15	ng/l
MCHC	30–34	g/dl	Rbc folate	160–640	ng/l
Reticulocytes	0.2–2.0	%	ESR < 50 years	<20	mm/h
Absolute count	10–100	10^9/l	ESR > 50 years	<30	mm/h
Total wbc	3.5–11.0	10^9/l	Prothrombin time	<3 s over control	
Differential wbc count:					
Neutrophils	2.0–7.5	10^9/l	Activated partial thromboplastin time	<7 s over control	
Lymphocytes	1.5–4.0	10^9/l	Thrombin time	<3 s over control	

Skin Disease

Table 26.1 Incidence of skin diseases*

Rates of consultation (general practice) per 1000/year	
All skin diseases	120.0
Dermatitis and eczema	45.6
'Rash'	13.3
Virus warts	14.3
Acne	9.6
Urticaria	8.6
Psoriasis	4.6
Chronic ulcer	2.4
Malignant neoplasms	0.8
Some comparisons	
Rheumatoid arthritis	5.6
Osteoarthritis	23.5
Back pain	32.8
Diseases of stomach	19.7
Irritable bowel	18.4

*Data from Office of Population Censuses and Surveys, Third National Study. HMSO, 1986.

Dermatology is the study of the skin and its diseases. Skin disorders are a common reason for seeking medical advice (Table 26.1). Diagnosis of skin disease depends to a great extent on recognition of the appearance of particular abnormalities. Apart from diseases which primarily affect the skin, many systemic diseases may produce dermatological manifestations. Examination of the skin is also of importance in deducing the overall state of health.

When a skin disease is widespread and interfering with skin functions, systemic consequences follow – sometimes, as in untreated pemphigus vulgaris, with fatal results. More limited skin diseases can cause distress or hardship. An example is loss of employment because of hand dermatitis. A blemish-free skin is constantly paraded by the media as desirable, and the psychological impact of readily visible skin lesions, even if biologically trivial, should not be underestimated. Another common problem associated with skin disorders is fear (often not expressed) that a skin disease is contagious, or a manifestation of cancer.

In this chapter there is a brief account of the biology of the skin, the principles of diagnosis and therapy, and then a description of those skin diseases which are either common or important. Diseases presenting as changes in the skin, but whose major impact is on other systems, are discussed in other chapters. Because of the great importance of the visual aspects of dermatology, a colour atlas, or whenever possible, patients, should be viewed in conjunction with the text. Therapy is considered in terms of general principles.

BIOLOGY OF THE SKIN

The skin is a protective barrier between a hostile environment and internal tissues. Its principal functions are to reduce the loss of water, electrolytes and other solutes, and the entry of unwanted molecules, microbes and radiation. It has a complex and specialised sensory innervation and contains a network of antigen-processing cells. The cutaneous vasculature and sweat glands are vital to heat regulation. Vitamin D is synthesised in the skin. By virtue of its smell, colour and texture, the skin has psychological and sexual roles.

Epidermis

Conventionally the skin is regarded as being composed of three layers: epidermis, dermis and fat. The epidermis is a stratified epithelium, the bulk of which is the keratinocyte population (Fig. 26.1). These cells are of ectodermal origin; they divide in the basal layer, where they are separated by the basal lamina from the dermis, progressively produce the sulphur-rich fibrous protein keratin, and become flattened and dead by the time they reach the surface. Keratinocytes are linked to one another by specialised cell junctions, notably the desmosomes, and in health the horny layer is tough, flexible and relatively impermeable. At the surface they are constantly shed as squames. Removal of the horny layer virtually destroys the barrier function of the skin with respect to water and solutes. The effectiveness of the horny layer is reduced if its production is faulty (e.g. in psoriasis), if the water content drops below a critical level (e.g. chapping), or if it is damaged (e.g. by detergents and lipid solvents).

Resident in the epidermis are the melanocytes, Langerhans cells, Merkel cells and some lymphocytes:

1. *Melanocytes* migrate early in fetal life from the neural crest and become established along the basal layer so that there is approximately 1 melanocyte per 10 keratinocytes. Via their dendritic processes, the yellow or brown pigmented protein melanin is passed in membrane-bound particles, called melanosomes, into the keratinocytes; here most of it is distributed over the surface of the nucleus which faces the sun. Melanin absorbs ultraviolet radiation and thus helps protect against DNA damage. In its absence, in albinism, skin cancer on exposed sites is common at an early age.

2. *Langerhans cells*, also dendritic, are of bone marrow origin. They are located in the mid-epidermis, function as antigen-presenting cells and can migrate to regional lymph nodes.

3. *Lymphocytes*, seen in small numbers in normal epidermis, are also of importance in the immune function of the skin.

4. *Merkel cells*, best recognised on electron microscopy by the possession of dense-cored granules, are closely associated with sensory nerve endings, and may represent a mechanoreceptor system.

The epidermis is separated from and attached to the dermis by a basal lamina, across which all nutrients must pass. A component of the basal lamina is the target of immunological attack in the blistering disease bullous pemphigoid (p. 1133).

Dermis

The dermis is a three-dimensional, fibrous tissue network of collagen and elastin associated with water-rich glycosaminoglycans, in which are embedded the blood and lymphatic vessels, neural elements and epidermal appendages – sweat glands, sebaceous glands and hair follicles (Fig. 26.1). The dermis is manufactured by fibroblasts, and other cells seen in normal tissue include dermal phagocytes and mast cells. The dermis has visco-elastic properties, allowing body movements without permanent distortion, yet considerable mechanical strength. It is essential to the well-being and repair of the epidermis. The superficial part of the dermis, containing capillaries and nerve endings, is more loosely woven than deeper layers, and projects into the undersurface of the epidermis as papillae.

Blood flow through the skin can be greatly in excess of nutritional demands, and skin vasculature contributes to thermoregulation and maintenance of blood pressure. There are networks of blood vessels at the levels of the deep fascia, the fat–dermis junction and in the papillary dermis, where capillary loops follow the contour of the dermo-epidermal junction. There are also numerous arterio-venous shunts which allow blood to bypass capillaries, conserving heat. Vascular control is by autonomic nerves and chemical mediators. The skin is also provided with an extensive plexus of lymphatics, distinguishable from veins by the fact that they do not possess valves, which act both as a drainage system for lymph and in the recirculation of lymphocytes.

There are afferent sensory nerves subserving touch, pain, temperature and itch, and also the specialised Meissner and Pacinian corpuscles, which are probably

Fig. 26.1   Cross-section of the skin.

Hair   Vein   Artery

Epidermis

Basal layer

Sebaceous gland

Dermis

Sweat gland

Subcutaneous fatty tissue

mechanoreceptors. The autonomic supply is sympathetic, with adrenergic, cholinergic and purinergic terminals.

Disorders of collagen and elastin are described on page 93.

Epidermal appendages

Eccrine sweat glands consist of secretory coils connected by straight ducts to the surface. There is a rich blood supply and a predominantly cholinergic sympathetic innervation. Because of the sodium resorptive properties of the ducts, sweat is hypotonic. The basal level of fluid loss through the skin of about 600 ml/day can be greatly increased in response to the need for heat loss.

Apocrine sweat glands are found in the axillae, ano-genital regions, on the breast and in the ear. They open into hair follicles and on to the skin surface. Their secretion is low in volume and after bacterial alteration it has a characteristic odour.

The pilosebaceous follicles produce both hairs and sebaceous glands. In man, hair (in the right place) is largely of cultural and sexual significance. A residual protective value is seen when its absence in bald males is accompanied in later life by sun-induced neoplasms. An important characteristic of hair follicles is their cyclical activity: for each follicle a period of active growth (anagen) is followed by a transition period (catagen) and then a resting phase (telogen), when the hair is shed and a new hair begins. Individual follicles are normally asynchronous, hence humans do not moult.

EXAMINATION OF THE SKIN

It is essential to examine all the skin, together with the mouth, genitalia, hair and nails, in a good light. If only the symptomatic parts proffered are examined, unsuspected or deliberately concealed lesions may be missed. The skin should be carefully palpated as well as inspected, to appreciate the thickness of lesions and of the whole skin.

Skin lesions should be described in terms of:

1. the individual characteristics of lesions (shape, colour, etc.)
2. their arrangement in relation to each other (if any)
3. their distribution.

The terms used have precise meanings and these are set out in Table 26.2.

Distribution

The following points regarding distribution should be noted:

1. Is the rash localised, regional or generalised?
2. Is there symmetry? Endogenous disorders are often symmetrical.

Table 26.2 Terms used to describe skin lesions

Skin lesion	Definition
Appearance	
Macule	Flat, circumscribed, impalpable area of colour change. There may be scaling, as in pityriasis versicolor
Papule	Small (less than 0.5 cm), solid, elevated lesion, most of which is above the plane of the skin
Plaque	Elevated lesion with relatively large surface area in relation to height
Nodule	Large (greater than 0.5 cm diameter) solid lesion
Purpura	Extravasated red cells (see Diascopy, p. 1112). Small purpuric lesions are called petechiae, large ones ecchymoses. They are not obliterated by pressure. The colour varies from red, through purple and brown, to yellow, depending on the age of the lesion
Weal	Elevation due to dermal oedema, lasting minutes to several hours
Angio-oedema	Massive oedematous reaction in loose dermis or subcutaneous tissue
Vesicle	Blister less than 0.5 cm diameter
Bulla	Blister greater than 0.5 cm diameter
Pustule	Elevation of the skin containing fluid and leucocytes, usually yellow or green in colour, but not necessarily infective
Erythema	Redness due to vasodilatation
Telangiectasia	Permanent dilatation of capillaries
Atrophy	Thinning, often with loss of normal skin markings, and increased transparency
Sclerosis	Hardening due to changes in the dermis
Ulcer	Loss of (at least) the epidermis
Excoriation	Scratch mark
Crust	Dried exudate
Scaling	Desquamating horny layer
Burrow	Irregular linear elevation of horny layer, characteristic of scabies
Shape and arrangement	
Linear	In a line
Annular	Ring-shaped
Target	Erythematous ring or rings separated by relative pallor with a purplish centre
Herpetiform	Clustered, like herpes simplex
Zosteriform	Clustered and following a dermatome
Reticular	Net-like

3. Is there localization by exposure to light, cold or some other environmental factor?
4. Has non-specific trauma, e.g. scratching, caused new lesions (Koebner phenomenon), as in psoriasis and lichen planus?
5. Is there an underlying anatomical basis, e.g. the vascular or nerve supply, the flexures or hair follicles?

Many conditions have characteristic patterns of distribution, the basis for which is obscure, e.g. dermatitis herpetiformis on elbows and knees, scalp, shoulders and buttocks.

DERMATOLOGICAL DIAGNOSIS

There is a great variety of dermatological diagnoses. However, the practised observer can describe changes in such a way as to suggest a diagnosis or differential diagnostic group. The history is important, narrowing the possibilities (Table 26.3). Certain diagnostic procedures and investigations may be used, as follows.

Table 26.3 Taking a history

History of the skin eruption
When and where did the problem start?
Has it spread, and how?
Has it changed in character? What was it like if different before?
Does it itch?
Does it come and go?
What has been used or taken for it (prescribed and self-medication)?
Have any other medications – oral, injected or topical – been used?
Is there any relation to sunlight?
Any past history of skin disease?
Does anyone the patient knows have anything similar?
What does the patient think is the cause?

Background
Age, sex, race. Pregnant? Pubertal?
Personal and family history of eczema, asthma or hay fever
Social history: occupation, hobbies, travel
Any known allergies?

Diascopy

Viewing the skin, having pressed it with a microscope slide or perspex spatula, helps to distinguish purpura (which does not blanch) from erythema (which does).

Nikolsky sign

The Nikolsky sign involves the production or extension of a blistering process by the combination of pressure with a sliding action. It is characteristic of pemphigus and some other blistering diseases.

Wood's light

Wood's light is a long-wave UV lamp which shows red fluorescence with erythrasma, green fluorescence with some common scalp fungal infections, and pale yellow fluorescence with pityriasis versicolor. It enhances the pallor of vitiligo, compared with other acquired conditions that produce pale patches, and is helpful in screening for the ash leaf macules of tuberose sclerosis.

Biopsy

Biopsies are carried out for histopathology and, when relevant, immunological studies, microbiological culture and electron microscopy.

Mycological techniques

Mycological techniques are described on page 1116.

Patch testing

Patch testing is described under 'Contact dermatitis' (p. 1126).

Scabies mite scraping

Scabies mite scraping is described on page 1121.

DERMATOLOGICAL THERAPY

Dermatological treatment includes *topical and systemic pharmacy*, *physical modalities* such as liquid nitrogen cryotherapy, ultraviolet radiation, radiotherapy, lasers and surgical procedures, and *dietary measures*. Topical therapy is the traditional province of the dermatologist.

Vehicles

Active ingredients are applied to the skin in a vehicle. Most vehicles can be regarded as one of the prototypes shown in Table 26.4.

A vehicle may be used therapeutically: a lotion to cool and dry, a cream to soothe, an ointment to moisturise dry skin and a paste to protect.

Table 26.4 Composition and properties of vehicles for topical treatment

Vehicle	Composition	Properties
Lotion	Liquid (water or alcohol)	Cools inflamed skin. Useful in hairy areas. Miscible with exudate
Shake lotion	Water + powder	Powder increases area for evaporation, so has cooling properties
Cream	Water + grease + emulsifier	Aqueous phase gives some cooling effect and miscibility with exudate. Grease increases hydration. Properties will vary depending on whether the emulsion is oil-in-water or water-in-oil
Ointment	Grease	Moisturises dry skin by trapping water passing through the epidermis. Hydrophobic (e.g. vaseline) or hydrophilic (e.g. lanolin)
Paste	Grease + powder	Moisturising and protective
Dusting powder	Powder	Reduces friction. Absorbs water

When an active ingredient is included, the vehicle must deliver it appropriately and maintain its integrity against oxidation and bacterial contamination. Therefore vehicles, especially creams, are liable to contain preservatives and stabilisers. Some preparations contain substances to enhance drug penetration, e.g. urea. When adverse reactions to topical agents occur, it should be remembered that not only the active ingredient but also the components of the vehicle should be considered as possible causes.

For most active ingredients the major barrier to penetration is the horny layer. Penetration is greater through facial and genital skin, flexures (e.g. axillae, crural folds) and is increased by occlusion (e.g. by rubber gloves), diseases altering the horny layer (e.g. eczema and psoriasis), and pharmaceutical penetration enhancers, such as urea. In contrast, when the horny layer is very thick, as on the palms and soles, there is reduced penetration.

Topical corticosteroids

Topical corticosteroids have anti-inflammatory and other actions, with useful suppressive effects in a number of skin disorders, but they do not cure disease. They can worsen skin infection and modify physical signs, and the more potent preparations easily produce side-effects, which can be permanent.

In general, the efficacy of topical steroids goes hand in hand with the ability to cause side-effects, and a preparation of the lowest potency that is effective should be used (Table 26.5). Applications are usually once or twice

Table 26.5 Potency of topical corticosteroids

Group	Potency	Examples
1	Very high	Clobetasol propionate
2	High	Betamethasone valerate
		Hydrocortisone butyrate
3	Moderate	Clobetasone butyrate
4	Low	Hydrocortisone

daily, with bland creams or ointments at other times if necessary. Efficacy is determined by the steroid molecule, its concentration, the vehicle, and also by factors favouring increased absorption.

Adverse effects are unlikely with topical 1% hydrocortisone. Adverse effects are listed in Table 26.6.

Other topically used drugs

A selection of some of the drugs used topically is shown in Table 26.7.

Cryotherapy

Many benign and some malignant skin lesions can be quickly and successfully treated by accurately applied low temperature. The most satisfactory agent is liquid nitrogen, whose temperature is $-196°C$, applied on a cotton-

Table 26.6 Adverse effects of topical steroids

Adverse effects	Factors increasing risk
Pituitary–adrenal axis suppression; growth suppression in children	Potency group 1*
	Potency group 2 with occlusion*
	Widespread skin inflammation
	Infancy
	Hepatic failure
Spread of skin infection	Overt infection
	Body folds
Atrophy (thin, red, fragile skin)	High risk sites, e.g. face, body folds
	Occlusion
	Prolonged use
Striae (stretch marks)	Potency groups 1 and 2*
	Body folds
Increased hair growth (hypertrichosis)	Potency groups 1 and 2*
	Prolonged use
Peri-oral dermatitis	Face
Exacerbation of skin disease on withdrawal	Psoriasis
	Facial dermatoses

* See Table 26.5.

Table 26.7 Some topical preparations used in skin diseases

Topical drug	Use
Tars	Chronic eczema, psoriasis
Dithranol	Psoriasis
Benzoyl peroxide	Acne
Calamine	Pruritus
Aminobenzoic acid esters	Sunscreens
Salicylic acid	Viral warts, other localised hyperkeratotic conditions
Podophyllin	Viral warts
Gamma benzene hexachloride	Scabies
Malathion	Pediculosis (lice)
Compound benzoic acid ointment	Some dermatophyte infections
Antifungal imidazoles	Some dermatophyte and yeast infections
Nystatin and amphotericin B	Candidiasis
Antibiotics, e.g. fusidic acid, mupirocin	Localised superficial Gram-positive bacterial infection
Acyclovir, idoxuridine	Some herpes simplex and zoster infections

wool swab, by a spray or a probe. The procedure can be painful and is often followed by swelling and blistering, but long-term cosmetic results are generally good. Hypopigmentation and some sensory loss can be troublesome consequences.

BACTERIAL DISEASES

Bacterial infection can produce skin lesions at or near the portal of entry, as in impetigo. Lesions may also occur as a manifestation of infection elsewhere. Thus, lesions may be due to organisms being deposited in the skin during septicaemia, blood-borne spread of a toxin; and hypersensitivity phenomena, such as the vasculitic Osler nodes and splinter haemorrhages of subacute bacterial endocarditis.

Normal intact skin is colonised by diphtheroids and non-pathogenic staphylococci, and in some sites such as the anterior nares, axilla and perineum, by potentially pathogenic *Staphylococcus aureus*. In moist areas there are often some Gram-negative bacilli.

Overt infection nearly always follows some kind of injury, albeit trivial. If it is associated with some obvious pre-existing skin lesions, such as eczema, it is referred to as secondary infection. Host factors, particularly the immunological status, are important in determining the degree and extent of infection.

Some skin diseases, such as hidradenitis suppurativa, are a non-specific reaction to bacteria, which, although contributory, are not the primary cause.

The types of staphylococcal and streptococcal skin infection are shown in Table 26.8.

Table 26.8 Staphylococcal and streptococcal bacterial infections of the skin

Due to direct bacterial infection	Due to toxin	Due to hypersensitivity
Staphylococcus aureus		
Impetigo	Staphylococcal scalded skin syndrome	
Ecthyma	Toxic shock syndrome	
Follicular infections	Staphylococcal scarlatina	
Streptococcus pyogenes		
Impetigo	Scarlet fever	Erythema
Ecthyma		Vasculitis
Erysipelas		
Cellulitis		
Necrotising fasciitis		

Impetigo

Impetigo (Plate 1, p. 1131) is a primary superficial bacterial skin infection, initially vesicular or bullous, later crusted. Impetigo may only involve the openings of hair follicles.

It is caused by *Staphylococcus aureus*, *Streptococcus pyogenes* group A, or both. In some tropical regions the streptococci can cause nephritis. Bullous impetigo is usually due to phage group II staphylococci.

Impetigo predominantly occurs among children and is highly contagious. Spread is mainly from skin to skin, although in streptococcal cases infected individuals may acquire the disease from pharyngeal colonisation. Trauma, for example from scratching insect bites, and infestation commonly predispose to the infection.

Exposed parts are mainly affected. The early lesions are clear or turbid blisters which soon become crusts, often golden yellow, with a surrounding zone of erythema. In bullous impetigo there are larger blisters with no erythema. The lesions tend to heal centrally but spread peripherally. Regional lymphadenopathy is common.

Diagnosis is by Gram stain and culture of a swab and this will help to distinguish impetigo from other lesions such as tinea and varicella.

Gentle removal of crusts is helpful. If localised, a topical antibiotic, such as fusidic acid or mupirocin, is adequate. For widespread impetigo, oral flucloxacillin (or erythromycin if the patient is allergic to penicillin) is required. Improvement of hygiene may be advisable – for example, not sharing towels.

Ecthyma

Ecthyma is a vesiculopurulent condition similar to impetigo, but the infection extends deeper, producing ulceration; it is caused by *Streptococcus pyogenes*, often with *Staphylococcus aureus*. The condition mainly affects children and the elderly, and is often associated with poor hygiene and/or insect bites. The initial vesicular lesion soon becomes a punched-out ulcer with overlying crust. The legs are commonly affected.

Treatment is with a penicillinase-resistant antibiotic, such as flucloxacillin or erythromycin. If there is surrounding cellulitis penicillin should be added.

The differential diagnosis includes ecthyma gangrenosum, due to *Pseudomonas septicaemia* (see below), and other causes of ulcers (p. 1146).

Staphylococcal scalded skin syndrome

Staphylococcal scalded skin syndrome is a generalised skin reaction to blood-borne staphylococcal epidermolytic toxins, which cause a split in the superficial epidermis; unlike impetigo there are no organisms in the accumulating fluid. It is caused by a focus of infection of *Staphylococcus pyogenes* of phage group II which may be cutaneous but can be elsewhere. Children, especially infants, are most susceptible.

A few days after the initiating staphylococcal infection there is a sudden onset of widespread tender erythema with fever. Twelve hours or so later there may be widespread flaccid bullae and the horny layer begins to detach in sheets.

Toxic epidermal necrolysis due to drugs (p. 1136) can be distinguished by the histology of a blister roof, which shows a deeper level of split in the epidermis in the drug-induced type, and by the history.

Treatment is with parenteral flucloxacillin (or equivalent), and careful attention to fluid balance and temperature regulation.

Erysipelas

Erysipelas (Plate 2, p. 1131) is a dermal infection, usually with group A streptococci.

There is often a recognisable portal of entry, such as a fungal infection between the toes or a fissure at the corner of the mouth. There may have been a previous upper respiratory tract streptococcal infection. The onset is often sudden, with fever, malaise and rigors, together with a bright red, tender swelling. The face and lower legs are common sites. The skin becomes oedematous and a well-defined, raised, sometimes blistering edge advances rapidly. There are often red streaks due to lymphangitis.

Acute contact dermatitis and angio-oedema of the face may simulate erysipelas but do not produce fever. Herpes zoster, before the outbreak of vesicles, is associated with pain or paraesthesiae. Erysipeloid (p. 1116) occurs in meat- and fish-handlers and systemic symptoms are much less severe.

Leucocytosis is usual. Surface culture is useless but the organism can sometimes be cultured from aspirated fluid. There is usually an antibody response to streptococcal proteins with rising titres of antideoxyribonuclease B; anti-streptolysin O is less often elevated.

Erysipelas is usually self-limited but can produce suppurative and widespread infection. There is involvement of lymphatics, and this predisposes to persistent swelling (lymphoedema) and recurrent attacks.

The treatment of choice is penicillin, parenterally in severe infections, unless contra-indicated by hyper-sensitivity.

Cellulitis

Cellulitis is a deeper dermal/subcutaneous infection than erysipelas, usually with group A streptococci. In practice there is no absolute distinction between erysipelas and cellulitis. There is usually an obvious portal, e.g. a leg ulcer or wound, or oedema of lymphatic, venous or renal origin.

There is spreading erythematous oedema as in erysipelas but without the sharply defined edge or vesiculation. There may be similar constitutional symptoms and lymphangitis. Untreated, gangrene may occur.

Treatment is the same as for erysipelas.

Necrotising fasciitis

Necrotising fasciitis (streptococcal gangrene) is a necrotising process usually due to group A streptococci, involving the deep fascia and vessels within it, with secondary death of overlying skin.

This uncommon process can occur in healthy subjects, but arterial insufficiency and diabetes predispose. Necrotising fasciitis usually begins like cellulitis, but after about 2 days the area becomes purplish, haemorrhagic bullae appear and there is evident tissue death. Untreated, there is a high mortality.

The diagnosis is often based on clinical suspicion alone, but streptococci can often be found in exudate or the blood.

Treatment by urgent and adequate surgical debridement is essential, together with parenteral penicillin or erythromycin if there is penicillin hypersensitivity.

Progressive bacterial synergistic gangrene

Progressive bacterial synergistic gangrene is gangrenous ulceration due to synergistic infection, with micro-aerophilic streptococci and *Staphylococcus aureus*, usually associated with an abdominal or thoracic operation wound.

One to two weeks after surgery there is a slowly spreading area of ulceration which has a rim of gangrenous skin surrounded by purplish erythema. The main differential diagnosis is pyoderma gangrenosum.

Treatment is by surgical débridement plus antibiotic therapy based on sensitivity tests.

Follicular infections

A furuncle (boil) is an acute necrotising infection of a follicle. A carbuncle is more extensive, involving contiguous follicles and the tissues around them. Infection of the hair follicle opening is termed superficial folliculitis.

The usual infecting organism is *Staphylococcus aureus*, and there is often nasal, axillary or perineal carriage of the organism. Friction, as at the nape of the neck, and moisture, as in the flexures, are important predisposing factors. Obesity, poor hygiene, widespread skin disease, immune deficiency and diabetes mellitus may predispose in severe cases. Superficial folliculitis can be non-infective; causes include contact with oils and other irritant chemicals.

Furuncles are tender red papules or nodules, which become pustular centrally and often heal with some scarring. Furunculosis may be chronic, as in sycosis barbae, a pustular eruption due to *Staphylococcus aureus* occurring on the male face. Carbuncles are often associated with fever and malaise, and with an underlying systemic illness such as diabetes or immune suppression.

Follicular infections can produce bacteraemia and, rarely, there may be serious consequences such as bony and cerebral abscesses, and endocarditis.

Swabs should be taken from pus and from the anterior nares, axilla and perineum of the patient and household contacts (potential reservoirs of infection) in chronic cases.

Furuncles and carbuncles may need incision and drainage. Superficial staphylococcal folliculitis should respond to flucloxacillin (or equivalent) for 1–2 weeks, but chronic cases may need treatment for longer, and treatment of reservoir sites – for example, chlorhexidine for the skin and mupirocin for the nose.

The differential diagnosis includes dermatophyte infection (the fungi can be demonstrated by microscopy and culture of hairs) and pseudofolliculitis, a non-infective papulopustular condition on the face and neck, due to cut hairs growing back into the skin. The latter is very common in negroes because their hair is tightly curled. Acne vulgaris (p. 1147) can usually be distinguished by the presence of comedones, and the pustules are sterile. Hidradenitis suppurativa is discussed on page 1147. In anthrax there is a haemorrhagic crust and vesicular margin and a swab will establish the diagnosis.

Erythrasma

Erythrasma is a common surface infection caused by *Corynebacterium minutissimum*. Sharply defined red or reddish-brown patches, sometimes with slight scaling, are seen in the axillae, groins, toe webs and sometimes other body folds. There are usually no symptoms.

The diagnosis is readily made with Wood's light; the affected skin fluoresces pink.

Most cases respond to a topical imidazole, e.g. clotrimazole, but if widespread, oral erythromycin for 10 days may be more effective.

Erysipeloid

Erysipeloid is an acute cutaneous infection with *Erysipelothrix insidiosa*. This Gram-positive bacillus causes infection in several animals and salt-water fish. Transfer to the skin occurs mainly to veterinary surgeons, butchers, fish-handlers and housewives.

The hand is the common site. A few days after inoculation there is a well-defined, slowly spreading, dusky erythematous oedema with little or no general upset (in contrast with erysipelas).

Treatment is with penicillin or tetracycline.

Pseudomonas infection of the skin

Pseudomonas aeruginosa is not normally found on the skin, but can become pathogenic, with production of a characteristic bluish-green pus and a fruity odour in circumstances of increased moisture. Examples may be found at the base of the nail in those whose hands are often immersed in water, toe spaces, beneath dressings for ulcers, and very importantly on raw surfaces following burns. Prior eradication of Gram-positive flora may also predispose. Localised infection usually responds to simple antiseptic measures, such as acetic acid, silver nitrate or silver sulphadiazine, together with drying.

Pseudomonas septicaemia can produce solitary or widespread vesicles with surrounding red haloes. Subsequent necrosis, often with haemorrhage into the tissues producing black crusts, is known as ecthyma gangrenosum. The lesions, as well as the blood, should yield *Pseudomonas* on culture, and prompt recognition and treatment can be life-saving.

Kawasaki's disease

Kawasaki's disease (mucocutaneous lymph node syndrome), described by Kawasaki in 1967, is most common in parts of Japan but probably has a worldwide distribution. The natural history of the illness suggests an infective aetiology but none has been identified. It is most common in toddlers and rare after 8 years of age; there is a slight male predominance among cases (1.6:1).

Characteristically the child is irritable and febrile and the limbs are tender peripherally. The rash is variable and may look like a severe measles eruption, but the sequence of appearance – on the head, followed by trunk and then limbs – is absent, and the swelling and tenderness of the hands and feet are not compatible with measles. Desquamation of a thick layer of skin starting around the nails and sometimes involving the whole hand and foot occurs later and this is a distinctive feature. It differs from staphylococcal toxin-induced desquamation in the thickness of the layer involved and from streptococcal desquamation, which is flaky. The natural history of the disease is that it resolves after 6–10 weeks.

About 20% of patients have some cardiac involvement, and myocarditis, with or without aneurysm of the proximal part of the coronary arteries, causes a mortality of 2% in Japanese series. Although small aneurysms have been demonstrated in 17% of patients investigated by coronary angiography, most of these resolve spontaneously. Postmortem pathology shows a small vessel angiitis with thrombus formation as the initiating lesion.

Aspirin has been shown to cause early resolution of symptoms and fever and it is used in low dose if thrombocytosis develops to inhibit platelet aggregation. Corticosteroids are not indicated; they may encourage aneurysm formation.

SUPERFICIAL FUNGAL DISEASES

Fungal infections involving the skin are broadly classified into superficial and deep. The former include the ringworm fungi (dermatophytes), candidiasis and pityriasis versicolor. Except for *Candida*, these fungi rarely invade deeper than the horny layer of the epidermis. Nails and hair, as well as the skin surface, may be involved (Plate 3, p. 1131). The clinical manifestations depend partly on the infecting species, on the part of the body affected and also on the host response to substances diffusing from the fungi into the skin. Deep fungal infections are discussed in Chapter 12.

Diagnosis is by microscopic examination of scrapings to show fungal hyphae, and species identification is by culture. The dermatophytes are grown on Sabouraud's medium. With skin lesions scale is collected by scraping with a blade, hair is plucked (or the surface scraped if hairs have broken off flush with the scalp) and clippings taken from nails. Material is sent to the laboratory dry in folded paper. Microscopy is performed on small samples after clearing with a few drops of 30% potassium hydroxide (KOH), a process speeded up by gentle warming. Careful pressure is exerted on the slide and coverslip between pieces of blotting paper to squeeze out surplus KOH. For some species of scalp dermatophyte infection and for pityriasis versicolor the Wood's light is valuable (p. 1112).

Tinea

The fungi causing the characteristic annular lesions known as tinea or ringworm (Fig. 26.2) are also known as the dermatophytes, for they have the ability to digest keratin.

Fig. 26.2 The annular lesions of tinea (ringworm).

There are three genera – *Trichophyton, Microsporum* and *Epidermophyton* – and numerous species which are recognised by their cultural characteristics. Humans are the primary host for some (the anthropophilic species), but with others the fungi are incidental pathogens to man, being primarily animal parasites (zoophilic) or found in soil (geophilic). The immune response is most marked against zoophilic species and these tend not to recur. With very inflammatory ringworm there can be so-called 'id' reactions, due to the immune response. These are widespread, often follicular, papular lesions which do not contain fungi. Probably for similar reasons, a vesicular eruption on the hands can be associated with ringworm of the feet. The distinctive appearance of ringworm infections can be greatly modified by topical steroids.

Successful treatment requires attention to sources of re-infection and measures to deal with acutely inflamed macerated skin, such as aluminium acetate soaks, as well as specific anti-fungal preparations. Topical agents, including Whitfield's ointment, and various imidazoles are suitable for localised skin infection. Oral griseofulvin is the treatment of choice for hair, nail, widespread skin and chronic infections. A weak topical steroid, together with antifungal therapy, may be useful if there is much inflammation.

Tinea pedis

Tinea pedis is a dermatophyte infection of the feet, sometimes with concurrent bacterial infection. This very common, often chronic condition is frequently acquired where bathing facilities are shared, and infection is favoured by maceration. It is much commoner in males.

The most common pattern is an itchy, inflamed, fissured, moist toe space, usually between the fourth and fifth toes. It is often unilateral. A vesicular pattern may occur involving the instep, dorsum of the foot or sides of the toes. A very chronic pattern may be seen, with hyperkeratosis and

fine white scaling accentuating skin creases on the soles. Tinea pedis may be accompanied by cellulitis.

Tinea pedis can resemble eczema, contact dermatitis, candidal infection and psoriasis. Endogenous eczema and psoriasis are more likely to be bilateral.

Most toe space infections respond to a topical antifungal agent, but extensive involvement of the soles needs prolonged treatment with griseofulvin. Regular cleansing of communal bathing facilities and prophylactic use of antifungal powders help reduce transmission of infection.

Tinea cruris

Tinea cruris is a dermatophyte infection of the groins and adjacent skin. Like tinea pedis, with which it is often associated, tinea cruris is much more common in males.

Itching is very common. There is inflammation with a well-defined margin which is scaly, vesicular or occasionally pustular, often with central clearing.

The differential diagnosis includes candidiasis, in which there is a less well defined edge and outlying tiny pustules. Erythrasma is not usually inflammatory. Intertrigo, an inflammatory process common in the obese, in which friction sweating and minor bacterial infection cause erythema in body folds, can mimic tinea cruris, but scrapings will be negative. Eczema and psoriasis can usually be recognised by their characteristic appearances on non-flexural skin elsewhere.

For limited infection treatment with a topical imidazole is sufficient. For extensive involvement, topical steroid treated cases or when therapy fails, however, oral griseofulvin will be needed, for 3–6 weeks.

Tinea corporis

Tinea corporis is often of animal origin, and is then self-limiting. Lesions are usually multiple and often, but not always, ring-shaped. Because the appearances are so variable, scrapings should be taken from any red, scaly rash that cannot be readily diagnosed. If the disease is limited in extent, a topical agent is usually sufficient; if widespread, then griseofulvin orally is preferable.

Tinea capitis

Many different fungal species can infect hair and scalp skin, with variable prevalence in different parts of the world. Affected hairs may break off a few millimetres above the scalp, producing short stubble, or flush with the scalp, giving bald patches which show black dots in dark-haired patients where hairs have broken off. When there is a marked degree of inflammation, producing an appearance like that of a carbuncle, the lesion is called a *kerion*, and in this circumstance there may be concurrent staphylococcal infection. An appearance known as *favus* is now very rare in the United Kingdom. In this form yellowish cup-shaped crusts develop, together with hair loss. Both kerion and favus can produce permanent alopecia. A summary of the different forms is given in Table 26.9.

Table 26.9 Types of tinea capitis

Clinical pattern	Representative species	Wood's light fluorescence	Source
Patchy baldness, with broken-off hairs and scaling of the scalp	*Microsporum canis*	Blue-green	Puppies, kittens
	Microsporum audouini	Green	Humans
Patchy baldness with black dots	*Trichophyton tonsurans*	–	Humans
	Trichophyton violaceum	–	Humans
Kerion	*Trichophyton verrucosum*	–	Cattle
Favus	*Trichophyton schoenleinii*	Dull green	Humans

Fig. 26.3 Candidiasis, a superficial fungal infection.

Distinction of fungal infection from other causes of patchy hair loss can be made by microscopy and culture.

Tinea of the hand

A diffuse hyperkeratosis with fine powdery accentuation of the palmar creases, usually of only one hand, is the commonest pattern of tinea of the hand. Other clinical pictures are seen, and resemble eczema and psoriasis, so if in doubt scrapings should be taken.

Tinea of nails

In many cases nail infection (onychomycosis) occurs in conjunction with fungal disease elsewhere. Predisposing factors include previous trauma and poor peripheral circulation. The toenails are more commonly affected than fingernails. The changes spread proximally from the free edge. The nail plate becomes discoloured and usually thickened, and may crumble away. It may also separate from the nail bed (onycholysis).

Confirmation of the diagnosis by microscopy and culture of clippings should precede treatment. The differential diagnosis includes psoriasis, in which there is often a distinctive pattern of fine pitting. Candidal infection produces changes that begin proximally. Eczema can simulate fungal infection.

Griseofulvin is the treatment of choice, but the response rate is low with toenails. Treatment may be required for 1–2 years. Concurrent topical tioconazole may improve the outcome.

Candidiasis

Most human candidal infection is caused by *Candida albicans* (Fig. 26.3). This yeast is a common commensal in the gastrointestinal tract, mouth and vagina, but not on the skin. It may become pathogenic in several circumstances. These are outlined in Table 26.10.

Unlike the dermatophyte fungi, *Candida* invades living

Table 26.10 Some factors facilitating candidal infection

Local	General
Maceration of skin	Debility
Topical steroids	Extremes of age
Dentures	Immunosuppression by drugs or
Poor oral hygiene	disease, particularly HIV
High oral carbohydrate levels	Broad-spectrum antibiotics
	Corticosteroids
	Diabetes mellitus
	Iron deficiency
	Cushing's syndrome
	Hypocalcaemia/hypoparathyroidism

tissue. In some circumstances serious systemic infection can occur (see also p. 286). Some of the clinical patterns of candidal infection of the skin and mucosal surfaces are shown in Table 26.11.

When infection is widespread and refractory to treatment this may be due to an immune deficiency syndrome, in which there is an abnormal response to other infections or occasionally a more or less isolated failure to eradicate *Candida*. The skin lesions in such patients often resemble ringworm, and nails as well as nail folds tend to be affected. There are several clinical/genetic types.

In *group I* there is a well-defined major primary immune defect, e.g. Swiss type agammaglobulinaemia. *Group II* comprises those cases without such a primary immune defect, although many do have some abnormality on investigation. Subgroups include:

1. the *Candida* endocrinopathy syndrome, with hypoparathyroidism and Addison's disease being the commoner associated organ-specific autoimmune diseases
2. autosomal recessive
3. autosomal dominant
4. diffuse (severe) mucocutaneous candidiasis
5. late onset candidiasis, in which thymoma and HIV infection should be considered.

Table 26.11 Clinical patterns of *Candida* infection

Type	Pattern of infection	Features
Oral		
Thrush	White patches	Can be scraped off to reveal inflamed mucous membrane
Atrophic candidiasis	Painful red atrophic mucous membrane	Common with antibiotic treatment and dentures
Chronic hyperplastic candidiasis	Thickened white adherent plaques	Needs differentiating from leukoplakia
Angular stomatitis	Soreness and fissuring at the angles	Occurs in folds, usually due to ill-fitting dentures
Skin		
Intertrigo	Sore, red, marginated skin, often with outlying pustules	Due to maceration
Ano-genital		
Vulvo-vaginitis	Itchy, sore with curd-like discharge	Commoner in pregnancy
Balanitis	Tiny red papules and pustules on glans and prepuce	Usually from sexual partner
Nails		
Paronychia	Painful swollen nail folds with loss of adhesion of cuticle	Maceration predisposes. May have poor peripheral circulation
Onychia	Thickened, discoloured nails	Uncommon, often associated with immune defects

Treatment of Candida *infections*

Any remediable predisposing factors should be dealt with. Locally active agents include nystatin, amphotericin B and the imidazoles. For chronic oral candidiasis prolonged treatment is often necessary. Oral ketoconazole is usually required for chronic mucocutaneous candidiasis, a relatively common problem in patients with symptomatic HIV infection.

Pityriasis versicolor

Pityriasis (tinea) versicolor is a superficial infection caused by the mycelial form of the commensal yeast *Pityrosporum orbiculare* (also known as *Malassezia furfur*).

For most patients who have the disorder it is assumed that there has been a change in the pathogenicity of their surface commensal yeasts. Young adults are the most affected and it is seen more in the tropics and subtropics. The distinctive hyper- and hypopigmentation is due to the diffusion into the epidermis of azelaic acid, a fatty acid from the fungus, which affects the melanocytes.

The upper trunk, arms and neck are the commonest sites. Lesions are macular and sharply demarcated, and have fine scaling. They may become confluent over large areas. On sun-protected Caucasian skin the patches are skin-coloured or pale brown, but after sun exposure and in darker races they are hypopigmented.

Scrapings show a mixture of clustered spherical yeasts and short mycelia. By Wood's light the affected areas fluoresce and it is often apparent that the infection is more widespread than can be seen by visible light.

Treatment by 2.5% selenium sulphide in a detergent base applied to affected areas and the scalp – a reservoir of yeasts, left on overnight and repeated a week later – usually clears the condition.

VIRAL DISEASES

Skin lesions are a common feature of many viral infections and may represent the direct consequences of virus replication (e.g. warts), the immune response to a virus, or interaction of the two. Only those where the skin or adjacent mucous membranes are the sole target are discussed here; the remainder, including herpes simplex and zoster, are considered in Chapter 12.

Warts

Warts are hypertrophies of the prickle cell layer of the skin (or adjacent mucous membranes) induced by human papilloma virus. Warts are transmissible, inoculation being favoured by mild trauma. They are commoner in children and young adults, and are usually self-limiting and benign. However, some subtypes of virus (defined by DNA hybridisation techniques), particularly those found in the rare condition epidermodysplasia verruciformis and in the genital tract, predispose to squamous carcinoma.

The hands, feet, face, around the knees, peri-anal and genital skin are the commonest sites. Table 26.12 gives the main clinical varieties.

Because most warts resolve spontaneously, caution is needed in assessing therapy, and methods such as scalpel

Table 26.12 Viral warts

Type of wart	Main site	Appearance
Common	Hand	Dome-shaped, papilliferous surface
Plane (flat)	Face and backs of hands	Flat-topped; smooth papules
Filiform	Face and neck	Elongated
Digitate	Scalp and neck	Elongated with horny cap
Plantar (verruca)	Soles	Circumscribed, often painful papules or nodules with altered surface pattern, sometimes with black dots
Mosaic plantar	Soles	Aggregation of numerous adjacent plantar warts
Ano-genital	Anal and genital regions	Soft, velvety, vegetative papules and plaques

surgery and radiotherapy should be abandoned. For many non-genital warts, salicylic acid paints (or plasters for large plantar warts) are effective. Cryotherapy (p. 1113) is uncomfortable but often more rapidly successful. In selected cases curettage and minimal cautery may be needed.

Venereal warts are frequently associated with other sexually transmitted diseases, requiring appropriate investigations. These lesions usually respond to liquid nitrogen cryotherapy or careful applications of podophyllin paint at weekly intervals, but this agent should be avoided during pregnancy because of the enhanced risk of absorption and fetal damage.

Molluscum contagiosum

Molluscum contagiosum (Fig. 26.4) is a contagious papular eruption caused by a DNA pox virus. It mainly occurs in children. The lesions are smooth, dome-shaped papules, often crater-like with a central keratinous plug or depression. When multiple, they are typically in groups. Lesions are ultimately self-limiting.

Direct microscopic examination of the cheesy contents or an entire curetted lesion reveals the characteristic egg-shaped molluscum bodies. (These are epidermal cells filled with virus particles.) Electron microscopy can also be used.

Single lesions can mimic benign or malignant epithelial tumours, e.g. keratoacanthoma or basal cell carcinoma.

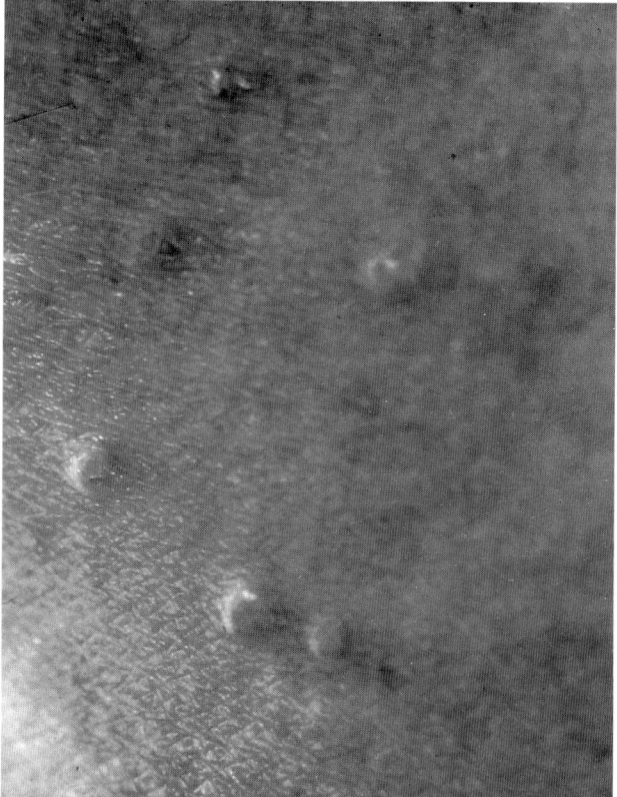

Fig. 26.4   Molluscum contagiosum: smooth papules with a keratinous core.

In young children it is often best to leave the lesions. Treatment is local destruction, e.g. with liquid nitrogen or by mildly traumatising the papules and then painting with iodine.

Orf and milkers' nodules

Orf is a pox viral disease of sheep, usually acquired directly from the peri-oral lesions occurring on lambs. Milkers' nodule is a similar condition acquired from infection of teats of cows and ulcers in the mouths of calves. It is caused by a parapox virus.

Several days after animal contact, a red papule appears, and evolves into a 1–2 cm diameter smooth, bluish-red nodule, the centre of which may develop a crusted surface. There is often a whitish ring around the central crust with orf nodules. There may be lymphangitis and lymphadenopathy, and sometimes a rash on the limbs resembling erythema multiforme (p. 1128). Resolution occurs in 3–4 weeks.

Diagnosis is usually evident from the history. Electron microscopy can confirm the diagnosis. No treatment is required.

Pityriasis rosea

Pityriasis rosea, a common self-limiting disorder, occurs mainly in children and young adults. Clustering of cases suggests an infective cause and a viral aetiology is likely but unproven.

The first lesion to appear, known as the herald patch, is red, circumscribed, slightly scaly and larger than those that will follow about 10 days later. The generalised eruption is maximal on the trunk and proximal aspect of the limbs, and usually includes distinctive ovoid patches whose long axes are parallel to the major skin creases. This produces a pattern somewhat like a Christmas tree on the back. The pink borders of these lesions are separated from the slightly brown centres by collarettes of scale. There is usually an admixture of smaller pink papules. Itching may occur, and occasionally there is malaise and lympadenopathy. The rash usually lasts 4–6 weeks. Recurrences are very unusual.

There are no diagnostic tests. Conditions that may resemble pityriasis rosea include drug eruption, seborrhoeic dermatitis, guttate psoriasis, tinea corporis and secondary syphilis.

Treatment with a mild topical steroid may be helpful.

ARTHROPODS AND THE SKIN

Numerous arthropods can inflict skin lesions on man, by the mechanisms listed below:

1. *mechanical trauma* (e.g. horse-fly, tungiasis)
2. *injection of toxins* (e.g. some spiders, bees, wasps, ants)
3. *hypersensitivity* (local and generalised) to injected materials (e.g. many arthropods, such as fleas, bedbugs); contact reactions (e.g. house dust mite); to an

invading parasite (e.g. scabies); to retained mouth-parts, etc. (e.g. tick bite granulomas)
4. *secondary infection* (e.g. many insect bites, scabies)
5. *transmission of disease* (e.g. leishmaniasis, erythema chronicum migrans – caused by a spirochaete, p. 1007).

Insect bite reactions should be suspected when there are grouped or linear arrays of itchy weals or papules. The lesions last longer than urticaria. Fleas and mites, often from domestic pets, mosquitoes, gnats, midges and bedbugs are frequent causes of this common problem. A careful history and examination of brushings from pets, their bedding, and house dust can help identify the cause.

Scabies

Scabies (Fig. 26.5) is an itchy dermatosis caused by the human mite *Sarcoptes scabiei*.

The spread of scabies requires close bodily contact, as between family members and sexual contacts. The female mite, just visible to the naked eye, makes the necessary journey from one human to another during close bodily contact and burrows into the horny layer, producing a serpiginous greyish elevation 1–10 mm long. Burrows are most commonly seen on the finger webs, wrists, elbows, around the nipples in women and on the male genitalia. In children the palms, soles and even face may be colonised and vesicles and pustules may be evident. In addition there is a widespread papular rash and extensive excoriation, probably the result of an allergic reaction to mite products.

Generally there are only a few burrows at a time, but

Fig. 26.5 Scabies: serpiginous burrow over back of hand.

in so-called crusted or Norwegian scabies there are vast numbers, particularly on the hands. This mainly occurs in mental defectives and the immunosuppressed.

With an initial attack there is a latent period of about 2 months before itching begins, but this is much less with subsequent episodes. The itching is often severe and tends to be worse at night. The distinctive burrows are usually overshadowed by widespread excoriations, eczematisation and secondary infection.

Mites can be extracted from burrows with a needle; somewhat easier is scraping the area after applying a drop of mineral oil or 30% potassium hydroxide and viewing the material microscopically for mites, eggs, faeces, etc.

The patient and all close contacts should be treated (after a hot bath) with a scabicide such as gamma benzene hexachloride (lindane), benzyl benzoate or malathion, from the neck downwards. Pruritus may continue for up to 2 weeks and can be helped by crotamiton (a less effective scabicide which also has antipruritic properties) or a topical steroid.

Other mites

Dogs, cats, birds, grain and stored foodstuffs are sometimes sources of mites that can attack man, producing itchy papules, often topped by tiny vesicles, and weals. Harvest mites, minute red creatures found in grass and other low vegetation, can produce similar and often very florid lesions. Diagnosis involves finding the offending mite, e.g. from brushings of pets.

Fleas

Fleas include varieties that can burrow into skin (e.g. *Tunga penetrans*, found only in the tropics) and those that feed on the skin. In general the human flea is unusual in the UK, but occurs in overcrowded communities with poor hygiene. Bites from fleas living on pets, birds and occasionally wild animals, such as hedgehogs, are very common.

The reaction to a flea bite is a hypersensitivity response. Individual lesions are like urticaria but often have a hae-morrhagic central punctum and last a week or two. They characteristically occur in groups, and often leave hyper-pigmentation as they resolve. Troublesome itching can be treated with an oral antihistamine and secondary infection with an antibiotic.

When the domestic pet is the source, the diagnosis can often be confirmed by examination of brushings from the animal. Flea faeces in this material stain damp white blot-ting paper red. The pet, and often the environment, need appropriate treatment.

Bedbugs

Bedbugs (*Cimex lectularius*) are nocturnal, wingless, blood-sucking insects, live in crevices in the walls, floor and furniture and can best be seen in the middle of the night. The lesions following their bites often do not appear until well into the next day. They mainly occur on the face and upper limbs. The environment should be treated with an insecticide.

Lice

Lice are obligate human parasitic wingless insects. The itchy reactions are a result of sensitisation. There are two species: *Pediculus humanus*, which occurs in two varieties – the head and body louse, and *Phthirus pubis* – the pubic or crab louse.

Head louse infection is very common in children, presenting as intense irritation, particularly at the back of the scalp. Secondary infection is frequent and may be mistakenly diagnosed as impetigo of the scalp. The insect is 3–4 mm long but usually the eggs and egg cases (nits) are much more easily seen, firmly cemented to the hairs. Treatment is with malathion or carbaryl. Contacts should also be treated.

The body louse is rare in developed countries, except in cases of self-neglect. There is widespread irritation with papules and excoriation. The lice and their eggs are best found on the clothing, particularly the seams. Treatment is with lindane.

Pubic lice have legs somewhat like crabs' pincers with which they are often found clinging to hairs. Secondary infection is common, and since these creatures are often acquired during sexual intercourse other venereal disease should be excluded. Treatment is with lindane.

PSORIASIS

Psoriasis is a non-infective, usually chronic inflammatory skin disease with a number of clinical manifestations, the most common of which is red plaques covered by silvery scales (Fig. 26.6). A distinctive arthritis may occur and nails are often involved. Genetic and environmental factors interact to account for the capricious natural history.

Psoriasis occurs in about 2% of the population in Britain, but is less common in other countries, notably West Africa and Japan. The condition may present at any age but onset is most common at puberty and the menopause. Additional triggering factors, both of onset and recurrence, are *infection*, especially streptococcal pharyngitis which characteristically provokes guttate psoriasis; *trauma* to the skin, generating new psoriatic lesions (the Koebner phenomenon, see below); and some *drugs*, notably lithium salts, systemic corticosteroids followed by their rapid withdrawal, and antimalarials. In some subjects UV radiation can initiate psoriasis on exposed skin. Rarely hypocalcaemia provokes psoriasis. The importance of stress is disputed but sudden psychological trauma can play a part in initiating the disease and causing relapse.

The tendency to develop psoriasis is genetically determined but the mode of inheritance remains unclear. There

Fig. 26.6 Psoriasis: the characteristic plaques covered by silvery scales.

is a close association with HLA-CW6 and HLA-DR7, the former conferring a 5–10-fold increased risk.

In the well-established psoriatic lesion there is epidermal thickening with increased mitoses, retention of nuclei in the horny layer (parakeratosis) accounting for the silvery scales, small collections of neutrophil polymorphs in the epidermis, tortuous dilated dermal capillaries and a dermal inflammatory infiltrate. Cell kinetic studies show that epidermal turnover is occurring in 5–7 days, compared with the normal 30–45 days. Epidermal maturation is also abnormal and not just as a consequence of the rapid throughput. At present there is no comprehensive theory to account for the many abnormalities that have been demonstrated in the epidermis, dermis and in circulating granulocytes, lymphocytes and the humoral immune system. From work in which psoriatic skin is explanted on to athymic nude mice it seems that the increased proliferative rate is intrinsic to the skin. It is likely that circulating factors determine the overall activity of the psoriasis and maintain the inflammatory process in the plaques.

The different patterns of psoriasis result from variations in expression of the disease (guttate, erythrodermic and pustular types) and modification of the features at certain sites, notably the scalp, flexures, palms and soles. The extent and duration are usually unpredictable, although some patterns are more likely to improve spontaneously, e.g. guttate psoriasis. Psoriasis means a condition (-iasis) of itching (psor-), but pruritus is not inevitable.

Discoid or plaque psoriasis. The well-defined, silvery-scaled red plaques may be found on any site, but knees and elbows, extensor surfaces of limbs and lower back are very commonly affected. Scratching the scales reveals many tiny bleeding points.

Flexural psoriasis. Psoriasis at sites such as the axillae, groins and beneath breasts is less readily recognised because the plaques are smooth, but usually remain more sharply defined than eczema. They are typically symmetrical.

Scalp psoriasis. Scaling often becomes very thick, beneath which are tell-tale areas of well-defined erythema.

Psoriasis of palms and soles. This may be more hyperkeratotic, without the silvery scale, but usually remains well defined.

Guttate psoriasis. There are numerous scaly papules and small plaques. This type of psoriasis mainly occurs in children and adolescents.

Erythrodermic psoriasis. Universal (or nearly so) involvement of the skin can produce metabolic consequences such as hypothermia and hypoproteinaemia (see also p. 1132).

Pustular psoriasis. Pustules occur when the neutrophil collections become clinically visible. The main varieties are a form localised to palms and soles (Plate 4, p. 1131), and a generalised type (Fig. 26.7). In the latter the patient is ill, with fever and leucocytosis, and large areas of erythema develop myriads of small sterile pustules which soon dry up and desquamate, to be followed by further waves of pustules. Systemic steroids, intensive topical steroid therapy, occasionally infections and hypocalcaemia may act as triggers. As with erythroderma, management entails rest, prevention of hypothermia, and maintenance of fluid, electrolyte and protein balance, as well as controlling the disease process. Localised pustular psoriasis of palms and soles is probably genetically distinct, there being no association with HLA-CW6 or HLA-DR7, and the condition often occurs without psoriasis elsewhere. Tar and dithranol are contra-indicated in generalised pustular psoriasis and generally unhelpful in palmo-plantar pustular psoriasis.

Psoriatic nail changes. The common patterns of psoriatic nail changes, often occurring together, are:

1. multiple small pits, resembling a thimble (Fig. 26.8)
2. onycholysis (separation of nail), often with an adjacent zone of orange discoloration
3. subungual (nail bed) keratosis
4. thickening and distortion of nails.

Nail changes are very common with psoriatic arthropathy involving the fingers.

Psoriatic arthropathy. Probably about 5% of psoriatics have a seronegative arthritis, although a much higher proportion have abnormalities detected by isotopic bone scans. Different patterns include:

1. distal arthritis – terminal interphalangeal joints of

Fig. 26.7 Generalised pustular psoriasis, showing pustules and desquamation.

Fig. 26.8 Psoriatic nails showing thimble-like pitting.

     fingers and interphalangeal joints of toes
2. simulation of rheumatoid arthritis, but more asymmetrical
3. sacroiliitis and ankylosing spondylitis
4. arthritis mutilans – involving multiple joints with marked bone resorption.

See page 999 for a full description of diagnosis and management.

Table 26.13 Treatment choices in psoriasis

Form	Site	First choice	Second choice	Third choice
Plaque	Face, flexures, genitalia	Topical steroid	Mild tar or weak dithranol	
	Scalp	Tar gel or pomade	Dithranol	Topical steroid
	Trunk, limbs: few plaques	Dithranol	Tar	Topical steroid
	Trunk, limbs: many plaques	Dithranol ± UVB UVB	PUVA	Systemic therapy, e.g. methotrexate
	Palms and soles	Topical steroid Tar Dithranol	PUVA	Oral retinoid
Guttate		Mild tar	UVB	Topical steroid
Erythrodermic with systemic complications		Oral retinoid	Methotrexate	Systemic steroid
Pustular psoriasis	Palms and soles	Topical steroid	PUVA	Oral retinoid
	Generalised	Oral retinoid	Methotrexate	Other systemic therapy

Treatment

The choice of treatment will depend on many factors. These include the capabilities and lifestyle of the patient as well as the type, location, extent and severity of the psoriasis. The options shown in Table 26.13 will not be appropriate for every patient, and are often used in combination. Some patients will prefer not to have any treatment. Nails do not respond well to topical therapy, but may improve with the rest of the psoriasis, especially when systemic treatments are used.

Topical therapy

Rest and bland applications are important in acutely inflamed psoriasis, erythrodermic and generalised pustular psoriasis. Many cases with discoid lesions respond well to tar and dithranol preparations, although, particularly with the latter, it is wise to begin with a weak preparation and gradually increase the potency to minimise irritation. Dithranol stains the skin but this fades after treatment is stopped. Topical steroids are less likely to clear psoriasis completely, but with due attention to their potential hazards they are useful for areas readily irritated, such as the flexures, genitalia, ears and face; they are often more effective on the palms and soles. The most potent preparations are best avoided, except on palms and soles, and even there they should be restricted to short courses.

Ultraviolet (UV) radiation and photochemotherapy

UVB (p. 1143) is used both alone, e.g. for guttate psoriasis, and together with other modalities. Photochemotherapy (also known as PUVA) is the combination of long-wave UVA and the photosensitising drug psoralen, usually taken orally 2 hours previously. It is a powerful treatment for psoriasis but prolonged use is likely to age the skin prematurely and to induce non-melanoma skin cancer. Photochemotherapy is restricted to specialist centres, but is valuable for extensive plaque psoriasis when topical therapy is poorly tolerated or has failed, and can be successful for erythrodermic and pustular forms.

Systemic therapy

For the most severe forms of psoriasis, drugs with antimitotic and immunosuppressant actions are used. Methotrexate is effective and reasonably safe. In long-term use hepatic fibrosis can occur and liver biopsies are recommended every 1–2 years to identify this before it is irreversible. Alcohol should be avoided. Cyclosporin A has recently been introduced for the treatment of cases where methotrexate is unsuitable. This drug is not antimitotic, and probably works by modulating the immune system. The main hazard is nephrotoxicity. Vitamin A derivatives (retinoids) with less toxicity than vitamin A itself have been found of value in pustular and erythrodermic psoriasis, and useful in combination with other treatments, e.g. photochemotherapy. Retinoids have a number of side-effects and, like methotrexate, are teratogenic, but they are not cytotoxic or immunosuppressant. They probably influence the disturbed maturation of the epidermis in psoriasis.

ECZEMA AND DERMATITIS

The word 'eczema' is derived from Greek and means 'the result of boiling out or over'. It is a pattern of inflammation with many possible causes rather than a disease. The different types are unified histopathologically by the presence of spongiosis in the epidermis.

The term 'dermatitis' is often used to imply an eczema of external origin, but it should always be qualified, as in 'contact allergic dermatitis', since 'dermatitis' is used in many other contexts, e.g. dermatitis artefacta, dermatitis herpetiformis, etc.

Eczema is usually itchy and red; when the inflammation is intense, vesicles are seen and there is oozing from the surface (Fig. 26.9). If the process continues, scaling and thickening occur, and with rubbing and scratching lichenification (development of leather-like plaques) is common.

The earliest and most distinctive pathological change is spongiosis, the accumulation of oedema fluid within and between keratinocytes. Viewed in microscopic section, this produces an appearance somewhat like a sponge. In acute eczema the process extends to produce intra-epidermal vesicles. In the dermis, and to a lesser extent the epidermis, there is an inflammatory infiltrate in which lymphocytes are prominent. With time, both the epidermis and dermis become thickened.

The aetiological factors in eczema include:

1. skin irritants
2. contact allergens
3. friction, low humidity, UV light
4. infections (bacterial, dermatophytes, yeasts)
5. atopic constitution
6. drugs and foods
7. local factors: venous stasis, ichthyosis.

Several may act in concert, particularly with eczema of the hand and lower leg, and not infrequently treatment is

Fig. 26.9 Eczema. With intense inflammation there are vesicles and oozing; if the process continues, scaling and thickening occur.

an inadvertent contributory factor. A careful history is essential in the evaluation of eczema. Several different clinical patterns of eczema and dermatitis (with eczematous features) are recognised. The basis for these patterns is well understood in some instances (e.g. contact allergic dermatitis) but obscure in others (e.g. discoid eczema). Since successful management depends upon recognising external factors that are contributing to the skin disease, it is helpful to classify according to whether the disease process is primarily exogenous or endogenous.

Whatever the cause, while active, eczema tends to spread, often beyond any recognisable stimulus such as a contact allergen. The face is often affected, even when not directly exposed to a causative agent.

EXOGENOUS ECZEMA

Irritant contact dermatitis

When the skin changes are a direct result of exposure and allergic mechanisms are not involved, the rash is termed irritant contact dermatitis. Not all reactions to irritants are eczematous; for example, the agent may produce necrosis or urticaria. Because obvious irritants tend to be avoided, the main problems occur with those which require prolonged and repeated contact, e.g. detergents, alkalis, mineral oils and organic solvents. Atopic individuals are particularly susceptible, as are housewives, hairdressers and those in a number of industrial occupations. Even when a period of avoidance produces healing, chronic irritant dermatitis tends to readily recur with re-exposure.

Allergic contact dermatitis

Allergic contact dermatitis is the response to a substance to which the individual has become sensitised. Most such substances are of low molecular weight and penetrate the skin to behave as haptens. There is conjugation with a skin protein, and the complete antigen is taken up by the Langerhans cells, which migrate to regional lymph nodes and act as antigen-presenting cells in a T lymphocyte mediated (type IV) immune response. All subsequent contact with the sensitiser then results in an acute eczematous reaction. This type of response is uncommon in children, although contact urticaria is frequent in atopics (see below).

Contact allergic dermatitis usually begins at the site of contact, but the clinical picture can at times be deceptive, e.g. nail varnish resin which causes no trouble locally but gives rise to eczematous patches where it is transferred to the face and neck by the fingers.

Many factors determine the acquisition of contact allergy. Some substances, e.g. epoxy resin and poison ivy, are inherently more likely to sensitise. Occlusion (e.g. a hand in a glove) and skin damage (e.g. from irritants) enhance penetration. It is possible that some individuals are more likely than others to be sensitised. The thick horny layer of the palms renders them less likely than the dorsa of the hands to be affected.

Once initiated, repeated exposure tends to produce increasingly severe and widespread dermatitis, and sites far removed, such as the eyelids, can be involved. Some common sensitisers are listed in Table 26.14.

Investigation: patch testing

The allergic state is reproduced in miniature by the application of a non-irritating dose of a suspected chemical beneath an occluding disc or patch placed on the back for 48 hours. Because some allergens are ubiquitous, a selection of common sensitisers is tested as well as any chosen on the basis of the patient's history. A positive reaction does not prove the cause of a patient's rash, but does help confirm suspicions and suggest unsuspected materials. Positive reactions may be only of past relevance.

Light-induced eczema

When eczema occurs on light-exposed skin the following should be considered:

1. *photo-contact allergy*, e.g. musk ambrette (a perfume in after-shave lotions); sunscreen medicaments
2. *photosensitive drug eruption*, e.g. chlorpromazine; sulphonamide; thiazide
3. *exacerbation of existing eczema*, e.g. atopic dermatitis.

Phototoxic reactions, which resemble sunburn rather than eczema, can occur following contact with tar and its derivatives, some dyes and plants, and with drugs (p. 1136).

Sensitivity to airborne allergens can closely mimic light reactions, but areas normally spared from sun exposure, such as the skin beneath the ears, under the chin and around the eyes, are involved. Dermatomyositis may occasionally mimic a light-induced eruption.

Summary 1   Classification of eczema

Exogenous	Endogenous
Irritant contact dermatitis	Atopic eczema/dermatitis
Allergic contact dermatitis	Discoid (nummular) eczema
Light-induced dermatitis	Seborrhoeic eczema/dermatitis
	Pompholyx
	Asteatotic eczema
	Gravitational eczema

ENDOGENOUS ECZEMA

Atopic eczema/dermatitis

Atopic eczema/dermatitis is closely associated with asthma, hay fever, urticaria and dry skin. There is usually a family history of one or more of these. The separate condition ichthyosis vulgaris (p. 1127) is probably more common in atopic individuals than the rest of the population. The skin readily becomes itchy in response to a number of allergic and non-allergic stimuli, and the pruritus may be dis-

Table 26.14   Some common sensitisers

Chemical	Source
Nickel	Jewellery, watch bands, silver coins
Chromate	Wet cement, many engineering processes
Epoxy resin	Two-part glues
Paraphenylenediamine	Blue-black hair dye
Rubber anti-oxidants	Gloves, shoes
Preservatives	Cosmetics and medicaments
Lanolin	Cosmetics and medicaments
Topical drugs	Neomycin, antihistamines, sulphonamides
Colophony	Sticking plasters

proportionate to the physical signs. High levels of circulating IgE antibodies are very common.

The disorder is very common, most cases beginning in infancy, and at least 5% of the population is affected to some degree. There is often a fluctuating course, but most cases clear up by adulthood, the majority within the first 5 years of life.

The fundamental basis for atopic eczema remains obscure. A number of immunological abnormalities have been described, including the overproduction of IgE, reduced numbers of suppressor/cytotoxic T lymphocytes, and cutaneous basophil hypersensitivity, e.g. to house dust mite antigen. Environmental factors are important determinants of fluctuations. These include ingested proteins (e.g. dairy products and eggs), and exposure to house dust mites, pollens and pet hair. Wool next to the skin frequently causes irritation. Extremes of climate often worsen the disease. Beyond a certain level of colonisation, *Staphylococcus aureus* may produce flares of erythema and pruritus.

Onset is often in the first 3 months of life. Itching is the major symptom and at times there may be little rash. In infancy the skin is often patchily dry and red, with episodes of vesiculation and crusting. By 1–2 years the elbow and knee flexures, wrists, hands and tops of the feet are typically involved. With prolonged rubbing and scratching, papules and then leathery plaques (lichenification) are seen. At any stage secondary infection may occur with superimposition of impetigo and follicular pustules. Urticaria from contact, e.g. with a pet or foods, is also common.

Eczema may be complicated by erythroderma (p. 1132). Severely affected children are often growth-retarded. Herpes simplex infection can be widespread (eczema herpeticum) and, particularly in the very young, may be disseminated to internal organs.

Treatment

The mainstays of treatment are avoidance of irritants, *mild* topical steroids, plentiful use of emollients when the skin is dry, antibiotics when necessary, tar preparations for the more chronic and less inflamed lesions, and a sedative antihistamine at night. Cotton clothes and use of a soap substitute, e.g. emulsifying ointment or aqueous cream BP, are helpful. Current evidence would suggest that children of atopic families should be breast-fed, at least up to 3 months if possible. Subsequent dietary manipulation may be helpful but should only be carried out with supervision.

Discoid eczema

Discoid (nummular) eczema involves discrete rounded patches of eczema, usually symmetrically distributed, for which there is no apparent cause. Discoid lesions may occur in atopic eczema and contact dermatitis, so these diagnoses should be excluded. The aetiology is unknown, and treatment is symptomatic.

Seborrhoeic eczema/dermatitis

Seborrhoeic eczema/dermatitis is of distinctive appearance and location. The cause is unknown but *Pityrosporum* yeasts play a part. There is usually no correlation with sebaceous activity although it is a disorder of areas where sebaceous glands are plentiful. Severe seborrhoeic dermatitis is an early feature in about one-third of AIDS patients.

There is less itching than with other eczemas. The lesions are yellowish-red, scaly away from flexures, and involve some or all of the following sites: scalp, eyelids, eyebrows, sides of nose, ears, axillae and groins, beneath the breasts, front of the chest, and upper back.

The differential diagnosis will depend on the sites affected. In the scalp, psoriasis can be very similar. In the flexures, psoriasis, contact allergic dermatitis, dermatophyte infections and candidiasis may need to be excluded; the truncal form can resemble pityriasis rosea and pityriasis versicolor (the latter diagnosed from a scraping). Methyldopa can produce a seborrhoeic dermatitis-like drug eruption.

The addition of sulphur, a mild tar, salicylic acid or an imidazole to a suitable topical steroid is often helpful. Shampoos containing selenium sulphide or zinc pyrithione are useful for scalp involvement.

Pompholyx

Pompholyx is an eruption of vesicles on the sides of fingers, palms and soles. Itching may be severe. The condition is usually episodic. Causes of pompholyx include: dermatitis or fungal infection of the feet (producing pompholyx of hands); ingestion of a contact allergen, e.g. nickel; and stress. Often no cause can be found. Treatment is symptomatic.

Asteatotic eczema

Asteatotic eczema is a mildly inflammatory condition which occurs mainly in the elderly on the shins, as erythema with a crazy paving-like pattern of superficial fissuring and scaling. It may be a result of reduced epidermal lipids. Hypothyroidism, uraemia, dehydration, low humidity and overzealous cleansing may contribute.

It often responds to less bathing and to emollients. A mild topical steroid ointment can be added if necessary.

Gravitational eczema

Eczema often occurs on the lower legs as a response to chronic venous hypertension, in association with haemosiderin staining, patchy atrophy, sclerosis, oedema and perhaps ulceration. It is commonest near the medial malleolus due to a previous deep vein thrombosis, but may also be seen in relation to varicose veins and incompetent perforating veins (p. 1145). Patches indistinguishable from discoid eczema may spread elsewhere.

Important in management are improvement of the venous hypertension, e.g. with support hosiery, and avoidance of potent topical steroids and potential sensitisers, such as neomycin.

Symptomatic treatment of eczema

Any causative and aggravating factors should be removed if at all possible. Acute weeping eczema can be soothed with wet compresses, e.g. aluminium acetate lotion BNF or 1:10 000 potassium permanganate solution, followed by a topical steroid cream. In some cases, particularly contact allergy, when a cause has been recognised and dealt with, a short course of systemic steroids is justified. For less acute eczema, a topical steroid of lowest effective potency is needed, often in a greasy base. If the surface is dry, additional applications of an emollient are helpful and reduce the likelihood of overuse of the steroid. For chronic lichenification, tar preparations (e.g. as impregnated bandages) are valuable.

ICHTHYOSIS

The term ichthyosis is used for a number of conditions in which there is either a disorder of keratinisation or shedding of the horny layer producing persistent, generalised, scaly skin. Most types of ichthyosis are inherited and present in infancy or childhood. Onset in adulthood can be associated with an underlying neoplasm (p. 1139).

Ichthyosis vulgaris is the only common type, occurring in about 1 per 300 of the population. It is inherited as an autosomal dominant trait, and has distinctive histology: absence of the granular cell layer of the epidermis. Individuals have rough skin with white scales, maximal on the extensor surfaces and sparing the antecubital and popliteal fossae. There are often rough follicular papules (keratosis pilaris) on the upper arms and thighs. The physical signs are worse in winter. Avoidance of soap and regular use of emollients are helpful measures.

Sex-linked recessive ichthyosis occurs in about 1 per 6000.

The female carrier may show mild changes, but the fully developed condition as seen in the male is more severe than ichthyosis vulgaris, with large brownish scales; the flexures are involved. The condition is characterised by steroid sulphatase deficiency.

Acquired ichthyosis has a similar clinical pattern to ichthyosis vulgaris. As well as being associated with neoplasia, particularly Hodgkin's disease, it can occur in gross nutritional deficiency.

REACTION PATTERNS

Despite the large number of named diseases, as an organ the skin has a limited range of reactions to noxious stimuli such as circulating immune complexes and infections. Some of these reaction patterns have sufficiently few common causes that their recognition can be a helpful step in arriving at a diagnosis. This may be particularly true when the patient has other symptoms, e.g. cough or malaise, for which there is no obvious cause.

A single aetiological factor may produce one or more of the reaction patterns described below. For example, the hepatitis B virus may lead to urticaria if the effect on dermal blood vessels is fully reversible, but purpuric vasculitis if the damage is more profound.

URTICARIA AND ANGIO-OEDEMA

The characteristic lesion in urticaria is a weal (Plate 5, p. 1131). This is due to oedema in the dermis, so weals are raised and often pallid, but surrounded by a zone of erythema. Urticaria is evanescent, usually lasting from minutes to a few hours (rarely more than 24 hours) and fades without trace. Itching may be severe. Lesions initially like urticaria may occur in vasculitis, arthropod bites and stings, and lupus erythematosus, but in these circumstances they are more long-lasting.

Angio-oedema occurs at a deeper level, in the subcutaneous tissues, particularly where they are rather loosely organised such as in and around the mouth (Fig. 26.10), around the eyes and on the scrotum. The lesions are larger, less well defined and not necessarily itchy.

The basis for urticaria and angio-oedema is vasodilation and extravasation of fluid due to release of mediators from mast cells and/or basophils. In some circumstances the

Fig. 26.10 Angio-oedema showing swelling of the upper lip.

mediators responsible can cause hypotension and bronchospasm, constituting anaphylactic shock (p. 110). Mechanisms include IgE and immune complex mediated reactions, and direct effects of chemicals, e.g. toxins and drugs. Symptomatic treatment is with antihistamines.

Hereditary angio-oedema is a rare but potentially life-threatening condition, in which non-pruritic swellings occur in the gastrointestinal and respiratory tracts as well as the skin and adjacent mucous membranes. The taking of a careful family history may suggest the diagnosis. There is either deficiency or an abnormality of the inhibitor of activated complement component C1. The best laboratory investigation is the measurement of C1 esterase inhibitor by antigenic activity or functional assay. Also useful is the demonstration of low C4 and C2, the substrates of activated and unopposed C1.

Common causes of urticaria and angio-oedema are listed in Table 26.15.

ERYTHEMA MULTIFORME

Erythema multiforme has a variety of causes, which include:

1. herpes simplex
2. other infections, e.g. mycoplasma
3. drugs, e.g. sulphonamides
4. pregnancy
5. collagen vascular disease, e.g. systemic lupus erythematosus.

The distinctive features of erythema multiforme are the target lesion, the distribution of the rash and the histology.

Summary 2   Reaction patterns

● Urticaria and angio-oedema

● Erythema multiforme

● Erythema nodosum

● Pyoderma gangrenosum

● Cutaneous vasculitis

● Erythroderma

Table 26.15 Common causes of urticaria and angio-oedema

Drugs	Plants
Penicillin, aspirin, X-ray contrast medium	Stinging nettles
Foods	**Systemic disease**
Azodyes, benzoate preservatives (chronic urticaria)	Hepatitis, B, other virus infections, systemic lupus erythematosus
Arthropod reactions	**Contact urticaria**
	Some foods and pet saliva on atopics
Transfusion of blood products and foreign proteins	**Inhalants**
	Grass pollens, house dust
Physical stimuli	
Light pressure (dermographism), cold, light, increase in body temperature (cholinergic urticaria)	

It is an acute eruption usually lasting about 3 weeks, maximally involving the hands and feet, forearms, elbows and knees. Among a variety of erythematous lesions there are usually some target lesions. These have a purplish or blistering centre inside one or more red rings. The mucosae of the mouth, genitalia and eyes may be involved (Stevens-Johnson syndrome) with blistering and haemorrhage. Sometimes internal organs, e.g. the kidney and lungs, are affected. There is an interval of about a week between the stimulus and the eruption, but this is shorter with recurrences. The pathogenesis is not fully understood.

ERYTHEMA NODOSUM

The plaques and nodules of erythema nodosum (Plate 6, p. 1131) are red, hot and tender. They typically occur over the shins but may be more widespread on the legs, on the outer aspect of the arms and sides of the neck. Erythema nodosum is often accompanied by fever, malaise and painful joints. Lesions disappear over 3–6 weeks, with the same colour changes as in a resolving bruise. It is mainly a condition of young adults.

Probably most cases are due to circulating immune complexes lodging in or near the venules in the deep dermis and subcutaneous fat. The causes of erythema nodosum include:

1. sarcoidosis
2. streptococcal infection
3. tuberculosis
4. other infections, e.g. yersinia, deep mycoses (where prevalent), chlamydia psittaci and lymphogranuloma venereum
5. drugs (uncommon), e.g. oral contraceptives, sulphonamides
6. ulcerative colitis and Crohn's disease
7. leukaemia and Hodgkin's disease.

Investigations should include haemoglobin, white blood cell count, erythrocyte sedimentation rate, antistreptolysin O titre, chest X-ray, and measurement of antibodies to likely infective agents, e.g. *Chlamydia psittaci* if there has

been exposure to birds. A tuberculin test will be strongly positive in tuberculosis but commonly negative in sarcoidosis (p. 510).

Similar but smaller nodules are seen in Behçet's disease (p. 1002). Erythema nodosum leprosum is clinically and histologically quite different (p. 278). The lesions of nodular vasculitis are more persistent and occur more on the calves. Thrombophlebitis and persistent insect bite reactions are usually asymmetrical.

Most cases last 4–6 weeks. Bed rest is advisable at first, and a non-steroidal anti-inflammatory drug may be helpful. Further action will depend on the cause.

PYODERMA GANGRENOSUM

Pyoderma gangrenosum (Fig. 26.11) is an uncommon, non-infective ulcerating condition frequently with an underlying systemic disease. The lower limbs and face are the most common sites but any part of the body may be affected. The necrotic area often begins as a sterile pustule which breaks down and spreads, sometimes to form a huge ulcer, with a characteristic ragged, purplish overhanging edge. Lesions may be multiple.

The pathogenesis is unclear, but many patients have evidence of a depressed immune system. Causes include:

1. ulcerative colitis
2. Crohn's disease
3. rheumatoid arthritis
4. other forms of arthritis
5. leukaemia, lymphomas, monoclonal gammopathies and myeloma.

The differential diagnosis includes infective causes of ulceration (e.g. postoperative gangrene, p. 1115) and vasculitic disorders (e.g. Wegener's granulomatosis). Cultures for aerobic and anaerobic bacteria and other organisms, and a biopsy should be taken before treatment.

Treatment of pyoderma gangrenosum is with high-dose corticosteroids, although for small lesions topical and intralesional corticosteroids can be effective.

Fig. 26.11 Pyoderma gangrenosum sometimes forms a huge ulcer, with a characteristic ragged, purplish overhanging edge.

CUTANEOUS VASCULITIS

Palpable purpura is the hallmark of cutaneous vasculitis (Fig. 26.12), but depending on the type and degree of vessel wall damage, other lesions, not all of which are purpuric, may occur; these include livedo reticularis, weals, papules, pustules, infarcts and ulcers.

Aetiological factors of cutaneous vasculitis include:

1. bacteria, e.g. streptococci, gonococci, *Mycobacterium tuberculosis* (erythema induratum) and *M. leprae* (erythema nodosum leprosum)
2. viruses, e.g. hepatitis B
3. neoplasia, e.g. lymphoma
4. drugs, e.g. sulphonamides, thiazides, captopril
5. food additives, e.g. tartrazine
6. autoimmune diseases, e.g. lupus erythematosus, polyarteritis nodosa, scleroderma.

The initial event is damage to the endothelium of the vessel. Both circulating and resident extravascular inflammatory cells are then activated to release mediators, some of which have destructive effects, while others contribute to repair. The net result depends on many factors: these include the nature of the initial insult, the type and location of the vessels affected and the adequacy of the collateral blood supply. One of the most common histological appearances is accumulation of neutrophils, their breakdown products, and nuclear debris around damaged

Fig. 26.12   Palpable purpura is the hallmark of cutaneous vasculitis, but other lesions may occur.

venules, an appearance termed *leucocytoclastic vasculitis*. Sometimes vasculitis occurs because there is inadequate clearance of a potential cause, such as circulating immune complexes, from the circulation, or there is a deficiency in repair mechanisms, e.g. removal of fibrin is too slow to maintain patency of affected vessels. A defect in the reticulo-endothelial system may account for the occurrence of vasculitis in lymphomas, other malignancies and sarcoidosis. Sometimes the localisation of vasculitic lesions can be explained by circumstances that slow blood flow, e.g. in the lower limbs and where skin is cooled by overlying fat.

As well as attempting to find the cause, it is of clinical importance to know whether other organs are being affected, especially the brain, heart, kidneys, lungs and gut.

There is no entirely satisfactory classification of vasculitis. Approaches used include:

1. cause (but often one cannot be found)
2. type of vessel and nature of the inflammatory infiltrate
3. clinical pattern.

For example, Henoch-Schönlein purpura is defined by the pattern of organ involvement. Some multisystem vasculitic syndromes are shown in Table 26.16.

Evaluation of vasculitis includes an assessment of:

1. what is being damaged (evidence of nervous system, heart, kidney or eye involvement requires more urgent action than involvement of the skin alone)
2. initiating factors, e.g. circulating immune complexes – the antigen might be an infectious agent, e.g. *Mycobacterium tuberculosis*, a drug or auto-antigen – and cryoproteins
3. perpetuating factors, e.g. a defect in the complement system, reticulo-endothelial system or fibrinolysis.

From this evaluation it may be possible to make a diagnosis and a plan for treatment.

Table 26.16   Some multisystem vasculitides that may involve the skin

Clinical patterns	Other organs commonly involved
Henoch-Schönlein purpura	Joints, gut, kidney
Polyarteritis nodosa	Kidneys, gut, cardiovascular system, nervous system, muscles and joints
Temporal arteritis	Eyes
Wegener's granulomatosis	Kidneys and respiratory tract
Malignant atrophic papulosis (Degos' disease)	Gut and brain
Lupus erythematosus	Widespread

Clinical features

Henoch-Schönlein purpura

Henoch-Schönlein purpura comprises arthralgia, abdominal pain and vasculitic rash, often with renal involvement. Children are predominantly affected. Streptococcal sore

1 Impetigo.

2 Erysipelas.

3 Fungal infection.

4 Pustular psoriasis.

5 Urticaria: arcuate weals.

6 Erythema nodosum.

7 Photosensitivity reaction.

8 Malignant melanoma.

9 Kaposi's sarcoma.

throat and upper respiratory virus infections are the most common recognisable causes. The rash is mainly on the buttocks and extensor surfaces of the limbs. As well as purpura there are usually erythematous macules and papules, and urticarial weals.

A small proportion of those who present with haematuria and proteinuria will progress to chronic progressive renal disease, but most will resolve in time. The intestinal involvement may result in bloody stools and occasionally obstruction.

The lesions are characterised by a leucocytoclastic vasculitis, and in many cases there is deposition of IgA around venules.

There is no specific treatment but some authorities use high-dose corticosteroids if there is severe renal disease.

Polyarteritis nodosa

Polyarteritis nodosa, or PAN (p. 1023), is a multisystem disorder in which there is necrotising vasculitis of small and medium-sized arteries. The distinctive feature in the skin is the occurrence of nodules along the course of subcutaneous arteries, best felt on the lower limb. In addition to nodules there are often purpuric papules, weals, or plaques of gangrene. Livedo reticularis, a net-like arrangement of bluish venules, is common.

Hypertension, renal disease and coronary artery disease are common. Abdominal pain may be due to bowel ischaemia or pancreatitis. The nervous system is often affected, with an asymmetrical polyneuritis the most distinctive feature. Muscle and joint pains are common and there is usually fever, leucocytosis and a high ESR.

The cause of PAN is usually unknown, but in some cases there is a preceding infection, e.g. streptococcal or hepatitis B, and occasionally a drug can be implicated, e.g. sulphonamides.

The differential diagnosis includes rheumatoid disease, lupus erythematosus, systemic sclerosis, Wegener's granulomatosis, allergic granulomatosis (Churg-Strauss syndrome), thrombotic thrombocytopenic purpura, cryoglobulinaemia, and in children, Kawasaki's disease (p. 1116). The disease is treated with high doses of corticosteroids.

Malignant atrophic papulosis

Malignant atrophic papulosis (Degos' disease) is a rare but very distinctive condition in which insignificant-looking red papules become slowly necrotic with a greyish-white central scale and heal with porcelain-like white scars.

Similar lesions occur internally, particularly in the intestine, and much of the high mortality is due to perforation or haemorrhage. The brain and kidney may also be affected.

Rheumatoid disease

Small purple or black spots around the nail folds are very characteristic of rheumatoid disease (p. 991), although also seen in other vasculitic diseases.

ERYTHRODERMA

Erythroderma, or exfoliative dermatitis, is redness of all or nearly all the skin. There is usually some degree of scaling. Most cases of erythroderma evolve from more limited eczema or psoriasis (p. 1122).

The principal causes include eczema; psoriasis; drugs, especially gold, allopurinol and sulphonamides; and lymphoma and leukaemia. The cause can usually be determined from the history and a skin biopsy, but in some cases no aetiology is found.

The skin is red, hot to the touch and often oedematous; itching can be severe and scaling is variable. Patients feel uncomfortably cold.

Erythroderma can have serious metabolic consequences, particularly in the elderly. The greatly increased blood flow through the skin, with loss of normal capacity for vasoconstriction, leads to hypothermia in a cold environment. Blood flow to other organs can be greatly diminished. There is increased fluid loss from the skin surface, with compensatory thirst and oliguria. Anaemia is common, and in part is due to a state of malabsorption secondary to the skin disease (dermatogenic enteropathy). Serum albumin falls due to loss from shed skin scales and reduced synthesis. The skin is more prone to infection and thrombophlebitis is common. Lymphadenopathy usually develops, even when the erythroderma is not due to lymphoma or leukaemia.

Systemic corticosteroids are needed for severe cases. Maintenance of fluid balance and body temperature is important and use of appropriate emollients can be helpful (p. 1112). More specific treatment will depend on the underlying cause.

BLISTERING DISEASES

Blisters are focal collections of free fluid in the skin. By convention small ones are called vesicles and larger ones bullae. They are the result of a defect or disturbance in the normal mechanisms that hold the components of the skin together. Extensive blistering produces a serious loss of normal skin function, and before effective treatment was available some of the bullous diseases had a high mortality.

Many different pathological processes can result in the clinical appearance of a blister. The diagnosis may be obvious from the history, such as in an insect bite reaction, but often there is a differential diagnosis and investigations are necessary. Light microscopy of an early blister, preferably one less than 24 hours old (before re-epithelialisation has begun), will provide useful evidence as to the level of the split in the skin and sometimes details of the pathogenetic mechanism, e.g. spongiosis. Electron microscopy allows a much more detailed analysis of blister formation and is of particular importance in the accurate diagnosis of epidermolysis bullosa, a heterogeneous group of inherited blistering disorders. Immunological phenomena are central to some of the bullous diseases, particularly pemphigus, pemphigoid and dermatitis herpetiformis, and these are best demonstrated on a sample of unfixed skin from just beyond the edge of a blister (peribullous skin). Other tests that may be indicated include serum for antibodies (see below), bacteriological and viral studies on blister fluid, and when appropriate porphyrin estimations and patch testing.

Pemphigus vulgaris

Pemphigus vulgaris is an uncommon, chronic, intra-epidermal blistering disease of unknown aetiology, characterised by the presence in affected skin and mucosa of an IgG antibody, which localises to the cell wall of keratinocytes (Fig. 26.13). A split forms within the epidermis.

The disease is most common in middle age and the Jewish race. The characteristic antibody is usually found in the bloodstream, and antibody titres approximately correlate with disease activity. Relapse is sometimes shown to be preceded by an increased titre. The pathology of pemphigus has been reproduced in vitro by the addition of high titre serum to skin explants. The pemphigus antibody probably brings about separation of keratinocytes by acti-

vating proteinases. Occasionally pemphigus is associated with other immunological diseases: thymoma, myasthenia gravis and systemic lupus erythematosus.

Pemphigus often begins in the mouth and sometimes other mucous membranes, with non-healing erosions. Blisters appear sooner or later on previously normal-looking skin, and when the disease is active, sideways pressure with a finger on unblistered skin can produce new blisters (Nikolsky sign). Increasing numbers of flaccid blisters appear, and when they burst, leave erosions. The resultant problems of infections and fluid loss are similar to the consequences of extensive burns.

The diagnosis is made from characteristic histology, showing a suprabasal split and free-floating keratinocytes (acantholysis). Immunohistochemical techniques show that the keratinocytes are coated with IgG. In all but localised or treated disease the pemphigus antibody can be demonstrated in the serum.

Treatment is with high doses of corticosteroids (about 80 mg prednisolone daily), together with an immunosuppressant agent such as azathioprine, with subsequent gradual reduction of the steroid. Gold salts have also been used with success but toxicity is a problem. Even with treatment, pemphigus remains a serious disorder, about 25% of patients dying from the disease or consequences of treatment. Most patients need maintenance therapy for lengthy periods, although in some a true remission occurs.

Bullous pemphigoid

Bullous pemphigoid (Fig. 26.14) is a fairly common subepidermal blistering disease characterised by an antibody

Fig. 26.13 The lesions of pemphigus vulgaris (A), pemphigoid (B) and dermatitis herpetiformis (C). (IF = immunofluorescence).

Fig. 26.14 The blisters of bullous pemphigoid are tense, clear or blood-stained, and often remain intact for several days.

which localises to the lamina lucida of the basement membrane (Fig. 26.13).

In pemphigoid the complement system is activated, and C3a and C5a attract and activate eosinophils. Eosinophil products and mast cell mediators contribute to the split which occurs in the basement membrane and the clinically evident inflammatory reaction.

Pemphigoid is mainly a disease of the elderly. It is usually preceded by an erythematous itchy rash, which can be mistaken for urticaria or eczema. It may be localised for some weeks before becoming generalised. The blisters are tense, clear or blood-stained, and often remain intact for several days. Unlike pemphigus, pemphigoid does not usually involve the mucous membranes, but when it does, there may be an associated malignancy. When blisters do break, the skin usually heals, and the prognosis is better than that of pemphigus.

Treatment of pemphigoid is also with prednisolone, but usually in somewhat lower doses than for pemphigus (40–60 mg daily initially), and azathioprine to facilitate steroid withdrawal.

Dermatitis herpetiformis

Dermatitis herpetiformis is an uncommon, chronic, intensely itchy disorder in which subepidermal blistering usually occurs.

There is a close association with HLA-B8 and DRW3, gluten-sensitive enteropathy and deposition of IgA in the dermal papillae throughout the skin. The enteropathy may not be symptomatic and there may be no biochemical abnormalities, but it is likely that absorbed products derived from gluten are important in the pathogenesis of the skin lesions. Abnormal immunity in patients with dermatitis herpetiformis is suggested by an increased incidence of organ-specific auto-immune disease, and a few patients (as with coeliac disease) develop small bowel lymphoma. The skin lesions are a result of activation of dense clusters of neutrophils in the dermal papillae, producing damage and then fluid accumulation (Fig. 26.13).

Dermatitis herpetiformis usually begins in young adults and can persist indefinitely. Initial lesions are very itchy grouped weals or papules, on which arise small blisters. Extensor surfaces are the characteristic sites, especially elbows, knees, shoulders, buttocks and scalp. Oral lesions are sometimes seen.

The diagnosis is best made from finding typical histology in an early lesion and IgA deposition in unaffected skin. (In the lesions the IgA can disappear as a result of the inflammatory infiltrate.) A jejunal biopsy usually shows subtotal villous atrophy. Potassium iodide, both systemically and topically, provokes dermatitis herpetiformis and has occasionally been used as a diagnostic test.

Dapsone has a dramatic beneficial effect in this condition, probably by modulation of the neutrophil myeloperoxidase enzyme system, and/or of the alternate pathway of complement activation. Haemolytic anaemia can occur. A gluten-free diet is helpful in most patients, and may reduce the likelihood of intestinal lymphoma.

MISCELLANEOUS DISORDERS OF UNKNOWN CAUSE

Lichen planus

Lichen planus (Fig. 26.15) is a fairly common disease which may affect skin, hair, nails and mucous membranes. The histology is distinctive and shows damage to the basal epidermal cells, with a dense band of lymphocytic infiltrate immediately beneath. There are close similarities to the changes seen in the skin in graft versus host disease.

The skin lesions are usually very itchy, and typically form purplish, polygonal, shiny, flat-topped papules. They are usually found on the flexor aspect of the wrists, the lower back and shins. Larger, more warty plaques are sometimes found on the lower legs. Induction of new lesions by injury to the skin, the Koebner phenomenon, is often seen. In the mouth lichen planus is mainly seen as a network of white lines on the buccal mucosa and white patches on the tongue. The scalp may be involved, producing patches of inflammation from which hair fall is usually permanent. Nails can also be affected, usually with longitudinal areas of thinning; in some cases nails also can be permanently lost.

Lichen planus often lasts a year or more and to some extent it is steroid-responsive. Post-inflammatory hyperpigmentation is common.

Fig. 26.15 The lesions of lichen planus typically form purplish, polygonal, shiny, flat-topped papules.

Granuloma annulare

There are two forms of granuloma annulare (Fig. 26.16), localised and generalised; both as a rule are asymptomatic. Histologically there is palisading granuloma formation around focal areas of dermal necrosis.

Localised granuloma annulare presents as rings of smooth firm papules. The backs of the hands and the tops of the feet are common sites. The commonest misdiagnoses

Table 26.17 Pathogenesis of drug eruptions – some examples

Mechanism	Drug	Clinical pattern
Direct effects		
Immunological		
IgE-mediated	Penicillin	Urticaria
Immune complex	Sulphonamides	Vasculitis
Effector pathway stimulation	Acetyl salicylic acid	Urticaria
Side-effect	Cytotoxic drugs	Alopecia
Overdosage	Anticoagulants	Purpura
Cumulative toxicity	Corticosteroids	Striae
Indirect effects		
Drug interaction	Aspirin-displacing warfarin	Purpura
Metabolic effects	Isoniazid	Pellagra
Ecological disturbance	Broad-spectrum antibiotics	Candidiasis
Exacerbation of existing disease	Hydralazine Lithium	Lupus erythematosus Psoriasis

Fig. 26.16 Granuloma annulare, localised form: note the ring-shaped arrangement of dermal papules.

are warts and fungal infection, in which epidermal changes are prominent in contrast to the smooth surface of granuloma annulare.

In generalised granuloma annulare the papules are much more widespread and not necessarily in ring-shaped configurations. This is often associated with diabetes mellitus. Diagnosis is confirmed by biopsy.

Necrobiosis lipoidica

This condition occurs in about 3 per 1000 diabetics, and more than half of patients with necrobiosis lipoidica are overtly diabetic. The pathology is similar to granuloma annulare but with more pronounced dermal necrosis.

The most common site is the shin. The lesion begins as a purplish plaque, which gradually enlarges and becomes atrophic with yellowish areas centrally. Ulceration is quite common. The condition is chronic, and when there is associated diabetes, careful control of blood glucose has no effect on the progress of the skin lesions.

DRUG ERUPTIONS

A 'drug' is taken to be a substance employed for the purposes of treatment, prevention or investigation of disease. This concept of a drug therefore includes substances such as radiological contrast media and immunisation materials. Drug eruptions are a frequent occurrence in hospital practice and can produce skin changes in many ways (Table 26.17). Some of these, such as the predisposition to can-

didal infection by a broad-spectrum antibiotic, or exacerbation of pre-existing disease, are not direct effects of drugs on the skin, but are none the less a consequence of drug exposure. Often the exact mechanism of a drug eruption is unknown.

Some drugs, such as antibiotics, thiazides and sulphonamides, gold, allopurinol, phenylbutazone and other non-steroidal anti-inflammatory drugs, are relatively common causes of rashes; others very rare, but in all patients who develop a rash the drug history is of great importance. Not only prescribed drugs, but also medicines and tablets bought over the counter must be considered.

Types of drug eruption

Urticaria

The mechanisms whereby a drug can cause urticaria include IgE-mediated immediate hypersensitivity, immune complex-mediated generation of activated complement components (serum sickness), a direct action on mast cells causing them to release histamine, and modulation of arachidonic acid metabolism. The drugs commonly implicated in urticaria are:

- penicillin and related antibiotics
- X-ray contrast media
- enzymes
- blood products
- opiates
- non-steroidal anti-inflammatory drugs
- pollen vaccines
- iodides.

Angio-oedema and anaphylaxis may accompany urticaria, particularly when the drug has been injected, and can be life-threatening.

Urticaria usually begins within minutes or hours of the

drug being given, but with immune complex-related urticaria it occurs several days after the challenge, and is often associated with fever, lymphadenopathy, joint symptoms and haematuria due to renal damage.

Morbilliform eruption

A widespread, symmetrical, blotchy, maculopapular, erythematous rash is probably the commonest drug eruption. There is often a mild fever, but serious consequences are uncommon. The mechanism is usually obscure but does involve delayed hypersensitivity in some cases, especially when the onset is within a few days of the drug being started. Morbilliform eruptions usually begin within a week of the onset of the drug, and may progress to erythroderma if the drug is continued.

Ampicillin, amoxycillin and derivatives, e.g. talampicillin, are common causes, especially when the patient has infectious mononucleosis or lymphatic leukaemia, or is also taking allopurinol, and can begin up to a few days after the antibiotic has been stopped. The common causes of morbilliform (exanthematic) drug eruptions are:

- allopurinol
- antituberculous drugs
- captopril
- carbamazepine
- gold salts
- H$_2$ antihistamines
- penicillamine
- penicillins
- phenothiazines
- phenylbutazone
- sulphonamides
- thiazides.

Erythroderma

When due to a drug, erythroderma, or exfoliative dermatitis (p. 1132), tends to begin several weeks after the drug has been started. Fever, malaise, poor temperature regulation and, in the elderly, high-output cardiac failure are common. Eczema (p. 1138) may progress to erythroderma. Common causes of drug-induced erythroderma are:

- allopurinol
- carbamazepine
- phenytoin
- isoniazid
- lithium
- gold salts
- chloroquine
- barbiturates
- P-aminosalicylic acid
- captopril
- sulphonamides
- methyldopa.

Erythema multiforme

Erythema multiforme (p. 1128) is a reaction distinguished by target lesions, which may have central bullae, and there can be mucous membrane involvement. (When severe this reaction constitutes the Stevens-Johnson syndrome.)

Most cases are not due to drugs. The commonest drugs to cause erythema multiforme are:

- sulphonamides
- phenytoin
- phenylbutazone
- barbiturates
- penicillins
- carbamazepine
- rifampicin
- gold salts.

Toxic epidermal necrolysis

Toxic epidermal necrolysis is a drug reaction which has a high mortality. There is often a brief prodrome of malaise and fever, followed by widespread, tender, erythematous areas which then blister. Large sheets of epidermis readily rub off with light pressure to leave painful denuded dermis. Mucous membranes as well as skin may be involved. Fluid imbalance, septicaemia and pneumonia are the most common problems.

Differentiation from staphylococcal scalded skin syndrome (p. 1114) can be made histologically on a blister roof because in toxic epidermal necrolysis the roof consists of the whole epidermis. Butazones, sulphonamides, allopurinol, gold salts and phenytoin are examples of drugs which can cause the syndrome, which can also be due to infections, graft versus host disease and lymphoma.

Management is similar to that of widespread burns with treatment of fluid and protein loss and of infection.

Photosensitivity

The most common photosensitivity drug reaction (Plate 7, p. 1131) resembles sunburn and is usually phototoxic, i.e. does not involve immunological mechanisms. Occasionally drugs produce photo-allergic reactions which may look like eczema in light-exposed skin. Drugs which can induce phototoxic and photo-allergic reactions include:

- phenothiazines
- thiazides
- sulphonamides
- tetracyclines
- sulphonylureas
- benoxaprofen (now discontinued)
- nalidixic acid
- amiodarone
- azapropazone
- protriptyline
- psoralens.

Drugs can also induce photosensitive diseases, e.g. procainamide can induce lupus erythematosus, and isoniazid, pellagra.

Fixed drug eruption

The characteristic feature of a fixed drug eruption is that inflammation occurs in exactly the same place or few places each time the drug is taken. The reaction is usually a round red patch, which may blister, and after the inflammation has subsided there is often prolonged hyperpigmentation. Unlike other drug reactions, the fixed drug eruption is only caused by a drug (or food, such as a colouring agent, or quinine in tonic water), and it is not seen in other contexts such as infection or autoimmune disease.

One of the commonest causes is phenolphthalein, widely used as a non-prescription laxative, and thus easily missed in the history. Sulphonamides, tetracyclines, barbiturates, phenylbutazone, chlordiazepoxide, quinine and dapsone are other common causes.

Vasculitis

Drug-induced vasculitis (p. 1130), usually in the form of palpable purpura, and often with urticarial and blistering lesions, can be accompanied by similar lesions in other organs and may be a serious illness. The commonest drugs to cause allergic vasculitis are:

- allopurinol
- thiazides
- phenytoin
- thiouracil
- non-steroidal anti-inflammatory drugs
- sulphonamides
- hydralazine
- quinidine
- captopril.

Erythema nodosum

Drugs are rarely responsible for erythema nodosum and other causes should be sought. Oral contraceptives and sulphonamides are the drugs most likely to be involved.

Pigmentation changes induced by drugs

Colour change can be produced by deposition of the drug in the skin and mucous membranes, stimulation of melanin production and alteration of the distribution of pigment so as to make it more apparent, as in post-inflammatory hyperpigmentation (p. 1143). The hyperpigmentation after fixed drug eruption may be the presenting feature. In some situations the pigmentation is only evident in light-exposed skin. In many examples of drug-related pigment change, the mechanism is unknown. A classification based on pigment colour is shown in Table 26.18.

Lichenoid drug eruption

The rash in lichenoid drug eruption is similar, but not usually identical, to lichen planus (p. 1134). It usually begins weeks to months after the drug is started. As in idiopathic lichen planus, hyperpigmentation is common. Common causes of lichenoid drug eruptions are:

- gold salts
- antimalarials
- thiazides
- phenothiazines
- methyldopa
- frusemide
- beta-blockers
- penicillamine
- chlorpropamide.

Drug-induced lupus erythematosus

Drug-induced lupus erythematosus has some differences from the naturally occurring condition (p. 1015). It is likely that individuals who become affected have a genetic predisposition. It has been best documented in association with hydralazine and procainamide. With hydralazine the probability of occurrence is broadly dose-related, being seen in 5% on 100 mg daily, 10% on 200 mg daily, but not in those on 50 mg daily. Other common causes include penicillamine, phenytoin, methyldopa, beta-blockers, sulphasalazine and oral contraceptives. In most cases drug-induced lupus erythematosus occurs after the drug has been taken for at least a few months. On discontinuation, the disease resolves in most cases, but may persist for years.

The condition is relatively less common in negroes and more common in the elderly; renal and central nervous system disease are less likely to occur than in idiopathic lupus erythematosus. Antihistone antibodies are characteristic, and antinative DNA antibodies are not found. Complement levels remain normal.

Purpura

When caused by a drug, purpura is usually a result of thrombocytopenia, vascular damage or both. Mechanisms include both toxic and allergic effects. (See p. 1098 for a full account.)

Pruritus

Itching without a rash is considered on page 1148. Drugs can cause generalised pruritus and the most common causes are:

- opiates
- CNS stimulants
- antidepressants
- oral contraceptives
- hepatotoxic drugs
- chloroquine.

For many drugs the mechanism is unknown, but some drugs produce intrahepatic cholestasis.

Table 26.18 Pigmentation caused by drugs

Pattern	Drug
Brown	
Similar to Addison's disease	ACTH
Similar to chloasma	Phenytoin / Oral contraceptives
Light-exposed areas	Phenothiazines / Psoralens / Cytotoxics
Generalised	Cytotoxics / Pyrimethamine
Generalised, with patchy pigmentation	Arsenic
Blue-grey	
Light-exposed areas	Minocycline / Amiodarone / Phenothiazines
Generalised, maximal on light-exposed areas	Gold / Silver / Bismuth
Shins, nails and palate (and sometimes light-exposed areas)	Antimalarials
Yellow	
Generalised	Mepacrine
Red	
Generalised	Clofazimine / Methysergide

Acne and acneform eruption

In true acne there are comedones, papules and pustules in a characteristic distribution (p. 1147). Drugs exerting an androgenic stimulus, such as testosterone and some progestogens, can exacerbate or induce acne.

An acne-like eruption, in which there are follicular lesions but in which the morphology or the distribution differ from true acne, is seen with a number of drugs, including corticosteroids and ACTH, halogens, anti-epileptic drugs, isoniazid and lithium salts.

Alopecia

Partial or complete hair loss is very common and appears early with cytotoxic drugs, but rarely and late with most of the other drugs listed below:

- cytotoxic agents (especially cyclophosphamide and anthracyclines)
- retinoids
- anticoagulants
- oral contraceptives
- antithyroid drugs
- phenytoin
- valproate.

Hypertrichosis

Corticosteroids and androgenic steroids can produce hirsutism, but some drugs can induce increased hair growth on areas not dependent on a sex hormone stimulus, such as the eyebrows and forearms. Minoxidil, cyclosporin A, diazoxide, phenytoin and penicillamine are the main causes.

Eczema

If sensitised via the skin to a 'drug' and then 'challenged' by an internal route, the patient can develop an often widespread eczematous eruption. Examples are given in Table 26.19.

Table 26.19 Eczema induced by topical drugs

Eliciting drug	Source of topical exposure
Antibiotics, e.g. penicillin, streptomycin	Contents of medical and veterinary ampoules
Antihistamines	In antipruritic creams, e.g. mepyramine
Aminophylline	Cross-reaction with ethylenediamine in Tri-adcortyl cream

Vesicular and bullous drug eruptions

Blistering can occur in several different types of drug eruption already described, e.g. fixed eruption, erythema multiforme, photosensitivity and vasculitis. Bullae are common at sites subjected to prolonged pressure in drug-induced coma. Porphyria (p. 780) can be precipitated by drugs, as occasionally can pemphigus (e.g. rifampicin) and acquired epidermolysis bullosa (e.g. frusemide).

Investigation and treatment of drug reaction

The evaluation of a possible drug reaction should include the following:

1. *A careful assessment of the risk to the patient*, from the rash itself and involvement of other organs, e.g. kidneys and brain in a vasculitis. An assessment of the airway and maintenance of adequate circulation in urticaria/anaphylaxis should be made.
2. *A full drug history*, including all present and recently completed treatments (tablets, mixtures, injections, suppositories, etc.) and their timing in relation to the onset of the rash. Some drugs can cause a rash several days after they were last given, e.g. ampicillin, gold and depot preparations.
3. *Past drug history and associated rashes.*
4. *Other possible explanations* for the rash, e.g. a virus infection.
5. *Consideration of which drugs can be stopped.* Non-essential drugs should be stopped and essential drugs changed to structurally different ones if possible.
6. *Laboratory investigations.* Except for the investigation of drug-induced blood dyscrasias, these are disappointing. Blood eosinophilia, if present, is supportive of drug eruption.
7. *A skin biopsy* may help in some cases.
8. *Treatment.* The most immediately serious drug reaction is anaphylaxis. Emergency treatment is with 1:1000 adrenalin, 1 ml im, or slowly iv if the patient is moribund. A parenteral antihistamine and hydrocortisone are also given, and if necessary the patient is intubated.

   Depending on severity, some patients with erythroderma, bullous erythema multiforme, toxic epidermal necrolysis and vasculitis will require treatment with systemic corticosteroids.

INTERNAL MALIGNANCY AND THE SKIN

A symptom or sign in the skin may be the first indicator of a systemic malignancy, and, when that possibility is high, may justify a careful search even before there have been any direct clues from the neoplasm itself. Some of the ways that internal malignancy and the skin interact are shown in Table 26.20.

In many instances the mechanism is unknown. Some of these manifestations with no known cause are described below.

1. *Generalised pruritus* without a primary rash (p. 1148).
2. *Dermatomyositis*, adult onset (p. 1021).
3. *Acanthosis nigricans.* The skin becomes hyperpigmented and warty, but feels soft. Body folds are maximally affected. There are other causes, such as obesity, some drugs and some inherited syndromes, but onset in a lean adult is highly likely to be associated with an adenocarcinoma or lymphoma.

Direct involvement
e.g. Direct spread from breast carcinoma; plaques and nodules from lymphoma

Genetic predisposition
e.g. Multiple cysts and benign skin tumours occurring with colonic carcinoma (Gardner's syndrome) with autosomal dominant inheritance

Carcinogen (also causing skin disease)
e.g. Vinyl chloride skin eruption and angiosarcoma of the liver following exposure to vinyl chloride monomer (used in plastic manufacture)

Metabolic products of tumour
e.g. Flushing due to malignant carcinoid; migratory necrolytic erythema with glucagonoma – partly due to essential amino acid deficiencies induced by metabolic abnormality

4. *Acquired hypertrichosis lanuginosa.* This is a rare condition but one that has a strong association with malignancy, especially Hodgkin's disease. The patient develops blond downy hair over the whole face and then elsewhere.

5. *Erythema gyratum repens.* Here the skin develops irregular wavy bands of erythema, the overall appearance resembling wood grain. Nearly all cases have an associated malignancy.

6. *Acquired ichthyosis.* The unexplained occurrence of dry, scaly but non-inflamed skin is often associated with lymphoma (p. 1128).

7. *Pachydermoperiostosis with finger clubbing.* The skin becomes thickened, with extra folds; the hands, elbows, knees and tongue enlarge and there may be painful periosteal new bone formation (see hypertrophic pulmonary osteoarthropathy, p. 459). These changes are associated with bronchial carcinoma.

8. *Pancreatic panniculitis.* Tender red nodules of distinctive histology, due to the effect on subcutaneous fat of circulating lipases from the pancreas, indicate either malignancy or inflammation in that organ. There is often arthritis and eosinophilia.

NAEVI AND TUMOURS OF THE SKIN

The terms 'tumour' and 'neoplasm' are used to denote a swelling composed of an excess of one or more cell types. Most primary tumours are either clearly benign or malignant, but occasionally some benign lesions evolve into malignant patterns of behaviour and are therefore termed pre-malignant. Some of the known causes of this are listed in Table 26.22 (p. 1141). A naevus is a circumscribed developmental defect, and the term has a similar meaning to hamartoma. Naevi are often, but not necessarily, evident at birth. There may be more than one cell type involved in the process.

Each of the cell types in the skin can proliferate to produce a tumour and the exact diagnosis usually rests with the pathologist. When the lesion is of epidermal origin, its superficial location often makes a clinical diagnosis easier than with a tumour of dermal origin; a tumour of the latter type usually presents as a lump with few distinctive features.

Many benign tumours and naevi are of little more than cosmetic importance, but in some instances they are pointers towards a genetic syndrome or multisystem disorder. They should thus at least be recognised and documented when patients are examined, and if causing distress removal may well be appropriate.

Malignant tumours of the skin can be fatal, and not infrequently come to attention during a routine medical examination. Malignant metastases in the skin can occasionally be the presenting feature of a cancer elsewhere and the histology can provide a valuable indication of the organ of origin.

Naevi

Pigmented naevi

Pigmented (melanocytic) naevi, or common moles, are occasionally evident at birth, but more commonly appear in childhood or adolescence. The naevus is initially brown, with clusters of proliferating melanocytes at the base of the epidermis. Melanocytic naevi that develop after birth are usually symmetrical in shape and colour and rarely grow to more than 1 cm in diameter. In time the cells migrate into the dermis and the lesion often becomes a flesh-coloured nodule.

The blue naevus is a slate-coloured lesion composed of a localised proliferation of melanocytes in the dermis which never reached the epidermis during development.

Malignant melanoma (p. 1142) may arise from a seemingly benign melanocytic naevus, but this is rare except from giant congenital pigmented naevi.

Vascular naevi

There are several types of vascular naevi, some of which resolve in infancy or childhood (e.g. the salmon patch and strawberry naevus). The port wine stain is an area of permanent vascular dilatation, often on the face, where it may produce a disfiguring purplish discoloration. When the area affected is in the distribution of the ophthalmic division of the trigeminal nerve, there may be an associated vascular anomaly in the brain or meninges which can cause epilepsy, hemiplegia or retardation (Sturge-Weber syndrome).

Naevi and multisystem disease

Tuberose sclerosis

Tuberose sclerosis is an autosomal dominantly inherited disorder in which mental deficiency is associated with abnormality of many other organs. The first skin lesions to appear, often in early infancy, are the 'ash leaf' macules. These well-circumscribed, often irregularly shaped, pale patches are best seen with Wood's light. From later childhood onwards, one or more of the following may appear: red angiofibromatous papules on the face (misnamed adenoma sebaceum), thickened plaques on the trunk (shagreen patches) and peri-ungual fibromas (smooth nodules beside the nails). The skin lesions can be important in recognising carriers of the gene.

Von Recklinghausen's disease

The many features of von Recklinghausen's disease, or neurofibromatosis (Fig. 26.17), an autosomal dominantly inherited condition, include acoustic neuroma, gliomas, spinal deformities and phaeochromocytoma. The skin shows multiple pale brown patches (*café au lait macules*), especially in the axillae (a pathognomic sign), and soft nodules (neurofibromas) composed of nerve sheath cells.

Benign tumours and cysts

The growth of these is usually slow, does not destroy normal tissues, and is eventually self-limiting. The lesion produced is usually symmetrical in shape. A classification is given in Table 26.21.

Fig. 26.17 Neurofibromatosis is associated with localised areas of hyperpigmentation.

Table 26.21 Some benign skin tumours

Tumour	Clinical features
Seborrhoeic wart (basal cell papilloma)	Onset from mid-adult life Pale brown through to black (due to melanin) Stuck-on appearance, with finely clefted surface Often multiple
Histiocytoma (dermatofibroma, sclerosing angioma)	May follow trauma, e.g. insect bite Reddish-brown (due to iron pigment) Hard, feels like a bean in the skin
Pyogenic granuloma	Often follows trauma Rapidly growing, may regress if not treated Red, easily bleeds
Skin tag	Usually on the sides of the neck and in major flexures Soft, pedunculated outpouchings of skin
Lipoma	Soft, often lobulated subcutaneous nodule May be multiple
Keratoacanthoma	Middle age onwards Sunlight, tar and mineral oil may be causes Rapidly growing Smooth nodule with keratin-filled centre Will resolve, with scarring
Keratinising cysts (epidermoid and pilar)	Smooth, firm swelling(s) within the skin May become inflamed and rupture When multiple, may be feature of Gardner's syndrome (colonic polyposis)

Precursors to squamous carcinoma

Actinic keratosis

Actinic (solar) keratosis is a lesion which arises on skin chronically damaged by the harmful effects of UV radiation, in particular UVB (p. 1143). The face, bald scalp, backs of hands and forearms are common sites. Actinic keratoses are often multiple; they are more likely on the blue-eyed, fair or red-haired and rare in dark-skinned people. The individual lesion usually presents as a papule or plaque of hard, often brownish keratin. Transformation to squamous carcinoma is uncommon.

Actinic keratoses can be treated by a number of modalities, e.g. cryotherapy, curettage and 5-fluorouracil cream.

Bowen's disease

Bowen's disease can be a consequence of previous ingestion of inorganic arsenic, usually given as a tonic many years ago. It is more common on covered than exposed sites. There is an association in some cases with internal malignancy. Bowen's disease presents as a slow-growing, well-defined, red scaly or crusted patch. It is often solitary, although it can be multiple. The major differential diagnosis is psoriasis.

Small lesions can be treated as for actinic keratosis, but excision is preferable for larger lesions.

Malignant and pre-malignant tumours

Squamous carcinoma

More than in other skin malignancies, there is likely to be an identifiable cause (Table 26.22) for squamous carcinoma (Fig. 26.18). The tumour often arises from a pre-malignant condition and is distinguished clinically by induration of

Table 26.22 Factors predisposing to primary skin malignancy

- Ultraviolet radiation
- X-rays
- Chemicals, e.g. hydrocarbons in mineral oil, inorganic arsenic
- Immunosuppression
- Genetic, e.g. xeroderma pigmentosum
- Scars, e.g. old burn scar
- Longstanding skin disease, e.g. lupus vulgaris, chronic leg ulcer
- Some human papilloma viruses (rare)

Fig. 26.18 Squamous carcinoma is characterised by induration of the base of the tumour and surrounding normal tissues; with growth, ulceration usually occurs.

the base and surrounding normal tissues. With growth, ulceration usually occurs.

Squamous carcinoma is much more liable to metastasise to regional lymph nodes than is basal cell carcinoma, and distant metastases can occur.

Diagnosis is by biopsy. Keratoacanthoma can be difficult to distinguish both clinically and histologically from squamous cell carcinoma.

Treatment will usually be by surgical excision, although in some circumstances radiotherapy may be preferable.

Basal cell carcinoma

Basal cell carcinoma (BCC), or rodent ulcer (Fig. 26.19), arises from cells which resemble the basal layer of the epidermis, and may have its origin from skin appendage epithelium.

It is the commonest malignant skin tumour in white races, and although sunlight exposure is clearly a major aetiological factor, unlike squamous cell carcinoma it is not often seen on the backs of the hands. The face is the commonest site, although when there has been exposure to a systemic carcinogen such as inorganic arsenic, BCC can be multiple and widespread.

The tumour is usually slow-growing, evolving from a translucent papule. Various growth patterns may occur, e.g. superficial spreading, nodular, infiltrative and sclerosing. Most nodular and infiltrative tumours ulcerate. Except for the sclerosing variety, BCC tends to retain a translucent raised margin as it extends into surrounding tissues. In some tumours there is an admixture of melanocytes and the resultant lesion can simulate malignant melanoma. Local

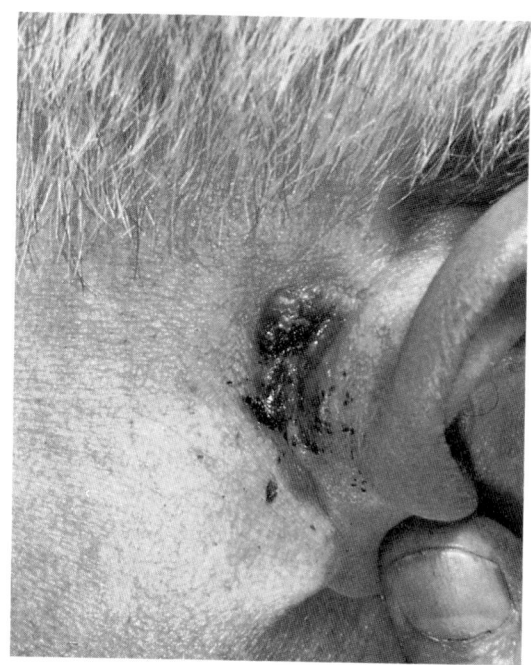

Fig. 26.19 Basal cell carcinoma evolves from a translucent papule and tends to retain a translucent raised margin as it extends into surrounding tissues.

destruction can be extreme, and very rarely BCC metastasises.

Treatment is usually by excision, radiotherapy, curettage or cryotherapy.

Malignant melanoma

Malignant melanoma (Plate 8, p. 1131) usually arises either from previously normal-looking skin, or a benign melanocytic naevus. It may also arise from a naevus in a nail bed, in a mucous membrane or from the choroid or the iris.

At present there is a rapidly rising incidence among Caucasians and, aetiologically, short bursts of sun exposure, as during a hot, sunny holiday, may be important. There is not the same association with chronic sun damage as with squamous cell carcinoma and to a lesser extent basal cell carcinoma. Conditions which can give rise to melanoma are lentigo maligna (Hutchinson's freckle) and dysplastic naevus. Lentigo maligna evolves as a flat, brown, variably pigmented patch, which slowly spreads on markedly sun-damaged skin. Dysplastic naevi are unusual-looking naevi, often larger than average, with a distinctive histology; they are sporadic or inherited as an autosomal dominant characteristic, and may be a precursor to melanoma.

Melanoma is often suspected when an enlarging pigmented lesion has one or more of the following features: irregular notched border, irregular pigmentation, often with red and white as well as brown/black areas, itching or prickling sensation, inflammatory halo, ulceration and bleeding.

The malignant cells spread laterally, in and just beneath the epidermis, and inwards. The prognosis depends on the depth of invasion, being excellent for completely excised, very superficial tumours. Metastasis occurs to both regional lymph nodes and distantly.

Lymphoma and leukaemia in the skin

B cell lymphoma, Hodgkin's disease and leukaemia may occasionally metastasise to the skin, or rarely present with cutaneous nodules. The skin is usually involved rather late in the course of the disease. The diagnosis is made from biopsy and other characteristic features of these diseases.

T lymphocytes have an affinity for the epidermis and its appendages, and therefore T cell neoplasia often involves the skin from the outset and may appear to be localised to the skin in some cases.

Mycosis fungoides is the best characterised T cell cutaneous neoplasm. There is often a long phase of poikilodermatous patches (poikiloderma is a combination of erythema, atrophy and reticulate pigmentation) before plaques and tumours appear. Itching usually occurs. Erythroderma (p. 1132) can develop, and if there are circulating neoplastic T cells, this constitutes the Sézary syndrome. Lymphadenopathy and visceral involvement occur late and indicate a poor prognosis.

Metastatic malignancy

Nodules, often ulcerating, may occur with many visceral malignancies.

Paget's disease of the nipple

The epidermis of the nipple becomes invaded by malignant cells arising from an underlying intraduct carcinoma of the breast tissue. The lesion is red, crusted and well defined, like Bowen's disease.

Kaposi's sarcoma

Kaposi's sarcoma (Plate 9, p. 1131) may well have a viral aetiology. The lesions of this multicentric vascular neoplasm are usually purplish patches, plaques or nodules. Leakage of blood readily produces purpura and brown staining of the skin. The lymphatics can be affected producing lymphoedema.

There are two major patterns of natural history: a slow, relatively benign course seen particularly in elderly Eastern European Jews, and a more rapid, aggressive evolution in parts of Africa, AIDS patients and occasionally following therapeutic immunosuppression. In the aggressive disease involvement of lymph nodes, mouth, gastrointestinal tract, lungs and other viscera may occur.

Among AIDS patients the male homosexual is particularly vulnerable to Kaposi's sarcoma. Initially the lesions may be insignificant-looking, flat, reddish-brown or purple patches. A distinctive feature of AIDS-related Kaposi's sarcoma is a tendency for ovoid lesions to orientate along major skin creases, which on the trunk resembles the arrangement seen in pityriasis rosea.

Skin and oral lesions are common features of patients with symptomatic HIV infection (Table 26.23).

Treatment, when indicated, is radiotherapy for localised lesions and, in some cases, cytotoxic chemotherapy for extensive disease.

Table 26.23   Skin and oral lesions in AIDS

Seborrhoeic dermatitis (early feature in 30%)	Severe drug eruptions
	Exacerbation of psoriasis
Itchy folliculitis	Vasculitis
Kaposi's sarcoma	Diffuse alopecia
Infections	Dry skin (late)
Molluscum contagiosum	Oral hairy leukoplakia
Peri-anal warts	Oral candidiasis
Superficial fungal infection	Oral Kaposi's sarcoma
Herpes zoster and simplex	
Atypical mycobacteria	

Primary sarcomas

Malignant tumours arising from the various mesenchymal elements in the skin are all rare and present as enlarging masses.

SUNLIGHT AND THE SKIN

For descriptive purposes, the continuum of electro-magnetic radiation emitted by the sun is divided into segments according to wavelengths (Table 26.24).

Of the energy reaching the earth's surface 99% is ultra-violet through to middle infra-red. The shorter wave-lengths of ultraviolet are filtered out by ozone in the stratosphere and by the atmosphere. The response of skin to solar radiation depends on the wavelength and on natural defences, the most important being melanin deposition. Ultraviolet B (UVB) is responsible for acute sunburn and the chronic changes of sun exposure: atrophy, dryness, blotchy pigmentation and wrinkling, solar keratoses and many skin cancers. The consequences of failure to repair damage inflicted on cellular DNA by UVB are seen in the rare autosomal recessively inherited condition xeroderma pigmentosum, in which sun-exposed skin becomes prema-turely aged and skin cancers can appear in childhood. UVA has a much less obvious effect on normal skin, but is often responsible for photosensitive drug reactions and polymorphic light eruption. A clinical clue that UVA is playing a part is the provocation of a sun-related skin disorder behind window glass, since this filters out UVB. The action spectrum, i.e. the determination of exactly which wavelengths are responsible for a photosensitivity disorder, is only known for a few diseases. Visible light does not produce reactions on normal skin, but is responsible for photosensitivity in some diseases, notably the porphyrias, where the maximal reactivity is around 400 nm.

Although most of the consequences of solar radiation on the skin appear harmful, one benefit is the synthesis of vitamin D_3. UV light is essential to break the steroid B ring and convert 7 dihydrocholesterol to pre-vitamin D_3 which then isomerises spontaneously to vitamin D_3.

The immune system in the skin is modified by ultraviolet exposure, and this may be important with regard to the development of skin cancer.

Table 26.24 Electromagnetic spectrum

Type	Wavelength
Gamma	0.1–100 A°
Vacuum UV	10–200 nm
Ultraviolet C (UVC)	200–290 nm
Ultraviolet B (UVB)	290–320 nm
Ultraviolet A (UVA)	320–400 nm
Visible light	400–760 nm
Near infra-red	0.74–1.5 m
Middle infra-red	1.5–5.6 m
Far infra-red	5.6–1000 m
Microwaves and radiowaves	>1 mm

Polymorphic light eruption

Polymorphic light eruption is a common disorder which mainly occurs in females. Usually in spring, a day or so after sun exposure, itchy red papules, plaques and sometimes vesicles appear on sun-exposed sites. The condition gradu-ally settles with continued sun exposure.

Drug photosensitivity

It is usually not known whether allergic or toxic mech-anisms are involved in drug photosensitivity. The drugs commonly responsible are given on page 1136.

Phytophotodermatitis

Psoralens, a group of chemicals found in many plants, can be activated by UVA to produce inflammation and hyperpigmentation; 8-methoxypsoralen with UVA is used therapeutically as PUVA (pp. 1124 and 1145). Contact with a plant containing a psoralen (e.g. common rue, giant hogweed), together with sun exposure, produces erythema, often blistering, and then considerable hyperpigmentation.

Photo-allergic contact dermatitis

A number of cosmetics and even sunscreens contain chemi-cals which are activated by UV and, in combination with skin constituents, generate photo-allergy. Investigation is by patch testing, using two sets of patches, one of which is exposed to UV after a period of contact with the skin. Photocontact allergy produces positive results only in the set which has been irradiated. In some patients the state of photosensitivity persists long after the allergen has been withdrawn.

Metabolic disorders with light sensitivity

Skin sensitivity to sunlight may occur in porphyrias (except the acute intermittent variety), pellagra, carcinoid syn-drome and Hartnup disease.

Disorders aggravated by sunlight

Many skin diseases may be worsened or triggered by sun-light. Common examples are lupus erythematosus and recurrent facial herpes simplex. Careful use of sunscreens can be helpful.

PIGMENTATION

Normal skin colour is determined by haemoglobin, both oxygenated (red) and reduced (blue), carotenoids (yellow) and melanin (brown).

Melanin is a polymer, synthesised from tyrosine in the melanocytes and distributed in cellular organelles called melanosomes via cell processes (dendrites) to the ker-atinocytes of the skin and hair. All races have the same number of melanocytes, about 1 per 36 keratinocytes, the differences in skin colour being due to the amount of melanin formation in the melanosomes (maximal in dark races) and the way these are dispersed (single in negroids; in membrane-bound packages in caucasoids). Apart from genetic factors, melanin production is stimulated by UV radiation and certain hormones, e.g. melanocyte stimulating hormones (MSH), the chemically related ACTH, and female sex hormones. Hyperpigmentation is a common sequel to many inflammatory skin diseases, especially those in which the lower epidermis is damaged. There is both stimulation of melanogenesis and passage of melanin into dermal macrophages. Sometimes hyperpigmentation is due to substances other than melanin, e.g. haemosiderin (brownish-red) and drugs, e.g. amiodarone (grey).

Many conditions associated with localised areas of hyperpigmentation are described elsewhere. These include neurofibromatosis (Fig. 26.17), xeroderma pigmentosum and Peutz-Jeghers disease. In practice the commonest are freckles, benign melanocytic naevi and post-inflammatory hyperpigmentation. The causes of generalised or extensive hyperpigmentation are given in Table 26.25.

Table 26.25 Causes of widespread hyperpigmentation

Condition	Cause	Pattern
Hypoadrenalism Cushing's syndrome	} ACTH excess	Maximal in flexures, creases of palms and soles, sites of friction and pressure, and buccal mucous membranes
Renal failure	MSH Carotenoids	Diffuse, maximal on hands and face
Haemochromatosis	Melanin Haemosiderin	Exposed skin and flexures
Vitamin B_{12} deficiency	Melanin	Widespread, accentuated over knuckles Hypomelanosis of hair
Any debilitating disease	Melanin	Generalised or Addisonian
Drugs	Melanin and sometimes the drug	See p. 1137
Acanthosis nigricans	Keratin	Flexures, sides of the neck

Loss of pigment

Complete or partial loss of melanin pigment can have many causes. It is helpful to consider localised and generalised loss of pigment separately (Table 26.26).

Vitiligo

Vitiligo (Fig. 26.20) is an acquired disorder in which melanocytes are lost from the basal layer of the epidermis. It probably occurs in about 0.4% of the population. A genetic

Table 26.26 Localised and generalised pigment loss

Condition	Cause	Clinical features
Localised hypopigmentation		
Vitiligo	Loss of melanocytes	Well-defined white patches, often with hyperpigmentation of the bordering skin Personal or family history of organ-specific auto-immune disease common
Pityriasis versicolor	Toxic effect on melanocytes	Slightly scaly macules mainly on the trunk, paler after sun exposure
Post-inflammatory		
(i)	Faulty melanin transfer to keratinoyctes	Pale patches with or after inflammation, e.g. Eczema
(ii)	Loss of melanocytes	e.g. Scarring after lupus erythematosus
Tuberose sclerosis	Poorly developed melanosomes	Leaf-shaped, pale macules
Leprosy	Decreased melanocytic activity	Pale patches are anaesthetic
Generalised pigment loss		
Albinism	Faulty production of melanin in skin, hair and eyes	Pale skin and hair, pink irises
Phenylketonuria	Competitive inhibition of tyrosinase by phenylalanine	Pale skin with mental deficiency
Hypopituitarism	ACTH and MSH deficiency	Associated endocrine deficiencies

basis is likely since about 40% have a family history. In the individuals and their families there is an increased frequency of organ-specific autoimmune diseases. The precise pathogenesis is unknown.

Vitiligo has often begun by the age of 20. It is characterised by sharply defined areas of pigment loss, sometimes with mild hyperpigmentation of the adjacent normal skin. The texture is normal and there is no scaling. In pale-skinned individuals their first awareness may be sunburn in the depigmented skin. Any site can be affected and symmetrical involvement is common. Occasionally vitiligo follows a dermatomal pattern. The face, axillae, groins, backs of hands, knees and elbows, and genitalia are common sites. The condition is usually progressive, but repigmentation can occur spontaneously.

Diagnosis is usually straightforward. By Wood's light pityriasis versicolor (which is scaly) fluoresces yellow, and vitiligo is more strikingly white than the other causes of hypopigmentation (Table 26.26). The pale macules of leprosy are anaesthetic.

No treatment is entirely satisfactory. Cosmetic camou-

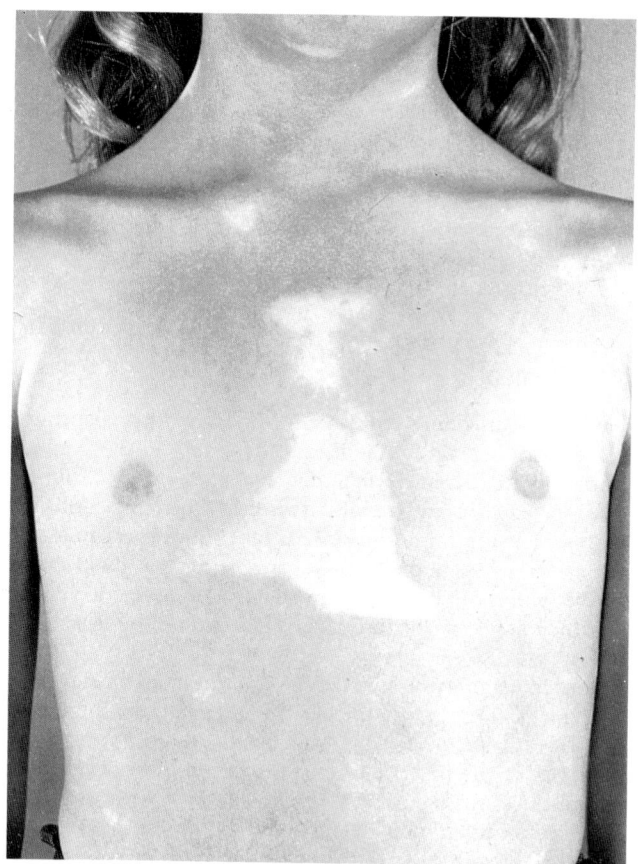

Fig. 26.20 Vitiligo shows sharply outlined areas of pigment loss.

flage is helpful in a few. Sunscreens should be used on exposed areas to prevent burning and chronic sun damage, and in the pale-skinned this measure can improve the appearance by reducing tanning of surrounding normal skin. Other measures used include psoralen and UVA (see PUVA treatment of psoriasis, p. 1124) and short-term application of potent topical corticosteroids.

PRESSURE SORES

A pressure sore (synonyms: bed sore, decubitus ulcer) is the consequence of sustained pressure to the tissues and is usually seen over a bony prominence, such as the ischial tuberosity, greater trochanter and elbow. The normal response to sustained pressure is movement to relieve that pressure. If discomfort is not felt or movement is not possible, then ischaemia is likely to occur. Friction (lateral pressure) exacerbates the tissue damage. Because fat and muscle are more susceptible, subcutaneous necrosis may be much greater than the surface changes suggest. Factors responsible for pressure sores are listed in Table 26.27.

The earliest clinical sign is redness on an area subjected to pressure, the erythema not fading within 30 minutes. Action at this stage may prevent further damage. Pro-

Table 26.27 Pathogenesis of pressure sores

Major factors	Contributory factors
Prolonged immobility	Anaemia
e.g. Paraplegia	Hypoproteinaemia
Arthritis	Severe weight loss
Operations and intensive care	
Plaster casts	
Apathy	
Loss of sensory stimuli	
e.g. Coma	
Multiple sclerosis	
Vascular disease	
e.g. Atherosclerosis	

gressive damage is manifested by blistering, ulceration and formation of slough.

For any patient at risk, prevention is the chief aim. Frequent changes of position, with care not to exert friction by dragging the skin, and careful choice of the surface on which the patient is lying or sitting, are crucial. For the established pressure sore, these measures are equally important. In addition, haemoglobin and nutrition should be improved if deficient, slough should be removed and the sore kept scrupulously clean. In some cases excision of the entire necrotic area, with closure or grafting, should be considered.

LEG ULCERATION

Ulceration of the lower leg can have many causes, some of which are shown in Table 26.28. In the UK most cases of leg ulceration are wholly or partly due to disorders of the venous system, but arterial insufficiency often co-exists and may be the major factor in many patients. In the tropics, infective causes are much more important. Particularly in the elderly there can be multiple aetiological factors. It is very important that the patient with a leg ulcer is given a full medical assessment, not only to determine the cause(s) as far as possible, but also to recognise other factors which may be contributory or delay healing.

VENOUS LEG ULCERATION

Venous leg ulceration is also known as stasis or gravitational ulceration. The skin changes are due to the consequences of raised pressure in the venous system.

Aetiology and pathogenesis

In most cases venous return is compromised by there having been a previous deep vein thrombosis. This may be apparent from the history, but in many other patients thrombosis can be demonstrated to have occurred by venography. In a few cases ulceration is associated with varicosity of the superficial veins, or defective communicating

Skin Disease

Table 26.28 Causes of leg ulceration

Cause	Example
Venous hypertension	Venous thrombosis
Arterial diseases	Atherosclerosis
Vasculitis	Rheumatoid disease, Wegener's granulomatosis
Pyoderma gangrenosum	See p. 1129
Trauma	Mechanical injury, burns, bites
Infections	Ecthyma, tuberculosis, syphilis, deep fungal infection
Diabetes mellitus	
Neuropathy	Leprosy
Blood disorders	Disseminated intravascular coagulation, platelet disorders, sickle cell anaemia and spherocytosis, polycythaemia
Plasma protein disorders	Cryoglobulinaemia
Scarring disorders	Radiodermatitis
Neoplasia	Cutaneous carcinomas, Kaposi's sarcoma

veins. Pressure in the venous system is raised because the valves are absent or destroyed, and this increased pressure is transmitted back to the capillary bed in the skin. There is extravascular deposition of fibrin, followed by fibrosis, and these changes are thought to impair transfer of oxygen and nutrients to the skin. It is also likely that venous distension produces reflex arteriolar constriction. This phenomenon occurs in normal individuals when standing still, but is promptly relieved in them by exercise, but not in those with persistently raised venous pressure. Patients who develop leg ulcers may also have decreased ability to lyse the fibrin and this may contribute to the pathogenesis.

Clinical features

Venous ulceration is most common in middle-aged and elderly women. Interestingly, leg ulcers occur frequently and early in Klinefelter's syndrome (p. 90).

Venous ulcers are usually preceded by varying combinations of oedema, prominent venules around the ankle, brown discoloration due to extravasation of red blood cells, eczema (p. 1127), fibrotic thickening of the dermis and subcutaneous fat, and white plaques stippled with telangiectases (*atrophie blanche*). These signs occur most commonly near the medial malleolus, but may be seen also on the lateral aspect of the ankle and over communicating veins. Another characteristic site is over the dorsum of the foot near the base of the toes. Ulceration may occur spontaneously or after trauma, which is often trivial. Unlike ulceration due to arterial disease or vasculitis, venous ulcers are often painless. The base of the ulcer

usually shows red granulation tissue and the edge is oedematous. The ulcer may be complicated by infection; cellulitis, usually due to *Staphylococcus aureus* and/or *Streptococcus pyogenes*, can develop rapidly. Another common complication is contact allergic dermatitis due to medicaments applied to the ulcer, e.g. antibiotics and antiseptics (p. 1125). In time the fibrotic process causes lymphoedema, and loss of movement at the ankle joint often occurs. Rarely, squamous and basal cell carcinoma can develop in chronic venous leg ulcers.

Management

Patients with venous leg ulcers often have other disorders, correction of which facilitates healing. These include nutritional deficiency, anaemia, diabetes, obesity, hypertension, cardiac and renal disease, myxoedema, and any disease causing immobility. It is most important to assess the arterial system in the legs, if necessary with a Doppler probe, since the compression that is valuable for venous insufficiency can be harmful if there is a poor arterial inflow.

Raised venous pressure can be counteracted by elevation of the legs at night and for periods of time during the day, and careful use of compression bandages combined with exercise. If the ulcer is due to incompetent superficial or communicating veins rather than deep vein thrombosis, surgical treatment may be indicated. Numerous treatments are available for the ulcer itself, and in most circumstances materials which do not contain potential sensitisers and maintain a moist surface should be used. There may be a role for desloughing agents, but for limited periods. Cellulitis requires systemic antibiotics.

When venous ulceration has been healed, the patient should continue to exercise and maintain compression with suitable stockings indefinitely.

ARTERIAL ULCERATION

When the arteriolar supply to a region of skin is insufficient or interrupted, necrosis occurs with resultant ulceration. The more profound process of gangrene is discussed on p. 448. In general, vascular occlusion can occur because of changes outside the vessel wall, within the wall itself (as in atherosclerosis and vasculitis), and due to changes in the blood (as in cryoglobulinaemia and platelet thrombi). The symptoms and signs will be determined by the size of the territory rendered ischaemic and the speed with which the process occurs. The most common cause of arterial ulceration is atheromatous disease of the aorta and its tributaries.

Clinical features of atherosclerosis ulceration

Arterial ulcers tend to be painful, sometimes severely so. There may be coldness, and pallor exaggerated by elevation of the limb, but cyanosis and blotchy erythema are also seen. Chronic ischaemia results in dryness and atrophy of the skin, loss of hair and thickened, distorted nails. Intermittent claudication may be present (p. 447). Common sites for arterial ulceration due to atherosclerosis are the front or lateral aspect of the ankle, and the toes. The ulcer tends to be well demarcated with a grey slough-covered base, which may expose deeper structures such as tendons.

The management of arterial ulceration is usually in the province of the vascular surgeon.

ACNE VULGARIS

Acne vulgaris is a disease that primarily involves the pilo-sebaceous follicles, i.e. the sebaceous glands, ducts and the distal part of the hair follicles into which they open. The lesions include keratinous plugs in the ducts (comedones), inflammatory papules, pustules, nodules, cysts and scars.

The best defined factors that determine the occurrence of acne vulgaris are androgenic stimulation of the sebaceous glands and the commensal anaerobic bacterium *Propionibacterium acnes* which heavily colonises active pilo-sebaceous follicles. Although the onset of acne around puberty is explained by the increased output of androgens at that time, it is much less clear why the disease becomes quiescent without any measurable change in the hormonal milieu or numbers of propionibacteria. The basis for the disorder of keratinisation in the sebaceous ducts which produces the comedones is uncertain. Inflammatory lesions are mainly derived from closed comedones (see below). Possible mediators of inflammation include free fatty acids, bacterial cell wall components and enzymes, and the patient's complement system. The pus in acne lesions is sterile and a consequence of inflammation, which is often so severe that scarring results.

Acne can occur in infants, but is usually mild and due to the influence of a transplacental hormonal stimulus. In older children, acne often represents the beginnings of puberty but may not occur until the mid-teens or beyond. The areas affected are those with maximal numbers of pilosebaceous follicles: the face, upper trunk and shoulders. Comedones are either open (blackheads) or closed (small whitish papules). The inflammatory lesions are erythematous, varying from papules through pustules to nodules and large collections of pus (wrongly) called cysts. The more destructive lesions heal with scarring, which is usually pitted, but hypertrophic or keloidal in those so predisposed. The course of acne can be erratic and there are often premenstrual exacerbations.

Lesions resembling acne can be provoked by halo-genated hydrocarbons, mineral oils, tars, greasy cosmetics, and drugs (p. 1138).

Treatment

Acne can have serious psychological effects and should never be ignored on the basis that it will get better sooner or later. Mild cases often respond to topical agents alone, e.g. benzoyl peroxide, 2.5–10% gel, or topical retinoic acid. The latter is more irritant, but often more effective when comedones are the predominant feature. If there is insufficient response after a few weeks' treatment, or if the acne is of moderate severity, an oral antibiotic should be used in addition (or instead, if topical therapy proves too irritant). Tetracyclines and erythromycin are equally effective, usually in a dose of 0.5 g twice daily for several months. Topical antibiotics can also be effective. For females with moderate acne hormonal modulation with the anti-androgen cyproterone acetate may be more effective. This drug must be given with an oestrogen, for mild cases in the form of a low-dose oral contraceptive pill. Patients with severe and destructive acne usually need treatment with oral isotretinoin. This vitamin A analogue is highly effective, but has a number of adverse effects, notably teratogenicity, so it is restricted to hospital use in the UK.

Other measures sometimes used include intralesional corticosteroids for inflammatory nodules and cysts, and dermabrasion, a surgical technique to improve scarring.

HIDRADENITIS SUPPURATIVA

Hidradenitis suppurativa is a chronic suppurative, inflammatory and scarring condition of blocked apocrine glands. There may be a genetic basis for this disorder, which has some similarity to acne vulgaris and may be associated with it. Following keratinous plugging of the apocrine glands there is bacterial infection, subsequent gland rupture, damage to surrounding tissues and healing with scarring and sinus tracts. The areas affected are the axillae, anogenital area and breasts. Tender inflammatory nodules, which discharge pus, are seen and blackheads are often present early on.

Because bacteria are playing a perpetuating role in this disorder, courses of antibiotics (if possible governed by sensitivity testing) are helpful but not curative. Incision, marsupialisation and even wide excision may be needed in chronic cases. Hormonal modulation, e.g. with anti-androgens in females, may have a role in treatment.

ROSACEA

Rosacea is a common condition of the middle-aged and elderly, in which there are varying combinations of redness of the face with telangiectasia, papules and sterile pustules. The facial erythema is often easily exacerbated by spicy foods, alcohol and emotional upset. Unlike acne there are no comedones and no elevation of sebum excretion rate. Common associations are eye disorders (e.g. conjunctivitis and keratitis), facial lymphoedema and rhinophyma, a hypertrophy of the nasal skin and its appendages. Despite the cause remaining unknown, treatment with oral oxy-tetracycline is effectively suppressive in most cases. It is usually helpful to minimise the effects of sun exposure.

Rosacea is slowly worsened by the use of topical steroids on the face, and a similar condition, *peri-oral dermatitis*, can be initiated by the more potent topical steroids/ preparations.

PRURITUS

Pruritus, or itching, is the distinctive sensation whose outward manifestation is the act of scratching. Except for the role of histamine in some disorders, and bile salts in obstructive liver disease, we know disappointingly little about the mechanisms of this common symptom.

When severe, pruritus can surpass pain in the distress it can cause, as patients who have scratched so much that they have substituted pain for itch can testify.

Many skin diseases can be itchy, and some, such as scabies, lichen planus and urticaria, severely so. Dry skin of whatever cause tends to be itchy, and this is a particularly common problem in the elderly and one of the reasons for pruritus in the atopic individual. Occasionally an external cause (such as fibreglass or scabies) can produce widespread pruritus with little to see. Itching can occur without any primary rash, the skin changes, if any, being those due to rubbing and scratching.

Generalised pruritus may be a pointer to systemic disease, which may be evident on examination but often requires investigation. Some commoner causes are shown in Table 26.29.

Wherever possible, the underlying cause of generalised pruritus should be treated. When symptomatic measures are called for, the use of emollients can be helpful, probably because dry skin has a lower threshold for pruritus. Although histamine release is not generally of much significance in generalised pruritus, oral H_1 antagonists can provide some relief, particularly when sedative anti-histamines are used. Uraemic pruritus can be helped by ultraviolet radiation (UVB). Pruritus due to cholestatic liver disease often responds to cholestyramine or colestipol. The itch in polycythaemia vera may respond to anti-serotonin agents, cyproheptadine or pizotifen.

Localised pruritus without primary signs of skin disease is common in the peri-anal and vulval areas. Sometimes there is a psychological basis for this, but not necessarily so. The causes are shown in Tables 26.30 and 26.31.

Table 26.29 Systemic causes of generalised pruritus

Hepatic disease	Haematological
Obstructive biliary disease	Iron deficiency
Pregnancy: oestrogen-induced	
cholestasis	Drugs
	Opiates
Endocrine disease	Subclinical drug sensitivity
Hyper- and hypothyroidism	
Diabetes mellitus (rare)	Psychiatric
	Neurosis
Renal	Psychosis, e.g. delusions of
Chronic renal failure	parasitosis
Parasitic	
Trichinosis	
Onchocerciasis	
Malignancy	
Hodgkin's disease	
Leukaemia and lymphoma	
Polycythaemia rubra vera	
Other neoplasms	

Table 26.30 Causes of pruritus ani

Ano-rectal disease
  Fissure
  Haemorrhoids
  Rectal carcinoma
  Faecal soiling

Skin disease
  Psoriasis
  Atopic dermatitis
  Irritant and allergic contact dermatitis (especially medicaments)

Infection
  Candidiasis

Infestation
  Threadworms

Psychogenic
  Anxiety
  Depression

Unknown

Table 26.31 Causes of pruritus vulvae

Diseases special to vulval skin
  Lichen sclerosus et atrophicus
  Leukoplakia
  Carcinoma

Skin disease
  Psoriasis
  Atopic dermatitis
  Irritant and allergic contact dermatitis (especially medicaments)

Infection
  Candidiasis
  Trichomonas

Infestation
  Pediculosis

Psychogenic
  Depression
  Anxiety

ALOPECIA

The evaluation of alopecia, or hair loss, takes account of:

1. the distribution
2. any abnormalities of the hair shafts
3. the scalp.

Androgenic alopecia (common baldness)

The prerequisites for this very common condition are: an inherited tendency, usually apparent in the family history; some degree of ageing; and post-pubertal androgen levels. The longer, coarser, pigmented terminal hairs on the scalp are progressively replaced by small, fine vellus hairs. In males there is recession of the anterior hairline and thinning over the crown, and ultimately terminal hair may only be present at the back and sides of the scalp. In an endocrinologically normal female there is thinning over the top of the scalp, but baldness to the extent seen in males is uncommon, except in the elderly, and if present warrants careful evaluation.

Diffuse alopecia

Diffuse alopecia is a decrease in hair density over the whole scalp without change in the skin or hair morphology. In some instances, e.g. a febrile illness, childbirth and severe emotional upset, the causative factor synchronises a proportion of the follicles so that hairs are shed 2–3 months later, a phenomenon called telogen effluvium. Regrowth usually takes place in about 6 months.

Normal hair growth requires an adequate nutrition, and diffuse alopecia accompanies malnutrition and wasting conditions. Iron deficiency, even in the absence of anaemia, has been associated with hair loss. Dry and progressively sparse hair is a feature of hypothyroidism. Many drugs (p. 1138) can produce diffuse alopecia, sometimes (as with cytotoxic agents) within days of administration, or after several weeks (as with anticoagulants, antithyroid drugs and the retinoids). Stopping the oral contraceptive has been associated with mild hair loss, similar to the effect of childbirth.

Alopecia areata

Alopecia areata (Fig. 26.21) is a common condition in which there is loss of hair in patches, typically with no skin changes. Hair on the face and body as well as scalp may be affected. A distinctive feature is the presence of shortened hairs which taper markedly where they emerge from the scalp (exclamation mark hairs). White hairs tend to be spared the process causing the hair loss. Alopecia areata is usually reversible, and when hair grows back it is often initially white. When the entire scalp becomes affected the condition is called *alopecia totalis*, and if all the body hair is lost as well the term *alopecia universalis* is applied. Regrowth usually occurs but is less likely with these more severe forms. Nails may show a distinctive pattern of pitting and ridging. There is sometimes an association with one or more organ-specific autoimmune diseases in the patient or family. The cause of alopecia areata is not known.

Inflammatory alopecia

Fungal (p. 1117) and bacterial infection can cause patchy hair loss with varying degrees of erythema, oedema and pustules. Lichen planus (p. 1134) and lupus erythematosus (p. 1015) may affect the scalp, and characteristically produce atrophy. Occasionally metastatic neoplasia presents as inflammatory alopecia.

Traumatic alopecia

Hair can be damaged by chemicals, e.g. those used in permanent waving, and physical trauma such as twisting between the fingers and pulling. Traumatic alopecia is a diagnostic possibility when the hair shafts are abnormal.

NAILS AND DISEASE

The nail is a specialised sheet of keratin largely produced by an invagination of the epidermis called the matrix, which is located beneath the posterior nail fold and extends beneath the nail plate as the lunule (half-moon). Disorders of the nails may result from local causes such as psoriasis, fungal infection and lesions beneath the nail (e.g. melanoma), or reflect a systemic disorder (see below).

Clubbing

Normally the angle between the nail and the posterior nail fold is less than 180°. In clubbing this angle increases, often becoming greater than 180°. The causes are discussed on page 459.

Koilonychia

Koilonychia is flattening or even depression of the normal slight convexity of the nail, and is usually due to iron deficiency.

Beau's lines

Beau's lines are transverse grooves in all the nails, reflecting

Fig. 26.21 A distinctive feature of alopecia areata is the presence of shortened 'exclamation mark' hairs which taper markedly where they emerge from the scalp.

a transient reduction in nail growth due to a severe illness. They may also occur after childbirth.

Yellow nail syndrome

In yellow nail syndrome the nails become yellow, thickened and excessively curved and virtually stop growing. Cuticular attachment is lost and there is usually some separation of nail from nail bed. The nail changes are associated with lymphoedema, bronchiectasis and pleural effusions.

It is more common to find yellow nails in circumstances such as psoriasis and dermatophyte fungal infection, these conditions being recognised by the associated skin changes and mycological investigations.

Splinter haemorrhages

Splinter haemorrhages are usually longitudinal or dot-shaped areas of haemorrhage beneath nails. Most are the result of minor trauma, are painless and appear beneath the distal third of the nail. Psoriasis and fungal infection of the nails may be associated with similar distal splinters. Painful and proximal splinter haemorrhages are much more likely to be associated with medical causes, of which the best established are subacute bacterial endocarditis, trichinosis, chronic mountain sickness and indwelling radial arterial catheters.

Paronychia

Paronychia is a painful swelling of the posterior nail fold. When acute, staphylococcal infection is likely. A more gradual onset and chronic course is usually associated with *Candida albicans*. Women are especially prone to chronic paronychia. Common predisposing factors are occupations in which the hands are frequently wet, diabetes mellitus and poor peripheral circulation.

PSYCHOLOGICAL CAUSES OF SKIN DISEASE

Many bona fide skin diseases, such as eczema and psoriasis, may worsen or be precipitated during periods of psychological stress. Similarly, anxiety and depression commonly accompany distressing skin disease, and can often be ameliorated by explanation, reassurance and encouragement. In such circumstances the psychological interplay may be contributory but is not causative.

There is a direct psychological cause, however, with dermatitis artefacta, many cases of delusions of infestation and psychogenic pruritus. A diagnosis of psychogenic pruritus rests on exclusion of an organic cause as well as association with other psychoneurotic symptoms and signs.

Dermatitis artefacta

Dermatitis artefacta is mainly seen in females. The lesions are self-inflicted but this is denied and they may indeed be produced subconsciously. They are often bizarre in appearance, resistant to therapy (except occlusive dressings, in which case lesions may appear at new sites), and often regarded with indifference. The patients tend to be immature or insecure but the motivation behind dermatitis artefacta is often difficult to elucidate, and the condition can be protracted.

Self-inflicted damage is also seen in psychotics and the Lesch Nyhan syndrome, a rare X-linked inherited disorder of purine metabolism associated with mental retardation and spasticity.

Delusions of infestation

This is the conviction that there are parasites on or in the skin, often supported by offerings of excoriated skin fragments. Such a delusion may be one element in a broader presentation of psychosis, including that due to organic disorders such as vitamin B_{12} deficiency, but can present in an isolated form (monosymptomatic delusional hypochondriasis). It is of course essential to exclude infestation such as scabies and pests in the home.

The monodelusional state responds well to the psychotropic drug pimozide.

Dermatological non-disease

The term 'dermatological non-disease' has been used to describe a disproportionate anxiety about minor and often physiological skin changes. Such patients are difficult to manage, but can be seriously disturbed and at risk of suicide.

Further reading

Braverman I M 1981 Skin signs of systemic disease. 2nd edn. W B Saunders, Philadelphia. *Single author, easy to read and well illustrated*

Fitzpatrick T B, Eisen A Z, Wolff K, Freedberg I W, Austen K F 1987 Dermatology in general medicine. 3rd edn. McGraw-Hill, New York. *A major, predominantly US text*

Levene G M, Calnan C D 1984 A colour atlas of dermatology. Wolfe Medical, London. *Minimal text, beautifully illustrated*

Rook A J, Wilkinson D S, Ebling F J G, Champion R H, Burton J L 1986 Textbook of dermatology. 4th edn. Blackwell, Oxford. *The comprehensive British textbook*

Du Vivier A 1987 Atlas of clinical dermatology. Churchill Livingstone, Edinburgh. *A good illustrated introduction*

Index

Note: alphabetisation is word-by-word: thus, Head injury before Headache; Anti-RNA antibody before Antibiotic.

Abbreviations are also listed.

A

Index

Index

1155

Index

Index

Index

H

Index

Index

Index

Index

Index

Index

1189

Index

Index

Index